DIAGNOSTIC IMAGING
ULTRASOUND

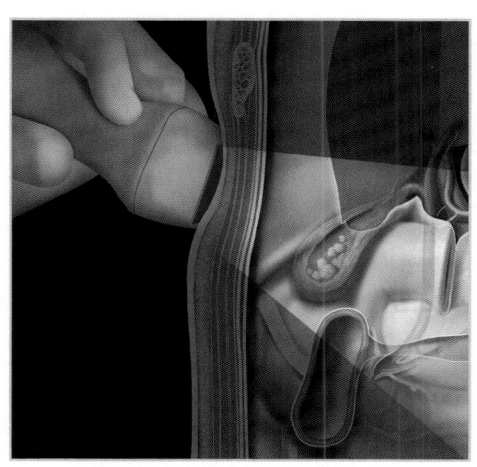

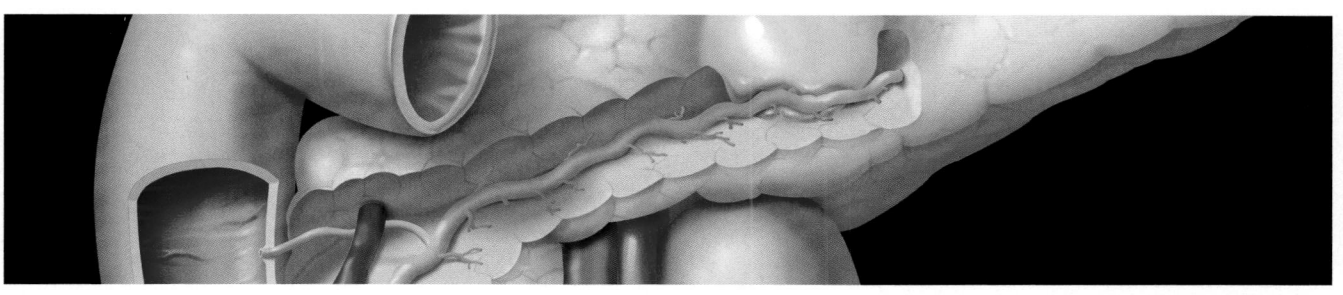

CONTRIBUTORS

Contributing Authors

Ravi Ramakantan, MD
Professor of Radiology
Department of Radiology
King Edward Memorial Hospital
Mumbai, India

Chander Lulla, MD, DMRD
Consultant Sonologist
RIA Clinic
Mumbai, India

David P.N. Chan, MBChB, FRCR
Honorary Clinical Assistant Professor
Department of Diagnostic Radiology and Organ Imaging
The Chinese University of Hong Kong
Hong Kong, China

Helen H.L. Chau, MBChB, FRCR
Honorary Clinical Assistant Professor
Department of Diagnostic Radiology and Organ Imaging
The Chinese University of Hong Kong
Hong Kong, China

Vivian Y.F. Leung, PhD, RDMS
Adjunct Assistant Professor
Department of Diagnostic Radiology and Organ Imaging
The Chinese University of Hong Kong
Hong Kong, China

Eric K.H. Liu, PhD, RDMS
Adjunct Assistant Professor
Department of Diagnostic Radiology and Organ Imaging
The Chinese University of Hong Kong
Hong Kong, China

Karen Y. Oh, MD
Assistant Professor of Radiology
Adjunct Assistant Professor of Obstetrics and Gynecology
University of Utah School of Medicine
Salt Lake City, Utah

Kathleen H. Puglia, MD
Clinical Instructor of Radiology
University of Utah School of Medicine
Salt Lake City, Utah

Steven A. Larsen, MD
Clinical Instructor
Oregon Health & Science University
Portland, Oregon

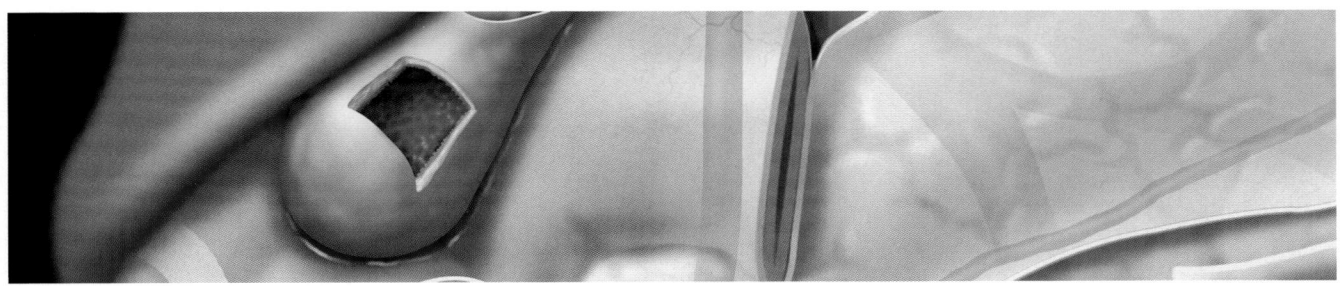

DIAGNOSTIC IMAGING: ULTRASOUND

We at Amirsys and Elsevier are proud to present **Diagnostic Imaging: Ultrasound**, the tenth volume in our acclaimed *Diagnostic Imaging (DI)* series. We began this precedent-setting, image- and graphic-rich series with David Stoller's <u>Diagnostic Imaging: Orthopaedics</u>. The next volumes, <u>DI: Brain, DI: Head and Neck, DI: Abdomen, DI: Spine, DI: Pediatrics, DI: Obstetrics, DI: Chest</u> and <u>DI: Breast</u> are now joined by Anil Ahuja's fabulous new textbook, <u>DI: Ultrasound</u>.

Worldwide, ultrasound is one of the most commonly performed imaging studies (perhaps second only to "plain film" radiography). Quick, widely-dispersed, and comparatively inexpensive, its diagnostic utility extends far beyond the abdomen and pelvis into less-familiar but very important areas such as the neck and extremities. Cross-sectional imagers who routinely and almost by reflex use CT and MR to image a broad spectrum of diseases will soon learn the remarkable utility of ultrasound as shown in Dr. Ahuja's newest text. He and his team have assembled elegant high-resolution studies using the most up-to-date ultrasound techniques available. Readers will see familiar diseases in a whole new "light" (no pun intended). They will also see diseases that are endemic in many parts of the world with which they may be less familiar. But with the worldwide translocations of large population groups, yesterday's "exotic" diseases are rapidly becoming today's diagnostic dilemmas. <u>DI: Ultrasound</u> shows you just what to look for and includes both common and less common presentations of many diseases that can be quickly and accurately diagnosed using this popular modality.

Again, the unique bulleted format of the DI series allows our authors to present approximately twice the information and four times the images per diagnosis compared to the old-fashioned traditional prose textbook. All the DI books follow the same format, which means that our many readers find the same information in the same place—every time! And in every body part! The innovative visual differential diagnosis "thumbnail" provides you with an at-a-glance look at entities that can mimic the diagnosis in question and has been highly popular (and much copied). "Key Facts" boxes provide a succinct summary for quick, easy review.

In summary, **Diagnostic Imaging: Ultrasound** is a product designed with you, the reader, in mind. Today's typical practice settings demand efficiency in both image interpretation and learning. We think you'll find this new volume a highly efficient and wonderfully rich resource that will significantly enhance your practice—and find a welcome place on your bookshelf. Enjoy!

Anne G. Osborn, MD
Executive Vice President & Editor-in-Chief, Amirsys, Inc.

H. Ric Harnsberger, MD
CEO & Chairman, Amirsys, Inc.

Paula J. Woodward, MD
Senior Vice President & Medical Director, Amirsys, Inc.

x

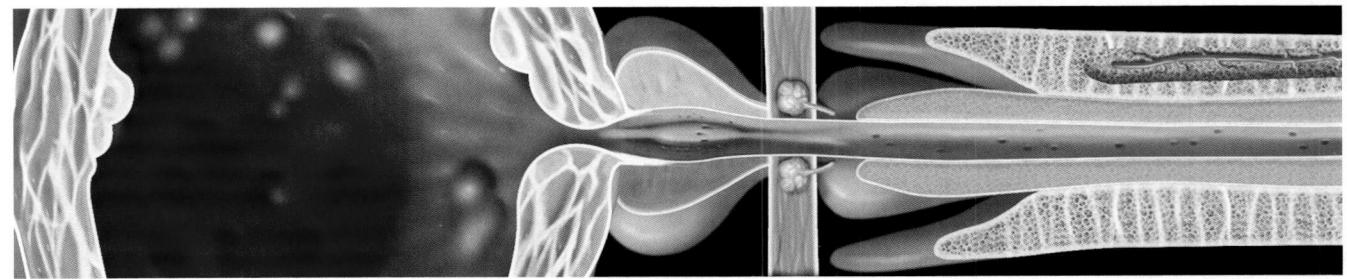

FOREWORD

It is a particular pleasure to be asked to provide a foreword for Anil Ahuja's timely contribution to the literature. I have long maintained that ultrasound is one of the most difficult of all imaging techniques, largely because the only person who can really assess the clinical problem is the operator who performed the study! Because of this it is critical that all those carrying out ultrasound are trained to an appropriate level. This book will help such training and provide a constant source of reference for workers faced with an unexpected lesion.

It is also pleasing to see a comprehensive text on ultrasound being developed at a time when many people wish to be trained in just one particular clinical subspecialty. While a musculoskeletal radiologist may become extremely competent in musculoskeletal ultrasound, there is still a pressing need for experts to be able to cover the whole range of ultrasound procedures. They will be the only people to advise on such developments as probe technology, ultrasound contrast agents, etc. There is no certainty that a patient presenting with a problem seemingly related to one body system may not have a lesion in another! Hence the importance of being able to switch from ultrasound of the hip to ultrasound of the iliac fossa. This book will assist such a comprehensive ultrasound approach.

With the rapidly increasing technical specifications of ultrasound machines and relative reduction in costs, it is not at all improbable that every ward of a hospital might soon "own" their own ultrasound machine. Indeed, in time, a personal ultrasound machine may become even more important than a stethoscope! These developments mean that ultrasound will have to be learned by a larger range of personnel and supervised to appropriate standards. This book will help all those participating in the wider scheme of ultrasound training. It will also be of enormous use to radiologists learning the technique and studying for postgraduate examinations.

The authors and the publisher have all done a superb job in making this book so attractive. I strongly believe that it will become *the* essential ultrasound text book and that Anil Ahuja's name will, as a result, become even more widely recognized within enlightened ultrasound departments. Congratulations to all.

Adrian K. Dixon, MD, FRCR, FRCP, FRCS, FMedSci
Professor of Radiology
University of Cambridge
Honorary Consultant Radiologist
Addenbrooke's Hospital
Cambridge, United Kingdom

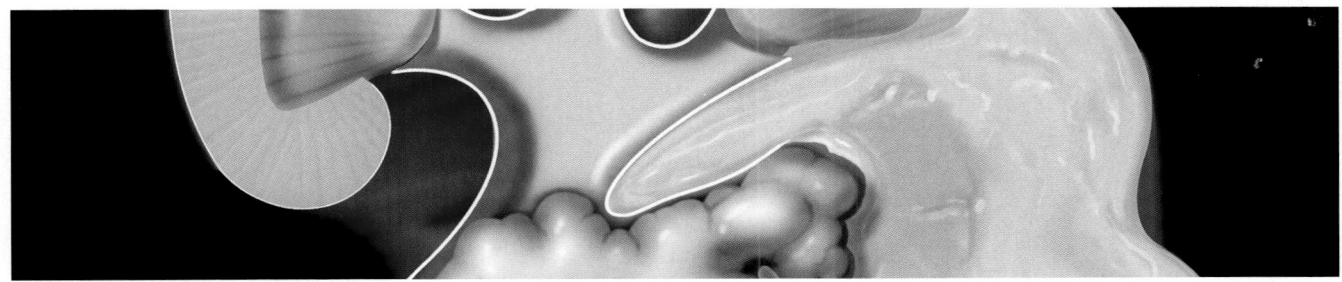

PREFACE

I have been fortunate to know Drs. Ric Harnsberger & Anne Osborn. What started as an academic relationship has over the years developed into a close friendship. I am privileged to have been asked to undertake this project and it is their vision, enthusiasm, and support that has helped me accomplish this task.

This book is unique in the Diagnostic Imaging series as it deals with a modality rather then a clinical specialty such as Head & Neck or Neuroradiology. Its scope is therefore wide, but this book is limited to clinical conditions that general sonologists, radiologists, clinicians, & residents commonly encounter in routine practice. The discussion of the role of ultrasound in Obstetric & Pediatric imaging has been restricted as these have been dealt with separately in other books in the Diagnostic Imaging series.

Although it is a book on ultrasound, you will find information & images from other modalities. In this era of multimodality imaging, techniques complement each other in diagnosis & management of patients. It is therefore essential to be familiar with the role of ultrasound in relation to other modalities. Each diagnosis contains common imaging appearances, basic pathology, treatment options and prognosis. The section introductions contain relevant information on anatomy, practical tips, technical parameters for optimal scanning. The protocol section includes indications where other imaging modalities may be necessary. The image annotation & key facts box crystallize relevant information and are ideal for those with short attention spans.

This book would not have been possible without the help of friends (authors and contributors) from various parts of the world. They have been generous with their images, expertise, time and patience, and I remain forever indebted. In particular I would like to acknowledge Dr. Chander Lulla & Prof. Ravi Ramakantan for their generosity with images and Prof. William Zwiebel & Prof. Paula Woodward for their help in preparing the table of contents. The team from Amirsys has been superb. Despite being in different continents & time zones they have patiently guided me along the entire process and none of this would have been possible without their help. Lastly, on behalf of all the authors I would like to thank sonographers in our respective departments for their dedication to this unique imaging modality.

The preparation of this book has brought members of my department closer, helped make new friendships, & consolidate old ones. I have enjoyed the process & hope you find this book useful.

Anil T. Ahuja, MD, FRCR
Professor
Department of Diagnostic Radiology and Organ Imaging
The Chinese University of Hong Kong
Hong Kong, China

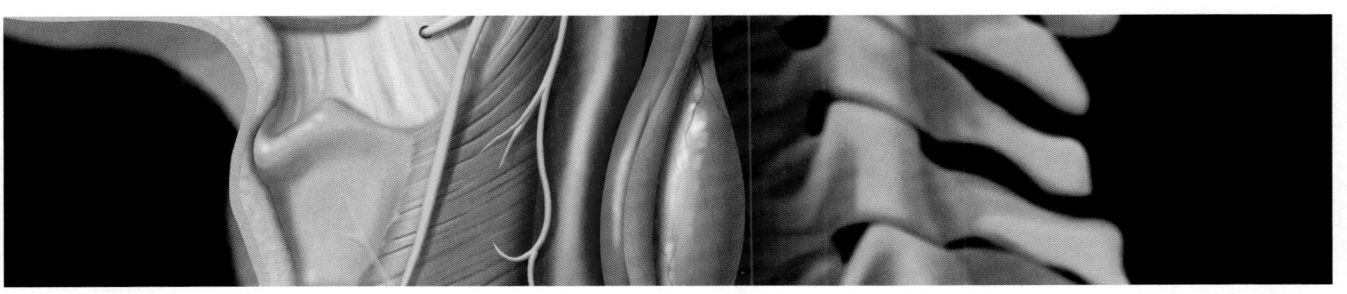

ACKNOWLEDGMENTS

Illustrations
Lane R. Bennion, MS
Richard Coombs, MS
Wes Price, MS

Image/Text Editing
Douglas Grant Jackson
Amanda Hurtado
Roth LaFleur

Medical Text Editing
Paula J. Woodward, MD
Anne Kennedy, MD
Daniel N. Sommers, MD
Marta E. Heilbrun, MD
Akram M. Shaaban, MBBCh

Case Management
Christopher Odekirk

Contributors
Jitendra Astekar
Nitin Chaubal
Avinash Gutte
Mukund Joshi
Sudheer Joshi
Arun Kinare
Ann King
William K.M. Kong
Aniruddha Kulkarni
Paul S.F. Lee
Tom W.K. Lee
Yolanda Y.P. Lee
Darshana Rasalkar
Rhian Rhys
Iain Stewart
Ki Wang
Simon C.H. Yu

Associate Editor
Kaerli Main

Production Lead
Melissa A. Hoopes

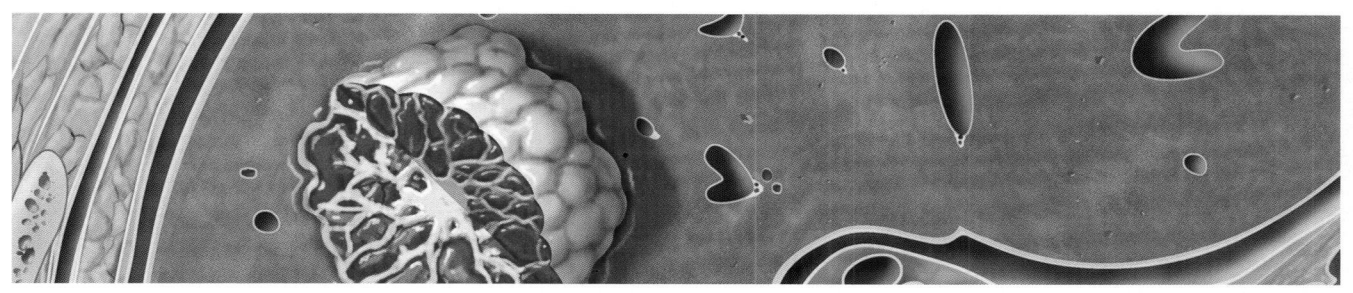

SECTIONS

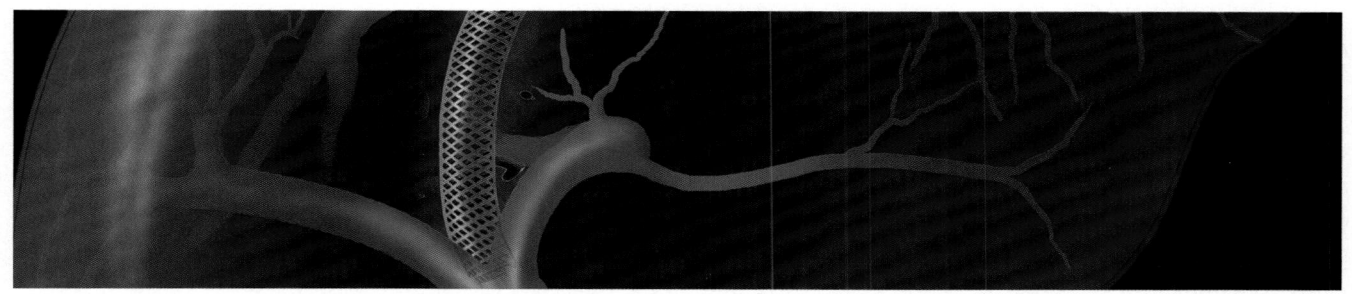

TABLE OF CONTENTS

SECTION 12
Breast

SECTION 13
Musculoskeletal

SECTION 14
Vascular

Introduction and Overview

Cerebrovascular

Abdominal Vessels

Extremities

DIAGNOSTIC IMAGING
ULTRASOUND

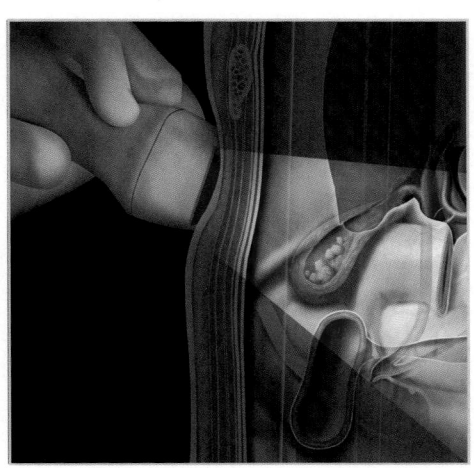

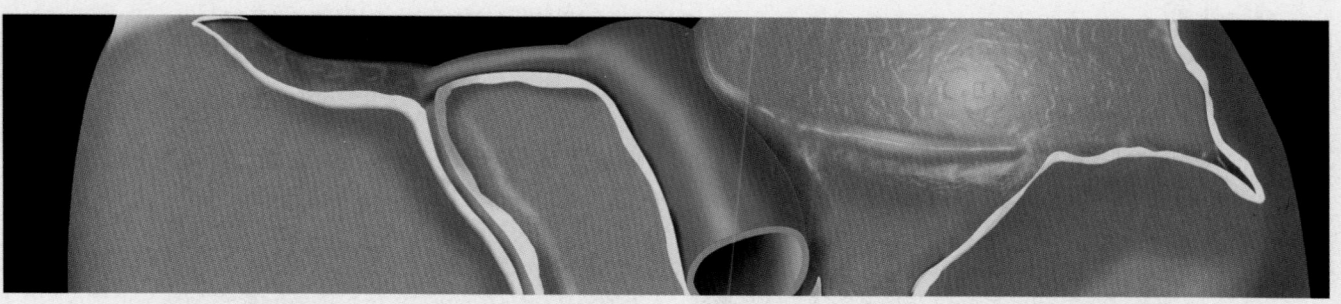

SECTION 1: Liver

HEPATIC SONOGRAPHY

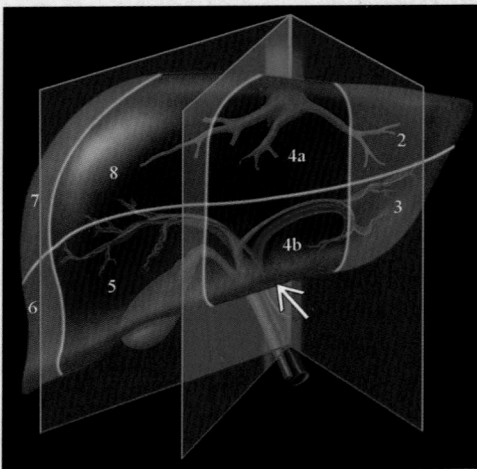

Graphic shows hepatic segments defined by vascular anatomy: 3 vertical planes along the hepatic veins & an oblique plane along the main portal branches. Segment 1 ➔ is between portal vein & IVC.

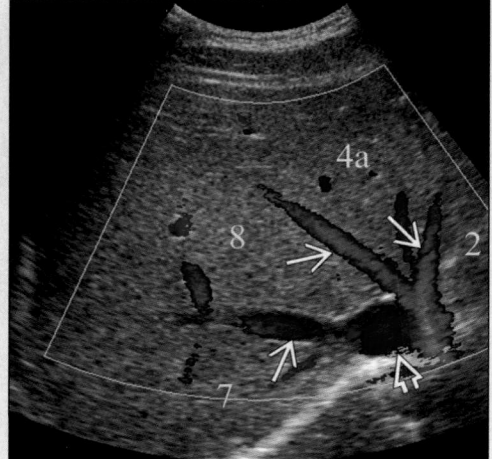

Transverse color Doppler ultrasound shows three hepatic veins ➔ draining into the IVC ➔. Vertical planes defined by 3 hepatic veins divide the liver into 4 segments.

IMAGING ANATOMY

Anatomic Relationships

- Liver lies in right hypochondrium (mostly protected by rib cage), epigastrium and left hypochondrium
- Superior: Both hemidiaphragm and the undersurface of heart
- Inferiorly: Gallbladder, porta hepatis, hepatic flexure, second part of duodenum
- Left: Esophagus and stomach

Histology

- Hepatic lobules (around 1 cm) form the liver parenchyma
- In each lobule there is a central hepatic vein from which branching plates of hepatocytes extend towards the periphery
- Plates of hepatocytes are separated by hepatic sinusoids through which portal venous blood flows towards central hepatic vein
- Hepatocytes extract metabolites from the portal venous blood, acting as a filter for nutrients, toxins
- Hepatocytes secrete bile into canaliculi which run within the plates of hepatocytes and drain in an opposite direction to portal venous blood and form hepatic ductules and eventually bile ducts

Vasculature

- Liver receives a dual blood supply from the portal vein and hepatic artery (which explains rarity of infarction)
- Intra-hepatic branches of the portal vein, hepatic artery and bile duct run together throughout the liver (portal triad)
- Portal vein
  - Receives venous blood from subdiaphragmatic part of esophagus, stomach, small and large bowel, gallbladder, pancreas and spleen
  - Forms by convergence of splenic and superior mesenteric veins behind the neck of the pancreas
  - Runs within the hepatoduodenal ligament posterior to the hepatic artery and common bile duct
  - Approximately 8 cm long

  - Divides at the porta hepatis into the left and right main portal veins
  - Right main portal vein gives cystic vein to gallbladder before entering right lobe of liver and dividing
  - Left main portal vein is joined by the ligamentum teres (obliterated left umbilical vein) and ligamentum venosum (obliterated ductus venosus) as it enters the left lobe
- Hepatic artery
  - Originates from celiac trunk (from aorta) as the common hepatic artery
  - Runs anterior to the portal vein and to the left of common bile duct in hepatoduodenal ligament
  - Divides at porta hepatis into left and right hepatic arteries, ramifies and accompanies portal veins and bile ducts
- Hepatic veins
  - Within liver, these run separate from portal triad
  - Sinusoids of hepatic lobules drain into intra- and sub-lobular veins then into hepatic veins
  - Typically three upper hepatic veins drain into the IVC: Right, middle (from caudate lobe) & left
  - Smaller, less consistent veins from the caudate lobe drain directly into a lower portion of IVC

Parenchymal Segmentation

- Couinaud's classification is the most commonly used
- Segment 1 (caudate lobe) lies between portal vein & inferior vena cava (IVC)
  - Unique in that it is supplied by the right and/or left portal vein(s), and drains directly into IVC
- Other segments are produced by four dividing planes
  - Vertically divided by the three planes along the three hepatic veins
  - Horizontally divided by the plane through the left and right main portal veins
  - 2: Left lateral superior segment
  - 3: Left lateral inferior segment
  - 4a: Left medial superior segment
  - 4b: Left medial inferior segment
  - 5: Right anterior inferior segment
  - 6: Right posterior inferior segment

Key Facts

- Unparalleled spatial resolution: Sonographic resolution of near- & mid-field hepatic lesions is unmatched by other imaging modalities
- Real-time imaging: Allows accurate guided biopsy/treatment of hepatic lesion(s)
- Limitations: Poor resolution of deep structures (penetration limited by acoustic attenuation) & inability to produce extended field-of-view image (due to overlying ribs & shape of liver)
  - Thus multiple views required for complete evaluation
- Key structures to identify
  - Hepatic parenchyma: Echotexture, distribution of vessels, surface contour
  - Portal and hepatic vessels (use Doppler study demonstrate patency and flow
  - Porta hepatis: Vessels, biliary ducts & lymph nodes
  - Gallbladder fossa: Gallbladder
  - Perihepatic: Fluid or mass
- Lesion localization: Record using hepatic segment classification (& record adjacent vessels) for follow-up examinations
  - Caudate lobe (segment 1)
  - Left lateral (2 superior & 3 inferior) segments
  - Left medial (4a superior & 4b inferior) segments
  - Right inferior (5 anterior & 6 posterior) segments
  - Right superior (7 posterior & 8 anterior) segments
- Vascularity: Use color &/or power Doppler to demonstrate lesion vascularity (may help shorten list of differential diagnosis)
  - Use spectral Doppler to interrogate for flow direction and velocity of blood within vessels

---

  - 7: Right posterior superior segment
  - 8: Right anterior superior segment

Ultrasound Appearance

- Normal liver parenchyma appears homogeneous and composed of fine echoes
  - As internal references for echogenicity
    - Liver is slightly more hyperechoic than normal renal cortex
    - Liver is more hypoechoic than spleen
- Wall of hepatic vein is not resolved with ultrasound, compared with wall of portal vein which is echogenic

ANATOMY-BASED IMAGING ISSUES

Key Concepts or Questions

- Liver is a large organ and there are many potential "blind spots" obscured by overlying anatomical structures, most of these can be overcome with different patient positions and interrogation planes
- Lower edge of the normal liver lies just below the subcostal margin, providing an acoustic window for interrogation of the liver
  - This acoustic window may be lost when obscured by bowel (with gas) and/or ribs; usually occurs if lower edge of liver is displaced superiorly (due to cirrhosis or a mass pushing up liver)

Imaging Approaches

- Supine, subcostal/subxiphoid
  - Good for left lobe and anterior segments of right lobe
- Right anterior oblique, subcostal
  - Good for posterior segments of right lobe and for looking behind calcified lesions
  - Good for subdiaphragmatic areas and porta hepatis (which may be obscured by anterior ribs or bowel gas in the supine position)
- Right lateral oblique, lower intercostal
  - Good for high-riding or small cirrhotic liver
  - Additional view of porta hepatis if anteriorly obscured by gas

Imaging Protocols

- Reduce bowel (gas) distention and increase gallbladder filling with a 4-6 hour fast prior to ultrasound
- All segments of the liver should be interrogated for a complete examination
- Interrogation with suspension of respiration in inspiration helps lower the liver
- Color Doppler interrogation of the main hepatic vein and main branches of the left and right portal vein
- Direction of flow of the main portal vein should be stated for patients with cirrhosis/portal hypertension
  - Normal portal venous flow is hepatopetal (from other organs towards the liver)
- Color Doppler and power Doppler interrogation of lesions

Imaging Pitfalls

- Missing liver
  - Situs inversus or hepatic hernia through diaphragm

Normal Measurements

- In midclavicular sagittal plane: Liver length should be less than 15 cm
  - Riedel lobe is a thin inferior extension from lateral aspect of right hepatic lobe

PATHOLOGY-BASED IMAGING ISSUES

Imaging Approaches

- Ultrasound is an inexpensive, fast, radiation-free and mobile examination
  - It is sensitive for the detection of most hepatic lesions
  - Spatial resolution of near- and mid-field hepatic lesions is unmatched by other imaging modalities
- Hepatic ultrasound is limited by poor resolution of deep structures (penetration limited by acoustic attenuation) and inability to produce an extended field-of-view image

HEPATIC SONOGRAPHY

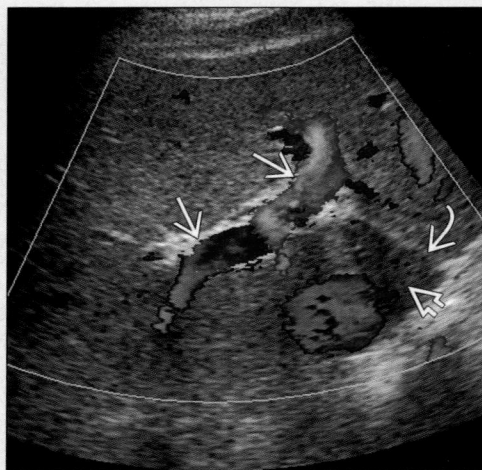

Oblique color Doppler ultrasound shows the portal vein bifurcation ➜. This plane divides superior & inferior hepatic segments. Note caudate lobe ➔ & fissure for ligamentum venosum ➔.

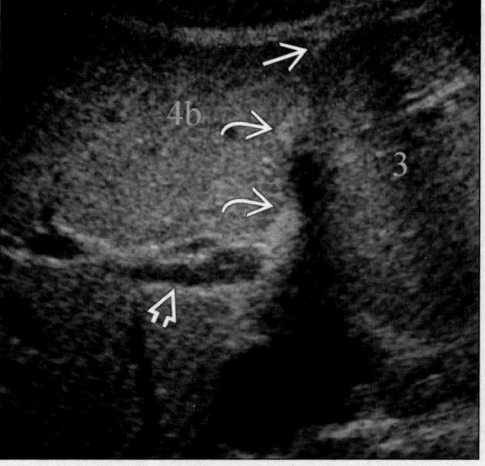

Transverse transabdominal ultrasound shows the ligamentum teres ➜ and related fissure ➜ which separates segment 4b from 3. Note fissure extends to left portal vein ➔.

- This makes relating a hepatic lesion to the surrounding anatomy difficult
- CT and MR may be more useful when such problems with ultrasound arise
• For imaging work-up of suspicious hepatic lesions
  - Ultrasound is good at locating the lesion and for monitoring progress
  - Real-time imaging capability of ultrasound allows accurate guided biopsy of lesion
  - Complimentary information of the lesion from CT and/or MR helps to reduce the need for biopsy
  - Intravenous ultrasound contrast agents are more sensitive in picking up subtle lesions and also demonstrate dynamic enhancing characteristics similar to CECT

Imaging Protocols
• Lesions detected by ultrasound should be further supplemented with color &/or power Doppler

Imaging Appearances of Focal Abnormalities
• Simple fluid: Through transmission (hypo-/anechoic); posterior acoustic enhancement
• Fluid with debris: Homogeneous low level echogenic content, fluid debris level when contents settle
  - Septae may be present
• Gas: Echogenic (in non-dependent position of cavity) and posterior ring down artifact
• Calcification: Echogenic and posterior acoustic shadowing

Differential Diagnosis for Focal Lesions
• Hyperechoic lesion
  - Fat-containing lesion
  - Hemangioma, adenoma, focal nodular hyperplasia
  - Hepatocellular carcinoma (HCC)
  - Hyperemic/hypervascular metastasis (gastrointestinal, ovarian, pancreatic, melanoma)
  - Calcification: Infection/infestation, neoplastic, vascular
  - Hematoma
• Hypoechoic lesion

- Cystic: Simple cyst, cystic neoplasm/metastases (ovarian, stomach, pancreas, colon)
- Fluid containing: Hydatid cyst, hematoma, abscess or necrotic neoplasm
• Lesion with internal septae
  - Cystic metastasis
  - Complicated simple cyst: Infection or hemorrhage into simple cyst
  - Infective collection: Pyogenic abscess, amebic abscess, hydatid cyst
  - Cavernous hemangioma, biliary cystadenoma, hepatic hamartoma
• Venous invasion
  - HCC
• Infiltrative lesion
  - HCC, lymphoma

EMBRYOLOGY

Embryologic Events
• Perinatal circulatory changes
  - In utero, blood returns from placenta via umbilical vein & ductus venosus to IVC
  - Umbilical vein is obliterated & forms ligamentum teres (free-edge of falciform ligament) after birth
  - Ductus venosus is obliterated & forms ligamentum venosum after birth

Practical Implications
• Circulatory/ligamentous structures
  - Portal hypertension may result in re-canalization of previously obliterated vessels as collaterals
  - Abscess and biloma may insinuate along these tissue/ligamentous planes

RELATED REFERENCES
1. Gray's Anatomy: The Anatomical Basis of Clinical Practice. Editor-in-Chief Susan Standring. 39th Ed. Elsevier, 2005

IMAGE GALLERY

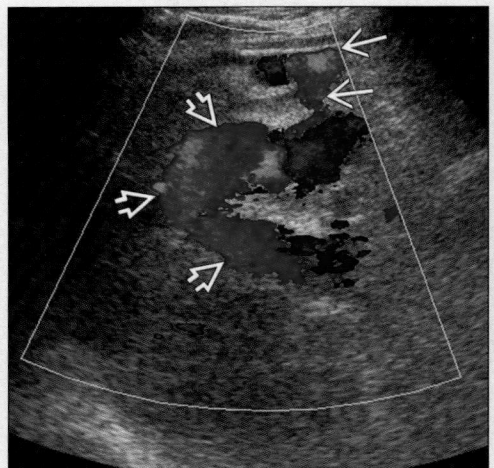
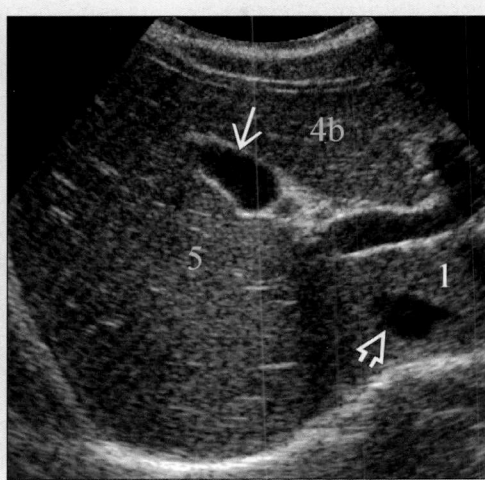

(Left) Transverse color Doppler ultrasound shows a recanalized umbilical vein ➡ (from ligamentum teres), channeling blood from the portal ➡ to the systemic circulation. *(Right)* Transverse transabdominal ultrasound shows the gallbladder ➡ & IVC ➡. A line joining these two structures represents the division between the left (segment 4b) and right (segment 5) lobes of liver.

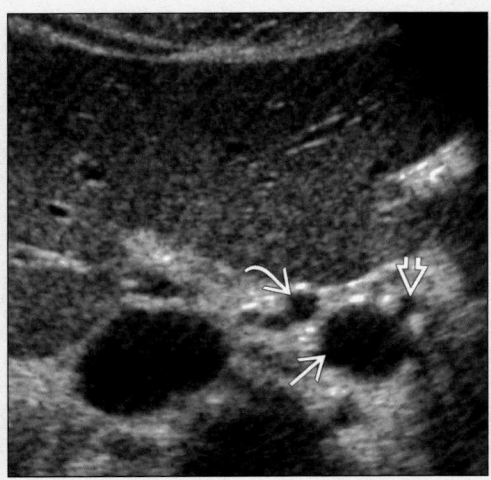
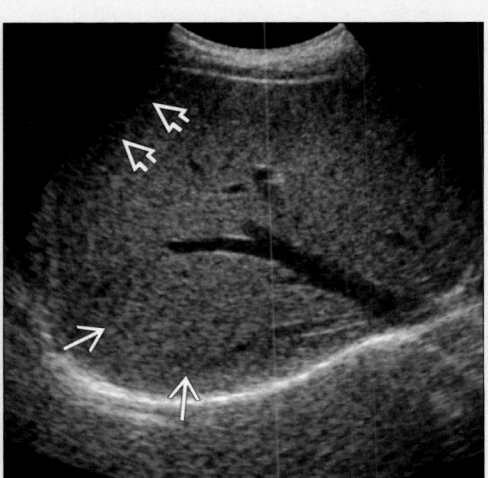

(Left) Transverse transabdominal ultrasound shows the portal vein ➡, common bile duct ➡, and hepatic artery ➡ in the hepatoduodenal ligament. *(Right)* Oblique transabdominal ultrasound in the right anterior oblique position is good for interrogating right upper segments ➡. Subcostal regions may still be obscured ➡.

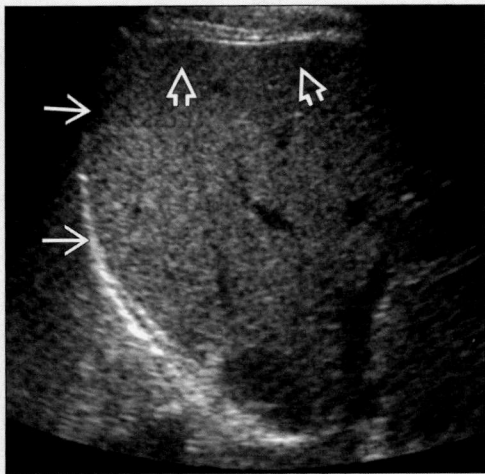
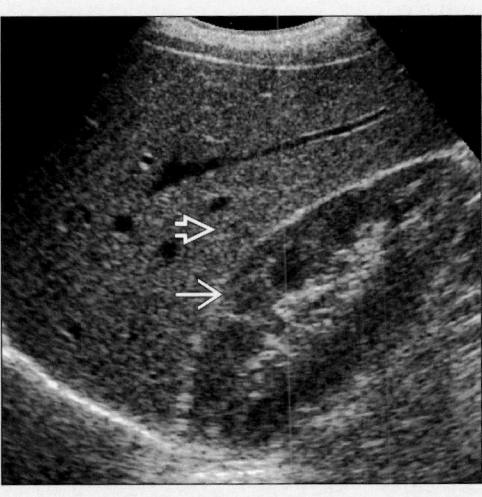

(Left) Oblique transabdominal ultrasound using an intercostal approach shows the upper part ➡ of the liver better, especially in high-riding or cirrhotic livers. Superficial regions are also better seen ➡. *(Right)* Longitudinal transabdominal ultrasound shows the right kidney ➡ is normally slightly hypoechoic compared to the liver ➡. The kidney is used as internal standard for echogenicity.

ACUTE HEPATITIS

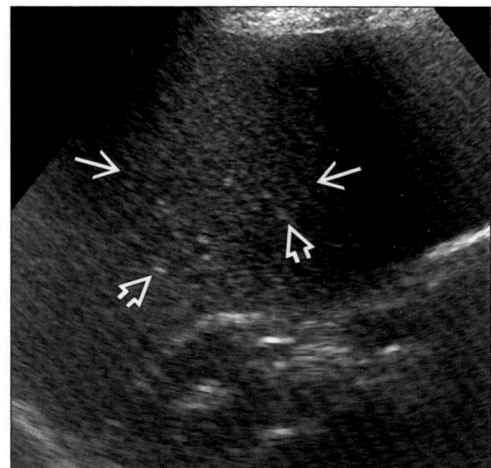

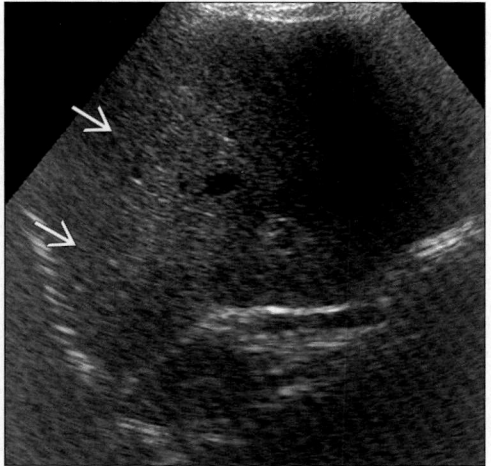

Oblique transabdominal ultrasound shows diffuse hypoechoic ➡ liver parenchyma in acute viral hepatitis. Against this, portal triad walls ➡ stand out as echogenic foci ("starry-sky").

Oblique transabdominal ultrasound shows decreased echogenicity of liver parenchyma ➡ in acute hepatitis, which becomes similar to that of kidney and spleen.

TERMINOLOGY

Definitions
- Nonspecific inflammatory response of liver to various agents

IMAGING FINDINGS

General Features
- Best diagnostic clue
  - Acute viral hepatitis on US
    - "Starry-sky" appearance: ↑ Echogenicity of portal triads against hypoechoic liver
    - Hepatomegaly and periportal lucency (edema)
- Location: Diffusely; involving both lobes
- Size
  - Acute: Enlarged liver
  - Chronic: Decrease in size of liver
- Other general features
  - Leading cause of hepatitis is viral infection
  - In medical practice, hepatitis refers to viral infection
  - Viral hepatitis

- Infection of liver by small group of hepatotropic viruses
- Stages: Acute, chronic active hepatitis (CAH) and chronic persistent hepatitis
- Responsible for 60% of cases of fulminant hepatic failure in US
  - Alcoholic hepatitis: Acute and chronic
  - Nonalcoholic steatohepatitis (NASH)
    - Significant cause of acute and progressive liver disease
    - May be an underlying cause of cryptogenic cirrhosis
  - Imaging of viral/alcoholic hepatitis done to exclude
    - Obstructive biliary disease/neoplasm
    - To evaluate parenchymal damage noninvasively

Ultrasonographic Findings
- Grayscale Ultrasound
  - **Acute viral hepatitis**
    - Hepatomegaly with diffuse decrease in echogenicity

DDx: Acute Hepatitis

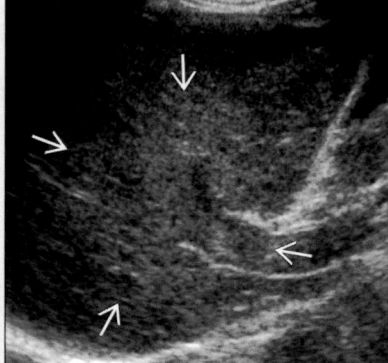

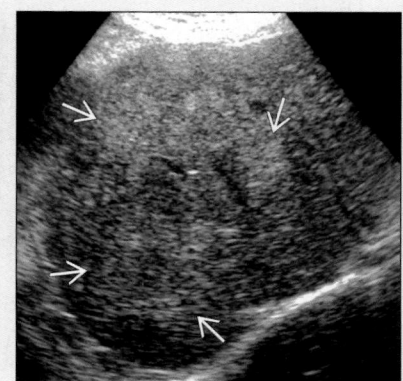

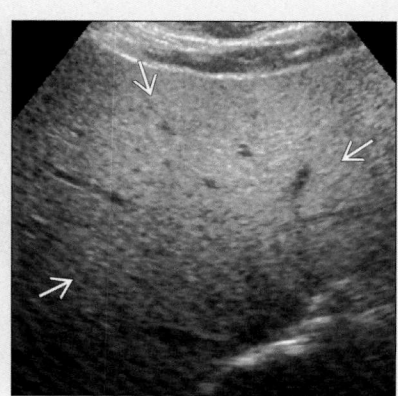

Infiltrative HCC

Diffuse Metastases

Fatty Liver

ACUTE HEPATITIS

Key Facts

Imaging Findings
- **Acute viral hepatitis**
- Hepatomegaly with diffuse decrease in echogenicity
- Splenomegaly and hepatic echogenicity diffusely becoming similar to spleen and renal cortex (normal liver is more echogenic than spleen and renal cortex)
- "Starry-sky" appearance: Increased echogenicity of portal triad walls against hypoechoic liver
- Periportal hypo-/anechoic area (hydropic swelling of hepatocytes)
- Thickening of GB wall; hypertonic GB, nontender
- Increase in echogenicity of fat in ligamentum venosum, falciform ligament, periportal tissues
- **Chronic active viral hepatitis**
- Increased echogenicity of liver

- "Silhouetting" of portal vein walls (loss of definition of portal veins)
- Heterogeneous parenchymal echotexture due to regenerating nodules
- Adenopathy in hepatoduodenal ligament
- Best imaging tool: Ultrasound to rule out biliary obstruction or other hepatic pathology

Top Differential Diagnoses
- Infiltrative Hepatocellular Carcinoma (HCC)
- Diffuse Metastases or Lymphoma
- Steatosis (Fatty Liver)

Diagnostic Checklist
- Ruling out other causes of "diffuse hepatomegaly"
- Two most consistent findings in acute hepatitis: Hepatomegaly and periportal edema

---

- Splenomegaly and hepatic echogenicity diffusely becoming similar to spleen and renal cortex (normal liver is more echogenic than spleen and renal cortex)
- "Starry-sky" appearance: Increased echogenicity of portal triad walls against hypoechoic liver
- Periportal hypo-/anechoic area (hydropic swelling of hepatocytes)
- Thickening of GB wall; hypertonic GB, nontender
- Increase in echogenicity of fat in ligamentum venosum, falciform ligament, periportal tissues
  - **Chronic active viral hepatitis**
    - Increased echogenicity of liver
    - "Silhouetting" of portal vein walls (loss of definition of portal veins)
    - Heterogeneous parenchymal echotexture due to regenerating nodules
    - Adenopathy in hepatoduodenal ligament
  - **Acute alcoholic hepatitis**
    - Hepatomegaly with diffuse increase in echogenicity
  - **Late stage of alcoholic hepatitis**
    - Atrophic liver with micronodular cirrhosis

CT Findings
- NECT
  - Acute viral hepatitis
    - Hepatomegaly, gallbladder wall thickening
    - Periportal hypodensity (fluid/lymphedema)
  - Chronic active viral hepatitis
    - Lymphadenopathy in porta hepatis/gastrohepatic ligament and retroperitoneum (in 65% of cases)
    - Hyperdense regenerating nodules
  - Acute alcoholic hepatitis
    - Hepatomegaly
    - Diffuse hypodense liver (due to fatty infiltration)
    - Fatty infiltration may be focal/lobar/segmental
  - Chronic alcoholic hepatitis
    - Mixture of steatosis and early cirrhotic changes
    - Steatosis: Liver-spleen attenuation difference will be less than 10 HU
    - Normal liver has slightly ↑ attenuation than spleen

- Nonalcoholic steatohepatitis (NASH)
  - Indistinguishable from alcoholic hepatitis
- CECT
  - Acute and chronic viral hepatitis
    - ± Heterogeneous parenchymal enhancement
  - Chronic hepatitis: Regenerating nodules may be isodense with liver

MR Findings
- Viral hepatitis
  - Increase in T1 and T2 relaxation times of liver
  - T2WI: High signal intensity bands paralleling portal vessels (periportal edema)
- Alcoholic steatohepatitis (diffuse fatty infiltration)
  - T1WI in-phase GRE image: Increased signal intensity of liver than spleen or muscle
  - T1WI out-of-phase GRE image: Decreased signal intensity of liver (due to lipid in liver)

Imaging Recommendations
- Best imaging tool: Ultrasound to rule out biliary obstruction or other hepatic pathology

DIFFERENTIAL DIAGNOSIS

Infiltrative Hepatocellular Carcinoma (HCC)
- Background cirrhosis
- Invasion of portal vein

Diffuse Metastases or Lymphoma
- Hepatomegaly due to diffuse infiltration
- Background vascular architecture may/may not be distorted
- Lymphoma more common in immune-suppressed patients
  - Examples: AIDS and organ transplant recipients

Steatosis (Fatty Liver)
- Hepatomegaly
- Diffuse, patchy or focal increase in echogenicity
- Normal vessels course through "lesion"

ACUTE HEPATITIS

PATHOLOGY

General Features
- General path comments
  - Different stages of hepatitis
    - Cellular dysfunction, necrosis, fibrosis, cirrhosis
  - HBV: Sensitized cytotoxic → T-cells hepatocyte necrosis → tissue damage
  - Alcoholic hepatitis: Inflammatory reaction leads to acute liver cell necrosis
- Etiology
  - Viral hepatitis: Caused by one of 5 viral agents
    - Hepatitis A (HAV), B (HBV), C (HCV) viruses
    - Hepatitis D (HDV), E (HEV) viruses
  - Other causes of hepatitis
    - Alcohol abuse
    - Bacterial or fungal
    - Autoimmune reactions; metabolic disturbances
    - Drug induced injury; exposure to environmental agents; radiation therapy
- Epidemiology
  - HBV (serum)
    - US incidence: 13.2 cases per 100,000 population
    - In US and Europe, carrier rate is < 1%
    - In Africa and Asia, carrier rate is 10%
    - Endemic areas: HCC accounts 40% of all cancers

Gross Pathologic & Surgical Features
- Acute viral hepatitis: Enlarged liver + tense capsule
- Chronic fulminant hepatitis: Atrophic liver
- Alcoholic steatohepatitis: Enlarged, yellow, greasy liver

Microscopic Features
- Acute viral: Coagulative necrosis with ↑ eosinophilia
- Chronic viral: Lymphocytes/macrophages/plasma cells/piecemeal necrosis
- Alcoholic hepatitis: Neutrophils/necrosis/Mallory bodies (alcoholic hyaline)

Staging, Grading or Classification Criteria
- Hepatitis A (HAV)
  - Virus: ssRNA
  - Transmission: Fecal-oral
  - Incubation period: 2-6 weeks
  - No carrier and chronic phase
- Hepatitis B (HBV)
  - Virus: DNA
  - Transmission: Parenteral + sexual
  - Incubation period: 1-6 months
  - Carrier and chronic phase present
- Hepatitis C (HCV)
  - Virus: RNA
  - Transmission: Blood transfusion
  - Incubation period: 2-26 weeks
  - Carrier and chronic phase present
- Hepatitis D (HDV)
  - Virus: RNA
  - Transmission: Parenteral + sexual
  - Incubation period: 1-several months
  - Carrier with HBV; chronic phase present
- Hepatitis E (HEV)
  - Virus: ssRNA
  - Transmission: Water-borne
  - Incubation period: 6 weeks
  - No carrier and chronic phase

CLINICAL ISSUES

Presentation
- Most common signs/symptoms
  - Acute and chronic hepatitis
    - Malaise/anorexia/fever/pain/hepatomegaly/jaundice
  - Acute HBV: May present with serum sickness-like syndrome
- Clinical Profile: Teenage or middle-aged patient with history of fever, RUQ pain, hepatomegaly & jaundice
- Lab data: ↑ Serologic markers; ↑ liver function tests
- Diagnosis: Based on
  - Serologic markers; virological; clinical findings

Demographics
- Age: Any age group (particularly teen-/middle-age)
- Gender: M = F

Natural History & Prognosis
- Hepatitis can be self-limited or more progressive and chronic in nature
- Complications
  - Relapsing and fulminant hepatitis
  - Of chronic viral (HBV, HCV) and alcoholic hepatitis
    - Cirrhosis: 10% of HBV and 20-50% of HCV
    - HCC: Particularly among carriers of HBsAg
- Prognosis
  - Acute viral and alcoholic: Good
  - Chronic persistent hepatitis: Good
  - Chronic active hepatitis (CAH): Not predictable
  - Fulminant hepatitis: Poor

Treatment
- Acute viral hepatitis: No specific treatment; prophylaxis-IG, HBIG, vaccine
- Chronic viral hepatitis: Interferon for HBV and HCV
- Alcoholic hepatitis: Alcohol cessation and good diet

DIAGNOSTIC CHECKLIST

Consider
- Ruling out other causes of "diffuse hepatomegaly"

Image Interpretation Pearls
- Two most consistent findings in acute hepatitis: Hepatomegaly and periportal edema

SELECTED REFERENCES

1. Mortele KJ et al: Imaging of diffuse liver disease. Semin Liver Dis. 21(2):195-212, 2001
2. Murakami T et al: Liver necrosis and regeneration after fulminant hepatitis: pathologic correlation with CT and MR findings. Radiology. 198(1):239-42, 1996
3. Okada Y et al: Lymph nodes in the hepatoduodenal ligament: US appearances with CT and MR correlation. Clin Radiol. 51(3):160-6, 1996

IMAGE GALLERY

Typical

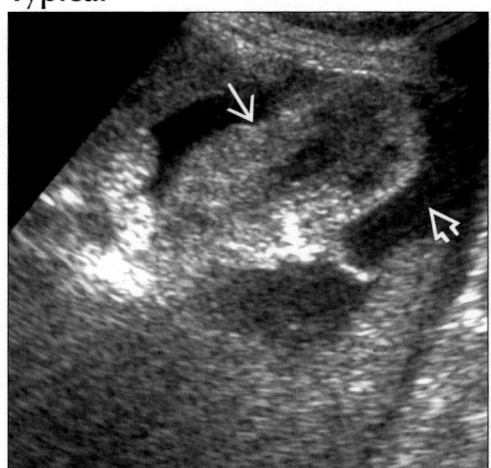
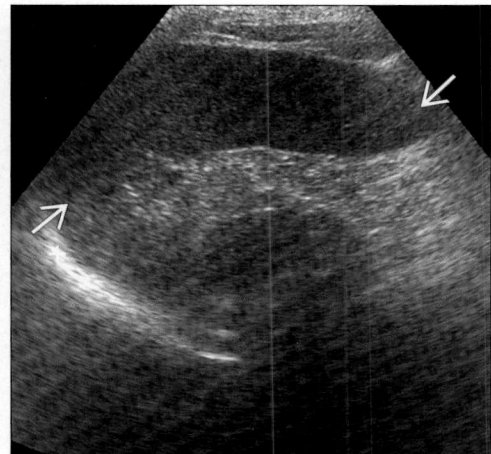

(Left) Oblique transabdominal ultrasound shows a markedly thickened gallbladder wall ➡ in acute hepatitis. There is near obliteration of the lumen. Note small amount of ascitic fluid ➡. *(Right)* Oblique transabdominal ultrasound shows splenomegaly ➡ in acute viral hepatitis. There is no splenic vein distension or evidence of collaterals.

Typical

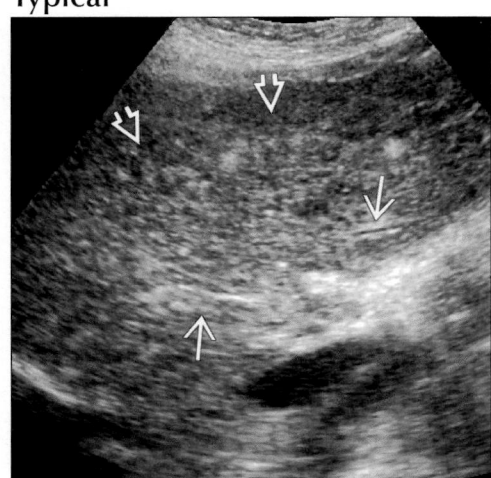
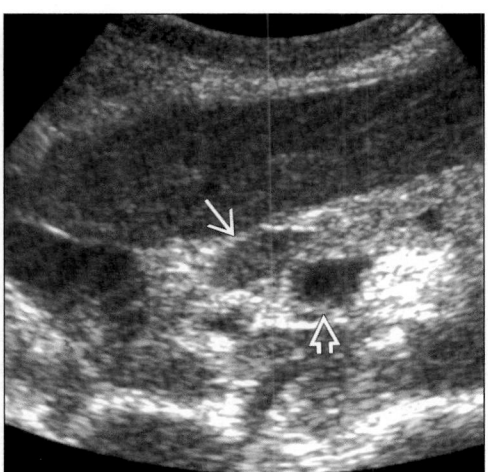

(Left) Oblique transabdominal ultrasound shows heterogeneous echogenicity ➡ of the liver in chronic active viral hepatitis. Portal vein walls ➡ are difficult to define. *(Right)* Transverse transabdominal ultrasound shows lymphadenopathy ➡ adjacent to the portal vein ➡ in a patient with viral hepatitis.

Typical

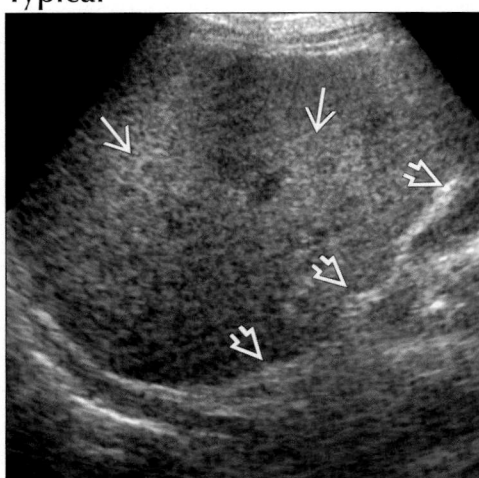
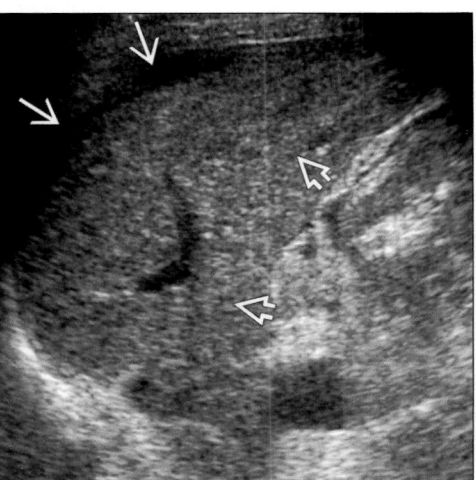

(Left) Transverse transabdominal ultrasound shows the rounded contour ➡ of hepatomegaly and diffuse increase in echogenicity ➡ in acute alcoholic hepatitis. *(Right)* Oblique transabdominal ultrasound shows cirrhosis in a patient with chronic viral hepatitis. Note atrophic liver bordered by ascites ➡. Note heterogeneous hepatic echo pattern ➡.

CIRRHOSIS, HEPATIC

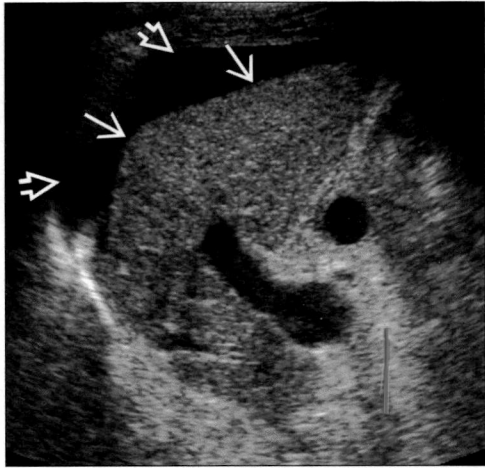 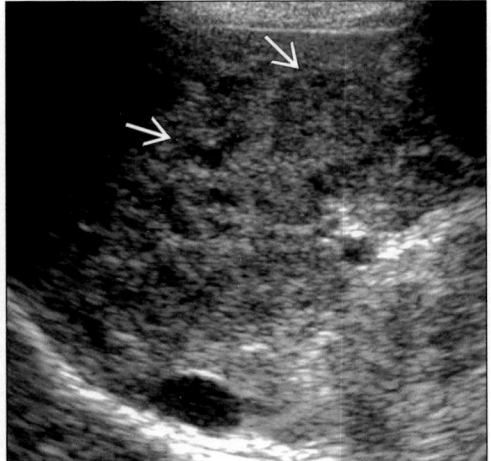

Longitudinal transabdominal ultrasound shows a small right hepatic lobe ➡ with coarsened echotexture and increased echogenicity. The liver is surrounded by ascites ➡.

Oblique transabdominal ultrasound shows macronodular cirrhosis ➡, with multiple solid heterogeneous nodules.

TERMINOLOGY

Definitions
- Chronic liver disease characterized by diffuse parenchymal necrosis with extensive fibrosis and regenerative nodule formation

IMAGING FINDINGS

General Features
- Best diagnostic clue: Nodular contour, coarse echotexture +/- hypoechoic nodules
- Location: Diffuse liver involving both lobes
- Size: General atrophy with relative enlargement of the caudate/left lobes
- Key concepts
  - Common end response of liver to a variety of insults and injuries
  - Classification of cirrhosis based on morphology, histopathology and etiology
  - Classification
    - Micronodular (Laennec) cirrhosis (< 1 cm diameter): Alcoholism (60-70% cases in US)
    - Macronodular (postnecrotic) cirrhosis: Viral hepatitis (10% in US; majority of cases worldwide)
    - Mixed cirrhosis
  - Alcohol abuse is most common cause in West; hepatitis B in Asia
  - One of 10 leading causes of death in Western world (6th in US)

Ultrasonographic Findings
- Grayscale Ultrasound
  - Nodular liver surface contour
  - Hepatomegaly (early stage)/normal size/shrunken
  - Enlarged caudate lobe & lateral segment of left lobe
  - Atrophy of right lobe & medial segment of left lobe
  - Increased echogenicity of fissures & portal structures
  - Coarsened echotexture, increase parenchymal echogenicity
  - Associated signs of fatty infiltration
  - Regenerating nodules (siderotic)
    - Iso-/hypoechoic nodules (regenerating nodules)
    - Hyperechoic rim (surrounding fibrosis)
  - Dysplastic nodules (> 1 cm)
    - Considered to be pre-malignant

DDx: Cirrhosis

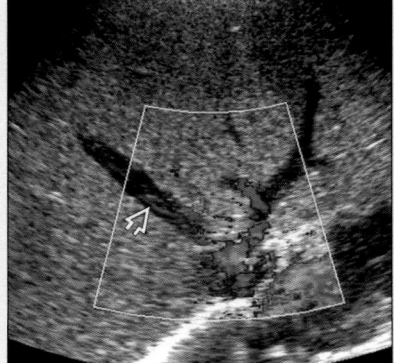 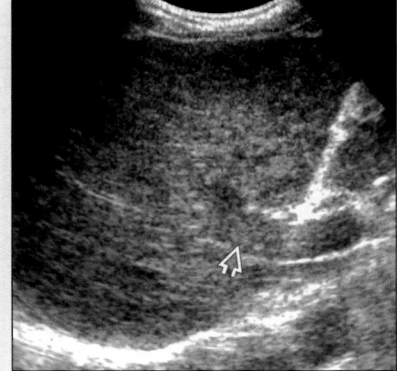 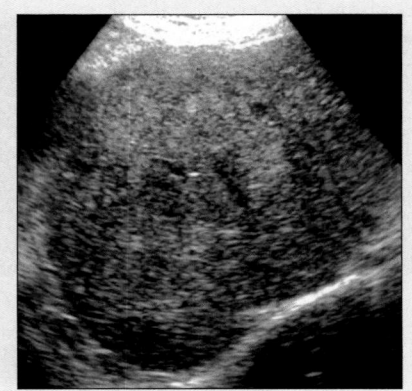

Budd Chiari   *Infiltrative HCC*   *Diffuse Mets*

CIRRHOSIS, HEPATIC

Key Facts

Imaging Findings
- Best diagnostic clue: Nodular contour, coarse echotexture +/- hypoechoic nodules
- Hepatomegaly (early stage)/normal size/shrunken
- Enlarged caudate lobe & lateral segment of left lobe
- Atrophy of right lobe & medial segment of left lobe
- Increased echogenicity of fissures & portal structures
- Regenerating nodules (siderotic)
- Signs of portal hypertension (PHT)
- Signs of hypo-albuminemia

Top Differential Diagnoses
- Budd-Chiari Syndrome
- Hepatocellular Carcinoma
- Treated Metastatic Disease

Pathology
- Micronodular (Laennec) cirrhosis: Alcohol
- Macronodular (postnecrotic) cirrhosis: Viral
- Steatosis → hepatitis → cirrhosis
- Alcohol (60-70%), chronic viral hepatitis B/C (10%)
- 3rd leading cause of death for men 34-54 years
- US: Hepatitis C (cirrhosis) causes 30-50% of HCC
- Japan: Hepatitis C (cirrhosis) 70% of HCC cases

Clinical Issues
- Fatigue, jaundice, ascites, encephalopathy
- Gynecomastia and testicular atrophy in males
- Virilization in females

Diagnostic Checklist
- Rule out other causes of "nodular dysmorphic liver"

- Difficult to differentiate from small hepatocellular carcinoma (HCC)
  - Compression of hepatic veins
  - Signs of portal hypertension (PHT)
    - Portal vein (> 13 mm), splenic (> 11 mm), superior mesenteric (> 12 mm), coronary (> 7 mm)
    - Dilated hepatic & splenic arteries with increased flow
    - Splenomegaly
    - Portal cavernoma (cavernous transformation of portal vein)
    - Portosystemic shunts: Lienorenal, gastrosplenic, paraumbilical
    - Ascites
  - Signs of hypo-albuminemia
    - Ascites
    - Edematous gallbladder wall and bowel wall
- Color Doppler
  - Hepatic vein: Portalization of hepatic vein
    - Loss of normal triphasic/flattened hepatic vein
    - Turbulence if hepatic vein compressed
  - Portal vein: Increased pulsatility, decreased velocity
    - Hepatofugal (away from liver) flow: Not candidate for splenorenal shunt/needs portacaval or mesocaval shunt
  - Hepatic artery: Dilatation of hepatic arteries with increased arterial flow

CT Findings
- Nodular contour & widened fissures
- Atrophy of right lobe & medial segment of left lobe
- Enlarged caudate lobe & lateral segment of left lobe
- Regenerative nodules; fibrotic & fatty changes
- Portal hypertension: Varices, ascites, splenomegaly
- Siderotic regenerative nodules
  - NECT: Increased attenuation due to iron content
  - CECT: Nodules disappear after contrast
    - Nodules & parenchyma enhance to same level
- Dysplastic regenerative nodules
  - NECT: Large nodules: Hyperdense (↑ iron + ↑ glycogen)
    - Small nodules: Isodense with liver (undetected)
  - CECT: Iso-/hyperdense to normal liver

- Fibrotic and fatty changes
  - NECT
    - Fibrosis: Diffuse lacework, thick bands & mottled areas of decreased density
    - Fatty changes: Mottled areas of low attenuation
  - CECT
    - Fibrosis: Less evident due to enhancement to same degree of liver
    - Confluent fibrosis: May show delayed persistent enhancement
    - Fatty changes: Areas of low attenuation

MR Findings
- Siderotic regenerative nodules: Paramagnetic effect of iron within nodules
  - T1WI: Hypointense
  - T2WI: Increased conspicuity of low signal intensity
  - T2 gradient-echo or FLASH: Markedly hypointense
  - Gamna-Gandy bodies (siderotic nodules in spleen)
    - Caused by hemorrhage (portal hypertension) into splenic follicles
    - T1 and T2WI: Hypointense
    - T2 GRE and FLASH images: Markedly hypointense
- Dysplastic regenerative nodules
  - T1WI: Hyperintense compared to liver parenchyma
  - T2WI: Hypointense relative to liver parenchyma
- Fibrotic and fatty changes
  - T1WI: Fibrosis: Hypointense; fat: Hyperintense
  - T2WI: Fibrosis: Hyperintense; fat: Hypointense
- MR angiography
  - Varices: Tortuous structures of high signal intensity

Imaging Recommendations
- Best imaging tool: Grayscale and color ultrasound

DIFFERENTIAL DIAGNOSIS

Budd-Chiari Syndrome
- Liver damaged, but no bridging fibrosis
- Occluded or narrowed hepatic veins ± IVC
- Collateral vessels extending to capsule
- Ascites

CIRRHOSIS, HEPATIC

- Acute phase: Hepatomegaly, hemorrhagic infarct
- Chronic phase: Fibrosis (post-infarct), "large regenerative nodules", collaterals
- Caudate lobe sparing (enlargement)

Hepatocellular Carcinoma
- Hypoechoic lesion within cirrhotic liver
- Portal vein thrombosis/invasion

Treated Metastatic Disease
- Example: Breast cancer metastases to liver
  - May shrink and fibrose with treatment
  - Simulating nodular contour of cirrhotic liver

Hepatic Sarcoidosis
- Systemic noncaseating granulomatous disorder
- Hypoattenuating nodules (size: Up to 2 cm)
- Hypointense nodules on T1 and T2WI MR

PATHOLOGY

General Features
- General path comments
  - Micronodular (Laennec) cirrhosis: Alcohol
  - Macronodular (postnecrotic) cirrhosis: Viral
  - Catalase oxidation of ethanol → damage cellular membranes & proteins
  - Cellular antigens → inflammatory cells → immune mediated cell damage
  - Steatosis → hepatitis → cirrhosis
  - Regenerative (especially siderotic) nodules → dysplastic nodules → HCC
    - Dysplastic nodules considered premalignant
- Etiology
  - Alcohol (60-70%), chronic viral hepatitis B/C (10%)
  - Primary biliary cirrhosis (5%)
  - Hemochromatosis (5%)
  - Primary sclerosing cholangitis, drugs, cardiac causes
  - Malnutrition, hereditary (Wilson), cryptogenic
  - In children: Biliary atresia, hepatitis, α-1 antitrypsin deficiency
- Epidemiology
  - 3rd leading cause of death for men 34-54 years
  - Risk of HCC
    - US: Hepatitis C (cirrhosis) causes 30-50% of HCC
    - Japan: Hepatitis C (cirrhosis) 70% of HCC cases
    - 2.5x higher in cirrhotic hepatitis B positive
    - Alcohol & primary biliary cirrhosis: 2-5 fold ↑ risk
  - Mortality due to complication
    - Ascites (50%), variceal bleeding (25%), renal failure (10%), bacterial peritonitis (5%), complications of ascites therapy (10%)

Gross Pathologic & Surgical Features
- Alcoholic cirrhosis
  - Early stage: Large, yellow, fatty, micronodular liver
  - Late stage: Shrunken, brown-yellow, hard organ with macronodules
- Postnecrotic cirrhosis
  - Macronodular (> 3 mm - 1 cm); fibrous scars

Microscopic Features
- Portal-central, portal-portal fibrous bands

- Micro & macronodules; mononuclear cells
- Abnormal arteriovenous interconnections

CLINICAL ISSUES

Presentation
- Most common signs/symptoms
  - Alcoholic cirrhosis: May be clinically silent (10-40% found at autopsy)
  - Nodular liver, anorexia, malnutrition, weight loss
  - Portal hypertension: Splenomegaly, varices, caput medusae
  - Fatigue, jaundice, ascites, encephalopathy
  - Gynecomastia and testicular atrophy in males
  - Virilization in females
- Clinical Profile: Patient with history of alcoholism, nodular liver, jaundice, ascites & splenomegaly
- Lab data: Abnormal liver function tests; anemia
  - Alcoholic cirrhosis: Severe increase in AST (SGOT)
  - Viral: Severe increase in ALT (SGPT)

Demographics
- Age: Middle and elderly age group
- Gender: Males more than females

Natural History & Prognosis
- Complications
  - Ascites, variceal hemorrhage, renal failure, coma
  - HCC: Due to hepatitis B, C and alcoholism
- Prognosis
  - Alcoholic cirrhosis: 5 year survival in less than 50%
  - Advanced disease: Poor prognosis

Treatment
- Alcoholic cirrhosis
  - Abstinence; decrease protein diet; multivitamins
  - Prednisone; diuretics (for ascites)
- Management limited to treating complications & underlying cause
- Advanced stage: Liver transplantation

DIAGNOSTIC CHECKLIST

Consider
- Rule out other causes of "nodular dysmorphic liver"

Image Interpretation Pearls
- Nodular liver contour; lobar atrophy & hypertrophy
- Regenerative nodules, ascites, splenomegaly, varices

SELECTED REFERENCES

1. Nicolau C et al: Gray-scale ultrasound in hepatic cirrhosis and chronic hepatitis: diagnosis, screening, and intervention. Semin Ultrasound CT MR. 23(1):3-18, 2002
2. Tchelepi H et al: Sonography of diffuse liver disease. J Ultrasound Med. 21(9):1023-32; quiz 1033-4, 2002
3. Dodd GD et al: Spectrum of imaging findings of the liver in end-stage cirrhosis: Part I, gross morphology and diffuse abnormalities. AJR. 173:1031-6, 1999
4. Zwiebel WJ: Sonographic diagnosis of diffuse liver disease. Semin Ultrasound CT MR. 16(1):8-15, 1995

IMAGE GALLERY

Typical

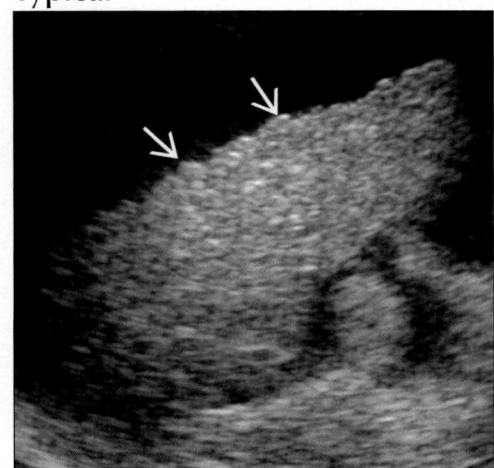
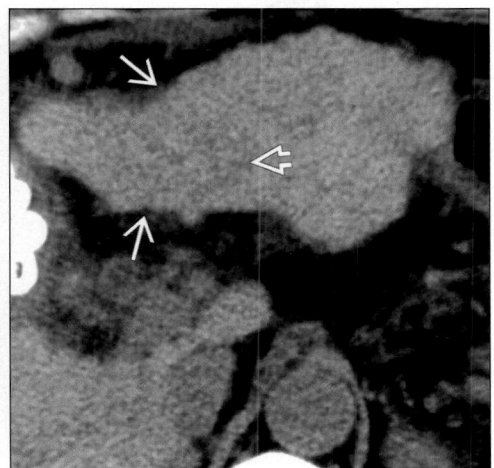

(Left) Longitudinal transabdominal ultrasound shows small right hepatic lobe with nodular surface ➡ highlighted by the surrounding ascites. Note coarsened echotexture of micronodular cirrhosis. *(Right)* Transverse NECT shows a magnified left hepatic lobe ➡ with irregular surface contour. The heterogeneity and nodularity of the cirrhotic liver parenchyma is subtle ➡.

Typical

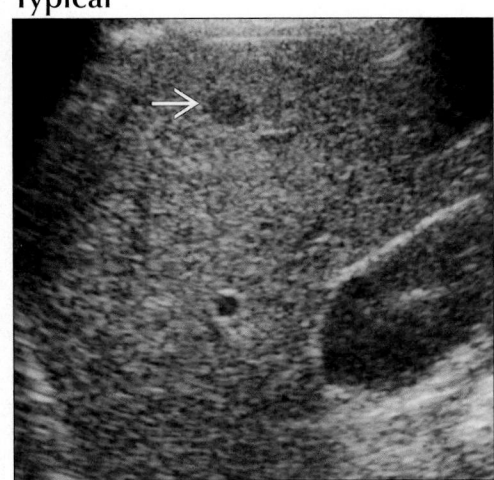
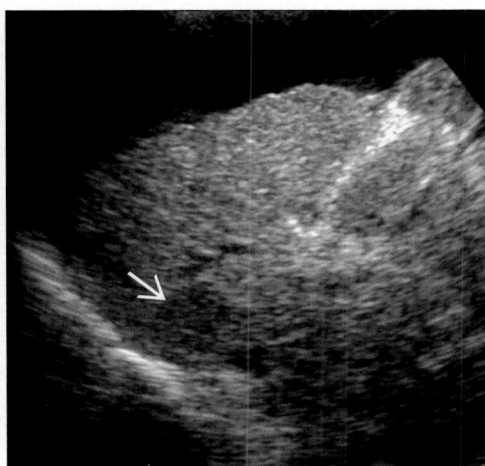

(Left) Transverse transabdominal ultrasound shows a well-defined hypoechoic nodule ➡ in a cirrhotic liver. This is the typical appearance of a regenerative nodule. *(Right)* Oblique transabdominal ultrasound shows a 2 cm hypoechoic nodule ➡ in a cirrhotic liver. Its large size was suspicious and subsequent biopsy showed it to be a dysplastic nodule.

Typical

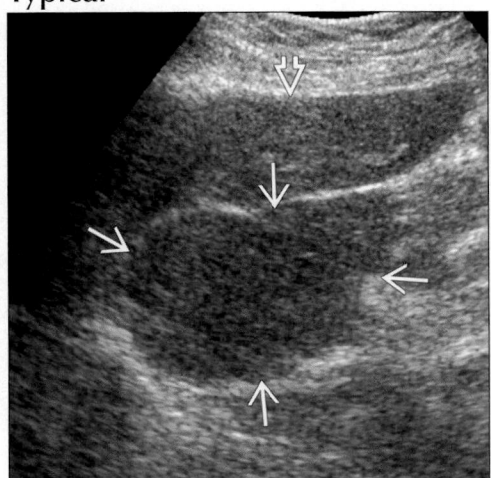
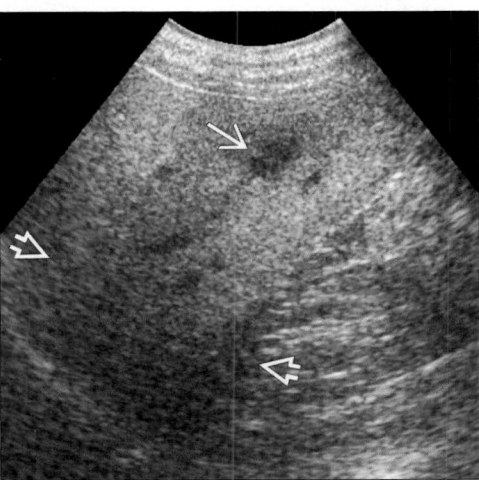

(Left) Longitudinal transabdominal ultrasound shows an enlarged caudate lobe ➡, compared to the atrophic medial segment of left lobe ➡. *(Right)* Oblique transabdominal ultrasound shows a hemangioma ➡ mimicking a regenerating nodule in a cirrhotic liver. Superimposed steatosis increased the echogenicity and caused acoustic attenuation ➡.

CIRRHOSIS, HEPATIC

(Left) Oblique transabdominal ultrasound shows diffuse gallbladder wall thickening ➡ in a cirrhotic patient, related to hypo-albuminemia or poor venous drainage. *(Right)* Oblique transabdominal ultrasound shows loops of small bowel with thickened walls ➡, floating within ascitic fluid ⬥➡. Mural edema may be due to portal hypertension or hypo-albuminemia.

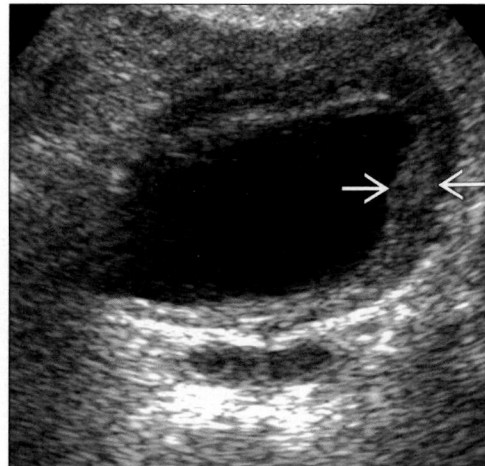
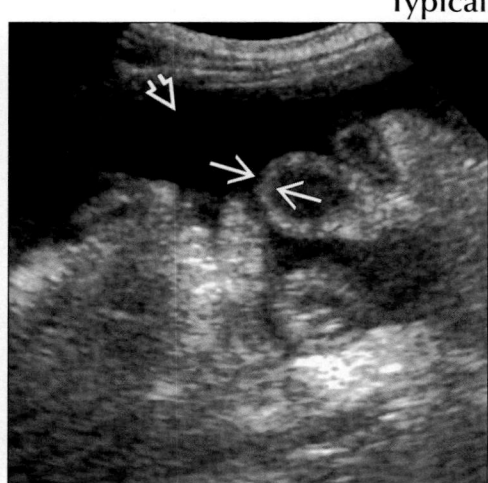

(Left) Oblique transabdominal ultrasound shows chronic ascites in a cirrhotic patient. Note fibrin strands ➡ running through the fluid. *(Right)* Oblique transabdominal ultrasound shows splenomegaly (16 cm between ⬥➡) and splenic varices ➡ due to portal hypertension.

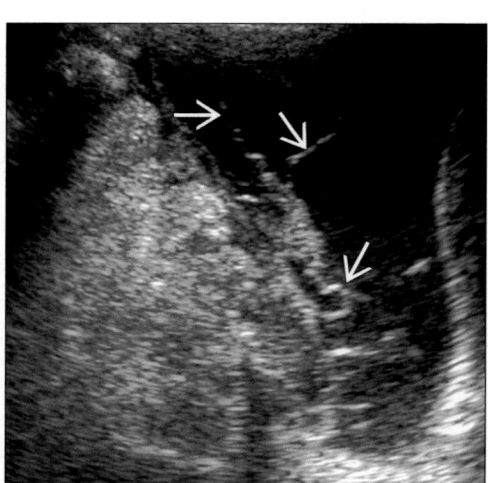
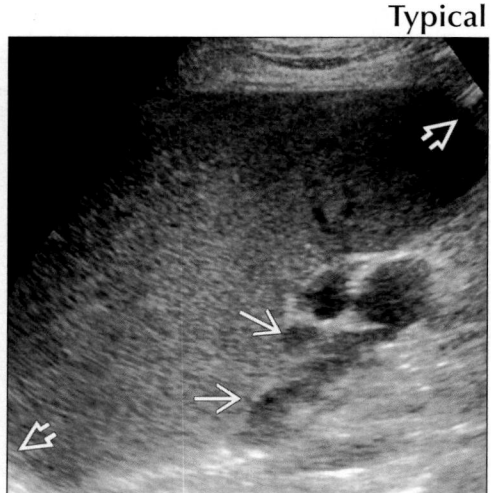

(Left) Oblique transabdominal ultrasound shows recanalization of the paraumbilical vein ➡, which acts as a portosystemic collateral to compensate for portal hypertension. *(Right)* Longitudinal color Doppler ultrasound shows flow in ectatic recanalized paraumbilical veins ➡ as a result of portal hypertension.

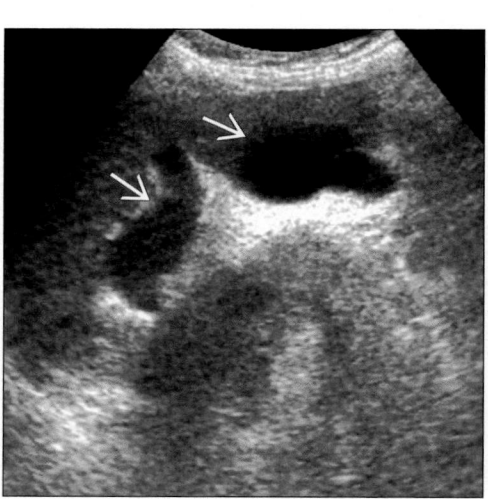
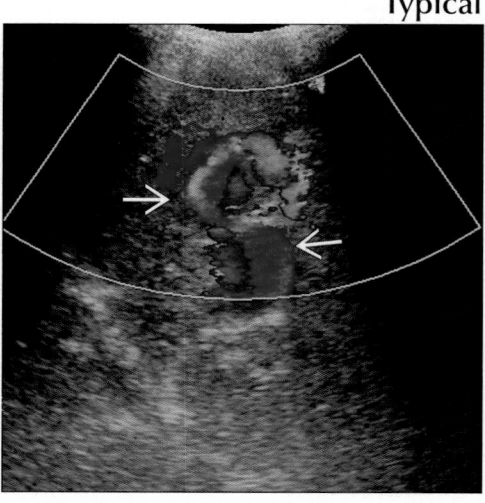

Typical

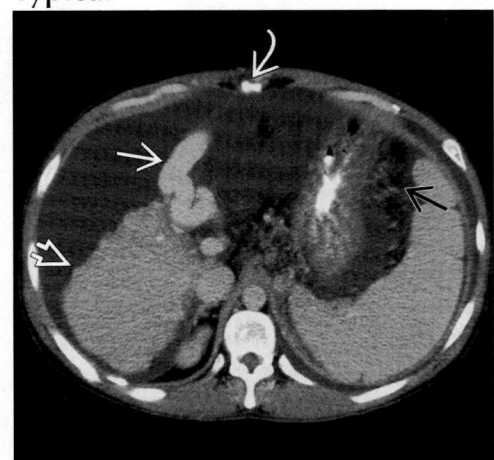
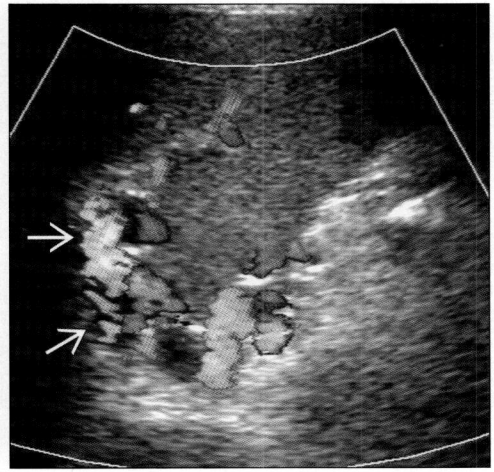

(Left) Transverse CECT shows ectatic recanalized paraumbilical vein ➡ & previous embolization ➡. Cirrhotic liver has a nodular surface ➡, prominent short gastric veins ➡ & splenomegaly. *(Right)* Oblique color Doppler ultrasound shows portal cavernoma ➡.

Typical

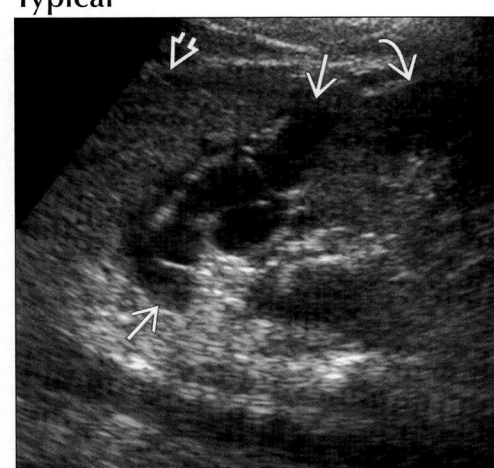
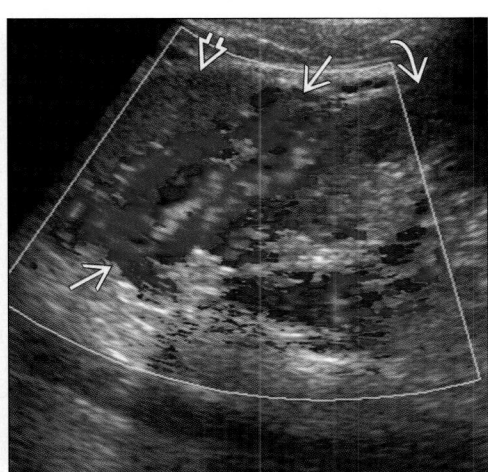

(Left) Oblique transabdominal ultrasound shows ectatic lienorenal collaterals ➡ between the spleen ➡ and superior pole of the left kidney ➡. *(Right)* Oblique color Doppler ultrasound shows flow ➡ within the lienorenal collaterals (demonstrated in the previous image) between the spleen ➡ and left kidney ➡.

Typical

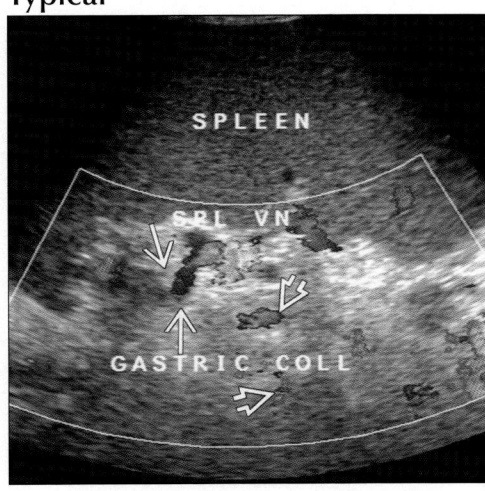
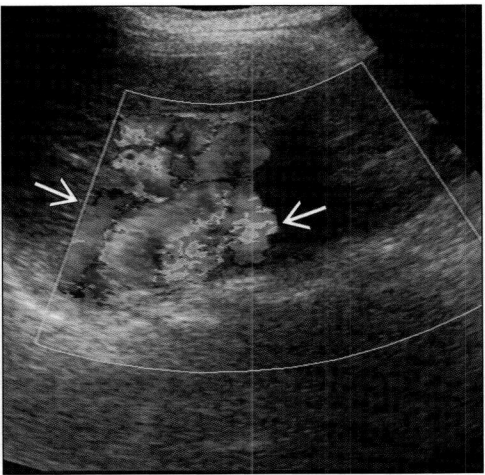

(Left) Oblique color Doppler ultrasound shows splenomegaly with splenic varices ➡ and gastric collaterals ➡. *(Right)* Oblique color Doppler ultrasound shows enlargement of short gastric veins ➡ and turbulent flow. These collaterals help decompress portal hypertension in a cirrhotic liver.

SCHISTOSOMIASIS, HEPATIC

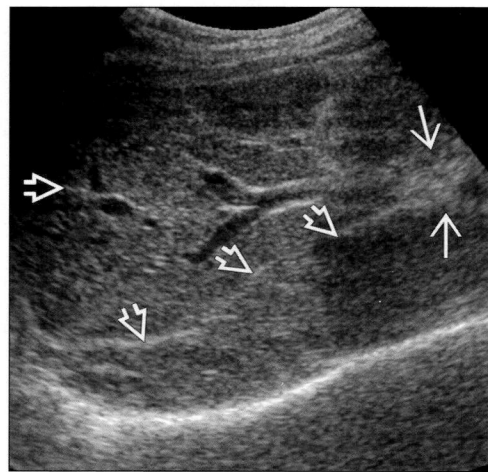

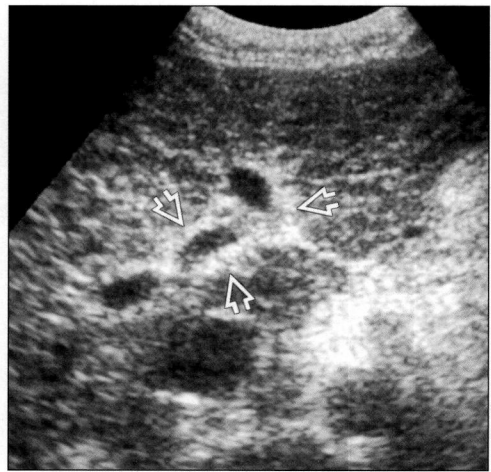

Oblique transabdominal ultrasound shows continuous, thickened, echogenic septa ➡, some of which can be traced back to porta hepatis where there is dense periportal fibrosis ➡.

Oblique transabdominal ultrasound shows thickening and hyperechogenicity around left main portal vein due to periportal fibrosis ➡.

TERMINOLOGY

Abbreviations and Synonyms
- Bilharzia, blood fluke

Definitions
- Hepatic parasitic infestation by Schistosoma species

IMAGING FINDINGS

General Features
- Best diagnostic clue: Echogenic periportal fibrotic bands
- Location
  - Periportal fibrosis initially around porta hepatis
  - May be panhepatic or localized to some lobes of the liver
- Morphology
  - Distortion of liver architecture and surface contour by extension of periportal fibrosis
  - Most common cause of hepatic fibrosis in the world

Ultrasonographic Findings
- Grayscale Ultrasound
  - Hepatomegaly in early stages
  - Atrophic liver in late stage (fibrosis and portal hypertension)
  - Irregular/notched liver surface
  - Echogenic granulomata
    - Peripheral/subcapsular location
    - Egg deposited in terminal portal venule resulting in inflammatory reaction
  - Periportal fibrosis
    - Periportal fibrosis is most severe at porta hepatis
    - Widened portal tracts
    - Hyperechoic and thickened walls of portal venules
    - Described as "clay-pipestem fibrosis"
    - "Bull's eye" lesion: Represents an anechoic portal vein surrounded by an echogenic mantle of fibrous tissue
  - Mosaic pattern
    - Network echogenic septa outlining polygonal areas of normal-appearing liver
    - Represents complete septal fibrosis (inflammation and fibrosis as a reaction to embolized eggs)

DDx: Schistosomiasis

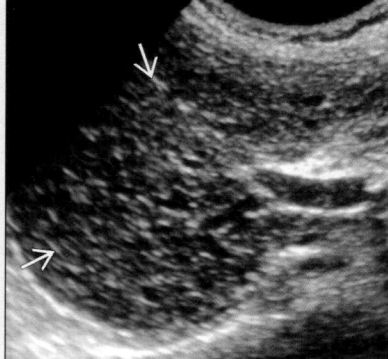

Cirrhosis

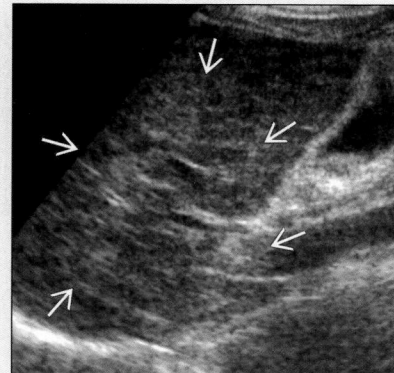

Infiltrative HCC

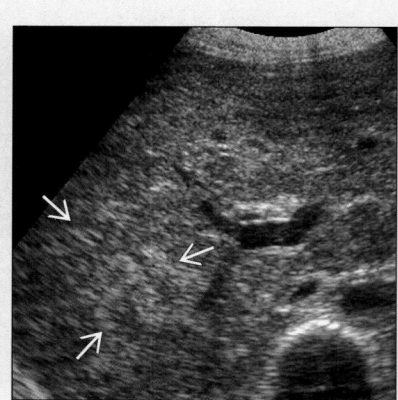

HELLP Syndrome

Key Facts

Imaging Findings
- Best diagnostic clue: Echogenic periportal fibrotic bands
- Periportal fibrosis initially around porta hepatis
- Distortion of liver architecture and surface contour by extension of periportal fibrosis
- Most common cause of hepatic fibrosis in the world
- Capsular calcification
- Hepatomegaly in early stages
- Atrophic liver in late stage (fibrosis and portal hypertension)
- Irregular/notched liver surface
- Echogenic granulomata
- Periportal fibrosis is most severe at porta hepatis
- Widened portal tracts
- Hyperechoic and thickened walls of portal venules

- "Bull's eye" lesion: Represents an anechoic portal vein surrounded by an echogenic mantle of fibrous tissue
- Network echogenic septa outlining polygonal areas of normal-appearing liver
- Hyperechoic gallbladder bed
- Associated signs of portal hypertension
- Cirrhosis in late stage
- Involvement of urinary tract
- Involvement of gastrointestinal tract
- Best imaging tool: Ultrasound for diagnosis and follow-up

Top Differential Diagnoses
- Cirrhosis
- Infiltrative Hepatocellular Carcinoma (HCC)
- HELLP (Hemolytic Anemia Elevated Liver Enzymes, Low Platelet Count) Syndrome

---

- May be discontinuous and appear mottled, nodular or sieve-like (partial septal fibrosis or calcification)
  - Hyperechoic gallbladder bed
  - Associated signs of portal hypertension
    - Portal vein dilation
    - Varices (gastric/esophageal)
    - Splenomegaly
    - Thickened gallbladder wall
    - Ascites
  - Cirrhosis in late stage
  - Involvement of urinary tract
    - Bladder and ureteric wall irregularities/calcification
    - Fibrotic bladder, ureteric strictures
    - Vesicoureteric reflux
    - Ureteritis cystica
    - Hydronephrosis, hydroureter
  - Involvement of gastrointestinal tract
    - Polypoid bowel mass
    - Bowel strictures
    - Granulomatous colitis

CT Findings
- NECT
  - Irregular hepatic contour
    - Junctional notches or depressions
  - Capsular calcification
  - "Tortoise shell" or "turtle back" appearance
    - Represents calcified septa, usually aligned perpendicular to the liver capsule
- CECT: Low attenuation rings around the portal vein branches throughout the liver, with marked enhancement following

Imaging Recommendations
- Best imaging tool: Ultrasound for diagnosis and follow-up

DIFFERENTIAL DIAGNOSIS

Cirrhosis
- Coarse echotexture
- Lack of echogenic fibrotic strands/periportal thickening

Infiltrative Hepatocellular Carcinoma (HCC)
- Background cirrhosis
- Portal vein invasion

HELLP (Hemolytic Anemia Elevated Liver Enzymes, Low Platelet Count) Syndrome
- Fibrin deposits and hemorrhagic necrosis predominantly develop in periportal areas
- Occurs during pregnancy

PATHOLOGY

General Features
- Etiology
  - S. japonicum: North Asia
  - S. mansoni: Africa, Egypt, Caribbean, South America (causes the most severe disease in the liver for this infestation)
  - S. hematobium: Mediterranean, Africa, Southeast Asia (typically affects urinary tract)
  - S. intercalatum and Schistosoma mekongi
- Epidemiology
  - Over 200 million infected worldwide
  - Concentrated in tropical and subtropical countries
- Associated abnormalities
  - Cercariae in infected water penetrate human/animal skin or buccal mucosa
  - Schistosomula (tailless Cercariae) travel via lymphatics to enter blood stream
  - Worm matures in venous blood
  - Adult male and female worms mate
  - Female worms lay eggs
  - Around 50% of eggs laid pass in urine/feces
  - Eggs hatch in water to release miracidia

SCHISTOSOMIASIS, HEPATIC

- ○ Miracidia infect snails (the intermediate host) and mature to become cercariae
- ○ Cercariae released by snails into water which infect humans/animals

Gross Pathologic & Surgical Features

- Adult worms live in pairs within portal veins for years
  - ○ S. japonicum in superior mesenteric vein
  - ○ S. mansoni in inferior mesenteric vein
  - ○ S. hematobium in vesical and ureteric venous plexuses
- Female worm releases eggs which travel in the blood to become trapped in tissues of different organs
- Trapped eggs stimulate a granulomatous reaction which is reversible in the early stages but becomes fibrotic later
- Fibrosis may lead to damage to the organ
  - ○ Liver: Periportal fibrosis, portal hypertension, gastrointestinal hemorrhage
  - ○ Urinary tract: Obstructive uropathy (renal failure), pyelonephritis/glomerulonephritis/amyloidosis
  - ○ Female genital tract (S. hematobium): Cervical/vulval/vaginal lesions
  - ○ Lungs: Cor pulmonale (S. mansoni)
  - ○ Nervous system: Brain (mainly S. japonicum), transverse myelitis (S. mansoni)
- Liver darkened by heme-derived pigments from schistosome gut

Microscopic Features

- Multiple tiny granulomas scattered in the periphery of the liver.
- Granuloma consists of an egg in the center surrounded by macrophages, lymphocytes, neutrophils, and eosinophils

CLINICAL ISSUES

Presentation

- Most common signs/symptoms
  - ○ Acute infection
    - ▪ Rash/dermatitis
    - ▪ Fever
    - ▪ Lethargy
    - ▪ Myalgia
    - ▪ Hepatosplenomegaly
  - ○ Signs and symptoms of chronic disease depend on Schistosome species, organ involved and host response
    - ▪ All schistosome species cause hepatic and intestinal disease (but rare with S. hematobium)
    - ▪ S. hematobium typically causes urinary tract disease
  - ○ Onset is usually insidious
  - ○ Hepatic: Dyspepsia, flatulence, abdominal pain; later (portal hypertension) with ascites, melena/hematemesis, peripheral edema
  - ○ Intestinal: Fatigue, abdominal pain, diarrhea, dysentery
  - ○ Urinary: Dysuria, frequency, terminal hematuria
  - ○ Pulmonary: Cough, wheeze, fatigue, dyspnea, hemoptysis
  - ○ Nervous: Seizures, headache, myeloradiculopathy

- ○ Female genital: Post-coital bleeding, genital ulceration, pelvic pain
- Other signs/symptoms: Co-infection with hepatitis B or C with S. Mansoni may lead to rapid disease progress
- Clinical Profile
  - ○ Eosinophilia (may be absent in chronic disease)
  - ○ Living eggs in stool/urine (need to perform egg viability test)
  - ○ Antibody specific to Schistosomes

Demographics

- Age: Maximum risk of exposure at 10-14 years
- Gender: Males more than females, may be related to increased activities in infected water

Natural History & Prognosis

- Treatment usually improves early disease especially liver function (due to large reserve)
- Schistosomiasis is the most common cause of hepatic fibrosis in the world
- Cirrhosis: especially with S. mansoni/S. japonicum
- Hepatocellular carcinoma: Especially with S. mansoni/S. japonicum
- Bladder carcinoma

Treatment

- Oral Praziquantel

DIAGNOSTIC CHECKLIST

Consider

- Excluding other causes of hepatic fibrosis/cirrhosis

Image Interpretation Pearls

- Mosaic/tortoise shell pattern of fibrosis is classic for this disease

SELECTED REFERENCES

1. Mortele KJ et al: The infected liver: radiologic-pathologic correlation. Radiographics. 24(4):937-55, 2004
2. Richter J et al: Ultrasound in tropical and parasitic diseases. Lancet. 362(9387):900-2, 2003
3. Ross AG et al: Schistosomiasis. N Engl J Med. 346(16):1212-20, 2002
4. WHO Expert Committee: Prevention and control of schistosomiasis and soil-transmitted helminthiasis. World Health Organ Tech Rep Ser. 912:i-vi, 1-57, back cover, 2002
5. Mortele KJ et al: Imaging of diffuse liver disease. Semin Liver Dis. 21(2):195-212, 2001
6. Cesmeli E et al: Ultrasound and CT changes of liver parenchyma in acute schistosomiasis. Br J Radiol. 70(835):758-60, 1997
7. Cheung H et al: The imaging diagnosis of hepatic schistosomiasis japonicum sequelae. Clin Radiol. 51(1):51-5, 1996
8. Cerri GG et al: Hepatosplenic schistosomiasis mansoni: ultrasound manifestations. Radiology. 153(3):777-80, 1984
9. Fataar S et al: Characteristic sonographic features of schistosomal periportal fibrosis. AJR Am J Roentgenol. 143(1):69-71, 1984
10. Hussain S et al: Ultrasonographic diagnosis of schistosomal periportal fibrosis. J Ultrasound Med. 3(10):449-52, 1984

IMAGE GALLERY

Typical

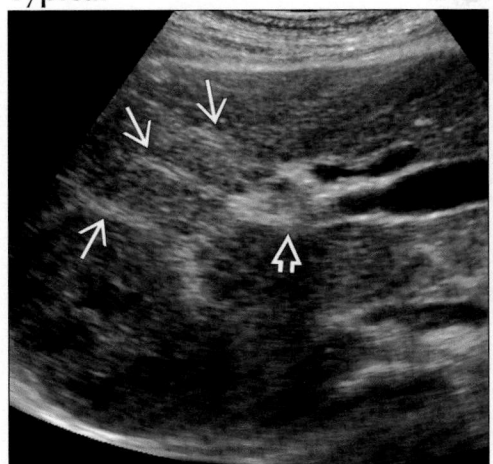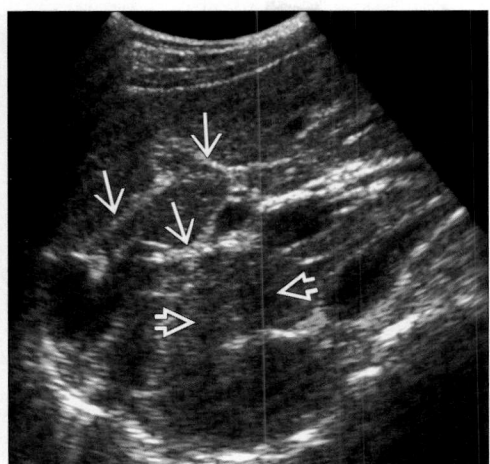

(Left) Oblique transabdominal ultrasound shows echogenic fibrotic septae ➡ extending peripherally from central periportal fibrosis ⇨. *(Right)* Oblique transabdominal ultrasound shows septal fibrosis ➡ with intermittent calcification causing posterior acoustic shadowing ⇨.

Typical

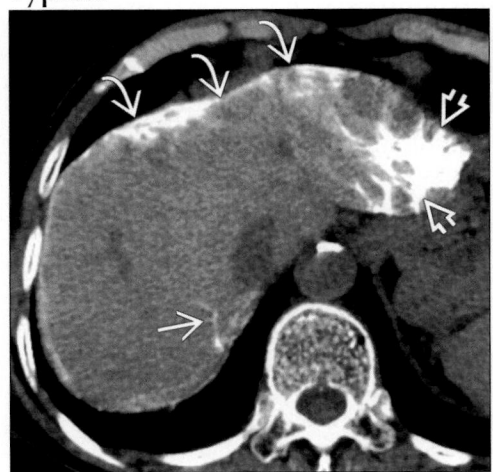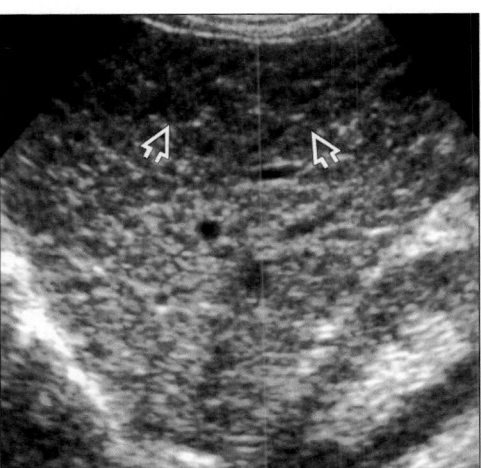

(Left) Transverse NECT of the liver shows thick band-like ⇨, and thin interrupted ➡ septal calcifications due to schistosomiasis. Note lobulation ➡ of liver contour. *(Right)* Oblique transabdominal ultrasound shows mottled appearance ⇨ of discontinuous periportal fibrosis in subcapsular region of liver.

Typical

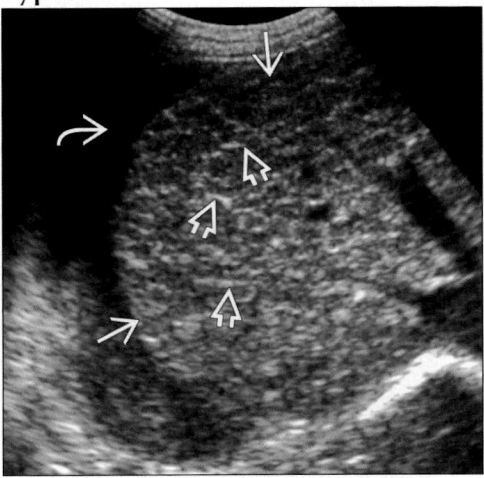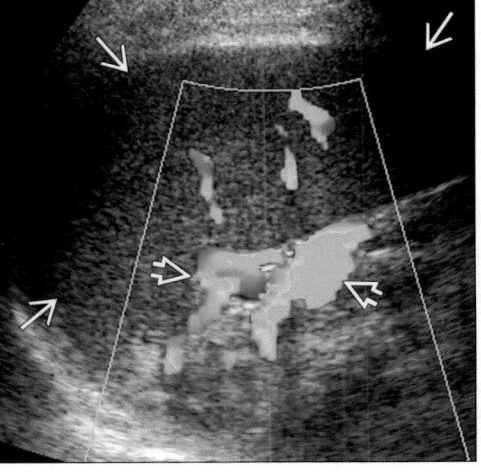

(Left) Transverse transabdominal ultrasound shows cirrhosis ➡ and ascites ⇨ in a patient with discontinuous septal thickening/fibrosis ⇨ due to schistosomiasis. *(Right)* Oblique color Doppler ultrasound shows splenomegaly ➡ in a patient with portal hypertension secondary to schistosomiasis. Note enlarged splenic hilar vessels ⇨.

STEATOSIS, HEPATIC

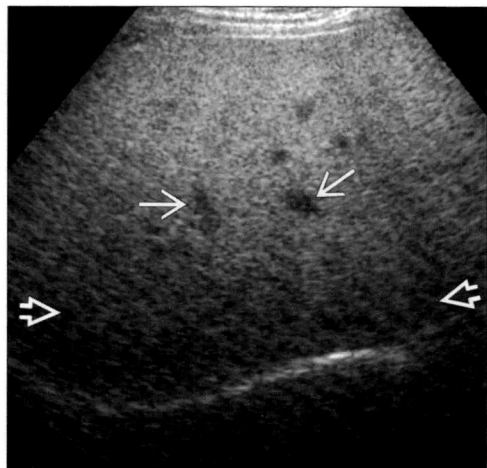

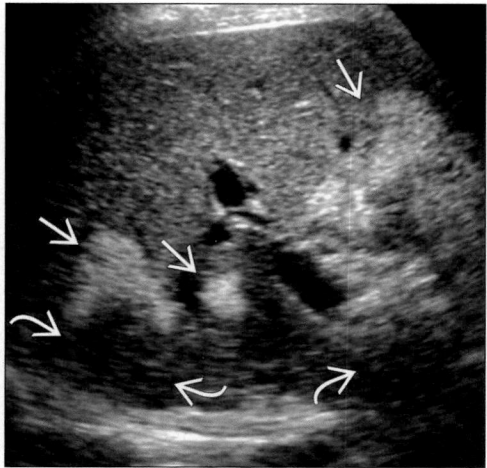

Transverse transabdominal ultrasound shows moderate steatosis with increased echogenicity, poor visualization of deep structures ➡ *and decreased resolution of vessel walls* ➡.

Transverse transabdominal ultrasound shows multiple areas of focal steatosis ➡, *showing posterior acoustic attenuation* ➡.

TERMINOLOGY

Abbreviations and Synonyms
- Hepatic steatosis or fatty metamorphosis/replacement

Definitions
- Steatosis is a metabolic complication of a variety of toxic, ischemic and infectious insults to liver

IMAGING FINDINGS

General Features
- Best diagnostic clue
  - Preservation of normal hepatic architecture
  - Decreased signal intensity of liver on T1W out-of-phase gradient echo images
- Imaging features depend on
  - Amount of fat deposited in liver
  - Presence of associated hepatic disease
  - Fat distribution within liver: Diffuse/focal

Ultrasonographic Findings
- Grayscale Ultrasound

- Diffuse fatty infiltration
  - Increased echogenicity, with liver significantly more echogenic than kidney
  - Smooth surface
  - Increase in size of liver and change in shape as volume of infiltration increases
  - Inferior margin of right lobe has rounded contours and the left lobe becomes biconvex
  - Posterior acoustic attenuation due to fatty infiltration
  - Margins of hepatic veins are blurred due to increased refraction and scattering of sound
  - With increasing infiltration, vessels are pushed apart and hepatic veins take a more curved course
- **Focal fatty infiltration**
  - Location: Right lobe, caudate lobe, perihilar region
  - Hyperechoic nodule/multiple confluent hyperechoic lesions
  - No mass effect, with vessels running undisplaced through the lesion
  - Fan-shaped lobar/segmental distribution
  - Lesions extend to edge of liver
- **Focal fatty sparing**

DDx: Steatosis

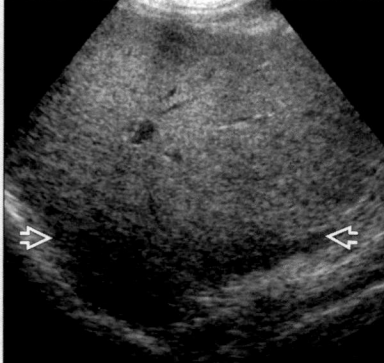

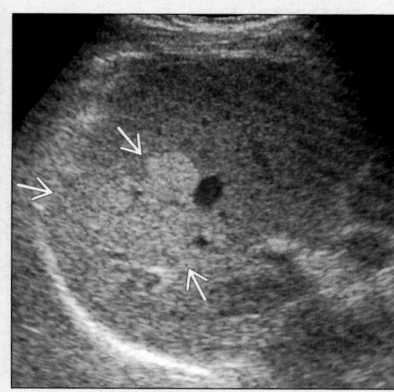

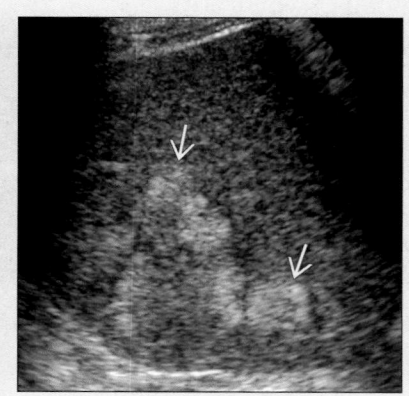

EtOH Hepatitis

Hemangioma

Hyperechoic Mets

Key Facts

Terminology
- Steatosis is a metabolic complication of a variety of toxic, ischemic and infectious insults to liver

Imaging Findings
- **Diffuse fatty infiltration**
- Increased echogenicity, with liver significantly more echogenic than kidney
- Increase in size of liver and change in shape as volume of infiltration increases
- Posterior acoustic attenuation due to fatty infiltration
- Margins of hepatic veins are blurred due to increased refraction and scattering of sound
- With increasing infiltration, vessels are pushed apart and hepatic veins take a more curved course
- **Focal fatty infiltration**
- Location: Right lobe, caudate lobe, perihilar region

- Hyperechoic nodule/multiple confluent hyperechoic lesions
- No mass effect, with vessels running undisplaced through the lesion
- Fan-shaped lobar/segmental distribution
- **Focal fatty sparing**
- Due to direct drainage of hepatic blood into systemic circulation
- Next to gallbladder bed (drained by cystic vein)
- Segment 4/anterior to portal bifurcation (drained by aberrant gastric vein)
- No mass effect (undisplaced vessels)

Top Differential Diagnoses
- Fatty Liver Hepatitis
- Hemangioma
- Metastases or Lymphoma

- Due to direct drainage of hepatic blood into systemic circulation
- Next to gallbladder bed (drained by cystic vein)
- Segment 4/anterior to portal bifurcation (drained by aberrant gastric vein)
- No mass effect (undisplaced vessels)
- Vessel architecture in the lesion resembles that of a normal liver
- Hypoechoic area within an echogenic liver

CT Findings
- NECT
  - Decreased attenuation of liver compared to spleen
    - Normal: Liver 8-10 HU more than spleen on NECT
  - Focal nodular fatty infiltration: Low attenuation
    - Common location: Adjacent to falciform ligament
- CECT
  - Detect fatty infiltration due to different degrees of liver & splenic relative enhancement
  - Normal vessels course through "lesion" (fatty infiltration)
  - CECT has lower sensitivity in detecting fatty liver

MR Findings
- T1 out-of-phase GRE: Decreased or loss of signal intensity of fatty liver
- T1 in-phase GRE: Increased signal intensity of fatty liver than spleen
- T1 C+ out-of-phase GRE: Paradoxical decreased signal intensity of liver
- STIR: Fatty areas as low signal intensity
- MR spectroscopy (MRS): For quantitative assessment

Nuclear Medicine Findings
- Technetium Tc-99m sulfur colloid
  - Differentiates true space occupying lesion from focal fat
  - Fat does not displace reticuloendothelial cells
  - Diffuse fatty infiltration
    - Inhomogeneous radionuclide uptake
- Xenon 133
  - Highly fat soluble
  - Accumulation of isotope in fatty areas of liver

- Specific sign of hepatic steatosis

DIFFERENTIAL DIAGNOSIS

Fatty Liver Hepatitis
- Diabetic fatty liver, alcoholic hepatitis (EtOH hepatitis), nonalcoholic steatohepatitis (NASH)
- Fatty liver + inflammatory change, fibrosis and necrosis
- Smooth surface, decreased plasticity
- Hepatic veins show a disjointed network-like appearance with blurred outline contrary to a curved course in simple fatty infiltration
- Increasing fibrosis and scarring

Fatty Cirrhosis
- Dense, firm liver
- Size of left lobe increases and right lobe decreases
- Prominent caudate lobe
- Heterogeneous, hyperechoic parenchyma
- Rarefaction of hepatic veins
- +/- Ascites, splenomegaly, portal venous collaterals

Hemangioma
- Typically hyperechoic nodule
- Posterior acoustic enhancement

Metastases or Lymphoma
- Hyperechoic metastases simulate focal steatosis
- Confluent tumor distorts vessels and bile ducts
- Diffuse lymphoma infiltration may be indistinguishable from normal liver or steatosis

PATHOLOGY

General Features
- General path comments
  - Ethanol increases hepatic synthesis of fatty acids
  - Carbon tetrachloride/high dose tetracycline decreases hepatic oxidation/utilization of fatty acids
  - Starvation, steroids & alcohol

STEATOSIS, HEPATIC

- Impairs release of hepatic lipoproteins
- Excessively mobilizes fatty acids from adipose tissue
  - Segmental areas of fatty infiltration occurs where glycogen is depleted from liver
    - Due to traumatic & ischemic insults
    - Decreased nutrients & insulin → decreased glycogen
    - Causes: Secondary to a mass, Budd-Chiari syndrome or tumor thrombus
- Etiology
  - Metabolic derangement
    - Obesity & hyperlipidemia, parenteral hyperalimentation
    - Poorly controlled diabetes mellitus (50%)
    - Severe hepatitis & protein malnutrition
    - Malabsorption (jejunoileal bypass)
    - Pregnancy, trauma, inflammatory bowel disease
    - Cystic fibrosis, Reye syndrome
  - Hepatotoxins
    - Alcohol (> 50%), carbon tetrachlorides, phosphorus
  - Drugs
    - Tetracycline, amiodarone, corticosteroids
    - Salicylates, tamoxifen, calcium channel blockers
- Epidemiology
  - Most frequently seen on liver biopsies of alcoholics
  - Seen in up to 50% of patients with diabetes mellitus
  - Quite prevalent in general population with obesity
  - Seen in 25% of nonalcoholics
    - Healthy adult males meeting accidental deaths
- Associated abnormalities
  - Nonalcoholic steatohepatitis
    - Seen in patients with hyperlipidemia & diabetes
    - May lead to "cryptogenic" cirrhosis

Gross Pathologic & Surgical Features
- Liver may weigh 4-6 kg
- Soft, yellow, greasy cut surface

Microscopic Features
- Macrovesicular fatty liver (most common type)
  - Hepatocytes with large cytoplasmic fat vacuoles displacing nucleus peripherally
    - Examples: Alcohol & diabetes mellitus
- Microvesicular
  - Fat is present in many small vacuoles
  - Example: Reye syndrome

Staging, Grading or Classification Criteria
- Sonographic grading for diffuse steatosis
  - Mild: Minimal increased parenchymal echogenicity & normal appearing intrahepatic vessel walls
  - Moderate: Further increased parenchymal echogenicity causing decreased resolution of intrahepatic vessel walls
  - Severe: Marked increased parenchymal echogenicity causing inability to resolve intrahepatic vessel walls

CLINICAL ISSUES

Presentation
- Most common signs/symptoms

- Asymptomatic, but often with abnormal liver function tests (LFTs)
- Enlarged liver in obese or diabetic patient
- Alcoholic patients
  - 2/3 alcoholics: Right upper quadrant (RUQ) pain, tenderness, hepatomegaly
- Clinical profile
  - Asymptomatic obese or diabetic patient with enlarged liver
- Lab data
  - Asymptomatic: Normal/mildly elevated LFTs
  - Alcoholic: Abnormal LFTs
  - Steatohepatitis may have markedly abnormal LFTs
- Diagnosis
  - Seldom require biopsy/histology

Natural History & Prognosis
- Alcoholics: Gradual disappearance of fat from liver after 4-8 weeks of adequate diet & abstinence from alcohol
- Resolves in 2 weeks after discontinuation of parenteral hyperalimentation
- Steatohepatitis may progress to acute or chronic liver failure

Treatment
- Removal of alcohol or offending toxins
- Correction of metabolic disorders
- Lipotropic agents like choline when indicated

DIAGNOSTIC CHECKLIST

Consider
- Rule out other liver pathologies which may mimic focal or diffuse steatosis (fatty liver)

Image Interpretation Pearls
- Key on all imaging modalities is presence of normal vessels coursing through "lesion" (fatty infiltration)

SELECTED REFERENCES

1. Brandt M: Liver. Differential Diagnosis in Ultrasound Imaging: a teaching atlas. Editor: Schmidt Guenter. 49-100. Thieme, Stuttgart, Germany, 2006
2. Rubaltelli L et al: Target appearance of pseudotumors in segment IV of the liver on sonography. AJR. 178: 75-7, 2002
3. Needleman L et al: Sonography of diffuse benign liver disease: accuracy of pattern recognition and grading. AJR Am J Roentgenol. 146(5):1011-5, 1986
4. Yates CK et al: Focal fatty infiltration of the liver simulating metastatic disease. Radiology. 159(1):83-4, 1986
5. Baker MK et al: Focal fatty infiltration of the liver: diagnostic imaging. Radiographics. 5(6):923-9, 1985
6. Quinn SF et al: Characteristic sonographic signs of hepatic fatty infiltration. AJR Am J Roentgenol. 145(4):753-5, 1985
7. Scatarige JC et al: Fatty infiltration of the liver: ultrasonographic and computed tomographic correlation. J Ultrasound Med. 3(1):9-14, 1984

IMAGE GALLERY

Typical

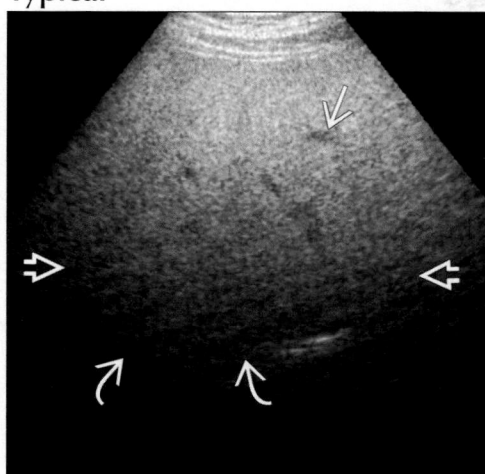

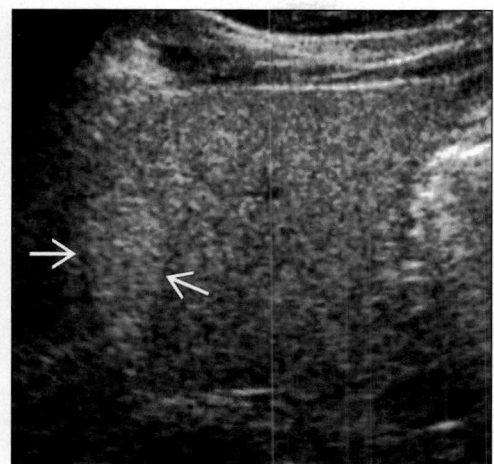

(Left) Transverse transabdominal ultrasound shows severe steatosis with poor visualization of deeper structures ➡ (e.g., diaphragm ➡; and unresolvable vessel walls ➡). Vessels still run normal course. (Right) Longitudinal transabdominal ultrasound shows subcapsular location of focal steatosis ➡.

Typical

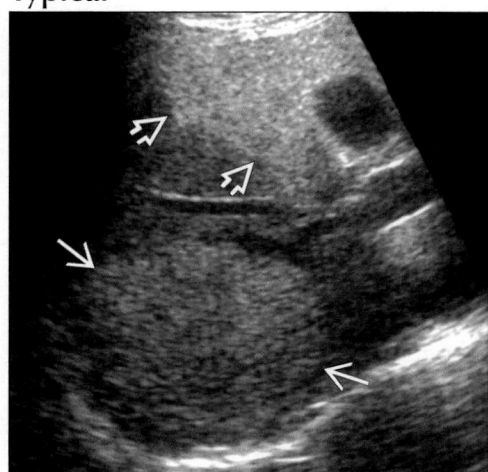

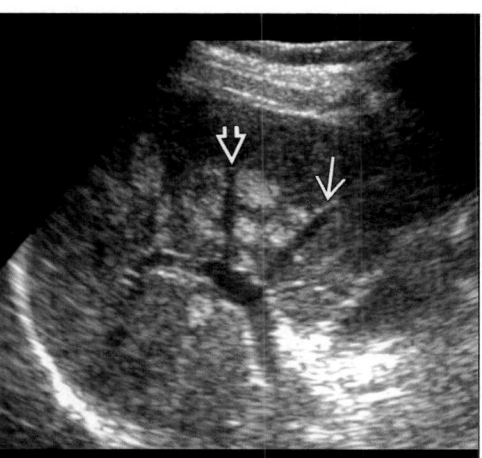

(Left) Transverse transabdominal ultrasound shows two areas of focal steatosis, a more superficial lesion showing geographic borders ➡ & a deeper lesion with round borders ➡. (Right) Oblique transabdominal ultrasound shows focal steatosis which does not distort the adjacent portal vein ➡. Another portal vein passes normally through one of the areas ➡.

Typical

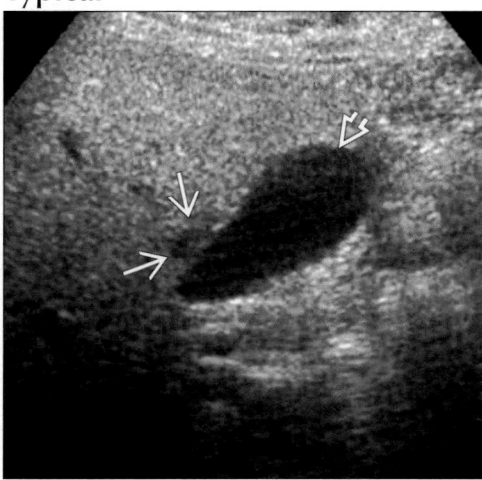

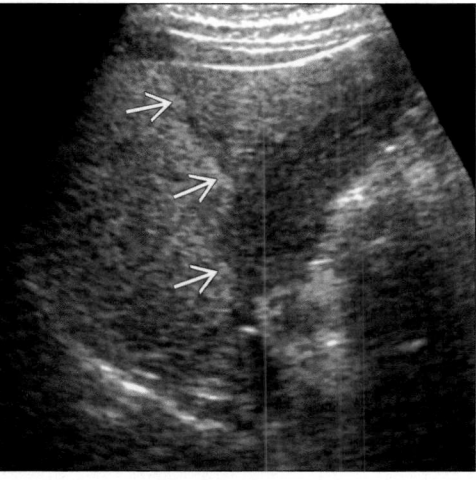

(Left) Oblique transabdominal ultrasound shows focal area of fatty sparing ➡ adjacent to the gallbladder ➡ and simulating a hypoechoic nodule. (Right) Longitudinal transabdominal ultrasound shows a large area of focal steatosis with a geographic border ➡.

PARENCHYMAL CALCIFICATION, HEPATIC

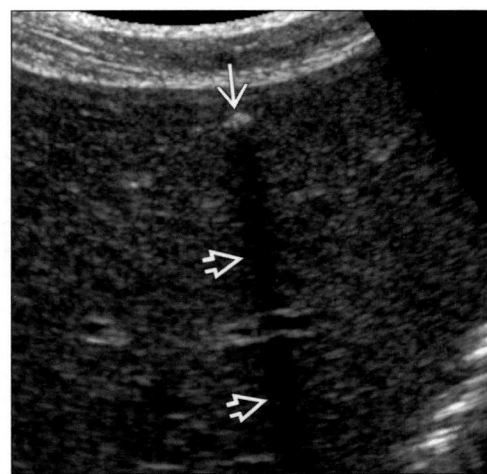

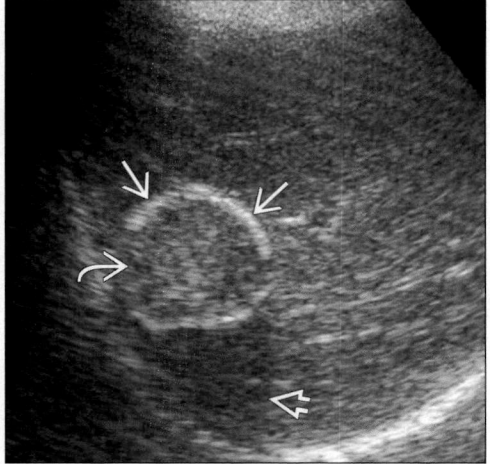

Oblique transabdominal ultrasound shows a small densely calcified granuloma ➡ with posterior acoustic shadowing ⧩. Note the amorphous appearance of the calcification.

Oblique transabdominal ultrasound shows a mildly calcified surface ➡ of an echinococcal cyst. Posterior acoustic shadow ⧩ is present but echogenic cyst content ➡ remains visible.

TERMINOLOGY

Definitions
- Calcification within the parenchyma of liver

IMAGING FINDINGS

General Features
- Best diagnostic clue: Posterior acoustic shadowing
- Location: Anywhere in the liver
- Size: Variable from a few mm to cm
- Morphology: Nodular, curvilinear or amorphous

Ultrasonographic Findings
- Grayscale Ultrasound
  - Hyperechoic interface
    - Specular reflection: Suggests a cyst wall
    - Lobulated: Nonspecific
    - Indistinct: Amorphous/intralesional calcification
  - Posterior acoustic shadowing
    - This may not be demonstrable for small lesions or mildly calcified lesions

- Posterior structures may still be visible if the superficial calcification is not dense
  - Increasing transducer frequency may help to demonstrate posterior shadowing

CT Findings
- NECT: Most sensitive in demonstrating calcification but requires additional scans prior to contrast
- CECT: Contrast-enhancement may mask underlying or adjacent calcification

MR Findings
- T1WI: Usually low signal
- T2WI: Variable signal intensity: Hyper-, iso-, hypo-intense
- T2* GRE: Susceptibility artifact may highlight lesion

Imaging Recommendations
- Best imaging tool: Ultrasound usually detects hepatic parenchymal calcification as an incidental finding
- Protocol advice
  - Using different ultrasound planes for interrogation to demonstrate posterior acoustic shadowing and alternatively contents posterior to calcification

DDx: Parenchymal Calcification

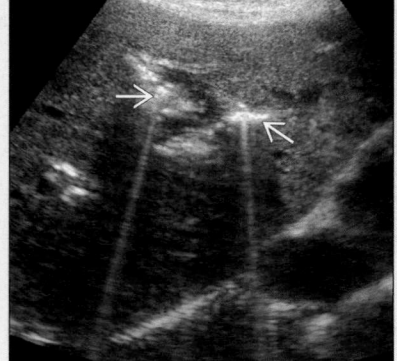

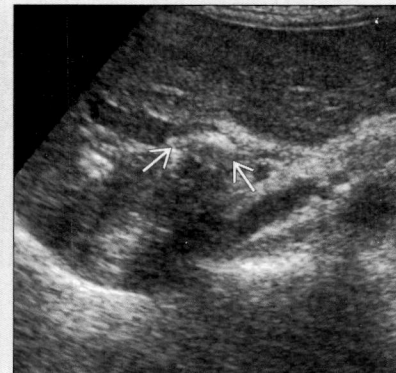

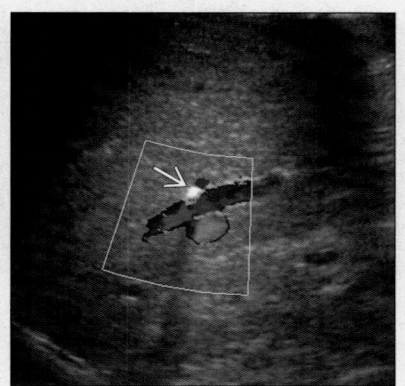

| Pneumobilia | Intraductal Stone | Vascular Calcification |

Key Facts

Imaging Findings
- Hyperechoic interface
- Posterior acoustic shadowing
- Increasing transducer frequency may help to demonstrate posterior shadowing
- Using different ultrasound planes for interrogation to demonstrate posterior acoustic shadowing and alternatively contents posterior to calcification

Top Differential Diagnoses
- Biliary Calcification
- Pneumobilia
- Vascular Calcification

Clinical Issues
- Calcification frequently considered to be a sign of decreased disease activity or response to treatment

---

○ Rule out malignancy, otherwise perform follow-up ultrasound in 3-6 months

DIFFERENTIAL DIAGNOSIS

Biliary Calcification
- Intrahepatic ductal calculi: Calcify much less frequently than gallbladder or common bile duct stones
- Parasite: Ascaris
- May have distal bile duct dilatation as a result of obstruction

Pneumobilia
- Ring down artifact posterior to gas

Vascular Calcification
- Mural: Hepatic artery aneurysm, degenerative calcification, vascular malformation
- Intraluminal: Chronic portal vein thrombosis
- Chronic hematoma

PATHOLOGY

General Features
- Etiology: Granuloma is most common incidental calcified lesion
- Epidemiology
  ○ Granulomatous infection: Tuberculosis, amoeba, histoplasmosis, pyogenic, TORCH, etc.

○ Infestation: Echinococcus, schistosomiasis
○ Neoplastic: Primary (hemangioma, hepatocellular carcinoma, cholangiocarcinoma, hepatoblastoma, hamartoma) or secondary (ovarian, mucinous carcinoma, osteosarcoma etc.)
○ Metabolic: Hemochromatosis
○ Degenerative i.e., granuloma, hematoma
○ Iatrogenic: Iron, thorotrast, thallium

CLINICAL ISSUES

Presentation
- Most common signs/symptoms: Usually an incidental finding

Natural History & Prognosis
- Calcification frequently considered to be a sign of decreased disease activity or response to treatment

DIAGNOSTIC CHECKLIST

Image Interpretation Pearls
- CT may be required for large densely calcified masses

SELECTED REFERENCES

1. Paley MR et al: Hepatic calcification. Radiol Clin North Am. 36(2):391-8, 1998

IMAGE GALLERY

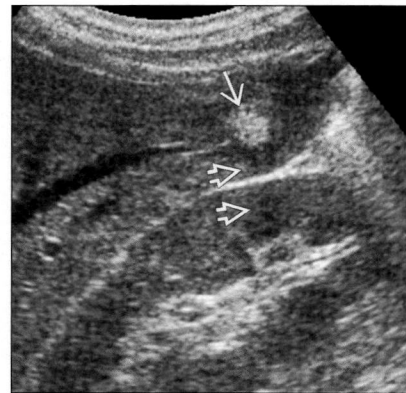 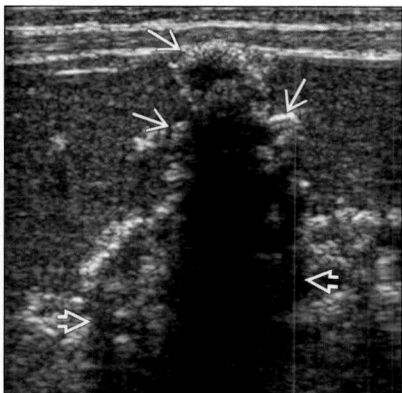 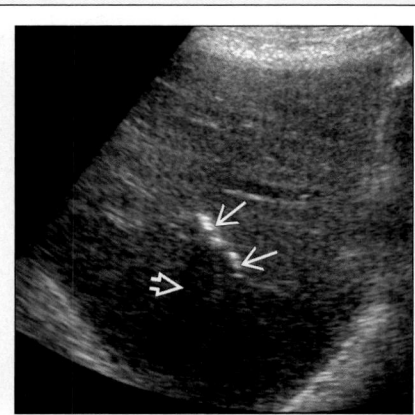

(Left) Oblique transabdominal ultrasound shows amorphous calcification ➡ within a treated metastatic deposit. Posterior acoustic shadowing ➡ is subtle. *(Center)* Oblique transabdominal ultrasound shows densely calcified metastases ➡ close to the liver surface, with posterior acoustic shadowing ➡. Note lobulated borders. *(Right)* Transverse transabdominal ultrasound shows curvilinear calcification ➡ in an old hematoma and posterior acoustic shadowing ➡. Note thin curvilinear appearance simulating duct/vessel.

DIFFUSE MICROABSCESSES, HEPATIC

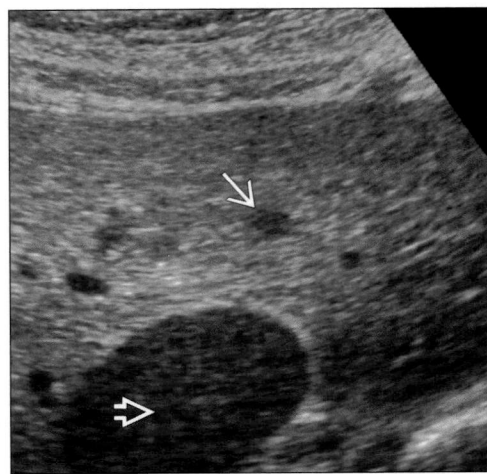

Oblique transabdominal ultrasound shows a hypoechoic microabscess ➡ with echogenicity similar to gallbladder contents ⇨.

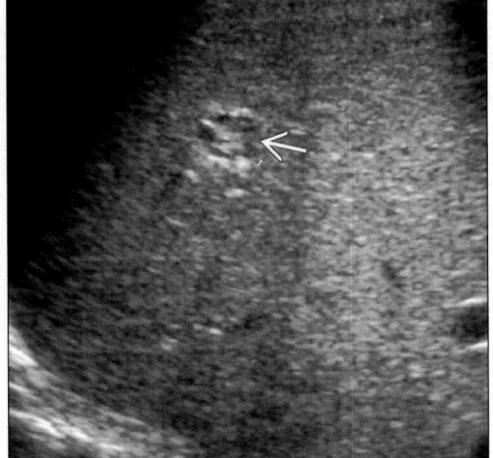

Oblique transabdominal ultrasound shows a microabscess with a "target" sign ➡ of central echogenic inflammation and surrounding hypoechoic fibrosis.

TERMINOLOGY

Definitions
- Hepatic parenchymal abscesses measuring around 1 cm in diameter
- Typically refers to hepatic candida abscesses in immunocompromised patients

IMAGING FINDINGS

General Features
- Best diagnostic clue: Multiple small lesions in the liver in a patient with neutropenic fever
- Location: Diffusely distributed in liver +/- spleen
- Size: Around 1 cm
- Morphology: Usually rounded

Ultrasonographic Findings
- Grayscale Ultrasound
  - Multiple small hypo-/iso-/hyper-echoic lesions
  - Target sign may be present
    - Central hyperechoic inflammation surrounded by hypoechoic halo of fibrosis

- "Wheel within a wheel" pattern may be present in larger fungal lesions
  - Hyperechoic nodule of inflammatory cells with surrounding hypoechoic halo of fibrosis
  - Central hypoechoic area of necrosis within hyperechoic lesion
- Lesions may disappear or calcify after successful treatment
- Similar lesions may be found in spleen

CT Findings
- CECT
  - Multiple small hypodense lesions in liver +/- spleen
  - Ill-defined margins
  - No contrast-enhancement

Imaging Recommendations
- Best imaging tool
  - Ultrasound is ideal for lesion detection, progress monitoring and guiding biopsy
  - Repeated imaging may be necessary to detect lesions (ultrasound being radiation-free is an advantage)

DDx: Diffuse Hepatic Microabscess

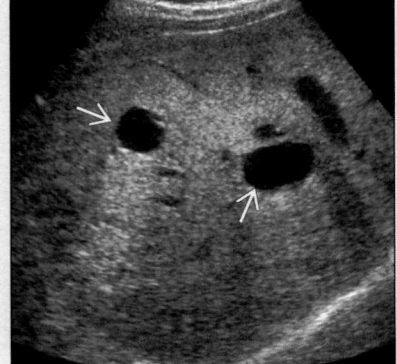

Simple Cysts

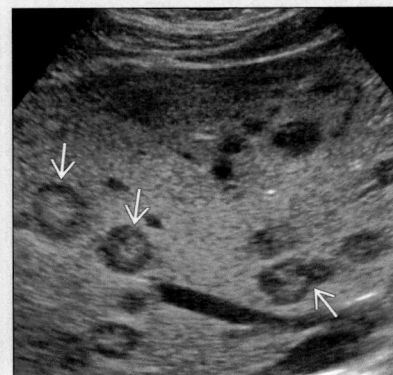

Metastases

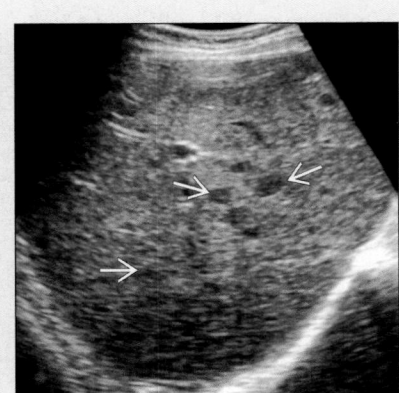

Lymphoma

Key Facts

Imaging Findings

- Best diagnostic clue: Multiple small lesions in the liver in a patient with neutropenic fever
- Multiple small hypo-/iso-/hyper-echoic lesions
- Target sign may be present
- "Wheel within a wheel" pattern may be present in larger fungal lesions
- Lesions may disappear or calcify after successful treatment

- Similar lesions may be found in spleen
- Protocol advice: Higher frequency transducer (e.g., 5 MHz) improves detection of small abscesses, this should be added to the examination in high risk patients

Top Differential Diagnoses

- Simple Cysts
- Necrotic Metastases
- Lymphomatous Infiltration

- Protocol advice: Higher frequency transducer (e.g., 5 MHz) improves detection of small abscesses, this should be added to the examination in high risk patients

- Mostly fungal: Candida albicans
- Pyogenic: Staphylococcus aureus

DIFFERENTIAL DIAGNOSIS

Simple Cysts

- Typical uniformly hypoechoic/anechoic content

Necrotic Metastases

- May also demonstrate the "target" sign (hypoechoic halo)
- Multiple
- Known primary tumor

Lymphomatous Infiltration

- Lymphadenopathy
- Hepatosplenomegaly

PATHOLOGY

General Features

- Etiology
  - Typically fungal infection in immunocompromised patients (leukemia, lymphoma, AIDS/post-transplant)
  - Pyogenic infections can also result in a similar appearance
- Epidemiology

CLINICAL ISSUES

Presentation

- Most common signs/symptoms
  - Fever unresponsive to antibiotic treatment
  - Abdominal pain
  - Deranged liver function

Treatment

- Antifungal agents: Amphotericin B, fluconazole

SELECTED REFERENCES

1. Verbanck J et al: Sonographic detection of multiple Staphylococcus aureus hepatic microabscesses mimicking Candida abscesses. J Clin Ultrasound. 27(8):478-81, 1999
2. Murray JG et al: Microabscesses of the liver and spleen in AIDS: detection with 5-MHz sonography. Radiology. 197(3):723-7, 1995
3. Gorg C et al: Ultrasound evaluation of hepatic and splenic microabscesses in the immunocompromised patient: sonographic patterns, differential diagnosis, and follow-up. J Clin Ultrasound. 22(9):525-9, 1994
4. Callen PW et al: Ultrasonography and computed tomography in the evaluation of hepatic microabscesses in the immunosuppressed patient. Radiology. 136(2):433-4, 1980

IMAGE GALLERY

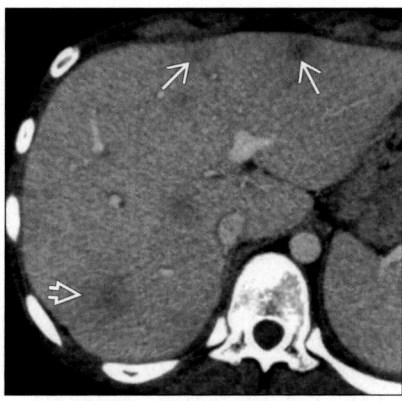 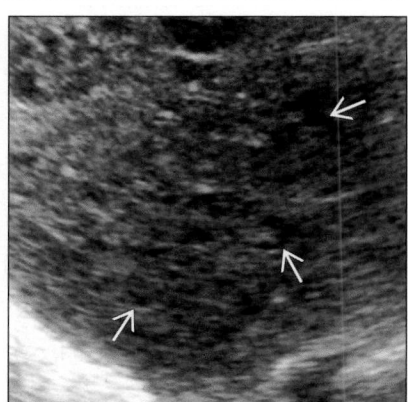 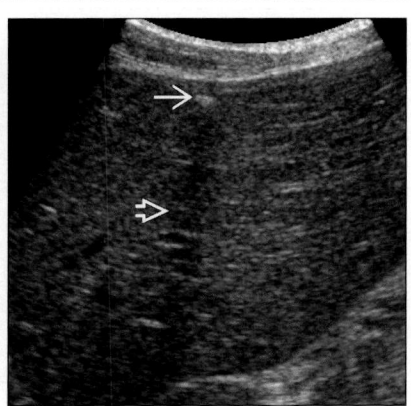

(Left) Transverse CECT shows multiple nonenhancing lesions ➡ of various sizes with ill-defined borders ➡. *(Center)* Oblique transabdominal ultrasound shows patchy hypoechoic pattern due to diffuse involvement ➡ of the parenchyma by candida. *(Right)* Oblique transabdominal ultrasound shows a calcified scar from microabscess ➡ after treatment. Note posterior acoustic shadowing ➡.

LYMPHOMA, HEPATIC

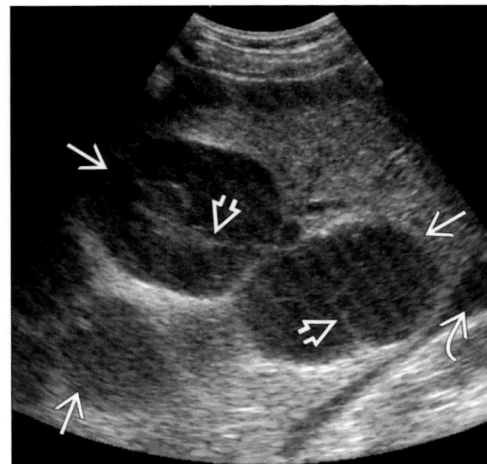

Oblique transabdominal ultrasound shows multiple lymphomatous deposits ➡, some with septae ⮥. Echogenicity similar to ascitic fluid ⬈, but no acoustic enhancement behind deposits.

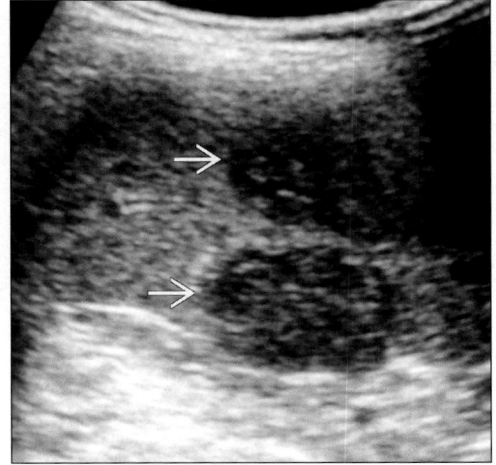

Transverse transabdominal ultrasound shows two hypoechoic lymphomatous deposits ➡ with heterogeneous echotexture in the spleen.

TERMINOLOGY

Abbreviations and Synonyms
- Hodgkin disease (HD), non-Hodgkin lymphoma (NHL)

Definitions
- Neoplasm of lymphoid tissues

IMAGING FINDINGS

General Features
- Best diagnostic clue: Uniformly hypoechoic masses
- Location
  - Lymphoma (HD and NHL) arises in periportal areas due to high content of lymphatic tissue
  - Liver is often a secondary site for lymphoma in HD and NHL
- Size: Variable; from few millimeters to centimeters
- Morphology
  - Discrete lesions (more likely to be primary NHL or AIDS associated lymphoma)
  - Diffuse infiltration (usually secondary site in HD or NHL) is difficult to detect on imaging

- Key concepts
  - Hepatic lymphoma is detected in vivo in less than 10% of cases
  - Primary hepatic lymphoma is rare and mostly seen in immunocompromised patients
  - Secondary is more common
    - Seen in more than 50% of patients with HD or NHL on autopsy
  - Lymphoma generally more common in immunosuppressed patients
    - Transplant recipients and AIDS patients are at high risk
  - Types of lymphoma
    - Hodgkin disease
    - Non-Hodgkin lymphoma

Ultrasonographic Findings
- Grayscale Ultrasound
  - Hepatomegaly
  - **Discrete form**
    - Multiple, well-defined, nodules/masses
    - Hypoechoic/anechoic (low echogenicity probably due to high cellular density and lack of background stroma)

DDx: Hepatic Lymphoma

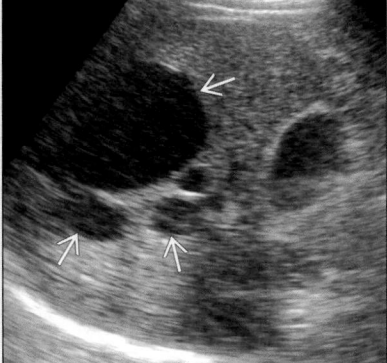

Multiple Cysts

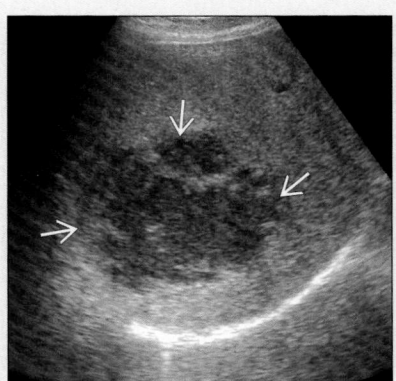

Abscesses

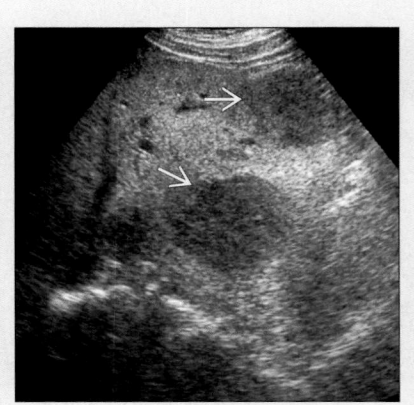

Hemangioma

Key Facts

Imaging Findings

- Lymphoma (HD and NHL) arises in periportal areas due to high content of lymphatic tissue
- Multiple, well-defined, nodules/masses
- Hypoechoic/anechoic (low echogenicity probably due to high cellular density and lack of background stroma)
- Large/conglomerate masses may appear to contain septae and mimic abscesses
- Innumerable subcentimeter hypoechoic foci, miliary in pattern and periportal in location
- Infiltrative pattern may be indistinguishable from normal liver
- Associated splenomegaly or splenic lesions
- Lymphadenopathy (periportal, para-aortic, mesenteric)

- Best imaging tool: Ultrasound for surveillance and monitoring lesion progress/treatment response
- Protocol advice: Ultrasound detection of lesion to be followed by CECT for disease staging

Top Differential Diagnoses

- Hepatic Cysts
- Liver Abscesses
- Hemangiomas

Diagnostic Checklist

- Rule out other multiple liver lesions like hepatic cysts, abscesses, hemangiomas
- Often the clue to the diagnosis is abnormal hepatic parenchymal echo pattern associated with splenomegaly and lymphadenopathy
- Confirmation with needle biopsy

  - Large/conglomerate masses may appear to contain septae and mimic abscesses
  - Diffuse/infiltrative form
    - Innumerable subcentimeter hypoechoic foci, miliary in pattern and periportal in location
    - Infiltrative pattern may be indistinguishable from normal liver
    - Most of these are missed and only diagnosed on autopsy
  - Other signs of lymphoma
    - Associated splenomegaly or splenic lesions
    - Lymphadenopathy (periportal, para-aortic, mesenteric)
    - Bowel wall thickening (infiltration)
    - Ascites

CT Findings

- NECT
  - May be normal
  - Primary lymphoma
    - Isodense or hypodense to liver
  - Secondary lymphoma
    - Multiple well-defined, large, homogeneous lobulated low density masses
    - Diffuse infiltration: Indistinguishable from normal liver or steatosis
- CECT
  - Poor contrast-enhancement
  - Usually homogeneous density
  - May have rim-enhancement

MR Findings

- T1WI
  - Discrete lesion: Hypointense masses
  - Diffuse infiltration: Indistinguishable from normal liver
- T2WI
  - Discrete lesion: Hyperintense masses
  - Diffuse infiltration: Indistinguishable from normal liver
- T1 C+
  - Poor gadolinium enhancement (similar to hypovascular metastases)

  - May have rim-enhancement
- Superparamagnetic iron oxide (SPIO)
  - Metastases: Bright signal on T2WI
    - Free of reticuloendothelial system (RES)
  - Rest of normal liver: Decreased signal
    - Due to SPIO particles phagocytized by RES of liver

Nuclear Medicine Findings

- PET
  - Hepatic lymphoma
    - Good concordance with other imaging modalities
    - Useful for staging disease

Imaging Recommendations

- Best imaging tool: Ultrasound for surveillance and monitoring lesion progress/treatment response
- Protocol advice: Ultrasound detection of lesion to be followed by CECT for disease staging

DIFFERENTIAL DIAGNOSIS

Hepatic Cysts

- Smooth contour
- Imperceptible walls
- May have increased density or intensity due to prior bleed or infection (e.g., polycystic liver)
- No mural nodules or debris

Liver Abscesses

- "Cluster sign" for pyogenic abscesses
- Often with atelectasis and right pleural effusion
- Typical systemic signs of infection

Hemangiomas

- Typically uniformly hyperechoic on US
- May be hypoechoic

Multifocal HCC

- Background cirrhotic liver, vascular invasion
- Hepatic vascular invasion/thrombosis

LYMPHOMA, HEPATIC

Metastases
• Difficult to differentiate without history of primary lesion

PATHOLOGY

General Features
• General path comments
  ○ Lymphoma
    ▪ Early disease: Miliary lesions
    ▪ Late disease: Multiple nodules
• Etiology: Viral cause suggested
• Epidemiology
  ○ Approximately 60,000 new cases of lymphoma diagnosed per year in the USA
  ○ Primary hepatic lymphoma is rare (around 100 cases described)
• Associated abnormalities
  ○ Immunocompromised patients are predisposed to lymphoma
    ▪ Congenital immunodeficiency
    ▪ Collagen vascular diseases
    ▪ HIV infection/AIDS
    ▪ Immunosuppressant therapy for organ transplant

Gross Pathologic & Surgical Features
• Lymphoma: Miliary, nodular or diffuse form

Microscopic Features
• Hodgkin disease
  ○ Typical Reed-Sternberg cells
• Non-Hodgkin lymphoma
  ○ Follicular small cleaved-cells (most common)
  ○ Small noncleaved cells (Burkitt lymphoma: Rare)

Staging, Grading or Classification Criteria
• Ann Arbor staging classification
• For NHL histology: Revised European American Lymphoma (REAL) classification or International Working Formulation

CLINICAL ISSUES

Presentation
• Most common signs/symptoms
  ○ Asymptomatic
  ○ Right upper quadrant pain
  ○ Hepatomegaly
  ○ Weight loss
  ○ Jaundice
  ○ Ascites
• Lab data: Elevated liver enzymes; may be normal in some patients
• Diagnosis: Imaging, occasionally fine needle aspiration biopsy

Demographics
• Age: Usually middle and older age group
• Gender: M > F

Natural History & Prognosis
• Depends on the histological classification and the stage of the disease
• Liver involvement may lead to fulminant hepatic failure with rapid progression of encephalopathy to coma and death

Treatment
• Chemotherapy may be hampered by hepatic insufficiency
• Radiotherapy or surgery

DIAGNOSTIC CHECKLIST

Consider
• Rule out other multiple liver lesions like hepatic cysts, abscesses, hemangiomas
• Often the clue to the diagnosis is abnormal hepatic parenchymal echo pattern associated with splenomegaly and lymphadenopathy
• Confirmation with needle biopsy

SELECTED REFERENCES

1. Helmberger T et al: New contrast agents for imaging the liver. Magn Reson Imaging Clin N Am. 9(4):745-66, 2001
2. Maher MM et al: Imaging of primary non-Hodgkin's lymphoma of the liver. Clin Radiol. 56(4):295-301, 2001
3. Rizzi EB et al: Non-hodgkin's lymphoma of the liver in patients with AIDS: sonographic, CT, and MRI findings. J Clin Ultrasound. 29(3):125-9, 2001
4. Coakley FV et al: Non-Hodgkin lymphoma as a cause of intrahepatic periportal low attenuation on CT. J Comput Assist Tomogr. 21(5):726-8, 1997
5. Kelekis NL et al: Focal hepatic lymphoma: magnetic resonance demonstration using current techniques including gadolinium enhancement. Magn Reson Imaging. 15(6):625-36, 1997
6. Munker R et al: Diagnostic accuracy of ultrasound and computed tomography in the staging of Hodgkin's disease. Verification by laparotomy in 100 cases. Cancer. 76(8):1460-6, 1995
7. Gazelle GS et al: US, CT, and MRI of primary and secondary liver lymphoma. J Comput Assist Tomogr. 18(3):412-5, 1994
8. Honda H et al: Hepatic lymphoma in cyclosporine-treated transplant recipients: sonographic and CT findings. AJR Am J Roentgenol. 152(3):501-3, 1989
9. Boechat MI et al: Primary liver tumors in children: comparison of CT and MR imaging. Radiology. 169(3):727-32, 1988
10. Nyberg DA et al: AIDS-related lymphomas: evaluation by abdominal CT. Radiology. 159(1):59-63, 1986
11. Weinreb JC et al: Magnetic resonance imaging of hepatic lymphoma. AJR Am J Roentgenol. 143(6):1211-4, 1984

LYMPHOMA, HEPATIC

IMAGE GALLERY

Typical

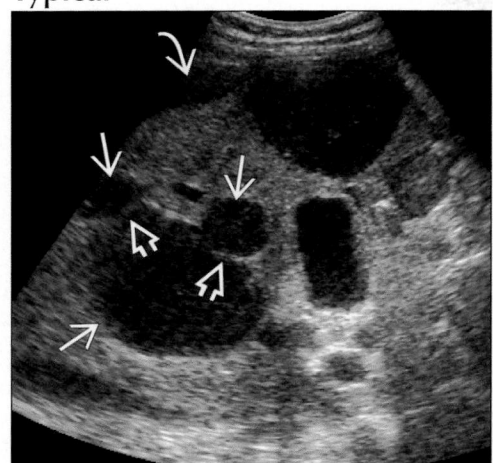

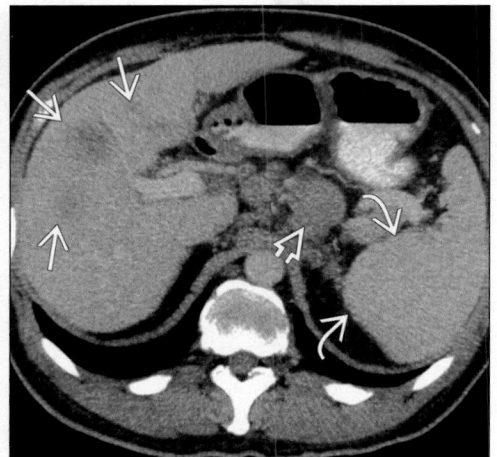

(Left) Oblique transabdominal ultrasound shows a conglomeration of multiple, hypoechoic lymphomatous deposits ➡, creating a lobulated contour (septae ⮡). The echogenicity is similar to ascitic fluid ➡. *(Right)* Transverse CECT shows several mildly hypoattenuating hepatic lymphomatous deposits ➡, lymphadenopathy ➡ and focal splenic deposit ➡ creating a bulge in the contour.

Typical

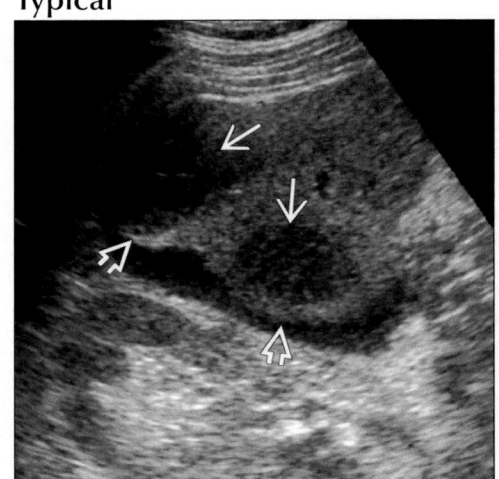

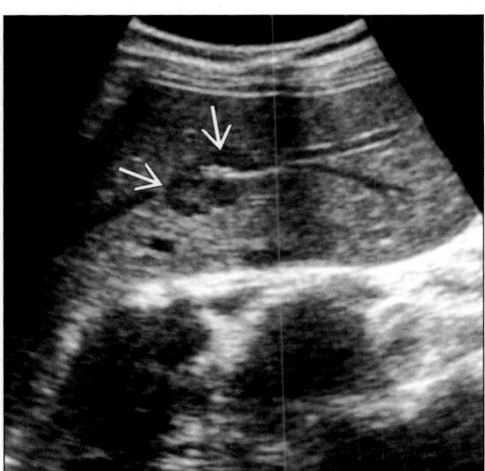

(Left) Oblique transabdominal ultrasound shows distortion of the hepatic surface contour ➡ by hypoechoic hepatic deposits ➡. *(Right)* Oblique transabdominal ultrasound shows small, hypoechoic, periportal lymphomatous deposits ➡.

Typical

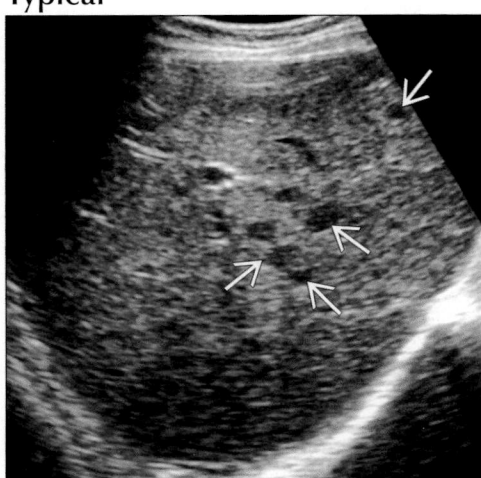

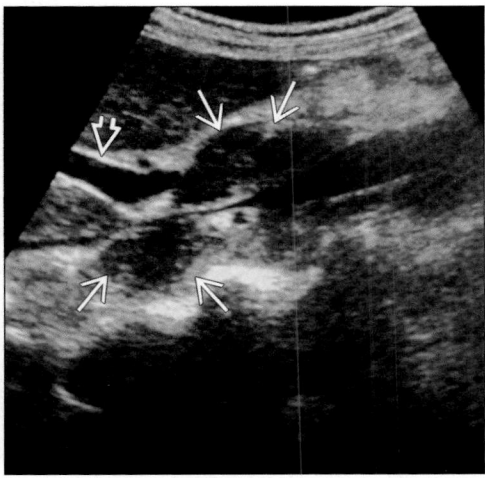

(Left) Oblique transabdominal ultrasound shows multiple, small, hypoechoic lymphomatous deposits ➡ periportal in distribution. *(Right)* Oblique transabdominal ultrasound shows enlarged lymph nodes ➡ (due to lymphomatous infiltration) in the porta hepatis region close to the portal vein ➡.

HEPATIC CYST

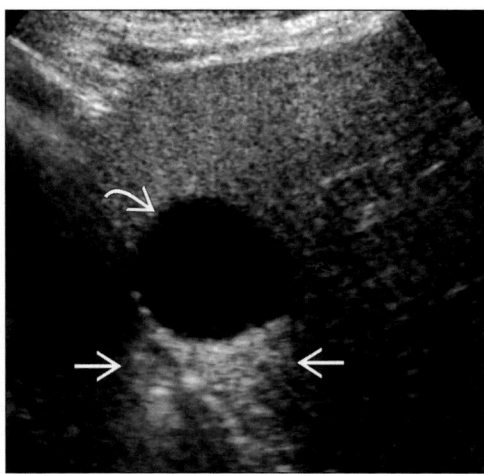

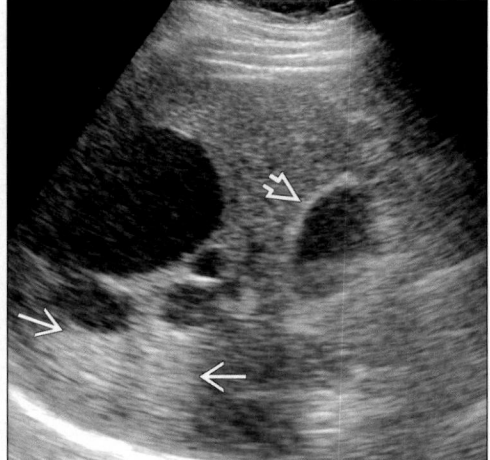

Oblique transabdominal ultrasound shows a simple cyst with smooth contour ➡ and through transmission ➡.

Transverse transabdominal ultrasound shows multiple cysts, all showing through transmission ➡. The gallbladder with sludge ➡ also shows similar through transmission.

TERMINOLOGY

Abbreviations and Synonyms
- Simple hepatic or bile duct cyst

Definitions
- Benign congenital or developmental fluid-filled space with wall derived from biliary endothelium

IMAGING FINDINGS

General Features
- Best diagnostic clue: Anechoic lesion with posterior enhancement & no mural nodularity on US, may cause bulge in hepatic contour
- Location
  - Simple cyst
    - Typically occurs beneath the surface of liver
    - Some may occur deeper
- Size: Varies from few mm to 10 cm
- Morphology
  - Typically unilocular with a thin smooth wall
  - Some may be multilocular or contain septae

- Typically contains clear fluid
- Some may have particulate content or old blood
- Key concepts
  - Current theory
    - True hepatic cysts arise from hamartomatous tissue
  - 2nd most common benign hepatic lesion after cavernous hemangioma
  - Congenital or developmental: Simple hepatic or bile duct cyst
    - Often solitary, occasionally multiple (less than 10) in clusters or disseminated
    - No communication with bile ducts
    - More prevalent in women
    - Usually asymptomatic
  - When more than 10 in number, one of fibropolycystic diseases must be considered
    - Example: Autosomal dominant polycystic liver disease (ADPLD) or biliary hamartomas
  - Acquired cyst-like hepatic lesions
    - Trauma (seroma or biloma)
    - Infection: Pyogenic or parasitic
    - Neoplasm: Primary or metastatic

DDx: Cystic Lesion

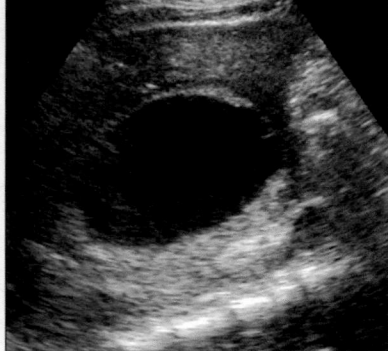

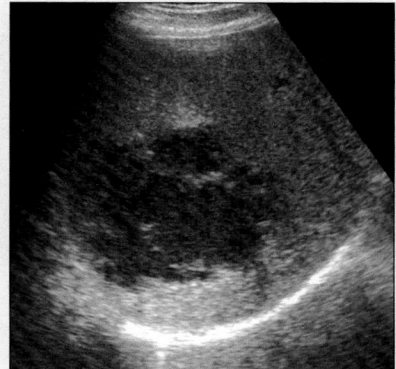

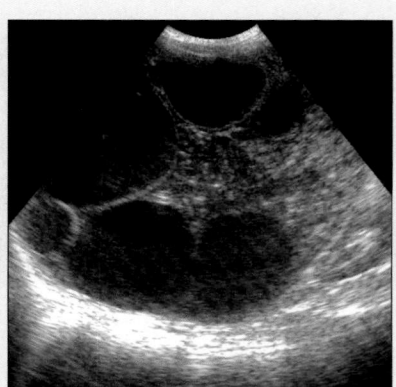

Cystic Metastasis

Pyogenic Abscess

Hydatid Cyst

HEPATIC CYST

Key Facts

Terminology
- Benign congenital or developmental fluid-filled space with wall derived from biliary endothelium

Imaging Findings
- Best diagnostic clue: Anechoic lesion with posterior enhancement & no mural nodularity on US, may cause bulge in hepatic contour
- Typically occurs beneath the surface of liver
- Typically unilocular with a thin smooth wall
- Some may be multilocular or contain septae
- Normal adjacent liver parenchyma
- Best imaging tool: Ultrasonography

Top Differential Diagnoses
- Cystic or Necrotic Metastases
- Pyogenic Abscess

- Hydatid Cyst
- Biliary Cystadenocarcinoma
- Hepatic Hemangioma

Pathology
- Defective development of intrahepatic biliary duct

Clinical Issues
- Usually asymptomatic, detected incidentally

Diagnostic Checklist
- Rule out cyst-like hepatic lesions (infection, neoplasm)
- Anechoic, thin wall, posterior enhancement
- Internal debris may settle under gravity, visible at the end of the examination

Ultrasonographic Findings
- Grayscale Ultrasound
  - Uncomplicated simple (bile duct) cyst
    - Anechoic mass
    - Smooth borders (occasionally lobulated)
    - Thin or non-detectable wall
    - No or few septations
    - No mural nodules or wall calcification
    - Do not cross segments
    - Normal adjacent liver parenchyma
  - Hemorrhagic or infected hepatic cyst
    - Septation/thickened wall
    - Solid appearing if internal debris (clots or fibrin strands) dispersed within cyst
    - Fluid-debris level if debris settles under gravity
    - With or without calcification
  - Autosomal dominant polycystic liver disease
    - Multiple cysts (more than 10); 1-10 cm size
    - Anechoic or with debris due to hemorrhage or infection
    - Calcification of some cyst walls
    - No septations or mural nodularity
    - Liver often distorted by innumerable cysts
    - In severe cases, hardly any hepatic parenchyma is seen, segmental liver anatomy and normal shape disappear
    - Also evaluate pancreas & kidneys for presence of cysts
- Color Doppler
  - Uncomplicated or complicated simple cyst
    - No internal or mural vascularity
    - Adjacent vessels may be distorted for large cysts

CT Findings
- NECT
  - Simple liver or bile duct cyst
    - Sharply defined margins with smooth, thin walls
    - Water density (-10 to +10 HU)
    - Usually no septations (rarely up to 2 thin septa)
    - No fluid-debris levels, mural nodularity or wall calcification

  - Hemorrhage into cyst may be indistinguishable from tumor
    - Mural nodularity
    - With or without calcification & fluid level
- CECT
  - Simple hepatic cyst or ADPLD
    - Uncomplicated or complicated (infected): No enhancement

MR Findings
- Simple hepatic cyst or ADPLD
  - T1WI: Hypointense
  - T2WI: Hyperintense
  - Heavily T2WI
    - Markedly increased signal intensity due to pure fluid content
    - Sometimes indistinguishable from a typical hemangioma
  - MRCP: No communication with bile duct
- Complicated (hemorrhagic) cyst
  - T1WI & T2WI
    - Varied signal intensity (due to mixed blood products)
    - With or without a fluid level
- T1 C+: No enhancement
- MRCP: No communication with bile duct walls

Imaging Recommendations
- Best imaging tool: Ultrasonography

DIFFERENTIAL DIAGNOSIS

Cystic or Necrotic Metastases
- No posterior acoustic enhancement
- Debris, mural nodularity or thick septa
- Wall vascularity

Pyogenic Abscess
- Complex cystic mass with debris
- Thick or thin multiple septations
- Mural nodularity & vascularity
- Adjacent parenchyma may be coarse & hypoechoic

HEPATIC CYST

Hydatid Cyst
- Large well-defined cystic liver mass with numerous peripheral daughter cysts
- Cyst within cyst appearance
- Unilocular, multilocular, multi-septated, heterogeneous
- Floating membrane and daughter cysts within
- With or without calcification & dilated bile ducts

Biliary Cystadenocarcinoma
- Usually large in size
- Homogeneous, anechoic, septated mass
- Rarely nonseptated
- May show fine mural or septal calcification
- Mural nodule or papillary excrescence with vascularity

Hepatic Hemangioma
- Well-defined margins
- Typically homogeneous & hyperechoic
- Some with posterior acoustic enhancement
- Atypical features: Hypoechoic center, irregular hyperechoic rim, calcification

PATHOLOGY

General Features
- Etiology
  - Congenital simple hepatic cyst
    - Defective development of intrahepatic biliary duct
  - Acquired hepatic cyst: Secondary to
    - Trauma, inflammation, neoplasia, infestation
- Epidemiology
  - Reported to occur in 2.5% of population
  - Incidence: 1-14% in autopsy series
- Associated abnormalities
  - Autosomal dominant polycystic liver disease
    - 50% have polycystic kidney disease; M:F = 1:2
  - Polycystic kidney disease: 40% have hepatic cysts
  - Tuberous sclerosis

Gross Pathologic & Surgical Features
- Cyst wall: ≤ 1 mm thick
- Usually beneath the surface of liver

Microscopic Features
- Single unilocular cyst with serous fluid
- Lined by cuboidal bile duct epithelium
- A thin underlying rim of fibrous stroma

CLINICAL ISSUES

Presentation
- Most common signs/symptoms
  - Uncomplicated simple cysts & ADPLD
    - Usually asymptomatic, detected incidentally
  - Complicated cyst: Pain &/or fever
  - Large cysts present with symptoms of mass effect
    - Abdominal pain (due to capsular distension), jaundice, palpable mass
  - Advanced disease of ADPLD patients present with
    - Hepatomegaly, liver failure (rarely), Budd-Chiari syndrome

- Clinical Profile
  - Asymptomatic patient with incidental detection of simple hepatic cyst on imaging or at time of autopsy
  - Patients with large hepatic cyst & mass effect: ↑ Direct bilirubin levels
  - Patients with advanced disease of ADPLD: ↑ LFTs
- Diagnosis
  - Fine needle aspiration & cytology (rarely necessary)

Demographics
- Age: Any (usually discovered incidentally in 5th-7th decades)
- Gender: M:F = 1:5

Natural History & Prognosis
- Complications
  - Infection or hemorrhage
  - Large cyst: Compression of IHBD & jaundice
- Prognosis
  - Small & large hepatic cysts: Good prognosis
  - Advanced disease of ADPLD: Good prognosis

Treatment
- Asymptomatic simple hepatic cyst & ADPLD
  - No treatment
- Large, symptomatic, infected hepatic cyst
  - Percutaneous aspiration & sclerotherapy with alcohol
  - Surgical resection or marsupialization
- Advanced disease of ADPLD
  - Partial liver resection, liver transplantation

DIAGNOSTIC CHECKLIST

Consider
- Rule out cyst-like hepatic lesions (infection, neoplasm)

Image Interpretation Pearls
- Anechoic, thin wall, posterior enhancement
- No internal or mural vascularity
- Internal debris may settle under gravity, visible at the end of the examination
- If multiple, evaluate kidneys, and pancreas to rule out ADPLD

SELECTED REFERENCES

1. Larssen TB et al: The occurrence of asymptomatic and symptomatic simple hepatic cysts. A prospective, hospital-based study. Clin Radiol. 60(9):1026-9, 2005
2. Liang P et al: Differential diagnosis of hepatic cystic lesions with gray-scale and color Doppler sonography. J Clin Ultrasound. 33(3):100-5, 2005
3. Mortele KJ et al: Cystic focal liver lesions in the adult: differential CT and MR imaging features. RadioGraphics. 21:895-910, 2001
4. Casillas VJ et al: Imaging of nontraumatic hemorrhagic hepatic lesions. RadioGraphics. 20:367-78, 2000
5. Gaines PA et al: The prevalence and characterization of simple hepatic cysts by ultrasound examination. Br J Radiol. 62(736):335-7, 1989

IMAGE GALLERY

Variant

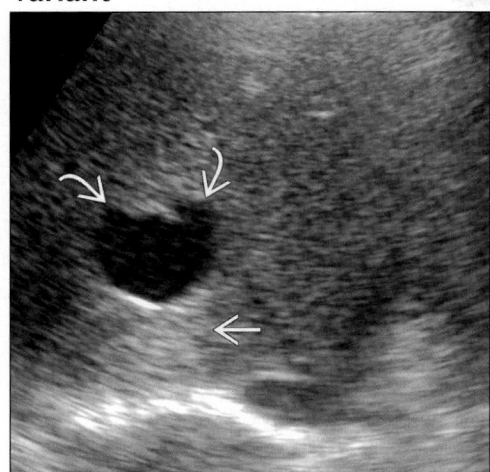
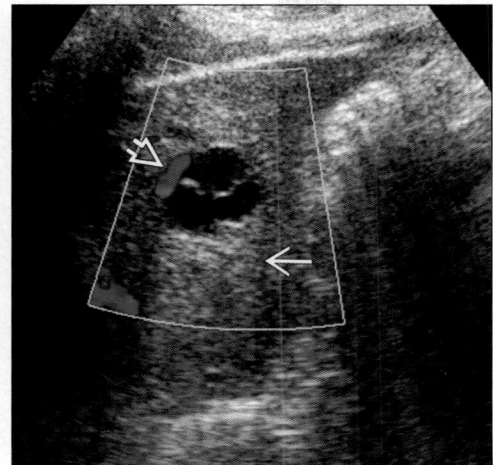

(Left) Transverse transabdominal ultrasound shows a simple cyst with a lobulated contour ➔ and posterior enhancement ➔. (Right) Longitudinal color Doppler ultrasound shows a septated cyst adjacent to a hepatic vein ➔. Posterior enhancement is present ➔ and there is no flow in the septae.

Typical

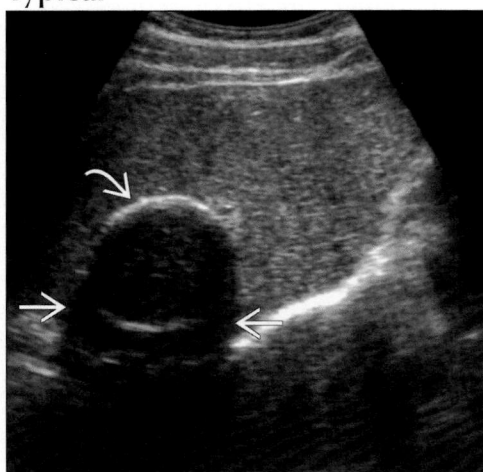
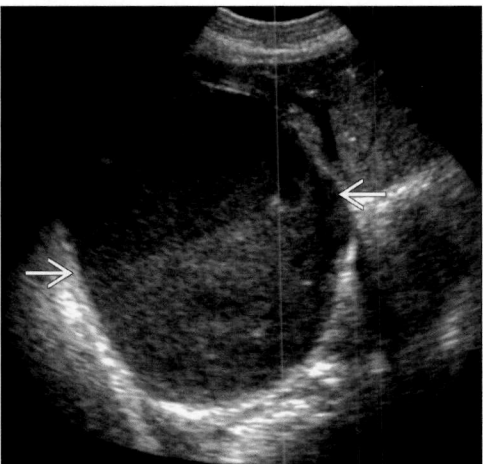

(Left) Transverse transabdominal ultrasound shows a cyst with smooth mural calcification ➔ and acoustic shadowing ➔. (Right) Longitudinal transabdominal ultrasound shows a large cyst with debris gravitating posteriorly ➔, suggesting a complicated cyst (i.e., previous hemorrhage/infection).

Typical

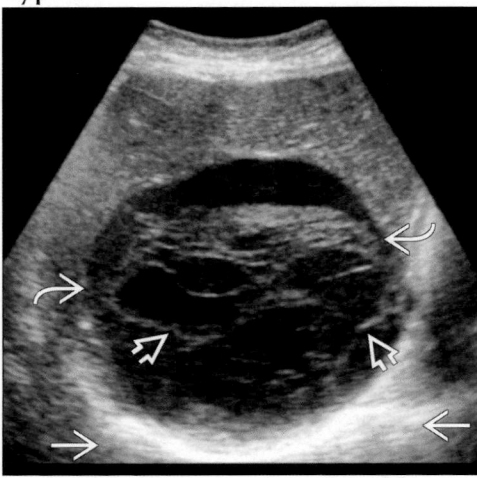
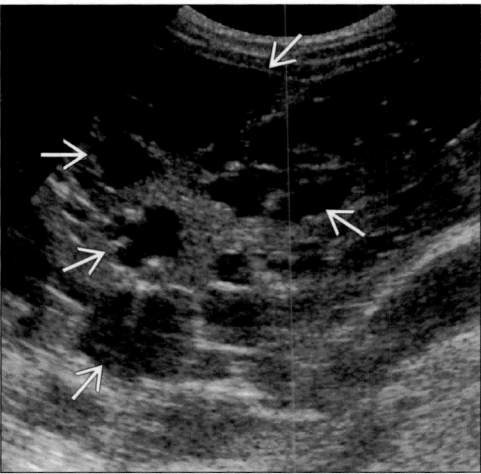

(Left) Transverse transabdominal ultrasound shows a cyst containing an organizing hematoma ➔ which is heterogeneous with fibrin strands ➔. Posterior enhancement is present ➔. (Right) Oblique transabdominal ultrasound shows multiple cysts ➔. When more than ten cysts are present, ADPLD should be considered, and the pancreas and kidneys should be reviewed.

CAROLI DISEASE

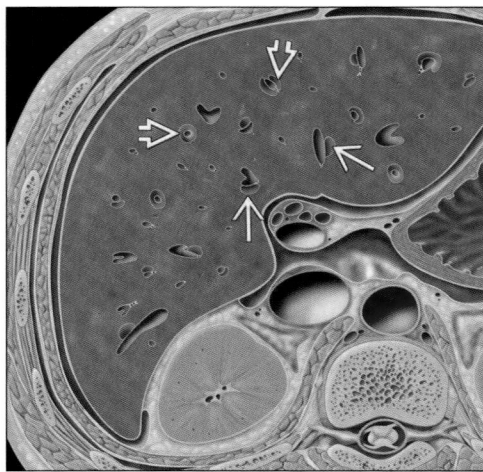

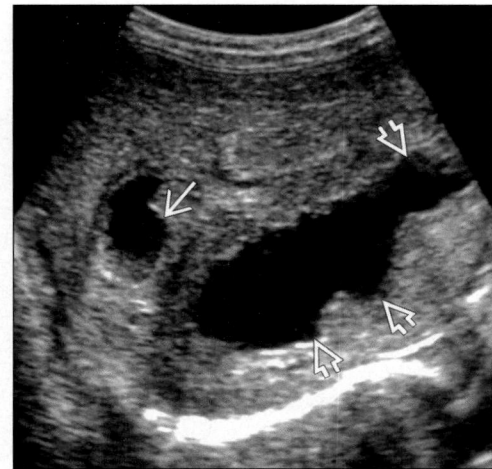

Transverse graphic shows focally dilated intrahepatic ductules ➡ running adjacent to portal venules, in Caroli disease. The dilated ductule may encircle ➡ the adjacent vein.

Oblique transabdominal ultrasound shows markedly dilated intrahepatic ducts ➡. The longitudinal profile shows a saccular configuration ➡, typical in Caroli disease.

TERMINOLOGY

Abbreviations and Synonyms
- Communicating cavernous biliary ectasia

Definitions
- Caroli disease: Congenital, multifocal, segmental, saccular dilatation of intrahepatic bile ducts (IHBD)
- Caroli syndrome: Cystic bile duct dilatation plus hepatic periportal fibrosis

IMAGING FINDINGS

General Features
- Best diagnostic clue: "Central dot" sign; portal radicles within dilated intrahepatic bile ducts on color Doppler ultrasound
- Location: Liver; diffuse, lobar, or segmental
- Size: Varies from few millimeters to few centimeters
- Morphology
  ○ One of the variants of fibropolycystic disease
  ○ Other variants of fibropolycystic disease
    ■ Congenital hepatic fibrosis

- Autosomal dominant polycystic liver disease
- Biliary hamartomas
- Choledochal cyst
  ○ Based on Todani classification
    ■ Type V: Represents Caroli disease
    ■ Cystic dilatation of intrahepatic bile ducts
  ○ Caroli disease is of two types
    ■ Simple type (Caroli disease), associated with renal tubular ectasia
    ■ Periportal fibrosis type (Caroli syndrome)
  ○ Associated with autosomal recessive polycystic disease
  ○ Usually manifests in adolescence, also seen in newborns & infants

Ultrasonographic Findings
- Grayscale Ultrasound
  ○ Dilated intrahepatic bile ducts
    ■ Focal or diffuse involvement in the liver
    ■ Saccular or fusiform configuration
    ■ Contains sludge due to biliary stasis
    ■ May contain calculi, which do not form casts of the ducts (compared to recurrent pyogenic cholangitis)

DDx: Caroli Disease

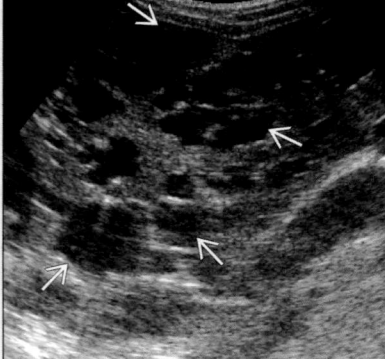

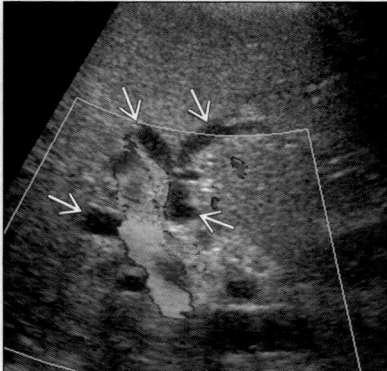

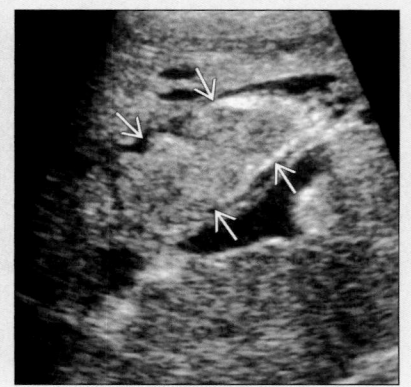

Multiple Cysts

Cholangitis

Recurrent Pyogenic Cholangitis

CAROLI DISEASE

Key Facts

Terminology
- Communicating cavernous biliary ectasia
- Caroli disease: Congenital, multifocal, segmental, saccular dilatation of intrahepatic bile ducts (IHBD)
- Caroli syndrome: Cystic bile duct dilatation plus hepatic periportal fibrosis

Imaging Findings
- Best diagnostic clue: "Central dot" sign; portal radicles within dilated intrahepatic bile ducts on color Doppler ultrasound
- Dilated intrahepatic bile ducts
- Focal or diffuse involvement in the liver
- Saccular or fusiform configuration
- Contains sludge due to biliary stasis
- May contain calculi, which do not form casts of the ducts (compared to recurrent pyogenic cholangitis)

- Echogenic septa completely or incompletely traversing dilated lumen of bile ducts (referred to as intraductal bridging)
- Signs of cirrhosis & portal hypertension if associated with hepatic fibrosis (rare)
- Ultrasound is ideal for suggesting diagnosis, follow-up and guiding interventional procedures

Top Differential Diagnoses
- Polycystic Liver Disease
- Ascending Cholangitis
- Recurrent Pyogenic Cholangitis (RPC)

Diagnostic Checklist
- Rule out other liver diseases which have hepatic cysts with or without dilated bile ducts

---

- Echogenic septa completely or incompletely traversing dilated lumen of bile ducts (referred to as intraductal bridging)
- "Central dot" sign
  - Small portal venous branches partially or completely surrounded by dilated IHBDs
- Abscess formation if complicated by cholangitis
- Signs of cirrhosis & portal hypertension if associated with hepatic fibrosis (rare)

Radiographic Findings
- Endoscopic retrograde cholangiopancreatogram (ERCP) findings
  - Saccular dilatations communicating with IHBDs, stones, strictures
  - May show communicating hepatic abscesses

CT Findings
- NECT: Multiple, rounded, hypodense areas inseparable from dilated IHBD
- CECT: Enhancing tiny dots (portal radicles) within dilated IHBD

MR Findings
- T1WI: Multiple, small, hypointense, saccular dilatations of IHBD
- T2WI: Hyperintense
- Coronal half-Fourier rapid acquisition with relaxation enhancement (rare)
  - Kidney: Multiple fluid-containing foci in papillae (e.g., medullary sponge kidney or renal tubular ectasia)
- T1 C+
  - Enhancement of portal radicles within dilated IHBD
- MR Cholangiopancreatography (MRCP)
  - Multiple hyperintense oval-shaped structures
  - Shows continuity with biliary tree
  - Luminal contents of bile ducts appear hyperintense in contrast to portal vein, which appears as signal void

Nuclear Medicine Findings
- Hepatobiliary scan

- Unusual pattern of retained activity throughout liver
- Technetium sulfur colloid
  - Multiple cold defects

Imaging Recommendations
- Best imaging tool
  - ERCP or 3D MRCP
  - Ultrasound is ideal for suggesting diagnosis, follow-up and guiding interventional procedures

DIFFERENTIAL DIAGNOSIS

Polycystic Liver Disease
- Hepatic cysts
  - Numerous (> 10, usually hundreds)
  - Do not communicate with each other or biliary tract
  - Do not demonstrate saccular configuration
  - Not associated with biliary ductal dilatation
- Patients with this disease often harbor renal cysts; not confined to medulla

Ascending Cholangitis
- Intrahepatic abscesses communicate with bile ducts
  - Mimics Caroli disease
- Margins of abscesses are irregular
- Extrahepatic bile duct dilatation
  - Due to an obstructing stone or tumor

Recurrent Pyogenic Cholangitis (RPC)
- Dilatation of both intra- & extrahepatic bile ducts; usually of cylindrical and not saccular type
- Biliary calculi of RPC
  - Cast-like (unlike Caroli disease)
  - Often fill ductal lumen

PATHOLOGY

General Features
- General path comments
  - Embryology-anatomy

CAROLI DISEASE

- Ductal plate malformation: Incomplete remodeling of ductal plate leads to persistence of embryonic biliary ductal structures
- Genetics: Inherited as an autosomal recessive pattern
- Etiology
  - Simple type
    - Malformation of ductal plate of large central IHBD
    - More common in adults
  - Periportal fibrosis type
    - Malformation of ductal plates of central IHBD & smaller peripheral bile ducts, latter leading to development of fibrosis
    - More common in infants & children
- Epidemiology: Rare disease
- Associated abnormalities
  - Medullary sponge kidney (renal tubular ectasia)
  - Autosomal dominant polycystic kidney disease

Gross Pathologic & Surgical Features
- Saccular dilatations of intrahepatic bile ducts
- Diffuse, lobar or segmental

Microscopic Features
- Simple type
  - Dilatation of segmental IHBD
  - Normal hepatic parenchyma
- Periportal fibrosis type
  - Segmental dilatation of IHBD
  - Proliferation of bile ductules & fibrosis

CLINICAL ISSUES

Presentation
- Most common signs/symptoms
  - Simple type
    - Right upper quadrant (RUQ) pain
    - Recurrent attacks of cholangitis, fever & jaundice
  - Periportal fibrosis type
    - Pain, hepatosplenomegaly
    - Hematemesis (due to varices)
  - Can be asymptomatic at an early stage
- Lab data
  - May show elevated liver enzymes & bilirubin levels
- Diagnosis
  - ERCP
  - MRCP

Demographics
- Age
  - Childhood and 2nd-3rd decade
  - Occasionally in infancy
- Gender: M:F = 1:1

Natural History & Prognosis
- Complications
  - Simple type
    - Stone formation (95%): Calcium bilirubinate
    - Recurrent cholangitis
    - Hepatic abscesses
  - Periportal fibrosis type
    - Cirrhosis & portal hypertension
    - Varices & hemorrhage
  - Cholangiocarcinoma in 7% of patients

- Prognosis
  - Long-term prognosis for Caroli disease is poor

Treatment
- Localized to lobe or segment
  - Hepatic lobectomy or segmentectomy
- Diffuse disease
  - Conservative
  - Decompression of biliary tract: External drainage or biliary-enteric anastomoses are effective
  - Extracorporeal shock wave lithotripsy
  - Oral bile salts
  - Liver transplantation

DIAGNOSTIC CHECKLIST

Consider
- Rule out other liver diseases which have hepatic cysts with or without dilated bile ducts

Image Interpretation Pearls
- Cholangiography: Bulbous dilatations of peripheral intrahepatic bile ducts
- ERCP: Saccular dilatations show communication with IHBD which differentiates Caroli from other variants of fibropolycystic disease

SELECTED REFERENCES

1. Guy F et al: Caroli's disease: magnetic resonance imaging features. Eur Radiol. 12(11):2730-6, 2002
2. Krause D et al: MRI for evaluating congenital bile duct abnormalities. J Comput Assist Tomogr. 26(4):541-52, 2002
3. Levy AD et al: Caroli's disease: radiologic spectrum with pathologic correlation. AJR Am J Roentgenol. 179(4):1053-7, 2002
4. Fulcher AS et al: Case 38: Caroli disease and renal tubular ectasia. Radiology. 220(3):720-3, 2001
5. Mortele KJ et al: Cystic focal liver lesions in the adult: differential CT and MR imaging features. Radiographics. 21(4):895-910, 2001
6. Akin O et al: An unusual sonographic finding in Caroli's disease. AJR Am J Roentgenol. 171(4):1167, 1998
7. Asselah T et al: Caroli's disease: a magnetic resonance cholangiopancreatography diagnosis. Am J Gastroenterol. 93(1):109-10, 1998
8. Gorka W et al: Value of Doppler sonography in the assessment of patients with Caroli's disease. J Clin Ultrasound. 26(6):283-7, 1998
9. Pavone P et al: Caroli's disease: evaluation with MR cholangiography. AJR Am J Roentgenol. 166(1):216-7, 1996
10. Miller WJ et al: Imaging findings in Caroli's disease. AJR Am J Roentgenol. 165(2):333-7, 1995
11. Rizzo RJ et al: Congenital abnormalities of the pancreas and biliary tree in adults. Radiographics. 15(1):49-68; quiz 147-8, 1995
12. Zangger P et al: MRI findings in Caroli's disease and intrahepatic pigmented calculi. Abdom Imaging. 20(4):361-4, 1995
13. Choi BI et al: Caroli disease: central dot sign in CT. Radiology. 174(1):161-3, 1990
14. Murphy BJ et al: The CT appearance of cystic masses of the liver. Radiographics. 9(2):307-22, 1989
15. Marchal GJ et al: Caroli disease: high-frequency US and pathologic findings. Radiology. 158(2):507-11, 1986

IMAGE GALLERY

Typical

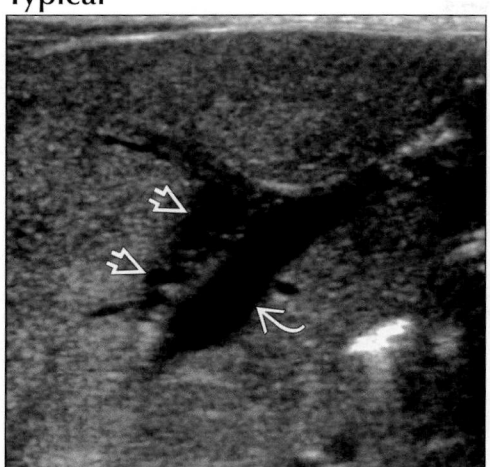

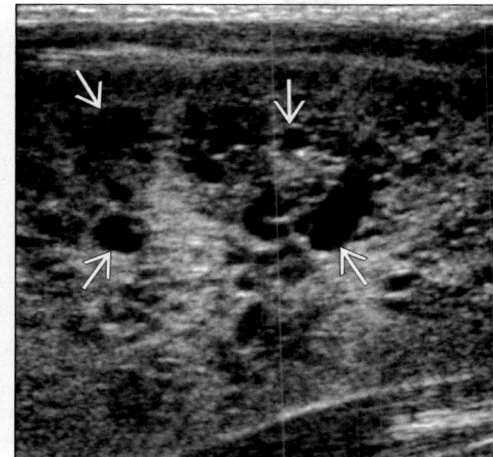

(Left) Transabdominal ultrasound shows saccular dilatation of the right intrahepatic duct ⮞, adjacent to the portal vein ⮞, in Caroli disease. (Right) Oblique transabdominal ultrasound shows multiple dilated intrahepatic ducts ⮞ diffusely involving the liver in Caroli disease.

Typical

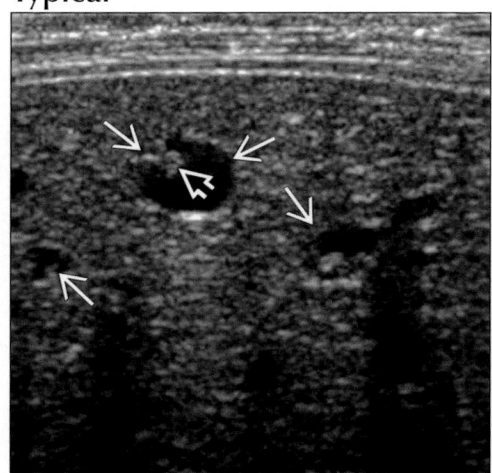

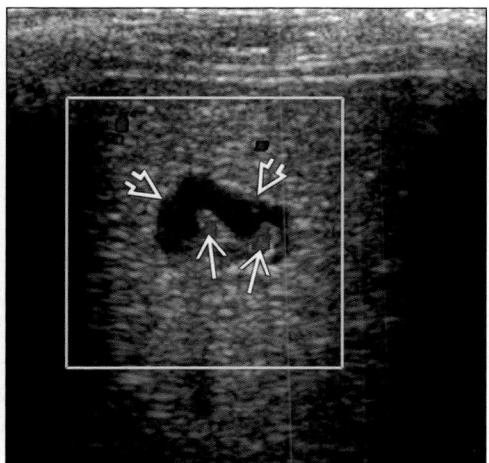

(Left) Oblique transabdominal ultrasound shows dilated ducts ⮞ in Caroli disease. One focus demonstrates a nodule ⮞ surrounded by dilated ducts, the "central dot" sign. (Right) Oblique color Doppler ultrasound shows color flow in portal radicles ⮞ surrounded by dilated intrahepatic ducts ⮞ in Caroli disease ("central dot" sign).

Typical

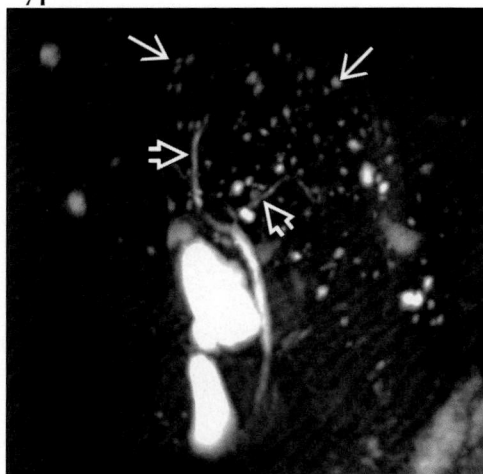

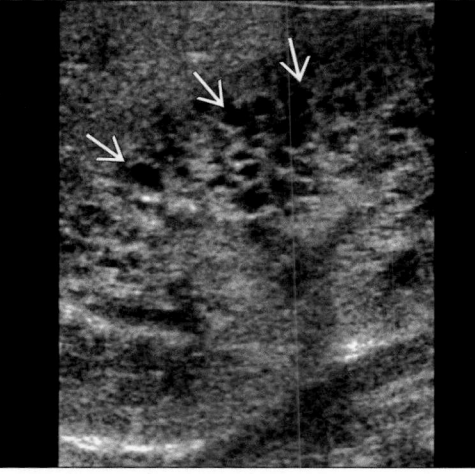

(Left) Oblique MRCP shows focally dilated intrahepatic ducts as fluid signal nodules ⮞ in Caroli disease. Some more central lesions can be seen continuous with the main branches of the bile duct ⮞. (Right) Longitudinal transabdominal ultrasound shows multiple small renal cortical cysts ⮞ in a patient with Caroli disease.

BILOMA

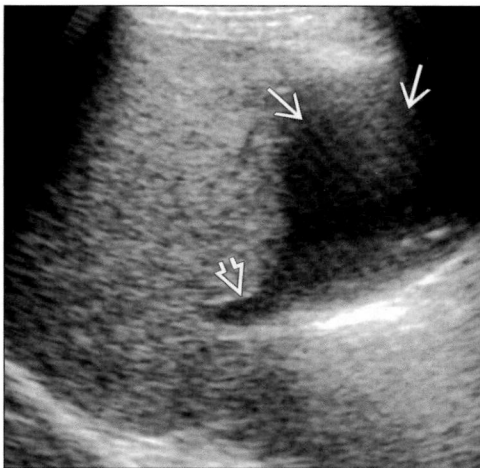 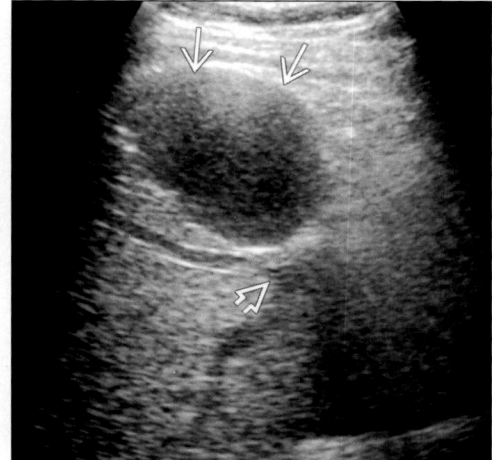

Oblique transabdominal ultrasound shows an anechoic biloma ➡ without appreciable capsule. Note its "neck" ➡ extending towards the porta hepatis.

Transverse transabdominal ultrasound shows an anechoic biloma ➡ with no appreciable capsule. Its deep surface is in contact with the porta hepatis ➡.

TERMINOLOGY

Definitions
- Encapsulated collection of bile outside the biliary tree

IMAGING FINDINGS

General Features
- Location
  - Intrahepatic
  - Extrahepatic: Intraperitoneal/extraperitoneal/scrotal

Ultrasonographic Findings
- Grayscale Ultrasound
  - Focal collection of fluid within the liver or close to the biliary tree
  - Round or oval in shape
    - Larger lesions may compress the adjacent liver surface/architecture
  - Usually unilocular
  - Thin capsule wall usually not discernible
  - Fluid content may be anechoic, suggesting fresh biloma
  - Fine internal septae may be present
    - Debris or septae suggests infected biloma
  - Posterior acoustic enhancement
- Color Doppler
  - No vascularity within the lesion
  - For infected biloma, there may be increased vascularity in adjacent tissue
- Needle aspiration under ultrasound guidance usually required to confirm diagnosis (detection of bilirubin in aspirate)

Nuclear Medicine Findings
- Hepatobiliary Scintigraphy: HIDA scan may demonstrate continual bile leakage into biloma

Imaging Recommendations
- Best imaging tool: Ultrasound is good at lesion detection & provides information on the site & size of lesion for progress monitoring or intervention

DIFFERENTIAL DIAGNOSIS

Perihepatic Collection/Seroma/Lymphocele
- May be anechoic or contain debris or loculations

DDx: Biloma

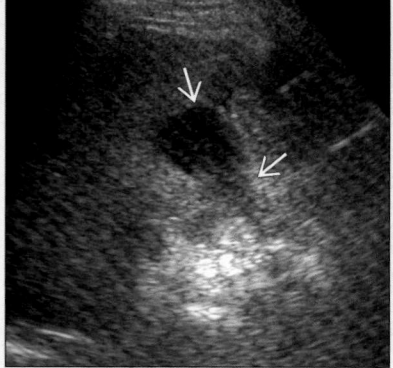 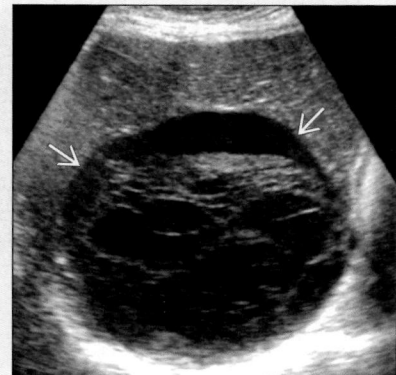 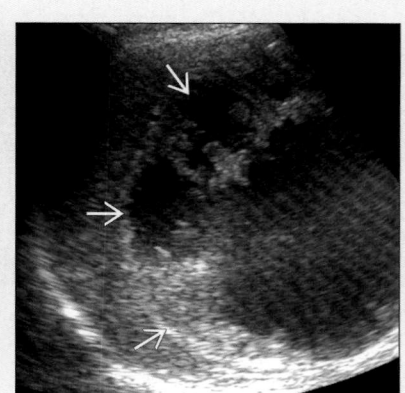

| *Seroma* | *Hemorrhagic Cyst* | *Hepatic Abscess* |

BILOMA

Key Facts

Imaging Findings
- Focal collection of fluid within the liver or close to the biliary tree
- Round or oval in shape
- Usually unilocular
- Thin capsule wall usually not discernible
- Fluid content may be anechoic, suggesting fresh biloma
- Debris or septae suggests infected biloma
- Posterior acoustic enhancement
- No vascularity within the lesion
- For infected biloma, there may be increased vascularity in adjacent tissue

Top Differential Diagnoses
- Perihepatic Collection/Seroma/Lymphocele
- Hepatic Cyst
- Hepatic Abscess

- Thick & irregular wall may be present
- Difficult to distinguish from biloma, aspiration biopsy may be required

Hepatic Cyst
- Variable appearance depending on whether it is sterile, infected or hemorrhagic

Hepatic Abscess
- Thick & irregular wall, surrounding vascularity

PATHOLOGY

General Features
- Etiology
  - Iatrogenic: Laparoscopic cholecystectomy, post-liver-transplant, ERCP or other instrumentation of biliary tree, liver biopsy
  - Posttraumatic: Blunt trauma, motor vehicle accident
  - Spontaneous rupture of bile duct

Gross Pathologic & Surgical Features
- Size of biloma depends on the difference between leakage rate and reabsorption rate of bile by the peritoneum/surroundings

CLINICAL ISSUES

Treatment
- Percutaneous drainage with/without pigtail catheter
- Surgical resection and repair reserved for complicated or cases unresponsive to drainage

DIAGNOSTIC CHECKLIST

Consider
- Other causes of fluid collection: Ascites, abscess, hematoma

SELECTED REFERENCES

1. Chiu WC et al: Ultrasonography for interval assessment in the nonoperative management of hepatic trauma. Am Surg. 71(10):841-6, 2005
2. Walker AT et al: Bile duct disruption and biloma after laparoscopic cholecystectomy: imaging evaluation. AJR Am J Roentgenol. 158(4):785-9, 1992
3. Vazquez JL et al: Evaluation and treatment of intraabdominal bilomas. AJR Am J Roentgenol. 144(5):933-8, 1985
4. Esensten M et al: Posttraumatic intrahepatic biloma: sonographic diagnosis. AJR Am J Roentgenol. 140:303-5, 1983
5. Kuligowska E et al: Bilomas: a new approach to the diagnosis and treatment. Gastroint Radiol. 8:237-43, 1983
6. Mueller PR et al: Detection and drainage of bilomas: special considerations. AJR Am J Roentgenol. 140(4):715-20, 1983
7. Gould L et al: Ultrasound detection of extrahepatic encapsulated bile: "biloma". AJR Am J Roentgenol. 132(6):1014-5, 1979

IMAGE GALLERY

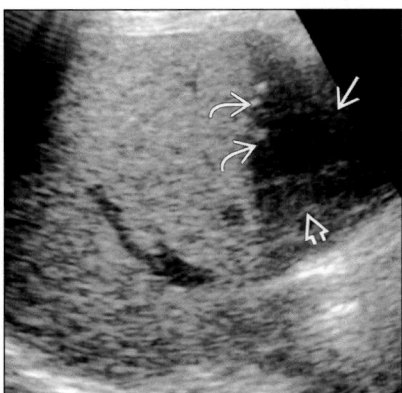 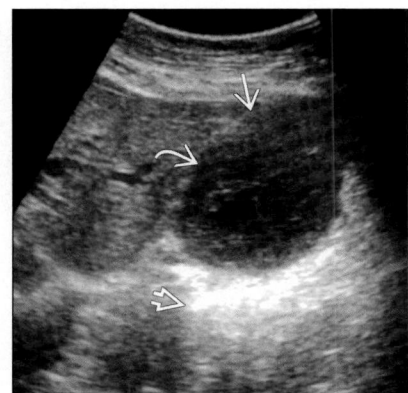 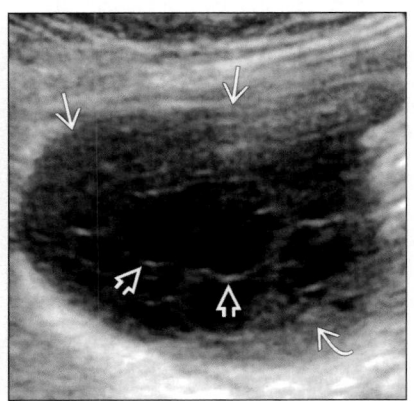

(Left) Oblique transabdominal ultrasound shows an infected biloma ➡ with internal debris gravitating to the dependent portion ➡. Note echogenic gas locules with posterior ring-down artifact ➡. (Center) Transverse transabdominal ultrasound shows a biloma ➡ compressing the surface of left hepatic lobe ➡. Note posterior acoustic enhancement ➡ reflecting fluid content in biloma. (Right) Oblique transabdominal ultrasound of an infected biloma ➡ shows fine internal septae ➡ and dependent debris ➡.

PYOGENIC HEPATIC ABSCESS

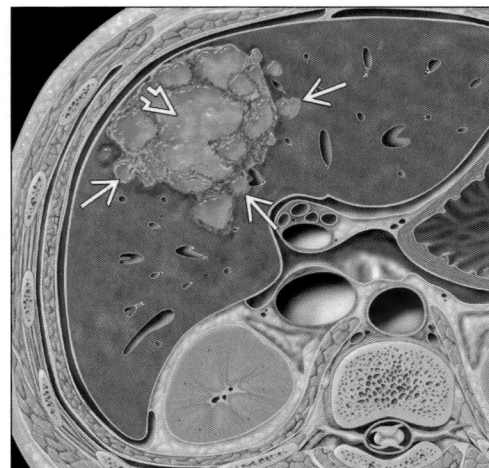

Transverse graphic shows a cluster of liver abscesses ➡ coalescing to form a larger lesion ➡.

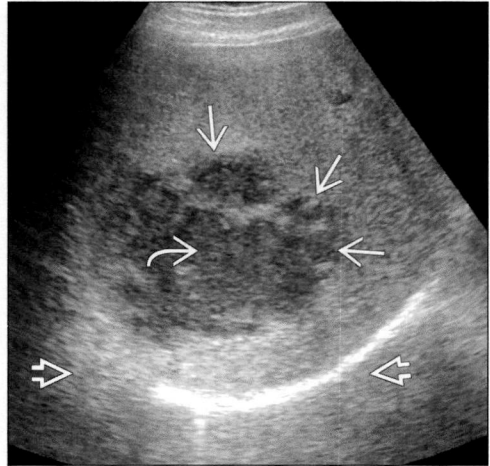

Oblique transabdominal ultrasound shows a cluster of coalescing abscesses ➡ within a liver segment. They have irregular walls, low level internal echoes ➡ & posterior enhancement ➡.

TERMINOLOGY

Abbreviations and Synonyms
- Liver pyogenic abscess

Definitions
- Localized collection of pus in liver due to bacterial infectious process with destruction of hepatic parenchyma and stroma

IMAGING FINDINGS

General Features
- Best diagnostic clue: "Cluster" sign: Cluster of small pyogenic abscesses coalesce into a single large cavity
- Location
  - Varies based on origin
    - Portal origin: Right lobe (65%); left lobe (12%); both lobes (23%)
    - Biliary tract origin: 90% involve both lobes, close to biliary ducts
      - If due to infection following an interventional procedure, the abscess is in the vicinity of the site of the procedure
- Size: Varies from few millimeters to 10 centimeters
- Other general features
  - In Western countries usually pyogenic (bacterial) in origin
    - Typically due to complication of infection elsewhere
  - Among all liver abscesses
    - Pyogenic: 88% (bacterial)
    - Amebic: 10% (Entamoeba histolytica)
    - Fungal: 2% (Candida albicans)
  - Most common causes of pyogenic abscess
    - Diverticulitis/ascending cholangitis/infection of infarcted tissue (e.g., post liver transplantation, necrotic tumor)
  - Pyogenic abscesses may be single or multiple
    - Biliary tract origin: Multiple small abscesses
    - Portal origin: Usually solitary larger abscess
    - Direct extension & trauma: Solitary large abscess
  - In developing countries mostly due to parasitic infestation

DDx: Pyogenic Abscess

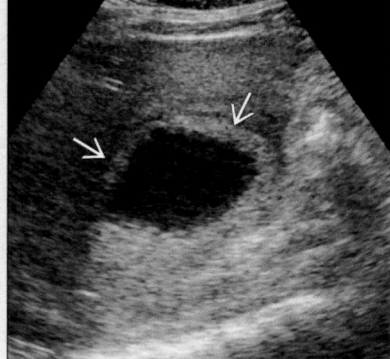

Cystic Metastasis

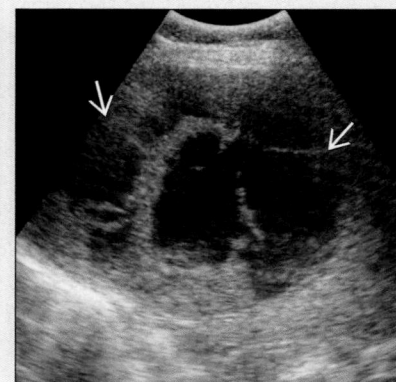

Hemorrhagic Cyst

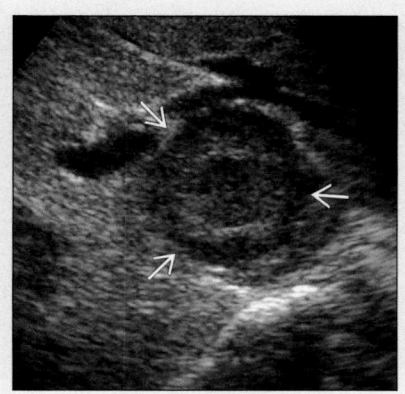

Amebic Abscess

PYOGENIC HEPATIC ABSCESS

Key Facts

Terminology
- Localized collection of pus in liver due to bacterial infectious process with destruction of hepatic parenchyma and stroma

Imaging Findings
- Best diagnostic clue: "Cluster" sign: Cluster of small pyogenic abscesses coalesce into a single large cavity
- Variable in shape & echogenicity
- Usually spherical or ovoid in shape
- Borders may be well-defined to irregular
- Wall may be thin/thick, hypoechoic/mildly echogenic
- Anechoic (50%), hyperechoic (25%), hypoechoic (25%)
- Fluid level or debris, internal septae and posterior acoustic enhancement

- Gas in an abscess seen as brightly echogenic foci with posterior reverberation artifact
- Early lesions tend to be echogenic & poorly demarcated
- May evolve into well-demarcated, nearly anechoic lesions
- The hepatic parenchyma in the vicinity of the abscess is heterogeneous & hypoechoic due to edema
- Vascularity may be demonstrable in thick wall portion
- Edematous parenchyma adjacent to abscess may be hypervascular

Top Differential Diagnoses
- Metastases (Especially After Treatment)
- Hemorrhagic Simple Cyst
- Amebic Abscess

- Amebic, echinococcal or other protozoal/helminthic

Ultrasonographic Findings
- Grayscale Ultrasound
  - Variable in shape & echogenicity
  - Usually spherical or ovoid in shape
  - Borders may be well-defined to irregular
  - Wall may be thin/thick, hypoechoic/mildly echogenic
  - Echogenicity of abscesses
    - Anechoic (50%), hyperechoic (25%), hypoechoic (25%)
  - Fluid level or debris, internal septae and posterior acoustic enhancement
  - Gas in an abscess seen as brightly echogenic foci with posterior reverberation artifact
  - Early lesions tend to be echogenic & poorly demarcated
  - May evolve into well-demarcated, nearly anechoic lesions
  - Associated right pleural effusion
  - The hepatic parenchyma in the vicinity of the abscess is heterogeneous & hypoechoic due to edema
- Color Doppler
  - Vascularity may be demonstrable in thick wall portion
  - Edematous parenchyma adjacent to abscess may be hypervascular

Radiographic Findings
- Radiography
  - Chest X-ray
    - Elevation of right hemidiaphragm
    - Right lower lobe atelectasis
    - Infiltrative lesions, right pleural effusion
  - Plain X-ray abdomen
    - Hepatomegaly, intrahepatic gas, air-fluid level
  - Contrast studies of bowel & urinary tract: May show cause of abscess
    - Diverticulitis, perforated ulcer & renal abscess
- ERCP: May define level & cause of biliary obstruction

CT Findings
- NECT
  - Simple abscess: Well-defined, round, hypodense mass (0-45 HU)
  - "Cluster" sign
    - Small abscesses aggregate to coalesce into a single big cavity, usually septated
  - Complex pyogenic abscess: "Target" lesion
    - Hypodense rim, isodense periphery
    - Decreased HU in center
  - Specific sign: Abscess with central gas
    - Seen as air bubbles or an air-fluid level
    - Present in less than 20% of cases
  - Large air-fluid or fluid-debris level
    - Often associated with bowel communication or necrotic tissue
- CECT
  - Sharply-defined, round, hypodense mass
  - Rim- or capsule- and septal-enhancement
  - Right lower lobe atelectasis & pleural effusion
  - Non-liquified infection may simulate hypervascular tumor

MR Findings
- T1WI: Hypointense
- T2WI: Hyperintense mass with perilesional edema
- T1 C+
  - Hypointense mass
  - Rim or capsule enhancement
  - Small abscesses less than 1 cm may show homogeneous enhancement, mimicking hemangiomas
- MRCP is highly specific in detecting obstructive biliary pathology

Nuclear Medicine Findings
- Hepato biliary & sulfur colloid scans
  - Rounded, cold areas
  - Occasionally, communication between abscess cavity & biliary system can be seen
- Gallium scan (Gallium citrate Ga-67)
  - Hot or mixed lesions (cold center & hot rim)

PYOGENIC HEPATIC ABSCESS

- White blood cell (WBC) scan
  - Hot lesions (due to WBC accumulation)
  - Highly specific for pyogenic abscesses compared to any nuclear or cross-sectional imaging

Imaging Recommendations
- Best imaging tool: Ultrasound for diagnosis, guiding aspiration and follow-up

DIFFERENTIAL DIAGNOSIS

Metastases (Especially After Treatment)
- Usually do not appear as a cluster or septated cystic mass
- Usually no elevation of diaphragm or atelectasis
- No fever or ↑ WBC with metastases
- Treated necrotic metastases may be indistinguishable from abscess

Hemorrhagic Simple Cyst
- Hemorrhage may produce internal debris/septae/wall thickening to a simple cyst
- Cyst may appear multiloculated

Amebic Abscess
- Compared to pyogenic: Amebic abscesses are
  - Usually peripheral, round or oval shape
  - Sharply-defined hypoechoic or low attenuation
- Most often solitary (85%)
- Right lobe more often (72%) than left (13%)
- Abuts liver capsule

Hydatid Cyst
- Large cystic liver mass + peripheral daughter cysts
- ± Curvilinear or ring-like pericyst calcification
- ± Dilated intrahepatic bile ducts: Due to mass effect and/or rupture into bile ducts

PATHOLOGY

General Features
- General path comments
  - Pyogenic abscess can develop via five major routes
  - Biliary: Ascending cholangitis from
    - Choledocholithiasis
    - Benign or malignant biliary obstruction
  - Portal vein: Pylephlebitis from
    - Appendicitis, diverticulitis
    - Proctitis, inflammatory bowel disease
    - Right colon infection spreads via: Superior mesenteric vein → portal vein → liver
    - Left colon infection via: Inferior mesenteric vein → splenic vein → portal vein → liver
  - Hepatic artery: Septicemia from bacterial endocarditis, pneumonitis, osteomyelitis
  - Direct extension
    - Perforated gastric or duodenal ulcer
    - Subphrenic abscess, pyelonephritis
  - Traumatic: Blunt or penetrating injuries or following interventional procedures
- Etiology
  - Pyogenic: Accounts for 88% of all liver abscesses

- Most commonly: E. coli (adults) & S. aureus (children)
- Epidemiology: Incidence rate is increasing in Western countries due to ascending cholangitis & diverticulitis
- Associated abnormalities: Diverticulitis, appendicitis; benign or malignant biliary obstruction; perforated gastric or duodenal ulcer; bacterial endocarditis, pneumonitis, osteomyelitis

Gross Pathologic & Surgical Features
- Pyogenic abscess: Multiple or solitary lesions

CLINICAL ISSUES

Presentation
- Most common signs/symptoms
  - Fever, RUQ pain, rigors, malaise
  - Nausea, vomiting, weight loss, tender hepatomegaly
  - If subphrenic then atelectasis & pleural effusion possible
- Clinical Profile
  - Middle-aged/elderly patient with history of
    - Fever, RUQ & usually left lower quadrant pain
    - Tender hepatomegaly & increased WBC count
- Lab data: Increased leukocytes & serum alk phosphatase
- Diagnosis: Fine needle aspiration cytology (FNAC)

Natural History & Prognosis
- Complications: Spread of infection to subphrenic space, causes atelectasis & pleural effusion
- Prognosis: Good after medical therapy & aspiration
  - Catheter drainage failure rate 8.4%
  - Recurrent abscess rate 8%

Treatment
- Antibiotics; percutaneous aspiration + parenteral antibiotics; percutaneous catheter/surgical drainage

DIAGNOSTIC CHECKLIST

Consider
- Rule out: Amebic/fungal liver abscesses; cystic tumors
  - Amebic: Entamoeba histolytica; fungal: Candida albicans; hepatic hydatid or simple cyst, biliary cystadenoma
- Check for history of transplantation or ablation/chemotherapy for liver tumor

Image Interpretation Pearls
- "Cluster" sign: Small abscesses coalesce into big cavity
- Specific sign: Presence of central gas or fluid level
- Non-liquified abscess may simulate solid tumor

SELECTED REFERENCES

1. Giorgio A et al: Pyogenic liver abscesses: 13 years of experience in percutaneous needle aspiration with US guidance. Radiology. 195: 122-4, 1995
2. Mendez RZ et al: Hepatic abscesses: MR imaging findings. Radiology. 190: 431-6, 1994
3. Jeffrey RB et al: CT small pyogenic hepatic abscesses: The cluster sign. AJR. 151(3): 487-9, 1988

IMAGE GALLERY

Typical

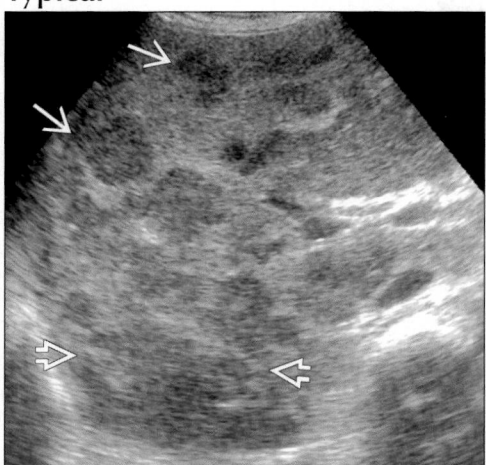 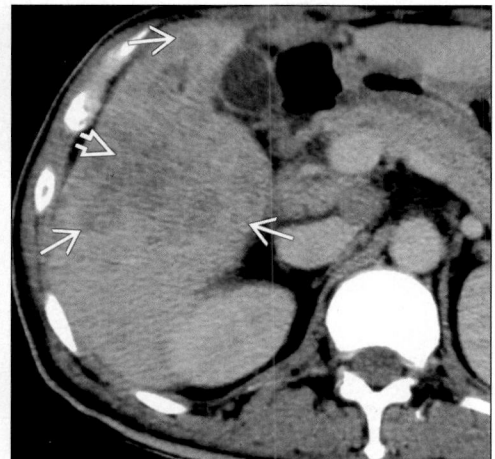

(Left) Transverse transabdominal ultrasound shows multiple abscesses ➡ in the right lobe of the liver, showing low-level internal echoes and irregular walls. The deeper lesions coalesce ⮞. *(Right)* Transverse CECT shows multiple abscesses ➡ in a cluster with some lesions coalescing ⮞. Mild rim enhancement is present around the lesions.

Typical

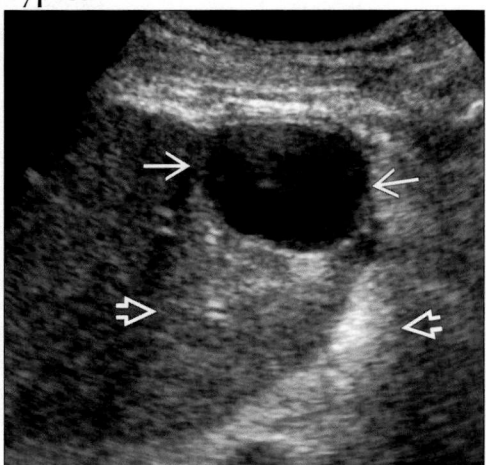 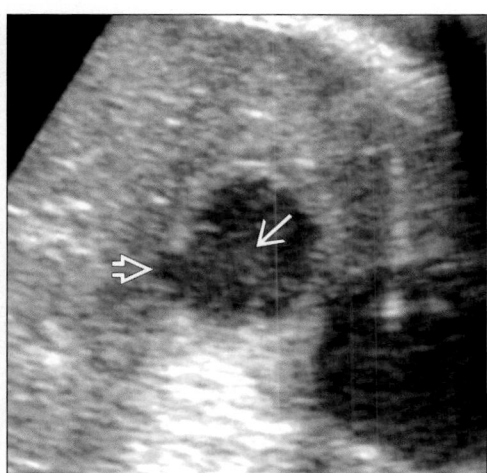

(Left) Oblique transabdominal ultrasound shows an anechoic abscess ➡ and posterior acoustic enhancement ⮞. This may be difficult to differentiate from a cyst. *(Right)* Oblique transabdominal ultrasound shows a hypoechoic abscess with low-level internal echoes ➡ and irregular shape ⮞.

Typical

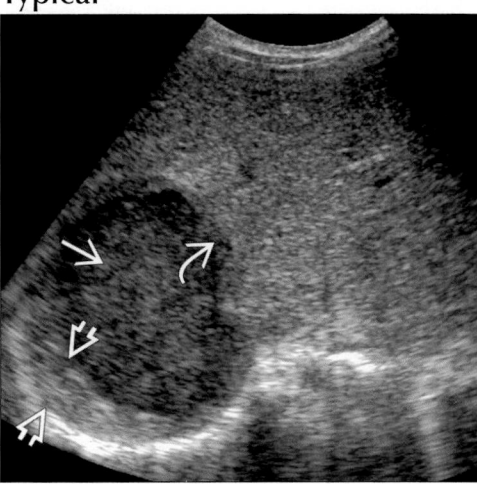 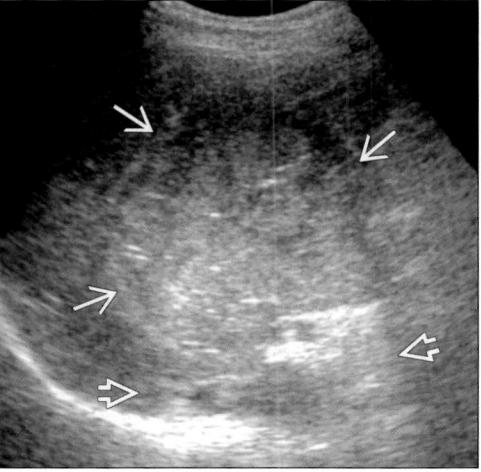

(Left) Transverse transabdominal ultrasound shows a hypoechoic abscess with uniform low-level debris ➡, irregular thick wall ⮞ and irregular contour ⮞. *(Right)* Oblique transabdominal ultrasound shows isoechoic contents within an abscess ➡ making it difficult to delineate from the liver parenchyma. Note posterior acoustic enhancement ⮞.

PYOGENIC HEPATIC ABSCESS

(Left) Transverse transabdominal ultrasound shows uniform internal debris ➡, hyperechoic to the liver parenchyma ➡. Note the posterior acoustic enhancement ⇨. *(Right)* Transverse transabdominal ultrasound shows a thick and irregular wall ➡, heterogeneous internal echoes ➡ and mass effect on the adjacent vein ⇨.

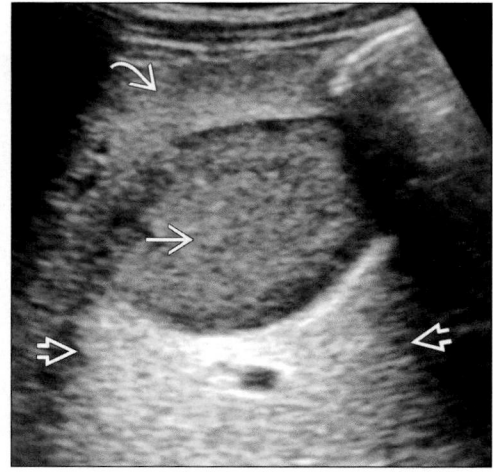
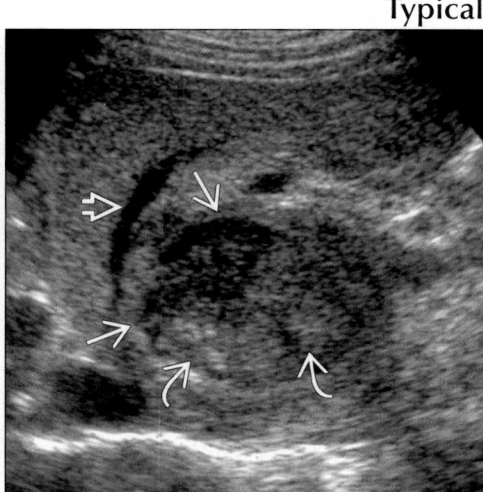

(Left) Longitudinal transabdominal ultrasound shows a fluid-debris level ➡ within a pyogenic abscess. The heavier debris (echogenic) ⇨ has settled in the dependent portion of the cavity. *(Right)* Transverse transabdominal ultrasound shows gas ➡ in the non-dependent portion of the abscess. Note reverberation artifact ⇨ posterior to the gas locules.

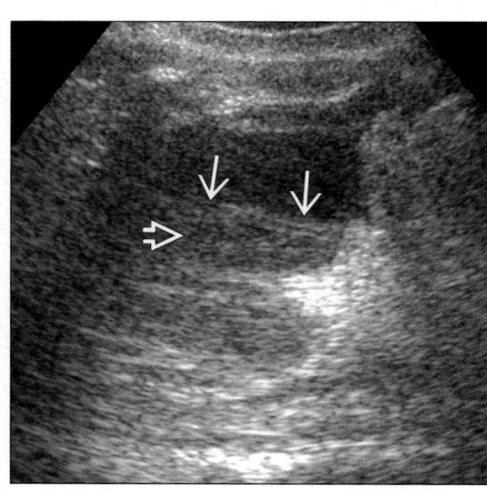
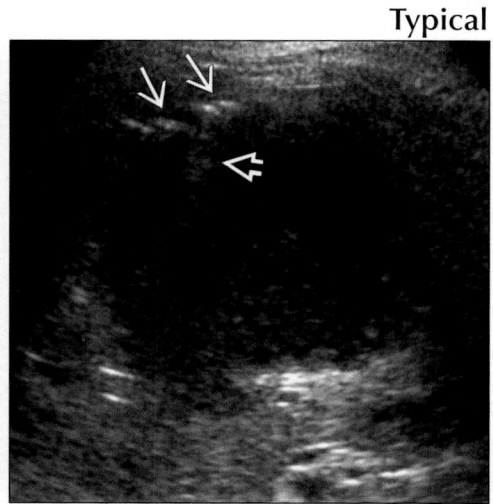

(Left) Longitudinal transabdominal ultrasound shows an abscess with multiple septae ➡ which have trapped locules of free gas ⇨, stopping them from rising to the non-dependent portion. *(Right)* Oblique ultrasound shows multiple septae ➡ within an abscess ⇨.

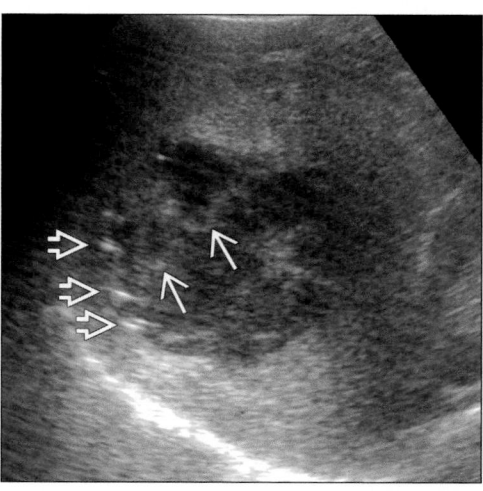
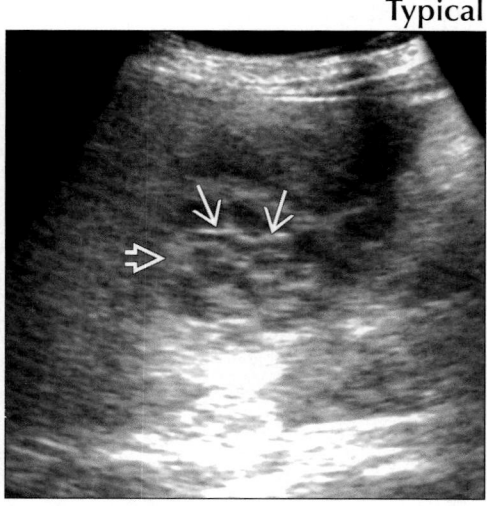

Typical

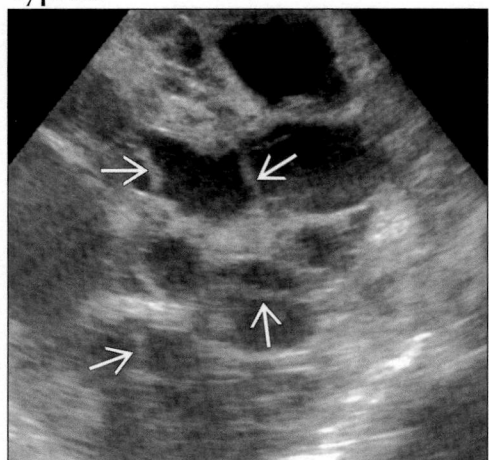

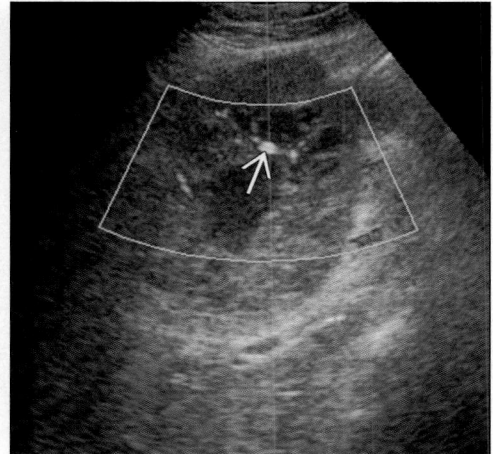

(Left) Transverse transabdominal ultrasound shows septae ➡ in multiple large abscesses. *(Right)* Oblique power Doppler ultrasound shows vascularity ➡ within a thick septum in an abscess.

Typical

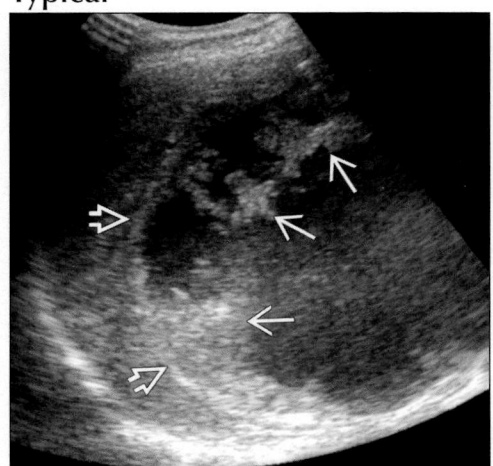

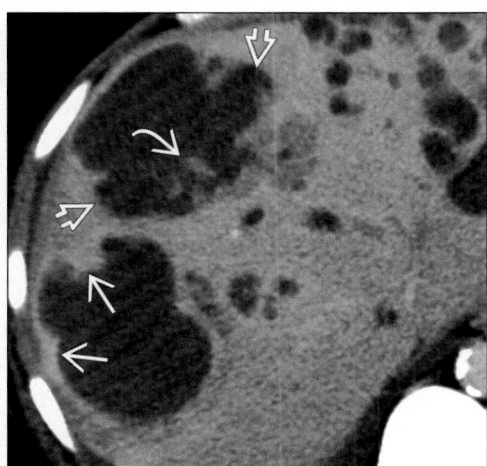

(Left) Oblique transabdominal ultrasound shows frond-like irregular septae/protrusions ➡ arising from the irregularly thickened wall ➡ of a pyogenic abscess. *(Right)* Transverse CECT shows large abscesses with irregularly thickened enhancing walls ➡, septae ➡ and lobulated margins ➡. Smaller abscesses are present in the rest of the liver.

Typical

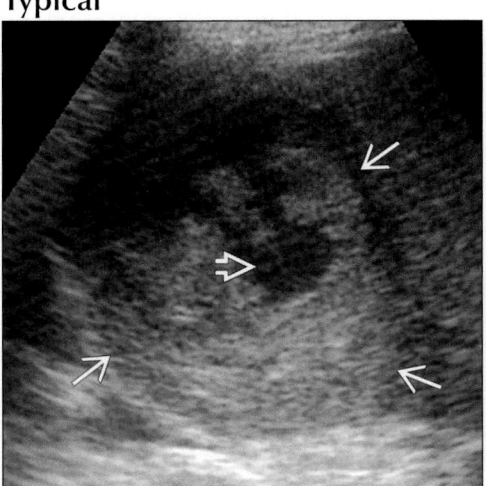

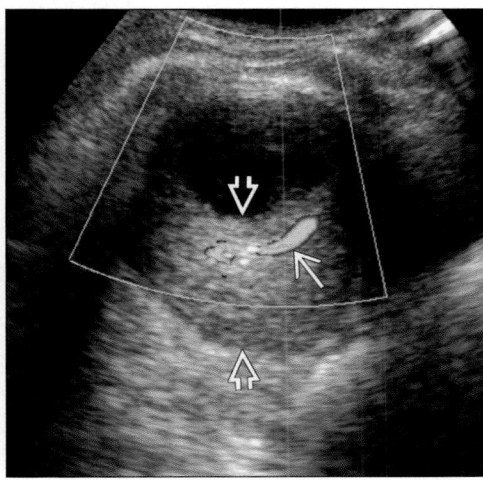

(Left) Oblique transabdominal ultrasound shows the thick irregular wall ➡ of a pyogenic abscess with only a small amount of fluid content ➡ in its center. *(Right)* Oblique power Doppler ultrasound shows vascularity ➡ within the thick wall ➡ of an abscess.

PYOGENIC PERI-HEPATIC ABSCESS

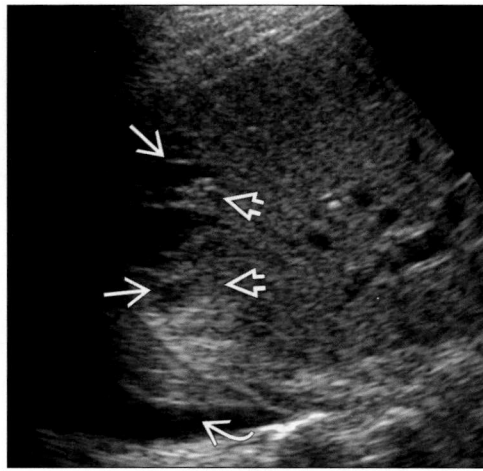

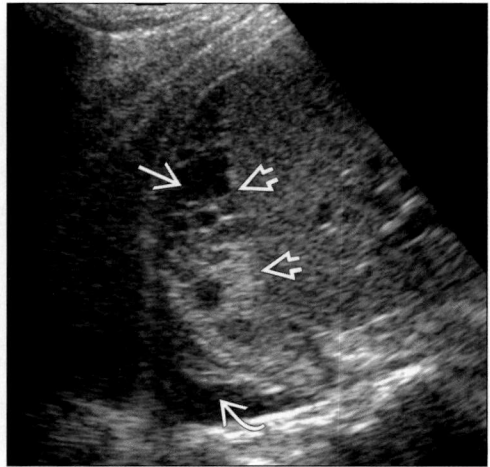

Longitudinal transabdominal ultrasound shows a heterogeneous subphrenic abscess ➡. Its interface ➡ with the liver is not well demonstrated. Note pleural effusion ➡ & atelectatic lung.

Oblique transabdominal ultrasound using the intercostal window shows a subphrenic abscess ➡ more clearly. Interface with the liver ➡ & pleural effusion ➡ are better demonstrated.

TERMINOLOGY

Definitions
- Abscess formation in one of the peri-hepatic spaces

IMAGING FINDINGS

General Features
- Best diagnostic clue: Fluid collection in contact with surface of liver
- Location
  - Subphrenic (peritoneal)
    - Superior to level of coronary ligament
  - Subhepatic (peritoneal)
    - Inferior to level of coronary ligament
  - Bare area (retroperitoneal)
    - Attachment of coronary ligament from peritoneum
- Morphology: Peri-hepatic ligaments divide the peri-hepatic spaces into several compartments where abscesses may form

Ultrasonographic Findings
- Grayscale Ultrasound
  - Crescentic/ovoid fluid collection on liver surface
  - Typical echogenic content
  - May contain gas (posterior ring-down artifact)
  - Subphrenic region may be easier to interrogate using an intercostal rather than subcostal window
  - Pleural effusion, adjacent lung atelectasis
  - Ascites
  - Associated liver/biliary tree pathology may be present

Nuclear Medicine Findings
- Ga-67 Scintigraphy: Shows activity and localizes the site of abscess

Imaging Recommendations
- Best imaging tool: Ultrasound is good for detection of lesion and guiding drainage
- Protocol advice
  - Lack of diagnostic features for infected collection often requires aspiration of contents for diagnosis
  - Aspirate facilitates microbiology culture

DDx: Pyogenic Peri-Hepatic Abscess

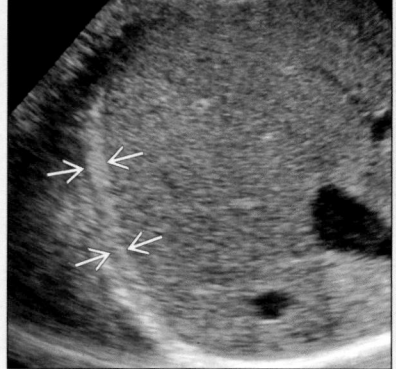

Hematoma

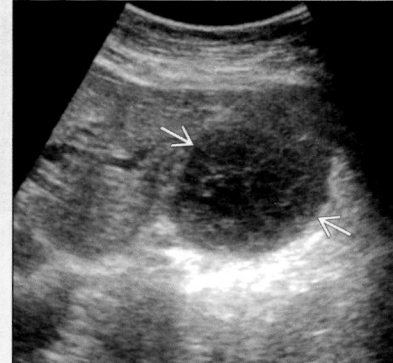

Biloma

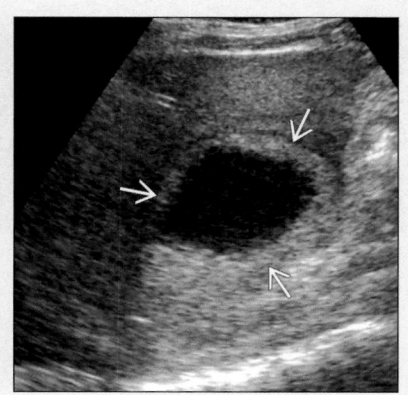

Metastasis

PYOGENIC PERI-HEPATIC ABSCESS

Key Facts

Imaging Findings
- Crescentic/ovoid fluid collection on liver surface
- Typical echogenic content
- May contain gas (posterior ring-down artifact)
- Subphrenic region may be easier to interrogate using an intercostal rather than subcostal window
- Pleural effusion, adjacent lung atelectasis
- Ascites
- Associated liver/biliary tree pathology may be present

- Best imaging tool: Ultrasound is good for detection of lesion and guiding drainage
- Lack of diagnostic features for infected collection often requires aspiration of contents for diagnosis

Top Differential Diagnoses
- Hematoma
- Biloma/Loculated Ascites
- Metastasis (On Hepatic Surface)

DIFFERENTIAL DIAGNOSIS

Hematoma
- Difficult to differentiate by morphology
- History of trauma or interventional procedure
- Gallium or white cell scan may help

Biloma/Loculated Ascites
- More likely to have clear content

Metastasis (On Hepatic Surface)
- More rounded contour (less likely to be crescentic)
- Thick irregular wall may be present
- More than one lesion may be present
- Tumor vascularity may be demonstrable

PATHOLOGY

General Features
- Etiology
  - Rupture of infected biliary tree: Cholecystitis or cholangitis
  - Rupture of liver abscess
  - Post-surgical: Liver or biliary tree surgery
  - Traumatic visceral injury

CLINICAL ISSUES

Presentation
- Most common signs/symptoms: Fever, chills, rigor

- Other signs/symptoms
  - Abdominal pain
  - Shoulder tip pain (subdiaphragmatic)
  - Raised white cell count

Treatment
- Ultrasound guided drainage of abscess
- Surgery for complicated anatomy or recurrent abscess

DIAGNOSTIC CHECKLIST

Consider
- Different positions of interrogation (intercostal, decubitus) to look for small collections in deep areas

SELECTED REFERENCES

1. Mori H et al: Exophytic spread of hepatobiliary disease via perihepatic ligaments: demonstration with CT and US. Radiology. 172(1):41-6, 1989
2. Lameris JS et al: Ultrasound-guided percutaneous drainage of intra-abdominal abscesses. Br J Surg. 74(7):620-3, 1987
3. Rubenstein WA et al: The perihepatic spaces: computed tomographic and ultrasound imaging. Radiology. 149(1):231-9, 1983
4. Whalen JP: Anatomy and radiologic diagnosis of perihepatic abscesses. Radiol Clin North Am. 14(3):406-28, 1976
5. Whalen JP et al: Classification of perihepatic abscesses. Radiology. 92(7):1427-37, 1969

IMAGE GALLERY

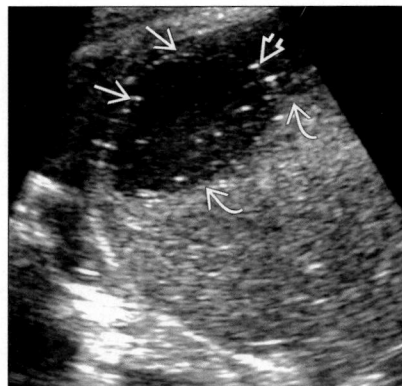 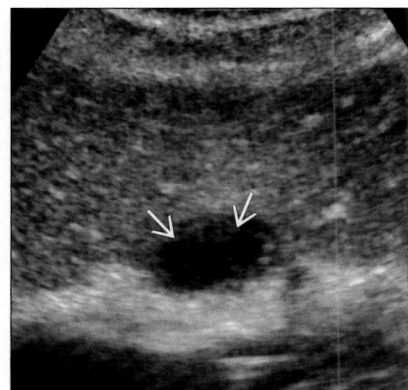 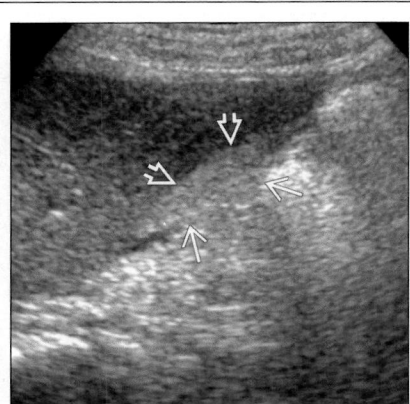

(Left) Oblique transabdominal ultrasound shows echogenic debris ➡ within a hypoechoic subphrenic abscess ➡. Note lobular indentation ➡ on liver surface. *(Center)* Oblique transabdominal ultrasound shows a hypoechoic abscess ➡ in the bare area of the liver (mainly posterior surface of right lobe). Note coronary ligaments are not discernible with imaging. *(Right)* Longitudinal transabdominal ultrasound shows a subhepatic abscess ➡. Uniform echogenic content makes detection difficult. Indentation of liver surface ➡ provides clue to diagnosis.

AMEBIC HEPATIC ABSCESS

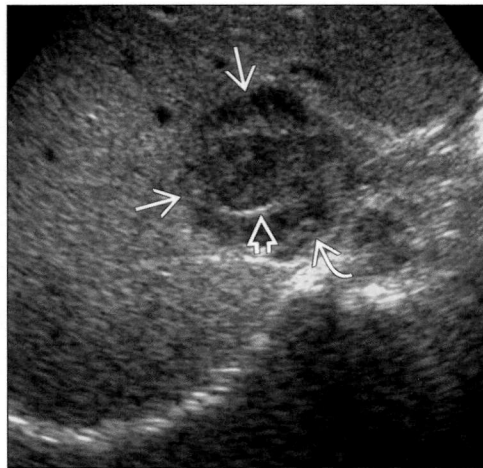

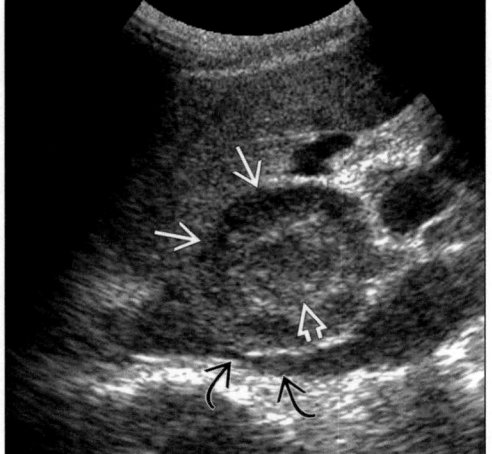

Transverse transabdominal ultrasound shows a round, hypoechoic amebic abscess ➡ with low-level internal echoes and septum ➱. Note abscess abuts posterior hepatic surface ➴.

Oblique transabdominal ultrasound shows same amebic abscess ➡ as previous image with low-level internal echoes ➱. The inferior vena cava ➷ is compressed by the protruding abscess.

TERMINOLOGY

Definitions
- Localized collection of pus in liver due to entamoeba histolytica with destruction of hepatic parenchyma & stroma

IMAGING FINDINGS

General Features
- Best diagnostic clue: Peripherally located, isoechoic mass, most often solitary (85%)
- Location
  - Right lobe: 72%
  - Left lobe: 13%
  - Usually peripheral
- Size: Varies from few millimeters to several centimeters
- Other general features
  - Most common extraintestinal manifestation of amebic infestation
  - Most common in developing countries
  - Western nations: High risk groups are recent immigrants, institutionalized & homosexuals

- Most often solitary (85%)
- Primary source of infection
  - Human carriers who pass amebic cysts into stool
- May become secondarily infected with pyogenic bacteria

Ultrasonographic Findings
- Grayscale Ultrasound
  - Usually solitary, peripherally located abscess
  - Abuts liver capsule, under diaphragm
  - Typically round or oval, sharply-defined hypoechoic
    - Amebic abscess is more likely to have a round or oval shape than pyogenic abscess (82:60%)
  - Imperceptible abscess wall, or wall nodularity in some
  - Homogeneous internal echoes
    - Hypoechoic with fine internal echoes is more common in amebic than pyogenic abscesses (58:36%)
    - No gas locules unless fistula formed with bowel
  - Internal septae may be present
  - No vascularity seen in wall or septa of amebic abscess
  - May show hypoechoic halo

DDx: Amebic Abscess

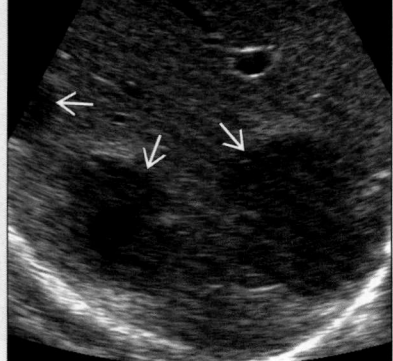

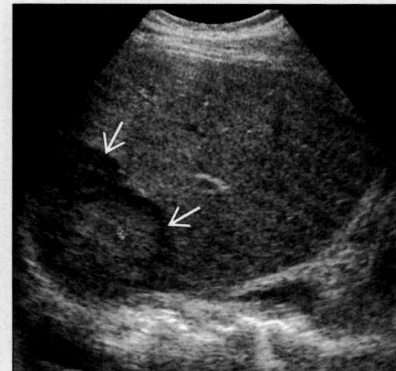

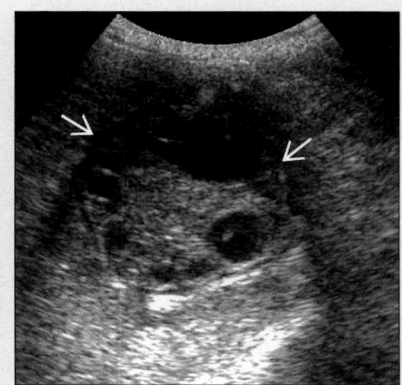

| *Pyogenic Abscess* | *Metastasis* | *Hydatid Cyst* |

Key Facts

Imaging Findings

- Best diagnostic clue: Membranes ± daughter cysts in a complex heterogeneous mass
- E. granulosus: Most common form of hydatid disease, unilocular form
- E. multilocularis (alveolaris): Less common but aggressive form
- **E. granulosus**
- Anechoic cyst with double echogenic lines separated by a hypoechoic layer
- Honeycombed cyst, multiple septations between daughter cysts in a mother cyst
- Detachment of endocyst from pericyst (partial or complete) results in varied appearances
- Undulating floating membrane within cyst
- "Water lily" sign: Complete detachment of membrane
- Anechoic cyst with internal debris, hydatid sand, "snowstorm pattern"
- **E. multilocularis**
- Single/multiple echogenic lesions
- Irregular necrotic regions & microcalcifications
- Ill-defined infiltrative solid masses
- Tend to spread to liver hilum
- Invasion of inferior vena cava (IVC) & diaphragm
- Evaluate lung, heart and brain for deposits

Top Differential Diagnoses

- Hemorrhagic or Infected Cyst
- Complex Pyogenic Abscess
- "Cystic" Metastases

Clinical Issues

- Serologic tests positive in more than 80% of cases

- ■ "Water lily" sign: Complete detachment of membrane
- ■ Anechoic cyst with internal debris, hydatid sand, "snowstorm pattern"
- ○ A densely calcified mass, curvilinear calcification
- ○ **E. multilocularis**
  - ■ Single/multiple echogenic lesions
  - ■ Irregular necrotic regions & microcalcifications
  - ■ Ill-defined infiltrative solid masses
  - ■ Tend to spread to liver hilum
  - ■ Invasion of inferior vena cava (IVC) & diaphragm
  - ■ Evaluate lung, heart and brain for deposits
- ○ US also used to monitor efficacy of
  - ■ Medical antihydatid therapy
- ○ Positive response findings include
  - ■ Reduction in cyst size
  - ■ Endocyst detachment
  - ■ Progressive increase in cyst echogenicity
  - ■ Mural calcification

Radiographic Findings

- Radiography
  - ○ E. granulosus: Curvilinear or ring-like pericyst calcification
    - ■ Seen in 20-30% of abdominal plain films
  - ○ E. multilocularis: Microcalcifications in 50% of cases
- ERCP
  - ○ Hydatid cyst may communicate with biliary tree
    - ■ Right hepatic duct 55%; left hepatic duct 29%, common hepatic duct 9%, gallbladder 6%, common bile duct 1%

CT Findings

- NECT
  - ○ E. granulosus
    - ■ Large unilocular/multilocular well-defined hypodense cysts
    - ■ Contains multiple peripheral daughter cysts of less density than mother cyst
    - ■ Curvilinear ring-like calcification
    - ■ Calcified wall: Usually indicates no active infection if completely circumferential

- ■ Dilated intrahepatic bile duct (IHBD): Due to compression/rupture of a cyst into bile ducts
- ○ Dilated ducts within vicinity of a cyst
- ○ E. multilocularis
  - ■ Extensive, infiltrative cystic and solid masses of low density (14-40 HU)
  - ■ Margins are irregular/ill-defined
  - ■ Amorphous type of calcification
  - ■ Can simulate a primary or secondary tumor
- CECT: Enhancement of cyst wall and septations

MR Findings

- T1WI
  - ○ Rim (pericyst): Hypointense (fibrous component)
  - ○ Mother cyst (hydatid matrix)
    - ■ Usually intermediate signal intensity
    - ■ Rarely hyperintense: Due to reduction in water content
  - ○ Daughter cysts: Less signal intensity than mother cyst (matrix)
  - ○ Floating membrane: Low signal intensity
  - ○ Calcifications: Difficult to identify on MR images
    - ■ Display low signal on both T1 & T2WI
- T2WI
  - ○ Rim (pericyst): Hypointense (fibrous component)
  - ○ First echo T2WI: Increased signal intensity
    - ■ Mother cysts more than daughter cysts
  - ○ Strong T2WI: Hyperintense
    - ■ Mother & daughter cysts have same intensity
  - ○ Floating membrane
    - ■ Low-intermediate signal intensity
- T1 C+: Enhancement of cyst wall and septations
- MRCP
  - ○ ± Demonstrate communication with biliary tree

Imaging Recommendations

- Best imaging tool: Ultrasound for diagnosis and follow-up

HEPATIC ECHINOCOCCUS CYST

DIFFERENTIAL DIAGNOSIS

Hemorrhagic or Infected Cyst
- Complex cystic heterogeneous mass
- Septations, fluid-levels & mural nodularity
- Calcification may or may not be seen

Complex Pyogenic Abscess
- "Cluster of grapes": Confluent complex cystic lesions

"Cystic" Metastases
- E.g., cystadenocarcinoma of pancreas or ovary
- May present with debris, mural nodularity, rim-enhancement

Biliary Cystadenocarcinoma
- Rare, multiseptated water density cystic mass
- No surrounding inflammatory changes

PATHOLOGY

General Features
- General path comments
  - Definitive host: Dog or fox
  - Intermediate host: Human, sheep or wild rodents
  - Germinal layer (endocyst) → scolices → larval stage
  - Hydatid sand: Free floating brood capsules & scolices form a white sediment
  - Larvae → portal vein → liver (75%)
    - Lungs (15%); other tissues (10%)
  - E. granulosus
    - Develop into hydatid stage (4-5 days) within liver
    - Hydatid cysts grow to 1 cm during first 6 months, 2-3 cm annually
  - E. multilocularis
    - Larvae proliferate & penetrate surrounding tissue
    - Cause a diffuse & infiltrative granulomatous reaction, simulating malignancy
    - Necrosis → cavitation → calcification
- Etiology
  - Caused by larval stage of Echinococcus tapeworm
    - E. granulosus & E. multilocularis
- Epidemiology
  - E. granulosus: Mediterranean region, Africa, South America, Australia & New Zealand
  - E. multilocularis: France, Germany, Austria, USSR, Japan, Alaska & Canada

Microscopic Features
- Cyst fluid content: Antigenic, pale yellow, neutral pH
- Endocyst: Gives rise to daughter vesicles/brood capsule, which may detach, form sediment or produce daughter cysts
- Ectocyst: Acellular substance secreted by parasite
- Pericyst: Host response forming a layer of granulation/fibrous tissue

CLINICAL ISSUES

Presentation
- Most common signs/symptoms
  - Cysts: Initially asymptomatic
    - Symptomatic when size ↑/infected/ruptured
  - Pain, fever, jaundice, hepatomegaly
  - Allergic reaction; portal hypertension
- Clinical Profile
  - Middle-aged patient with right upper quadrant pain, palpable mass, jaundice
    - Eosinophilia, urticaria + anaphylaxis
- Lab data
  - Eosinophilia; ↑ serologic titers
  - ± ↑ Alkaline phosphatase/Gamma-glutamyl transpeptidase (GGTP)
- Diagnosis
  - Serologic tests positive in more than 80% of cases
  - Percutaneous aspiration of cyst fluid
    - Danger of peritoneal spill & anaphylactic reaction

Demographics
- Age
  - Hydatid disease usually acquired in childhood
  - Not diagnosed until 30-40 years of age
- Gender: M = F

Natural History & Prognosis
- Complications
  - Compression/infection or rupture into biliary tree
  - Rupture into peritoneal or pleural cavity
  - Spread of lesions to lungs, heart, brain & bone
- Prognosis: E. granulosus (good); E. multilocularis (fatal in 10-15 years untreated)

Treatment
- E. granulosus
  - Medical: Albendazole/mebendazole
  - Direct injection of scolicidal agents
  - Percutaneous aspiration & drainage of cyst
  - Surgical: Segmental or lobar hepatectomy
- E. multilocularis
  - Partial hepatectomy/hepatectomy + liver transplant

DIAGNOSTIC CHECKLIST

Consider
- Rule out other complex or septate cystic liver masses
  - Biliary cystadenoma, pyogenic liver abscess, cystic metastases & hemorrhagic or infected cyst
  - E. multilocularis imaging and clinical behavior simulates solid malignant neoplasm

Image Interpretation Pearls
- Daughter cysts can float freely within mother cyst
  - Altering patient's position may change position of daughter cysts

SELECTED REFERENCES

1. Haddad MC et al: Unilocular hepatic echinococcal cysts: sonography and computed tomography findings. Clin Radiol. 56(9):746-50, 2001
2. Pedrosa I et al: Hydatid disease: radiologic and pathologic features and complications. RadioGraphics. 20:795-817, 2000
3. Lewall DB et al: Hepatic echinococcal cysts: sonographic appearance and classification. Radiology. 155(3):773-5, 1985

IMAGE GALLERY

Typical

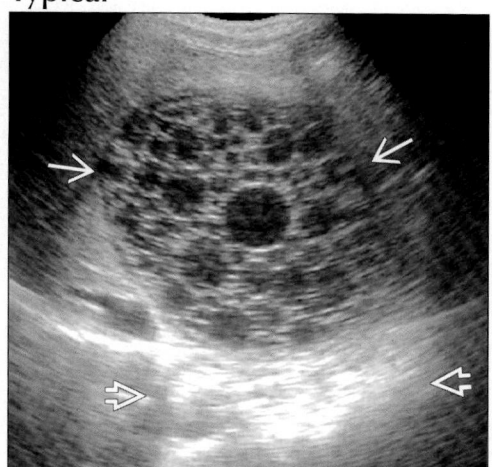

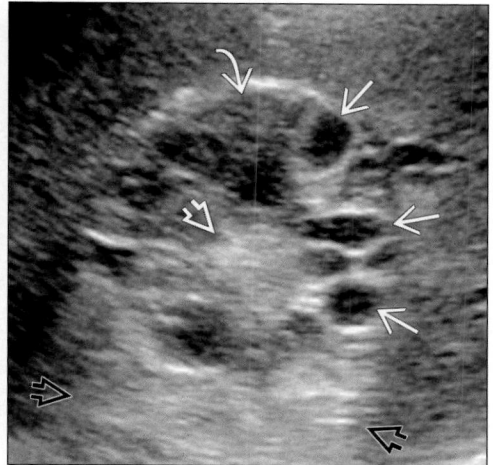

(Left) Oblique transabdominal ultrasound shows an echinococcal cyst ➡ containing multiple daughter cysts. Note the posterior acoustic enhancement ➡. *(Right)* Oblique transabdominal ultrasound shows an echinococcal cyst with multiple daughter cysts ➡ and mixed isoechoic ➡ and hyperechoic ➡ content. Note the posterior enhancement ➡.

Typical

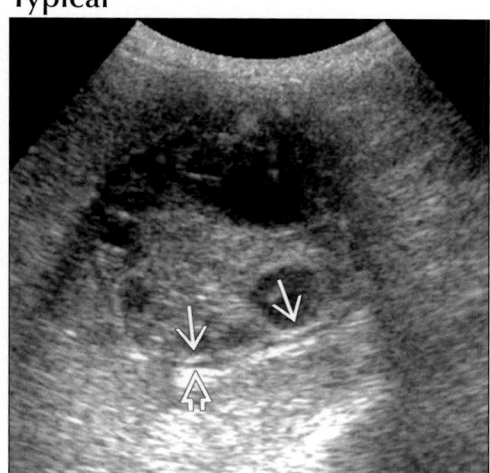

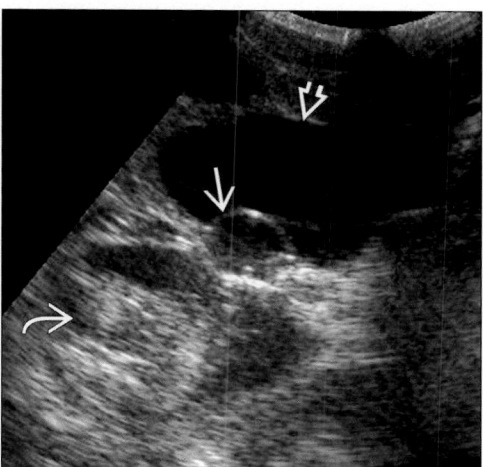

(Left) Oblique transabdominal ultrasound shows a hypoechoic rim ➡ outside the ectocyst ➡ of an echinococcal cyst. *(Right)* Oblique transabdominal ultrasound shows a single daughter cyst ➡ in the wall of an echinococcal cyst ➡. Another cyst shows a collapsed endocyst ➡.

Typical

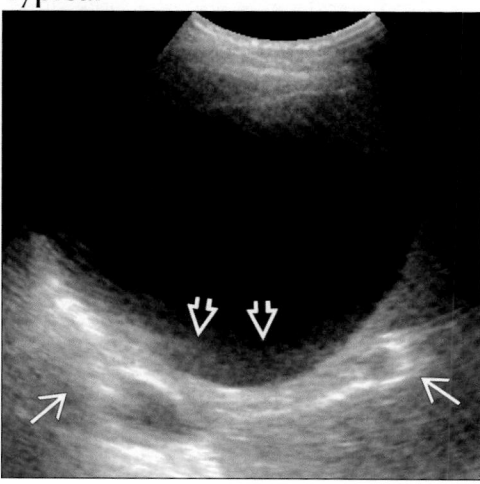

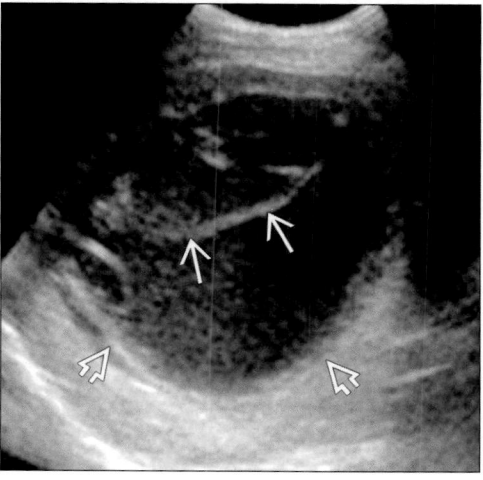

(Left) Oblique transabdominal ultrasound shows hydatid sand ➡ gravitating to the dependent portion of the cyst. Note the posterior acoustic enhancement ➡. *(Right)* Oblique transabdominal ultrasound shows a detached endocyst ➡ floating within an echinococcal cyst (water lily sign). The outer ectocyst ➡ holds up the shape of the cyst.

HEPATIC ECHINOCOCCUS CYST

(Left) Oblique transabdominal ultrasound shows a ruptured hydatid cyst with multiple septae ➡ and fine echogenic hydatid sand ➡. (Right) Oblique transabdominal ultrasound shows a ruptured echinococcal cyst ➡ with multiple septae (some of which are thick ➡) and dispersed echogenic hydatid sand ➡.

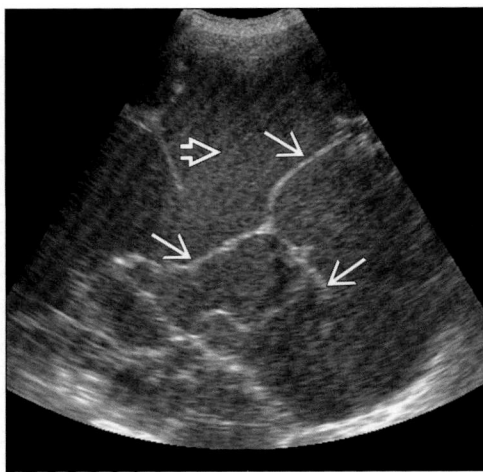
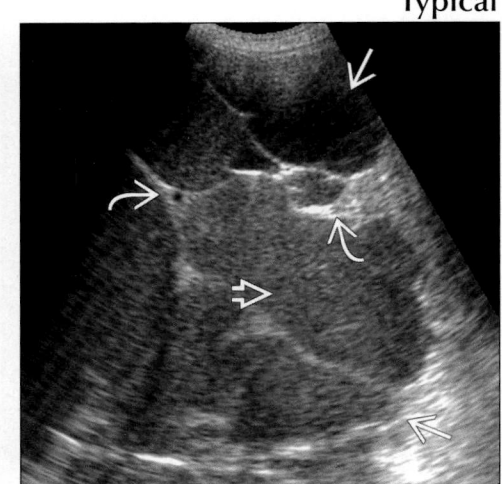

(Left) Oblique color Doppler ultrasound shows vascularity ➡ within the thick septae of the ruptured echinococcal cyst seen in the previous image. (Right) Oblique transabdominal ultrasound shows an oval-shaped hydatid cyst ➡ containing daughter cysts & echogenic material. A larger ruptured cyst ➡ shows a floating endocyst ➡.

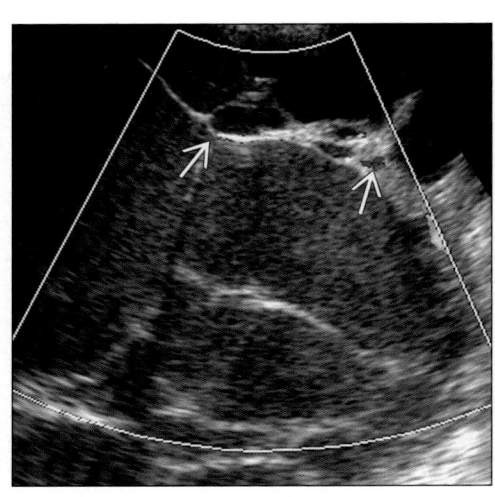
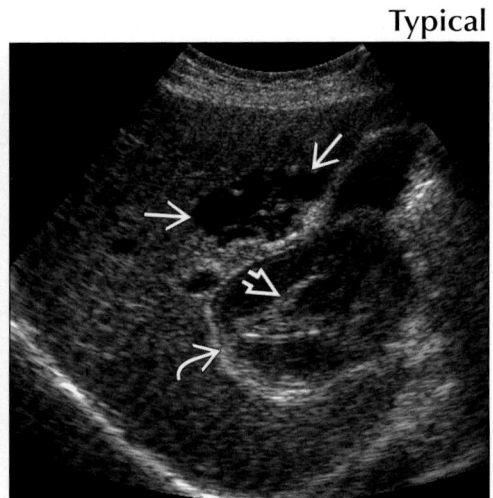

(Left) Oblique transabdominal ultrasound shows three echinococcal cysts, one with hydatid sand ➡, one with a collapsed endocyst ➡ and one with clear content ➡. (Right) Oblique transabdominal ultrasound shows common bile duct dilatation causesd by small cysts ➡ and fine echogenic material (hydatid sand) that was released after echinococcal cyst rupture.

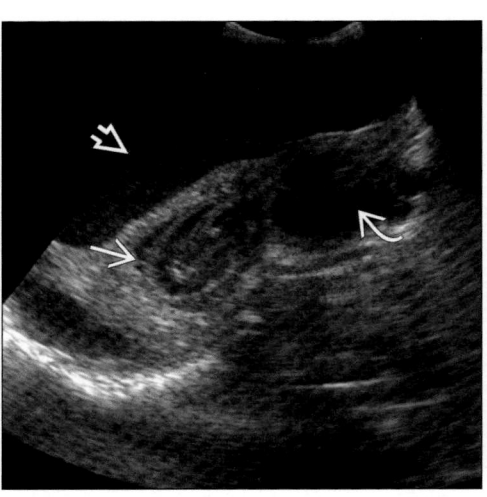
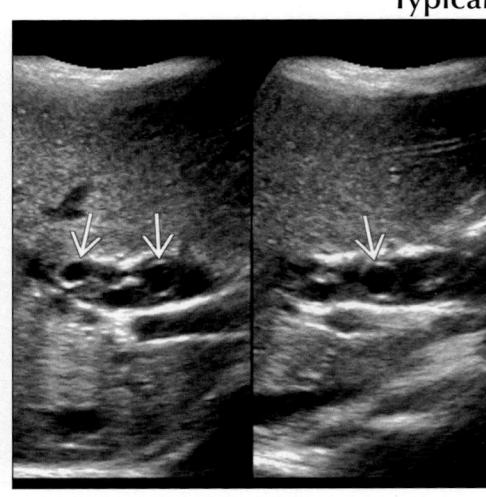

Typical

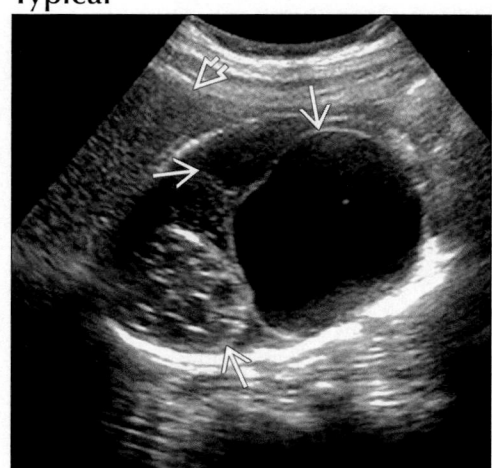
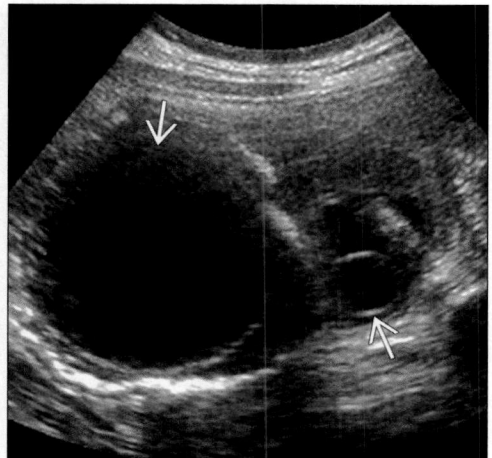

(Left) Longitudinal transabdominal ultrasound shows echinococcal cysts ➡ (with different appearances) in the right kidney behind the liver ⮞, disseminated after hepatic cyst rupture. *(Right)* Transverse transabdominal ultrasound shows echinococcal cysts ➡ (with different appearances) in the right kidney. These were disseminated after hepatic cyst rupture.

Typical

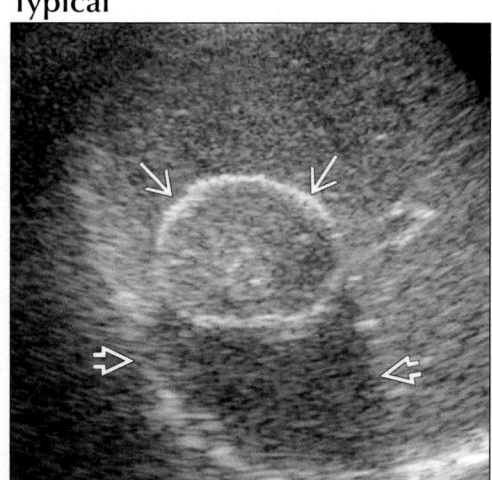
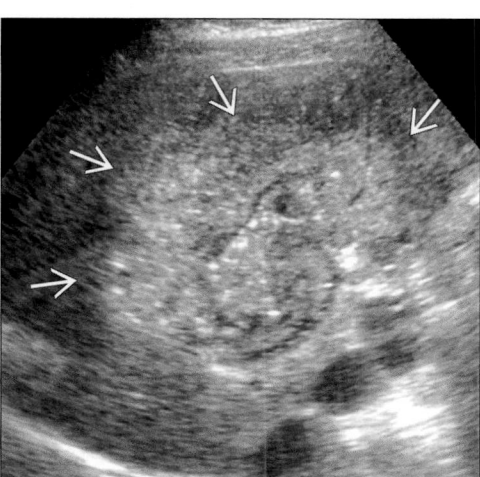

(Left) Oblique transabdominal ultrasound shows curvilinear calcification of ectocyst of an echinococcal cyst ➡ with posterior acoustic attenuation ⮞ obscuring underlying liver parenchyma. *(Right)* Oblique transabdominal ultrasound shows irregular and indistinct borders ➡ in an invasive form of hydatid disease (E. multilocularis).

Typical

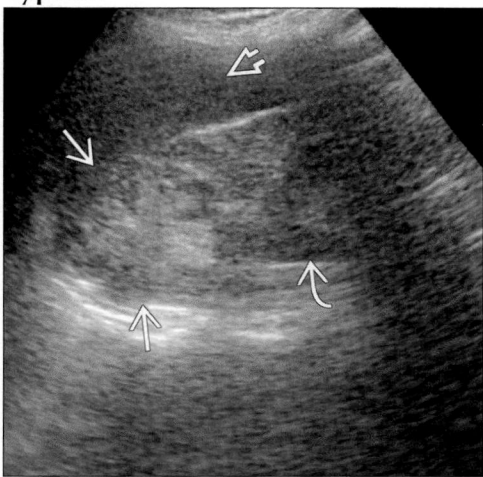
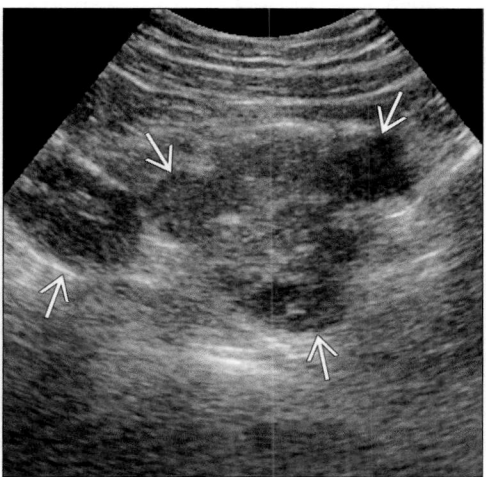

(Left) Longitudinal transabdominal ultrasound shows an echinococcal (E. multilocularis) cyst ➡ in the right adrenal gland behind the liver ⮞ and above the right kidney ➡. *(Right)* Oblique transabdominal ultrasound shows hydatid cysts ➡ in the left side of the pelvis in the same patient as the previous two images with disseminated E. multilocularis infection.

HEPATIC TRAUMA

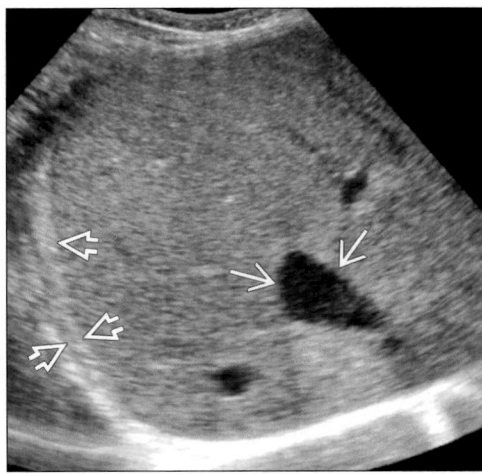

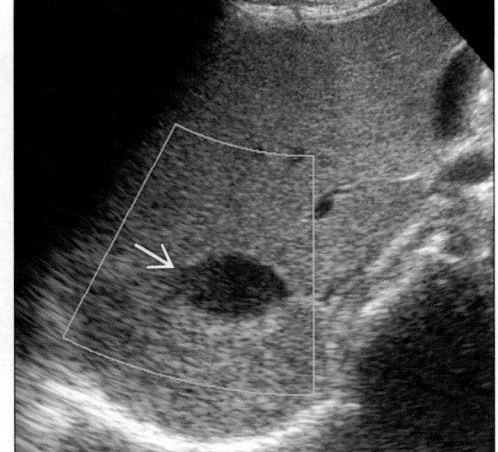

Oblique transabdominal ultrasound shows a hypoechoic organizing hepatic hematoma ➡. Note the hyperechoic curvilinear subcapsular hematoma ➡ in a different phase of evolution.

Oblique color Doppler ultrasound shows the same organizing hematoma ➡ as in previous image. There is lack of vascularity within or around the organizing hematoma.

TERMINOLOGY

Abbreviations and Synonyms
- Liver or hepatic injury

IMAGING FINDINGS

General Features
- Best diagnostic clue: Irregular hepatic lesion and perihepatic hematoma in a patient with abdominal trauma
- Location
  - Right lobe (75%); left lobe (25%)
  - Intraparenchymal or subcapsular
- Key concepts
  - Liver 2nd most frequently injured solid intra-abdominal organ after spleen
    - Due to its anterior & partially subcostal location
  - Most common causes of hepatic trauma
    - Blunt (more common), penetrating and iatrogenic injuries
  - Iatrogenic injury due to liver biopsy

    - Most common cause of subcapsular hematoma in US
  - Abdominal trauma
    - Leading cause of death in United States (< 40 yrs)

Ultrasonographic Findings
- Grayscale Ultrasound
  - Lesions are common in segments 6, 7 and 8 which may be difficult to image in a trauma setting
  - Helpful ancillary signs: Subcapsular hematoma, hemoperitoneum, right renal or splenic laceration/hematoma
  - Subcapsular hematoma: Lentiform or curvilinear fluid collection
    - Initially: Echogenic
    - After 4-5 days: Hypoechoic
  - After 1-4 weeks: Internal echoes and septation may develop within hematoma
  - Rate of hematoma evolution depends on vascularity of region, slower for intraperitoneal or subcapsular regions, faster for parenchymal hematomas
  - Diffuse heterogeneous liver echo pattern with absence of normal hepatic vessels suggests diffuse parenchymal injury

DDx: Hepatic Trauma

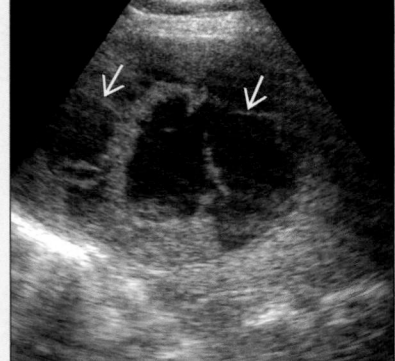

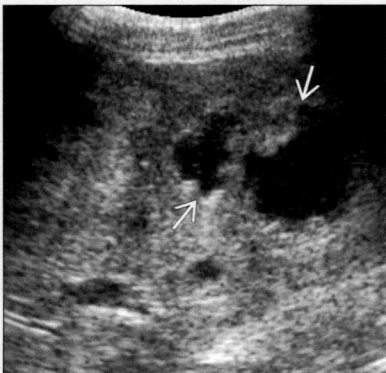

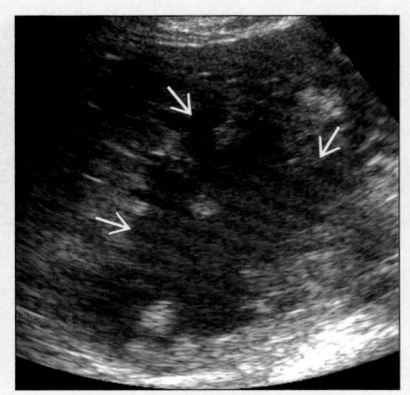

| *Cyst Hemorrhage* | *Necrotic Met* | *Hepatic Abscess* |

Key Facts

Imaging Findings

- Best diagnostic clue: Irregular hepatic lesion and perihepatic hematoma in a patient with abdominal trauma
- Lesions are common in segments 6, 7 and 8 which may be difficult to image in a trauma setting
- Helpful ancillary signs: Subcapsular hematoma, hemoperitoneum, right renal or splenic laceration/hematoma
- Subcapsular hematoma: Lentiform or curvilinear fluid collection
- Rate of hematoma evolution depends on vascularity of region, slower for intraperitoneal or subcapsular regions, faster for parenchymal hematomas
- Diffuse heterogeneous liver echo pattern with absence of normal hepatic vessels suggests diffuse parenchymal injury
- Parenchymal laceration: Irregular shaped hematoma which may point towards capsular surface
- Parenchymal laceration may show direct extension to surface
- Hepatic fracture is seen as laceration extending across two surfaces
- Ultrasound: For early assessment e.g., in focused assessment with sonography for trauma (FAST) & for monitoring progression

Top Differential Diagnoses

- Hemorrhagic Cyst
- Necrotic Neoplasm (Primary or Secondary)
- Hepatic Abscess

- Intraparenchymal hematoma
  - Rounded echogenic or hypoechoic foci
- Parenchymal laceration
  - Parenchymal laceration: Irregular shaped hematoma which may point towards capsular surface
  - Parenchymal laceration may show direct extension to surface
  - Abnormal echotexture relative to normal liver due to hematoma which would evolve with time
- Hepatic fracture
  - Hepatic fracture is seen as laceration extending across two surfaces
  - May result in infarction
- Biloma
  - Rounded/ellipsoid, anechoic, loculated structures
  - Well-defined sharp margins, close to bile ducts

CT Findings

- Lacerations
  - Simple or stellate (parallel to portal/hepatic vein branches)
    - Simple: Hypodense solitary linear laceration
    - Stellate: Hypodense branching linear lacerations
- Parenchymal and subcapsular hematomas (lenticular configuration)
  - Unclotted blood (35-45 HU) soon after injury
    - NECT: May be hyperdense relative to normal liver
    - CECT: Hypodense compared to enhancing normal liver tissue
  - Clotted blood (60-90 HU)
    - More dense than unclotted blood & normal liver
    - May be more dense than unenhanced liver
- Active hemorrhage or pseudoaneurysm
  - CECT: Active hemorrhage
    - Isodense to enhanced vessels
    - Seen as contrast extravasation (85-350 HU)
    - Extravasated contrast material and surrounding decreased attenuation clot
- Hemoperitoneum: Perihepatic and peritoneal recess collections of blood
- Periportal tracking: Linear, focal or diffuse periportal zones of decreased HU

- Due to dissecting blood, bile or dilated periportal lymphatics
  - DDx: Overhydration (check for distended IVC)
    - Elevated venous pressure & transudation
- Areas of infarction
  - Small or large areas of low attenuation
  - Usually wedge-shaped; segmental or lobar
  - Intrahepatic/subcapsular gas (due to hepatic necrosis)
- CT diagnosis of liver trauma
  - Accuracy: 96%
  - Sensitivity: 100%
  - Specificity: 94%

MR Findings

- T1WI and T2WI
  - Varied signal intensity depending on
    - Degree and age of hemorrhage or infarct

Angiographic Findings

- Conventional
  - Demonstrate
    - Active extravasation, pseudoaneurysm
    - A-V, arteriobiliary or portobiliary fistulas

Imaging Recommendations

- Best imaging tool
  - Ultrasound: For early assessment e.g., in focused assessment with sonography for trauma (FAST) & for monitoring progression
  - CECT: In hemodynamically stable cases
  - Angiography: To localize active hemorrhage and embolization
- Protocol advice: CECT: Include lung bases and pelvis

DIFFERENTIAL DIAGNOSIS

Hemorrhagic Cyst

- Usually round/oval smooth contour
- No accessory findings of hepatic trauma

Necrotic Neoplasm (Primary or Secondary)

- Irregular wall may show vascularity

HEPATIC TRAUMA

- May have multiple lesions
- May invade hepatic vasculature/lymph nodes

Hepatic Abscess
- Irregular wall may show vascularity
- May have internal gas locules

PATHOLOGY

General Features
- Etiology
  - Blunt trauma (more common)
    - Motor vehicle accidents (more common)
    - Falls and assaults
  - Penetrating injuries
    - Gunshot and stab injuries
  - Iatrogenic
    - Liver biopsy, chest tubes, transhepatic cholangiography
- Epidemiology
  - 5-10% blunt abdominal trauma have liver injury
  - Mortality from hepatic trauma: 10-20%
- Associated abnormalities
  - Splenic injury (45%); bowel injury (5%); rib fractures
  - Left hepatic lobe laceration often associated with bowel or pancreatic injury

Gross Pathologic & Surgical Features
- Laceration or contusion
- Subcapsular or intraparenchymal hematoma

Staging, Grading or Classification Criteria
- Clinical classification based on American Association for Surgery of Trauma (AAST)
  - Grade I
    - Subcapsular hematoma: Less than 10% surface area
    - Laceration: Capsular tear, less than 1 cm parenchymal depth
  - Grade II
    - Subcapsular hematoma: 10-50% surface area
    - Intraparenchymal hematoma: Less than 10 cm diameter
    - Laceration: 1-3 cm parenchymal depth, less than 10 cm in length
  - Grade III
    - Subcapsular hematoma: More than 50% surface area; expanding/ruptured subcapsular or parenchymal hematoma
    - Intraparenchymal hematoma: More than 10 cm or expanding
    - Laceration: Parenchymal fracture more than 3 cm deep
  - Grade IV
    - Laceration: Parenchymal disruption involving 25-75% of hepatic lobe or 1-3 Couinaud segments within a single lobe
  - Grade V
    - Laceration: Parenchymal disruption involving > 75% of hepatic lobe or > 3 Couinaud segments within a single lobe
    - Vascular: Juxtahepatic venous injuries (retrohepatic vena cava, major hepatic veins)
  - Grade VI
    - Vascular: Hepatic avulsion

CLINICAL ISSUES

Presentation
- Most common signs/symptoms
  - Right upper quadrant (RUQ) pain, tenderness, guarding, rebound tenderness
  - Hypotension, tachycardia, jaundice
  - Hematemesis or melena (due to hemobilia)
- Clinical Profile: Patient with history of motor vehicle accident, RUQ tenderness, guarding and hypotension
- Lab data
  - Decreased hematocrit (not acutely)
  - Increased direct/indirect bilirubin
  - Increased alkaline phosphatase levels

Natural History & Prognosis
- Complications
  - Hemobilia, biloma, A-V fistula, pseudoaneurysm
- Prognosis
  - Grade I, II and III: Good
  - Grade IV, V and VI: Poor
  - May not necessarily correlate with AAST grading
  - Mortality: 10-20%
    - 50% due to liver injury itself
    - Rest from associated injuries

Treatment
- Grade I, II and III
  - Conservative management for almost all injuries diagnosed on CT
    - Implies some degree of clinical stability
- Grade IV, V and VI
  - Surgical intervention for shock and peritonitis
    - Control hemorrhage, drainage and repair
  - Embolization for active extravasation

DIAGNOSTIC CHECKLIST

Image Interpretation Pearls
- Laceration of left hepatic lobe often associated with bowel and pancreatic injury

SELECTED REFERENCES

1. Poletti PA et al: Blunt abdominal trauma: does the use of a second-generation sonographic contrast agent help to detect solid organ injuries? AJR Am J Roentgenol. 183(5):1293-301, 2004
2. Rose JS: Ultrasound in abdominal trauma. Emerg Med Clin North Am. 22(3):581-99, vii, 2004
3. Poletti PA et al: CT criteria for management of blunt liver trauma: correlation with angiographic and surgical findings. Radiology. 216(2):418-27, 2000
4. Richards JR et al: Sonographic detection of blunt hepatic trauma: hemoperitoneum and parenchymal patterns of injury. 47(6):1092-7, 1999
5. Becker CD et al: Blunt hepatic trauma in adults: correlation of CT injury grading with outcome. Radiology. 201(1):215-20, 1996

IMAGE GALLERY

Typical

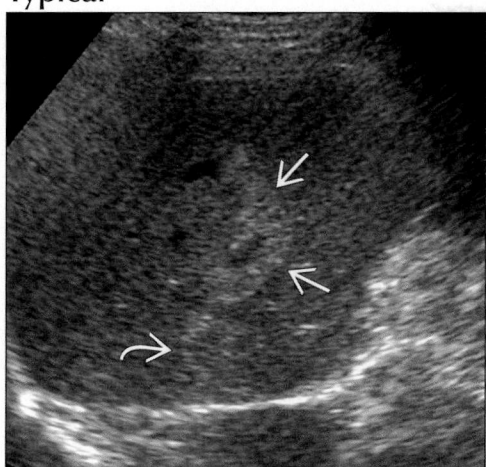
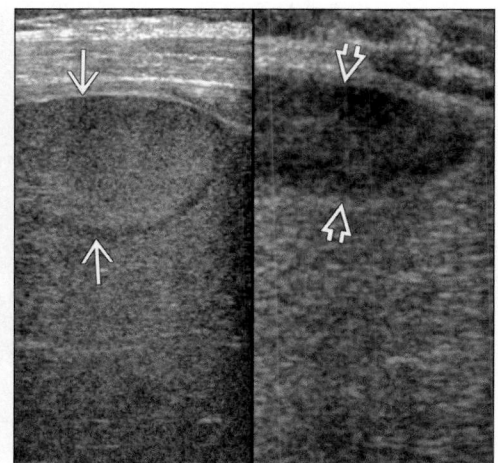

(Left) Oblique transabdominal ultrasound shows an acute hepatic hematoma ➡ hyperechoic compared to the parenchyma. There is subtle extension ➡ to the posterior surface. *(Right)* Oblique transabdominal ultrasound shows evolution of a lentiform subcapsular hematoma from isoechoic ➡ to hypoechoic ➡ with respect to the liver parenchyma.

Typical

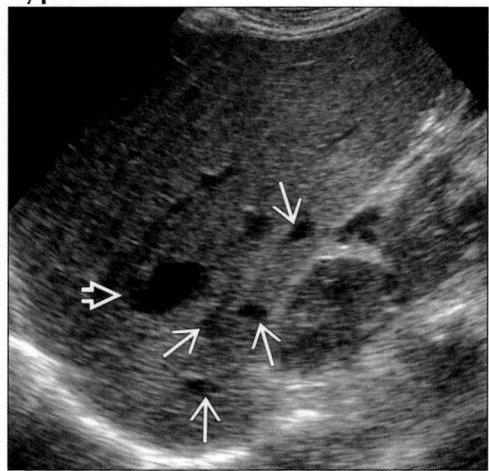
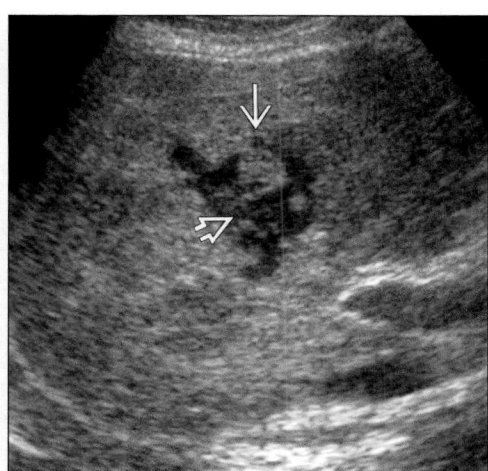

(Left) Oblique transabdominal ultrasound shows a resolving complex hepatic laceration ➡ with branching extensions ➡ to the posterior surface. *(Right)* Oblique transabdominal ultrasound shows an irregularly shaped hypoechoic organizing hematoma ➡ with irregular walls & internal echoes ➡.

Typical

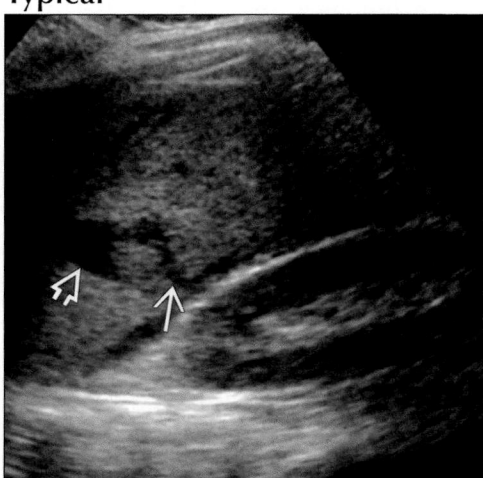
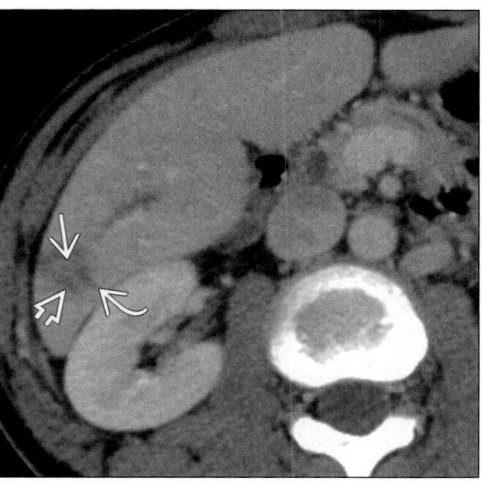

(Left) Oblique transabdominal ultrasound shows an organizing hepatic hematoma ➡ with extension ➡ to the posterior surface of liver confirming a laceration. *(Right)* Transverse CECT shows a hepatic hematoma ➡, with hypodense rim ➡ and extension to the posterior hepatic surface ➡.

HEPATIC ADENOMA

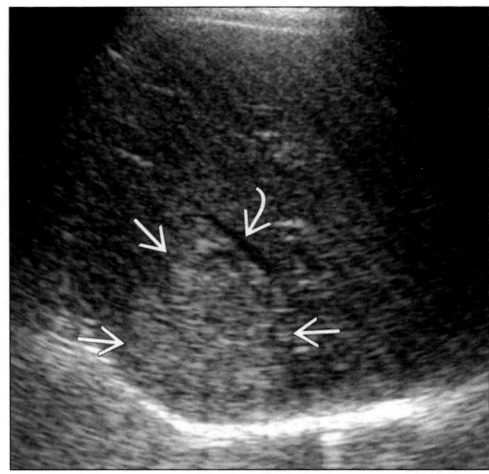 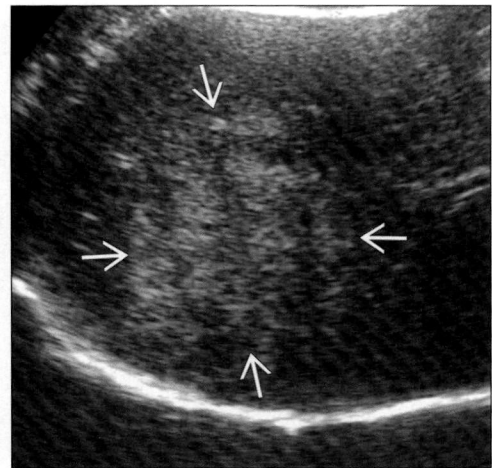

Transverse transabdominal ultrasound shows a well-defined, homogeneous, hyperechoic hepatic adenoma ➡ adjacent to the left hepatic vein ➡.

Oblique transabdominal ultrasound shows a large hyperechoic adenoma ➡. Note contour is slightly lobulated.

TERMINOLOGY

Abbreviations and Synonyms
- Hepatocellular adenoma (HCA) or liver cell adenoma

Definitions
- Benign tumor that arises from hepatocytes arranged in cords that occasionally form bile

IMAGING FINDINGS

General Features
- Best diagnostic clue: Heterogeneous, hypervascular mass with hemorrhage in a young woman, often with contraceptive use
- Location
  ○ Subcapsular region of right lobe of liver (75%)
  ○ Intraparenchymal or pedunculated (10%)
- Size
  ○ Varies between 6-30 cm
  ○ Average size: 8-10 cm
- Key concepts
  ○ Rare benign neoplasm

- ○ Second most frequent hepatic tumor in young women after focal nodular hyperplasia (FNH)
  ○ Associated with oral contraceptive steroids
  ○ Usually single (adenoma); rarely multiple (adenomatosis)

Ultrasonographic Findings
- Grayscale Ultrasound
  ○ Well-defined borders
  ○ Round or mildly lobulated contour
  ○ Hypo-/iso-/hyperechoic mass
  ○ Complex hyper & hypoechoic heterogeneous mass with anechoic areas
    ▪ Due to fat, hemorrhage, necrosis & calcification
  ○ Hypoechoic halo of compressed liver tissue with multiple vessels
  ○ Hemorrhage: Intratumoral or retroperitoneal hemorrhage
- Color Doppler
  ○ Hypervascular tumor, supplied by hepatic artery
  ○ Large peripheral arteries & veins
  ○ Intratumoral veins present
    ▪ Absent in FNH
    ▪ Useful discriminating feature for HCA

DDx: Liver Cell Adenoma

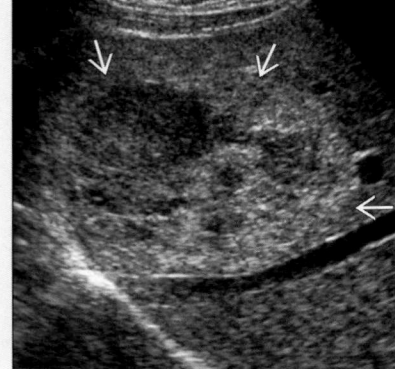 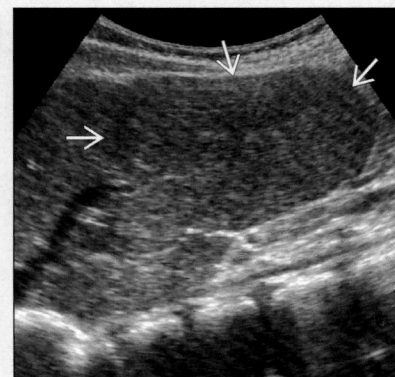 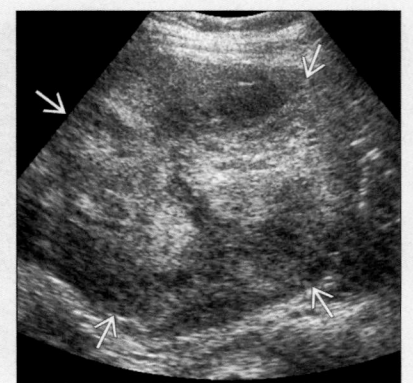

Hemangioma   *Focal Nodular Hyperplasia*   *Hepatocellular Carcinoma*

HEPATIC ADENOMA

Key Facts

Terminology
- Hepatocellular adenoma (HCA) or liver cell adenoma
- Benign tumor that arises from hepatocytes arranged in cords that occasionally form bile

Imaging Findings
- Best diagnostic clue: Heterogeneous, hypervascular mass with hemorrhage in a young woman, often with contraceptive use
- Subcapsular region of right lobe of liver (75%)
- Average size: 8-10 cm
- Well-defined borders
- Round or mildly lobulated contour
- Hypo-/iso-/hyperechoic mass
- Complex hyper & hypoechoic heterogeneous mass with anechoic areas
- Hypoechoic halo of compressed liver tissue with multiple vessels
- Hemorrhage: Intratumoral or retroperitoneal hemorrhage
- Best imaging tool: Ultrasound is good for lesion detection, guiding biopsy and monitoring size

Top Differential Diagnoses
- Hemangioma
- Focal Nodular Hyperplasia (FNH)
- Hepatocellular Carcinoma (HCC)

Diagnostic Checklist
- Rule out other benign & malignant liver tumors which have similar imaging features, particularly HCC or FNH

CT Findings
- NECT
  - Well-defined, spherical mass
  - Isodense to hypodense (due to lipid)
  - Hemorrhage: Intratumoral, parenchymal or subcapsular
  - Fat or calcification seen (less often than on MR)
- CECT
  - Arterial phase
    - Heterogeneous, hyperdense enhancement
  - Portal venous phase
    - Less heterogeneous
    - Hyper-/iso-/hypodense to liver
  - Delayed phase (10 min)
    - Homogeneous, hypodense
    - Enhancement does not persist (due to arteriovenous shunting)
    - Pseudocapsule: Hyperattenuated to liver & adenoma
  - Large adenomas
    - More heterogeneous than smaller lesions

MR Findings
- T1WI
  - Mass: Heterogeneous signal intensity
    - Increased signal intensity (due to fat & recent hemorrhage), more evident on MR than CT
    - Decreased signal intensity (necrosis, calcification, old hemorrhage)
  - Rim (fibrous pseudocapsule): Hypointense
- T2WI
  - Mass: Heterogeneous signal intensity
    - Increased signal intensity (old hemorrhage/necrosis)
    - Decreased signal intensity (fat, recent hemorrhage)
  - Rim (fibrous pseudocapsule): Hypointense
- T1 C+
  - Gadolinium arterial phase
    - Mass: Heterogeneous enhancement
  - Delayed phase
    - Pseudocapsule: Hyperintense to liver & adenoma

Nuclear Medicine Findings
- Technetium sulfur colloid
  - Usually "cold" (photopenic): In 80%
  - Uncommonly "warm": In 20%
    - Due to uptake in sparse Kupffer cells
- HIDA scan
  - Increased activity
- Gallium scan
  - No uptake

Angiographic Findings
- Conventional
  - Hypervascular mass with centripetal flow
  - Enlarged hepatic artery with feeders at tumor periphery (50%)
  - Hypovascular; avascular regions
    - Due to hemorrhage & necrosis

Imaging Recommendations
- Best imaging tool: Ultrasound is good for lesion detection, guiding biopsy and monitoring size
- T2WI; T1WI with dynamic enhanced multiphasic; GRE in-and opposed-phase images

DIFFERENTIAL DIAGNOSIS

Hemangioma
- Hyperechoic mass with/without posterior acoustic shadowing
- Large lesions may be heterogeneous
- May contain calcification

Focal Nodular Hyperplasia (FNH)
- No malignant degeneration or hemorrhage
- Central scar may be present
- When small (≤ 3 cm), FNH without scar may be indistinguishable from adenoma

Hepatocellular Carcinoma (HCC)
- May have identical imaging features as hepatic adenoma
- Background cirrhosis usually present

HEPATIC ADENOMA

- Histologically: May be difficult to distinguish well-differentiated HCC from adenoma
- Biliary, vascular, nodal invasion & metastases establish that lesion is malignant

Fibrolamellar Hepatocellular Carcinoma
- Large, lobulated mass with scar & septa
- Heterogeneous architecture on all imaging
- Vascular, biliary, nodal invasion may be present

Metastases
- Usually multiple & look for primary tumors
  ○ Breast, thyroid, kidney and endocrine

PATHOLOGY

General Features
- General path comments
  ○ HCA: Surrounded by a fibrous pseudocapsule
    ▪ Due to compression of adjacent liver tissue
  ○ High incidence of
    ▪ Hemorrhage, necrosis & fatty change
  ○ No scar within tumor
- Etiology
  ○ ↑ Risk in oral contraceptives & anabolic steroid users
  ○ Pregnancy
    ▪ Increased tumor growth rate and tumor rupture
  ○ Diabetes mellitus
  ○ Von-Gierke type Ia glycogen storage disease
    ▪ Multiple adenomas: 60%
- Epidemiology
  ○ Estimated incidence in oral contraceptive users
    ▪ 4 adenomas per 100,000 users

Gross Pathologic & Surgical Features
- Well-circumscribed mass on external surface of liver
- Soft, pale or yellow tan
- Frequently bile-stained nodules
- Large areas of hemorrhage or infarction
- "Pseudocapsule" & occasional "pseudopods"

Microscopic Features
- Sheets or cords of hepatocytes
- Absence of portal & central veins & bile ducts
- Increased amounts of glycogen & lipid
- Scattered, thin-walled, vascular channels

Staging, Grading or Classification Criteria
- Typical hepatocellular adenoma (HCA)
  ○ Type I: Estrogen associated HCA
  ○ Type II: Spontaneous HCA in women
  ○ Type III: Spontaneous HCA in men
  ○ Type IV: Spontaneous HCA in children
  ○ Type V: Metabolic disease associated HCA
- Anabolic steroid-associated HCA
- Multiple hepatocellular adenomas (adenomatosis)

CLINICAL ISSUES

Presentation
- Most common signs/symptoms
  ○ RUQ pain (40%): Due to hemorrhage
  ○ Asymptomatic (20%)
  ○ May be mistaken clinically/pathologically for HCC
- Clinical Profile: Woman on oral contraceptives
- Lab data: Usually normal liver function tests
- Diagnosis: Biopsy & histology

Demographics
- Age
  ○ Young women of childbearing age group
  ○ Predominantly in 3rd & 4th decades
- Gender
  ○ 98% seen in females (M:F = 1:10)
  ○ Not seen in males unless on anabolic steroids or with glycogen storage disease

Natural History & Prognosis
- Complications
  ○ Hemorrhage: Intrahepatic or intraperitoneal (40%)
  ○ Rupture: Increased risk in pregnancy
  ○ Risk of malignant transformation
    ▪ When size is more than 10 cm (in 10%)
- Prognosis
  ○ Usually good
    ▪ After discontinuation of oral contraceptives
    ▪ After surgical resection of large/symptomatic
  ○ Poor
    ▪ Intraperitoneal rupture
    ▪ Rupture during pregnancy
    ▪ Adenomatosis (> 10 adenomas)
    ▪ Malignant transformation

Treatment
- Adenoma less than 6 cm
  ○ Observation & discontinue oral contraceptives
- Adenoma more than 6 cm & near surface
  ○ Surgical resection
- Pregnancy should be avoided due to increased risk of rupture

DIAGNOSTIC CHECKLIST

Consider
- Rule out other benign & malignant liver tumors which have similar imaging features, particularly HCC or FNH
- Percutaneous biopsy is associated with high risk of bleeding
- Check for history of oral contraceptives & glycogen storage disease (in case of multiple adenomas)

Image Interpretation Pearls
- Spherical well-defined hypervascular & heterogeneous mass due to hemorrhage & fat

SELECTED REFERENCES

1. Grazioli L et al: Hepatic adenomas: imaging and pathologic findings. RadioGraphics. 21:877-94, 2001
2. Grazioli L et al: Liver adenomatosis: clinical, pathologic and imaging findings in 15 patients. Radiology. 216:395-402, 2000
3. Ichikawa T et al: Hepatocellular adenoma:multiphasic CT and histopathologic findings in 25 patients. Radiology. 214:861-8, 2000

IMAGE GALLERY

Typical

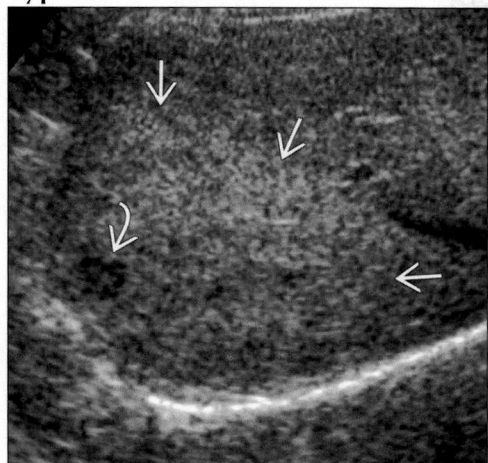
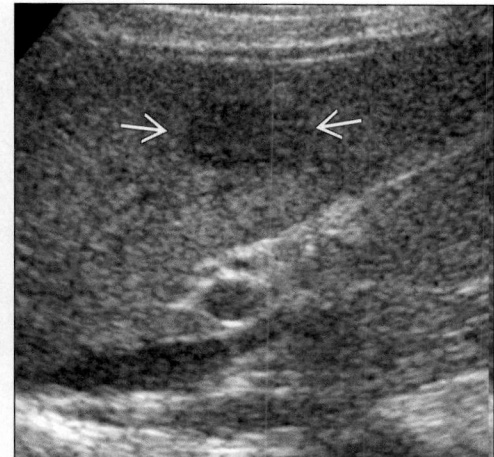

(Left) Oblique transabdominal ultrasound shows a large hyperechoic adenoma ⮕ containing a hypoechoic focus ⮕, which may represent hemorrhage or necrosis. (Right) Oblique transabdominal ultrasound shows a hypoechoic adenoma ⮕. This appearance is nonspecific and carries a long differential diagnosis (hemangioma, metastasis, HCC, etc.)

Typical

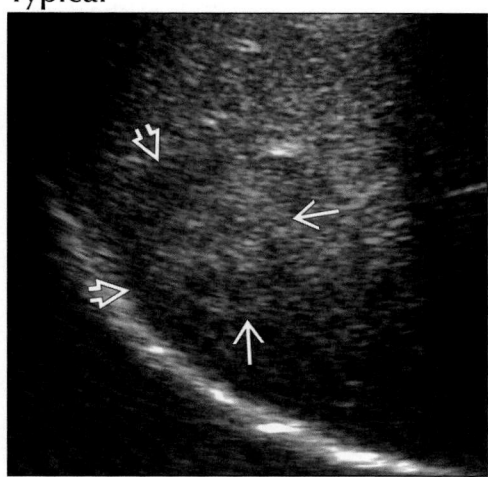
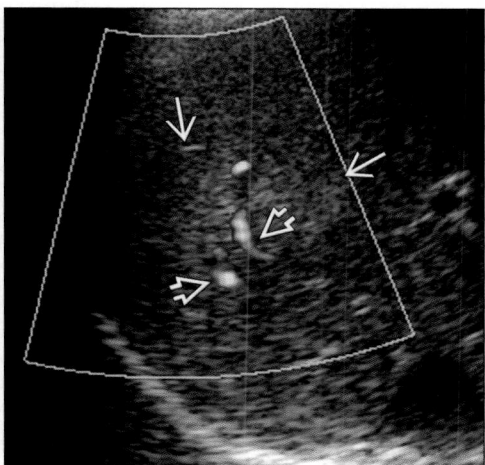

(Left) Oblique transabdominal ultrasound shows a heterogeneous iso-echoic adenoma ⮕ adjacent to diaphragm. Note incomplete hypoechoic halo ⮕ which represents the surrounding compressed liver. (Right) Oblique power Doppler ultrasound shows flow in intratumoral veins ⮕ of the adenoma ⮕. Power Doppler is useful for demonstrating slow flow.

Typical

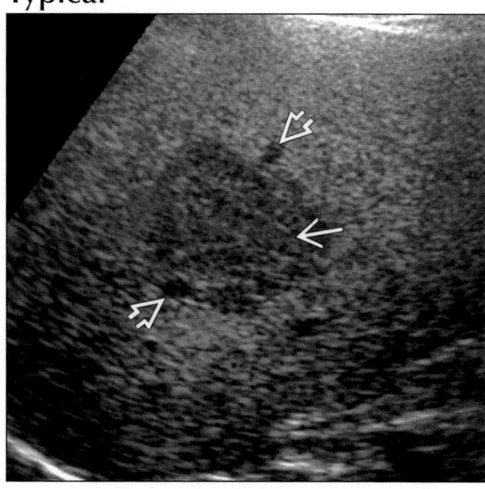
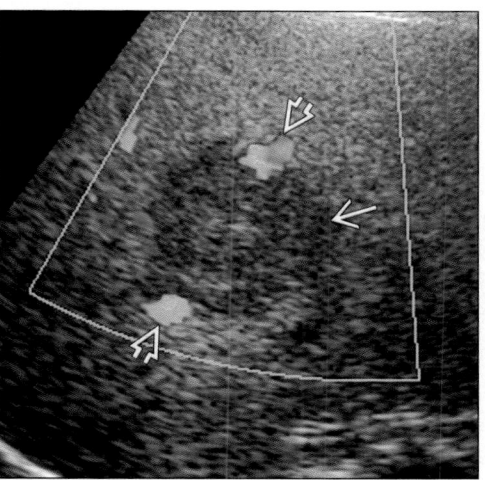

(Left) Oblique transabdominal ultrasound shows large vessels ⮕ at the periphery of a hypoechoic hepatic adenoma ⮕. (Right) Oblique color Doppler ultrasound confirms flow in these large peripheral vessels ⮕ surrounding the hepatic adenoma ⮕.

FOCAL NODULAR HYPERPLASIA

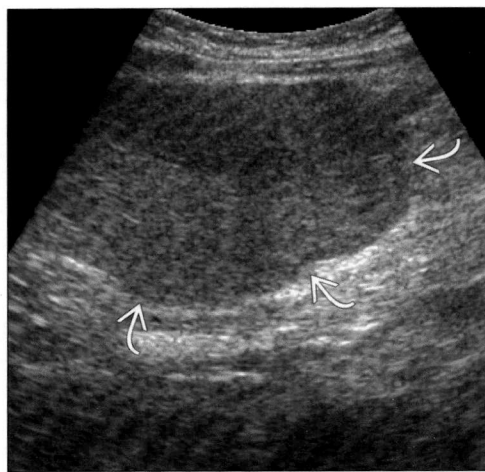

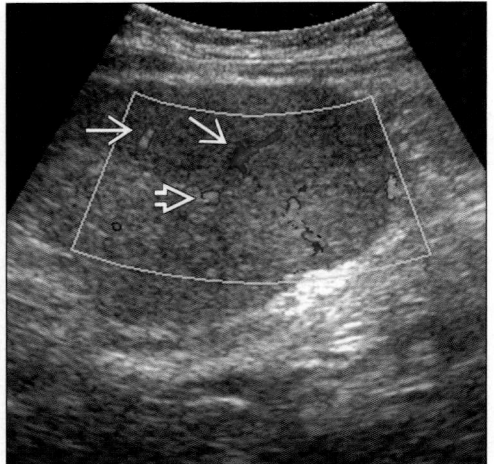

Transverse ultrasound shows the lateral segment of the left lobe of the liver with bulging surface contours ➤. The lesion is isoechoic to liver parenchyma making it difficult to detect.

Transverse color Doppler ultrasound shows centrifugal blood flow away ➡ from center ⬌ of the lesion. This may sometimes give a "spoke-wheel" pattern. Note the lesion itself is subtle.

TERMINOLOGY

Abbreviations and Synonyms
- Focal nodular hyperplasia (FNH)

Definitions
- Benign tumor of liver caused by hyperplastic response to a localized vascular abnormality

IMAGING FINDINGS

General Features
- Best diagnostic clue: Homogeneously isoechoic mass with central scar
- Location
  - More common in right lobe
  - Right lobe to left lobe: 2:1
  - Usually subcapsular & rarely pedunculated
- Size
  - Majority are smaller than 5 cm (85%)
  - Mean diameter at time of diagnosis is 3 cm
- Key concepts

- 2nd most common benign tumor of liver after hemangioma
- Benign congenital hamartomatous malformation
- Accounts for 8% of primary hepatic tumors in autopsy series
- Usually a solitary lesion (80%); multiple in 20%
- Multiple FNHs associated with multiorgan vascular malformations and with certain brain neoplasms

Ultrasonographic Findings
- Grayscale Ultrasound
  - Histologically FNH is sometimes referred to as circumscribed cirrhosis
    - Sonographically it may simulate normal liver making detection difficult if there is no significant mass effect or bulge in liver contour
    - Usually homogeneous and isoechoic, occasionally hypoechoic or hyperechoic
  - Mass effect: Displacement of normal hepatic vessels and ducts
  - Central scar: Seen in some lesions
    - Mostly hypoechoic but may be hyperechoic in 18%

DDx: Focal Nodular Hyperplasia

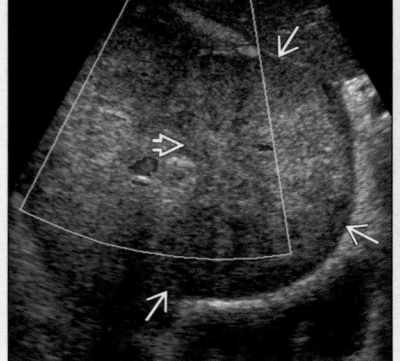

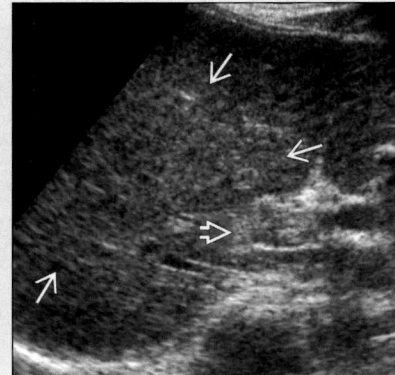

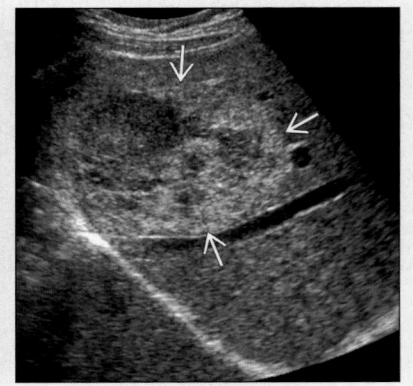

Fibrolamellar HCC

Infiltrative HCC

Hemangioma

FOCAL NODULAR HYPERPLASIA

Key Facts

Terminology
- Benign tumor of liver caused by hyperplastic response to a localized vascular abnormality

Imaging Findings
- Histologically FNH is sometimes referred to as circumscribed cirrhosis
- Sonographically it may simulate normal liver making detection difficult if there is no significant mass effect or bulge in liver contour
- Usually homogeneous and isoechoic, occasionally hypoechoic or hyperechoic
- Central scar: Seen in some lesions
- Central scar may contain calcification (of central feeding artery) but calcification of tumor parenchyma is rare

- Large central feeding artery with multiple small vessels radiating peripherally: "Spoke-wheel" pattern
- Large draining veins at tumor margins
- Highly vascular tumor but hemorrhage is rare

Top Differential Diagnoses
- Fibrolamellar Hepatocellular Carcinoma (HCC)
- Infiltrative HCC
- Cavernous Hemangioma

Diagnostic Checklist
- Radiologically FNH may mimic fibrolamellar HCC, which is usually a large lesion (> 12 cm), has evidence of calcification (in 68%) & metastases in 70% cases

---

- Central scar may contain calcification (of central feeding artery) but calcification of tumor parenchyma is rare
  - Prominent draining veins seen as hypoechoic nodules around the lesion
- Color Doppler
  - Large central feeding artery with multiple small vessels radiating peripherally: "Spoke-wheel" pattern
  - Large draining veins at tumor margins
  - Highly vascular tumor but hemorrhage is rare
  - High-velocity Doppler signals
    - Due to increased blood flow or arteriovenous shunts

CT Findings
- NECT: Isodense or hypodense to normal liver
- CECT
  - Hepatic arterial phase (HAP) scan
    - Transient intense hyperdensity
  - Portal venous phase (PVP) scan
    - Hypodense or isodense to normal liver
  - Delayed scans
    - Mass: Isodense to liver
    - Central scar: Hyperdense
    - Scar visible in 2/3rd of large & 1/3rd of small FNH

MR Findings
- T1WI
  - Mass: Isointense to slightly hypointense
  - Central scar: Hypointense
- T2WI
  - Mass: Slightly hyperintense to isointense
  - Central scar: Hyperintense
- T1 C+
  - Arterial phase: Hyperintense (homogeneous)
  - Portal venous: Isointense
  - Delayed phase: Isointense mass with hyperintense central scar
- Specific hepatobiliary MR contrast agents
  - T2WI with superparamagnetic iron oxide (SPIO)
    - FNH shows decreased signal due to uptake of iron oxide particles by Kupffer cells within lesion

- Degree of signal loss in FNH is greater than other focal liver lesions (metastases, adenoma & HCC)
  - Gadobenate dimeglumine (Gd-BOPTA)
    - Bright homogeneous enhancement of FNH
    - Prolonged enhancement of FNH on delayed scan (due to malformed bile ductules)
    - Delayed scan: Significant enhancement of scar

Nuclear Medicine Findings
- Technetium sulfur colloid
  - Normal or increased uptake
  - Only FNH has both Kupffer cells & bile ductules
  - Almost pathognomonic in 60% of cases
- Tc-HIDA scan (hepatic iminodiacetic acid)
  - Normal or increased uptake
  - Prolonged enhancement (80%)
- Tc-99m tagged red blood cell scan (not useful)
  - Early isotope uptake & late defect

Angiographic Findings
- Conventional
  - Arterial phase: Hypervascular mass with hypovascular central scar
    - Enlargement of main feeding artery with a centripetal blood supply
    - "Spoke-wheel" pattern" as on color Doppler
  - Venous phase: Large draining veins
  - Capillary phase: Intense & nonhomogeneous stain
    - No avascular zones

Imaging Recommendations
- Best imaging tool
  - Ultrasound for surveillance
  - CECT or contrast-enhanced MR for diagnosis

DIFFERENTIAL DIAGNOSIS

Fibrolamellar Hepatocellular Carcinoma (HCC)
- Large (more than 12 cm) heterogeneous mass
- Fibrous central scar

- Large & central or eccentric with fibrous bands & calcification (68%)
- Biliary, vascular & nodal invasion may be present
- Metastases (70% of cases)

Infiltrative HCC
- Mass within cirrhotic liver
- Necrosis & hemorrhage may be present
- Vascular invasion

Cavernous Hemangioma
- Isoechoic or heterogeneous lesions may simulate FNH
- No central scar

Hepatic Adenoma
- Usually heterogeneous echogenicity due to hemorrhage, necrosis or fat
- Symptomatic due to hemorrhage in 50%, scar atypical

Isoechoic Metastasis
- Multiple lesions, older patient, known primary tumor

PATHOLOGY

General Features
- Genetics
  - In genetic hemochromatosis patients, FNH cells were homozygous for Cys282Tyr mutation
  - Ki-67 antigen positive in 4% of FNH hepatocytes
- Etiology
  - Ischemia caused by an occult occlusion of intrahepatic vessels
  - Localized arteriovenous shunting caused by anomalous arterial supply
  - Hyperplastic response to abnormal vasculature
  - Oral contraceptives don't cause FNH, but have trophic effect on growth
- Epidemiology
  - 4% of all primary hepatic tumors in pediatric population
  - 3-8% in adult population
- Associated abnormalities
  - Hepatic hemangioma (in 23%)
  - Multiple lesions of FNH are associated with
    - Brain neoplasms: Meningioma, astrocytoma
    - Vascular malformations of various organs

Gross Pathologic & Surgical Features
- Localized, well-delineated, usually solitary (80%), subcapsular mass
- No true capsule, frequently central fibrous scar
- No intratumoral calcification, hemorrhage or necrosis
- Multiple masses (in 20%), rarely pedunculated
- Size: Less than 5 cm (in 85%)

Microscopic Features
- Normal hepatocytes with large amounts of fat, triglycerides & glycogen
- Thick-walled arteries in fibrous septa radiating from center to periphery
- Proliferation & malformation of bile ducts lead to slowing of bile excretion
- Absent portal triads & central veins

- Difficult differentiation from regenerative cirrhotic nodule & liver adenoma

CLINICAL ISSUES

Presentation
- Most common signs/symptoms
  - Often asymptomatic (in 50-90% incidental finding)
  - Vague abdominal pain (10-15%) due to mass effect
  - Other signs/symptoms
    - Hepatomegaly & abdominal mass (very rare)
  - Lab data: Usually normal liver function tests
  - Diagnosis
    - Suggestive imaging findings
    - Core needle biopsy (include central scar)

Demographics
- Age
  - Common in young to middle-aged women
  - Range: 7 months to 75 years
- Gender: M:F = 1:8

Natural History & Prognosis
- Excellent

Treatment
- Discontinuation of oral contraceptives
- FNH seldom requires surgery

DIAGNOSTIC CHECKLIST

Consider
- To rule out other benign & malignant liver lesions particularly fibrolamellar hepatocellular carcinoma

Image Interpretation Pearls
- On CECT immediate, intense, homogeneously enhancing lesion on arterial phase followed rapidly by isodensity on venous phase with delayed enhancement of scar
- Classic FNH looks like a cross-section of an orange (central "scar", radiating septa)
- Radiologically FNH may mimic fibrolamellar HCC, which is usually a large lesion (> 12 cm), has evidence of calcification (in 68%) & metastases in 70% cases
- Atypical FNH (telangiectatic FNH): Lack of central scar, heterogeneous lesion, hyperintense on T1WI, markedly hyperintense on T2WI & has persistent contrast-enhancement on delayed CECT & T1 C+
  - Probably can not make this diagnosis by imaging

SELECTED REFERENCES

1. Attal P et al: Telangiectatic focal nodular hyperplasia: US, CT, and MR imaging findings with histopathologic correlation in 13 cases. Radiology. 228(2):465-72, 2003
2. Vilgrain V et al: Prevalence of hepatic hemangioma in patients with focal nodular hyperplasia: MR imaging analysis. Radiology. 229(1):75-9, 2003
3. Brancatelli G et al: Focal nodular hyperplasia: CT findings with emphasis on multiphasic helical CT in 78 patients. Radiology. 219: 61-8, 2001

IMAGE GALLERY

Typical

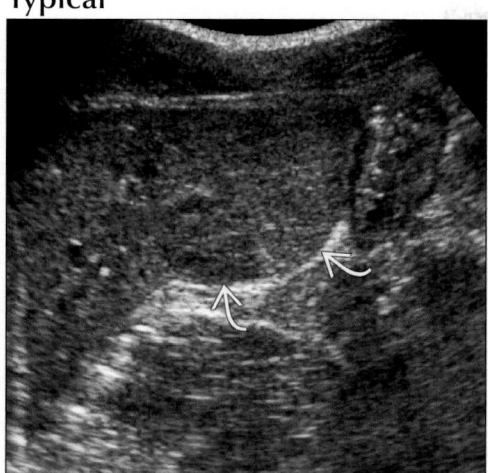

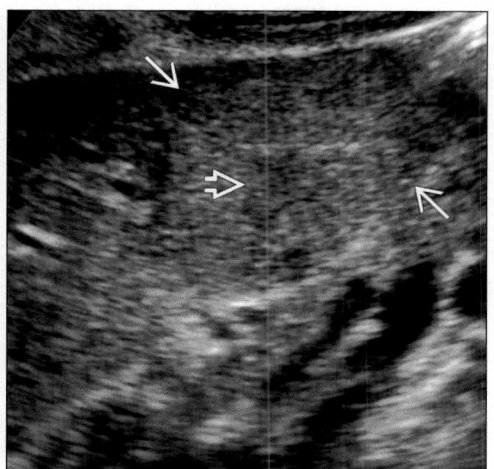

(Left) Transverse transabdominal ultrasound shows a well-defined mass causing contour deformity ➡. Without contour change the isoechoic lesion is not distinguishable from the surrounding liver. Doppler may show displaced vessels. *(Right)* Oblique transabdominal ultrasound shows a hypoechoic central scar ➡ in center of an isoechoic mass (FNH) ➡. The scar may show vascular calcification but the tumor itself rarely calcifies.

Typical

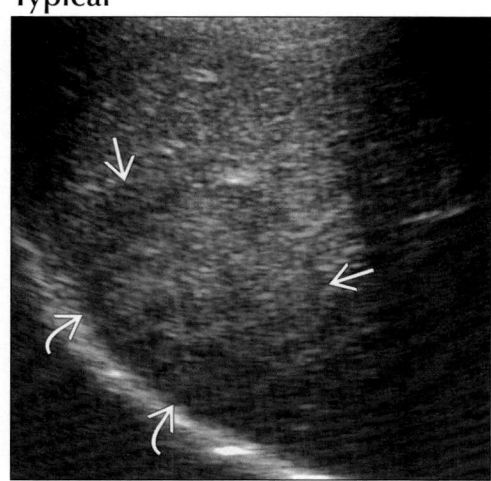

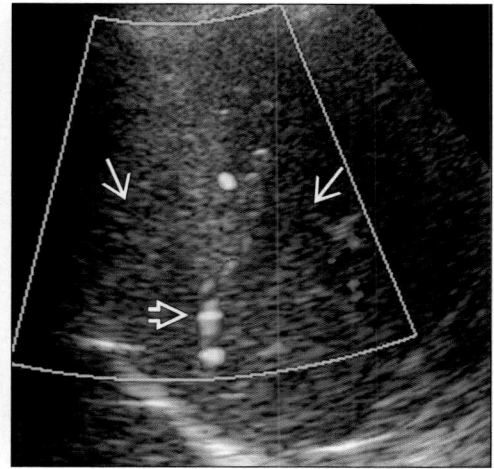

(Left) Transverse transabdominal ultrasound shows a mildly heterogeneous lesion ➡ with ill-defined borders, beneath the liver capsule ➡ without any contour change. Such isoechoic lesions may be missed. *(Right)* Oblique power Doppler ultrasound (same patient as in previous image) shows feeding vessel ➡ entering the center of the lesion ➡. The typical "spoke-wheel" pattern is not often seen.

Typical

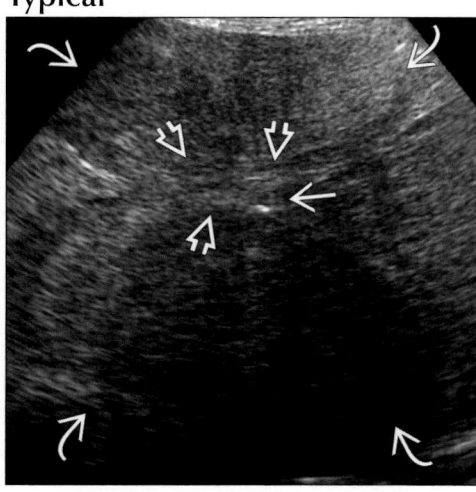

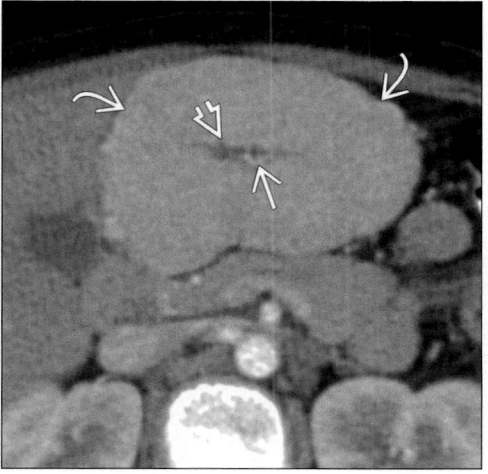

(Left) Transverse transabdominal ultrasound shows calcification ➡ within the central scar ➡ of an FNH ➡. Note there is no intratumoral parenchymal calcification, which is rarely seen in FNH. *(Right)* Transverse CECT shows the FNH ➡ (same patient as in previous image) enhancing homogeneously (arterial phase) except for a hypodense central scar ➡ with a feeding artery ➡ within (calcification not shown on this image).

HEPATOCELLULAR CARCINOMA

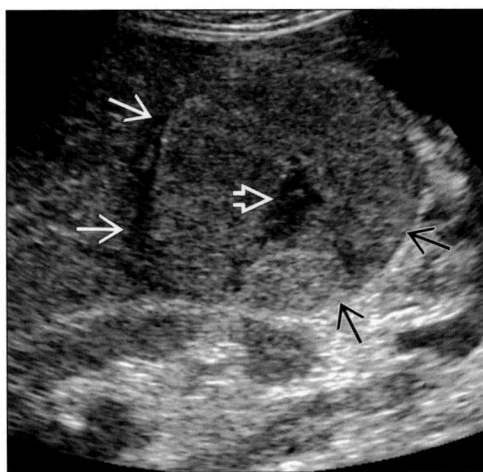

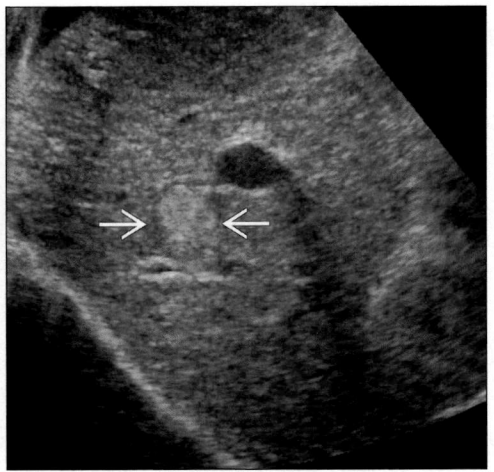

Transverse transabdominal ultrasound shows an isoechoic HCC with a thin medial hypoechoic halo ➡ and central necrosis ➤. Note the bulging contour ⇾ due to the mass.

Oblique transabdominal ultrasound shows a small slightly hyperechoic HCC ➡. This is difficult to distinguish this from other hyperechoic lesions such as a hemangioma.

TERMINOLOGY

Abbreviations and Synonyms
- Hepatocellular carcinoma (HCC); hepatoma or primary liver cancer

Definitions
- Malignant neoplasm originating from hepatocytes

IMAGING FINDINGS

General Features
- Best diagnostic clue: Large heterogeneous mass with vascular invasion (portal or hepatic vein)
- Location
  - More commonly right lobe of liver (solitary)
  - Both hepatic lobes (multicentric small nodules)
  - Throughout liver in a diffuse manner (diffuse small foci)
- Size
  - Small tumors: Less than 3 cm
  - Large tumors: More than 5 cm
  - Diffuse or cirrhotomimetic: Subcentimeter to several cms
- Key concepts
  - Most frequent primary visceral malignancy in world
    - Accounts for 80-90% of all adult primary liver malignancies
    - Usually arising in cirrhotic liver, due to chronic viral hepatitis (HBV, HCV) or alcoholism
  - 2nd most common malignant liver tumor in children after hepatoblastoma
  - Growth patterns of HCC: Three major types
    - Solitary, often large mass
    - Multinodular or multifocal
    - Diffuse or cirrhotomimetic
    - Metastases to lung, adrenal
    - Lymph nodes & bone

Ultrasonographic Findings
- Grayscale Ultrasound
  - **Hypoechoic**: Most common appearance, especially for small HCC
    - Indicates a solid tumor
    - May be surrounded by a thin hypoechoic halo (capsule)

DDx: Hepatocellular Carcinoma

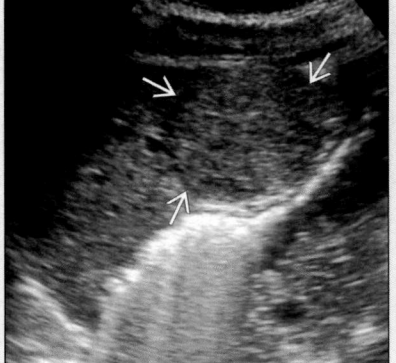

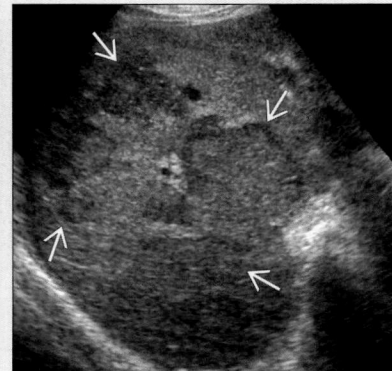

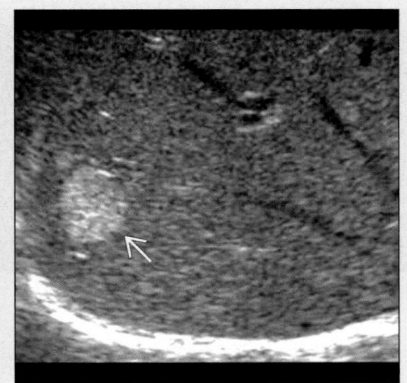

Focal Nodular Hyperplasia

Cirrhosis + Mets

Hemangioma

HEPATOCELLULAR CARCINOMA

Key Facts

Imaging Findings
- Best diagnostic clue: Large heterogeneous mass with vascular invasion (portal or hepatic vein)
- More commonly right lobe of liver (solitary)
- **Hypoechoic**: Most common appearance, especially for small HCC
- Indicates a solid tumor
- **Hyperechoic**: Sometimes in small HCC
- Indicates fatty metamorphosis/hypervascularity
- **Mixed echogenicity**: More common in larger HCC
- Indicates tumor necrosis/fibrosis
- Invasion of portal vein & less commonly hepatic vein may occur

Top Differential Diagnoses
- Focal Nodular Hyperplasia (FNH)
- Metastases

- Hepatic Hemangioma
- Cholangiocarcinoma

Pathology
- Cirrhosis (60-90%): Due to chronic viral hepatitis (HBV, HCV) or alcoholism
- High incidence: Africa & Asia; low in Western hemisphere

Clinical Issues
- Clinical Profile: Elderly patient with history of cirrhosis, ascites, weight loss, right upper quadrant pain & ↑ alpha-fetoprotein (AFP)

Diagnostic Checklist
- Any mass detected in a cirrhotic liver is regarded as HCC until proven otherwise
- HCC: Hypervascular mass invading portal vein

- **Hyperechoic**: Sometimes in small HCC
  - Indicates fatty metamorphosis/hypervascularity
  - Simulates hemangioma/focal steatosis
- **Mixed echogenicity**: More common in larger HCC
  - Indicates tumor necrosis/fibrosis
- Background cirrhosis (except for fibrolamellar HCC)
- Focal fat may be found within some large HCCs
- Calcification is rare unless treated
- Invasion of portal vein & less commonly hepatic vein may occur
- Hilar lymphadenopathy (rare)
- Hemoperitoneum if subcapsular HCC ruptures
- Associated signs of portal hypertension: Ascites, splenomegaly, portosystemic collaterals
- Fibrolamellar HCC
  - Well-defined partially/completely encapsulated mass
  - Prominent central fibrous scar
  - Calcification within scar
  - Intralesional necrosis/hemorrhage
  - Regional adenopathy and metastases to lung and peritoneum
  - Evidence of background cirrhosis or hepatitis in < 5% of patients
  - AFP usually negative or mildly elevated
- Pulsed Doppler
  - High velocity (arterial type) flow & low resistance (tumor vessels)
  - Tumor thrombus neo-vascularity show arterial flow
- Color Doppler
  - Shows irregular hypervascularity within neoplasm
  - Tumor thrombus (portal vein) shows hypervascularity

CT Findings
- NECT
  - In noncirrhotic liver
    - Solitary HCC: Large hypodense mass; ± necrosis, fat, calcification
    - Multifocal HCC: Multiple hypodense lesions rarely with a central necrotic portion
    - Dominant hypodense mass with decreased attenuation satellite nodules

- Encapsulated HCC: Well-defined, rounded, hypodense mass
  - In cirrhotic liver
    - Iso-/hypodense mass
    - Cirrhotic liver, ascites and portal hypertension
- CECT
  - Hepatic arterial phase
    - Heterogeneous enhancement
    - THAD (transient hepatic attenuation differences): Wedge-shaped areas of increased density due to perfusion abnormality from portal vein tumor thrombus occlusion and increased arterial flow
  - Portal venous phase: Decreased attenuation with heterogeneous enhancement
  - Delayed scan: Hypodense to surrounding liver
  - Small hypervascular HCC
    - Early and late arterial phases: Hyperattenuating, more on late phase
    - CT hepatic arteriography: Lesions show intense enhancement
    - CT during arterial portography: No enhancement

MR Findings
- Variable intensity depending on degree of fatty change, fibrosis, necrosis
- T1WI
  - Non-cirrhotic liver
    - hypo-/iso-/hyperintense
  - Cirrhotic liver
    - HCC: Hypointense
    - Cirrhotic nodules: Increased signal intensity
- T2WI
  - Noncirrhotic liver: Slightly hyperintense
  - Cirrhotic liver: Hyperintense HCC
    - Cirrhotic nodules: Iso to hypointense
  - HCC arising within a siderotic nodule
    - "Nodule within a nodule" pattern
    - HCC appears as a small focus of increased signal intensity within decreased signal intensity nodule
- T1 C+ (gadolinium)
  - Large HCC in noncirrhotic liver: Nonspecific
    - Central or peripheral enhancement
    - Homogeneous or rim-enhancement

HEPATOCELLULAR CARCINOMA

○ HCC nodules (hypervascular)
  ▪ Arterial phase: Hyperintense

Nuclear Medicine Findings
- Hepatobiliary scan: Uptake in 50%
- Technetium sulfur colloid
  ○ HCC in a cirrhotic liver: Seen as a defect
  ○ HCC in a noncirrhotic liver: Heterogeneous uptake
- Gallium scan: Gallium-avid in 90% of cases

Angiographic Findings
- Conventional
  ○ Hypervascular tumor
    ▪ Marked neovascularity and AV shunting
    ▪ Large hepatic artery and vascular invasion
  ○ "Threads and streaks" sign: Portal vein tumor thrombus

Imaging Recommendations
- Best imaging tool: Ultrasound for serial screening of high risk patients (chronic hepatitis)
- Helical triphasic CT (NE, arterial & venous phases) or MR & CEMR; angiography

DIFFERENTIAL DIAGNOSIS

Focal Nodular Hyperplasia (FNH)
- Homogeneous hypo/iso/hyperechoic mass with central scar
- On nonenhanced & delayed CECT & CEMR almost isodense/isointense to liver

Metastases
- Mimic nodular or multifocal HCC
- Less likely to invade portal vein
- Lower incidence in cirrhotic livers

Hepatic Hemangioma
- Well-defined, spherical nodule
- Typically hyperechoic

Cholangiocarcinoma
- Peripheral tumor often obstructs bile ducts leading to ductal dilatation
- Capsular retraction; volume loss
- Less likely to invade portal vein

PATHOLOGY

General Features
- General path comments
  ○ Invasion: Vascular (common) & biliary (uncommon)
  ○ Fibrolamellar HCC: Young patients without underlying liver disease (cirrhosis or hepatitis)
- Genetics: HBV DNA integrated into host's genomic DNA in tumor cells
- Etiology
  ○ Cirrhosis (60-90%): Due to chronic viral hepatitis (HBV, HCV) or alcoholism
  ○ Carcinogens: Aflatoxins, siderosis, thorotrast, androgens
  ○ α-1-antitrypsin deficiency, hemochromatosis, Wilson

- Epidemiology
  ○ High incidence: Africa & Asia; low in Western hemisphere
  ○ Worldwide highest incidence is in Japan (4.8%)
  ○ HCC in cirrhosis due to hepatitis C virus
    ▪ 30-50% of HCC in US; 70% in Japan
  ○ North America: 40% of HCC in non-cirrhotic livers

Gross Pathologic & Surgical Features
- Soft tumor with or without necrosis, hemorrhage, calcification, fat, vascular invasion

Microscopic Features
- Solid (cellular) or acinar with increased cytoplasmic fat & glycogen

CLINICAL ISSUES

Presentation
- Clinical Profile: Elderly patient with history of cirrhosis, ascites, weight loss, right upper quadrant pain & ↑ alpha-fetoprotein (AFP)
- Lab data: Increased AFP and liver function tests
- Diagnosis: Biopsy and histology

Demographics
- Age
  ○ Low incidence areas: 6th-7th decade
  ○ High incidence areas: 30-45 years
- Gender
  ○ Low incidence areas (M:F = 2.5:1)
  ○ High incidence areas (M:F = 8:1)

Natural History & Prognosis
- Complications: Spontaneous rupture & hemoperitoneum
- 30% 5 year survival

Treatment
- Surgical resection limited by inadequate hepatic reserve
- Radiofrequency/alcohol ablation for small isolated tumors
- Intraarterial chemoembolization for multifocal unresectable tumor

DIAGNOSTIC CHECKLIST

Image Interpretation Pearls
- Any mass detected in a cirrhotic liver is regarded as HCC until proven otherwise
- HCC: Hypervascular mass invading portal vein

SELECTED REFERENCES

1. Rapaccini GL et al: Hepatocellular carcinomas <2 cm in diameter complicating cirrhosis: ultrasound and clinical features in 153 consecutive patients. Liver Int. 24(2):124-30, 2004
2. Yu SC et al: Imaging features of hepatocellular carcinoma. Clin Radiol. 59(2):145-56, 2004
3. Nisenbaum HL et al: Ultrasound of focal hepatic lesions. Semin Roentgenol. 30(4):324-46, 1995

IMAGE GALLERY

Typical

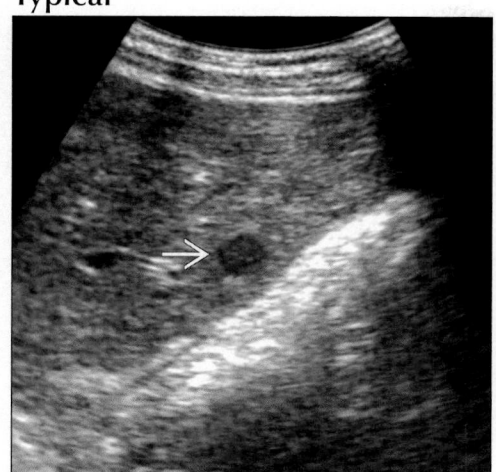 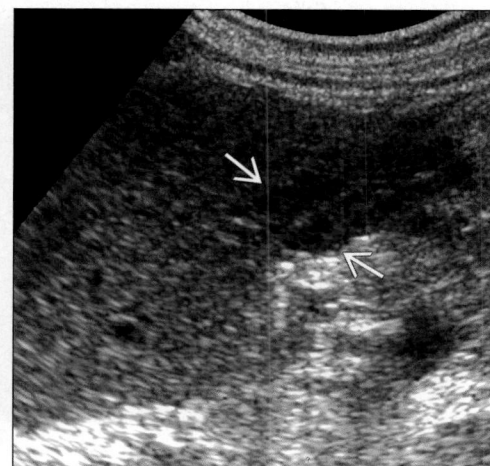

(Left) Oblique transabdominal ultrasound shows a hypoechoic nodule ➡ in a patient with raised AFP, which was found to be HCC on biopsy. (Right) Transverse transabdominal ultrasound shows a small slightly hypoechoic nodule ➡ which was confirmed to be HCC on biopsy.

Typical

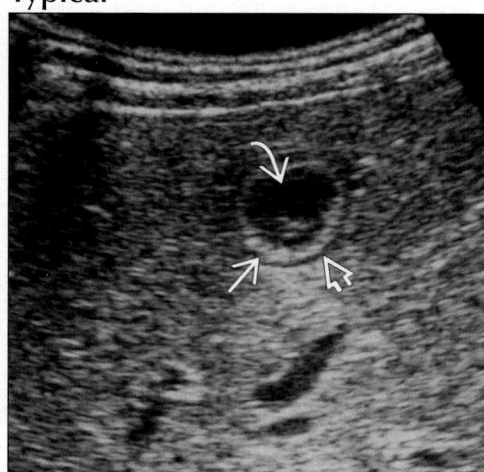 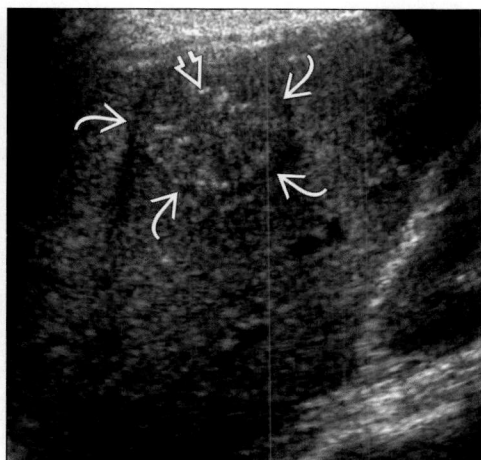

(Left) Transverse transabdominal ultrasound shows a small echogenic HCC ➡ with a necrotic hypoechoic center ➡ and thin hypoechoic halo ➡. (Right) Longitudinal transabdominal ultrasound shows a small isoechoic HCC with hypoechoic halo ➡ and internal calcification ➡.

Typical

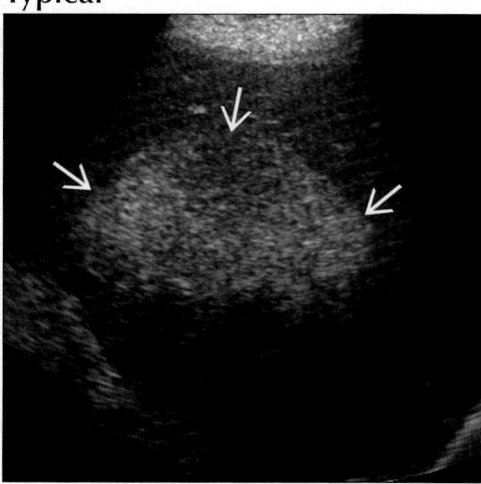 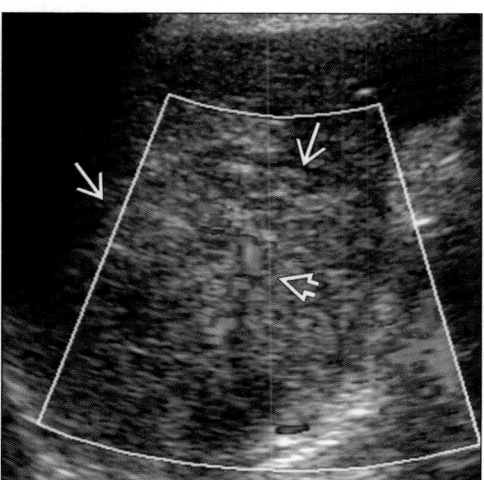

(Left) Oblique transabdominal ultrasound shows a hyperechoic HCC with well-defined borders ➡. (Right) Oblique color Doppler ultrasound shows internal vascularity ➡ in an isoechoic HCC with a thin halo ➡.

(Left) Oblique transabdominal ultrasound shows a large fibrolamellar HCC with a bulging surface contour ⇨ and a slightly echogenic central scar ⇨. *(Right)* Transverse transabdominal ultrasound shows a large infiltrative HCC with lobulated borders ➡. A portal vein branch is displaced ⇨ in a wide arc by the lesion's posterior border.

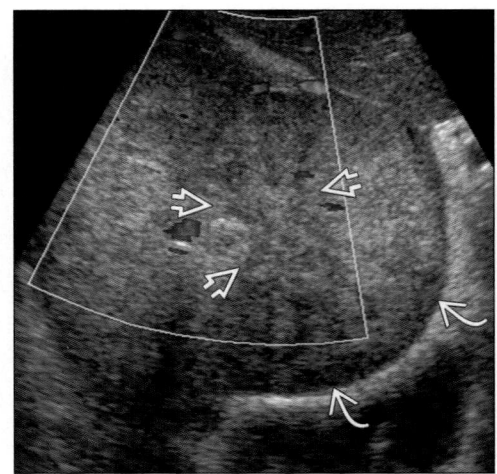
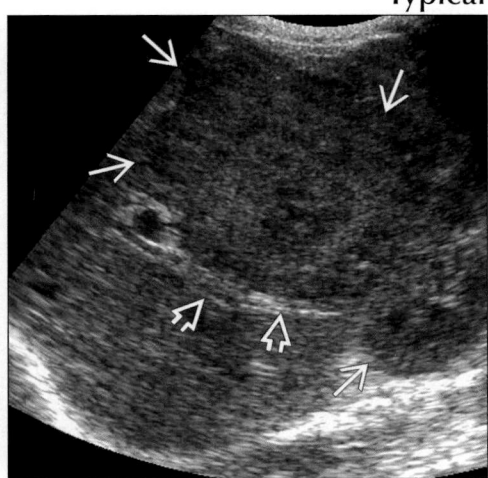

(Left) Transverse transabdominal ultrasound shows a small, mildly hyperechoic HCC ➡, with obliteration of the hepatic vein lumen ⇨. *(Right)* Transverse power Doppler ultrasound of the same mass ➡ as previous image with no color flow in the hepatic vein ⇨ due to compression/infiltration. Hepatic veins are less frequently involved than the portal vein.

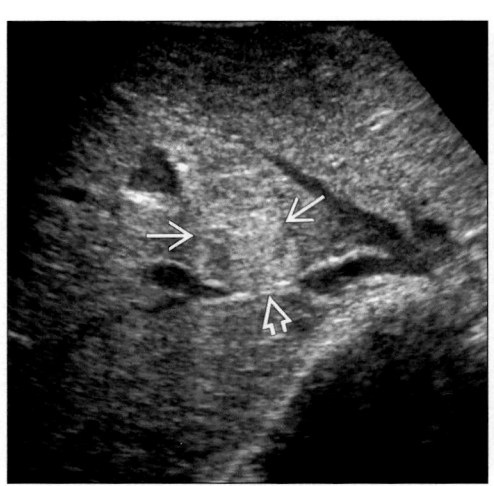
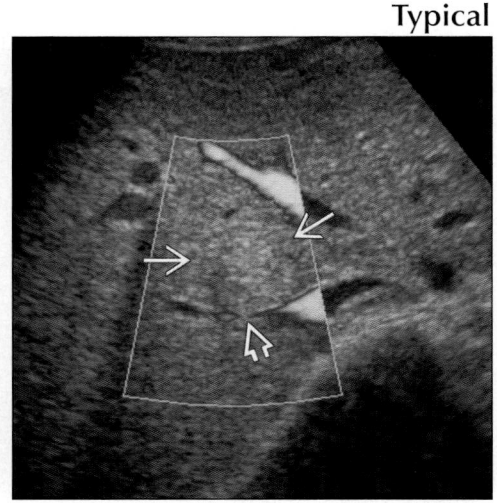

(Left) Transverse transabdominal ultrasound shows a multifocal HCC with small, echogenic ➡ and large, heterogeneous ⇨ masses. *(Right)* Transverse transabdominal ultrasound shows a large isoechoic HCC with bulging borders ⇨ and invasion ➡ into the right portal vein ➡.

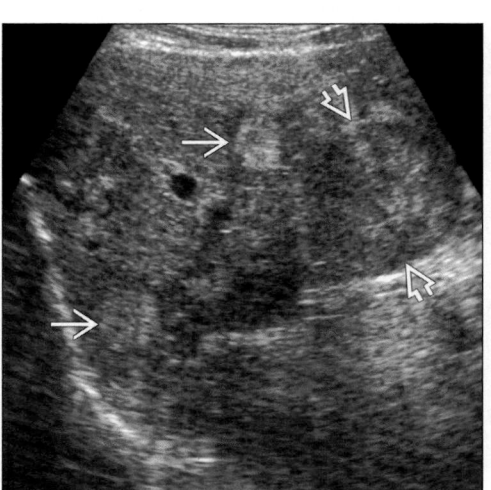
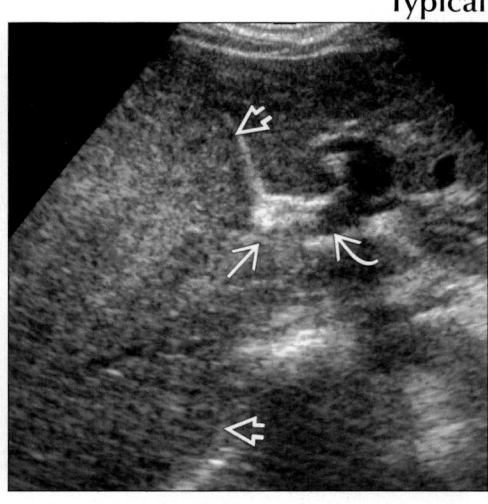

Typical

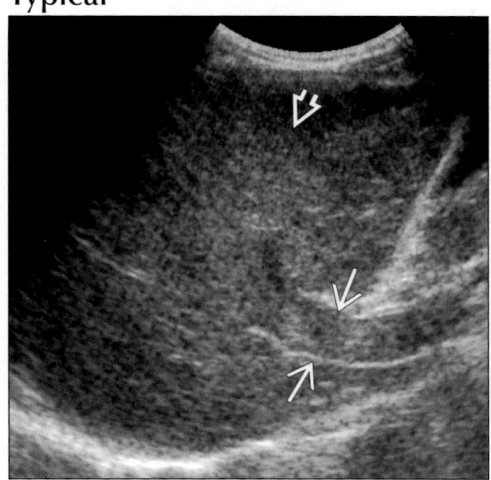 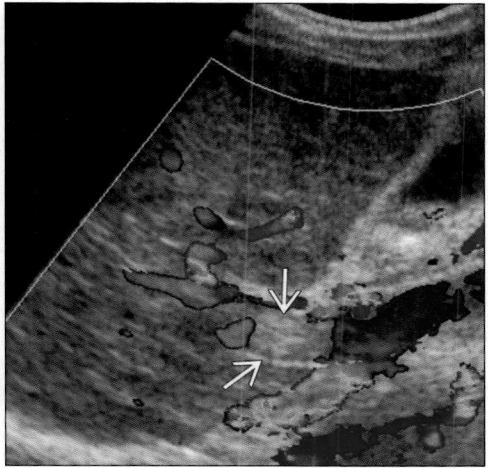

(Left) Oblique transabdominal ultrasound shows an isoechoic HCC with invasion into the portal vein ➡. The HCC ➡ itself is difficult to discern from the cirrhotic liver. *(Right)* Longitudinal color Doppler ultrasound (same patient in the previous image) shows lack of color flow within the portal vein thrombus ➡.

Typical

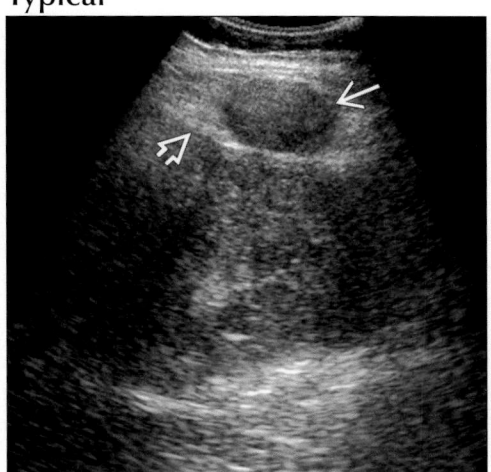 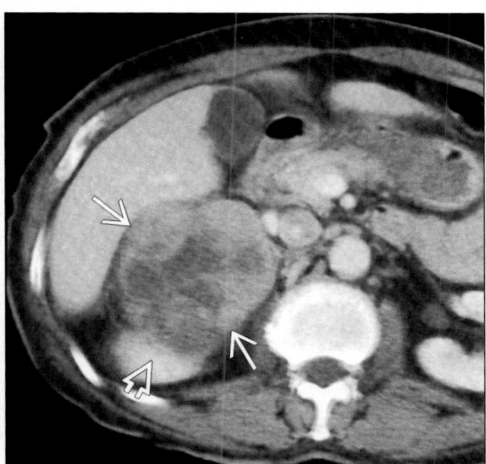

(Left) Longitudinal transabdominal ultrasound shows an intraperitoneal metastasis ➡ from HCC on the surface ➡ of the right lobe. *(Right)* Transverse CECT shows an intraperitoneal metastasis ➡ on Gerota fascia anterior to the upper pole of the right kidney ➡.

Typical

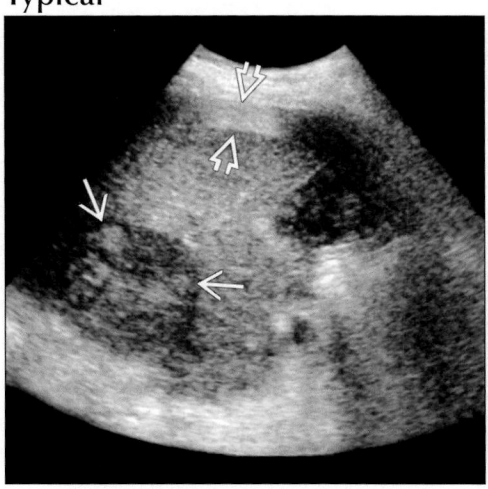 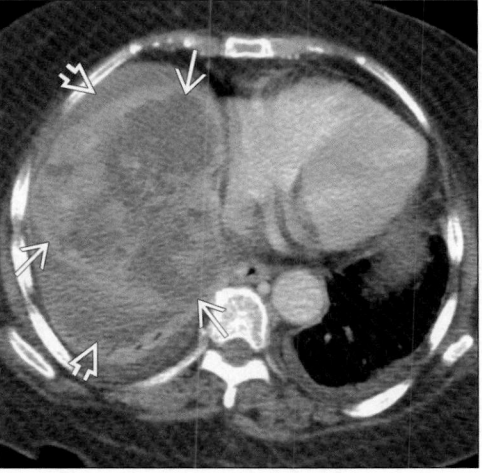

(Left) Oblique transabdominal ultrasound (intercostal window) shows a hyperechoic layer of blood ➡ on the lateral surface of the liver, which contains an HCC ➡. *(Right)* Transverse CECT (same patient as previous image) shows a higher more superficial aspect of the HCC ➡, with dense blood ➡ outside the capsule. This is probably the tumor rupture site.

HEPATIC CAVERNOUS HEMANGIOMA

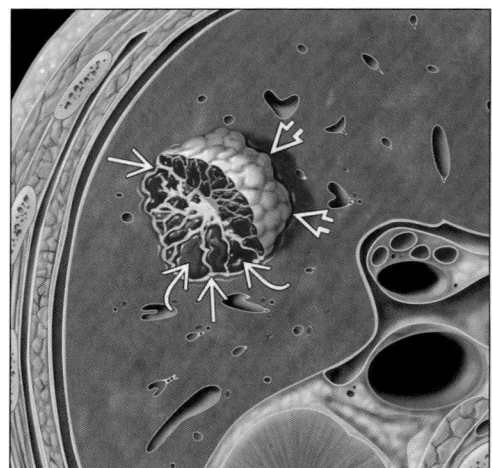

Transverse graphic shows a solitary hemangioma, illustrating the lobular contour ➡, multiple internal fibrous septae ➡ separating vascular channels ➡.

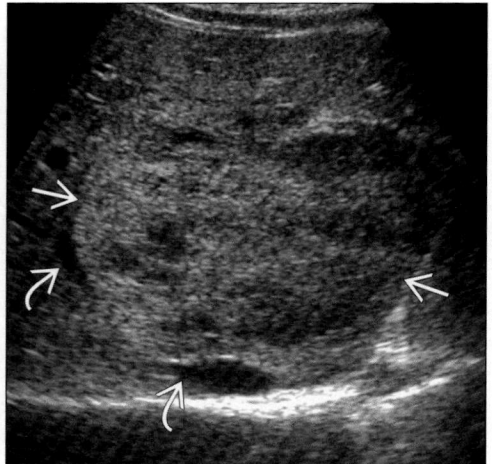

Transverse transabdominal ultrasound shows a hemangioma ➡ with geographic borders, partly indistinguishable from surrounding parenchyma. Adjacent vessels are displaced ➡.

TERMINOLOGY

Abbreviations and Synonyms
- Cavernous hemangioma of liver; capillary hemangioma (small lesion)

Definitions
- Benign tumor composed of multiple vascular channels lined by a single layer of endothelial cells supported by thin fibrous stroma

IMAGING FINDINGS

General Features
- Best diagnostic clue: Well-defined, uniformly hyperechoic mass
- Location: Common in subcapsular area in posterior right lobe of liver
- Size
  - Vary from few millimeters to more than 20 cm
  - Small (capillary) hemangioma: < 2 cm
  - Typical hemangioma: 2-10 cm
  - Giant hemangioma: > 10 cm (an arbitrary cutoff)

- Morphology
  - Most common benign tumor of liver
  - Second most common liver tumor after metastases
  - More commonly seen in postmenopausal women
  - Usually solitary & grow slowly
  - May be multiple in up to 10% of cases
  - Calcification is rare (less than 10%)
    - Usually in scar of giant hemangioma

Ultrasonographic Findings
- Grayscale Ultrasound
  - Variable echogenicity and appearance
  - Echogenicity depends on plane of scanning, direction & angle of insonation
  - Always found next to a vessel which it displaces but does not infiltrate
  - Blood supply is from the hepatic artery
  - Hyperechoic mass (in over two-thirds of patients)
    - Probably due to slow blood flow rather than multiple interfaces
    - Echogenicity may change with the time of scanning e.g., with exercise
    - Occasionally see hypoechoic center with hyperechoic rim

DDx: Hepatic Hemangioma

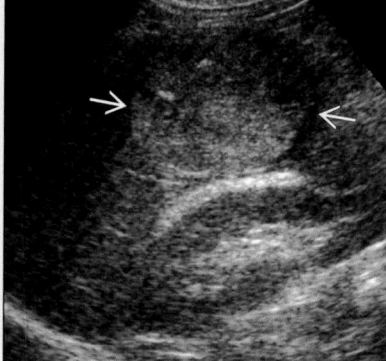

Hepatocellular Carcinoma

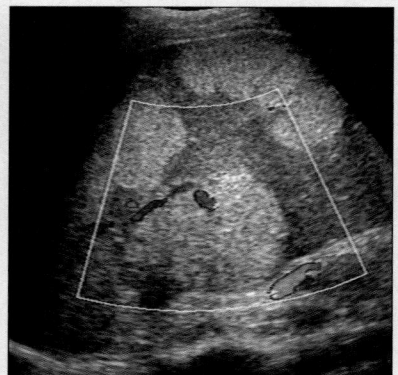

Metastases

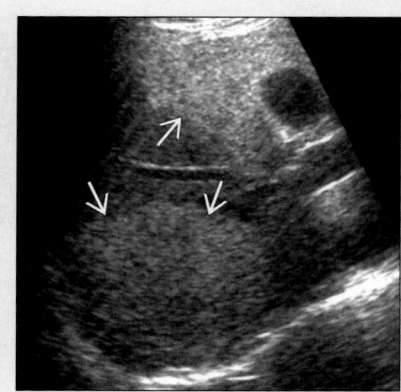

Focal Steatosis

Key Facts

Imaging Findings
- Best diagnostic clue: Multiple lesions randomly distributed throughout the liver
- Most common malignant tumor of liver
- Liver is second only to regional lymph nodes as a site of metastatic disease
- Round or oval, with smooth or irregular borders
- Causes architectural distortion if large or numerous
- No portal vein invasion
- Most metastases are hypovascular, except those from neuroendocrine tumors
- Contrast-enhanced US increases detectability of hepatic metastases

Top Differential Diagnoses
- Cysts (vs. Hypoechoic Metastases)
- Abscesses (vs. Hypoechoic Metastases)

- Hemangiomas (vs. Hyperechoic Metastases)
- Hepatocellular Carcinoma (vs. Target Lesion)
- Steatosis (vs. Hypo or Hyperechoic Metastasis)

Clinical Issues
- Asymptomatic, RUQ pain, tender hepatomegaly
- Weight loss, jaundice or ascites
- Lab data: Elevated LFTs; normal in 25-50% of patients

Diagnostic Checklist
- Rule out other multiple liver lesions like hepatic cysts, abscesses, hemangiomas which can mimic metastases
- Always correlated with clinical history and look for evidence of a primary tumor
- Target lesion suggests malignancy: Metastasis or HCC

- Mural nodules, thick walls, fluid-fluid levels, internal septae/debris distinguish them from simple cysts
- Necrotic center may be lined with irregular walls and contain debris
- Cystic primaries: Cystadenocarcinoma of pancreas/ovary; colon
- Necrosis/treated metastases: Sarcomas; squamous cell carcinoma
  - **Calcified metastases**
    - Markedly echogenic interface with acoustic shadowing or diffuse small echogenic foci
    - Mucinous primaries: Colon, ovary
    - Calcific/ossific primaries: Osteosarcoma, chondrosarcoma, neuroblastoma, malignant teratoma
    - Treated metastases
  - **Infiltrative/diffuse metastases**
    - Lung or breast primary
    - May simulate cirrhosis
- Color Doppler
  - Most metastases are hypovascular, except those from neuroendocrine tumors
  - Contrast-enhanced US increases detectability of hepatic metastases
    - Chaotic/bizarre vascularity in tumor bed

CT Findings
- NECT
  - May be normal
  - Isodense, hypodense or hyperdense
  - Calcified: Mucinous adenocarcinoma (colon), treated metastases (breast), malignant teratoma
  - Cystic metastases (less than 20 HU)
    - Fluid levels, debris, mural nodules
    - Thickened walls or septations may be seen
    - Usually cystadenocarcinoma or sarcoma (pancreatic, GI or ovarian primaries)
- CECT
  - Hypovascular metastases
    - Low attenuation center with peripheral rim-enhancement (e.g., epithelial metastases)

- Indicates vascularized viable tumor in periphery & hypovascular or necrotic center
- Rim-enhancement may also be due to compressed normal parenchyma
  - Hypervascular metastases
    - Hyperdense in late arterial phase images
    - May have internal necrosis without uniform hyperdense enhancement
    - Hypo- or isodense on NECT & portal venous phase images
    - Examples: Islet cell, carcinoid, thyroid, renal carcinomas & pheochromocytoma

MR Findings
- T1WI: Multiple low signal lesions
- T2WI
  - Moderate to high signal
  - "Light bulb" sign: Very high signal intensity (e.g., cystic & neuroendocrine metastases)
  - Mimic cysts or hemangiomas due to high signal "light bulb" appearance
- T1 C+
  - Hypovascular metastases
    - Similar with gadolinium-enhancement to CECT
    - Low signal in center and peripheral rim-enhancement
  - Hypervascular metastases
    - Hyperintense enhancement on arterial phase
- Superparamagnetic iron oxide (SPIO)
  - Metastases: Bright signal on T2WI
    - Free of reticuloendothelial system (RES)
  - Rest of normal liver: Decreased signal
    - Due to SPIO particles phagocytized by RES of liver

Nuclear Medicine Findings
- PET
  - Metastases
    - Multiple increased metabolic foci
    - Fluorodeoxyglucose (18-FDG) avid

Imaging Recommendations
- Best imaging tool: Ultrasound: Inexpensive, fast, radiation free, high sensitivity

HEPATIC METASTASES

- Protocol advice
  - Ultrasound for metastasis screening or surveillance
  - NE + CECT or MR + CEMR for equivocal cases or treatment planning

DIFFERENTIAL DIAGNOSIS

Cysts (vs. Hypoechoic Metastases)
- May have internal debris if bled or infected
- No mural nodule, thick wall, internal septae
- Posterior acoustic enhancement
- No rim or central vascularity/contrast-enhancement

Abscesses (vs. Hypoechoic Metastases)
- May be solid or cystic (internal debris/septae, thick irregular wall)
- Often with atelectasis & right pleural effusion
- Typical systemic signs of infection
- "Cluster sign" on CT for pyogenic abscesses

Hemangiomas (vs. Hyperechoic Metastases)
- Classically uniformly hyperechoic on US
- If in doubt, follow-up US in 3 months or CECT/MR
- Typical peripheral nodular discontinuous enhancement on CECT or CEMR
- Markedly hyperintense on T2WI

Hepatocellular Carcinoma (vs. Target Lesion)
- Cirrhotic liver, ascites, portal hypertension
- Portal vein invasion/thrombosis
- In cirrhotic livers, metastases from non-hepatic primaries are rare
  - Decreased portal blood flow
  - Decreased levels of lecithin receptors which are necessary to bind tumor cells to hepatocytes
- Thus any mass in a cirrhotic liver is highly suspicious for HCC rather than metastasis

Steatosis (vs. Hypo or Hyperechoic Metastasis)
- Focal fatty sparing: Hypoechoic area in hyperechoic liver
- Focal fatty infiltration: Hyperechoic area
- Segment 4 around the porta hepatis, subcapsular or gallbladder fossa
- Geometric borders
- No architectural distortion: Vessels course through undistorted, no mass effect
- Low density on CT
- Focal signal dropout on opposed-phase T1 GRE MR

PATHOLOGY

General Features
- Etiology
  - Hypovascular liver metastases
    - Lung, GI tract, pancreas & most breast cancers
    - Lymphoma, bladder & uterine malignancy
  - Hypervascular liver metastases
    - Endocrine tumors, renal & thyroid cancers
    - Some breast cancers, sarcomas & melanoma

Staging, Grading or Classification Criteria
- Liver metastases indicate stage IV tumor

CLINICAL ISSUES

Presentation
- Most common signs/symptoms
  - Asymptomatic, RUQ pain, tender hepatomegaly
  - Weight loss, jaundice or ascites
- Lab data: Elevated LFTs; normal in 25-50% of patients
- Diagnosis: Imaging, core or fine needle aspiration biopsy

Demographics
- Age: Usually middle & older age group
- Gender: Depends on underlying primary tumor

Natural History & Prognosis
- Depends on primary tumor site
- 20-40% have good 5 year survival rate if resectable
- In patients with metastatic colon cancer
  - 3 year survival rate
    - In 21% of patients with solitary lesions
    - In 6% with multiple lesions in one lobe
    - In 4% with widespread disease

Treatment
- Resection or ablation for colorectal liver metastases
- Chemoembolization: Carcinoid/endocrine metastases
- Chemotherapy for all others

DIAGNOSTIC CHECKLIST

Consider
- Rule out other multiple liver lesions like hepatic cysts, abscesses, hemangiomas which can mimic metastases
- Always correlated with clinical history and look for evidence of a primary tumor

Image Interpretation Pearls
- Target lesion suggests malignancy: Metastasis or HCC
- Epithelial metastases: Vascular wall/rim-enhancement

SELECTED REFERENCES

1. Helmberger T et al: new contrast agents for imaging the liver. Magn Reson Imaging Clin N Am. 9(4):745-66, 2001
2. Valls C et al: Hepatic metastases from colorectal cancer: preoperative detection and assessment of resectability with helical CT. Radiology. 218(1):55-60, 2001
3. Blake SP et al: Liver metastases from melanoma: detection with multiphasic contrast-enhanced CT. Radiology. 213(1):92-6, 1999
4. Nazarian LN et al: Size of colorectal liver metastases at abdominal CT: comparison of precontrast and postcontrast studies. Radiology. 213(3):825-30, 1999
5. Paulson EK et al: Carcinoid metastases to the liver: role of triple-phase helical CT. Radiology. 206(1):143-50, 1998
6. Wernecke K et al: The distinction between benign and malignant liver tumors on sonography: value of a hypoechoic halo. AJR Am J Roentgenol. 159(5):1005-9, 1992

IMAGE GALLERY

Typical

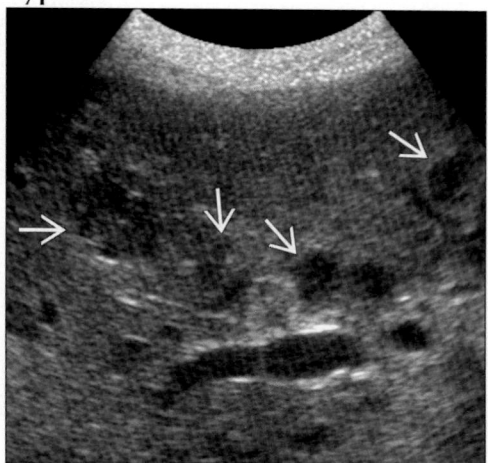
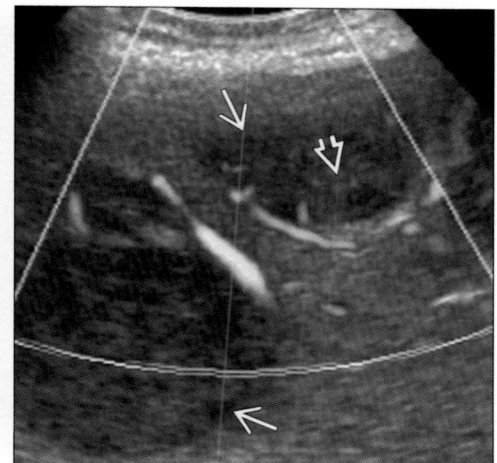

(Left) Transverse transabdominal ultrasound shows multiple hypoechoic metastases ➡ with irregular walls. There is no anechoic center or posterior acoustic enhancement (compared with cystic metastases). *(Right)* Oblique power Doppler ultrasound shows multiple hypoechoic metastases ➡. Faint vascularity ➡ is demonstrated within the more superficial lesion.

Typical

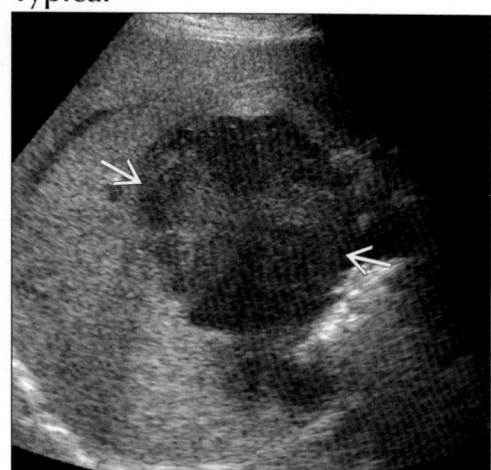
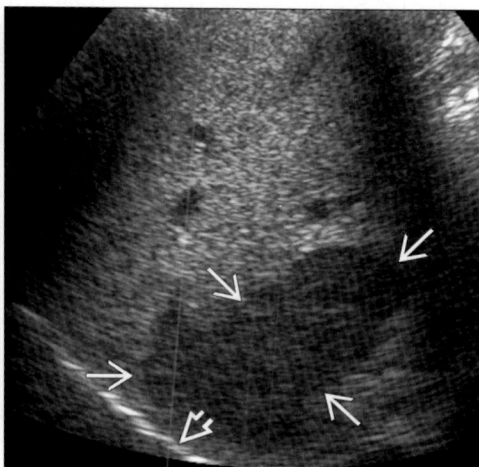

(Left) Longitudinal transabdominal ultrasound shows a hypoechoic metastasis ➡, which contains internal echoes. The margins are irregular. *(Right)* Oblique transabdominal ultrasound shows a hypoechoic metastasis with a smooth lobulated border ➡, just under the diaphragm ➡.

Typical

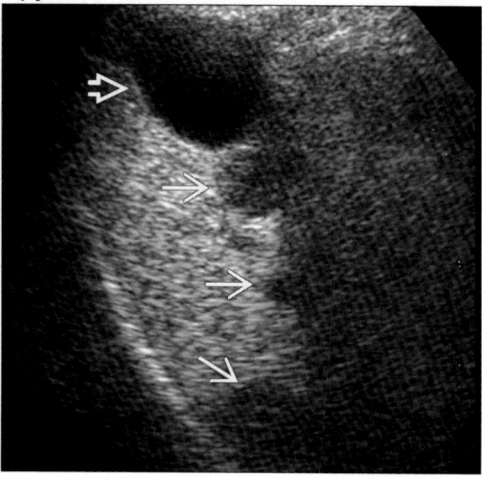
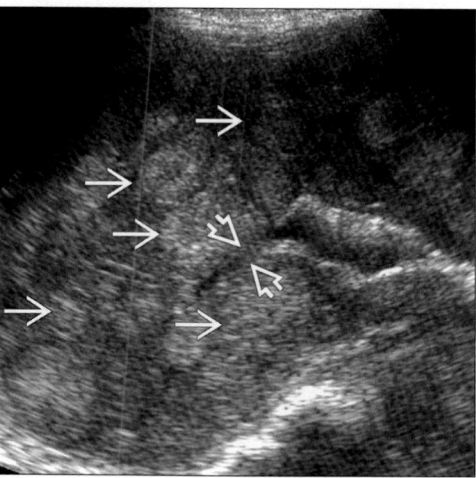

(Left) Oblique transabdominal ultrasound shows hypoechoic infiltrative metastases with a broad irregular border ➡ situated behind the gallbladder ➡. *(Right)* Transverse transabdominal ultrasound shows multiple hyperechoic metastases ➡. There is distortion and compression of the right portal vein ➡.

Typical

(Left) Transverse transabdominal ultrasound shows typical multiple target lesions in the liver representing metastases ➡ from lung carcinoma. The echogenic core may be irregular ➡. (Right) Oblique transabdominal ultrasound shows large target metastasis with a lobulated hypoechoic rim ➡.

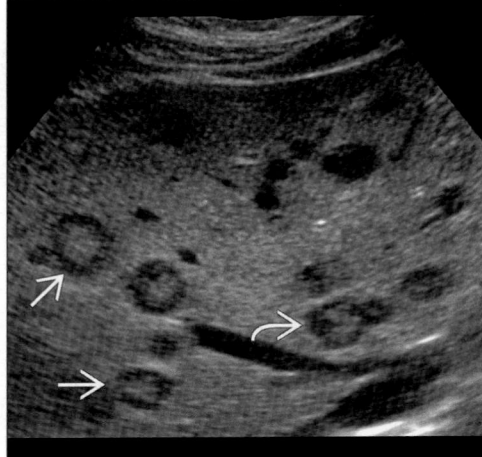
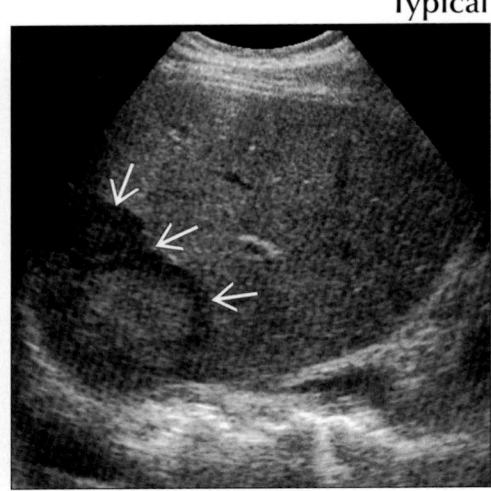

Typical

(Left) Longitudinal transabdominal ultrasound shows several hypoechoic metastases ➡. Mural irregularity ➡ is best demonstrated in the larger lesion, which also has posterior enhancement ➡. (Right) Oblique transabdominal ultrasound shows a thick walled, cystic metastasis ➡ with posterior acoustic enhancement ➡.

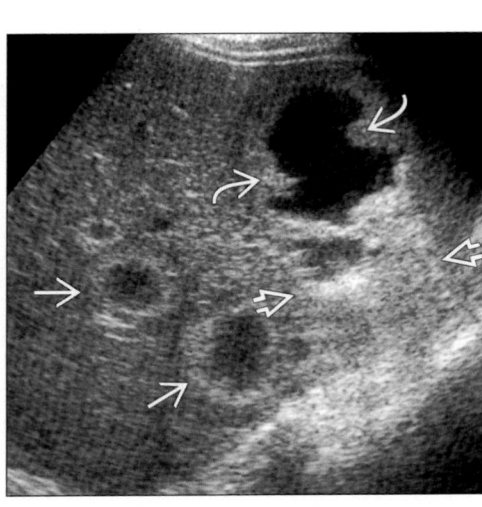
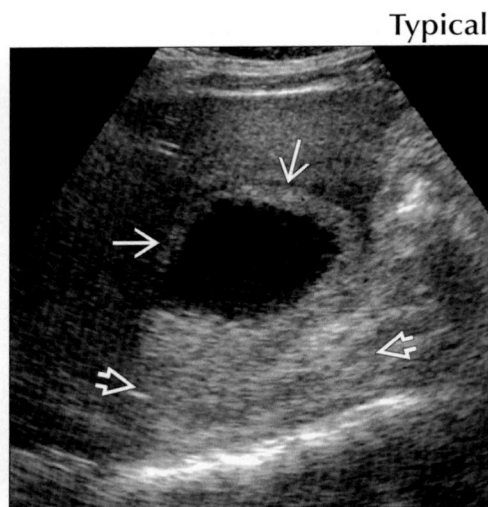

Typical

(Left) Oblique color Doppler ultrasound shows a subcapsular cystic lesion ➡ with a thick, vascular wall ➡. (Right) Longitudinal power Doppler ultrasound shows a vascular ➡ mural nodule ➡ in a cystic metastasis.

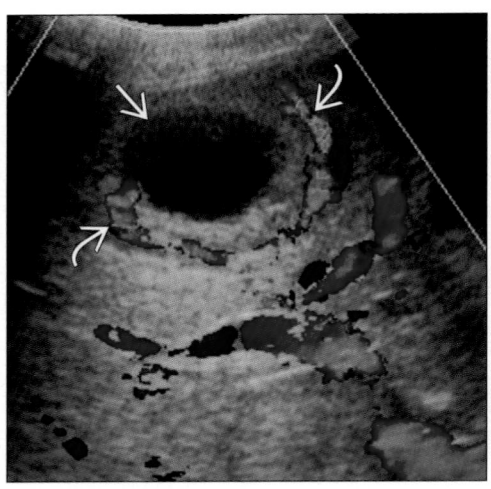
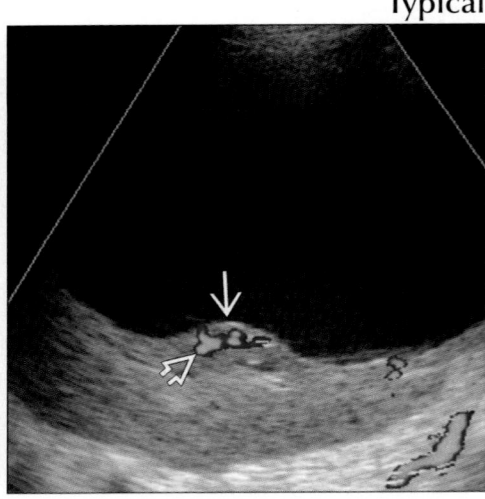

Typical

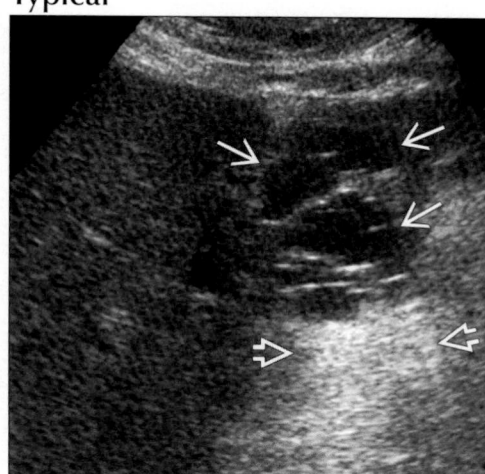

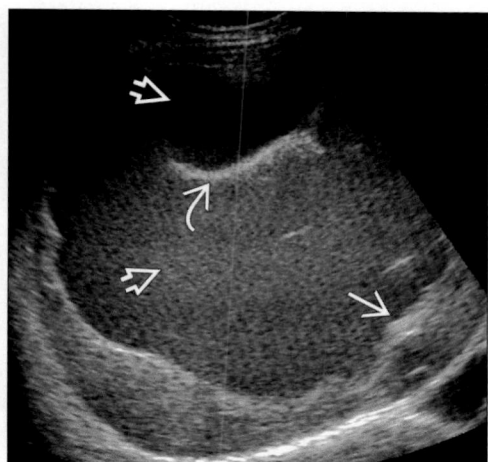

(Left) Transverse transabdominal ultrasound shows a cystic metastasis with multiple locules ➡ and posterior acoustic enhancement ➡ due to the lesion's fluid content. (Right) Transverse transabdominal ultrasound shows a large cystic metastasis with an internal septum ➡ separating two compartments ➡ with different content. Note the mural nodularity ➡.

Variant

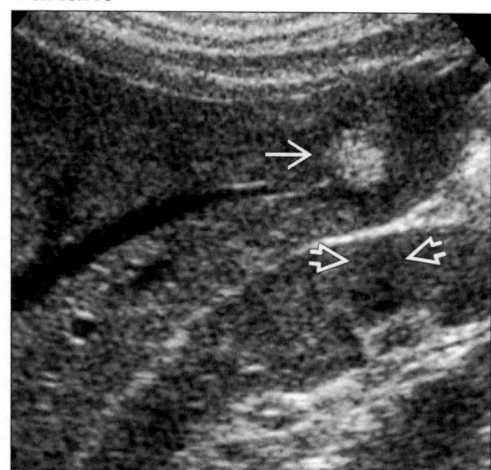

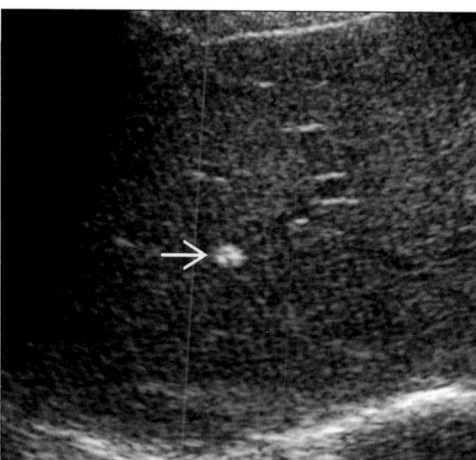

(Left) Oblique transabdominal ultrasound shows calcified metastasis ➡ with mild posterior acoustic shadowing ➡. (Right) Oblique transabdominal ultrasound shows a tiny calcified metastasis ➡ with no posterior shadowing due to its small size. This is difficult to differentiate from a calcified granuloma (needs clinical correlation).

Variant

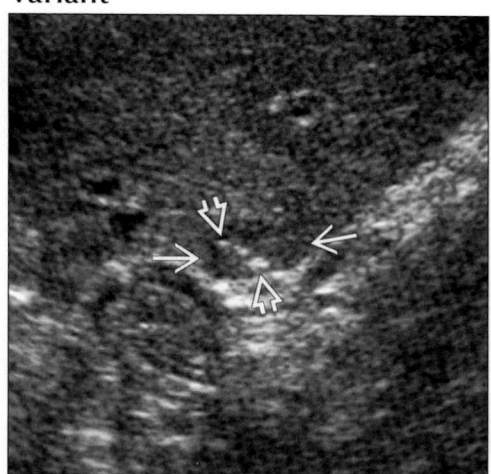

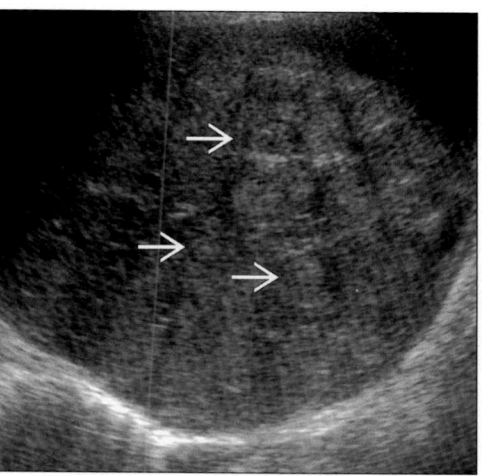

(Left) Oblique transabdominal ultrasound shows "target" metastasis ➡ containing specks of calcification ➡. (Right) Oblique transabdominal ultrasound shows multiple isoechoic metastases ➡, which are difficult to discern from the background.

PORTAL HYPERTENSION

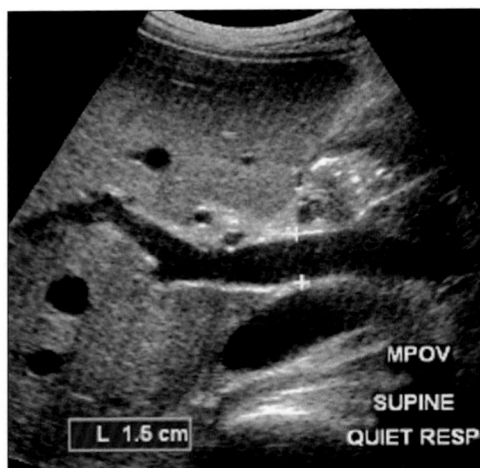

Oblique ultrasound shows the main portal vein (MPOV, cursors) measures 15 mm with the patient supine and quiet respiration. Maximum normal diameter is 13 mm.

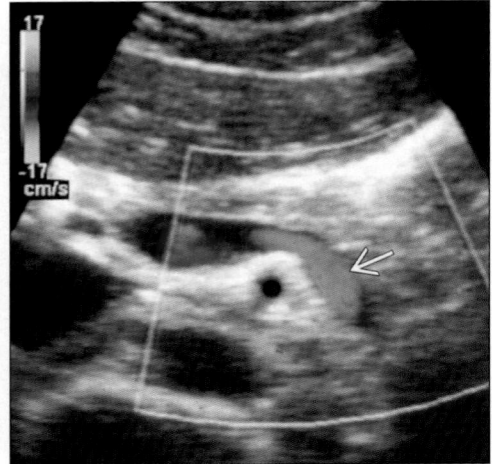

Transverse color Doppler ultrasound shows reversed (hepatofugal) blood flow in splenic vein ➜ in a patient with cirrhosis-related portal hypertension.

TERMINOLOGY

Abbreviations and Synonyms
- Portal hypertension (PH)

Definitions
- Portal venous pressure > 10 mm Hg above inferior vena cava (IVC) pressure

IMAGING FINDINGS

General Features
- Best diagnostic clue
  - Distended portal vein (PV)
  - Portosystemic collaterals
- Location: Portal venous system carries blood from gut to liver
- Size
  - Normal PV diameter, up to 13 mm
    - Adjacent to IVC
    - Supine, quiet respiration
  - Normal PV diameter in inspiration, up to 16 mm

- Normal respiratory variation in splenic vein/superior mesenteric vein (SMV): 50-100% diameter increase from quiet respiration to deep inspiration

Ultrasonographic Findings
- Grayscale Ultrasound
  - PV diameter > 13 mm is abnormal (specific, not sensitive); in supine quiet respiration at site where PV crosses anterior to IVC
  - < 20% increase in splenic vein or SMV diameter from quiet respiration to deep inspiration (more sensitive than PV measurement)
  - Hepatic cirrhosis
    - Liver surface nodularity
    - Small right lobe, enlarged caudate/left lobes
    - Microscopic or macroscopic cirrhotic changes = PH with 100% certainty
  - Portal or splenic vein aneurysm
    - Usually occur in context of PH
    - Other causes uncommon; e.g., chronic pancreatitis/trauma
  - Nonspecific associated findings
    - Coarse liver texture
    - Splenomegaly

DDx: Portal Hypertension

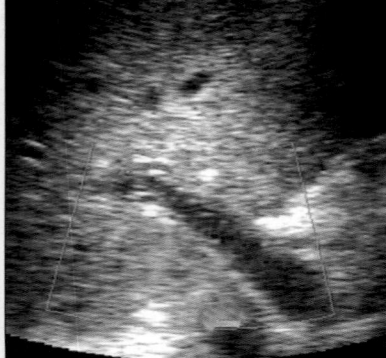

Portal Vein Thrombosis

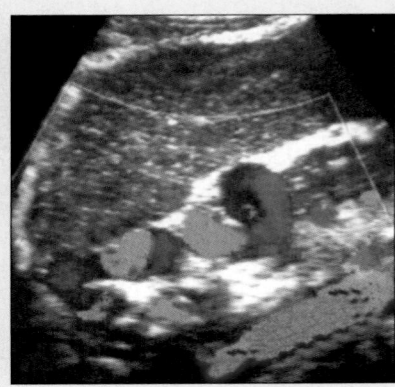

Splenic Vein Thrombosis/Collaterals

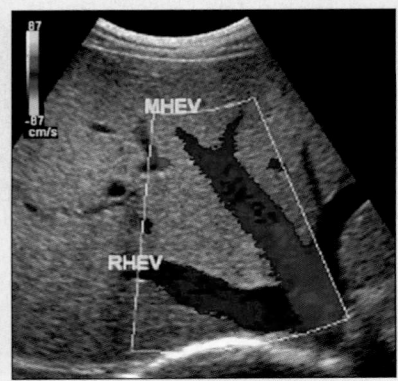

Congestive Heart Failure

PORTAL HYPERTENSION

Key Facts

Imaging Findings
- PV diameter > 13 mm is abnormal (specific, not sensitive); in supine quiet respiration at site where PV crosses anterior to IVC
- < 20% increase in splenic vein or SMV diameter from quiet respiration to deep inspiration (more sensitive than PV measurement)
- Hepatic cirrhosis
- Microscopic or macroscopic cirrhotic changes = PH with 100% certainty
- Portal or splenic vein aneurysm
- Reversed (hepatofugal) blood flow in portal vein, splenic vein, SMV on pulsed Doppler (PD)
- Lack of respirophasisity in PV flow on PD
- Slow PV flow velocity or to-and-fro PV flow on PD
- Portosystemic collaterals

- Color Doppler US as primary tool for PH diagnosis
- Contrast-enhanced CT or MR best for detailed assessment of collateralization

Top Differential Diagnoses
- Portal Vein Occlusion
- Splenic Vein Occlusion
- Congestive Heart Failure (Passive Venous Congestion)
- Hepatic Vein or IVC Occlusion/Budd Chiari Syndrome

Diagnostic Checklist
- PH when portal vein is dilated and spleen is enlarged without underlying cause
- PH may be silent clinically and is an important incidental diagnosis with US, CT, or MR

- Ascites
- Pulsed Doppler
  - Reversed (hepatofugal) blood flow in portal vein, splenic vein, SMV on pulsed Doppler (PD)
  - Lack of respirophasisity in PV flow on PD
  - Slow PV flow velocity or to-and-fro PV flow on PD
- Color Doppler
  - Reversed (hepatofugal) blood flow in portal vein, splenic vein, SMV
  - Portosystemic collaterals
    - Gastroesophageal: Coronary/right gastric, left gastric/splenogastric
    - Lienorenal
    - Umbilical vein (recanalized/paraumbilical)
    - Mesenteric/retroperitoneal
    - Intrahepatic: PV to PV; PV to systemic veins; PV to hepatic veins
  - Portal or splenic vein aneurysm

Imaging Recommendations
- Best imaging tool: Color/spectral Doppler US
- Protocol advice
  - Color Doppler US as primary tool for PH diagnosis
  - Contrast-enhanced CT or MR best for detailed assessment of collateralization
    - Confirmation/assessment of vascular complications; e.g., PV thrombosis
    - Planning for intervention/transplantation

DIFFERENTIAL DIAGNOSIS

Portal Vein Occlusion
- May have causes other than liver disease
- May cause flow reversal in splenic vein/SMV
- Produces porto-systemic collateralization

Splenic Vein Occlusion
- Splenomegaly
- Large lienorenal/splenogastric collaterals
- Commonly cause upper gastrointestinal bleeding
- **Note:** Think of this diagnosis with isolated, left sided collaterals

Congestive Heart Failure (Passive Venous Congestion)
- Reversible postsinusoidal PH
- Distended hepatic veins, IVC, portal vein
- Hepatomegaly
- Ascites

Hepatic Vein or IVC Occlusion/Budd Chiari Syndrome
- Hepatomegaly
- Liver dysfunction
- Ascites

Splenomegaly
- Neoplastic/hematologic disorders
- Reactive splenomegaly
- Hypersplenism

PATHOLOGY

General Features
- Genetics: Several genetic causes of liver disease causing PH; e.g., congenital hepatic fibrosis/biliary cirrhosis
- Etiology
  - Presinusoidal
    - Portal vein occlusion
    - Schistosomiasis
    - Congenital hepatic fibrosis
  - Sinusoidal
    - Cirrhosis (most common)
    - Chronic active hepatitis (common)
    - Numerous less common causes: e.g., hemochromatosis, primary sclerosing cholangitis
  - Postsinusoidal
    - Passive venous congestion (usually due to heart failure)
    - Hepatic vein occlusion (see "Budd-Chiari Syndrome")
    - IVC occlusion
- Epidemiology

- Large geographical variation in PH/liver disease etiology
  - Alcohol, hepatitis C: Western nations
  - Hepatitis B: Asia
  - Schistosomiasis: Africa, middle east
- Associated abnormalities
  - Portal vein thrombosis (related to sluggish flow)
  - Portal and splenic venous aneurysm
  - Gastrointestinal hemorrhage (from collateralization and clotting dysfunction)
  - Elevated splanchnic arterial flow in cirrhosis (aggravates PH)

Gross Pathologic & Surgical Features

- Cirrhosis
  - Right lobe most severely injured/scarred
  - Compensatory enlargement of left and caudate lobes
  - Nodular regeneration of liver tissue produces surface nodularity
- High portal pressure → visceral edema → ascites
- Dilated submucosal porto-systemic gastrointestinal collaterals subject to erosion → bleeding
- Ascites is predominantly a result of portal hypertension and resulting visceral edema, complicated by hypoalbuminemia

Microscopic Features

- Cirrhosis: Lobular scarring and regeneration due to toxins (especially alcohol) or chronic infection (hepatitis B/C)

CLINICAL ISSUES

Presentation

- Most common signs/symptoms
  - PH often is asymptomatic
    - Important incidental diagnosis on US, CT
  - Gastrointestinal bleeding/hemorrhage
  - Hepatic dysfunction/liver failure
- Other signs/symptoms
  - Ascites
  - Pleural fluid
  - Splenomegaly

Demographics

- Age: Much more common in adults than children

Natural History & Prognosis

- Most causes of PH are progressive
- Prognosis guarded, due to progression of liver disease/therapeutic failure

Treatment

- Endoscopic sclerotherapy for gastroesophageal hemorrhage
- Transjugular intrahepatic portocaval shunt (TIPS)
- Liver transplantation

DIAGNOSTIC CHECKLIST

Consider

- PH when portal vein is dilated and spleen is enlarged without underlying cause

Image Interpretation Pearls

- PH may be silent clinically and is an important incidental diagnosis with US, CT, or MR
- Cirrhotic liver morphology/nodularity = PH with 100% certainty

SELECTED REFERENCES

1. Shi B et al: Regional portal hypertension diagnosed by ultrasonography: imaging findings and diagnostic values. Hepatogastroenterology. 52(64):1062-5, 2005
2. Zwiebel WJ: Ultrasound assessment of the hepatic vasculature. IN: Zwiebel WJ and Pellerito: Introduction to vascular ultrasonography 5th ed. Philadelphia, Saunders/Elsevier. 585-610, 2005
3. Bolondi L et al: Doppler flowmetry in portal hypertension. J Gastroenterol Hepatol. 5(4):459-67, 1990
4. Duerinckx AJ et al: The pulsatile portal vein in cases of congestive heart failure: correlation of duplex Doppler findings with right atrial pressures. Radiology. 176(3):655-8, 1990
5. Goyal AK et al: Ultrasonic measurements of portal vasculature in diagnosis of portal hypertension. A controversial subject reviewed. J Ultrasound Med. 9(1):45-8, 1990
6. Hosoki T et al: Portal blood flow in congestive heart failure: pulsed duplex sonographic findings. Radiology. 174(3 Pt 1):733-6, 1990
7. Ralls PW: Color Doppler sonography of the hepatic artery and portal venous system. AJR Am J Roentgenol. 155(3):517-25, 1990
8. Di Lelio A et al: Cirrhosis: diagnosis with sonographic study of the liver surface. Radiology. 172(2):389-92, 1989
9. Gibson RN et al: Identification of a patent paraumbilical vein by using Doppler sonography: importance in the diagnosis of portal hypertension. AJR Am J Roentgenol. 153(3):513-6, 1989
10. Patriquin H et al: Duplex Doppler examination in portal hypertension: technique and anatomy. AJR Am J Roentgenol. 149(1):71-6, 1987
11. Giorgio A et al: Cirrhosis: value of caudate to right lobe ratio in diagnosis with US. Radiology. 161(2):443-5, 1986
12. Bolondi L et al: Ultrasonographic study of portal venous system in portal hypertension and after portosystemic shunt operations. Surgery. 95(3):261-9, 1984
13. Subramanyam BR et al: Sonography of portosystemic venous collaterals in portal hypertension. Radiology. 146(1):161-6, 1983
14. Bolondi L et al: Ultrasonography in the diagnosis of portal hypertension: diminished response of portal vessels to respiration. Radiology. 142(1):167-72, 1982
15. Weinreb J et al: Portal vein measurements by real-time sonography. AJR Am J Roentgenol. 139(3):497-9, 1982

IMAGE GALLERY

Typical

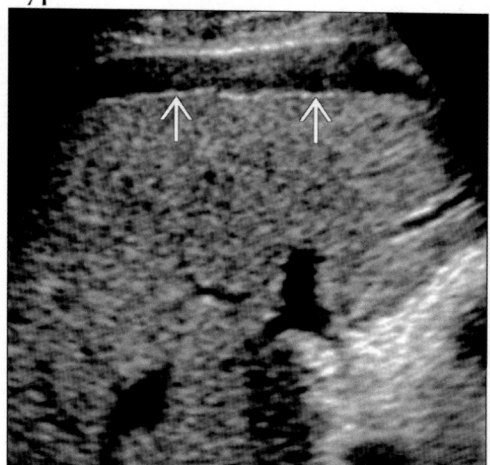 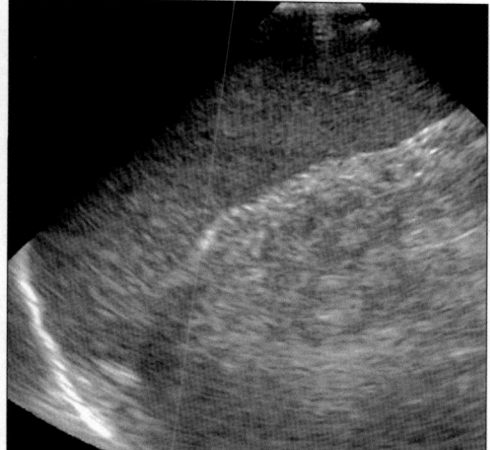

(Left) Longitudinal ultrasound shows liver surface nodularity ➡ due to regeneration, coarse liver texture, and ascites, in a patient with alcohol-related cirrhosis. *(Right)* Oblique ultrasound (same patient as previous image) shows splenomegaly (cephalocaudad dimension 17.5 cm).

Typical

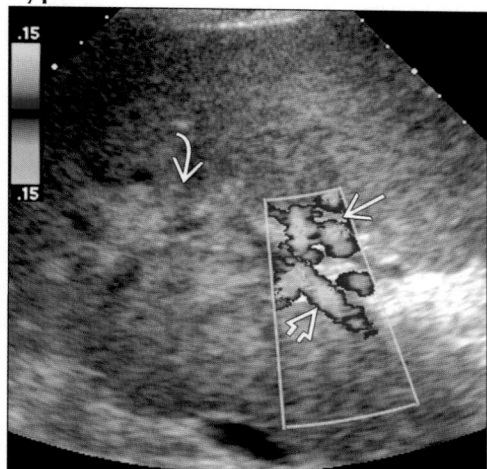 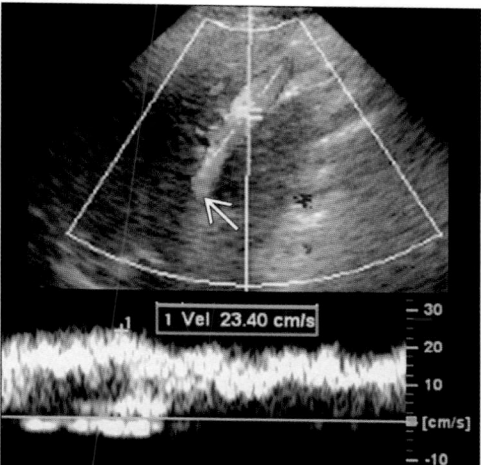

(Left) Oblique color Doppler ultrasound shows collateral veins ➡ in the porta hepatis. The portal vein ➡ is patent. Note a hepatocellular carcinoma ➡ in the right lobe. *(Right)* Longitudinal color Doppler ultrasound shows a huge umbilical vein collateral (peak velocity 23 cm/sec) arising from the left portal vein ➡, coursing along inferior border of the liver, and heading for the anterior abdominal wall.

Typical

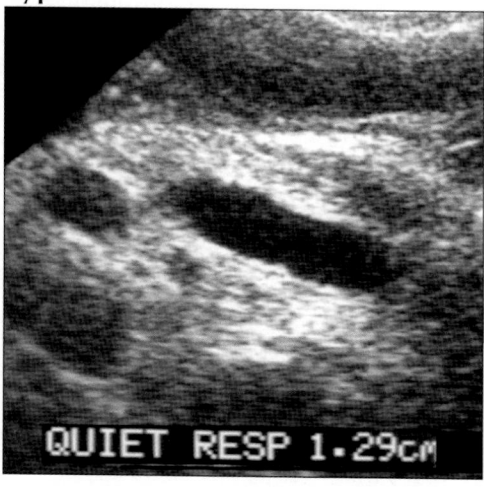 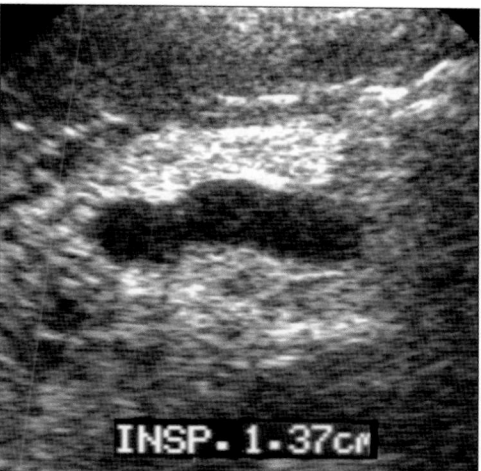

(Left) Transverse ultrasound shows absence of respiratory response in a patient with portal hypertension. In quiet respiration, the splenic vein measures 13 mm. *(Right)* Transverse ultrasound in deep inspiration, the splenic vein size increases only minimally, to 14 mm. Change in diameter < 20% indicates portal hypertension.

PORTO-SYSTEMIC COLLATERALS

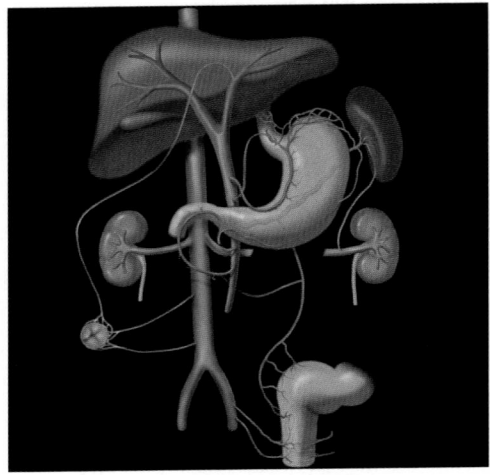

Graphic shows multiple pathways of porto-systemic blood flow.

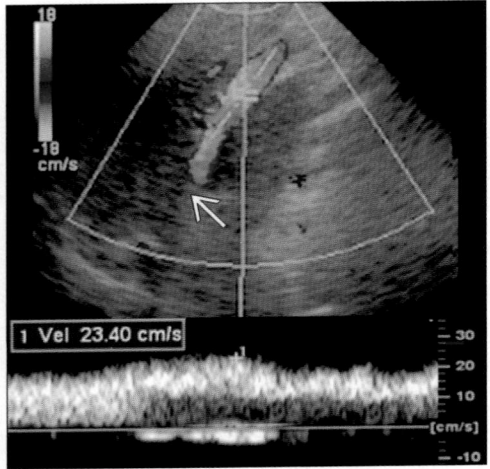

Longitudinal color Doppler ultrasound shows an umbilical vein collateral extending anteriorly from left portal vein branch ➡. High velocity suggests high volume flow.

TERMINOLOGY

Abbreviations and Synonyms
- Porto-systemic collaterals

Definitions
- Collateral pathways through which portal blood flow is diverted to the systemic circulation in response to elevated portal venous pressure

IMAGING FINDINGS

General Features
- Best diagnostic clue: Prominent, anomalous epigastric blood vessels with venous Doppler flow signals
- Location: Usually seen in the epigastrium
- Size: Few mm-cm or more
- Morphology: Usually tortuous, often multiple

Ultrasonographic Findings
- Grayscale Ultrasound
  - **Prominent, anomalous vascular channels oriented as follows**
    - From left portal vein, following ligamentum teres to the anterior abdominal wall; continues to umbilicus (peri-umbilical vein collateral)
    - Cephalad from porto-splenic confluence to gastroesophageal junction ("coronary" or left gastric vein collateral): Normal coronary vein ≤ 7 mm
    - Posterior to lower liver margin (left gastroepiploic vein collaterals)
    - In wall of gallbladder
    - Cephalad from splenic hilum to gastroesophageal area (short gastric [splenogastric] collaterals)
    - Adjacent to gastroesophageal junction, deep to left hepatic lobe (gastroesophageal collaterals)
    - Caudad from splenic hilum to left kidney (lienorenal collaterals)
    - In porta hepatis, with patent portal vein (coronary or left gastric collaterals)
    - Within hepatic parenchyma (porto-hepatic, porto-caval collaterals; other routes possible)
- Pulsed Doppler
  - Venous Doppler flow signal in above-described vessels

DDx: Porto-Systemic Collaterals

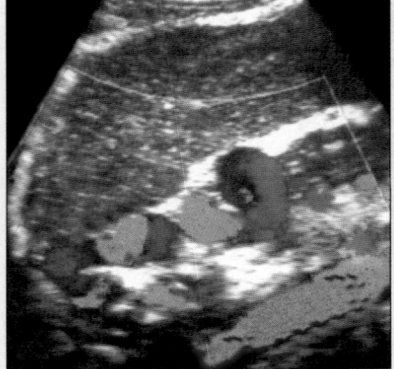

Splenic Vein Occlusion

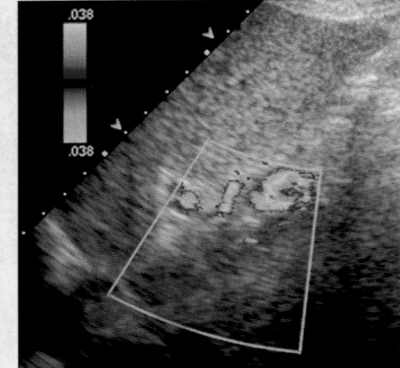

Inferior Vena Cava Occlusion

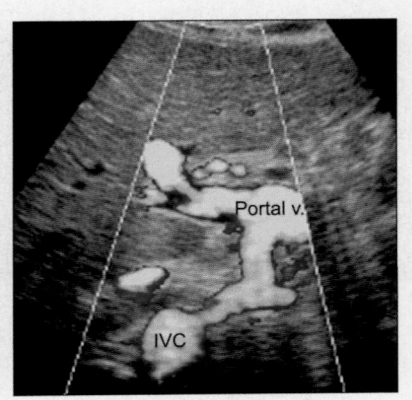

Surgical Porto-Systemic Shunts

Key Facts

Imaging Findings

- **Prominent, anomalous vascular channels oriented as follows**
- Cephalad from porto-splenic confluence to gastroesophageal junction ("coronary" or left gastric vein collateral): Normal coronary vein ≤ 7 mm
- Posterior to lower liver margin (left gastroepiploic vein collaterals)
- In wall of gallbladder
- Cephalad from splenic hilum to gastroesophageal area (short gastric [splenogastric] collaterals)
- Adjacent to gastroesophageal junction, deep to left hepatic lobe (gastroesophageal collaterals)
- Caudad from splenic hilum to left kidney (lienorenal collaterals)
- Within hepatic parenchyma (porto-hepatic, porto-caval collaterals; other routes possible)
- Color Doppler: Low-velocity flow in above-described collaterals, directed away from portal system
- Color Doppler sonography: Identifies large collaterals accessible through epigastric "acoustic windows"
- Contrast-enhanced CT or MR: Comprehensive evaluation of porto-systemic collaterals

Diagnostic Checklist

- Large branch from left portal vein to anterior abdominal wall continuing to umbilicus = peri-umbilical vein collateral
- Large collaterals isolated to left epigastrium suggests splenic vein occlusion

---

- ▪ Flow away from the portal venous system (i.e., hepatofugal)
- ▪ Flow usually continuous (i.e., no respiratory variation)
- Color Doppler: Low-velocity flow in above-described collaterals, directed away from portal system

Imaging Recommendations

- Best imaging tool
  - ○ Color Doppler sonography: Identifies large collaterals accessible through epigastric "acoustic windows"
  - ○ Contrast-enhanced CT or MR: Comprehensive evaluation of porto-systemic collaterals
    - ▪ Not restricted to acoustic windows
    - ▪ "Global" perspective
    - ▪ Potential visualization of small collaterals
- Protocol advice
  - ○ Proper adjustment of Doppler controls is essential
  - ○ Systematic search of usual collateral locations

DIFFERENTIAL DIAGNOSIS

Splenic Vein Occlusion

- No portal venous hypertension
- Large venous collaterals but only in left epigastrium
  - ○ Lienorenal
  - ○ Splenogastric (short gastric)
- Associated with gastroesophageal variceal hemorrhage

Inferior Vena Cava (IVC) Occlusion

- Causes extensive systemic-to-systemic venous collaterals, possibly seen with US
- May follow similar routes to portal hypertension-related collaterals

Left Renal Vein Occlusion

- Collateralization from left kidney to splenic hilum/retroperitoneum
- Blood flow is **toward** spleen
  - ○ Opposite portal hypertension/splenic vein occlusion

Superior Mesenteric Vein (SMV) Occlusion

- Predominantly mesenteric collateralization from SMV branches to portal system
- Collaterals not likely seen with US

Surgical Porto-Systemic Shunt

- Seldom used in era of transjugular intrahepatic portocaval shunts
- Mimic spontaneous portosystemic collaterals
- Portocaval, lienorenal, mesocaval

IVC Anomalies

- e.g., Azygous continuation of IVC
- Large, anomalous epigastric veins seen with ultrasound
- Usually US-identifiable

Left Renal Vein Anomalies

- Retroaortic or circumaortic renal veins
- Usually US-identifiable

Congenital Intrahepatic Porto-Systemic Shunts

- Result of vitello-umbilical venous plexus during embryogenesis
- Often asymptomatic early in infancy and present later with hepatic encephalopathy
- May spontaneously regress

Intrahepatic Arteriovenous Malformations

- Example: Hereditary hemorrhagic telangiectasia
- Prominent intrahepatic arteries communicating with hepatic veins
- Most noticeable US finding: Large hepatic artery branches/strong arterial signals (differentiates from venous collaterals)

Anomalous Origin/Course of Epigastric Arteries

- e.g., Replaced right hepatic artery
- May be mistaken for venous collateral
- Arterial flow differentiates from porto-systemic collaterals

Epigastric Arterial Occlusive Disease
- Splenic, celiac, superior mesenteric artery
- Possibly large epigastric collateral vessels
- Arterial flow differentiates from porto-systemic collaterals

PATHOLOGY

General Features
- Etiology
  - Portal hypertension (portal venous pressure > 10 mm Hg ↑ IVC pressure)
  - Causes of portal hypertension
    - Cirrhosis and other primary liver disease
    - Portal vein occlusion
    - Hepatic vein occlusion
    - IVC occlusion obstructing hepatic vein outflow
- Epidemiology: Related to underlying conditions causing portal hypertension
- Associated abnormalities
  - Portal or splenic venous aneurysms resulting from elevated portal pressure
  - Veno-occlusive disease

Microscopic Features
- Origin of umbilical vein collateralization debated
  - Is it a persistent or recanalized umbilical vein, or a paraumbilical vein?

CLINICAL ISSUES

Presentation
- Most common signs/symptoms
  - Gastroesophageal hemorrhage
    - Large submucosal varicose veins
    - Gastritis/esophagitis → inflammation, venous wall injury
    - Venous rupture, hemorrhage
  - Incidental diagnosis of collaterals on US, CT, MR
    - May be mistaken for other pathology
    - Important indicator of portal hypertension
- Other signs/symptoms
  - Splenomegaly
    - Related to portal hypertension
    - Possible congestion from veno-occlusive disease

Demographics
- Age: Related to age range of underlying disorders
- Gender: Related to demographics of underlying disorders

Natural History & Prognosis
- Guarded
  - Significant risk of gastroesophageal hemorrhage
  - Significant risk of progression of underlying disorder

Treatment
- Transjugular intrahepatic portocaval shunt (TIPS)
- Surgical portocaval shunt
- Endoscopic sclerotherapy for variceal hemorrhage

DIAGNOSTIC CHECKLIST

Consider
- Porto-systemic collaterals when large, anomalous vessels are seen in the epigastrium

Image Interpretation Pearls
- Large branch from left portal vein to anterior abdominal wall continuing to umbilicus = peri-umbilical vein collateral
- Large collaterals isolated to left epigastrium suggests splenic vein occlusion

SELECTED REFERENCES

1. Henseler KP et al: Three-dimensional CT angiography of spontaneous portosystemic shunts. Radiographics. 21(3):691-704, 2001
2. Matsumoto A et al: Three-dimensional portography using multislice helical CT is clinically useful for management of gastric fundic varices. AJR Am J Roentgenol. 176(4):899-905, 2001
3. Kim M et al: Portosystemic collaterals of the upper abdomen: review of anatomy and demonstration on MR imaging. Abdom Imaging. 25(5):462-70, 2000
4. von Herbay A et al: Color Doppler sonographic evaluation of spontaneous portosystemic shunts and inversion of portal venous flow in patients with cirrhosis. J Clin Ultrasound. 28(7):332-9, 2000
5. Nilsson A et al: Colour Doppler imaging of shunts from the left portal branch in portal hypertension. Description of a typical pattern. Acta Radiol. 39(5):564-7, 1998
6. Grattagliano A et al: Spontaneous intrahepatic portosystemic venous shunt in a patient with cirrhosis: diagnosis by combined color Doppler and pulsed Doppler ultrasonography. Liver. 17(6):307-10, 1997
7. Riehl J et al: [Spontaneous portasystemic shunt in liver cirrhosis: imaging with color-coded duplex ultrasonography] Ultraschall Med. 18(6):272-6, 1997
8. Rathi PM et al: Gallbladder varices: diagnosis in children with portal hypertension on duplex sonography. J Clin Gastroenterol. 23(3):228-31, 1996
9. Kudo M et al: Intrahepatic portosystemic venous shunt: diagnosis by color Doppler imaging. Am J Gastroenterol. 88(5):723-9, 1993
10. Sie A et al: Color Doppler sonography in spontaneous splenorenal portosystemic shunts. J Ultrasound Med. 10(3):167-9, 1991
11. Mostbeck GH et al: Hemodynamic significance of the paraumbilical vein in portal hypertension: assessment with duplex US. Radiology. 170(2):339-42, 1989
12. Di Candio G et al: Ultrasound detection of unusual spontaneous portosystemic shunts associated with uncomplicated portal hypertension. J Ultrasound Med. 4(6):297-305, 1985
13. Lafortune M et al: The recanalized umbilical vein in portal hypertension: a myth. AJR Am J Roentgenol. 144(3):549-53, 1985

IMAGE GALLERY

Typical

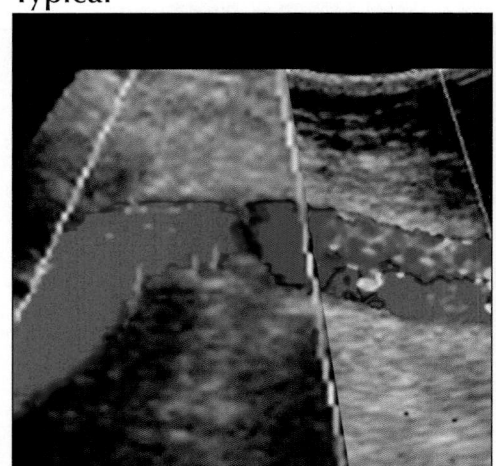
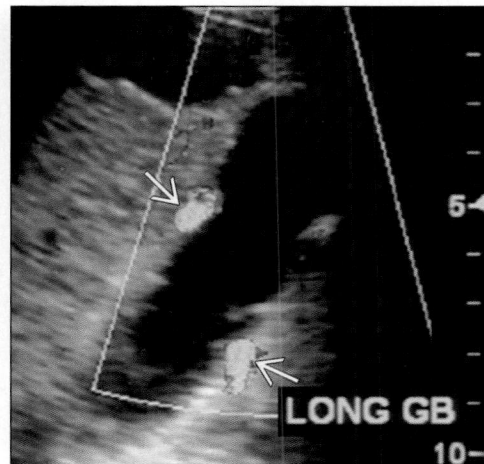

(Left) Longitudinal color Doppler ultrasound composite of two images shows continuation of umbilical vein as it turns inferiorly along abdominal wall. *(Right)* Oblique color Doppler ultrasound shows gallbladder wall varicosities ➡ in patient with portal hypertension.

Typical

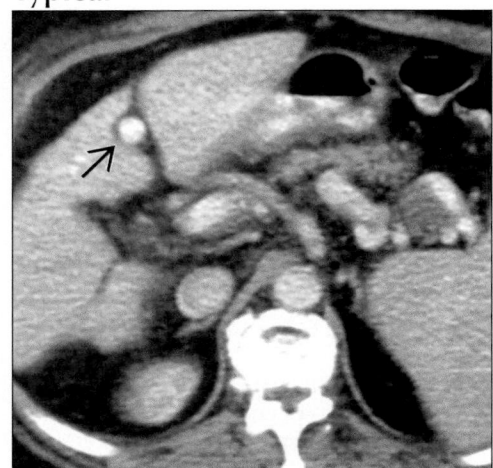
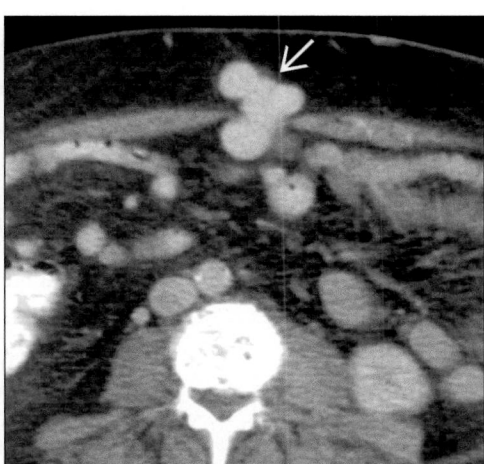

(Left) Transverse CECT shows umbilical vein collateral ➡ in the ligamentum teres. *(Right)* Transverse CECT of the same patient as previous image shows a varicose collateral vein ➡ exiting abdomen at umbilicus, ultimately to arborize into superficial veins connected to systemic circulation.

Typical

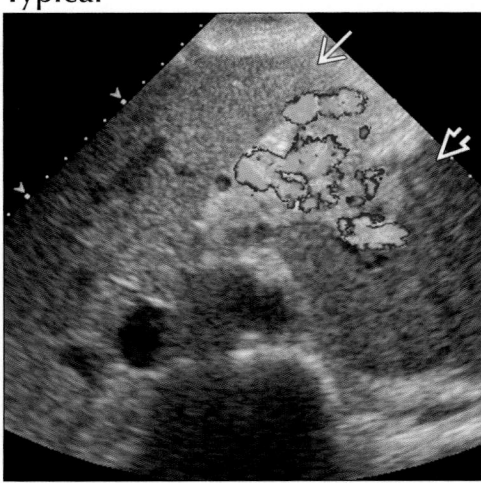
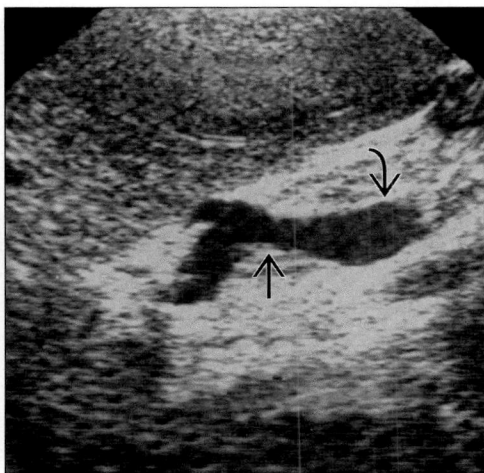

(Left) Transverse color Doppler ultrasound shows large left gastric collateral veins between the liver ➡ and spleen ➡. *(Right)* Longitudinal ultrasound shows a dilated coronary (left gastric) vein ➡ at its origin from the portal vein ➡, which is seen in cross-section.

TIPS SHUNTS

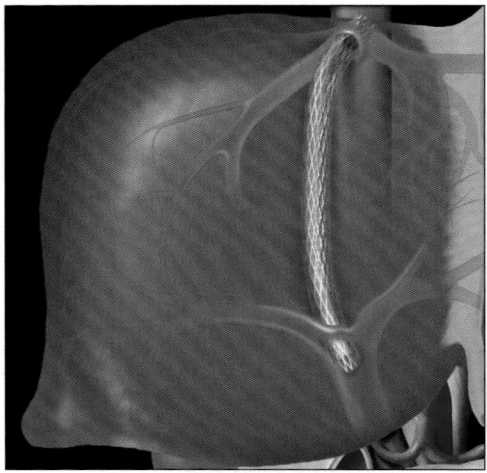

Graphic of TIPS shunt creation. The hepatic vein is punctured within 2 cm of the IVC. It extends to the right portal vein, adjacent to its junction with the main portal vein.

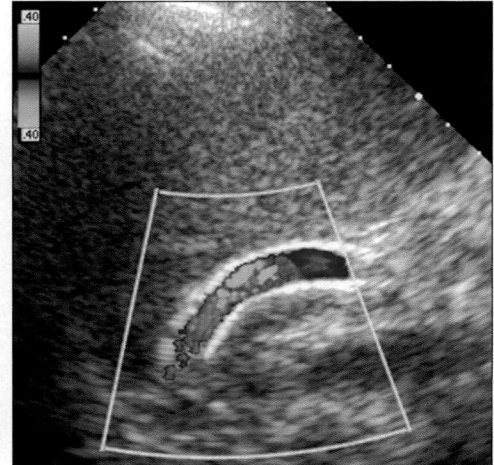

Longitudinal color Doppler ultrasound shows the mid portion of a normally patent TIPS shunt. Although the stent is highly echogenic, it does not obstruct sonographic visualization.

TERMINOLOGY

Abbreviations and Synonyms
- Transjugular intrahepatic portocaval shunt (TIPS)
- Hepatopetal blood flow: Toward liver
- Hepatofugal blood flow: Away from liver

Definitions
- Shunt between main portal vein and a hepatic vein created with balloon-expandable metallic stent

IMAGING FINDINGS

General Features
- Location: Most common route: Right hepatic vein to right portal vein, then to main portal vein
- Size: 10-12 mm diameter
- Morphology
  - Typically follows a curved course through hepatic parenchyma
  - Portal end slightly proximal to main portal vein bifurcation
  - Hepatic end at, or slightly cephalad to, hepatic vein/inferior vena cava (IVC) junction

Ultrasonographic Findings
- Grayscale Ultrasound
  - Stents are echogenic; easily seen on grayscale images, yet do not block sound transmission
  - Stent typically curved but **not** kinked
  - Normally uniform stent caliber
  - Hepatic and portal ends "squarely" within veins (best seen with grayscale)
- Pulsed Doppler
  - **Portal vein, satisfactory function**
    - Hepatopetal flow
    - Flow velocity > > pre-TIPS value; **at least 35 cm/sec**; typically about 43 cm/sec
    - Flow toward shunt in right and left portal branches (occasionally away in left branch)
  - **Portal vein, shunt malfunction**
    - Hepatofugal or bidirectional flow
    - Peak velocity < 35 cm/sec
    - Flow away from the shunt (hepatopetal) in right and left portal branches
  - **Within shunt, satisfactory function**

DDx: TIPS Shunt

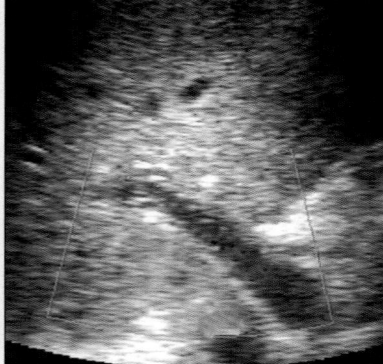
Portal Vein Thrombosis

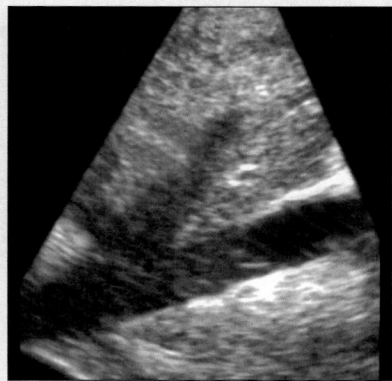
Hepatic Vein, IVC Thrombosis

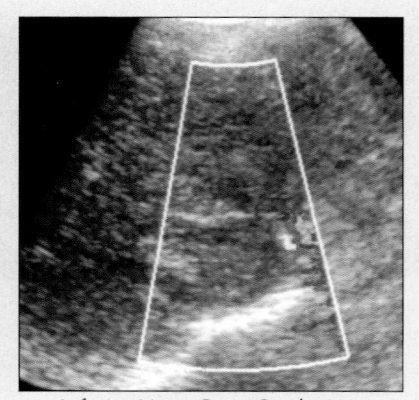
Inferior Vena Cava Occlusion

Key Facts

Imaging Findings

- **Portal vein, satisfactory function**
- Hepatopetal flow
- Flow velocity > > pre-TIPS value; **at least 35 cm/sec;** typically about 43 cm/sec
- **Portal vein, shunt malfunction**
- Hepatofugal or bidirectional flow
- Peak velocity < 35 cm/sec
- **Within shunt, satisfactory function**
- Peak velocity at any location, **at least 90 cm/sec**
- Similar velocity throughout shunt; not > 50 cm/sec point-to-point variation
- Similar velocity temporally; not > 50 cm/sec change, study-to-study
- **Within shunt, malfunction**
- Shunt velocity < 90 cm/sec at any point
- Temporal drop in velocity ≥ 50 cm/sec
- Point-to-point increase in velocity ≥ 50 cm/sec (indicating focal stenosis)
- Absence of flow (indicating occlusion); **always confirm angiographically**

Pathology

- Primary patency (no intervention): 1 yr = 25-66%; 2 yr = 5-42%
- Secondary (assisted) patency: 1 yr = 85%; 2 yr = 61%; 5 yr = 55%
- **Goal of US: Detect stenosis before shunt occludes or symptoms recur**

Diagnostic Checklist

- TIPS malfunction with shunt velocity < 90 cm/sec or portal vein velocity < 35 cm/sec

---

- Flow slightly turbulent, slight pulsatility, possible slight respiratory variation
- Peak velocity at any location, **at least 90 cm/sec**
- Similar velocity throughout shunt; not > 50 cm/sec point-to-point variation
- Similar velocity temporally; not > 50 cm/sec change, study-to-study
  - **Within shunt, malfunction**
    - Continuous flow (no pulsatility or respiratory change)
    - Shunt velocity < 90 cm/sec at any point
    - Temporal drop in velocity ≥ 50 cm/sec
    - Point-to-point increase in velocity ≥ 50 cm/sec (indicating focal stenosis)
    - Focal, severe turbulence (post-stenosis)
    - Absence of flow (indicating occlusion); **always confirm angiographically**
- Color Doppler
  - **Portal/splenic vein, satisfactory function**
    - Widely patent, with hepatopetal flow
    - Flow toward shunt in right and left portal branches (occasionally away in left branch)
  - **Within shunt, satisfactory function**
    - Color flow extends to stent margins (i.e., no flow void indicating stenosis)
    - Uniform, velocity (color scale) throughout shunt
    - Mild turbulence
  - **Within shunt, malfunction**
    - Visible stenosis, either focal or diffuse
    - Focal color change indicative of high velocity
    - Focal severe flow disturbance (post-stenosis)
    - Absence of flow (occlusion): Check with spectral Doppler (more sensitive); **always confirm angiographically**

Other Modality Findings

- CTA, MRA
  - Anatomic depiction of stenosis/occlusion/collateralization
  - Less technically dependent
  - Not limited by available "acoustic windows"
  - Multiplanar reconstruction possible
  - More expensive than US

- Contrast-enhancement essential for CTA, generally required for MRA

Imaging Recommendations

- Best imaging tool
  - Controversial as to whether CTA/MRA are superior to US for TIPS shunt surveillance
  - Use US as primary TIPS surveillance tool
  - CTA/MRA
    - For technically compromised/equivocal US
    - To get a "global" view
- Protocol advice
  - Pre-TIPS assessment (grayscale, color Doppler, spectral Doppler)
    - Assess liver morphology
    - Search for hepatic masses (very important)
    - Document volume of ascites and pleural fluid, if any
    - Document patency and flow direction in portal, splenic veins
    - Look for portal vein bifurcation outside of liver (if so, puncture can → exsanguination)
    - Measure flow velocity in portal vein
    - Document patency and flow direction in right and left portal vein branches
    - Document patency and flow direction in three major hepatic vein trunks
    - Document IVC patency
  - Post-TIPS assessment (grayscale, color Doppler, spectral Doppler)
    - Search for hepatic masses
    - Document volume of ascites and pleural fluid, if any
    - Examine stent configuration/position
    - Confirm patency and flow direction in splenic and portal veins
    - Confirm patency and flow direction in portal vein branches (easiest way: Show opposite flow color in vein/adjacent artery; e.g., red/blue)
    - Measure velocity mid portal vein (**not** adjacent to shunt)
    - Assess shunt color Doppler

TIPS SHUNTS

- Record Doppler waveforms/peak velocities: Proximal, mid, distal shunt
- Compare findings with prior results **before** discharging patient (re-check if needed)
- Stenosis present? document peak stenosis velocity/post-stenotic turbulence
- Document patency, flow direction, Doppler waveforms in hepatic veins

DIFFERENTIAL DIAGNOSIS

Portal Vein, Hepatic Vein or IVC Thrombosis
- Mimic signs/symptoms of shunt failure

PATHOLOGY

General Features
- General path comments
  - Causes of TIPS shunts failure
    - Technical problems: Malposition, kinks, incomplete deployment
    - Venous trauma during stent insertion: Usually hepatic vein → fibrosis/stenosis
    - Neointimal hyperplasia (may be ameliorated by covered stents but insufficient data exists)
    - Thrombosis: Coagulopathy; intercurrent illness, due to above problems
- Epidemiology
  - Maintaining TIPS shunt patency is major problem
    - Primary patency (no intervention): 1 yr = 25-66%; 2 yr = 5-42%
    - Secondary (assisted) patency: 1 yr = 85%; 2 yr = 61%; 5 yr = 55%
    - **Goal of US: Detect stenosis before shunt occludes or symptoms recur**
    - Covered stents may improve primary patency, but insufficient data exists
- Associated abnormalities: TIPS may cause hepatic encephalopathy: Portal flow bypasses liver

CLINICAL ISSUES

Presentation
- Clinical Profile
  - Primary TIPS uses
    - Recurrent or intractable (life threatening) variceal bleeding
    - Intractable ascites due to cirrhosis/portal hypertension
    - Temporizing measure, pre-liver transplantation
  - Other TIPS uses
    - Acute or chronic hepatic vein thrombosis with Budd-Chiari syndrome
    - Acute portal vein thrombosis (TIPS followed by thrombectomy/thrombolysis)

Demographics
- Age: Generally adults/also children
- Gender: Male and female

Natural History & Prognosis
- Guarded
  - Maintaining shunt patency is difficult
  - Inevitable liver disease progression
  - High risk of cirrhosis-related hepatocellular carcinoma

DIAGNOSTIC CHECKLIST

Consider
- TIPS malfunction with shunt velocity < 90 cm/sec or portal vein velocity < 35 cm/sec

Image Interpretation Pearls
- Low flow is difficult to detect with US; confirm shunt occlusion angiographically (CTA, MRA, DSA)

SELECTED REFERENCES

1. Benito A et al: Doppler ultrasound for TIPS: does it work? Abdom Imaging. 29(1):45-52, 2004
2. Middleton WD et al: Doppler evaluation of transjugular intrahepatic portosystemic shunts. Ultrasound Q. 19(2):56-70; quiz 108 - 10, 2003
3. Bodner G et al: Color and pulsed Doppler ultrasound findings in normally functioning transjugular intrahepatic portosystemic shunts. Eur J Ultrasound. 12(2):131-6, 2000
4. Ong JP et al: Transjugular intrahepatic portosystemic shunts (TIPS): a decade later. J Clin Gastroenterol. 30(1):14-28, 2000
5. Kerlin RK Jr: TIPS technique: Techniques in Vascular and Interventional Radiology. 1(2):68-79, 1998
6. Murphy TP et al: Long-term follow-up after TIPS: use of Doppler velocity criteria for detecting elevation of the portosystemic gradient. J Vasc Interv Radiol. 9(2):275-81, 1998
7. Ducoin H et al: Histopathologic analysis of transjugular intrahepatic portosystemic shunts. Hepatology. 25(5):1064-9, 1997
8. Haskal ZJ et al: elevated portosystemic gradients and loss of shunt function. J Vasc Interv Radiol. 8(4):549-56, 1997
9. Kanterman RY et al: Doppler sonography findings associated with transjugular intrahepatic portosystemic shunt malfunction. AJR Am J Roentgenol. 168(2):467-72, 1997
10. Feldstein VA et al: Transjugular intrahepatic portosystemic shunts: accuracy of Doppler US in determination of patency and detection of stenoses. Radiology. 201(1):141-7, 1996
11. Dodd GD 3rd et al: Detection of transjugular intrahepatic portosystemic shunt dysfunction: value of duplex Doppler sonography. AJR Am J Roentgenol. 164(5):1119-24, 1995
12. Kerlan RK Jr et al: Transjugular intrahepatic portosystemic shunts: current status. 164(5):1059-66, 1995
13. Surratt RS et al: Morphologic and hemodynamic findings at sonography before and after creation of a transjugular intrahepatic portosystemic shunt. AJR Am J Roentgenol. 160(3):627-30, 1993
14. Foshager MC et al: Duplex sonography after transjugular intrahepatic portosystemic shunts (TIPS):normal hemodynamic findings and efficacy in predicting shunt patency and stenosis.AJR Am J Roentgenol. 1995 Jul;165(1):1-7.

IMAGE GALLERY

Typical

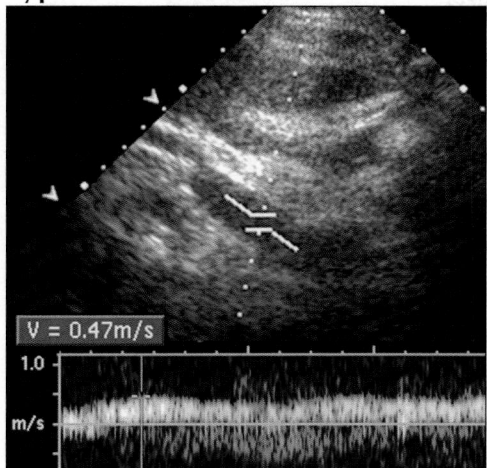 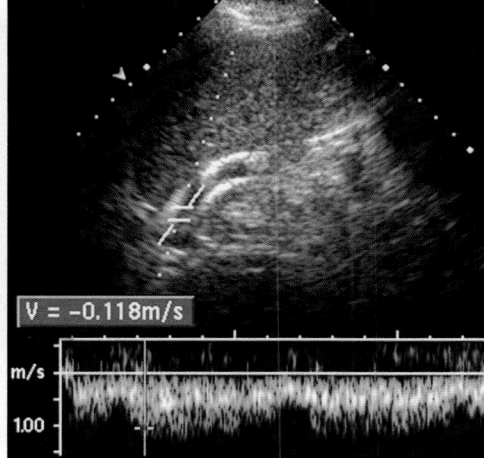

(Left) Oblique pulsed Doppler ultrasound shows peak velocity of 47 cm/sec in portal vein, consistent with normal shunt function. (Right) Longitudinal pulsed Doppler ultrasound (in same patient as previous image) shows peak shunt velocity of 118 cm/sec, also consistent with normal shunt function.

Typical

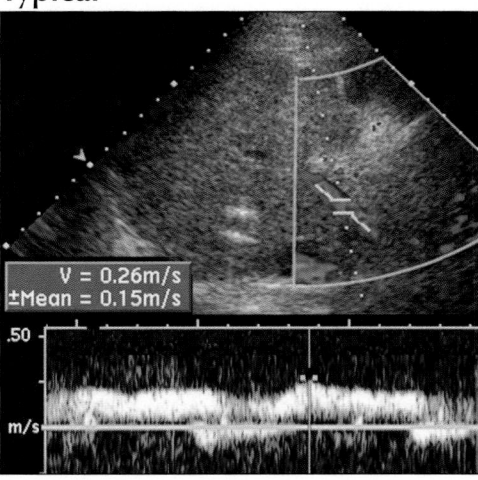 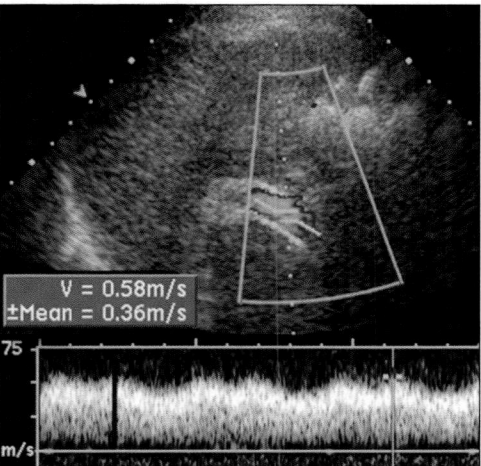

(Left) Oblique pulsed Doppler ultrasound in patient with recurrent ascites, shows low portal vein velocity (26 cm/sec), well below expected velocity of > 35 cm/sec. (Right) Oblique pulsed Doppler ultrasound near portal end of shunt, in same patient as previous image, shows an abnormally low shunt velocity of 58 cm/sec; well below expected level of > 90 cm/sec.

Typical

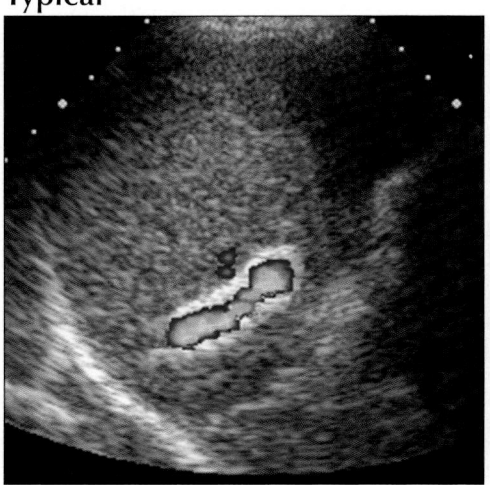 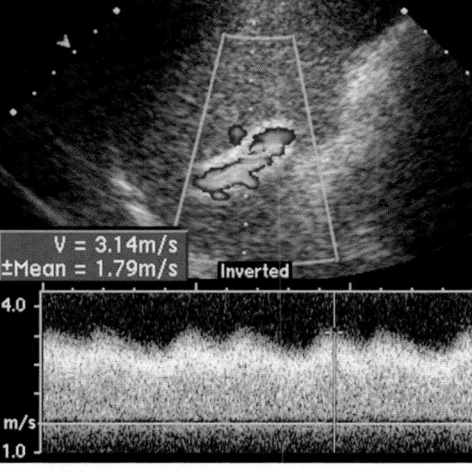

(Left) Longitudinal color Doppler ultrasound in same patient as previous image, shows focal narrowing and high velocity (blue shades) near hepatic end of shunt. (Right) Longitudinal pulsed Doppler ultrasound shows markedly elevated flow velocity (300 cm/sec) in narrowed area, In conjunction with other findings, this clearly is flow limiting stenosis.

PORTAL VEIN OCCLUSION

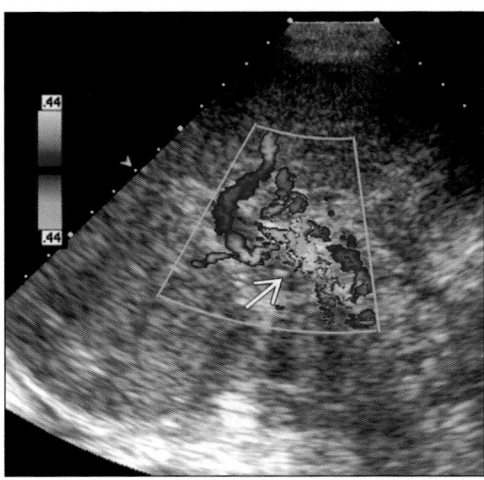

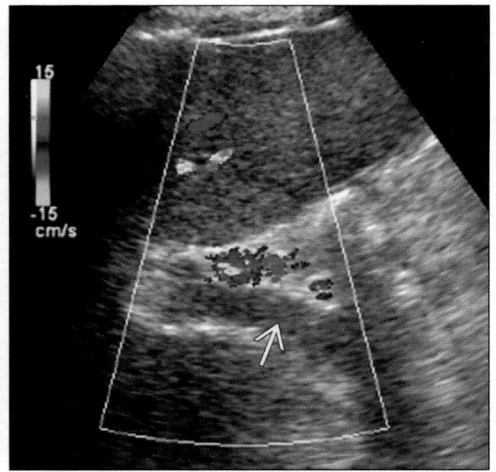

Oblique color Doppler ultrasound shows porta hepatis collateralization in patient with subacute portal vein thrombosis. Note absence of portal vein flow ➡️. Right and left branches (not shown) were patent.

Oblique color Doppler ultrasound shows absent flow in portal vein ➡️, in cirrhotic patient who presented with abdominal pain.

TERMINOLOGY

Abbreviations and Synonyms
- Portal vein (PV)
- Hepatopetal: Toward liver
- Hepatofugal: Away from liver

Definitions
- Obstruction of the portal vein, most commonly due to thrombosis

IMAGING FINDINGS

General Features
- Best diagnostic clue
  - Visualized PV with absent blood flow on color or spectral Doppler US
  - Cavernous transformation of the PV (i.e., collateralization)
- Location: Main portal vein and/or right and left branches
- Size
  - Acute thrombosis; PV may be enlarged
  - Chronic occlusion; PV small, not visible

Ultrasonographic Findings
- Grayscale Ultrasound
  - Normal PV readily seen; non-visualization suggests occlusion
  - Faintly echogenic material within PV lumen (thrombus or tumor)
  - Cavernous transformation of the PV
    - Multiple tubular channels along usual course of PV
    - Portal vein not seen
    - Subacute and especially chronic occlusion
  - Possible soft tissue mass, if PV occlusion due to extrinsic tumor invasion
  - Possible findings of pancreatitis if PV thrombosis due to this condition
- Pulsed Doppler
  - Absent Doppler signals in PV
  - Reversed flow in splenic vein; possibly superior mesenteric vein
  - Continuous flow in collaterals (no respiratory variation)
- Color Doppler

DDx: Portal Vein Occlusion

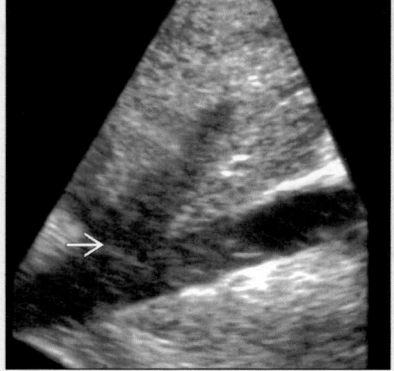

Hepatic Vein/IVC Occlusion

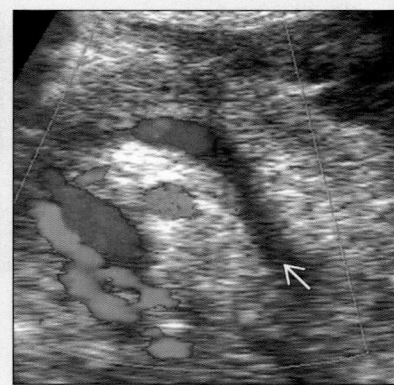

Splenic Vein Occlusion

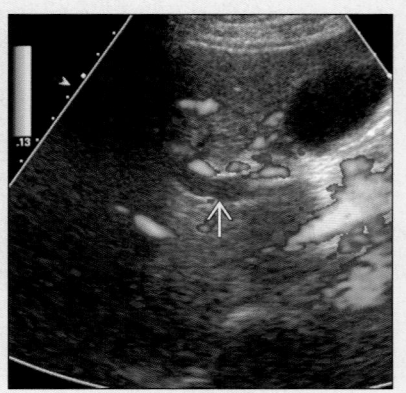

False Positive

Key Facts

Imaging Findings
- Normal PV readily seen; non-visualization suggests occlusion
- Faintly echogenic material within PV lumen (thrombus or tumor)
- Cavernous transformation of the PV
- Absent Doppler signals in PV
- Reversed flow in splenic vein; possibly superior mesenteric vein
- Continuous flow in collaterals (no respiratory variation)
- No color (flow) in PV
- Possible tumor vessels in PV
- Reversed flow in splenic vein; possibly SMV
- Hepatofugal flow in porto-systemic collaterals (due to portal hypertension)

- Color/spectral Doppler sonography: For surveillance and initial diagnosis
- CECT/MR: Comprehensive evaluation; extent of occlusion/collateralization

Top Differential Diagnoses
- Hepatic Vein/IVC Occlusion
- Splenic Vein Occlusion
- False positive occlusion: Poor technique
- False positive occlusion: Slow flow states
- False negative occlusion: Poor technique
- False negative occlusion: Non-occlusive thrombus

Diagnostic Checklist
- PV readily seen; non-visualization suggests occlusion
- False + and - diagnoses are a problem; good Doppler technique essential

○ No color (flow) in PV
○ Possible tumor vessels in PV
  - If occluding material is propagating tumor thrombus
  - Tiny vessels producing a dot-dash pattern
  - Low resistance arterial flow in tumor vessels
  - Not consistently seen
○ Reversed flow in splenic vein; possibly SMV
○ Hepatopetal flow in cavernous transformation
○ Hepatofugal flow in porto-systemic collaterals (due to portal hypertension)
○ Absent flow in hepatic vein or inferior vena cava if PV occlusion secondary to these conditions

Imaging Recommendations
- Best imaging tool
  ○ Color/spectral Doppler sonography: For surveillance and initial diagnosis
  ○ CECT/MR
    - CECT/MR: Comprehensive evaluation; extent of occlusion/collateralization
    - Search for cause
    - Evaluate underlying condition
- Protocol advice
  ○ Technical errors are a major diagnostic impediment
    - Check to see if you can detect flow in other vessels at equivalent depth

DIFFERENTIAL DIAGNOSIS

Hepatic Vein/IVC Occlusion
- Causes slow flow in PV
- Possible secondary PV occlusion

Splenic Vein Occlusion
- No flow/non-visualization of splenic vein
- Extensive left sided collaterals
- Confirm that portal vein is patent

False Positive Occlusion
- False positive occlusion: Poor technique
  ○ Inadequate Doppler angle

○ Wrong velocity scale
○ Insufficient color/spectral Doppler gain
- False positive occlusion: Slow flow states
  ○ Very slow, or to-and-fro PV flow
  ○ Can't detect flow with color Doppler, sometimes spectral Doppler also
  ○ Usually due to cirrhosis

False Negative Occlusion
- False negative occlusion: Poor technique
  ○ False negative occlusion: Non-occlusive thrombus
  ○ Too much color gain > "blooming" of color beyond flow stream
  ○ Blooming over-writes grayscale image, obscuring thrombus
  ○ Less likely with tumor invasion, which typically is occlusive

Non-Occlusive Thrombosis
- Variable degree of obstruction
- May be inapparent clinically

Dilated Bile Duct
- Patent adjacent PV seen with color Doppler

PATHOLOGY

General Features
- Genetics: Inherited hypercoagulability may be causative factor in PV thrombosis
- Etiology
  ○ Thrombosis
    - Combination of etiologic factors is common
    - Stasis: Sinusoidal obstruction as in cirrhosis; hepatic vein or IVC obstruction
    - Severe dehydration (especially in children)
    - Hypercoagulable states (genetic/neoplasm-related)
    - Pancreatitis: Portal/splenic vein inflammation (phlebitis) → thrombosis
    - Abdominal sepsis → seeding of portal vein → phlebitis → thrombosis (e.g., appendicitis/Crohn disease)

PORTAL VEIN OCCLUSION

- Hepatic vein or IVC occlusion → secondary PV thrombosis
- Complication of surgery/liver transplantation
  - Tumor propagation
    - Hepatocellular carcinoma; most common
    - Cholangiocarcinoma
    - Metastatic disease
  - Direct neoplastic invasion
    - Usually pancreatic carcinoma
    - Rarely other neoplasms, usually metastatic
- Epidemiology: Most cases of PV occlusion are cirrhosis or pancreatitis related
- Associated abnormalities: PV occlusion may be secondary to hepatic vein or IVC occlusion

Gross Pathologic & Surgical Features
- Acute thrombosis
  - Lumen partially filled with thrombus; flow maintained
  - Lumen entirely filled with thrombus; occlusion
  - Possible associated thrombosis of splenic vein/superior mesenteric vein
- Subacute/chronic thrombosis
  - PV replaced by tangle of collateral veins; cavernous transformation
  - Appearance 6-20 days after occlusion
  - Maturation gradual, most prominent chronically
  - Two collateral routes
    - Porto-portal along usual PV course
    - Porto-systemic: Left gastric veins or splenogastric, splenorenal
- Tumor propagation
  - Tumor grows along vein lumen
  - Vein wall intact
- Tumor invasion
  - Tumor directly invades through vein wall
  - Wall destroyed

Microscopic Features
- Vein wall inflammation is essential component of thrombosis (thrombophlebitis)

CLINICAL ISSUES

Presentation
- Most common signs/symptoms
  - Abdominal pain and distention
    - If phlebitis/inflammation → causes pain
    - Obstruction → bowel edema → pain
    - Bowel edema/congestion may cause ileus
    - Bowel edema possibly → ascites
  - Abnormal liver function tests
- Other signs/symptoms
  - Rare acute abdomen from venous bowel infarction
  - Asymptomatic incidental diagnosis (acute)
    - Non-occlusive thrombus
    - PV blood flow maintained
    - Questionable clinical relevance
    - Need for anticoagulation also questionable
  - Asymptomatic incidental diagnosis (chronic)
    - Cavernous transformation found on US, CT, MR
    - Possibly in otherwise healthy individual
    - Possibly in patient with cirrhosis

- Remote disorder → PV thrombosis → effective collateralization
  - Gastrointestinal hemorrhage from porto-systemic collaterals

Demographics
- Age: Usually adult, childhood also
- Gender: Male and female

Natural History & Prognosis
- Guarded
  - Usually related to underlying condition
  - Possible gastroesophageal varices → hemorrhage
- Good prognosis if asymptomatic/incidental,

Treatment
- Anticoagulation
- Supportive
- TIPS plus PV thrombectomy/thrombolysis

DIAGNOSTIC CHECKLIST

Consider
- PV occlusion when PV is not readily seen with US

Image Interpretation Pearls
- PV readily seen; non-visualization suggests occlusion
- False + and - diagnoses are a problem; good Doppler technique essential
- Tangle of veins in porta hepatis & absent portal vein = cavernous transformation

SELECTED REFERENCES

1. Grisham A et al: Deciphering mesenteric venous thrombosis: imaging and treatment. Vasc Endovascular Surg. 39(6):473-9, 2005
2. Hidajat N et al: Imaging and radiological interventions of portal vein thrombosis. Acta Radiol. 46(4):336-43, 2005
3. Hidajat N et al: Portal vein thrombosis: etiology, diagnostic strategy, therapy and management. Vasa. 34(2):81-92, 2005
4. Zwiebel WJ: Ultrasound Assessment of the Hepatic Vasculature. In, Zwiebel WJ, Pellerito J S: Introduction to Vascular Ultrasonography, 5th ed. Philadelphia, Saunders/Elsevier. 585-611, 2005
5. Ganger DR et al: Transjugular intrahepatic portosystemic shunt (TIPS) for Budd-Chiari syndrome or portal vein thrombosis: review of indications and problems. Am J Gastroenterol. 94(3):603-8, 1999
6. De Gaetano AM et al: Splanchnic collateral circulation detected with Doppler sonography. AJR Am J Roentgenol. 165(5):1151-5, 1995
7. Tanaka K et al: Diagnosis of portal vein thrombosis in patients with hepatocellular carcinoma:efficacy of color Doppler sonography compared with angiography. AJR Am J Roentgenol. 160(6):1279-83, 1993
8. Tessler FN et al: Diagnosis of portal vein thrombosis: value of color Doppler imaging. AJR Am J Roentgenol. 157(2):293-6, 1991
9. Wang LY et al: Duplex pulsed Doppler sonography of portal vein thrombosis in hepatocellular carcinoma. J Ultrasound Med. 10(5):265-9, 1991
10. Atri M et al: Incidence of portal vein thrombosis complicating liver metastasis as detected by duplex ultrasound. J Ultrasound Med. 9(5):285-9, 1990

IMAGE GALLERY

Typical

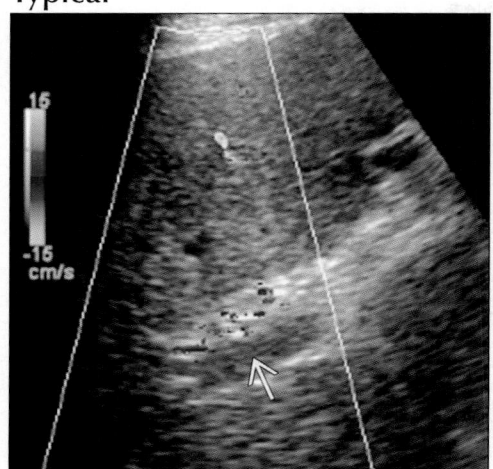 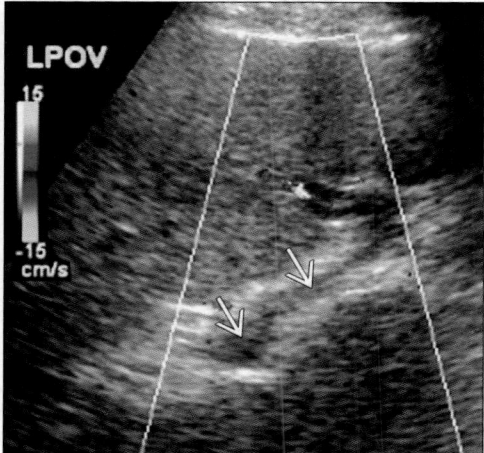

(Left) Oblique color Doppler ultrasound shows occlusion of the right portal branch ➡. *(Right)* Transverse color Doppler ultrasound shows occlusion of the left portal branch ➡, in the same cirrhotic patient with main portal vein occlusion.

Typical

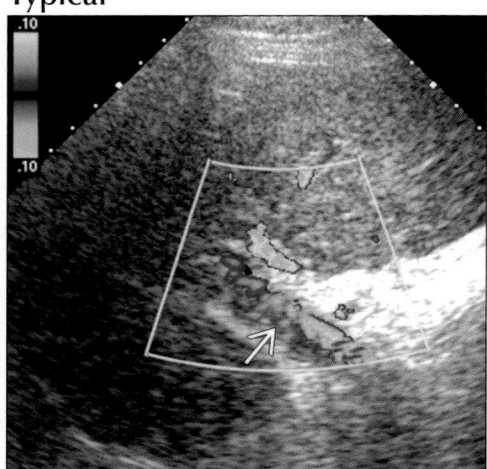 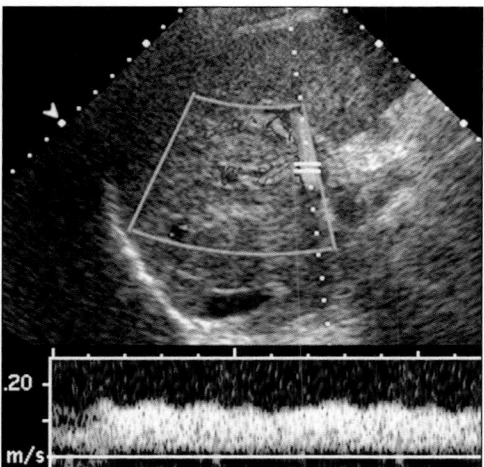

(Left) Oblique color Doppler ultrasound shows non-occlusive portal vein thrombus ➡. *(Right)* Oblique pulsed Doppler ultrasound in the same patient as previous image shows patency of the right portal branch with normal flow velocity, indicating that portal vein thrombus was not substantially occlusive. Left portal branch (not shown) also had substantial flow.

Typical

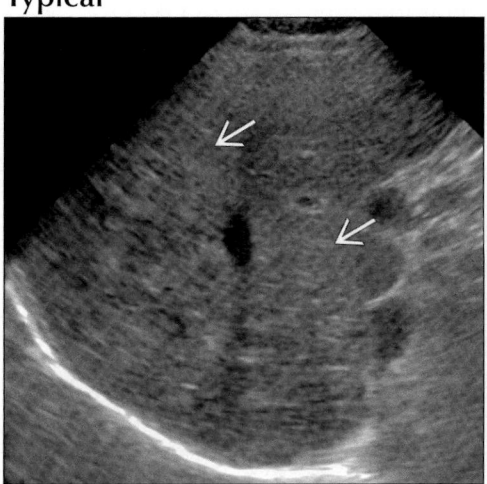 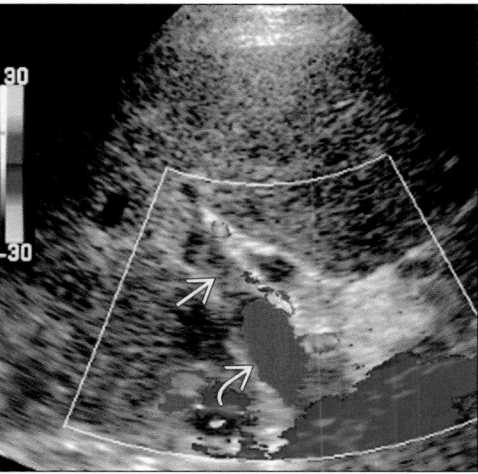

(Left) Longitudinal ultrasound shows abnormal, heterogeneous hepatic architecture ➡ in a large portion of the right hepatic lobe due to infiltrating hepatocellular carcinoma. *(Right)* Oblique color Doppler ultrasound in the same patient as previous image shows coarse echogenic tumor ➡ in the right portal branch. The main portal vein ➡ is patent. Findings were confirmed with MR.

BUDD-CHIARI SYNDROME

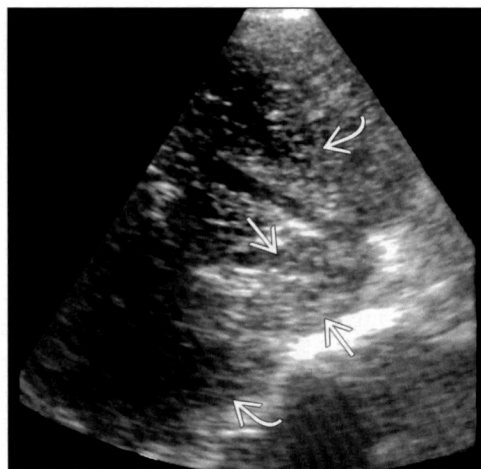

Transverse ultrasound shows echogenic material filling the IVC ➡. Hepatic parenchyma is hypoechoic peripherally ➢ due to edema.

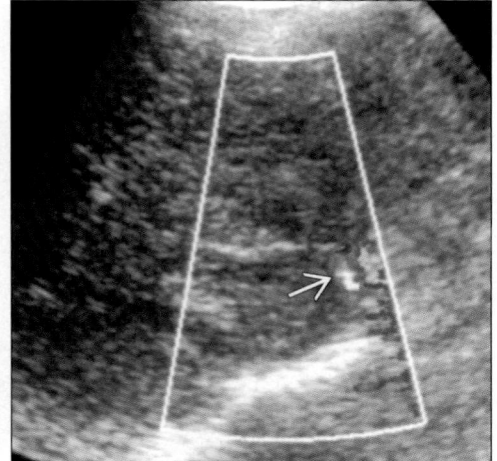

Transverse color Doppler ultrasound in nearly same position as previous image, shows small area of blood flow ➡ (color) in periphery of IVC.

TERMINOLOGY

Definitions
- Budd-Chiari: Clinical syndrome caused by obstruction of hepatic venous outflow
  - Abdominal pain
  - Hepatic dysfunction
  - Ascites
  - Lower extremity edema [with inferior vena cava (IVC) obstruction]

IMAGING FINDINGS

General Features
- Best diagnostic clue: Hepatic veins (HVs) or IVC visualized, but without flow on color Doppler examination
- Location: Obstruction may be in hepatic veins, IVC, sinusoidal (parenchymal) veins

Ultrasonographic Findings
- Grayscale Ultrasound
  - **Acute**

- HVs visualized, possibly distended
- HVs/IVC partially or completely filled with low echogenicity material
- Involved parenchyma may be hypoechoic due to edema
  - **Chronic**
    - Findings depend on severity of injury
    - Compensatory hypertrophy of caudate lobe, unaffected segments/lobes
    - Atrophy of involved segments/lobes
    - Regenerative nodules, possibly large
- Color Doppler
  - **Color Doppler acute**
    - Absent or severely restricted flow in HVs/IVC
    - Continuous (non-pulsatile) flow in patent portions of HVs proximal to obstruction
    - Intrahepatic collateralization, "bicolored HVs": Flow in opposite direction in HV branches with a common trunk
    - Reversed flow in patent portions of IVC
    - Reduced velocity, continuous flow in portal vein, possibly hepatofugal flow
    - Possible tiny tumor vessels in HVs/IVC (low resistance arterial flow)

DDx: Budd-Chiari Syndrome

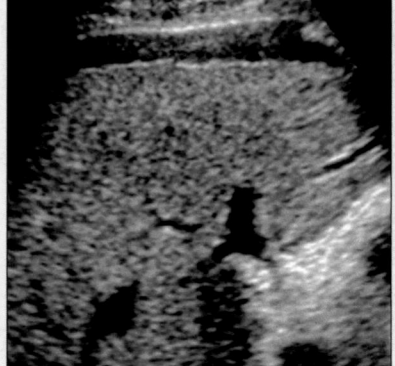

Cirrhosis

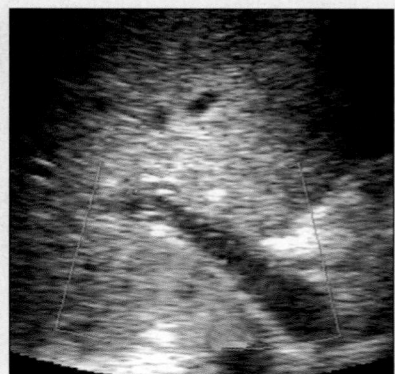

Portal Vein Thrombosis

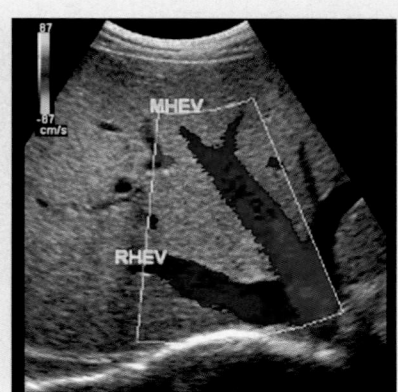

Passive Venous Congestion

BUDD-CHIARI SYNDROME

Key Facts

Terminology
- Budd-Chiari: Clinical syndrome caused by obstruction of hepatic venous outflow

Imaging Findings
- **Acute**
- HVs visualized, possibly distended
- HVs/IVC partially or completely filled with low echogenicity material
- Involved parenchyma may be hypoechoic due to edema
- **Chronic**
- Compensatory hypertrophy of caudate lobe, unaffected segments/lobes
- Atrophy of involved segments/lobes
- **Color Doppler acute**
- Absent or severely restricted flow in HVs/IVC

- Continuous (non-pulsatile) flow in patent portions of HVs proximal to obstruction
- Intrahepatic collateralization, "bicolored HVs": Flow in opposite direction in HV branches with a common trunk
- Reversed flow in patent portions of IVC
- Reduced velocity, continuous flow in portal vein, possibly hepatofugal flow
- **Color Doppler chronic**
- Stenotic or non-visualized (occluded) HVs/IVC
- Intrahepatic and/or extrahepatic collateralization

Top Differential Diagnoses
- Hepatic Cirrhosis
- Acute, Severe Passive Venous Congestion
- Acute Hepatitis

- ○ Color Doppler chronic
  - Stenotic or non-visualized (occluded) HVs/IVC
  - Intrahepatic and/or extrahepatic collateralization

Other Modality Findings
- Acute CT findings
  - NECT: Stenosis or occlusion of hepatic veins/IVC; hyperdense thrombus; hypodense affected parenchyma, hepatomegaly
  - CECT: Early central enhancement, late peripheral enhancement in affected portions
- Chronic CT findings
  - Obliteration or stenosis of HVs/IVC; atrophy affected segments, collateralization, large regenerative nodules
- MR findings
  - Analogous to CT; high water content affected areas acutely, similar enhancement pattern
- Angiographic findings: Classic "spider web" pattern on wedge hepatic venography

Imaging Recommendations
- Best imaging tool
  - Color Doppler sonography for initial diagnosis/exclusion of Budd-Chiari
  - CECT or MR for comprehensive assessment

DIFFERENTIAL DIAGNOSIS

Hepatic Cirrhosis
- Hypertrophy of caudate lobe and lateral segment of left lobe
- Patent HVs and IVC
- Atrophy of right lobe and medial segment of left lobe
- Porto-systemic collaterals, ascites, splenomegaly
- Regenerative nodules that are usually small in size compared to post HV occlusion nodules

Portal Vein Thrombosis
- Liver dysfunction, ascites, porto-systemic collaterals, splenomegaly
- HVs/IVC patent

Acute, Severe Passive Venous Congestion
- Usually congestive heart failure: Hepatic congestion/enlargement
- Ascites: HV, IVC dilated, but patent

Acute Hepatitis
- Hepatomegaly, liver dysfunction, +/- ascites; HVs and IVC patent

PATHOLOGY

General Features
- Etiology
  - Thrombotic occlusion of HVs or IVC
    - Cirrhosis-related (immediate cause uncertain)
    - Hypercoagulable states dehydration/shock/sepsis
  - HV/IVC tumor propagation
    - Hepatocellular carcinoma (most common); also cholangiocarcinoma and rarely metastases
    - Rare primary angiosarcoma of IVC
  - Extrinsic HV/IVC compression (stasis and/or thrombosis)
    - Budd-Chiari due to stasis, possibly > thrombosis
    - Hepatocellular carcinoma, hepatic metastasis, adrenal tumor, adenopathy
  - Centrilobular HV obstruction
    - Obstruction of tiny centrilobular veins ("hepatic veno-occlusive disease")
    - Etiology: Bone marrow transplantation, antineoplastic drugs, radiation therapy
  - "Congenital-membranous" IVC obstruction
    - Etiology is unclear: Congenital, injury, infection all hypothesized
    - Tapered or membrane-like IVC obstruction
    - May present in adulthood; "congenital" questioned
    - Japan, India, Israel, South Africa

Gross Pathologic & Surgical Features
- Acute phase

BUDD-CHIARI SYNDROME

- ○ Acute findings due to venous outflow obstruction > hepatic congestion
- ○ Chronic findings due to ischemia, necrosis, regeneration
- • Chronic phase
  - ○ Liver: Nodular, shrunken, may be cirrhotic
  - ○ Atrophy of affected lobes and hypertrophy of caudate lobe

Microscopic Features
- • Acute: Centrilobular congestion, dilated sinusoids
- • Chronic: Fibrosis, necrosis and cell atrophy

CLINICAL ISSUES

Presentation
- • Most common signs/symptoms
  - ○ Classical acute Budd-Chiari presentation
    - ▪ Rapid onset of abdominal pain, liver tenderness, hepatic dysfunction
    - ▪ Possible abdominal distention from ascites, hypotension
    - ▪ Acute signs/symptoms are variable: Depend on rapidity of obstructive process, extent of HV involvement, severity of obstruction, collateralization
  - ○ Chronic signs/symptoms
    - ▪ RUQ pain, hepatomegaly, hepatic dysfunction
    - ▪ Splenomegaly, ascites, varicosities
- • Other signs/symptoms: Acute or chronic lower extremity edema, if IVC obstructed

Demographics
- • Age: Any group
- • Gender: Females more than males

Natural History & Prognosis
- • Complications
  - ○ Acute: Liver failure, shock, pulmonary embolization from IVC
  - ○ Chronic
    - ▪ Regeneration/liver dysfunction/failure: Portal hypertension/variceal bleeding/cirrhosis
  - ○ Congenital-membranous IVC obstruction
    - ▪ Complicated by hepatocellular carcinoma in 20-40% of cases in Japan & South Africa
- • Prognosis
  - ○ Variable; depends on etiology, extent of liver damage, collateralization, HV revascularization
    - ▪ Mild and moderate venous obstruction: Good prognosis
    - ▪ Severe, extensive venous obstruction: Poor prognosis
    - ▪ Neoplastic obstruction: Usually fatal
    - ▪ Centrilobular obstruction; variable prognosis: Mild with complete recovery to fulminant hepatic failure and death

Treatment
- • Medical management
  - ○ Anticoagulation, steroids, nutritional therapy
- • Transjugular intrahepatic portosystemic shunt (TIPS)
  - ○ Ameliorates intractable ascites

- ○ Controls intractable, recurrent gastrointestinal hemorrhage
- • Congenital-membranous IVC occlusion
  - ○ Balloon angioplasty, stent insertion
- • Liver transplantation, controversial

DIAGNOSTIC CHECKLIST

Image Interpretation Pearls
- • Classical finding: Flow in opposite directions in hepatic vein branches from a common trunk = intrahepatic collateralization

SELECTED REFERENCES

1. Bargallo X et al: Sonography of Budd-Chiari syndrome. AJR Am J Roentgenol. 187(1):W33-41, 2006
2. Camera L et al: Triphasic helical CT in Budd-Chiari syndrome: patterns of enhancement in acute, subacute and chronic disease. Clin Radiol. 2006
3. Chaubal N et al: Sonography in Budd-Chiari syndrome. J Ultrasound Med. 25(3):373-9, 2006
4. Zwiebel WJ: Ultrasound assessment of the hepatic vasculature. In: Introduction to Vascular Ultrasonography. 5th ed. Philadelphia, Saunders/Elsevier. 585-611, 2005
5. Brancatelli G et al: Benign regenerative nodules in Budd-Chiari syndrome and other vascular disorders of the liver: radiologic-pathologic and clinical correlation. Radiographics. 22(4):847-62, 2002
6. Noone TC et al: Budd-Chiari syndrome: spectrum of appearances of acute, subacute, and chronic disease with magnetic resonance imaging. J Magn Reson Imaging. 11(1):44-50, 2000
7. Singh V et al: Budd-Chiari syndrome: our experience of 71 patients. J Gastroenterol Hepatol. 15(5):550-4, 2000
8. Vilgrain V et al: Hepatic nodules in Budd-Chiari syndrome: imaging features. Radiology. 210(2):443-50, 1999
9. Cho OK et al: Collateral pathways in Budd-Chiari syndrome: CT and venographic correlation. AJR Am J Roentgenol. 167(5):1163-7, 1996
10. Blum U et al: Budd-Chiari syndrome: technical, hemodynamic, and clinical results of treatment with transjugular intrahepatic portosystemic shunt. Radiology. 197(3):805-11, 1995
11. Kane R et al: Diagnosis of Budd-Chiari syndrome: comparison between sonography and MR angiography. Radiology. 195(1):117-21, 1995
12. Millener P et al: Color Doppler imaging findings in patients with Budd-Chiari syndrome: correlation with venographic findings. AJR Am J Roentgenol. 161(2):307-12, 1993
13. Hommeyer SC et al: Venocclusive disease of the liver: prospective study of US evaluation. Radiology. 184(3):683-6, 1992
14. Ralls PW et al: Budd-Chiari syndrome: detection with color Doppler sonography. AJR Am J Roentgenol. 159(1):113-6, 1992

IMAGE GALLERY

Typical

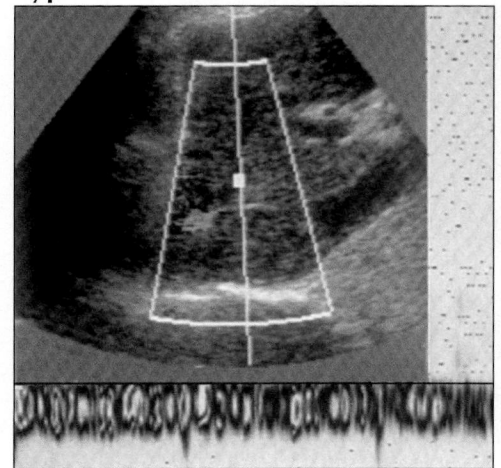

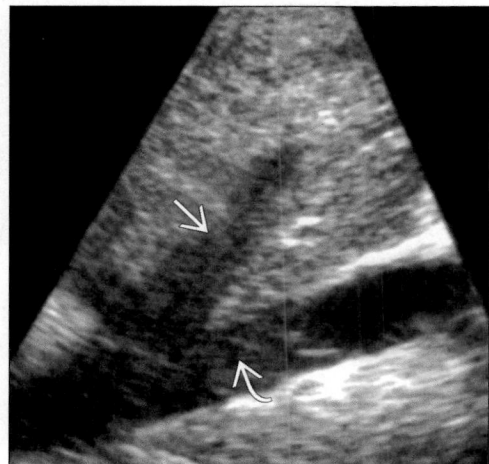

(Left) Transverse color Doppler ultrasound shows continuous venous flow in IVC region. (Right) Longitudinal ultrasound in same patient as previous image more clearly shows echogenic material within right hepatic vein ⇒ and IVC ⇉. Diagnosis: Hepatocellular carcinoma.

Typical

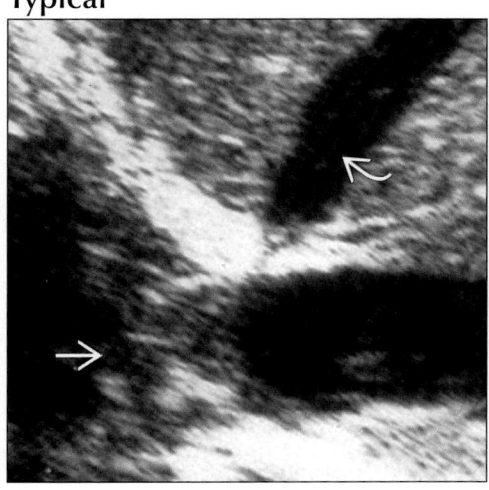

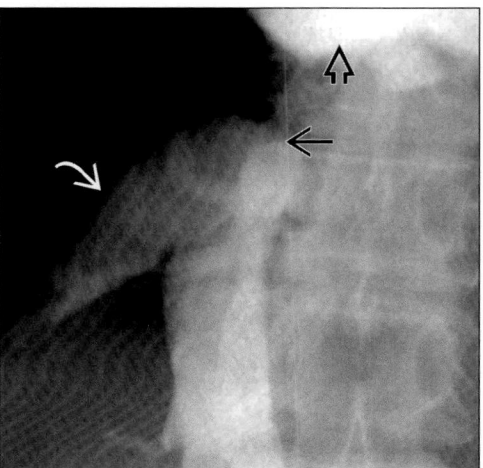

(Left) Longitudinal ultrasound shows echogenic material obstructing the IVC ⇒ at level of diaphragm, with a patent right hepatic vein ⇉. IVC flow reversal was visible in real time. (Right) Longitudinal angiography in same patient as previous image, shows focal IVC occlusion ⇒ and hepatic vein patency ⇉. Right atrium ⇶.

Typical

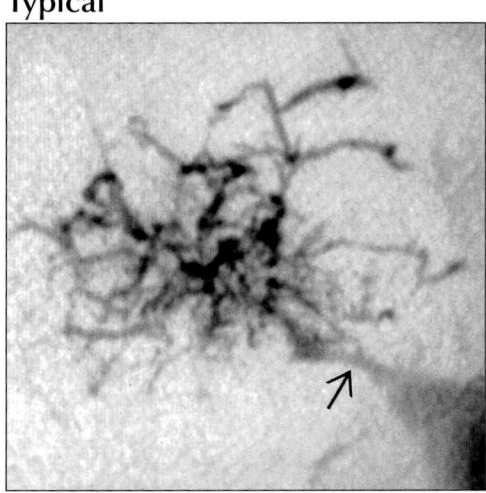

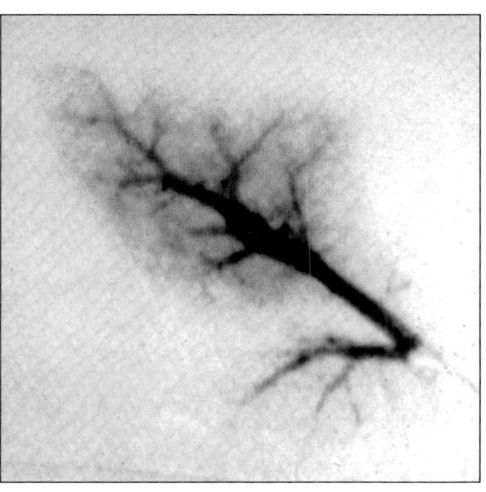

(Left) Oblique angiography shows "spider web" pattern of intrahepatic collateralization caused by hepatic vein obstruction. Note tight hepatic vein stenosis ⇒. (Right) Oblique angiography shows normal hepatic vein arborization for comparison with previous image.

PORTAL VEIN GAS

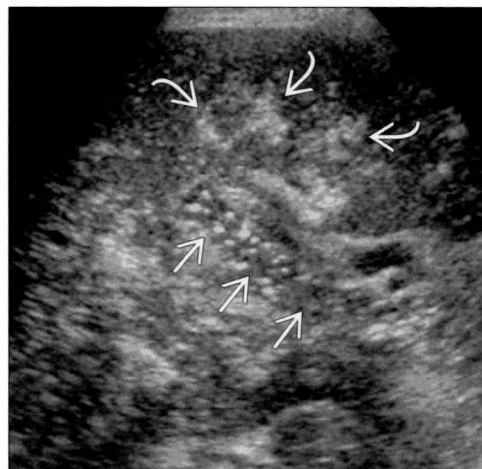

Oblique ultrasound of liver shows innumerable round echogenic foci in portal vein ➡ representing gas bubbles. Brightly echogenic patches ➡ are parenchymal gas.

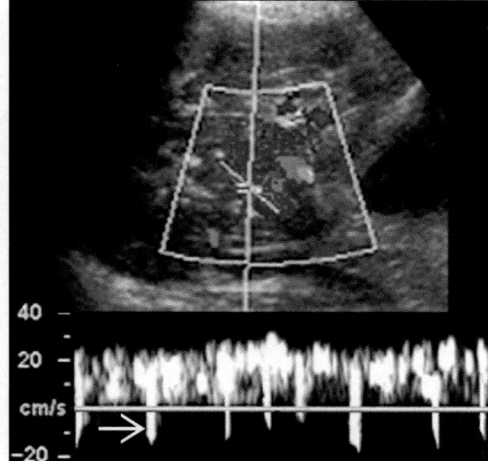

Oblique color Doppler ultrasound shows strong transient signals ➡ superimposed on portal vein waveform, consistent with gas. Most are registered in direction of flow but some are bidirectional.

TERMINOLOGY

Abbreviations and Synonyms
- Portal vein (PV)

Definitions
- Gas within the portal venous system

IMAGING FINDINGS

General Features
- Best diagnostic clue: Bright reflectors in portal veins on grayscale or color Doppler
- Location: Portal venous system, hepatic parenchyma

Ultrasonographic Findings
- Grayscale Ultrasound
  - Highly reflective foci in portal venous system
    - Move along with blood; not fast, not slow
    - Few to numerous, related to amount of gas
  - Poorly defined, highly reflective parenchymal foci
    - Scattered small patches to numerous or large areas
- Pulsed Doppler
  - High intensity transient signals (HITS)
    - Strong, commonly bidirectional spikes superimposed on portal venous flow pattern
    - Pinging sound from audible Doppler output
- Color Doppler
  - Bright reflectors in portal venous system
  - Possibly multicolored (twinkle)

Imaging Recommendations
- Best imaging tool
  - Grayscale or color Doppler for initial detection
  - NECT/CECT to determine source of gas

DIFFERENTIAL DIAGNOSIS

Biliary Tract Gas
- Bright reflections adjacent to, but not in, PV branches
- Central concentration, near porta hepatis
- No parenchymal patches
- Stationary; move only with altered patient position

Parenchymal Abscess
- May produce ill-defined echogenic patch
- Localized, not multifocal

DDx: Portal Vein Gas

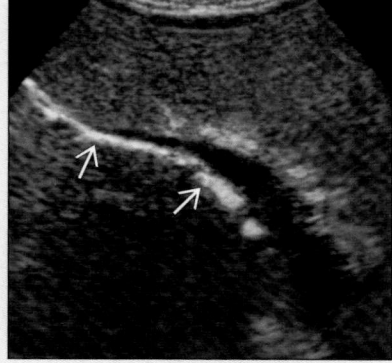

Biliary Tract Gas

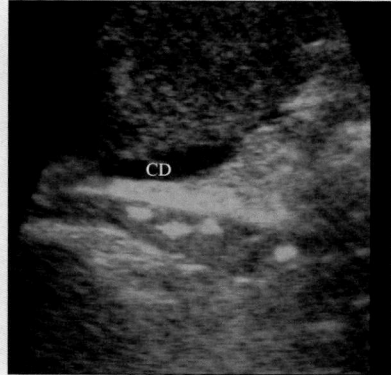

Gallstones in Common Duct (CD)

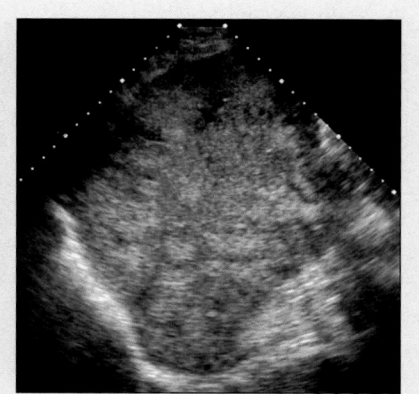

Echogenic Liver Metastases

PORTAL VEIN GAS

Key Facts

Imaging Findings
- Highly reflective foci in portal venous system
- Move along with blood; not fast, not slow
- Poorly defined, highly reflective parenchymal foci
- Scattered small patches to numerous or large areas
- High intensity transient signals (HITS)
- Strong, commonly bidirectional spikes superimposed on portal venous flow pattern
- Bright reflectors in portal venous system

Top Differential Diagnoses
- Biliary Tract Gas
- Parenchymal Abscess
- Biliary Calculi/Parenchymal Calcifications
- Echogenic Hepatic Metastases

Pathology
- Gas under pressure
- Intravasation through injured mucosa
- Gas forming organisms

Biliary Calculi/Parenchymal Calcifications
- Not in portal venous system
- Sharply defined, immobile

Echogenic Hepatic Metastases
- Well defined margins

PATHOLOGY

General Features
- Etiology
  - Three basic gas sources
    - Gas under pressure
    - Intravasation through injured mucosa
    - Gas forming organisms
  - "Benign" causes
    - Bowel distention, especially stomach, colon
    - Inflammatory bowel disease
    - Gastric ulcer
    - Interventions: Endoscopic biopsy, liver mass ablation, gastric tube, post surgery
    - Benign pneumatosis intestinalis: e.g., Emphysema
  - Serious, even life-threatening causes
    - Bacterial colitis/necrotizing enterocolitis
    - Bowel ischemia/infarction (especially colon)
    - Peritoneal space abscess/infected gallbladder/liver abscess
    - Necrotizing pancreatitis
    - Malignancies involving bowel

CLINICAL ISSUES

Presentation
- Most common signs/symptoms: Related to underlying disorder
- Other signs/symptoms: May be asymptomatic

Demographics
- Age: Newborns to adults

Natural History & Prognosis
- Usually sign of serious condition
- Sometimes an inconsequential finding

Treatment
- Related to underlying disorder

SELECTED REFERENCES

1. Chiu HH et al: Hepatic portal venous gas. Am J Surg. 189(4):501-3, 2005
2. Peloponissios N et al: Hepatic portal gas in adults: review of the literature and presentation of a consecutive series of 11 cases. Arch Surg. 138(12):1367-70, 2003
3. Schulze CG et al: Hepatic portal venous gas. Imaging modalities and clinical significance. Acta Radiol. 36(4):377-80, 1995
4. Lafortune M et al: Air in the portal vein: sonographic and Doppler manifestations. Radiology. 180(3):667-70, 1991

IMAGE GALLERY

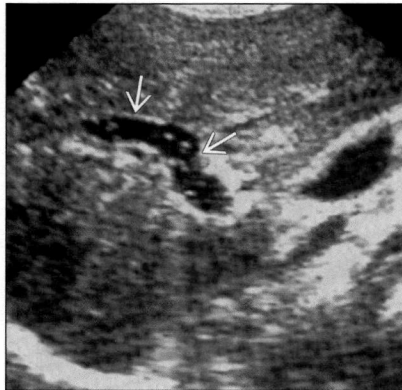 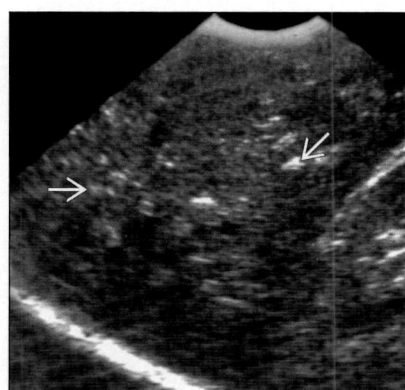 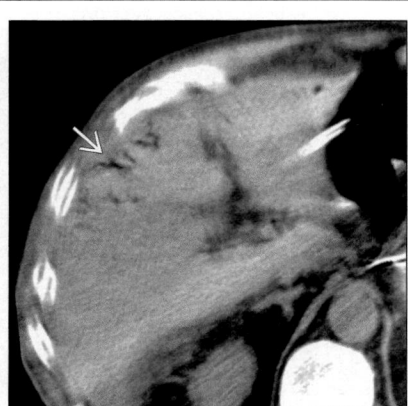

(Left) Oblique ultrasound shows bright dots, representing gas bubbles, within portal vein ➡. *(Center)* Longitudinal ultrasound in same patient as previous image shows bright patches in hepatic parenchyma ➡ due to gas accumulation. *(Right)* Transverse NECT shows gas accumulation in peripheral portal radicles ➡ in a patient with acute mesenteric ischemia.

POST-TRANSPLANT LIVER

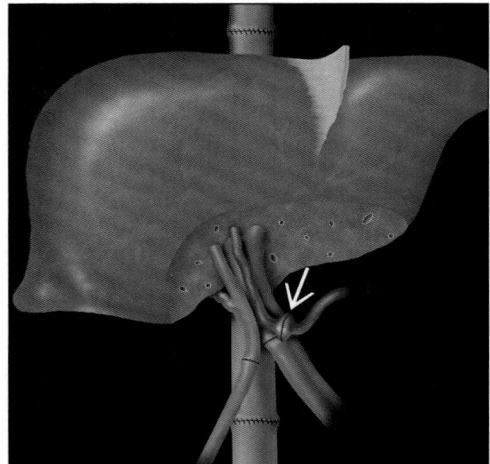

Graphic shows the typical anastomoses in a liver transplant. There are end-to-end anastomoses for the IVC, PV and CBD. The HA is reconstructed creating a "fish-mouth" anastomosis ➡.

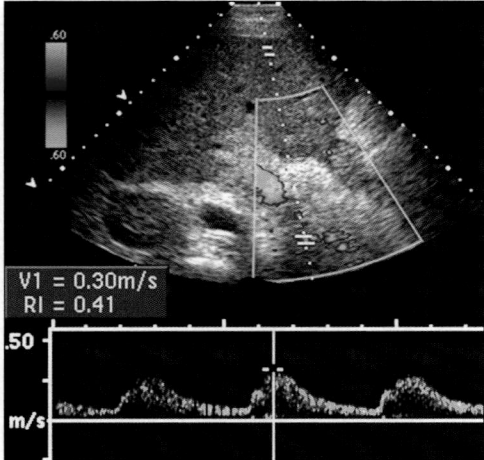

Oblique pulsed Doppler ultrasound two days post-transplant shows damped hepatic arterial Doppler waveforms due to stenosis. Peak systolic velocity is 30 cm/sec. Resistive index 0.41.

TERMINOLOGY

Abbreviations and Synonyms
- Inferior vena cava (IVC)
- Portal vein (PV)
- Hepatic vein (HV)
- Hepatic artery (HA)

Definitions
- Whole liver transplant (cadaver)
  - Included: Intact IVC, PV; HA (possibly with aortic "patch"), bile duct
  - Anastomosis of IVC, PV and bile duct: Usually end-to-end
  - Anastomosis of HA: End-to-end, "fish mouth" to celiac axis, or aortic patch to recipient aorta
- Split liver transplant (cadaver)
  - Right lobe, IVC, PV, HA and bile duct to adult
  - Left lobe to pediatric recipient (complicated PV, HA and bile duct hook-up)
- Living donor transplant
  - Modification of split liver method
  - Right lobe if adult recipient; left lobe if child
  - Complicated PV, HA and bile duct hook-up

IMAGING FINDINGS

General Features
- Best diagnostic clue
  - Vascular flow abnormalities
  - Biliary dilatation
- Size
  - Whole liver: Normal hepatic size
  - Split liver: Smaller, but hypertrophies with time
- Morphology
  - Whole liver: Usual hepatic morphology
  - Split liver: Varies with lobe transplanted

Ultrasonographic Findings
- Grayscale Ultrasound
  - Normally functioning transplant: Same appearance as normal, native liver
  - Hepatic artery pseudoaneurysm
    - Looks like cyst without color
  - Biliary dilatation
    - US detection specific, relatively insensitive
    - Prominent extrahepatic bile duct: Compare size to baseline measurement

---

DDx: Post-Transplant Liver

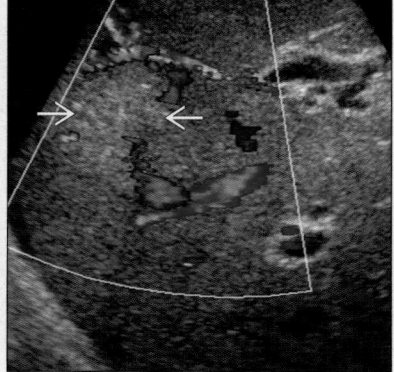

Hepatocellular Carcinoma

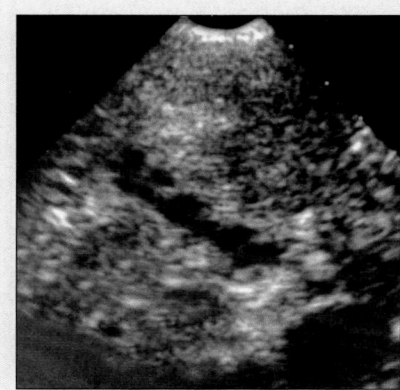

Sclerosing Cholangitis

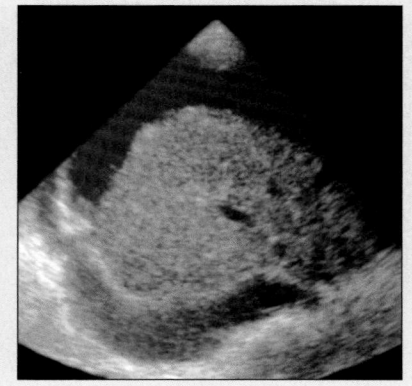

Cirrhosis

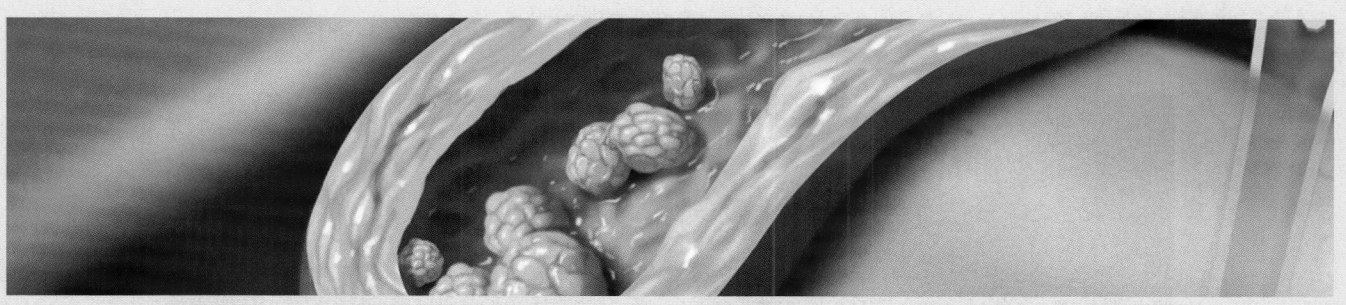

SECTION 2: Biliary System

BILIARY SONOGRAPHY

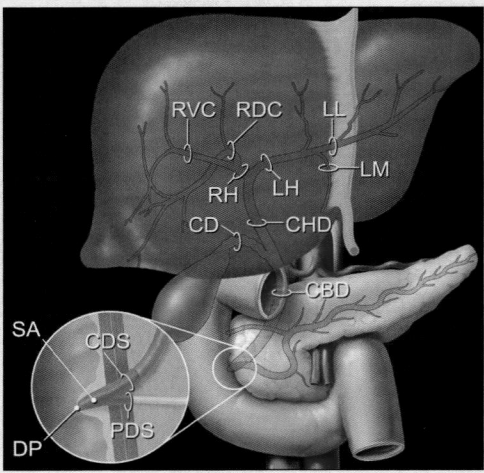

Graphic shows the branching system of the normal biliary tree, with a detailed view of the papilla of Vater. (See text for abbreviation keys).

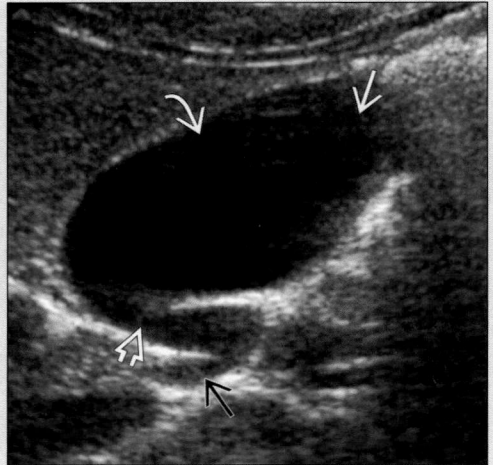

Oblique transabdominal ultrasound shows the normal globular configuration of the GB: Fundus ➡; body ➡; neck ➡ and cystic duct ➡.

TERMINOLOGY

Abbreviations
- Extrahepatic biliary structures
  - Gallbladder (GB)
  - Cystic duct (CD)
  - Right hepatic (RH) and left hepatic (LH) ducts
  - Common hepatic duct (CHD)
  - Common bile duct (CBD)
  - Papilla of Vater, choledochal sphincter (CDS), pancreatic duct sphincter (PDS), sphincter of ampulla (SA), duodenal papilla (DP)
- Intrahepatic duct
  - Right dorsal-caudal (RDC) duct/right posterior duct (RPD)
  - Right ventral-cephalic (RVC) duct/right anterior duct (RAD)
  - Left lateral (LL) duct and left medial (LM) duct

Definitions
- Proximal/distal biliary tree
  - Proximal represents portion of biliary tree that is in relative proximity to liver and hepatocytes
  - Distal refers to caudal end closer to bowel
- Central/peripheral
  - Central denotes biliary ducts close to porta hepatis
  - Peripheral refers to higher order branches of intrahepatic biliary tree extending to hepatic parenchyma

IMAGING ANATOMY

General Anatomic Considerations
- GB is located in GB fossa, an indentation on the undersurface of liver at the junction between left and right lobe of liver
  - Attached to liver by short veins and bile ducts (of Luschka) and covered by parietal peritoneum
  - Divided into fundus, body and neck
  - GB fundus
    - Rounded inferior tip projected below the liver edge
    - "Phrygian cap": Part of GB fundus partially septated and folded upon itself
  - GB body
    - Midportion of GB
    - Often in contact with duodenum and hepatic flexure of colon
  - GB neck
    - Lies between GB body and cystic duct
    - Constant relationship with the main interlobar fissure and undivided right portal vein
- Cystic duct (CD)
  - Variable length; usually 2-4 cm long
  - Contains tortuous spiral folds (valves of Heister)
  - Highly variable point of entry into CHD
    - May join the CHD along its lateral, posterior or medial border
    - May run a parallel course to CHD and insert into lower 1/3 of CBD close to ampulla of Vater
- Common hepatic duct (CHD)
  - Formed by union of right hepatic (RH) and left hepatic (LH) ducts
  - Together with RH and LH ducts: Form the hilar/central portion of extrahepatic bile duct at porta hepatis
- Common bile duct (CBD)
  - Formed by union of CHD and CD
  - Extends caudally within the hepatoduodenal ligament
    - Lying anterior to portal vein and to the right of hepatic artery
  - Passes posterior to first part of duodenum and head of pancreas
  - Usually joins pancreatic duct as a common channel within the duodenal wall
  - Finally drains to second part of duodenum via ampulla of Vater
- Normal branching pattern of biliary tree
  - Division usually in accordance with Couinaud functional anatomy of liver

BILIARY SONOGRAPHY

Key Facts

Imaging Approach
- Transabdominal ultrasound is an ideal initial investigation for suspected biliary tree or GB pathology
- Supplemented by various imaging modalities including MR/MRCP and CT, US plays a key role in the multimodality evaluation of complex biliary problems

Imaging Protocol
- Patient should be fasted for at least 4 hours prior to US examination
- Complete assessment includes evaluating the liver, porta hepatis region and pancreas in sagittal, transverse and oblique views

- Subcostal and right intercostal views to align bile ducts and GB along imaging plane for optimal visualization
- Usually structures are better assessed and imaged with patient in full suspended inspiration and in left lateral oblique position
- Harmonic imaging provides improved contrast between bile ducts and adjacent tissues, leading to improved visualization of bile ducts, its luminal content and wall

Common Indications for US for Biliary and GB Diseases Include
- Right upper quadrant/epigastric pain
- Deranged liver function test or jaundice
- Suspected gallstone disease

- RH duct forms from RAD (drains segments 5 & 8) and RPD (drains segments 6 & 7)
- LH duct forms from LM duct (drains segments 1 & 4) and LL duct (drains segment 2 & 3)
  - This normal pattern occurs in 56-58% of normal population
- Normal variants mainly due to the variability of site of insertion of the RPD
  - RPD extends more to the left and joins the junction of RH and LH ducts (trifurcation pattern): ~ 8%
  - RPD extends more to the left and joins the LH duct: ~ 13%
  - RPD extends in a caudo-medial direction to join the CHD/CBD directly: ~ 5%
- Anomalous drainage of various segmental hepatic ducts directly into CHD is less common
- Normal measurement limits of bile ducts
  - CBD/CHD
    - < 6-7 mm in patients without history of biliary disease in most studies
    - Controversy about dilatation related to previous cholecystectomy and old age
  - Intrahepatic ducts
    - Normal diameter of first and higher order branches < 2 mm or < 40% of the diameter of adjacent portal vein
    - First (i.e., LH duct and RH duct) and second order branches are normally visualized
    - Visualization of third and higher order branches is often abnormal and indicates dilatation

ANATOMY-BASED IMAGING ISSUES

Imaging Approaches
- Transabdominal ultrasound is an ideal initial investigation for suspected biliary tree or GB pathology
  - Cystic nature of bile ducts and GB, especially if these are dilated, provides an inherently high contrast resolution

- Acoustic window provided by liver and modern state-of-art ultrasound technology provides good spatial resolution
- Common indications of US for biliary and GB diseases include
  - Right upper quadrant/epigastric pain
  - Deranged liver function test or jaundice
  - Suspected gallstone disease
- Supplemented by various imaging modalities including MR/MRCP and CT
- US plays a key role in the multimodality evaluation of complex biliary problems

Imaging Protocols
- Patient should be fasted for at least 4 hours prior to US examination
  - Ensure GB is not contracted after meal
- Complete assessment includes scanning the liver, porta hepatis region and pancreas in sagittal, transverse and oblique views
- Subcostal and right intercostal views to align bile ducts and GB along imaging plane for optimal visualization
- Usually structures are better assessed and imaged with patient in full suspended inspiration and in left lateral oblique position
- Harmonic imaging provides improved contrast between bile ducts and adjacent tissues, leading to improved visualization of bile ducts, its luminal content and wall
- For imaging of gallstone disease, special maneuvers are recommended
  - Move patient from supine to left lateral decubitus position
    - Demonstrates mobility of gallstones
    - Gravitates small gallstones together to appreciate posterior acoustic shadowing
  - Set the focal zone at the level of gallstone
    - Maximizes the effect of posterior acoustic shadowing

Imaging Pitfalls
- Common pitfalls in US evaluation of GB

BILIARY SONOGRAPHY

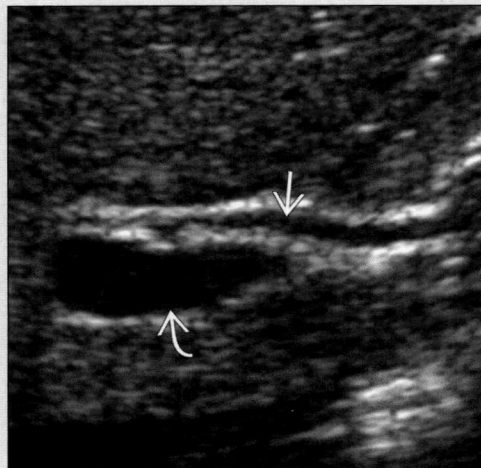

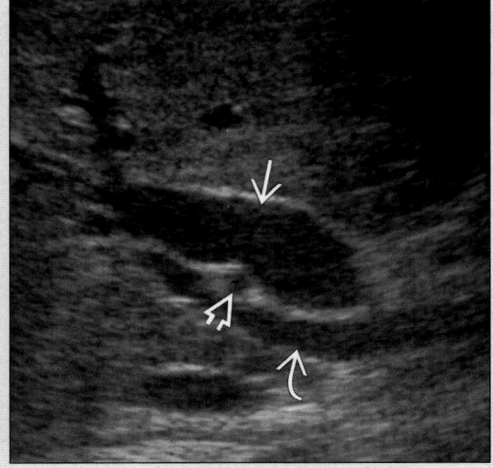

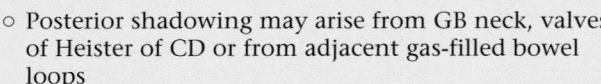

Oblique transabdominal ultrasound shows the normal position and size of the CBD ➡ relative to the main portal vein (MPV) ↗. The CBD is anterior to and of smaller caliber than the MPV.

Oblique transabdominal ultrasound shows the normal anatomical relationship of the CBD ➡ anterior to MPV ↗ and hepatic artery ↘ at the porta hepatis. The CBD is dilated due to distal obstruction.

- ○ Posterior shadowing may arise from GB neck, valves of Heister of CD or from adjacent gas-filled bowel loops
  - ▪ Mimics cholelithiasis
  - ▪ Scan after repositioning patient in prone or left lateral decubitus positions
- ○ Food material within gastric antrum/duodenum
  - ▪ Mimics GB filled with gallstones or GB containing milk-of-calcium
  - ▪ On real time, carefully evaluate peristaltic activity of involved bowel ± oral administration of water
- ○ Presence of slice-thickness or side-lobe artifacts
  - ▪ May mimic intraluminal, dependent, low level echoes within GB
  - ▪ Minimize by changing US settings and scanning after repositioning patient
- • Common pitfalls in US evaluation of biliary tree
  - ○ Redundancy, elongation or folding of GB neck on itself
    - ▪ Mimics dilatation of CHD or proximal CBD
    - ▪ Avoided by scanning patient in full suspended inspiration
    - ▪ Careful real-time scanning allows separate visualization of CHD/CBD medial to GB neck
  - ○ Presence of gas-filled bowel loops adjacent to distal extrahepatic bile ducts
    - ▪ Obscure distal biliary tree and render detection of choledocholithiasis difficult
    - ▪ Scan with patient in decubitus positions or after oral intake of water
  - ○ Gas/particulate material in adjacent duodenum and pancreatic calcification
    - ▪ Mimic choledocholithiasis within CBD
  - ○ Presence of gas within biliary tree
    - ▪ May mimic choledocholithiasis, differentiated by presence of reverberation artifacts
    - ▪ Limits US detection of biliary calculus

CLINICAL IMPLICATIONS

Clinical Importance
- • In patients with obstructive jaundice, US plays a key role
  - ○ Differentiates biliary obstruction from liver parenchymal disease
  - ○ Determines the presence, level and cause of biliary obstruction
- • Level and causes of biliary obstruction
  - ○ Intrahepatic causes
    - ▪ Primary sclerosing cholangitis
    - ▪ Liver mass with extrinsic compression of bile ducts
  - ○ Porta hepatis/hepatic confluence
    - ▪ Cholangiocarcinoma
    - ▪ Choledocholithiasis
    - ▪ Primary sclerosing cholangitis
    - ▪ GB carcinoma
  - ○ Distal extrahepatic/intrapancreatic
    - ▪ Pancreatic ductal carcinoma
    - ▪ Cholangiocarcinoma
    - ▪ Chronic/acute pancreatitis
    - ▪ Choledocholithiasis in CBD
    - ▪ Ampullary tumor/stricture
- • Criteria for malignant obstruction
  - ○ Abrupt transition from dilatation to narrowing
  - ○ Eccentric ductal wall thickening with contour irregularity
  - ○ Mass in or around duct
  - ○ Presence of enlarged regional lymph nodes, liver metastases or vascular invasion

RELATED REFERENCES

1.   Khalili K et al: Diagnostic ultrasound. 3rd ed. Elsevier Mosby, St. Louis. 171-212, 2005
2.   Koeller KK et al: Radiologic pathology. 2nd ed. Armed Forces Institute of Pathology, Washington DC, 2003

IMAGE GALLERY

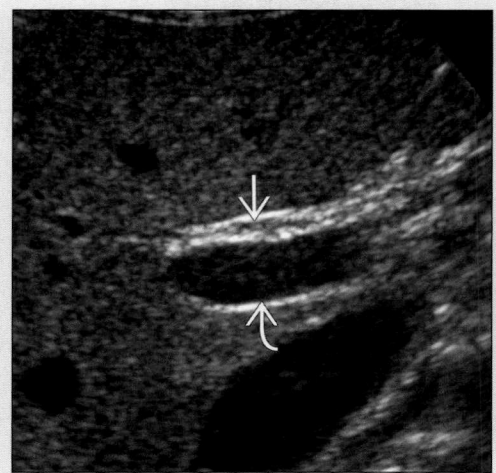

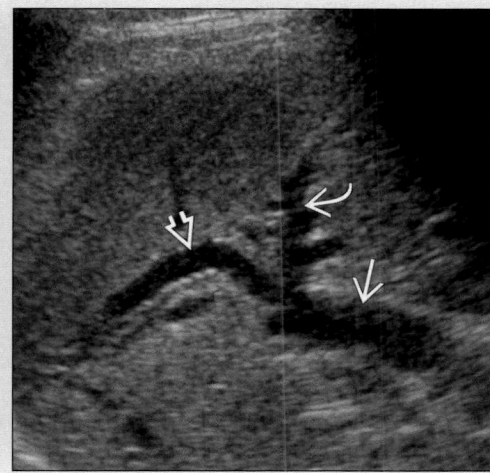

(Left) Oblique transabdominal ultrasound shows the normal position of the RH duct ➡ anterior to the right portal vein (RPV) ➡. Caliber of the RH duct is normally smaller than that of the RPV. *(Right)* Oblique transabdominal ultrasound shows branching of the RH duct ➡ into the RAD ➡ and RPD ➡. All of them are dilated due to an obstructing CBD stone.

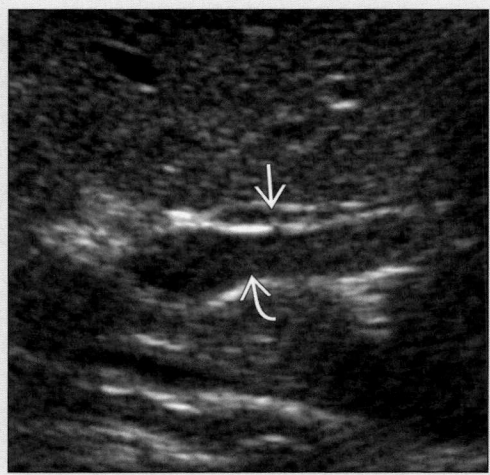

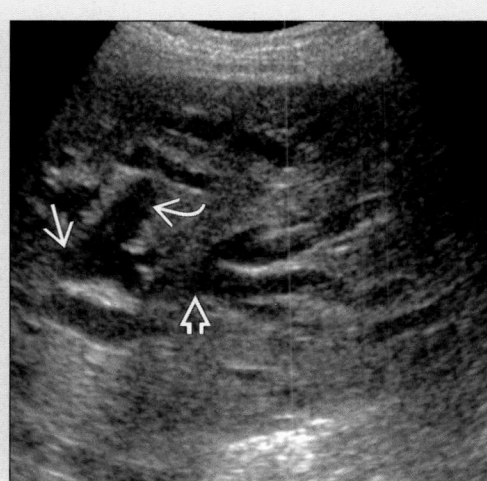

(Left) Transverse transabdominal ultrasound shows the normal position of the LH duct ➡ anterior to the left portal vein (LPV) ➡. A non-dilated LH duct is smaller than LPV. *(Right)* Transverse transabdominal ultrasound shows branching of the LH duct ➡ into the LM duct ➡ and the LL duct ➡. These are markedly dilated due to distal extrahepatic obstruction.

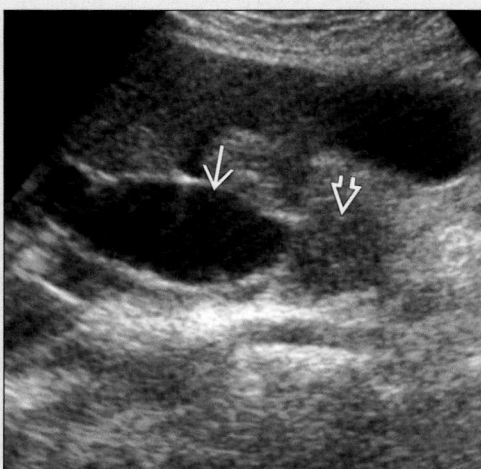

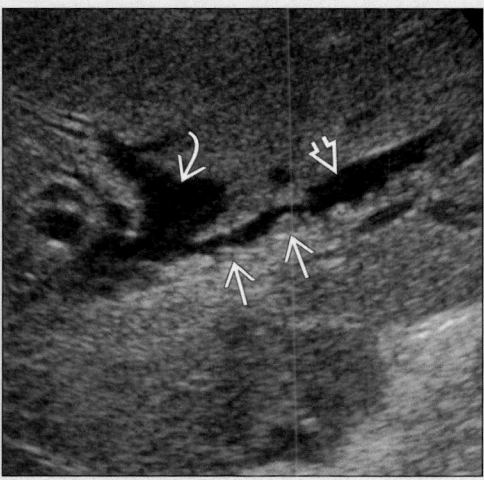

(Left) Oblique transabdominal ultrasound shows abrupt truncation of a dilated CBD ➡ by an obstructing ductal carcinoma ➡ at the pancreatic head. *(Right)* Transverse transabdominal ultrasound shows presence of echogenic biliary sludge ➡ within a dilated LL duct ➡ and its branches. Note the LM duct ➡ is also dilated but free of sludge.

CHOLELITHIASIS

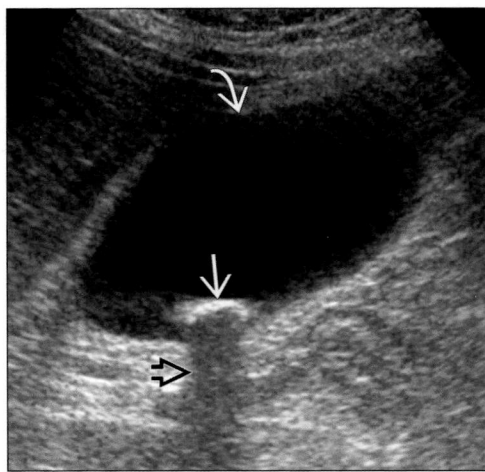

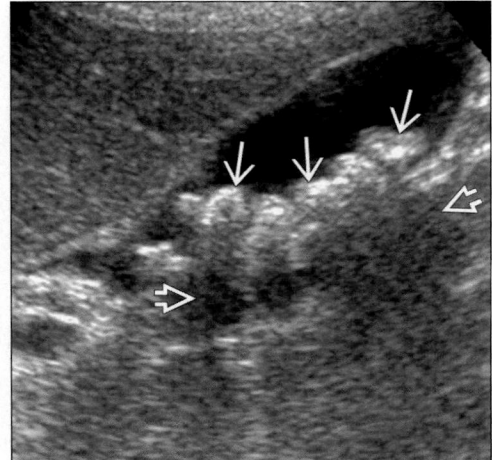

Oblique transabdominal ultrasound shows an echogenic focus ➡ casting marked posterior acoustic shadowing ⧁ within the dependent position of a non-distended gallbladder ➡.

Oblique transabdominal ultrasound shows multiple echogenic foci ➡ within the gallbladder representing gallstones. Note the posterior acoustic shadow ⧁.

TERMINOLOGY

Abbreviations and Synonyms
- Gallstone, cholecystolithiasis

IMAGING FINDINGS

General Features
- Best diagnostic clue
  - Ultrasound of gallbladder (GB)
    - Highly reflective echoes
    - Posterior acoustic shadowing
    - Mobile on changing patient's position
- Location: Gallbladder
- Size: Variable

Ultrasonographic Findings
- Grayscale Ultrasound
  - High reflective echogenic focus within gallbladder lumen
  - Prominent posterior acoustic shadow
  - Gravity dependent movement on change of patient position

  - Reverberation artifact
  - Variant ultrasound features
    - Non-visualization of gallbladder with large collection of bright echoes with acoustic shadowing (GB packed with stones), may be mistaken for duodenal bulb
    - Double-arc shadow sign or wall-echo-shadow (WES) sign: Two echogenic curvilinear lines separated by sonolucent line (anterior GB wall, bile, stone)
    - Non-shadowing gallstone (stone < 5 mm in size)
    - Immobile adherent stone or impacted in GB neck
  - Associated ultrasound findings if superimposed complications
    - Acute cholecystitis: Thick walled and distended gallbladder, positive sonographic Murphy sign, pericholecystic fluid
    - Acute cholangitis: Obstructing common bile duct (CBD) stones, biliary dilatation
    - Acute pancreatitis: Ill-defined swelling of pancreatic parenchyma, inflammatory change in adjacent soft tissue
    - Biliary fistula
    - Gallstone ileus

DDx: Cholelithiasis

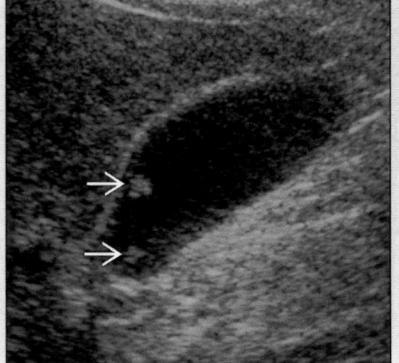

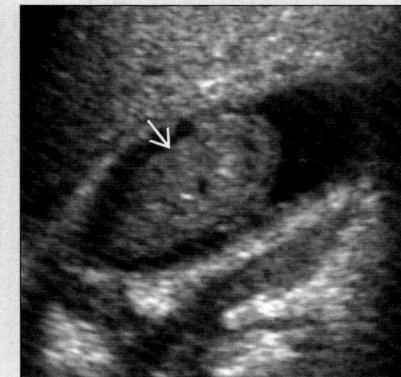

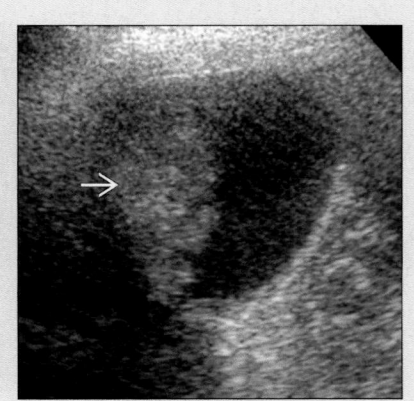

Gallbladder Polyp

Sludge Ball

Gallbladder Carcinoma

CHOLELITHIASIS

Key Facts

Terminology
- Gallstone, cholecystolithiasis

Imaging Findings
- High reflective echogenic focus within gallbladder lumen
- Prominent posterior acoustic shadow
- Gravity dependent movement on change of patient position
- False negative ultrasound: Small contracted GB full of stones, small gallstones, GB in ectopic/unusual position, obese/uncooperative patient
- Examine patient in supine and left decubitus/oblique position to demonstrate mobility of gallstone
- In supine position stones are highly likely to be found in GB neck and in the left decubitus position they gravitate towards the fundus

- Always evaluate for signs of cholecystitis, cholangitis or pancreatitis

Top Differential Diagnoses
- Gallbladder Polyp
- Gallbladder Sludge
- Gallbladder Carcinoma

Diagnostic Checklist
- Ultrasound is the best imaging tool for evaluation of patients with upper abdominal pain/discomfort
- Consider cholelithiasis in patients with RUQ pain/discomfort after fatty meal, especially in obese middle-age female

---

- Power Doppler
  - No color flow demonstrated
  - "Twinkling" artifact
  - Increased flow in pericholecystic region in cholelithiasis complicated by acute cholecystitis
- False negative ultrasound: Small contracted GB full of stones, small gallstones, GB in ectopic/unusual position, obese/uncooperative patient

Radiographic Findings
- Radiography
  - Radio-opaque in 10-20%
    - Cholesterol stone: Only about 5% radio-opaque
    - Pigmented stone: About 50% radio-opaque
  - Laminated appearances
  - Faceted outline
  - Mercedes-Benz sign: Radio-opaque outline with lucent center

CT Findings
- NECT
  - Calcified gallstones are hyperdense to bile
  - Pure cholesterol stone is hypodense
    - There is an inverse relationship between cholesterol content and CT attenuation
  - Some gallstones may be isodense to bile and may be missed by CT

Non-Vascular Interventions
- ERCP
  - Mobile filling defects inside contrast-filled gallbladder
  - +/- Stones in extra-hepatic bile ducts

MR Findings
- T2WI: Small focus of signal void or low signal outlined by markedly hyperintense bile within gallbladder
- MRCP: Focus of signal void inside gallbladder

Other Modality Findings
- Oral cholecystogram
  - Filling defects within contrast-filled gallbladder
  - Shows contracted GB after fatty meal
  - Shows cystic duct patency

Nuclear Medicine Findings
- Hepatobiliary Scintigraphy
  - Tracer activity demonstrated in gallbladder
    - Except in stone impaction or obstruction at cystic duct
  - Free tracer excretion and drainage to small bowel

Imaging Recommendations
- Best imaging tool: Ultrasound
- Protocol advice
  - Transabdominal ultrasound
    - Examine patient in supine and left decubitus/oblique position to demonstrate mobility of gallstone
    - In supine position stones are highly likely to be found in GB neck and in the left decubitus position they gravitate towards the fundus
    - Set depth of focal zone and time-gain compensation curve to maximize visualization of posterior acoustic shadowing
    - Always evaluate for signs of cholecystitis, cholangitis or pancreatitis

DIFFERENTIAL DIAGNOSIS

Gallbladder Polyp
- Small round mass with smooth contour arising from gallbladder wall
- Low/medium echogenicity, usually multiple
- Not mobile, may have a short stalk or may be sessile
- No posterior acoustic shadowing
- Normal GB wall

Gallbladder Sludge
- Mass in gallbladder lumen, sludge ball
- Low/medium echogenicity
- Mobile
- Lack of posterior acoustic shadowing
- Fluid-sludge level

Gallbladder Carcinoma
- Ill-defined mass from gallbladder wall

- Infiltrates adjacent liver parenchyma
- Not mobile
- Increased vascularity within the lesion on color Doppler
- Associated lymphadenopathy

Focal Adenomyomatosis
- Focal wall thickening due to hypertrophied Rokitansky-Aschoff sinuses
- Gallbladder fundus
- Reverberation/comet-tail artifacts due to co-existent cholesterol deposits

Parasite Infestation in Gallbladder
- Tubular configuration
- Double parallel echogenic lines
- Active movement in viable worm, gravity dependent movement in dead worm

PATHOLOGY

General Features
- Genetics: Familial in some racial groups: Navaho, Pima, Chippewa Indians
- Etiology
  - Hemolytic diseases: Sickle cell disease, thalassemia, hereditary spherocytosis
  - Metabolic disorders: Obesity, cystic fibrosis, diabetes mellitus, pancreatic diseases, hyperlipidemia
  - Cholestasis: Biliary tree malformation such as choledochal cyst, Caroli disease
  - Intestinal malabsorption: Crohn disease, bypass surgery, ileal resection
  - Genetic predisposition
- Epidemiology: 10% of population, most common in obese female in their forties

Gross Pathologic & Surgical Features
- Three types according to stone composition
  - Cholesterol stone, main component of most calculi containing < 25% cholesterol by definition
  - Pigmented stone
  - Mixed stone: Mixture of cholesterol and calcium carbonate/bilirubinate as main composition

Microscopic Features
- Various degree of acute/chronic inflammatory changes within gallbladder wall

CLINICAL ISSUES

Presentation
- Most common signs/symptoms: Right upper quadrant (RUQ) pain/discomfort after fatty meal
- Other signs/symptoms
  - Asymptomatic, incidental finding on imaging
  - Biliary colic
  - Present with complications including acute cholecystitis, cholangitis, pancreatitis, gallstone ileus or cancer of gallbladder

Demographics
- Age: Peak: 5th to 6th decade

- Gender: M:F = 1:3
- Gallstones are rare in neonates without predisposing causes such as obstructive congenital biliary lesion, dehydration, infection, hemolytic anemia
- Gallstones in older children are associated with sickle cell disease, cystic fibrosis, hemolytic anemia, Crohn disease

Natural History & Prognosis
- May remain asymptomatic all along
- On and off symptom if left untreated
- Excellent prognosis unless complication occur

Treatment
- Conservative management if asymptomatic
- If symptomatic, consider laparoscopic/open cholecystectomy or extracorporeal shock wave lithotripsy (ESWL)

DIAGNOSTIC CHECKLIST

Consider
- Ultrasound is the best imaging tool for evaluation of patients with upper abdominal pain/discomfort
- Consider cholelithiasis in patients with RUQ pain/discomfort after fatty meal, especially in obese middle-age female

Image Interpretation Pearls
- Nonshadowing calculi may be mistaken for other lesions in GB such as polyp, sludge, carcinoma
- Important to demonstrate posterior acoustic shadowing and mobility on changing patient's position

SELECTED REFERENCES

1. Bellows CF et al: Management of gallstones. Am Fam Physician. 72(4):637-42, 2005
2. Guraya SY: Reappraisal of the management of cholelithiasis in diabetics. Saudi Med J. 26(11):1691-4, 2005
3. Palazzo L et al: Biliary stones: including acute biliary pancreatitis. Gastrointest Endosc Clin N Am. 15(1):63-82, viii, 2005
4. Hanbidge AE et al: From the RSNA refresher courses: imaging evaluation for acute pain in the right upper quadrant. Radiographics. 24(4):1117-35, 2004
5. Gandolfi L et al: The role of ultrasound in biliary and pancreatic diseases. Eur J Ultrasound. 16(3):141-59, 2003
6. Adusumilli S et al: MR imaging of the gallbladder. Magn Reson Imaging Clin N Am. 10(1):165-84, 2002
7. Baron RL et al: Imaging the spectrum of biliary tract disease. Radiol Clin North Am. 40(6):1325-54, 2002
8. Bar-Meir S: Gallstones: prevalence, diagnosis and treatment. Isr Med Assoc J. 3(2):111-3, 2001
9. Kalloo AN et al: Gallstones and biliary disease. Prim Care. 28(3):591-606, vii, 2001
10. Kratzer W et al: Prevalence of gallstones in sonographic surveys worldwide. J Clin Ultrasound. 27(1):1-7, 1999
11. Chan FL et al: Modern imaging in the evaluation of hepatolithiasis. Hepatogastroenterology. 44(14):358-69, 1997
12. Leung JW et al: Hepatolithiasis and biliary parasites. Baillieres Clin Gastroenterol. 11(4):681-706, 1997

CHOLELITHIASIS

IMAGE GALLERY

Typical

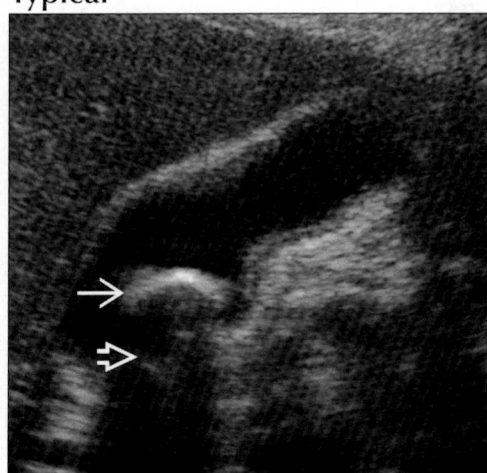 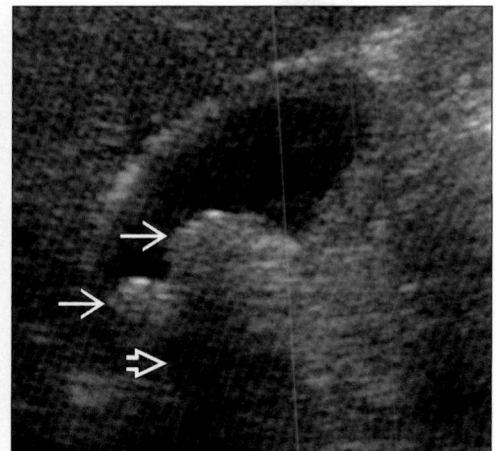

(Left) Oblique transabdominal ultrasound shows an echogenic focus ➡ within the dependent part of the gallbladder lumen casting marked posterior acoustic shadowing ➡. (Right) Oblique transabdominal ultrasound shows multiple calcified gallstones ➡, which are echogenic and gravitate to the dependent part of the gallbladder casting posterior acoustic shadow ➡.

Typical

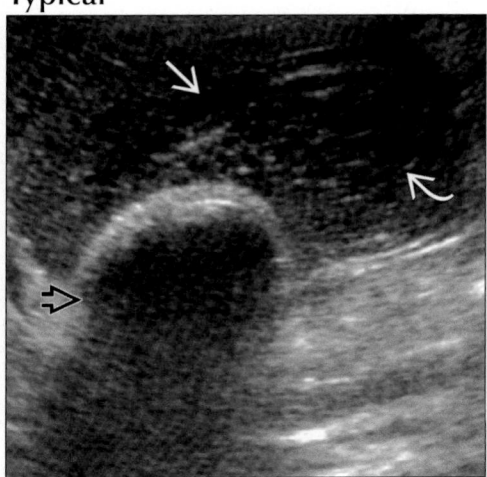 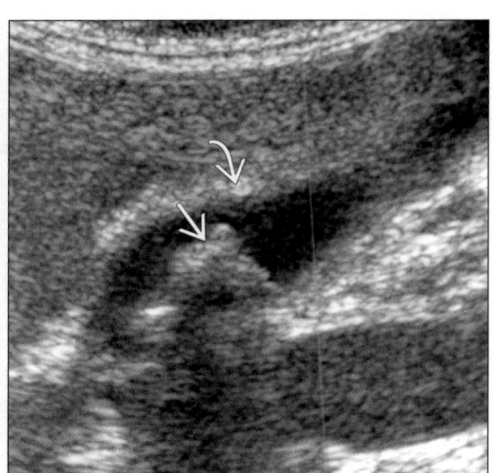

(Left) Oblique transabdominal ultrasound shows a gallstone ➡, associated inflamed and thickened GB wall ➡, and sludge ➡ in the GB lumen. Features are suggestive of calculus cholecystitis. (Right) Oblique transabdominal ultrasound shows a large gallstone ➡ inside a contracted gallbladder with wall thickening ➡ consistent with chronic cholecystitis.

Variant

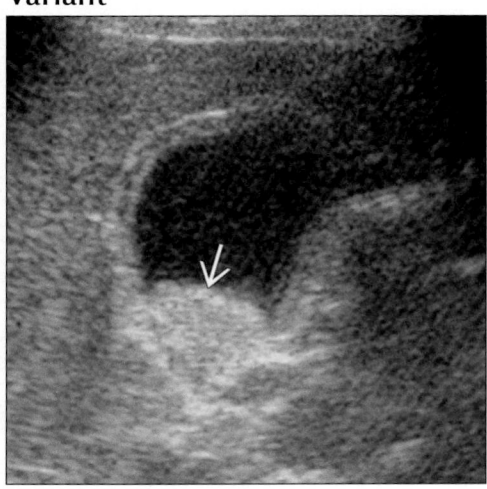 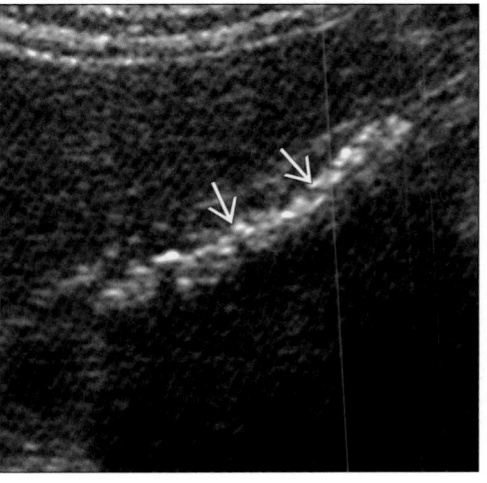

(Left) Oblique transabdominal ultrasound shows a large echogenic gallstone ➡ in the dependent part of the gallbladder. Note the absence of posterior acoustic shadowing. Color Doppler would be important in this case to rule out mass. (Right) Oblique transabdominal ultrasound shows a gallbladder packed with small shadowing echogenic stones ➡. This may sometimes be mistaken for gas in the duodenal bulb.

CHOLELITHIASIS

(Left) Abdominal radiograph showing a large, well-defined calcified ➡ opacity in the RUQ. Ultrasound confirmed this to be a gallstone. *(Right)* Transverse NECT shows a large stone ➡ occupying the whole GB lumen. Note the whorled internal pattern of the stone.

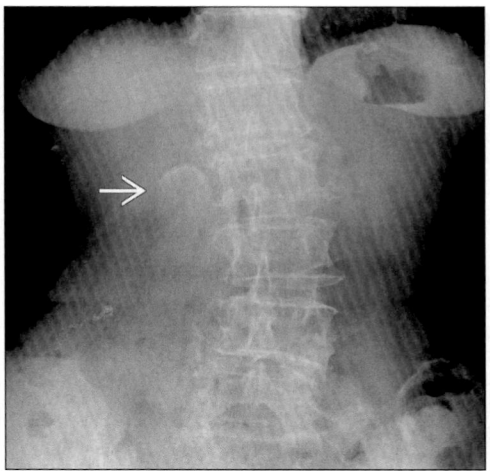
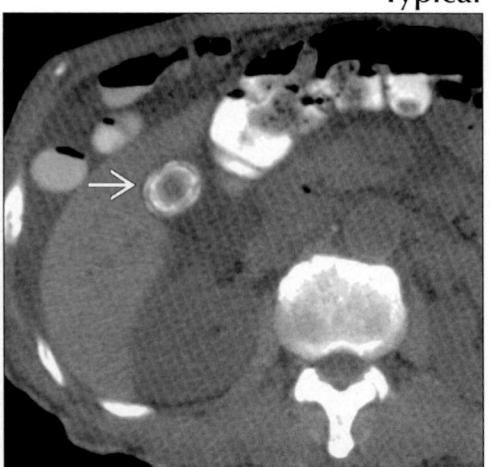

(Left) Transverse NECT shows multiple, incidental gallstones ➡. The GB wall appears normal ➡. Note the right adrenal lesion ➡ for which the CT was performed. *(Right)* Transverse CECT shows multiple incidental gallstones ➡. Note the wedge-shaped perfusion defect noted in the right lobe of liver ➡ for which the CT was performed.

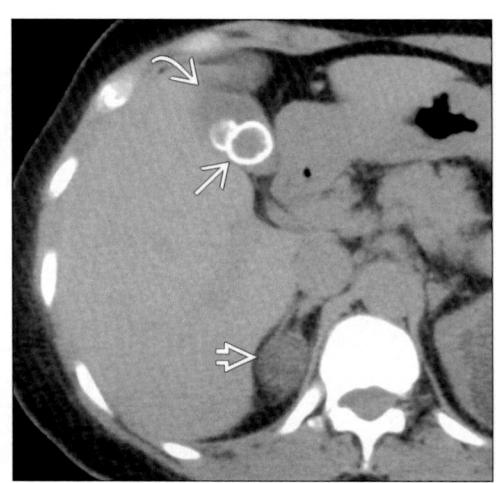
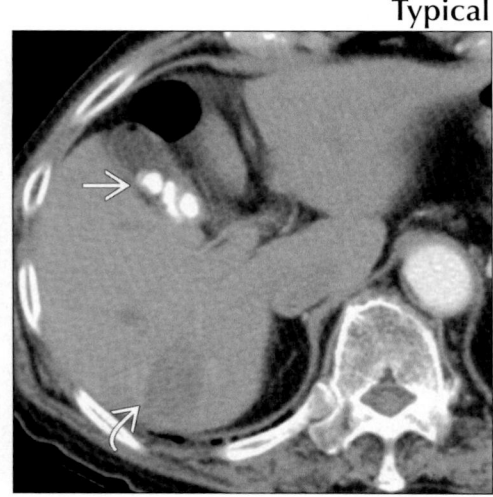

(Left) Supine abdominal radiograph showing features of small bowel obstruction due to a migrated gallstone ➡ impacted at the distal ileum. Note the air in the gallbladder ➡ due to fistula formation. *(Right)* Small bowel follow through study shows the level of obstruction ➡ coincides with the position of the gallstone shown in the adjoining plain radiograph.

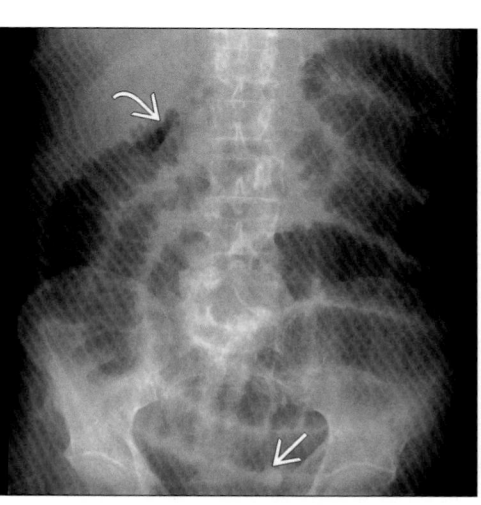
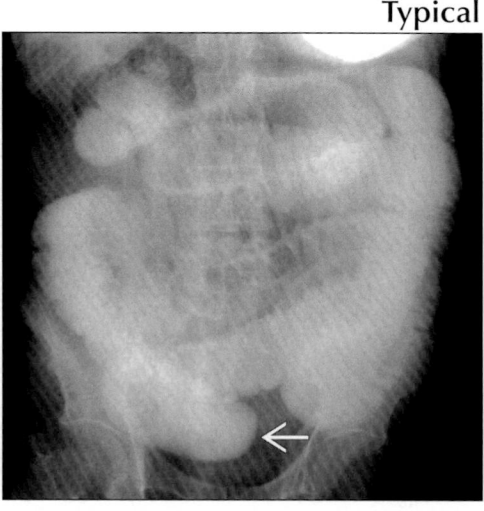

Typical

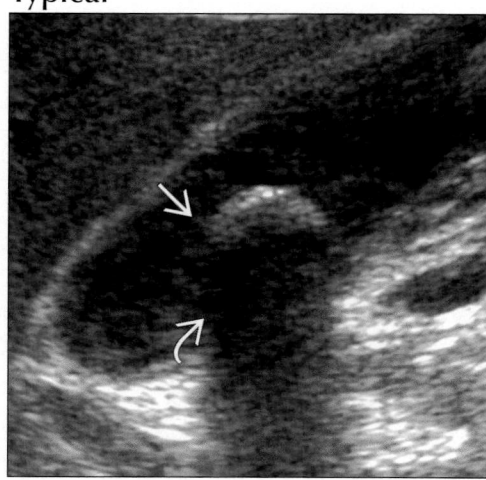

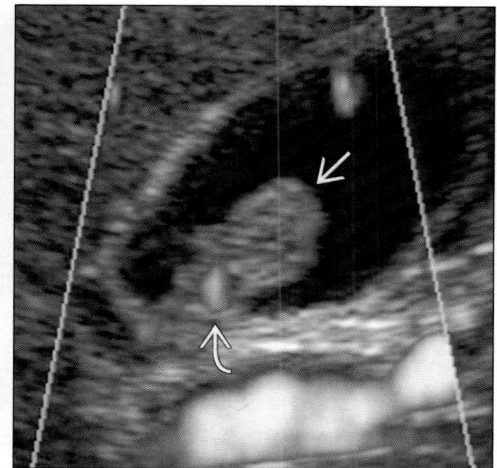

(Left) Oblique transabdominal ultrasound shows a solitary echogenic gallstone ➡ with marked posterior acoustic shadowing ➡ (normal GB wall, no pericholecystic fluid). *(Right)* Oblique power Doppler ultrasound shows a large, sessile, nonshadowing, soft tissue lesion in GB lumen ➡. It shows mild vascularity ➡; features suggestive of a sessile GB polyp. Dopplers helps to differentiate polyps from gallstone.

Typical

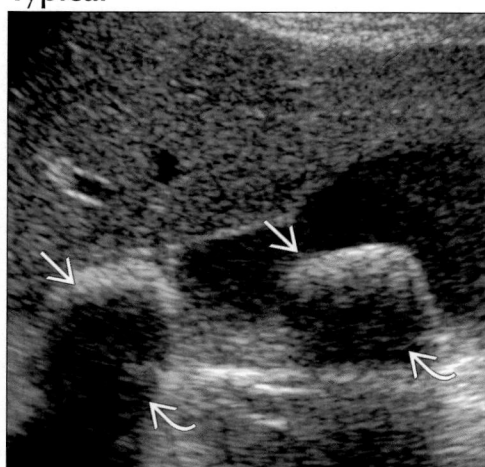

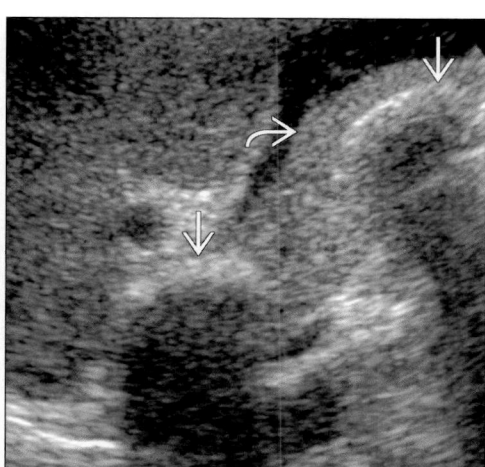

(Left) Oblique transabdominal ultrasound shows two echogenic foci ➡ in the GB lumen casting marked posterior acoustic shadowing ➡, suggestive of GB stones. *(Right)* Oblique transabdominal ultrasound shows two echogenic gallstones ➡ within the GB lumen with sludge ➡ overlying them. Sludge and stones are often associated.

Typical

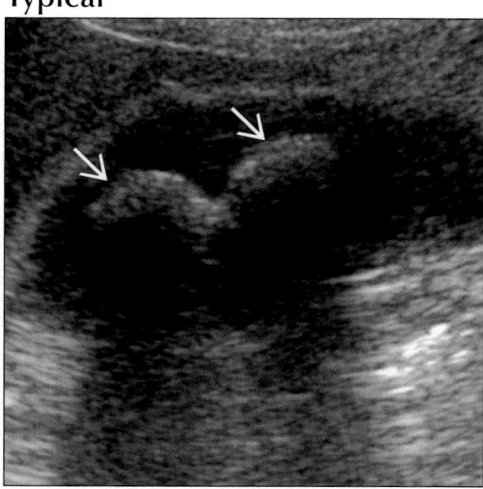

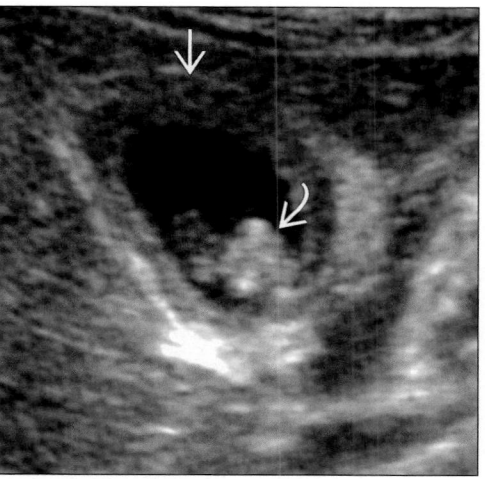

(Left) Oblique transabdominal ultrasound shows two echogenic ➡ floating gallstones. Note the marked posterior acoustic shadowing, and lack of any changes to suggest associated cholecystitis. *(Right)* Transverse transabdominal ultrasound shows a thickened and edematous GB wall ➡ with echogenic sludge ➡ within the lumen; features suggestive of cholecystitis.

ECHOGENIC BILE, BLOOD CLOTS, PARASITES

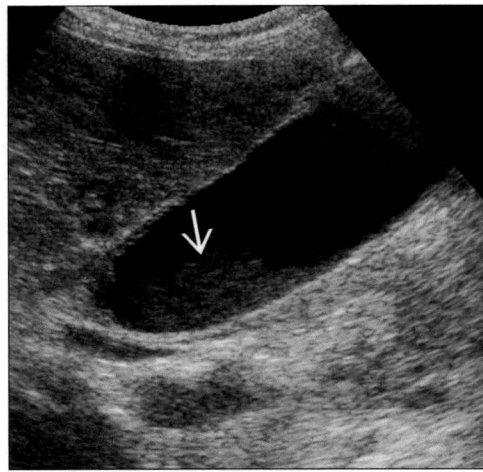

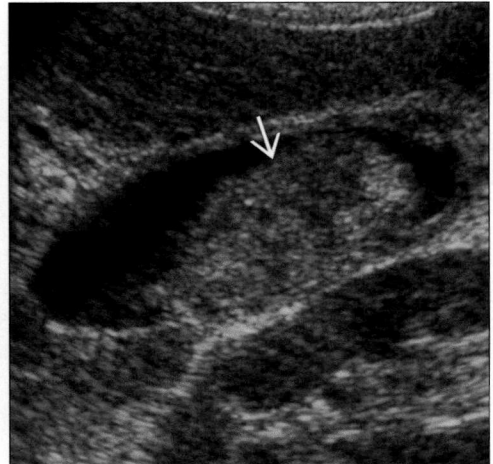

Oblique transabdominal ultrasound shows a "mass" with medium level echoes ➡ in the dependent position of the gallbladder. Note the absence of posterior acoustic shadowing.

Oblique transabdominal ultrasound shows a mobile echogenic "lesion" ➡ with globular contour within the gallbladder, consistent with sludge ball. Note absence of posterior acoustic shadowing.

TERMINOLOGY

Abbreviations and Synonyms
- Biliary sludge, tumefactive sludge, biliary sand, microlithiasis

Definitions
- Presence of particulate material (calcium bilirubinate +/- cholesterol crystals) in bile

IMAGING FINDINGS

General Features
- Best diagnostic clue
  - Echogenic bile: Mobile "mass" within gallbladder (GB) with mid/high level echoes, lack of posterior acoustic shadowing
  - Blood clot: Heterogeneous low-level echoes floating within GB, mobile
  - Parasites: Elongated, tubular, mobile structures, parallel echogenic walls
- Location: Within gallbladder, occasionally parasite found within intrahepatic/extrahepatic bile ducts

- Size: Variable

Ultrasonographic Findings
- Grayscale Ultrasound
  - Echogenic bile
    - Amorphous, mid/high level echoes within GB
    - Floating echoes, mobile echoes
    - Sediment in dependent positions
    - Lack of posterior acoustic shadowing
    - "Hepatization" of gallbladder: Sludge-filled GB with same echotexture as the liver
    - Lack of internal vascularity
  - Tumefactive sludge
    - Round low to intermediate level mass-like "lesion"
    - No posterior acoustic shadowing
    - Gravitates to dependent position on changing patient position
    - Lack of intralesional vascularity on color Doppler examination
  - Blood clot
    - Echogenic/mixed echoes within GB
    - Occasional retractile and conforms to configuration of GB
    - Blood-fluid level within GB

DDx: Filling Defect in Gallbladder

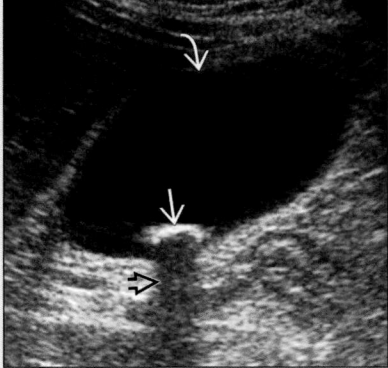

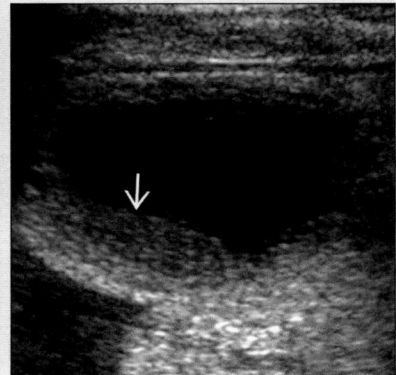

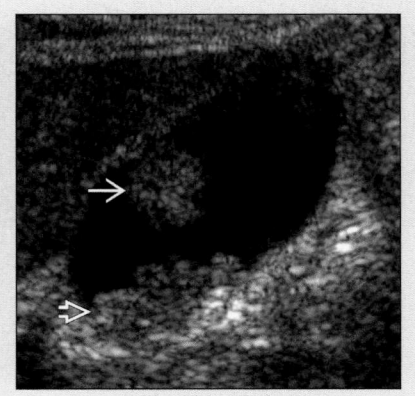

Cholelithiasis

Fundal Adenomyomatosis

Gallbladder Polyps

ECHOGENIC BILE, BLOOD CLOTS, PARASITES

Key Facts

Terminology
- Biliary sludge, tumefactive sludge, biliary sand, microlithiasis
- Presence of particulate material (calcium bilirubinate +/- cholesterol crystals) in bile

Imaging Findings
- Echogenic bile: Mobile "mass" within gallbladder (GB) with mid/high level echoes, lack of posterior acoustic shadowing
- Blood clot: Heterogeneous low-level echoes floating within GB, mobile
- Parasites: Elongated, tubular, mobile structures, parallel echogenic walls
- Amorphous, mid/high level echoes within GB
- Sediment in dependent positions
- Blood-fluid level within GB

- Power Doppler: No internal vascularity in "mass-like" GB filling defects
- Best imaging tool: Transabdominal ultrasound
- Use high frequency transducer (if possible) for better detail of intraluminal filling defect/echoes
- Change patient position to demonstrate mobility of intraluminal material to dependent portion

Top Differential Diagnoses
- Cholelithiasis
- Focal Adenomyomatosis
- Gallbladder Polyp

Diagnostic Checklist
- Consider biliary sludge or blood clot within GB when mobile medium/high level echoes without acoustic shadowing are seen

---

- Hemobilia +/- aerobilia inside biliary ducts if originates from instrumentation of biliary tree
  - Parasitic infestation
    - Ascariasis: Tubular or echogenic parallel lines within bile duct or gallbladder, sonolucent center, active movement of the worm
    - Daughter hydatid cysts: Round anechoic cysts within bile duct/gallbladder, mother cyst in liver
- Power Doppler: No internal vascularity in "mass-like" GB filling defects

CT Findings
- NECT
  - Medium density material within GB
  - No wall thickening or pericholecystic inflammatory change
- CECT
  - Lack of contrast-enhancement
  - Intact GB wall without evidence of invasion of adjacent structures

Non-Vascular Interventions
- ERCP
  - Filling defects within gallbladder
  - Gravitate to dependent position

MR Findings
- MRCP
  - Hypointense filling defect against markedly hyperintense bile within GB
  - Non-dilated biliary and pancreatic ducts

Imaging Recommendations
- Best imaging tool: Transabdominal ultrasound
- Protocol advice
  - Use high frequency transducer (if possible) for better detail of intraluminal filling defect/echoes
  - Focal zone should be adjusted to level of gallbladder to maximize sonographic visualization
  - Change patient position to demonstrate mobility of intraluminal material to dependent portion

DIFFERENTIAL DIAGNOSIS

Cholelithiasis
- Densely echogenic material within GB
- Marked posterior acoustic shadowing
  - Occasionally GB stone may be non-shadowing
- Mobile and gravitate to dependent position
- No GB wall thickening or pericholecystic fluid if uncomplicated

Focal Adenomyomatosis
- Most common at GB fundus
- Mass-like filling defect arising from wall of GB
- No posterior acoustic shadowing
- Not mobile on changing patient position
- Lack of internal vascularity
- May have associated features of adenomyomatosis in the rest of GB (e.g., echogenic foci with comet-tail artifacts)

Gallbladder Polyp
- Small (usually < 1 cm) smooth polypoidal mass in GB wall
- Smooth contour, immobile
- Usually avascular, occasionally with increased internal vascularity

Gallbladder Empyema
- Heterogeneous echoes within GB due to presence of pus/inflammatory exudate
- Distended GB
- Presence of impacted gallstones in GB neck
- GB wall thickening, pericholecystic fluid collection, positive sonographic Murphy sign
- Clinically septic with localized peritoneal signs in right upper quadrant

Gallbladder Carcinoma
- If large, can completely occupy GB with heterogeneous echoes
- Infiltrative mass with early invasion of adjacent liver parenchyma
- Increased internal vascularity

- Regional nodal metastases
- Presence of gallstones

PATHOLOGY

General Features
- Etiology
  - Predisposing factors for formation of echogenic bile
    - Prolonged fasting/on total parenteral nutrition
    - Rapid weight loss
    - Presence of critical illness
    - Ceftriaxone or prolonged octreotide therapy
    - Post-bone marrow transplantation
  - Cause of blood clot inside GB
    - Usually originates from hemorrhage of bile duct, mostly related to recent instrumentation/intervention (such as ERCP/PTBD)
    - Occasionally due to presence of hemorrhagic cholecystitis; associated with finding of acute gangrenous cholecystitis
    - Rarely due to blunt abdominal trauma
  - Parasitic infestation
    - Most common organism: Ascaris lumbricoides
    - Other possible causative agents: Clonorchis sinensis, biliary rupture of hepatic hydatid cysts
- Epidemiology
  - Biliary sludge
    - Similar epidemiology to cholelithiasis
    - M < F
    - More common in middle age, obese, female
  - Ascaris infestation
    - Most frequent helminthic infestation in humans
    - Estimated ~ 25% of world population infected
    - Endemic in Africa, South America and parts of Asia

Gross Pathologic & Surgical Features
- Thick crystalized bile sediment within normal-looking GB
- If long-standing disease +/- superimposed inflammation
  - GB wall thickening with variable extent of chronic inflammatory infiltrate

CLINICAL ISSUES

Presentation
- Most common signs/symptoms
  - Mostly asymptomatic
  - May have clinical symptoms when complications occur
    - Stone formation
    - Biliary colic
    - Acute acalculous/calculous cholecystitis
    - Pancreatitis

Natural History & Prognosis
- Biliary sludge
  - Approximately 50% of cases resolve spontaneously over 3 year period
  - 20% persist and remain asymptomatic

- 5-15% develop gallstones
- 10-15% become symptomatic
- Blood clot inside GB
  - Resolve spontaneously if left untreated
- Parasitic infestation
  - Most cases are asymptomatic
  - May cause complication such as biliary obstruction, biliary colic, intestinal obstruction
  - High rate of eradication with good prognosis after appropriate medical therapy

Treatment
- Biliary sludge
  - No treatment is required in vast majority of cases
  - Elective cholecystectomy if complications occur (e.g., stone formation)
- Parasitic infestation
  - Medical therapy for parasite eradication
  - Mebendazole for Ascariasis

DIAGNOSTIC CHECKLIST

Consider
- Consider biliary sludge or blood clot within GB when mobile medium/high level echoes without acoustic shadowing are seen
- Long tubular structures with parallel echogenic lines and lucent center with active movement indicate Ascaris infestation

SELECTED REFERENCES

1. Choi D et al: Sonographic findings of active Clonorchis sinensis infection. J Clin Ultrasound. 32(1):17-23, 2004
2. Green MH et al: Haemobilia. Br J Surg. 88(6):773-86, 2001
3. Ko CW et al: Biliary sludge. Ann Intern Med. 130(4 Pt 1):301-11, 1999
4. Nishiwaki M et al: Posttraumatic intra-gallbladder hemorrhage in a patient with liver cirrhosis. J Gastroenterol. 34(2):282-5, 1999
5. Campani R et al: The latest in ultrasound: three-dimensional imaging. Part II. Eur J Radiol. 27 Suppl 2:S183-7, 1998
6. Schulman A: Ultrasound appearances of intra- and extrahepatic biliary ascariasis. Abdom Imaging. 23(1):60-6, 1998
7. Barton P et al: Biliary sludge after liver transplantation: 1. Imaging findings and efficacy of various imaging procedures. AJR Am J Roentgenol. 164(4):859-64, 1995
8. Aslam M et al: Ultrasonographic diagnosis of hepatobiliary ascariasis. J Ultrasound Med. 12(10):573-6, 1993
9. Zargar SA et al: Intrabiliary rupture of hepatic hydatid cyst: sonographic and cholangiographic appearances. Gastrointest Radiol. 17(1):41-5, 1992
10. Lee SP: Pathogenesis of biliary sludge. Hepatology. 12(3 Pt 2):200S-203S; discussion 203S-205S, 1990

IMAGE GALLERY

Typical

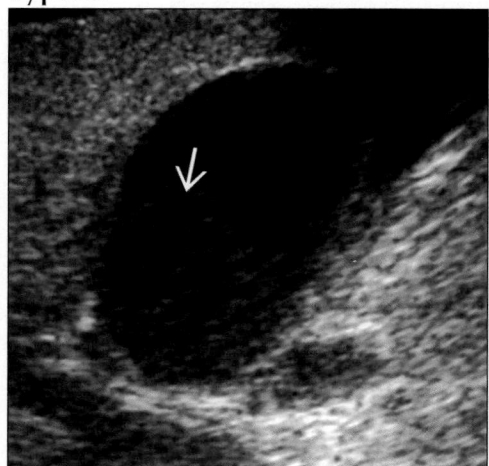
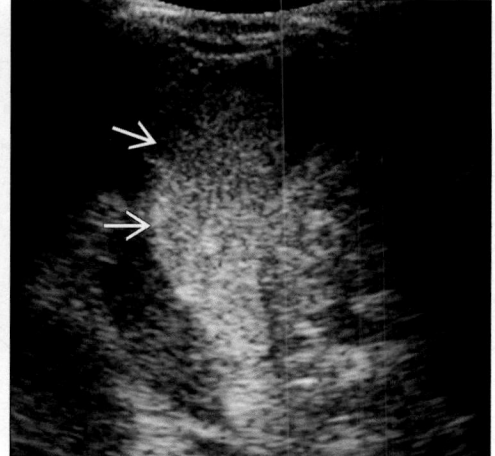

(Left) Oblique transabdominal ultrasound shows heterogeneous echogenic material ➡ *in the gallbladder lumen due to a blood clot, following a percutaneous transhepatic biliary drainage. (Right) Oblique transabdominal ultrasound shows markedly echogenic material* ➡*, almost completely filling the gallbladder (hepatization of gallbladder). Note absence of posterior acoustic shadowing.*

Typical

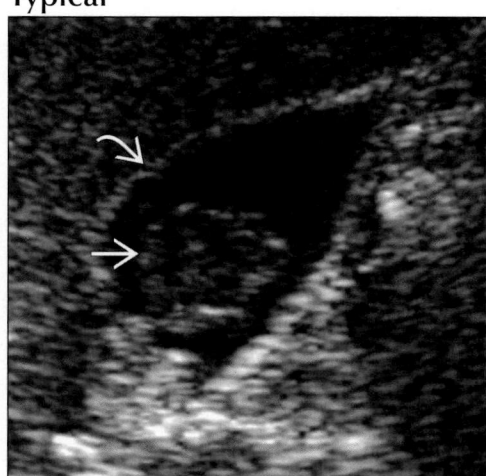
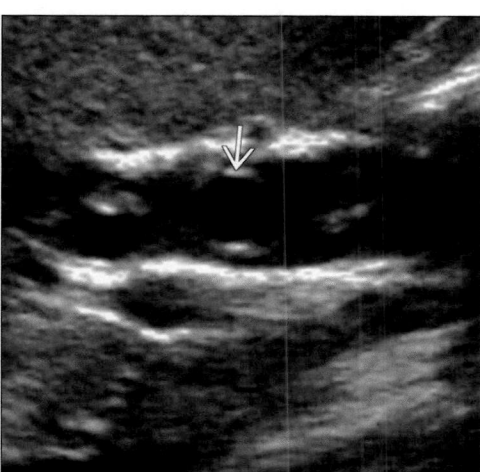

(Left) Oblique transabdominal ultrasound shows a mildly hyperechoic sludge ball ➡ *within the gallbladder. Note absence of posterior acoustic shadowing. Note GB wall* ➡ *is normal in thickness. (Right) Oblique transabdominal ultrasound shows a daughter cyst* ➡ *within the dilated common bile duct due to a rupture of a hepatic hydatid cyst into the biliary tree.*

Typical

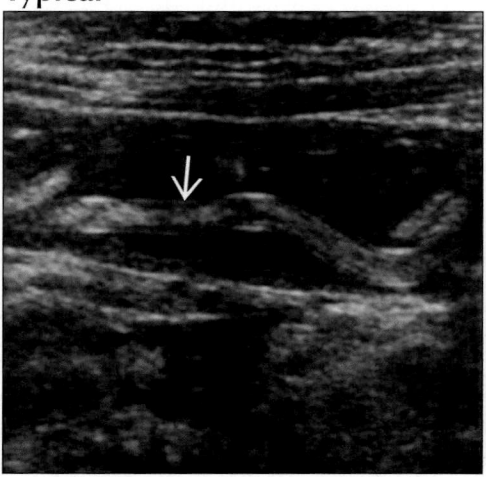
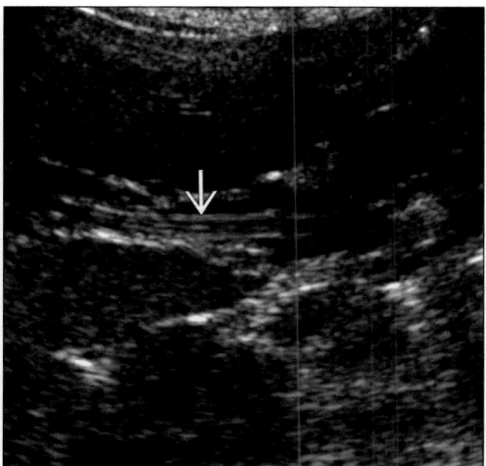

(Left) Oblique transabdominal ultrasound shows a tubular, mobile structure ➡*, with parallel echogenic lines, within the GB suggestive of parasitic infestation by Ascaris lumbricoides. (Right) Oblique transabdominal ultrasound shows another long, tubular structure* ➡*, with parallel echogenic lines, within the dilated common bile duct. It showed active movement on real time ultrasound, compatible with viable worm infestation.*

GALLBLADDER CHOLESTEROL POLYP

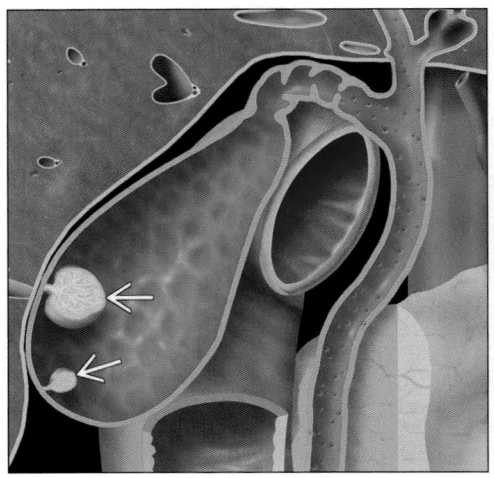

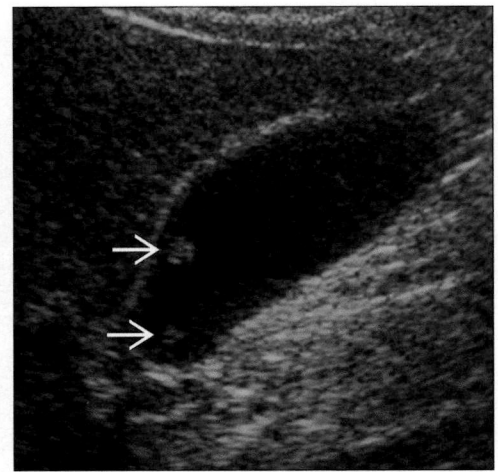

Graphic shows well-circumscribed, pedunculated nodules ➜ arising from the gallbladder wall suggestive of cholesterol polyps. Note the preserved GB wall without invasion to the adjacent liver parenchyma.

Oblique transabdominal US shows small, non-shadowing, well-defined, round, slightly hyperechoic nodules ➜ adherent to the gallbladder wall, characteristic of gallbladder polyps.

TERMINOLOGY

Abbreviations and Synonyms
- Focal gallbladder (GB) cholesterosis, polypoid cholesterosis

Definitions
- Abnormal deposit of cholesterol ester producing a villous-like structure covered with a single layer of epithelium and attached via a delicate stalk

IMAGING FINDINGS

General Features
- Best diagnostic clue: Multiple, small, non-shadowing lesions attached to gallbladder wall
- Location
  - Anywhere on GB wall
  - Most commonly in middle 1/3 of gallbladder
- Size: Usually 2-10 mm in size
- Morphology
  - More than one half of all polypoidal gallbladder lesions are cholesterol polyps

- Well-circumscribed, ovoid/round in configuration

Ultrasonographic Findings
- Grayscale Ultrasound
  - Transabdominal ultrasound is the most sensitive technique for detecting small cholesterol polyps
  - Polypoidal mass arising from GB wall
    - Small, usually in the range of 2-10 mm in size
    - Multiple lesions: Occasionally appear solitary and only the dominant is detected
    - Medium to high level internal echoes
    - Smooth in contour, sometimes multi-lobulated outline
    - Round or ovoid shape, broad-base with gallbladder wall
    - Does not cast posterior acoustic shadow (vs. gallstone)
    - Not mobile on changing patient's position (vs. biliary sludge)
    - Overlying GB wall is intact & normal
    - No invasion of adjacent liver parenchyma or regional nodal metastases
  - Variation of US appearances

DDx: Gallbladder Cholesterol Polyp

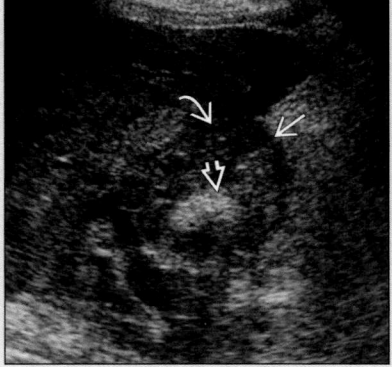

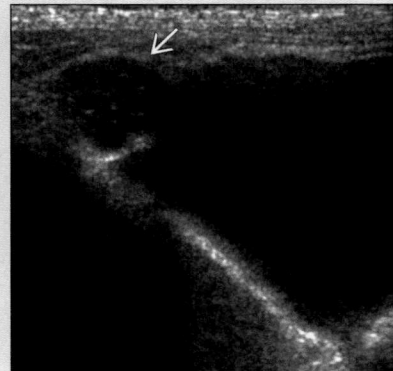

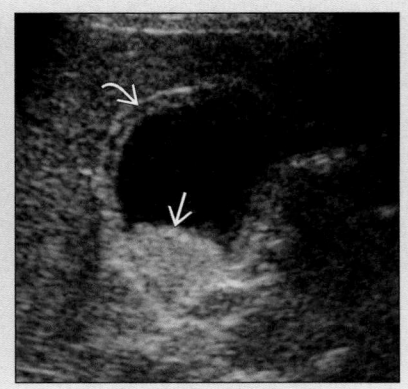

Gallbladder Carcinoma *Hyperplastic Cholecystosis* *Non-Shadowing Cholelithiasis*

GALLBLADDER CHOLESTEROL POLYP

Key Facts

Imaging Findings
- Best diagnostic clue: Multiple, small, non-shadowing lesions attached to gallbladder wall
- Most commonly in middle 1/3 of gallbladder
- More than one half of all polypoidal gallbladder lesions are cholesterol polyps
- Overlying GB wall is intact & normal
- No invasion of adjacent liver parenchyma or regional nodal metastases
- Avascular or hypovascular on Doppler examination
- Larger lesions may have slight internal vascularity
- Scan in supine, decubitus and lateral positions to demonstrate immobility of GB polyp
- Set depth of focal zone at level of GB mass maximize accuracy of mass characterization

- For lesion < 10 mm with no suspicious features, serial follow-up to monitor size
- For lesion > 10 mm with atypical features (sessile appearance, singularity, internal vascularity), further evaluation with CECT or proceed to surgery to exclude the possibility of malignancy

Top Differential Diagnoses
- Gallbladder Carcinoma
- Hyperplastic Cholecystosis
- Non-Shadowing Cholelithiasis

Diagnostic Checklist
- Easily differentiated from non-shadowing cholelithiasis or biliary sludge by demonstrating immobility of polyp

---

- Large size: Lesions up to 20 mm have been described
- Pedunculated with well-defined stalk from GB wall
- Fine pattern of echogenic foci within larger lesions
- Power Doppler
  - Avascular or hypovascular on Doppler examination
  - Larger lesions may have slight internal vascularity

CT Findings
- NECT
  - Small soft tissue density nodule on GB wall
  - Intact GB wall
  - No calcification or fat component
- CECT
  - Mild enhancement
  - Multiplicity usually better assessed after IV contrast administration

MR Findings
- T1WI
  - Small, round nodule in GB wall
  - Homogeneous, intermediate signal intensity
- T2WI: Homogeneous intermediate signal intensity
- MRCP
  - Low signal intensity filling defect attached to GB wall
  - Contrast against markedly hyperintense bile within GB lumen

Imaging Recommendations
- Best imaging tool: Transabdominal US
- Protocol advice
  - Adequate fasting prior to US is essential for detection and characterization of GB polypoidal mass
  - Scan in supine, decubitus and lateral positions to demonstrate immobility of GB polyp
  - Set depth of focal zone at level of GB mass maximize accuracy of mass characterization
  - Imaging algorithm for polypoid GB mass

- For lesion < 10 mm with no suspicious features, serial follow-up to monitor size
- For lesion > 10 mm with atypical features (sessile appearance, singularity, internal vascularity), further evaluation with CECT or proceed to surgery to exclude the possibility of malignancy

DIFFERENTIAL DIAGNOSIS

Gallbladder Carcinoma
- Irregular soft tissue thickening of GB wall
- Destruction of GB wall
- Evidence of invasion to adjacent liver parenchyma and regional nodal metastases
- Increased chaotic internal vascularity
- Presence of gallstones

Hyperplastic Cholecystosis
- Focal (fundal) form
- Smooth sessile mass in fundal region
- Non-shadowing & immobile
- Comet-tail artifacts from the GB wall

Adenoma/Adenomyoma
- True benign neoplasm of gallbladder
- Account for < 5% of gallbladder polyp
- Solitary lesion
- Larger size (> 10 mm)
- Usually pedunculated in appearances

Non-Shadowing Cholelithiasis
- Densely echogenic
- Mobile on changing patient's position
- Gravitate to dependent portion of GB lumen

Biliary Sludge
- Medium to high level echogenicity
- Mobile on changing patient's position
- No posterior acoustic shadowing
- Fluid sediment level

Inflammatory Polyp
- Comprise 5-10% of gallbladder polyps

- Multiple in 50% of cases
- Background of gallstone disease and chronic cholecystitis

GB Metastases

- Most common from melanoma and adenocarcinoma of GI origin
- Hyperechoic, broad-based polypoidal mass
- Usually > 10 mm in size
- Clinical history of known primary malignancy

PATHOLOGY

General Features

- Genetics: No documented genetic predisposition
- Etiology
  - Uncertain
  - May be attributed to absorption of cholesterol from supersaturated bile
  - Does not predispose to cholecystitis or functional derangement
- Epidemiology
  - Polypoidal lesions of gallbladder affect ~ 5% of adult population
  - Mostly asymptomatic, incidental finding during ultrasound for unrelated conditions
- Associated abnormalities: Occasionally associated with cholelithiasis

Gross Pathologic & Surgical Features

- Multiple nodules on cut sections
- Sessile/pedunculated smooth mucosal projections
- Intact mucosal surface
- GB wall is not thickened (unless complicated with chronic cholecystitis) or inflamed

Microscopic Features

- Focal accumulation of lipid-laden macrophages underneath the columnar epithelium
- Fibrous stroma
- Infiltrated with variable degree of chronic inflammatory cells
- Intact mucosa with smooth projections
- No evidence of muscularis layers infiltration

CLINICAL ISSUES

Presentation

- Most common signs/symptoms: Asymptomatic, incidental finding on US for other purposes
- Other signs/symptoms: Mild non-specific right upper abdominal discomfort

Demographics

- Age: More common in middle age
- Gender: M < F

Natural History & Prognosis

- No malignant potential
- No interval increase in size on serial follow-up US

Treatment

- Treatment is not required, cholecystectomy only indicated if
  - Symptomatic
  - Possibility of malignant polyp cannot be excluded
    - Patient's age > 60 years
    - Size > 10 mm (37-88% polyp > 10 mm is malignant)
    - Serial increase in size on follow-up US
    - Sessile morphology
    - Solitary polypoid GB mass
    - Doppler features of malignancy: Flow velocity > 20 cm/s, resistive index < 0.65
    - Associated with gallstone disease

DIAGNOSTIC CHECKLIST

Consider

- Consider neoplastic or malignant GB polyp if size > 10 mm, irregular outline, growth on serial US examinations and invasion to adjacent structures

Image Interpretation Pearls

- Multiple, small, round/ovoid masses attached to GB wall with no posterior acoustic shadowing
- Easily differentiated from non-shadowing cholelithiasis or biliary sludge by demonstrating immobility of polyp

SELECTED REFERENCES

1. Chattopadhyay D et al: Outcome of gall bladder polypoidal lesions detected by transabdominal ultrasound scanning: a nine year experience. World J Gastroenterol. 11(14):2171-3, 2005
2. Kaido T et al: Large cholesterol polyp of the gallbladder mimicking gallbladder carcinoma. Abdom Imaging. 29(1):100-1, 2004
3. Owen CC et al: Gallbladder polyps, cholesterolosis, adenomyomatosis, and acute acalculous cholecystitis. Semin Gastrointest Dis. 14(4):178-88, 2003
4. Sandri L et al: Gallbladder cholesterol polyps and cholesterolosis. Minerva Gastroenterol Dietol. 49(3):217-24, 2003
5. Myers RP et al: Gallbladder polyps: epidemiology, natural history and management. Can J Gastroenterol. 16(3):187-94, 2002
6. Csendes A et al: Late follow-up of polypoid lesions of the gallbladder smaller than 10 mm. Ann Surg. 234(5):657-60, 2001
7. Mainprize KS et al: Surgical management of polypoid lesions of the gallbladder. Br J Surg. 87(4):414-7, 2000
8. Furukawa H et al: Small polypoid lesions of the gallbladder: differential diagnosis and surgical indications by helical computed tomography. Arch Surg. 133(7):735-9, 1998
9. Furukawa H et al: CT evaluation of small polypoid lesions of the gallbladder. Hepatogastroenterology. 42(6):800-10, 1995
10. Sugiyama M et al: Large cholesterol polyps of the gallbladder: diagnosis by means of US and endoscopic US. Radiology. 196(2):493-7, 1995
11. Levy AD et al: From the archives of the AFIP. Benign tumors and tumorlike lesions of the gallbladder and extrahepatic bile ducts: radiologic-pathologic correlation. Armed Forces Institute of Pathology.

GALLBLADDER CHOLESTEROL POLYP

IMAGE GALLERY

Typical

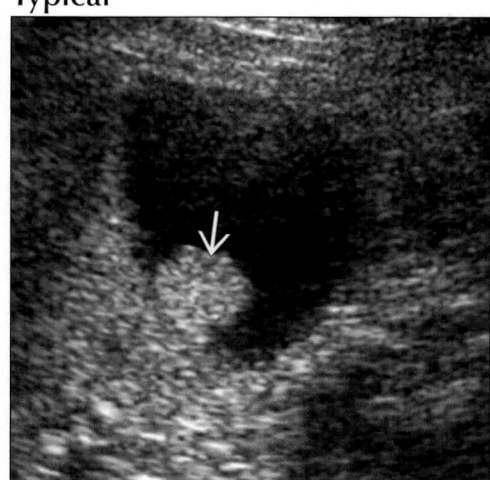
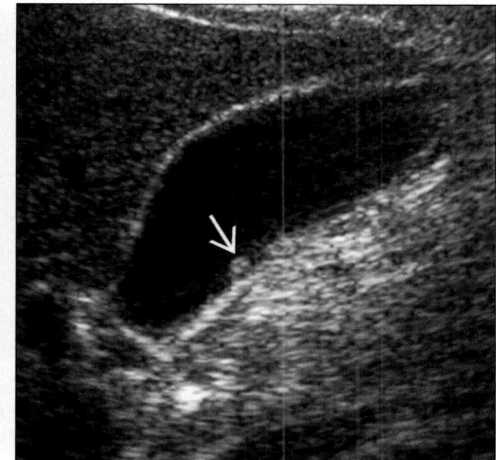

(Left) Oblique transabdominal ultrasound shows a well-circumscribed, homogeneously hyperechoic mass ➡ with a smooth margin, arising from the gallbladder wall compatible with a gallbladder polyp. (Right) Oblique transabdominal ultrasound shows a small, well-defined, echogenic nodule ➡ adherent to the gallbladder wall. The nodule was immobile and not casting posterior acoustic shadow.

Typical

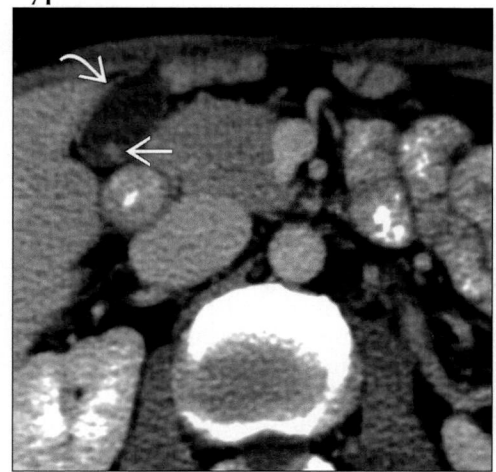
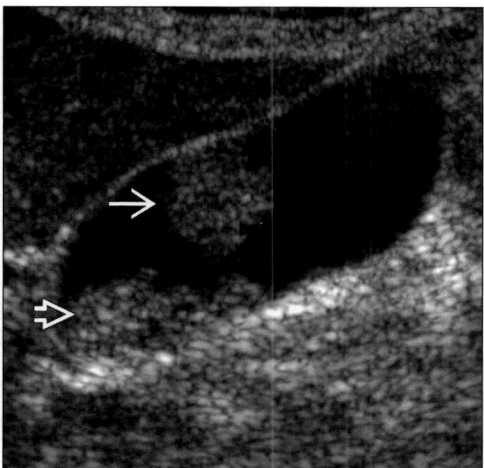

(Left) Transverse CECT shows a well-defined gallbladder polyp ➡. Note normal gallbladder wall ➡. (Right) Oblique transabdominal ultrasound shows a large polypoid growth ➡ with a slightly lobulated contour, arising from the anterior gallbladder wall. A similar lesion with a sessile appearance ➡ is present on the posterior GB wall.

Variant

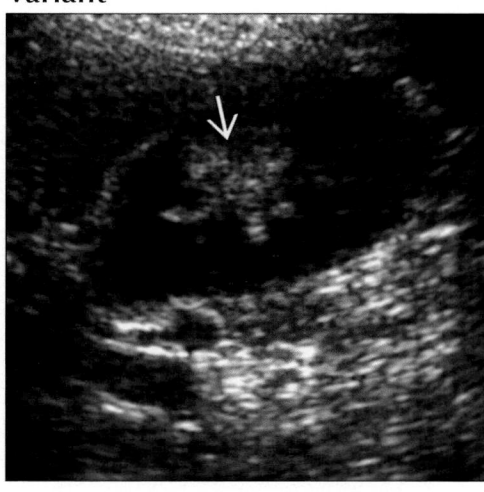
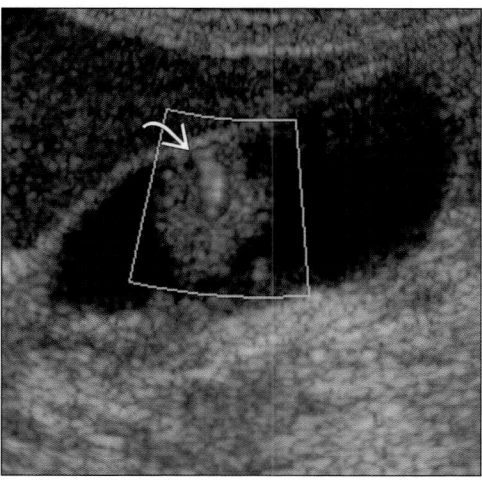

(Left) Oblique transabdominal ultrasound shows a large papilliform hyperechoic mass ➡ in the non-dependent wall of the gallbladder. Note surface irregularities and lack of posterior acoustic shadowing. (Right) Oblique power Doppler ultrasound shows presence of internal vascularity ➡ within a large gallbladder polyp. The gallbladder wall is intact with no invasion to adjacent liver parenchyma.

THICKENED GALLBLADDER WALL

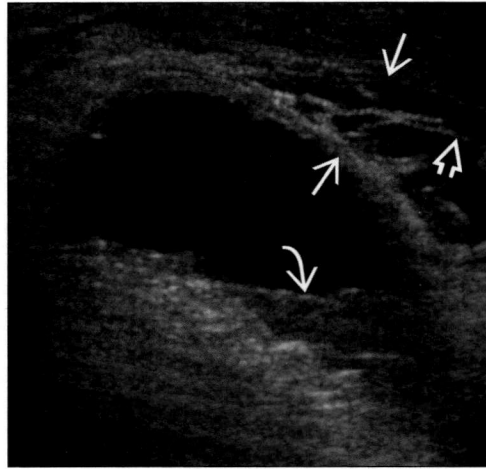 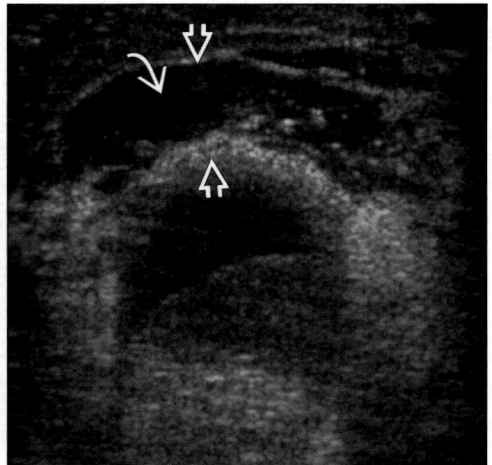

Oblique transabdominal ultrasound shows diffuse gallbladder wall thickening ➡, with echogenic striations ➡. Note presence of biliary sludge ➡ within the GB.

Transverse transabdominal ultrasound shows diffuse gallbladder wall thickening (between the two echogenic lines ➡), with heterogeneous hypoechoic areas ➡.

TERMINOLOGY

Abbreviations and Synonyms
- Diffuse gallbladder (GB) wall thickening; edematous gallbladder wall

Definitions
- Gallbladder wall thickness > 3 mm

IMAGING FINDINGS

General Features
- Best diagnostic clue: Diffuse GB wall thickening with striated appearance
- Location: Gallbladder wall
- Size: Variable degree of severity

Ultrasonographic Findings
- Grayscale Ultrasound
  - Diffuse GB wall thickening (> 3 mm, especially over anterior wall)
  - Smooth contour
  - Homogeneous/heterogeneous, hypoechoic thickening
  - Diffuse/patchy hypoechoic region between two echogenic lines
  - Linear echogenic striations within the hypoechoic area
  - GB lumen obliteration in severe GB wall thickening
    - Distension of GB lumen in thickening due to acute cholecystitis
  - Lack of invasion of adjacent structures (e.g., liver parenchyma) in non-neoplastic conditions
  - Findings related to underlying causes
    - Ascites in liver cirrhosis or hypoalbuminemia
    - Change in hepatic parenchymal echogenicity in cirrhosis/hepatitis
    - Gallstones/positive sonographic Murphy sign in acute cholecystitis
    - Regional lymph nodes/liver invasion in malignancy
- Power Doppler
  - Avascular if thickening due to systemic causes
  - Hyperemic in acute cholecystitis

DDx: Diffuse Gallbladder Wall Thickening

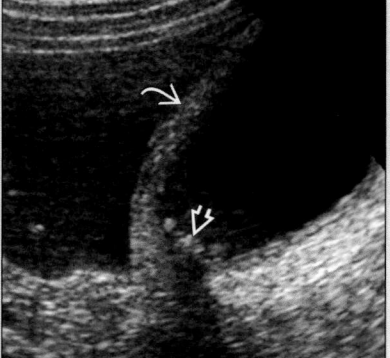 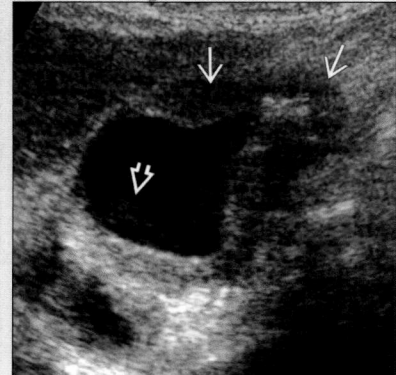 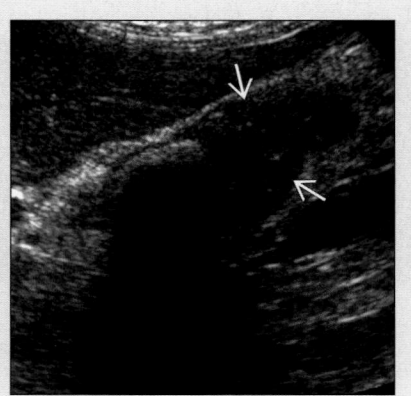

Acute Calculous Cholecystitis   *Hyperplastic Cholecystosis*   *Gallbladder Carcinoma*

THICKENED GALLBLADDER WALL

Key Facts

Terminology
- Gallbladder wall thickness > 3 mm

Imaging Findings
- Diffuse GB wall thickening (> 3 mm, especially over anterior wall)
- Homogeneous/heterogeneous, hypoechoic thickening
- Linear echogenic striations within the hypoechoic area

- GB lumen obliteration in severe GB wall thickening
- Make sure patient is adequately fasted to avoid false positive findings
- Look for any clues towards underlying cause

Top Differential Diagnoses
- Acute Calculous Cholecystitis
- Hyperplastic Cholecystosis
- Gallbladder Carcinoma with Diffuse Wall Infiltration

CT Findings
- CECT
  - Homogeneous soft tissue thickening of GB wall
  - Increased streakiness of adjacent peri-cholecystic fat

Imaging Recommendations
- Best imaging tool: Transabdominal ultrasound
- Protocol advice
  - Make sure patient is adequately fasted to avoid false positive findings
  - Look for any clues towards underlying cause

DIFFERENTIAL DIAGNOSIS

Acute Calculous Cholecystitis
- Impacted gallstone in distended, tender gallbladder
- Pericholecystic fluid collection
- Positive sonographic Murphy sign

Hyperplastic Cholecystosis
- Fundal type: Focal wall thickening in GB fundus
- Diffuse type: Hour-glass appearance
- Presence of comet-tail artifacts

Gallbladder Carcinoma with Diffuse Wall Infiltration
- Irregular wall thickening
- Tumor invasion of adjacent liver parenchyma, nodes
- Increased intra-tumoral vascularity

PATHOLOGY

General Features
- Etiology
  - Inflammatory conditions
    - Primary: Acute calculous/acalculous cholecystitis, chronic cholecystitis, AIDS-related cholangiopathy
    - Secondary: Acute hepatitis, perforated peptic ulcer, pancreatitis
  - Systemic diseases
    - Congestive heart failure
    - Renal failure
    - Liver cirrhosis
    - Hypoalbuminemia
  - Neoplastic infiltration
    - Gallbladder carcinoma
    - Leukemic/lymphomatous infiltration

DIAGNOSTIC CHECKLIST

Consider
- Gallbladder inflammatory conditions and systemic illnesses in patients with diffuse gallbladder wall thickening

SELECTED REFERENCES

1. Rubens DJ: Hepatobiliary imaging and its pitfalls. Radiol Clin North Am. 42(2):257-78, 2004

IMAGE GALLERY

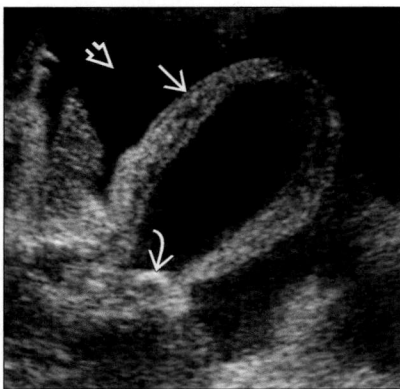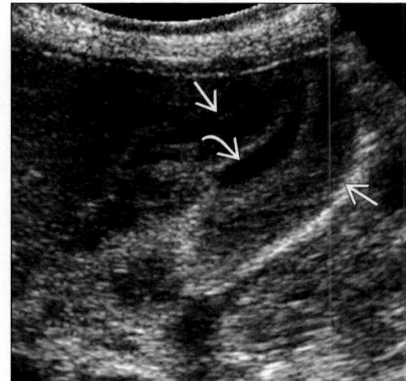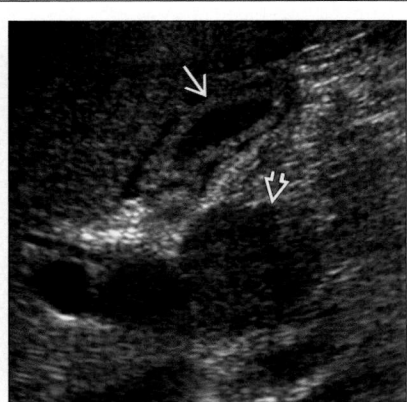

(Left) Oblique transabdominal ultrasound shows a diffusely thickened gallbladder wall ➡ with a small gallstone ➡ in the gallbladder neck. Note ascites ➡ related to liver cirrhosis. *(Center)* Oblique transabdominal ultrasound shows marked diffuse hypoechoic gallbladder wall thickening ➡ obliterating the gallbladder lumen ➡ in a patient with acute hepatitis. *(Right)* Oblique transabdominal ultrasound shows a diffusely thickened gallbladder wall ➡ due to lymphomatous infiltration. Note abnormal lymph node ➡ in porta hepatis.

ACUTE CALCULOUS CHOLECYSTITIS

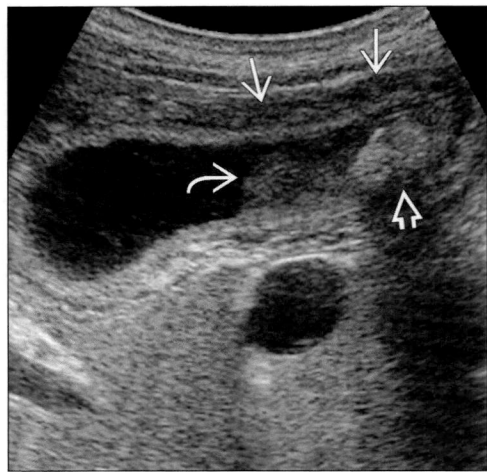

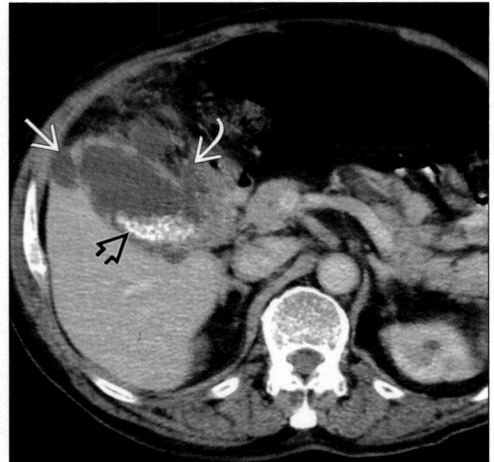

Oblique transabdominal ultrasound shows a distended gallbladder, wall thickening ➡, stones ⊳ and sludge ⊳. The patient had a positive sonographic Murphy sign.

Transverse CECT shows a pericholecystic collection ➡ with perigallbladder stranding ➡ and multiple intraluminal calculi ⊳.

TERMINOLOGY

Abbreviations and Synonyms
- Acute cholecystitis

Definitions
- Acute inflammation of gallbladder (GB) secondary to calculus obstructing cystic duct

IMAGING FINDINGS

General Features
- Best diagnostic clue
  - Impacted gallstone in cystic duct
  - Gallbladder wall thickening
  - Pericholecystic collection
  - Positive sonographic Murphy sign
- Location: Stone impacted in GB neck or cystic duct
- Size: Distended GB (> 5 cm transverse diameter)
- Morphology: Distended GB more rounded in shape than normal "pear-shaped" configuration

Ultrasonographic Findings
- Grayscale Ultrasound
  - Uncomplicated cholecystitis
    - Gallstones +/- impaction in GB neck or cystic duct
    - Hazy delineation of GB wall
    - GB wall lucency "halo sign", sonolucent middle layer (edema)
    - Positive sonographic Murphy sign
    - Diffuse GB wall thickening (> 4 mm)
    - Striated wall thickening: Several alternating irregular discontinuous lucent and echogenic bands with GB wall
    - GB hydrops: Distension with AP diameter > 5 cm
    - Sludge inside GB
    - Clear pericholecystic fluid
    - Crescent-shaped/loculated pericholecystic fluid: Inflammatory intraperitoneal exudate/abscess
  - Complicated cholecystitis
    - Gallbladder perforation: Pericholecystic abscess
    - Gangrenous cholecystitis: Asymmetric wall thickening, marked wall irregularities, intraluminal membrane

---

DDx: Acute Calculous Cholecystitis

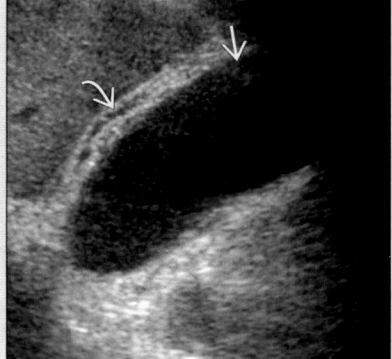

Acalculous Cholecystitis

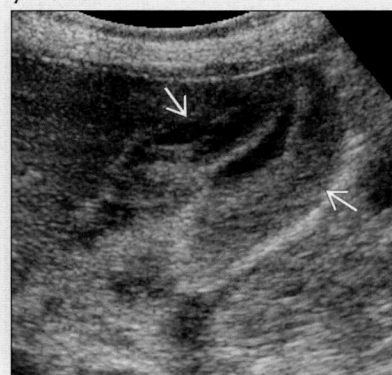

GB Wall Thickening

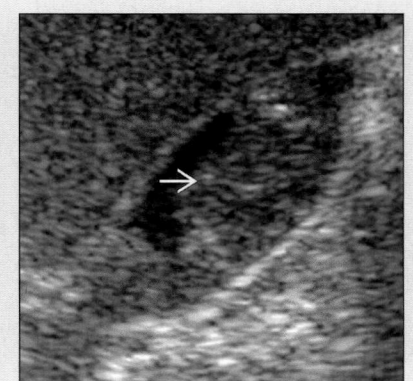

Gallbladder Sludge

ACUTE CALCULOUS CHOLECYSTITIS

Key Facts

Terminology
- Acute inflammation of gallbladder (GB) secondary to calculus obstructing cystic duct

Imaging Findings
- Gallstones +/- impaction in GB neck or cystic duct
- Positive sonographic Murphy sign
- Diffuse GB wall thickening (> 4 mm)
- Sludge inside GB
- Clear pericholecystic fluid
- Protocol advice: In order to detect impacted/immobile calculus, the patient is best scanned in the left posterior oblique position; evaluate the region of the GB, its neck, cystic duct and adjacent soft tissues in multiple planes

Top Differential Diagnoses
- Acute Acalculous Cholecystitis
- Nonspecific GB Wall Thickening
- Gallbladder Sludge/Echogenic Bile
- Acute Pancreatitis

Clinical Issues
- Acute right upper quadrant (RUQ) pain
- Fever
- May progress to gangrenous cholecystitis and perforation if untreated
- Excellent prognosis in uncomplicated cases or with prompt surgery
- Mirizzi syndrome: Stone in cystic duct causing common bile duct obstruction

---

- Emphysematous cholecystitis: Gas in GB wall/lumen
- Empyema of gallbladder: Highly reflective intraluminal echoes without shadowing, purulent exudate/debris
- Gallstone ileus
- Bouveret syndrome: Gallstone erodes in to duodenum leading to duodenal obstruction

Radiographic Findings
- Radiography: Calcified stones in only 15-20% of patients with cholecystitis
- ERCP
  - No filling of gallbladder
  - Sharply-defined filling defect in contrast-material filled lumen of cystic duct

CT Findings
- CECT
  - Uncomplicated cholecystitis
    - GB wall thickening
    - Increased mural enhancement
    - Pericholecystic fat stranding, pericholecystic fluid
    - Gallstones inside GB neck or cystic duct
  - Complicated cholecystitis
    - Intramural or pericholecystic abscesses leading to asymmetric GB wall thickening
    - Gas in lumen and/or wall of gallbladder
    - High attenuation gallbladder hemorrhage

Nuclear Medicine Findings
- Hepato biliary scan
  - Tc-99m iminodiacetic acid derivatives
  - Non-visualization of GB at 4 hours has 99% specificity
  - Increased uptake in gallbladder fossa during arterial phase due to hyperemia in 80% of patients
  - "Rim sign" seen in 34% of patients is due to increased uptake in gallbladder fossa
    - Positive predictive value of 57% for gangrenous cholecystitis

Imaging Recommendations
- Best imaging tool: US or biliary scintigraphy
- Protocol advice: In order to detect impacted/immobile calculus, the patient is best scanned in the left posterior oblique position; evaluate the region of the GB, its neck, cystic duct and adjacent soft tissues in multiple planes

DIFFERENTIAL DIAGNOSIS

Acute Acalculous Cholecystitis
- Thickened GB wall > 4-5 mm
- Distended GB
- Absence of gallstone
- Pericholecystic fluid in absence of ascites
- Positive Murphy sign: Pain and tenderness with transducer pressure over the gallbladder
- Subserosal edema

Nonspecific GB Wall Thickening
- Negative sonographic Murphy sign
- Lack of gallstone
- Clinical evidence of underlying etiology: Congestive heart failure, hypoalbuminemia

Gallbladder Sludge/Echogenic Bile
- Echogenic material within gallbladder
- Mobile, gravity dependent
- No GB wall thickening or pericholecystic collection
- Negative sonographic Murphy sign

Acute Pancreatitis
- Gallbladder distension and thickening secondary to peri-pancreatic inflammation
- Enlarged hypoechoic pancreas
- Peripancreatic fluid or inflammatory changes

Liver Abscess
- Irregular, hypoechoic mass with thick walls and posterior enhancement

ACUTE CALCULOUS CHOLECYSTITIS

PATHOLOGY

General Features
- General path comments
  - Distended GB
  - Thickened, inflamed GB wall
  - Pericholecystic adhesions to omentum
- Genetics
  - Increased incidence of gallstones in selected population
    - Hispanics, Pima Native Americans
- Etiology
  - 95% of acute cholecystitis due to calculous cholecystitis (5% acalculous)
    - Obstructing stone in cystic duct
- Epidemiology
  - Incidence parallels prevalence of gallstones
    - M:F = 1:3

Gross Pathologic & Surgical Features
- Gallstones in gallbladder neck or cystic duct
- Thickened GB wall with hyperemia of wall
- Omental adhesions

Microscopic Features
- Lumen: Gallstones, sludge
- GB mucosa: Ulcerations
- GB wall: Acute polymorphonuclear (PMN) infiltration
- Bacterial cultures positive in 40-70% of patients

Staging, Grading or Classification Criteria
- Non-perforated
  - GB wall intact on CT and/or US
- Gangrenous
  - Positive Murphy sign
  - Shaggy, irregular, asymmetric wall (mucosal ulcers, intraluminal hemorrhage, necrosis)
  - Hypoechoic foci in GB wall (microabscesses in Rokitansky- Aschoff sinuses)
  - Intraluminal pseudomembranes
- Perforated
  - US: Pericholecystic abscess, GB wall necrosis
  - Gallstone lying free in peritoneal cavity
  - Sonolucent/complex collection surrounding GB
  - Collection in liver adjacent to GB

CLINICAL ISSUES

Presentation
- Most common signs/symptoms
  - Acute right upper quadrant (RUQ) pain
  - Fever
- Other signs/symptoms: Positive Murphy sign
- Clinical Profile
  - Increased white blood cell (WBC)
  - May have mild elevation in liver enzymes

Demographics
- Age: Typically > 25 years
- Gender: M:F = 1:3

Natural History & Prognosis
- May progress to gangrenous cholecystitis and perforation if untreated
- Excellent prognosis in uncomplicated cases or with prompt surgery
- Complications
  - Mirizzi syndrome: Stone in cystic duct causing common bile duct obstruction
  - Bouveret syndrome: Gallstone erodes into duodenum causing obstruction

Treatment
- Prompt cholecystectomy
  - Laparoscopic surgery for uncomplicated cases
- Percutaneous cholecystectomy
  - Useful for poor operative risk patients with GB empyema
- Percutaneous drainage
  - Well-defined, well-localized pericholecystic abscesses

DIAGNOSTIC CHECKLIST

Consider
- Acalculous cholecystitis, perforated ulcer or acute pancreatitis with secondary GB wall thickening

Image Interpretation Pearls
- Stone impacted in cystic duct
- Diffuse GB wall thickening, pericholecystic fluid
- Sonographic Murphy sign must be unequivocal to be considered positive

SELECTED REFERENCES

1. Makela JT et al: Acute cholecystitis in the elderly. Hepatogastroenterology. 52(64):999-1004, 2005
2. Mills LD et al: Association of clinical and laboratory variables with ultrasound findings in right upper quadrant abdominal pain. South Med J. 98(2):155-61, 2005
3. Hanbidge AE et al: From the RSNA refresher courses: imaging evaluation for acute pain in the right upper quadrant. Radiographics. 24(4):1117-35, 2004
4. Menakuru SR et al: Current management of gall bladder perforations. ANZ J Surg. 74(10):843-6, 2004
5. Bennett GL et al: Ultrasound and CT evaluation of emergent gallbladder pathology. Radiol Clin North Am. 41(6):1203-16, 2003
6. Browning JD et al: Gallstone disease and its complications. Semin Gastrointest Dis. 14(4):165-77, 2003
7. Cheema S et al: Timing of laparoscopic cholecystectomy in acute cholecystitis. Ir J Med Sci. 172(3):128-31, 2003
8. Gandolfi L et al: The role of ultrasound in biliary and pancreatic diseases. Eur J Ultrasound. 16(3):141-59, 2003
9. Ko CW et al: Gastrointestinal disorders of the critically ill. Biliary sludge and cholecystitis. Best Pract Res Clin Gastroenterol. 17(3):383-96, 2003
10. Oh KY et al: Limited abdominal MRI in the evaluation of acute right upper quadrant pain. Abdom Imaging. 28(5):643-51, 2003
11. Ozaras R et al: Acute viral cholecystitis due to hepatitis A virus infection. J Clin Gastroenterol. 37(1):79-81, 2003
12. Pazzi P et al: Biliary sludge: the sluggish gallbladder. Dig Liver Dis. 35 Suppl 3:S39-45, 2003

ACUTE CALCULOUS CHOLECYSTITIS

IMAGE GALLERY

Typical

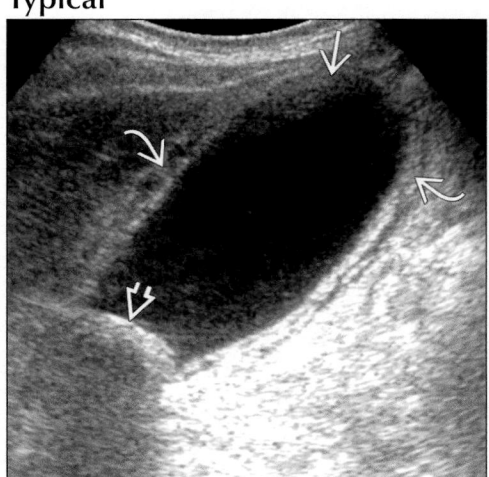
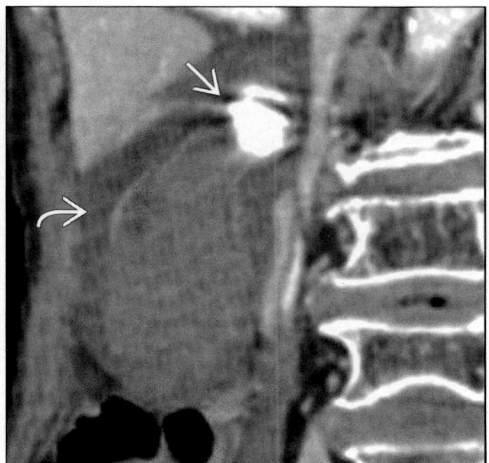

(Left) Oblique transabdominal ultrasound shows a distended gallbladder ➡, with an impacted gallstone ➡ at the gallbladder neck and diffuse wall thickening ➡. *(Right)* CECT with coronal reformation shows a distended gallbladder with an impacted stone at its neck ➡, with thickened wall and pericholecystic fluid ➡.

Typical

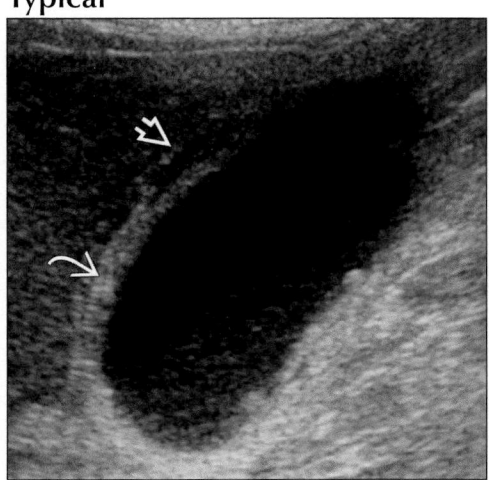
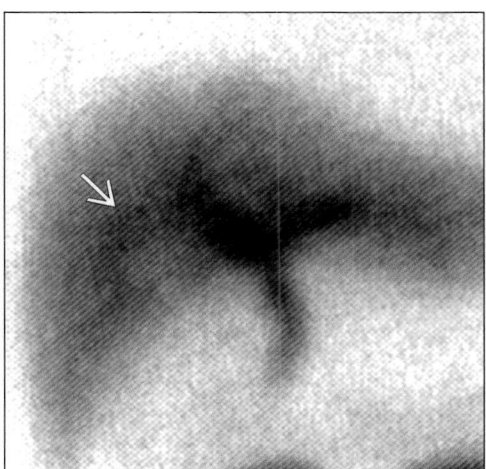

(Left) Oblique transabdominal ultrasound shows pericholecystic fluid ➡ adjacent to a distended and thick-walled gallbladder ➡ containing sludge. *(Right)* Radionuclide scan with tracer uptake in the GB fossa showing a classical "rim sign" ➡. Non-visualization of the GB at 4 hours has a 99% specificity. This can be a helpful study when the ultrasound findings are equivocal.

Typical

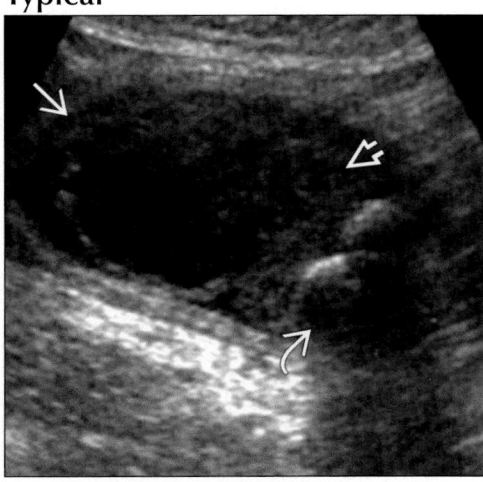
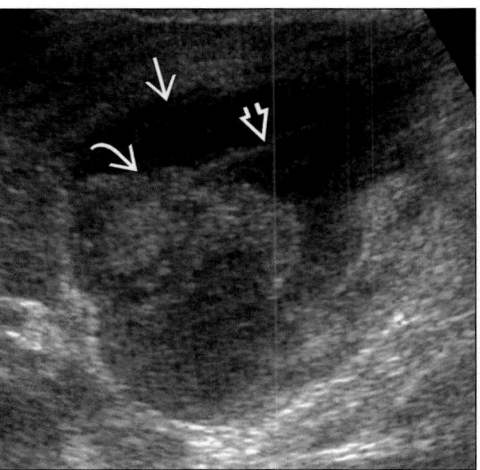

(Left) Oblique transabdominal ultrasound shows a gangrenous gallbladder with asymmetric wall thickening, sloughed mucosa ➡, impacted stones at the gallbladder neck ➡, and sludge ➡. *(Right)* Oblique transabdominal ultrasound shows a distended gangrenous gallbladder ➡ containing echogenic debris ➡, irregular wall, and intraluminal membrane ➡ due to sloughing of mucosa.

ACUTE ACALCULOUS CHOLECYSTITIS

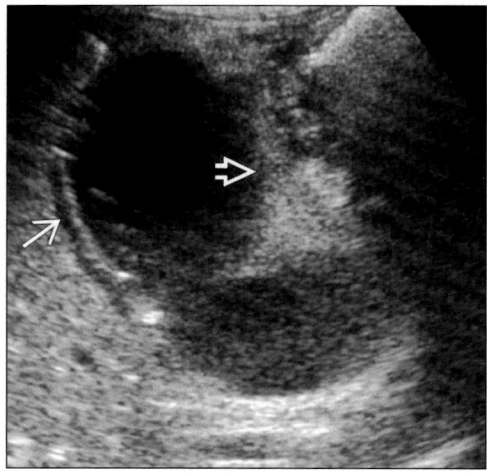
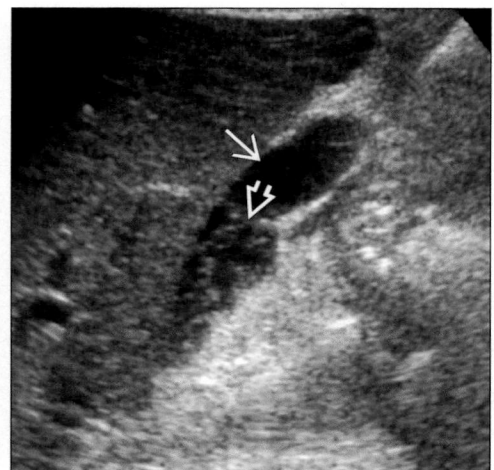

Transabdominal ultrasound shows a distended GB with hypoechoic wall thickening ➡. Part of the GB wall appears irregular ⬥ & asymmetric due to sloughed mucosa. Note absence of impacted gallstone.

Oblique transabdominal ultrasound shows focal fluid ➡ in the right pericholecystic region in a patient with acute acalculous cholecystitis. Note presence of internal echoes in the GB ⬥ due to inflammatory debris.

TERMINOLOGY

Definitions
- Acute inflammation of gallbladder (GB) not related to gallstone, usually secondary to ischemia

IMAGING FINDINGS

General Features
- Best diagnostic clue
  - Gallbladder wall thickening without impacted gallstone
  - Positive sonographic Murphy sign

Ultrasonographic Findings
- Grayscale Ultrasound
  - US features of acute acalculous cholecystitis are similar to acute calculous cholecystitis except for absence of impacted gallstone
  - GB wall thickening (> 4 mm)
    - Hypoechoic, layered/striated appearances
  - GB distension
    - Commonly filled with sludge
  - Pericholecystic fluid collection
  - Positive sonographic Murphy sign
  - Complication
    - Gangrenous cholecystitis: Irregular/asymmetric GB wall thickening, intraluminal membrane and echogenic material due to sloughed mucosa
    - GB perforation: Collapsed GB; wall defect with adjacent heterogeneous hypoechoic fluid collection
- Color Doppler: Hyperemia within thickened/inflamed GB wall

CT Findings
- CECT
  - Distended GB with wall thickening, enhancing wall and pericholecystic fat stranding
  - Complication: Pericholecystic fluid collection, gas within GB lumen/wall

MR Findings
- T2WI: Distended GB, high signal pericholecystic fat
- T1 C+: "Rim sign" of increased hepatic enhancement

Imaging Recommendations
- Best imaging tool: US

DDx: Acute Acalculous Cholecystitis

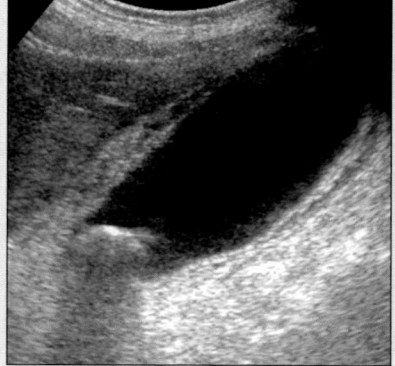
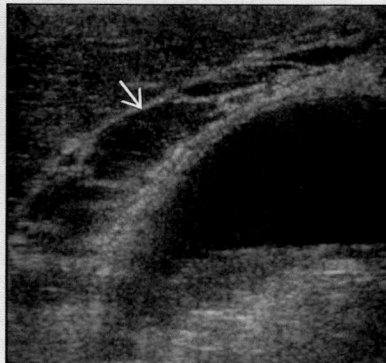
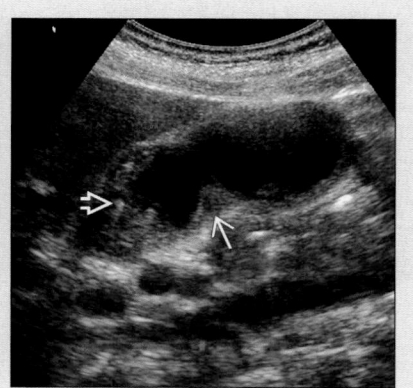

Acute Calculous Cholecystitis

Sympathetic GB Wall Thickening

Hyperplastic Cholecystosis

ACUTE ACALCULOUS CHOLECYSTITIS

Key Facts

Terminology
- Acute inflammation of gallbladder (GB) not related to gallstone, usually secondary to ischemia

Imaging Findings
- US features of acute acalculous cholecystitis are similar to acute calculous cholecystitis except for absence of impacted gallstone
- GB wall thickening (> 4 mm)
- GB distension
- Pericholecystic fluid collection
- Positive sonographic Murphy sign
- Color Doppler: Hyperemia within thickened/inflamed GB wall

Clinical Issues
- Most common signs/symptoms: Acute RUQ pain, fever in critically ill patient
- In general has worse prognosis than acute calculous cholecystitis

DIFFERENTIAL DIAGNOSIS

Acute Calculous Cholecystitis
- US features similar to acalculous cholecystitis
- Presence of impacted gallstone

Sympathetic GB Wall Thickening
- Smooth diffuse GB wall thickening
- Clinically not septic, underlying causes (e.g., hypoalbuminemia, cirrhosis, congestive heart failure)

Hyperplastic Cholecystosis
- Focal (fundal/mid body) or diffuse GB wall thickening
- Comet-tail artifacts, intramural cystic spaces

PATHOLOGY

General Features
- Etiology
  - Acalculous cholecystitis constitutes ~ 5% of acute cholecystitis
    - Pathogenesis: Ischemia with secondary inflammation/infection
  - More commonly seen in critically ill patients with underlying risk factors
    - Post major surgery, severe trauma, sepsis, diabetes, atherosclerotic disease
    - AIDS patients have opportunistic GB infection
    - Obstruction of cystic duct by extrinsic compression by metastases, lymphadenopathy

CLINICAL ISSUES

Presentation
- Most common signs/symptoms: Acute RUQ pain, fever in critically ill patient
- Clinical Profile: Raised white cell count

Natural History & Prognosis
- In general has worse prognosis than acute calculous cholecystitis
- May progress to gangrenous cholecystitis and perforation if untreated

Treatment
- Prompt cholecystectomy
- Percutaneous cholecystostomy
  - Useful in poor operative risk patients

DIAGNOSTIC CHECKLIST

Image Interpretation Pearls
- US features of acute calculous cholecystitis without impacted gallstone in critically ill patients

SELECTED REFERENCES
1. Barie PS et al: Acute acalculous cholecystitis. Curr Gastroenterol Rep. 5(4):302-9, 2003

IMAGE GALLERY

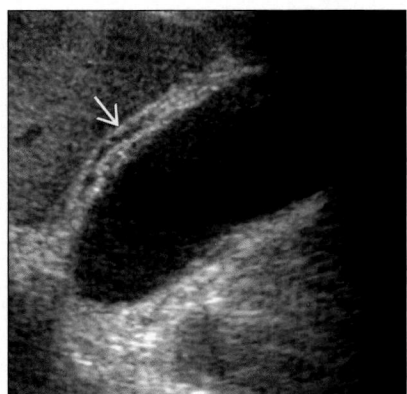 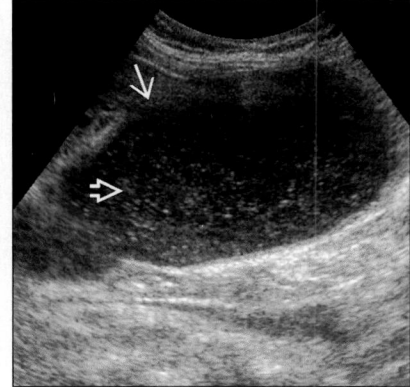 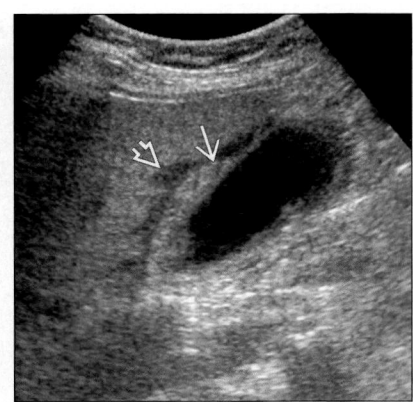

(Left) Oblique ultrasound shows a distended GB with diffuse wall thickening & a striated hypoechoic appearance ➡. Sonographic Murphy sign was positive & there was no impacted gallstone. *(Center)* Oblique ultrasound shows marked GB distension ➡ with mild wall thickening & presence of floating low level echoes ▷ due to GB empyema. *(Right)* Oblique ultrasound shows diffuse GB wall thickening ➡ in acute acalculous cholecystitis. Note layer of hypoechoic inflammatory change in adjacent liver parenchyma ▷ due to extension of GB inflammation.

CHRONIC CHOLECYSTITIS

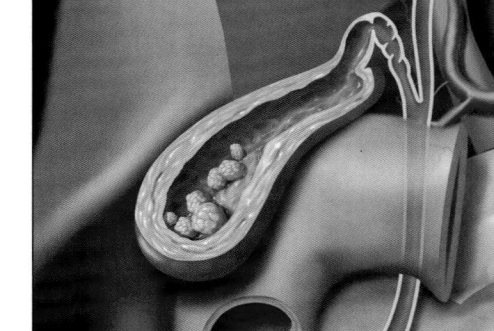

Graphic shows multiple gallstones inside a contracted thick-walled gallbladder, which are characteristic features of chronic cholecystitis.

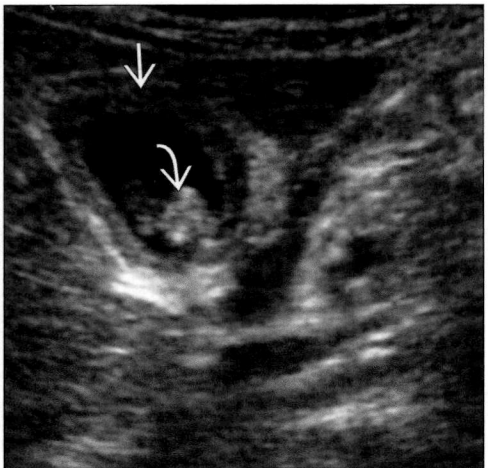

Transverse transabdominal ultrasound shows a contracted GB with diffuse wall thickening ➡ and containing an echogenic sludge ball and gallstones ➡. Note absence of pericholecystic inflammation.

TERMINOLOGY

Definitions
- Thickening and fibrosis of gallbladder (GB) wall due to chronic inflammation

IMAGING FINDINGS

General Features
- Best diagnostic clue: Thick-walled contracted GB with gallstones
- Location: Gallbladder
- Morphology: Smooth thickening of GB wall

Ultrasonographic Findings
- Grayscale Ultrasound
  - Diffuse GB wall thickening
    - Mean thickness ~ 5 mm
    - Smooth/irregular contour
  - Contracted gallbladder
    - Gallbladder lumen may be obliterated in severe cases
  - Presence of gallstones in nearly all cases
  - Absence of pericholecystic inflammation
  - Xanthogranulomatous cholecystitis
    - Rare form of chronic cholecystitis
    - Hypoechoic nodules or bands within thickened GB wall
    - Occasionally wall thickening may appear irregular and infiltrative; mimics GB carcinoma
- Power Doppler: Lack of hyperemic changes within thickened GB wall

CT Findings
- CECT
  - Contracted GB with diffuse wall thickening
  - High density gallstones within GB
  - Lack of pericholecystic inflammation

Nuclear Medicine Findings
- Hepatobiliary Scintigraphy
  - Delayed GB visualization (up to 1-4 hours)
  - Visualization of bowel activity prior to GB activity

Imaging Recommendations
- Best imaging tool: US is the initial and most sensitive imaging tool for diagnosis
- Protocol advice

DDx: Chronic Cholecystitis

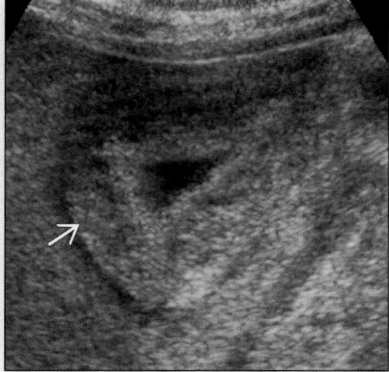

Sympathetic GB Wall Thickening

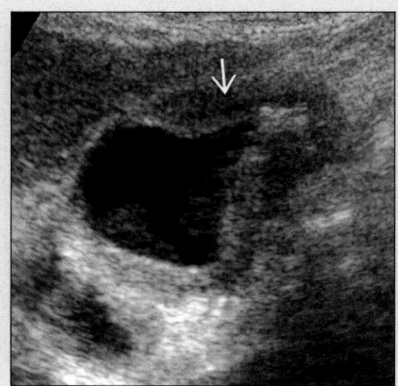

Gallbladder Adenomyomatosis

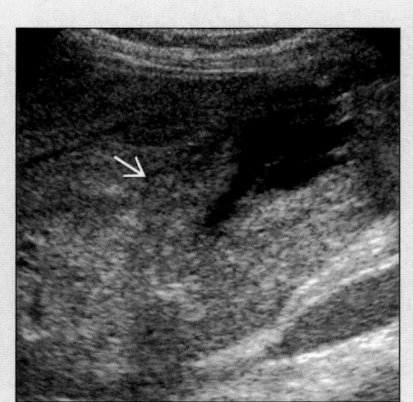

Gallbladder Carcinoma

CHRONIC CHOLECYSTITIS

Key Facts

Imaging Findings
- Diffuse GB wall thickening
- Contracted gallbladder
- Gallbladder lumen may be obliterated in severe cases
- Presence of gallstones in nearly all cases
- Absence of pericholecystic inflammation
- Power Doppler: Lack of hyperemic changes within thickened GB wall

- Ensure adequate fasting (> 6 hours) prior to US examination to avoid false positive finding of thickened GB due to post-prandial status
- Examine patient in multiple planes/positions to detect gallstone in a severely contracted GB

Top Differential Diagnoses
- Sympathetic/Reactive GB Wall Thickening
- Adenomyomatosis of Gallbladder
- Gallbladder Carcinoma

○ Ensure adequate fasting (> 6 hours) prior to US examination to avoid false positive finding of thickened GB due to post-prandial status
○ Examine patient in multiple planes/positions to detect gallstone in a severely contracted GB

DIFFERENTIAL DIAGNOSIS

Sympathetic/Reactive GB Wall Thickening
- Known underlying causes (e.g., hypoalbuminemia, cirrhosis, congestive heart failure etc.) usually detected clinically
- Smooth hypoechoic wall thickening ± linear striations

Adenomyomatosis of Gallbladder
- Comet-tail artifacts
- More commonly affects fundus or mid GB with focal thickening rather than diffuse involvement

Gallbladder Carcinoma
- Ill-defined infiltrative wall thickening/mass
- Invasion of adjacent liver parenchyma and regional nodal metastases

PATHOLOGY

General Features
- Etiology: ~ 100% associated with gallstone disease
- Epidemiology: Same as gallstone disease (i.e., male < female, middle age, obesity etc.)

CLINICAL ISSUES

Presentation
- Most common signs/symptoms
  ○ Mostly asymptomatic
  ○ Mild RUQ pain/discomfort after meal

Demographics
- Age: Middle and older age groups
- Gender: M < F

Natural History & Prognosis
- Good prognosis with minimal symptoms
- Bouts of acute cholecystitis may complicate chronic cholecystitis

Treatment
- Conservative management for symptom free and mildly symptomatic cases
- Cholecystectomy in symptomatic cases or complication of acute cholecystitis

DIAGNOSTIC CHECKLIST

Image Interpretation Pearls
- Gallstones within thick-walled contracted GB

SELECTED REFERENCES

1. Bortoff GA et al: Gallbladder stones: imaging and intervention. Radiographics. 2000;20(3):751-66

IMAGE GALLERY

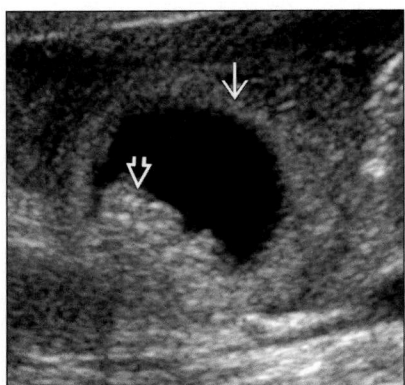 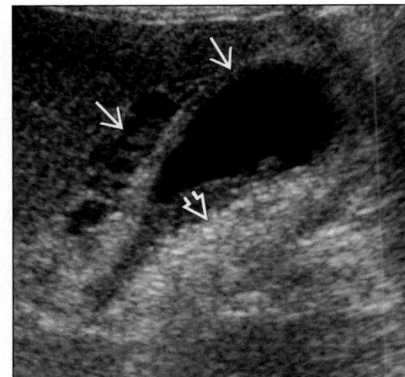 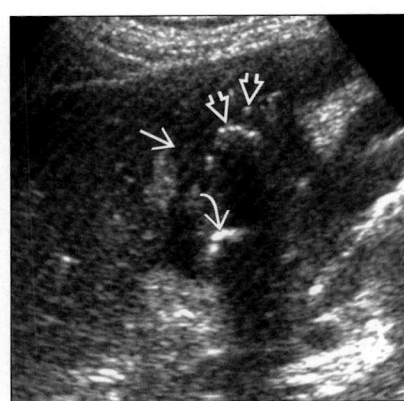

(Left) Transverse transabdominal ultrasound shows diffuse wall thickening ➡ within contracted gallbladder. Note presence of echogenic sludge & stones ➡ within GB. (Center) Oblique transabdominal ultrasound shows diffuse wall thickening ➡, with a striated hypoechoic appearance & multiple stones ➡ within a contracted gallbladder. (Right) Oblique transabdominal ultrasound shows ill-defined thickening of the GB wall ➡, which contains stones ➡. Note presence of echogenic band & foci ➡ within thickened GB wall. Dx: Xanthogranulomatous cholecystitis.

PORCELAIN GALLBLADDER

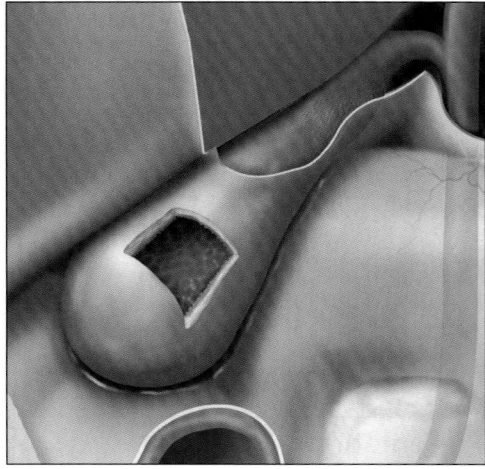

Graphic shows diffuse calcifications of the gallbladder walls in a porcelain gallbladder.

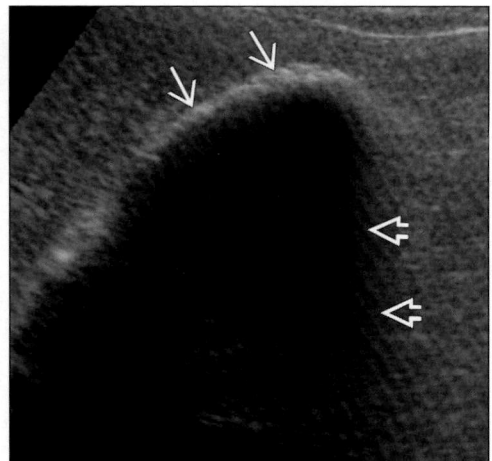

Transabdominal ultrasound shows a curvilinear echogenicity in the GB wall ➡ casting dense posterior acoustic shadowing ➡. Absence of wall-echo-shadow sign suggests porcelain GB, rather than large gallstone.

TERMINOLOGY

Abbreviations and Synonyms
- Calcified gallbladder (GB), calcifying cholecystitis, cholecystopathia chronica calcarea

Definitions
- Calcification of gallbladder wall

IMAGING FINDINGS

General Features
- Best diagnostic clue: Rim of calcification in right upper quadrant conforming to shape of the gallbladder
- Location: Gallbladder wall
- Size: Diffuse or focal involvement of GB wall
- Morphology: Two patterns: Selective mucosal calcification and diffuse intramural calcification

Ultrasonographic Findings
- Grayscale Ultrasound
  - Degree and pattern of calcification determines the ultrasound appearance

  - Thick diffuse GB wall calcification
    - Echogenic curvilinear line in GB fossa
    - Dense posterior acoustic shadowing
  - Segmental GB wall calcification
    - Coarse echogenic foci in GB wall with acoustic shadowing
    - Interrupted echogenic line on anterior GB wall
    - Scattered irregular clumps of high echoes within GB wall
- Color Doppler: Avascular over-calcified GB wall

Radiographic Findings
- Radiography: Curvilinear or granular calcification in GB wall

CT Findings
- NECT
  - Calcification in GB wall
    - Diffuse or segmental in distribution

Imaging Recommendations
- Best imaging tool: CT, US
- Protocol advice

DDx: Porcelain Gallbladder

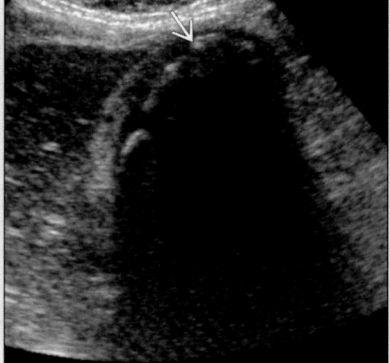

Large Gallstone

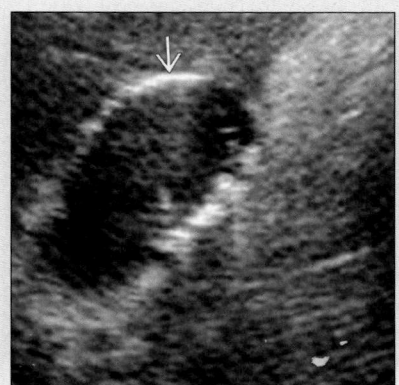

Emphysematous Cholecystitis

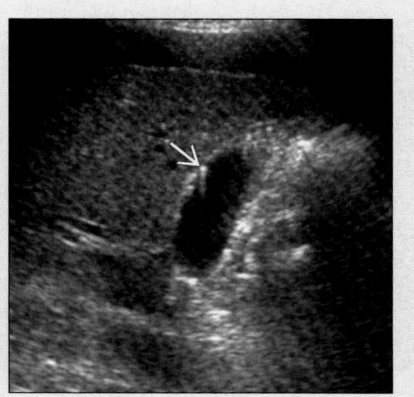

Gallbladder Adenomyomatosis

PORCELAIN GALLBLADDER

Key Facts

Terminology
- Calcification of gallbladder wall

Imaging Findings
- Echogenic curvilinear line in GB fossa
- Dense posterior acoustic shadowing
- Coarse echogenic foci in GB wall with acoustic shadowing
- Interrupted echogenic line on anterior GB wall

Top Differential Diagnoses
- Large Gallstone
- Emphysematous Cholecystitis
- Hyperplastic Cholecystosis

Diagnostic Checklist
- Look for gallbladder mass if porcelain GB identified
- WES sign on ultrasound helps to differentiate gallstones from porcelain GB

- Set focus at the level of GB to maximize depiction of high amplitude echoes and dense posterior acoustic shadowing
- Pay attention to presence of associated GB soft tissue mass indicating presence of GB carcinoma

DIFFERENTIAL DIAGNOSIS

Large Gallstone
- Wall-echo-shadow (WES) complex appearance
- Mobile on changing patient's position

Emphysematous Cholecystitis
- Echogenic crescent in gallbladder, reverberation artifacts
- Clinical information of fulminant biliary sepsis

Hyperplastic Cholecystosis
- Diffuse or focal GB wall thickening
- Echogenic foci with comet-tail artifacts

PATHOLOGY

General Features
- Epidemiology: Rare: 0.06-0.8% of cholecystectomy specimens
- Associated abnormalities: Gallstones in 90-95%
- Risk factor for GB carcinoma

CLINICAL ISSUES

Presentation
- Usually asymptomatic, occasional RUQ discomfort

Demographics
- Age: Occurs in 6th decade; mean age = 54 years
- Gender: M:F = 1:5

Natural History & Prognosis
- Risk of gallbladder cancer: ~ 0-5% incidence

Treatment
- Prophylactic cholecystectomy is current consensus recommendation

DIAGNOSTIC CHECKLIST

Consider
- Look for gallbladder mass if porcelain GB identified

Image Interpretation Pearls
- WES sign on ultrasound helps to differentiate gallstones from porcelain GB

SELECTED REFERENCES

1. Gore RM et al: Imaging benign and malignant disease of the gallbladder. Radiol Clin North Am. 40(6): 1307-23, vi, 2002

IMAGE GALLERY

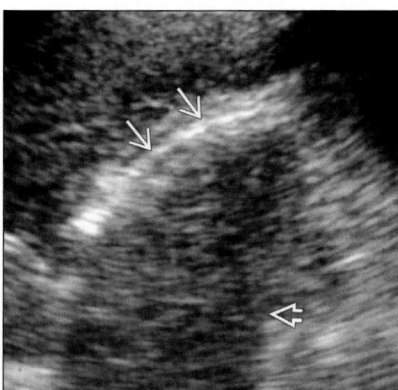 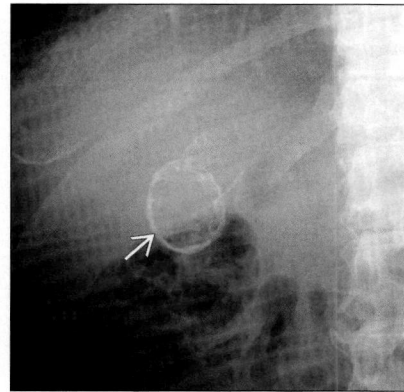 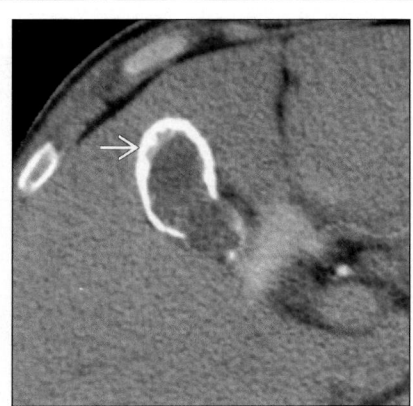

(Left) Oblique transabdominal ultrasound shows diffuse GB wall calcification, which appears as an echogenic band ➡ with dense posterior acoustic shadowing ➡. *(Center)* Plain radiograph of the abdomen shows a globular, curvilinear calcification ➡ projected over the right upper abdomen suggestive of a porcelain gallbladder. *(Right)* Transverse CECT shows heavily calcified GB wall ➡. There is no associated enhancing soft tissue mass to suggest GB carcinoma.

HYPERPLASTIC CHOLECYSTOSIS

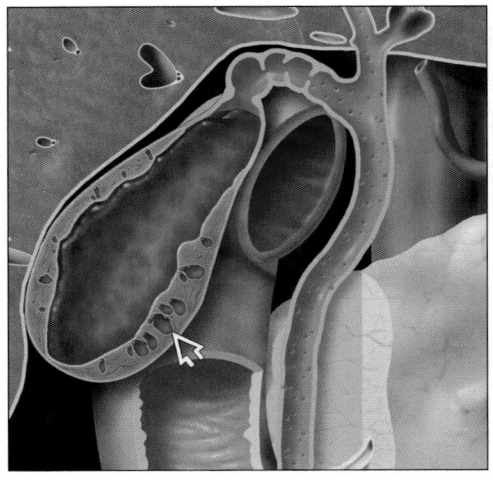

Graphic shows characteristic features of adenomyomatosis. Note thickened gallbladder wall with multiple intramural cystic spaces ➡.

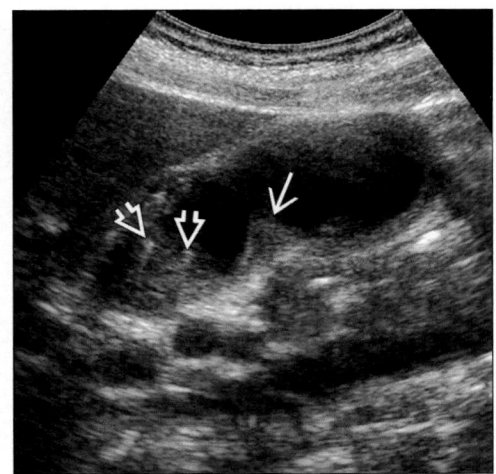

Oblique transabdominal ultrasound shows a thickened GB wall, with "comet-tail" artifacts ➡ *and focal mid GB wall constriction* ➡ *(hourglass appearance).*

TERMINOLOGY

Abbreviations and Synonyms

- Hyperplastic cholecystosis is collective term for two conditions
  - Cholesterolosis; strawberry gallbladder (GB)
  - Adenomyomatosis

Definitions

- General: Idiopathic non-neoplastic & non-inflammatory proliferative disorders resulting in GB wall thickening
- Adenomyomatosis: Mural GB wall thickening secondary to exaggeration of normal luminal epithelial folds (Rokitansky-Aschoff sinuses) in conjunction with smooth muscle proliferation
- Cholesterolosis: Deposition of foamy cholesterol-laden histiocytes in subepithelium of GB; numerous small accumulations (strawberry GB) or larger polypoid deposit (cholesterol polyp)

IMAGING FINDINGS

General Features

- Best diagnostic clue
  - Adenomyomatosis: Fundal, diffuse or mid-body GB wall thickening with intramural high amplitude echoes & "comet-tail" reverberation artifacts
  - Cholesterolosis: Multiple GB polyps
- Location
  - GB wall
  - Focal or diffuse type of involvement
- Size: Polyps typically 5-10 mm

Ultrasonographic Findings

- Grayscale Ultrasound
  - **Cholesterolosis**
    - Not related to serum cholesterol levels
    - Multiple small GB polyps with no posterior acoustic shadowing or "comet-tail" artifact
    - Usually ~ 5-10 mm in size
    - Well-defined, smooth margin
    - Occasionally pedunculated
    - Occasionally pedunculated
    - Low to medium level of echoes

DDx: Hyperplastic Cholecystosis

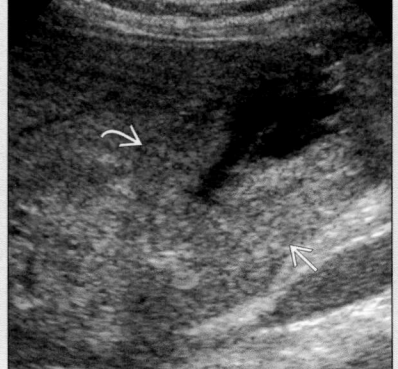

Gallbladder Carcinoma

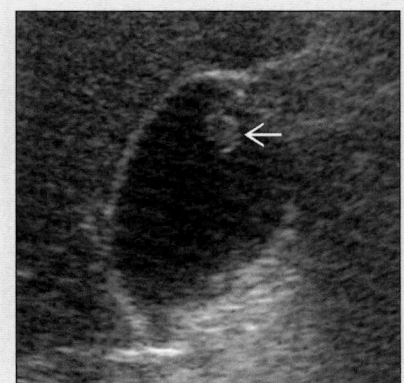

Adenomatous Polyp

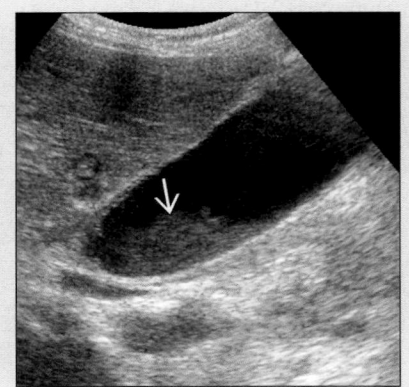

Echogenic Bile

GALLBLADDER CARCINOMA

Key Facts

Terminology
- Malignant epithelial neoplasm arising from gallbladder (GB) mucosa

Imaging Findings
- Large GB mass infiltrating gallbladder fossa extending into liver
- Polypoid intraluminal mass of irregular shape
- Diffuse or focal irregular mural thickening or destruction of GB wall
- Regional metastatic lymphadenopathy
- Best imaging tool: US, CECT
- Any polypoid mass of irregular shape within the GB lumen and every infiltrating lesion destroying GB wall is suspicious of GB carcinoma
- GB carcinoma produces lymph node metastases and invasion of adjacent structures early in disease

Top Differential Diagnoses
- GB Polyp
- Adenomyomatosis
- Xanthogranulomatous Cholecystitis
- Chronic Cholecystitis
- Metastatic Disease to GB Fossa

Clinical Issues
- Most common signs/symptoms: Right upper quadrant (RUQ) pain, weight loss, jaundice
- Very poor prognosis; 4% 5 year survival rate, 75% of patients have mets at time of diagnosis

Diagnostic Checklist
- Mass infiltrating GB fossa with liver invasion
- Large polypoid GB mucosal mass with flow

- Non-visualization of GB
- Common hepatic duct obstruction
- Dilated intrahepatic ducts

CT Findings
- CECT
  - Hypovascular mass infiltrating GB fossa, invading liver along main lobar fissure; porta hepatis with adenopathy
  - Calcified stones or porcelain GB

MR Findings
- T1WI: Iso- or hypointense GB fossa mass with increased signal compared to normal liver
- T2WI: Mass slightly increased in signal intensity compared to liver
- T1 C+: Hypovascular GB fossa mass invading liver
- MRCP
  - Dilated bile ducts due to common hepatic duct obstruction

Nuclear Medicine Findings
- Hepato biliary scan
  - Non-filling of GB

Imaging Recommendations
- Best imaging tool: US, CECT
- Protocol advice
  - Longitudinal & transverse ultrasound scan of GB fossa with grayscale and color Doppler
  - Any polypoid mass of irregular shape within the GB lumen and every infiltrating lesion destroying GB wall is suspicious of GB carcinoma
  - GB carcinoma produces lymph node metastases and invasion of adjacent structures early in disease

DIFFERENTIAL DIAGNOSIS

GB Polyp
- Non-shadowing, mucosal mass
  - Moderately echogenic without shadowing
- Non-mobile, attached to wall
- Typically < 1 cm for cholesterol polyp

- No vascularity detected on Doppler

Adenomyomatosis
- Localized fundal GB wall thickening, hyperechoic tumorous thickening due to hypertrophy of Rokitansky-Aschoff sinuses
- Focal thickening of midportion of GB ("hourglass GB")
- May demonstrate diffuse wall thickening
- Intramural cholesterol crystals as bright echoes with "comet-tail" reverberation echoes
- No adjacent infiltration or lymph node metastases

Xanthogranulomatous Cholecystitis
- Gallstones
- Ill-defined, infiltrative GB wall thickening
- Indistinguishable from gallbladder carcinoma, diagnosis is usually made following surgery
- No lymph node enlargement

Chronic Cholecystitis
- Contracted gallbladder
- Gallstone
- Wall thickening

Metastatic Disease to GB Fossa
- Most often nodal distribution around portal vein
- Melanoma may directly metastasize to GB mucosa
- Hepatoma and other hepatic tumors may secondarily spread to GB via duct invasion
- Porta hepatis lymphadenopathy
  - Lymphoma and GI tract carcinoma most common

PATHOLOGY

General Features
- General path comments
  - 90% adenocarcinoma
    - Early stage: Polypoid mucosal mass
    - Late stage: Mass infiltrating GB fossa
  - 10% squamous or anaplastic carcinoma
- Genetics: No known association
- Etiology

GALLBLADDER CARCINOMA

- Associated with porcelain GB & chronic inflammation 2° to gallstones; malignant degeneration of adenomatous mucosal polyps
  - 75% have gallstones
  - Porcelain GB predisposes to GB carcinoma
- Epidemiology
  - Most common type of biliary cancer
  - 75% are women
  - Average age of presentation is 70 years
  - Fifth most common GI cancer, 9x more common than extrahepatic cholangiocarcinoma
- Associated abnormalities
  - Gallstones in > 65%
  - Chronic cholecystitis
  - Porcelain GB (4-60%)
  - Ulcerative colitis; rarely Crohn disease
  - Primary sclerosing cholangitis
  - Familial polyposis coli

Gross Pathologic & Surgical Features
- Scirrhous infiltrating mass extending from GB wall to obliterate GB fossa & invade liver; porta hepatis adenopathy
- Direct invasion of liver, duodenum, stomach, bile duct, pancreas, right kidney
- Lymphatic spread to porta hepatis, peripancreatic & retroperitoneal nodes
- Intraperitoneal spread common with ascites, omental nodules & peritoneal implants
- Hematogenous spread (late in clinical course) to lungs, liver & bones
- Perineural invasion common

Microscopic Features
- Adenocarcinoma (90%)
- Squamous or anaplastic carcinoma (10%)

Staging, Grading or Classification Criteria
- Stage I: Carcinoma confined to mucosa
- Stage II: Carcinoma involves mucosa & muscularis
- Stage III: Carcinoma extends to serosa
- Stage IV: Transmural involvement with positive nodes
- Stage V: Liver or distant metastases

CLINICAL ISSUES

Presentation
- Most common signs/symptoms: Right upper quadrant (RUQ) pain, weight loss, jaundice
- Clinical Profile: Elevated bilirubin, elevated alkaline phosphatase with biliary obstruction

Demographics
- Age: Mean 70 years
- Gender: M:F = 1:3

Natural History & Prognosis
- Spreads by local invasion to liver, nodal spread to porta hepatis and para-aortic nodes, hematogenous spread to liver
- Very poor prognosis; 4% 5 year survival rate, 75% of patients have mets at time of diagnosis

Treatment
- Cholecystectomy for lesions confined to GB wall without liver invasion
- Radical cholecystectomy and/or partial hepatectomy with regional node dissection for lesions infiltrating porta hepatis

DIAGNOSTIC CHECKLIST

Consider
- Adenomyomatosis with GB wall thickening
  - Benign adenomatous polyp < 2 cm

Image Interpretation Pearls
- Porcelain GB
- Mass infiltrating GB fossa with liver invasion
- Large polypoid GB mucosal mass with flow
- Associated adjacent lymphadenopathy

SELECTED REFERENCES

1. Enomoto T et al: Xanthogranulomatous cholecystitis mimicking stage IV gallbladder cancer. Hepatogastroenterology. 50(53):1255-8, 2003
2. Goindi G et al: Risk factors in the aetiopathogenesis of carcinoma of the gallbladder. Trop Gastroenterol. 24(2):63-5, 2003
3. Kokudo N et al: Strategies for surgical treatment of gallbladder carcinoma based on information available before resection. Arch Surg. 138(7):741-50; dis 750, 2003
4. Misra S et al: Carcinoma of the gallbladder. Lancet Oncol. 4(3):167-76, 2003
5. Pandey M: Risk factors for gallbladder cancer: a reappraisal. Eur J Cancer Prev. 12(1):15-24, 2003
6. Yamamoto T et al: Early gallbladder carcinoma associated with primary sclerosing cholangitis and ulcerative colitis. J Gastroenterol. 38(7):704-6, 2003
7. Yun EJ et al: Gallbladder carcinoma and chronic cholecystitis: differentiation with two-phase spiral CT. Abdom Imaging. 29(1):102-8, 2003
8. Corvera CU et al: Role of laparoscopy in the evaluation of biliary tract cancer. Surg Oncol Clin N Am. 11(4):877-91, 2002
9. Cunningham CC et al: Primary carcinoma of the gall bladder: a review of our experience. J La State Med Soc. 154(4):196-9, 2002
10. Doty JR et al: Cholecystectomy, liver resection, and pylorus-preserving pancreaticoduodenectomy for gallbladder cancer: report of five cases. J Gastrointest Surg. 6(5):776-80, 2002
11. Gore RM et al: Imaging benign and malignant disease of the gallbladder. Radiol Clin North Am. 40(6):1307-23, vi, 2002
12. Varshney S et al: Incidental carcinoma of the gallbladder. Eur J Surg Oncol. 28(1):4-10, 2002
13. Xu AM et al: Multi-slice three-dimensional spiral CT cholangiography: a new technique for diagnosis of biliary diseases. Hepatobiliary Pancreat Dis Int. 1(4):595-603, 2002
14. Dixit VK et al: Aetiopathogenesis of carcinoma gallbladder. Trop Gastroenterol. 22(2):103-6, 2001
15. Donohue JH: Present status of the diagnosis and treatment of gallbladder carcinoma. J Hepatobiliary Pancreat Surg. 8(6):530-4, 2001
16. Kaushik SP: Current perspectives in gallbladder carcinoma. J Gastroenterol Hepatol. 16(8):848-54, 2001

GALLBLADDER CARCINOMA

IMAGE GALLERY

Typical

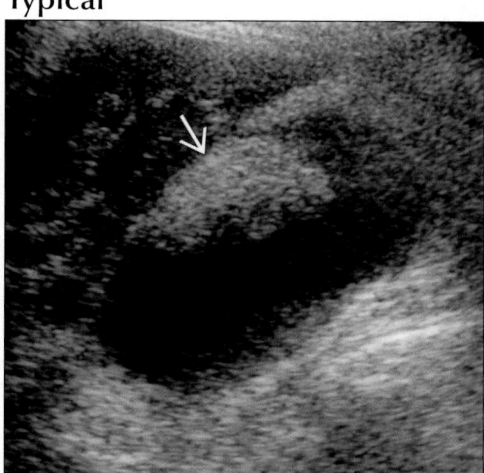
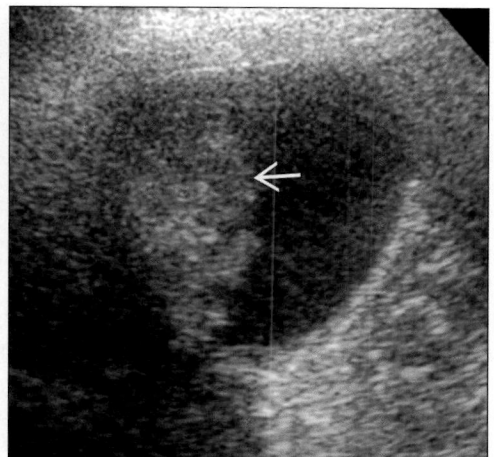

(Left) Oblique transabdominal ultrasound shows a focal eccentric mildly echogenic wall thickening ➡ arising from the anterior wall of the gallbladder. *(Right)* Transverse transabdominal ultrasound shows a polypoidal intraluminal mass ➡ of medium echogenicity in the right lateral wall of the gallbladder.

Typical

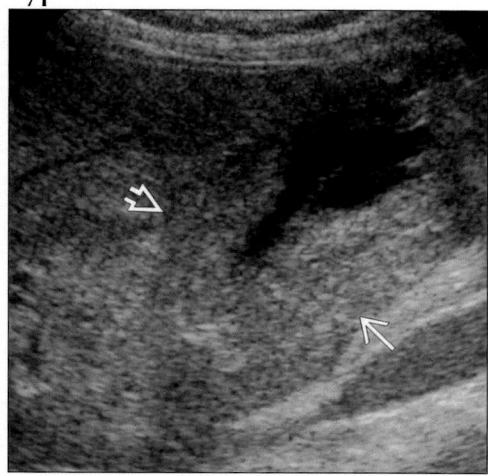
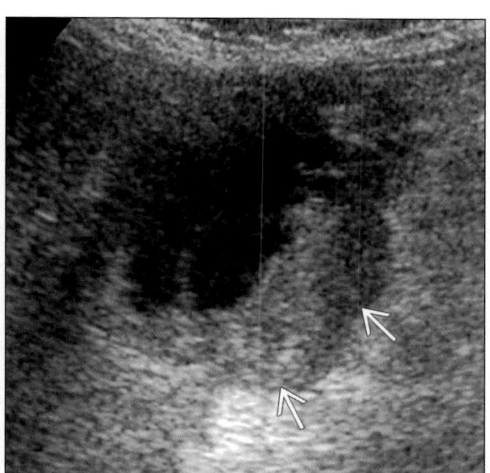

(Left) Oblique transabdominal ultrasound shows a large, mildly echogenic gallbladder mass ➡ with an irregular margin. The tumor infiltrates into the adjacent liver parenchyma ➡. *(Right)* Transverse transabdominal ultrasound shows marked, ill-defined, circumferential wall thickening of the gallbladder wall ➡, with medium echogenicity.

Typical

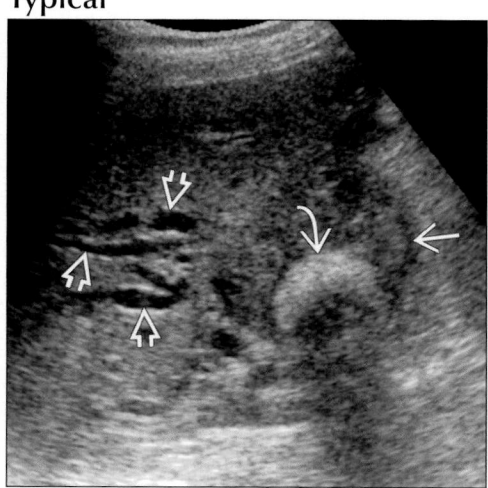
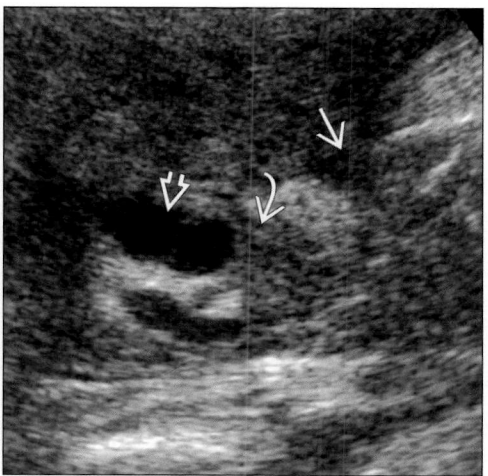

(Left) Oblique transabdominal ultrasound shows an ill-defined gallbladder mass ➡ with adjacent liver infiltration at the hepatic confluence, right intrahepatic ductal dilatation ➡, and gallstone ➡. *(Right)* Oblique transabdominal ultrasound shows an irregular gallbladder mass ➡ with tumor infiltration to the proximal common bile duct ➡ and extrahepatic ductal dilatation ➡.

BILIARY DUCTAL DILATATION

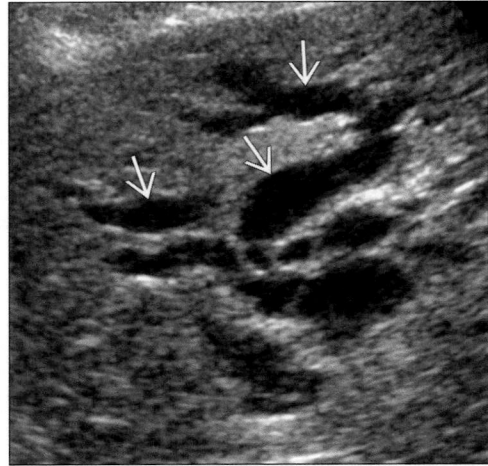

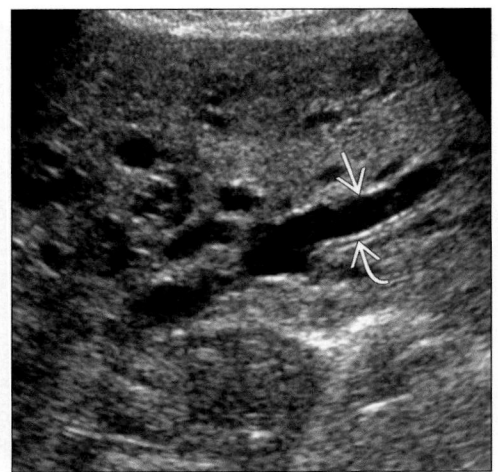

Transverse transabdominal ultrasound of the right lobe shows marked dilatation of the intrahepatic ducts ➜ due to malignant biliary obstruction at proximal extrahepatic bile duct.

Transverse transabdominal ultrasound shows dilatation of intrahepatic duct ➜ in left lobe. Note normal looking accompanying portal vein ➜ in parallel with the dilated left intrahepatic duct.

IMAGING FINDINGS

General Features
- Best diagnostic clue: Tubular anechoic fluid-filled structures accompanying portal veins in extrahepatic and intrahepatic segments
- Location: Intrahepatic +/- extrahepatic bile ducts

Ultrasonographic Findings
- Grayscale Ultrasound
  - Intrahepatic ductal dilatation
    - Dilatation of ductal diameter > 2 mm
    - Tubular anechoic branching structures accompanying portal veins
    - Irregularity and tortuosity of dilated ductal walls
    - Central stellate confluence of tubular structures proximally at liver hilum
    - Acoustic enhancement posterior to dilated ducts
  - Extrahepatic ductal dilatation
    - Dilatation of common hepatic/bile duct > 6-7 mm
    - Anechoic tubular structure related to main portal vein and hepatic artery in porta hepatis
    - Can trace its communication with intrahepatic ducts
  - Underlying causes of ductal dilatation may be found
- Power Doppler: Helpful to distinguish dilated ducts (no color flow) from adjacent vascular branches of hepatic artery and portal veins

CT Findings
- CECT: Water density tubular/serpiginous structures within liver parenchyma adjacent to intrahepatic portal veins

MR Findings
- MRCP: Hyperintense serpiginous structures within the liver parenchyma, communicate with extrahepatic ducts

Imaging Recommendations
- Best imaging tool
  - Transabdominal ultrasound as initial investigation for assessment of level, cause of biliary obstruction & guide interventional procedure
  - For better anatomical evaluation of underlying pathology, CT/MR provides supplementary information
- Protocol advice
  - US scanning technique

DDx: Biliary Ductal Dilatation

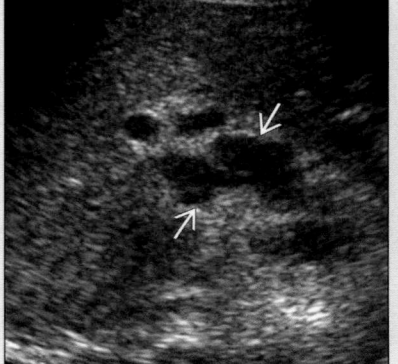

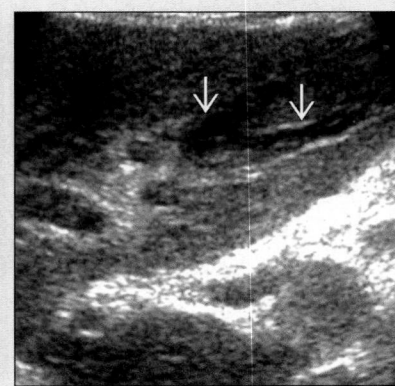

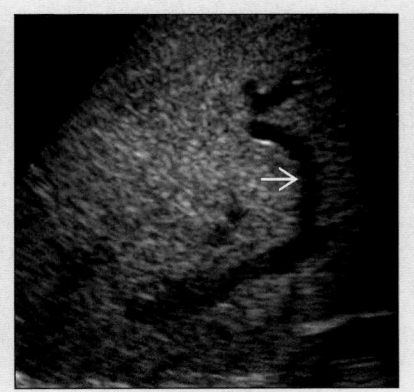

Portal Vein Cavernoma

Thrombosed Portal Vein Branch

Veno-venous Collaterals

BILIARY DUCTAL DILATATION

Key Facts

Imaging Findings
- Tubular anechoic branching structures accompanying portal veins
- Irregularity and tortuosity of dilated ductal walls
- Central stellate confluence of tubular structures proximally at liver hilum
- Acoustic enhancement posterior to dilated ducts
- Dilatation of common hepatic/bile duct > 6-7 mm

- Transabdominal ultrasound as initial investigation for assessment of level, cause of biliary obstruction & guide interventional procedure

Top Differential Diagnoses
- Portal Vein Cavernoma
- Thrombosed Portal Vein Branch
- Veno-Venous Collaterals

- Include comprehensive assessment on sagittal, transverse and oblique planes, intercostal and subcostal approach
- Intrahepatic ducts are better visualized on deep inspiration
- Oblique plane with patient in left decubitus position to minimize obscuration by overlying bowel gas to assess common hepatic/bile duct
- Harmonic imaging allows better visualization of the dilated ductal wall and its content

DIFFERENTIAL DIAGNOSIS

Portal Vein Cavernoma
- Cavernous transformation of portal vein; racemose conglomerate of collateral veins
- Doppler: Portal venous flow

Thrombosed Portal Vein Branch
- Hypoechoic (acute) or echogenic (chronic) filling defect within main portal vein & its branches
- Color Doppler: Patchy flow or complete absence of flow

Veno-Venous Collaterals
- Collateral between thrombosed/stenosed hepatic veins & normal hepatic veins/portal veins
- Color Doppler: Venous flow
- Seen in Budd Chiari syndrome

PATHOLOGY

General Features
- Etiology
  - Non-obstructive causes
    - Advanced age
    - Previous cholecystectomy
    - Congenital disease (e.g., choledochal cyst)
  - Obstructive causes
    - Intrahepatic obstruction: Calculus, recurrent pyogenic cholangitis, sclerosing/AIDS cholangitis, intrahepatic cholangiocarcinoma etc.
    - Extrahepatic obstruction: Intrapancreatic level (e.g., ductal carcinoma of pancreatic head), suprapancreatic level (e.g., extrahepatic cholangiocarcinoma), porta hepatis level (e.g., extrinsic lymph node compression)

CLINICAL ISSUES

Presentation
- Depends on underlying cause (e.g., acute cholangitis: RUQ pain, fever and chills)
- Obstructive jaundice: Painless or RUQ pain

SELECTED REFERENCES

1. Gandolfi L et al: The role of ultrasound in biliary and pancreatic diseases. Eur J Ultrasound. 16(3):141-59, 2003

IMAGE GALLERY

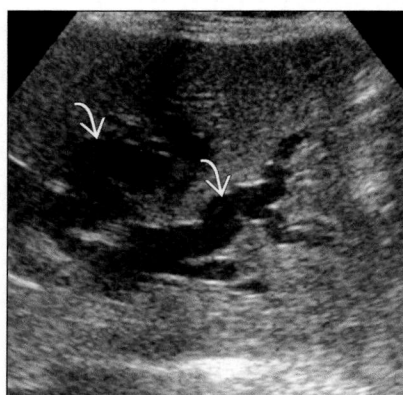 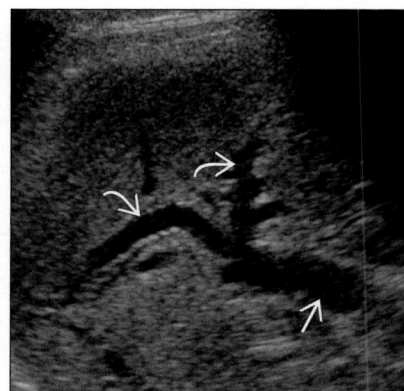 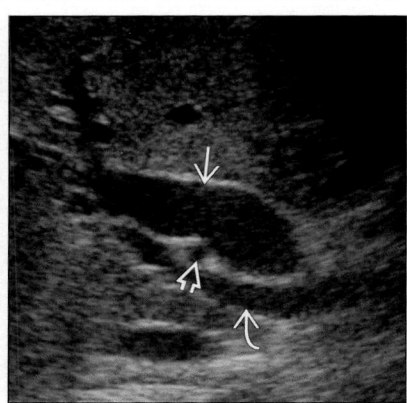

(Left) Oblique transabdominal ultrasound shows tortuous dilatation of the left intrahepatic ducts ⊇ due to a large stone impacted at the distal common bile duct. The stone was fragmented and removed via ERCP. *(Center)* Oblique transabdominal ultrasound shows dilatation of the right intrahepatic ducts ⊇, which is continuous with dilated proximal extrahepatic bile duct ⊇. *(Right)* Oblique transabdominal ultrasound shows dilatation of common duct ⊇ due to obstructing CBD stone. Note normal caliber of accompanying main portal vein ⊇ and hepatic artery ⊇.

CHOLEDOCHAL CYST

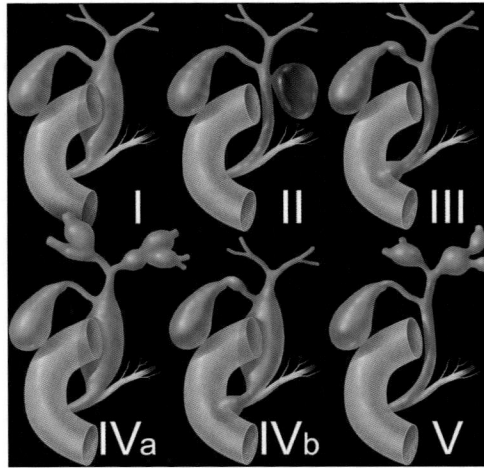

Graphic shows Todani classification of choledochal cyst: Type I: Extrahepatic involvement; II: Diverticulum; III: Choledochocele; IV: Multiple extrahepatic (IVa with intrahepatic involvement); V: Caroli disease.

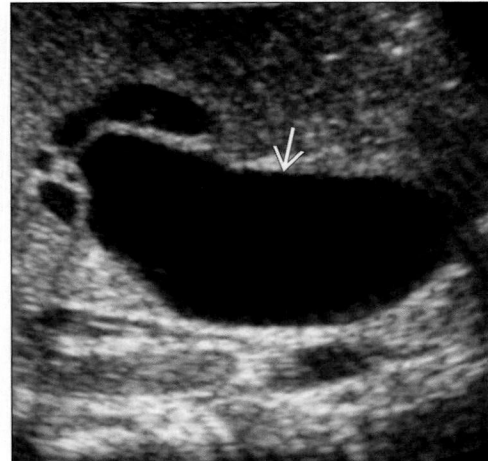

Oblique transabdominal ultrasound shows fusiform cystic dilatation of the extrahepatic biliary duct ➡ continuous with non-dilated intrahepatic ducts; typical appearances of type 1 lesion.

TERMINOLOGY

Abbreviations and Synonyms
- Choledochal malformations, common bile duct cyst/diverticulum, choledochocele

Definitions
- Spectrum of extrahepatic and intrahepatic bile ducts malformations characterized by fusiform dilatation

IMAGING FINDINGS

General Features
- Best diagnostic clue: Fusiform dilation of biliary tree
- Location: May involve intrahepatic bile ducts, extrahepatic ducts, or both
- Morphology: Refer to Todani classification of 5 types discussed in pathology section

Ultrasonographic Findings
- Grayscale Ultrasound
  - Best first test to demonstrate dilated biliary tree and extent of ductal involvement

  - Antenatal ultrasound (25 weeks): Right-sided cyst in fetal abdomen +/- dilated hepatic ducts
  - Uncomplicated choledochal cyst
    - Cystic extrahepatic mass separated from gallbladder and communicates with common hepatic or intrahepatic ducts
    - Fusiform dilatation of extrahepatic bile duct
    - Abrupt change of caliber at junction of dilated segment to normal ducts
    - Intrahepatic ductal dilatation due to simultaneous involvement or secondary to stenosis
  - Choledochal cyst with complications
    - Choledocholithiasis: Highly reflective echoes casting posterior acoustic shadow within dilated bile duct
    - Acute pancreatitis: Ill-defined, hypoechoic swelling of pancreatic parenchyma, adjacent soft tissue inflammation
    - Biliary cirrhosis: Coarse liver echotexture, nodular hepatic contour, decreased compliance
    - Malignant transformation: Ill-defined soft tissue mass within dilated bile duct, local tumor invasion, lymphadenopathy

DDx: Choledochal Cyst

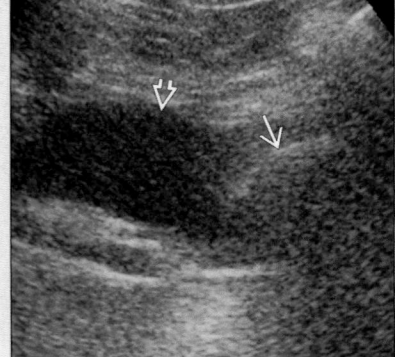

Cholangitis

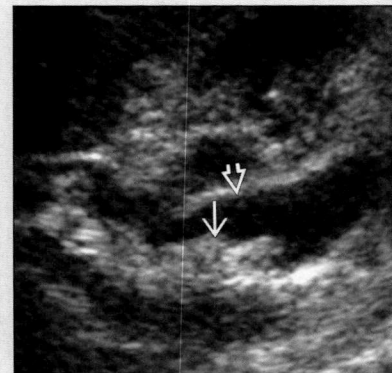

Choledocholithiasis

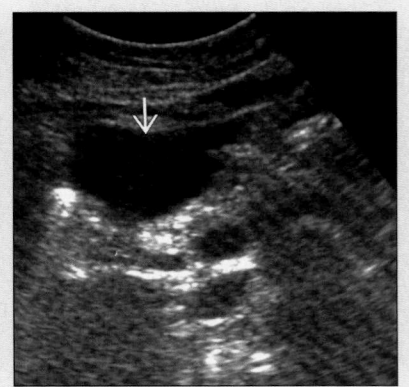

Pancreatic Pseudocyst

CHOLEDOCHAL CYST

Key Facts

Terminology
- Spectrum of extrahepatic and intrahepatic bile ducts malformations characterized by fusiform dilatation

Imaging Findings
- Location: May involve intrahepatic bile ducts, extrahepatic ducts, or both
- Cystic extrahepatic mass separated from gallbladder and communicates with common hepatic or intrahepatic ducts
- Best imaging tool: Ultrasound/MRCP

Top Differential Diagnoses
- Acute Cholangitis
- Biliary Obstruction of Various Causes
- Pancreatic Pseudocyst

Pathology
- Type I: Segmental or diffuse fusiform dilatation of common bile duct; 75-95% of cases
- Type II: Diverticulum of extrahepatic duct
- Type III: Choledochocele
- Type IV: Multiple extrahepatic bile duct cysts; alone (IVb) or with intrahepatic biliary involvement (IVa)
- Type V: Cystic dilatation of the intrahepatic bile ducts

Clinical Issues
- Age: 2/3 of all choledochal malformations are diagnosed before 10 years of age
- Complications: Bile duct perforation, biliary stone formation, bacterial cholangitis, development of bile duct carcinomas

---

- Color Doppler: Useful for demonstrating position and displacement of adjacent vessels

CT Findings
- CECT
  - Fusiform dilatation of extra- and/or intrahepatic bile ducts
  - Helpful to delineate its relationship with adjacent structures such as pancreas and duodenum
  - Contrast-enhancing soft tissue within dilated biliary tree would raise the suspicion of malignant transformation

MR Findings
- MRCP
  - Replacing percutaneous cholangiogram in pre-operative planning
  - Heavily T2 weighted imaging
  - Allow clear visualization of extent of biliary dilatation and the length of common trunk of distal common bile duct and pancreatic duct

Other Modality Findings
- Endoscopic retrograde cholangiopancreatography (ERCP) and percutaneous cholangiogram usually reserved for difficult or complex cases

Nuclear Medicine Findings
- Hepatobiliary Scintigraphy
  - Photopenic area in right upper quadrant within the liver that fills within 60 minutes
  - Stasis of tracer within the cyst
  - Prominent intrahepatic ductal tracer activity
  - Absence of tracer passage into small bowel

Imaging Recommendations
- Best imaging tool: Ultrasound/MRCP
- Protocol advice
  - Scan the patient in both supine and right oblique position to ensure optimal anatomical delineation of dilated biliary tree
  - Diagnostic pitfall
    - Overlying bowel gas precludes accurate assessment of extent of involvement

- Difficult to ascertain nature if cyst is too large and its relationship with the rest of biliary tree cannot be well established
  - MR/MRCP for additional anatomic detail
  - Hepatobiliary scans for functional evaluation and if diagnosis not certain on ultrasound (e.g., large cyst)

DIFFERENTIAL DIAGNOSIS

Acute Cholangitis
- Ductal wall thickening
- Obstructing choledocholithiasis

Biliary Obstruction of Various Causes
- Ectatic (rather than fusiform) dilatation
- Degree of dilatation less than choledochal cyst
- Primary lesion identifiable (e.g., choledocholithiasis, cholangiocarcinoma/pancreatic head tumor)

Pancreatic Pseudocyst
- Well-defined, cystic lesion related to pancreatic head
- Previous history of acute pancreatitis
- May be associated with changes of chronic pancreatitis

Caroli Disease
- Technically classified as type V choledochal cyst
- Congenital nonobstructive dilatation of the large intrahepatic bile ducts
- Localized saccular ectasia, producing multiple cyst-like structures of varying size

PATHOLOGY

General Features
- Etiology
  - Most prevalent of the current theories involves the anomalous junction of the common biliary and pancreatic ducts which provides conduit for mixing of pancreatic juices and bile

CHOLEDOCHAL CYST

- Activation of pancreatic enzymes within the common bile duct of patients with an anomalous junction
- Additional theories: Decrease in the number of ganglion cells in the narrow portion of the bile duct causing increased intraluminal pressure, reovirus infection, familial pattern of inheritance, failure of recanalization, and duodenal duplication
- Epidemiology
  - More common in the far East (Orientals) than in Western countries
  - Approximately 1/3 of all reported cases occur in Japanese patients

Gross Pathologic & Surgical Features

- Range in diameter from a few centimeters to over 15 cm
- Cyst wall is thickened, fibrotic, and occasionally calcified in adults

Microscopic Features

- Histologically: Varying degrees of chronic inflammation and scattered elastic and smooth muscle fibers
- Biliary epithelium lining the cyst is often intact in infants
- Goblet-cell metaplasia and epithelial dysplasia with nuclear hyperchromasia, irregularity, and loss of polarity have been described and may play a role in subsequent development of carcinoma
- Type III cysts (choledochocele) are usually lined by duodenal mucosa, but occasionally may have biliary epithelium

Staging, Grading or Classification Criteria

- Classification modified by Todani in 1977
- Type I: Segmental or diffuse fusiform dilatation of common bile duct; 75-95% of cases
- Type II: Diverticulum of extrahepatic duct
- Type III: Choledochocele
- Type IV: Multiple extrahepatic bile duct cysts; alone (IVb) or with intrahepatic biliary involvement (IVa)
- Type V: Cystic dilatation of the intrahepatic bile ducts

CLINICAL ISSUES

Presentation

- Most common signs/symptoms
  - Neonate/newborn
    - Prolonged neonatal jaundice (i.e., obstructive cholangiopathy)
    - Incidental finding on antenatal ultrasound screening
  - Infant
    - Jaundice, acholic stools, hepatomegaly, palpable abdominal mass
  - Adult
    - Upper abdominal pain, jaundice, recurrent cholangitis/pancreatitis, biliary cirrhosis
- Other signs/symptoms: Adult patients tend to present with recurrent cholangitis, pancreatitis, or rarely portal hypertension

Demographics

- Age: 2/3 of all choledochal malformations are diagnosed before 10 years of age
- Gender: More common in females; 3 or 4:1 ratio

Natural History & Prognosis

- Low grade biliary obstruction may develop and can potentially result in cirrhosis and portal hypertension
- Prevalence of cancer, usually adenocarcinoma, arising in choledochal cysts varies from 2-18%, corresponding to roughly 5-35x increased risk
- Complications: Bile duct perforation, biliary stone formation, bacterial cholangitis, development of bile duct carcinomas

Treatment

- Type I: Complete surgical excision followed by biliary drainage procedure, typically Roux-en-Y choledochojejunostomy
- Type II: Cysts can usually be surgically excised entirely
- Type III: Choledochocele < 3 cm may be approached endoscopically with sphincterotomy; > 3 cm are excised surgically by using a transduodenal approach
- Type IV: Dilatated extrahepatic duct is completely excised with biliary-enteric drainage procedure, intrahepatic involvement is left untreated
- Type V: When limited to a single hepatic lobe, may be resected; diffuse disease is streaked with liver transplantation when liver failure develops

SELECTED REFERENCES

1. Kishino T et al: Choledochocele demonstrated on conventional sonography. J Clin Ultrasound. 34(4):199-202, 2006
2. Chen CP et al: Prenatal diagnosis of choledochal cyst using ultrasound and magnetic resonance imaging. Ultrasound Obstet Gynecol. 23(1):93-4, 2004
3. Hamada Y et al: Magnetic resonance cholangiopancreatography on postoperative work-up in children with choledochal cysts. Pediatr Surg Int. 20(1):43-6, 2004
4. Haliloglu M et al: Choledochal cysts in children: evaluation with three-dimensional sonography. J Clin Ultrasound. 31(9):478-80, 2003
5. Sugiyama M et al: Anomalous pancreaticobiliary junction shown on multidetector CT. AJR Am J Roentgenol. 180(1):173-5, 2003
6. Zhong L et al: Imaging diagnosis of pancreato-biliary diseases: a control study. World J Gastroenterol. 9(12):2824-7, 2003
7. Benya EC: Pancreas and biliary system: imaging of developmental anomalies and diseases unique to children. Radiol Clin North Am. 40(6):1355-62, 2002
8. Casaccia G et al: Cystic anomalies of biliary tree in the fetus: is it possible to make a more specific prenatal diagnosis? J Pediatr Surg. 37(8):1191-4, 2002
9. de Vries JS et al: Choledochal cysts: age of presentation, symptoms, and late complications related to Todani's classification. J Pediatr Surg. 37(11):1568-73, 2002
10. Guy F et al: Caroli's disease: magnetic resonance imaging features. Eur Radiol. 12(11):2730-6, 2002
11. Krause D et al: MRI for evaluating congenital bile duct abnormalities. J Comput Assist Tomogr. 26(4):541-52, 2002
12. Gubernick JA et al: US approach to jaundice in infants and children. Radiographics. 20(1):173-95, 2000

CHOLEDOCHAL CYST

IMAGE GALLERY

Typical

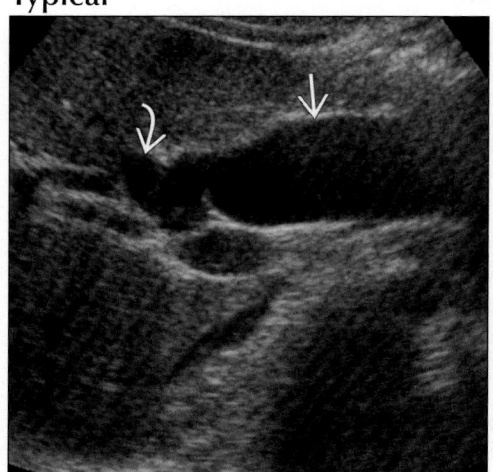
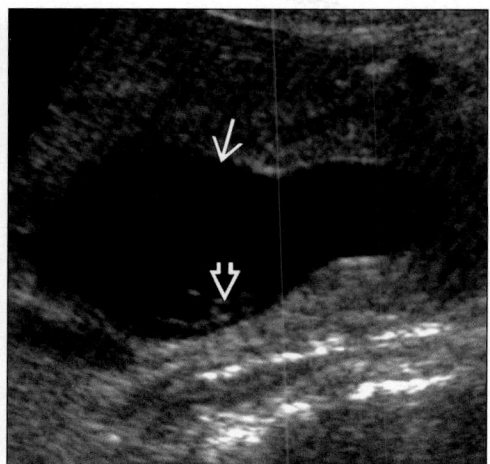

(Left) Oblique transabdominal ultrasound shows fusiform dilatation of the common bile duct ➡, which is continuous with mildly dilated intrahepatic ducts ➡. *(Right)* Oblique transabdominal ultrasound shows fusiform dilatation of the intrahepatic bile duct ➡ in the left lobe of liver. Note the presence of biliary sludge ➡ in its dependent part.

Typical

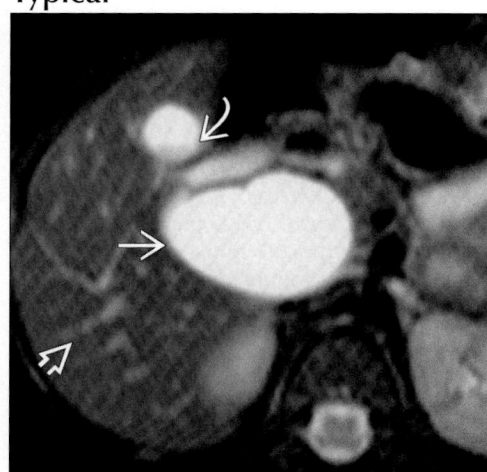
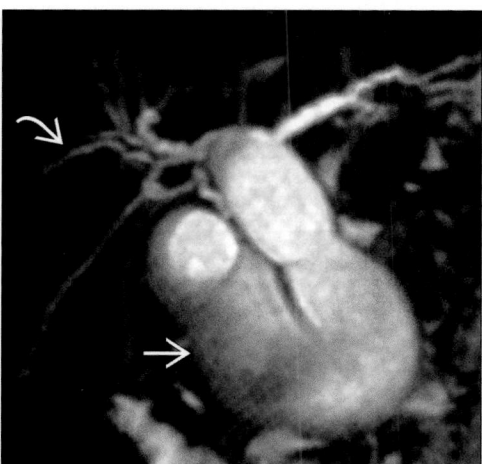

(Left) Axial MRCP shows a large choledochal cyst ➡. The normal gallbladder shows layering of sludge ➡, note the non-dilated intrahepatic biliary ducts ➡. *(Right)* Reformatted MRCP image showing the choledochal cyst ➡. Note the relatively non dilated intrahepatic biliary ducts ➡.

Typical

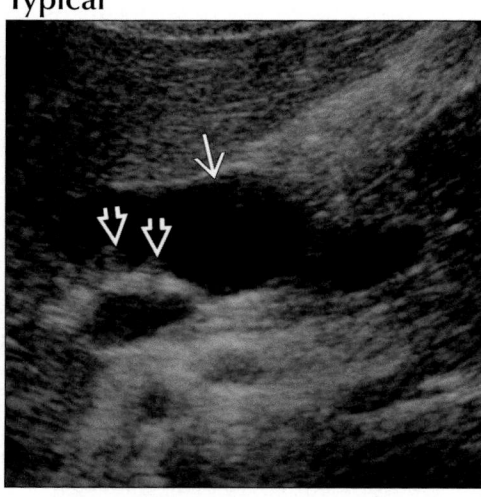
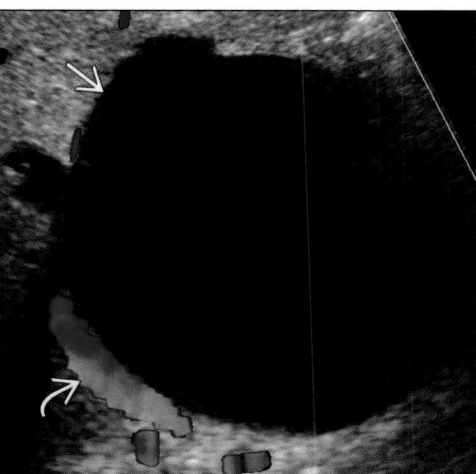

(Left) Oblique transabdominal ultrasound of a choledochal cyst shows fusiform dilatation of the common bile duct ➡ with non-shadowing stones ➡ in its dependent portion. *(Right)* Oblique color Doppler ultrasound shows a grossly dilated, globular appearance of the common bile duct ➡ anterior to the main portal vein ➡ with normal hepatopetal blood flow.

CHOLEDOCHOLITHIASIS

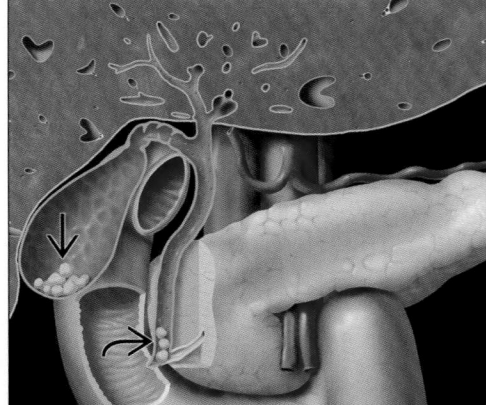

Graphic shows multiple, non-obstructive stones in the distal CBD ➚ and gallbladder ➘.

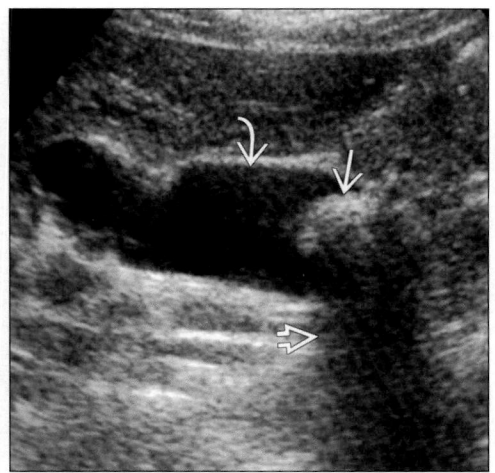

Oblique transabdominal ultrasound shows an echogenic focus ➡ within the distal portion of a dilated CBD ➘, with posterior acoustic shadowing ➭ suggesting extrahepatic choledocholithiasis.

TERMINOLOGY

Abbreviations and Synonyms
- Cholangiolithiasis, biliary calculi

Definitions
- Intra- &/or extrahepatic ductal stones/calculi

IMAGING FINDINGS

General Features
- Best diagnostic clue: High level echogenic focus within biliary ducts casting posterior acoustic shadowing
- Location: Intra- & extrahepatic bile ducts (more common in CBD)
- Size: Variable
- Morphology
  - Classified into two types based on etiology
    - Primary choledocholithiasis: de novo formation within bile duct
    - Secondary choledocholithiasis: Gallstone migration from GB to bile ducts

Ultrasonographic Findings
- Grayscale Ultrasound
  - Appearances depend on the site, size and composition of stones
  - Intrahepatic stones
    - Majority appear as highly echogenic foci with posterior acoustic shadowing
    - Located in region of portal triads paralleling the course of intrahepatic portal veins
    - Small (< 5 mm) or soft pigmented stones may not produce posterior shadowing
    - Larger stone may cause biliary obstruction with focal intrahepatic ductal dilatation
    - If affected duct filled with stones appears as linear echogenic structure with posterior acoustic shadowing
  - Extrahepatic biliary stones
    - Most commonly seen within CBD
    - Classic appearances: Rounded echogenic lesion with posterior acoustic shadowing
    - Most often found within lumen of periampullary region/distal portion of CBD

DDx: Choledocholithiasis

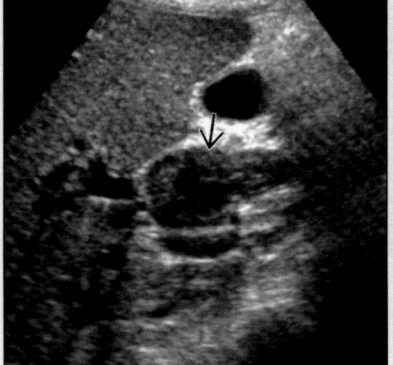

Cholangiocarcinoma

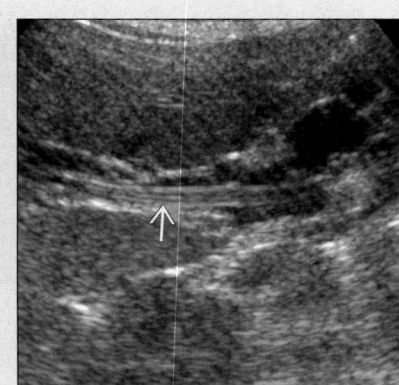

Parasitic Infestation

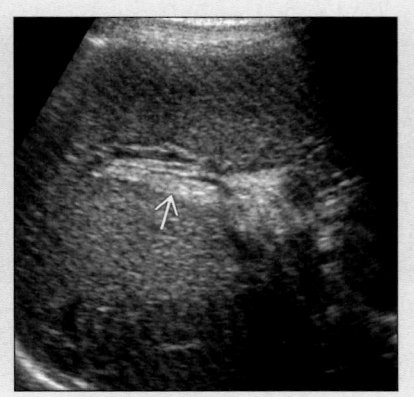

Acute Cholangitis

CHOLEDOCHOLITHIASIS

Key Facts

Imaging Findings

- Appearances depend on the site, size and composition of stones
- Majority appear as highly echogenic foci with posterior acoustic shadowing
- Small (< 5 mm) or soft pigmented stones may not produce posterior shadowing
- Larger stone may cause biliary obstruction with focal intrahepatic ductal dilatation
- Best imaging tool: US, MRCP
- CBD stones are most commonly located in the region of ampulla of Vater, high chance of being obscured by bowel gas
- Examine patient in different positions: Supine, left lateral oblique, standing

- Use multiple scanning sites for optimal acoustic window
- Use compression by firm probe pressure to collapse superficial bowel and its content
- Perform a detailed assessment of the region of head of pancreas

Top Differential Diagnoses

- Cholangiocarcinoma
- Biliary Parasitic Infestation
- Pancreatic or Ampullary Cancer

Diagnostic Checklist

- Rule out other causes of "CBD obstruction"
- Echogenic filling defects casting posterior acoustic shadowing associated with dilatation of CBD/intrahepatic bile ducts

---

- Associated extrahepatic and intrahepatic ductal dilatation
- Small stones may lack posterior shadowing
  - 10% stones: No posterior acoustic shadow
    - Small size, soft & porous composition
    - DDx: Intraductal clot, infection, sludge ball, tumor, parasite
  - CBD/intrahepatic bile duct dilatation (IHBD) based on stone size, degree & duration of obstruction
    - CBD: 4-6 mm (normal size); 6-7 mm (equivocal); more than 8 mm (dilatation)
    - Common hepatic duct: 4-5 mm (normal size)
    - IHBD: 1-2 mm (usually not visible)
- Color Doppler
  - Echogenic focus is avascular
  - Aids definition of dilated biliary ducts against background intrahepatic parenchymal vessels

Radiographic Findings

- ERCP
  - Radiolucent filling defects within intrahepatic +/- extrahepatic bile ducts
  - Faceted/angular border (compared with smooth round contour for gas bubbles)
  - Portal for stone retrieval or internal stent insertion
- Intra-operative & post-operative (T tube) cholangiography
  - Direct tests for detection of CBD stones
  - Meniscus of contrast material clearly outlines margins of stones

CT Findings

- NECT
  - Attenuation of calculi varies from less than water density, through soft tissue, to dense calcification
  - Typically high density filling defect within biliary duct
  - Abrupt termination of CBD (complete obstruction by a large stone)
    - Stone isodense to bile or pancreas (DDx: Malignant stricture & carcinoma of ampulla)
  - CBD &/or IHBD dilatation

- Varies depending on stone size, degree & duration of obstruction
- Water density tubular branching structures

MR Findings

- MRC (MR cholangiography)
  - Bile: Very bright signal
  - Ductal stones: Decreased signal intensity foci
  - Low-signal filling defects within increased signal intensity bile

Nuclear Medicine Findings

- Hepatobiliary scan (HIDA)
  - Delayed bowel activity beyond 2 hours
  - Persistent hepatic and common bile duct activity up to 24 hours

Imaging Recommendations

- Best imaging tool: US, MRCP
- Protocol advice
  - CBD stones are most commonly located in the region of ampulla of Vater, high chance of being obscured by bowel gas
  - Practical advice to optimize detection
    - Examine patient in different positions: Supine, left lateral oblique, standing
    - Use multiple scanning sites for optimal acoustic window
    - Use compression by firm probe pressure to collapse superficial bowel and its content
    - Perform a detailed assessment of the region of head of pancreas
  - Postcholecystectomy patients with persistent RUQ pain: CBD imaged
    - After fasting & 45 min to 1 hr after a fatty meal
    - CBD dilates more than 2 mm above baseline in partial stone obstruction
  - If gas obscures CBD; have patient drink 6-12 oz of water
    - Keep patient in right decubitus position for 2-3 minutes & rescan in semierect position

CHOLEDOCHOLITHIASIS

DIFFERENTIAL DIAGNOSIS

Cholangiocarcinoma
- Infiltrative mass at hepatic confluence
- Soft tissue growth within ductal lumen
- Obstruction & dilatation of CBD/IHBD
- Regional nodal and liver metastases

Biliary Parasitic Infestation
- Most common infestation: Ascaris, Clonorchis
- Parallel echogenic tubular structures with sonolucent centre within bile duct
- Active movement of the parasite
- Lack of posterior acoustic shadowing

Pancreatic or Ampullary Cancer
- Hypodense mass in head of pancreas or ampulla
- Ill-defined infiltrative margin
- "Double duct" sign
  - Obstruction & dilatation of pancreatic duct/CBD
- Vascular encasement
- Contiguous organ invasion/regional nodal metastases may be seen

Acute Bacterial Cholangitis
- Clinical information suggesting biliary sepsis
- Ductal wall thickening
- Presence of CBD stone obstruction with proximal extra- and intra-hepatic ductal dilatation
- Echogenic biliary sludge within ducts

Primary Sclerosing Cholangitis (PSC)
- Idiopathic or autoimmune reaction or genetic
- CBD always involved; IHBD & extrahepatic (68-89%)
- ERCP: Classic "beaded appearance"

PATHOLOGY

General Features
- General path comments
  - Mechanism of stones in CBD & IHBD
    - Obstruction, dilatation, sclerosis, stricture
    - Bile stasis/infection: Bilirubinate stone formation
    - Infection: E. coli, Klebsiella & other gram negative organisms with β-glucuronidase activity
- Etiology
  - Primary choledocholithiasis (5%): de novo formation of stones within bile ducts
    - Chronic hemolytic disease, recurrent cholangitis
    - Congenital anomalies of bile ducts (e.g., Caroli disease)
    - Prior biliary surgery, foreign body (suture material)
    - Parasites: Clonorchis sinensis & ascaris (major causes in Asia)
  - Secondary duct stones (95%): Gallstones migrate into CBD
    - Obesity, Crohn disease & ileal resection
    - Hemolytic anemias (sickle cell anemia & hereditary spherocytosis)
    - Increased triglycerides, hyperalimentation, Native American heritage
- Associated abnormalities: Gallstones

CLINICAL ISSUES

Presentation
- Most common signs/symptoms
  - RUQ pain, pruritus, jaundice
  - May be asymptomatic
- Other signs/symptoms: May present with complication: Acute cholangitis, acute pancreatitis
- Clinical Profile: Fat, fertile, middle aged female with history of acute or intermittent RUQ pain & jaundice
- Lab data
  - Increased alkaline phosphatase & direct bilirubin

Demographics
- Age: Usually adults; can be seen in any age group
- Gender: Females (middle age) more than males

Natural History & Prognosis
- Small stones may pass spontaneously without causing any symptoms
- Complications: Cholangitis, obstructive jaundice, pancreatitis, secondary biliary cirrhosis

Treatment
- Stones < 3 mm: Usually pass spontaneously, surgery usually not required
- Stones 3-10 mm: Endoscopic sphincterotomy
  - Stone retrieval balloon to sweep duct
  - Basket to snare stones
- Stones more than 10-15 mm
  - Require fragmentation by mechanical lithotripsy
  - May require operative removal (i.e., cholecystectomy with exploration of CBD)

DIAGNOSTIC CHECKLIST

Consider
- Rule out other causes of "CBD obstruction"

Image Interpretation Pearls
- Echogenic filling defects casting posterior acoustic shadowing associated with dilatation of CBD/intrahepatic bile ducts

SELECTED REFERENCES

1. Freitas ML et al: Choledocholithiasis: evolving standards for diagnosis and management. World J Gastroenterol. 12(20):3162-7, 2006
2. Hanbidge AE et al: From the RSNA refresher courses: imaging evaluation for acute pain in the right upper quadrant. Radiographics. 24(4):1117-35, 2004
3. Baron RL et al: Imaging the spectrum of biliary tract disease. Radiol Clin North Am. 40(6):1325-54, 2002
4. Fulcher AS: MRCP and ERCP in the diagnosis of common bile duct stones. Gastrointest Endosc. 56(6 Suppl):S178-82, 2002
5. Mark DH et al: Evidence-based assessment of diagnostic modalities for common bile duct stones. Gastrointest Endosc. 56(6 Suppl):S190-4, 2002
6. Vilgrain V et al: Choledocholithiasis: role of US and endoscopic ultrasound. Abdom Imaging. 26(1):7-14, 2001
7. Pickuth D: Radiologic diagnosis of common bile duct stones. Abdom Imaging. 25(6):618-21, 2000

CHOLEDOCHOLITHIASIS

IMAGE GALLERY

Typical

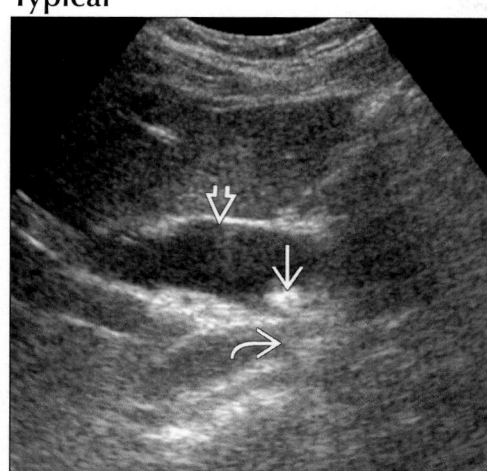
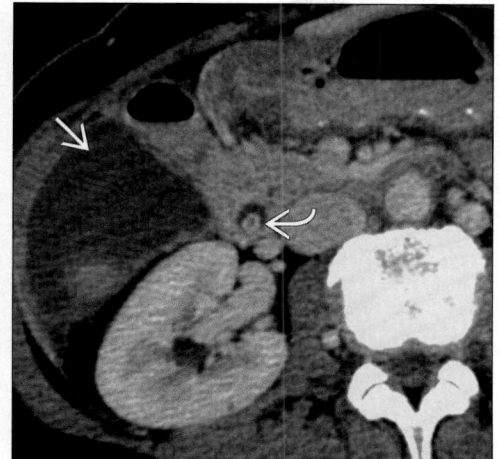

(Left) Oblique transabdominal ultrasound shows a small echogenic stone ➡ with faint acoustic shadowing ⇻ within the dependent portion of the dilated common bile duct ⇶. (Right) Transverse CECT shows an impacted stone ➡ at the terminal portion of the CBD at the head of the pancreas. Note ascites ➡ in the subhepatic region.

Typical

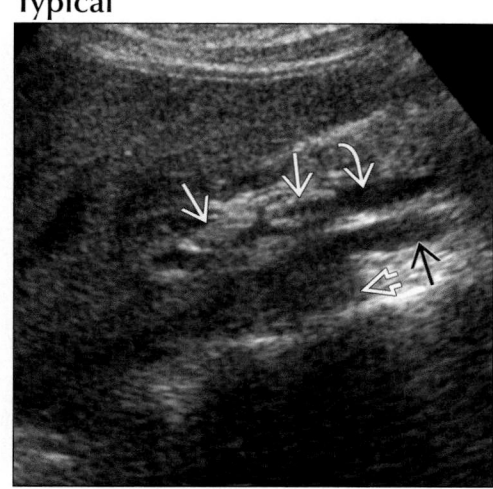
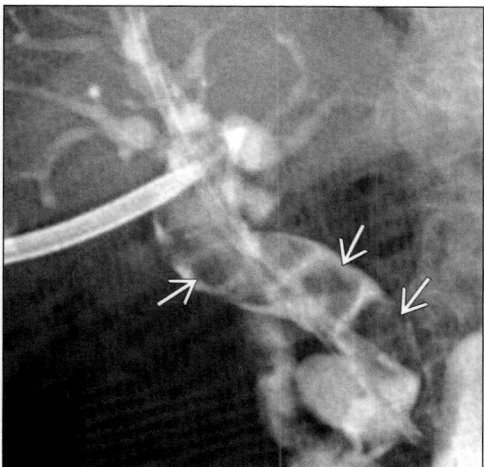

(Left) Oblique transabdominal ultrasound shows two intraductal stones ➡ within the mid portion of a non-dilated CBD ⇻. Note the presence of posterior acoustic shadowing ⇶. Main portal vein ➡. (Right) Transhepatic cholangiography shows multiple filling defects ➡ with a faceted contour within the dilated CBD compatible with extrahepatic choledocholithiasis. The patient underwent tract dilatation for percutaneous stone extraction.

Typical

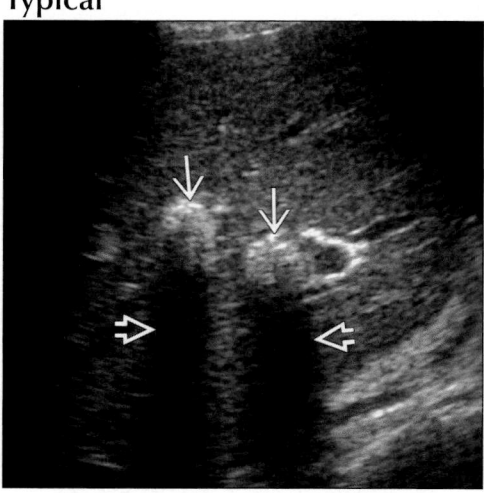
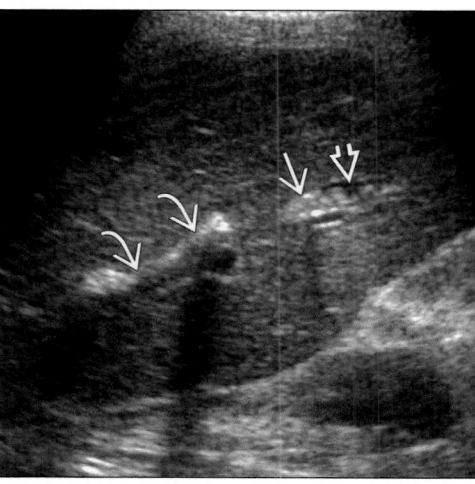

(Left) Oblique transabdominal ultrasound shows large, intrahepatic ductal stones ➡, with strong posterior acoustic shadowing ⇶, in the intrahepatic bile ducts of the right lobe of the liver. (Right) Oblique transabdominal ultrasound shows intrahepatic ductal stones ➡ in a dilated intrahepatic duct ⇶. Note hyperechogenicity along the portal triad ➡ representing an intrahepatic duct packed with stones.

BILIARY DUCTAL GAS

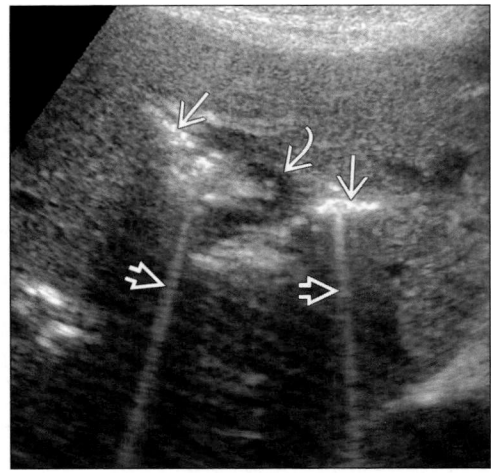

Transverse transabdominal ultrasound shows echogenic foci ➡ in a linear configuration adjacent to the left portal vein ➡, casting posterior acoustic shadowing and reverberation artifact ➡.

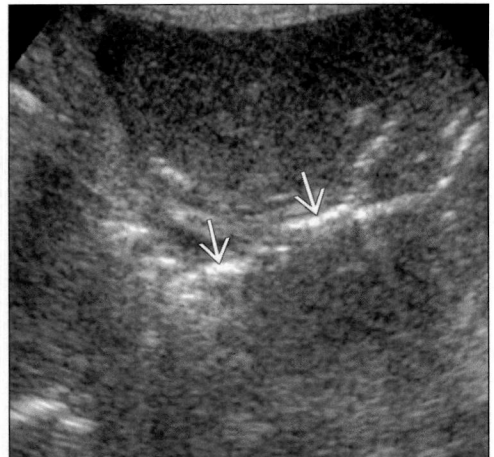

Transverse transabdominal ultrasound shows an abundant amount of biliary ductal gas within the left intrahepatic ducts ➡, casting posterior acoustic shadowing. Patient underwent ERCP two days prior.

TERMINOLOGY

Abbreviations and Synonyms
- Pneumobilia, aerobilia

Definitions
- Gas within biliary tree including bile ducts or gallbladder

IMAGING FINDINGS

General Features
- Best diagnostic clue: Bright echogenic foci in linear configuration following portal triads casting posterior acoustic shadowing
- Location: Most commonly seen within intrahepatic bile ducts, occasionally involving extrahepatic bile ducts and gallbladder

Ultrasonographic Findings
- Grayscale Ultrasound
  - Gas within intrahepatic bile duct
    - Bright echogenic foci in linear configuration
    - Follows the location of portal triads
    - In non-dependent position: Left lobe biliary ducts with patient in supine position
    - Associated with posterior acoustic shadowing
    - Reverberation artifacts with large quantities of air
    - Movement of gas, best demonstrated following change in patient's position
  - Gas within extrahepatic bile duct
    - Echogenic foci in linear configuration casting posterior acoustic shadowing
    - Within extrahepatic bile ducts adjacent to major structures in porta hepatis
  - Gas within gallbladder
    - Band-like echogenic layer in least dependent portion within gallbladder
    - Prominent reverberation artifacts obscuring luminal content

CT Findings
- CECT: Linear/serpiginous gas density adjacent to well opacified portal venous radicles and portal veins

Imaging Recommendations
- Best imaging tool: Ultrasound
- Protocol advice

DDx: Biliary Ductal Gas

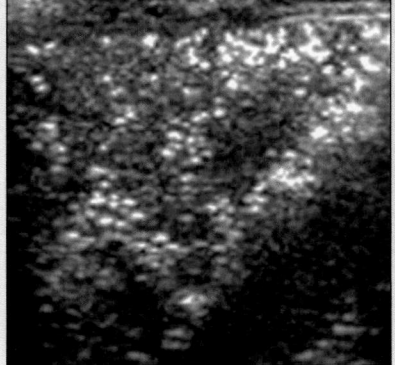

Portal Venous Gas

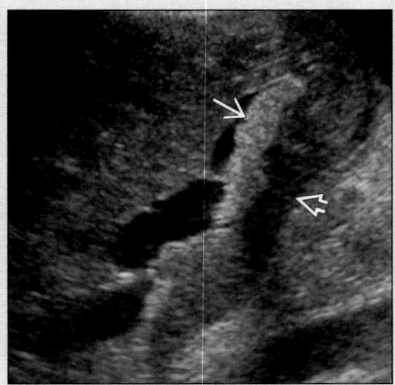

Intrahepatic Echogenic Sludge

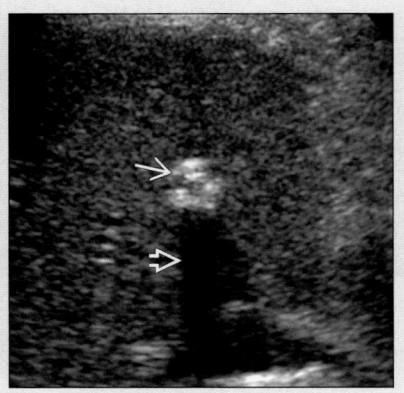

Calcified Hepatic Granuloma

BILIARY DUCTAL GAS

Key Facts

Terminology
- Pneumobilia, aerobilia

Imaging Findings
- Best diagnostic clue: Bright echogenic foci in linear configuration following portal triads casting posterior acoustic shadowing
- In non-dependent position: Left lobe biliary ducts with patient in supine position

Top Differential Diagnoses
- Portal Venous Gas
- Intrahepatic Ductal Stones/Sludge
- Calcified Hepatic Granuloma

Pathology
- Previous biliary intervention
- Cholecysto-enteric/choledocho-enteric fistula
- Biliary infection with gas-forming organism

- ○ Examine patient in supine and oblique positions to demonstrate movement of gas
- ○ Set appropriate focus level to optimize visualization of reverberation artifacts or posterior acoustic shadowing

DIFFERENTIAL DIAGNOSIS

Portal Venous Gas
- Branching echogenic foci in periphery of liver parenchyma within portal venous radicle
- Gas in mesenteric vessels

Intrahepatic Ductal Stones/Sludge
- Echogenic foci casting dense posterior acoustic shadowing, ± fluid level
- In region of portal triad or within dilated intrahepatic ducts

Calcified Hepatic Granuloma
- Coarse echogenic focus with marked posterior shadowing, solitary/multiple
- Not related to portal triad

PATHOLOGY

General Features
- Etiology
  - ○ Previous biliary intervention
    - ■ Recent ERCP +/- sphincterotomy

- ■ Biliary-enteric anastomosis
- ■ Presence of internal biliary stent or external biliary drainage catheter
- ○ Cholecysto-enteric/choledocho-enteric fistula
  - ■ Prolonged acute cholecystitis +/- superimposed gallstone ileus (in 20%)
  - ■ Perforated duodenal ulcer
  - ■ Erosion by biliary malignancy (e.g., carcinoma of gallbladder)
- ○ Biliary infection with gas-forming organism
  - ■ Emphysematous cholecystitis
  - ■ Acute bacterial cholangitis

CLINICAL ISSUES

Natural History & Prognosis
- Majority will resolve spontaneously
- Prognosis depends on the underlying etiology

DIAGNOSTIC CHECKLIST

Image Interpretation Pearls
- Echogenic foci in linear configuration at portal triads with reverberation artifacts

SELECTED REFERENCES

1. Yarmenitis SD: Ultrasound of the gallbladder and the biliary tree. Eur Radiol. 12(2):270-82, 2002

IMAGE GALLERY

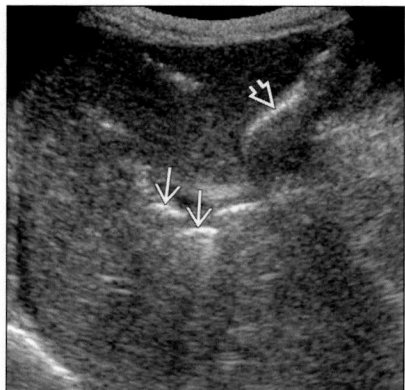 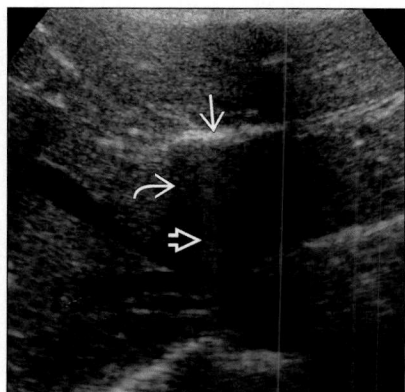 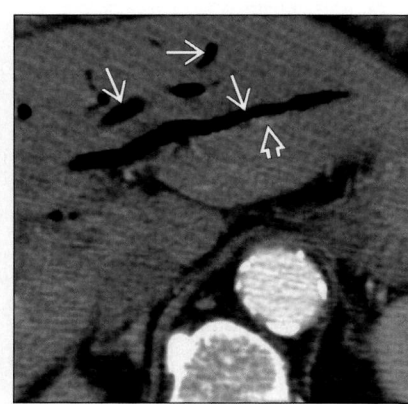

(Left) Oblique transabdominal ultrasound shows gas within the proximal right intrahepatic ducts ➡ and collapsed gallbladder ➡ due to presence of cholecystoduodenal fistula following prolonged cholecystitis. (Center) Transverse transabdominal ultrasound shows linear echogenicity in portal triad ➡ with posterior acoustic shadowing ➡ and reverberation artifacts ➡. (Right) Transverse CECT shows biliary ductal gas ➡ within intrahepatic bile ducts in left lobe of liver. Note accompanying left portal venous radicle ➡.

CHOLANGIOCARCINOMA

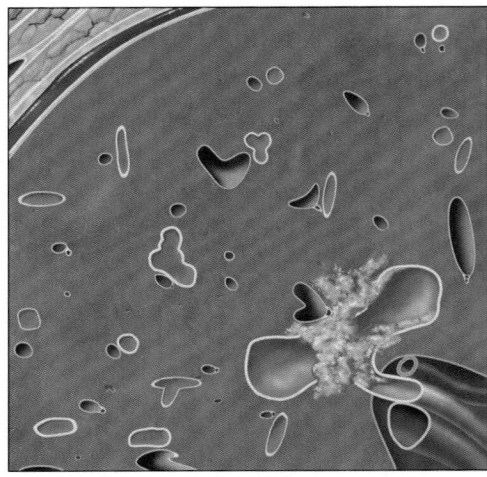

Graphic shows an infiltrative mass at the confluence of the right and left hepatic ducts (Klatskin tumor). It is invading the adjacent liver parenchyma and hepatic veins, a common finding with cholangiocarcinoma.

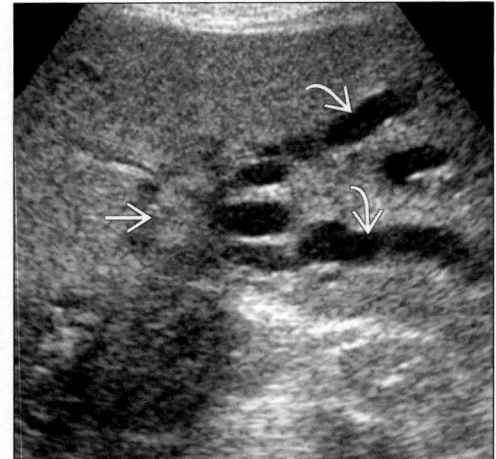

Transverse transabdominal ultrasound shows an ill-defined isoechoic mass ➡ at the hepatic confluence associated with marked intrahepatic ductal dilatation ➡.

TERMINOLOGY

Abbreviations and Synonyms
- Cholangiocellular carcinoma, bile duct carcinoma

Definitions
- Malignancy that arises from intrahepatic bile duct (IHBD) or extrahepatic bile duct epithelium

IMAGING FINDINGS

General Features
- Best diagnostic clue: Intra- or extra-hepatic mass with infiltrative margins and dilatation of biliary ducts
- Location
  - Extrahepatic cholangiocarcinoma (EHC) (~ 90%); 2/3 found in common bile duct (CBD)/common hepatic duct (CHD)
    - Distal common bile duct (30-50%) most common extrahepatic location
    - Proximal CBD (15-30%)
    - Common hepatic duct (14-37%)
    - Confluence of hepatic ducts (10-26%)
  - Intrahepatic cholangiocarcinoma (IHC) ~ 10%
    - Peripheral/central hepatic ducts
- Size: Intrahepatic mass (5-20 cm); extrahepatic, smaller (present with obstructive jaundice earlier)
- Morphology
  - 2nd most common primary hepatic tumor after hepatocellular carcinoma (HCC)
  - Manifests with various histologic types and growth patterns
  - Different types of morphological appearances
    - Peripheral (IHBD) may be exophytic, polypoid or infiltrative
    - Central or hilar (confluence of right & left hepatic ducts and proximal CBD): Small mass in liver hilus: Klatskin tumor
    - Extrahepatic ductal tumor: Obstructive, stenotic or polypoid type

Ultrasonographic Findings
- Grayscale Ultrasound
  - Appearances depend on the anatomical site of primary tumor and local tumor extension
  - **Intrahepatic cholangiocarcinoma**

DDx: Cholangiocarcinoma

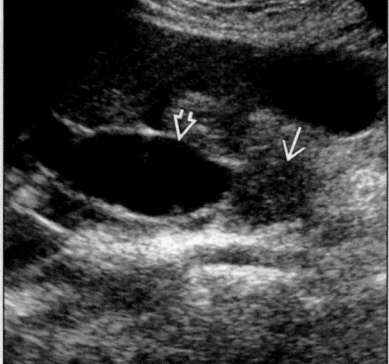

Pancreatic Head Ductal Carcinoma

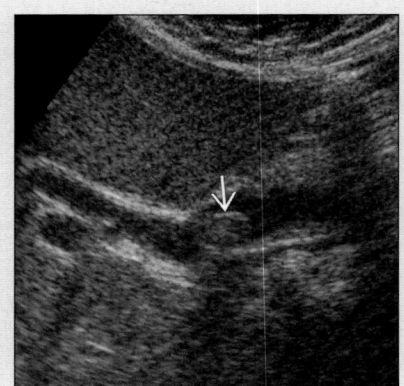

Choledocholithiasis

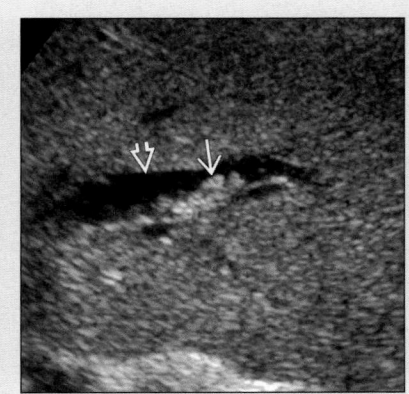

Recurrent Pyogenic Cholangitis

ASCENDING CHOLANGITIS

Key Facts

Imaging Findings

- Dilatation of intra- and extrahepatic bile ducts (in 75% of cases)
- In cases of early cholangitis or intermittent CBD obstruction, bile ducts may not be dilated
- Circumferential thickening of bile duct wall
- Periportal hypo-/hyper-echogenicity adjacent to dilated intrahepatic ducts
- Presence of obstructing choledocholithiasis
- Presence of purulent bile/sludge
- Multiple small hepatic cholangitic abscesses
- Pneumobilia is a rare finding
- Color Doppler: May show increased periportal vascularity related to reactive hyperemia
- US is ideal tool for initial evaluation

- In difficult or equivocal cases, MRCP or contrast cholangiography (ERCP, PTC) may be indicated
- ERCP/PTC serve as portal for biliary drainage (internal/external biliary drainage)
- Subtle US features (such as ductal dilatation, ductal wall thickening) may be difficult to appreciate
- Scan patient in different positions (supine, oblique, lateral) using multiple acoustic windows (intercostal, oblique subcostal) to detect subtle ductal change

Top Differential Diagnoses

- Cholangiocarcinoma
- Ductal Pancreatic Carcinoma
- Choledocholithiasis
- Due to overlap in ultrasound features of various cholangitis, clinical correlation & laboratory data are essential to suggest correct diagnosis

---

- ○ Presence of purulent bile/sludge
  - Intraluminal echogenic material, usually within dilated intrahepatic ducts
  - Usually not casting acoustic shadow
- ○ Multiple small hepatic cholangitic abscesses
  - Anatomically clustered in a lobe or segment of liver
  - Represent liquefaction of biliary inflammation, late finding
  - Hypoechoic cystic lesions with floating homogeneous/heterogeneous internal echoes and debris
- ○ Pneumobilia is a rare finding
  - Due to ascending infection by gas-forming organisms or presence of choledochoenteric fistula
  - Echogenic foci in linear configuration along/adjacent to portal triad
  - Presence of reverberation artifacts
- Color Doppler: May show increased periportal vascularity related to reactive hyperemia

Radiographic Findings

- Cholangiography
  - ○ Ascending (bacterial) cholangitis
    - Stone: Radiolucent filling defect
    - Irregular bile duct lumen/wall
    - Ductal stricture, obstruction & proximal dilatation
    - IHBD may show communicating hepatic abscesses

CT Findings

- Obstructing stone: Calcific/soft tissue/water density
- "Bull's eye" sign: Rim of bile surrounding a stone
- Dilatation of intra-/extrahepatic bile ducts
- High density intraductal material (purulent bile)
- Multiple small rim-enhancing cystic lesions indicate development of cholangitic abscesses

MR Findings

- T2WI: Stones (hypointense); bile (hyperintense)
- MRCP
  - ○ Low signal filling defects (stones) within increased signal bile
  - ○ Irregular strictures, proximal dilatation of bile ducts

- ○ Multiple small hyperintense hepatic lesions - cholangitic abscesses

Imaging Recommendations

- Best imaging tool
  - ○ US is ideal tool for initial evaluation
  - ○ In difficult or equivocal cases, MRCP or contrast cholangiography (ERCP, PTC) may be indicated
  - ○ ERCP/PTC serve as portal for biliary drainage (internal/external biliary drainage)
- Protocol advice
  - ○ Subtle US features (such as ductal dilatation, ductal wall thickening) may be difficult to appreciate
  - ○ Scan patient in different positions (supine, oblique, lateral) using multiple acoustic windows (intercostal, oblique subcostal) to detect subtle ductal change

DIFFERENTIAL DIAGNOSIS

Cholangiocarcinoma

- Ill-defined infiltrative mass
- Commonly at hepatic confluence
- Dilated intrahepatic ducts with non-dilated extrahepatic ducts distal to site of tumor
- Regional metastatic lymph node and liver metastases

Ductal Pancreatic Carcinoma

- Infiltrative hypoechoic mass in pancreatic head
- Dilatation of intra- and extrahepatic and pancreatic ducts
- Vascular encasement
- Regional nodal and liver metastases

Choledocholithiasis

- Clinically patient is not septic
- Echogenic focus casting posterior acoustic shadowing
- +/- Biliary ductal dilatation

Primary Sclerosing Cholangitis (PSC)

- Segmental strictures, beaded and pruned ducts
- Involves both intrahepatic & extrahepatic ducts
- End-stage: Liver (lobular, hypertrophy & atrophy)

ASCENDING CHOLANGITIS

Recurrent Pyogenic Cholangitis (RPC)
- Mainly intrahepatic ductal involvement
- Intrahepatic ductal stones/sludge
- Presence of multifocal intrahepatic ductal strictures with segmental dilatation
- Clinical information of ethnic origin and recurrent attacks of cholangitis help in suggesting etiology

Other Forms of Secondary Cholangitis
- AIDS-related cholangitis
- Chemotherapy-induced cholangitis
- Ischemic cholangitis
- Due to overlap in ultrasound features of various cholangitis, clinical correlation & laboratory data are essential to suggest correct diagnosis

PATHOLOGY

General Features
- Etiology
  - Due to bile duct calculi, stricture & papillary stenosis
  - Pathogenesis: Stone/obstruction/bile stasis/infection
  - Usually secondary to gallstones & infection in industrialized countries
  - Often due to poor nutrition & parasitic infestation in developing countries
  - Classification of cholangitis (etiology/pathogenesis)
    - Primary sclerosing cholangitis (PSC)
    - Secondary sclerosing cholangitis
    - Secondary nonsclerosing cholangitis
  - Secondary sclerosing cholangitis
    - Ascending (bacterial) cholangitis
    - Recurrent pyogenic (parasitic) cholangitis (RPC)
    - AIDS-related cholangitis
    - Chemotherapy-induced cholangitis
    - Ischemic cholangitis
  - Secondary nonsclerosing cholangitis
    - Malignant or benign liver/biliary pathology
  - Based on onset, classified into acute & chronic
- Epidemiology: Most common type of cholangitis in Western countries
- Associated abnormalities: Gallstone disease

Gross Pathologic & Surgical Features
- Inflamed mucosal lining of bile ducts with thickening
- Pus/inflammatory debris within bile ducts
- Formation of multiple small abscess cavities within periductal liver parenchyma

Microscopic Features
- Acute inflammatory infiltrates involving ductal mucosa/submucosa
- Periductal aggregates of leucocytes with edema
- Liquefied necrosis in cholangitic abscesses

CLINICAL ISSUES

Presentation
- Most common signs/symptoms: Charcot triad (RUQ pain, fever, jaundice)
- Other signs/symptoms
  - Septicemia, septic shock
  - Lethargy, mental confusion (especially in elderly patients)
- Lab data
  - Increased WBC count & bilirubin levels
  - Increased alkaline phosphatase
  - Positive blood cultures in toxic phase

Demographics
- Age: More common in middle age or elderly
- Gender: Slight female predominance

Natural History & Prognosis
- Complications: Cholangitic liver abscesses & septicemia
- Majority improved with antibiotics treatment
- High mortality if not decompressed
- Overall mortality significantly improved with antibiotics treatment and biliary decompression

Treatment
- Antibiotics to cover gram negative organisms
- Biliary decompression for uncontrolled sepsis and failed medical therapy
  - ERCP sphincterotomy + stone extraction
  - Internal biliary stent via ERCP
  - External biliary drainage via percutaneous transhepatic biliary drainage (PTBD)
  - Fulminant cases and failed non-operative biliary decompression, may require surgical decompression

DIAGNOSTIC CHECKLIST

Consider
- Correlate with clinical & laboratory data to achieve accurate imaging interpretation

Image Interpretation Pearls
- Biliary ductal dilatation and thickening related to obstructing choledocholithiasis in appropriate clinical setting

SELECTED REFERENCES
1. Ciocirlan M et al: Diagnostic endoscopic retrograde cholangiopancreatography. Endoscopy. 36(2):137-46, 2004
2. Arai K et al: Dynamic CT of acute cholangitis: early inhomogeneous enhancement of the liver. AJR Am J Roentgenol. 181(1):115-8, 2003
3. Baron RL et al: Imaging the spectrum of biliary tract disease. Radiol Clin North Am. 40(6):1325-54, 2002
4. Menu Y et al: Non-traumatic abdominal emergencies: imaging and intervention in acute biliary conditions. Eur Radiol. 12(10):2397-406, 2002
5. Hanau LH et al: Acute (ascending) cholangitis. Infect Dis Clin North Am. 14(3):521-46, 2000
6. Song HH et al: Eosinophilic cholangitis: US, CT, and cholangiography findings. J Comput Assist Tomogr. 21(2):251-3, 1997
7. Balthazar EJ et al: Acute cholangitis: CT evaluation. J Comput Assist Tomogr. 17(2):283-9, 1993
8. Goldberg HI et al: Diagnostic and interventional procedures for the biliary tract. Curr Opin Radiol. 3(3):453-62, 1991

ASCENDING CHOLANGITIS

IMAGE GALLERY

Typical

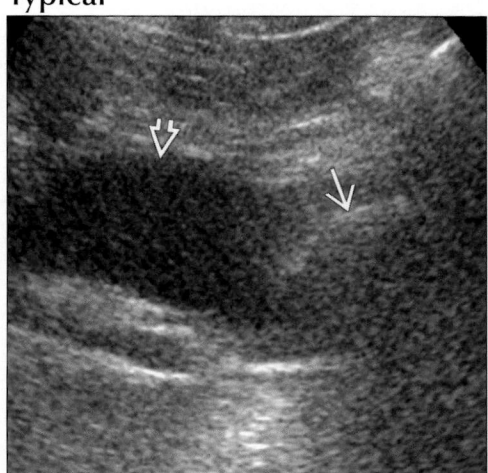 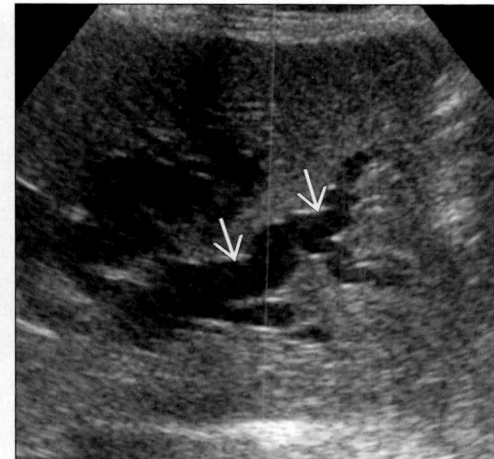

(Left) Oblique transabdominal ultrasound shows a large echogenic calculus ➜ casting marked posterior acoustic shadowing within the dilated common bile duct ➜. Subsequent ERCP drained pus. *(Right)* Transverse transabdominal ultrasound shows an irregular contour and mild degree of wall thickening of dilated intrahepatic ducts ➜ in left lobe of liver.

Typical

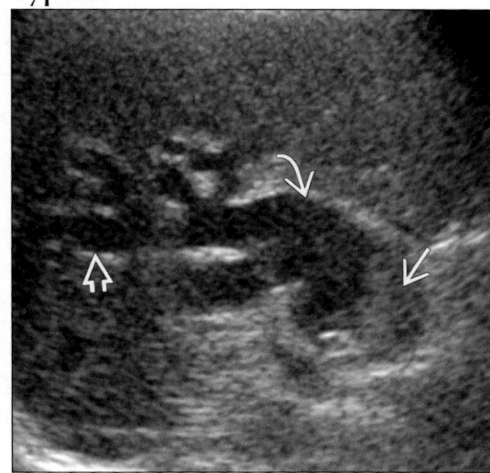 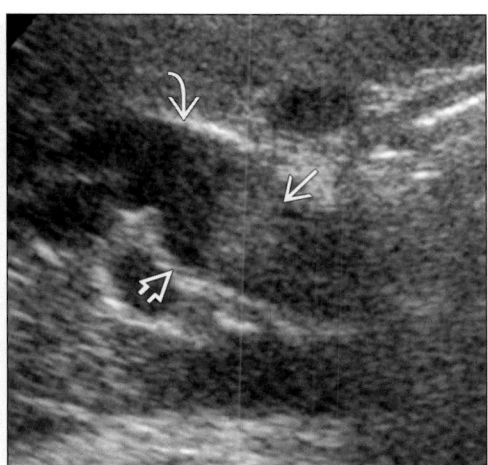

(Left) Oblique transabdominal ultrasound shows a dilated common hepatic duct ➜, containing echogenic material ➜ within its distal portion. Note intrahepatic ductal dilatation ➜. *(Right)* Oblique transabdominal ultrasound shows a markedly dilated common bile duct ➜ the wall is mildly thickened ➜ and it is filled with echogenic material ➜ due to infected bile.

Typical

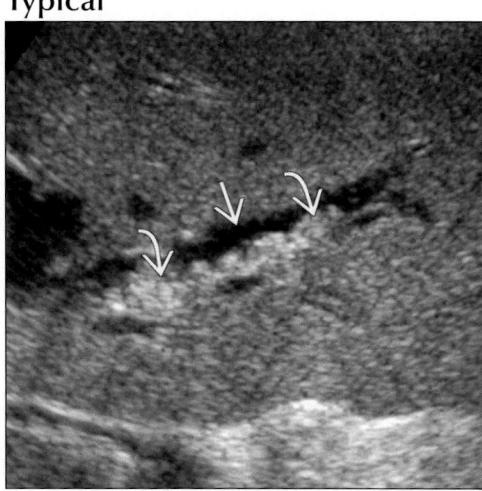 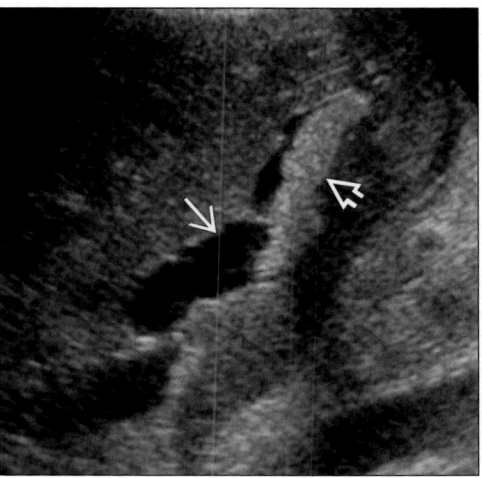

(Left) Transverse transabdominal ultrasound shows dilatation of intrahepatic ducts ➜ in the left lobe of the liver. Echogenic material ➜ within the dilated ducts represents infected biliary sludge. *(Right)* Oblique transabdominal ultrasound shows a grossly dilated intrahepatic duct ➜ in the right lobe of the liver containing echogenic material ➜ due to infected biliary sludge.

RECURRENT PYOGENIC CHOLANGITIS

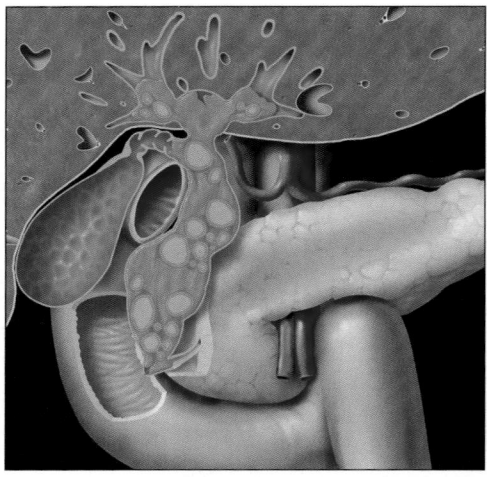

Graphic shows marked dilation of intrahepatic bile ducts with multiple common bile duct and intrahepatic stones.

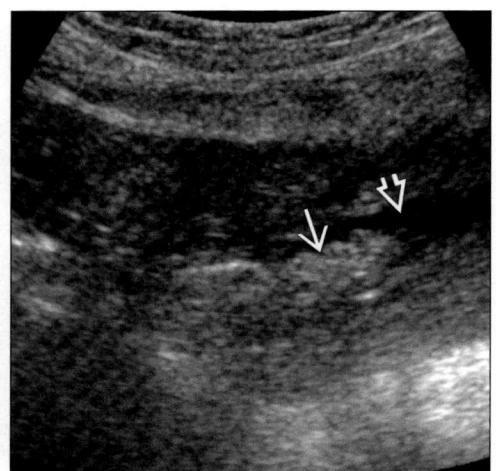

Transverse transabdominal ultrasound in a patient with RPC shows echogenic filling defects ➡ within dilated intrahepatic ducts ⧁ of the lateral segment of the left lobe.

TERMINOLOGY

Abbreviations and Synonyms
- Recurrent pyogenic cholangitis (RPC), hepatolithiasis, oriental cholangiohepatitis

Definitions
- Recurrent episodes of acute pyogenic cholangitis with intra- and extrahepatic biliary pigment stones

IMAGING FINDINGS

General Features
- Best diagnostic clue
  - Intra- and extrahepatic biliary stones within dilated biliary ducts
  - No gallbladder stone
- Location
  - Any segment of the liver may be affected
  - Lateral segment of the left lobe is most commonly involved
- Size: Stones are typically 1-4 cm in size

Ultrasonographic Findings
- Grayscale Ultrasound
  - Ultrasound is commonly used for screening and monitoring disease
  - Ultrasound findings depend on the stage of the disease and presence of any associated complication
  - Early disease without biliary sepsis
    - Dilated intrahepatic and extrahepatic bile ducts
    - Presence of echogenic sludge/stones with posterior acoustic shadowing
    - May appear as multiple echogenic masses in serpiginous configuration along portal triads if stones/sludge fills the dilated ducts
    - Occasionally intrahepatic ductal stones may not cast any posterior acoustic shadow
  - Early disease with active biliary sepsis
    - Periportal hypo- or hyper-echogenicity due to periductal inflammation
    - Biliary ductal thickening related to edematous inflammation
    - Floating echoes within dilated ducts due to inflammatory debris

DDx: Recurrent Pyogenic Cholangitis

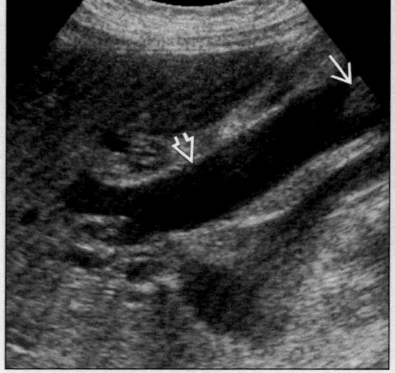

Ascending Cholangitis

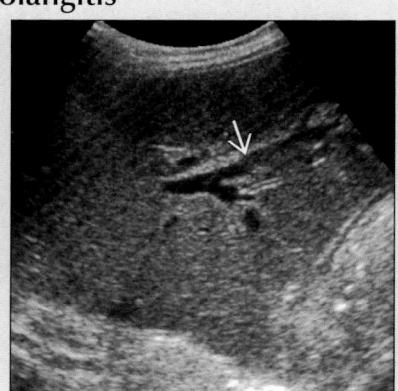

Sclerosing Cholangitis

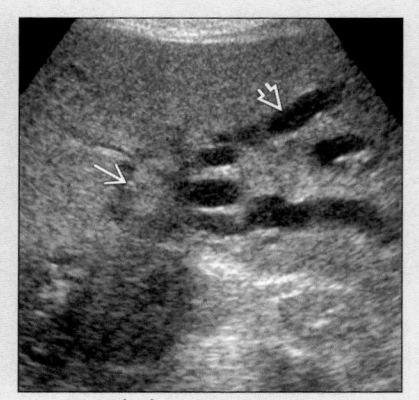

Cholangiocarcinoma

AIDS-RELATED CHOLANGIOPATHY

Key Facts

Terminology
- Spectrum of biliary inflammatory lesions caused by AIDS-related opportunistic infections leading to biliary stricture/obstruction or cholecystitis

Imaging Findings
- Bile duct wall thickening
- May involve both extra- and intrahepatic bile ducts
- Focal biliary strictures and dilatation

- Dilatation of common bile duct due to inflamed/stenosed papilla of Vater
- Diffuse GB wall thickening
- Clinically and radiologically indistinguishable from acute acalculous cholecystitis

Top Differential Diagnoses
- Acute Bacterial Cholangitis
- Cholangitis (Sclerosing/Recurrent Pyogenic)
- Cholangiocarcinoma

Imaging Recommendations
- Best imaging tool
  - US as initial imaging test
    - Negative US scan rules out the diagnosis
  - MRCP/ERCP for patients with equivocal findings on US and serves as portal for sphincterotomy

DIFFERENTIAL DIAGNOSIS

Acute Bacterial Cholangitis
- Obstructing CBD stone
- Intrahepatic ductal dilatation, biliary wall thickening and periportal changes

Cholangitis (Sclerosing/Recurrent Pyogenic)
- Multiple intrahepatic strictures and stones
- Stricture formation in extrahepatic ducts

Cholangiocarcinoma
- Infiltrative mass along ductal epithelium
- Invades hepatic parenchyma and regional lymph node metastases

PATHOLOGY

General Features
- Epidemiology: Late stage AIDS patients (CDC stage IV AIDS based on T4 counts)

- Opportunistic infection of GB, bile ducts from cryptosporidium & CMV; periductal inflammation, acalculous cholecystitis

CLINICAL ISSUES

Presentation
- Most common signs/symptoms: Epigastric/RUQ pain ± fever
- Clinical Profile: Elevated alkaline phosphatase with normal bilirubin level

Natural History & Prognosis
- Poor prognosis due to advanced AIDS presentation

Treatment
- Asymptomatic: Conservative pain relief
- Symptomatic: Sphincterotomy for pain relief, does not alter intrahepatic disease

DIAGNOSTIC CHECKLIST

Image Interpretation Pearls
- AIDS patient with distal ampullary stenosis, intrahepatic strictures or acalculous cholecystitis

SELECTED REFERENCES
1. Cello JP: AIDS-Related biliary tract disease. Gastrointest Endosc Clin N Am. 8(4):963, 1998

IMAGE GALLERY

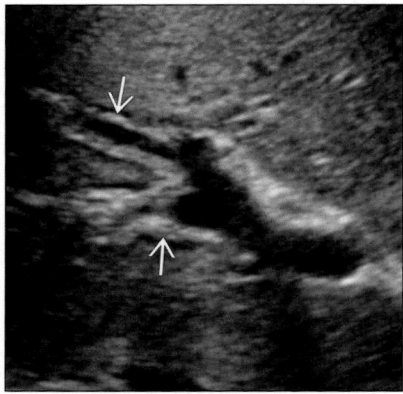 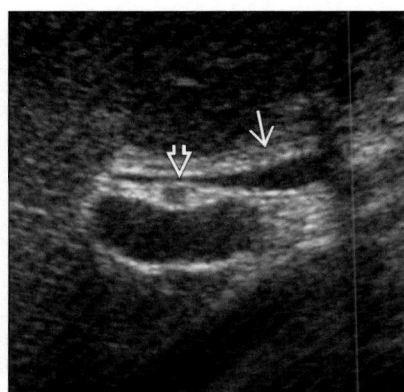 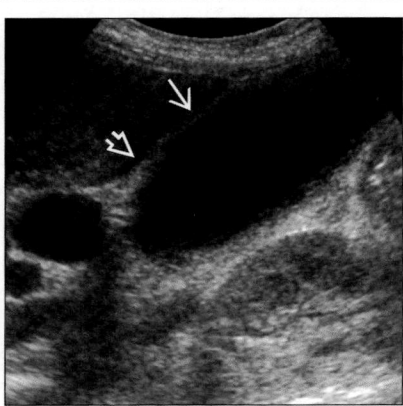

(Left) Oblique transabdominal ultrasound in an AIDS-infected patient with impaired liver function shows mild intrahepatic ductal dilatation, with diffuse echogenic wall thickening ➡. *(Center)* Oblique transabdominal ultrasound shows marked wall thickening of an extrahepatic bile duct ➡, with focal extrinsic narrowing of the common duct ➡ at the porta hepatis. *(Right)* Oblique transabdominal ultrasound shows diffuse wall thickening ➡ in a distended GB. Note the presence of trace pericholecystic fluid ➡ and absence of an impacted gallstone.

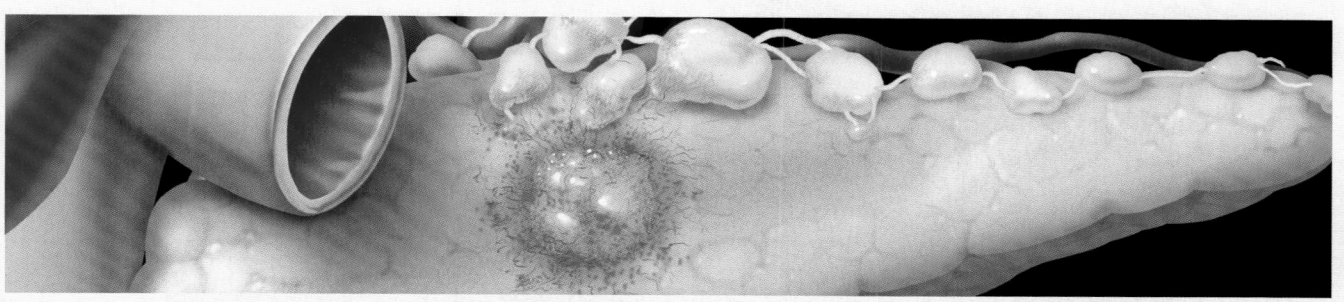

SECTION 3: Pancreas

PANCREATIC SONOGRAPHY

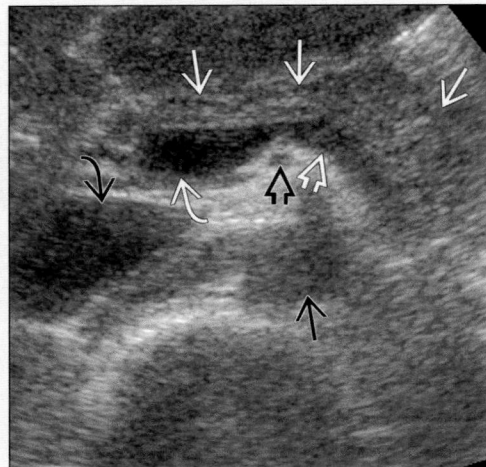

Transverse transabdominal ultrasound shows anatomical relationship of the pancreas ➡ to the splenic vein ➡, SMA ➡, portal vein confluence ➡, abdominal aorta ➡ and IVC ➡.

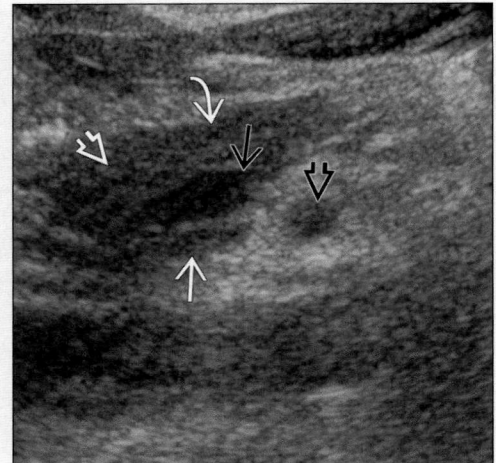

Transverse transabdominal ultrasound shows the normal anatomical relationship of the uncinate process ➡ which is medial extension of pancreatic head ➡ behind the SMV ➡. (➡ SMA, ➡ pancreatic neck).

IMAGING ANATOMY

General Anatomic Considerations

- Pancreas is non-encapsulated, retroperitoneal structure that lies in anterior pararenal space
- Obliquely in transverse plane spanning between duodenal loop and splenic hilum
- Level changes on respiratory movement
  - Craniocaudal shifting of 2-8 cm may occur on respiration
- Length ~ 12-15 cm across
- Pancreas can be identified & localized on ultrasound by
  - Typical parenchymal architecture, homogeneously isoechoic/hyperechoic echotexture
  - Surrounding anatomical landmarks: Anterior to splenic vein, SMA

Critical Anatomic Structures

- Anatomical division
  - Head: Parenchyma to the right of superior mesenteric vessels
  - Uncinate process: Represents medial extension of head
    - Lies posterior to superior mesenteric vessels
  - Neck: Narrow portion anterior to superior mesenteric vessels
    - Serves as dividing line between pancreatic head and body
  - Body: Parenchyma to left of superior mesenteric vessels
    - Constitute main bulk of pancreatic parenchyma
  - Tail: Most distal portion of pancreatic parenchyma
    - No clear anatomic landmark separates tail from body
- Histological division
  - Functionally the pancreas comprised of exocrine and endocrine tissues
    - 80% exocrine tissue; ductal and acinar cells
    - 2% endocrine tissue; islet cell of Langerhans
    - 18% fibrous stroma containing blood vessels, nerves and lymphatics

Anatomic Relationships

- Pancreas is closely related to several important structures/organs
  - Gastrointestinal tract & peritoneal spaces
    - Anteriorly: Stomach, transverse colon and root of transverse mesocolon, lesser sac
    - Right: Duodenal loop (esp. second part of duodenum)
  - Major vessels
    - Abdominal aorta: Posterior to body of pancreas
    - Coeliac axis: Related to superior border of pancreas
    - Common hepatic artery: Branch of coeliac axis, related to superior border of pancreatic neck and head
    - Gastroduodenal artery: Branch of coeliac axis, coursing inferiorly anterior to pancreatic head
    - Splenic artery: Branch of coeliac axis, towards the left in tortuous course along superior border of pancreatic body and tail
    - Superior mesenteric artery (SMA): Arises from abdominal aorta just caudal to inferior border of pancreas, descends anterior to uncinate process
    - Inferior vena cava: Posterior to head of pancreas
    - Splenic vein: Coursing transversely from splenic hilum to portal vein confluence posterior to pancreatic tail and body
    - Superior mesenteric vein: Ascends to right of SMA anterior to uncinate process
    - Portal vein: Confluence posterior to pancreatic neck, proximal portion above superior margin of pancreatic head
  - Common bile duct
    - Distal portion posterior to or embedded within pancreatic head
    - Forms common trunk with pancreatic duct in 80% to drain into ampulla of Vater

PANCREATIC SONOGRAPHY

Key Facts

Relevant Anatomy
- Pancreas is a non-encapsulated, retroperitoneal structure that lies in anterior pararenal space
  - Anatomical division: Head, uncinate process, neck, body and tail
- Identified and localized on ultrasound by:
  - Typical parenchymal architecture: Homogeneously isoechoic/hyperechoic echotexture
  - Anatomical landmarks: Anterior to splenic vein, SMA

Imaging Protocol
- Transabdominal ultrasound serves as a useful initial imaging modality for suspected pancreatic lesion
  - Technical limitation: Obscuration by bowel gas, inadequate US penetration in obese patients
- Scanning with patient in various positions (erect, sitting, both obliques and decubituses) may help
- Ask patient to drink plenty of water to distend the stomach which acts as an acoustic window
- Cross-sectional imaging techniques including CT and MR are usually required for further characterization of pancreatic lesion detected on US
- Endoscopic US (EUS) or intra-operative US (IOU) help detect small pancreatic tumors (e.g., islet cell tumor) not apparent on transabdominal US, CT or MR

Common Pathologies
- Pancreatitis: Acute or chronic
- Cysts/cystic neoplasm: Pancreatic pseudocyst, congenital cyst, serous/mucinous cystic tumor
- Solid tumor: Ductal carcinoma, islet cell tumor, solid and papillary neoplasm, metastases, lymphoma

ANATOMY-BASED IMAGING ISSUES

Key Concepts or Questions
- Transabdominal ultrasound serves as a useful initial imaging modality for suspected pancreatic lesion
- Advantages of US
  - Readily available
  - Relatively inexpensive imaging technique
  - Does not involve ionizing radiation
  - Supplemented with Doppler US to identify abnormal flow (thrombosis, tumor encasement) or abnormal vascularity (tumor vascularity)
  - Use as real time imaging guide for interventional procedures
- Disadvantages of US
  - Pancreas is retroperitoneal structure and considered "deep" intra-abdominal organ for imaging with transabdominal ultrasound
  - Limited US beam penetration in obese patient with thick subcutaneous and omental fat
  - Often entire pancreatic parenchyma cannot be completely examined due to overlying bowel gas
  - Operator-dependent imaging technique
- Technical consideration in transabdominal US for assessment of pancreatic lesion
  - Examination should begin in transverse plane in midline below xiphisternum, using vascular landmarks to identify pancreas
    - Longitudinal view for further evaluation particularly if lesion is detected
  - Pancreatic body can usually be better delineated by transducer pressure to displace overlying bowel gas
  - If there is abundant bowel gas obscuring pancreatic parenchyma
    - Scanning with patient in various positions including erect, sitting, both obliques and decubitus may help
    - Ask patient to drink plenty of water to distend the stomach which acts as an acoustic window
  - Using left kidney/spleen as acoustic window, pancreatic tail can be visualized in left coronal view
  - Head can be better assessed through right lateral/decubitus approach in a coronal plane
  - Place area of interest within the focal zone of transducer
  - Always examine the rest of the abdomen in detail
  - Doppler US to aid assessment of patency and flow characteristics of vessels
- Special US techniques such as endoscopic US (EUS) or intra-operative US (IOU) are useful in detecting small pancreatic tumors (e.g., islet cell tumor) which are not apparent on transabdominal US, CT or MR
- Cross-sectional imaging techniques including CT and MR are usually required for further characterization of pancreatic lesion detected on US
- Advantages of CT
  - Fast scanning in era of multi-detector CT, thus more practical in critically ill patients
  - Shows calcifications better than other imaging modalities
  - Less prone to technical and interpretative errors
- Advantages of MR
  - No ionizing radiation is involved
  - Does not require iodinated contrast agent
  - Multiplanar capability
  - Allows easy evaluation of common bile duct and pancreatic duct using MRCP sequences

PATHOLOGY-BASED IMAGING ISSUES

Key Concepts or Questions
- Two main categories to differentiate on imaging include neoplasm (most commonly ductal pancreatic carcinoma) and pancreatitis
  - Ductal pancreatic carcinomas typically cause narrowing or obstruction of vessels and ducts, and extend dorsally to coeliac axis and SMA origins
  - Acute pancreatitis causes fluid exudation and fat infiltration, extends ventrally and laterally to mesentery and anterior pararenal space, less common cause for ductal obstruction

PANCREATIC SONOGRAPHY

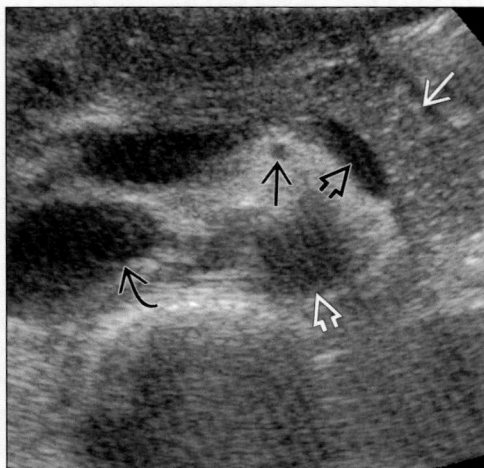

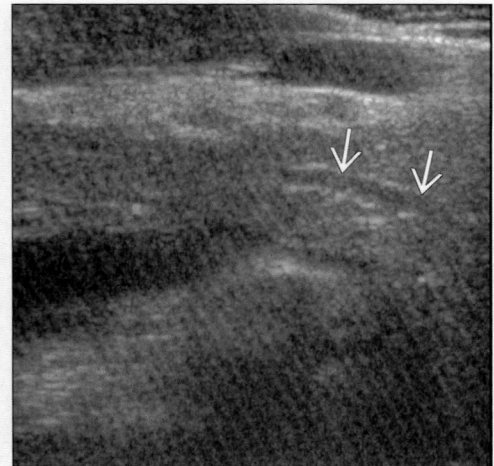

Transverse transabdominal ultrasound shows normal pancreatic tail ➤ with homogeneous echotexture. Note splenic vein ➤, SMA ➤, abdominal aorta ➤ and IVC ➤.

Transverse transabdominal ultrasound performed with a high-frequency transducer in a thin patient shows a non-dilated pancreatic duct ➤ within the pancreatic body.

- Differential diagnoses of cystic pancreatic mass
  - Common
    - Pseudocyst
    - Mucinous cystic tumor
    - Serous cystadenoma
    - Necrotic pancreatic ductal carcinoma
    - Intraductal papillary mucinous tumor (IPMT)
  - Uncommon
    - Simple/congenital cyst (e.g., Von Hippel Lindau syndrome, adult polycystic kidney disease)
    - Solid and papillary neoplasm of pancreas
    - Lymphangioma
    - Cystic metastases/lymphoma
- Conditions to consider if dilated pancreatic duct is seen
  - Chronic pancreatitis: Parenchymal or intraductal calcification, atrophic pancreas
  - Pancreatic ductal carcinoma: Common bile and pancreatic ductal dilatation for most common lesions in pancreatic head
  - Periampullary tumor
  - IPMT
  - Obstructing distal common bile duct (CBD) stone

EMBRYOLOGY

Embryologic Events
- Embryologically, pancreas is developed from dorsal and ventral pancreatic buds
  - Body-tail segment developed from dorsal pancreatic bud
  - Head-uncinate segment developed from ventral pancreatic bud
- During normal development, ventral bud migrates dorsally around fetal duodenum to merge with dorsal bud to form pancreatic substance and branching pancreatic and bile ducts

Practical Implications
- Failure or anomalies of rotation or fusion may result in congenital lesions such as annular pancreas, pancreas divisum, agenesis of dorsal pancreas

- Ventral (head-uncinate) and dorsal (body-tail) segments may have different echotexture that may be misinterpreted as pathology
- Pancreatic ductal obstruction of either dorsal or ventral buds may lead to dilatation of involved portion with sparing of uninvolved segments

CLINICAL IMPLICATIONS

Clinical Importance
- Ductal pancreatic carcinoma: Usually presents late with poor overall prognosis, surgically not operable in most cases
- Serous cystadenoma: No malignant potential, microcystic/macrocystic in appearances
- Mucinous cystic pancreatic tumor: Regarded as pre-malignant lesion, predominantly cystic with septations +/- solid component
- Islet cell tumor: Hypervascular primary tumor and liver metastases, most common
  - Insulinoma, functional tumors small at presentation
  - Non-functional tumors large at diagnosis
- Solid and papillary neoplasm, metastases, lymphoma; rare lesions

RELATED REFERENCES

1. Koeller KK et al (eds): Radiologic Pathology. 2nd ed. Washington D.C., Armed Forces Institute of Pathology, 2003
2. Bennett GL et al: Pancreatic ultrasonography. Surg Clin North Am. 81(2):259-81, 2001

PANCREATIC SONOGRAPHY

IMAGE GALLERY

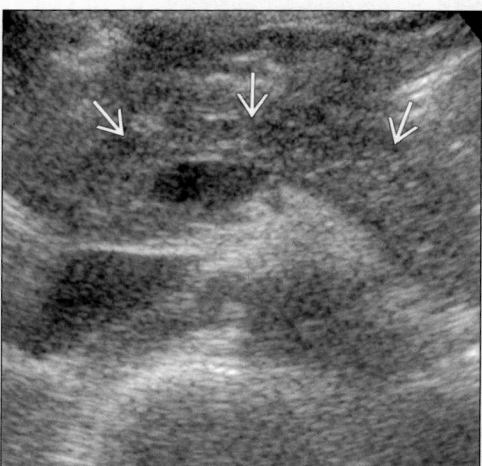

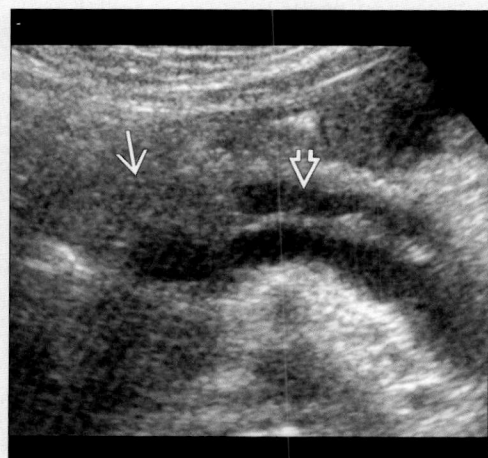

(Left) Transverse transabdominal ultrasound shows the homogeneous echotexture of the pancreas ➡ in a healthy patient. Note the lack of pancreatic ductal dilatation and parenchymal mass/calcification. *(Right)* Transverse transabdominal ultrasound shows an ill-defined hypoechoic carcinoma in the pancreatic head ➡ causing obstruction and dilatation of the pancreatic duct ➡.

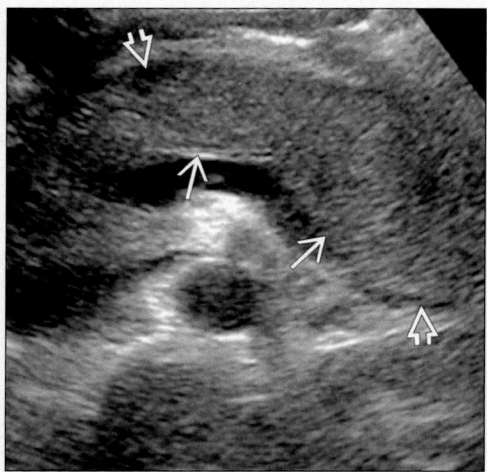

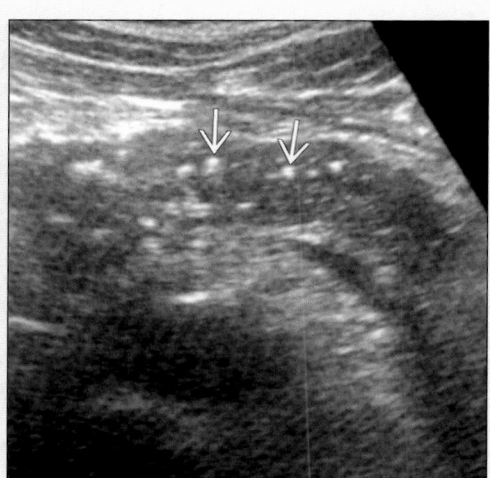

(Left) Transverse transabdominal ultrasound shows global swelling with a diffusely hypoechoic echo pattern of the pancreas ➡ suggestive of acute pancreatitis. Note presence of small peri-pancreatic fluid ➡. *(Right)* Transverse transabdominal ultrasound shows calcifications ➡ within the pancreatic parenchyma in patient with chronic pancreatitis related to alcohol abuse.

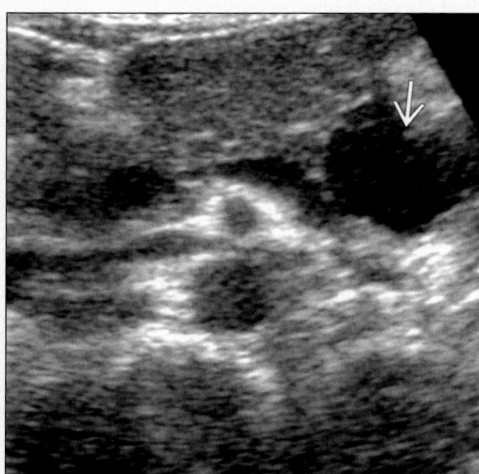

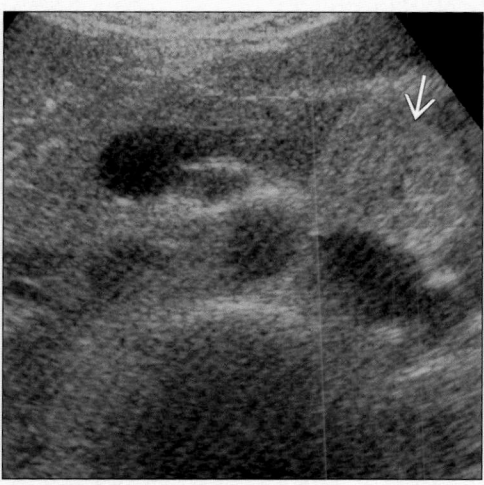

(Left) Transverse transabdominal ultrasound shows the well-circumscribed, unilocular, cystic lesion ➡ in the pancreatic tail. The rest of the pancreas is unremarkable. Pathology: Pseudocyst. *(Right)* Transverse transabdominal ultrasound shows a well-circumscribed, solid, hyperechoic mass ➡ in pancreatic tail.

ACUTE PANCREATITIS

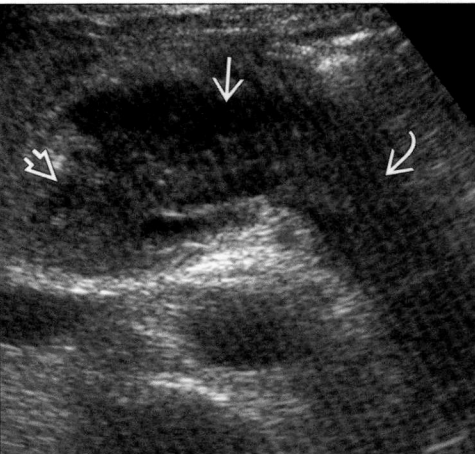
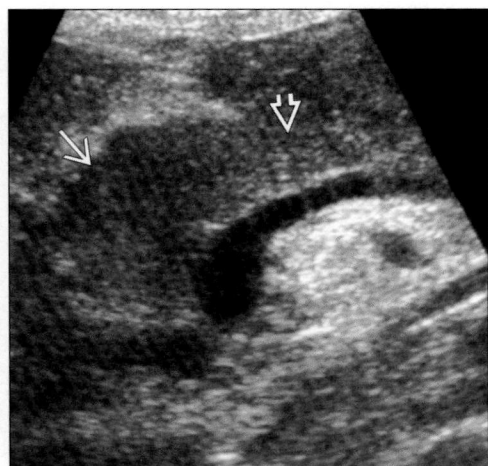

Transverse transabdominal ultrasound shows a swollen pancreatic body ➡ with ill-defined heterogeneous hypoechoic echo pattern. The pancreatic head ⊳ and tail ⇗ are less severely affected.

Transverse transabdominal ultrasound shows focal enlargement of pancreatic head ➡ with homogeneous hypoechoic echo pattern in focal pancreatitis. Note normal echo pattern of pancreatic body ⊳.

TERMINOLOGY

Abbreviations and Synonyms
- Acute edematous pancreatitis, acute necrotizing pancreatitis

Definitions
- Acute inflammatory process of pancreas with variable involvement of other regional tissues or remote organ systems

IMAGING FINDINGS

General Features
- Best diagnostic clue: Enlarged pancreas, fluid collections & obliteration of fat planes
- Location: Pancreas and peripancreatic tissue
- Size: Pancreas increased in size, focal or diffuse involvement

Ultrasonographic Findings
- Grayscale Ultrasound

  ○ In mild pancreatitis sonographic signs may be subtle or normal
  ○ Enlarged, hypoechoic pancreas: Due to interstitial edema
  ○ Blurred pancreatic outline/margin: Due to pancreatic edema and peripancreatic exudate
  ○ Enlarged heterogeneous pancreas in patients with intrapancreatic necrosis or hemorrhage
  ○ Dilated pancreatic duct due to duct compression by edematous pancreas
  ○ Inflammatory change in soft tissues around pancreas/kidneys
  ○ Gallstone or intraductal calculi
  ○ Complications
    ■ Pancreatic pseudocyst: Well-circumscribed, unilocular cystic lesion within pancreas or peri-pancreatic tissue
    ■ Pancreatic/peri-pancreatic fluid collection
    ■ Pancreatic abscess or infected collections: Thick-walled, mostly anechoic with internal echoes and debris
    ■ Vascular complications: Pseudoaneurysm formation and portosplenic venous thrombosis, Doppler USG helps for diagnosis

DDx: Acute Pancreatitis

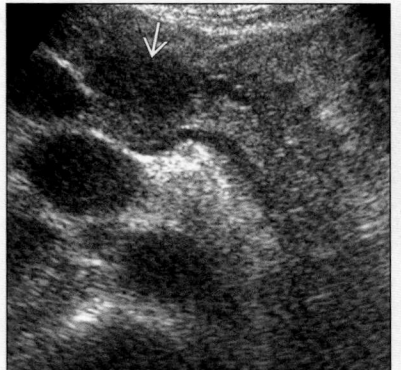

Pancreatic Carcinoma

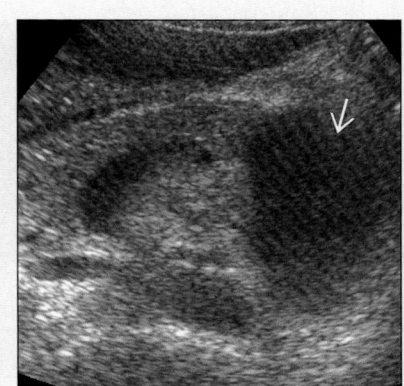

Pancreatic Lymphoma

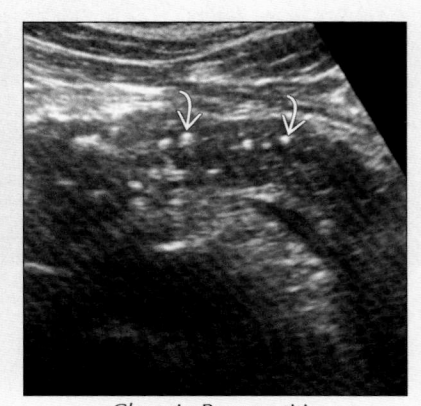

Chronic Pancreatitis

ACUTE PANCREATITIS

Key Facts

Terminology
- Acute inflammatory process of pancreas with variable involvement of other regional tissues or remote organ systems

Imaging Findings
- In mild pancreatitis sonographic signs may be subtle or normal
- Enlarged, hypoechoic pancreas: Due to interstitial edema
- Blurred pancreatic outline/margin: Due to pancreatic edema and peripancreatic exudate
- Enlarged heterogeneous pancreas in patients with intrapancreatic necrosis or hemorrhage
- Dilated pancreatic duct due to duct compression by edematous pancreas

- Inflammatory change in soft tissues around pancreas/kidneys
- Gallstone or intraductal calculi
- Pancreatic pseudocyst: Well-circumscribed, unilocular cystic lesion within pancreas or peri-pancreatic tissue
- Pancreatic/peri-pancreatic fluid collection
- Pancreatic abscess or infected collections: Thick-walled, mostly anechoic with internal echoes and debris

Top Differential Diagnoses
- Infiltrating Pancreatic Carcinoma
- Lymphoma & Metastases
- Chronic Pancreatitis
- Perforated Duodenal Ulcer
- "Shock" Pancreas

  - Pancreatic ascites and pleural effusion (usually left-sided)

Radiographic Findings
- Radiography
  - Sentinel loop: Mildly dilated, gas-filled segment of small bowel with or without air-fluid levels
  - "Colon cutoff" sign
    - Markedly distended transverse colon with air
    - Absence of gas distal to splenic flexure caused by colonic spasm due to spread of pancreatic inflammation to proximal descending colon

CT Findings
- CECT
  - Focal or diffuse enlargement of pancreas with ill-defined margin
  - Heterogeneous enhancement: Areas of nonenhancement indicates necrotic element
  - Infiltration of peripancreatic fat
  - Detection of complications
    - Pancreatic/peripancreatic collection +/- infection: Rim-enhancing fluid density
    - Pseudoaneurysm: Cystic vascular lesion, enhances like adjacent blood vessels
    - Portal/splenic venous thrombosis: Nonenhancement of thrombosed vein
    - Chest: Pleural effusions & basal atelectasis

MR Findings
- T2WI FS
  - Fluid collections, pseudocyst, necrotic areas: Hyperintense
  - Gallstones or intraductal calculi: Hypointense
- T1 C+
  - Heterogeneous enhancement pattern
    - Nonenhancing decreased signal areas (necrosis/fluid collection/pseudocyst)
    - Vascular occlusions can be easily demonstrated
- MRCP
  - All fluid-containing structures: Hyperintense
  - Dilated or normal main pancreatic duct (MPD)

Imaging Recommendations
- Best imaging tool: CECT, ultrasound
- Protocol advice
  - Role of ultrasound in acute pancreatitis: Although ultrasound is an ideal initial examination in acutely ill patient, it has certain diagnostic limitations in early acute pancreatitis
    - Changes of pancreatitis may be quite subtle and the pancreas may initially appear normal
    - Transducer pressure cannot be applied on the abdomen as the patient often has severe abdominal pain
    - Associated distended colon, and small bowel obscures visualization of pancreas and peripancreatic soft tissues
  - Ultrasound is useful in
    - Detection of gallstone/choledocholithiasis
    - Survey of potential complications such as pseudocyst/pancreatic abscess formation
    - Provide real time guidance for interventional procedures (e.g., aspiration of peri-pancreatic collection/abscess)
  - CECT helps in better delineation of extent of pancreatitis, detection of pancreatic necrosis and complications, prediction of clinical outcome

DIFFERENTIAL DIAGNOSIS

Infiltrating Pancreatic Carcinoma
- Irregular, heterogeneous, hypoechoic mass
- Abrupt obstruction & dilatation of pancreatic duct
- Regional nodal metastases: Splenic hilum & porta hepatis
- Contiguous organ invasion
  - Duodenum, stomach & mesenteric root

Lymphoma & Metastases
- Nodular, bulky, enlarged pancreas due to infiltration
- Retroperitoneal adenopathy
- Peripancreatic infiltration (obliteration of fat planes)
- Primary may be seen in case of metastatic infiltration

ACUTE PANCREATITIS

Chronic Pancreatitis
- Atrophic pancreatic parenchyma
- Intraductal/parenchymal calcifications
- Lack of peri-pancreatic fluid collection
- Functional pancreatic exocrine/endocrine insufficiency

Perforated Duodenal Ulcer
- Penetrating ulcers may infiltrate anterior pararenal space, simulating pancreatitis
- Less than 50% of cases have evidence of extraluminal gas or contrast medium collections
- Pancreatic head may be involved

"Shock" Pancreas
- Infiltration of peripancreatic & mesenteric fat planes following hypotensive episode (e.g., blunt trauma)
- Pancreas itself looks normal or diffusely enlarged

PATHOLOGY

General Features
- General path comments
  - Embryology-anatomy
    - Congenital anomalies may cause pancreatitis
    - Annular pancreas: Failure of migration of ventral bud to contact dorsal
    - Pancreas divisum: Ventral & dorsal pancreatic buds fail to fuse; relative block at minor papilla
- Genetics
  - Hereditary pancreatitis
    - Autosomal dominant & incomplete penetrance
- Etiology
  - Alcohol/gallstones/metabolic/infection/trauma/drugs
  - Pathogenesis: Due to reflux of pancreatic enzymes, bile, duodenal contents & increased ductal pressure
    - MPD or terminal duct blockage
    - Edema; spasm; incompetence of sphincter of Oddi

Gross Pathologic & Surgical Features
- Bulky pancreas, necrosis, fluid collection & pseudocyst

Microscopic Features
- Acute edematous pancreatitis
  - Edema, congestion, leukocytic infiltrates
- Acute hemorrhagic pancreatitis
  - Tissue destruction, fat necrosis & hemorrhage

Staging, Grading or Classification Criteria
- CT classification: Five grades based on severity
  - Grade A: Normal pancreas
  - Grade B: Focal or diffuse enlargement of gland, contour irregularities & heterogeneous attenuation, no peripancreatic inflammation
  - Grade C: Intrinsic pancreatic abnormalities & associated inflammation in peripancreatic fat
  - Grade D: Small & usually single, ill-defined fluid collection
  - Grade E: Two or more large fluid collections, presence of gas in pancreas or retroperitoneum
- Most important criterion: Presence & extent of necrotizing pancreatitis (nonenhancing parenchyma)

CLINICAL ISSUES

Presentation
- Most common signs/symptoms
  - Acute onset epigastric pain, often radiating to back
  - Tenderness, fever, nausea, vomiting
- Lab data
  - Increased serum amylase & lipase
  - Other: Hyperglycemia, increased lactate dehydrogenase (LDH), leukocytosis, hypocalcemia, fall in hematocrit, rise in blood urea nitrogen (BUN)

Demographics
- Age: Usually young & middle age group
- Gender: Males more than females

Natural History & Prognosis
- Complications
  - Pancreatic
    - Fluid collections, pseudocyst, necrosis, abscess
  - Gastrointestinal
    - Hemorrhage, infarction, obstruction, ileus
  - Biliary: Obstructive jaundice
  - Vascular: Pseudoaneurysm, porto-splenic vein thrombosis, hemorrhage
  - Disseminated intravascular coagulation (DIC), shock, renal failure
- Prognosis
  - Early detection with minor complications: Good
  - Late detection with major complications: Poor
  - Ranson criteria/APACHE II criteria help predict prognosis
  - Infected pancreatic necrosis: Almost 50% mortality even with surgical debridement

Treatment
- Conservative
  - Nil by mouth (NPO), gastric tube decompression, analgesics, antibiotics
- Treat complications of acute pancreatitis
  - Infected or obstructing pseudocysts require drainage: Surgical or percutaneous routes
  - Infected necrosis needs surgery/catheter drainage

DIAGNOSTIC CHECKLIST

Consider
- Rule out other pathologies which can cause "peripancreatic infiltration"

Image Interpretation Pearls
- Bulky, irregularly enlarged pancreas with obliteration of peripancreatic fat planes, fluid collections, pseudocyst or abscess formation

SELECTED REFERENCES
1. Gandolfi L et al: The role of ultrasound in biliary and pancreatic diseases. Eur J Ultrasound. 16(3):141-59, 2003
2. Balthazar EJ: Acute pancreatitis: assessment of severity with clinical and CT evaluation. Radiology. 223(3):603-13, 2002
3. Balthazar EJ: Staging of acute pancreatitis. Radiol Clin North Am. 40(6):1199-209, 2002

ACUTE PANCREATITIS

IMAGE GALLERY

Typical

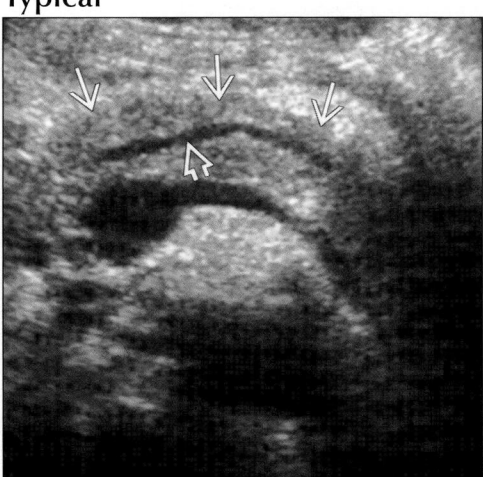

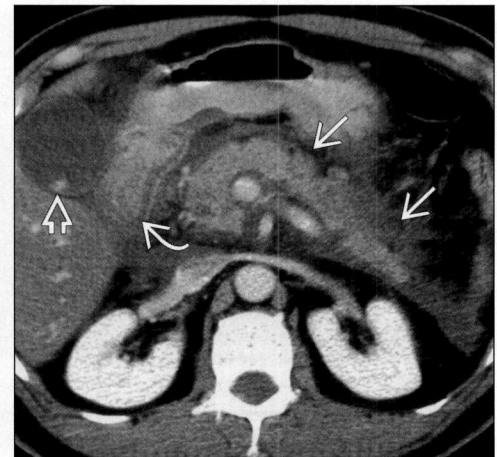

(Left) Transverse transabdominal ultrasound shows diffuse, hypoechoic, enlarged pancreatic parenchyma ➡. Note the presence of mild pancreatic ductal dilatation ➡. (Right) Transverse CECT shows an inflamed pancreas with peripancreatic stranding ➡. The adjoining duodenum appears inflamed with an edematous wall ➡. Note a calculus in the gallbladder ➡.

Typical

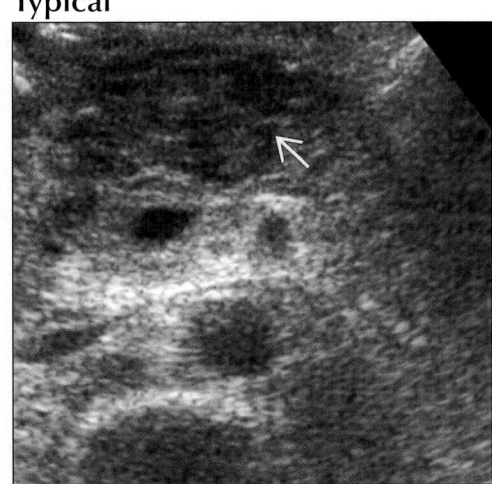

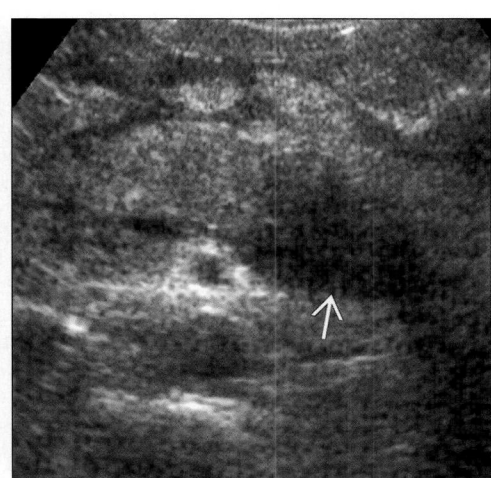

(Left) Transverse transabdominal ultrasound shows a large heterogeneous collection ➡ involving the pancreatic head and body compatible with abscess formation, resulting from infected phlegmon. (Right) Transverse transabdominal ultrasound shows subtle swelling with hypoechoic echo pattern ➡ of the pancreatic tail, compatible with focal pancreatic necrosis.

Typical

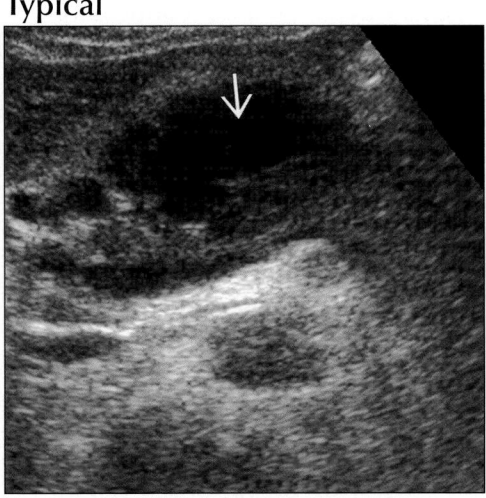

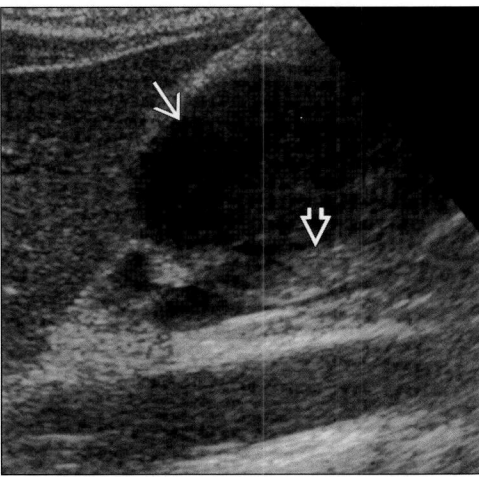

(Left) Transverse transabdominal ultrasound shows a large, ill-defined, anechoic/hypoechoic collection ➡ in the pancreatic body in acute pancreatitis. (Right) Longitudinal transabdominal ultrasound shows a large heterogeneous fluid collection ➡ in the anterior peripancreatic area. Note the pancreatic body ➡ is compressed by the fluid collection.

PANCREATIC PSEUDOCYSTS

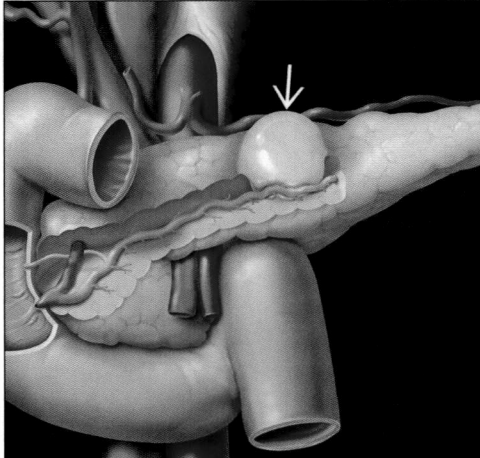

Graphic shows well-circumscribed cystic lesion ➡ in the pancreatic body suggestive of pancreatic pseudocyst. The adjacent pancreatic duct is not compressed or displaced.

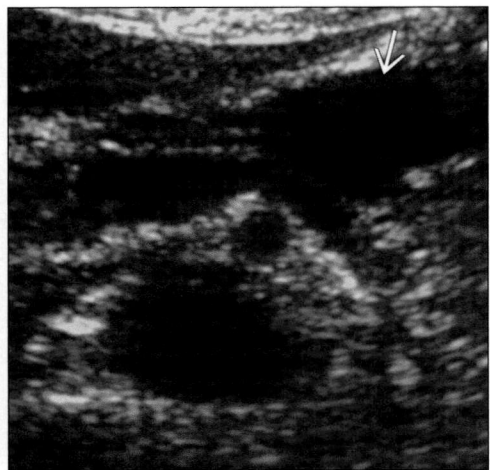

Transverse transabdominal ultrasound shows well-circumscribed unilocular pseudocyst ➡ in pancreatic body. No pancreatic parenchymal calcification or ductal dilatation is seen.

TERMINOLOGY

Definitions
- Collection of pancreatic fluid & inflammatory exudate encapsulated by non-epithelialized fibrous tissue

IMAGING FINDINGS

General Features
- Best diagnostic clue: Well-defined cystic mass with infiltration of peripancreatic fat planes
- Location
  - Two thirds within pancreas
    - Body & tail (85%); head (15%)
  - One third in extra-pancreatic location
    - Juxtasplenic, retroperitoneum, intraperitoneal & mediastinum
    - Intraparenchymal: Left lobe of liver, spleen, kidney
- Size: Varies from 2-10 cm
- Morphology
  - One of the complications of acute pancreatitis

- Seen in approximately 15% of patients with acute pancreatitis
  - Develop over a period of 4-6 weeks after onset of acute pancreatitis
- Can also be seen with chronic pancreatitis
- In contrast to true cysts, pseudocysts lack a true epithelial lining

Ultrasonographic Findings
- Grayscale Ultrasound
  - Uncomplicated pseudocyst
    - Well-circumscribed, smooth-walled, unilocular anechoic mass with posterior acoustic enhancement
    - Most common in pancreatic body and tail
  - Variant/complicated pseudocyst
    - Multilocular in 6% of cases
    - Fluid-debris level, internal echoes and septations (due to hemorrhage/infection)
    - Solid or complex in morphology (during initial phase of cyst formation)
    - Wall calcification: May make it difficult to assess details of pseudocyst

DDx: Pancreatic Pseudocyst

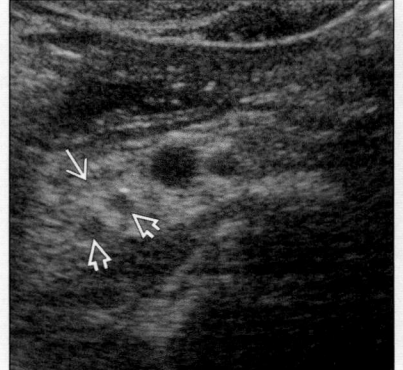

Serous Cystadenoma

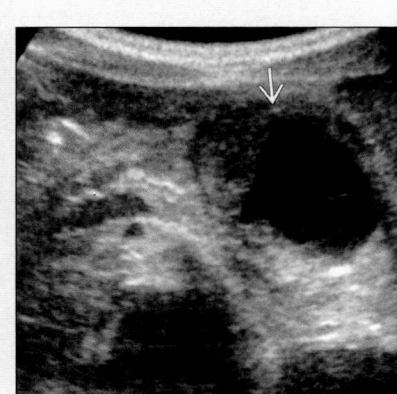

Mucinous Pancreatic Tumor

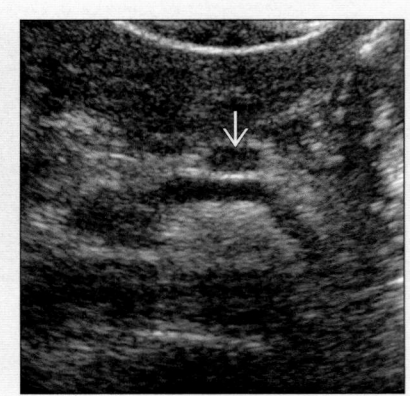

Congenital Cyst

CHRONIC PANCREATITIS

Key Facts

Terminology
- Progressive, irreversible inflammatory damage of pancreas evident on imaging or functional testing

Imaging Findings
- Atrophic gland: Gland may be enlarged in early part of chronic pancreatitis & during an acute on chronic episode, enlargement may be focal or diffuse
- Patchy hypoechoic (due to inflammatory change) and hyperechoic (combination of fibrosis and calcification) echo pattern
- Irregular pancreatic contour
- Dilated MPD (irregular, smooth or beaded)
- Pancreatic calcifications
- Focal mass/enlargement in 40%
- Pseudocyst: 25-40%, intra/peripancreatic
- Dilatation of common bile duct: 5-10%

- Portosplenic venous thrombosis: 5%
- Arterial pseudoaneurysm formation
- Ascites/pleural effusion
- Peripancreatic inflammatory change
- Areas of focal intraparenchymal necrosis
- Best imaging tool: Ultrasound, MRCP, ERCP

Top Differential Diagnoses
- Pancreatic Carcinoma
- Acute Pancreatitis
- IPMT of Pancreas

Diagnostic Checklist
- Glandular atrophy, dilated MPD and ductal calculi/parenchymal calcifications are best signs for chronic pancreatitis

---

- Parenchymal calcifications
  - Focal mass/enlargement in 40%
  - Pseudocyst: 25-40%, intra/peripancreatic
    - Unilocular, anechoic & sharply defined
  - Dilatation of common bile duct: 5-10%
    - Smooth gradual tapering
  - Portosplenic venous thrombosis: 5%
  - Arterial pseudoaneurysm formation
  - Ascites/pleural effusion
  - Peripancreatic inflammatory change
  - Areas of focal intraparenchymal necrosis

Radiographic Findings
- Radiography
  - Plain X-ray abdomen
    - Pancreatic calcification
    - Small, irregular calcifications (local or diffuse)
- Barium (UGI series)
  - Changes seen in second part of duodenum
    - Thickened, irregular & spiculated mucosal folds
    - Stricture & proximal dilatation
    - Enlarged papilla of Vater (Poppel papillary sign)
- ERCP
  - Dilated & beaded MPD plus radicles
  - MPD filling defects: Intraductal calculi
  - Common bile duct (CBD) may appear dilated with distal narrowing

CT Findings
- NECT
  - Glandular atrophy
  - Dilated MPD with ductal calculi
  - Intra and peripancreatic cysts
  - Thickening of peripancreatic fascia
  - Hypodense focal mass (fibrosis and fat necrosis)
- CECT
  - Heterogeneous enhancement of pancreas
  - Mass due to chronic pancreatitis: Varied enhancement due to presence or absence of fibrosis

MR Findings
- T1WI GEI
  - Decreased or loss of signal intensity

- Fat suppressed T2WI
  - Pseudocyst, necrotic areas: Hyperintense
  - Gallstones, intraductal calculi: Hypointense
- T1 C+ GEI
  - Heterogeneous enhancement pattern
    - Nonenhancing decreased signal areas: Necrosis, pseudocyst
    - Pancreatic pseudocyst contiguous with dilated MPD is well depicted
    - Vascular occlusions can be demonstrated
- MRCP
  - Fluid-containing structures are well depicted
    - Dilated MPD plus radicles
    - Pseudocyst contiguous with MPD
    - CBD may be dilated with smooth distal tapering

Imaging Recommendations
- Best imaging tool: Ultrasound, MRCP, ERCP

DIFFERENTIAL DIAGNOSIS

Pancreatic Carcinoma
- Irregular, heterogeneous mass
- Location: Head (60% of cases); body (20%); tail (15%)
- Obstruction causing dilatation of MPD and/or CBD
- Extensive local invasion & regional metastases
  - Local invasion to medial wall of duodenum, liver & regional nodal metastases early in course of disease
- 65% of patients present with advanced local disease & distant metastases
- Some cases of chronic pancreatitis & pancreatic cancer are impossible to differentiate without surgical excision & histology

Acute Pancreatitis
- Diffuse/focal parenchymal enlargement
- Hypoechoic echogenicity in inflamed parenchyma
- No pancreatic ductal dilatation
- Lack of pancreatic calcification
- Peripancreatic fluid collection

CHRONIC PANCREATITIS

IPMT of Pancreas

- IPMT: Intraductal papillary mucinous tumor
- Low grade malignancy arises from main pancreatic duct or branch pancreatic duct (BPD)
- Involvement of main pancreatic duct may simulate chronic pancreatitis
- Dilated MPD and parenchymal atrophy

PATHOLOGY

General Features

- General path comments
  - Embryological consideration
    - Congenital anomalies may predispose to chronic pancreatitis
    - Pancreas divisum: Ducts too small to adequately drain pancreatic secretions leading to chronic stasis
    - Annular pancreas: Pancreatic ductal obstruction and stasis of secretions
  - Chronic calcifying pancreatitis (alcoholism)
    - Diffuse involvement
  - Chronic obstructive pancreatitis (gallstones)
    - Lesions are more prominent in head of pancreas
    - Pattern does not have a lobular distribution
- Genetics
  - Hereditary pancreatitis
    - Autosomal dominant with incomplete penetrance
- Etiology
  - Chronic pancreatitis usually caused by alcohol abuse
  - Gallstones, hyperlipidemia, trauma, drugs often cause acute but rarely chronic pancreatitis
  - Pathogenesis: Due to chronic reflux of pancreatic enzymes, bile, duodenal contents & increased ductal pressure
    - MPD or terminal duct blockage
    - Edema, spasm or incompetent sphincter of Oddi
    - Periduodenal diverticulum or tumor
- Epidemiology: More common in developing countries

Gross Pathologic & Surgical Features

- Hard atrophic pancreas with intraductal calculi & dilated MPD
- Areas of multiple parenchymal calcifications
- Pseudocysts may be seen

Microscopic Features

- Atrophy & fibrosis of acini with dilated ducts
- Mononuclear inflammatory reaction
- Occasionally squamous metaplasia of ductal epithelium

CLINICAL ISSUES

Presentation

- Most common signs/symptoms
  - Recurrent attacks of epigastric pain, typically radiates to back
  - Jaundice, steatorrhea & diabetes mellitus
  - Endocrine & exocrine deficiencies due to progressive destruction of gland

  - Weight loss
- Clinical Profile: Patient with history of chronic alcoholism, recurrent attacks of epigastric pain radiating to back, jaundice, steatorrhea & diabetes
- Lab data
  - Elevated serum amylase & lipase
  - Increased blood glucose levels & fat in stool
  - Secretin test: Decreased amylase & bicarbonate

Demographics

- Age: Usually middle age group
- Gender: Males more than females

Natural History & Prognosis

- Complications
  - Diabetes mellitus
  - Malabsorption
  - Biliary obstruction; jaundice
  - GI bleeding & splenic vein thrombosis
  - Significant increase incidence of pancreatic cancer
- Prognosis
  - Poor

Treatment

- Surgical or endoscopic intervention
  - Ductal & GI obstruction
  - GI bleeding
  - Large pseudocyst or persistently symptomatic
- Conservative treatment if no major complication (e.g., pain control, medical therapy for diabetes mellitus, etc.)

DIAGNOSTIC CHECKLIST

Consider

- Differentiate from other conditions which can cause "MPD dilatation & glandular atrophy"
- May be very difficult to distinguish chronic pancreatitis with a focal fibrotic mass (in head) from pancreatic carcinoma

Image Interpretation Pearls

- Glandular atrophy, dilated MPD and ductal calculi/parenchymal calcifications are best signs for chronic pancreatitis

SELECTED REFERENCES

1. Bruno MJ: Chronic pancreatitis. Gastrointest Endosc Clin N Am. 15(1):55-62, viii, 2005
2. Lankisch PG: The problem of diagnosing chronic pancreatitis. Dig Liver Dis. 35(3):131-4, 2003
3. Matos C et al: MR imaging of the pancreas: a pictorial tour. Radiographics. 22(1):e2, 2002
4. Remer EM et al: Imaging of chronic pancreatitis. Radiol Clin North Am. 40(6):1229-42, v, 2002
5. Varghese JC et al: Value of MR pancreatography in the evaluation of patients with chronic pancreatitis. Clin Radiol. 57(5):393-401, 2002
6. Forsmark CE: The diagnosis of chronic pancreatitis. Gastrointest Endosc. 52(2):293-8, 2000
7. Johnson PT et al: Pancreatic carcinoma versus chronic pancreatitis: dynamic MR imaging. Radiology. 212(1):213-8, 1999

CHRONIC PANCREATITIS

IMAGE GALLERY

Typical

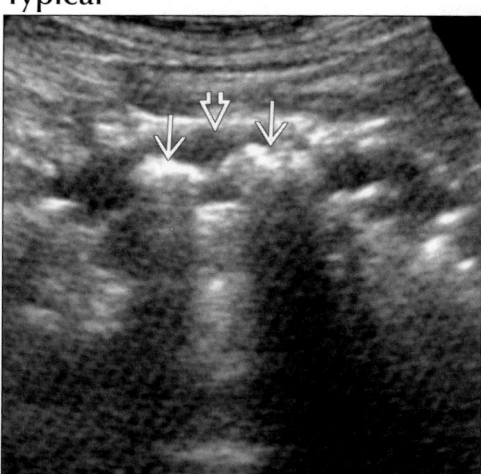 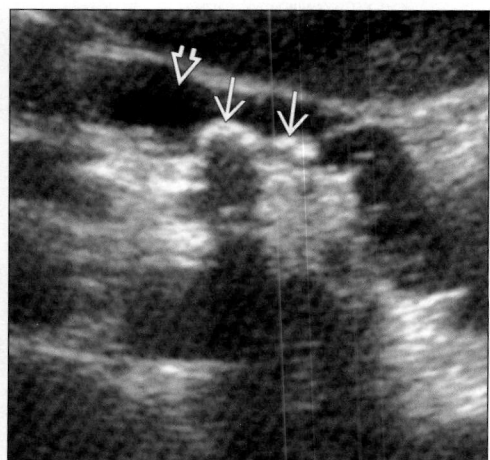

(Left) Transverse transabdominal ultrasound shows atrophic pancreatic parenchyma containing multiple intraductal stones ➡ within a markedly dilated pancreatic duct ➡. *(Right)* Transverse transabdominal ultrasound shows multiple echogenic intraductal stones ➡ within a dilated pancreatic duct ➡. Note the atrophic parenchyma.

Typical

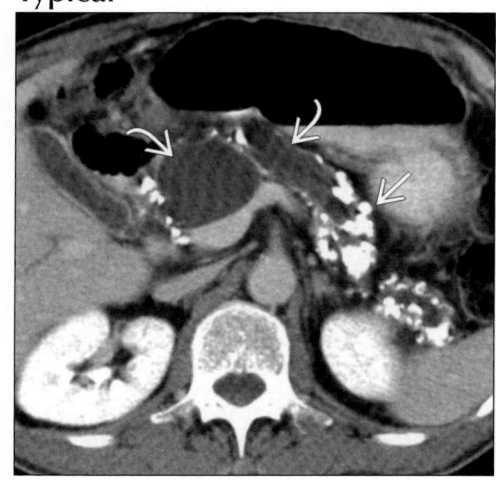 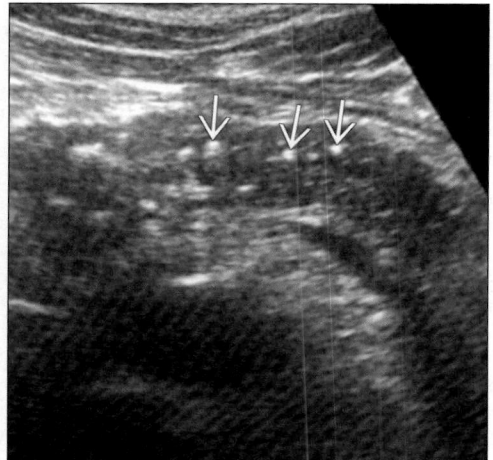

(Left) Transverse CECT shows an atrophied pancreas with parenchymal calcification ➡. Note the dilatation of the pancreatic duct ➡ in the head and body of the pancreas. *(Right)* Transverse transabdominal ultrasound of a case of chronic pancreatitis shows multiple small parenchymal calcifications ➡ affecting the pancreatic body. Note the blurred pancreatic outlines.

Typical

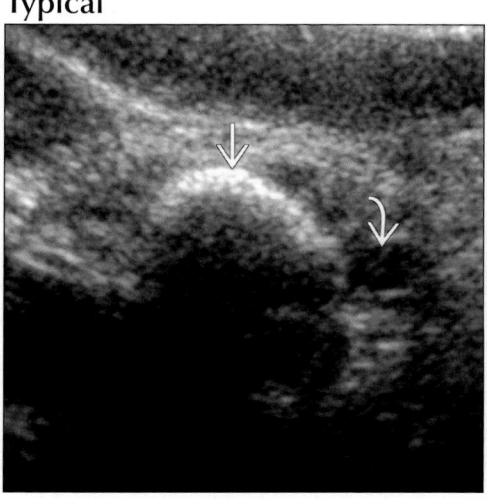 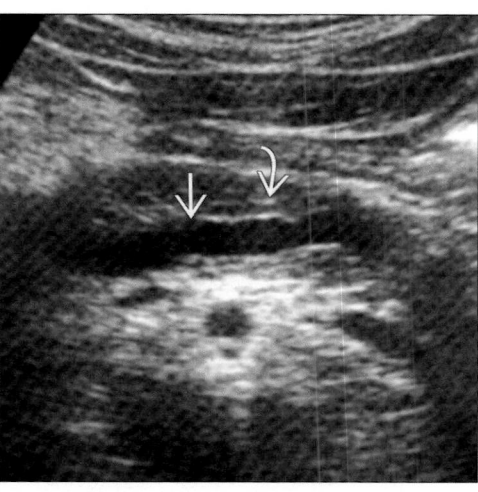

(Left) Transverse transabdominal ultrasound shows a large calcified focus ➡ within the atrophic pancreas. Also note a small cystic lesion ➡ in the pancreatic tail due to a pancreatic pseudocyst. *(Right)* Transverse transabdominal ultrasound shows markedly a dilated pancreatic duct ➡ and tiny pancreatic parenchymal calcification ➡. No intraductal stones are seen in this case.

MUCINOUS CYSTIC PANCREATIC TUMOR

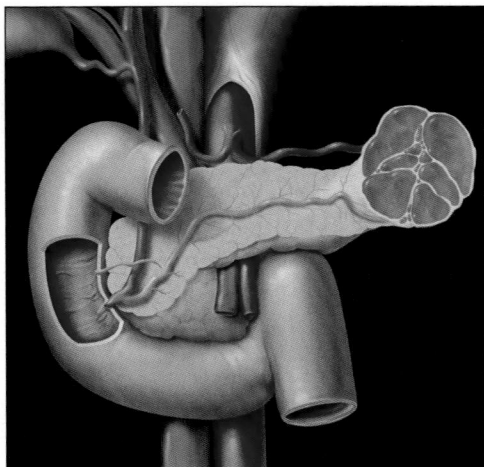

Graphic shows a multiseptated mucin-filled cystic mass in tail of pancreas. The pancreatic duct is displaced, not obstructed. The appearances are suggestive of mucinous cystic tumor.

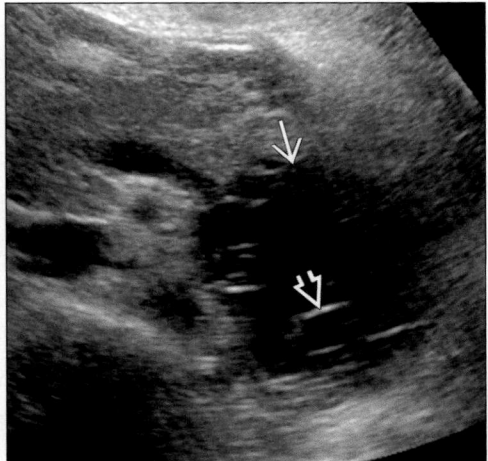

Transverse transabdominal ultrasound shows a well-defined, predominantly cystic mass ➡ in the pancreatic tail. Note presence of internal septations ⬌ within the lesion.

TERMINOLOGY

Abbreviations and Synonyms
- Mucinous macrocystic neoplasm, mucinous cystadenoma or cystadenocarcinoma

Definitions
- Thick-walled, uni-/multilocular low grade malignant tumor composed of large, mucin-containing cysts

IMAGING FINDINGS

General Features
- Best diagnostic clue: Multiseptated mass in body or tail of pancreas, particularly in women
- Location: Tail of pancreas (more common)
- Size: Varies from 2 cm to more than 10 cm in diameter

Ultrasonographic Findings
- Grayscale Ultrasound
  - Well-demarcated thick-walled cystic mass, commonly in pancreatic tail
  - Unilocular/multilocular cysts

- Separated by thick echogenic septae
    - Cyst contents may be clearly anechoic, echogenic with debris +/- solid component
  - Solid papillary tissue protruding into tumor suggests malignancy
    - May contain mural calcification
    - Do not communicate with ductal system
    - Has a tendency to invade adjacent structures
  - Liver metastases: Thick-walled cystic liver lesions
- Color Doppler
  - Hypovascular mass, scant vascularity
  - May encase splenic vein
  - Displacement of surrounding vessels

CT Findings
- CECT
  - Multilocular/unilocular low attenuation cystic lesion
  - Enhancement of internal septa and cyst wall

MR Findings
- Predominantly cystic signal, mixed signal of internal septae and solid component
- Enhancement of septations and cyst wall on fat suppression technique

DDx: Mucinous Cystic Pancreatic Neoplasm

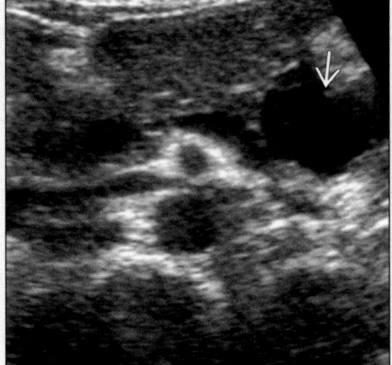

Pancreatic Pseudocyst

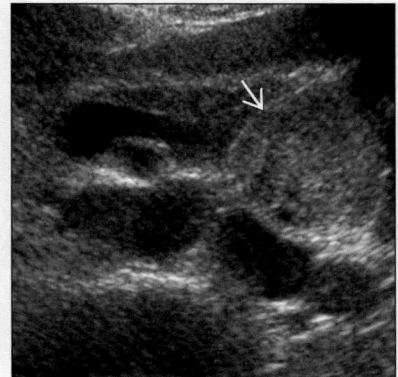

Serous Cystadenoma

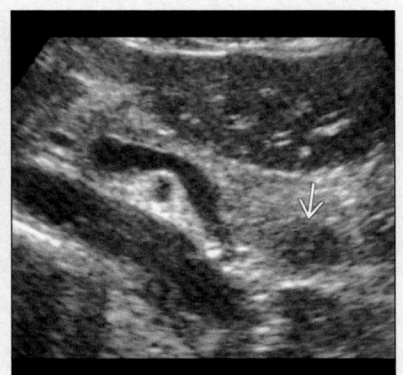

Islet Cell Pancreatic Tumor

MUCINOUS CYSTIC PANCREATIC TUMOR

Key Facts

Terminology
- Thick-walled, uni-/multilocular low grade malignant tumor composed of large, mucin-containing cysts

Imaging Findings
- Best diagnostic clue: Multiseptated mass in body or tail of pancreas, particularly in women
- Cyst contents may be clearly anechoic, echogenic with debris +/- solid component

- Solid papillary tissue protruding into tumor suggests malignancy
- May contain mural calcification
- Has a tendency to invade adjacent structures
- Hypovascular mass, scant vascularity
- May encase splenic vein

Top Differential Diagnoses
- Pseudocyst
- Serous Cystadenoma of Pancreas

Imaging Recommendations
- Best imaging tool: US, CECT, T1 C+ MR

- Cystic cavity may be filled with thick mucoid material/clear/green/blood-tinged fluid
- Solid papillary projections protrude into the tumor

DIFFERENTIAL DIAGNOSIS

Pseudocyst
- Unilocular anechoic cyst with no septa or solid component

Serous Cystadenoma of Pancreas
- Macrocystic variant of serous cystadenoma: Usually has thinner wall, located in pancreatic head

Cystic Islet Cell Tumor
- CECT/angiography: Hypervascular primary & secondary lesions

Variant of Ductal Adenocarcinoma
- Pancreatic and common bile duct obstruction & dilatation

PATHOLOGY

General Features
- Epidemiology: 10% of pancreatic cysts; 1% of pancreatic neoplasms

Gross Pathologic & Surgical Features
- Large encapsulated mass by thick fibrous capsule

CLINICAL ISSUES

Presentation
- Most common signs/symptoms: Asymptomatic, epigastric pain, palpable mass

Demographics
- Age: Mean age: 50 years (range of 20-95 years)
- Gender: M:F = 1:19

Natural History & Prognosis
- Completely excised: Good prognosis
- 5 year survival rate with malignancy regardless of surgery (74%)
- Invariably transforms into cystadenocarcinoma

DIAGNOSTIC CHECKLIST

Image Interpretation Pearls
- Large, multiloculated cystic mass with enhancing septa & cyst wall in pancreatic body or tail

SELECTED REFERENCES
1.   Hara T et al: Mucinous cystic tumors of the pancreas. Surg Today. 32(11):965-9, 2002

IMAGE GALLERY

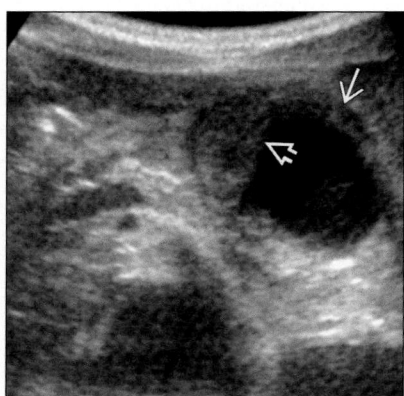 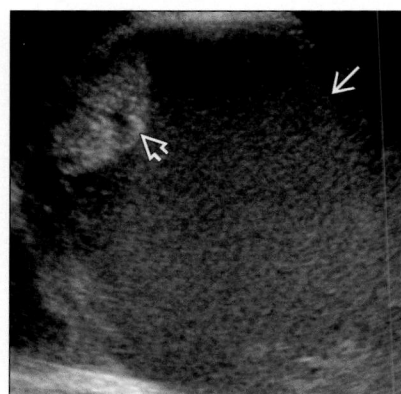 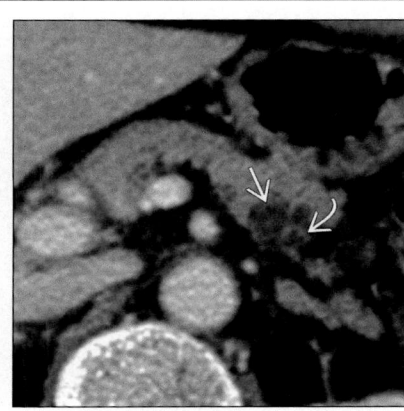

(Left) Transverse transabdominal ultrasound shows a well-defined cystic mass ➡ with eccentric solid component ➡ in pancreatic tail. Note absence of ductal dilatation. (Center) Transverse transabdominal ultrasound shows a large well-circumscribed cystic mass ➡ involving pancreatic body & tail with low level homogeneous echoes & eccentric hyperechoic solid component ➡. (Right) Transverse CECT shows a well-circumscribed cystic mass ➡ in pancreatic tail with thin enhancing internal septations ➡, suggestive of mucinous cystic pancreatic tumor.

SEROUS CYSTADENOMA

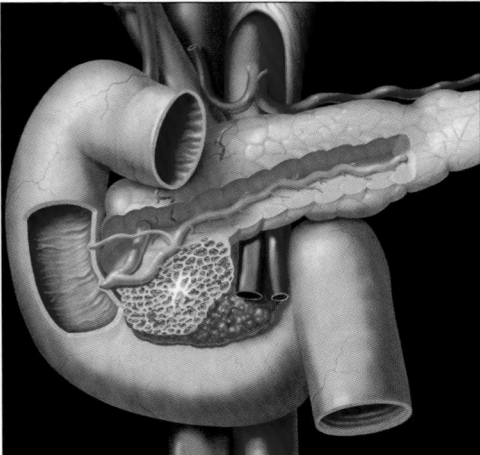

Graphic shows a sponge-like or honeycombed mass in the pancreatic head. Note presence of innumerable small cysts and central scar. The pancreatic duct (PD) is not obstructed.

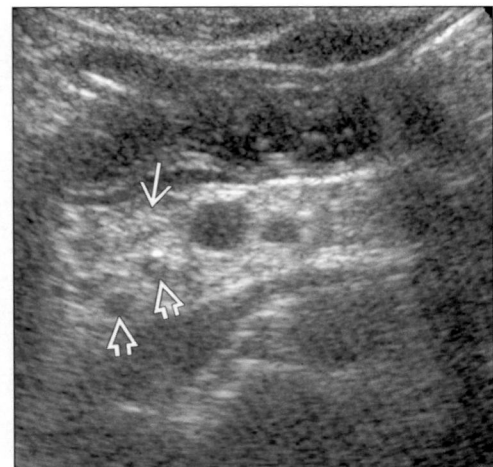

Transverse transabdominal ultrasound shows a well-defined, solid, slightly hyperechoic mass ➡ in the pancreatic head. Note the presence of microcysts ➡ within the lesion. The PD is not dilated.

TERMINOLOGY

Abbreviations and Synonyms
- Glycogen-rich cystadenoma, microcystic adenoma of pancreas

Definitions
- Benign pancreatic neoplasm arises from acinar cells, composed of innumerable small cysts containing proteinaceous fluid separated by connective tissue septae

IMAGING FINDINGS

General Features
- Best diagnostic clue: Honeycomb or sponge-like mass in pancreatic head (microcystic serous cystadenoma)
- Location
  ○ Head of pancreas: 30%
  ○ Can be seen in any part of pancreas, predominantly in the pancreatic head
- Size: Variable sizes
- Morphology
  ○ Slowly growing tumors which may become large masses
  ○ Innumerable small cysts (1-20 mm) within cystadenoma
  ○ Calcification is more common in serous than mucinous tumor (38%:16%)
  ○ Based on WHO subclassification: Two types
    ▪ Serous microcystic adenomas (more common)
    ▪ Serous oligocystic ("macrocystic" variant) adenoma

Ultrasonographic Findings
- Grayscale Ultrasound
  ○ Well-demarcated mass with external lobulations
  ○ Appearances depend on size of individual cysts
    ▪ Slightly echogenic, solid-appearing mass (small cysts depicted as interfaces)
    ▪ Partly solid-looking mass with anechoic cystic areas: Cysts usually in periphery
    ▪ Multicystic mass with septae and solid component
  ○ Central stellate scar: Characteristic feature
    ▪ Appears as central, stellate-shaped echogenic area within the mass
    ▪ Present in up to 20% of cases

DDx: Serous Cystadenoma

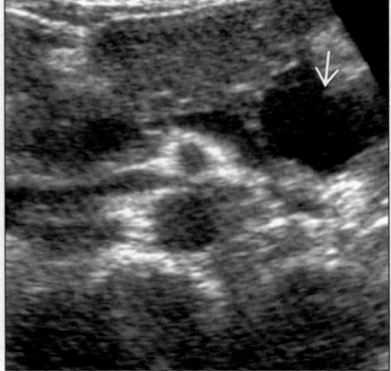

Pancreatic Pseudocyst

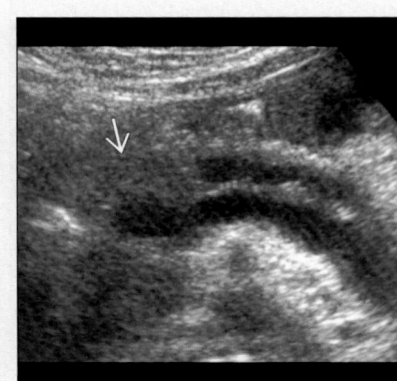

Ductal Pancreatic Carcinoma

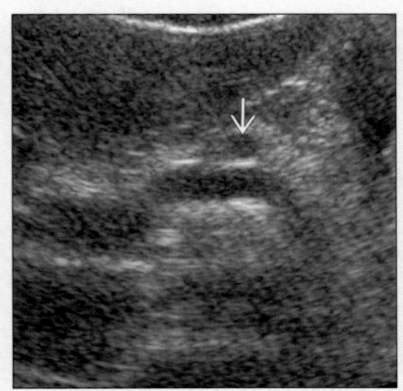

Congenital Cyst

SEROUS CYSTADENOMA

Key Facts

Terminology
- Glycogen-rich cystadenoma, microcystic adenoma of pancreas

Imaging Findings
- Well-demarcated mass with external lobulations
- Appearances depend on size of individual cysts
- Slightly echogenic, solid-appearing mass (small cysts depicted as interfaces)
- Partly solid-looking mass with anechoic cystic areas: Cysts usually in periphery
- Multicystic mass with septae and solid component
- Central stellate scar: Characteristic feature
- Amorphous central calcification
- Pancreatic and common bile duct dilatation is rare
- In patients with thin body habitus, higher frequency transducer help to depict small cysts within the mass

- Careful examination for presence of subtle pancreatic calcification

Top Differential Diagnoses
- Pancreatic Pseudocyst
- Ductal Pancreatic Carcinoma
- Congenital Pancreatic Cysts

Diagnostic Checklist
- Rule out other "cystic pancreatic masses" such as pseudocysts, congenital cysts and cystic malignant neoplasms
- Large, well-demarcated, lobulated cystic lesion composed of innumerable small cysts (1-20 mm) separated by thin septa located in head of pancreas

---

- ○ Amorphous central calcification
  - ▪ Echogenic foci with "sunburst" appearance
  - ▪ Dense posterior acoustic shadowing distal to pancreatic head mass
- ○ Pancreatic and common bile duct dilatation is rare
  - ▪ Due to soft consistency of the tumor, contrary to ductal pancreatic carcinoma
- Color Doppler
  - ○ Increased vascularity in peripheral portion and within septae
  - ○ No vascular encasement

Radiographic Findings
- ERCP
  - ○ Displacement, narrowing & dilatation of adjacent MPD and/or CBD

CT Findings
- Microcystic adenoma: Honeycomb pattern
  - ○ Enhancement of septa delineating small cysts
  - ○ Honeycomb pattern
  - ○ Calcification within central scar
- Macrocystic serous cystadenoma (usually unilocular)
  - ○ One or few cystic components (locules)
  - ○ Thin nonenhancing imperceptible wall

MR Findings
- T1WI
  - ○ Tumor: Hypointense
  - ○ Blood within cysts: Varied intensity
  - ○ Central scar & calcification: Hypointense
- T2WI
  - ○ Tumor: Hyperintense
  - ○ Central scar & calcification: Hypointense
- T1 C+
  - ○ Capsular enhancement
  - ○ Enhancement of septa delineating small cysts
  - ○ Central scar: Enhancement on delayed scan

Angiographic Findings
- Conventional
  - ○ Highly vascular tumor due to extensive capillary network within septa

- ○ Neovascularity & dense tumor blush
- ○ Dilated feeding arteries
- ○ Prominent draining veins

Imaging Recommendations
- Best imaging tool: CECT, US
- Protocol advice
  - ○ In patients with thin body habitus, higher frequency transducer help to depict small cysts within the mass
  - ○ Careful examination for presence of subtle pancreatic calcification

DIFFERENTIAL DIAGNOSIS

Pancreatic Pseudocyst
- Collection of pancreatic fluid encapsulated by fibrous tissue
- Location: More common in body or tail
- Usually unilocular
- Classically lack of septae, solid component or central calcification
- Peripancreatic fat plane infiltration
- Clinical information is important: History of previous pancreatitis

Ductal Pancreatic Carcinoma
- More common than serous cystadenoma
- May contain cystic component due to tumor necrosis
- Lack of tumoral calcification
- Pancreatic and common bile ductal dilatation
- Evidence of vascular encasement and regional/distant metastases

Congenital Pancreatic Cysts
- Well-circumscribed anechoic pancreatic lesion
- Lack of solid component, septa or calcification
- No pancreatic ductal dilatation
- May have underlying clinical conditions: von Hippel-Lindau & ADPKD

Mucinous Cystadenoma of Pancreas
- Most consider this tumor as premalignant

SEROUS CYSTADENOMA

- Location: Tail of pancreas (more common)
- Multiloculated cystic mass with echogenic internal septa
- Malignant tumor: Internal solid component
- May be indistinguishable from macrocystic serous cystadenoma of pancreas by imaging alone

Intraductal Papillary Mucinous Tumor (IPMT)
- Low grade malignancy arises from main pancreatic duct (MPD) or branch pancreatic duct (BPD)
- BPD type lesion simulate serous microcystic adenoma due to presence of dilated small branch ducts in pancreatic head
  ○ Appear as "grape-like" clusters or small cysts
- Marked pancreatic ductal dilatation

Cystic Islet Cell Tumor
- Usually non-insulin producing & nonfunctioning
- Mixed cystic and solid tumor
- No pancreatic ductal dilatation
- Angiography: Hypervascular primary & secondary

PATHOLOGY

General Features
- General path comments
  ○ Cell of origin: Centroacinar cell
  ○ Positive staining for epithelial membrane antigen & cytokeratin of low and high molecular weights
  ○ Composed of smaller cysts (1-20 mm)
  ○ In general no malignant potential
- Epidemiology
  ○ Cystic pancreatic neoplasms are rare
  ○ Accounts 10-15% of all pancreatic cysts
  ○ Accounts only 1% of all pancreatic neoplasms
- Associated abnormalities: Associated with von Hippel-Lindau disease

Gross Pathologic & Surgical Features
- Well-circumscribed, round/ovoid, cystic, multilocular
- Lobulated edges secondary to bulging cysts
- Macroscopic cut section
  ○ Honeycombed or spongy appearance (due to small, innumerable cysts)
  ○ Fluid in cysts
    ▪ Typically clear with no mucoid plugs
    ▪ Rarely hemorrhagic in nature
  ○ Thin fibrous septa radiating from central scar
  ○ Dystrophic calcification within central scar

Microscopic Features
- Cysts lined by cuboidal/flat epithelial cells separated by fibrous septa
- Cells are glycogen-rich
- No cytologic atypia nor mitotic figures
- Pancreatic tissue adjacent to tumor is normal or focally atrophic

CLINICAL ISSUES

Presentation
- Most common signs/symptoms

○ Asymptomatic or vague nonspecific epigastric pain
○ Weight loss, jaundice, palpable mass
○ Other signs/symptoms of mass effect on adjacent structures (stomach & bowel)
- Diagnosis
  ○ Endoscopic US with cyst aspiration & cytology

Demographics
- Age
  ○ Middle & elderly age group (more common)
  ○ Mean age 65 years
- Gender: M:F = 1:4

Natural History & Prognosis
- Most lesions remain static over time without causing any complication
- Potential complications
  ○ Obstructive jaundice: CBD obstruction
  ○ Bowel obstruction: Obstruction of second part of duodenum
  ○ Atrophy of pancreas distal to the tumor
- Prognosis
  ○ No malignant potential
  ○ Completely excised if symptomatic: Good prognosis

Treatment
- Asymptomatic & small tumors
  ○ No surgical excision if confidently diagnosed
  ○ Routine clinical and imaging follow-up
- Symptomatic & large tumors
  ○ Complete surgical excision & follow-up

DIAGNOSTIC CHECKLIST

Consider
- Rule out other "cystic pancreatic masses" such as pseudocysts, congenital cysts and cystic malignant neoplasms

Image Interpretation Pearls
- Large, well-demarcated, lobulated cystic lesion composed of innumerable small cysts (1-20 mm) separated by thin septa located in head of pancreas

SELECTED REFERENCES

1. Sand J et al: The differentiation between pancreatic neoplastic cysts and pancreatic pseudocyst. Scand J Surg. 94(2):161-4, 2005
2. Goldsmith JD: Cystic neoplasms of the pancreas. Am J Clin Pathol. 119 Suppl:S3-16, 2003
3. Anderson MA et al: Nonmucinous cystic pancreatic neoplasms. Gastrointest Endosc Clin N Am. 12(4):769-79, viii, 2002
4. Sheth S et al: Imaging of uncommon tumors of the pancreas. Radiol Clin North Am. 40(6):1273-87, vi, 2002
5. Yeh HC et al: Microcystic features at US: a nonspecific sign for microcystic adenomas of the pancreas. Radiographics. 21(6):1455-61, 2001
6. Curry CA et al: CT of primary cystic pancreatic neoplasms. AJR. 175: 99-103, 2000
7. Kato T et al: Ultrasonographic and endoscopic ultrasonographic angiography in pancreatic mass lesions. Acta Radiol. 36(4):381-7, 1995

IMAGE GALLERY

Typical

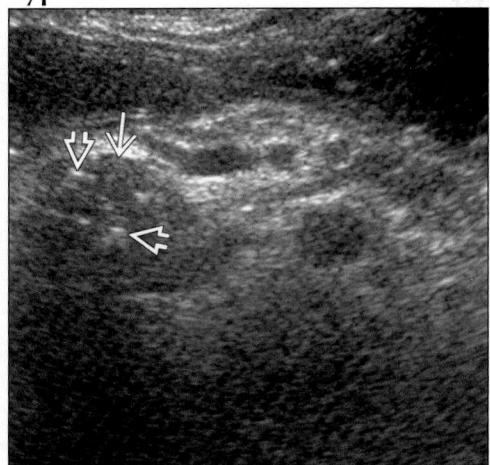
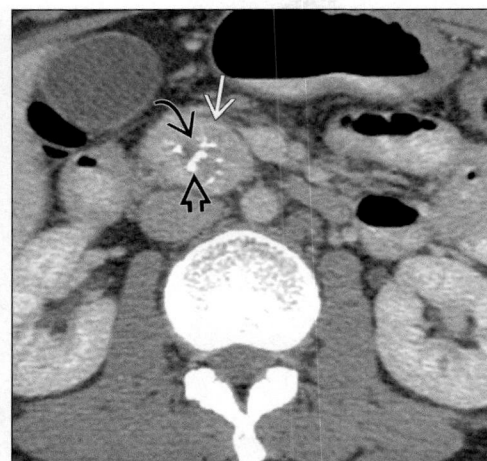

(Left) *Transverse transabdominal ultrasound shows a well-defined, solid, hypoechoic mass* ➡ *in the pancreatic head. Note the presence of echogenic calcification* ➡ *with posterior acoustic shadow.* *(Right)* *Transverse CECT shows well-defined enhancing soft tissue mass* ➡ *in the pancreatic head. Foci of calcification* ➡ *and hypodense center* ➡ *(scar/cystic component) noted within the lesion.*

Typical

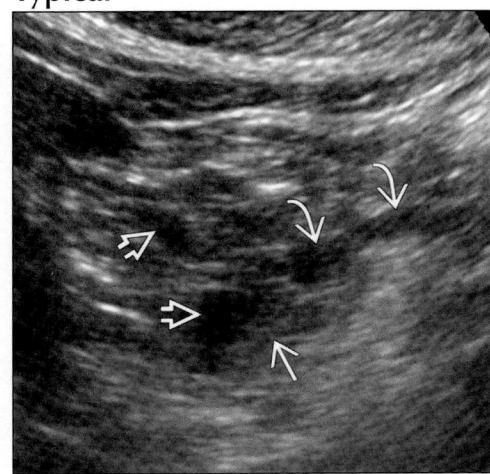
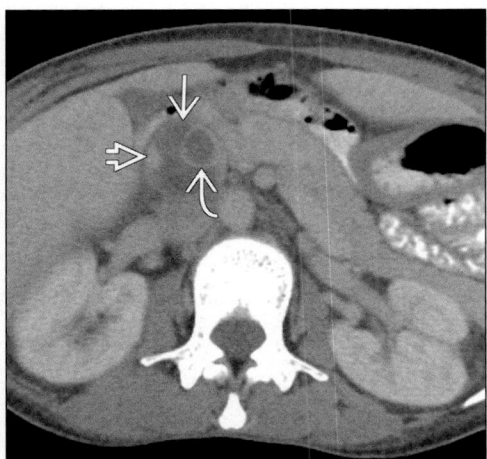

(Left) *Transverse transabdominal ultrasound shows an ill-defined hypoechoic mass* ➡ *in the pancreatic head containing small microcysts* ➡. *Note portal vein and splenic vein confluence* ➡. *(Right)* *Transverse CECT shows a well-circumscribed cystic mass* ➡ *in the head of the pancreas. Note the presence of an enhancing solid component* ➡ *and septae* ➡ *within the lesion.*

Variant

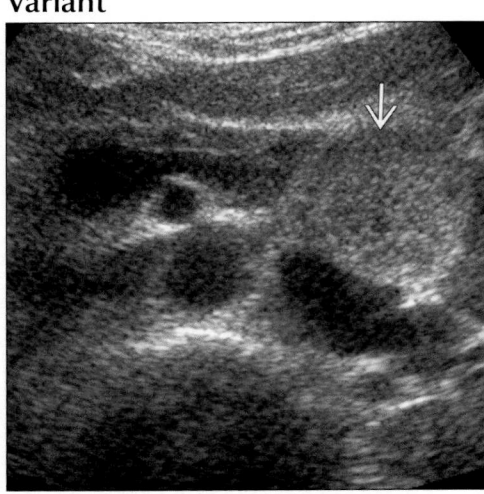
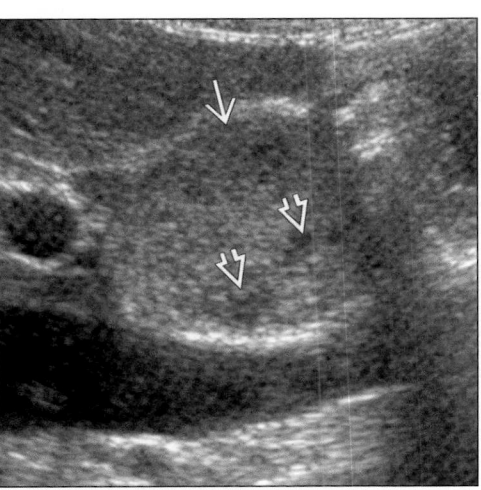

(Left) *Transverse transabdominal ultrasound shows a well-circumscribed, solid, slightly hyperechoic mass* ➡ *in the pancreatic tail. Note the absence of pancreatic ductal dilatation or calcification within the lesion.* *(Right)* *Longitudinal transabdominal ultrasound shows small cystic components* ➡ *within the solid, slightly hyperechoic mass* ➡ *in the pancreatic tail. Biopsy confirmed the diagnosis.*

DUCTAL PANCREATIC CARCINOMA

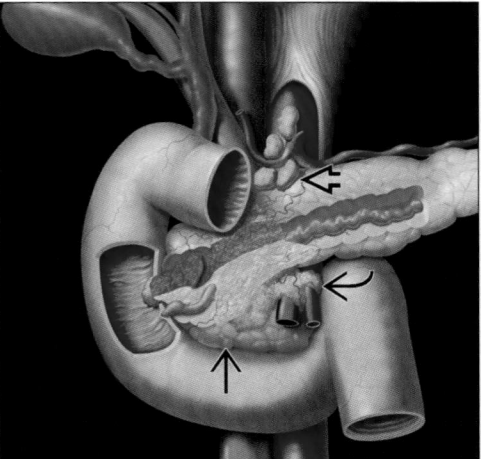

Graphic shows an infiltrative mass ➡ in the pancreatic head partially obstructing the common bile duct and pancreatic duct. Superior mesenteric vessels are encased ➡; celiac nodes ⋑ present.

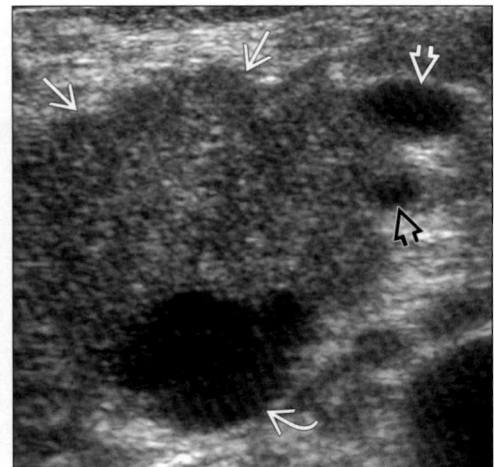

Transverse transabdominal ultrasound shows an infiltrative mass ➡ in the pancreatic head and uncinate process, close to the portal vein ➡ and SMA ⋑. Note pancreatic duct dilatation ⋑.

TERMINOLOGY

Abbreviations and Synonyms
- Pancreatic ductal adenocarcinoma, pancreatic cancer

Definitions
- Malignancy arises from ductal epithelium of exocrine pancreas

IMAGING FINDINGS

General Features
- Best diagnostic clue: Irregular, heterogeneous pancreatic mass with abrupt obstruction of pancreatic and/or common bile duct ("double duct sign")
- Location: Head (60-70%), body (20%), diffuse (15%), tail (5%)
- Size
  - Varies; average diameter is 2-3 cm
  - Large tumor can be up to 8-10 cm
- Morphology
  - Most common primary malignant tumor of exocrine pancreas
  - Accounts for 80-95% of nonendocrine pancreatic neoplasms
  - Ill-defined tumor with extensive local invasion into soft tissues, duodenum, stomach, left adrenal, spleen
  - Rarely resectable for cure at the time of presentation
  - Metastatic involvement of liver, portal hilar nodes, peritoneum, lungs, pleura, bone

Ultrasonographic Findings
- Grayscale Ultrasound
  - Poorly-defined, homogeneous/heterogeneous, hypoechoic mass in the pancreas or pancreatic fossa
    - Usually > 2 cm at presentation
    - Mostly hypoechoic relative to homogeneous hyperechoic echotexture of normal parenchyma in uninvolved area
    - Necrosis/cystic component: Rarely seen
    - Diffuse glandular tumor involvement: Difficult to differentiate from acute pancreatitis on USG
  - Small isoechoic tumor: Appears as focal contour deformity of gland (e.g., in uncinate process)
  - Pancreatic ductal dilatation distal to tumor
    - > 3 mm in diameter
    - Loses its parallel nature

DDx: Ductal Pancreatic Carcinoma

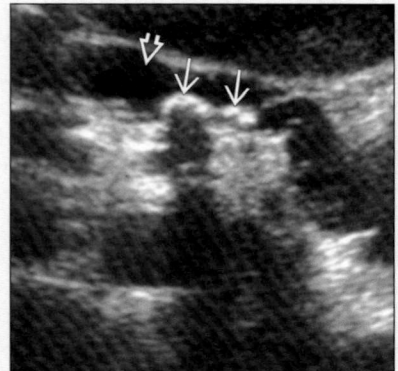

Chronic Pancreatitis

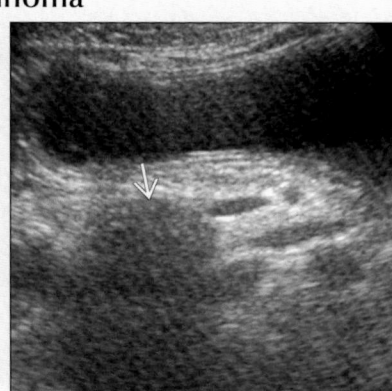

Serous Cystadenoma

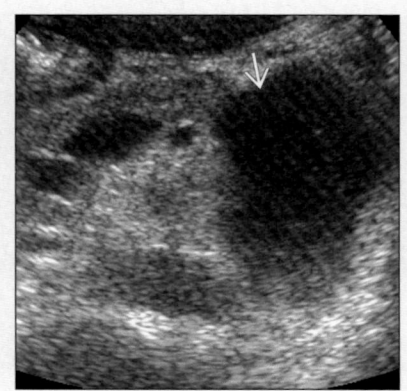

Pancreatic Lymphoma

DUCTAL PANCREATIC CARCINOMA

Key Facts

Terminology
- Malignancy arises from ductal epithelium of exocrine pancreas

Imaging Findings
- Best diagnostic clue: Irregular, heterogeneous pancreatic mass with abrupt obstruction of pancreatic and/or common bile duct ("double duct sign")
- Location: Head (60-70%), body (20%), diffuse (15%), tail (5%)
- Ill-defined tumor with extensive local invasion into soft tissues, duodenum, stomach, left adrenal, spleen
- Metastatic involvement of liver, portal hilar nodes, peritoneum, lungs, pleura, bone
- Poorly-defined, homogeneous/heterogeneous, hypoechoic mass in the pancreas or pancreatic fossa
- Pancreatic ductal dilatation distal to tumor

- Bile duct dilatation
- Displacement/encasement of adjacent vascular structures (superior mesenteric artery, splenic artery, hepatic artery, gastroduodenal artery)
- Mild increase in color flow within the tumor
- Best imaging tool: CECT, US +/- endoscopic US
- CECT helps predict resectability better than US

Top Differential Diagnoses
- Chronic Pancreatitis
- Serous Cystadenoma
- Mucinous Cystic Pancreatic Tumor

Diagnostic Checklist
- Irregular heterogeneous mass in head of pancreas with eccentric ductal obstruction/dilatation & extensive local invasion & regional metastases

- Tortuous in configuration
- Abrupt tapering at the site of obstruction
  - Bile duct dilatation
    - Common in pancreatic head ductal carcinoma
    - Level of obstruction can be at pancreatic head, above head or porta hepatis, depending on tumor size and associated regional lymphadenopathy
    - +/- Dilatation of cystic duct and gallbladder (Courvoisier sign)
  - Displacement/encasement of adjacent vascular structures (superior mesenteric artery, splenic artery, hepatic artery, gastroduodenal artery)
  - Associated findings: Atrophy/pancreatitis proximal to pancreatic ductal obstruction, ascites due to peritoneal metastasis
  - Liver and regional lymph node metastases
- Color Doppler
  - Mild increase in color flow within the tumor
  - Helps to assess vascular encasement or venous obstruction

Radiographic Findings
- Barium (UGI) study
  - "Frostberg 3" sign
    - "Inverted 3" contour to medial part of duodenal sweep
  - Spiculated duodenal wall, traction & fixation
  - "Antral padding"
    - Extrinsic indentation of posteroinferior margin of antrum
- ERCP
  - Irregular, nodular, rat-tailed eccentric obstruction
  - Localized encasement with prestenotic dilatation
  - "Double duct" sign: Obstruction of pancreatic and common bile duct at same level

CT Findings
- CECT
  - Heterogeneous, poorly-enhancing mass
  - Pancreatic ductal dilatation distal to tumor
  - Lesion in head may cause common bile duct (CBD) obstruction & dilatation of bile ducts

  - Vascular invasion: "Tear drop" shaped superior mesenteric vein (SMV)
    - Encasement of more than half circumference of vessel, narrowing or occlusion
  - Contiguous organ invasion
    - Duodenum, splenic hilum, porta hepatis, stomach & mesenteric root
  - Distant metastases
    - Liver, peritoneum & regional lymph nodes

MR Findings
- T1WI
  - Low signal intensity relative to normal parenchyma due to fibrous nature of tumor
  - Fat suppressed T1WI
    - Hypointense lesion compared to high signal intensity of normal pancreatic parenchyma
- T1 C+: Poor or no enhancement on dynamic study
- T2 GRE & T1WI spin-echo sequences
  - Detects vascular invasion

Angiographic Findings
- Conventional
  - Hypovascular tumor
  - Displacement, encasement or occlusion by tumor

Imaging Recommendations
- Best imaging tool: CECT, US +/- endoscopic US
- Protocol advice
  - On US the pancreas may be better visualized by distending stomach with water or scanning in sitting/standing position
  - Clue to detection of small tumor: Focal contour irregularity, subtle pancreatic ductal or bile duct dilatation
  - CECT helps predict resectability better than US

DIFFERENTIAL DIAGNOSIS

Chronic Pancreatitis
- Focal or diffuse atrophy of gland, fibrotic mass in head
- Dilated main pancreatic duct with ductal calculi

DUCTAL PANCREATIC CARCINOMA

- Parenchymal calcification
- Distal CBD long stricture causes prestenotic dilatation
- Thickening of peripancreatic fascia & fat necrosis
- May be indistinguishable from cancer on imaging

Serous Cystadenoma
- Mixed cystic/solid pancreatic head lesion
- Central scarring with calcification
- No pancreatic ductal dilatation

Mucinous Cystic Pancreatic Tumor
- Multiseptated cystic mass with solid component
- More common in pancreatic tail
- No pancreatic or bile duct dilatation

Lymphoma
- Focal or diffuse glandular enlargement of pancreas
- Rarely obstructs pancreatic/bile ducts
- Associated intra-abdominal lymphadenopathy/splenic involvement

Islet Cell Carcinoma
- Hypervascular primary & secondary tumors
- No pancreatic ductal dilatation
- Usually functioning tumors are small in size & non-functioning tumors are large in size

Metastases
- Solitary/multiple pancreatic masses
- Presence of concomitant intra-abdominal metastases: Liver, adrenal glands, lymph nodes
- Rarely obstruct pancreatic and biliary ducts

PATHOLOGY

General Features
- General path comments
  - Scirrhous infiltrative adenocarcinoma with dense cellularity and sparse vascularity
  - 99% arises from exocrine ductal epithelium, 1% from acinic pancreatic gland
  - Spread: Local, peripancreatic, perivascular, perineural & lymphatic invasion
- Genetics: Mutations in K-ras genes & p16INK4 gene on chromosome 9p2, abnormal high levels of p53 gene
- Associated abnormalities
  - Heritable syndromes
    - Hereditary pancreatitis, ataxia telangiectasia
    - Familial colon cancer, Gardner syndrome
    - Familial aggregation of pancreatic cancer
- Risk Factors: Cigarette smoking, diabetes mellitus, chronic pancreatitis, high-fat diet

Gross Pathologic & Surgical Features
- Hard nodular mass obstructing pancreatic duct/CBD
- Hypovascular, locally invasive, desmoplastic response

Microscopic Features
- White fibrous lesion, dense cellularity, nuclear atypia
- Most ductal cancers are mucinous adenocarcinomas

Staging, Grading or Classification Criteria
- Stage I: Confined to pancreas +/- extension into peripancreatic tissues
- Stage II: Stage I plus regional lymph node metastases
- Stage III: Stage I & II plus distant metastases

CLINICAL ISSUES

Presentation
- Most common signs/symptoms
  - Usually asymptomatic until late in its course
  - Clinical presentation depends on site of primary tumor within the pancreas
    - Pancreatic head: Obstructive jaundice
    - Body & tail: Weight loss & massive metastases to liver
  - At presentation
    - 65% patients: Advanced local disease/metastases
    - 20%: Localized disease with spread to regional lymph nodes
    - 15%: Tumor confined to pancreas

Demographics
- Age: Mean age at onset: 55 years, peak age: 7th decade
- Gender: M:F = 2:1

Natural History & Prognosis
- Prognosis
  - In general, poor prognosis due to unresectable disease at presentation
  - With surgery: 5 year survival rate is about 20%
  - Without surgery: 5 year survival rate is less than 5%

Treatment
- Complete surgical resection for potentially curative tumor (< 15%): Pancreaticoduodenectomy ("Whipple resection")
- Palliative/adjuvant therapy
  - External beam radiotherapy/chemotherapy
  - Endoscopic stenting: Palliates obstructive jaundice
  - Gastric bypass: Palliates duodenal obstruction
  - Chemical splanchnicectomy or celiac nerve block to palliate abdominal pain

DIAGNOSTIC CHECKLIST

Consider
- Differentiate from other solid pancreatic masses with or without main pancreatic duct dilatation

Image Interpretation Pearls
- Irregular heterogeneous mass in head of pancreas with eccentric ductal obstruction/dilatation & extensive local invasion & regional metastases

SELECTED REFERENCES

1. Kitano M: Clinical significance of vascular assessment by contrast-enhanced harmonic ultrasonography of pancreatic carcinomas. J Gastroenterol. 40(6):666-8, 2005
2. Delbeke D et al: Pancreatic tumors: role of imaging in the diagnosis, staging, and treatment. J Hepatobiliary Pancreat Surg. 11(1):4-10, 2004
3. Yusoff IF et al: Preoperative assessment of pancreatic malignancy using endoscopic ultrasound. Abdom Imaging. 28(4):556-62, 2003

DUCTAL PANCREATIC CARCINOMA

IMAGE GALLERY

Typical

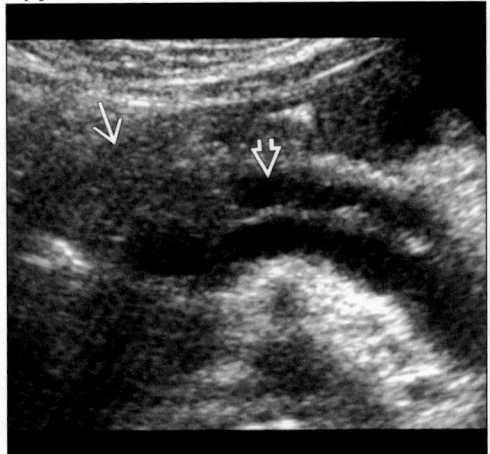 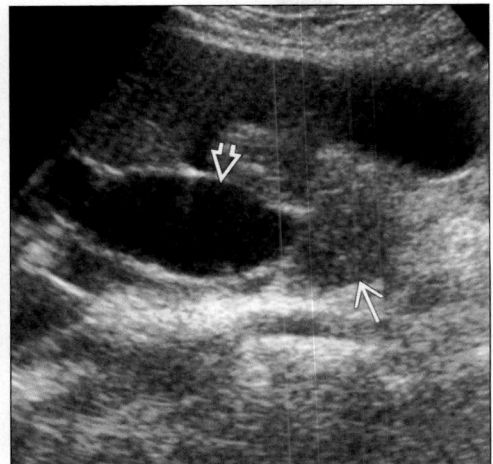

(Left) Transverse transabdominal ultrasound shows an ill-defined, solid, isoechoic mass ➡ in the pancreatic head, with pancreatic duct dilatation ➡ in the body and tail. (Right) Oblique transabdominal ultrasound shows an ill-defined, solid, hypoechoic mass ➡ in the pancreatic head causing truncation of the terminal portion of the common bile duct, with proximal dilatation ➡.

Typical

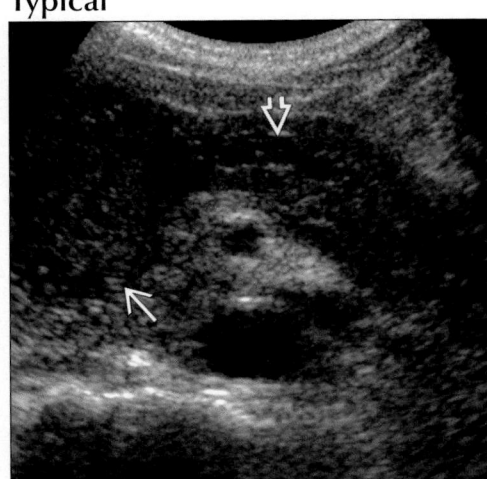 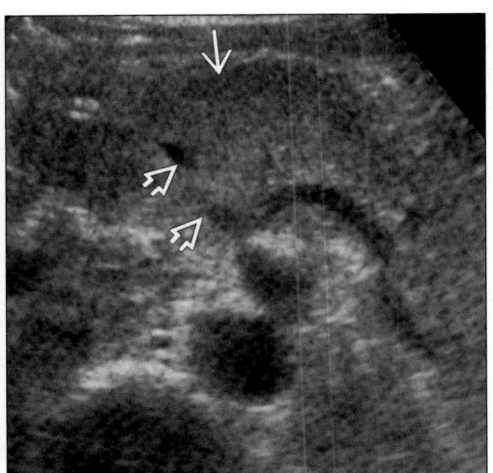

(Left) Transverse transabdominal ultrasound shows an ill-defined, solid, hypoechoic mass ➡ in the head of pancreas with associated distal pancreatic ductal dilatation ➡. (Right) Transverse transabdominal ultrasound shows an ill-defined, slightly hypoechoic, solid mass ➡ in the head and body of the pancreas. Note vascular encasement of the common hepatic artery ➡.

Typical

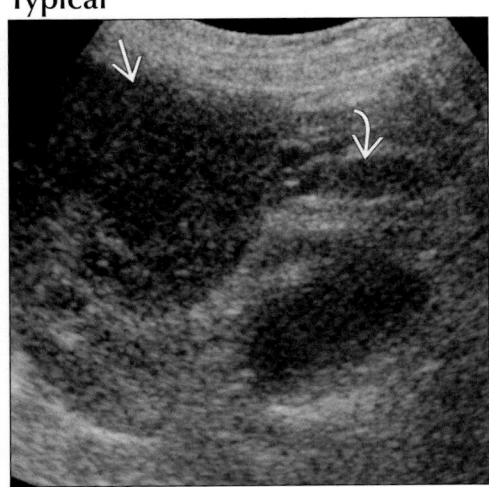 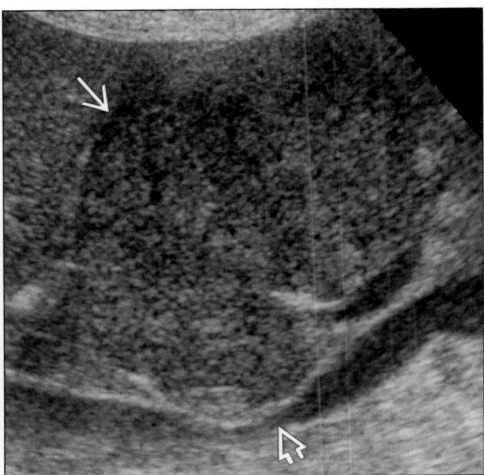

(Left) Transverse transabdominal ultrasound shows a heterogeneous, hypoechoic, solid mass ➡ in the pancreatic head. The pancreatic duct is dilated ➡ distal to the obstruction. (Right) Oblique transabdominal ultrasound shows a large, heterogeneous, hypoechoic, solid mass ➡ in the pancreatic head, causing posterior displacement and compression of the adjacent main portal vein ➡.

ISLET CELL TUMORS

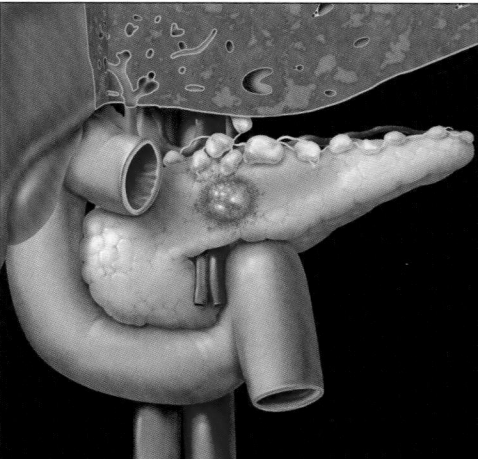
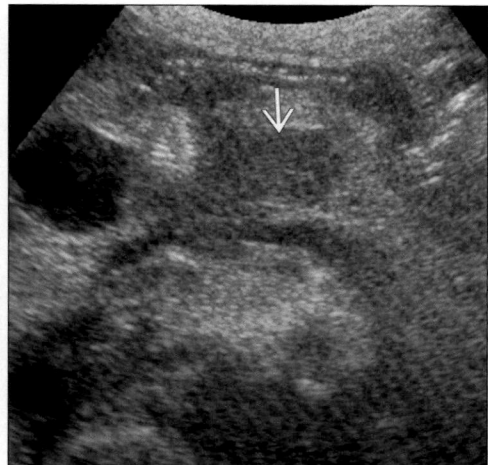

Graphic shows a small hypervascular lesion in the pancreatic body with regional metastatic lymphadenopathy. Note the absence of pancreatic ductal dilatation.

Transverse transabdominal ultrasound shows a solid hypoechoic mass ➡ in the body of the pancreas. No associated pancreatic duct dilatation or intratumoral calcification is seen.

TERMINOLOGY

Abbreviations and Synonyms
- Pancreatic/gastroenteropancreatic neuroendocrine tumor (NET)

Definitions
- Tumors arising from pancreatic endocrine cells (islets of Langerhans)

IMAGING FINDINGS

General Features
- Best diagnostic clue: Hypervascular mass(es) in pancreas (primary) & liver (metastases)
- Location
  - Pancreas (85%); ectopic (15%)
    - Ectopic: Duodenum, stomach, nodes, ovary
- Size: Varies from few millimeters to 10 centimeters
- Morphology
  - Single or multiple (with different cell types)
    - Functioning tumors: Secrete one/multiple pancreatic hormones, with dominant single defining clinical presentation, small at presentation
    - Nonfunctioning tumors: Larger than functioning tumors at diagnosis
    - Cystic islet cell tumor: Usually non-insulin producing & nonfunctioning

Ultrasonographic Findings
- Grayscale Ultrasound
  - Transabdominal ultrasound
    - Detection of islet cell tumor is generally difficult due to small tumor size and obesity (high oral intake due to repeated hypoglycemic attacks)
    - Reported sensitivity ~ 25-60%
    - Most common appearances: Small, solid, hypoechoic pancreatic mass, lack of calcification or necrosis
    - Occasional isoechoic mass: Seen as focal bulge of contour
    - Large tumor (mostly non-functional): May be echogenic and contain calcification and internal necrosis

DDx: Islet Cell Pancreatic Tumor

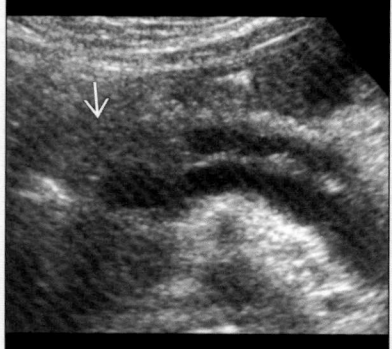
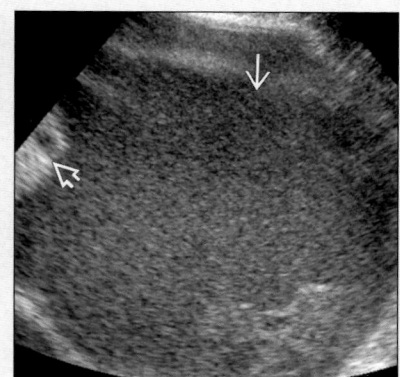
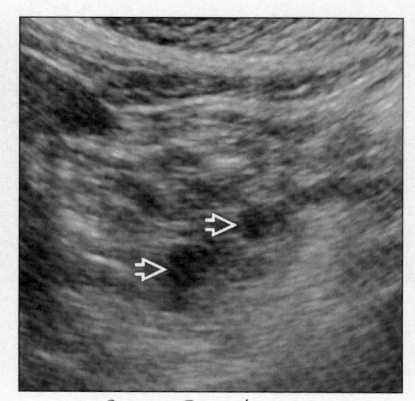

Ductal Pancreatic Carcinoma　　　*Mucinous Cystadenoma*　　　*Serous Cystadenoma*

ISLET CELL TUMORS

Key Facts

Imaging Findings
- Best diagnostic clue: Hypervascular mass(es) in pancreas (primary) & liver (metastases)
- Pancreas (85%); ectopic (15%)
- Most common appearances: Small, solid, hypoechoic pancreatic mass, lack of calcification or necrosis
- Occasional isoechoic mass: Seen as focal bulge of contour
- Large tumor (mostly non-functional): May be echogenic and contain calcification and internal necrosis
- Liver and regional lymph node metastases: 60-90% at clinical presentation
- Hyperechoic hepatic metastases are suggestive of islet cell tumors rather than adenocarcinoma

- Transabdominal US has limited role in detection of islet cell tumor (small tumor size, patient's body habitus)

Top Differential Diagnoses
- Ductal Pancreatic Carcinoma
- Mucinous Cystic Tumor of Pancreas
- Serous Cystadenoma of Pancreas

Diagnostic Checklist
- Hypervascular pancreatic tumor & liver metastases suggests islet cell tumor
- Contrast-enhanced CT and endoscopic US offers better diagnostic accuracy
- Intra-operative has highest sensitivity and is useful to ensure complete resection of tumor

---

- Intratumoral calcification is highly suggestive of malignancy
- Liver and regional lymph node metastases: 60-90% at clinical presentation
- Hyperechoic hepatic metastases are suggestive of islet cell tumors rather than adenocarcinoma
  - Endoscopic ultrasound (EUS)
    - Detects small islet cell tumors
    - Detection rate increased to ~ 80%
    - Small homogeneously hypoechoic mass
    - Helps detect regional lymph node metastases
  - Intra-operative ultrasound (IOUS)
    - Detects very small lesions
    - Highest sensitivity (75-100%)
    - Similar to ultrasound appearances on transabdominal and endoscopic US
- Color Doppler: Increased vascular flow within the pancreatic mass and liver metastases

CT Findings
- CECT
  - Usually hypervascular in arterial and portovenous phases
  - Nonenhancing cystic or necrotic areas
  - Enhancing liver metastases
- Large functional & nonfunctional tumors: Highly malignant
  - Calcification
  - Local invasion
  - Early invasion of portal vein leads to liver metastases

MR Findings
- T1WI SE image
  - Small tumors: Isointense
  - Large tumors: Heterogeneous (cystic & necrotic)
- T1 C+
  - Fat-saturated delayed enhanced T1WI SE: Hyperintense (small)
  - Nonenhancing (cystic + necrotic areas) & increased enhancing viable tumor
- T2WI SE image
  - Small tumors: Isointense
  - Large tumors: Hyperintense (cystic & necrotic)

Angiographic Findings
- Conventional
  - Functioning & nonfunctioning tumors
    - Hypervascular (primary & secondary)
  - Hepatic venous sampling after intra-arterial stimulation of pancreas
    - Functioning tumors: Elevated levels of hormones
    - Nonfunctioning: Decreased levels or absent

Imaging Recommendations
- Transabdominal US has limited role in detection of islet cell tumor (small tumor size, patient's body habitus)
  - If definite biochemical evidence, further imaging studies essential even if initial US is negative
- Endoscopic ultrasound
- CECT
- MR & T1 C+ (including fat suppressed delayed images)
- Intra-operative ultrasound is useful to ensure complete resection for small functional pancreatic islet tumor

DIFFERENTIAL DIAGNOSIS

Ductal Pancreatic Carcinoma
- Location: Head (60%)
- Ill-defined heterogeneous hypoechoic mass
- Pancreatic and common bile duct obstruction
- Vascular encasement
- Extensive local invasion & regional metastases
- Obliteration of retropancreatic fat

Mucinous Cystic Tumor of Pancreas
- Can be similar to cystic islet cell tumor
- Location: Tail of pancreas (more common)
- Multiloculated cystic mass with septations and solid component
- Predominantly avascular
- Lack of pancreatic ductal dilatation

Serous Cystadenoma of Pancreas
- Honeycomb or sponge appearance
- Location: Head of pancreas (more common)

ISLET CELL TUMORS

- Microcystic type: Microcysts with pancreatic head mass, central scarring + calcifications
- Macrocystic type: Thin wall/septa than cystic islet cell
- No pancreatic or biliary ductal dilatation

Metastases
- Common primary: Renal cell carcinoma & melanoma
- Small, well-defined, round hypervascular lesions
- May be solitary or multiple
- Indistinguishable from islet cell tumor metastases

Lymphoma
- Solid hypoechoic mass
- Presence of intra-abdominal lymphadenopathy
- Lymphomatous involvement in the rest of body

PATHOLOGY

General Features
- General path comments
  - Embryology-anatomy
    - Originate from embryonic neuroectoderm
- Etiology
  - Neoplasms arise from amine precursor uptake & decarboxylation (APUD) cells
  - Pathogenesis
    - Insulinoma: β-cell tumor → hyperinsulinemia → hypoglycemia
    - Gastrinoma: Islet cell tumor → increased gastrin → increased gastric acid → peptic ulcer
    - Glucagonoma: α-cell tumor → increased glucagon → erythema migrans & diabetes mellitus
    - Nonfunctioning: Derived from α & β cells
- Epidemiology
  - Insulinoma: Most common islet cell tumor
    - Solitary benign (90%); malignant (10%)
  - Gastrinoma: 2nd common
    - Multiple & malignant (60%); MEN I (20-60%)
  - Nonfunctioning: 3rd common
    - Accounts 20-45% of all islet cell tumors
    - Malignant (80-100%)
- Associated abnormalities
  - Gastrinoma (Zollinger-Ellison syndrome)
    - Associated with MEN type I

Gross Pathologic & Surgical Features
- Small tumor: Encapsulated & firm
- Large tumor: ± Cystic, necrotic, calcified

Microscopic Features
- Sheets of small round cells, uniform nuclei/cytoplasm
- Electron microscopy: Neuron specific enolase ("neuro-endocrine")

CLINICAL ISSUES

Presentation
- Most common signs/symptoms
  - Insulinoma: Whipple triad (hypoglycemia + low fasting glucose + relief by IV glucose)
    - Palpitations, sweating, tremors, headache, coma
  - Gastrinoma (Zollinger-Ellison syndrome)

- Peptic ulcer, increased acidity & diarrhea
  - Glucagonoma
    - Necrolytic erythema migrans, diarrhea, diabetes, weight loss
  - Nonfunctional tumor
    - Mostly asymptomatic or constitutional symptoms
    - Pain, jaundice, variceal bleeding

Demographics
- Age: Peak: 4th-6th decade
- Gender
  - Insulinoma: M < F
  - Gastrinoma: M > F

Natural History & Prognosis
- Complications
  - Insulinoma: Recurrent symptomatic hyperglycemia
  - Gastrinoma: Bleeding/perforated peptic ulcers
  - Glucagonoma: Deep venous thrombosis (DVT) & pulmonary embolism

Treatment
- Acute phase: Octreotide (potent hormonal inhibitor)
- Insulinoma: Surgery curative
- Gastrinoma
  - Medical: Omeprazole, 5-fluorouracil
  - Surgery curative in 30% cases
- Nonfunctional: Resection/embolization
- Transarterial chemoembolization for liver metastases

DIAGNOSTIC CHECKLIST

Consider
- Differentiate from other solid, cystic, vascular tumors
- Correlate with clinical & biochemical information

Image Interpretation Pearls
- Hypervascular pancreatic tumor & liver metastases suggests islet cell tumor
- Ultrasound serves good screening investigation, technical failure due to small tumor size and body habitus
- Contrast-enhanced CT and endoscopic US offers better diagnostic accuracy
- Intra-operative has highest sensitivity and is useful to ensure complete resection of tumor

SELECTED REFERENCES

1. Proye CA et al: Current concepts in functioning endocrine tumors of the pancreas. World J Surg. 28(12):1231-8, 2004
2. Marcos HB et al: Neuroendocrine tumors of the pancreas in von Hippel-Lindau disease: spectrum of appearances at CT and MR imaging with histopathologic comparison. Radiology. 225(3):751-8, 2002
3. Ichikawa T et al: Islet cell tumor of the pancreas: biphasic CT versus MR imaging in tumor detection. Radiology. 216(1):163-71, 2000
4. Thoeni RF et al: Detection of small, functional islet cell tumors in the pancreas: selection of MR imaging sequences for optimal sensitivity. Radiology. 214(2):483-90, 2000
5. Vazquez Sequeiros E et al: The role of endoscopic ultrasonography in diagnosis, staging, and management of pancreatic disease states. Curr Gastroenterol Rep. 2(2):125-32, 2000

ISLET CELL TUMORS

IMAGE GALLERY

Typical

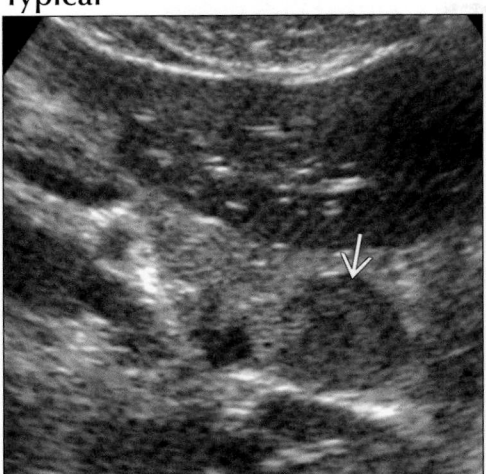
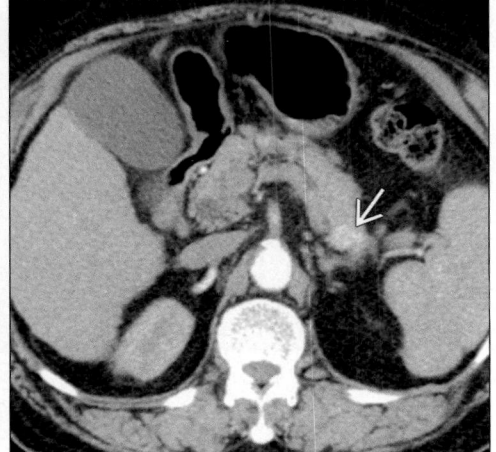

(Left) Transverse transabdominal ultrasound shows a well-defined, solid, hypoechoic mass ➡ in the pancreatic tail. Patient presented with hypoglycemia. *(Right)* Transverse CECT (same patient as previous image) shows a well-defined hypervascular mass ➡ in the pancreatic tail. Surgery confirmed a pancreatic insulinoma.

Typical

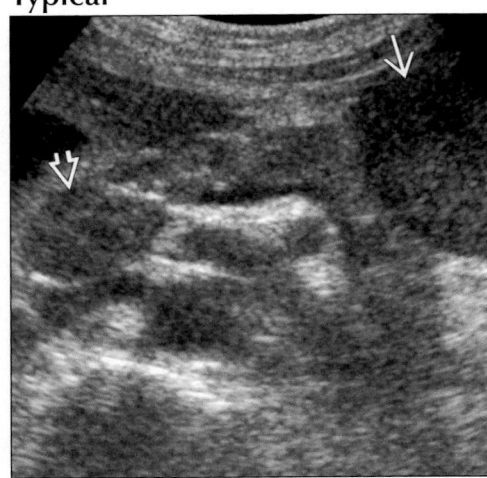
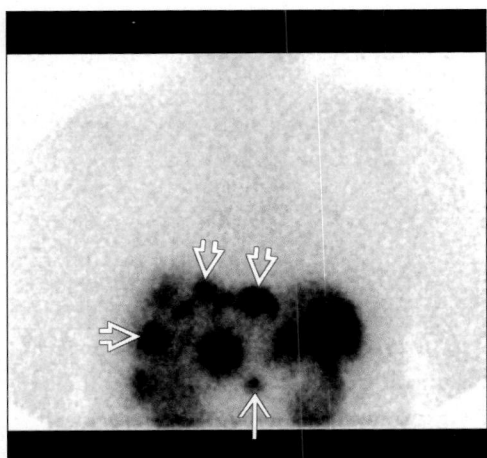

(Left) Transverse transabdominal ultrasound shows large, solid, hypoechoic mass ➡ in the pancreatic tail with a metastatic lymph node ➡ in the peripancreatic head region. Note no pancreatic duct dilatation. *(Right)* Octreotide scintigraphy shows small focus of increased tracer uptake in pancreas ➡ with multiple hot spots ➡ involving both lobes of liver. Pathology: Gastrinoma, with liver metastasis.

Typical

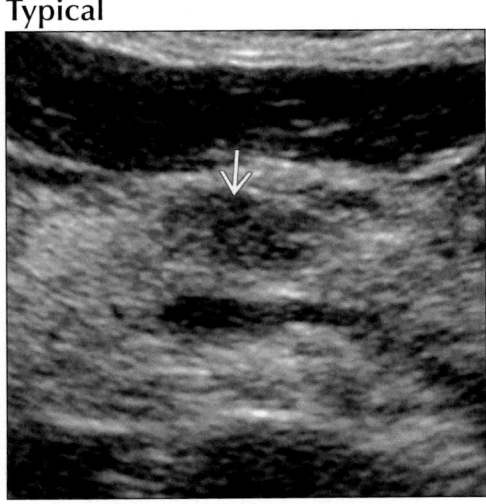
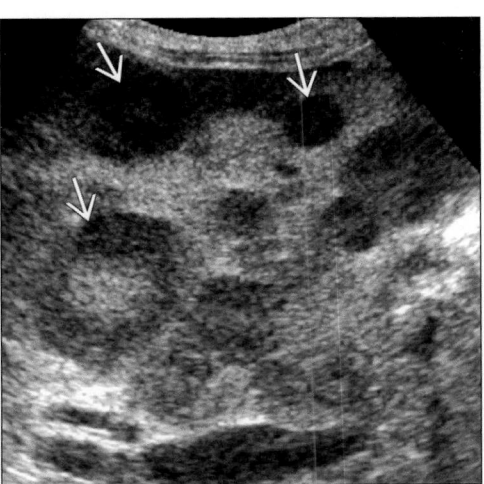

(Left) Transverse transabdominal ultrasound shows an ill-defined hypoechoic mass ➡ in the body of the pancreas. The patient had recurrent peptic ulcer with raised gastrin level suggestive of gastrinoma. *(Right)* Transverse transabdominal ultrasound shows multiple, well-defined, hypoechoic and hyperechoic liver metastases ➡.

SOLID AND PAPILLARY NEOPLASM

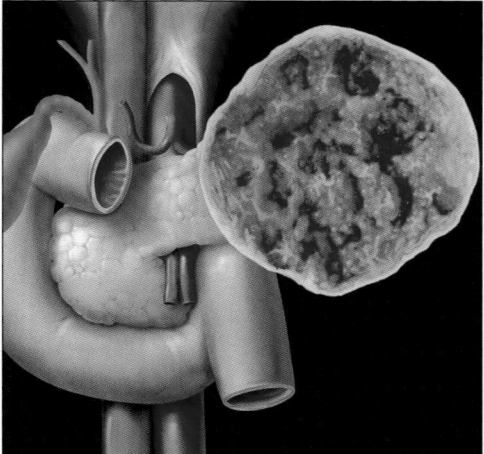

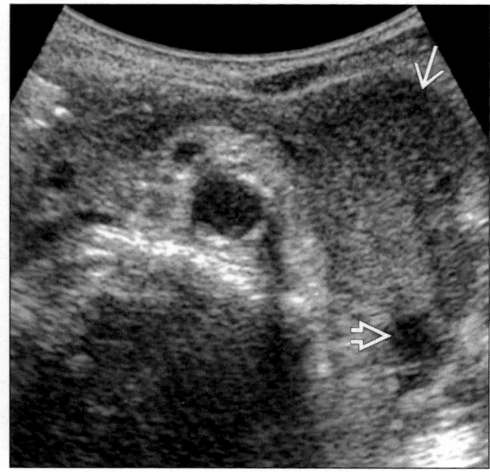

Graphic shows a large mass in the pancreatic tail with mixed solid and cystic/hemorrhagic components.

Transverse transabdominal ultrasound shows a large, solid, slightly hypoechoic mass ➡ in the tail of pancreas. Note presence of a small cystic component ➡ in the posterior portion of mass.

TERMINOLOGY

Abbreviations and Synonyms
- Solid and papillary epithelial neoplasm; papillary cystic carcinoma; solid and cystic tumor of pancreas

Definitions
- Pancreatic mass of low malignant potential with solid and cystic features

IMAGING FINDINGS

General Features
- Best diagnostic clue: Well-demarcated large mass with solid and cystic areas in pancreatic tail
- Location: Tail/body of pancreas
- Size: Average 10 cm, range of 2.5-20 cm

Ultrasonographic Findings
- Well-defined heterogeneous mass in pancreatic tail
  - Solid and cystic components
  - Hypoechoic center due to tumor necrosis, hemorrhage
  - Cystic portion may show fluid level
  - Dystrophic calcification occasionally seen
- No pancreatic ductal dilatation
- Liver metastases in ~ 4%: Well-defined hypoechoic solid hepatic masses
- Color Doppler: Hypovascular pattern

CT Findings
- CECT
  - Heterogeneous, mixed solid/cystic large mass
  - Low density areas of variable size within the lesion; depends on degree of hemorrhage and necrosis
  - Hypovascular with no contrast-enhancement

MR Findings
- T1WI
  - Large well-demarcated mass with central areas of low and high signal intensity
  - High signal intensity secondary to hemorrhage

Angiographic Findings
- Avascular/hypovascular; depends on necrosis

Imaging Recommendations
- Best imaging tool: US, CECT

DDx: Solid and Papillary Neoplasm

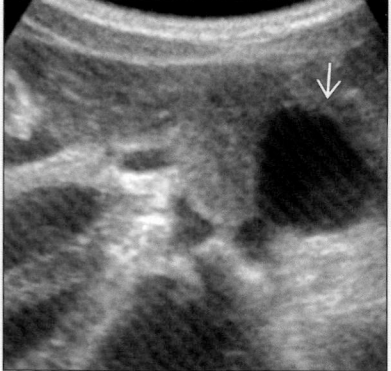

Mucinous Cystic Tumor

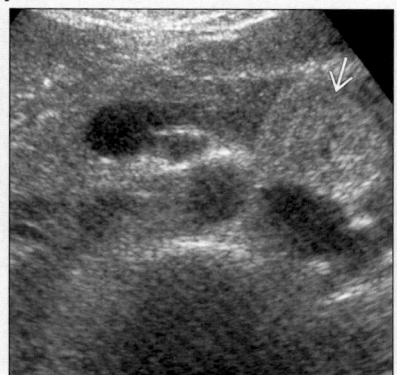

Serous Cystic Tumor

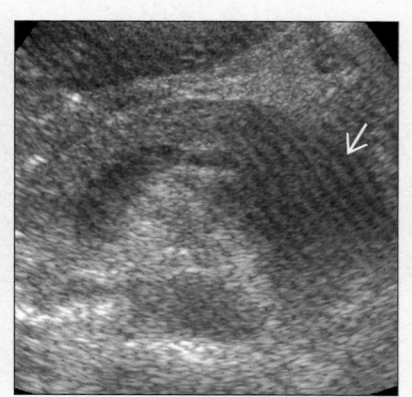

Pancreatic Lymphoma

SOLID AND PAPILLARY NEOPLASM

Key Facts

Imaging Findings
- Well-defined heterogeneous mass in pancreatic tail
- Solid and cystic components
- Hypoechoic center due to tumor necrosis, hemorrhage
- Cystic portion may show fluid level
- Dystrophic calcification occasionally seen
- No pancreatic ductal dilatation
- Color Doppler: Hypovascular pattern

Top Differential Diagnoses
- Mucinous Cystic Pancreatic Tumor
- Serous Cystadenoma of Pancreas
- Pancreatic Lymphoma/Metastases

Diagnostic Checklist
- Well-demarcated encapsulated pancreatic tail mass with mixed cystic and solid components and low malignant potential

DIFFERENTIAL DIAGNOSIS

Mucinous Cystic Pancreatic Tumor
- Middle age to elderly women
- Cystic spaces separated by septa and solid component

Serous Cystadenoma of Pancreas
- Usually located in head of pancreas
- "Sponge" appearance with innumerable small cysts

Pancreatic Lymphoma/Metastases
- Solitary/multiple pancreatic masses
- Intra-abdominal lymph nodes for lymphoma

Pancreatic Ductal Carcinoma
- Ill-defined infiltrative hypoechoic mass
- Pancreatic and common bile ductal dilatation

PATHOLOGY

General Features
- General path comments
  - 0.13-2.7% of all pancreatic tumors
  - Low malignant potential

Gross Pathologic & Surgical Features
- Thick, fibrous, hypervascular capsule surrounding a mixture of solid and cystic areas

CLINICAL ISSUES

Presentation
- Asymptomatic or non specific abdominal pain
- Palpable abdominal mass

Demographics
- Age: < 35 years of age, M:F = 1:9
- Ethnicity: African-Americans or non-Caucasian groups

Natural History & Prognosis
- Metastases in ~ 4%
- Prognosis: Good after surgical resection; rarely recurs

Treatment
- Complete surgical excision

DIAGNOSTIC CHECKLIST

Image Interpretation Pearls
- Well-demarcated encapsulated pancreatic tail mass with mixed cystic and solid components and low malignant potential

SELECTED REFERENCES

1.   Buetow PC et al: Solid and papillary epithelial neoplasm of the pancreas: imaging-pathologic correlation on 56 cases. Radiology. 199(3):707-11, 1996

IMAGE GALLERY

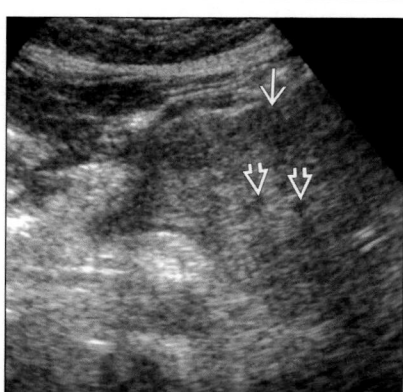 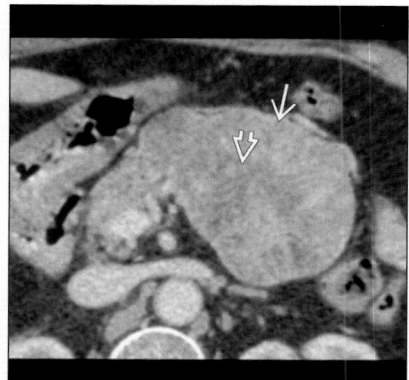 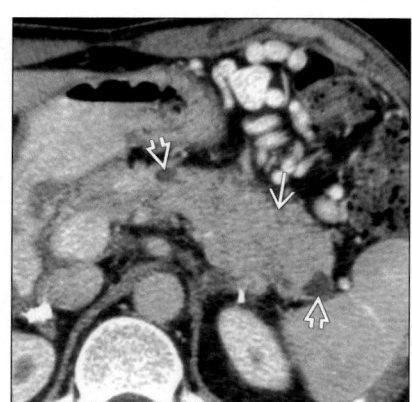

(Left) Transverse transabdominal ultrasound shows a large, ill-defined, heterogeneous hypoechoic mass ➡ occupying the pancreatic body and tail with small cysts ➡. *(Center)* Transverse CECT shows a large, heterogeneously enhancing mass ➡ in the pancreatic body and tail. Note presence of hypodense components ➡ due to tumor necrosis. *(Right)* Transverse CECT shows an ill-defined, mildly enhancing, soft tissue mass ➡ in the pancreatic tail, containing small cysts ➡ in its periphery. Note absence of calcification and ductal dilatation.

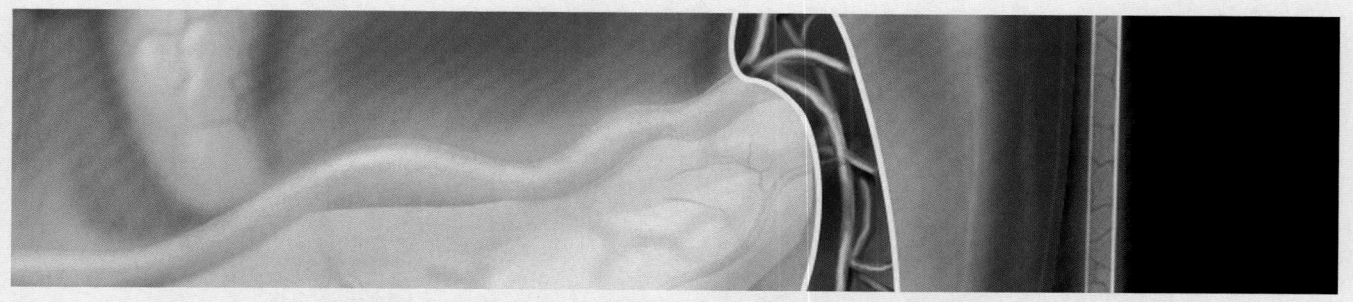

SECTION 4: Spleen

SPLENIC SONOGRAPHY

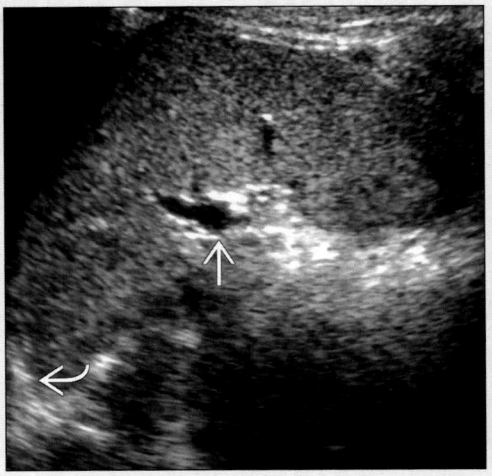

Oblique transabdominal ultrasound shows normal spleen with homogeneous parenchymal echoes. Note splenic hilum with splenic vein ➡ & diaphragm ➡.

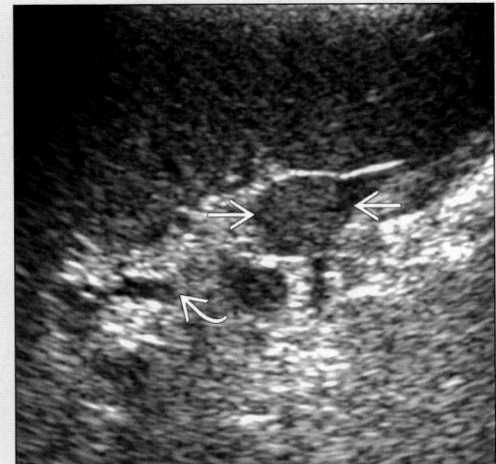

Oblique transabdominal ultrasound shows accessory spleen ➡ isoechoic to splenic parenchyma, situated close to splenic hilum ➡.

IMAGING ANATOMY

General Anatomic Considerations
- Location
  - Usually left upper quadrant
  - Intraperitoneal
  - Supported by gastrosplenic & lienorenal ligaments
  - Long axis is along the left 10th rib
  - Diaphragmatic surface: Convex & usually situated between the ninth & eleventh ribs
- Ultrasound appearance
  - Homogeneous parenchyma with uniform mid to low level echogenicity
  - Normal splenic parenchyma is hyperechoic to liver & hypoechoic to kidney

Critical Anatomic Structures
- Splenic hilum; splenic vein & artery

Anatomic Relationships
- Diaphragm
  - Supero-laterally
- Left kidney
  - Postero-medially
- Pancreas
  - Medially
  - Tail of pancreas inserts into lieno-renal ligament
- Stomach
  - Antero-medially

ANATOMY-BASED IMAGING ISSUES

Imaging Approaches
- Patient scanning position: Supine or right decubitus position
- Scanning plane: Coronal & oblique (along intercostal space)
  - Angulation of transducer to visualize entire spleen

Imaging Protocols
- Respiration: Modest to deep inspiration, central portion of hemi-diaphragm depresses the spleen inferiorly for better visualization
- Acoustic window can be provided by left lobe of liver (if enlarged), distended stomach (fluid), large pancreatic pseudocyst or mass
  - Free intraperitoneal fluid or left pleural effusion improves splenic evaluation using anterolateral approach

Imaging Pitfalls
- Distended stomach may mimic a splenic mass
- Enlarged left lobe of liver may mimic a perisplenic or subcapsular collection/hematoma/mass
- Retrorenal spleen may mimic a renal mass
- Small spleen high up under the costal margin may be difficult to visualize

Normal Measurements
- Average adult spleen is 12 cm in length, 7 cm in width & 4 cm in thickness
- Splenic index: Normally 120-480 cm³ (length x width x depth)
- Average weight is 150 g, ranges between 80-300 g
- Increases slightly during digestion and can vary in size depending on nutritional status of body
- Normal spleen decreases in size & weight with advancing age
- Shape: Typically "fat inverted comma" shape with convex superolateral (diaphragmatic) surface & concave inferomedial (visceral) surface
- Spleen frequently has notches or indentations on the surface
  - May simulate laceration on imaging
    - Key differentiating feature is absence of peri-splenic fluid/hemorrhage
- Structure: Branching trabeculae subdivide the spleen into communicating compartments
  - Branches of arteries, veins, nerves, lymphatics travel through trabeculae
- Splenic red pulp

SPLENIC SONOGRAPHY

Key Facts

Anatomy
- Location: Usually left upper quadrant
- Intraperitoneal, supported by gastrosplenic & splenorenal ligaments
- Size: Average adult spleen is 12 cm in length, 7 cm in breadth & 3-4 cm in thickness

Normal Echogenicity
- Homogeneous parenchyma with uniform mid to low level echogenicity
- Normal splenic parenchyma is hyperechoic to liver & hypoechoic to kidney

Patient Scanning Position
- Supine or right decubitus position
- Scanning plane: Coronal & oblique (along intercostal space)
- Anterior & posterior angulation of the transducer to visualize entire splenic volume
- Respiration: Modest to deep inspiration (spleen pushed inferiorly for better visualization)

Imaging Pitfalls
- A distended stomach may mimic a splenic mass
- Enlarged left lobe of liver may mimic a subcapsular collection/hematoma/mass
- Small spleen high up under the costal margin may be difficult to visualize

Key Concepts or Questions
- Is the spleen enlarged? Is the echogenicity altered?
- Is there a focal discrete mass or multiple lesions within the spleen?
- Is the spleen injured in a case of abdominal trauma?

○ Comprises the vascular tissue of the spleen
  ▪ Composed of sinusoids which are divided by plates of cells (splenic cords)
  ▪ Red pulp vein drains sinusoids
○ Most common source of non-hematological or non-lymphoid tumors
○ Mottled enhancement on CT/MR due to variable flow through cords & sinuses of red pulp
- Splenic white pulp
  ○ Lymphatic tissue of spleen
  ○ Gives rise to lymphatic tumors
- Other features
  ○ Splenic tissue: Soft & pliable
    ▪ Easily indented & displaced by masses and adjacent loculated fluid collections
  ○ Changes position in response to resection of adjacent organs; e.g., post-nephrectomy

PATHOLOGIC ISSUES

General Pathologic Considerations
- Splenomegaly
  ○ In adults ≥ 13 cm or longer
  ○ In children; if spleen > 1.25 times longer than left kidney
  ○ Congestion: Portal hypertension, splenic vein occlusion or thrombosis, sickle cell disease
  ○ Space occupying lesion: Tumor, abscess, cysts
  ○ Deposition: Hemosiderosis, storage disorders (Gaucher disease, amyloidosis, hemochromatosis)
  ○ Infection: Malaria, "kala azar", tuberculosis, fungal, bacterial
- Splenic lymphatic tumors
  ○ Most common
  ○ Lymphoma, leukemia (often massive in chronic lymphatic leukemia)
- Splenic metastases
  ○ Usually multiple & part of disseminated disease
  ○ Variety of sources, especially melanoma
- Primary vascular tumors
  ○ Hemangioma

  ▪ Variable size & echogenicity, well-defined hyperechoic solid to mixed to purely cystic lesion
○ Hamartoma
  ▪ Well-defined homogeneous echogenic mass, good acoustic transmission & posterior enhancement
○ Lymphangioma
  ▪ Multicystic with septation
○ Peliosis
  ▪ Multifocal heterogeneous echo pattern
- Incidental splenic mass
  ○ Patient with a known malignancy
    ▪ Very aggressive tumor (e.g., melanoma), or tumor draining into splenic vein (retrograde spread); suspect metastases
  ○ No known primary tumor
    ▪ Patients with high risk for lymphoma (e.g., AIDS, transplant recipient, associated lymphadenopathy); suspect lymphoma
    ▪ Immunosuppressed: Suspect opportunistic infection, peliosis, lymphoma
  ○ Asymptomatic, healthy adult
    ▪ Echogenic mass, probably hemangioma
    ▪ Subcapsular multicystic mass; probably lymphangioma
- Splenic infection
  ○ Histoplasmosis & tuberculosis (TB) commonly affect spleen
  ○ Otherwise, uncommon, except in immunocompromised patients
    ▪ AIDS, transplant recipients, leukemia, alcoholism
  ○ Multiple small abscesses: Candida (and other fungal infection), TB, pneumocystis
  ○ Single large abscess: Usually bacterial
  ○ Calcification: Seen in treated abscess/granulomas (TB, fungal, pneumocystis)
- Splenic infarction
  ○ Relatively common cause of acute left upper quadrant pain
  ○ Appears as sharply marginated, wedge-shaped, hypoechoic lesion abutting splenic capsule
  ○ Etiologies
    ▪ Sickle cell and other hemoglobinopathies

SPLENIC SONOGRAPHY

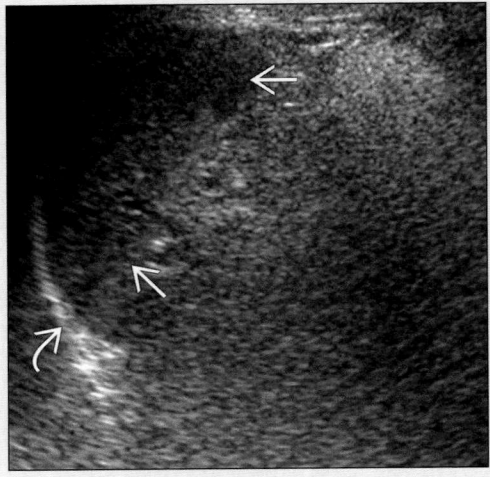

Oblique transabdominal ultrasound shows a small atrophied spleen (6 cm) ➡ in an elderly woman. Note the echogenic diaphragm ➡ superiorly.

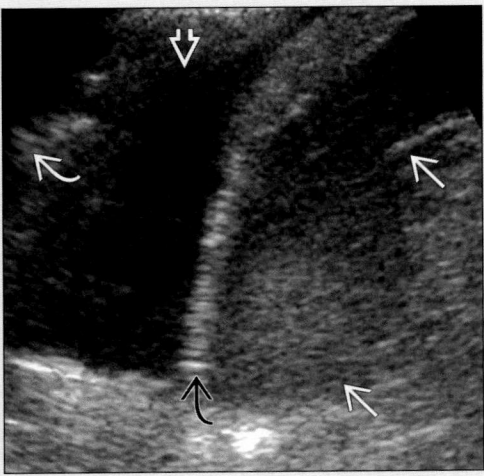

Oblique transabdominal ultrasound shows a small spleen ➡ seen through the acoustic window of a left pleural effusion ➡. Note underlying left lung consolidation ➡ & echogenic diaphragm ➡.

- "Spontaneous" in any cause of splenomegaly
- Embolic (e.g., i.v. drug abuse, endocarditis, atrial fibrillation)
- Calcified lesions
  - Granulomas (multiple or solitary); TB, histoplasmosis, sarcoidosis, brucellosis
  - Hamartoma, calcified wall (cyst/abscess/old hematoma) & vascular calcification (linear)
- Pancreatitis involving tail may spread directly to the spleen, leading to intrasplenic pseudocyst formation
- Small spleen: Atrophy, infarction, irradiation, hereditary hypoplasia, polysplenia syndrome

PATHOLOGY-BASED IMAGING ISSUES

Key Concepts or Questions
- Is the spleen enlarged?
- Is the echogenicity altered?
- Is there a focal discrete mass or multiple lesions within the spleen?
- Is there an infiltrative lesion in the spleen?
- Is the spleen injured in a case of abdominal trauma?

Imaging Pitfalls
- "Wandering spleen" (spleen with a long mesentery)
  - May be intraperitoneal in location & simulate mass
  - May undergo torsion & lead to splenic infarction
- Splenosis: Traumatic rupture of spleen with implantation & growth of heterotopic splenic tissue
  - May appear as solid masses in the abdomen
  - Splenic tissue can be confirmed on sulfur colloid isotope scan
- Bright echoes simulating calcification may be seen along the cyst wall
  - Represent reflection artifact, when sound beam hits cyst wall at right angles
- Often it is difficult to distinguish perisplenic collection from subcapsular hematoma
  - Subcapsular hematoma may indent the contour of the spleen

EMBRYOLOGY

Embryologic Events
- Arises from dorsal mesogastrium during fifth week of fetal life
- Normally develops as a single mass of tissue & rotates to left
- Usually fixed by peritoneal reflections to left hemi-diaphragm, abdominal wall, kidney, stomach

Practical Implications
- Accessory spleen
  - Incidence 10-30% on autopsy
  - Usually small & located near the hilum
  - May be aberrant in location, may increase in size, especially after splenectomy
    - Enlarged or ectopic accessory spleen may simulate lymph nodes, pancreatic tail mass, renal tumor
    - Confirmed by radionuclide sulfur colloid or tagged RBC scan (more sensitive)
- Asplenia: Failure to develop
  - Asplenia often associated with other congenital anomalies including situs inversus and cardiac anomalies
    - High early mortality, especially from sepsis
- Polysplenia
  - Associated with cardiac & other anomalies
  - Associated with early mortality
  - May simulate splenosis

RELATED REFERENCES

1. Fried AM. Related Articles et al: Spleen and retroperitoneum: the essentials. Ultrasound Q. 21(4):275-86, 2005
2. Li PS et al: The reproducibility and short-term and long-term repeatability of sonographic measurement of splenic length. Ultrasound Med Biol. 30(7):861-6, 2004
3. Gorg C et al: The small spleen: sonographic patterns of functional hyposplenia or asplenia. J Clin Ultrasound. 31(3):152-5, 2003

SPLENOMEGALY

Key Facts

Imaging Findings
- Normal spleen in adult measures up to 12 cm; enlarged if it is 13 cm or longer
- In children, splenomegaly should be suspected if the spleen is more than 1.25x longer than the adjacent kidney
- Splenomegaly with altered parenchymal echogenicity is seen in different etiological conditions
- **SMG with normal echogenicity**
- Infection, congestion (portal hypertension), early sickle cell disease
- Hereditary spherocytosis, hemolysis, Felty syndrome - rheumatoid arthritis (RA) and splenomegaly
- **SMG with hyperechoic pattern**
- Metastases, leukemia, post-chemotherapy, post-radiation therapy
- Malaria, tuberculosis, sarcoidosis, polycythemia
- **SMG with hypoechoic pattern**
- Metastases, lymphoma, multiple myeloma, chronic lymphocytic leukemia
- Best imaging tool: Ultrasound for confirmation of SMG and detection of focal lesions, CT allows better characterization of some lesions while MR preferred for hemorrhage or siderosis

Top Differential Diagnoses
- Large splenic abscess
- Hemangioma
- Lymphangioma
- Lymphoma
- Leukemia and myeloproliferative disorders
- Large solitary metastasis or lymphoma deposit

  - Metastases, leukemia, post-chemotherapy, post-radiation therapy
  - Malaria, tuberculosis, sarcoidosis, polycythemia
  - Hereditary spherocytosis, portal vein thrombosis, hematoma
  - **SMG with hypoechoic pattern**
    - Metastases, lymphoma, multiple myeloma, chronic lymphocytic leukemia
    - Congestion from portal hypertension, non-caseating granulomatous infection
    - Sickle cell disease: Immediately after sequestration, peripheral hypoechoic areas
    - Gaucher disease: Multiple, well-defined, discrete hypoechoic lesions; fibrosis or infarction
  - **SMG with mixed echogenic pattern**
    - Abscesses, metastases, hemorrhage/hematoma in different stages of evolution (liquefaction, necrosis, gas, calcification)
- Color Doppler: Portal hypertension: Dilated splenic vein, splenic vein thrombus, splenic hilar collaterals, lieno-renal collaterals, recanalized umbilical vein

Radiographic Findings
- Radiography
  - Splenic tip below 12th rib
  - Severe SMG may displace stomach & splenic flexure of colon (splenic flexure usually anterior to spleen)

CT Findings
- SMG: Medial margin of spleen is convex on CT
- Congestive SMG
  - Portal hypertension: SMG with varices, nodular shrunken liver, ascites
  - Splenic vein occlusion or thrombosis (often secondary to pancreatitis or pancreatic tumors)
  - Sickle-cell disease: Splenic sequestration
    - Peripheral low and high attenuation areas, represent areas of infarct & hemorrhage
- Space occupying lesions: Cysts, abscess, tumor
  - Cysts: Hypodense on NECT, no enhancement on CECT
  - Abscess: Hypodense on NECT with irregular, shaggy margin enhancing on CECT

  - Tumor: Hyperdense/hypodense on NECT & variable enhancement on CECT
- Hemosiderosis
  - Increased attenuation of spleen (hemosiderin deposition), due to multiple blood transfusions (thalassemia, hemophilia)
- Storage disorders
  - Gaucher disease
    - Spleen may have abnormal low attenuation
    - Severe SMG, often extending into pelvis
  - Amyloidosis
    - NECT & CECT: Generalized or focal low attenuation
  - Primary hemochromatosis
    - Density of spleen is normal (unlike that of liver)
  - Secondary hemochromatosis
    - Increased attenuation values of liver & spleen
- Extramedullary hematopoiesis
  - Spleen may be diffusely enlarged
  - CECT: Focal masses of hematopoietic tissue of similar attenuation to normal splenic tissue
- Splenic trauma
  - Splenic laceration or subcapsular hematoma, surrounding perisplenic hematoma (> 30 HU)

MR Findings
- Congestive SMG
  - Portal hypertension
    - Multiple tiny (3-8 mm) foci of decreased signal, hemosiderin deposits; organized hemorrhage (Gamna-Gandy bodies or siderotic nodules)
  - Sickle cell disease
    - Areas of abnormal signal intensity, hyperintense with dark rim on T1WI (subacute hemorrhage)
  - Hemochromatosis
    - Primary: Normal signal & size of spleen
    - Secondary: Marked signal loss; enlarged spleen
  - Gaucher disease: Increased signal intensity on T1WI
  - Infarction
    - Peripheral, wedge-shaped areas of hypointensity resulting from iron deposition
  - Hemosiderosis

SPLENOMEGALY

- Reduced signal intensity of spleen on both T1 & T2WI

Nuclear Medicine Findings
- Chromium 51-labeled RBCs or platelets
  - Hypersplenism: Injected RBCs exhibit shortened half-life (average half-life of 25-35 days)
- Tc-99m sulfur colloid scan: Measure of splenic function

Imaging Recommendations
- Best imaging tool: Ultrasound for confirmation of SMG and detection of focal lesions, CT allows better characterization of some lesions while MR preferred for hemorrhage or siderosis
- Protocol advice: On sonography spleen is best visualized following deep inspiration with the patient in right lateral decubitus position

DIFFERENTIAL DIAGNOSIS

Solitary Splenic Masses
- Large splenic abscess
  - Irregular wall, well-defined, hypoechoic to anechoic depending on degree of liquefaction and necrosis
- Benign primary tumor
  - Hemangioma
    - Solid, echogenic mass with or without cystic component
    - Central punctate or peripheral calcification
  - Lymphangioma
    - Thin-walled hypoechoic foci sharp margins with variable vascularity
    - Usually subcapsular in location; ± calcification
- Malignant primary tumor
  - Lymphoma
    - Both Hodgkin and Non-Hodgkin lymphoma
    - Primary lymphoma arising within the spleen can invade the capsule and extend beyond the spleen
    - Pattern: Diffuse involvement (seen as splenomegaly) or focal hypoechoic lesions (with out posterior acoustic enhancement)
  - Leukemia and myeloproliferative disorders
    - Diffuse enlargement of spleen with variable echogenicity, very rarely focal hypoechoic nodular lesions
- Secondary tumor
  - Large solitary metastasis or lymphoma deposit
  - Well-defined hypoechoic lesions

Other LUQ Masses
- e.g., gastric, renal, adrenal tumor: Extrasplenic in location, usually splenic capsule intact

PATHOLOGY

General Features
- Etiology
  - Congestive SMG: Heart failure, portal HT, cirrhosis, cystic fibrosis, splenic vein thrombosis, sickle cell (SC) sequestration

  - Neoplasm: Leukemia, lymphoma, metastases, primary neoplasm, Kaposi sarcoma
  - Storage disease: Gaucher, Niemann-Pick, gargoylism, amyloidosis, DM, hemochromatosis, histiocytosis
  - Infection: Hepatitis, malaria, mononucleosis, TB, typhoid, kala-azar, schistosomiasis, brucellosis
  - Hemolytic anemia: Hemoglobinopathy, hereditary spherocytosis, primary neutropenia, thrombocytopenic purpura
  - Other causes of extramedullary hematopoiesis like: Osteopetrosis, myelofibrosis
  - Collagen disease: Systemic lupus erythematosus, RA, Felty syndrome

CLINICAL ISSUES

Presentation
- Most common signs/symptoms
  - Asymptomatic, abdominal fullness and discomfort, dragging pain
  - Signs & symptoms related to underlying cause
- Lab data: Abnormal complete blood count, liver function tests, antibody titers, cultures or bone marrow exam

Natural History & Prognosis
- Complications
  - Splenic rupture can occur spontaneously or following minor trauma
- Hypersplenism: Usually develops as a result of SMG
  - Hyperfunctioning spleen removes normal RBC, WBC & platelets from circulation
- Prognosis
  - Depends on primary disease

Treatment
- Treatment varies based on underlying condition
- Splenectomy in symptomatic & complicated cases

DIAGNOSTIC CHECKLIST

Consider
- SMG, most common cause of left upper quadrant mass
- SMG, secondary to underlying condition

Image Interpretation Pearls
- US can confirm presence of enlarged spleen or space occupying lesions within spleen
- CT & MR can further characterize abnormalities
- Radioisotope scanning can provide functional information

SELECTED REFERENCES
1. Peck-Radosavljevic M: Hypersplenism. Eur J Gastroenterol Hepatol. 13(4):317-23, 2001
2. Paterson A et al: A pattern-oriented approach to splenic imaging in infants and children. Radiographics. 19(6):1465-85, 1999
3. Mittelstaedt CA et al: Ultrasonic-pathologic classification of splenic abnormalities: gray-scale patterns. Radiology. 134(3):697-705, 1980

SPLENOMEGALY

IMAGE GALLERY

Typical

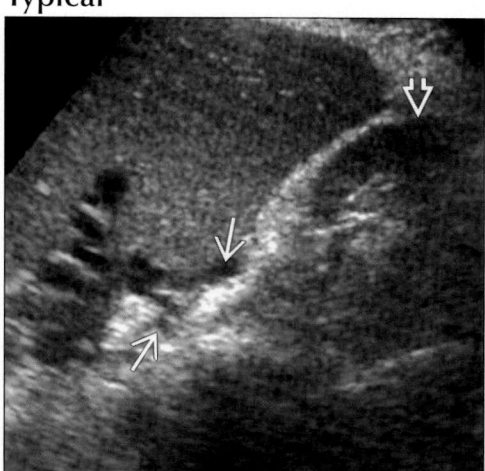

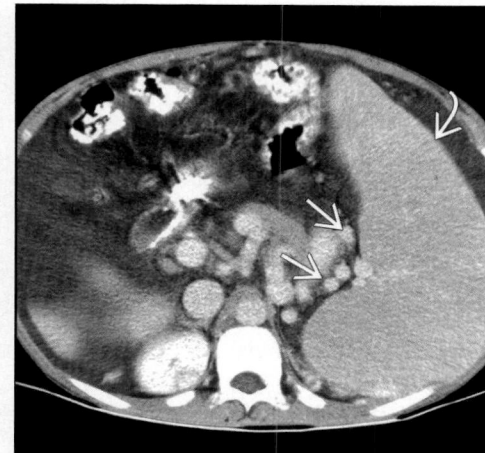

(Left) Transverse transabdominal ultrasound shows splenomegaly with lienorenal collaterals ➡, secondary to portal hypertension. Left kidney ➡. *(Right)* Transverse CECT shows massive splenomegaly ➡, with multiple splenic hilar collaterals ➡.

Typical

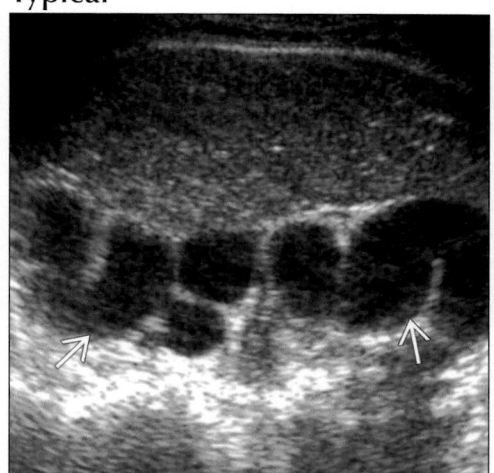

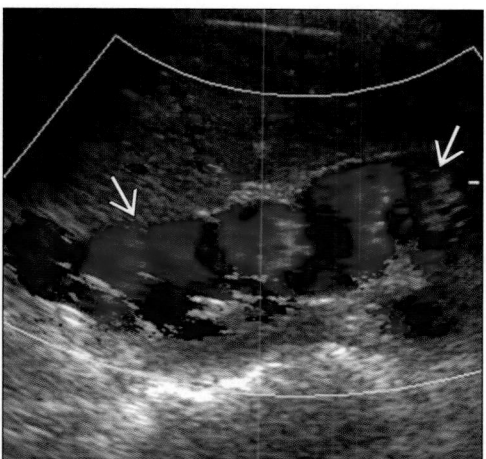

(Left) Transverse transabdominal ultrasound shows moderate splenomegaly with dilated splenic hilar collaterals ➡. *(Right)* Transverse color Doppler ultrasound shows dilated splenic hilar collaterals ➡ in a patient with portal hypertension.

Typical

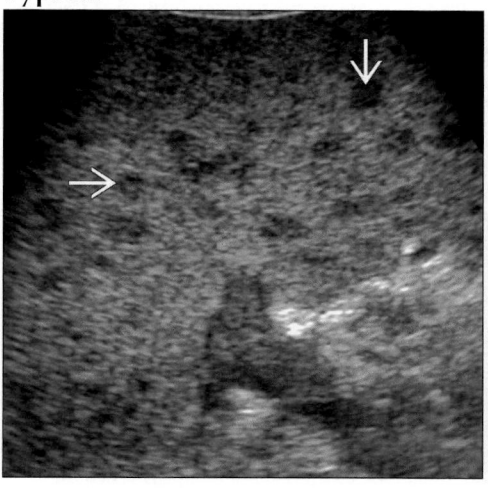

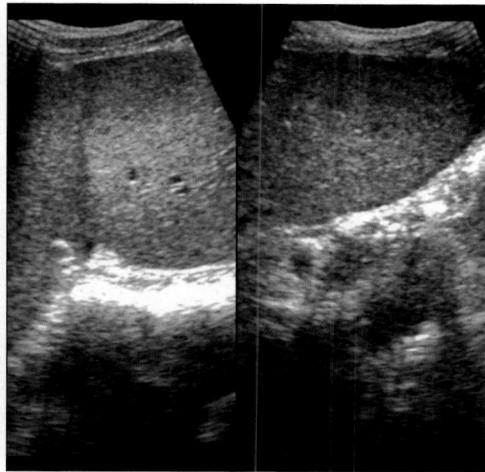

(Left) Transverse transabdominal ultrasound shows marked splenomegaly with multiple focal hypoechoic granulomas ➡. *(Right)* Oblique transabdominal ultrasound shows marked splenomegaly due to malaria, splenic span (27 cm).

CYSTS & CYST-LIKE SPLENIC LESIONS

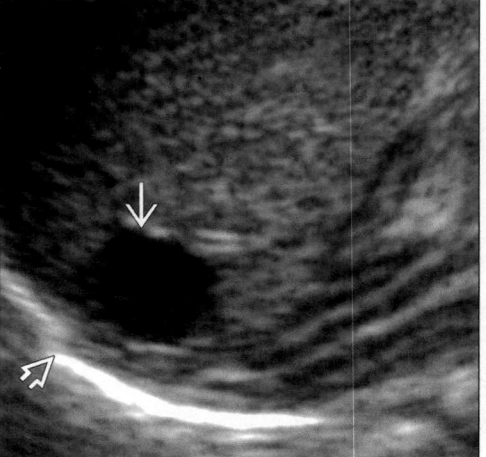

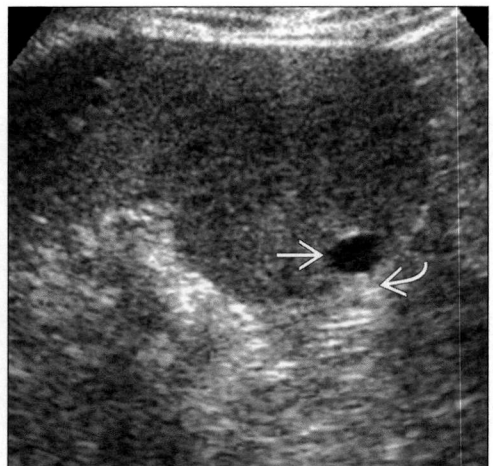

Transverse transabdominal ultrasound shows a well-defined, anechoic splenic cyst ➡️ close to the linear echogenic diaphragm ➡️.

Longitudinal transabdominal ultrasound shows an incidentally detected, clearly demarcated, small, anechoic splenic cyst ➡️, with posterior acoustic enhancement ➡️.

TERMINOLOGY

Definitions
- Cystic parenchymal masses of spleen

IMAGING FINDINGS

General Features
- Best diagnostic clue: Anechoic sharply-defined spherical lesion with posterior acoustic enhancement
- Location: Usually subcapsular (65%)
- Size: Variable
- Key concepts
  - Cystic masses do not commonly occur in spleen
    - "Simple" cysts like those found in the liver or kidney, do not occur in the spleen
  - Classification of splenic cysts based on etiology
    - Congenital cyst (primary or true)
    - Acquired cyst (secondary)
  - Congenital cyst: Epidermoid
    - Inner cellular lining (epithelial lining), account for minority of splenic cysts
  - Acquired cyst (secondary): As splenic infarcts/trauma are relatively common, the incidence of acquired cysts is much larger than congenital cysts
    - Pseudocysts, liquefied hematoma, abscess, cystic metastases, cystic degeneration of infarct
    - Epithelial lining absent, but has fibrous wall, accounts for 80% of splenic cysts
    - Wall calcification seen in 38-50% of cases; cystic nature: Due to liquefactive necrosis

Ultrasonographic Findings
- Grayscale Ultrasound
  - Well-defined anechoic or hypoechoic lesion ± posterior acoustic enhancement
  - Congenital (primary or true) cyst: Epidermoid
    - Congenital: Anechoic, smooth borders, epithelial or endothelial lining, non-detectable walls ± trabeculation (36%), posterior enhancement
    - Endothelial lined cysts: Lymphangiomas (rare) and cystic hemangiomas (very rare)
    - No septations or nodules

DDx: Cystic Splenic Lesions

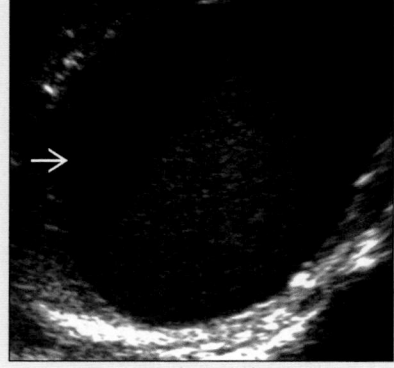

Large Splenic Abscess

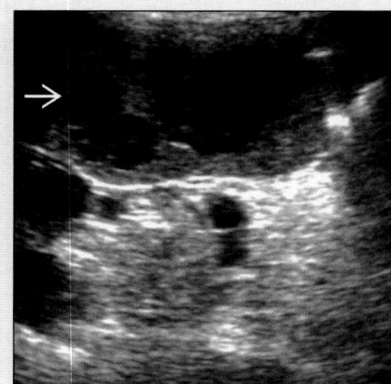

Lymphoma Deposits

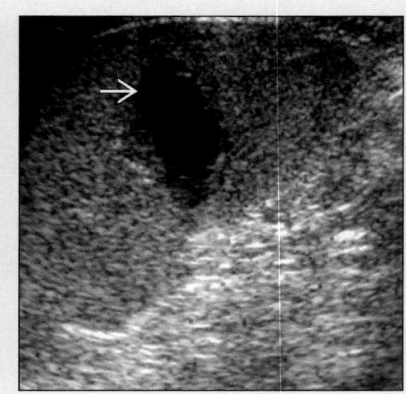

Splenic Hematoma

CYSTS & CYST-LIKE SPLENIC LESIONS

Key Facts

Imaging Findings
- Best diagnostic clue: Anechoic sharply-defined spherical lesion with posterior acoustic enhancement
- Location: Usually subcapsular (65%)
- Congenital: Anechoic, smooth borders, epithelial or endothelial lining, non-detectable walls ± trabeculation (36%), posterior enhancement
- Post-traumatic: No cellular lining, small, anechoic or mixed with internal echoes, echogenic wall, ± calcification, ± trabeculation of cyst wall (15%)
- Infectious cysts (echinococcus cyst ± internal small daughter cysts & floating membranes ± calcification, hydatid sand)
- Other: Pancreatic pseudocyst extending into spleen, liquified hematoma, liquified splenic abscess (solitary or multiple)

- Reliable differentiation between true cysts and acquired cysts is not always possible by ultrasound
- Ultrasound guided diagnostic aspiration can be safely performed: Aspiration yields clear watery fluid or brownish fluid due to previous hemorrhage

Top Differential Diagnoses
- Inflammatory or Infection
- Neoplastic
- Hematoma or laceration

Diagnostic Checklist
- Congenital: Large, well-defined with thin wall & no rim
- Acquired (post-traumatic): Usually small, sharply-defined, often anechoic with thick wall ± calcification

---

- Complicated: Septations, internal echoes (cholesterol crystals, hemorrhage, inflammatory debris) - floating debris within the cyst may produce moving uniform internal echoes - "snowstorm"/"pseudosolid" appearance, thickened wall ± calcification
  - Acquired (false or pseudo) cyst
    - Post-traumatic: No cellular lining, small, anechoic or mixed with internal echoes, echogenic wall, ± calcification, ± trabeculation of cyst wall (15%)
    - Infectious cysts (echinococcus cyst ± internal small daughter cysts & floating membranes ± calcification, hydatid sand)
    - Other: Pancreatic pseudocyst extending into spleen, liquified hematoma, liquified splenic abscess (solitary or multiple)
  - Reliable differentiation between true cysts and acquired cysts is not always possible by ultrasound
  - Ultrasound guided diagnostic aspiration can be safely performed: Aspiration yields clear watery fluid or brownish fluid due to previous hemorrhage

Radiographic Findings
- Large acquired splenic cysts
  - Curvilinear or plaque-like wall calcification

CT Findings
- Congenital cyst: Epidermoid
  - Solitary, well-defined, spherical, unilocular, cystic lesion (water HU)
  - Thin wall + sharp interface to normal splenic tissue
  - Hemorrhagic, infected, ↑ protein: ↑ Attenuation
  - No rim or intracystic enhancement, may rarely have calcified wall
- Acquired cyst
  - Hematoma (evolving)
    - ↓ HU, sharply-defined margins, nonspecific cystic lesion
    - CECT: No enhancement of contents
  - False or pseudocyst (end stage of splenic hematoma)
    - Usually small, solitary, sharply-defined, water HU, ± wall calcification (may resemble eggshell)
  - Liquefied abscess

- Hypodense lesions, with peripheral enhancement on CECT

MR Findings
- Congenital (primary or true) cyst: Epidermoid
  - T1WI: Hypointense, variable intensity if infected or hemorrhagic
  - T2WI: Hyperintense
- Acquired (false or pseudo) cyst: Post-traumatic
  - T1WI: Hypointense; variable intensity (blood)
  - T2WI: Hyperintense
  - Calcification or hemosiderin deposited in wall
    - Hypointense (both T1 & T2WI)
  - Hematoma: Varied intensity based on age & evolution of blood products
    - After 3 weeks appears as a cystic mass: T1WI hypointense; T2WI hyperintense

Imaging Recommendations
- Best imaging tool: Ultrasound for initial evaluation followed by CT or MR for further characterization
- Protocol advice: The patient is best scanned in supine or right lateral decubitus position following deep inspiration with USG transducer along the long axis of spleen

DIFFERENTIAL DIAGNOSIS

Inflammatory or Infection
- Pyogenic abscess
  - Solitary, multiple, well-defined, ± irregular borders, hypoechoic to anechoic depending on the stage of liquefaction/necrosis, ± gas within abscess
- Fungal abscess
  - e.g., Candida, Aspergillus, Cryptococcal
  - Usually microabscesses: Multiple, small, well-defined, hypoechoic to echogenic, distributed throughout the parenchyma
- Granulomatous abscesses
  - e.g., Mycobacterium & atypical tuberculosis (TB); cat-scratch

○ Multiple, small, well-defined, hypoechoic lesions involving the entire splenic parenchyma

Neoplastic

- Benign: e.g., hemangioma & lymphangioma
  ○ Hemangioma
    ▪ Variable size & echogenicity lesions, solid & cystic areas, rarely solitary large lesion involving entire spleen
  ○ Lymphangioma
    ▪ Heterogeneous/multicystic appearance, intracystic echoes: Proteinaceous material
- Malignant: e.g., lymphoma & metastases
  ○ Lymphoma
    ▪ Hypoechoic/anechoic type of lymphomatous nodules: May resemble cysts, however reveal "indistinct boundary" echo pattern
    ▪ Posterior acoustic enhancement is absent
  ○ Metastases: Necrotic/cystic
    ▪ Relatively common; e.g., malignant melanoma, adenocarcinoma of breast, pancreas, ovaries & endometrium may cause "cystic" splenic metastases
    ▪ Multiple focal cystic lesion of variable size

Vascular

- Hematoma or laceration
  ○ Hypo/iso/hyperechoic blood filled cleft
  ○ Hematoma echogenicity depends on the stage of bleed; fresh blood echo-free initially, later becomes echogenic
  ○ Occasionally cystic degeneration of intrasplenic hematoma results in formation of a false/pseudocyst (80% splenic pseudocyst: Post-traumatic in etiology)
- Infarction (arterial or venous)
  ○ Acute phase: Well-defined wedge-shaped areas of decreased echogenicity
  ○ Subacute & chronic phases: Anechoic (due to liquefactive necrosis)
- Peliosis
  ○ Multiple, indistinct areas of hypo- or hyperechogenicity that may involve entire spleen

Intrasplenic Pseudocyst

- In 1.1-5% of patient with pancreatitis → intrasplenic pseudocyst or abscess
- Pathogenesis
  ○ Direct extension of pancreatic pseudocyst: Secondary to digestive effects of enzymes on splenic vessels or parenchyma along lienorenal ligament
- Imaging
  ○ Well-defined rounded cystic lesion involving the spleen
  ○ Associated inflammatory changes of pancreas, peripancreatic fluid collection (especially near tail)

PATHOLOGY

General Features

- Etiology
  ○ Congenital (true) epidermoid: Genetic defect of mesothelial migration

○ Post-traumatic: End stage of splenic hematoma/infarction
  ▪ Pathogenesis: Liquefactive necrosis, cystic change

Gross Pathologic & Surgical Features

- Congenital (true) epidermoid cyst
  ○ Usually large, glistening smooth walls
- Post-traumatic (false or pseudocyst)
  ○ Smaller than true cysts, debris, wall calcification

Microscopic Features

- Congenital (true) cyst: Endothelial lining present
- Post-traumatic (false) cyst: Endothelial lining absent

CLINICAL ISSUES

Presentation

- Most common signs/symptoms
  ○ Asymptomatic; mild pain, palpable mass in the left upper quadrant (LUQ)
  ○ Tenderness in LUQ; splenomegaly

Demographics

- Age: 2/3rd below 40 years old
- Gender: M:F = 2:3

Natural History & Prognosis

- Complications: Hemorrhage, rupture, infection
- Prognosis
  ○ Good: Uncomplicated cases; after surgical removal
  ○ Poor: Complicated cases

Treatment

- Small & asymptomatic: No treatment
- Small & symptomatic: Surgery
- Large (> 6 cm): Surgical removal (debatable)
- Ultrasound-guided drainage with injection of sclerosing agent is an alternative option

DIAGNOSTIC CHECKLIST

Consider

- Rule out infectious, vascular & neoplastic cystic lesions

Image Interpretation Pearls

- Congenital: Large, well-defined with thin wall & no rim
- Acquired (post-traumatic): Usually small, sharply-defined, often anechoic with thick wall ± calcification
- Differentiation by imaging alone is often impossible & may require ultrasound guided aspiration

SELECTED REFERENCES

1. Urrutia M et al: Cystic masses of the spleen: radiologic-pathologic correlation. Radiographics. 16(1):107-29, 1996
2. Shirkhoda A et al: Imaging features of splenic epidermoid cyst with pathologic correlation. Abdom Imaging. 20(5):449-51, 1995

CYSTS & CYST-LIKE SPLENIC LESIONS

IMAGE GALLERY

Typical

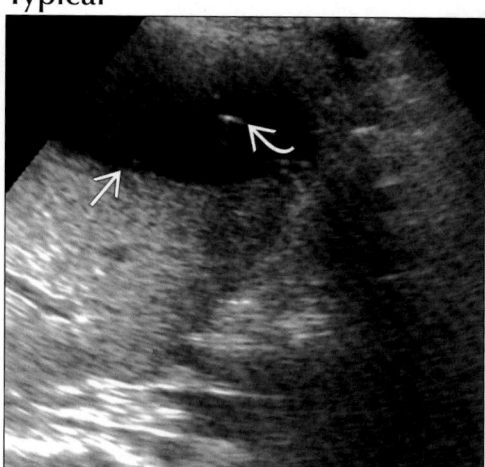
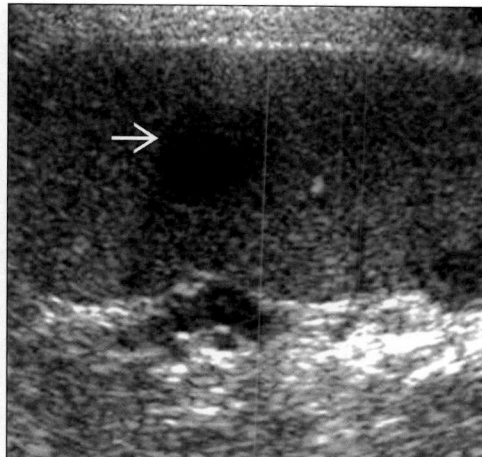

(Left) Transverse transabdominal ultrasound shows a well-defined splenic cyst ➡, with some internal echoes ➡. (Right) Longitudinal transabdominal ultrasound shows a well-defined, anechoic splenic cyst ➡.

Typical

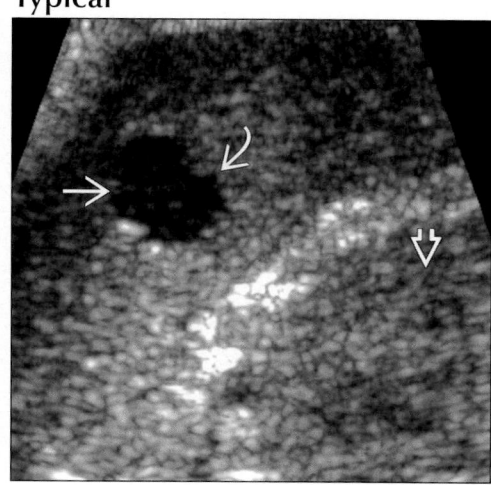
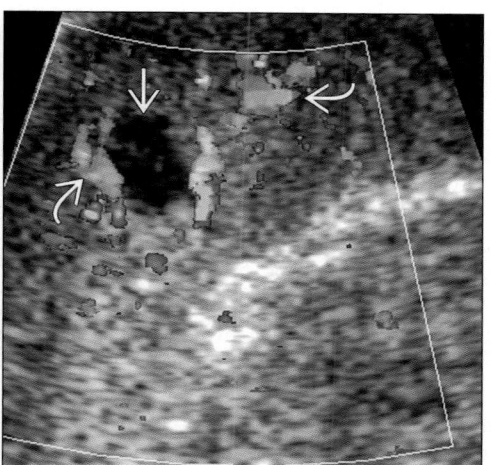

(Left) Transverse transabdominal ultrasound shows a splenic cyst ➡ with slightly irregular walls ➡. Left kidney ➡. (Right) Transverse color Doppler ultrasound (same patient as in previous image) shows the avascular nature of the splenic cyst ➡. The surrounding splenic parenchymal vascularity ➡ is normal.

Typical

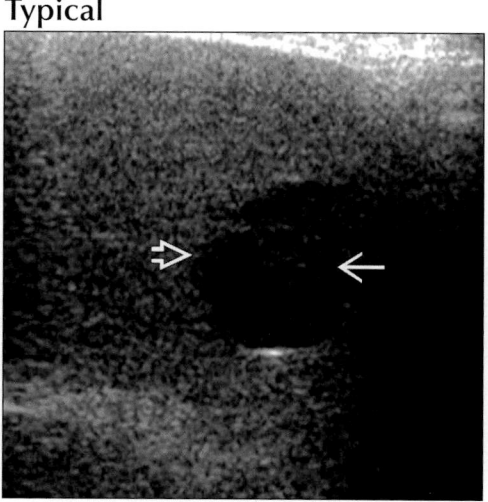
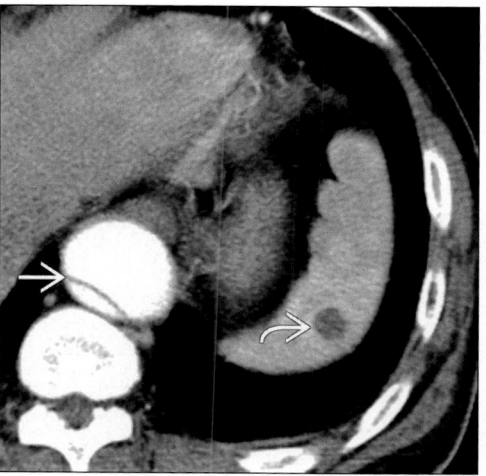

(Left) Transverse transabdominal ultrasound shows an incidentally detected small splenic cyst ➡, with fine internal echoes ➡. (Right) Transverse CECT (same patient as in previous image) shows the small, nonenhancing, hypodense splenic cyst ➡, and an aortic dissection (intimal flap ➡).

SPLENIC TUMORS

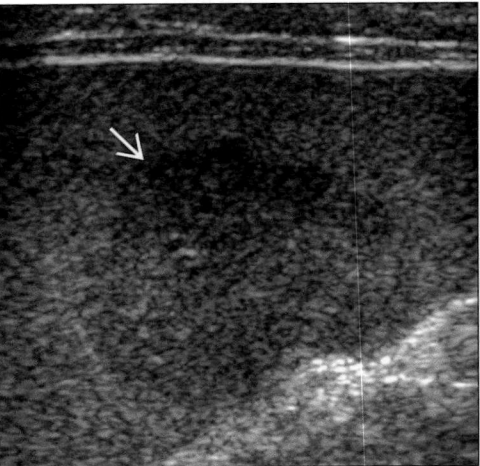 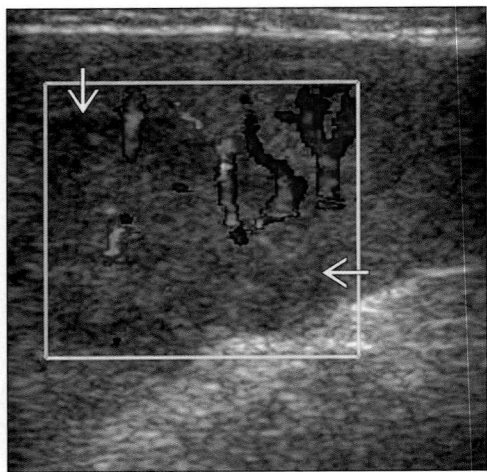

Longitudinal transabdominal ultrasound shows a large, solitary, hypoechoic lymphomatous mass ➡ in the lower pole of the spleen.

Transverse color Doppler ultrasound (same patient as previous image) shows peripheral vascularity within the lymphomatous mass ➡.

TERMINOLOGY

Abbreviations and Synonyms
- Splenic mass or lesion

Definitions
- Space occupying benign or malignant tumor of spleen

IMAGING FINDINGS

General Features
- Best diagnostic clue: Solitary or multiple, solid or cystic splenic masses
- Key concepts
  - Classification based on pathology & histology
    - Benign & malignant tumors
  - Benign tumors
    - Hemangioma, hamartoma, lymphangioma
  - Hemangioma
    - Most common incidentally detected primary benign neoplasm of spleen
    - Multiple as part of a generalized angiomatosis (Klippel-Trenaunay-Weber & Beckwith-Wiedemann syndrome)
    - Hemangiomatosis: Diffuse splenic hemangiomas
  - Hamartoma
    - Rare benign tumor of spleen; incidentally detected at autopsy or imaging
    - Contains anomalous mixture of normal elements of splenic tissue
    - May be associated with hamartomas elsewhere as in tuberous sclerosis
  - Lymphangioma
    - Rare benign splenic neoplasm, solitary/multiple; usually subcapsular in location
    - Lymphangiomatosis: Diffuse lymphangiomas
    - Most lymphangiomas occur in childhood
  - Malignant tumors
    - Lymphoma, AIDS-related lymphoma, leukemia, myeloproliferative disorders
    - Metastases, angiosarcoma
    - Rare malignant splenic tumors: Malignant fibrous histiocytoma, leiomyosarcoma & fibrosarcoma
  - Lymphoma

DDx: Splenic Masses

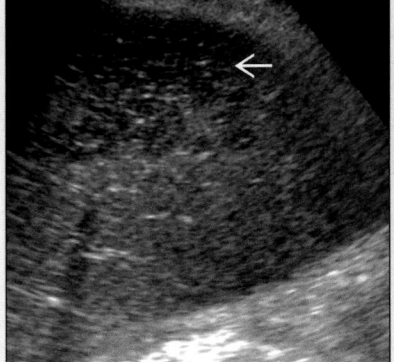 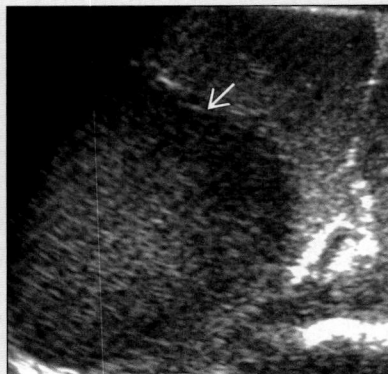 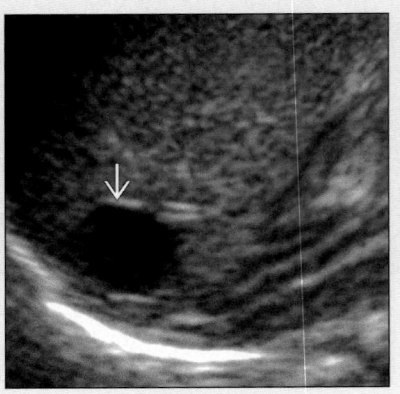

Subcapsular Infarct

Large Abscess

Splenic Cyst

SPLENIC TUMORS

Typical

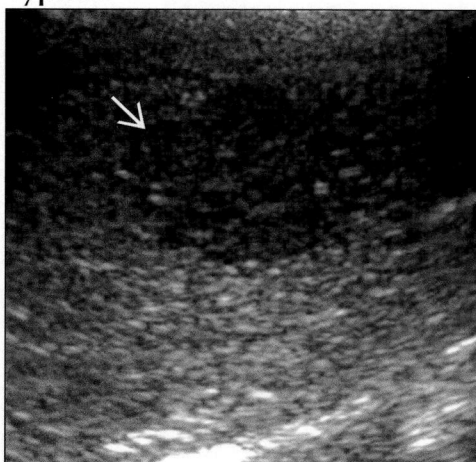

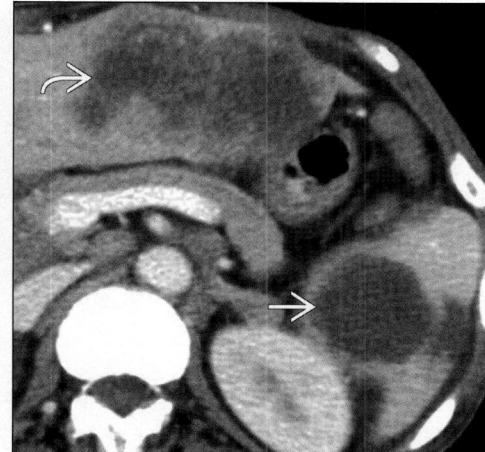

(Left) Transverse transabdominal ultrasound shows a solitary, hypoechoic splenic metastasis ➡. Metastases may vary from a target appearance to a uniform iso/hypo/hyperechoic lesion or heterogeneous mass. (Right) Transverse CECT shows multiple, nonenhancing, hypodense splenic metastases ➡. Note the associated left liver lobe metastases ➡.

Typical

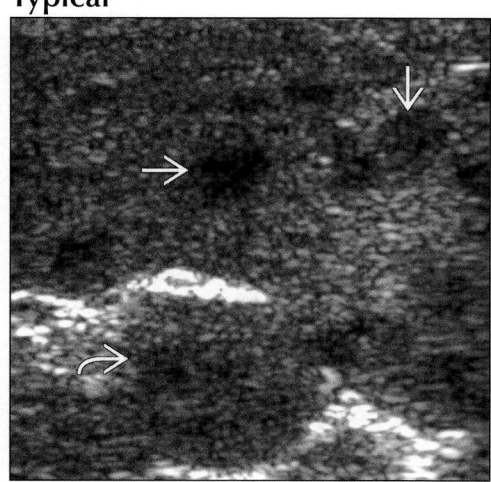

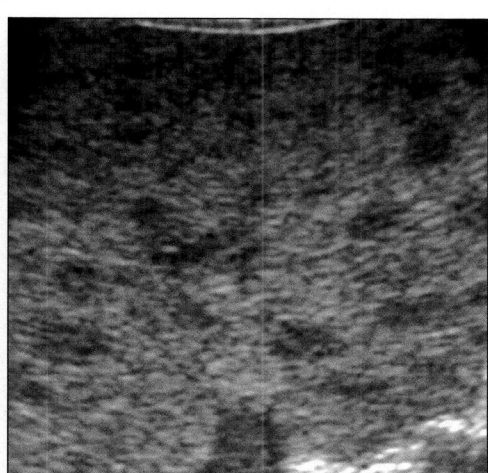

(Left) Transverse transabdominal ultrasound shows multiple, small, hypoechoic, nodular, splenic lymphomatous deposits ➡ with an enlarged splenic hilar lymph node ➡. Hyperechoic lesions are rare. (Right) Longitudinal transabdominal ultrasound shows multiple, small, hypoechoic splenic tuberculous granulomas. In chronic disease these granulomas may be calcified.

Typical

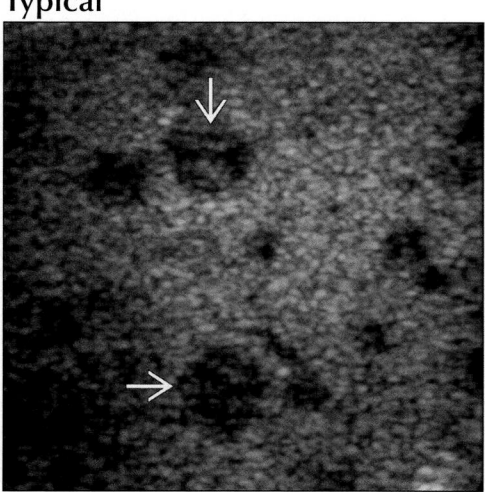

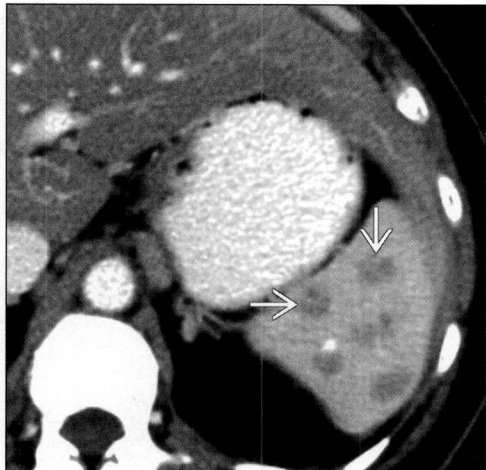

(Left) Oblique transabdominal ultrasound shows multiple, well-defined, hypoechoic splenic granulomas ➡. The differential will include TB, fungal infection, and sarcoid. (Right) Transverse CECT (same patient as in previous image) shows no enhancement within the hypodense splenic granulomas ➡.

SPLENIC TRAUMA

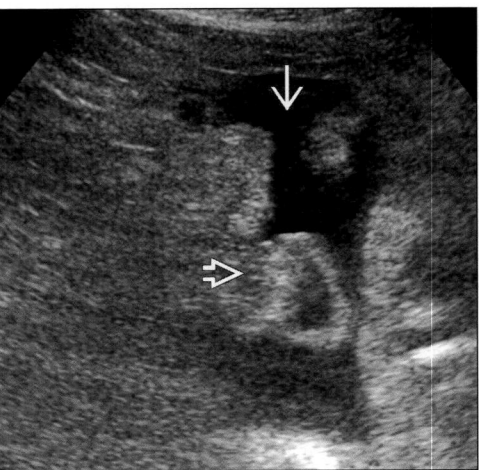

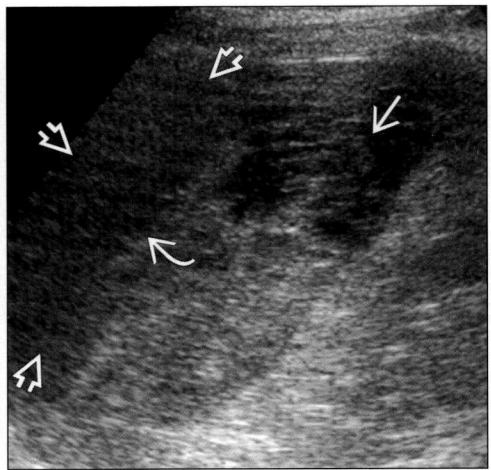

Longitudinal transabdominal ultrasound "FAST" protocol shows intra-peritoneal free fluid ➡ in a patient with blunt abdominal trauma. Note the floating bowel loops ➡.

Oblique transabdominal ultrasound (same patient as previous image) shows a hypoechoic subcapsular hemorrhage ➡ flattened spleen ➡, with associated splenic parenchymal hematoma ➡.

TERMINOLOGY

Abbreviations and Synonyms
- Splenic laceration, splenic fracture, subcapsular hematoma of spleen
- FAST protocol: Focused abdominal sonography in trauma

Definitions
- Parenchymal injury to spleen with or without capsular disruption

IMAGING FINDINGS

General Features
- Best diagnostic clue: Hypoechoic splenic laceration with echogenic acute bleeding
- Morphology
  - Lacerations: Linear or jagged edges
  - Subcapsular hematoma: Flattened contour of splenic parenchyma
  - Splenic fracture: Laceration extending from outer cortex to hilum

Ultrasonographic Findings
- Grayscale Ultrasound
  - Splenic trauma can result in
  - Hemoperitoneum: Intraperitoneal, perisplenic, perihepatic fluid/blood and fluid/blood in pouch of Douglas, hepatorenal pouch
  - Subcapsular hematoma: Collection of blood between the splenic parenchyma & splenic capsule
    - Subcapsular hematoma: Crescentic, hypoechoic collection with sharp margins indenting the splenic parenchyma & closely applied to splenic margins; may calcify at a later stage
    - Subcapsular hematoma: Hyperechoic initially & can easily be missed as it imperceptibly merges along splenic outline
  - Splenic laceration/rupture
    - Splenic laceration/rupture: Hypo/iso/hyperechoic blood filled cleft within spleen
    - Splenic laceration/rupture: Loss of normal splenic contour/fragmented spleen
    - Splenic laceration/rupture: Generalized heterogeneous echo pattern suggesting diffuse splenic injury, blood in perisplenic tissue

DDx: Splenic Trauma

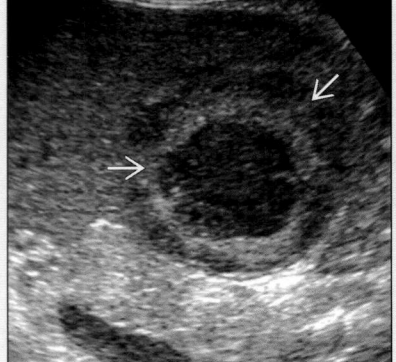

Splenic Abscess

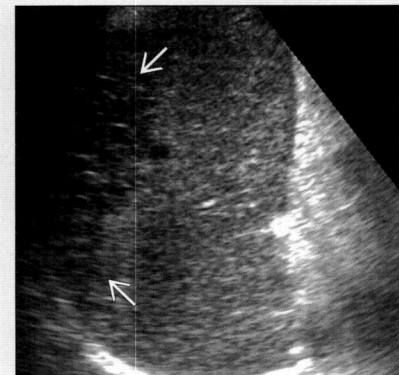

Splenic Infarct

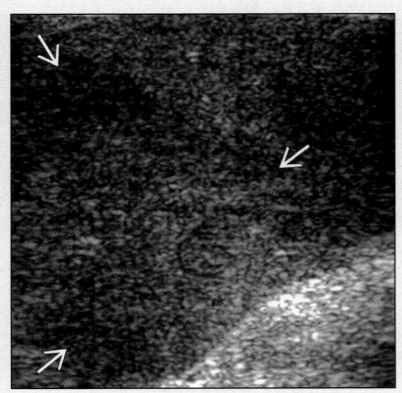

Lymphoma

SPLENIC TRAUMA

Key Facts

Terminology
- Parenchymal injury to spleen with or without capsular disruption

Imaging Findings
- Hemoperitoneum: Intraperitoneal, perisplenic, perihepatic fluid/blood and fluid/blood in pouch of Douglas, hepatorenal pouch
- Subcapsular hematoma: Crescentic, hypoechoic collection with sharp margins indenting the splenic parenchyma & closely applied to splenic margins; may calcify at a later stage
- Subcapsular hematoma: Hyperechoic initially & can easily be missed as it imperceptibly merges along splenic outline
- Splenic laceration/rupture: Hypo/iso/hyperechoic blood filled cleft within spleen
- Splenic laceration/rupture: Loss of normal splenic contour/fragmented spleen
- Splenic laceration/rupture: Generalized heterogeneous echo pattern suggesting diffuse splenic injury, blood in perisplenic tissue
- Absent vascularity in splenic infarct
- Rarely pseudoaneurysm of splenic artery & its branches may develop as a delayed complication (10%)

Top Differential Diagnoses
- Splenic Abscess
- Splenic Infarct
- Lymphoma
- Splenic Cyst

4

23

- Follow-up of splenic lacerations/hematoma
  - Different stages of resolution; progressively liquefies, contracts & finally resorbs with or without scarring, of variable echogenicity on ultrasound
  - Occasionally, cystic degeneration of an intrasplenic hematoma results in a false cyst; (80% splenic cysts: Post-traumatic in origin)
  - Secondary infection/abscess: Ill-defined collection with internal debris & thick irregular wall
- Splenic infarction: Rare, if splenic artery is thrombosed following trauma, wedge-shaped hypoechoic area - broad base towards periphery and apex towards hilum
- Color Doppler
  - Laceration/hematoma: Absent vascularity
  - Absent vascularity in splenic infarct
  - Rarely pseudoaneurysm of splenic artery & its branches may develop as a delayed complication (10%)

CT Findings
- NECT: Hyperdense (> 30 HU) hemoperitoneum or perisplenic clot (> 45 HU)
- CECT
  - Subcapsular hematoma: Crescentic region of low attenuation along splenic margin flattening/indenting/compressing the normal parenchyma
  - Parenchymal laceration: Jagged linear area of nonenhancement due to hematoma, almost always associated with hemoperitoneum
  - Splenic fracture: Deep laceration traversing two capsular surfaces through splenic hilum with complete separation of splenic fragments
  - Shattered spleen: Multiple splenic lacerations
  - Contusion: Mottled splenic parenchymal enhancement pattern
  - Intrasplenic hematoma: Round hypodense inhomogeneous region +/- hyperdense clot

- Active arterial extravasation/pseudoaneurysm: Hyperdense focus isodense with aorta (80-350 HU); surrounded by a hypodense clot or hematoma: Usually requiring surgical intervention
- "Sentinel clot"; perisplenic hematoma: Hyperdense area (> 60 HU) adjacent to spleen is a sensitive predictor of splenic injury

Angiographic Findings
- Avascular parenchymal laceration; flattened lateral contour secondary to subcapsular hematoma
- Rounded contrast collections (pseudoaneurysms); amorphous parenchymal extravasation

Imaging Recommendations
- Best imaging tool
  - Ultrasound (FAST protocol) in a hemodynamically unstable patient
  - CECT if patient is hemodynamically stable
- Protocol advice
  - Limitations of ultrasound in abdominal trauma
    - A unstable patient in pain with multiple tubes, lines, wound dressings, spinal injuries cannot be placed in a optimal scanning position
    - Subtle splenic trauma such as a small hematoma may be missed on ultrasound
    - Other organ/parts of the patient (brain, thorax, spine) may be injured & may require imaging by CT which provides a quick global overview in a patient with blunt abdominal trauma
    - Associated ileus causing gaseous distension obscures larger portion of abdomen on ultrasound

DIFFERENTIAL DIAGNOSIS

Splenic Abscess
- Rounded, hypoechoic well-defined lesions
- Usually with thick irregular wall/margin,
- Echogenicity of internal content may vary from hypoechoic to anechoic: Depending on the stage of liquefaction/necrosis
- Accompanied by clinical signs of infection

SPLENIC TRAUMA

Splenic Infarct
- Wedge-shaped hypoechoic area, broad base towards the capsule and apex towards the splenic hilum
- Associated with splenomegaly; systemic emboli
- Avascular area on color Doppler

Lymphoma
- Single or multiple hypoechoic nodular lesions; splenomegaly
- "Indistinct boundary" echo pattern, without posterior acoustic enhancement

Splenic Cyst
- Rounded hypoechoic or anechoic lesion; posterior acoustic enhancement; well-defined cyst wall
- +/- Internal septations, internal echoes, thick wall with or with out calcification

PATHOLOGY

General Features
- General path comments: Laceration, fractures, intraparenchymal or subcapsular hematoma
- Etiology
  - Penetrating injuries or blunt trauma with blow to left upper quadrant (LUQ)
  - Patients on anticoagulants or those with marked splenomegaly; prone to splenic injury on minor trauma
  - Spontaneous splenic rupture: Sickle cell disease, patients with bleeding diathesis
- Epidemiology: Most common abdominal organ injury requiring surgery
- Associated abnormalities: Injuries to left thorax, tail of pancreas, left kidney, left liver lobe and/or mesentery

Gross Pathologic & Surgical Features
- Varies according to extent of injury

Microscopic Features
- Necrotic injured tissue with surrounding hematoma

Staging, Grading or Classification Criteria
- Grading may be misleading; minor injuries may lead to devastating delayed bleed
  - Grade 1: Subcapsular hematoma or laceration < 1 cm
  - Grade 2: Subcapsular hematoma or laceration 1-3 cm
  - Grade 3: Capsular disruption; hematoma > 3 cm; parenchymal hematoma > 3 cm
  - Grade 4A: Active parenchymal or subcapsular bleeding, pseudoaneurysm or arteriovenous fistula; shattered spleen
  - Grade 4B: Active intraperitoneal bleed

CLINICAL ISSUES

Presentation
- Most common signs/symptoms: Blunt abdominal trauma; LUQ pain; hypotension

Natural History & Prognosis
- Prone to develop delayed hemorrhage; excellent prognosis with early diagnosis & intervention (surgery or embolization)

Treatment
- Non-operative management for minor injuries: 48%
- Angiographic embolization if active arterial extravasation on CT
- Splenectomy or splenorrhaphy when surgery required: 52%

DIAGNOSTIC CHECKLIST

Consider
- Congenital cleft/normal lobulation (smoothly contoured, medially located) if no hemoperitoneum
- Perisplenic fluid from ascites/urine/bile/lavage

Image Interpretation Pearls
- Innocuous injury may lead to life-threatening delayed hemorrhage, especially in patients on anticoagulant treatment
- In cases of splenic trauma ultrasound examination should primarily be aimed at detecting perisplenic fluid/blood collection, followed by CECT evaluation if patient is hemodynamically stable

SELECTED REFERENCES

1. Gorg C et al: Colour Doppler ultrasound patterns and clinical follow-up of incidentally found hypoechoic, vascular tumours of the spleen: evidence for a benign tumour. Br J Radiol. 79(940):319-25, 2006
2. Blaivas M et al: Feasibility of FAST examination performance with ultrasound contrast. J Emerg Med. 29(3):307-11, 2005
3. Doody O et al: Blunt trauma to the spleen: ultrasonographic findings. Clin Radiol. 60(9):968-76, 2005
4. Fried AM. Related Articles et al: Spleen and retroperitoneum: the essentials. Ultrasound Q. 21(4):275-86, 2005
5. Lutz N et al: The significance of contrast blush on computed tomography in children with splenic injuries. J Pediatr Surg. 39(3):491-4, 2004
6. Richards JR et al: Sonographic patterns of intraperitoneal hemorrhage associated with blunt splenic injury. J Ultrasound Med. 23(3):387-94, quiz 395-6, 2004
7. Sato M et al: Reevaluation of ultrasonography for solid-organ injury in blunt abdominal trauma. J Ultrasound Med. 23(12):1583-96, 2004
8. Sirlin CB et al: Blunt abdominal trauma: clinical value of negative screening US scans. Radiology. 230(3):661-8, 2004
9. Minarik L et al: Diagnostic imaging in the follow-up of nonoperative management of splenic trauma in children. Pediatr Surg Int. 18(5-6):429-31, 2002
10. Stengel D et al: Discriminatory power of 3.5 MHz convex and 7.5 MHz linear ultrasound probes for the imaging of traumatic splenic lesions: a feasibility study. J Trauma. 51(1):37-43, 2001
11. Krupnick AS et al: Use of abdominal ultrasonography to assess pediatric splenic trauma. Potential pitfalls in the diagnosis. Ann Surg. 225(4):408-14, 1997
12. Jeffrey RB Jr et al: Detection of active intraabdominal arterial hemorrhage: value of dynamic contrast-enhanced CT. AJR Am J Roentgenol. 156(4):725-9, 1991

SPLENIC TRAUMA

IMAGE GALLERY

Typical

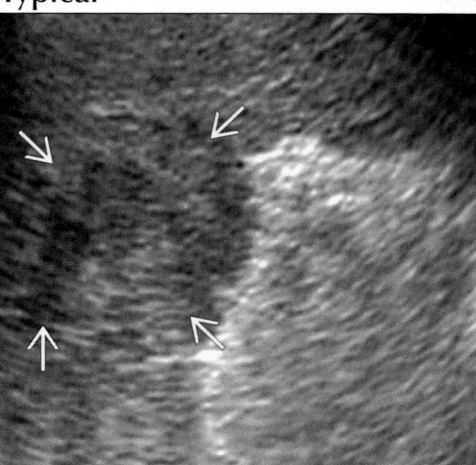
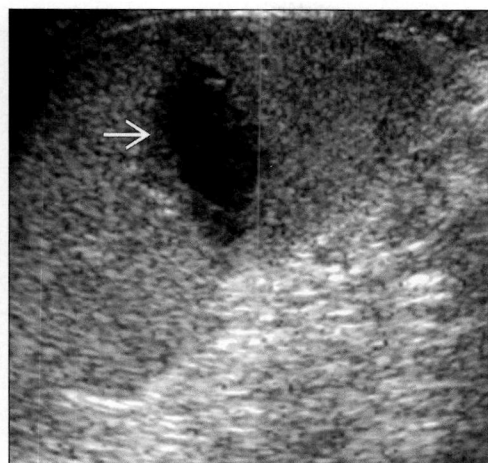

(Left) Oblique transabdominal ultrasound shows a focal area of ill-defined, heterogeneous echo pattern ➡ representing a subacute intrasplenic hematoma. *(Right)* Longitudinal transabdominal ultrasound shows a well-defined, hypoechoic, liquefied chronic splenic parenchymal hematoma ➡.

Variant

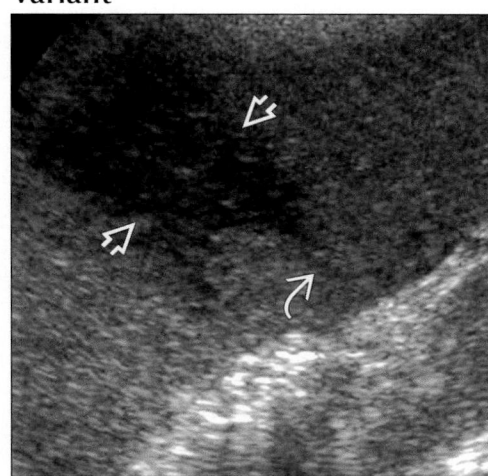
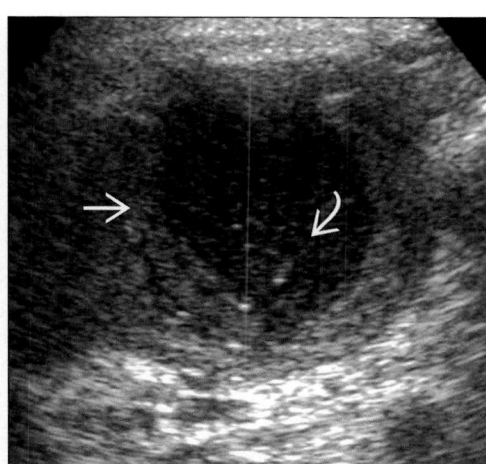

(Left) Longitudinal transabdominal ultrasound shows a well-defined, hypoechoic splenic parenchymal laceration ➡ extending to the subcapsular region ➡. *(Right)* Transverse transabdominal ultrasound shows a well-defined, thick walled infected splenic hematoma ➡, with echogenic internal debris ➡.

Typical

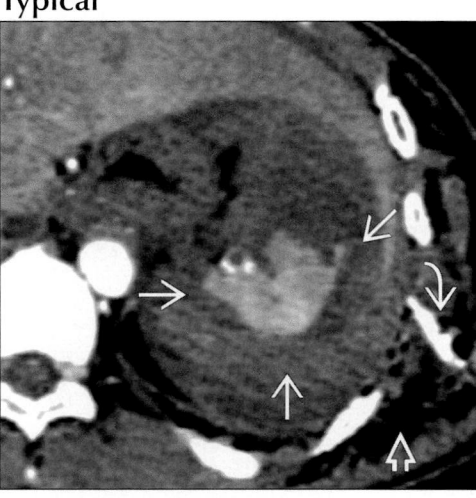
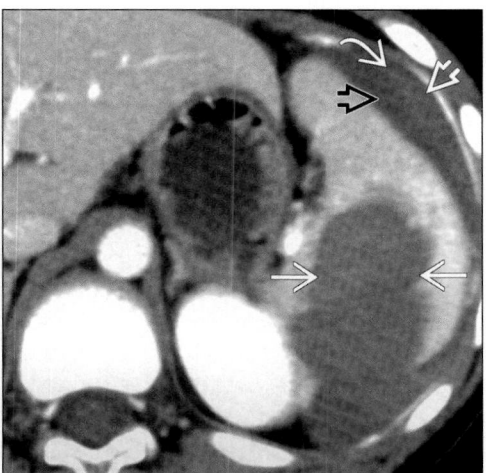

(Left) Transverse CECT shows a lacerated spleen ➡ with perisplenic hemorrhage. Note the adjacent fractured rib ➡ and subcutaneous emphysema ➡. *(Right)* Transverse CECT shows a large, hypodense, nonenhancing, intra-parenchymal splenic hematoma ➡. Note the faintly visible splenic capsule ➡ separating the subcapsular ➡ & perisplenic hemorrhage ➡.

SPLENIC CALCIFICATIONS

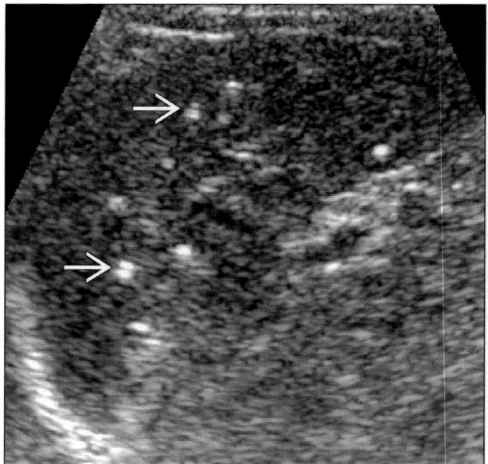

Longitudinal transabdominal ultrasound shows multiple small hyperechoic calcific foci ➡ representing old calcified splenic granulomas.

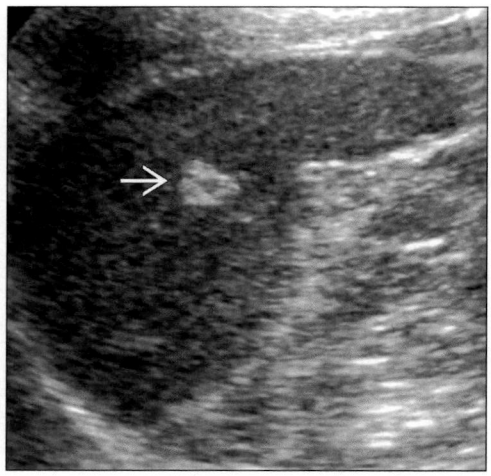

Transverse transabdominal ultrasound shows a solitary well-defined calcified splenic hamartoma ➡.

TERMINOLOGY

Definitions
- Focal nodular (micro/macronodular) or linear hyperechoic foci with or without posterior acoustic shadowing

IMAGING FINDINGS

General Features
- Location: Splenic parenchyma or subcapsular region
- Size: Variable; usually small or punctate, occasionally large or chunky
- Morphology: Nodular or linear

Ultrasonographic Findings
- Grayscale Ultrasound
  - Hyperechoic foci with posterior acoustic shadowing
  - Early calcification may or may not produce shadowing
  - Calcified lesions represent benign etiology: Chronic granuloma, hamartomas, organized hematoma, cyst
  - Curvilinear wall/rim calcification: Hydatid cyst, simple cyst
  - Calcified intrasplenic pseudoaneurysm (rare)
  - Vascular calcification: Linear along the vessel wall/calcified thrombus
- Color Doppler
  - Color flow along linear vascular calcification
  - "Twinkling" artifact: Color signals posterior to calcification

Imaging Recommendations
- Best imaging tool: USG for screening and follow-up
- Protocol advice: Patient best scanned in supine or right decubitus position following deep inspiration with the transducer along long axis of spleen

DIFFERENTIAL DIAGNOSIS

Siderosis
- Diffuse; sickle cell anemia, multiple blood transfusions

Gamma Gandy Bodies
- Echogenic foci of hemosiderin and calcium deposition - secondary to intraparenchymal hemorrhage

DDx: Splenic Calcification

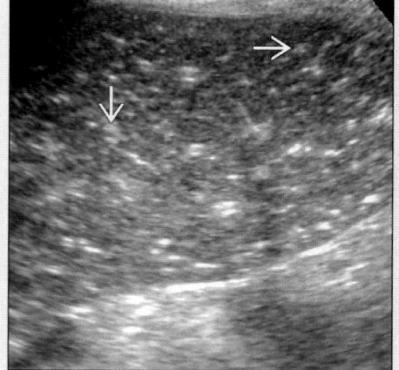

Siderosis

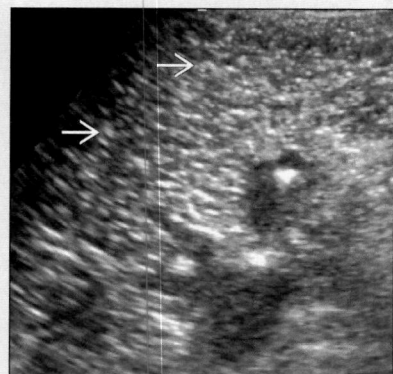

Gamma Gandy Bodies

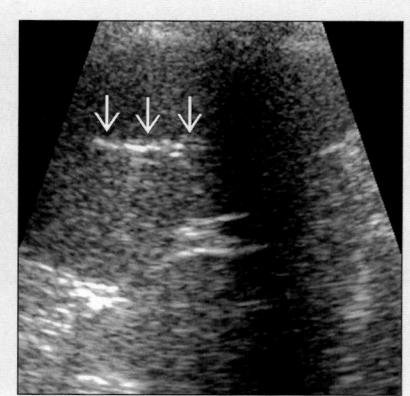

Vascular Calcification

SPLENIC CALCIFICATIONS

Key Facts

Imaging Findings

- Hyperechoic foci with posterior acoustic shadowing
- Early calcification may or may not produce shadowing
- Calcified lesions represent benign etiology: Chronic granuloma, hamartomas, organized hematoma, cyst
- Curvilinear wall/rim calcification: Hydatid cyst, simple cyst
- Calcified intrasplenic pseudoaneurysm (rare)

- Vascular calcification: Linear along the vessel wall/calcified thrombus
- Color flow along linear vascular calcification
- "Twinkling" artifact: Color signals posterior to calcification

Top Differential Diagnoses

- Siderosis
- Gamma Gandy Bodies
- Splenic Vascular Calcification

- Most commonly seen in liver cirrhosis with portal hypertension, splenic vein thrombosis, hemolytic anemia, hemochromatosis

Splenic Vascular Calcification

- Splenic artery calcification, splenic vein calcification (rare); linear echogenic wall calcification
- Calcified splenic artery aneurysm; nodular rim/wall calcification
- Embolic material used for splenic arteriovenous malformation (AVM) or pseudoaneurysm embolization

PATHOLOGY

General Features

- Etiology
  - Disseminated
    - Granuloma (most common): Tuberculosis, histoplasmosis, brucellosis, sarcoidosis
    - Phlebolith: Visceral angiomatosis
  - Capsular and parenchymal
    - Pyogenic/non pyogenic abscess
    - Pneumocystis carinii infection
    - Infarction (multiple), hematoma
    - Splenic hamartoma, inflammatory pseudotumor
    - Lymphoma (post-radiotherapy), metastasis (rare)
    - Splenic infarct
  - Calcified cyst wall
    - Congenital cyst
    - Post-traumatic cyst

- Echinococcal cyst
- Cystic dermoid

CLINICAL ISSUES

Presentation

- Most common signs/symptoms: Asymptomatic; usually an incidental finding

Natural History & Prognosis

- Benign/inactive condition
- Prognosis: Excellent

Treatment

- No treatment necessary

DIAGNOSTIC CHECKLIST

Image Interpretation Pearls

- Calcified splenic lesions may be safely followed up with serial USG examinations as they are unlikely to represent lesions requiring treatment

SELECTED REFERENCES

1. Andrews MW. Related Articles et al: Ultrasound of the spleen. World J Surg. 24(2):183-7, 2000
2. Goerg C et al: Splenic lesions: sonographic patterns, follow-up, differential diagnosis. Eur J Radiol. 13(1):59-66, 1991

IMAGE GALLERY

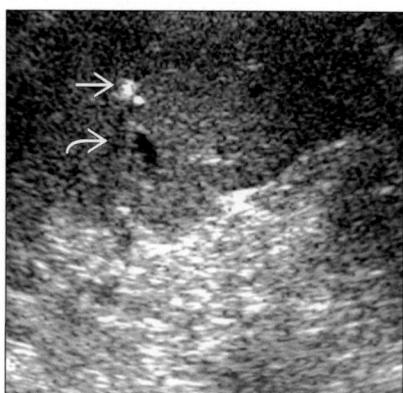 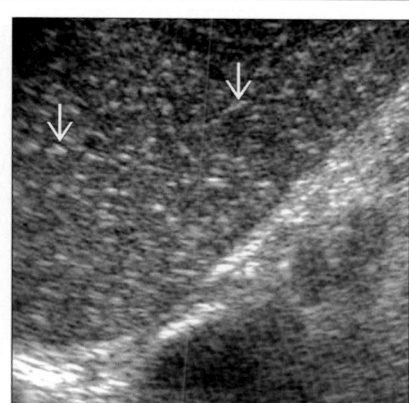 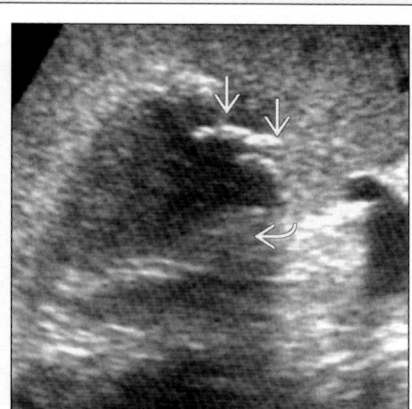

(Left) Longitudinal transabdominal ultrasound shows a solitary calcified splenic granuloma ➜, with minimal posterior acoustic shadowing ➜. *(Center)* Oblique transabdominal ultrasound shows splenomegaly and multiple punctate calcified granulomas ➜ due to splenic sarcoidosis. *(Right)* Transverse transabdominal ultrasound shows a calcified splenic cyst wall ➜, with dense posterior acoustic shadowing ➜.

SPLENIC VASCULAR DISORDERS

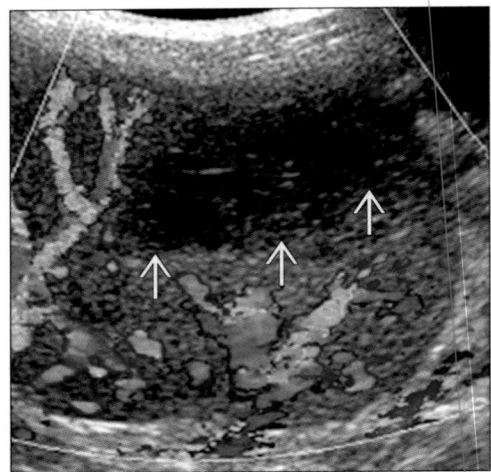

Oblique color Doppler ultrasound shows a hypoechoic zone of infarction ➡ in the periphery of the spleen. Note absence of blood flow in the affected area.

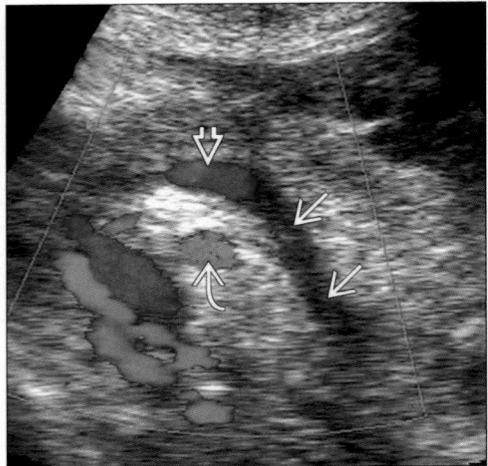

Transverse color Doppler ultrasound shows acute thrombotic occlusion of the splenic vein ➡. The proximal part of vein ⟴ remains patent. Superior mesenteric artery ➡.

TERMINOLOGY

Abbreviations and Synonyms
- Splenic infarction (abbreviated "infarction")
- Splenic artery (SA) occlusion
- Splenic vein (SV) thrombosis

Definitions
- Infarction: Loss of viability of part or all of the splenic parenchyma due to ischemia
- SA occlusion: Complete blockage of SA blood flow
- SV thrombosis: Complete blockage of SV blood flow

IMAGING FINDINGS

General Features
- Best diagnostic clue
  - Infarction: Hypoechoic region within splenic parenchyma on grayscale US; absent blood flow on color Doppler (CD) examination
  - SA occlusion: Absent flow in SA on CD examination, possibly with collateralization

- SV thrombosis: Acute, SV visualized with no flow on CD exam; chronic, non-visualization of SV with large gastric or left renal collaterals
- Location
  - Infarction: Classically in periphery of splenic parenchyma but may be located anywhere
  - SA occlusion: Usually entire artery; or distal only
  - SV thrombosis: Entire vein or distal only (near hilum)
- Size: Infarction ranges from focal area to entire spleen
- Morphology: Acute infarct: Classically wedge shaped, broad base at periphery; may be rounded

Ultrasonographic Findings
- Grayscale Ultrasound
  - **Acute infarct**: Hypoechoic region in splenic parenchyma with absent flow on CD exam
    - Grayscale findings may not appear for 24-48 hrs after loss of blood flow
  - **Chronic infarct**: Linear or rounded echogenic region with "divot" on surface of spleen, scarring
  - **Acute SA occlusion**: Grayscale diagnosis unlikely
  - **Chronic SA occlusion**: Absence of SA (scarred)

DDx: Splenic Vascular Disorders

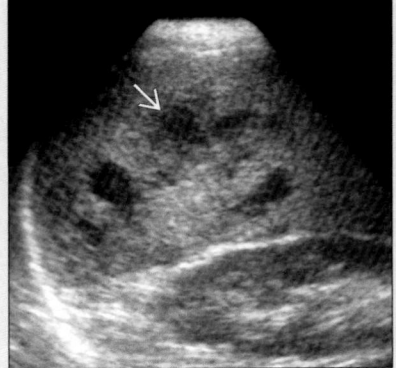

Splenic Abscesses

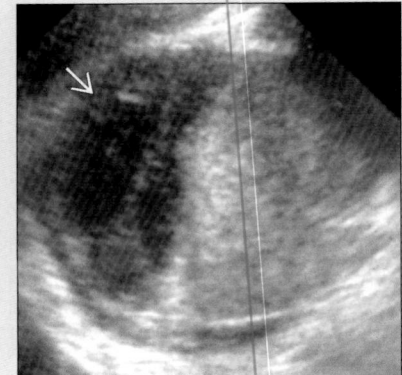

Splenic Hematoma

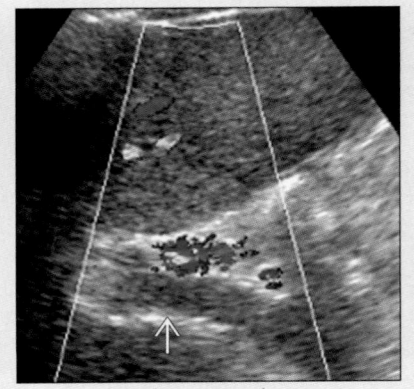

Portal Vein Occlusion

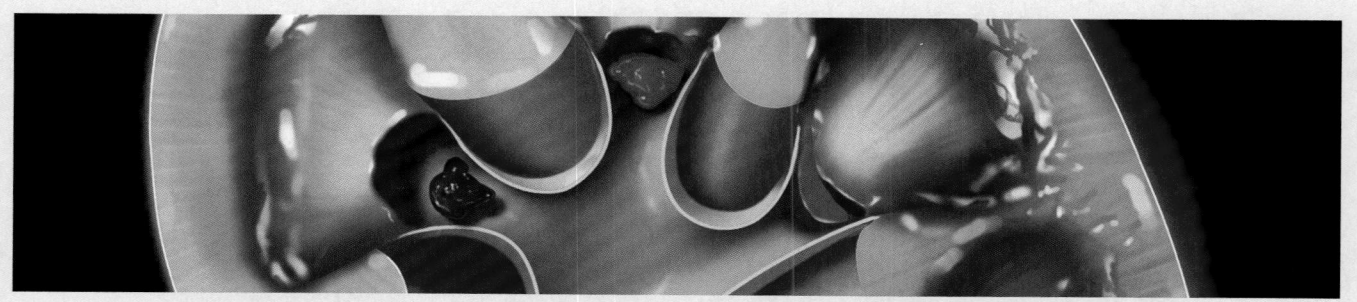

SECTION 5: Urinary Tract

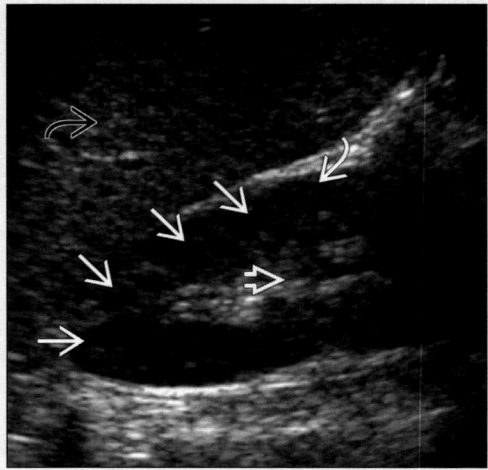

Longitudinal ultrasound of adult kidney shows central echogenic renal sinus ⮀ and peripheral renal cortex ⮀, slightly hypoechoic compared to liver ⮀. Between the sinus and cortex are hypoechoic pyramids ⮀.

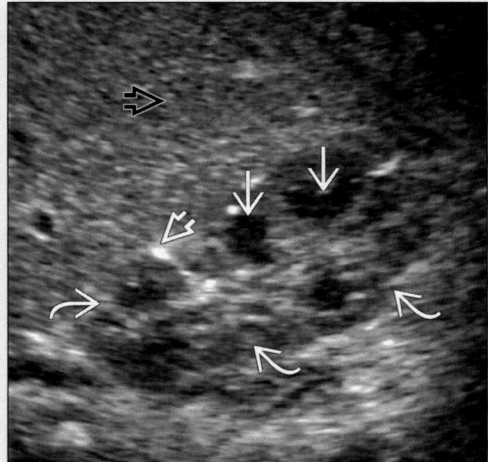

Transabdominal ultrasound of an infant kidney shows prominent hypoechoic pyramids ⮀. Note fetal lobulation ⮀ & echogenic junction line ⮀ at anterior 1/3 of kidney. The renal cortex is isoechoic to liver ⮀.

IMAGING ANATOMY

General Anatomic Considerations

- Kidneys: Retroperitoneal, near posterior body wall
  - Periphery: Renal parenchyma: Consists of medullary pyramids and cortex
    - Cortex: Peripheral portion; column of Bertin → extend between medullary pyramids
    - Medullary pyramid: Contains renal tubules, supporting tissue, blood vessels
  - Central: Collecting system: Calyces, infundibula and renal pelvis
  - Surrounded by renal capsule, then by perirenal fat of variable thickness
- Ureter
  - Tubular retroperitoneal structure connecting renal pelvis with bladder
- Bladder: Central pelvic cavity
  - Shape varies with degree of distension
  - Ureters enter bladder and urethra leaves bladder at three corners of the trigone

Critical Anatomic Structures

- Anatomical division: Kidney
  - Medullary pyramid: Tightly packed tissue with few reflecting interfaces
    - Lower echogenicity than cortex
    - Corticomedullary differentiation is poor in large patients
  - Cortex: Contains glomeruli: Moderately powerful reflectors
    - Higher echogenicity than medulla
    - Adult: Slightly lower or equal echogenicity to liver and spleen
  - Renal sinus complex: Highest echogenicity
    - Children or slim adult: Little sinus fat: Uroepithelium appears as a narrow echogenic band
    - Adult with more sinus fat: Uroepithelium has similar echogenicity and merges with it
  - Collecting system

- Normally narrow urine-filled space usually invisible
- Renal pelvis: Variable appearance, ranging from hardly discernible small intrarenal structure to large anechoic extrarenal structure
  - Renal capsule: Interface between perinephric tissue and cortex
    - Sharp echogenic line around kidney
  - Perinephric fat: Variable in thickness and echogenicity
    - Usually medium high echogenicity
    - Occasion of low echogenicity, may simulate perinephric fluid collection
- Anatomical structures related to bladder
  - Trigone: Triangular area of bladder wall, smoother than surrounding muscle
    - No definite distinguishing feature, sometimes appears slightly thicker than rest of bladder wall
  - Ureteric orifices
    - Occasionally identified as small out pouching on bladder wall
    - Ureteric jet: Intermittent hyperechoic jet directed obliquely into bladder lumen on grayscale US, best seen by color Doppler
  - Urethra
    - Small depression at bladder base, best seen on sagittal views

Anatomic Relationships

- Right kidney
  - Anteriorly: Liver and hepatic flexure
- Left kidney
  - Anterosuperiorly: Spleen, colon
- Right renal artery
  - Posterior to inferior vena cava (IVC)
- Left renal artery
  - Posterior to left renal vein
- Ureter
  - Abdominal portion: Lies on medial edge of psoas muscle
  - Terminal portion: At level of ischial spine, turns anteriorly and medially to enter bladder
    - Male: Lies above seminal vesicles

URINARY TRACT SONOGRAPHY

Key Facts

Imaging Protocol
- Most important role of US: Determine nature of renal masses
- Scan kidneys in multiple longitudinal & transverse planes to ensure entire renal parenchyma imaged
- Use graded compression technique to visualize level of obstruction in dilated ureter
- Use high-frequency transducer/different angulation to delineate anterior & lateral bladder wall

Common Pathologies
- Solid renal masses
  - Primary malignant tumors: Renal cell carcinoma, Wilms tumor (pediatrics), renal sarcoma
  - Secondary malignant tumors: Lymphoma, metastasis, invasive transitional cell carcinoma
  - Benign tumor: Angiomyolipoma, oncocytoma
  - Inflammatory masses: Acute bacterial nephritis, renal abscess, xanthogranulomatous pyelonephritis, tuberculoma
  - Pseudotumor: Column of Bertin, dromedary hump, fetal lobulation
- Complex cystic masses
  - Complicated cortical cyst: Hemorrhagic cyst, infected cyst, multiseptated cyst
  - Benign: Abscess, hematoma
  - Tumor: Cystic renal cell carcinoma, multilocular cystic nephroma, cystic Wilms tumor
- Bladder wall masses
  - Congenital: Simple/ectopic ureterocele
  - Bladder tumors: Transitional cell, squamous cell
  - Inflammatory: cystitis, schistosomiasis, tuberculosis
  - Hematoma

- Female: Lies close to lateral fornices of vagina
- Bladder
  - Male: Prostate causes impression on bladder base
  - Female: Uterus bulges into posterior wall of bladder

ANATOMY-BASED IMAGING ISSUES

Key Concepts or Questions
- Renal shape and outline varies, depending on angle of scan
  - Anterior approach: Narrow outline with sinus complex lying centrally
  - Oblique posterolateral plane: Wider outline with renal pelvis at lower end
- Difference in sonographic features between neonatal and adult kidneys
  - Neonatal kidney
    - Higher cortical echogenicity due to greater concentration of glomeruli; cortex may be more echogenic than liver
    - Prominent hypoechoic pyramids, larger in relation to cortex, may be mistaken as dilated calices in hydronephrosis
    - Little or no renal sinus fat: Consists solely of narrow structures of calyceal system
    - Relatively distended calyceal system: 75% with calyces and infundibula seen as fluid-filled structures
  - Cortical changes persist until 6-24 months, then it acquires adult pattern
- Doppler signal in renal arteries
  - Low resistance signal: Rapid systolic rise, continuing high-velocity flow throughout diastole
- Doppler signal in renal vein
  - Slightly undulating with respiration in main veins; continuous in smaller vein

Imaging Approaches
- Important to choose sonographic scan plane which matches the anatomic planes to achieve true longitudinal and transverse scans of kidney
- Upper pole of right kidney may be imaged through liver on anterior plane
- Lower pole of right kidney imaged via oblique approach, as it is obscured by hepatic flexure on anterior approach
- Left kidney: Posterior oblique approach
- Bladder: Best to delineate bladder wall thickness at full distension

Imaging Protocols
- Patient requires to be turned into varying degrees of obliquity to complete examination of kidneys
- Scan kidneys in multiple longitudinal and transverse planes to ensure entire renal tissue is examined
- Measure the anteroposterior diameter of renal pelvis on transverse plane if there is evidence of hydronephrosis
- Right kidney
  - Start with anterolateral approach using liver as acoustic window
  - Additional posterior approach to image lower pole
  - Examine in full inspiration → moves kidney below ribs and away from overlying bowel gas
- Left kidney
  - Posterior approach: Scanned through lumbar muscle
  - Occasionally, scan upper pole of kidney through spleen
- Ureter
  - Use graded compression technique to visualize dilated ureter, which is usually obscured by bowel gas
  - Color Doppler to demonstrate ureteric jets; presence of strong jet excludes ureteric obstruction
- Bladder
  - Angulation of transducer helps to show lateral wall and bladder base
  - Use higher frequency transducer to reduce reverberation from anterior bladder wall
  - Transrectal scanning better delineates lower anterior bladder wall

Imaging Pitfalls
- Kidney

URINARY TRACT SONOGRAPHY

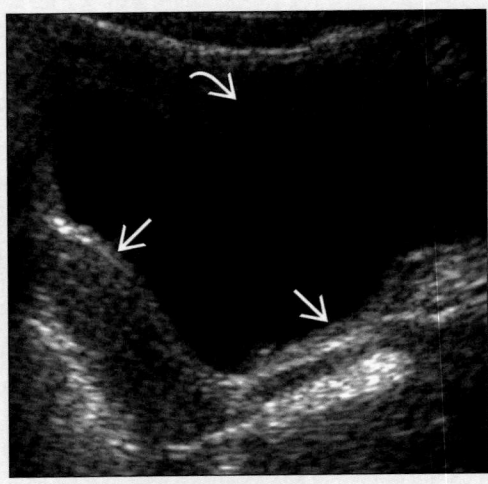

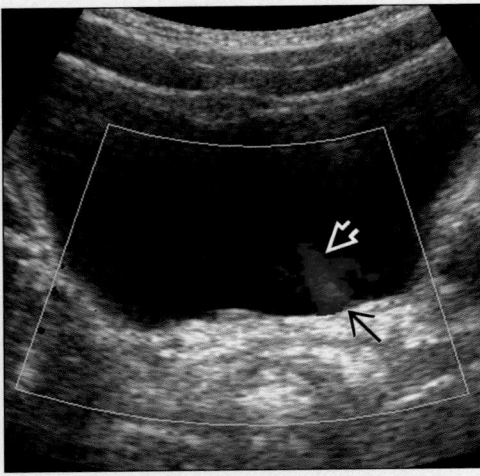

Longitudinal ultrasound shows normal configuration of the urinary bladder, with even thickness of the posterior bladder wall ➡. Note anterior wall ➡ is less defined due to reverberation artifact.

Transverse color Doppler ultrasound shows a ureteric jet ➡, exiting the left ureteral orifice ➡ and entering the bladder. Angle of flow is typically oblique.

○ More posterior the scan plane, greater muscle bulk between kidney and transducer → less well-defined tissue plane within kidney: Loss of cortico-medullary differentiation
• Bladder: "Blind spot" on conventional imaging plane
○ Lateral wall: Beam nearly parallel to wall
○ Base: Lies behind symphysis pubis
○ Anterior bladder wall: Image degraded by reverberation artifact

Normal Measurements
• Renal length
○ < 1 year old: 4.98 + 0.155 x age (month)
○ > 1 year old: 6.79 + 0.22 x age (years)
○ Adulthood: Right kidney: 10.74 ± 1.35 (SD), left kidney: 11.10 ± 1.15 (SD)
• Renal Doppler indices of main renal artery and branches
○ Peak systolic velocity: 0.6-1.4 m/s
○ Resistive index (RI): 0.56-0.7
○ Pulsatility index (PI): 0.7-0.14
○ Systolic rise time: 0.11 ± 0.06
• AP diameter of renal pelvis
○ 5 mm, < 20 week gestation
○ < 8 mm, 20-30 week gestation
○ < 10 mm, > 30 week gestation

PATHOLOGY-BASED IMAGING ISSUES

Key Concepts or Questions
• If renal masses detected clinically or in intravenous pyelography
○ Exclude hydronephrosis or cortical renal cysts (most common causes)
○ Large solid renal mass: Needs further investigation/biopsy
• If dilated collecting system detected, trace distally for level of obstruction

○ Common cause: Obstruction: Ureteric stone, inflammatory stricture, extrinsic compression, congenital abnormalities such as ureteropelvic junction (UPJ) obstruction
○ Uncommon cause: Active diuresis, diabetes insipidus, reflux nephropathy

Imaging Pitfalls
• Distended bladder, pregnancy causes dilatation of collecting system mimicking obstruction
• Extrarenal pelvis and parapelvic cyst simulate hydronephrosis

EMBRYOLOGY

Embryologic Events
• Kidney: Formed by fusion of two embryonic parenchymatous masses (= ranunculi)
• Line of fusion runs obliquely forward and upward

Practical Implications
• Renal junction line: Normal variant
○ Echogenic line at upper and middle thirds of kidney without disruption of renal contour
• Column of Bertin: Normal variant
○ Hypertrophic medial bands of cortical tissue that separate pyramids of renal medullae
○ At junction of upper and middle thirds of kidney
○ May mimic renal tumor
• Fetal lobulation; persistent cortical lobation
○ 14 individual lobes with centrilobar cortex located around calices

RELATED REFERENCES

1. Sty JR et al: Genitourinary imaging techniques. Pediatr Clin North Am. 53(3):339-61, 2006
2. Dahnert W: Radiology review manual. 4th ed. Philadelphia, lippincott, Williams and Wilkins, 723-56, 2000
3. McGahan JP et al: Diagnostic ultrasound: a logical approach. Lippincott-Raven, 1998

IMAGE GALLERY

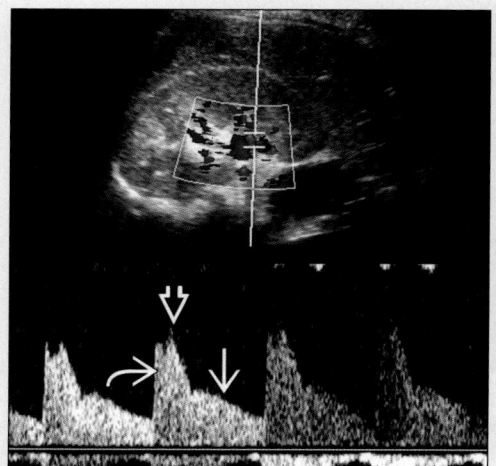

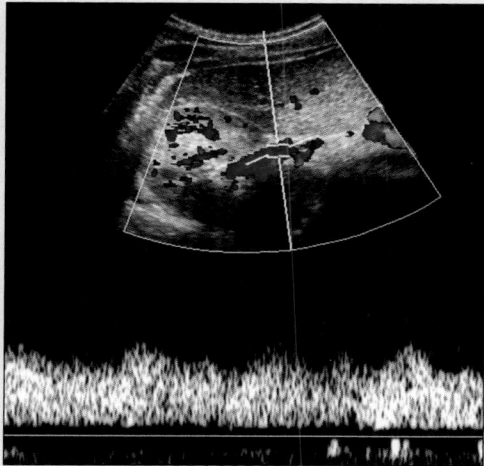

(Left) Pulsed Doppler ultrasound shows a normal renal artery spectral signal. Note rapid systolic rise ➡ and persistent high flow during diastole ➡. Diastolic velocity is about half of peak systolic velocity ➡. *(Right)* Pulsed Doppler ultrasound shows a normal flow pattern of the renal vein, with continuous flow throughout systole and diastole.

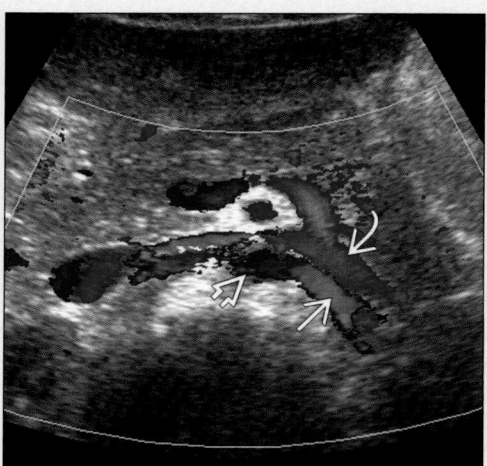

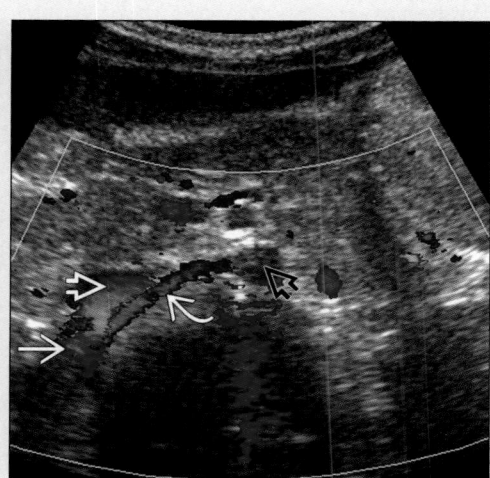

(Left) Color Doppler ultrasound shows the normal relationship of the left renal artery ➡ behind the left renal vein ➡ (aorta ➡). The left renal vein passes behind the superior mesenteric artery to enter the IVC. *(Right)* Color Doppler ultrasound shows the short course of the right renal vein ➡, before entering IVC ➡. The right renal artery ➡ passes behind the IVC ➡ and joins the aorta ➡.

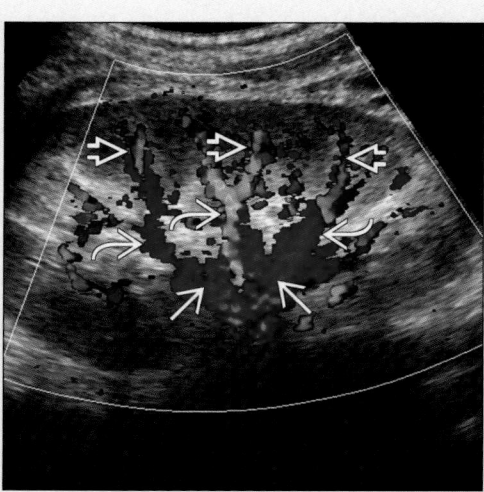

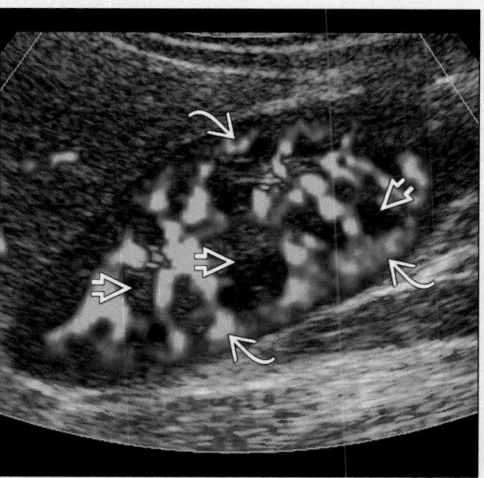

(Left) Longitudinal color Doppler ultrasound shows the division of the main renal artery into anterior and posterior branches ➡ within the renal hilum. They further divide into segmental ➡ and interlobar ➡ arteries. *(Right)* Power Doppler ultrasound shows homogeneous intense cortical vascularity ➡ and no detectable flow in the renal pyramids ➡.

COLUMN OF BERTIN, KIDNEY

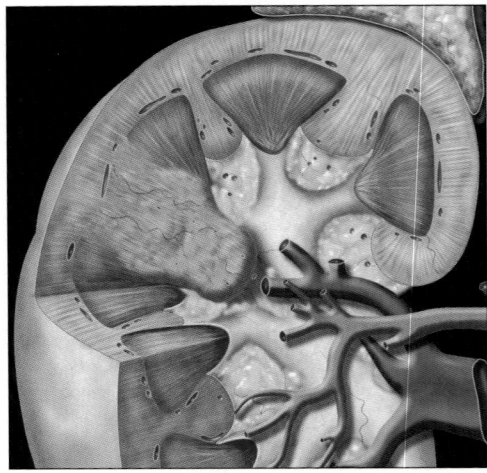

Graphic shows a column of Bertin, which is not a real mass but an extension of renal cortical tissue between the pyramids.

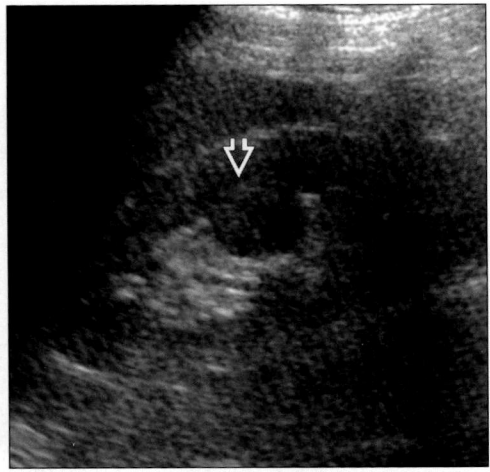

Longitudinal transabdominal ultrasound shows a column of Bertin ➡, which is isoechoic and continuous with renal cortex. Note the smooth renal outline.

TERMINOLOGY

Abbreviations and Synonyms

- Septal cortex, hypertrophied or enlarged column of Bertin, focal cortical hyperplasia, benign cortical rest, cortical island, focal renal hypertrophy, junctional parenchyma

Definitions

- Hypertrophic medial bands of cortical tissue that separate the pyramids of the renal medulla

IMAGING FINDINGS

General Features

- Best diagnostic clue
  - Isoechoic and continuous with renal cortex, protruding into renal sinus
  - No abnormal vascularity
- Location
  - At junction of upper and middle thirds of kidney
  - Left side > right side
  - Unilateral > bilateral (18% of cases)

Ultrasonographic Findings

- Grayscale Ultrasound
  - Normal renal outline
  - Isoechoic with renal cortex
  - Contains renal pyramids
  - Bordered by junctional parenchymal defect
  - Indentation of renal sinus
- Color Doppler
  - Arcuate artery seen within
  - Normal perfusion indicating normal renal tissue

Radiographic Findings

- IVP
  - Splaying and abnormal separation of upper and lower pole of collecting system
  - Mass effect on pelvicaliceal system, always at level of emerging renal vein

CT Findings

- CECT
  - Absence of a mass
  - Similar enhancement as normal renal cortex on corticomedullary phase

DDx: Column of Bertin

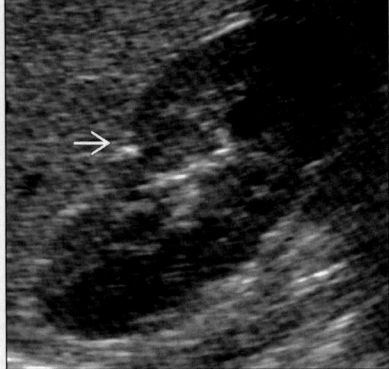

Renal Scarring

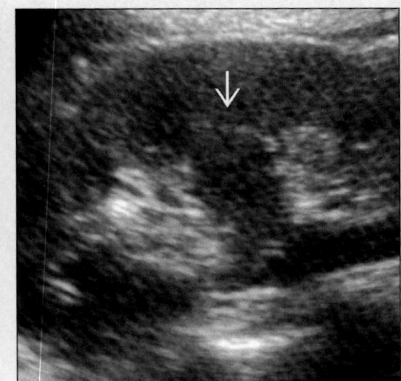

Duplex Kidney

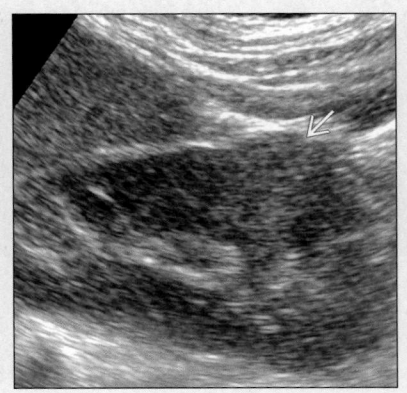

Dromedary Hump

COLUMN OF BERTIN, KIDNEY

Key Facts

Terminology
- Hypertrophic medial bands of cortical tissue that separate the pyramids of the renal medulla

Imaging Findings
- Isoechoic and continuous with renal cortex, protruding into renal sinus
- At junction of upper and middle thirds of kidney
- Normal renal outline
- Contains renal pyramids

Top Differential Diagnoses
- Renal Scarring
- Renal Duplication
- Dromedary Hump
- Renal Tumor

Diagnostic Checklist
- Pseudotumor, extension of cortical tissue between pyramids
- Arcuate artery demonstrated on Doppler

DIFFERENTIAL DIAGNOSIS

Renal Scarring
- Reduced thickness of the cortex at the site of scarring
- Nodular compensatory hypertrophy of unaffected tissue

Renal Duplication
- Two central echogenic renal sinuses separated by intervening bridging renal parenchyma

Dromedary Hump
- Hypoechoic pseudotumor composed of normal renal tissue
- Bulge on renal cortex

Renal Tumor
- e.g., Renal cell carcinoma, metastases, lymphoma, angiomyolipoma etc.
- Mass is usually round or oval, may be heterogeneous in echogenicity
- Doppler: Hypervascular mass or displaced arcuate artery

PATHOLOGY

General Features
- General path comments: Embryology: Unresorbed polar parenchyma of one or both of two sub-kidneys that fuse to form a normal kidney

CLINICAL ISSUES

Presentation
- Most common signs/symptoms: Asymptomatic, normal variant
- Diagnosis
  - Usually found incidentally on imaging
  - Most likely to simulate a mass on sonography

DIAGNOSTIC CHECKLIST

Consider
- Pseudotumor, extension of cortical tissue between pyramids

Image Interpretation Pearls
- Isoechoic and continuous with renal cortex
- Arcuate artery demonstrated on Doppler
- Absence of a mass on CECT

SELECTED REFERENCES
1. Yeh HC et al: Junctional parenchyma: revised definition of hypertrophic column of Bertin. Radiology. 185(3):725-32, 1992
2. Seppala RE et al: Sonography of the hypertrophied column of Bertin. AJR Am J Roentgenol. 148(6):1277-8, 1987
3. Lafortune M et al: Sonography of the hypertrophied column of Bertin. AJR Am J Roentgenol. 146(1):53-6, 1986
4. Leekam RN et al: The sonography of renal columnar hypertrophy. J Clin Ultrasound. 11(9):491-4, 1983

IMAGE GALLERY

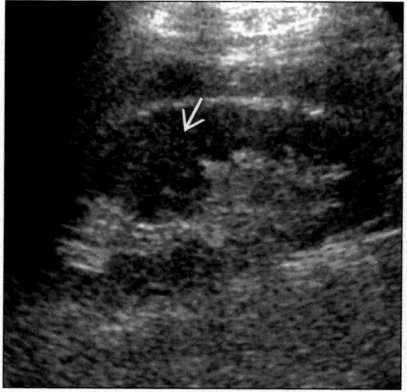 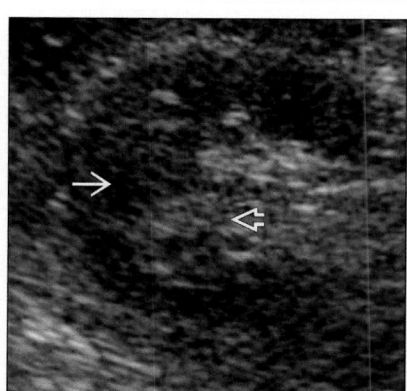 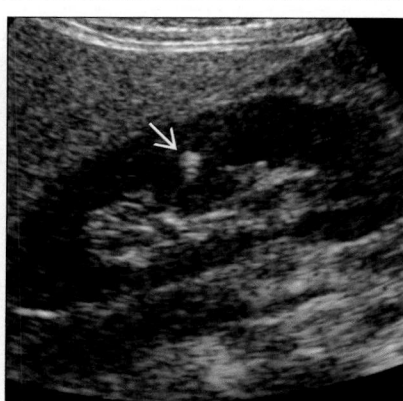

(Left) Longitudinal transabdominal ultrasound shows the classic appearance of a column of Bertin ➡. Note the smooth renal outline. *(Center)* Transverse transabdominal ultrasound shows a column of Bertin ➡. It is isoechoic and continuous with the adjacent cortex, indenting into the central renal sinus ➡. *(Right)* Longitudinal transabdominal ultrasound shows a classical column of Bertin, with a milk-of-calcium cyst ➡ present within it.

RENAL JUNCTION LINE

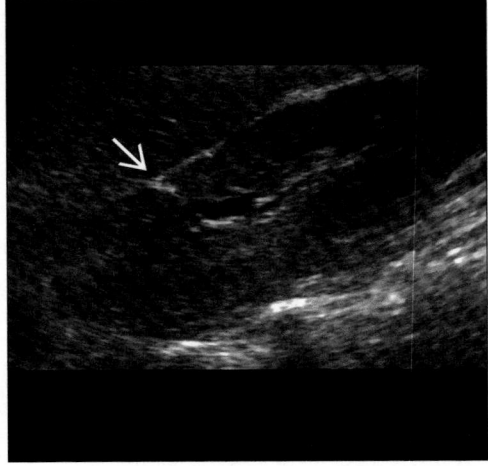

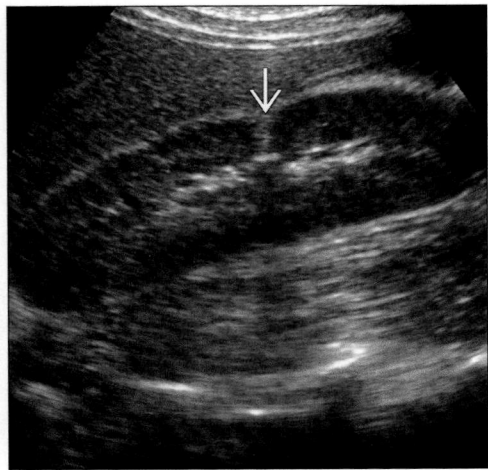

Longitudinal transabdominal ultrasound shows the typical appearance of a renal junction line ➡ *at the anterosuperior aspect of right kidney.*

Longitudinal transabdominal ultrasound shows a renal junction line ➡ *at the middle third of the right kidney. This location is less common than the one shown in the previous image.*

TERMINOLOGY

Abbreviations and Synonyms
- Junctional parenchymal defect and interrenuncular septum
- Intraparenchymal component of parenchymal junctional line
- Oddono sulcus

Definitions
- Line which represents plane of embryologic fusion between fetal renal lobes

IMAGING FINDINGS

General Features
- Best diagnostic clue
  - Echogenic line at upper and middle thirds of kidney without disruption of renal contour
  - Characteristic location at anterosuperior aspect of kidney
- Location
  - Junction of upper and middle thirds of the kidney

- More often seen on right than left side
- Uncommonly at posteroinferior surface of either kidney on posterior approach
- Size
  - Variable size of fusion defect
    - Small linear indentation or sulcus on renal surface
    - Deep fissure of varying depth
    - Hilar asymmetry as lateral wedge-shaped extension of anterosuperior recess of renal hilum
    - Complete cleft in continuity with lobar sulcus that opens into renal sinus

Ultrasonographic Findings
- Grayscale Ultrasound
  - Junctional parenchymal defect
    - Triangular echogenic focus at cortex
  - Interrenuncular septum
    - Echogenic line between upper and lower poles of kidney
    - Connects perirenal space with renal sinus
    - Occasionally may indent cortex

CT Findings
- Superficial notch containing fat at anterosuperior aspect of kidney

---

DDx: Renal Junctional Line

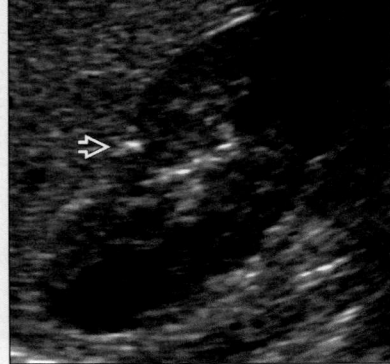

Scar

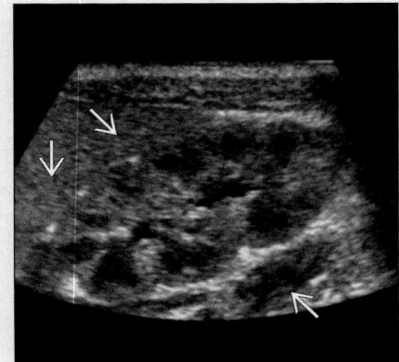

Fetal Lobulation

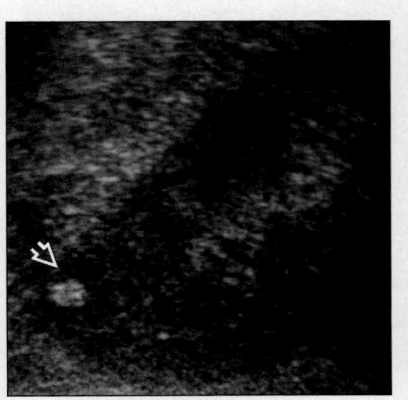

Angiomyolipoma

RENAL JUNCTION LINE

Key Facts

Terminology
- Line which represents plane of embryologic fusion between fetal renal lobes

Imaging Findings
- Echogenic line at upper and middle thirds of kidney without disruption of renal contour
- Characteristic location at anterosuperior aspect of kidney
- Triangular echogenic focus at cortex
- Overlays column of Bertin
- May extend as complete cleft crossing entire thickness of renal parenchyma into renal sinus

- Connects perirenal space with renal sinus

Top Differential Diagnoses
- Scar
- Fetal Lobulation
- Angiomyolipoma

Diagnostic Checklist
- Absence of parenchymal loss useful to differentiate it from cortical scar

DIFFERENTIAL DIAGNOSIS

Scar
- Focal indentation directly over calyces, associated with parenchymal thinning

Fetal Lobulation
- Indentations lie between renal pyramids or calyces

Angiomyolipoma
- Discrete echogenic mass, roundish in shape, intraparenchymal in location

PATHOLOGY

General Features
- General path comments: Layer of connective tissue trapped when proportion of kidneys form from fusion of two metanephric elements

Gross Pathologic & Surgical Features
- Deep diagonal groove extending from anterior surface of upper pole of kidney backward and downward into hilum

CLINICAL ISSUES

Natural History & Prognosis
- Normal variant

Treatment
- None

DIAGNOSTIC CHECKLIST

Image Interpretation Pearls
- Absence of parenchymal loss useful to differentiate it from cortical scar

SELECTED REFERENCES

1. Currarino G et al: The Oddono's sulcus and its relation to the renal "junctional parenchymal defect" and the "interrenicular septum". Pediatr Radiol. 27(1):6-10, 1997
2. Yeh HC et al: Junctional parenchyma: revised definition of hypertrophic column of Bertin. Radiology. 185(3):725-32, 1992
3. Kenney IJ et al: The renal parenchymal junctional line in children: ultrasonic frequency and appearances. Br J Radiol. 60(717):865-8, 1987
4. Hoffer FA et al: The interrenicular junction: a mimic of renal scarring on normal pediatric sonograms. AJR Am J Roentgenol. 145(5):1075-8, 1985
5. Hiromura T et al: Lobar dysmorphism of the kidney: reevaluation of junctional parenchyma using helical CT.

IMAGE GALLERY

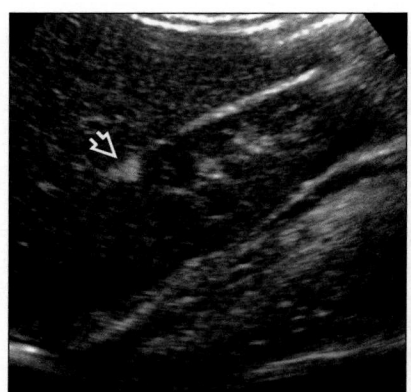 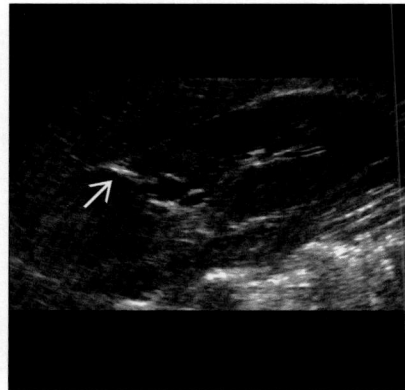 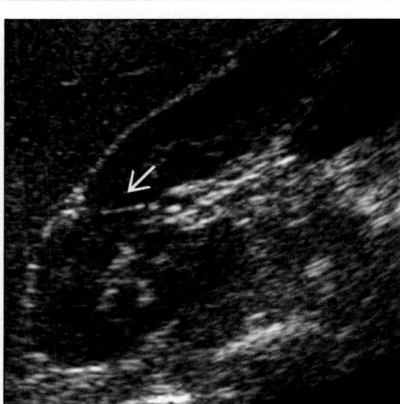

(Left) Longitudinal transabdominal ultrasound shows a junctional parenchymal defect as a triangular echogenic focus ➢ near the junction of the upper and middle third of the kidney. (Center) Longitudinal transabdominal ultrasound shows the interrenuncular septum ➡ as an echogenic line running from the cortex into the renal hilum. Note contour of renal outline is smooth. (Right) Oblique transabdominal ultrasound shows an echogenic line ➡ between the upper and middle thirds of the right kidney without disruption of the renal contour.

RENAL ECTOPIA

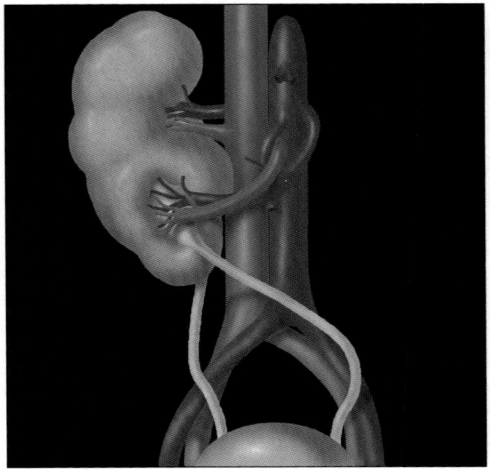

Graphic shows crossed inferior fused renal ectopia. Note the attendant left ureter inserts on the opposite side in its normal location.

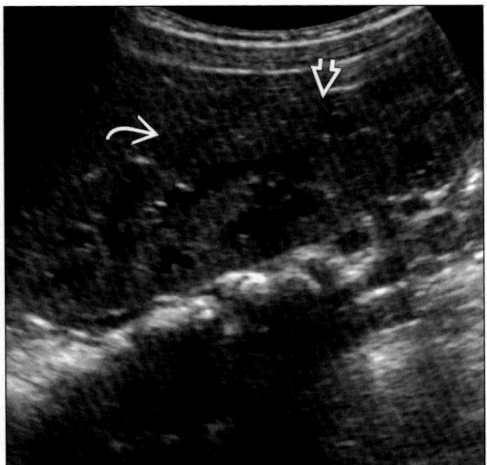

Longitudinal transabdominal ultrasound shows fusion of the upper pole of the crossed ectopic left kidney ⮞ to the lower pole of right kidney ⮞.

TERMINOLOGY

Abbreviations and Synonyms
- Renal ectopia (RE)

Definitions
- Abnormal location of kidney due to developmental anomaly

IMAGING FINDINGS

General Features
- Best diagnostic clue: Abnormal location of kidney
- Location
  - Kidneys normal location: 1st-3rd lumbar vertebrae
  - Ipsilateral RE: Kidney on same side of body as orifice of its attendant ureter
    - Cranial (superior RE): Above normal position; intrathoracic; or below eventrated diaphragm
    - Caudal (simple RE): Below normal position; abdominal, iliac or pelvic
    - Abdominal: Kidney lies above iliac crest, below L2
    - Iliac: Kidney located opposite iliac crest or in iliac fossa
    - Pelvic (sacral): Kidney located in true pelvis; below iliopectineal line
  - Crossed RE: Kidney located on opposite side of midline from its ureteral orifice
- Size: Ectopic kidneys vary in size
- Other general features
  - Caudal RE: Unilateral (more common), involvement of both kidneys (rare), solitary kidney (least common)
  - Crossed RE: With fusion (most common), without fusion (10-15%), solitary kidney (least common)
  - Classification of unilateral fused kidney or crossed fused RE
    - Superior RE: Kidney crosses over midline; lies superior to resident kidney
    - Inferior RE: Crossed kidney inferior to resident; its upper pole fused to lower pole of resident kidney
    - Sigmoid (S-shaped): Crossed kidney lies inferiorly
    - Unilateral lump kidney: Both kidneys completely fused; large irregular lump
    - Unilateral L-shaped: Crossed kidney inferior & transverse; resident kidney normally oriented

DDx: Ectopic Kidney

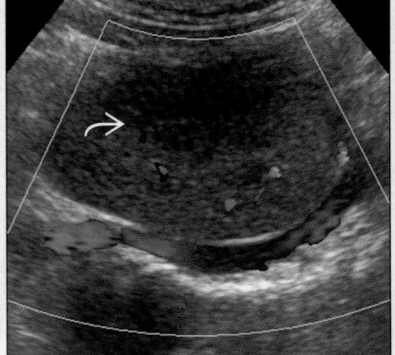

Transplant Kidney

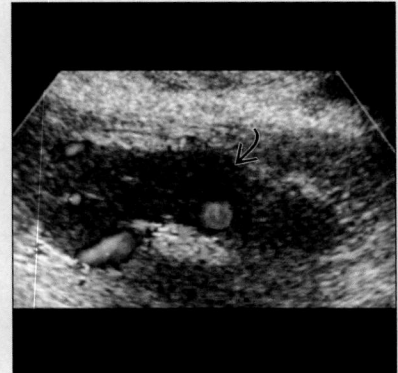

Horseshoe Kidney

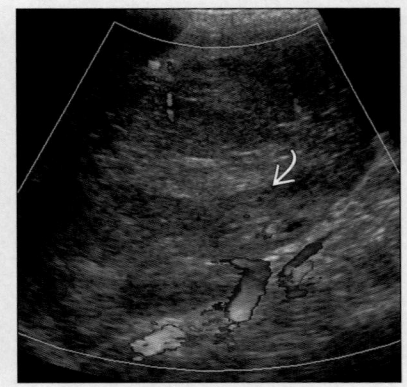

Displaced Kidney

RENAL ECTOPIA

Key Facts

Terminology
- Renal ectopia (RE)
- Abnormal location of kidney due to developmental anomaly

Imaging Findings
- Best diagnostic clue: Abnormal location of kidney
- Cranial RE: Kidney lies just below an eventrated diaphragm
- Caudal RE (abdominal, iliac, or pelvic): Renal sinus echo complex: Eccentric or absent
- Crossed RE: Both kidneys on the same side with separable outline
- Crossed fused RE: Fused lower pole unit positioned medially, extending anterior to spine

Top Differential Diagnoses
- Renal Allograft: Transplanted Kidney in Iliac Fossa
- Renal Autotransplantation
- Horseshoe Kidney
- Acquired Renal Displacement

Diagnostic Checklist
- Important not to confuse RE with renal ptosis
- Make sure no other intra-abdominal mass present to displace kidney to simulate crossed unfused RE
- Look for associated features with RE: Obstructive hydronephrosis, infection, calculus formation
- CECT helps in detecting RE & cause of displacement
- MR urography demonstrates the relative positions of RE and ureteric insertion

---

- Unilateral disc: Each kidney fused to other along medial concave border

Ultrasonographic Findings
- Grayscale Ultrasound
  - Cranial RE: Kidney lies just below an eventrated diaphragm
    - Passing through defect in diaphragm
  - Caudal RE (abdominal, iliac, or pelvic): Renal sinus echo complex: Eccentric or absent
    - Kidney commonly small, malrotated or dysmorphic
  - Crossed RE: Both kidneys on the same side with separable outline
    - Absence of kidney in expected site of renal fossa
    - Kidneys move separately from each other during respiration
  - Crossed fused RE: Fused lower pole unit positioned medially, extending anterior to spine
    - 85-90% cases of crossed ectopia
    - Usually fusion of upper pole of ectopic kidney to lower pole of normal positioned kidney
    - Apparent elongated kidney with anterior or posterior notches in renal parenchyma
    - Both kidneys more caudally located than normal
    - Two renal sinuses lie in different planes and different orientation
- Color Doppler
  - Pelvic kidney
    - Arterial supply from common iliac or internal iliac arteries
  - Crossed RE and crossed fused RE
    - Separate vascular supply to each kidney, invariably aberrant renal arteries
    - Aberrant arteries may cross ureter and cause obstruction
    - Ureteric jets from ureterovesical junctions located in their normal position

Radiographic Findings
- IVP
  - Cranial RE: Kidney lies partially or completely in thorax

- Length of attendant ureter longer than normal
  - Abdominal or iliac RE: Kidney in either abdominal or iliac area
    - Kidney usually smaller & ureter shorter than normal
    - Bizarre pattern of calyces; extrarenal calyces (common)
  - Pelvic kidney: Left (70%) > right; if bilateral, left usually lower than right kidney & generally fused
    - Ureter is frequently too high as it exits renal pelvis ("high insertion")
    - May see ectopic ureter, extrarenal calyces, calyceal diverticula
  - Crossed RE: Distal ureter inserts into trigone on side of origin
    - Superior RE, inferior RE and unilateral lump kidney: Both pelvises rotated anteriorly
    - Sigmoid (S-shaped): Resident kidney pelvis is medial; lateral in crossed kidney
    - Unilateral disc: Resident kidney pelvis is anteromedial, pelvis of other is anterolateral
  - Bilateral crossed RE: Both kidneys on wrong side but their attendant ureters arise normally

CT Findings
- Cranial RE: Kidney residing in thorax; differentiate from a mediastinal mass
  - Adrenal gland may lie above, behind or below ectopic kidney
- Abdominal or iliac RE
  - Adrenal gland in normal place; appears linear on CT
  - Colonic flexures, duodenum, loops of small bowel, spleen, tail of pancreas in abnormal position
- Pelvic RE: Differentiate RE from various pelvic masses
- Crossed RE: CT with thin (4-5 mm) slices may show degree of separation of kidneys

MR Findings
- Cross RE
  - MR urography
    - Maximum Intensity Projection (MIP) image shows relative position of both kidneys

RENAL ECTOPIA

- Fusion of collecting system clearly demonstrated in fused RE
- Contrast-enhanced image shows the course of ureters and normal position of ureterovesical junctions

Nuclear Medicine Findings
- Tc99m-DMSA or Tc99m-glucoheptonate scan
  - Detects ectopic kidney by outlining kidney shape
  - Crossed fused renal ectopia: Isotope excretion or localization by a kidney, with no contralateral isotope excretion or localization

DIFFERENTIAL DIAGNOSIS

Renal Allograft: Transplanted Kidney in Iliac Fossa
- Small echogenic native kidneys visible in renal beds
- Renal vessels anastomosed to external iliac artery, vein
- Ureter reimplanted into bladder via submucosal tunnel; variable axis of pelvis

Renal Autotransplantation
- Surgically repositioning patient's own kidney

Horseshoe Kidney
- Fusion of lower poles of kidneys in low mid-abdomen

Acquired Renal Displacement
- Due to large liver, splenic or any retroperitoneal tumor

PATHOLOGY

General Features
- Etiology
  - Cranial RE: Kidney herniated into thorax through lumbocostal triangle or foramen of Bochdalek
  - Caudal RE: Diminished ureteral growth; umbilical arteries block cranial ascent of kidney; asymmetry in level of development of 2 kidneys
  - Crossed RE: Mesonephric ducts & ureteral buds may stray from normal course
  - RE inherited as autosomal recessive trait; reported in monozygotic twins
- Epidemiology
  - Cranial RE: 1 in 15,000 autopsies
  - Abdominal or iliac RE: 1 in 600 on intravenous pyelogram (IVP)
  - Pelvic kidney: 1 in 725 live births
  - Unilateral crossed fused RE: 1 in 1,300 to 1 in 7,600
- Associated abnormalities
  - Genitourinary (50%): Malrotation, hypospadias, high insertion of ureter into renal pelvis, ectopic ureter, extrarenal calyces, calyceal diverticula, bladder extrophy
  - Skeletal (40%): Anomalies of ribs, vertebral bodies; skull asymmetry & absence of radius
  - Cardiovascular (40%): Valvular & septal defects
  - Gastrointestinal (33%): Anorectal malformations, malrotation.
  - Ears, lips, palate (33%): Low-set or absent ears; hare lip; cleft palate
  - Hematopoietic (7%): Fanconi anemia
  - Cranial RE: Omphalocele
  - Pelvic kidney: Vesicoureteral reflux, contralateral renal agenesis, absent or hypoplastic vagina
  - Crossed ectopia: Megaureter, cryptorchidism, urethral valves, multicystic dysplasia

CLINICAL ISSUES

Presentation
- Most common signs/symptoms
  - May be asymptomatic, incidental finding
  - May present with signs & symptoms of obstruction, urolithiasis, reflux & infection

Demographics
- Gender: Cranial RE (M > F); crossed fused RE (M < F)

Natural History & Prognosis
- Complications
  - Obstruction, urolithiasis, reflux, infection
  - Pelvic kidneys: ↓ Function & may obstruct labor
  - Aberrant arteries may cross & obstruct ureter
  - Abdominal & iliac ectopic kidneys more injury prone; prone to vascular injury during aortic surgery
- Prognosis
  - Recurrent obstruction, reflux, infection: Poor

Treatment
- Treat complications of renal ectopia

DIAGNOSTIC CHECKLIST

Image Interpretation Pearls
- Important not to confuse RE with renal ptosis
  - Kidney drops further down in abdomen from its normal position, but attendant ureter of normal length & renal arteries arise from normal site
- Make sure no other intra-abdominal mass present to displace kidney to simulate crossed unfused RE
  - Retroperitoneal mass, huge renal cyst, gigantic renal pelvis secondary to ureteropelvic obstruction
- Look for associated features with RE: Obstructive hydronephrosis, infection, calculus formation
- CECT helps in detecting RE & cause of displacement
- MR urography demonstrates the relative positions of RE and ureteric insertion

SELECTED REFERENCES

1. Guarino N et al: The incidence of associated urological abnormalities in children with renal ectopia. J Urol. 172(4 Pt 2):1757-9; discussion 1759, 2004
2. Birmole BJ et al: Crossed renal ectopia. J Postgrad Med. 39(3):149-51, 1993
3. Goodman JD et al: Crossed fused renal ectopia: sonographic diagnosis. Urol Radiol. 8(1):13-6, 1986
4. McCarthy S et al: Ultrasonography in crossed renal ectopia. J Ultrasound Med. 3(3):107-12, 1984
5. Hertz M et al: Crossed renal ectopia: clinical and radiological findings in 22 cases. Clin Radiol. 28(3):339-44, 1977

RENAL ECTOPIA

IMAGE GALLERY

Typical

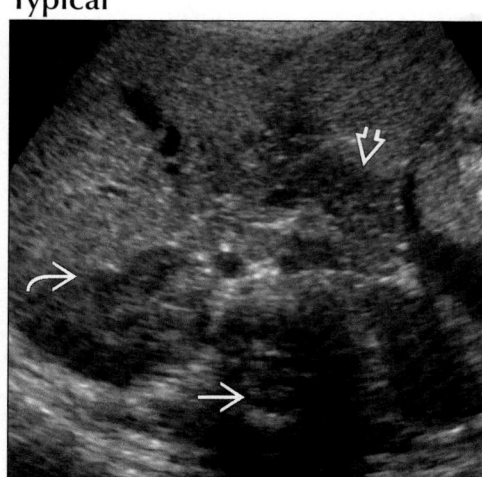

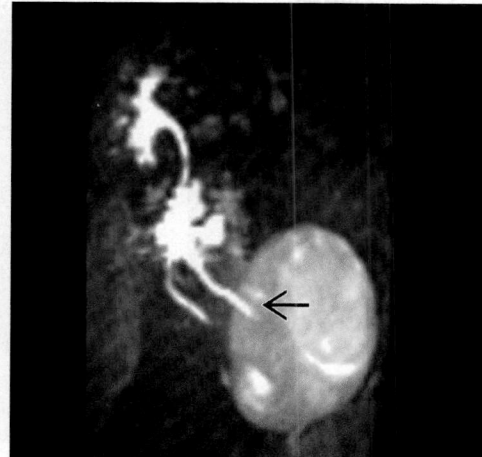

(Left) Transverse transabdominal ultrasound shows the left kidney ⇒ located inferomedial to the right kidney ⇒, anterior to spine ⇒. *(Right)* Oblique MR urography shows relative positions of both kidneys. Note collecting systems are separated. The left ureter ⇒ inserts at its normal position at the vesicoureteric junction.

Typical

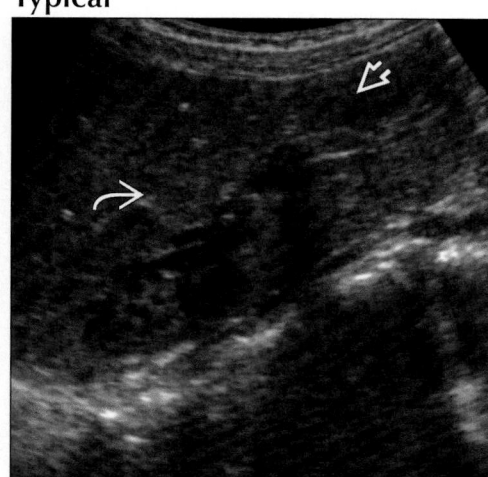

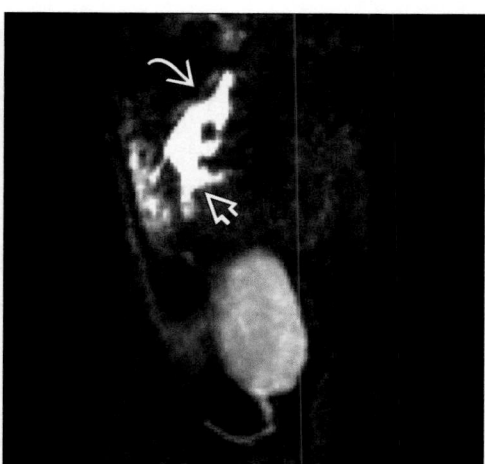

(Left) Longitudinal transabdominal ultrasound shows fusion of the upper pole of crossed ectopic left kidney ⇒ to the lower pole of the right kidney ⇒. The fused renal complex is longer than a normal single kidney. *(Right)* Longitudinal T1 C+ MR shows fusion of the collecting system of the ectopic left kidney ⇒ to the right kidney ⇒.

Typical

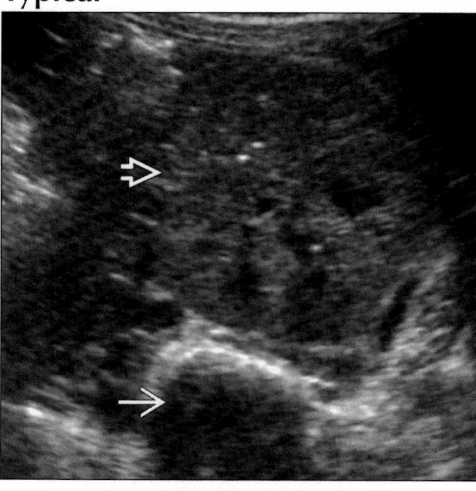

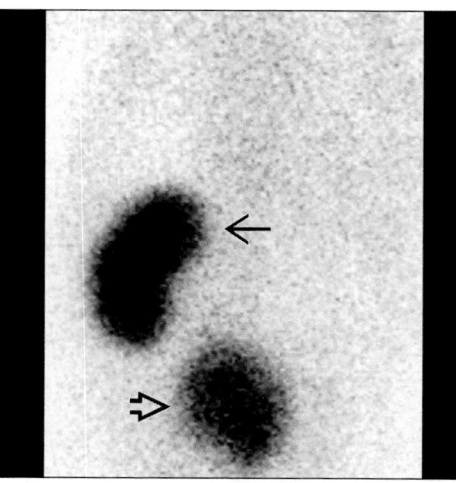

(Left) Transverse transabdominal ultrasound shows an ectopic kidney ⇒ in the left iliac fossa, just anterior to spine ⇒. *(Right)* Longitudinal DMSA radio-isotope scan shows the ectopic left kidney ⇒ in the pelvis, much lower in position than the right kidney ⇒.

HORSESHOE KIDNEY

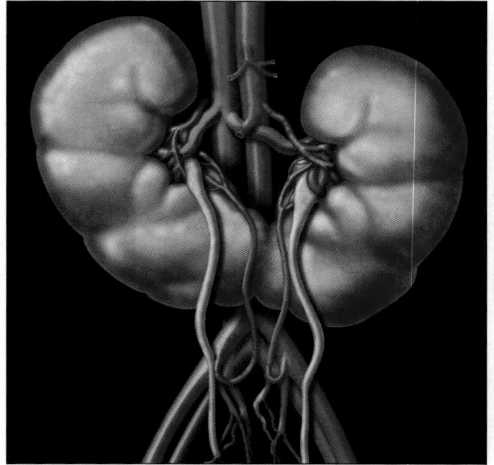

Graphic shows a horseshoe kidney with the isthmus anterior to the aorta and inferior vena cava and fusion of the lower poles.

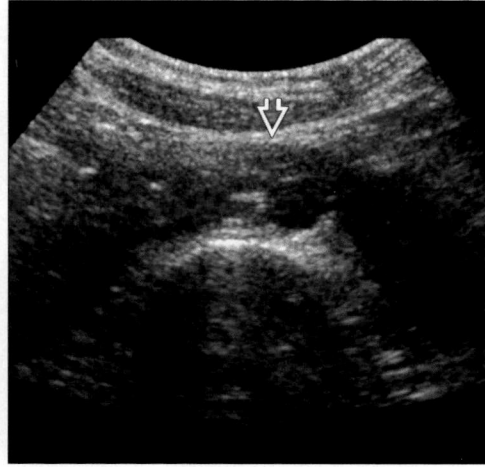

Transverse transabdominal ultrasound shows a classic horseshoe kidney with an isthmus of renal tissue ➡ *crossing the midline, anterior to the spine, inferior vena cava and aorta.*

TERMINOLOGY

Definitions
- Congenital anomaly of the kidney where 2 kidneys are fused by isthmus at the lower poles

IMAGING FINDINGS

General Features
- Best diagnostic clue: 2 kidneys on opposite sides of the body with the lower poles fused in midline
- Location
  - Ectopic, lies lower than normal kidney
  - Isthmus usually anterior to aorta and inferior vena cava (IVC) at L4/L5 level
  - Rarely, isthmus is posterior or in between aorta (posterior) and IVC (anterior)
- Morphology
  - 2 types of fusion
    - Midline or symmetrical fusion (90% of cases)
    - Lateral or asymmetrical fusion

Ultrasonographic Findings
- Grayscale Ultrasound
  - May be missed on US, therefore pay careful attention to identification of lower poles of kidneys
  - Kidneys usually lower than normal
  - Renal long axis medially orientated
  - Lower poles with curved configuration, elongation and poorly-defined
  - Inverted triangular or pyriform shape (longitudinal scan)
  - Isthmus crosses midline anterior to spine and great vessels
  - Difficult to visualize isthmus in subjects with large body habitus, or if isthmus is composed of fibrous tissue
  - Look for associated pelvocaliectasis and calculus

Radiographic Findings
- Radiography
  - Kidney appears too close to the spine
  - Vertical long axis of kidney may be seen, lower poles lie closer to spine
  - Visualize the isthmus of the 2 kidneys
- IVP

DDx: Horseshoe Kidney

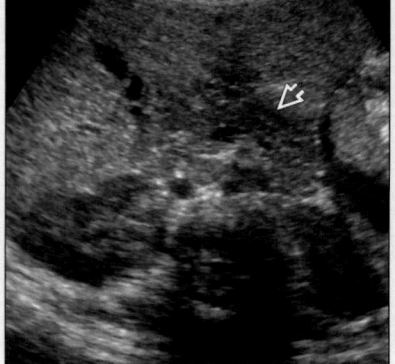

Cross Renal Ectopia

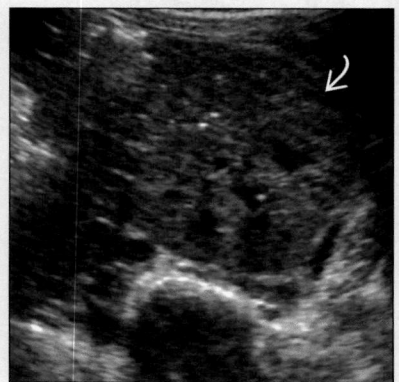

Pelvic Kidney

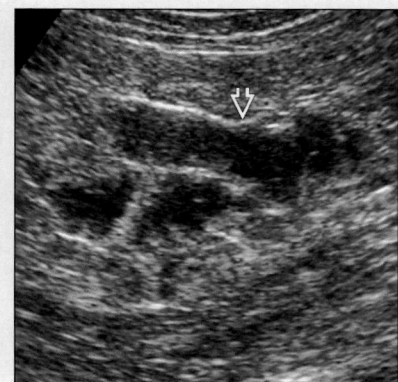

Small Bowel Loop

HORSESHOE KIDNEY

Key Facts

Terminology
- Congenital anomaly of the kidney where 2 kidneys are fused by isthmus at the lower poles

Imaging Findings
- Best diagnostic clue: 2 kidneys on opposite sides of the body with the lower poles fused in midline
- Midline or symmetrical fusion (90% of cases)
- May be missed on US, therefore pay careful attention to identification of lower poles of kidneys
- Renal long axis medially orientated
- Lower poles with curved configuration, elongation and poorly-defined
- Isthmus crosses midline anterior to spine and great vessels
- US for diagnosis in utero

- IVP followed by CT or scintigraphy for pre-operative assessment

Top Differential Diagnoses
- Renal Ectopia (RE)
- Crossed renal ectopia: 2 kidneys are on the same side of the body (right side > left)
- Small Bowel Loop
- Para-Aortic Lymphadenopathy

Clinical Issues
- Asymptomatic or associated abnormalities
- Gender: M:F = 2:1

Diagnostic Checklist
- Associated abnormalities and other complications in imaging, treatment and prognosis
- Kidney appears U-shaped with isthmus in midline

- Midline fusion
  - Hand holding calyces: Lower calyces descend toward midline near isthmus
  - Nephrogram is U-shaped
- Lateral fusion
  - Lower calyces crosses midline and drain part of renal parenchyma on opposite kidney
  - Nephrogram is L-shaped
  - One part crosses midline and lies in transverse position, renal pelvis lies anteriorly or laterally
  - Remaining part lies in vertical position, renal pelvis lies anteriorly or medially
- Renal pelvis often large and flabby; ureter inserts abnormally high in renal pelvis
- Rarely, kidney is fused at the upper poles (5%)
- Ipsilateral lower calyces medial to ureter; may simulate renal malrotation without fusion
- Ureteropelvic (more common) or ureterovesical junction obstruction with delayed clearing of contrast
- "Flower-vase" appearance: Each ureter crosses isthmus and curves laterally and continues medially, assuming a normal course distally

CT Findings
- CTA
  - Variant arterial supply
    - Multiple, bilateral renal arteries
    - Inferior mesenteric artery always crosses the isthmus
    - Arteries arising from aorta or common iliac, internal iliac, external iliac or inferior mesenteric arteries
- CECT
  - Define structural abnormalities
    - Degree and site of fusion: Midline or lateral fusion
    - Degree of renal malrotation
    - Renal parenchymal changes (e.g., scarring, cystic disease)
    - Collecting system abnormalities (e.g., duplex system, hydronephrosis)
  - Differentiate composition of isthmus between fibrous or normal parenchymal tissue

Nuclear Medicine Findings
- Demonstrate fusion with functional parenchymal tissue

Angiographic Findings
- Conventional: Variant arterial supply

Imaging Recommendations
- Best imaging tool
  - US for diagnosis in utero
  - IVP followed by CT or scintigraphy for pre-operative assessment
- Protocol advice: CTA: Use 3D volume-rendered CT to better define the vessels

DIFFERENTIAL DIAGNOSIS

Renal Ectopia (RE)
- Kidney congenitally in abnormal position
- Ipsilateral or simple ectopia: Kidney on proper side of body as its ureter
  - Abdominal: Kidney lies above iliac crest but below L2
  - Iliac: Kidney is located opposite iliac crest or in iliac fossa
  - Pelvic (sacral): Kidney in true pelvis
- Crossed renal ectopia: 2 kidneys are on the same side of the body (right side > left)
  - With fusion (90%): 2 fused kidneys lie on the same side of spine; ureter of crossed kidney crosses midline to insert into bladder
  - Without fusion: 2 kidneys lie on the same side of spine without fusion; ureter of crossed kidney crosses midline to insert into bladder
  - Solitary: 1 kidney arises on the wrong side, ureter crosses midline to insert into bladder
  - Bilateral: Left and right kidneys arise on the wrong side, both ureters crosses midline to insert into bladder

HORSESHOE KIDNEY

Small Bowel Loop
- Collapsed or fluid-filled small bowel loop crossing midline
- Peristalsis/change in configuration on real-time scanning

Para-Aortic Lymphadenopathy
- Soft tissue mass at midline anterior to spine
- May extend lateral to kidneys but no fusion seen
- Both kidneys normal in axis and alignment

PATHOLOGY

General Features
- General path comments: Most common renal fusion anomaly
- Genetics: Reported in identical twins, but no clear evidence
- Epidemiology: 1:400 people
- Associated abnormalities
  - Congenital disorders
    - Chromosomal abnormalities: Turner syndrome, trisomy 18
    - Hematological abnormalities: Fanconi anemia, dyskeratosis congenita with pancytopenia
    - Laurence-Biedl-Moon syndrome
    - Thalidomide embryopathy
  - Anomalies (most common to least common)
    - Ureteropelvic junction (UPJ) obstruction
    - Vesicoureteral reflux
    - Unilateral or bilateral duplication
    - Megaureter
    - Ectopic ureter
    - Unilateral triplication
    - Renal dysplasia
    - Retrocaval ureter
    - Supernumerary kidney
    - Anorectal malformation
    - Esophageal atresia
    - Rectovaginal fistula
    - Omphalocele
    - Cardiovascular, vertebral, neurological, peripheral skeletal or facial anomalies

Gross Pathologic & Surgical Features
- Isthmus is composed of normal parenchyma or connective tissue

CLINICAL ISSUES

Presentation
- Most common signs/symptoms
  - Asymptomatic or associated abnormalities
  - Vague abdominal pain, radiating to the back
  - Nausea and vomiting
  - Rovsing sign, palpable abdominal mass

Demographics
- Age
  - Any age
- Still births > infants > children > adults; ↓ with age because many diagnosed based on associated abnormalities
- Gender: M:F = 2:1

Natural History & Prognosis
- Complications
  - Trauma injury: Isthmus lies anteriorly without protection by ribs → split by hard blow to abdomen
  - UPJ obstruction: High "insertion" of ureter
  - Recurrent infections: Vesicoureteral reflux and UPJ obstruction
  - Urolithiasis: 75% metabolic calculi, 25% struvite calculi
  - Wilms tumors in children: 2-8x more common
  - Primary renal carcinoid tumor: ↑ Prevalence
- Prognosis
  - Poor, with associated abnormalities causing significant morbidity and mortality
  - Good, without other abnormalities

Treatment
- Surgical separation in symptomatic patients

DIAGNOSTIC CHECKLIST

Consider
- Associated abnormalities and other complications in imaging, treatment and prognosis

Image Interpretation Pearls
- Kidney appears U-shaped with isthmus in midline
- In any patient when soft tissue is seen anterior to the spine, aorta, IVC, always carefully identify lower poles of both kidneys to rule out a horseshoe kidney

SELECTED REFERENCES

1. Strauss S et al: Sonographic features of horseshoe kidney: review of 34 patients. J Ultrasound Med. 19(1):27-31, 2000
2. Pozniac MA et al: Three-dimensional computed tomographic angiography of a horseshoe kidney with ureteropelvic junction obstruction. Urology 49:267-268, 1997
3. Banerjee B et al: Ultrasound diagnosis of horseshoe kidney. Br J Radiol. 64(766):898-900, 1991
4. Mesrobian HG et al: Wilms tumor in horseshoe kidneys: a report from the National Wilms Tumor Study. J Urol. 133(6):1002-3, 1985
5. Grainger R et al: Horseshoe kidney--a review of the presentation, associated congenital anomalies and complications in 73 patients. Ir Med J. 76(7):315-7, 1983
6. Evans WP et al: Horseshoe kidney and urolithiasis. J Urol. 125(5):620-1, 1981
7. Pitts WR Jr et al: Horseshoe kidneys: a 40-year experience. J Urol. 113(6):743-6, 1975
8. Whitehouse GH: Some urographic aspects of the horseshoe kidney anomaly-a review of 59 cases. Clin Radiol. 26(1):107-14, 1975
9. Boatman DL et al: Congenital anomalies associated with horseshoe kidney. J Urol. 107:205-7, 1973
10. Kolln CP et al: Horseshoe kidney: a review of 105 patients. J Urol. 107(2):203-4, 1972
11. Segura JW et al: Horseshoe kidney in children. J Urol. 108:333-6, 1972

IMAGE GALLERY

Typical

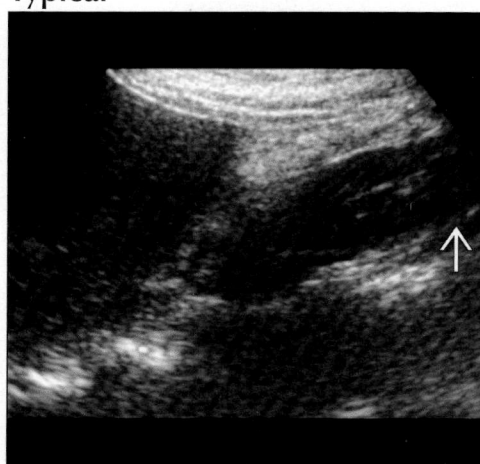
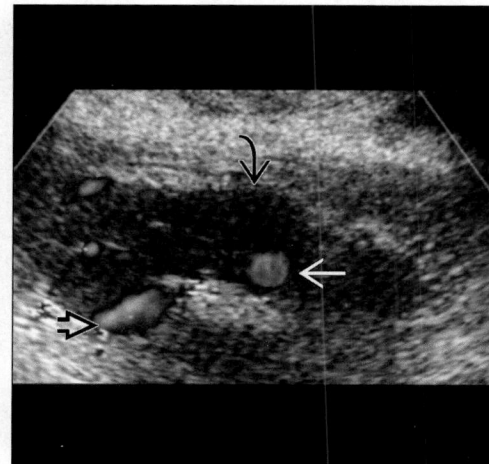

(Left) Longitudinal transabdominal ultrasound shows a low-lying right kidney with an elongated and poorly-defined lower pole ➡. (Right) Transverse color Doppler ultrasound shows the isthmus ➔ crossing the midline anterior to the inferior vena cava ▷ and aorta ➡.

Typical

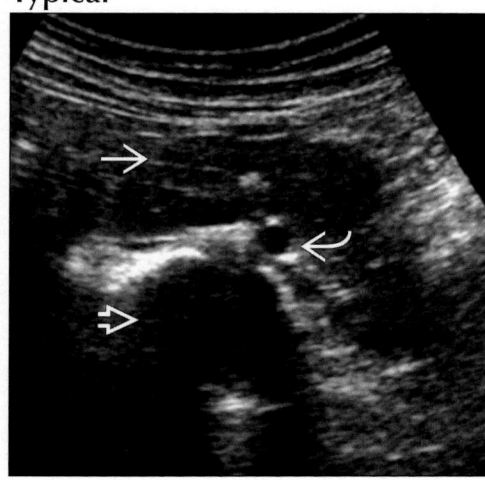
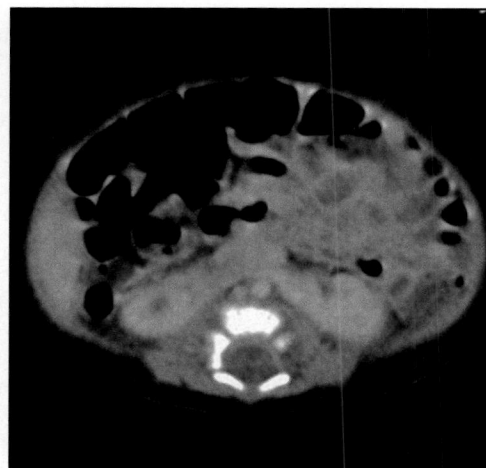

(Left) Transverse transabdominal ultrasound shows fusion of the lower poles of both kidneys with an isthmus of renal tissue crossing the midline ➡ anterior to the aorta ➔ and spine ➡. (Right) Transverse CECT shows enhancing parenchymal isthmus crossing the midline and connecting the lower poles of both kidneys.

Typical

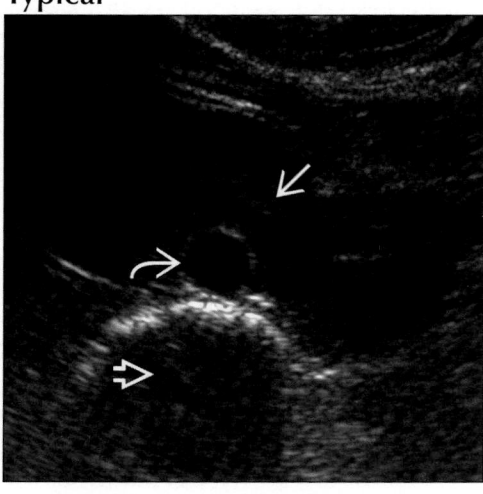
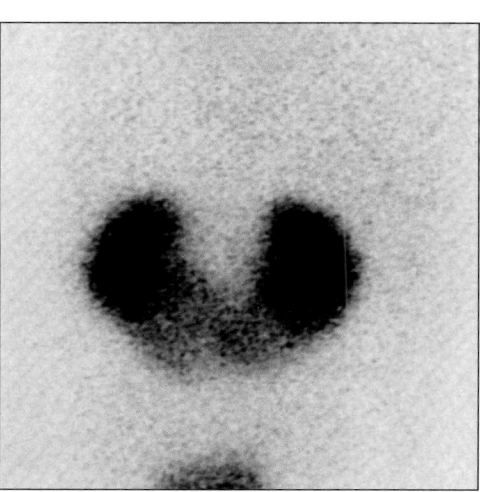

(Left) Transverse transabdominal ultrasound shows fusion of the lower poles of both kidneys with an isthmus of renal tissue ➡ crossing the midline anterior to the aorta ➔ and spine ➡. (Right) Tc-99m DMSA scan shows symmetrical midline fusion of a horseshoe kidney with a characteristic U-shape.

URETERAL DUPLICATION

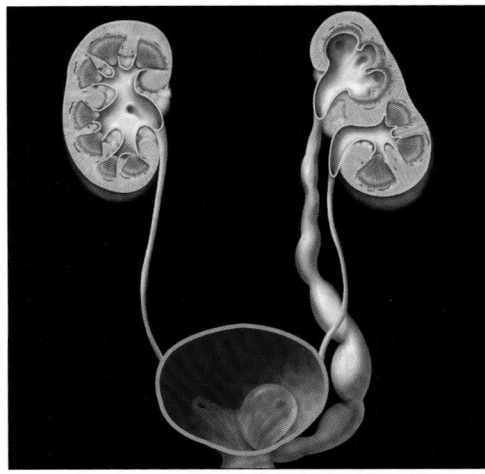

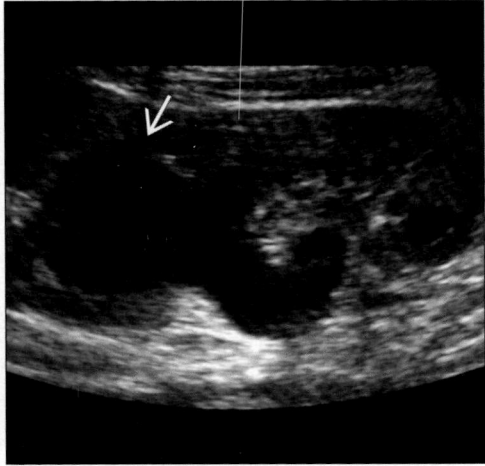

Graphic shows a left duplex kidney. Upper moiety is hydronephrotic with a hydroureter draining into an ectopic ureterocele. Note upper moiety ureter inserts medial and caudal to lower moiety ureter.

Longitudinal transabdominal ultrasound shows a duplex kidney with a dilated upper moiety collecting system ➡, associated with cortical thinning. The lower moiety is unremarkable.

TERMINOLOGY

Abbreviations and Synonyms
- Double ureters, duplex collecting system, bifid collecting system, duplicate pyelocalyceal system

Definitions
- 2 ureters drain a duplex kidney and remain separate to bladder or beyond

IMAGING FINDINGS

General Features
- Best diagnostic clue
  - Look for two distinct renal pelves in a kidney
  - Two central echogenic renal sinuses with intervening bridging renal parenchyma
  - One or two dilated ureters on ipsilateral side
- Other general features
  - 85% obey Weigert-Meyer rule: Upper moiety ureter inserts medial & caudal to lower moiety ureter
  - 15% upper moiety ureter inserts anywhere along ectopic pathway
  - Most commonly, upper moiety ureter is ectopic & obstructed due to ectopic insertion, ectopic ureterocele or abnormal vessel crossing it
  - Lower moiety ureter subjected to reflux due to its shortened ureteric tunnel at bladder insertion
  - Kidney & ureter may be normal, except duplicated
  - 20% of contralateral ureter is also duplicated

Ultrasonographic Findings
- Grayscale Ultrasound
  - Non-hydronephrotic duplex collecting system
    - Two central echogenic renal sinuses with intervening bridging renal parenchyma
    - Course of duplicated, non-dilated ureters cannot be traced by US, best seen by IVP or CT urography
    - Renal enlargement
  - Hydronephrotic duplex collecting system
    - Commonly hydronephrotic upper pole moiety with hydroureter
    - Occasional dysplastic small upper pole moiety with hydroureter
    - Upper moiety ureter inserts more medial and inferior than lower moiety ureter

DDx: Ureteric Duplication

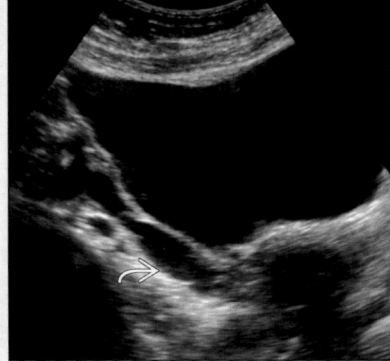

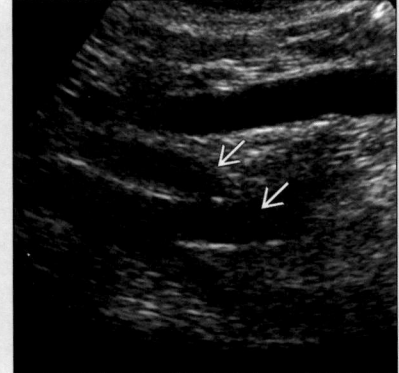

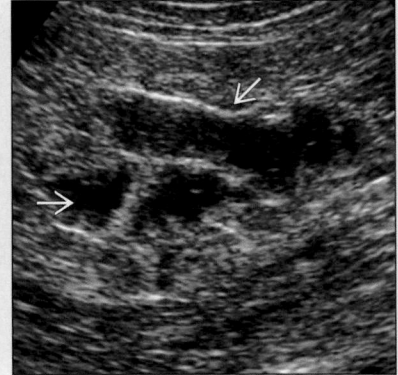

Hydrosalpinx

Iliac Vessels

Fluid in Bowel

URETERAL DUPLICATION

Key Facts

Terminology
- 2 ureters drain a duplex kidney and remain separate to bladder or beyond

Imaging Findings
- Look for two distinct renal pelves in a kidney
- Two central echogenic renal sinuses with intervening bridging renal parenchyma
- 85% obey Weigert-Meyer rule: Upper moiety ureter inserts medial & caudal to lower moiety ureter
- Commonly hydronephrotic upper pole moiety with hydroureter
- Occasional dysplastic small upper pole moiety with hydroureter
- Upper moiety ureter inserts more medial and inferior than lower moiety ureter
- Upper moiety ureter associated with ureterocele, cystic structure within bladder
- Lower moiety can be hydronephrotic due to reflux
- Transrectal or transvaginal US may identify ectopic ureteric insertion into prostate or vagina

Top Differential Diagnoses
- Hydrosalpinx
- Iliac Vessels
- Fluid-Filled Bowel
- Ureterocele

Diagnostic Checklist
- 2 distinct ureters
- IVP or CT urography are imaging modalities of choice
- US does not clearly demonstrate course of non-dilated ureters

- ■ Upper moiety ureter associated with ureterocele, cystic structure within bladder
- ■ Lower moiety can be hydronephrotic due to reflux
- ■ Upper moiety ureter with extravesicle insertion can be traced as hydroureter beyond bladder neck
- ■ Transrectal or transvaginal US may identify ectopic ureteric insertion into prostate or vagina
- Color Doppler: Ureteric jets can be located to identify vesicoureteric junction of both upper and lower moieties

Radiographic Findings
- IVP (or CT urography)
  - Duplex kidney with double ureters; 2 jets of contrast
  - Poor or no excretion by upper pole of duplex kidney
  - "Drooping lily" sign: Hydronephrosis and ↓ function of obstructed upper pole → downward displacement of lower pole calyces
  - "Nubbin" sign: Scarring, atrophy and ↓ function of lower pole moiety; may simulate renal mass
  - Fewer calyces & infundibula of lower pole collecting system; shortened upper pole infundibulum
  - Single or diffuse calyceal clubbing, thin overlying parenchyma ± scarring in lower pole
  - ± Ureteropelvic junction obstruction of lower pole
- Voiding cystourethrogram
  - ± Reflux, ureterocele, diverticulum of urethra
  - Best to demonstrate ectopic ureter of a nonfunctioning moiety when vesicoureteral reflux present

CT Findings
- "Faceless kidney": No renal sinus or collecting system at junction of upper & lower pole of a duplex kidney
- ± Obstruction in either pole of a duplex kidney

MR Findings
- T1WI
  - Low signal intensity duplicated ureter, tortuous and dilated if obstructed
  - Severe hydronephrosis or dysplastic upper moiety depending on degree of obstruction
  - Can detect parenchymal scarring due to reflux

- T2WI
  - High signal intensity ureter, tortuous or dilated to level of insertion if obstructed
  - Superior to demonstrate ectopic ureter extending from poorly functioning moiety of duplex kidney invisible on other imaging
  - Maximum intensity projection (MIP) image, demonstrate relative positions of upper and lower moiety ureters
- T1 C+
  - Variable degree of function of obstructed upper moiety can be seen
  - Delayed image can demonstrate whole course of non-dilated ureter
  - Ureteroceles can sometimes be demonstrated within bladder

Nuclear Medicine Findings
- ± Reflux up ureter in nonfunctioning duplex kidney with ureteral duplication
- Assess relative function, important for surgical planning
- Detect parenchymal scarring

Imaging Recommendations
- Best imaging tool: IVP or CT urography

DIFFERENTIAL DIAGNOSIS

Hydrosalpinx
- Obstructed fallopian tube, usually caused by pelvic inflammatory disease
- Look for polypoid projections/fold, internal debris, wall hyperemia
- Usually associated with fluid in cul-de-sac, uterine enlargement, endometrial fluid and thickening

Iliac Vessels
- Pulsate, confirmed by color Doppler

Fluid-Filled Bowel
- May simulate tortuous ureter, peristalsis/change in configuration on real time scanning

URETERAL DUPLICATION

Ureterocele
• Can be isolated finding

PATHOLOGY

General Features
• General path comments: Both ureters pass through bladder wall through a common tunnel
• Etiology
  ○ Genetics: Autosomal dominant with low penetrance
  ○ Environment: Geographic areas → ↑ prevalence
• Epidemiology: 1 per 500 persons
• Associated abnormalities
  ○ Solitary or dysplastic kidney, hypoplastic kidneys, all types of fused kidneys or posterior urethral valves
  ○ Complex congenital anomalies: VATER, VACTERL (vertebral, anal, cardiovascular, tracheoesophageal, renal and limb)

CLINICAL ISSUES

Presentation
• Most common signs/symptoms
  ○ Diagnosed in utero on antenatal ultrasound
  ○ Usually asymptomatic
  ○ Ureteropelvic junction obstruction more common in duplex kidney, present as huge abdominal mass
  ○ Incontinence in females due to insertion of upper pole ureteral orifice below bladder sphincter
  ○ No enuresis in males as insertion is always above external sphincter
  ○ Epididymitis/orchitis in pre adolescent males
  ○ Urge incontinence in males due to insertion of ureter into posterior urethra
  ○ Intermittent or persistent urinary tract infections ± acute pyelonephritis, due to reflux
  ○ Urethral obstruction in either male or female due to prolapsed ureterocele associated with duplicated ureter
• Other signs/symptoms: Transitional cell carcinoma of duplicated ureter occurs in elderly population

Demographics
• Gender: M:F = 1:10

Natural History & Prognosis
• Complications: Urolithiasis, abscess, renal failure

Treatment
• Lower grades of reflux: Medical treatment
• Higher grades of reflux, upper pole obstruction, ectopy, poor renal function: Surgical treatment

DIAGNOSTIC CHECKLIST

Consider
• Young females with recurrent urinary tract infections
• Young females with continuous dribbling urinary incontinence

Image Interpretation Pearls
• 2 distinct ureters
• IVP or CT urography are imaging modalities of choice
• US does not clearly demonstrate course of non-dilated ureters

SELECTED REFERENCES

1. Zissin R et al: Renal duplication with associated complications in adults: CT findings in 26 cases. Clin Radiol. 56(1):58-63, 2001
2. Fernbach SK et al: Ureteral duplication and its complications. Radiographics. 17(1):109-27, 1997
3. Ulchaker J et al: The spectrum of ureteropelvic junction obstructions occurring in duplicated collecting systems. J Pediatr Surg. 31(9):1221-4, 1996
4. Bellah RD et al: Ureterocele eversion with vesicoureteral reflux in duplex kidneys: findings at voiding cystourethrography. AJR Am J Roentgenol. 165(2):409-13, 1995
5. Fernbach SK et al: Complete duplication of the ureter with ureteropelvic junction obstruction of the lower pole of the kidney: imaging findings. AJR Am J Roentgenol. 164(3):701-4, 1995
6. Husmann DA et al: Ureterocele associated with ureteral duplication and a nonfunctioning upper pole segment: management by partial nephroureterectomy alone. J Urol. 154(2 Pt 2):723-6, 1995
7. Share JC et al: The unsuspected double collecting system on imaging studies and at cystoscopy. AJR Am J Roentgenol. 155(3):561-4, 1990
8. Winters WD et al: Importance of prenatal detection of hydronephrosis of the upper pole. AJR Am J Roentgenol. 155(1):125-9, 1990
9. Share JC et al: Ectopic ureterocele without ureteral and calyceal dilatation (ureterocele disproportion): findings on urography and sonography. AJR Am J Roentgenol. 152(3):567-71, 1989
10. Ahmed S et al: Vesicoureteral reflux in complete ureteral duplication: surgical options. J Urol. 140(5 Pt 2):1092-4, 1988
11. Bisset GS 3rd et al: The duplex collecting system in girls with urinary tract infection: prevalence and significance. AJR Am J Roentgenol. 148(3):497-500, 1987
12. Mesrobian HG: Ureteropelvic junction obstruction of the upper pole moiety in complete ureteral duplication. J Urol. 136(2):452-3, 1986
13. Nussbaum AR et al: Ectopic ureter and ureterocele: their varied sonographic manifestations. Radiology. 159(1):227-35, 1986
14. Amis ES Jr et al: Lower moiety hydronephrosis in duplicated kidneys. Urology. 26(1):82-8, 1985
15. Lavallee G et al: Obstructed duplex kidney in an adult: ultrasonic evaluation. J Clin Ultrasound. 13(4):281-3, 1985
16. Gartell PC et al: Renal dysplasia and duplex kidneys. Eur Urol. 9(2):65-8, 1983
17. Inamoto K et al: Duplication of the renal pelvis and ureter: associated anomalies and pathological conditions. Radiat Med. 1(1):55-64, 1983
18. Gates GF: Ultrasonography of the urinary tract in children. Urol Clin North Am. 7(2):215-22, 1980
19. Morgan CL et al: Ultrasonic diagnosis of obstructed renal duplication and ureterocele. South Med J. 73(8):1016-9, 1980
20. Rose JS et al: Ultrasound diagnosis of ectopic ureterocele. Pediatr Radiol. 8(1):17-20, 1979
21. Mascatello VJ et al: Ultrasonic evaluation of the obstructed duplex kidney. AJR Am J Roentgenol. 129(1):113-20, 1977

IMAGE GALLERY

Typical

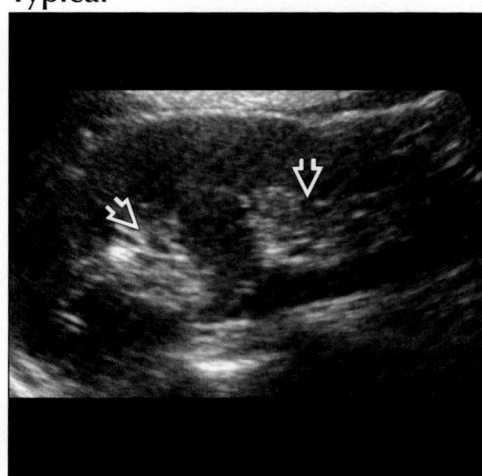
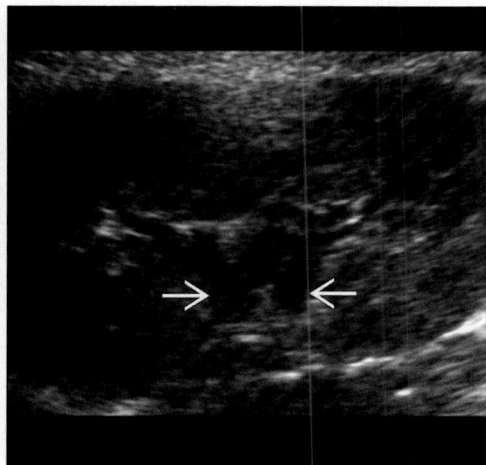

(Left) Longitudinal transabdominal ultrasound shows duplex kidney with two echo complexes ➡ and intervening cortical tissue. No evidence of obstructive hydronephrosis in either moiety. *(Right)* Longitudinal transabdominal ultrasound shows partial ureteral duplication with two central echo complexes. There is a bifid renal pelvis ➡ but no obstructive hydronephrosis.

Typical

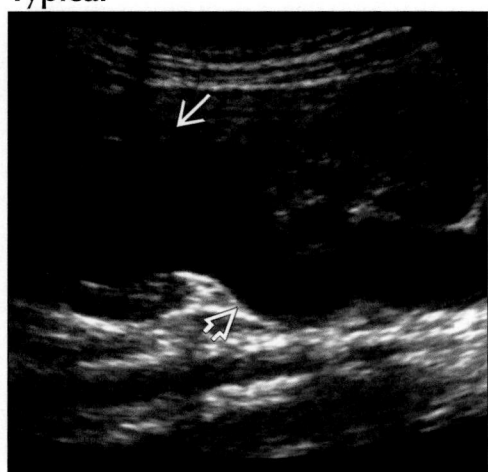
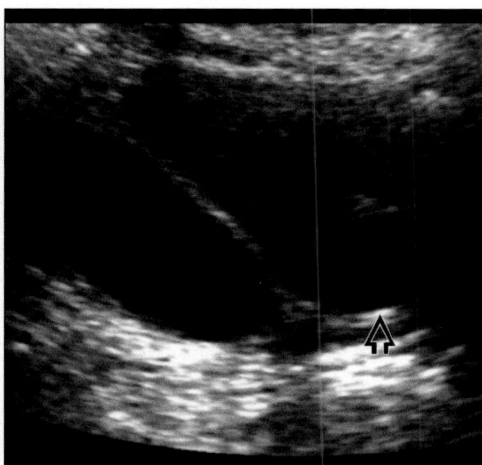

(Left) Longitudinal transabdominal ultrasound shows a typical case of ureteropelvic duplication. Upper moiety collecting system ➡ is dilated and connected to a dilated ureter ➡. *(Right)* Oblique transabdominal ultrasound of a ureterocele ➡ at the vesicoureteric junction, accounting for the ureteric obstruction.

Typical

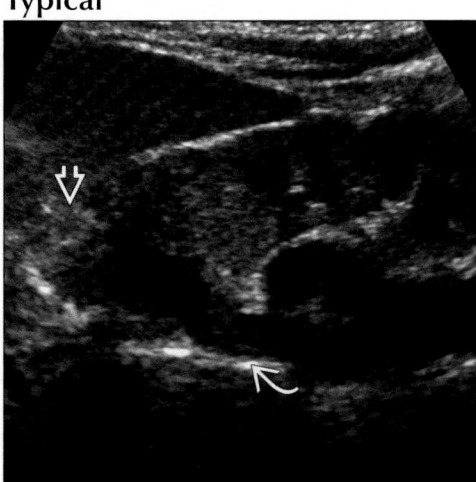
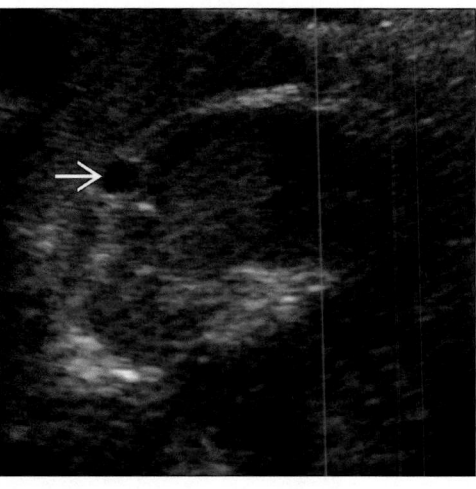

(Left) Longitudinal transabdominal ultrasound shows a typical renal duplication with a hydronephrotic, dysplastic upper moiety ➡ connected to a tortuous hydroureter ➡. *(Right)* Transverse ultrasound shows a dysplastic upper moiety, with loss of corticomedullary differentiation and a tiny cortical cyst ➡.

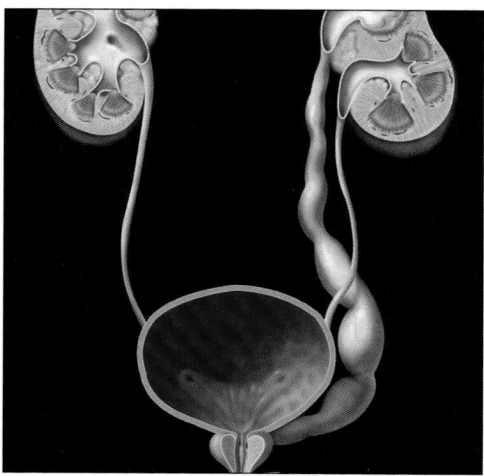

Graphic shows a dilated upper moiety ureter of a left duplex kidney, with extravesicle ectopic insertion into the prostatic urethra.

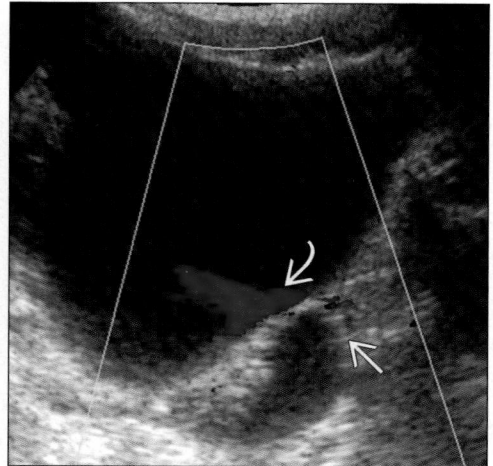

Transverse color Doppler ultrasound shows an ectopic insertion of a ureter into the prostate ➡ beyond the trigone of the bladder. A ureteric jet on the contralateral side is noted ➡.

TERMINOLOGY

Abbreviations and Synonyms
- Ectopic ureter (EU), ureteral ectopia

Definitions
- Ureter that does not terminate at bladder trigone
  - Ectopic insertion within bladder: Usually no significant pathology
- Common usage: Ureter that terminates outside bladder

IMAGING FINDINGS

General Features
- Best diagnostic clue: 70-80% associated with complete ureteral duplication
- Location
  - Usually extravesicular insertion; males always above external sphincter
  - Males: Vas deferens 10%, seminal vesicle 28%, prostatic urethra 54%, ejaculatory duct 8%
    - Prostatic urethra most common insertion site in male
  - Females: Uterus or cervix 3%, vagina 27%, urethra 32%, vestibule 38%
    - Urethra or vestibule most common insertion site in female
  - 5-17% of ectopic ureters are bilateral
- Morphology
  - Complete duplication: Ectopic ureter drains upper moiety
  - Orifice commonly stenotic, leading to obstruction of upper pole moiety

Ultrasonographic Findings
- Grayscale Ultrasound
  - Dilated ureter extends beyond bladder trigone
  - Ureterocele may be present if intravesicular insertion
  - Look for hydronephrotic or dysplastic upper moiety in complete ureteral duplication
  - Small dysplastic and non-functional kidney if single ureter system
  - Transrectal/transvaginal US clearly delineates site of insertion of ectopic ureter
- Color Doppler

DDx: Ectopic Ureter

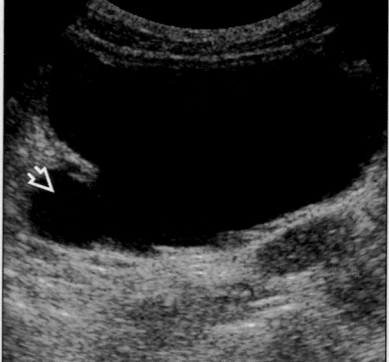

Diverticulum

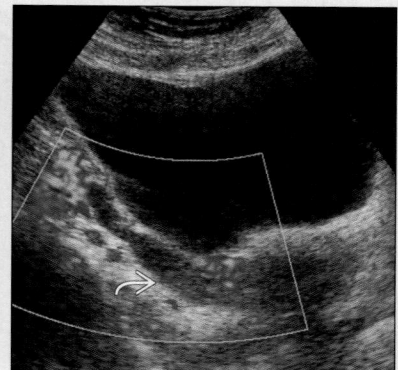

Hydrosalpinx

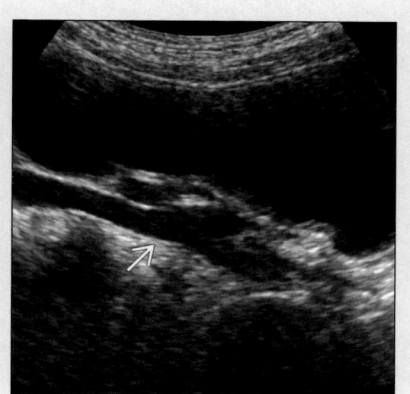

Iliac Vessels

URETERAL ECTOPIA

Key Facts

Terminology
- Common usage: Ureter that terminates outside bladder

Imaging Findings
- Best diagnostic clue: 70-80% associated with complete ureteral duplication
- Prostatic urethra most common insertion site in male
- Urethra or vestibule most common insertion site in female
- Dilated ureter extends beyond bladder trigone
- Ureterocele may be present if intravesicular insertion
- Look for hydronephrotic or dysplastic upper moiety in complete ureteral duplication
- Small dysplastic and non-functional kidney if single ureter system

- Protocol advice: Trace dilated ureter on US to its termination below bladder

Top Differential Diagnoses
- Bladder Diverticulum
- Hydrosalpinx
- Iliac Vessels
- Fluid-Filled Bowel Loop

Clinical Issues
- Females: Continual dribbling urinary incontinence (50%)
- Males: No incontinence because ectopic ureteral orifice always above external sphincter

Diagnostic Checklist
- Weigert-Meyer rule: Upper moiety ureter inserts inferior and medial to lower moiety ureter

---

- o Ureteral jet from the ectopic intravesicular insertion
- o Normal position of contralateral ureteral jet at interureteric bar

Radiographic Findings
- IVP
  - o Dilated upper pole collecting system
  - o Non-visualization of upper pole moiety with severe obstruction/dysplasia
    - Visualized lower pole moiety: Fewer calyces than normal for whole kidney
    - Lower pole displaced infero-laterally ("drooping-lily" sign)
  - o Ectopic insertion of single system ureter: Involved kidney usually small, dysplastic and nonfunctional

CT Findings
- CECT
  - o Hydronephrotic upper pole moiety with variable function
  - o Dilated, tortuous ureter to level of insertion
  - o Males with single ectopic ureters: Non-functional kidney and dilated ipsilateral seminal vesicle

MR Findings
- T1WI
  - o Tortuous low signal intensity ureter dilated to level of ectopic insertion
  - o Severe hydronephrosis of upper pole moiety
- T2WI
  - o Tortuous high signal intensity ectopic ureter dilated to level of insertion
  - o High signal cystic dysplasia of ipsilateral upper pole moiety
- T1 C+: Variable degree of function in obstructed upper pole moiety

Fluoroscopic Findings
- Voiding cystourethrogram (VCUG): Reflux into either moiety
- VCUG useful to locate insertion of ectopic ureter if within urinary tract

- o Will not visualize ectopic insertion if outside urinary tract

Nuclear Medicine Findings
- Renal scintigraphy
  - o Variable function of moiety drained by ectopic ureter

Imaging Recommendations
- Best imaging tool
  - o Ultrasound
  - o CT may be useful to locate small poorly functioning dysplastic kidney with single ectopic ureter
  - o MR urography can display ectopic ureteral insertions even if outside urinary tract
- Protocol advice: Trace dilated ureter on US to its termination below bladder

DIFFERENTIAL DIAGNOSIS

Bladder Diverticulum
- Outpouching sac from bladder with a neck

Hydrosalpinx
- Obstructed and dilated fallopian tube, associated with other features or pelvic inflammatory disease

Iliac Vessels
- Mistaken as dilated ureters behind bladder
- Pulsate, confirmed by color Doppler

Fluid-Filled Bowel Loop
- Peristalsis and change in configuration on real-time scanning

PATHOLOGY

General Features
- General path comments
  - o Ectopic ureters opening to bladder neck or posterior urethra may reflux

URETERAL ECTOPIA

○ Ectopic ureters terminating outside urinary tract: Usually obstructed
- Etiology
  ○ Congenital: Abnormal ureteral bud migration
    - Failure of separation of ureteral bud from Wolffian duct results in caudal ectopia
- Epidemiology
  ○ Incidence: At least 1 in 1,900
  ○ True incidence uncertain since many cases asymptomatic
- Associated abnormalities
  ○ Hypoplasia or dysplasia of renal moiety drained by ectopic ureter
  ○ Degree of ureteral ectopia correlates with degree of renal abnormality
  ○ Imperforate anus, tracheo-esophageal fistula

Gross Pathologic & Surgical Features

- Single system ectopic ureter: Absent ipsilateral hemitrigone
- Distance from trigone correlates with degree of ipsilateral renal dysplasia
  ○ More distal the ureter, the greater the dysplasia
  ○ Very distal insertions ⇒ usually very poor renal function

Microscopic Features

- Muscularis of ectopic ureteral wall may have ultrastructural abnormalities

CLINICAL ISSUES

Presentation

- Most common signs/symptoms
  ○ Recurrent or chronic urinary tract infections (UTIs)
  ○ Females: Continual dribbling urinary incontinence (50%)
    - Males: No incontinence because ectopic ureteral orifice always above external sphincter
  ○ Males: Chronic or recurrent epididymitis
- Clinical Profile
  ○ Girl with continuous dribbling urinary incontinence
  ○ Prepubertal boy with epididymitis or UTI

Demographics

- Age
  ○ Age at diagnosis varies widely; some cases not detected during life
  ○ Many cases diagnosed with prenatal ultrasound
- Gender
  ○ M:F = 1:6
  ○ Single system ectopic ureters more common in males
  ○ Ectopic ureters in males usually drain single systems
  ○ Females: 80% of ectopic ureters are duplicated systems

Natural History & Prognosis

- Most ectopic ureters drain single kidneys or upper pole moieties with minimal function

Treatment

- Options, risks, complications

○ Ectopic ureter with duplicated system: Surgical upper pole nephrectomy
○ Single system: Nephrectomy if minimal function
○ If renal function preserved or dx made prenatally: Ureteropyelostomy or common sheath ureteral implantation

DIAGNOSTIC CHECKLIST

Image Interpretation Pearls

- Weigert-Meyer rule: Upper moiety ureter inserts inferior and medial to lower moiety ureter

SELECTED REFERENCES

1. Wille S et al: Magnetic resonance urography in pediatric urology. Scand J Urol Nephrol. 37(1):16-21, 2003
2. Berrocal T et al: Anomalies of the distal ureter, bladder, and urethra in children: embryologic, radiologic, and pathologic features. Radiographics. 22(5):1139-64, 2002
3. Damry N et al: Ectopic vaginal insertion of a duplicated ureter: demonstration by magnetic resonance imaging (MRI). JBR-BTR. 84(6):270, 2001
4. Staatz G et al: Magnetic resonance urography in children: evaluation of suspected ureteral ectopia in duplex systems. J Urol. 166(6):2346-50, 2001
5. Engin G et al: MR urography findings of a duplicated ectopic ureter in an adult man. Eur Radiol. 10(8):1253-6, 2000
6. Gylys-Morin VM et al: Magnetic resonance imaging of the dysplastic renal moiety and ectopic ureter. J Urol. 164(6):2034-9, 2000
7. Cabay JE et al: Ectopic ureter associated with renal dysplasia. JBR-BTR. 82(5):228-30, 1999
8. Komatsu K et al: Single ectopic vaginal ureter diagnosed by computed tomography. Urol Int. 63(2):147-50, 1999
9. Carrico C et al: Incontinence due to an infrasphincteric ectopic ureter: why the delay in diagnosis and what the radiologist can do about it. Pediatr Radiol. 28(12):942-9, 1998
10. Amatulle P et al: Ureteral duplication anomaly with ectopic intraprostatic insertion. J Ultrasound Med. 16(3):231-3, 1997
11. Dunnick NR et al: Textbook of uroradiology. 2nd ed. Baltimore, Williams and Wilkins, 29-33, 1997
12. Fernbach SK et al: Ureteral duplication and its complications. Radiographics. 17(1):109-27, 1997
13. Yanagisawa N et al: Diagnostic magnetic resonance-urography in an infant girl with an ectopic ureter associated with a poorly functioning segment of a duplicated collecting system. Int J Urol. 4(3):314-7, 1997
14. Gharagozloo AM et al: Detection of a poorly functioning malpositioned kidney with single ectopic ureter in girls with urinary dribbling: imaging evaluation in five patients. AJR Am J Roentgenol. 164(4):957-61, 1995
15. Rothpearl A et al: MR urography: technique and application. Radiology. 194(1):125-30, 1995
16. Jelen Z: The value of ultrasonography as a screening procedure of the neonatal urinary tract: a survey of 1021 infants. Int Urol Nephrol. 25(1):3-10, 1993
17. Herman TE et al: Radiographic manifestations of congenital anomalies of the lower urinary tract. Radiol Clin North Am. 29(2):365-82, 1991

IMAGE GALLERY

Typical

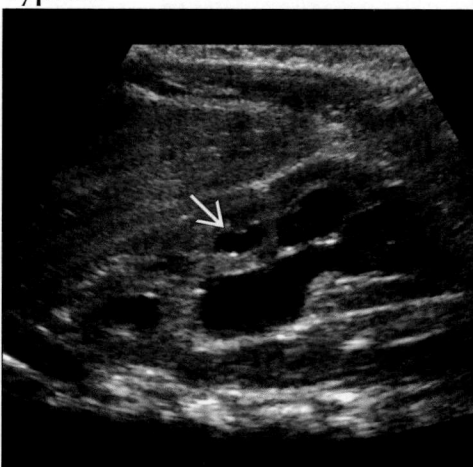

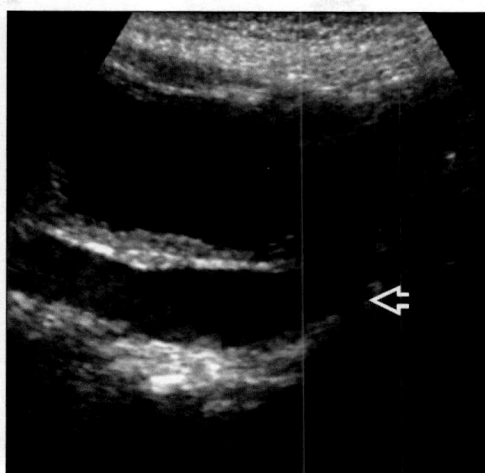

(Left) Longitudinal transabdominal ultrasound shows a dilated single collecting system of the right kidney ➡. (Right) Longitudinal transabdominal ultrasound shows a dilated ureter coursing behind and distal to the bladder trigone, into the vagina ➡.

Typical

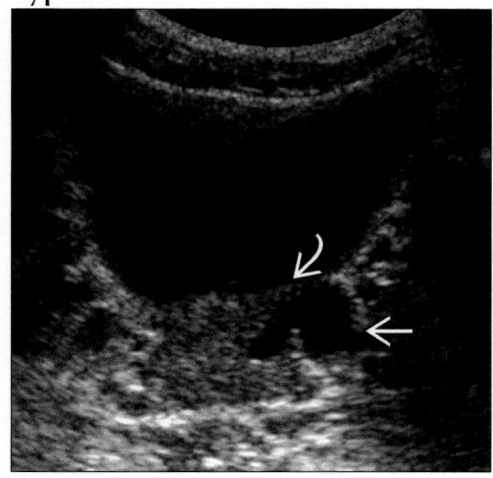

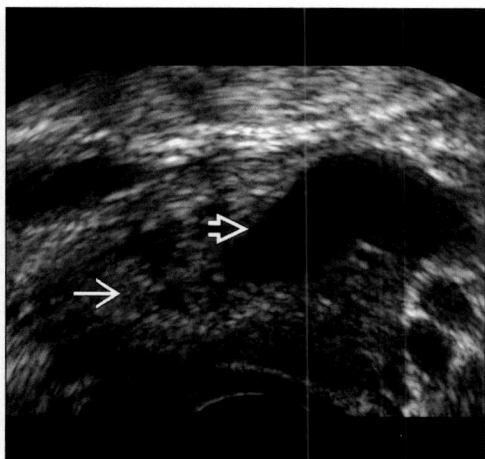

(Left) Transverse transabdominal ultrasound shows a hydronephrotic distal left ureter inserting into the prostate ➡, beyond the trigone of the urinary bladder ➡. (Right) Oblique transrectal ultrasound clearly shows the ectopic insertion of the ureter ➡ into the prostate ➡.

Typical

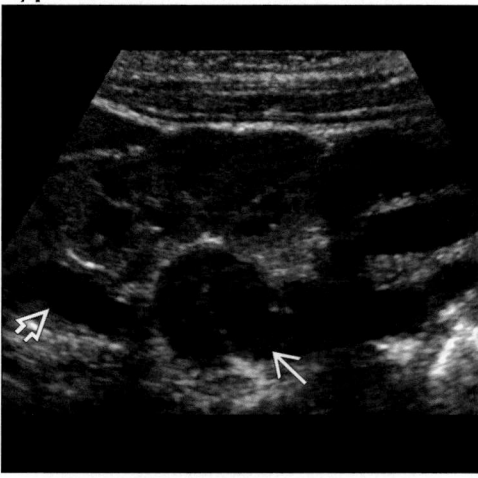

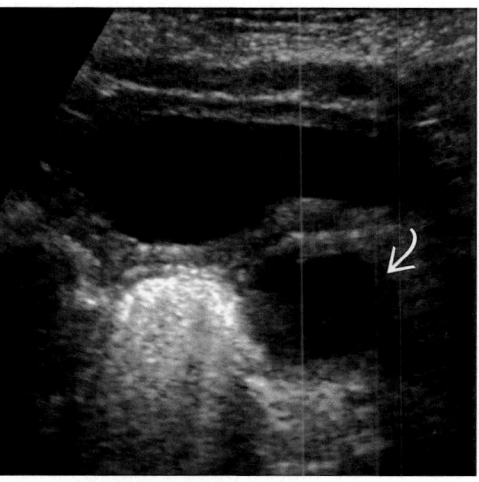

(Left) Oblique transabdominal ultrasound shows a tortuous hydroureter ➡ arising from a dysplastic upper moiety ➡ of a duplex kidney. (Right) Transverse transabdominal ultrasound shows the ectopic insertion of the upper moiety ureter ➡ below the urinary bladder into the vagina.

URETEROPELVIC JUNCTION OBSTRUCTION

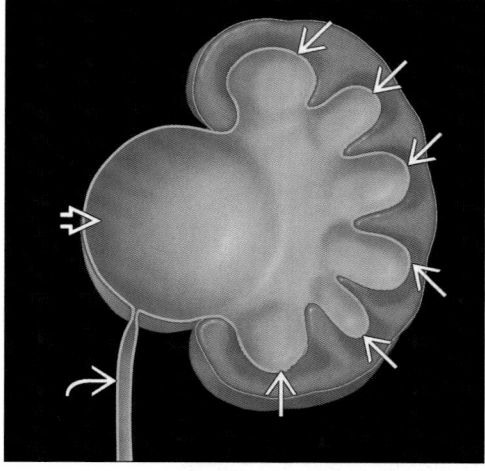

Graphic shows a markedly dilated renal pelvis ⇨ and calices ⇨ in a ureteropelvic junction obstruction. The ureter ⇨ is not dilated.

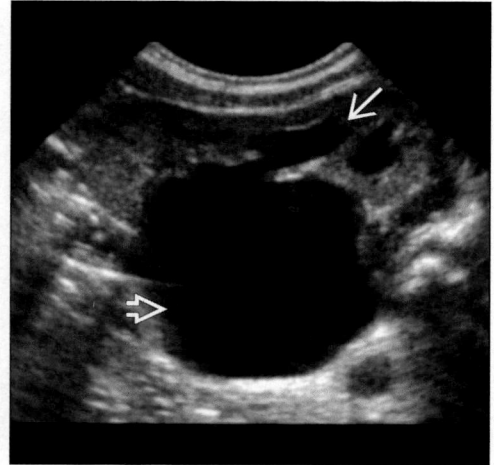

Transverse transabdominal ultrasound shows a markedly dilated renal pelvis ⇨ communicating with dilated calices ⇨. No dilated ureter evident.

TERMINOLOGY

Abbreviations and Synonyms

- Ureteropelvic junction (UPJ) obstruction, pelviureteric junction obstruction, idiopathic, pelvic or congenital hydronephrosis

Definitions

- Obstructed urine flow from renal pelvis to proximal ureter → pressure increase in renal pelvis

IMAGING FINDINGS

General Features

- Best diagnostic clue: Pyelocaliectasis down to the level of UPJ without ureterectasis
- Location
  - Left kidney (2 times) > right kidney
  - Unilateral > bilateral obstruction (10-30% of cases)

Ultrasonographic Findings

- Grayscale Ultrasound
  - Use US in both prenatal and postnatal evaluation
  - Prenatal findings
    - Grade II/III fetal hydronephrosis: Anteroposterior (AP) pelvic diameter > 10 mm +/- slight caliectasis, 50% require postnatal urologic surgery
    - Mild pyelectasis (pelvic diameter 4-10 mm in < 20 weeks of gestation and 5-10 mm in 20-24 weeks): 10-15% obstructed
    - Grade IV fetal hydronephrosis: Moderate dilatation of calices, preserved renal cortex
    - Grade V fetal hydronephrosis: Severe dilatation of calices with atrophic cortex, requires neonatal corrective surgery
    - Large urinoma or urine ascites if severely dilated collecting system
    - Oligo-, poly- or euhydroamnios
  - Postnatal findings
    - Dilatation of renal pelvis and calices down to level of ureteropelvic junction
    - Marked ballooning of the renal pelvis
    - Assess severity and level of obstruction
    - Renal parenchymal atrophy if long-standing
    - Ureter of normal caliber, bladder normal in size and contour

DDx: UPJ Obstruction

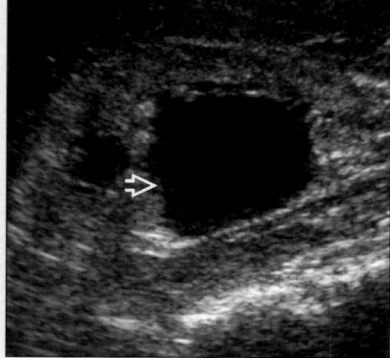

Parapelvic Cyst

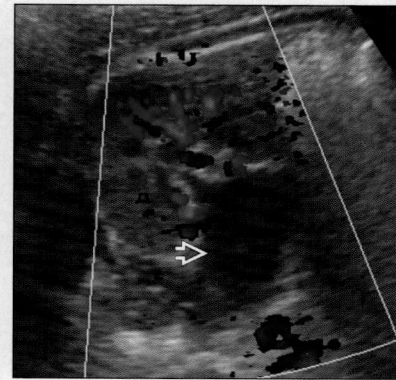

Extrarenal Pelvis

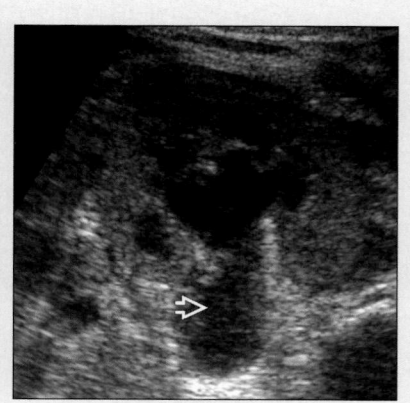

Pyonephrosis

URETEROPELVIC JUNCTION OBSTRUCTION

Key Facts

Terminology
- Obstructed urine flow from renal pelvis to proximal ureter → pressure increase in renal pelvis

Imaging Findings
- Best diagnostic clue: Pyelocaliectasis down to the level of UPJ without ureterectasis
- Left kidney (2 times) > right kidney
- Unilateral > bilateral obstruction (10-30% of cases)
- Dilatation of renal pelvis and calices down to level of ureteropelvic junction
- Marked ballooning of the renal pelvis
- Renal parenchymal atrophy if long-standing
- Ureter of normal caliber, bladder normal in size and contour
- Associated contralateral renal anomalies: Multicystic dysplastic kidney, renal duplication, agenesis

- Endoureteral US: Demonstrates crossing vessels in more than 50% of UPJ obstruction

Top Differential Diagnoses
- Pararenal Cyst
- Extrarenal Pelvis
- Pyonephrosis

Diagnostic Checklist
- Use CT or MR to evaluate potential acquired etiologies of UPJ obstruction
- Use endoureteric US to guide site of endopyelotomy, to avoid damage to adjacent vessels
- IVP shows significant obstruction only during acute pain episode for UPJ obstruction caused by lower-pole renal vessel

5

27

- Hypertrophy of normal kidney contralateral to hydronephrotic kidney
- Associated contralateral renal anomalies: Multicystic dysplastic kidney, renal duplication, agenesis
- Endoureteral US: Demonstrates crossing vessels in more than 50% of UPJ obstruction
  - Crossing vessel at all sites adjacent to UPJ, most common anteromedial in location
  - Demonstrate septum between ureteral and renal pelvic lumen in UPJ with high insertion of ureter
  - Useful to guide site of endopyelotomy to avoid damage to adjacent vessels

Radiographic Findings
- IVP
  - Marked pyelocaliectasis; UPJ narrowing
  - Giant hydronephrosis; may displace, rotate and obstruct contralateral kidney and ureter
  - Incomplete visualization of normal caliber ureter
  - Delayed clearing of contrast from collecting system
  - Chronic changes: Diminished opacification, loss of cortical thickness
  - "Linear band" sign: Linear oblique crossing defect in proximal end of ureter
  - Intermittent UPJ obstruction caused by crossing vessel
    - No obstruction between episodes of pain
    - Marked obstruction with contrast trapped in segment of proximal ureter during acute episode
  - Diuresis IVP as adjunct
    - Delayed clearing (> 10 min) of contrast, pyelocaliectasis and flank pain; suggest intermittent UPJ obstruction
- Voiding cystourethrography
  - Exclude severe vesicoureteral reflux in infants
- Retrograde ureteropyelography
  - Assess ureter if not visualized in other studies

CT Findings
- CTA: Use 3D reconstruction to better define vessels prior to endoscopic pyelotomy
- NECT

- Hydronephrosis ± ureterectasis
- Level of obstruction
- ± Acquired etiologies (e.g., crossing vessels, neoplasm, retroperitoneal inflammatory conditions) and associated abnormalities (e.g., renal malformation)

MR Findings
- MRA: Detect crossing vessels
- MR urography
  - Demonstrate narrowing at UPJ
  - Delayed contrast excretion and contrast stasis at UPJ on dynamic scan
  - No contrast excretion into ureter

Nuclear Medicine Findings
- Diuresis renography
  - Separates obstructive from nonobstructive dilatation
  - Localize level of obstruction
  - Assess renal function, often pre-operatively
  - "Homsy" sign: Delayed double-peak pattern; suggests intermittent UPJ obstruction

Imaging Recommendations
- Best imaging tool: IVP: Adult; US: Neonates and children
- Protocol advice
  - IVP
    - Visualize UPJ with prone oblique view; left/right anterior oblique for left/right UPJ, respectively
    - Diuresis IVP: Furosemide IV 0.5 mg/kg 15-20 min into IVP; film at 5, 10, 15 min after injection
  - CTA or MRA: Define vessels and their relation to UPJ
  - US: Serial US should be done several days postnatally due to relative neonatal oliguria
  - Diuresis Renography: Tc-99m labeled mercaptoacetyltriglycine (MAG3) is preferred due to lower radiation burden

URETEROPELVIC JUNCTION OBSTRUCTION

DIFFERENTIAL DIAGNOSIS

Pararenal Cyst
- Lymphatic in orgin or develops from embryologic rests
- Well-defined anechoic renal sinus mass not communicating with calices

Extrarenal Pelvis
- Prominent renal pelvis beyond the contour of kidney on axial image
- Much smaller in size than ureteropelvic junction obstruction

Pyonephrosis
- Internal echoes within the dilated renal pelvis
- Associated urothelial thickening

PATHOLOGY

General Features
- General path comments: Obstruction caused by spectrum of pathophysiological processes of varying etiologies
- Genetics: Familial occurrences in some cases
- Etiology
  - Congenital (most common)
    - Partial replacement of UPJ muscle by collagen
    - Abnormal arrangement of junction muscles causing dysmotility
    - Crossing vessels near UPJ
    - High ureteric insertion
    - Valves and folds
    - Kinks or angulations
  - Acquired
    - Scarring: Inflammation, surgery, trauma
    - Vesicoureteral reflux
    - Malignant neoplasm: Transitional cell carcinoma, squamous cell carcinoma, metastasis
    - Benign neoplasm: Polyp, mesodermal tumor
    - Intraluminal lesion: Stone, clot, papilla, fungus ball, cholesteatoma, bullet, miscellaneous
- Epidemiology: Neonates: 40% of all significant neonatal hydronephrosis (1/500 pregnancies)
- Associated abnormalities
  - Cystic renal dysplasia, primary megaureter
  - Lower or upper segment of duplex kidney
  - Ectopic, malrotated, pelvic and horseshoe kidneys
  - Complex congenital anomaly: VATER (vertebral, anus, tracheoesophageal, renal and radial)

CLINICAL ISSUES

Presentation
- Most common signs/symptoms
  - Neonates
    - Asymptomatic, diagnosed by prenatal screening
    - Palpable, sometimes visible abdominal mass
  - Children and adults
    - Intermittent abdominal or flank pain, nausea, vomiting
    - Hematuria, renovascular hypertension (rare)

Demographics
- Age: Any age; less common in adults
- Gender
  - Overall, M:F = 2:1
  - In infants, M:F = 5:1

Natural History & Prognosis
- Complications: Failure to thrive, renal insufficiency, urinary tract infection, urolithiasis, gastroduodenal obstruction, traumatic or spontaneous kidney rupture
- Prognosis: Good, after treating unilateral obstruction

Treatment
- Indicated when patient has symptoms, stones, infection or renal function is impaired or at risk
  - Infants and children: Open pyeloplasty
  - Adults: Endopyelotomy
- Follow-up: 3-6 months with diuresis renography

DIAGNOSTIC CHECKLIST

Consider
- Use CT or MR to evaluate potential acquired etiologies of UPJ obstruction
- Use endoureteric US to guide site of endopyelotomy, to avoid damage to adjacent vessels

Image Interpretation Pearls
- IVP shows significant obstruction only during acute pain episode for UPJ obstruction caused by lower-pole renal vessel
- IVP can be normal between episodes of pain

SELECTED REFERENCES

1. McDaniel BB et al: Dynamic contrast-enhanced MR urography in the evaluation of pediatric hydronephrosis: Part 2, anatomic and functional assessment of uteropelvic junction obstruction. AJR Am J Roentgenol. 185(6):1608-14, 2005
2. Khaira HS et al: Helical computed tomography for identification of crossing vessels in ureteropelvic junction obstruction-comparison with operative findings. Urology. 62(1):35-9, 2003
3. Keeley FX Jr et al: A prospective study of endoluminal ultrasound versus computerized tomography angiography for detecting crossing vessels at the ureteropelvic junction. J Urol. 162(6):1938-41, 1999
4. Rouviere O et al: Ureteropelvic junction obstruction: use of helical CT for preoperative assessment--comparison with intraarterial angiography. Radiology. 213(3):668-73, 1999
5. Wolf JS Jr et al: Imaging for ureteropelvic junction obstruction in adults. J Endourol. 10(2):93-104, 1996
6. Bagley DH et al: Endoluminal sonography in evaluation of the obstructed ureteropelvic junction. J Endourol. 8(4):287-92, 1994
7. Grignon A et al: Ureteropelvic junction stenosis: antenatal ultrasonographic diagnosis, postnatal investigation, and follow-up. Radiology. 160(3):649-51, 1986
8. Grignon A et al: Urinary tract dilatation in utero: classification and clinical applications. Radiology. 160(3):645-7, 1986
9. Hoffer FA et al: Intermittent hydronephrosis: a unique feature of ureteropelvic junction obstruction caused by a crossing renal vessel. Radiology. 156(3):655-8, 1985

URETEROPELVIC JUNCTION OBSTRUCTION

IMAGE GALLERY

Typical

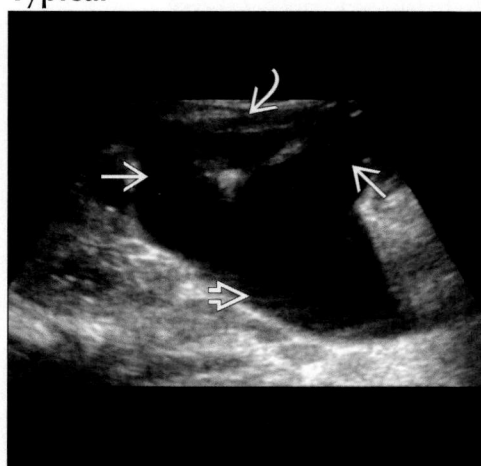
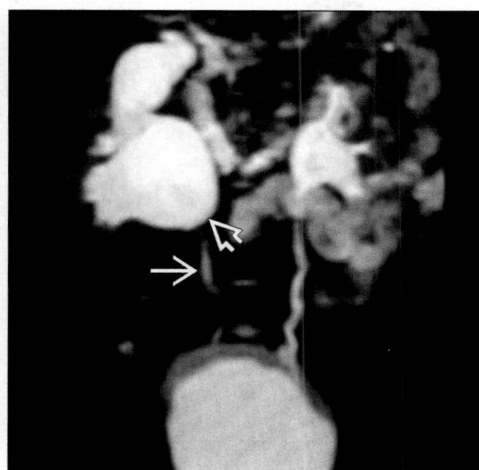

(Left) Oblique transabdominal ultrasound shows marked dilatation of the renal pelvis down to the UPJ ➡, with moderate caliectasis ➡ and generalized cortical thinning ➡. (Right) MR urography shows dilatation of the calyces and renal pelvis down to a narrowing at the UPJ ➡ of the right kidney. The right ureter ➡ is not dilated.

Typical

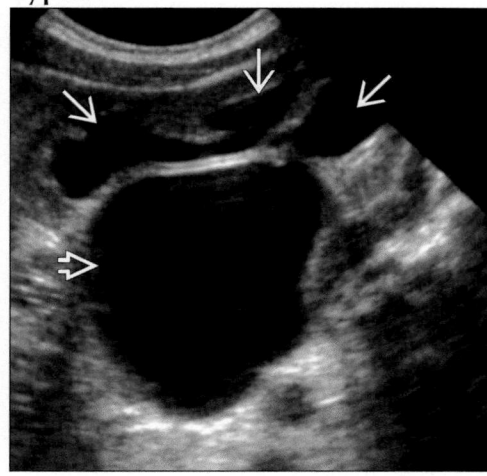
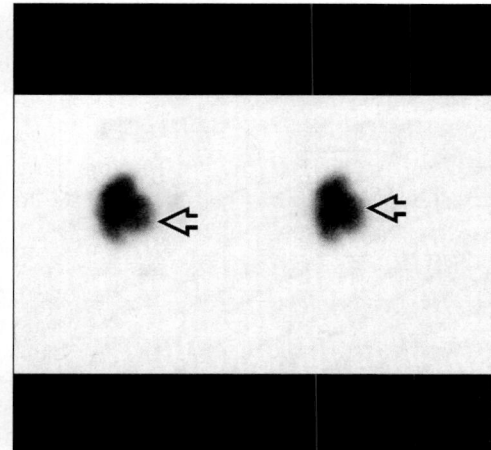

(Left) Transverse transabdominal ultrasound shows a markedly dilated renal pelvis ➡ and generalized caliectasis ➡. (Right) Delayed static image of a diuresis MAG 3 radioisotope scan shows stasis of the tracer within a dilated collecting system above the UPJ ➡ in both 1 hour (left) and 3 hour (right) delayed scan.

Typical

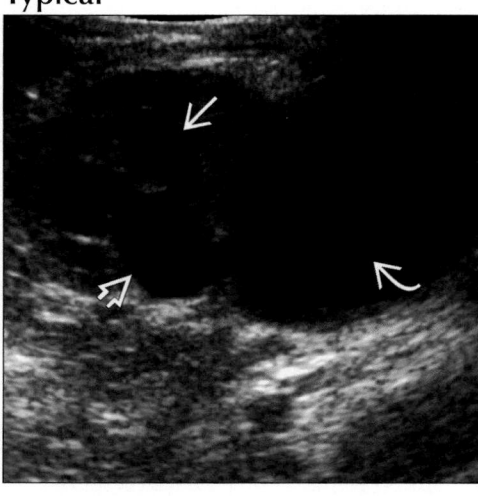
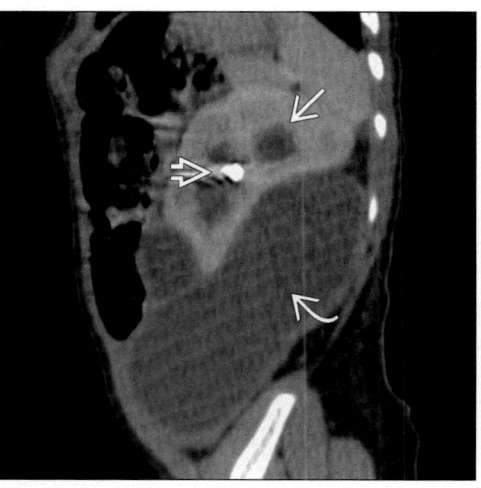

(Left) Transverse transabdominal ultrasound shows a moderately dilated renal pelvis ➡ and calyces ➡ in a child with UPJ obstruction associated with a perirenal urinoma ➡. (Right) CECT with oblique sagittal reformat shows residual caliectasis ➡ after insertion of a percutaneous nephrostomy tube ➡. Note the kidney is compressed by the adjacent perirenal urinoma ➡.

UROLITHIASIS

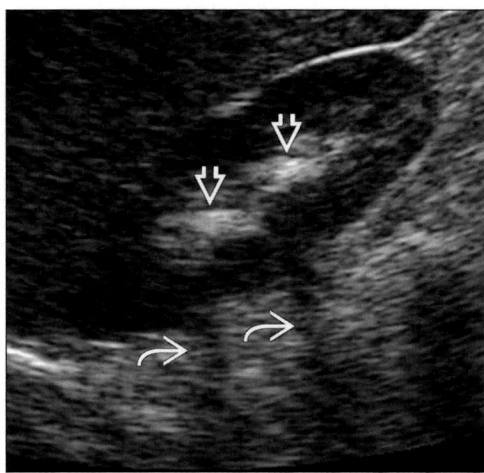
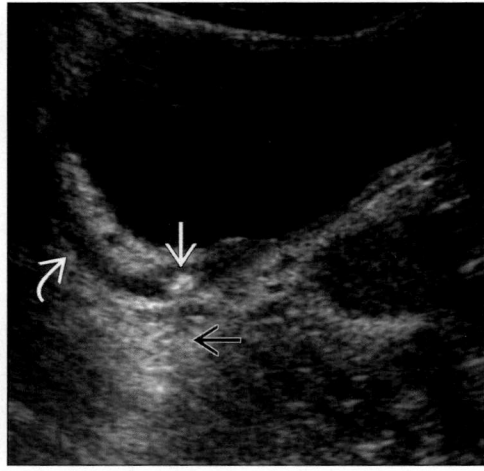

Longitudinal transabdominal ultrasound shows two non-obstructive renal calculi ➡ associated with strong posterior acoustic shadowing ➡. Note normal cortical thickness and outline.

Longitudinal transabdominal ultrasound shows an obstructive lower ureteric calculus ➡. Note the dilatation of the ureter ➡ proximal to the calculus and faint posterior shadowing ➡.

TERMINOLOGY

Abbreviations and Synonyms
- Calculous disease; nephrolithiasis; kidney, renal or urinary stones

Definitions
- Concretions within the urinary system

IMAGING FINDINGS

General Features
- Location
  - Upper urinary tract (UT): Calyceal, renal pelvis or ureteropelvic junction (UPJ)
  - Ureteral calculi: Ureter or ureterovesicle junction (UVJ)
  - Lower UT: Bladder, urethral, prostatic
- Other general features
  - Types of stones
    - Calcium stones (75-80%): Calcium oxalate and/or calcium phosphate
    - Struvite stones (15-20%): Magnesium ammonium phosphate (struvite), magnesium ammonium phosphate + calcium phosphate (triple phosphate)
    - Uric acid stones (5-10%)
    - Cystine stones (1-3%)
    - Matrix stones (rare): Mucoproteins
    - Xanthine stones (extremely rare)
    - Milk-of-calcium: Calcium carbonate + calcium phosphate (carbonate apatite)
    - Protease inhibitor stones: Indinavir-induced

Ultrasonographic Findings
- Grayscale Ultrasound
  - Calculi seen as crescent-shaped echogenic foci with sharp distal acoustic shadowing
  - Non-obstructive calculi may have similar echogenicity as central sinus echo, distinguished by their acoustic shadowing
  - Acoustic shadowing varies according to size and composition of stone
  - Very small stones may not show obvious posterior acoustic shadowing, which can be enhanced by tissue harmonics
  - Calculi best visualized in kidney and at UVJ

DDx: Renal Calculi

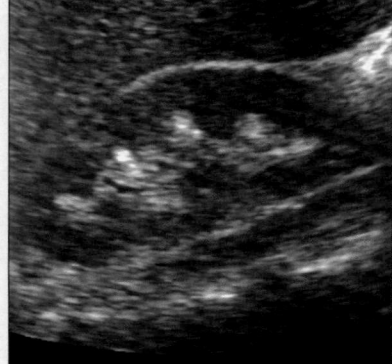
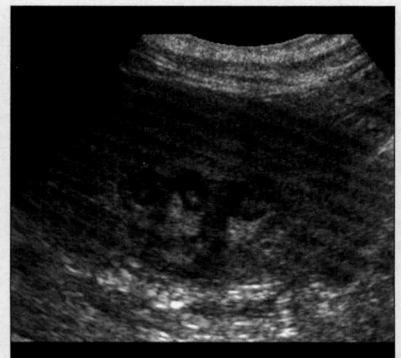
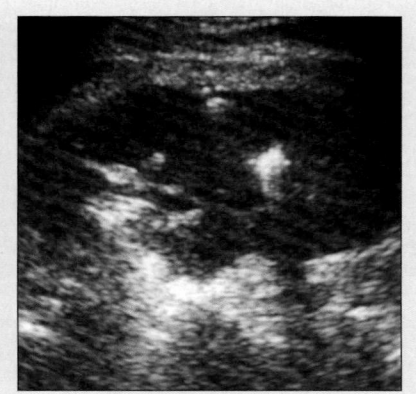

Nephrocalcinosis

Papillary Necrosis

Emphysematous Pyelonephritis

UROLITHIASIS

Key Facts

Terminology
- Calculous disease; nephrolithiasis; kidney, renal or urinary stones

Imaging Findings
- Calculi seen as crescent-shaped echogenic foci with sharp distal acoustic shadowing
- Calculi best visualized in kidney and at UVJ
- Stone in ureter visualized if ureter is dilated
- Stones in non-dilated ureter poorly visualized due to overlying bowel gas and deep location
- Most urinary tract stones show twinkling artifacts: Useful ancillary finding in equivocal cases
- Ureteric jet: visualization of "jet" of urine into bladder excludes obstructing distal stone
- Resistive index > 0.7 in symptomatic kidney

Top Differential Diagnoses
- Nephrocalcinosis
- Papillary Necrosis
- Emphysematous Pyelonephritis (EP)

Clinical Issues
- Acute colicky flank pain radiating to groin (60-95% with these symptoms have stones)
- Spontaneous passage through ureter: 80% (< 4 mm), 50% (4-6 mm), 20% (> 8 mm)

Diagnostic Checklist
- Use tissue harmonics to enhance posterior acoustic shadowing if small calculi suspected
- CT more sensitive for calculi in course of ureter with perinephric stranding ± hydronephrosis

- Stone in ureter visualized if ureter is dilated
- Stones in non-dilated ureter poorly visualized due to overlying bowel gas and deep location
  - Improved detection rate by transvaginal or transperineal scanning
- Color Doppler
  - Most urinary tract stones show twinkling artifacts: Useful ancillary finding in equivocal cases
    - Rapidly changing color posterior to stone with a comet tail
  - Ureteric jet: visualization of "jet" of urine into bladder excludes obstructing distal stone
  - High grade ureteric obstruction: Complete absence jet or low level flow
  - Low grade ureteric obstruction: May or may not have jet asymmetry
  - Resistive index > 0.7 in symptomatic kidney

Radiographic Findings
- Radiography
  - Pre-CT belief
    - Radiography detects 90% of calcium stones, some struvite and "misses" uric acid stones
  - Based on CT correlation: Radiography "misses" majority of calculi
    - Due to small size, insufficient radiopacity, overlying bones, bowel, etc.
  - Calcium oxalate or phosphate stones
    - Usually very opaque, visible if large
  - Struvite and cystine stones
    - Staghorn calculi: Shape may conform to pelvicaliceal system
    - Usually opaque, detectible if large
  - Uric acid and xanthine stones
    - Rarely opaque or detectible (when mixed with calcium salts)
  - Milk-of-calcium
    - Moderately opaque
  - Protease inhibitor stones
    - Nonopaque
- IVP
  - Lucent (uric acid, cystine, matrix): Filling defects

- Opaque (calcium, milk-of-calcium): Obscured by contrast-opacified urine
  - ± PC diverticula, UPJ obstruction, tubular ectasia (medullary sponge kidney), urinary diversion
  - Ureteral calculi: Nephrographic phase
    - Delayed ("obstructive", peak at 6 hrs.); prolonged
    - Dense; striated; absent ("negative")
  - Ureteral calculi: Pyelographic phase
    - Delayed opacification (≥ 24 hours)
    - Hydronephrosis; stone in ureter
    - ↓ Contrast density in collecting system
    - Contrast extravasation; ± forniceal rupture
    - Asymmetry of ureteral caliber to obstructed level
    - "Standing column" of contrast to obstructed level
    - Interureteric ridge or edema (pseudoureterocele)
  - Ureteral calculi: Late phase
    - Vicarious excretion of contrast (to gallbladder)

CT Findings
- NECT
  - Stones are uniformly dense except matrix & indinavir stones
  - Radiopacity (most to least): Calcium oxalate and/or phosphate > cystine > struvite > uric acid
  - Matrix stones
    - Soft tissue attenuation (pure)
    - Laminated peripheral calcification, diffuse ↑ density or round faintly opaque nodules with densely calcified center (when mixed with calcium salts)
  - Milk-of-calcium: Layered opaque suspension; stone movement
  - Indinavir stones: Not or faintly opaque; deduced from secondary findings (obstruction)
  - Ureteral calculi: Visualize stone and secondary signs
    - "Soft tissue rim" sign: Ureteral wall edema at stone
    - Pseudoureterocele: UVJ edema around calculus
    - Hydronephrosis; hydroureter; perinephric or periureteral stranding
- CECT: Lucent (matrix and indinavir stones): Filling defects

UROLITHIASIS

MR Findings
- No signal (no mobile protons); large: Signal voids
- Ureteral calculi: Abrupt change in ureteral caliber indicates obstruction level; secondary signs

DIFFERENTIAL DIAGNOSIS

Nephrocalcinosis
- Calcification within parenchyma: Cortex & medulla (most common)
- Indistinguishable except by location

Papillary Necrosis
- Calcified sloughed papilla
- Cystic collections within medullary pyramids
- Clubbing of adjacent calices

Emphysematous Pyelonephritis (EP)
- Intrarenal gas associated with distal shadowing obscuring deeper structures

PATHOLOGY

General Features
- General path comments: Majority are mixed composition; > 50% contain calcium salts
- Etiology
  o Calcium stones
    - Idiopathic (85%): Idiopathic hypercalciuria
    - Acquired (15%): Hyperparathyroidism, sarcoidosis, renal tubular acidosis, hyperoxaluria, steroids, Cushing syndrome, immobilization, ↑ vitamin D
  o Struvite stones: Urinary tract infections (UTI) (Proteus, Klebsiella, Pseudomonas; urea-splitting)
  o Uric acid stones: Hyperuricosuria (25% with gout), ileostomy, chemotherapy, acidic & concentrated urine, adenine phosphoribosyltransferase deficiency
  o Cystine stones: Cystinuria (autosomal recessive)
  o Matrix stones: Chronic UTI, urine stasis, obstruction
  o Xanthine stones: Xanthine oxidase deficiency
  o Milk-of-calcium: Pelvicaliceal diverticula, ureteroceles
  o Risk factors
    - Environment: Warm climates, summer
    - Medications: Acetazolamide, indinavir
    - Anatomical abnormalities: UPJ obstruction (horseshoe or ectopic kidney), PC diverticula, tubular ectasia, urinary diversion
  o Pathogenesis
    - Supersaturated solution → crystal formation in urine (excessive excretion & precipitation theory)
    - Lack of substances that inhibit crystal deposition, stone formation & growth (inhibitor theory)
    - Presence of specific macromolecules that are essential for stone formation (matrix theory)
- Epidemiology
  o Prevalence: 2-3%; 40-60 years of age (in Caucasians)
  o Incidence: 1-2 per 1,000; peak at 20-40 years of age

Gross Pathologic & Surgical Features
- Matrix stones: Gelatinous or soft putty texture; tan to red-brown

Microscopic Features
- Crystals dependent on type of stones

CLINICAL ISSUES

Presentation
- Most common signs/symptoms
  o Upper UT: Asymptomatic, flank pain, fever
  o Ureteral calculi
    - Acute colicky flank pain radiating to groin (60-95% with these symptoms have stones)
  o Lower UT: Asymptomatic, dysuria, dull/sharp pain radiating to penis, buttocks, perineum or scrotum
- Lab data
  o Urinalysis: Hematuria, crystals ± bacteruria or pyuria

Demographics
- Age: 1:8 have stones by 70 years of age
- Gender: M:F = 3:1

Natural History & Prognosis
- Spontaneous passage through ureter: 80% (< 4 mm), 50% (4-6 mm), 20% (> 8 mm)
- Complications: Obstruction, infection, abscess and renal insufficiency
- Prognosis: Recurrence without treatment: 10% at 1 year, 35% at 5 years, 50% at 10 years

Treatment
- ↑ Hydration (2L urine/day), restrict diet (protein, sodium, calcium) & drugs (thiazides or allopurinol)
- Extracorporeal shock wave lithotripsy (ESWL), percutaneous nephrostolithotomy, endoscopic retrieval or suprapubic cystolithotomy
- Follow-up recurrence only: 4-6 weeks after treatment, 24 hour urine (volume, calcium, phosphorus, uric acid, creatine, oxalate, citrate, cystine screen)

DIAGNOSTIC CHECKLIST

Image Interpretation Pearls
- Use tissue harmonics to enhance posterior acoustic shadowing if small calculi suspected
- CT more sensitive for calculi in course of ureter with perinephric stranding ± hydronephrosis

SELECTED REFERENCES
1. Palmer JS et al: Diagnosis of pediatric urolithiasis: role of ultrasound and computerized tomography. J Urol. 174(4 Pt 1):1413-6, 2005
2. Yang JM et al: Transvaginal sonography in the assessment of distal ureteral calculi. Ultrasound Obstet Gynecol. 26(6):658-62, 2005
3. Tack D et al: Low-dose unenhanced multidetector CT of patients with suspected renal colic. AJR Am J Roentgenol. 180(2):305-11, 2003

IMAGE GALLERY

Typical

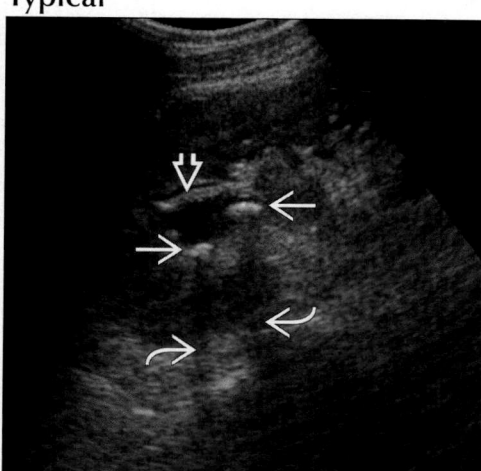

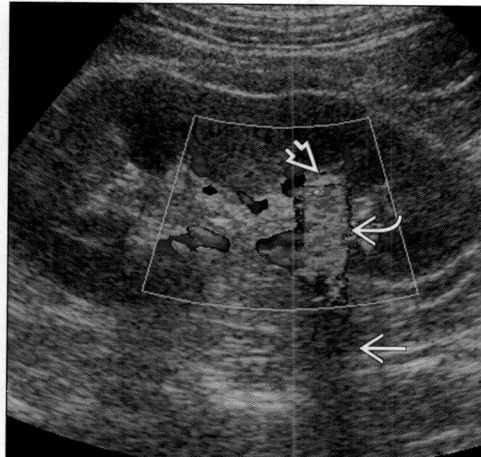

(Left) Oblique transabdominal ultrasound shows two small echogenic calculi ➡ with strong posterior acoustic shadowing ➡ within a dilated calyx ➡. *(Right)* Longitudinal color Doppler ultrasound shows twinkling artifact ➡ immediately behind an echogenic calculus ➡ in the lower pole of the kidney. Posterior acoustic shadowing ➡ is also evident.

Typical

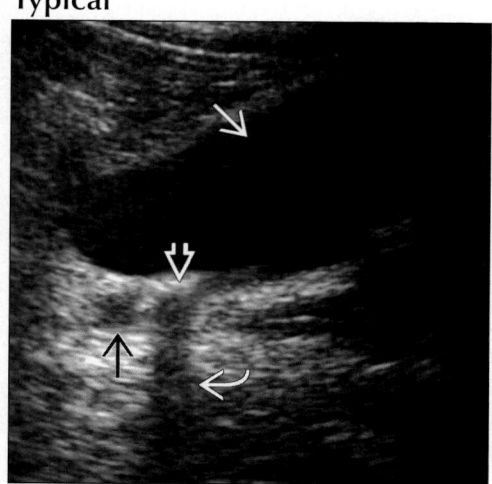

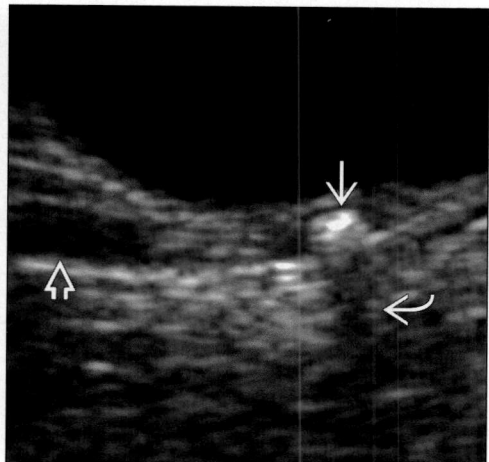

(Left) Oblique transabdominal ultrasound shows an echogenic calculus ➡ with strong acoustic shadowing ➡ at the vesicoureteric junction just before the distal ureter ➡ inserts into the bladder ➡. *(Right)* Longitudinal transabdominal ultrasound shows a vesico-ureteric junction calculus ➡. Note the posterior acoustic shadowing ➡ and dilatation of the proximal ureter ➡.

Typical

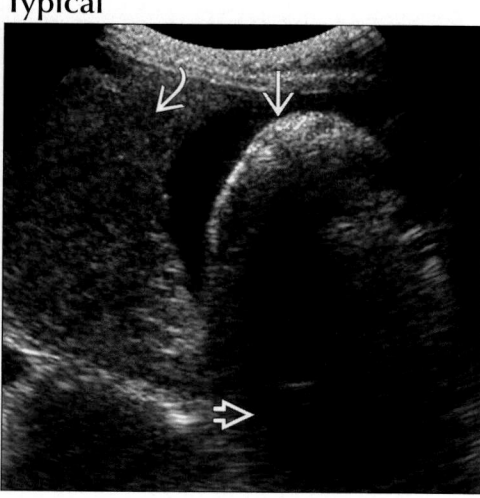

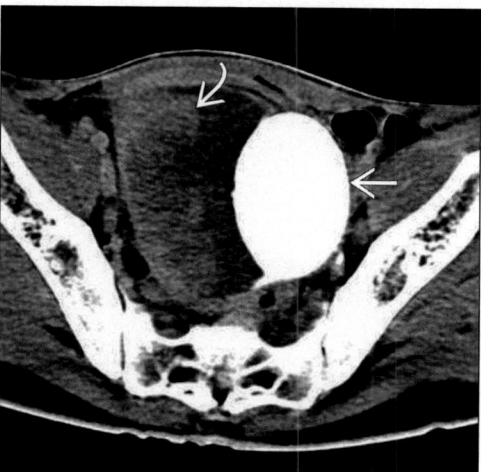

(Left) Transverse transabdominal ultrasound shows a large stone ➡ in the urinary bladder with strong posterior acoustic shadowing ➡. Note the large squamous cell carcinoma ➡ of the bladder wall. *(Right)* Transverse CECT of the same patient as in previous image clearly shows the large bladder calculus ➡ and the moderately enhancing squamous cell carcinoma of the bladder ➡.

5

34

Typical

(Left) Supine abdominal radiograph shows a well-defined, rounded radio-opacity in the right renal region ➡ *consistent with a renal calculus. (Right) Intravenous urogram (same patient as in previous image) shows a filling defect in the right renal pelvis* ➡ *. Note the fullness of the pelvicaliceal system* ➡ *with cupped calyces.*

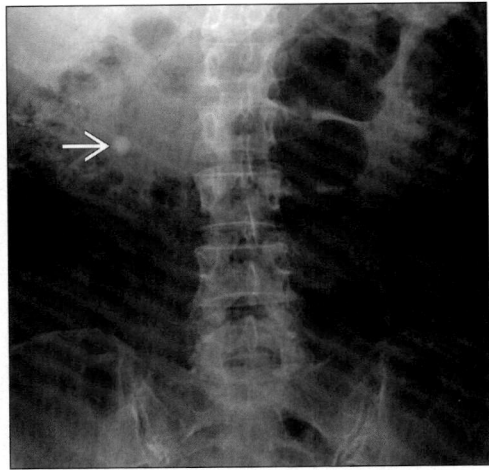

Typical

(Left) Longitudinal transabdominal ultrasound shows a large calculus in the renal pelvis ➡ *with strong posterior acoustic shadowing* ⇒ *. Note the dilatation of the pelvicaliceal system* ➡ *. (Right) Longitudinal transabdominal ultrasound shows a small, non-obstructive, echogenic calculus in the lower pole calyx* ➡ *, associated with acoustic shadowing* ➡ *. The pelvicaliceal system* ⇒ *and renal cortex appear normal.*

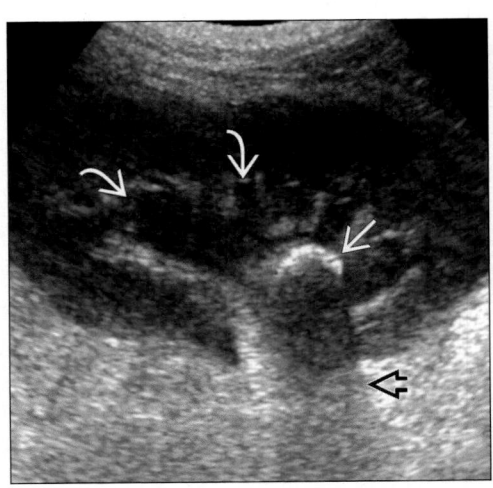
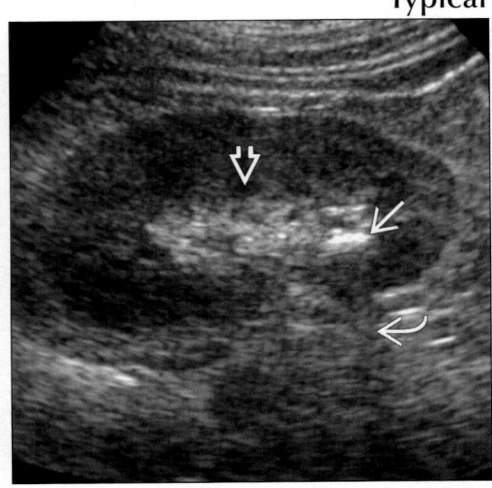

Typical

(Left) Longitudinal transabdominal ultrasound shows a large obstructing calculus ➡ *in the renal pelvis with posterior acoustic shadowing* ⇒ *. Note hydronephrosis* ➡ *and a thin renal cortex* ⇒ *. (Right) Longitudinal transabdominal ultrasound shows an echogenic calculus in the lower pole* ➡ *. The calyceal system is asymmetrically dilated with debris within* ➡ *suggesting pyonephrosis.*

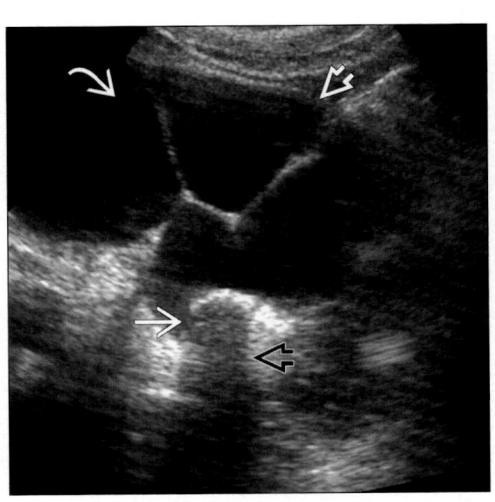
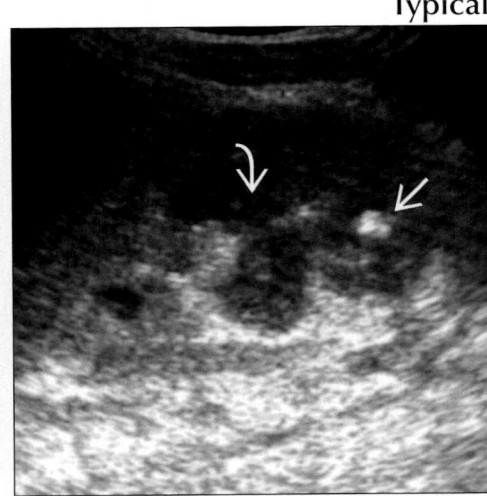

UROLITHIASIS

Typical

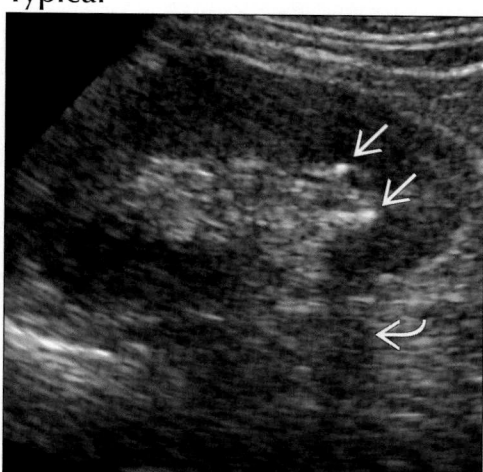 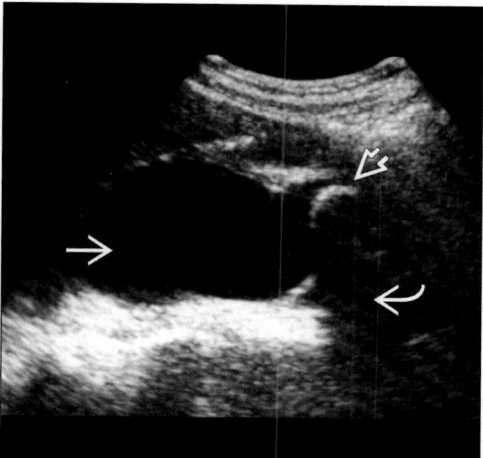

(Left) *Longitudinal transabdominal ultrasound shows multiple, small, shadowing ➡ calculi ➡ in the lower pole calyx with no dilatation of the pelvicaliceal system and normal cortical outline.* *(Right)* *Oblique transabdominal ultrasound shows a large calculus ➡ in the proximal ureter with strong posterior acoustic shadowing ➡. Note marked dilatation of the renal pelvis ➡ but no internal debris.*

Typical

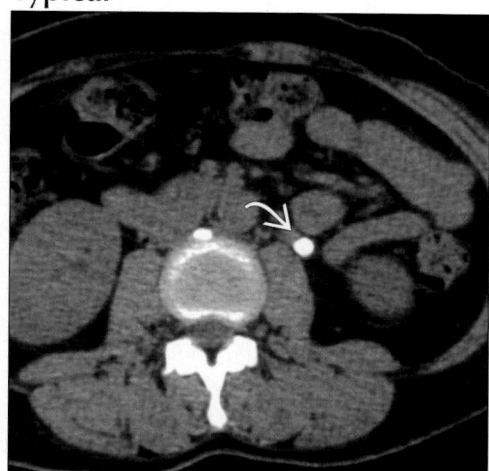 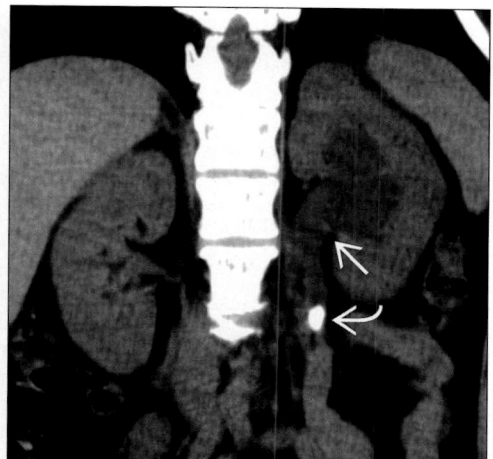

(Left) *Transverse NECT shows well-defined calculus in the proximal left ureter ➡. On US small ureteric calculi, in the absence of ureteral dilatation are often obscured by feces and bowel gas.* *(Right)* *NECT with coronal reformat shows an obstructing calculus in the left ureter at the junction of upper and middle third ➡. Note the dilatation of proximal ureter and pelvicaliceal system ➡.*

Typical

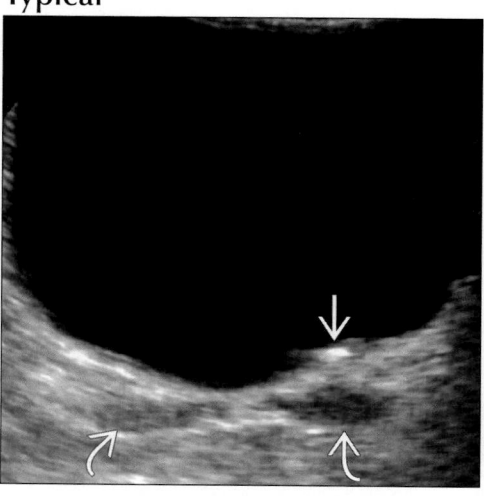 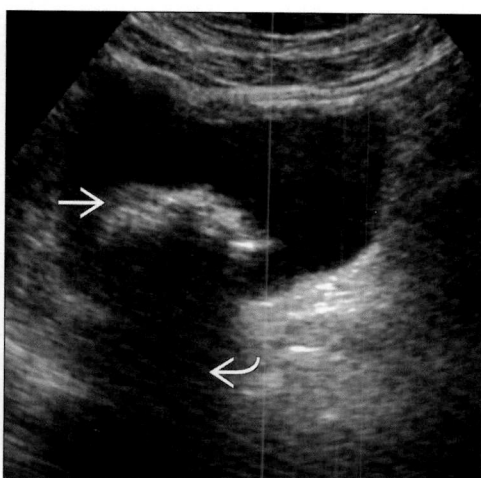

(Left) *Longitudinal transabdominal ultrasound shows a small echogenic calculus at the vesicoureteric junction ➡. Note dilatation of the ureter proximal to it ➡ and lack of dense shadowing.* *(Right)* *Transverse transabdominal ultrasound shows a large echogenic calculus in the bladder lumen ➡ with marked posterior acoustic shadowing ➡.*

NEPHROCALCINOSIS

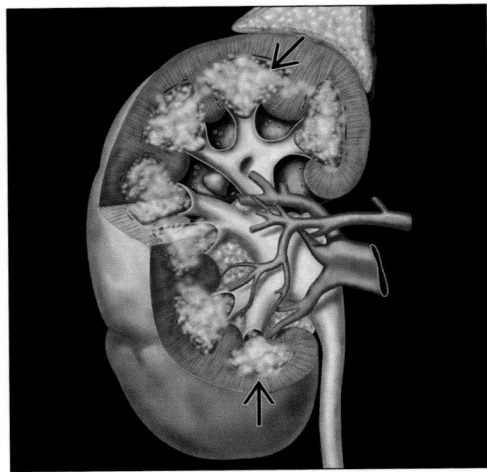

Graphic shows diffuse calcification ➡ in renal the pyramids, representing nephrocalcinosis.

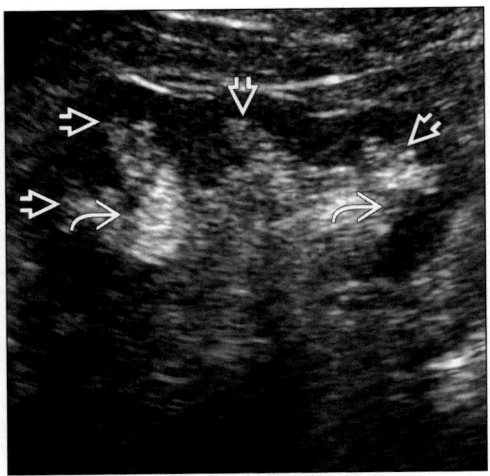

Longitudinal transabdominal ultrasound shows diffuse nephrocalcinosis, with marked increase in echogenicity of the renal pyramids ➡. Posterior acoustic shadowing is present in some regions ➡.

TERMINOLOGY

Abbreviations and Synonyms
- Medullary nephrocalcinosis, cortical nephrocalcinosis

Definitions
- Radiologically detectable diffuse calcium deposition within the renal substance

IMAGING FINDINGS

General Features
- Best diagnostic clue: Calcification within renal parenchyma
- Location
  - Renal parenchyma
    - Medullary nephrocalcinosis: 95%
    - Cortical nephrocalcinosis: 5%
    - Both cortical and medullary: Rare
- Size: Kidneys often normal size and contour
- Morphology
  - Variable patterns of calcification
    - Scattered punctate calcification in renal medullae
    - Dense, confluent medullary calcification: Common in renal tubular acidosis
    - "Tram line" calcification or punctate calcifications in renal cortex

Ultrasonographic Findings
- Grayscale Ultrasound
  - **Medullary nephrocalcinosis**
    - Earliest sign of medullary nephrocalcinosis: Absence of hypoechoic papillary structures
    - Solitary focus of hyperechogenicity at tip of pyramid near fornix
    - Hyperechoic rim at corticomedullary junction and along periphery of pyramids
    - Generalized increased echogenicity of renal pyramids +/- shadowing
    - Acoustic shadowing may be absent with small and light calcifications
  - **Cortical nephrocalcinosis**, less common
    - Homogeneously increased echogenicity of renal parenchyma
    - In cortical nephrocalcinosis kidney is more echogenic than liver

---

DDx: Nephrocalcinosis

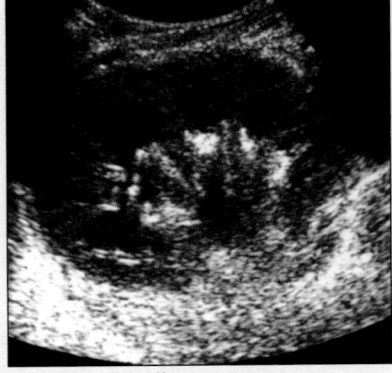

Papillary Necrosis

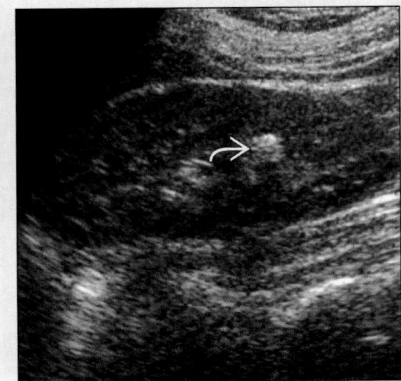

Renal Calculus

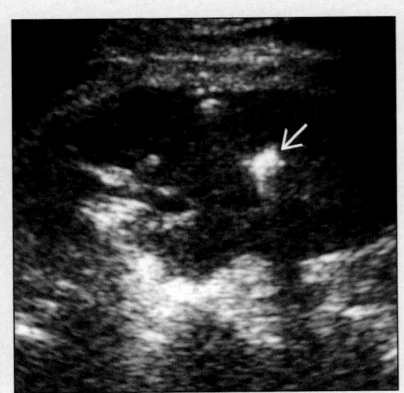

Emphysematous Pyelonephritis

NEPHROCALCINOSIS

Key Facts

Terminology
- Radiologically detectable diffuse calcium deposition within the renal substance

Imaging Findings
- Medullary nephrocalcinosis: 95%
- Cortical nephrocalcinosis: 5%
- Earliest sign of medullary nephrocalcinosis: Absence of hypoechoic papillary structures
- Solitary focus of hyperechogenicity at tip of pyramid near fornix
- Hyperechoic rim at corticomedullary junction and along periphery of pyramids
- Generalized increased echogenicity of renal pyramids +/- shadowing
- **Cortical nephrocalcinosis**, less common

- In cortical nephrocalcinosis kidney is more echogenic than liver
- US is sensitive for screening of early nephrocalcinosis in children with known predisposing metabolic conditions, such as RTA, hyperoxaluria

Top Differential Diagnoses
- Papillary Necrosis
- Renal Calculus
- Emphysematous Pyelonephritis

Diagnostic Checklist
- Focal areas of dystrophic calcification in masses or infection are not considered nephrocalcinosis

Radiographic Findings
- Radiography
  - Fine stippled calcification in renal pyramids
  - Coarse, confluent calcification
  - Punctate or "tramline" cortical calcification
- IVP
  - Medullary: Calcification in renal pyramids on preliminary films
  - May see linear striations and/or cystic spaces in papillae in patients with underlying medullary sponge kidney

CT Findings
- NECT
  - Stippled or confluent calcifications in renal parenchyma
  - May see ring-like pattern due to relatively increased calcification at corticomedullary junction

Imaging Recommendations
- Best imaging tool: Noncontrast CT
- Protocol advice
  - Detection of nephrocalcinosis on plain films is improved by low kV technique
  - US is sensitive for screening of early nephrocalcinosis in children with known predisposing metabolic conditions, such as RTA, hyperoxaluria

DIFFERENTIAL DIAGNOSIS

Papillary Necrosis
- Common in analgesic nephropathy
- Cystic collections within medullary pyramids
- Sloughed papilla seen as echogenic nonshadowing structure at the pyramids
- Clubbing of adjacent calyces
- Calcified sloughed papilla with distal acoustic shadowing

Renal Calculus
- Discrete echogenic focus with sharp distal acoustic shadowing

Emphysematous Pyelonephritis
- Gas within renal parenchyma associated with distal dirty shadowing

PATHOLOGY

General Features
- General path comments
  - Calcium stones grow on papillae
    - Most break loose and enter collecting system → urolithiasis
    - If calcium stones remain in place → medullary nephrocalcinosis
- Genetics
  - Type I renal tubular acidosis: Familial form
    - Autosomal dominant inheritance pattern most common
    - May be due to defect in chloride-bicarbonate exchange gene AE1
  - Hyperoxaluria: Familial form
    - Autosomal recessive
- Etiology
  - Medullary nephrocalcinosis
    - 40%: Hyperparathyroidism
    - 20%: Renal tubular acidosis type I
    - 20%: Medullary sponge kidney
  - Cortical nephrocalcinosis
    - Chronic glomerulonephritis
    - Renal cortical necrosis
    - Transplant kidney: Chronic rejection
  - Three primary mechanisms for calcium deposition
    - Metastatic: Metabolic abnormality leads to calcium deposition in the medullae of morphologically normal kidneys
    - Urinary stasis: Calcium salts precipitate in dilated collecting ducts containing static urine

NEPHROCALCINOSIS

- Dystrophic: Calcium deposition in damaged renal tissue
  - Entities causing metastatic calcification
    - Medullary: Renal tubular acidosis type I (distal)
    - Medullary: Hyperparathyroidism
    - Medullary: Hypercalcuria
    - Medullary: Hyperoxaluria
  - Nephrocalcinosis due to urinary stasis
    - Medullary sponge kidney (MSK): Cystic or fusiform dilation of collecting ducts in renal pyramids
  - Nephrocalcinosis due to dystrophic calcification
    - Acute cortical necrosis secondary to shock, placental abruption, nephrotoxins
    - Cortical: Chronic glomerulonephritis
- Epidemiology
  - Incidence: 0.1-6%
  - Medullary sponge kidney: Seen in 0.5% of excretory urograms
- Associated abnormalities: Urolithiasis when calculi formed in renal medulla erode into collecting system

Gross Pathologic & Surgical Features
- Depends on underlying etiology of nephrocalcinosis

Microscopic Features
- Calcium deposition in the interstitium, tubule epithelial cells, along basement membranes
- Calcium deposition within lumina of tubules

CLINICAL ISSUES

Presentation
- Most common signs/symptoms
  - Most often asymptomatic
  - Other signs/symptoms
    - Flank pain, hematuria if associated with urolithiasis
- Clinical profile: Cortical nephrocalcinosis
  - Acute cortical necrosis
    - Nephrotoxic drugs (ethylene glycol, methoxyflurane anesthesia, amphotericin B)
    - Acute vascular insult (shock, placental abruption)
  - Chronic glomerulonephritis
  - Alport syndrome: Hereditary nephritis and nerve deafness
- Clinical profile: Medullary nephrocalcinosis
  - Skeletal deossification
    - Primary and secondary hyperparathyroidism
    - Bony metastases
    - Prolonged immobilization
  - Increased intestinal absorption of calcium
    - Sarcoidosis
    - Milk-alkali syndrome
  - Medullary sponge kidney
  - Hyperoxaluria
    - Hereditary type
    - Acquired: Secondary to small bowel disease or bariatric surgery
  - Renal tubular acidosis type I (distal RTA)
    - May be primary or secondary to other systemic disease (Sjögren, lupus, others)
    - Distal tubule unable to secrete hydrogen ions

- Metabolic acidosis with urinary pH > 5.5
- Type II (proximal) RTA never causes nephrocalcinosis

Demographics
- Age: Any
- Gender: M > F

Natural History & Prognosis
- Depends on underlying cause of nephrocalcinosis

Treatment
- Options, risks, complications: Medullary nephrocalcinosis often complicated by urolithiasis

DIAGNOSTIC CHECKLIST

Consider
- Focal areas of dystrophic calcification in masses or infection are not considered nephrocalcinosis

Image Interpretation Pearls
- Massive, dense medullary nephrocalcinosis usually due to RTA type I
- Unilateral or segmental medullary nephrocalcinosis → medullary sponge kidney

SELECTED REFERENCES

1. Aziz S et al: Rapidly developing nephrocalcinosis in a patient with end-stage liver disease who received a domino liver transplant from a patient with known congenital oxalosis. J Ultrasound Med. 24(10):1449-52, 2005
2. Lin CC et al: Renal sonographic findings of type I glycogen storage disease in infancy and early childhood. Pediatr Radiol. 35(8):786-91, 2005
3. Sakamoto H et al: Bilateral nephrocalcinosis associated with distal renal tubular acidosis. Intern Med. 44(1):81-2, 2005
4. Diallo O et al: Type 1 primary hyperoxaluria in pediatric patients: renal sonographic patterns. AJR Am J Roentgenol. 183(6):1767-70, 2004
5. Hoppe B et al: Diagnostic and therapeutic approaches in patients with secondary hyperoxaluria. Front Biosci. 8:e437-43, 2003
6. Peacock M: Primary hyperparathyroidism and the kidney: biochemical and clinical spectrum. J Bone Miner Res. 17 Suppl 2:N87-94, 2002
7. Kim YG et al: Medullary nephrocalcinosis associated with long-term furosemide abuse in adults. Nephrol Dial Transplant. 16(12):2303-9, 2001
8. Sayer JA et al: Diagnosis and clinical biochemistry of inherited tubulopathies. Ann Clin Biochem. 38(Pt 5):459-70, 2001
9. Unwin RJ et al: The renal tubular acidoses. J R Soc Med. 94(5):221-5, 2001
10. Schepens D et al: Images in Nephrology. Renal cortical nephrocalcinosis. Nephrol Dial Transplant. 15(7):1080-2, 2000
11. Campfield T et al: Nephrocalcinosis in premature infants: variability in ultrasound detection. J Perinatol. 19(7):498-500, 1999
12. Chen MY et al: Abnormal calcification on plain radiographs of the abdomen. Crit Rev Diagn Imaging. 40(2-3):63-202, 1999
13. Dyer RB et al: Abnormal calcifications in the urinary tract. Radiographics. 18(6):1405-24, 1998

NEPHROCALCINOSIS

IMAGE GALLERY

Typical

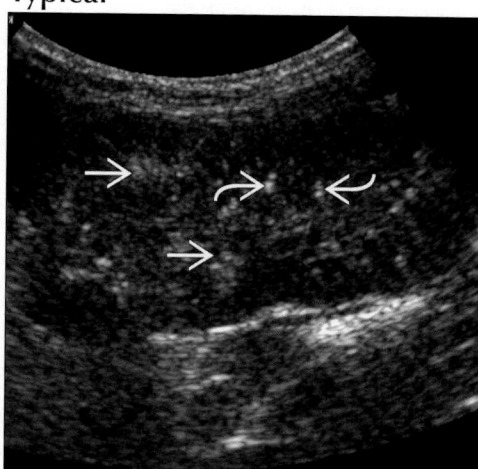

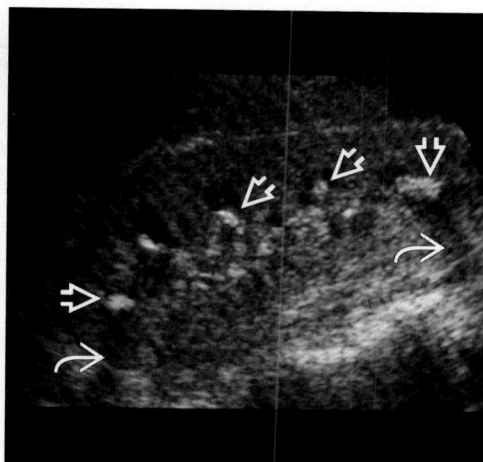

(Left) Longitudinal transabdominal ultrasound shows early nephrocalcinosis with loss of the normal hypoechoic papillary structures ➡. Tiny foci of echogenicity ➡ are found in some pyramids. *(Right)* Longitudinal transabdominal ultrasound shows hyperechogenicity present at the tip of the pyramids ➡, associated with posterior acoustic shadowing ➡.

Typical

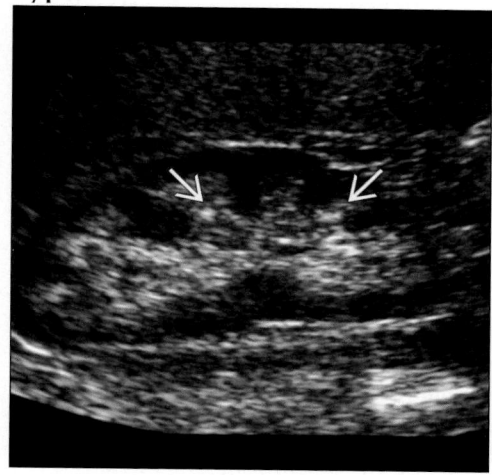

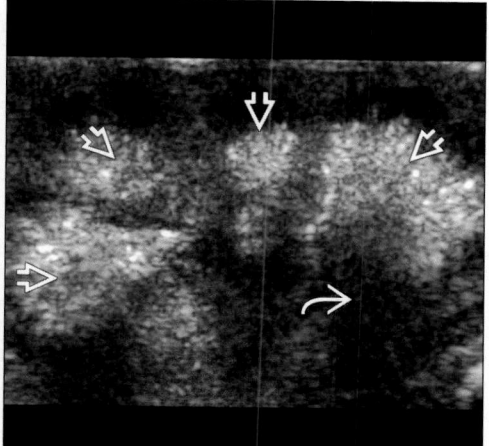

(Left) Longitudinal transabdominal ultrasound shows early nephrocalcinosis with tiny echogenic foci ➡ present in some pyramids. *(Right)* Longitudinal transabdominal ultrasound shows an advanced stage of nephrocalcinosis, with generalized increased echogenicity of the renal pyramids ➡ and associated posterior acoustic shadowing ➡.

Typical

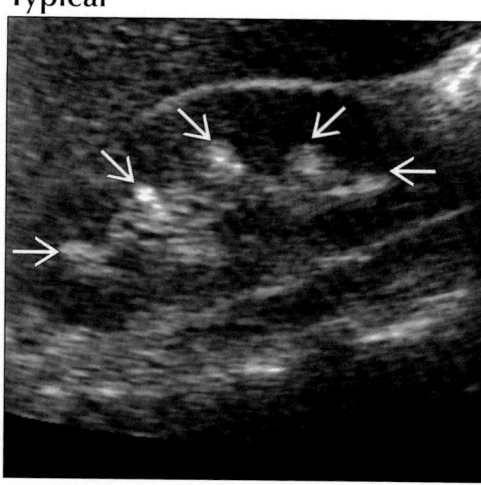

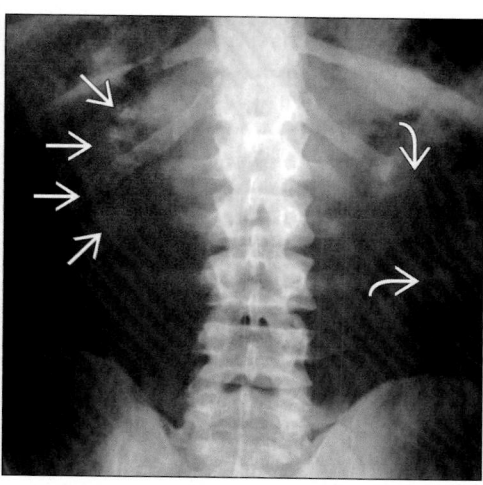

(Left) Longitudinal transabdominal ultrasound shows diffuse echogenic renal pyramids ➡. *(Right)* Posteroanterior radiography shows diffuse, densely calcified pyramids ➡ in the right kidney. Nephrocalcinosis in the left kidney ➡ is less well seen as it is partially obscured by bowel gas.

HYDRONEPHROSIS

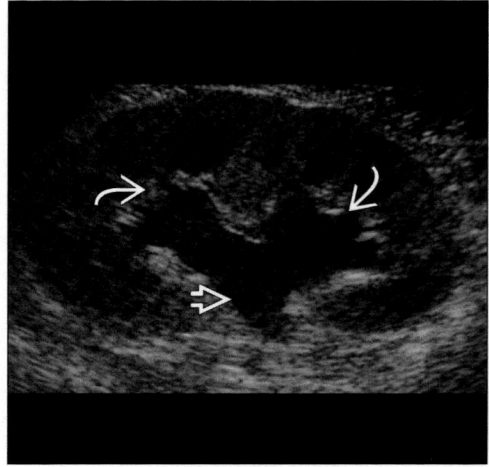

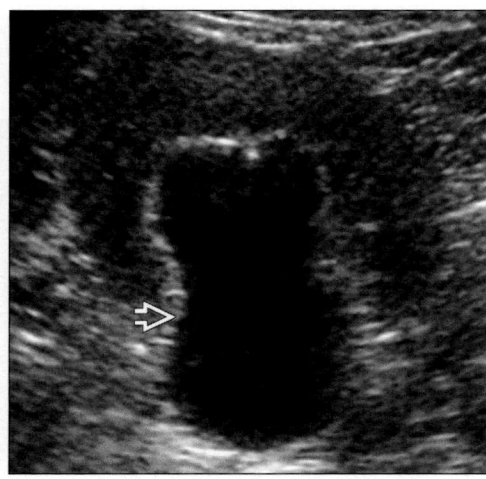

Longitudinal transabdominal ultrasound shows dilated upper and lower pole calyces ➡ communicating with the renal pelvis ➡.

Transverse transabdominal ultrasound shows moderate dilatation of the renal pelvis ➡. The cortical thickness is normal.

TERMINOLOGY

Abbreviations and Synonyms
- Pelvicaliectasis, pelvicaliceal dilatation

Definitions
- Calyceal dilatation of any cause

IMAGING FINDINGS

General Features
- Best diagnostic clue: Dilated renal pelvis communicating with anechoic fluid-filled calyces
- Size
  - Degree of collecting system dilatation depends on
    - Duration of obstruction
    - Renal output
    - Presence of spontaneous decompression

Ultrasonographic Findings
- Grayscale Ultrasound
  - General features

- Group of anechoic fluid-filled spaces within sinus complex, communicating
- Renal enlargement
- Mild hydronephrosis: Small separation of calyceal pattern (splaying), normal bright sinus echoes, normal parenchymal thickness
- Moderate hydronephrosis: Ballooning of major and minor calyces, diminished sinus echoes, normal or thinned parenchymal thickness
- Severe hydronephrosis: Massive dilatation of renal pelvis and calyces, associated with cortical thinning and loss of normal renal sinus echogenicity
  - Ultrasound grading
    - Grade 0: Homogeneous central renal sinus complex without separation
    - Grade 1: Separation of central sinus echoes of ovoid configuration, continuity of echogenic sinus periphery
    - Grade 2: Separation of central sinus echoes of rounded configuration, dilated calycesces connecting with renal pelvis; continuity of echogenic sinus periphery

DDx: Hydronephrosis

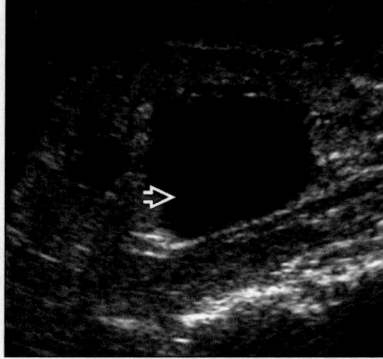

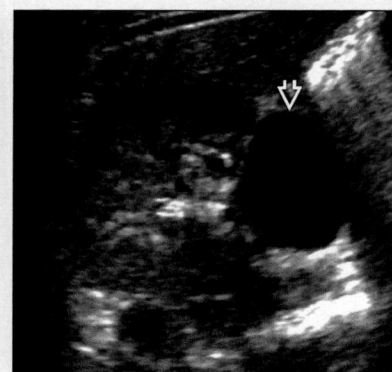

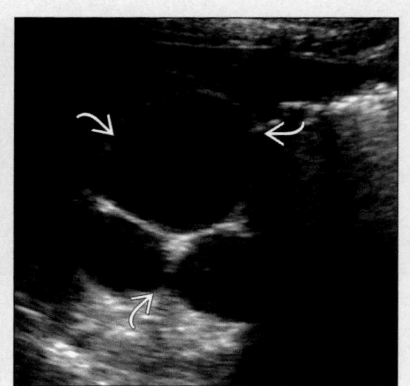

Parapelvic Cyst

Extrarenal Pelvis

Multicystic Dysplastic Kidney

HYDRONEPHROSIS

Key Facts

Terminology
- Calyceal dilatation of any cause

Imaging Findings
- Best diagnostic clue: Dilated renal pelvis communicating with anechoic fluid-filled calyces
- Mild hydronephrosis: Small separation of calyceal pattern (splaying), normal bright sinus echoes, normal parenchymal thickness
- Moderate hydronephrosis: Ballooning of major and minor calyces, diminished sinus echoes, normal or thinned parenchymal thickness
- Fetal renal pelvis diameter ≥ 8 mm at 20-30 week or ≥ 10 mm beyond 30 week gestation requires post natal follow-up

Top Differential Diagnoses
- Parapelvic Cyst
- Extrarenal Pelvis
- Multicystic Dysplastic (MCD) Kidney

Clinical Issues
- Complicated by spontaneous urinary extravasation from forniceal/pelvic tear if acute obstruction
- Superimposed infection, calculus formation if chronic obstruction
- Parenchymal atrophy if chronic obstruction, leading to renal impairment

- - Grade 3: Replacement of major portions of renal sinus; discontinuity of echogenic sinus periphery
  - ○ Antenatal US: Renal pelvis anterior-posterior (AP) diameter ≥ 5 mm prior to 20 week gestation
    - Fetal renal pelvis diameter ≥ 8 mm at 20-30 week or ≥ 10 mm beyond 30 week gestation requires post natal follow-up
  - ○ Postnatal US: Increased renal parenchymal echogenicity is predictor of impaired relative renal function
  - ○ Intermittent hydronephrosis secondary to ureteropelvic junction obstruction
    - Clearly demonstrable obstruction of renal pelvis during acute attack
    - Renal pelvis obstruction diminishes/resolves during symptom-free intervals
    - Renal pelvic wall thickening on convalescence
  - ○ Focal hydronephrosis (hydrocalyx): Congenital, infectious stricture
    - Anechoic cystic lesion with smooth margin, commonly upper pole
- Pulsed Doppler
  - ○ RI normal in non-obstructed dilatation in pregnancy or chronic obstruction
  - ○ Obstructive hydronephrosis: RI > 0.7 or RI 0.1 higher than opposite side in unilateral obstruction
  - ○ Arteriolar vasoconstriction in obstruction, hence reduces diastolic arterial flow velocity
- Color Doppler: Ureteric jet not detectable/at low level in acute obstruction

Radiographic Findings
- IVP
  - ○ Increasingly dense nephrogram in acute obstruction
  - ○ Diminished nephrographic density in chronic hydronephrosis
  - ○ Delayed opacification of collecting system
  - ○ Dilated collecting system +/- ureter
  - ○ Widening of forniceal angles
  - ○ Site of obstruction demonstrated at end of persistent column of contrast in dilated system
  - ○ Reduced parenchymal thickness in chronic hydronephrosis

CT Findings
- NECT
  - ○ Dilatation of renal collecting system +/- ureter
  - ○ Inflammation or perinephric or periureteral fat
  - ○ Ureteral rim sign: Thickening of ureteral wall secondary to edema from stone impaction

Nuclear Medicine Findings
- DMSA scan: Central photopenic area +/- cortical scar
- MAG 3/DTPA scan: Central photopenic area at vascular phase, tracer accumulation within hydronephrotic collecting system with delayed drainage

Imaging Recommendations
- Best imaging tool: IVP or contrast-enhanced CT helps differentiate hydronephrosis or multiple parapelvic cysts
- Protocol advice
  - ○ Work-up of prenatal diagnosed hydronephrosis
    - Post natal US for serial monitoring
    - Voiding cystourethrogram to evaluate vesicoureteric reflux or posterior urethral valves in severe cases
    - Diuretic renography to evaluate degree of obstruction and determine differential renal function
  - ○ Post natal US to be performed 4-7 days after birth because relative dehydration in first days of life: False negative sign of hydronephrosis

DIFFERENTIAL DIAGNOSIS

Parapelvic Cyst
- Lymphatic in origin or develop from embryologic rests
- Well-defined anechoic renal sinus mass
- May have internal echoes if hemorrhage
- Does not communicate with the collecting system

Extrarenal Pelvis
- Calyces not dilated
- Beyond renal outline on transverse scans

HYDRONEPHROSIS

Multicystic Dysplastic (MCD) Kidney
- Developmental anomaly, also known as renal dysplasia, renal dysgenesis, multicystic kidney
- Small kidney with multiple non-communicating cysts
- Absence of both normal parenchyma and normal renal sinus complex

Prominent Renal Vasculature
- Mimics dilated renal pelvis on transverse scans
- Vascular flow demonstrated on color Doppler

Renal Medullae in Infant/Children
- Prominent subcortical hypoechoic medullae mimic hydrocalices

Autosomal Dominant Polycystic Kidney
- Bilateral enlarged kidneys with multiple asymmetrical cysts of varying size
- Cysts with internal echoes if hemorrhage or infected

PATHOLOGY

General Features
- Etiology
  - Obstruction: Stone, blood clot, sloughed papilla, crossing of iliac vessels, stricture
    - +/- Ureteric dilatation, depending on level of obstruction
    - Confirmed by IVP, isotope renogram, antegrade/retrograde pyelography
    - Hydronephrosis may be absent in acute obstruction
    - In long-standing obstruction, calyceal dilatation usually occurs except in retroperitoneal fibrosis
  - Relieved obstruction
    - If obstruction severe or prolonged, dilatation may not return to normal
  - Reflux nephropathy
    - Upper pole calyces more often affected, associated with scar
  - Pregnancy
    - More marked on right side, may become permanent after multiple pregnancies
  - Congenital hydronephrosis
    - Ureteropelvic obstruction, posterior urethral valve, ectopic ureterocele, prune belly syndrome, vesicoureteric junction obstruction
    - Mostly isolated malformation
  - Papillary necrosis
    - Calyces with sloughed papillae become clubbed
  - Post infective/prolonged pyelonephritis
    - Calyceal clubbing and scar
- Associated abnormalities: Amount of residual renal cortex is of prognostic significance

CLINICAL ISSUES

Presentation
- Most common signs/symptoms
  - Diagnosed on antenatal US
  - Abdominal mass
  - Flank pain/hematuria for renal or ureteric stone

Natural History & Prognosis
- Complicated by spontaneous urinary extravasation from forniceal/pelvic tear if acute obstruction
- Superimposed infection, calculus formation if chronic obstruction
- Parenchymal atrophy if chronic obstruction, leading to renal impairment

DIAGNOSTIC CHECKLIST

Consider
- If normal pattern of fornices disturbed in US/IVP

Image Interpretation Pearls
- False positive sign of hydronephrosis
  - Full bladder may cause distension of calyces, reverts to normal when bladder empty
  - Increased urine flow: Overhydration, medication, following urography

SELECTED REFERENCES

1. Becker A et al: Obstructive uropathy. Early Hum Dev. 82(1):15-22, 2006
2. Belarmino JM et al: Management of neonatal hydronephrosis. Early Hum Dev. 82(1):9-14, 2006
3. Chi T et al: Increased echogenicity as a predictor of poor renal function in children with grade 3 to 4 hydronephrosis. J Urol. 175(5):1898-901, 2006
4. Pates JA et al: Prenatal diagnosis and management of hydronephrosis. Early Hum Dev. 82(1):3-8, 2006
5. Sidhu G et al: Outcome of isolated antenatal hydronephrosis: a systematic review and meta-analysis. Pediatr Nephrol. 21(2):218-24, 2006
6. Tsai JD et al: Intermittent hydronephrosis secondary to ureteropelvic junction obstruction: clinical and imaging features. Pediatrics. 117(1):139-46, 2006
7. Riccabona M et al: Hydronephrotic kidney: pediatric three-dimensional US for relative renal size assessment--initial experience. Radiology. 236(1):276-83, 2005
8. Wollenberg A et al: Outcome of fetal renal pelvic dilatation diagnosed during the third trimester. Ultrasound Obstet Gynecol. 25(5):483-8, 2005
9. Cheng AM et al: Outcome of isolated antenatal hydronephrosis. Arch Pediatr Adolesc Med. 158(1):38-40, 2004
10. Moon DH et al: Value of supranormal function and renogram patterns on 99mTc-mercaptoacetyltriglycine scintigraphy in relation to the extent of hydronephrosis for predicting ureteropelvic junction obstruction in the newborn. J Nucl Med. 44(5):725-31, 2003
11. Hertzberg BS et al: Doppler US assessment of maternal kidneys: analysis of intrarenal resistivity indexes in normal pregnancy and physiologic pelvicaliectasis. Radiology. 186(3):689-92, 1993
12. Kamholtz RG et al: Obstruction and the minimally dilated renal collecting system: US evaluation. Radiology. 170(1 Pt 1):51-3, 1989
13. Scola FH et al: Grade I hydronephrosis: pulsed Doppler US evaluation. Radiology. 171(2):519-20, 1989
14. Laing FC et al: Postpartum evaluation of fetal hydronephrosis: optimal timing for follow-up sonography. Radiology. 152(2):423-4, 1984

HYDRONEPHROSIS

IMAGE GALLERY

Typical

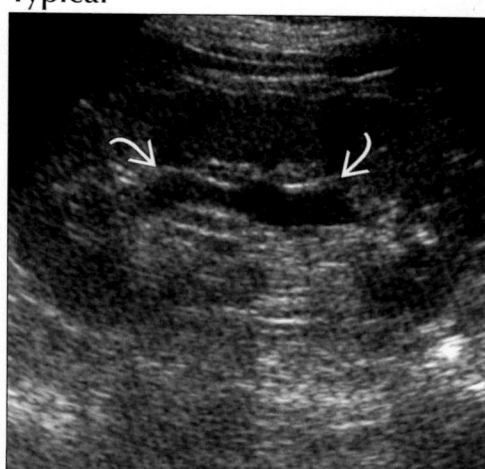

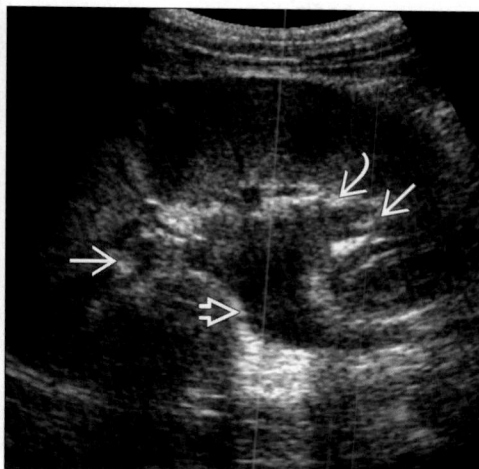

(Left) Longitudinal transabdominal ultrasound shows splaying of calyces ➡ in mild hydronephrosis. *(Right)* Longitudinal transabdominal ultrasound shows a dilated renal pelvis ➡ and mild caliectasis ➡ in a patient with a full bladder. The normal pattern of fornices ➡ is still preserved.

Typical

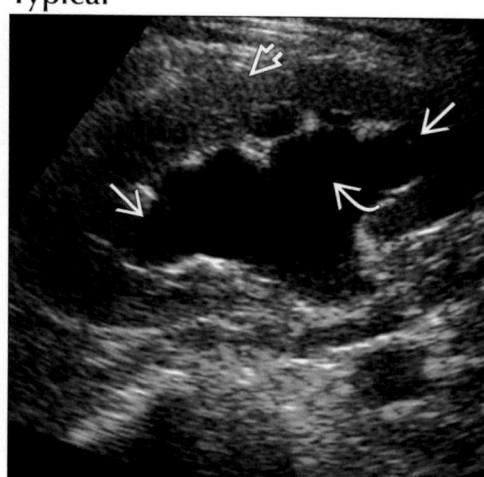

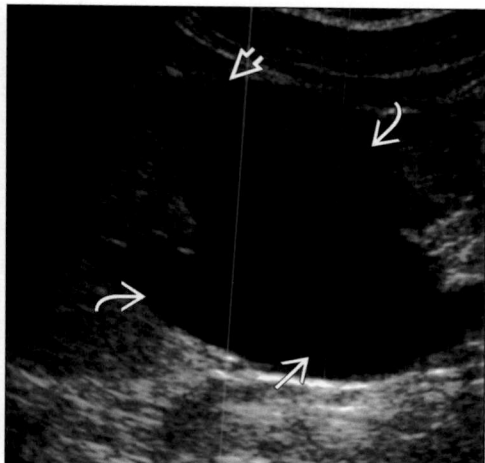

(Left) Longitudinal transabdominal ultrasound shows ballooning of the major ➡ and minor calyces ➡ in moderate hydronephrosis. Note normal renal cortical thickness ➡. *(Right)* Longitudinal transabdominal ultrasound shows marked dilatation of the renal pelvis ➡ and calyces ➡ in severe hydronephrosis. There is a focal cortical scar ➡ at mid pole.

Typical

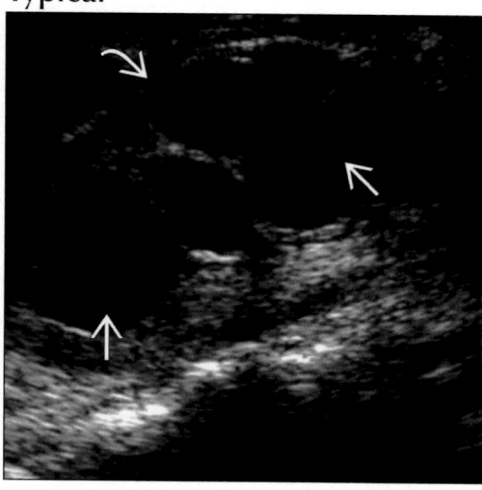

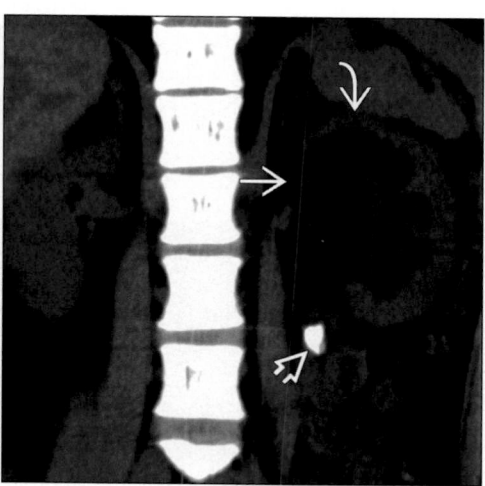

(Left) Longitudinal transabdominal ultrasound shows a dilated calyceal system ➡ with cortical thinning ➡ in chronic hydronephrosis. *(Right)* NECT with coronal reformation shows hydronephrosis ➡ on the left side due to an obstructing upper ureteric calculus ➡. Note the upper pole cortical thinning ➡ due to chronic obstruction.

SIMPLE RENAL CYST

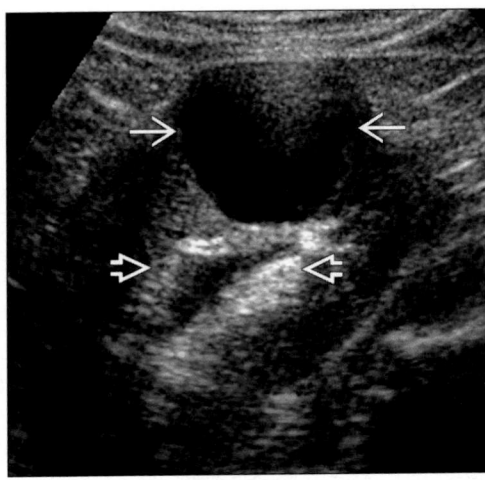

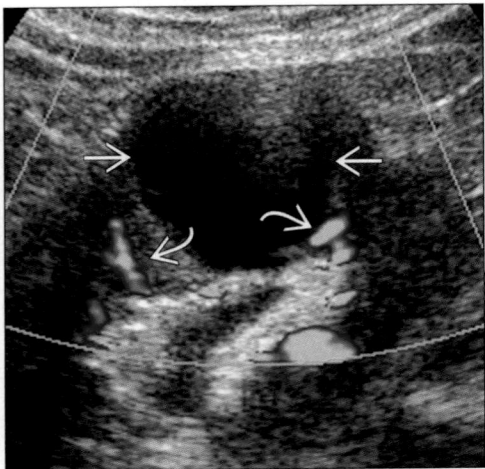

Longitudinal transabdominal ultrasound shows a simple renal cortical cyst ➡. The cyst is round, thin-walled, without internal solid material and with posterior accoustic enhancement ➡.

Longitudinal color Doppler ultrasound of the same renal cyst ➡ as previous image. Note the avascular nature of this lesion, with splaying of the adjacent blood vessels ➡.

TERMINOLOGY

Definitions
- A benign, fluid-filled, nonneoplastic renal lesion
- Most common renal lesion, usually detected incidentally on imaging
- Occurs as single or multiple lesions and rarely unilateral if multiple
- Uncommon in children and young adults, except for those with chronic renal disease undergoing renal dialysis
- Incidence increases with age
- Rarely associated with tuberous sclerosis, von Hippel-Lindau disease, neurofibromatosis or Caroli disease

IMAGING FINDINGS

General Features
- Best diagnostic clue: Well-defined, round or oval, smooth thin-walled renal lesion with or without displacement of central calyceal system
- Location: Renal cortex (deep or superficial)

- Size: Diameter ranges from few mm to more than 10 cm
- Other general features
  - Simple renal cyst classification
    - Typical or uncomplicated
    - Complicated: Hemorrhagic, infected, ruptured, neoplasm from cystic wall
    - Atypical: Calcified, hyperdense, septated, multiple simple, localized cystic disease, milk of calcium

Ultrasonographic Findings
- Grayscale Ultrasound
  - Typically appears as anechoic, unilocular, thin-walled, round/oval renal lesion
  - Has good sound transmission giving rise to characteristic distal acoustic enhancement
  - Has no internal echoes, septum or solid component
  - Small cysts (< 3 mm in diameter) may appear as echo-free lesions without posterior acoustic enhancement
  - US is more accurate than CT in demonstrating internal cyst morphology
  - If multiple simple cysts are found, it is important to rule out polycystic kidney disease

DDx: Renal Simple Cyst

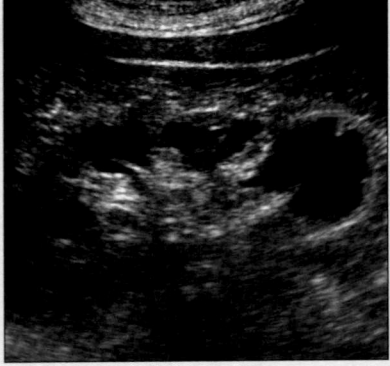

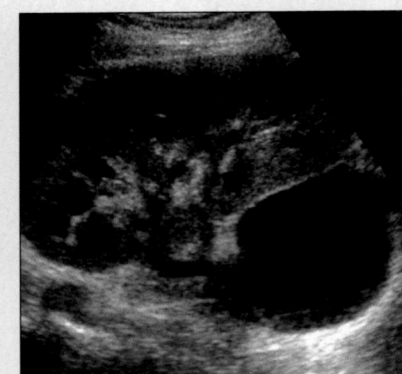

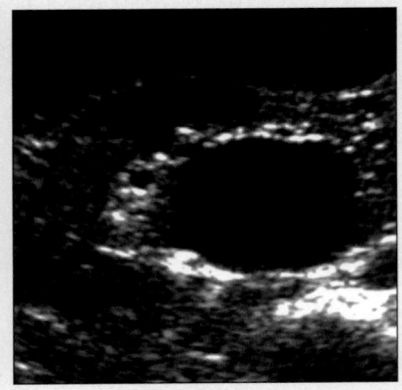

Hydrocalyces

Perinephric Collection

Parapelvic Cyst

SIMPLE RENAL CYST

Key Facts

Terminology
- A benign, fluid-filled, nonneoplastic renal lesion

Imaging Findings
- Typically appears as anechoic, unilocular, thin-walled, round/oval renal lesion
- Has good sound transmission giving rise to characteristic distal acoustic enhancement
- Has no internal echoes, septum or solid component
- Small cysts (< 3 mm in diameter) may appear as echo-free lesions without posterior acoustic enhancement
- US is more accurate than CT in demonstrating internal cyst morphology
- If multiple simple cysts are found, it is important to rule out polycystic kidney disease
- Lack of intracystic color signal
- Adjacent blood vessels seen to be displaced
- Best imaging tool: Ultrasound is ideal for characterizing simple or complex renal cysts

Top Differential Diagnoses
- Hydrocalyx or Hydronephrosis
- Perinephric Collections
- Parapelvic Cyst
- Prominent Pyramids
- Pyelogenic Cyst
- Extrarenal Pelvis

Diagnostic Checklist
- Anechoic intracystic content with good through transmission, no internal septation
- Always distinguish simple renal cyst from other complex cystic renal lesions

- Color Doppler
  - Lack of intracystic color signal
  - Adjacent blood vessels seen to be displaced

Radiographic Findings
- Radiography: Abdominal radiographs occasionally show cortical bulge projecting into perinephric fat
- IVP
  - Well-defined nonenhancing radiolucent mass in renal parenchyma
  - Large cyst distorts renal contour and splays or obliterates calyces
  - "Beak or claw" sign may be seen if cysts extend beyond renal capsule

CT Findings
- CT: Water density, spherical/oval nonenhancing lesion with no visible wall
- Categorized as class I cyst in Bosniak classification system
  - Benign cyst that contains no septum or calcifications
  - Homogeneous, lucent mass of water density (< 20 HU) with a thin or invisible, nonenhancing wall
- Small (< 1 cm): Cannot measure region of interest; if less than blood density on NECT, probably cyst

MR Findings
- T1WI: Round/oval, homogeneous, hypointense mass
- T2WI: Homogeneous, hyperintense mass with imperceptible wall; smooth & distinct inner margin
- CEMR: No enhancement

Imaging Recommendations
- Best imaging tool: Ultrasound is ideal for characterizing simple or complex renal cysts
- Protocol advice: Once diagnosis of simple renal cyst is established, no further imaging or monitoring of the cyst is warranted

DIFFERENTIAL DIAGNOSIS

Polycystic Kidney Disease (PCKD)
- Both kidneys are grossly enlarged with renal parenchyma largely replaced by cysts of varying size
- May have hepatic and pancreatic cystic involvement
- Usually no appreciable renal tissue on ultrasound
- Important to detect atypical features of cysts which may represent hemorrhage, infection or tumor growth

Hydrocalyx or Hydronephrosis
- Dilated calyces coalesce centrally appearing like fingers of a glove
- May be confused with multiple simple renal cysts
- Can be differentiated from cysts by demonstrating communication with collecting system

Perinephric Collections
- Loculated perinephric fluid collections may indent or distort renal contour
- Seromas or urinomas invariably simulate simple renal cysts

Parapelvic Cyst
- Lymphangiectases of renal hilum
- Appears as medially located cystic lesion with surrounding echogenic walls
- Rarely extend to corticomedullary junction or involve renal capsule
- Lack of communication of cyst with collecting system
- Can be isolated, multiple, unilateral, or bilateral
- Most are asymptomatic, but may cause hematuria, hypertension, hydronephrosis, become infected or hemorrhagic

Prominent Pyramids
- Prominent pyramids may be observed in normal pediatric kidneys, acute glomerulonephritis, transplant acute rejection and acute tubular necrosis

Pyelogenic Cyst
- Also referred to as pyelocalyceal diverticulum

SIMPLE RENAL CYST

- Is urine-containing eventration of upper collecting system
- Appears as cystic lesion, sometimes thick-walled arising from renal parenchyma
- Mimics simple renal cyst or obstructed hydrocalyx
- Ultrasound and CT are nonspecific unless intracystic milk of calcium or mobile calculi are present
- IVP is modality of choice

Extrarenal Pelvis

- Can be demonstrated to communicate with collecting system

PATHOLOGY

General Features

- Etiology
  - Exact etiology is uncertain
  - Is believed to be caused by obstruction of ducts or tubules or may arise in embryonic rests

Gross Pathologic & Surgical Features

- Unilocular; arise in cortex (superficial) and bulge from renal surface; less common from medulla
- Clear or straw-colored fluid; up to several liters
- Smooth, yellow-white, thin and translucent wall
- Rarely calcified; no communication to renal pelvis

Microscopic Features

- Cyst wall is composed of fibrous tissue and is lined by flattened cuboidal epithelium
- Cyst fluid contains plasma transudate

CLINICAL ISSUES

Presentation

- Most common signs/symptoms
  - Mostly asymptomatic
  - May present with palpable mass
  - Local pain due to large cyst wall distention or spontaneous intracystic hemorrhage
  - Flank pain, malaise and fever due to infected cyst
- Other signs/symptoms
  - Occasionally, severe abdominal pain and hematuria caused by spontaneous, iatrogenic or traumatic rupture of cyst
  - Rarely, hypertension may occur secondary to renal segmental ischemia as a result of cyst obstruction

Demographics

- Age
  - Occur in 50% of patients > 50 years of age
  - Rare in individuals < 30 years of age
- Gender: Most reports show no gender predilections but some suggest incidence M > F

Natural History & Prognosis

- Low malignant potential
- Slow-growing and increases in size by 5% annually
- Complications include hydronephrosis, hemorrhage, infection or rupture

- Spontaneous cyst rupture into collecting system or perinephric space may occur due to buildup of pressure within cyst secondary to either intracystic hemorrhage or change in cyst fluid content
- Following rupture, cyst may regress or disappear completely
- In general, prognosis is very good

Treatment

- Indications for surgical intervention reserved solely for symptomatic cysts that affect renal function
- Cyst rupture is managed conservatively
- Treatment options include
  - Percutaneous needle aspiration of cyst +/- injection of sclerosing agent
  - Retrograde marsupialization and flexible ureteroscopy: Nephroscopy
  - Laparoscopic marsupialization or excision

DIAGNOSTIC CHECKLIST

Consider

- Characterize simple from complex cysts
- If multiple simple cysts found, exclude findings of polycystic kidney disease

Image Interpretation Pearls

- Anechoic intracystic content with good through transmission, no internal septation
- Always distinguish simple renal cyst from other complex cystic renal lesions

SELECTED REFERENCES

1. Israel GM et al: An update of the Bosniak renal cyst classification system. Urology. 66(3):484-8, 2005
2. Bisset RAL, Khan AN (ed). Differential Diagnosis in Abdominal Ultrasound. WB Saunders. 334-335, 2002
3. Terada N et al: The natural history of simple renal cysts. J Urol. 167(1):21-3, 2002
4. Rathaus V et al: Pyelocalyceal diverticulum: the imaging spectrum with emphasis on the ultrasound features. Br J Radiol. 74(883):595-601, 2001
5. Bosniak MA: Diagnosis and management of patients with complicated cystic lesions of the kidney. AJR. 169: 819, 1997
6. Davidson AJ et al: Radiologic assessment of renal masses: Implication for patient care. Radiology. 202: 297, 1997
7. Siegel CL et al: CT of cystic renal masses: Analysis of diagnostic performance and interobserver variation. AJR. 169: 813, 1997
8. Bosniak MA: Difficulties in classifying cystic lesions of the kidney. Urol Radiol. 13(2):91-3, 1991
9. Luscher TF et al: Simple renal cyst and hypertension: cause or coincidence? Clin Nephrol. 26(2):91-5, 1986
10. Papanicolaou N et al: Spontaneous and traumatic rupture of renal cysts: diagnosis and outcome. Radiology. 160(1):99-103, 1986
11. Chan JC et al: Hypertension and hematuria secondary to parapelvic cyst. Pediatrics. 65(4):821-3, 1980

SIMPLE RENAL CYST

IMAGE GALLERY

Typical

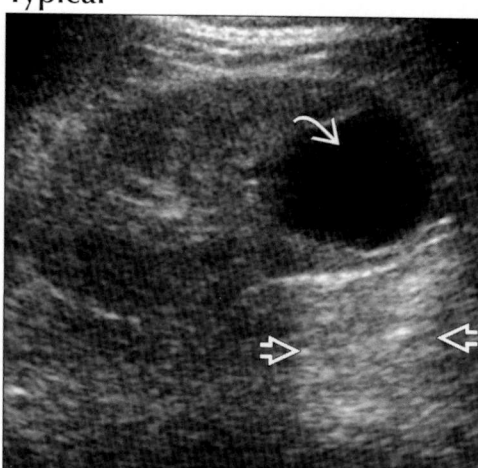 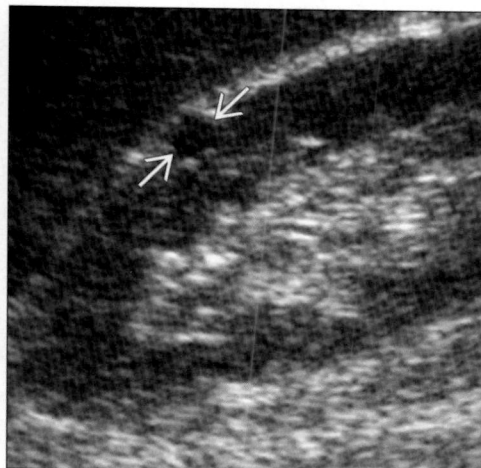

(Left) Longitudinal transabdominal ultrasound shows a typical renal cyst embedded within the renal parenchyma. Note distal acoustic enhancement ➡, which is typical of a simple cyst ➡. (Right) Longitudinal transabdominal ultrasound shows a small renal cortical cyst ➡ with no distal acoustic enhancement. Absence of this typical feature may cause confusion of small cysts with solid tumors.

Typical

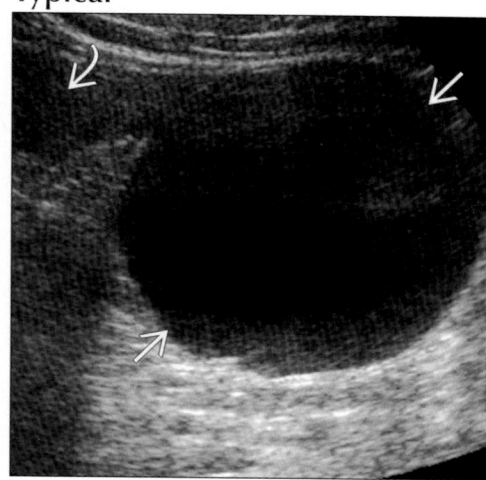 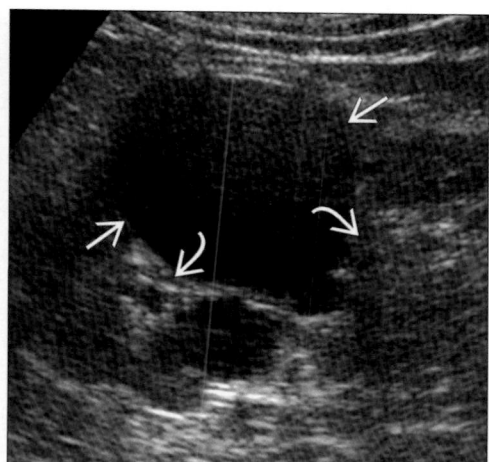

(Left) Longitudinal transabdominal ultrasound shows a large renal cyst ➡ arising from the lower pole of the kidney ➡. Large cysts may produce distension, pain or spontaneous hemorrhage. (Right) Longitudinal transabdominal ultrasound shows a large renal cyst ➡ displacing the central sinus echo complex ➡.

Variant

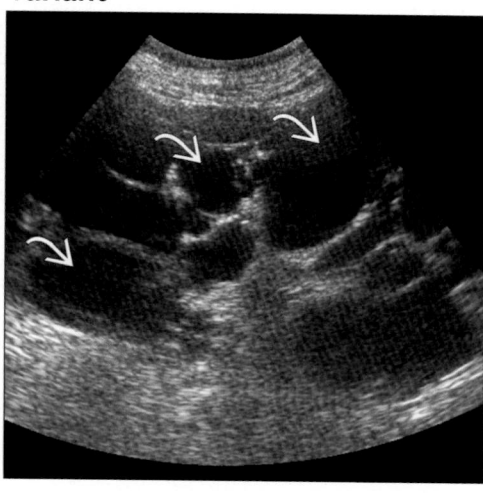 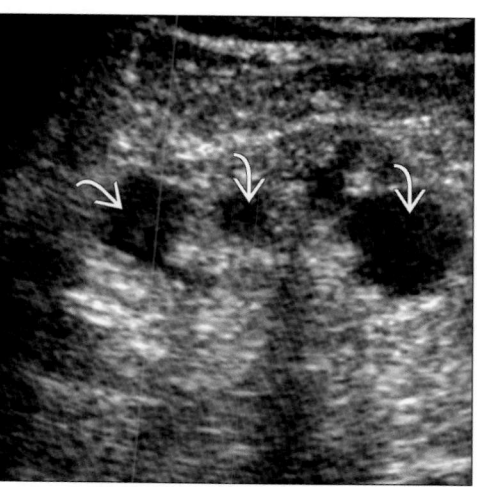

(Left) Longitudinal transabdominal ultrasound shows multiple simple cysts ➡ in PCKD. Note the kidney is grossly enlarged and replaced by cysts of variable size. Minimal renal tissue can be seen. (Right) Longitudinal transabdominal ultrasound shows multiple cysts ➡ in a non-functioning kidney due to chronic renal disease. Renal cystic change is common in patients undergoing dialysis.

COMPLEX RENAL CYST

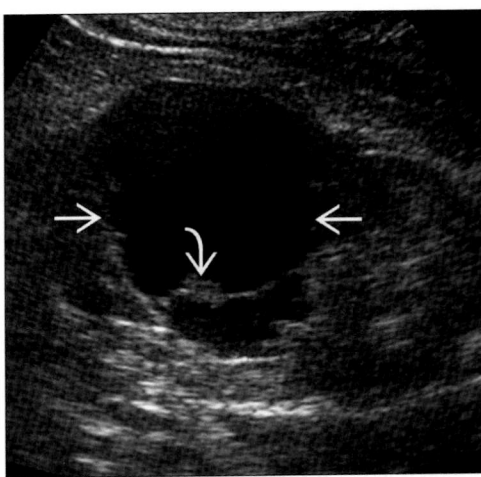

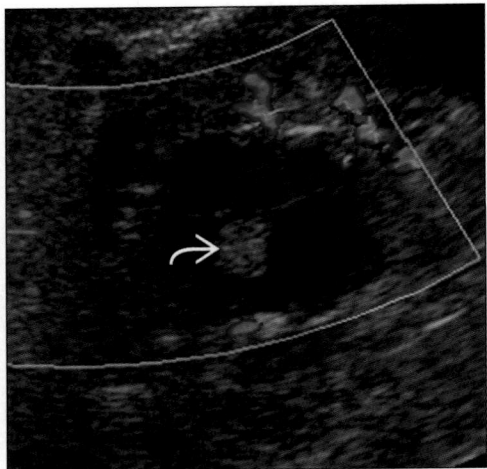

Longitudinal transabdominal ultrasound shows a mid-pole complex renal cyst ➡ with a nodule ➡ arising from the thick septum. Nodularity and thick septum are features that may be seen in RCC.

Transverse color Doppler ultrasound of the nodule ➡ in the previous image. Although no nodular vascularity is seen, contrast-enhanced CT is recommended to exclude malignancy.

TERMINOLOGY

Abbreviations and Synonyms
- Renal cystic mass

Definitions
- Related to simple cyst complications: Hemorrhage, infection, ischemia and cystic renal cell carcinoma (RCC)
- Bosniak CT classification for renal cysts
  - Class I: Benign cysts (well-defined, round, homogeneous, lucent (< HU 20), avascular, thin-walled)
  - Class II: Minimally complicated cysts; benign (well-marginated, mildly irregular, calcified, septated, avascular, hyperdense, usually ≤ 3 cm)
  - Class IIF: Possibly benign (hyperdense, thick or nodular calcifications in wall or septa, vaguely enhanced, may be ≥ 3 cm)
  - Class III: Indeterminate
  - Class IV: Malignant lesions with large cystic or necrotic components (irregular wall thickening or enhancing mass)

IMAGING FINDINGS

General Features
- Best diagnostic clue: Fluid-filled renal lesion shows either calcification, septations, turbid internal content, internal nodules, vascularity, or wall thickening
- Size: Usually 2-5 cm diameter (up to 10 cm)
- Morphology: Depends on histology

Ultrasonographic Findings
- Grayscale Ultrasound
  - May appear as round, oval or irregular shaped hypoechoic fluid-filled lesion
  - Infected cyst: Thick wall with scattered internal echoes ± debris-fluid level representing pus
  - Hydatid cyst: Simple; multiloculated with endocyst and membranes; calcified or solid (chronic)
    - Mural nodularity suggests scolices
    - Membrane of endocyst detaches and precipitates to form "hydatid sand"
    - Calcification may resemble "egg-shell" or reticular in pattern
  - Hemorrhagic cyst: Appearance varies with age of blood

DDx: Mimickers of Complex Cysts

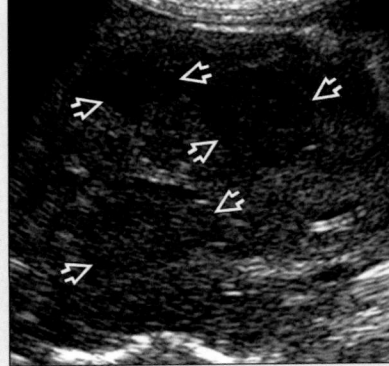

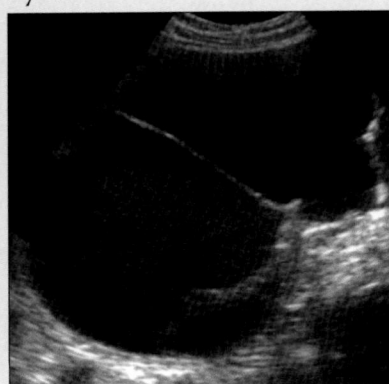

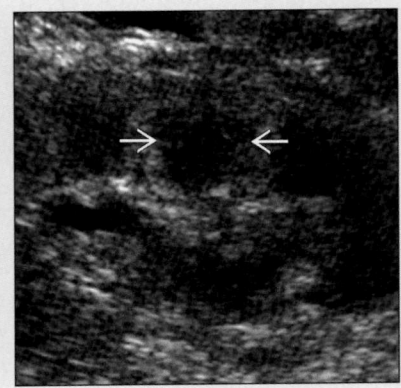

Renal Lymphoma

Gross Hydronephrosis

Medullary Pyramid

COMPLEX RENAL CYST

Key Facts

Imaging Findings

- Best diagnostic clue: Fluid-filled renal lesion shows either calcification, septations, turbid internal content, internal nodules, vascularity, or wall thickening
- Infected cyst: Thick wall with scattered internal echoes ± debris-fluid level representing pus
- Hydatid cyst: Simple; multiloculated with endocyst and membranes; calcified or solid (chronic)
- Hemorrhagic cyst: Appearance varies with age of blood
- Proteinaceous cysts: May contain low level echoes, with bright reflectors or even layers of echoes
- Calcified cyst: Wall or septal calcification ± shadowing

- Milk-of-calcium cyst: "Comet-tail" artifact + line of calcium debris
- Neoplastic wall: Tumor nodule or wall thickening
- Cystic RCC: Thick septa, septal or peripheral calcification, wall or septal nodularity
- Localized cystic disease: Conglomerate of simple cysts simulating multiloculated cystic mass
- Cyst vascularity greatly ↑ risk of malignancy
- Contrast-enhanced ultrasound + harmonic imaging: ↑ Sensitivity and useful in characterizing complex renal cysts

Top Differential Diagnoses

- Renal Metastasis
- Renal Lymphoma
- Hydronephrosis

- Appears as anechoic, solid, septate lesion or contains fluid-debris level
- Thick calcified wall ± multiloculated (chronic)
- Proteinaceous cysts: May contain low level echoes, with bright reflectors or even layers of echoes
  - May simulate renal abscess
  - Variant of hemorrhagic cyst
- Calcified cyst: Wall or septal calcification ± shadowing
  - Milk-of-calcium cyst: "Comet-tail" artifact + line of calcium debris
  - Wall nodularity may be obscured by wall or diffuse calcification of cystic mass
- Neoplastic wall: Tumor nodule or wall thickening
- Cystic RCC: Thick septa, septal or peripheral calcification, wall or septal nodularity
  - Unilocular: Debris-filled, thick and irregular wall which may be calcified
  - Multilocular: Multiple thick internal septations > 2 mm, nodular and calcified
  - Cystic necrosis: Debris-filled; appearance varies with degree of necrosis
  - Tumor originating in simple cyst: rare, mural tumor nodule arising from cyst base
- Localized cystic disease: Conglomerate of simple cysts simulating multiloculated cystic mass
  - Presence of renal parenchyma between cysts; usually unilateral
  - Lack of well-defined pseudocapsule around aggregate of cysts
  - Can simulate multilocular cystic nephroma, cystic neoplasm or autosomal dominant polycystic kidney disease
- Color Doppler
  - Cyst vascularity greatly ↑ risk of malignancy
  - Sensitivity is low to show cyst perfusion
  - Contrast-enhanced ultrasound + harmonic imaging: ↑ Sensitivity and useful in characterizing complex renal cysts
    - Benign neoplasm, inflammatory and traumatic lesions may enhance due to granulation tissue including inflammatory neovascularization

CT Findings

- Benign cysts: Change of < 10 HU from pre- to post-contrast images
- Infected cyst: Thick wall, septated, heterogeneous enhancing fluid, debris- or gas-fluid level; ± calcification (chronic)
- Hemorrhagic cyst: Nonenhancing
  - NECT: Hyperdense & CECT: Hypodense, homogeneous (70-90 HU) (acute)
  - Heterogeneous (clot or debris), ↑ wall thickness & ↓ attenuation ± calcification (chronic)
- Ruptured cyst: Retroperitoneal or perinephric fluid collection, blood (varied density)
- Neoplastic wall: Focal thickening or enhancing nodule
  - Insensitive to characterize small cyst < 3 cm

MR Findings

- Contrast-enhanced MR is useful to detect intracystic enhancement
- MR is as good as ultrasound to demonstrate multiple septa within cyst
- Infected cyst: T1WI: ↑ Intensity, less homogeneous than simple cyst; ↓ intensity than subacute hemorrhage (similar to chronic); ± thickened wall
- Hemorrhagic cyst
  - Variable signal intensity due to age of hemorrhage
  - T1WI: Highest intensity in subacute (< 72 hours)
  - T2WI: High intensity (< simple cyst); fluid-debris level; ± heterogeneous mass and lobulation of contour
- Neoplastic wall: Focal mass or wall thickening; fluid simulates uncomplicated or hemorrhagic cyst
- Proteinaceous cyst: ↑ Protein simulates hemorrhage
- Calcified cyst: MR is insensitive to detect calcification but is superior than CT to detect enhancement within calcified cyst

Imaging Recommendations

- Best imaging tool: Ultrasound, as initial investigation for characterizing simple or minimally complex renal cysts + monitoring of complex renal cysts (Bosniak Class IIF)

COMPLEX RENAL CYST

- Protocol advice: High grade renal complex cysts should be evaluated with CT or MR for decision of surgical intervention

DIFFERENTIAL DIAGNOSIS

Renal Metastasis
- Common in patients with advanced malignancy
- Primary sites include lung, breast, melanoma, stomach, cervix, colon, pancreas, prostate and contralateral kidney
- May appear as isoechoic, hypoechoic or hyperechoic masses

Renal Lymphoma
- Primary renal lymphoma is rare but renal involvement is common
- May manifest as diffuse renal enlargement, bilateral multiple hypoechoic renal masses, direct infiltration from retroperitoneum and perirenal space
- Perinephric extension with vascular and ureteral encasement is common

Hydronephrosis
- Marked hydronephrosis with cortical thinning easily confused with multiloculated cysts
- In hydronephrosis, communication can be demonstrated between "cystic lobules"
- Debris within dilated collecting system can mimic bleeding into cyst

Medullary Pyramids
- Prominent medullary pyramids are commonly seen in children, transplant kidneys with acute rejection and acute tubular necrosis

Renal Abscess
- May extend into calices and perinephric space
- Appears as thick-walled, complex cystic mass with internal debris
- Septations may be present

PATHOLOGY

General Features
- General path comments
  - Most common renal mass in adults (62%)
  - Hemorrhagic cyst: 6% all cysts; calcified cyst: 1-3%
- Etiology
  - Infected cyst: Hematogenous spread, vesicoureteric reflux, surgery or cyst puncture
  - Hemorrhagic cyst: Unknown, trauma, bleeding diathesis or varicosities in simple cyst
  - Calcified cyst: Hemorrhage, infection or ischemia

Gross Pathologic & Surgical Features
- Infected cyst: Markedly thickened wall ± calcification; varying pus, fluid and calcified or noncalcified debris
- Hemorrhagic cyst: Rust-colored putty-like material surrounded by thick fibrosis and plates of calcification
- Neoplastic wall: Discrete nodule at base of cyst

Microscopic Features
- Hemorrhagic cyst: Uni- or multilocular, thickened wall
- Neoplastic wall: Well-differentiated clear/granular cell
- Septated cyst: Compressed normal parenchyma or nonneoplastic connective tissue

CLINICAL ISSUES

Presentation
- Most common signs/symptoms
  - Asymptomatic or palpable mass and flank pain
  - Infected cyst: Pain in flank, malaise and fever
  - Hemorrhagic cyst: Abrupt and severe pain
  - Ruptured cyst: Severe abdominal pain, hematuria

Demographics
- Age: 50% > 50 years of age; rare in < 30 years of age
- Gender: M > F but cysts in females tend to be benign

Natural History & Prognosis
- Complications: Hydronephrosis, hemorrhage, infection, cyst rupture or carcinoma
- Prognosis: Very good

Treatment
- Bosniak class II: No treatment
- Bosniak class IIF: Follow-up by imaging
- Bosniak class III and IV: Surgical excision
- Follow-up: Changes size, configuration & internal consistency; excision if changes suggest carcinoma

DIAGNOSTIC CHECKLIST

Consider
- Imaging generally more reliable than clinical correlation

Image Interpretation Pearls
- Image evaluation and classification of cystic masses is key to management

SELECTED REFERENCES

1. Israel GM et al: An update of the Bosniak renal cyst classification system. Urology. 66(3):484-8, 2005
2. Hartman DS et al: From the RSNA refresher courses: a practical approach to the cystic renal mass. Radiographics. 24 Suppl 1:S101-15, 2004
3. Laven BA et al: Malignant B-cell lymphoma in renal cyst wall. Urology. 64(3):590, 2004
4. Ho VB et al: Renal masses: quantitative assessment of enhancement with dynamic MR imaging. Radiology. 224(3):695-700, 2002
5. Jamis-Dow CA et al: Small (< or = 3-cm) renal masses: detection with CT versus US and pathologic correlation. Radiology. 198(3):785-8, 1996
6. Rosenberg ER et al: The significance of septations in a renal cyst. AJR Am J Roentgenol. 144(3):593-5, 1985
7. Fishman MC et al: High protein content: another cause of CT hyperdense benign renal cyst. J Comput Assist Tomogr. 7(6):1103-6, 1983
8. Diamond HM et al: Echinococcal disease of the kidney. J Urol. 115(6):742-4, 1976

COMPLEX RENAL CYST

IMAGE GALLERY

Typical

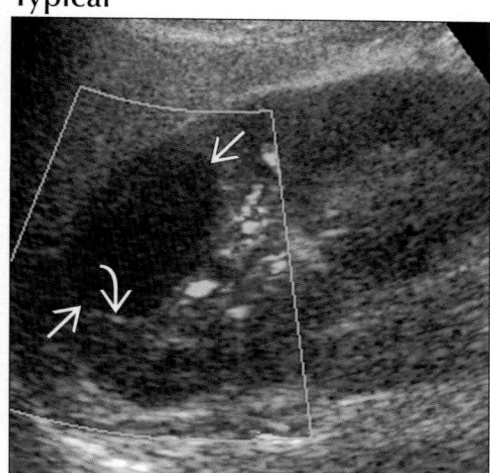
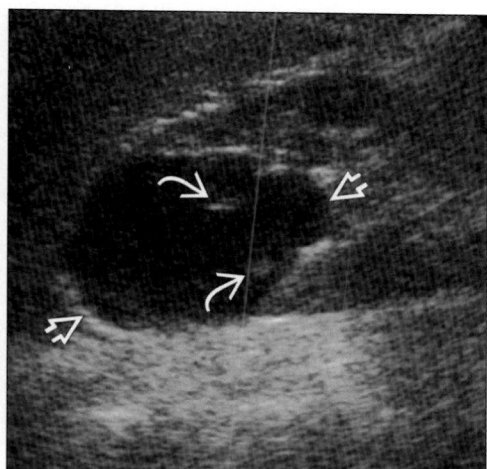

(Left) Longitudinal power Doppler ultrasound shows a benign cyst ➡. The cyst is oval, well-defined, avascular, without internal septation or solid component with a barely visible thin wall ➡. (Right) Longitudinal transabdominal ultrasound shows a minimally complex cyst ➡. It is well-defined with a mildly irregular wall and internal echoes ➡. Appearance may represent hemorrhagic cyst.

Typical

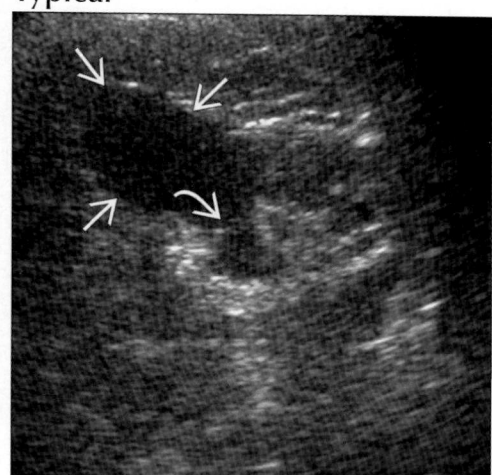
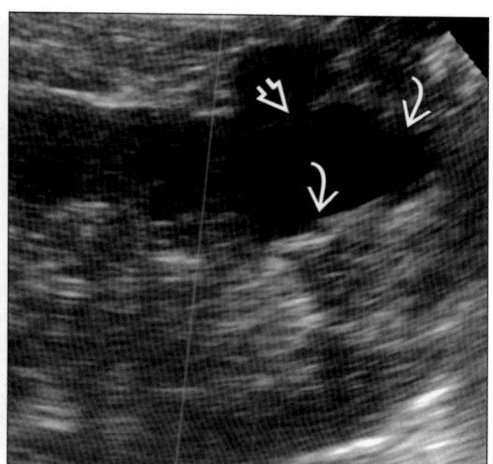

(Left) Transverse transabdominal ultrasound shows an exophytic, elongated cyst ➡. Apart from its unusual shape and thin septum ➡, no other features seen to suggest malignancy. (Right) Longitudinal transabdominal ultrasound shows a septated renal cyst with a thin septum ➡, slightly irregular wall ➡ and absent nodularity. Follow-up scan is suggested to prove benignity.

Typical

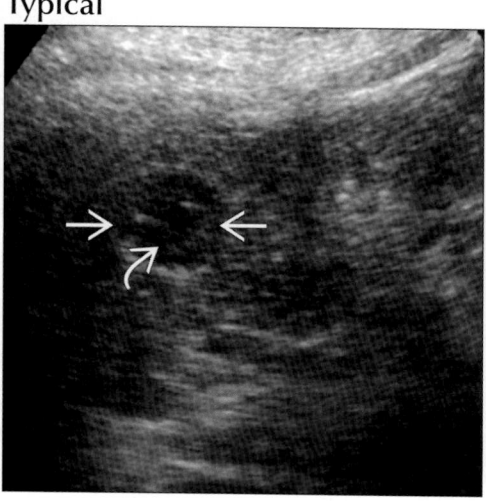
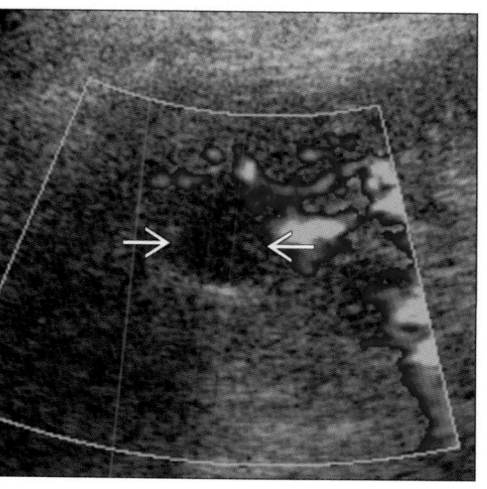

(Left) Longitudinal transabdominal ultrasound shows a small renal hemorrhagic cyst ➡ with internal echoes ➡ mimicking RCC. (Right) Oblique power Doppler ultrasound shows same cystic lesion ➡ in previous image devoid of vascularity. Although the cyst is avascular on ultrasound, definitive diagnosis must be made by CT, MR or biopsy.

Typical

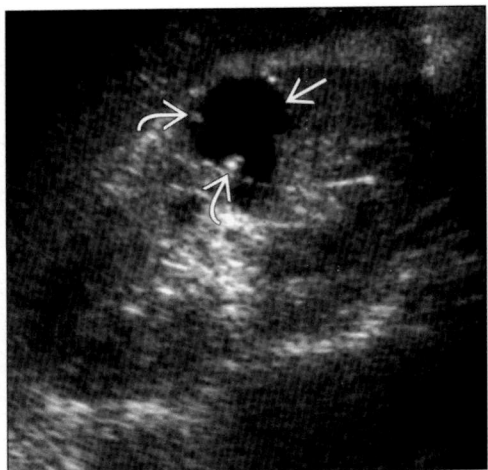 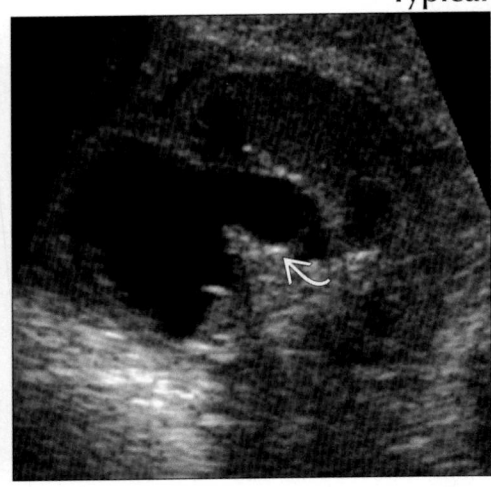

(Left) Longitudinal transabdominal ultrasound shows a cyst ➡ with an irregular wall and nodular thickening ➡. The cyst is > 3 cm and slightly more complicated than a simple cyst. **(Right)** Transverse transabdominal ultrasound shows the same cyst. Note its irregular shape and thin wall calcification ➡. This cyst warrants a CT scan to rule out malignancy and follow-up imaging if not resected.

Typical

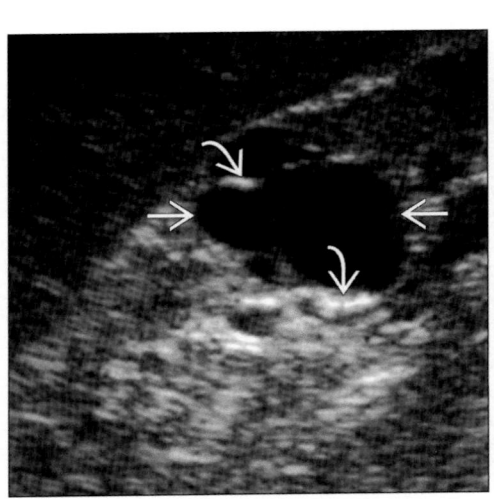 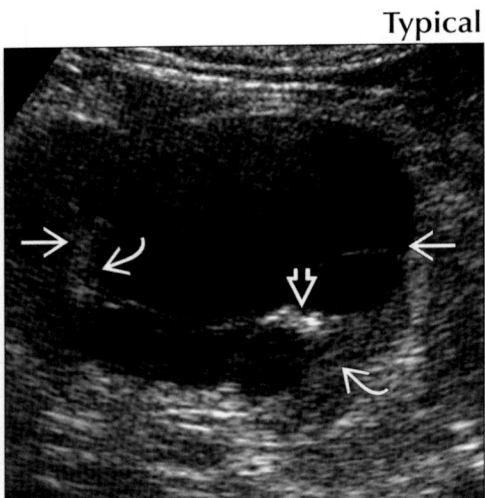

(Left) Longitudinal transabdominal ultrasound shows localized renal cystic disease, with multiple small thin-wall cysts forming a cystic mass ➡. Note the walls of some cysts are calcified ➡. **(Right)** Oblique transabdominal ultrasound shows a large, septated renal cyst ➡. The cyst wall is thickened ➡, with septal calcification ➡. This is a surgical lesion if cyst vascularity is present.

Typical

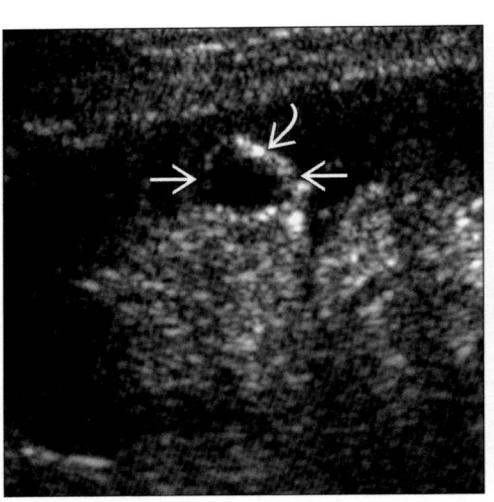 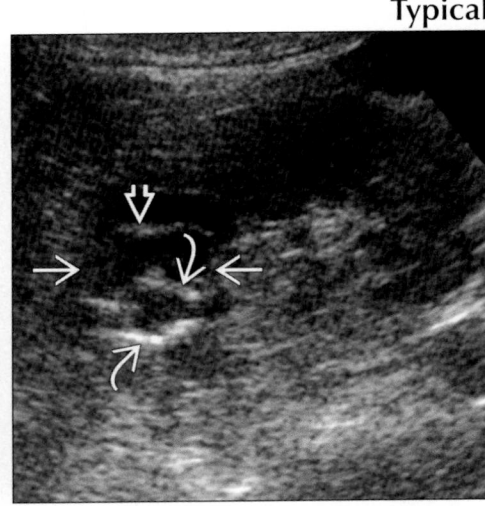

(Left) Longitudinal transabdominal ultrasound shows a small renal cyst ➡ with a calcified wall ➡. Wall calcification may obscure wall nodularity. CT may be required for cyst characterization. **(Right)** Longitudinal transabdominal ultrasound shows a multiseptated cyst ➡ with thick septae ➡ and calcification ➡. This cyst has an equivocal appearance and warrants CT scan for characterization.

Typical

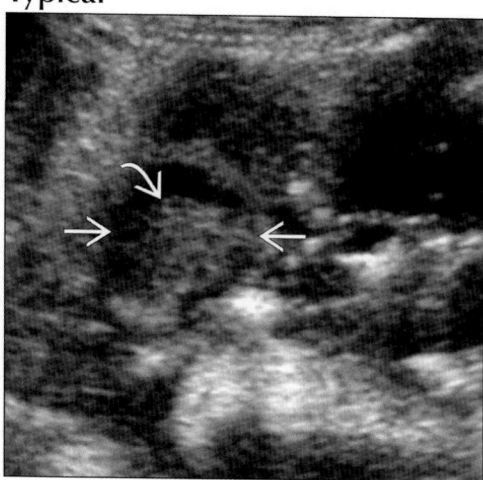
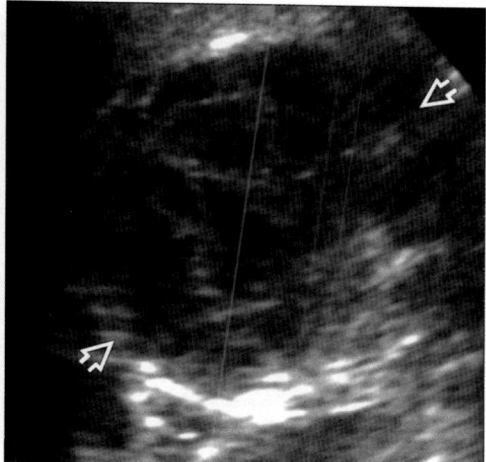

(Left) Longitudinal transabdominal ultrasound shows a small, hemorrhagic, renal cyst ➡ containing a debris-fluid level ➡. The appearance of a hemorrhagic cyst is variable depending on the age of the blood. *(Right)* Transverse transabdominal ultrasound shows a hemorrhagic renal cyst ➡ with organized clot forming an internal reticular pattern. The cyst was avascular on color Doppler suggesting benignity.

Variant

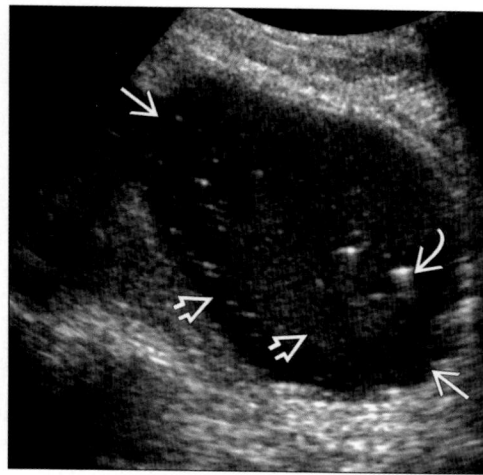
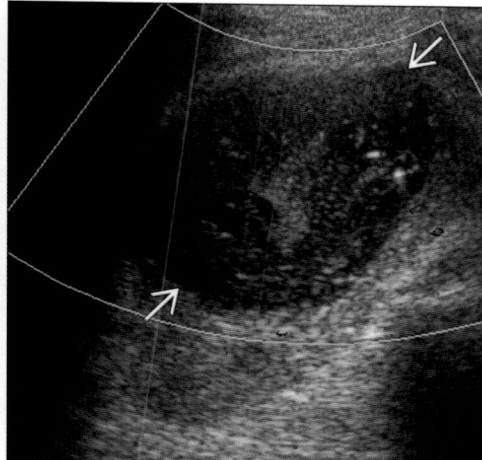

(Left) Oblique transabdominal ultrasound shows a large, complex renal cyst ➡ containing layers of echoes (hypo- & hyper-) ➡ with bright reflectors ➡. These features suggest a proteinaceous cyst. *(Right)* Longitudinal color Doppler ultrasound of the same cyst ➡ in the previous image. The cyst is avascular and has turbid echoes resembling a renal abscess. Cyst aspirate was thick and jelly-like.

Typical

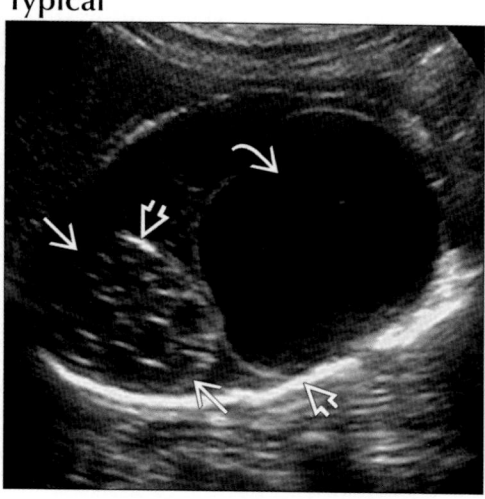
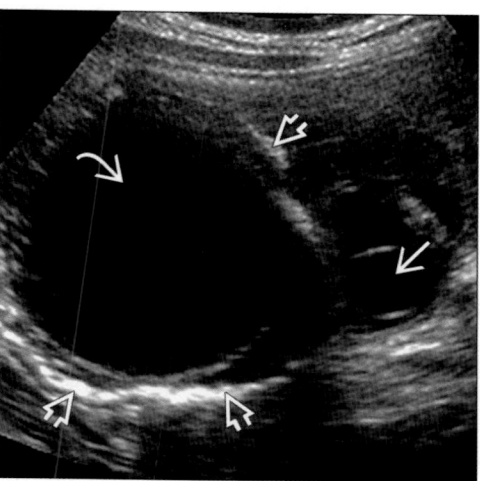

(Left) Longitudinal transabdominal ultrasound shows renal hydatid cyst as multiloculated cyst with an endocyst ➡ and daughter cysts ➡. Egg-shell and cyst wall calcification ➡ are noted. *(Right)* Transverse transabdominal ultrasound shows the same well-developed hydatid cyst as the previous image, with an endocyst ➡ embedded in the calcified wall ➡ adjacent to a daughter cyst ➡.

CYSTIC DISEASE OF DIALYSIS

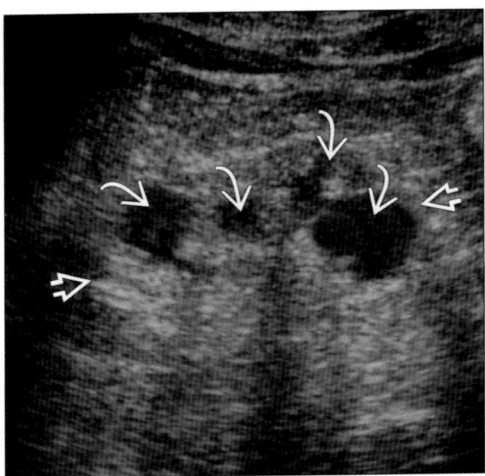

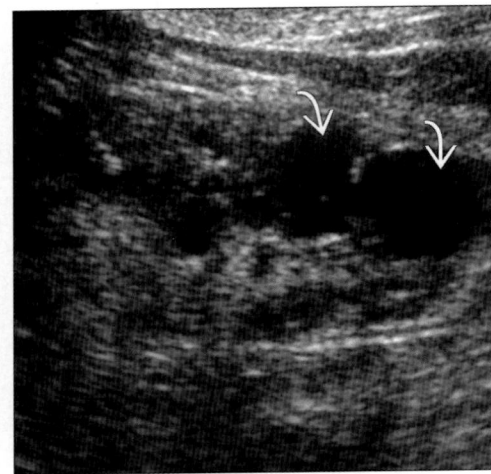

Longitudinal transabdominal ultrasound shows small echogenic kidney ➡ in a patient with ACKD. Multiple cysts ➡ of varying size are randomly distributed throughout the cortex and medulla.

Longitudinal transabdominal ultrasound shows a small native kidney in a dialysis patient. Note large cysts ➡ in a small kidney may actually increase renal volume.

TERMINOLOGY

Abbreviations and Synonyms
- Acquired cystic kidney disease (ACKD)

Definitions
- Occurs in patients with chronic renal disease and those on long-term dialysis
- Kidneys are usually of small to normal size
- Presence of at least 1-5 renal cysts
- Pathologically, extension of cysts involves > 25% of renal parenchyma
- Cyst rupture, cyst hemorrhage and malignant transformation into renal cell carcinoma (RCC) are well-known complications
- Risk of RCC is higher in patients with cysts enlarging renal volume
- Successful transplant may prevent development of new cysts but does not affect malignant potential

IMAGING FINDINGS

General Features
- Best diagnostic clue
  - Early stage: Small kidneys with few cysts
  - Advanced stage: Large kidneys + multiple small cysts
- Location: Bilateral; in areas of scarring throughout cortex and medulla
- Size: Cysts: Variable in size between 0.5-3.0 cm demonstrated on imaging

Ultrasonographic Findings
- Grayscale Ultrasound
  - One or more small cysts < 3 cm seen in small kidneys
  - Renal size may be enlarged due to acquired cysts
  - Cysts scattered in both renal cortex and medulla
  - Cysts usually present in areas of renal scarring
  - If advanced, appearance resembles small kidney affected by adult polycystic kidney disease (ADPKD)
  - Hemorrhagic cysts may contain low level internal echoes or hemorrhagic material mimicking neoplasm

DDx: Mimics of ACKD

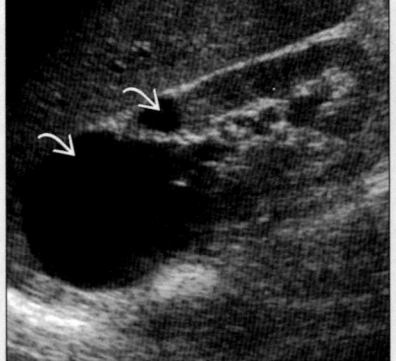

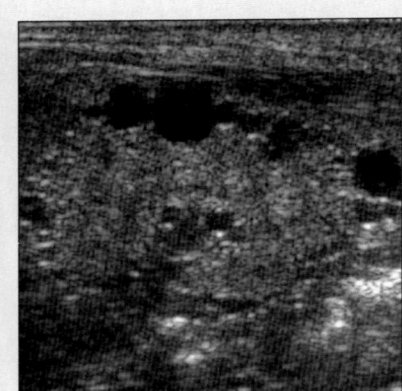

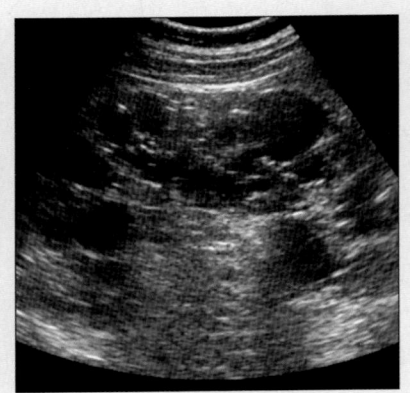

Simple Cysts

Multicystic Dysplastic Kidney

Polycystic Kidney

CYSTIC DISEASE OF DIALYSIS

Key Facts

Imaging Findings
- One or more small cysts < 3 cm seen in small kidneys
- Renal size may be enlarged due to acquired cysts
- Cysts scattered in both renal cortex and medulla
- Cysts usually present in areas of renal scarring
- If advanced, appearance resembles small kidney affected by adult polycystic kidney disease (ADPKD)
- Hemorrhagic cysts may contain low level internal echoes or hemorrhagic material mimicking neoplasm
- Cyst rupture may bleed into pelvis or retroperitoneum resulting in hemoperitoneum or retroperitoneal hematoma, respectively
- Malignant transformation of cysts typically manifest as papillary growth within the cyst
- Cysts depicted as well-defined avascular lesions

- Cystic tumors show intratumoral color signal while hemorrhagic cysts do not
- Power Doppler: Is more sensitive than color Doppler to detect slow flow signals in small RCC
- Best imaging tool: Ultrasound as initial investigation for evaluating patients on dialysis for 3 years
- CT considered if suspicious renal lesions are found on ultrasound
- Screening of dialysis patients annually after 3 years of dialysis is controversial because no significant effect demonstrated on patient outcome

Top Differential Diagnoses
- Multiple Simple Cysts
- Adult Polycystic Kidneys Disease (ADPKD)
- Multicystic Dysplastic Kidney (MCDK)

- ○ Cyst rupture may bleed into pelvis or retroperitoneum resulting in hemoperitoneum or retroperitoneal hematoma, respectively
- ○ Malignant transformation of cysts typically manifest as papillary growth within the cyst
- Color Doppler
  - ○ Cysts depicted as well-defined avascular lesions
  - ○ Cystic tumors show intratumoral color signal while hemorrhagic cysts do not
- Power Doppler: Is more sensitive than color Doppler to detect slow flow signals in small RCC

CT Findings
- Cysts appear as well-defined, thin-walled, nonenhancing lesions with HU < 20
- Tumors enhance with contrast and often have irregular appearance
- Main role is to assess malignant transformation and detect small tumors
- Superior to ultrasound to detect small tumors and differentiate from them from cysts ± hemorrhage
- Not recommended if patient cannot tolerate ionic contrast

MR Findings
- MR performed to rule out RCC if patient cannot tolerate ionic contrast
- Similar to CT findings, tumors enhance after injection of gadolinium while cysts do not

Angiographic Findings
- DSA: Only warranted for renal artery embolization in cases of persistent or severe cyst hemorrhage

Imaging Recommendations
- Best imaging tool: Ultrasound as initial investigation for evaluating patients on dialysis for 3 years
- Protocol advice
  - ○ CT considered if suspicious renal lesions are found on ultrasound
  - ○ Screening of dialysis patients annually after 3 years of dialysis is controversial because no significant effect demonstrated on patient outcome

DIFFERENTIAL DIAGNOSIS

Multiple Simple Cysts
- Renal function not impaired
- Incidence increases with increasing age
- Arise from renal cortex
- Rarely as numerous as in ADPKD
- Usually not associated with nephromegaly

Adult Polycystic Kidneys Disease (ADPKD)
- Differential features favoring ADPKD
  - ○ Family history; presence of renal failure
  - ○ Cysts (other organs): Liver, pancreas, spleen, ovaries
  - ○ Intracranial aneurysms
- Fourth leading cause of chronic renal failure in the world
- Hereditary disorder characterized by multiple renal cysts & various systemic manifestations
- Well-defined, round or oval cysts + thin imperceptible or calcified wall
- Kidneys (100%); liver (75%); pancreas (10%); ovaries & testis

Multicystic Dysplastic Kidney (MCDK)
- Also known as renal dysplasia, renal dysgenesis
- Sonographically, appears as small kidney consisting of multiple cysts or echogenic kidney if cysts are too tiny to be visualized
- Usually unilateral affecting entire kidney
- Bilateral, segmental or focal involvement possible but rare
- 30% associated with contralateral pelviureteric junction obstruction

Von Hippel-Lindau Disease
- Autosomal dominant; multiple renal cysts & cysts in other organs
- Renal cysts are usually less numerous than in ADPKD
- Hemangioblastomas: Cerebellar, spinal & retinal
- Multifocal renal cell carcinomas, pheochromocytomas

Tuberous Sclerosis
- Multiple bilateral renal cysts

CYSTIC DISEASE OF DIALYSIS

- Small fat-containing renal angiomyolipomas
- Cerebral paraventricular calcifications

Medullary Cystic Disease
- Nephronophthisis or salt wasting nephropathy
- Two types based on age related & inherited patterns
  - Childhood nephronophthisis: Autosomal recessive + associated eye, CNS, hepatic, skeletal abnormalities
  - Adult form: Autosomal dominant + no associated
- Kidneys are almost invariably small in size
- Clinically, progressive renal failure in young patients
- Imaging
  - Renal cysts may be too small to be seen
  - Visible cysts occur only in renal medulla

PATHOLOGY

General Features
- Etiology
  - Cyst formation may be due to obstruction of tubules by oxalate crystals, interstitial fibrosis or hyperplasia
  - Cyst formation also believed to be due to compensatory hypertrophy of normal nephrons secondary to nephron loss
- Epidemiology
  - ACKD is common in men and African-Americans
  - M:F = 7:1
  - RCC: Incidence is 30x greater in patients with ACKD than in normal population
- Associated abnormalities
  - RCC (small, multiple, bilateral with cysts; usually papillary)
  - Hemorrhagic cyst
  - Hemoperitoneum
  - Retroperitoneal hematoma

Gross Pathologic & Surgical Features
- Moderately enlarged kidneys with cysts up to 3 cm in cortex and medulla containing clear fluid, often with calcium oxalate crystals, papillary hyperplasia common

Microscopic Features
- Cysts lined by flattened to hyperplastic cuboidal or columnar epithelium
- Residual renal tissue exhibits fibrotic cortex, sclerotic glomeruli, atrophic tubules and interstitial fibrosis

CLINICAL ISSUES

Presentation
- Most common signs/symptoms: Asymptomatic
- Other signs/symptoms
  - Hematuria
  - Flank pain
  - Renal colic
  - Palpable renal mass
  - Hemoglobin drop

Natural History & Prognosis
- ACKD seen in 40% of patients on dialysis for 3 years, 80% on dialysis for 8 years

- Complications: Cyst rupture and hemorrhage into pelvis and retroperitoneum
- 4-7% of patients with ACKD develop RCC over a 7-10 years period
- RCC developed are less aggressive as classical RCC with infrequent metastasis (5-7%)
- Prognosis for ACKD ± complications is fair because of poor patient renal function

Treatment
- Mild bleeding into cysts, managed with bed rest and analgesics
- Persistent and severe hemorrhage necessitates nephrectomy or renal artery embolization
- RCC requires nephrectomy
- Asymptomatic simple cysts require no treatment
- Bosniak category III & IV cysts require surgical exploration and biopsy or nephrectomy
  - ~ 50% of category III cysts are malignant

DIAGNOSTIC CHECKLIST

Consider
- Duration of dialysis
- Differentiate from other multiple renal cystic diseases

Image Interpretation Pearls
- Bilateral, multiple small cysts in small and echogenic kidneys
- Large cysts with solid components highly suspicious of RCC

SELECTED REFERENCES

1. Ishikawa I et al: Twenty-year follow-up of acquired renal cystic disease. Clin Nephrol. 59(3):153-9, 2003
2. Neureiter D et al: Dialysis-associated acquired cystic kidney disease imitating autosomal dominant polycystic kidney disease in a patient receiving long-term peritoneal dialysis. Nephrol Dial Transplant. 17(3):500-3, 2002
3. Chatha RK et al: Von Hippel-Lindau disease masquerading as autosomal dominant polycystic kidney disease. Am J Kidney Dis. 37(4):852-8, 2001
4. Nascimento AB et al: Rapid MR imaging detection of renal cysts: age-based standards. Radiology. 221(3):628-32, 2001
5. Slywotzky CM et al: Localized cystic disease of the kidney. AJR Am J Roentgenol. 176(4):843-9, 2001
6. Tantravahi J et al: Acquired cystic kidney disease. Semin Dial. 13(5):330-4, 2000
7. Hughson MD et al: Renal cell carcinoma of end-stage renal disease: an analysis of chromosome 3, 7, and 17 abnormalities by microsatellite amplification. Mod Pathol. 12(3):301-9, 1999
8. Fick GM et al: Natural history of autosomal dominant polycystic kidney disease. Annual Review of Medicine. 45: 23-9, 1994
9. Matson MA et al: Acquired cystic kidney disease: occurrence, prevalence, and renal cancers. Medicine (Baltimore). 69(4):217-26, 1990
10. Parfrey PS et al: The diagnosis and prognosis of autosomal dominant polycystic kidney disease. N Engl J Med. 323(16):1085-90, 1990
11. Sanders RC et al: The sonographic distinction between neonatal multicystic kidney and hydronephrosis. Radiology. 151(3):621-5, 1984

CYSTIC DISEASE OF DIALYSIS

IMAGE GALLERY

Typical

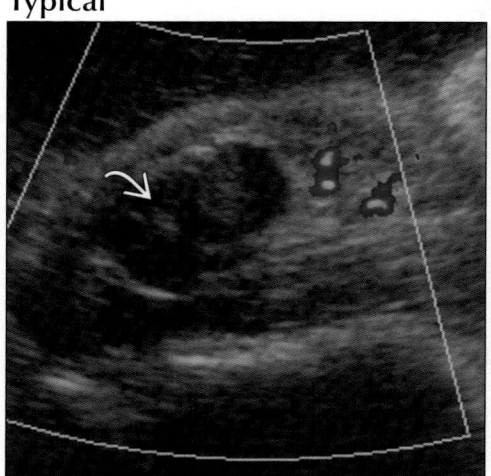 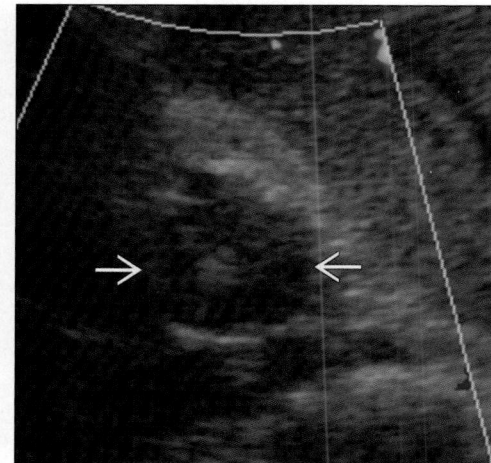

(Left) Longitudinal color Doppler ultrasound shows a small kidney in a patient with ACKD. A cyst with internal echoes ➔ is suggestive of hemorrhage. No color signal is detected within the cyst. (Right) Transverse color Doppler ultrasound shows the same cyst ➔ as in previous image. Note bleeding into cyst is a common complication in patients with ACKD; others include cyst rupture and RCC.

Typical

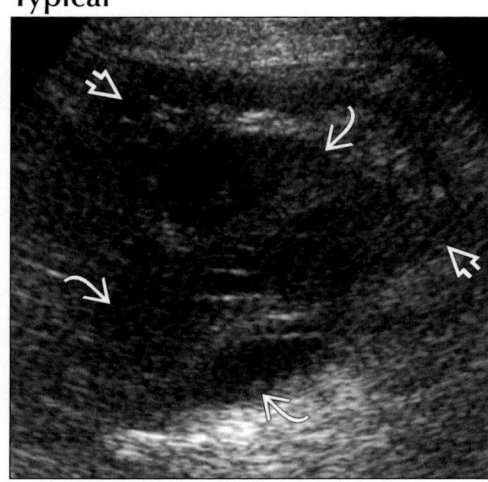 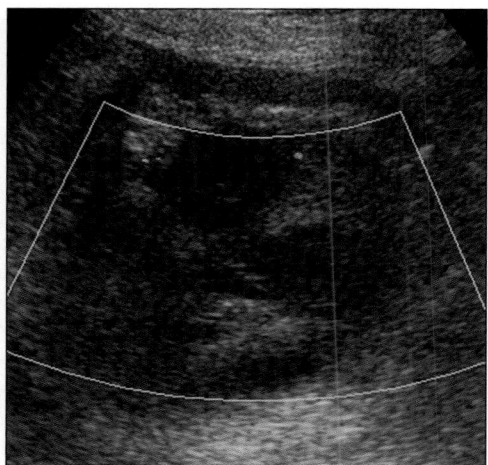

(Left) Longitudinal transabdominal ultrasound shows ACKD with a neoplasm. A large cystic mass ➔ with complex internal content arises from the mid-pole of the kidney ➔ and extends into the retroperitoneum. (Right) Transverse color Doppler ultrasound (same patient as in previous image) shows scarce color signal in this mass. Surgical findings revealed a RCC with extensive hemorrhage. Note RCC in ACKD is usually small unless it bleeds.

Typical

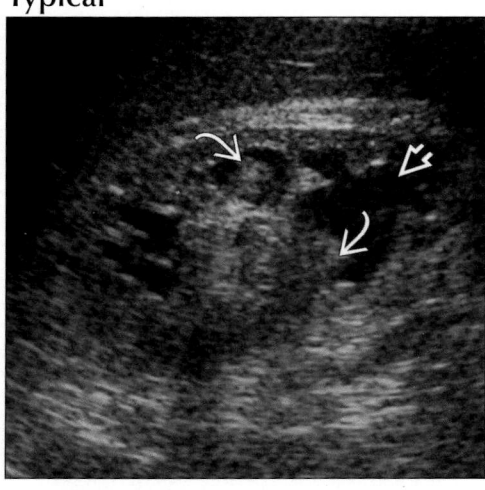 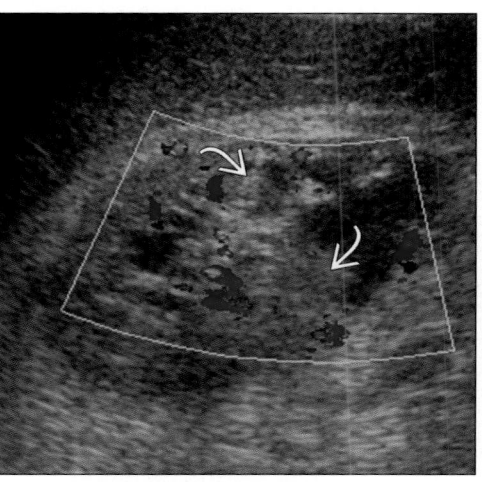

(Left) Longitudinal transabdominal ultrasound of ACKP shows echogenic material ➔ in a cyst and of the renal pelvis, causing a hydrocalyx in lower pole ➔. Features suggest neoplasms such as RCC or TCC. (Right) Longitudinal color Doppler ultrasound in the same patient as previous image, shows echogenic material in the kidney devoid of color signal. Ureteroscopy and biopsy confirmed it to be organized blood clot ➔.

MULTILOCULAR CYSTIC NEPHROMA

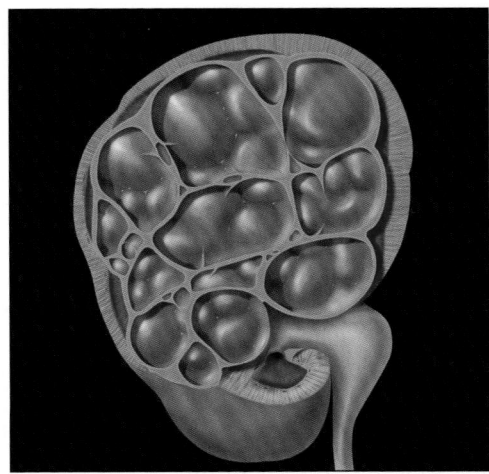

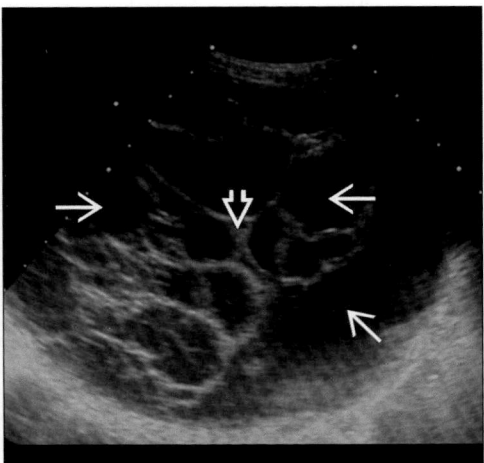

Graphic shows multiple non-communicating cysts separated by thick septae. The multiloculated cystic mass herniates into the renal hilum but shows no communication with collecting system.

Transverse transabdominal ultrasound shows a typical multilocular cystic nephroma, with multiple non-communicating anechoic cysts ➡ of varying size, separated by echogenic septae ➡.

TERMINOLOGY

Abbreviations and Synonyms
- Multilocular cystic nephroma (MLCN), cystic nephroma, cyst adenoma

Definitions
- Best classified as one of the two types of multilocular cystic renal tumor
  - Cystic nephroma: MLCN
  - Cystic partially differentiated nephroblastoma (CPDN)
- Rare nonhereditary benign cystic renal neoplasm

IMAGING FINDINGS

General Features
- Best diagnostic clue: Unilateral, large multilocular cystic renal mass
- Location: Typically solitary intraparenchymal cyst
- Morphology: Well-circumscribed cystic mass with a thick fibrous capsule ± herniation into renal pelvis

Ultrasonographic Findings
- Grayscale Ultrasound
  - Variable appearance depending on number and size of cystic locules
  - Tumor with large locules
    - Multiple, non-communicating anechoic cysts within a well-defined mass
    - Hyperechoic septa and fibrous capsule which may be calcified
    - Fine vessels may be seen within the septae on Doppler
    - No intracystic mural nodule
  - Tumor with small locules
    - Occasionally more solid-looking due to numerous tiny cysts causing acoustic interfaces

CT Findings
- CECT
  - Large, well-defined multiloculated cystic mass, +/- calcification, +/- capsular enhancement
  - Small locules/proteinaceous material within cysts → may appear as solid mass, nonenhancing
  - May herniate into renal hilum, distort collecting system, ± obstruction

DDx: Multilocular Cystic Nephroma

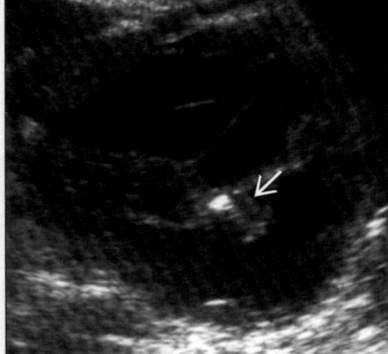

Cystic RCC

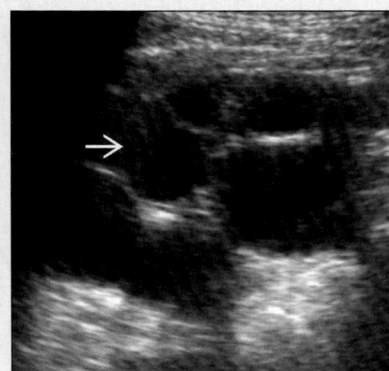

Multicystic Dysplastic Kidney

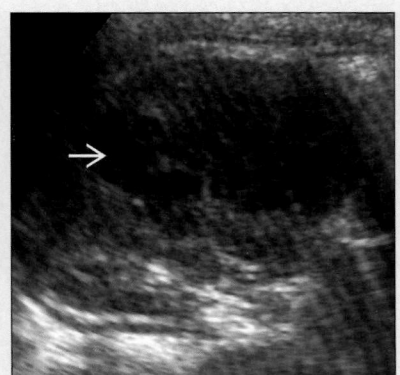

Renal Abscess

MULTILOCULAR CYSTIC NEPHROMA

Key Facts

Terminology
- Cystic nephroma: MLCN
- Cystic partially differentiated nephroblastoma (CPDN)

Imaging Findings
- Multiple, non-communicating anechoic cysts within a well-defined mass
- Hyperechoic septa and fibrous capsule which may be calcified

- Fine vessels may be seen within the septae on Doppler
- No intracystic mural nodule
- Occasionally more solid-looking due to numerous tiny cysts causing acoustic interfaces

Top Differential Diagnoses
- Cystic Renal Cell Carcinoma (RCC)
- Multicystic Dysplastic Kidney (MCDK)
- Renal Abscess

MR Findings
- T1WI: Multiloculated hypointense mass (clear fluid) with variable signal intensity (blood or protein)
- T2WI: Hyperintense (clear fluid) or variable (blood or protein) with hypointense capsule and septa (fibrous tissue)
- T1 C+: Enhancement of thin septa

DIFFERENTIAL DIAGNOSIS

Cystic Renal Cell Carcinoma (RCC)
- More irregular septae or with intracystic solid component

Multicystic Dysplastic Kidney (MCDK)
- Usually involves whole kidney, present in newborn and neonate

Renal Abscess
- Ill-defined complex fluid collection with internal echoes

PATHOLOGY

General Features
- Etiology: Arises from metanephric blastema
- Epidemiology: Rare tumor

Gross Pathologic & Surgical Features
- Thick fibrous capsule

- "Honeycombed" cystic areas of varied sizes

CLINICAL ISSUES

Presentation
- Most common signs/symptoms
  ○ Children: No pain; palpable abdominal/flank mass
  ○ Adults: Abdominal/flank pain; ± palpable mass

Demographics
- Age
  ○ M > F: 3 months to 2 years (mostly CPDN)
  ○ F > > M: 5th & 6th decades (mostly MLCN)

Natural History & Prognosis
- Prognosis
  ○ Cured with complete excision
    ▪ Malignant transformation extremely rare
  ○ Local recurrence usually due to incomplete excision

SELECTED REFERENCES
1. Hopkins JK et al: Best cases from the AFIP: cystic nephroma. Radiographics. 24(2):589-93, 2004
2. Agrons GA et al: Multilocular cystic renal tumor in children: radiologic-pathologic correlation. Radiographics. 15(3):653-69, 1995

IMAGE GALLERY

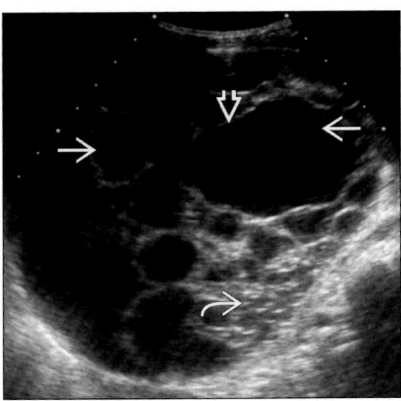 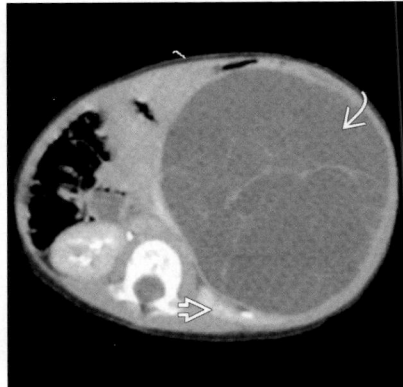 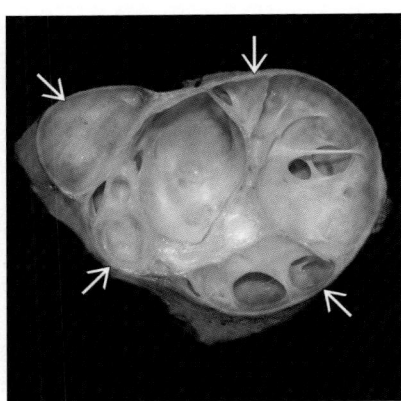

(Left) Longitudinal transabdominal ultrasound shows multiple anechoic cysts ➡, separated by echogenic septae ➡. Portions of lesion appear more solid ➡ due to acoustic interfaces of numerous tiny cysts. *(Center)* Transverse CECT shows a multiloculated, septated cystic mass ➡ occupying almost the entire left kidney with minimal residual functioning parenchymal tissue ➡. *(Right)* Gross pathology of a MLCN shows a multiloculated, septated cystic mass, containing cysts of varying sizes. The mass is well-circumscribed with a fibrous capsule ➡.

RENAL PAPILLARY NECROSIS

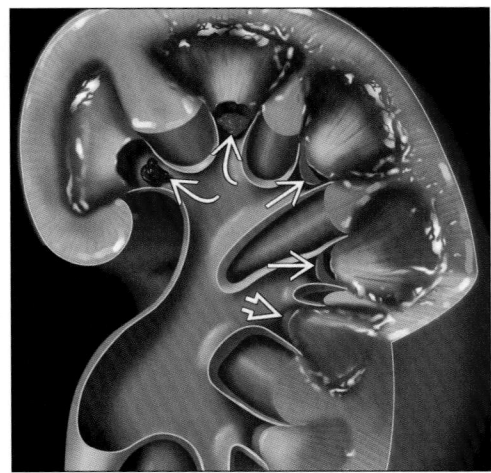

Longitudinal graphic shows RPN. Variable degrees of severity are noted with early necrosis in-situ ➡, necrosis and cavitation at the rim of the papillae ➡ and finally sloughed papillae ➡.

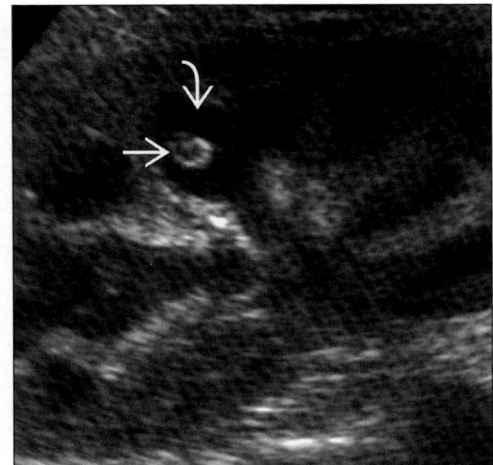

Longitudinal transabdominal ultrasound shows RPN with a necrotic papilla appearing as an echogenic focus ➡ with "ring" calcification in the medullary pyramid surrounded by fluid ➡.

TERMINOLOGY

Abbreviations and Synonyms
- Renal papillary necrosis (RPN)

Definitions
- Necrosis of renal papilla within medulla secondary to interstitial nephritis or ischemia

IMAGING FINDINGS

General Features
- Best diagnostic clue: Echogenic papilla with ring calcification, surrounded by fluid in medulla
- Location
  - Bilateral (analgesics, diabetes and sickle cell disease)
  - Unilateral (obstruction, infection, venous thrombus)

Ultrasonographic Findings
- Grayscale Ultrasound
  - Ultrasound: Insensitive for early necrotic changes
  - **Early stage**
    - Apparent pelvicaliceal dilatation
    - Echogenic "rings" in medulla (necrotic papillae)
    - Rim of fluid around necrotic papillae
  - **Late stage**
    - Single/multiple cystic cavities in medullary pyramids continuous with calyces ± calcification
    - Sloughed papillae appear as echogenic lesions in collecting system simulating calculi
    - Hydronephrosis is a common association

Radiographic Findings
- IVP
  - Subtle streak of contrast from fornix to papilla
  - Triangular or bulbous papillary cavitation
  - Widened fornix and clubbed calyces
  - Calcified filling defect in calyces/renal pelvis
  - "Ring shadow": Outlining detached papilla

CT Findings
- Early: ↓ Enhancement in medullary tip with circumscribed, ill-defined rim
- Ring-shaped medullary calcification
- Hematoma, lobar infarct, scarring (sickle cell)
- Contrast filled clefts in renal parenchyma
- Filling defects: Renal pelvis/ureter (sloughed papillae)

DDx: Renal Papillary Necrosis

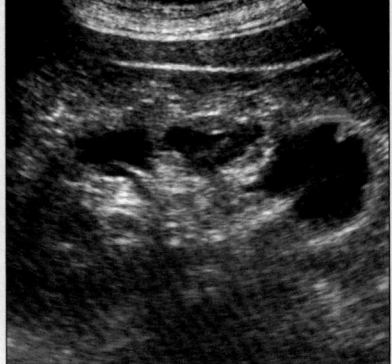

Hydrocalyx

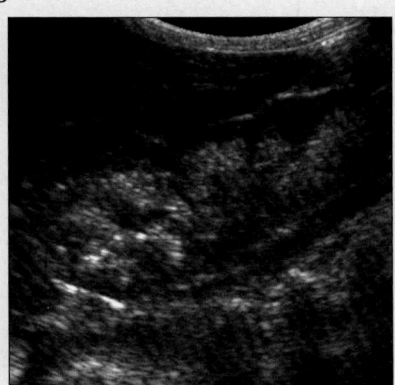

Medullary Sponge Kidney

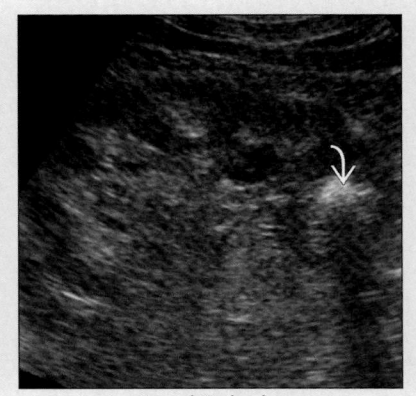

Renal Calculus

RENAL PAPILLARY NECROSIS

Key Facts

Imaging Findings
- Best diagnostic clue: Echogenic papilla with ring calcification, surrounded by fluid in medulla
- Ultrasound: Insensitive for early necrotic changes
- Apparent pelvicaliceal dilatation
- Echogenic "rings" in medulla (necrotic papillae)
- Rim of fluid around necrotic papillae
- Single/multiple cystic cavities in medullary pyramids continuous with calyces ± calcification

- Sloughed papillae appear as echogenic lesions in collecting system simulating calculi
- Hydronephrosis is a common association

Top Differential Diagnoses
- Renal Calculus
- Medullary Sponge Kidney
- Hydronephrosis or Hydrocalyx

Imaging Recommendations
- Best imaging tool: CT
- Protocol advice: Ultrasound: Initial scan; CT or IVP: Further investigation

DIFFERENTIAL DIAGNOSIS

Renal Calculus
- Echogenic lesion with posterior shadowing

Medullary Sponge Kidney
- Multiple small cystic cavities or tubular ectasia
- Associated with medullary nephrocalcinosis

Hydronephrosis or Hydrocalyx
- Mimic of early RPN; common association of late RPN

PATHOLOGY

General Features
- General path comments
  - Necrosis in situ of papillae ± Ca++ or ossification
  - Central cavitation of papillae extending from fornix
  - Necrosis & cavitation at periphery of papillae → sloughing of papillae
- Etiology
  - Analgesic abuse, diabetes mellitus, sickle cell disease
  - Urinary tract infection & obstruction, renal transplant

CLINICAL ISSUES

Presentation
- Most common signs/symptoms
  - Flank pain, dysuria, fever, ureteral colic
  - Pyuria, hematuria, acute oliguric renal failure

Natural History & Prognosis
- Complications: Obstruction, infection, renal failure, transitional cell carcinoma
- Prognosis: Early stage (good); advanced stage (poor)

Treatment
- Early stage: Antibiotic treatment
- Advanced stage: Ureteral stent, surgery

DIAGNOSTIC CHECKLIST

Consider
- Correlate imaging with patient's clinical history

Image Interpretation Pearls
- Echogenic "rings" in medullary pyramids ± obstruction

SELECTED REFERENCES

1. Lang EK et al: Detection of medullary and papillary necrosis at an early stage by multiphasic helical computerized tomography. J Urol. 170(1):94-8, 2003
2. Hoffman JC et al: Demonstration of renal papillary necrosis by sonography. Radiology. 145(3):785-7, 1982

IMAGE GALLERY

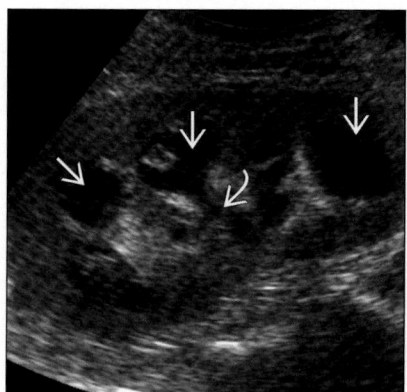 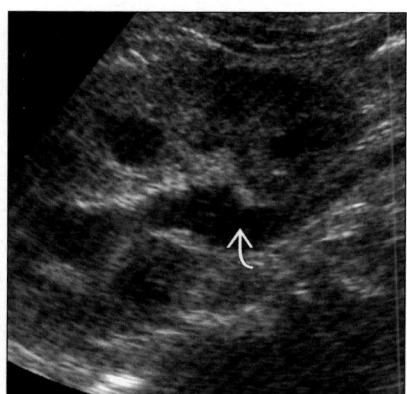 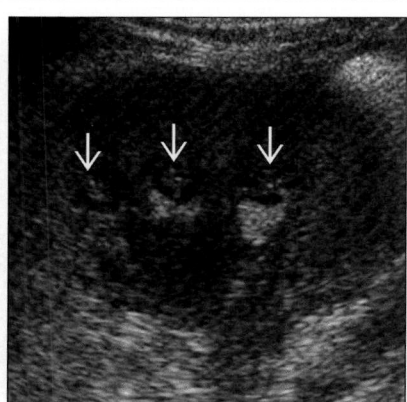

(Left) Longitudinal transabdominal ultrasound shows RPN with multiple cystic lesions ➡ representing dilated, clubbed calyces. A narrow infundibulum ➡ connecting to the renal pelvis noted. *(Center)* Oblique transabdominal ultrasound shows corresponding kidney with associated mild hydronephrosis ➡. Hydronephrosis may be due to obstruction by the sloughed papilla and is common in late RPN. *(Right)* Longitudinal transabdominal ultrasound shows early RPN with echogenic medullary tips representing necrotic papillae ➡, which are outlined by rim of fluid.

RENAL TRAUMA

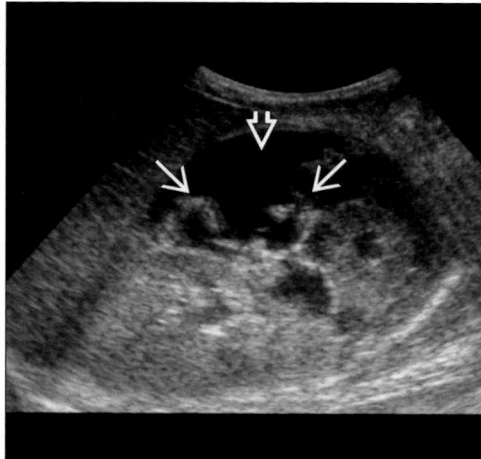

Longitudinal transabdominal ultrasound shows a fractured kidney with fragmented renal tissues ➡ and subcapsular hematoma ➡.

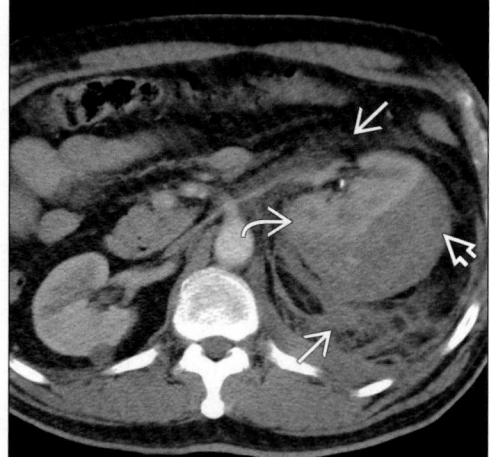

Transverse CECT shows laceration of the left kidney ➡, which is compressed by a large subcapsular hematoma ➡. Increased streakiness ➡ also present in perinephric space.

TERMINOLOGY

Definitions
- Injury to the kidney

IMAGING FINDINGS

General Features
- Best diagnostic clue: Renal parenchymal defect with perirenal hemorrhage ± extravasation of blood/urine
- Other general features
  - Seen in 8-10% of patients with blunt or penetrating abdominal injuries
  - 80-90% of cases involve blunt rather than penetrating injury
  - Serious renal injuries usually associated with multi-organ involvement
  - 98% of isolated renal injuries are minor and require no specific therapy
  - Radiologic classification of renal injuries
    - Grade I-IV
  - Grade I: 75-85% of all renal injuries
    - Minor injury (contusion; intrarenal or subcapsular hematoma)
    - Minor laceration + limited perinephric hematoma
    - No extension to collecting system or medulla
    - Small subsegmental cortical infarct
  - Grade II: 10% of all renal injuries
    - Major injury (major cortical laceration + extension to medulla and collecting system)
    - With or without urine extravasation or segmental renal infarct
  - Grade III: 5% of cases
    - Catastrophic injury (multiple renal lacerations and vascular injury involving renal pedicle)
  - Grade IV: Rare consequence
    - Ureteropelvic junction injury: Complete transection or laceration

Ultrasonographic Findings
- Grayscale Ultrasound
  - Best used in follow-up of patients with known renal parenchymal injury
  - Useful in isolated renal injury due to iatrogenic causes such as post renal biopsy or lithotripsy (ESWL)

DDx: Renal Trauma

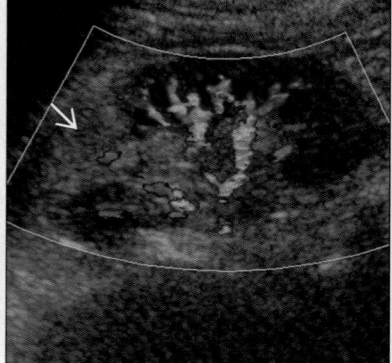

Pyelonephritis

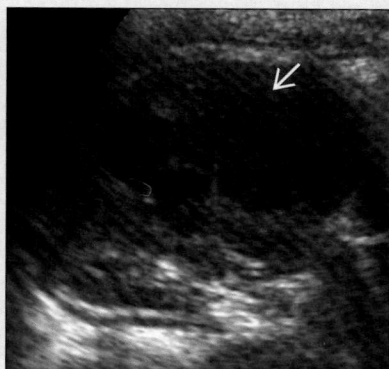

Renal Abscess

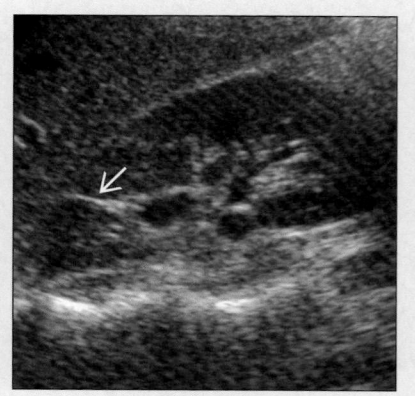

Junction Line

RENAL TRAUMA

Key Facts

Imaging Findings
- Best diagnostic clue: Renal parenchymal defect with perirenal hemorrhage ± extravasation of blood/urine
- Useful in isolated renal injury due to iatrogenic causes such as post renal biopsy or lithotripsy (ESWL)
- Look for regional distortion of corticomedullary differentiation
- Hematoma: Can be hypoechoic, hyperechoic or heterogeneous
- Laceration: Linear defect extending through kidney
- Perirenal collection: Associated with renal laceration
- Subcapsular hematoma: Localized perirenal fluid collection flattens renal contour
- Shattered kidney: Multiple fragments of disorganized tissue with blood and urine collections

- Ultrasound: For early assessment in focused assessment with sonography for trauma (FAST) and for monitoring progress
- CT has the advantage of assessing concomitant injuries to other organs

Top Differential Diagnoses
- Focal Pyelonephritis
- Renal Abscess
- Renal Junction Line

Diagnostic Checklist
- Look for concomitant injury in liver, spleen and bowel if free fluid present
- Negative US finding does not exclude renal injury
- US more likely to be abnormal with severe (grade II or greater) renal injury

---

- Look for regional distortion of corticomedullary differentiation
- Hematoma: Can be hypoechoic, hyperechoic or heterogeneous
- Laceration: Linear defect extending through kidney
- Perirenal collection: Associated with renal laceration
- Subcapsular hematoma: Localized perirenal fluid collection flattens renal contour
- Shattered kidney: Multiple fragments of disorganized tissue with blood and urine collections
- Color Doppler: Assessment of vascular pedicle injuries

Radiographic Findings
- IVP
  - Grade I: Normal
  - Grade II-IV
    - Delayed, absent excretion or extravasation

CT Findings
- Grade I lesions
  - Intrarenal hematoma or contusion
    - Parenchymal phase: ↓ Enhancement relative to normal kidney
    - Delayed phase: Hyperdense due to urine stasis + clot filled tubules
  - Subcapsular hematoma
    - Round or elliptic fluid collection (40-70 HU clotted blood)
  - Minor lacerations: Small linear hypodense areas in periphery
  - Limited perinephric hematoma: Adjacent to laceration
  - Subsegmental cortical infarct
    - Small, sharply demarcated, wedge-shaped decreased attenuation area → scar
- Grade II lesions
  - Major laceration through cortex extending to medulla
    - Long irregular or linear hypodense area
  - When laceration extends into collecting system
    - Nephrographic phase: Large, distracted renal fracture (hypodense)

- Excretory phase: Contrast extravasation into perinephric space
  - Segmental renal infarct: Sharply demarcated, wedge-shaped area of decreased enhancement
- Grade III lesions
  - Multiple renal lacerations and vascular injury
    - Nephrographic phase: Several irregular, linear or band-like interpolar hypodense areas ± areas of active arterial contrast extravasation
  - Subacute infarction
    - "Cortical rim" sign: Preserved capsular or subcapsular enhancement (reliable sign)
    - Seen 6-8 hours after infarction
  - "Shattered kidney"
    - Segmental infarction: Nonenhancing wedge-shaped area (devitalized upper or lower renal pole branch)
    - Global infarction (non- enhancement) + no perinephric hematoma (renal artery thrombosis)
    - Global infarction (non- enhancement) + perinephric hematoma (renal artery avulsion)
- Grade IV lesions
  - Ureteropelvic junction: Complete transection (avulsion) or laceration
    - Good excretion of contrast + medial perinephric extravasation
    - A circumferential urinoma may be seen around affected kidney

Imaging Recommendations
- Best imaging tool
  - Ultrasound: For early assessment in focused assessment with sonography for trauma (FAST) and for monitoring progress
    - Limitations of ultrasound: An unstable patient with wound dressing, multiple tubes and lines cannot be placed in optimal scanning position
    - Other parts of the body (brain, thorax, spine) may be injured and require imaging: CT provides a quick global overview in a patient with multitrauma

RENAL TRAUMA

- Associated ileus causing gaseous distension obscures large portion of the abdomen and ultrasonography
  - CT has the advantage of assessing concomitant injuries to other organs
- Protocol advice: For any renal laceration evident on CT, must obtain 8-10 minute delayed scans to evaluate for urinary extravasation
- Helical CECT: Gold standard imaging
- IVU: Limited urography (to evaluate hemodynamically unstable patient)
  - Take a plain film abdomen and administer 100-150 ml of 60% contrast IV; obtain immediate "cone down" nephrogram film + full film after 8 minutes
  - "One-shot IVU": To assess the normal kidney
- Retrograde pyelography
  - To assess ureteral and renal pelvic injuries
- US: To assess hemoperitoneum in a hemodynamically unstable patient

DIFFERENTIAL DIAGNOSIS

Focal Pyelonephritis
- Either increased or decreased areas of echogenicity, reduced focal vascularity

Renal Abscess
- Ill-defined complex fluid collection with low-amplitude internal echoes, disruption of corticomedullary junction

Renal Junction Line
- Echogenic line at upper and middle thirds of kidney without disruption of renal contour
- Normal parenchymal echogenicity and vascularity

Renal Tumor
- Spontaneous bleed or may be seen in renal tumors
- Perinephric fluid collection of blood density
- Look for underlying renal mass lesion, such as renal cell carcinoma, angiomyolipoma

PATHOLOGY

General Features
- Etiology
  - Motor vehicle accidents (MVA), falls, fights, assaults
    - Blunt, penetrating and deceleration injuries
  - Adults: Kidneys protected by ribs, heavy musculature of back and flank
  - Children: Kidneys relatively large, more mobile and more vulnerable to trauma
- Epidemiology: Renal trauma incidence; 8-10% of abdominal injuries
- Associated abnormalities
  - Other organ injuries in 75% of cases
    - Liver, spleen, bowel, pancreas

Gross Pathologic & Surgical Features
- Contusion, laceration, hematoma, infarction, vascular or ureteropelvic injury

CLINICAL ISSUES

Presentation
- Most common signs/symptoms
  - Flank pain, tenderness, hematuria or ecchymosis
  - Poor correlation between degree of hematuria and severity of renal injury
    - 14% of major and 10% of minor injuries may not have hematuria
- Lab data
  - Blood in urine (> 5 red blood cells/high power field)
- Diagnosis: Clinical and classic imaging features are diagnostic of renal trauma

Demographics
- Age: Any (children more vulnerable than adults)

Natural History & Prognosis
- Complications
  - Early: Urinoma, perinephric abscess, sepsis, arteriovenous fistula, pseudoaneurysm
  - Late: Hydronephrosis, HTN, calculus formation, chronic pyelonephritis, renal failure and atrophy
- Prognosis
  - Grade I and II: Good
  - Grade III and IV
    - Unilateral after treatment: Good, Bilateral: Poor

Treatment
- Grade I and II: Conservative therapy
- Grade III and IV
  - Active bleeding: Angioembolization
  - Renal artery thrombosis: Anticoagulants; stenting
  - Active urinary extravasation
    - Consider ureteral stent and catheter drainage
  - Indications for surgery
    - Vascular (renal pedicle) injury
    - Shattered kidney
    - Expanding or pulsatile hematoma
    - Shocked multitrauma patient

DIAGNOSTIC CHECKLIST

Consider
- Acute injuries of kidney from blunt abdominal trauma often associated with significant splenic, hepatic or bowel trauma
- 65% isolated renal injuries have no free fluid
- Look for concomitant injury in liver, spleen and bowel if free fluid present

Image Interpretation Pearls
- Negative US finding does not exclude renal injury
- US more likely to be abnormal with severe (grade II or greater) renal injury

SELECTED REFERENCES

1. McGahan PJ et al: Ultrasound detection of blunt urological trauma: a 6-year study. Injury. 36(6):762-70, 2005
2. Nural MS et al: Diagnostic value of ultrasonography in the evaluation of blunt abdominal trauma. Diagn Interv Radiol. 11(1):41-4, 2005

Typical

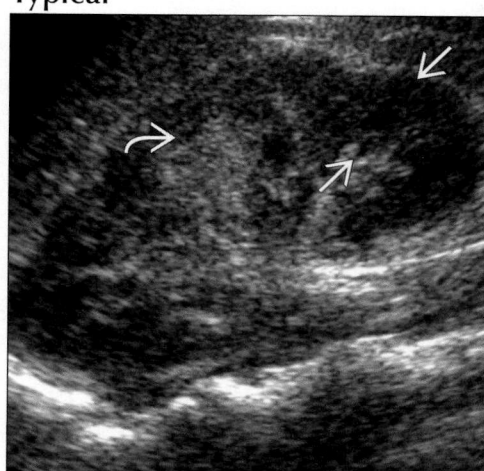
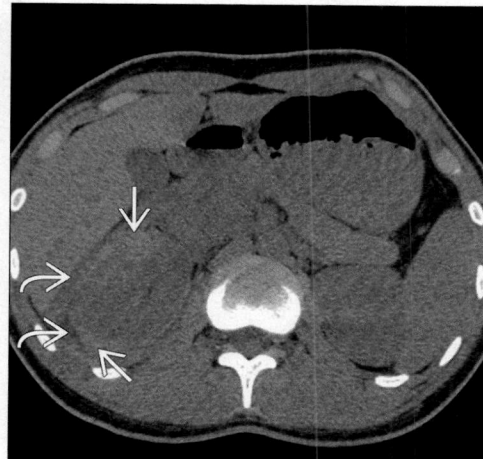

(Left) Longitudinal transabdominal ultrasound shows a focal poorly-defined area of hyperechogenicity ➡ present at the mid-pole of the kidney compatible with a contusion. Note there is loss of corticomedullary differentiation at the mid-pole when compared with lower pole ➡. *(Right)* Transverse NECT shows hyperdense hemorrhagic contusions ➡ in the right kidney, surrounded by a thin rim of perinephric fluid ➡.

Typical

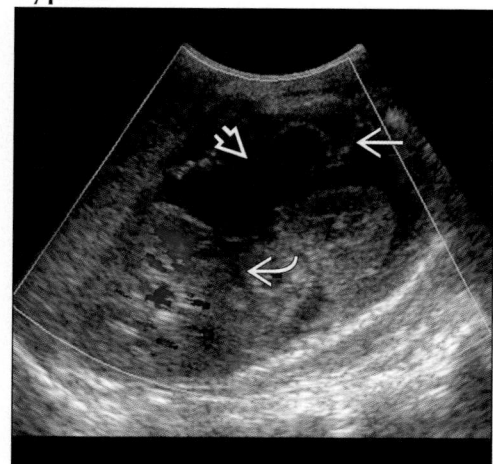
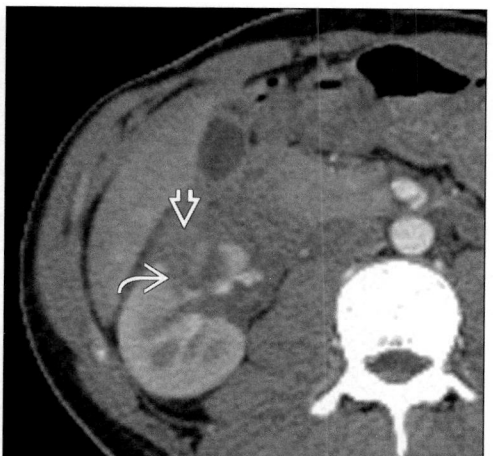

(Left) Longitudinal color Doppler ultrasound shows a cortical laceration extending into the caliceal system ➡. The lower pole is distorted with fragments ➡ floating within a subcapsular hematoma ➡. Vascularity is preserved in the intact upper pole of kidney. *(Right)* Transverse CECT shows complete cortical laceration of the right kidney ➡ and adjacent subcapsular hematoma ➡.

Typical

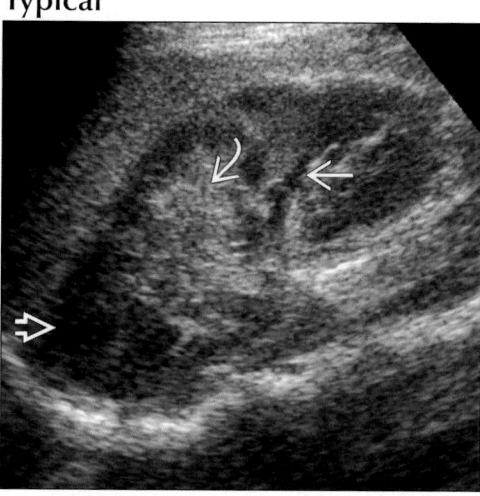
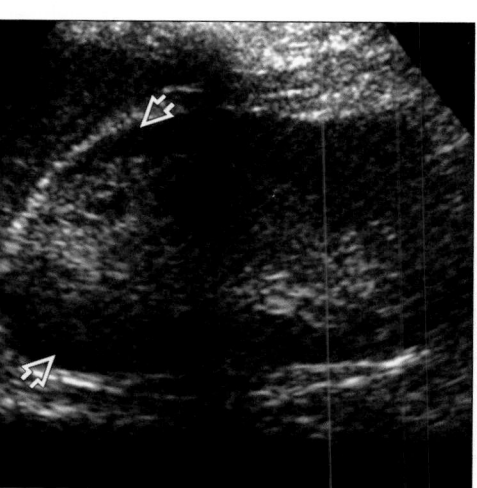

(Left) Longitudinal transabdominal ultrasound shows an ill-defined hyperechoic area ➡ at the mid-pole compatible with contusion. Mild caliectasis ➡, and thin rim of subcapsular fluid ➡ present. *(Right)* Longitudinal transabdominal ultrasound demonstrates a small to moderate amount of perinephric fluid ➡ around a contused kidney. This is only clue of renal injury on this US.

PERINEPHRIC FLUID COLLECTIONS

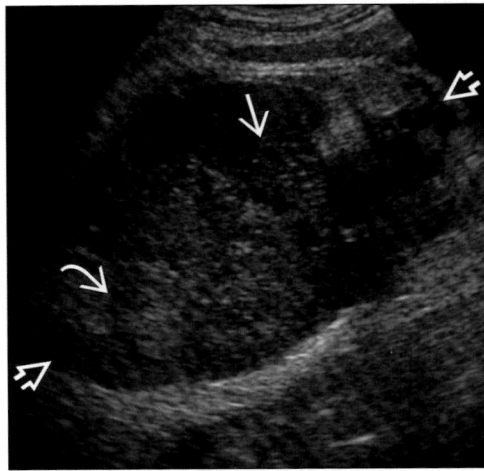

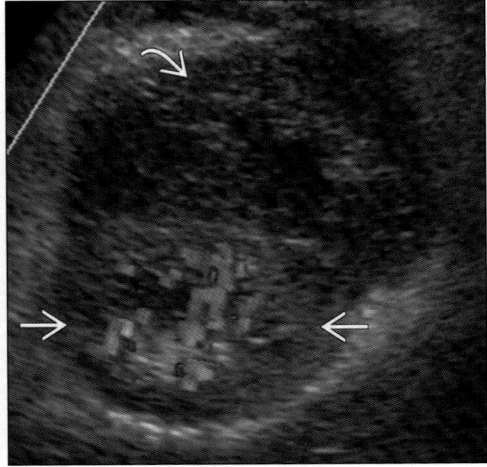

Longitudinal transabdominal ultrasound shows a large perirenal abscess ⊟. The abscess is encapsulating the kidney ⊟ and appears as a heterogeneous mass with internal debris ⊟ and a thick wall.

Transverse color Doppler ultrasound of the previous perirenal abscess ⊟ shows echogenic debris ⊟ within the abscess. Sonographically, it may not be possible to differentiate abscess from hematoma.

TERMINOLOGY

Definitions
- Fluid collection in perinephric spaces: Subcapsular, perirenal, anterior and posterior pararenal
- Urinoma is uriniferous perirenal pseudocyst secondary to tear in collecting system with continuing renal function

IMAGING FINDINGS

General Features
- Best diagnostic clue: Cystic masses in one or more perinephric spaces
- Location
  - Urinoma: Localized (most common); diffuse (filling entire perirenal space); subcapsular; may extend to pararenal spaces and intrarenal tissue or even into pleural cavity (urothorax)
  - Hematoma: Variable depending on site of bleeding
  - Abscess: Variable depending on route of infection
  - Pancreatic pseudocyst: Pararenal spaces (frequent)
- Size: Variable

Ultrasonographic Findings
- Grayscale Ultrasound
  - Appearance depends on nature of fluid collection
  - Urinoma usually localized, well-defined, thin-walled, anechoic with no septations
  - Hematoma: Sonographic features vary with time
    - Acute hematoma: Echogenic internal echoes
    - Hematoma may become anechoic or cystic containing low level echoes ± septations
    - Hematoma may resemble urinoma or abscess depending on stage of formation or liquefaction
    - Subcapsular hematoma may mimic or mask neoplasms
  - Abscess: Depicted as hypoechoic or nearly anechoic mass displacing kidney ± fluid-debris level and thick irregular wall
  - Echogenicity of abscesses ↑ if gas-containing
  - Lymphocele: Well-defined, anechoic ± septations
  - Pancreatic pseudocyst: Well-defined, loculated, anechoic ± debris-fluid level, depicted as complex masses if hemorrhagic or infected
  - Ultrasound: Sensitive to reveal perinephric fluid collections but nonspecific to characterize them

DDx: Perinephric Fluid Collection

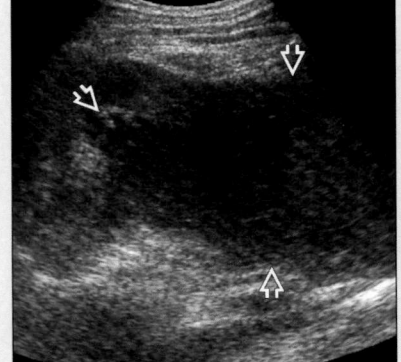

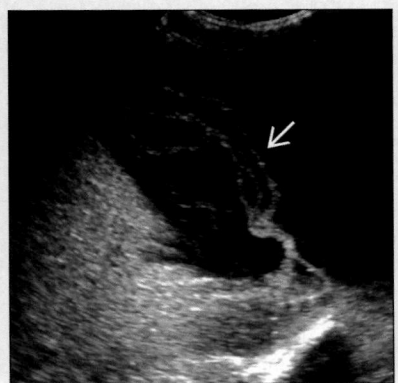

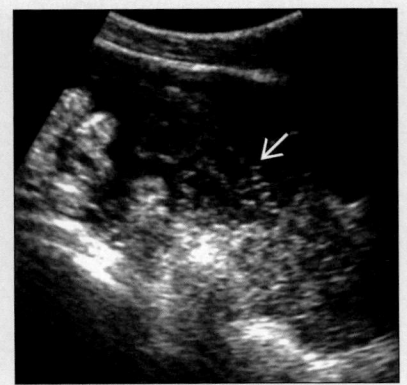

Lymphoma Infiltration

TB Peritonitis

Pseudomyxoma Peritionei

PERINEPHRIC FLUID COLLECTIONS

Key Facts

Imaging Findings
- Appearance depends on nature of fluid collection
- Urinoma usually localized, well-defined, thin-walled, anechoic with no septations
- Hematoma: Sonographic features vary with time
- Acute hematoma: Echogenic internal echoes
- Hematoma may become anechoic or cystic containing low level echoes ± septations
- Hematoma may resemble urinoma or abscess depending on stage of formation or liquefaction
- Subcapsular hematoma may mimic or mask neoplasms
- Abscess: Depicted as hypoechoic or nearly anechoic mass displacing kidney ± fluid-debris level and thick irregular wall
- Echogenicity of abscesses ↑ if gas-containing

- Lymphocele: Well-defined, anechoic ± septations
- Pancreatic pseudocyst: Well-defined, loculated, anechoic ± debris-fluid level, depicted as complex masses if hemorrhagic or infected
- Ultrasound: Sensitive to reveal perinephric fluid collections but nonspecific to characterize them
- Color Doppler: May be helpful to identify soft tissue component in subcapsular hematoma due to tumor rupture; arteriovenous fistula in bleeding angiomyolipoma
- Ultrasound is initial investigation for perinephric fluid collection and guided aspiration

Top Differential Diagnoses
- Lymphoma Infiltration
- Peritonitis
- Pseudomyxoma Peritonei

- Color Doppler: May be helpful to identify soft tissue component in subcapsular hematoma due to tumor rupture; arteriovenous fistula in bleeding angiomyolipoma

Radiographic Findings
- Radiography
  - Normal in 40% of patients
    - Absent psoas margin
    - Apparent renal mass
    - Absent renal outline with ↑ opacity in renal region in 50% of patients
    - Renal displacement
    - Scoliosis with concavity to involved side
    - Bowel displacement due to mass effect of large fluid collection
    - Abscesses: Retroperitoneal or perinephric gas formation (mottled appearance)
- IVP
  - Abnormal in 80% of patients
  - Circumferential perirenal urinoma mimics nephromegaly
  - Abscess associated with calicectasis or calyceal stretching in 39% of cases ± renal displacement

CT Findings
- CECT
  - Highly sensitive for detection of perinephric fluid collection, its extent and underlying causes
  - For traumatic large perinephric fluid collection, especially medially or deep laceration: Delayed images to evaluate for urinary extravasation
  - Hematoma: High attenuation (> 28 HU)
  - Lymphocele: Medium attenuation (18-24 HU)
  - Abscess or chronic hematoma: (> 28 HU) on delayed images

Angiographic Findings
- Main role is for superselective embolization of bleeding artery in active hemorrhage into perinephric space

Imaging Recommendations
- Best imaging tool
  - CT is diagnostic method of choice
  - Ultrasound is ideal adjunct to CT and guided aspiration
- Protocol advice
  - Ultrasound is initial investigation for perinephric fluid collection and guided aspiration
  - CT is required to identify cause of perinephric hematoma or characterize fluid collections
  - Angiography is offered for superselective embolization of bleeding tumor
  - For suspected occult renal cell carcinoma (RCC) as cause of hematoma, consider follow-up ± biopsy by ultrasound or CT

DIFFERENTIAL DIAGNOSIS

Lymphoma Infiltration
- Malignant renal infiltration may be remarkably hypoechoic and is well-known to mimic fluid, particularly lymphoma with extensive retroperitoneal and renal involvement
- Lymphoma may completely encircle a kidney producing a hypoechoic collar

Peritonitis
- Defined as diffuse inflammation of parietal or visceral peritoneum caused by infectious and non-infectious etiologies
- Infectious (common): Bacterial (tuberculosis), fungal, parasital, viral
- Non-infectious (less common): Sclerosing, granulomatous, chemical
- Infectious peritonitis sonographically appears as particulate or loculated ascites

Pseudomyxoma Peritonei
- Rare condition characterized by intraperitoneal accumulation of gelatinous material owing to rupture of mucinous appendiceal or ovarian tumor

PERINEPHRIC FLUID COLLECTIONS

- Appearance variable ranging from loculated, anechoic ascites to complex echogenic, thick ascites
- Bowel loops may be depressed by mucus rather than floating in it
- Scalloping of hepatic outline may be seen

Cystic Lymphangioma
- Appears as uni- or multilocular cysts which are clear or contain low level echoes
- Occurs anywhere in perirenal, pararenal or pelvic extraperitoneal spaces

PATHOLOGY

General Features
- Etiology
  - Urinoma is due to trauma, surgery, calculus erosion, urinary obstruction
  - Hematoma secondary to trauma, renal biopsy, renal tumor rupture, renal cyst rupture, anticoagulant therapy, aortic aneurysm rupture
  - Abscess caused by infection, sinus or fistula related to pyelonephritis or hematogenous spread
  - Lymphocele or lymphatic collection from trauma or malignant obstruction
  - Pseudocyst caused by acute pancreatitis may track into perinephric spaces
  - Subcapsular transudate associated with renal parenchymal disease caused by nephropathies: "Floating kidney"

CLINICAL ISSUES

Presentation
- Most common signs/symptoms
  - Abscess: Fever, flank pain, chills, dysuria, weight loss, lethargy and gastrointestinal symptoms
  - Hematoma: Flank pain, often severe, palpable mass, shock
- Other signs/symptoms: Abscess: Pleuritic pain, pelvic or thigh pain

Natural History & Prognosis
- Abscess: Life-threatening if remains undetected with mortality rate as high as 56%, prognosis is otherwise good
- Subcapsular or perinephric hematoma without underlying significant pathology usually resolves spontaneously with good prognosis
- Urinoma has good prognosis after surgical repair

Treatment
- Abscess: Percutaneous needle aspiration and catheter drainage as first line of therapy with antibiotics as adjunct + close monitoring with serial imaging such as CT or ultrasound
- Small abscess < 5 cm may be treated solely by antibiotics
- Subcapsular or perinephric hematoma: Treatment varies with etiology
  - Extrafascial nephrectomy for malignant tumors or extensive hemorrhage

- Superselective embolization for active bleeding in benign tumors or traumatic renal rupture
- Managed conservatively for self-limiting bleeding in benign entities
- For suspected occult RCC, monitor closely by CT
- Perinephric or intrarenal urinoma: Percutaneous aspiration or surgical repair

DIAGNOSTIC CHECKLIST

Consider
- Characterization of perinephric fluid should be made by CT or percutaneous needle aspiration
- Must identify underlying etiology in spontaneous perinephric hematoma to exclude malignancy

Image Interpretation Pearls
- Ultrasound along with clinical characteristics may facilitate specific diagnosis and treatment

SELECTED REFERENCES

1. Lekha V Chandrasekharan et al: An unexpected cause of spontaneous perinephric urinoma: a case report. The Internet Journal of Radiology. Vol. 4, Number 1, 2005
2. Iqbal N et al: Management of blunt renal trauma: a profile of 65 patients. J Pak Med Assoc. 54(10):516-8, 2004
3. Shu T et al: Renal and perirenal abscesses in patients with otherwise anatomically normal urinary tracts. J Urol. 172(1):148-50, 2004
4. Yang DM et al: Retroperitoneal cystic masses: CT, clinical, and pathologic findings and literature review. Radiographics. 24(5):1353-65, 2004
5. Smith JK et al: Imaging of renal trauma. Radiol Clin North Am. 41(5):1019-35, 2003
6. Haddad MC et al: Radiology of perinephric fluid collections. Clin Radiol. 57(5):339-46, 2002
7. Haddad MC et al: Perirenal fluid in renal parenchymal medical disease ('floating kidney'): clinical significance and sonographic grading. Clin Radiol. 56(12):979-83, 2001
8. Shih WJ et al: Spontaneous subcapsular and intrarenal hematoma demonstrated by various diagnostic modalities and monitored by ultrasonography until complete resolution. J Natl Med Assoc. 92(4):200-5, 2000
9. Dalla Palma L et al: Medical treatment of renal and perirenal abscesses: CT evaluation. Clin Radiol. 54(12):792-7, 1999
10. Farman J et al: CT of pancreatitis with renal and juxtarenal manifestations. Clin Imaging. 21(3):183-8, 1997
11. Sebastia MC et al: CT evaluation of underlying cause in spontaneous subcapsular and perirenal hemorrhage. Eur Radiol. 7(5):686-90, 1997
12. Brkovic D et al: Aetiology, diagnosis and management of spontaneous perirenal haematomas. Eur Urol. 29(3):302-7, 1996
13. Tien R et al: Circumferential perirenal urinoma mimicking nephromegaly on urography. Urol Radiol. 11(2):92-6, 1989
14. Griffin JF et al: Computed tomography of pararenal fluid collections in acute pancreatitis. Clin Radiol. 35(3):181-4, 1984

PERINEPHRIC FLUID COLLECTIONS

Typical

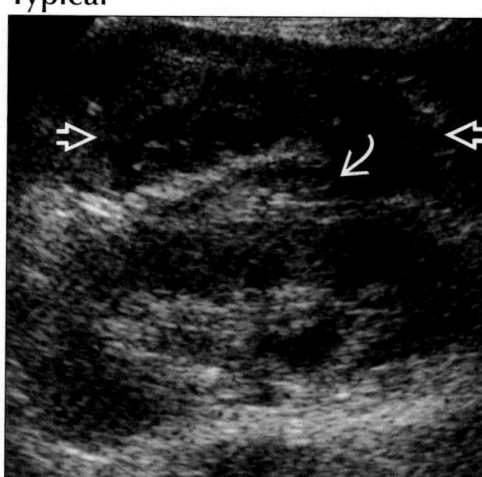
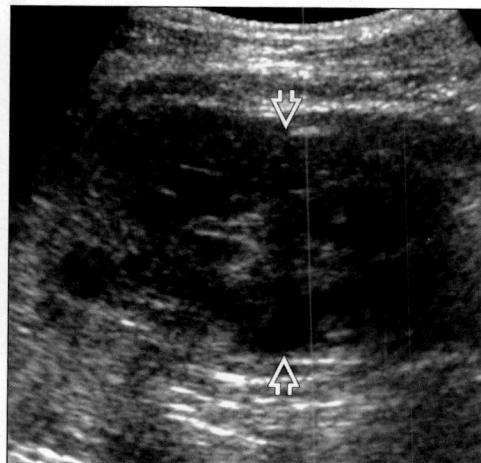

(Left) Longitudinal transabdominal ultrasound shows a large, anterior pararenal hematoma ⇒ in a patient with a recent percutaneous nephrostomy. Note its communication ➔ with the perirenal space. (Right) Transverse transabdominal ultrasound shows a complex perinephric hematoma ⇒. It is irregular, thick-walled and septated, with features mimicking abscess. Clinical features help to distinguish the two.

Typical

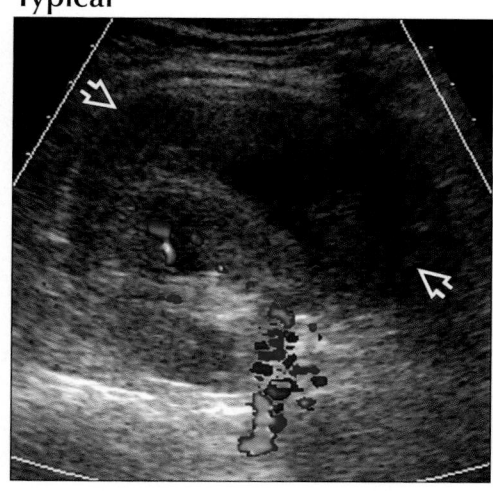
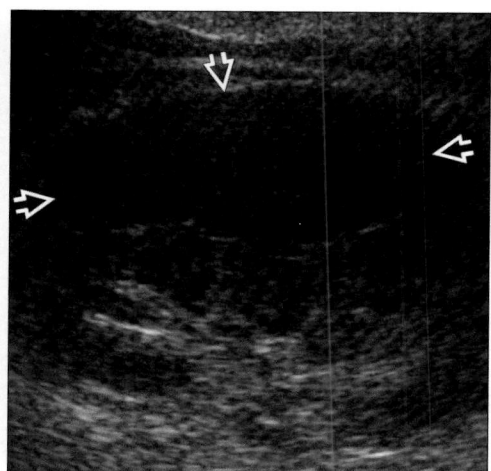

(Left) Transverse color Doppler ultrasound shows a large, spontaneous subcapsular perinephric hematoma ⇒. Note occult RCC must be considered in a spontaneous perinephric hematoma. (Right) Longitudinal transabdominal ultrasound shows an anechoic hematoma immediately after biopsy ⇒. Note a fresh hematoma may resemble a urinoma and can be confirmed only by percutaneous aspiration.

Typical

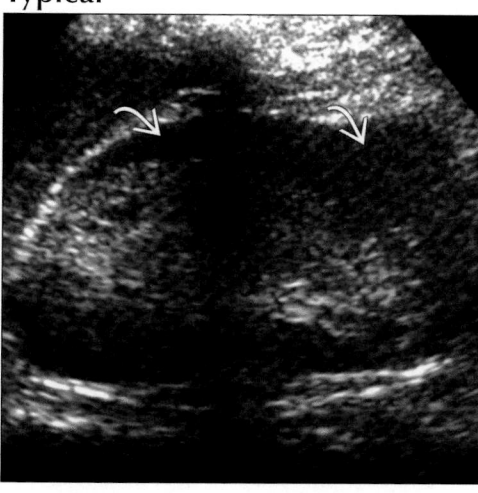
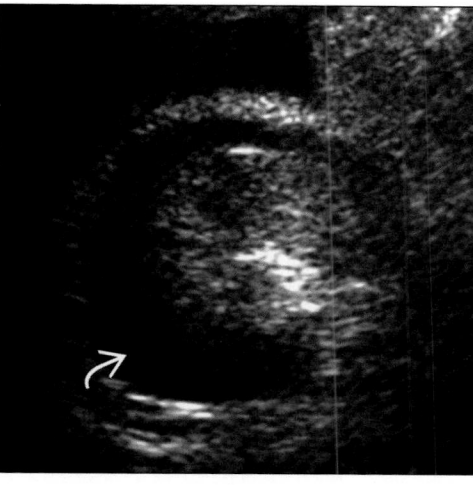

(Left) Longitudinal transabdominal ultrasound shows a post-traumatic subcapsular urinoma ➔ surrounding the kidney. Urinomas are typically anechoic and mimick fresh blood. (Right) Transverse transabdominal ultrasound shows the sickle-shaped, subcapsular urinoma in the previous patient ➔. Urinomas can be localized, subcapsular, intrarenal, pararenal or intrathoracic.

ACUTE PYELONEPHRITIS

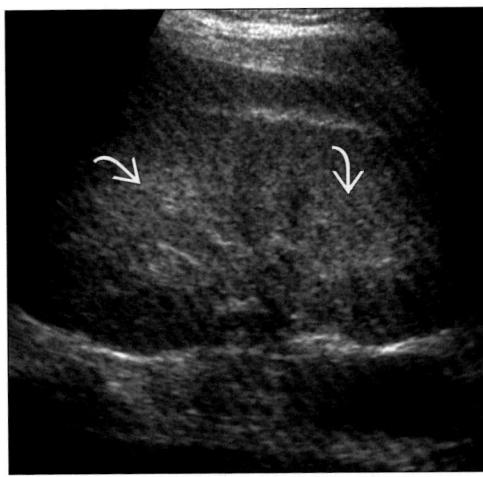

Longitudinal transabdominal ultrasound shows AP. The kidney is swollen with loss of CM differentiation and ↑ parenchymal heterogenicity ➡, which may be due to microabscesses and necrosis.

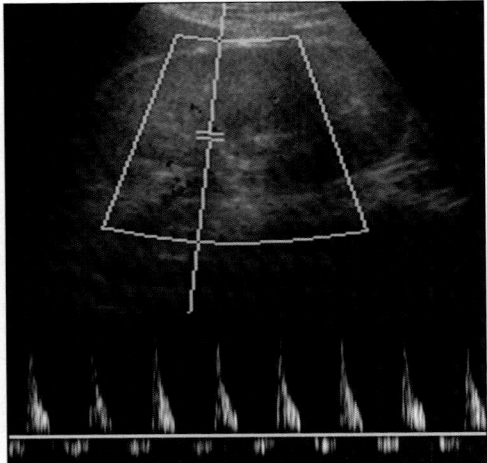

Longitudinal color Doppler ultrasound in a patient with AP shows high-RI in an intrarenal vessel. This may be due to vascular obstruction due to edema, microabscesses or necrosis.

TERMINOLOGY

Abbreviations and Synonyms
- Acute Pyelonephritis (AP)

Definitions
- Renal infection of pelvis, calyces & interstitium
- Predisposed by obstruction, ureteric reflux, diabetes, pregnancy, urinary tract infection (UTI)

IMAGING FINDINGS

General Features
- Best diagnostic clue: Renal enlargement with thickened urothelium and microabscesses
- Location: Usually unilateral

Ultrasonographic Findings
- Grayscale Ultrasound
  - Normal or swollen kidney & ↓ renal echogenicity
  - Loss of corticomedullary (CM) differentiation ± effacement of sinus echoes
  - Thickened renal pelvic urothelium
  - Microabscesses or areas of necrosis
- Power Doppler: May show ↓ renal vascularity or vascular defect due to vasoconstriction

CT Findings
- Renal enlargement, focal swelling, sinus obliteration
- Diffuse absent, "patchy" or striated nephrogram
- Loss of normal CM differentiation
- Calyceal effacement, dilated renal pelvis & ureter
- Thickening of walls of renal pelvis, calyces, ureter

Nuclear Medicine Findings
- Cortical scintigraphy evaluates renal scars (children)

Imaging Recommendations
- Best imaging tool: Ultrasound is useful to rule out abscess or obstruction particularly in children
- Protocol advice: Initial investigation by ultrasound followed by CT for delineation of complication

DIFFERENTIAL DIAGNOSIS

Acute Tubular Necrosis
- Due to ischemia or nephrotoxicity

DDx: Acute Pyelonephritis

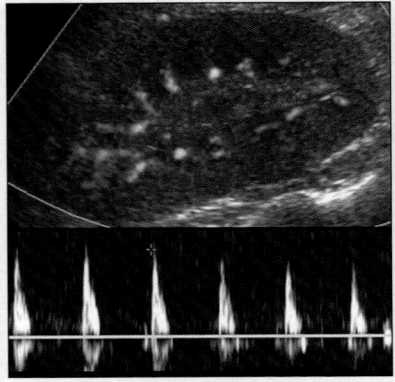

Acute Tubular Necrosis

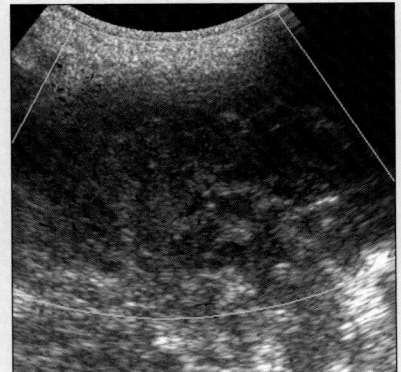

Renal Lymphoma

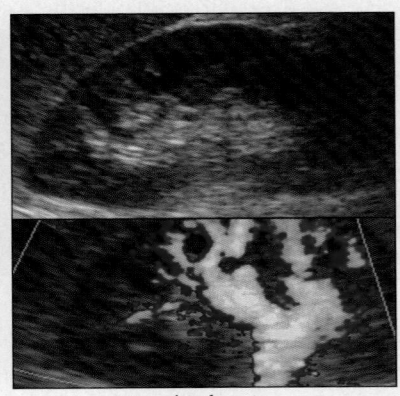

Renal Infarction

ACUTE PYELONEPHRITIS

Key Facts

Terminology
- Renal infection of pelvis, calyces & interstitium

Imaging Findings
- Best diagnostic clue: Renal enlargement with thickened urothelium and microabscesses
- Normal or swollen kidney & ↓ renal echogenicity
- Loss of corticomedullary (CM) differentiation ± effacement of sinus echoes
- Thickened renal pelvic urothelium

- Microabscesses or areas of necrosis
- Power Doppler: May show ↓ renal vascularity or vascular defect due to vasoconstriction
- Protocol advice: Initial investigation by ultrasound followed by CT for delineation of complication

Top Differential Diagnoses
- Acute Tubular Necrosis
- Lymphoma
- Acute Renal Infarction

- ↑ Renal size & pyramids & resistivity index (RI > 0.8)

Lymphoma
- Diffuse: Enlarged kidney & ↓ echogenicity
- Multifocal: Enlarged kidney & hypoechoic masses

Acute Renal Infarction
- Global or segmental vascular defect on color Doppler imaging in normal/enlarged kidney

PATHOLOGY

General Features
- Etiology
  - Most common organism: Escherichia coli
  - Route: Ascending > hematogenous infection
- Epidemiology: ↑ Incidence: M > 65 years, F < 40 years

Gross Pathologic & Surgical Features
- "Polar abscesses": Microabscesses on renal surface
- Narrowed calyces & enlarged kidney

Microscopic Features
- Mononuclear cell infiltrate & fibrosis
- Interstitial or tubular necrosis

CLINICAL ISSUES

Presentation
- Most common signs/symptoms: Fever, malaise, dysuria, flank pain & tenderness

- Lab data
  - ↑ ESR; ↑ WBC; ↑ proteinuria
  - Positive urine culture for bacilli

Demographics
- Age: Common in adults (also seen in children)
- Gender: M < F

Natural History & Prognosis
- Complications: Abscess formation or pyonephrosis
- Prognosis: Good

Treatment
- Acute: Antibiotic therapy

DIAGNOSTIC CHECKLIST

Consider
- Clinical correlation for equivocal imaging findings

Image Interpretation Pearls
- Swollen kidney & poor CM differentiation & sinus echoes effacement ⇒ usually AP

SELECTED REFERENCES

1. Dacher JN et al: Power Doppler sonographic pattern of acute pyelonephritis in children: comparison with CT. AJR Am J Roentgenol. 166(6):1451-5, 1996
2. Talner LB et al: Acute pyelonephritis: can we agree on terminology? Radiology. 192(2):297-305, 1994

IMAGE GALLERY

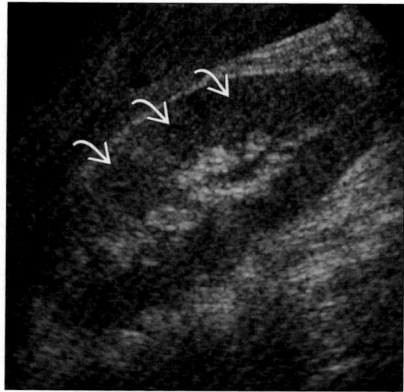 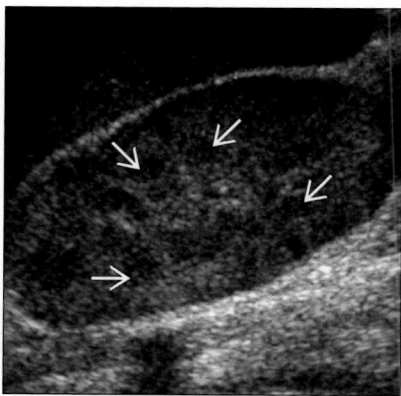 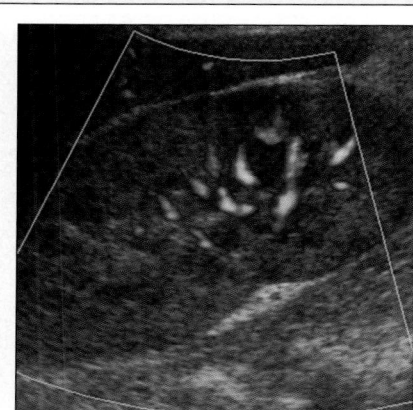

(Left) Longitudinal transabdominal ultrasound shows AP in which the affected kidney is of normal size but with poor CM differentiation ⇒. *(Center)* Longitudinal transabdominal ultrasound shows a swollen kidney with multiple small hypoechoic lesions ➡ representing abscesses. Note the infected kidney has lost CM differentiation and sinus echoes. *(Right)* Longitudinal power Doppler ultrasound in a patient with AP shows ↓ in parenchymal vascularity probably due to formation of microabscesses or necrosis.

FOCAL BACTERIAL NEPHRITIS

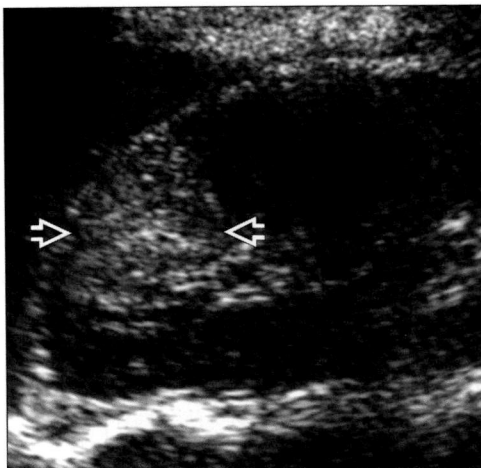

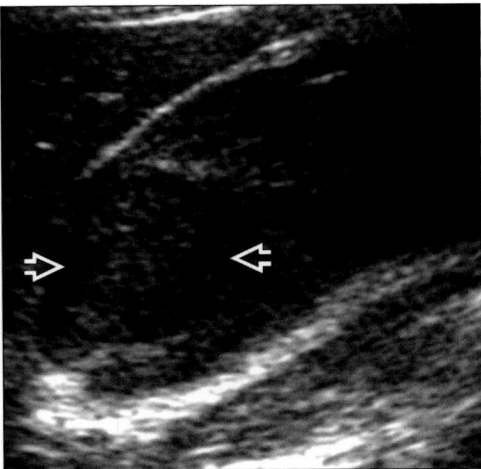

Longitudinal transabdominal ultrasound shows FBN seen as a wedge-shaped echogenic mass ➡ in a febrile patient with flank pain. ↑ Echogenicity in FBN may be due to hemorrhage.

Longitudinal transabdominal ultrasound shows FBN ➡ after antibiotic therapy (same patient as left). Note FBN becomes hypoechoic, which may be due to either resolving FBN or progressing FBN with liquefaction.

TERMINOLOGY

Abbreviations and Synonyms
- Focal bacterial nephritis (FBN); lobar nephronia; focal pyelonephritis

Definitions
- Presents as acute pyelonephritis but is distinguishable by presence of focal inflammatory mass without frank abscess formation

IMAGING FINDINGS

General Features
- Best diagnostic clue: Renal enlargement + focal ↑/↓ parenchymal echogenicity
- Location: Kidney, unilateral

Ultrasonographic Findings
- Grayscale Ultrasound
  - Normal or enlarged kidney (due to edema)
  - Urothelial thickening of renal pelvis
  - FBN: Localized ↑/↓ parenchymal echogenicity
    - ↑ Echogenicity (related to hemorrhage)
    - ↓ Echogenicity (liquefaction of FBN with abscess formation or resolving FBN after therapy)
  - FBN: Usually wedge-shaped, poorly defined margin
  - FBN: Focal renal enlargement simulating mass lesion
  - Multi-FBN ⇒ patchy heterogeneous renal parenchyma
  - Multi-FBN ⇒ ↓ corticomedullary (CM) distinction
  - Multi-FBN ⇒ obliteration of sinus echoes
  - ± Hydronephrosis or calculus
  - ± Renal or perinephric abscess formation
  - US cannot differentiate FBN from abscess or tumor
- Power Doppler
  - FBN: Focal ↓ in vascularity
  - Multi-FBN: Multiple areas of hypovascularity

CT Findings
- NECT
  - Typical: Triangular mass with iso- or hypodensity
  - Hyperdense lesion ⇒ hemorrhagic FBN
  - Irregularly marginated; lobar in distribution
- CECT
  - Depicted as nephrographic defect
  - Patchy and inhomogeneous enhancement in FBN

DDx: Focal Bacterial Nephritis

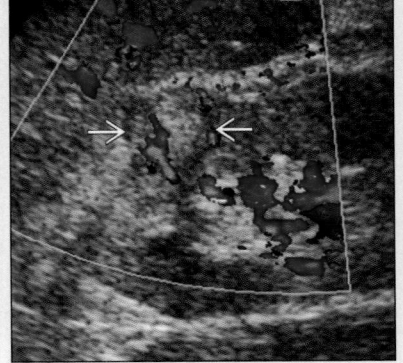

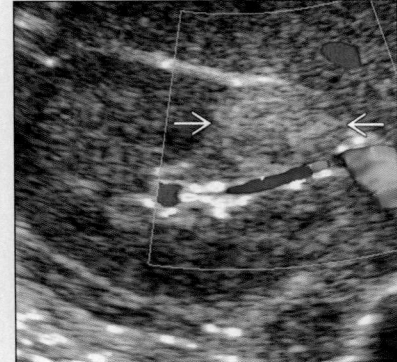

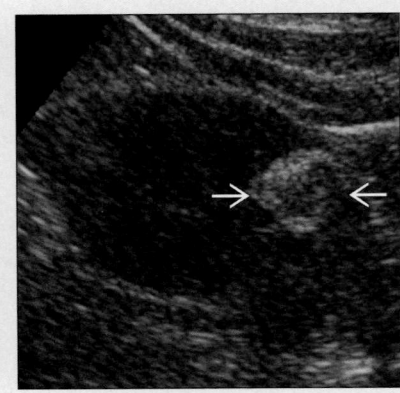

Renal Cell Carcinoma

Renal Metastasis

Angiomyolipoma

FOCAL BACTERIAL NEPHRITIS

Key Facts

Imaging Findings
- Normal or enlarged kidney (due to edema)
- Urothelial thickening of renal pelvis
- FBN: Localized ↑/↓ parenchymal echogenicity
- FBN: Usually wedge-shaped, poorly defined margin
- FBN: Focal renal enlargement simulating mass lesion
- Multi-FBN ⇒ patchy heterogeneous renal parenchyma
- Multi-FBN ⇒ ↓ corticomedullary (CM) distinction

- Multi-FBN ⇒ obliteration of sinus echoes
- ± Hydronephrosis or calculus
- ± Renal or perinephric abscess formation
- FBN: Focal ↓ in vascularity
- Multi-FBN: Multiple areas of hypovascularity

Top Differential Diagnoses
- Renal Cell Carcinoma (RCC)
- Renal Metastasis
- Renal Angiomyolipoma (AML)

  ○ ± CM abscess; renal or perinephric abscess

Imaging Recommendations
- Best imaging tool: CT is method of choice; better than ultrasound in delineation of FBN and its progression
- Protocol advice: Initial investigation or follow-up by ultrasound; CT for suspected complication

DIFFERENTIAL DIAGNOSIS

Renal Cell Carcinoma (RCC)
- May be solid, cystic or mixed; usually hypervascular
- Typically echogenic cortical mass with hypoechoic rim

Renal Metastasis
- Variable echogenicity, typically hypoperfused masses

Renal Angiomyolipoma (AML)
- Benign renal tumor composed of abnormal blood vessels, smooth muscle and fatty components
- Majority are hyperechoic with high fat content

PATHOLOGY

General Features
- Etiology: Ascending bacterial infection from bladder via ureter to kidney by Escherichia coli (75%)

Microscopic Features
- Heavy polymorphonuclear infiltrate at tip of papilla with distortion of glomeruli and renal tubules

CLINICAL ISSUES

Presentation
- Most common signs/symptoms: Fever and pyuria

Natural History & Prognosis
- FBN → multi-FBN → corticomedullary abscess → cortical abscess → perinephric abscess
- Prognosis: Generally good except in patients with UT abnormalities, advanced disease and ↓ renal function

Treatment
- Antimicrobial therapy ± surgical intervention/percutaneous abscess drainage

DIAGNOSTIC CHECKLIST

Consider
- Ultrasound-guided needle aspiration in doubtful cases

Image Interpretation Pearls
- Renal enlargement with hypoperfused, wedge-shaped lesion involving CM region

SELECTED REFERENCES

1. Kawashima A et al: Radiologic evaluation of patients with renal infections. Infect Dis Clin North Am. 17(2):433-56, 2003
2. Nosher JL et al: Acute focal bacterial nephritis. Am J Kidney Dis. 11(1):36-42, 1988

IMAGE GALLERY

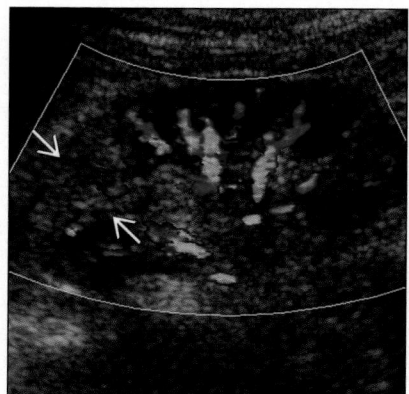 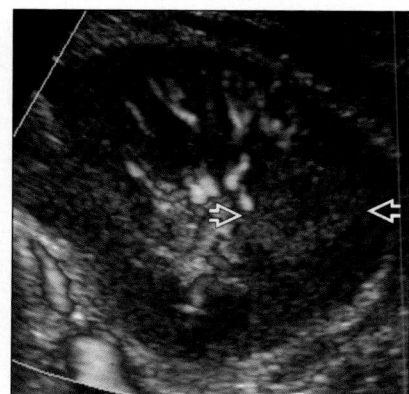 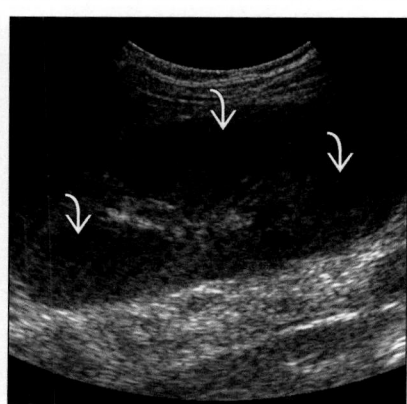

(Left) Longitudinal color Doppler image shows a wedge-shaped area of echogenic FBN ➡ with a parenchymal vascular defect. With proper clinical correlation, sonographic findings are diagnostic of FBN. *(Center)* Transverse power Doppler image shows echogenic FBN ➡ simulating a mass lesion. Sonographic findings overlap with those of renal metastasis & AML. *(Right)* Longitudinal ultrasound shows multi-FBN ➡ producing a patchy, heterogeneous appearance in the kidney. This appearance may be confused with multifocal renal lymphoma or metastases.

EMPHYSEMATOUS PYELONEPHRITIS

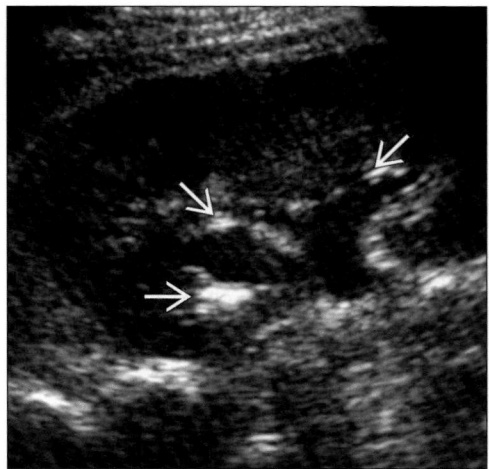

Longitudinal transabdominal ultrasound shows multiple foci of echogenic gas ➡ around the renal pelvis.

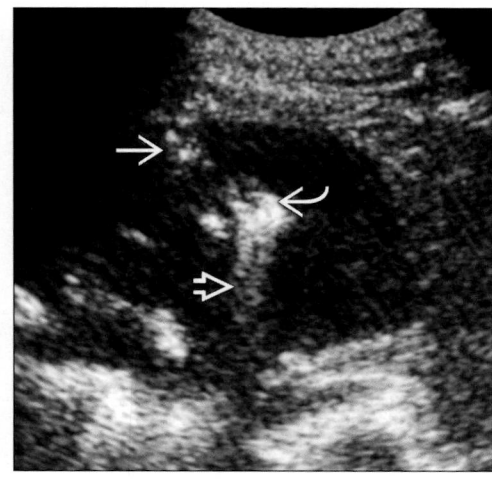

Transverse transabdominal ultrasound shows echogenic gas within the renal cortex ➡ and deep parenchyma ➡, with ring down artifacts ➡.

TERMINOLOGY

Abbreviations and Synonyms
- Emphysematous pyelonephritis (EPN)

Definitions
- Life-threatening, fulminant, necrotizing upper urinary tract infection (UTI) associated with gas within kidney

IMAGING FINDINGS

General Features
- Location
  - Unilateral > bilateral (5-7% of cases)
  - Left (52%) > right (43%)

Ultrasonographic Findings
- Grayscale Ultrasound
  - Highly echogenic areas within renal sinus and parenchyma with unsharp shadowing
  - Ring-down artifacts: Air bubbles trapped in fluid
  - Gas in perinephric space; may obscure kidney

Radiographic Findings
- Radiography: Gas in parenchyma ± paranephric space

CT Findings
- 2 types of EPN
  - Type I (33%) (true EPN)
    - Parenchymal destruction without fluid; streaky or mottled gas radiating from medulla to cortex
    - ± Crescent of subcapsular or perinephric gas
  - Type II (66%)
    - Renal or perirenal fluid abscesses with bubbly gas pattern ± gas within renal pelvis
- Intraparenchymal, intracaliceal and intrapelvic gas
- Gas often extends into subcapsular, perinephric, pararenal, contralateral retroperitoneal spaces

MR Findings
- T1WI, T2WI: Void of signal

Imaging Recommendations
- Best imaging tool: CT is ideal to determine location and extent of renal and perirenal gas

---

DDx: Emphysematous Pyelonephritis

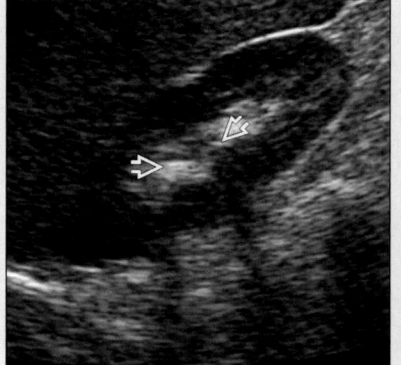

Renal Calculus

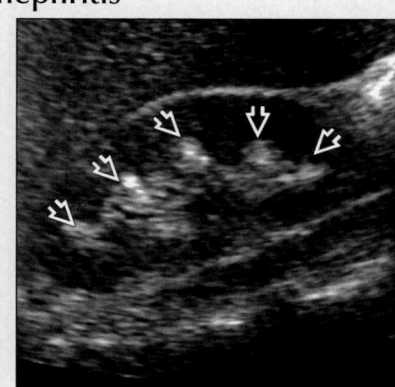

Nephrocalcinosis

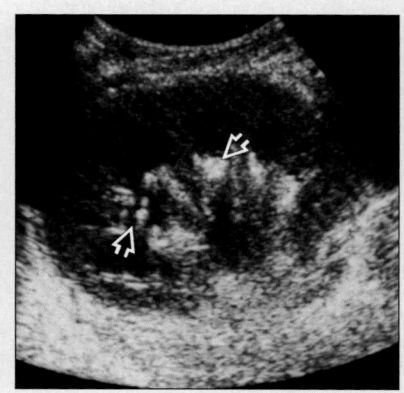

Papillary Necrosis

EMPHYSEMATOUS PYELONEPHRITIS

Key Facts

Imaging Findings
- Highly echogenic areas within renal sinus and parenchyma with unsharp shadowing
- Ring-down artifacts: Air bubbles trapped in fluid
- Gas in perinephric space; may obscure kidney
- Best imaging tool: CT is ideal to determine location and extent of renal and perirenal gas

Top Differential Diagnoses
- Renal Calculus
- Nephrocalcinosis
- Papillary Necrosis

Pathology
- Suppurative necrotizing infection of renal parenchyma and perirenal tissue with multiple cortical abscesses

Clinical Issues
- Complications: Generalized sepsis

DIFFERENTIAL DIAGNOSIS

Renal Calculus
- Discrete echogenic focus with sharp distal acoustic shadowing

Nephrocalcinosis
- Generalized increased echogenicity of renal pyramid ± shadowing

Papillary Necrosis
- Single or multiple cystic cavities in medullary pyramids continuous with calices
- Sloughed papillae seen as echogenic nonshadowing structures at pyramids

PATHOLOGY

General Features
- Etiology
  - Single or mixed organism(s) infection
    - E. coli (68%), Klebsiella pneumoniae (9%)
    - Proteus mirabilis, pseudomonas, enterobacter, candida, clostridia species
  - Risk factor
    - Recurrent or chronic UTIs
    - Immunocompromised: Diabetes mellitus (87-97%)
    - Ureteral obstruction (20-40%): Calculi, stenosis
    - Renal failure: Polycystic kidney, end-stage
  - Pathogenesis
    - Pyelonephritis → ischemia and low oxygen tension → anaerobe proliferation in an anaerobic environment → CO_2 production

Gross Pathologic & Surgical Features
- Suppurative necrotizing infection of renal parenchyma and perirenal tissue with multiple cortical abscesses

CLINICAL ISSUES

Presentation
- Most common signs/symptoms: Extremely ill at presentation: Fever, flank pain, hyperglycemia, acidosis, dehydration and electrolyte imbalance

Natural History & Prognosis
- Complications: Generalized sepsis
- Prognosis: Poor
  - Mortality: 66% with type I, 18% with type II

Treatment
- Antibiotic therapy; nephrectomy for type I
- CT-guided drainage procedures for type II

SELECTED REFERENCES

1. Grayson DE et al: Emphysematous infections of the abdomen and pelvis: a pictorial review. Radiographics. 22(3):543-61, 2002
2. Joseph RC et al: Genitourinary tract gas: imaging evaluation. Radiographics. 16(2):295-308, 1996

IMAGE GALLERY

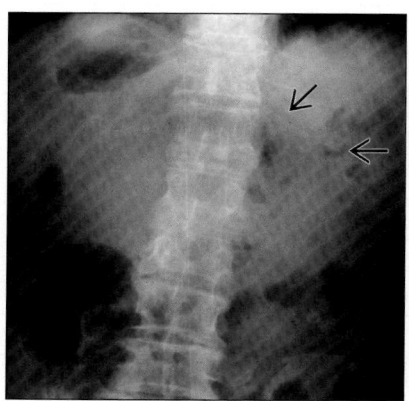 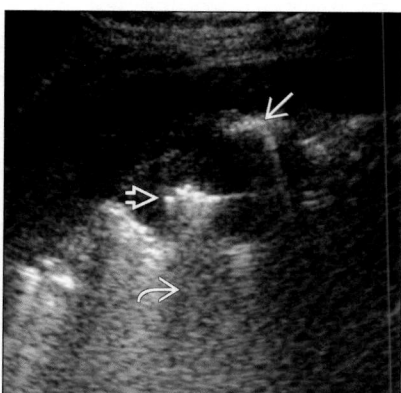 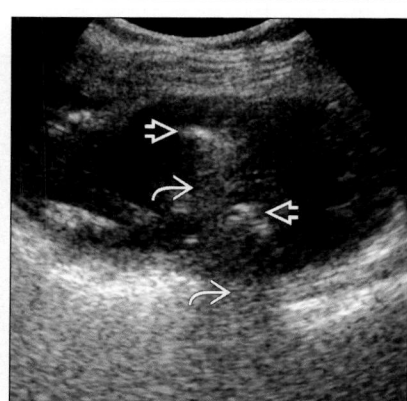

(Left) Plain radiograph shows a mottled gas pattern ➡ over the left renal fossa in emphysematous pyelonephritis. *(Center)* Transverse transabdominal ultrasound shows echogenic gas ➡ within the renal parenchyma, associated with distal shadowing ➡. Normal bowel gas ➡ is noted in the peri-renal region. *(Right)* Longitudinal transabdominal ultrasound show multiple foci of echogenic gas ➡ present within the renal parenchyma with associated distal shadowing ➡.

PYONEPHROSIS

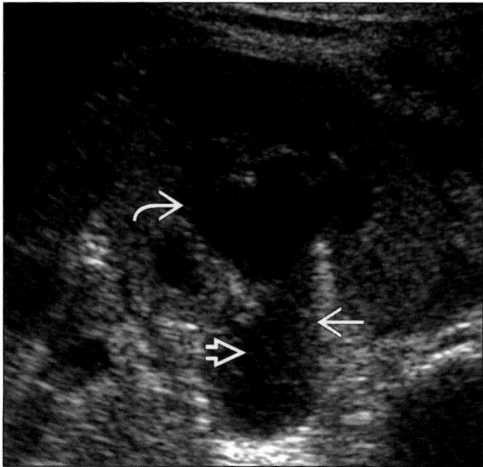

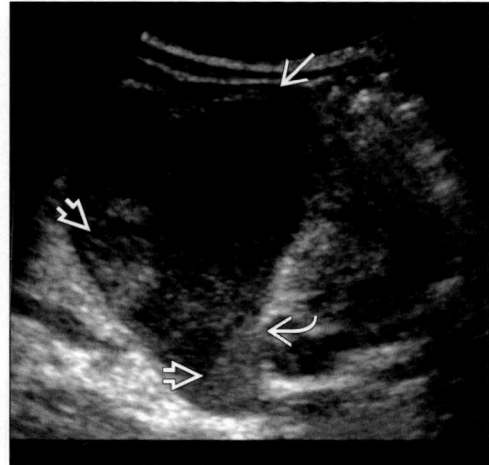

Transverse transabdominal ultrasound shows low-level echoes ➡ suggesting debris within a dilated renal pelvicaliceal system ➡. Urothelial thickening is also present ➡.

Transverse transabdominal ultrasound shows echogenic pus ➡ in the dependent portion of the dilated renal pelvis ➡. Note marked cortical thinning due to chronic obstruction ➡.

TERMINOLOGY

Definitions
• Distention of renal collecting system with pus or infected urine

IMAGING FINDINGS

General Features
• Best diagnostic clue: Presence of mobile debris and layering of low-amplitude echoes in hydronephrotic kidney

Ultrasonographic Findings
• Grayscale Ultrasound
  ○ Hydronephrosis, with or without hydroureter, in conjunction with debris within
  ○ Most consistent finding: Low level mobile echoes
  ○ Echogenic pus layering in dependent portion of collecting system
  ○ Associated stone or gas may be seen sometimes
  ○ Thickening of urothelial lining of the renal pelvis or ureter

DIFFERENTIAL DIAGNOSIS

Hydronephrosis
• Echo-free dilated collecting system, no dependent internal echoes

Transitional Cell Carcinoma (TCC)
• Solid tumor with vascularity within dilated collecting system

Complex Renal Cyst
• Echoes/solid component/septum within the cyst
• No communication with renal pelvis or adjacent calices

PATHOLOGY

General Features
• Etiology
  ○ Long-standing ureteric obstruction
    ▪ Calculus or ureteropelvic junction in young adult
    ▪ Malignant ureteral stricture in elderly

DDx: Pyonephrosis

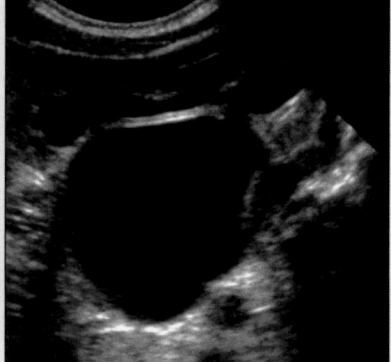

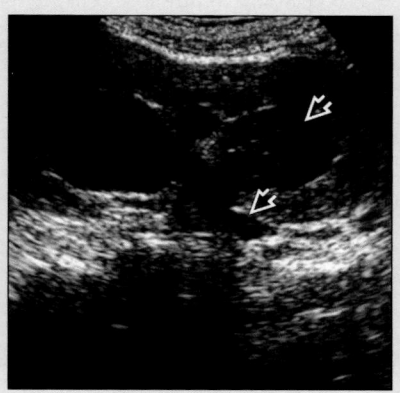

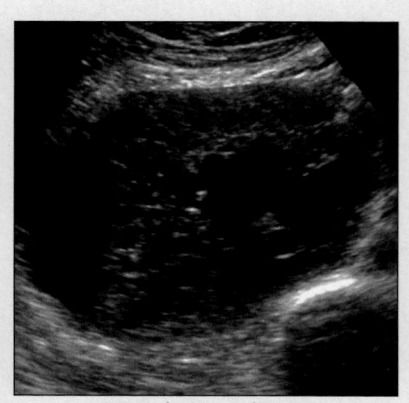

Hydronephrosis

Transitional Cell Carcinoma

Complex Renal Cyst

PYONEPHROSIS

Key Facts

Terminology
- Distention of renal collecting system with pus or infected urine

Imaging Findings
- Best diagnostic clue: Presence of mobile debris and layering of low-amplitude echoes in hydronephrotic kidney
- Thickening of urothelial lining of the renal pelvis or ureter

Top Differential Diagnoses
- Hydronephrosis
- Transitional Cell Carcinoma (TCC)
- Complex Renal Cyst

Diagnostic Checklist
- May be indistinguishable from non-infected hydronephrosis
- Proceed to percutaneous nephrostomy for urine microscopy and culture if patient clinically septic

---

- Stagnant urine becomes infected, filled with white blood cells, bacteria, debris and pus
  - Ascending urinary tract infection
  - Blood-borne bacterial pathogen
- Epidemiology: Most common organism: E. Coli
- Associated abnormalities: Complications: Renal abscess, perinephric abscess, xanthogranulomatous pyelonephritis, fistula to duodenum, colon or pleura

Microscopic Features
- Purulent exudate composed of sloughed urothelium and inflammatory cells from early formation of microabscesses and necrotizing papillitis

CLINICAL ISSUES

Presentation
- Most common signs/symptoms: Fever, chills, flank pain
- Other signs/symptoms: Pyuria, leukocytosis, bacteriuria

Natural History & Prognosis
- Progress to bacteremia or septic shock leads to 25-50% mortality
- Delay in diagnosis and treatment leads to irreversible renal parenchymal damage and renal failure

Treatment
- Early diagnosis and drainage are crucial to prevent bacteremia and septic shock

DIAGNOSTIC CHECKLIST

Image Interpretation Pearls
- May be indistinguishable from non-infected hydronephrosis
  - Proceed to percutaneous nephrostomy for urine microscopy and culture if patient clinically septic

SELECTED REFERENCES

1. Gopaldas R et al: A case of pyonephrosis secondary to ureteral stent calculus. Int Urol Nephrol. 37(3):467-70, 2005
2. Browne RF et al: Imaging of urinary tract infection in the adult. Eur Radiol. 14 Suppl 3:E168-83, 2004
3. Noble VE et al: Renal ultrasound. Emerg Med Clin North Am. 22(3):641-59, 2004
4. Paterson A: Urinary tract infection: an update on imaging strategies. Eur Radiol. 14 Suppl 4:L89-100, 2004
5. Sharma S et al: Neonatal pyonephrosis--a case report. Int Urol Nephrol. 36(3):313-5, 2004
6. Wah TM et al: Lower moiety pelvic-ureteric junction obstruction (PUJO) of the duplex kidney presenting with pyonephrosis in adults. Br J Radiol. 76(912):909-12, 2003
7. Wang IK et al: The use of ultrasonography in evaluating adults with febrile urinary tract infection. Ren Fail. 25(6):981-7, 2003

IMAGE GALLERY

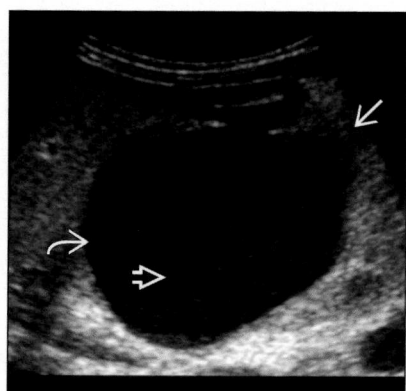 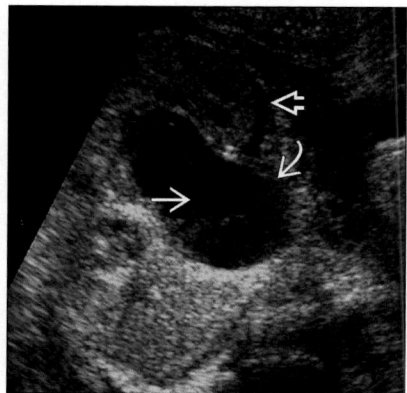 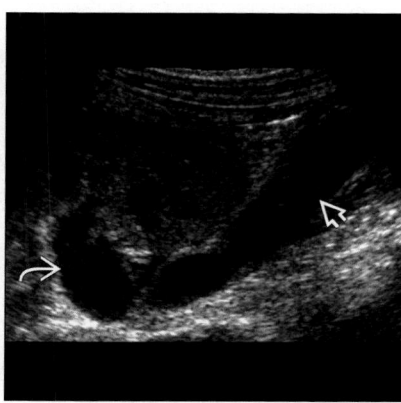

(Left) Longitudinal transabdominal ultrasound shows low-level echoes ➡ in a markedly dilated collecting system ➡, in a case of ureteropelvic junction obstruction. There is minimal residual cortical tissue ➡. (Center) Transverse transabdominal ultrasound shows low-amplitude echoes layering ➡ within a dilated renal pelvis ➡. A small rim of perinephric fluid is also present ➡. (Right) Oblique transabdominal ultrasound shows diffuse low-level echoes within a dilated renal pelvis ➡ and ureter ➡, due to distal ureteric obstruction by calculus.

RENAL ABSCESS

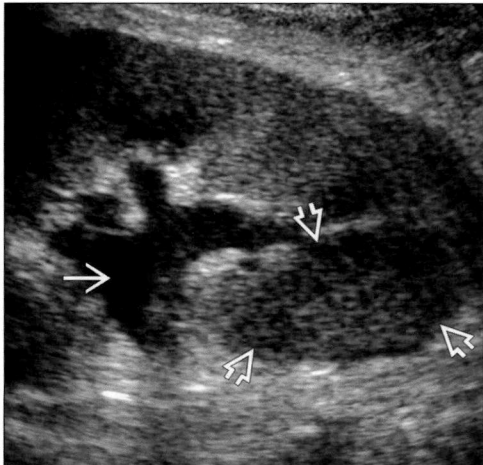

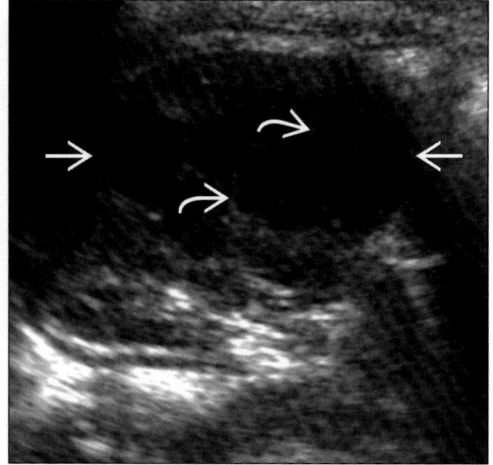

Longitudinal transabdominal ultrasound shows an oval renal abscess ➤ with echogenic internal debris and weak acoustic enhancement. Mild associated hydronephrosis is also noted ➤.

Oblique transabdominal ultrasound shows a large renal abscess ➤ with irregular wall and internal septations ➤. On ultrasound the abscess is indistinguishable from a hemorrhagic cyst or RCC.

TERMINOLOGY

Definitions
- Develops from unresolved focal pyelonephritis which progresses to parenchymal necrosis

IMAGING FINDINGS

General Features
- Best diagnostic clue: Well-defined hypoechoic area with irregular wall and internal debris
- Location: Single > multiple; unilateral > bilateral

Ultrasonographic Findings
- Grayscale Ultrasound
  - Round or thick/smooth-walled complex cystic mass
  - Anechoic/hypoechoic ± weak acoustic enhancement
  - May contain echogenic internal debris
  - Internal echogenic foci with "comet-tail" may represent gas-forming organisms within abscess
  - ± Internal septations or loculations
  - ± Renal sinus obliteration or calyceal effacement
  - ± Calculus or hydronephrosis

- Perinephric extension in para- or perirenal spaces
- ± Loss of cleavage plane with Gerota fascia

CT Findings
- NECT
  - Round, well-defined, low-attenuation masses
  - ± Gas within collection
- CECT
  - Focal hypodense area ± wall enhancement
  - Renal sinus obliteration or calyceal effacement
  - Perinephric reaction or extension
    - Edema or obliteration of perinephric fat
    - Thickened Gerota fascia and perinephric septa

Imaging Recommendations
- Best imaging tool: CT for perinephric extension; ultrasound for guided aspiration
- Protocol advice: Initial examination (ultrasound); further investigation (CT)

DIFFERENTIAL DIAGNOSIS

Renal Carcinoma (RCC)
- Hypervascular mass; usually asymptomatic

DDx: Renal Abscess

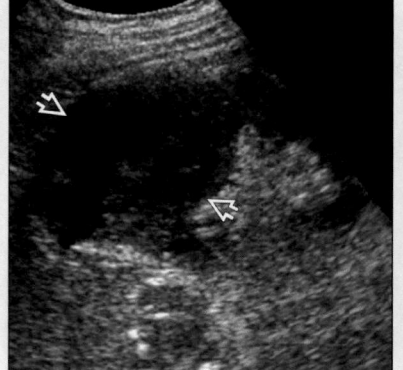

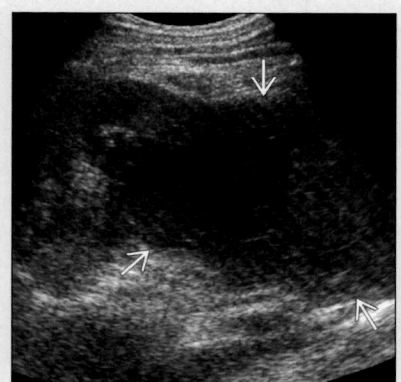

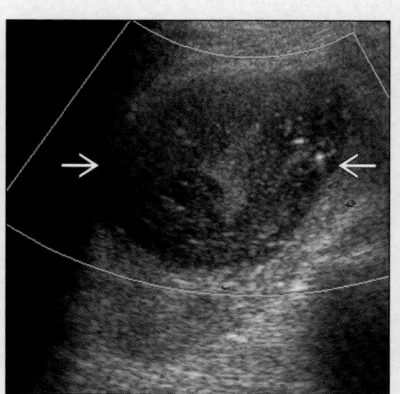

Renal Cell Carcinoma

Renal Lymphoma

Proteinaceous Cyst

RENAL ABSCESS

Key Facts

Imaging Findings
- Round or thick/smooth-walled complex cystic mass
- Anechoic/hypoechoic ± weak acoustic enhancement
- May contain echogenic internal debris
- Internal echogenic foci with "comet-tail" may represent gas-forming organisms within abscess
- ± Internal septations or loculations
- ± Renal sinus obliteration or calyceal effacement
- ± Calculus or hydronephrosis
- Perinephric extension in para- or perirenal spaces
- ± Loss of cleavage plane with Gerota fascia

Top Differential Diagnoses
- Renal Carcinoma (RCC)
- Metastases and Lymphoma
- Hemorrhagic Cyst or Proteinaceous Cyst

Diagnostic Checklist
- Ultrasound guided aspiration in equivocal cases

- 25-40% diagnosed incidentally on CT or ultrasound

Metastases and Lymphoma
- Metastases: Hypovascular with variable echogenicity
- Lymphoma: Hypovascular; multiple distinct hypoechoic masses (common)

Hemorrhagic Cyst or Proteinaceous Cyst
- Appearance indistinguishable from abscess
- Proteinaceous cyst: Variant of hemorrhagic cyst; contains thick layers of internal debris

PATHOLOGY

General Features
- Etiology
  - Ascending urinary tract infections (80%)
    - Corticomedullary abscess by E. coli/Proteus species
  - Hematogenous spread (20%)
    - Cortical abscess by Staphylococcus aureus
- Associated abnormalities: Urolithiasis (20-60%)

Microscopic Features
- Necrotic glomeruli & polymorphonuclear infiltration

CLINICAL ISSUES

Presentation
- Most common signs/symptoms: Fever, flank/abdominal pain, chills and dysuria

Demographics
- Age: All; M = F

Natural History & Prognosis
- Complications: Abscess rupture
  - Into calyceal system (pyonephrosis)
  - Into perinephric space (perinephric abscess)
  - Beyond Gerota fascia (paranephric abscess)
  - Into peritoneum (subdiaphragmatic/pelvic abscess)
  - Compression or obstruction → renal atrophy
- Prognosis
  - Good (early therapy); poor (delayed therapy)

Treatment
- Antibiotic therapy ± percutaneous/open surgical drainage ± nephrectomy

DIAGNOSTIC CHECKLIST

Consider
- Clinical history & urinalysis for work-up of diagnosis
- Ultrasound guided aspiration in equivocal cases

Image Interpretation Pearls
- Hypoechoic mass & irregular wall & internal debris

SELECTED REFERENCES

1. Yen DH et al: Renal abscess: early diagnosis and treatment. Am J Emerg Med. 17(2):192-7, 1999

IMAGE GALLERY

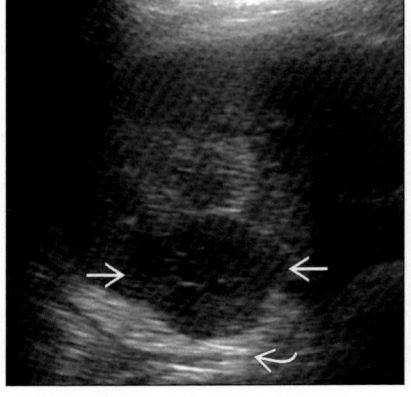 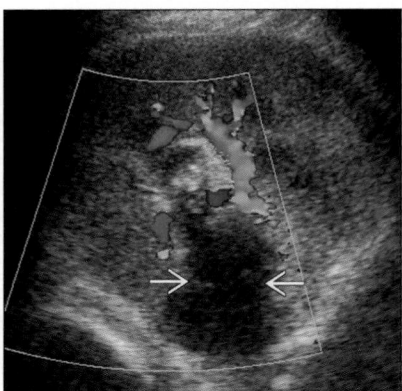 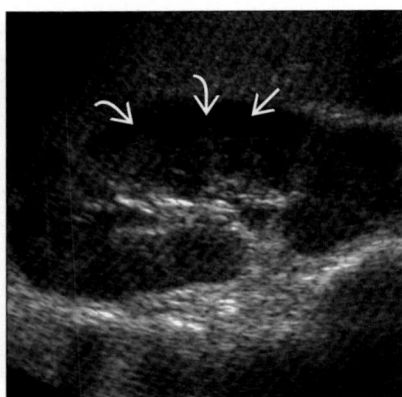

(Left) Oblique transabdominal ultrasound shows a hypoechoic, semi-solid renal abscess ➡. Note weak posterior enhancement ➡. *(Center)* Transverse color Doppler ultrasound shows a renal abscess ➡ extending from the central calyx to the cortex. Appearance may mimic metastasis or lymphoma which is typically hypoechoic and avascular. *(Right)* Longitudinal transabdominal ultrasound shows an anechoic perinephric fluid collection ➡. Note that the renal outline is irregular with adhesions ➡. Features are consistent with a perinephric abscess.

XANTHOGRANULOMATOUS PYELONEPHRITIS

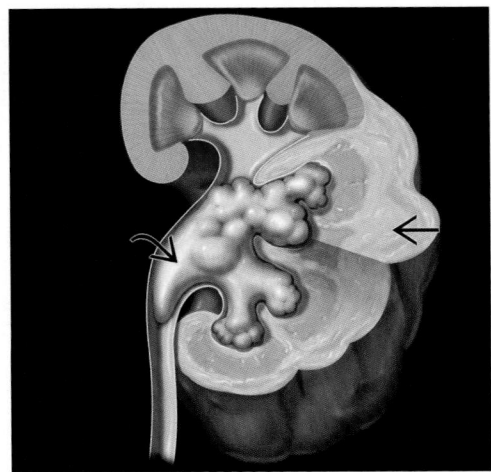

Graphic shows XGP with a long-standing ureteropelvic obstruction by a large staghorn stone ⇗, causing perirenal fibrofatty proliferation ⇥.

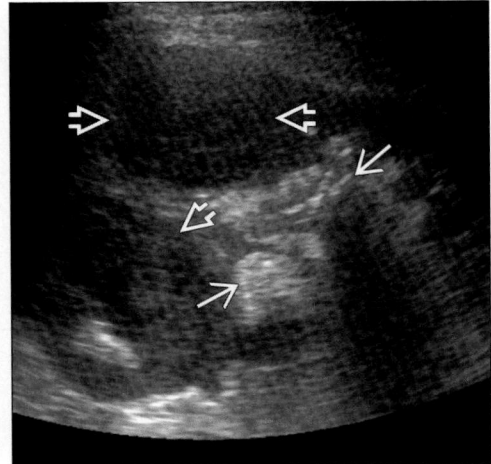

Longitudinal transabdominal ultrasound shows diffuse XGP. Note that the kidney is enlarged and the parenchyma is replaced by round hypoechoic masses ⇥. Calculi ⇥ are seen obstructing the renal pelvis.

TERMINOLOGY

Abbreviations and Synonyms
- Xanthogranulomatous pyelonephritis (XGP/XGPN)

Definitions
- Chronic renal inflammation usually associated with long-standing urinary calculus obstruction (75%)
- Characterized by destruction and replacement of renal parenchyma by lipid-laden macrophages
- Manifested either diffusely (> 80%) or focally (< 20%)
  - Diffuse: Due to obstruction at ureteropelvic junction
  - Focal or segmental: Due to obstruction of single infundibulum or one moiety of duplex system
- Three stages of XGP: Intrarenal ⇒ perirenal ⇒ perinephric ± retroperitoneal involvement

IMAGING FINDINGS

General Features
- Best diagnostic clue: Staghorn calculus with renal enlargement and perirenal fibrofatty proliferation
- Location: Unilateral (most cases) > bilateral

Ultrasonographic Findings
- Grayscale Ultrasound
  - Appearance varies depending on pattern of XGP
  - Diffusely enlarged kidney; highly reflective central echocomplex containing calculus
  - Anechoic or hypoechoic round masses replacing normal parenchyma
  - Echogenicity depends on amount of debris and necrosis within masses
  - Contracted pelvis due to fibrosis
  - Parenchymal thinning ± hydrocalyces
  - Pyonephrosis, pus-filled calyces or renal abscesses may be present
  - Segmental XGP: Anechoic or hypoechoic masses surrounding calculus-obstructing calyx
  - Perinephric inflammatory tissue ± fluid collection

CT Findings
- Multiple focal low attenuating renal masses with rim-enhancement
- Poor or no contrast excretion into collecting system
- Renal sinus fat obliterated with large central calculus
- Perinephric extension ± adjacent organs or structures

DDx: Xanthogranulomatous Pyelonephritis

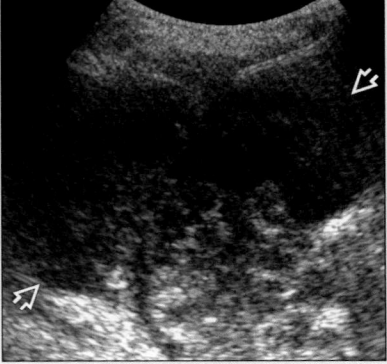

Renal Lymphoma

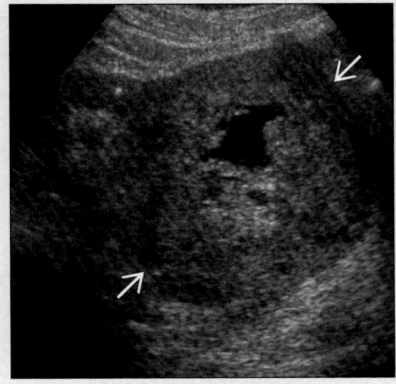

Renal Cell Carcinoma

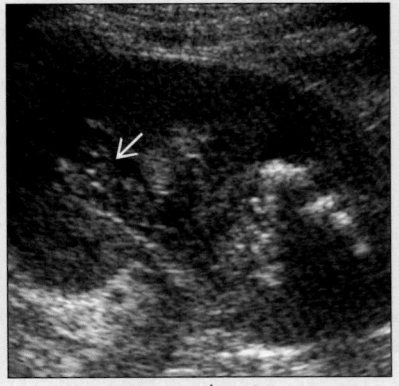

Pyonephrosis

XANTHOGRANULOMATOUS PYELONEPHRITIS

Key Facts

Imaging Findings

- Diffusely enlarged kidney; highly reflective central echocomplex containing calculus
- Anechoic or hypoechoic round masses replacing normal parenchyma
- Echogenicity depends on amount of debris and necrosis within masses
- Contracted pelvis due to fibrosis
- Parenchymal thinning ± hydrocalyces
- Pyonephrosis, pus-filled calyces or renal abscesses may be present
- Segmental XGP: Anechoic or hypoechoic masses surrounding calculus-obstructing calyx
- Perinephric inflammatory tissue ± fluid collection

Top Differential Diagnoses

- Renal Neoplasm
- Pyonephrosis or Renal Abscess
- Papillary Necrosis

Imaging Recommendations

- Best imaging tool: Ultrasound ideal at initial investigation; CT good for assessing renal function and retroperitoneal involvement

DIFFERENTIAL DIAGNOSIS

Renal Neoplasm

- XGP may simulate renal cell carcinoma, transitional cell carcinoma and renal metastasis
- Lymphoma may appear very similar to XGP

Pyonephrosis or Renal Abscess

- Pyonephrosis: Echoes within collecting system
- Renal abscess: Ill-defined hypoechoic masses

Papillary Necrosis

- Due to analgesic abuse, diabetes mellitus, chronic pyelonephritis, and sickle cell anemia

PATHOLOGY

General Features

- Etiology
  - Chronic infection and obstruction of ureteropelvic junction by long-standing calculus
  - Pyonephrosis ⇒ mucosal destruction and extension into adjacent cortex & medulla ⇒ papillary necrosis
- Epidemiology: Peak age: 40-50 years; M < F

Microscopic Features

- Lipid-laden "foamy" macrophages, diffuse infiltration of plasma cells and histiocytes

CLINICAL ISSUES

Presentation

- Most common signs/symptoms: Flank pain, fever, palpable mass & weight loss

Natural History & Prognosis

- Urinary symptoms ± complications: Hepatic dysfunction, extrarenal extension, fistulas
- Good prognosis and rare mortality

Treatment

- Antibiotic treatment and nephrectomy

DIAGNOSTIC CHECKLIST

Consider

- Histologic diagnosis in equivocal XGP

SELECTED REFERENCES

1. Kim JC: US and CT findings of xanthogranulomatous pyelonephritis. Clin Imaging. 25(2):118-21, 2001
2. Fan CM et al: Xanthogranulomatous pyelonephritis. AJR Am J Roentgenol. 165(4):1008, 1995

IMAGE GALLERY

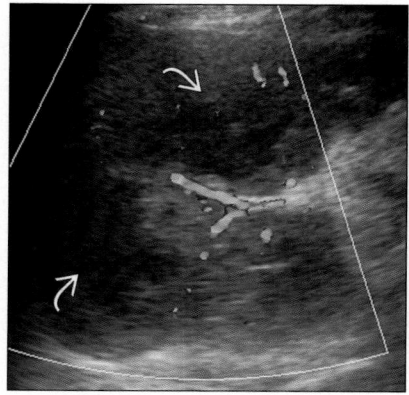 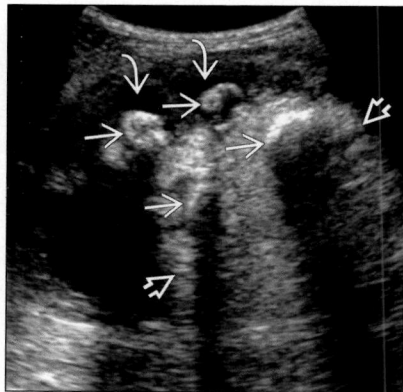 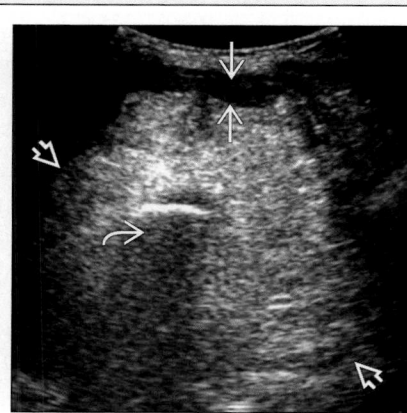

(Left) Longitudinal color Doppler ultrasound shows multiple hypoechoic masses ➡ which are avascular and may represent debris-filled calyces, renal abscesses or foci of parenchymal destruction. *(Center)* Longitudinal ultrasound shows extensive peripelvic fat infiltration secondary to XGP ➡. Note calculi ➡ in the renal pelvis and calyces with associated hydrocalycosis ➡. *(Right)* Transverse ultrasound in XGP shows renal parenchyma replaced by echogenic xanthogranulomatous tissue ➡ with large central calculus ➡. Cortical thinning ➡ is evident.

URINARY TRACT TUBERCULOSIS

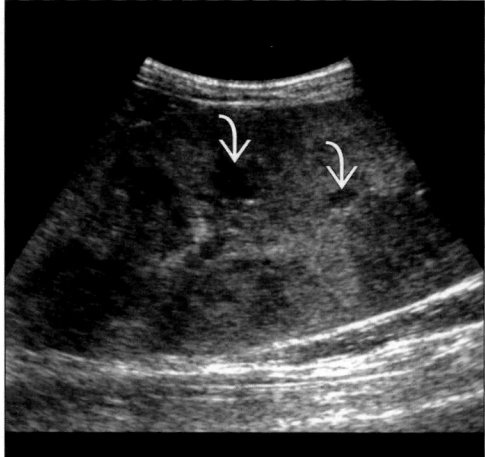

Longitudinal transabdominal ultrasound shows renal TB, with distorted renal parenchyma. There are small, irregular, hypoechoic lesions ➥ which represent cavities connecting to the collecting system.

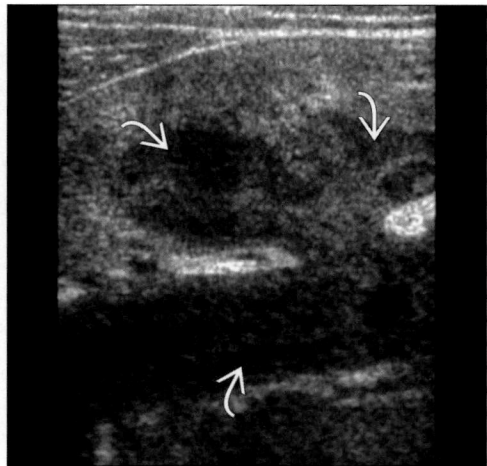

Longitudinal high-resolution ultrasound shows gross mucosal thickening ➥ in the collecting system of a patient with fulminant renal TB. The appearance may mimic pyonephrosis or neoplasm.

TERMINOLOGY

Abbreviations and Synonyms
- Urinary tract TB
- Renal tuberculosis (renal TB)

Definitions
- Urinary tract infection (UTI) by mycobacterium TB via hematogenous spread from primary focus, usually lungs
- Ureteral and bladder disease are secondary to renal involvement
- Earliest form of bladder TB starts around ureteral orifice

IMAGING FINDINGS

General Features
- Best diagnostic clue: Calcification, cavities and strictures in urinary tract (UT)
- Location
  - Kidney, ureter and bladder

  - Usually bilateral involvement but can also be unilateral
  - Right kidney > left kidney
  - Upper pole > lower pole

Ultrasonographic Findings
- Grayscale Ultrasound
  - Appearance is non-specific and variable
  - Useful to demonstrate non-excreting kidney on IVP
  - Useful to reveal extrarenal spread to adnexa in females and testes in males
  - May detect intra-abdominal lymphadenopathy
  - **Early:** Normal kidney or small focal cortical lesions with poorly defined border ± calcification
  - **Progressive**
    - Papillary destruction with echogenic masses near calyces
    - Distorted renal parenchyma
    - Irregular hypoechoic masses connecting to collecting system; no renal pelvic dilatation
    - Mucosal thickening ± ureteric and bladder involvement
    - Small, fibrotic thick-walled bladder

DDx: Urinary Tract Tuberculosis

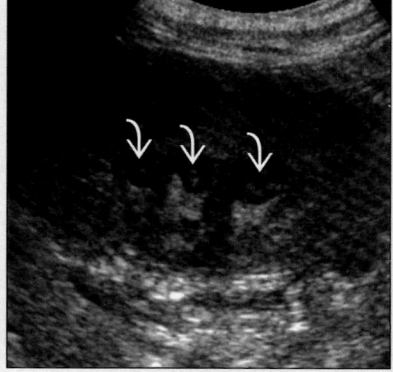

Papillary Necrosis

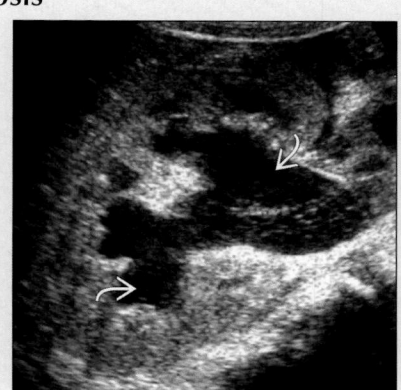

Pyonephrosis

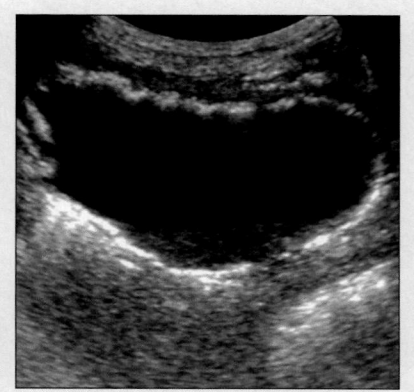

Emphysematous Cystitis

URINARY TRACT TUBERCULOSIS

Key Facts

Imaging Findings

- Best diagnostic clue: Calcification, cavities and strictures in urinary tract (UT)
- Appearance is non-specific and variable
- Useful to demonstrate non-excreting kidney on IVP
- Useful to reveal extrarenal spread to adnexa in females and testes in males
- May detect intra-abdominal lymphadenopathy
- **Early:** Normal kidney or small focal cortical lesions with poorly defined border ± calcification
- **Progressive**
- Papillary destruction with echogenic masses near calyces
- Distorted renal parenchyma
- Irregular hypoechoic masses connecting to collecting system; no renal pelvic dilatation

- Mucosal thickening ± ureteric and bladder involvement
- Small, fibrotic thick-walled bladder
- Echogenic foci or calcification (granulomas) in bladder wall near ureteric orifice
- Localized or generalized pyonephrosis
- **Late**
- Small, shrunken kidney, "paper-thin" cortex & dense dystrophic calcification in collecting system
- May resemble chronic renal disease
- US unable to evaluate renal function

Top Differential Diagnoses

- Papillary Necrosis
- Pyonephrosis
- Xanthogranulomatous Pyelonephritis (XGP)

- Echogenic foci or calcification (granulomas) in bladder wall near ureteric orifice
- Localized or generalized pyonephrosis
- **Late**
  - Small, shrunken kidney, "paper-thin" cortex & dense dystrophic calcification in collecting system
  - May resemble chronic renal disease
- Less sensitive than CT in detection of
  - Calyceal, pelvic or ureteral abnormalities
  - Isoechoic parenchymal masses
  - Small calcifications
  - Small cavities that communicate with collecting system
- US unable to evaluate renal function

Radiographic Findings

- IVP
  - Early: Irregular caliceal contour
  - Progressive
    - Irregular tract formation from calyx to papilla
    - Large irregular cavities with extensive destruction due to papillary necrosis
    - Hydrocalices or "phantom calyx" proximal to infundibular stricture
    - "Moth-eaten" calices
    - Atrophic "hiked-up" renal pelvis with no dilatation
    - Delayed excretion
    - Fibrosis and stricture of renal pelvis or ureter ⇒ beaded ureter, focal calcification or hydronephrosis
    - Small volume bladder
  - Late
    - Heavily calcified caseous mass surrounded by thin parenchymal shell ⇒ "putty kidney"
    - Small, shrunken, scarred, nonfunctioning kidney & dystrophic calcification (autonephrectomy)

CT Findings

- CECT
  - Renal parenchymal masses, cavities and scarring
  - "Moth-eaten" calices
  - Amputated infundibulum due to stricture

- Hydrocalycosis, hydronephrosis or hydroureter due to stricture
- UT calcifications
- UT wall thickening
- Small, poorly or non-enhanced kidney & calcification
- Pararenal and retroperitoneal spread
- Advanced disease: Better than IVP to delineate renal parenchymal masses, scarring, thick urinary tract walls & extra-urinary tubercular manifestations

Imaging Recommendations

- Best imaging tool
  - IVP: Detection of early calyceal changes
  - CT: Investigation of advanced urinary TB
  - Ultrasound: Monitoring of disease progress if iodinated contrast administration is contraindicated
- Protocol advice: IVP as primary investigation, followed-up by either US or CT to rule out obstructive uropathy

DIFFERENTIAL DIAGNOSIS

Papillary Necrosis

- Sonographically, necrotic papilla depicted as echogenic nonshadowing lesion surrounded by fluid in medulla

Pyonephrosis

- Dependent echoes within collecting system
- Shifting fluid-debris level
- Gas within collecting system
- Echoes throughout pelvicaliceal system

Xanthogranulomatous Pyelonephritis (XGP)

- Enlarged kidney with highly reflective central echocomplex containing calculus
- Both XGP and renal TB show thickening of perirenal fasciae and spread of inflammation into adjacent organs

URINARY TRACT TUBERCULOSIS

Cystitis
- US: Irregularly thickened bladder wall & reduced bladder volume
- Emphysematous cystitis: Highly reflective intramural gas in bladder wall

PATHOLOGY

General Features
- General path comments
  - Reactivation of dormant mycobacterium TB which spread into medulla causing papillitis
  - Necrotizing papillae sloughed into calyces can both infect and obstruct calyces, ureters and bladder
  - Ulceration of calyx gives typical ulcerocavernous lesion
  - Fibrosis causes obstructive strictures leading to hydronephrosis or pyonephrosis
  - Infundibular stricture may result in chronic renal abscesses
  - Healing results in fibrous tissue and calcium salts being deposited, producing calcified lesion
  - Diffuse renal involvement with parenchymal destruction and calcification
- Etiology
  - Infection by mycobacterium TB by hematogenous spread from pulmonary TB
  - Reactivation of prior blood-borne metastatic dormant tubercle bacilli
- Epidemiology
  - < 2% in developed countries
  - > 20% in developing countries
  - M:F = 2:1
- Associated abnormalities
  - Males: Prostatitis, epididymitis or orchitis
  - Females: Salpingitis, endometritis or oophoritis

Gross Pathologic & Surgical Features
- Small, irregular fibrocalcific kidney

Microscopic Features
- Cortical granulomas consist of Langerhans giant cells surrounded by lymphocytes and fibroblasts
- Papillary destruction extending into collecting system with extensive fibrosis
- Infundibular, pelvic and ureteric strictures
- Diffuse parenchymal destruction and calcification

CLINICAL ISSUES

Presentation
- Most common signs/symptoms
  - Asymptomatic common
  - Earliest symptom: Frequency
  - Recurrent UTI: Flank pain, dysuria, fever
  - Sterile pyuria; gross painless hematuria
- Other signs/symptoms
  - Malaise, anorexia, weight loss, night sweats, hypertension
  - Prostatic enlargement ± tenderness (male)

- Infertility, pelvic pain, or abnormal menstrual bleeding (female)

Demographics
- Age: Most cases occur in sexually active adults aged 20–69 years

Natural History & Prognosis
- Renal infection → obstructive uropathy → renal failure or extrarenal organ involvement
- Obstructive complication common leading to variable degree of renal functional losses
- Complications: Hydronephrosis, abscess formation, hypertension, extrarenal spread
- Low mortality but high morbidity
- High relapse rate in patients with poor nutritional status and social condition

Treatment
- Antituberculosis chemotherapy usually followed by surgical intervention after 8 weeks of therapy
- Surgical intervention
  - Percutaneous balloon stenting to correct strictures
  - Partial or total nephrectomy to remove large foci of infection in renal calcifications or for extensive renal damage
  - Cystectomy & substitution cystoplasty for extensive bladder damage

DIAGNOSTIC CHECKLIST

Consider
- TB if concurrent multiple abnormalities exist in UT
- Chest radiography to look for primary TB focus
- Biopsy of lesions, urinalysis & culture

Image Interpretation Pearls
- Abnormalities in multiple sites: Renal parenchymal mass/cavitation ± hydrocalices/hydronephrosis ± UT calcifications ± small and thick-walled bladder

SELECTED REFERENCES

1. Altintepe L et al: Urinary tuberculosis: ten years' experience. Ren Fail. 27(6):657-61, 2005
2. Muttarak M et al: Tuberculosis of the genitourinary tract: imaging features with pathological correlation. Singapore Med J. 46(10):568-74; quiz 575, 2005
3. Vijayaraghavan SB et al: Spectrum of high-resolution sonographic features of urinary tuberculosis. J Ultrasound Med. 23(5):585-94, 2004
4. Wang LJ et al: Imaging findings of urinary tuberculosis on excretory urography and computerized tomography. J Urol. 169(2):524-8, 2003
5. Wise GJ et al: Genitourinary manifestations of tuberculosis. Urol Clin North Am. 30(1):111-21, 2003
6. Izbudak-Oznur I et al: Renal tuberculosis mimicking xanthogranulomatous pyelonephritis: ultrasonography, computed tomography and magnetic resonance imaging findings. Turk J Pediatr. 44(2):168-71, 2002
7. Wang LJ et al: CT features of genitourinary tuberculosis. J Comput Assist Tomogr. 21(2):254-8, 1997
8. Premkumar A et al: CT and sonography of advanced urinary tract tuberculosis. AJR Am J Roentgenol. 148(1):65-9, 1987

IMAGE GALLERY

Typical

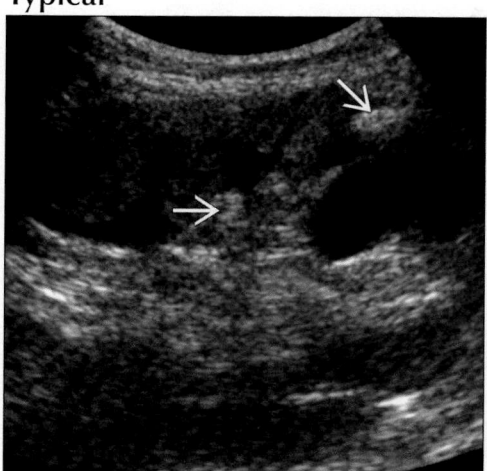 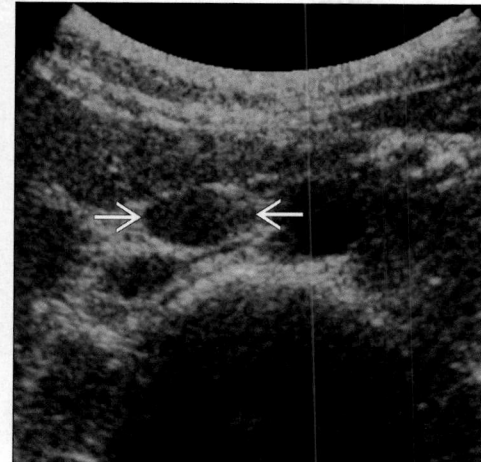

(Left) Longitudinal transabdominal ultrasound shows renal TB with papillary involvement. Echogenic nonshadowing lesions ➡ surrounded by fluid in renal medulla suggest papillary necrosis. (Right) Transverse transabdominal ultrasound shows an enlarged, para-aortic lymph node ➡ in a patient with renal TB. Associated lymphadenopathy is common and may be either reactive or infective.

Typical

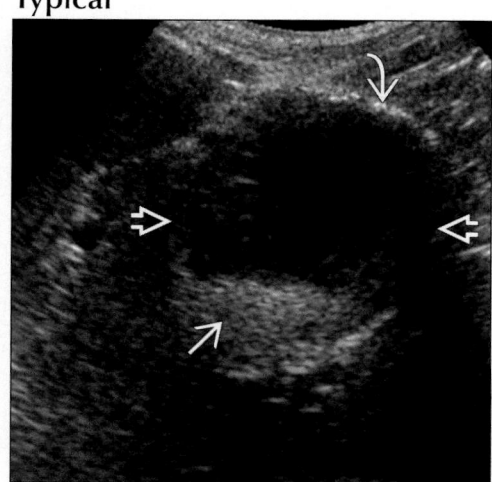 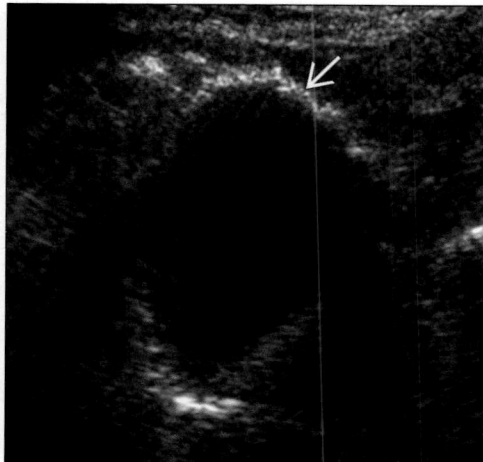

(Left) Transverse transabdominal ultrasound shows a renal TB abscess ➡, with internal debris ➡ and a calcified wall ➡. Abscess formation is secondary to stricture at the calyceal stem. (Right) Transverse transabdominal ultrasound shows a previous abscess with a calcified wall ➡. However, a gas-producing abscess with gas bubbles rising to the anterior wall may produce a similar appearance.

Typical

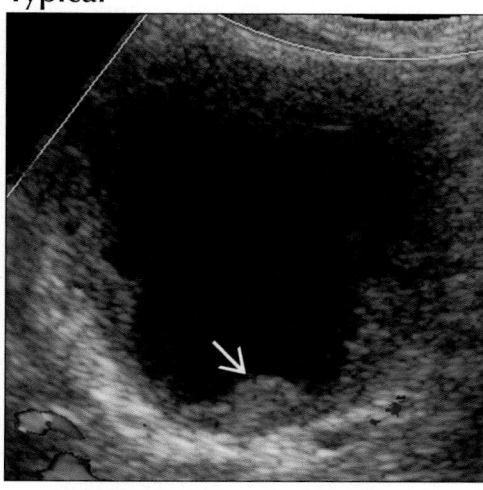 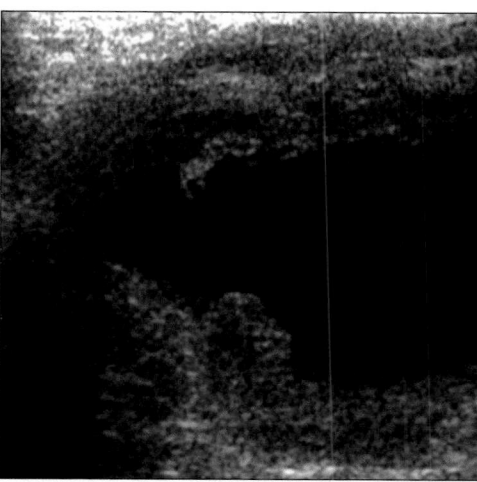

(Left) Longitudinal transabdominal ultrasound shows a urinary bladder infected by TB. There is irregular mucosal thickening near the ureteric orifice ➡, which is the earliest site for onset of disease. (Right) Transverse transabdominal ultrasound shows TB of the bladder with an irregularly thickened bladder wall. Its appearance may be indistinguishable from other forms of bacterial cystitis.

RENAL CELL CARCINOMA

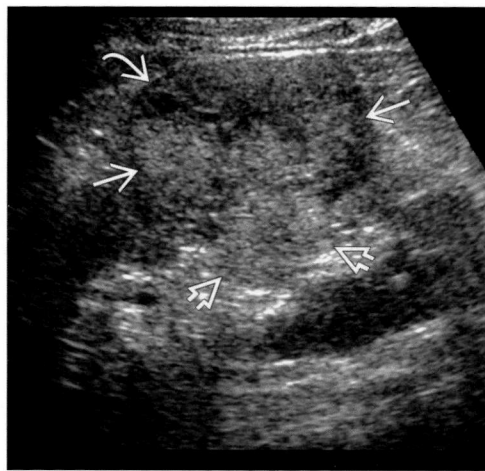

Longitudinal transabdominal ultrasound shows exophytic RCC ➡ with mixed echogenicity. Note that the tumor disrupts central sinus echoes ⏩ and has a hypoechoic "pseudocapsule" ↝.

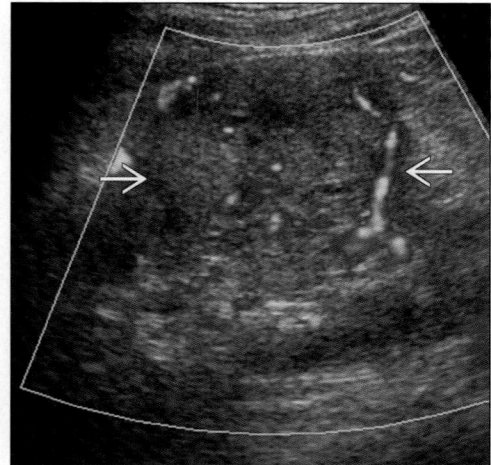

Corresponding longitudinal power Doppler ultrasound shows RCC ➡ with rich internal vascularity. RCC is typically hypervascular unlike renal metastasis, lymphoma, or transitional cell carcinoma (TCC).

TERMINOLOGY

Abbreviations and Synonyms
- Renal cell carcinoma (RCC)
- Hypernephroma, renal carcinoma

Definitions
- Malignant renal tumor arises from tubular epithelium
- Most common primary renal malignancy
- Most RCC are sporadic but can be hereditary (~ 4%)
- Papillary RCC is slow-growing, less aggressive than non-papillary RCC
- Different manifestations of RCC
  - Bilateral synchronous multifocal tumors
  - Small RCC with synchronous adrenal metastasis
  - RCC associated with large abdominal lymphoma
  - Multiseptated cystic mass
  - Occult RCC with paraaortic lymphadenopathy
  - RCC causing arteriovenous fistula (AVF)
  - RCC simulating angiomyolipoma (AML)
  - RCC with renal vein (RV) or inferior vena cava (IVC) thrombosis

IMAGING FINDINGS

General Features
- Best diagnostic clue
  - Hypervascular cortical renal mass
  - Presence of fat within tumor excludes RCC
- Location
  - 2% of sporadic RCC are bilateral and 16-25% of sporadic RCC are multicentric in same kidney
  - Renal cortex (most common)
- Morphology: Usually solid mass; variants are cystic
- Other general features
  - 25-40% found incidentally on abdominal CT or US

Ultrasonographic Findings
- Grayscale Ultrasound
  - Variable appearance: Solid, cystic or complex
  - Hyperechoic (48%), isoechoic (42%), or hypoechoic (10%)
  - Most common appearance: Hyperechoic and vascular
  - Small tumors are usually hyperechoic; simulate AML
  - Large tumors tend to be hypoechoic, exophytic with anechoic necrotic areas

DDx: Mimickers of RCC

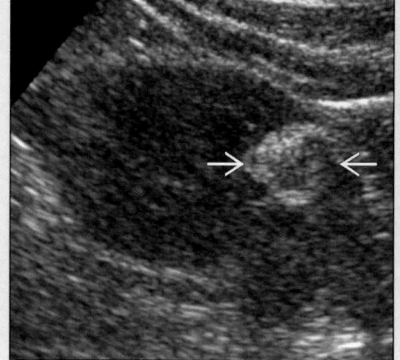

Angiomyolipoma

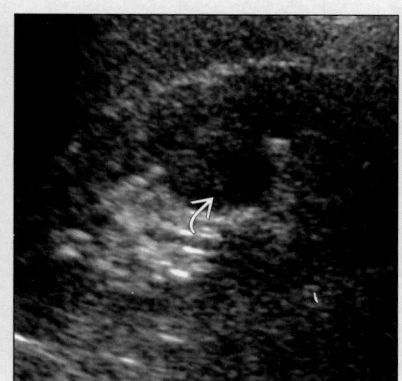

Column of Bertin

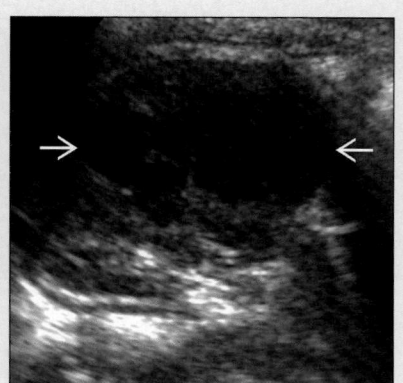

Renal Abscess

RENAL CELL CARCINOMA

Key Facts

Imaging Findings
- Variable appearance: Solid, cystic or complex
- Hyperechoic (48%), isoechoic (42%), or hypoechoic (10%)
- Most common appearance: Hyperechoic and vascular
- Small tumors are usually hyperechoic; simulate AML
- Large tumors tend to be hypoechoic, exophytic with anechoic necrotic areas
- Hypoechoic rim resembling "pseudocapsule"
- Papillary RCC: Unilocular, often hypoechoic; calcification common (30%)
- Cystic RCC: Unilocular; hypoechoic mass with fluid-debris levels (hemorrhage and necrosis) + thick and irregular wall
- Cystic RCC: Multilocular; multiple thick septations with nodules ± calcification

- Calcifications may be detected (6-20%)
- Discernible tumor vascularity; most prominent around tumor periphery
- RV thrombosis (23%) and IVC tumor extension (7%)
- May show high velocity signal from AVF
- US ideal for screening RCC and surveillance of tumor recurrence after nephrectomy

Top Differential Diagnoses
- Renal Angiomyolipoma
- Column of Bertin
- Renal Abscess

Diagnostic Checklist
- Rule out RCC in all solid renal lesions
- Hyperechoic renal lesions with calcifications and hypoechoic rim ⇒ RCC

- Hypoechoic rim resembling "pseudocapsule"
- Papillary RCC: Unilocular, often hypoechoic; calcification common (30%)
  - Intracapsular (85%)
- Cystic RCC: Rare (< 5%); unilocular or multilocular
  - Cystic RCC: Unilocular; hypoechoic mass with fluid-debris levels (hemorrhage and necrosis) + thick and irregular wall
  - Cystic RCC: Multilocular; multiple thick septations with nodules ± calcification
- Calcifications may be detected (6-20%)
- Detect 85% of mass > 3 cm, ≤ 60% < 2 cm
- Nodal ± organ metastases may be present
- Color Doppler
  - Discernible tumor vascularity; most prominent around tumor periphery
  - Vascularity: RCC < renal parenchyma
  - RV thrombosis (23%) and IVC tumor extension (7%)
  - May show high velocity signal from AVF

CT Findings
- NECT
  - Hyperdense, isodense or hypodense mass compared to normal renal tissue
  - Heterogeneous mass (hemorrhage and necrosis)
  - Alteration of renal contour
  - ± Calcifications (10% of cases); amorphous
  - Intratumoral fat density is rare
  - Cystic RCC
    - Uni- or multilocular cystic mass with thick wall
    - Calcification of septa or tumor capsule
- CECT
  - Enhancement: RCC < normal renal tissue
  - Small (≤ 3 cm), hypervascular mass better seen on nephrographic phase
  - Heterogeneous enhancement ⇒ hemorrhage and necrosis
  - Lucent rim (pseudocapsule); ± infiltration of collecting system
  - Subcapsular ± perinephric hemorrhage (hyperdense)
  - Direct extension to adjacent muscles & viscera
  - Nodal metastases (≥ 1 cm) and organ metastases (often hypervascular)

- Cystic RCC: Enhancing, smooth or nodular septa

MR Findings
- Isointense (60%) on T1 & T2WI or hyperintense (40%) on T2WI
- Hypointense band/rim on T1WI (25%) & T2WI (60%)
- T1 C+: Enhances, usually less than renal tissue
- Multiplanar ideal for renal venous & IVC extension

Imaging Recommendations
- Best imaging tool
  - US ideal for screening RCC and surveillance of tumor recurrence after nephrectomy
  - Multiphase CT is best for diagnosis and staging
  - MR: Staging is equal or better than CT
- Protocol advice
  - Equivocal renal mass on ultrasound evaluated by CECT
  - CT angiography & 3D mapping for tumor staging

DIFFERENTIAL DIAGNOSIS

Renal Angiomyolipoma
- Tumor mixed with vessels, muscle and fat
- Classical appearance: Homogeneous, well-defined, echogenic cortical mass
- Exceedingly rare to have calcification
- Distinguishable features from RCC: Fat-containing and absence of calcification

Column of Bertin
- Renal cortical tissue protruding into renal sinus
- Isoechoic; located in mid 1/3 of kidney
- May contain pyramids

Renal Abscess
- Secondary to pyelonephritis or renal infection
- Renal enlargement with complex cystic mass
- Differentiated by clinical history and urinalysis

Complex Renal Cyst
- Septated cyst ± calcification ± nodularity ± thick wall

RENAL CELL CARCINOMA

Renal Metastases & Lymphoma
- Metastases: Usually hypovascular; infiltrative
- Lymphoma
  - Usually multiple or bilateral; hypovascular
  - Focal, hypoechoic lymphoma indistinct from RCC
  - Biopsy warranted for diagnosis

Renal Oncocytoma
- Renal adenoma with large epithelial cells
- Overlapping sonographic features with RCC
- CT: Characteristic stellate central scar

Transitional Cell Carcinoma (TCC)
- Infiltrative tumor involving renal parenchyma indistinct from RCC
- Renal pelvic filling defect, irregular narrowing of collecting system
- Usually hypovascular

PATHOLOGY

General Features
- Etiology
  - Risk factors
    - Advanced age
    - Genetics: Von Hippel-Lindau (VHL) disease
    - Environmental: Smoking, long-term dialysis
    - Chemical: Diethylstilbestrol, fluoroacetamide, dimethylnitrosamine, lead, cadmium
- Epidemiology
  - Accounts for 2% of all cancers
  - 24-45% VHL patients develop RCC which are mostly bilateral and multifocal

Gross Pathologic & Surgical Features
- Completely solid to cystic mass with irregular lobulated margins
- Heterogeneous appearance with hemorrhage and necrosis (cut section)

Microscopic Features
- Clear cell (70%), papillary (10-15%), granular cell (7%), chromophobe cell (5%), sarcomatoid (1.5%), collecting duct (< 1%)
- Cell type: Clear cell or glanular cytoplasm
- Cellular organization: Papillary, tubular or medullary

Staging, Grading or Classification Criteria
- Robson classification of RCC with TNM correlation
  - Stage I: Tumor confined to kidney
  - Stage II: Invasion of perinephric fat
  - Stage IIIA: Tumor spread to renal vein and/or inferior vena cava
  - Stage IIIB: Regional lymph node metastasis
  - Stage IIIC: Venous and nodal involvement
  - Stage IVA: Invasion of adjacent organs (except ipsilateral adrenal gland)
  - Stage IVB: Distant metastases

CLINICAL ISSUES

Presentation
- Most common signs/symptoms
  - Gross hematuria (60%), flank pain (40%), palpable flank mass (30-40%), (classical triad < 10%)
  - Fever, anorexia, weight loss, malaise, nausea, vomiting, constipation
- Other signs/symptoms
  - Hypertension, hepatopathy, and hypercalcemia
  - Distant metastases may cause symptoms of cough, hemoptysis, bone pain

Demographics
- Age: 50-70 years of age
- Gender: M:F = 2:1

Natural History & Prognosis
- Prognosis
  - 5, 10 year survival rate
    - Stage I: 67%, 56%
    - Stage II: 51%, 28%
    - Stage III: 33.5%, 20%
    - Stage IV: 13.5%, 3%
  - Bilateral or multiple RCC have poorer survival rate; solitary RCC or metastasis has better survival rate
  - Tumor recurrence after nephrectomy: 20-30% in 15-18 months

Treatment
- Radical nephrectomy is the standard treatment
- Partial nephrectomy is a common alternative
  - Requires ≤ 5 cm tumor size, peripheral location, exophytic extension and no invasion of vessels or lymph nodes
- Chemotherapy and radiotherapy: Ineffective
- Immunotherapy: 15% complete/partial response

DIAGNOSTIC CHECKLIST

Consider
- Rule out RCC in all solid renal lesions
- Hyperechoic renal lesions with calcifications and hypoechoic rim ⇒ RCC
- Complex cystic masses with thick septa, calcifications, irregular wall or mural nodules ⇒ RCC

Image Interpretation Pearls
- Renal lesions with internal vascularity highly suggestive of malignancy

SELECTED REFERENCES

1. Prando A et al: Renal cell carcinoma: unusual imaging manifestations. Radiographics. 26(1):233-44, 2006
2. Catalano C et al: High-resolution multidetector CT in the preoperative evaluation of patients with renal cell carcinoma. AJR Am J Roentgenol. 180(5):1271-7, 2003
3. Herts BR et al: Triphasic helical CT of the kidneys: contribution of vascular phase scanning in patients before urologic surgery. AJR. 173:1273-7, 1999
4. Motzer RJ et al: Renal-cell carcinoma. N Engl J Med. 335(12):865-75, 1996

RENAL METASTASES

Key Facts

Imaging Findings
- Usually small and round, occasionally wedge-shaped mimicking infarction
- Usually intraparenchymal; rarely disrupts renal contour or capsule
- May be isoechoic, hypoechoic or hyperechoic
- Majority are hypoechoic
- Perinephric hemorrhage may be seen in melanoma
- Insensitive to detect small metastatic lesions
- Mostly avascular or hypovascular
- Melanoma metastasis: Hypervascular; may stimulate renal cell carcinoma (RCC)

Top Differential Diagnoses
- Primary Renal Neoplasm
- Renal Angiomyolipoma
- Renal Cysts

- Transitional cell carcinoma: Infiltrative into renal cortex + irregular narrowing of collecting system

Renal Angiomyolipoma
- Majority are echogenic due to intratumoral fat content

Renal Cysts
- Simple, hemorrhagic, septated or calcified; may simulate renal pyramids

Renal Infarction
- Avascular, wedged-shaped renal lesion

Renal Infection
- Nephritis or phlegmon simulating metastasis

PATHOLOGY

General Features
- Etiology: Dissemination of advanced primary malignancy; hematogenous > direct spread
- Epidemiology
  - Autopsy: Renal metastasis > renal primaries
  - 7-13 % in large autopsy studies

Microscopic Features
- Renal metastases: Varies based on primary cancer

CLINICAL ISSUES

Presentation
- Most common signs/symptoms: Usually asymptomatic; may have hematuria or flank pain
- Diagnosis
  - CT or US-guided percutaneous biopsy

Natural History & Prognosis
- Silent with low clinical detection
- Complications: Perinephric hemorrhage
- Prognosis is very poor

Treatment
- Chemotherapy or palliative treatment
- Nephrectomy if metastasis is small and isolated

DIAGNOSTIC CHECKLIST

Consider
- Renal metastasis in presence of extrarenal primary cancer and widespread systemic metastasis
- Biopsy for suspected lesions

SELECTED REFERENCES

1. Rendon RA et al: The natural history of small renal masses. J Urol. 164(4):1143-7, 2000
2. Mitnick JS et al: Metastatic neoplasm to the kidney studied by computed tomography and sonography. J Comput Assist Tomogr. 9(1):43-9, 1985

IMAGE GALLERY

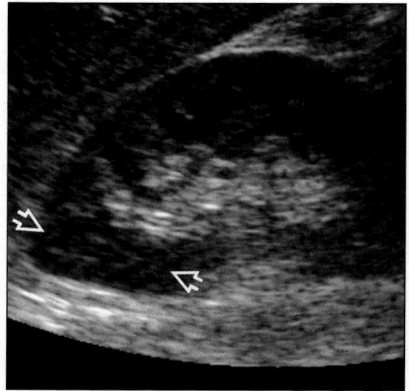 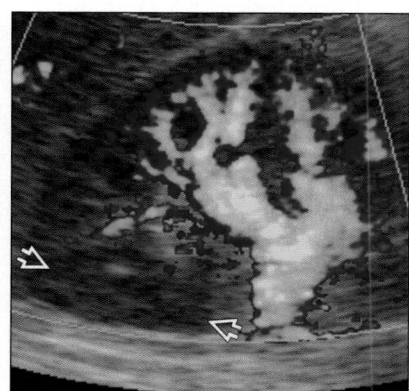 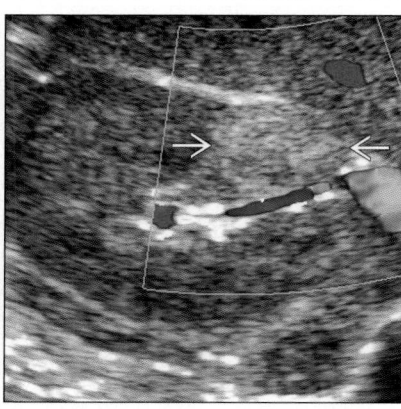

(Left) Longitudinal ultrasound shows isoechoic renal metastasis ➔ in patient with known lung carcinoma. Mass is ill-defined & easily overlooked on grayscale imaging. *(Center)* Power Doppler in same patient as left shows an avascular renal mass ➔, typical of renal metastases. Lymphoma, infarct & phlegmon may show a similar appearance. *(Right)* Color Doppler ultrasound shows an echogenic renal metastasis ➔ which is intraparenchymal & avascular with no disruption of the renal contour. Renal metastases are often small & remain undetected except at autopsy.

RENAL ANGIOMYOLIPOMA

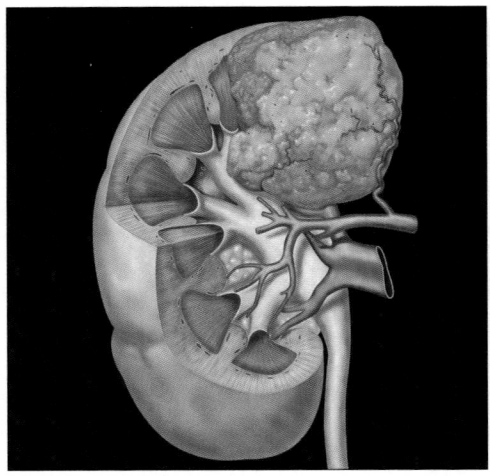

Graphic shows a vascular renal mass containing adipose and soft tissue components.

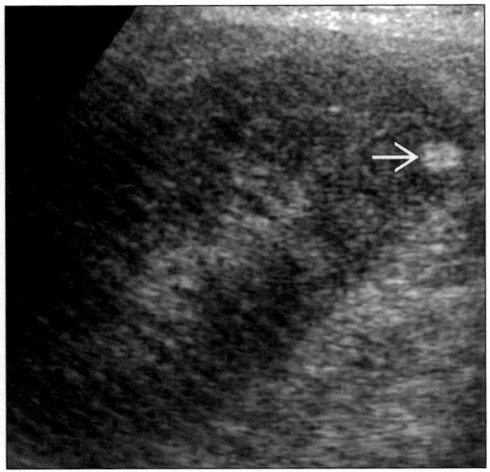

Longitudinal transabdominal ultrasound shows a typical small round AML in the renal cortex ➡.

TERMINOLOGY

Abbreviations and Synonyms
- Angiomyolipoma (AML), renal hamartoma or choristoma

Definitions
- Benign renal tumor composed of abnormal blood vessels, smooth muscle & fatty components in varying proportions

IMAGING FINDINGS

General Features
- Best diagnostic clue: Intrarenal fatty mass
- Location: Intrarenal (cortex) or exophytic in location
- Size
  - Varies in size
    - May range from few mm to 25 cm or more
- Morphology
  - Usually discrete, rarely diffuse, parenchymal mass
  - Bleeding into large AMLs > 4 cm is common
- Other general features
  - Most common benign renal tumor
  - 80% of cases are detected as incidental finding on imaging
  - Isolated: Usually solitary & unilateral; occasionally multiple & bilateral
  - If multiple & bilateral, usually associated with tuberous sclerosis (TS)
  - 80% of tuberous sclerosis have renal AMLs

Ultrasonographic Findings
- Grayscale Ultrasound
  - Fat-rich AMLs are characteristically hyperechoic
  - Tumor echogenicity similar to that of renal sinus
  - When small < 3 cm, appear as round, discrete, hyperechoic renal cortical lesions
  - When large, tumor outline may be lobulated
  - About 25% of AMLs are exophytic
  - Tumor echogenicity depends on its constituents
    - Fatty tissue
    - Smooth muscle
    - Blood vessels
  - May resemble small (< 3 cm) renal cell carcinoma (RCC)
    - 32% of small RCC are echogenic

DDx: Renal Angiomyolipoma

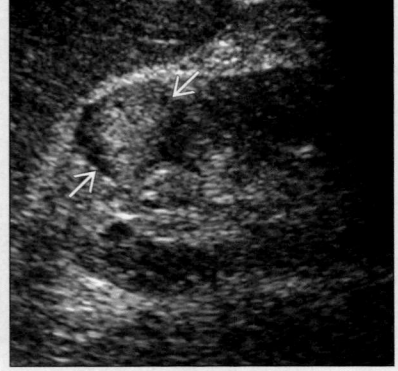

RCC

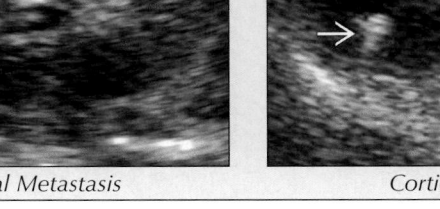

Renal Metastasis

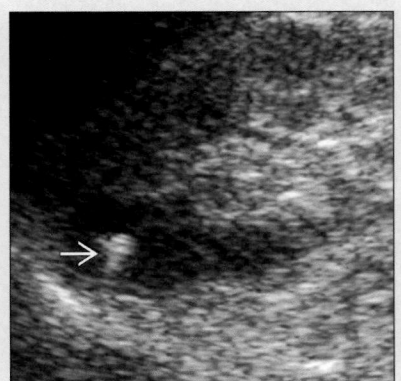

Cortical MCC

RENAL ANGIOMYOLIPOMA

Key Facts

Terminology
- Benign renal tumor composed of abnormal blood vessels, smooth muscle & fatty components in varying proportions

Imaging Findings
- Best diagnostic clue: Intrarenal fatty mass
- Fat-rich AMLs are characteristically hyperechoic
- May resemble small (< 3 cm) renal cell carcinoma (RCC)
- Intratumoral cystic areas: Potential pitfall for false negative results
- Fluid in perinephric space and retroperitoneum: Evidence of tumor rupture

Top Differential Diagnoses
- Renal Cell Carcinoma

- Renal Metastases and Lymphoma
- Cortical Milk of Calcium Cyst (MCC)

Clinical Issues
- Slow growing tumors with no malignant potential.
- Only AML associated with TS may undergo malignant transformation and warrant annual follow up with US or CT

Diagnostic Checklist
- Ultrasound is good for screening and monitoring of AML
- Well-circumscribed, discrete fatty renal mass
- Presence of posterior shadowing from renal lesion is more suggestive of AML than RCC

- Hypoechoic rim and intratumoral cysts rarely depicted in AML but common in RCC
- Calcification is rarely seen in AML but common in RCC
- Shadowing present in 1/3 of AMLs but none in RCC
  - Intratumoral cystic areas: Potential pitfall for false negative results
    - May represent hemorrhage, necrosis and dilated calyces
  - Fluid in perinephric space and retroperitoneum: Evidence of tumor rupture
- Color Doppler: Detects arteriovenous fistula or pseudoaneurysm in hemorrhagic AML, renal vein involvement and inferior vena cava extension

Radiographic Findings
- Radiography: Radiolucent mass: When lesion contains large amount of fat
- IVP
  - Small tumor: Well-defined radiolucent defect
  - Large tumor: Distortion of collecting system

CT Findings
- CTA: Aneurysmal renal vessels may be seen
- NECT
  - Well-marginated cortical heterogeneous tumor, predominantly of fat density (-30 to -100 HU)
  - Renal mass with fat is almost diagnostic of AML
  - When multiple AML seen, suspect TS
  - ~ 5% have no detectable fat on CT, such AML cannot be diagnosed by CT or other imaging modalities
  - Calcification rarely seen; if present suspect RCC
- CECT
  - Varied enhancement pattern based on amount of fat & vascular components
  - Benign satellite deposits may be seen in regional lymph nodes, liver & spleen
  - Extension of tumor into IVC is rare

MR Findings
- Varied signal intensity due to vessels, muscle & fat

- Tumor with increased fat content
  - T1WI: Hyperintense
  - Fat suppression sequences: Signal loss
- T1 C+
  - Tumor with increased fat content: Minimal enhancement
  - Tumor with high vascular component: Significant enhancement

Angiographic Findings
- Tumor with increased vascular component
  - Multisacculated pseudoaneurysms
  - Presence of arteriovenous shunts
  - "Sunburst" appearance of capillary nephrogram
  - "Onion peel" appearance of peripheral vessels in venous phase

Imaging Recommendations
- Best imaging tool
  - Ultrasound is ideal for screening and monitoring of AML
  - CT is useful for diagnosis

DIFFERENTIAL DIAGNOSIS

Renal Cell Carcinoma
- Rarely reported to contain fat (engulfed renal sinus fat)
- Calcification within tumor highly suggestive of RCC

Renal Metastases and Lymphoma
- Renal metastases
  - Occasionally, present as a large solitary mass, but devoid of fat
- Renal lymphoma
  - Primary very rare; secondary from generalized spread (more common)
  - Bilateral involvement is seen in 40-60% of cases

Renal Oncocytoma
- Rare benign renal tumor; rarely contains fat
- Well-defined homogeneous hypoechoic to isoechoic masses

RENAL ANGIOMYOLIPOMA

- Central scar cannot be confidently identified on ultrasound
- CT and Angiography: Typical spoke-wheel vascular pattern
- Diagnosis: Requires entire tumoral resection

Perirenal Liposarcoma
- Large exophytic AML may simulate retroperitoneal liposarcoma (both contain fat)
  - Renal parenchymal defect & enlarged vessels favor AML
  - Smooth compression of kidney & extension beyond perirenal space favor liposarcoma
- Diagnosis: Requires entire tumoral resection

Wilms Tumor
- Pediatric renal tumor that may contain fat

Deep Cortical Scar
- Echogenic line, may associated with hydrocalyx

Cortical Milk of Calcium Cyst (MCC)
- Echogenic focus within anechoic cyst, with ring-down artifact

PATHOLOGY

General Features
- Etiology
  - Benign mesenchymal tumor of kidney
  - Hamartoma: Benign tumor consisting of tissues that normally occur in organ of origin
  - Choristoma: Benign tumor composed of tissues not normally occurring within organ of origin
- Epidemiology
  - 0.3-3% in autopsy series
  - 80% isolated (sporadic) AML
  - 20% AML associated with TS
- Associated abnormalities: TS; lymphangiomyomatosis

Gross Pathologic & Surgical Features
- Round, lobulated, yellow-to-gray color secondary to fat content

Microscopic Features
- Variable amounts of angioid (vascular), myoid (smooth muscle), & lipoid (fatty) components

CLINICAL ISSUES

Presentation
- Most common signs/symptoms
  - Often asymptomatic, incidental finding or detected during screening of tuberous sclerosis for RCC
  - Hematuria, flank pain or palpable flank mass
  - Acute abdomen (spontaneous hemorrhage, rupture)
- Other signs/symptoms: Occasionally, hypertension & chronic renal failure
- Diagnosis: Imaging & biopsy

Demographics
- Age: Usually beyond 40 years old
- Gender

  - More common in females than males (M:F = 1:4)
  - AML associated with TS (M:F = 1:1)

Natural History & Prognosis
- Slow growing tumors with no malignant potential.
- Only AML associated with TS may undergo malignant transformation and warrant annual follow up with US or CT
- Complications: Hemorrhage and rupture
- Prognosis
  - Usually good: After partial or complete nephrectomy
  - Poor: With hemorrhage, rupture, no treatment

Treatment
- If asymptomatic, conservative treatment unless there are complications
- Tumor size < 4 cm: Conservative treatment with follow-up
- Tumor size > 4 cm: Partial nephrectomy often recommended
- Patients presenting with spontaneous bleeding treated with embolization initially
  - Surgery postponed until patient stabilizes

DIAGNOSTIC CHECKLIST

Consider
- Ultrasound is good for screening and monitoring of AML
- AML with minimal fat and with cystic component may result in false negatives
- Cortical scars and MCC may give false positive results

Image Interpretation Pearls
- Well-circumscribed, discrete fatty renal mass
- Presence of posterior shadowing from renal lesion is more suggestive of AML than RCC

SELECTED REFERENCES

1. Kim JK et al: Angiomyolipoma with minimal fat: differentiation from renal cell carcinoma at biphasic helical CT. Radiology. 230(3):677-84, 2004
2. Israel GM et al: CT differentiation of large exophytic renal angiomyolipomas and perirenal liposarcomas. AJR Am J Roentgenol. 179(3):769-73, 2002
3. Wilson SS et al: Angiomyolipoma with vena caval extension. Urology. 60(4):695-6, 2002
4. Yamakado K et al: Renal angiomyolipoma: relationships between tumor size, aneurysm formation, and rupture. Radiology. 225(1):78-82, 2002
5. Katz DS et al: Massive renal angiomyolipoma in tuberous sclerosis. Clin Imaging. 21(3):200-2, 1997
6. Lemaitre L et al: Imaging of angiomyolipomas. Semin Ultrasound CT MR. 18(2):100-14, 1997
7. Siegel CL et al: Angiomyolipoma and renal cell carcinoma: US differentiation. Radiology. 198(3):789-93, 1996
8. Forman HP et al: Hyperechoic renal cell carcinomas: increase in detection at US. Radiology. 188(2):431-4, 1993
9. Curry NS et al: Intratumoral fat in a renal oncocytoma mimicking angiomyolipoma. AJR Am J Roentgenol. 154(2):307-8, 1990
10. Bosniak MA et al: CT diagnosis of renal angiomyolipoma: the importance of detecting small amounts of fat. AJR Am J Roentgenol. 151(3):497-501, 1988

RENAL ANGIOMYOLIPOMA

IMAGE GALLERY

Variant

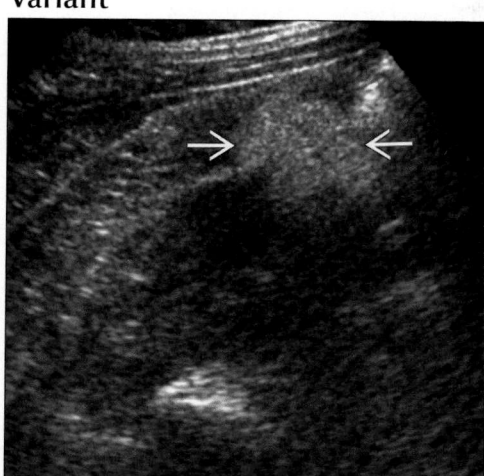
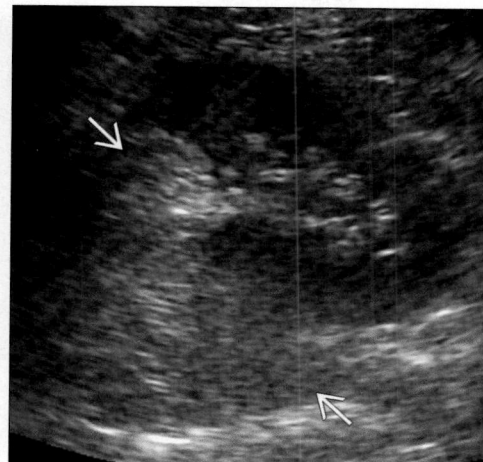

(Left) Longitudinal transabdominal ultrasound shows an exophytic AML with irregular outline ➡ arising from the lower pole of the kidney. *(Right)* Oblique transabdominal ultrasound shows a large exophytic echogenic tumor ➡ arising from the mid-upper pole left kidney and extending into the retroperitoneum.

Variant

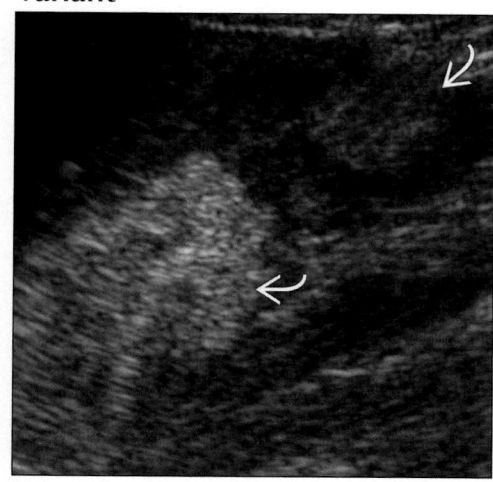
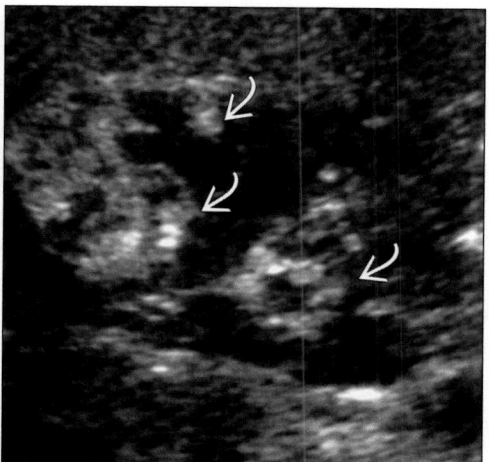

(Left) Longitudinal transabdominal ultrasound shows two medium sized AMLs ➡ with different echogenicity. The difference is probably due to a difference in fat content in the two lesions. *(Right)* Longitudinal transabdominal ultrasound shows multiple irregular echogenic AMLs of varying sizes ➡ in tuberous sclerosis. These have potential to turn malignant and require annual follow-up.

Variant

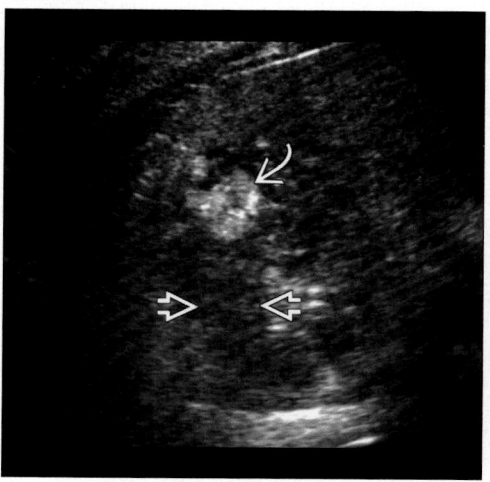
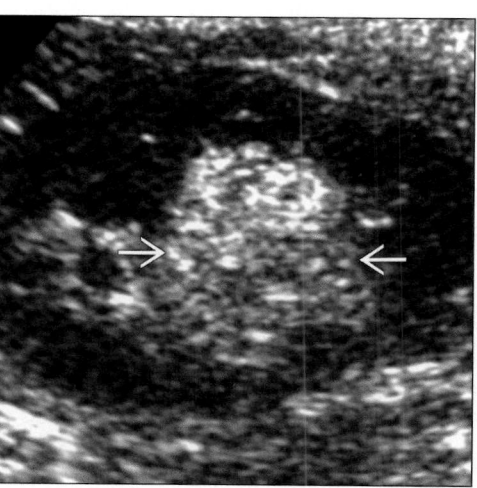

(Left) Transverse transabdominal ultrasound shows a small hyperechoic lesion ➡ in the lower pole of the kidney. Note the acoustic shadowing ➡ posterior to it suggestive of AML. *(Right)* Longitudinal transabdominal ultrasound depicts a large hyperechoic AML ➡ distorting renal sinus complex.

TRANSITIONAL CELL CARCINOMA

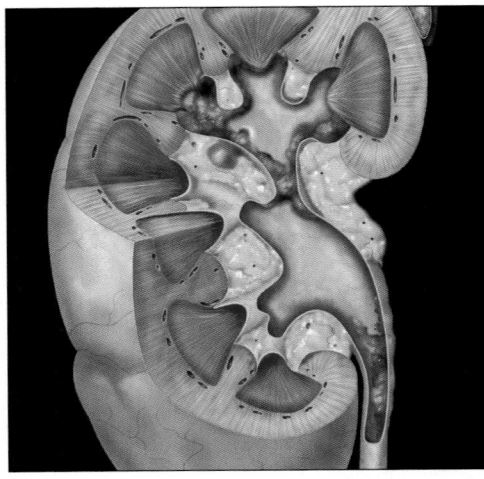

Graphic shows a multifocal TCC involving the upper pole calices and the proximal ureter. Hydronephrosis ± hydrocalices are commonly associated with upper tract TCC.

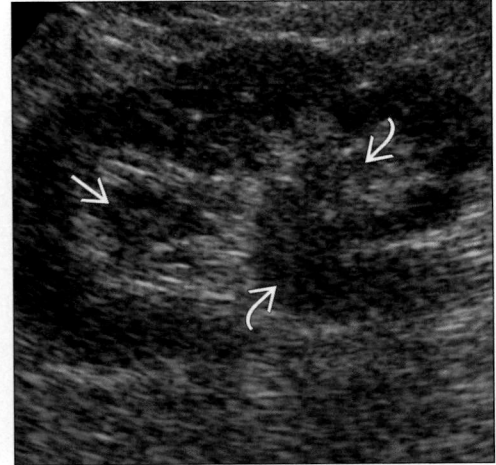

Longitudinal transabdominal ultrasound shows a hypoechoic TCC ➡ in the renal sinus filling the lower pole calices and the proximal ureter. Upper caliectasis may be due to a blood clot or synchronous TCC ➡.

TERMINOLOGY

Abbreviations and Synonyms
- Transitional cell carcinoma (TCC)

Definitions
- Often multiple and may involve any part of collecting system; 10% have bilateral metachronous or synchronous primary tumors
- Papillary: Exophytic polypoid masses; low grade; less aggressive; slow-growing
- Non-papillary: Nodular or flat tumors appearing as focal urothelial thickening; high grade; infiltrative

IMAGING FINDINGS

General Features
- Best diagnostic clue: Intraluminal mass or focal urothelial thickening in collecting system, ureter or bladder on imaging
- Location: Risk of TCC: Bladder (90%) > renal pelvis (8%) > ureter (2%)

Ultrasonographic Findings
- Grayscale Ultrasound
  - Renal pelvis
    - Small non-obstructing tumor hard to visualize
    - Small renal, ureteric and TCC in bladder diverticulum may be missed on ultrasound
    - Ultrasound (US) is useful in demonstration of obstructive uropathy
    - Renal TCC: Intraluminal hypoechoic mass or focal urothelial thickening
    - Renal TCC: Papillary tumor seen as discrete, solid, central hypoechoic renal sinus mass ± splitting of central echo complex ± proximal caliectasis
    - Renal TCC: Infiltrative tumor distorts renal architecture but preserves renal shape
    - Renal TCC: Focal hypoechogenicity of adjacent renal cortex reflects local invasion
    - Renal TCC rarely invades inferior vena cava (IVC)
    - Infiltrative tumor involving renal parenchyma: Indistinguishable from renal cell carcinoma (RCC), metastasis or lymphoma
    - High grade TCC: Densely echogenic; mimics calculus or fungus ball

DDx: Mimickers of TCC

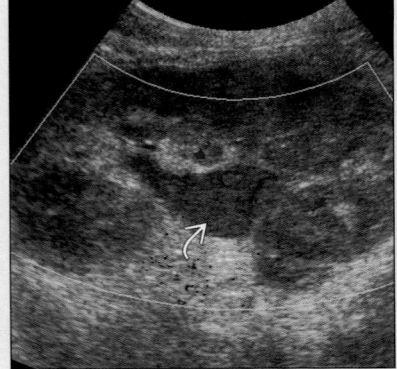
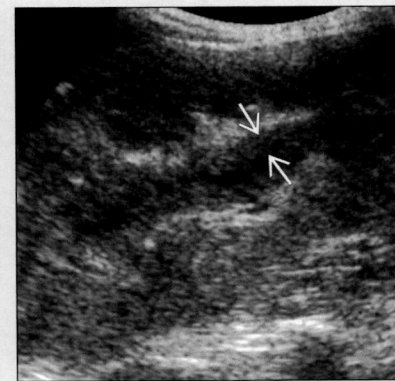
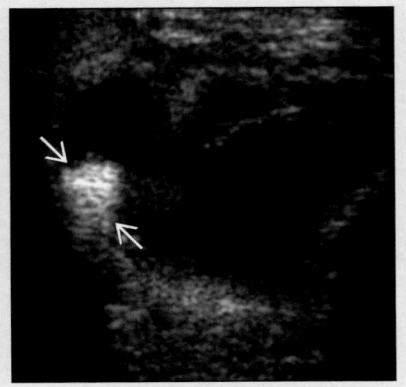

| Hemonephrosis | Urothelial Thickening | Fungus Ball |

TRANSITIONAL CELL CARCINOMA

Key Facts

Imaging Findings
- Small non-obstructing tumor hard to visualize
- Small renal, ureteric and TCC in bladder diverticulum may be missed on ultrasound
- Renal TCC: Intraluminal hypoechoic mass or focal urothelial thickening
- Renal TCC: Papillary tumor seen as discrete, solid, central hypoechoic renal sinus mass ± splitting of central echo complex ± proximal caliectasis
- Renal TCC: Infiltrative tumor distorts renal architecture but preserves renal shape
- Renal TCC: Focal hypoechogenicity of adjacent renal cortex reflects local invasion
- Renal TCC rarely invades inferior vena cava (IVC)

- Infiltrative tumor involving renal parenchyma: Indistinguishable from renal cell carcinoma (RCC), metastasis or lymphoma
- High grade TCC: Densely echogenic; mimics calculus or fungus ball
- Bladder TCC: Majority are fixed, polypoid masses arising along bladder wall
- Detection of internal vascularity excludes blood clot, fungus ball, pus, echolucent calculi
- Doppler is useful to document IVC patency in infiltrative TCC

Top Differential Diagnoses
- Blood Clot or Hemonephrosis
- Urothelial Thickening
- Fungus Ball

- Increased TCC echogenicity is due to squamous metaplasia with formation of keratin pearls: Very echogenic but not shadowing
  - Ureter
    - Hydronephrosis ± hydroureter
    - Solid ureteral mass occasionally depicted
  - Bladder
    - Bladder TCC: Majority are fixed, polypoid masses arising along bladder wall
    - Infiltrative tumors with diffuse or localized wall thickening are less common
    - Punctate calcification in tumor may be depicted
    - Ultrasound is sensitive to detect tumor arising from bladder diverticulum, which is inaccessible by cystoscopy
- Color Doppler
  - Detection of internal vascularity excludes blood clot, fungus ball, pus, echolucent calculi
  - No tumor vascularity does not exclude TCC
  - Doppler is useful to document IVC patency in infiltrative TCC

Radiographic Findings
- IVP
  - Single or multiple discrete filling defects; surface is usually irregular, stippled, serrated or frond-like
  - Renal pelvis
    - "Stipple sign": Contrast within interstices of tumor
    - "Oncocalyx": Ballooned tumor-filled calyx
    - "Phantom calyx": Unopacified calyx from obstruction of calyceal infundibulum
  - Ureter
    - Normal or delayed excretion (partial obstruction) ± hydroureter
    - Irregularly narrowed lumen + non-tapering margins
  - Bladder
    - Irregular filling defect with broad base and frond-like projections
- Retrograde pyelography
  - Renal pelvis
    - Pyelotumoral backflow: Contrast in interstices

- Opacification of phantom calyces; irregular papillary or nodular mucosa
  - Ureter
    - Champagne glass sign: Cup-shaped contrast collection distal to intraluminal filling defect

CT Findings
- CT urography: Detect UT tumors and calculi; assess perirenal tissues; enable staging of TCC
- CECT: Hypovascular infiltrative tumor with minimal enhancement (43-82 HU); preserved renal shape
- Renal pelvis
  - Sessile, flat or polypoid solid mass ± hydronephrosis ± calcification
  - Compression or invasion of renal sinus fat and parenchyma
  - Crust-like rims: Contrast in curvilinear calyceal spaces around periphery of the tumor
- Ureter
  - Eccentric or circumferential wall thickening ± hydronephrosis
- Bladder
  - Focal wall thickening and mass protruding into lumen; ± enhancement

MR Findings
- Comparable to CT for evaluation of perivesical fat involvement
- Better than CT in detection of adjacent organ invasion
- Renal pelvis and ureter
  - T2WI: Same or slightly ↑ versus normal parenchyma
  - T1 C+: ↓ or ↑ Enhancement
- Bladder: MR is staging modality of choice
  - T2WI: Hyperintense to normal bladder wall; ± perivesical invasion
  - T1 C+: Mild enhancement (primary, perivesical, nodal or bone invasion)

Imaging Recommendations
- Best imaging tool
  - Ultrasound and IVP: Renal TCC
  - Cystoscopy: Bladder TCC

TRANSITIONAL CELL CARCINOMA

○ Retrograde pyelography and/or CT urography: Renal or ureter TCC
○ CT and MR: For staging
• Protocol advice
○ Vigilant monitoring for metachronous lesions and recurrence by imaging
○ Annual imaging for 2 years after initial diagnosis or treatment of TCC

DIFFERENTIAL DIAGNOSIS

Blood Clot or Hemonephrosis
• Has same echogenicity as tumors; mobile, avascular and resolves over time

Urothelial Thickening
• Occurs in renal transplant rejection, UT infection, reflux, chronic obstruction, malignancies such as lymphoma, metastasis

Fungus Ball
• Echogenic, avascular, non-shadowing masses within calyces
• Associated with disseminated fungal infection

Pus or Pyonephrosis
• Has echogenic debris within calyces

Calculus
• Echogenic foci with or without posterior shadowing

Sloughed Papilla or Prominent Papilla
• Destruction of the apex of the pyramid → irregular cavitation and sinus formation between papilla and calyx
• In hydronephrosis, prominent papillae appear as filling defects in the calices

Renal Cell Carcinoma (RCC)
• May be infiltrative extending into renal pelvis
• Indistinguishable from infiltrative TCC

PATHOLOGY

General Features
• General path comments
○ Uroepithelial cancers
  ■ TCC: 90% of renal pelvic and 97% of ureteral Ca
○ Synchronous or metachronous (multicentricity)
• Etiology: Smoking (≥ 3-fold); occupational exposure; abuse of analgesics; immunosuppressive therapy; Balkan nephritis; recurrent or chronic UT infection
• Epidemiology: TCC ~ 90% of all urothelial tumors

Gross Pathologic & Surgical Features
• ≥ 85% papillary (low grade); ± infiltrative (high grade)

Microscopic Features
• Transitional epithelium
• Epithelial atypia or dysplasia; abnormal fibrovascular core of lamina propria

Staging, Grading or Classification Criteria
• Carcinoma in situ (pTis)

• Non-invasive papillary TCC (pTa)
• Minimally invasive TCC (pT1)
• Muscle invasive tumors (pT2 -pT4)
• N1-3: Pelvic nodes; N4: Above iliac bifurcation
• M1 distant metastases

CLINICAL ISSUES

Presentation
• Most common signs/symptoms: Gross hematuria (70-80%); dull or colicky pain (50%)

Demographics
• Age: > 60 years of age (M:F = 4:1)

Natural History & Prognosis
• Renal pelvis and ureter: 5 year survival rate
○ ≤ T1 (77-80%); T2 (44%); ≥T3 (0-20%)
• Bladder: Overall 5 year survival rate is 30%

Treatment
• Renal pelvis and ureter
○ Total nephroureterectomy and bladder cuff excision
○ Metastases: Chemotherapy ± radiation
• Bladder
○ Superficial: Transurethral resection + bacillus Calmette-Guérin
○ Deep: Partial/radical cystectomy (with "neobladder" or ileal conduit) or radiation ± chemotherapy
○ Metastases: Surgery or radiation ± chemotherapy

DIAGNOSTIC CHECKLIST

Consider
• Synchronous or metachronous TCC
• Cystoscopy still necessary to diagnose bladder cancer

Image Interpretation Pearls
• Intraluminal mass in UT with vascularity

SELECTED REFERENCES

1. Browne RF et al: Transitional cell carcinoma of the upper urinary tract: spectrum of imaging findings. Radiographics. 25(6):1609-27, 2005
2. Akbar SA et al: Multidetector CT urography: techniques, clinical applications, and pitfalls. Semin Ultrasound CT MR. 25(1):41-54, 2004
3. Yossepowitch O et al: Transitional cell carcinoma of the bladder in young adults: presentation, natural history and outcome. J Urol. 168(1):61-6, 2002
4. Dibb MJ et al: Ultrasonographic analysis of bladder tumors. Clin Imaging. 25(6):416-20, 2001
5. Szopinski K et al: Magnetic resonance urography: initial experience of a low-dose Gd-DTPA-enhanced technique. Eur Radiol. 10(7):1158-64, 2000
6. Wong-You-Cheong JJ et al: Transitional cell carcinoma of the urinary tract: radiologic-pathologic correlation. Radiographics. 18:123-42, 1998
7. Oba K et al: Transitional cell carcinoma of the renal pelvis with vena caval tumor thrombus. Int J Urol. 4(3):307-10, 1997
8. Nicolet V et al: Thickening of the renal collecting system: a nonspecific finding at US. Radiology. 168(2):411-3, 1988

Typical

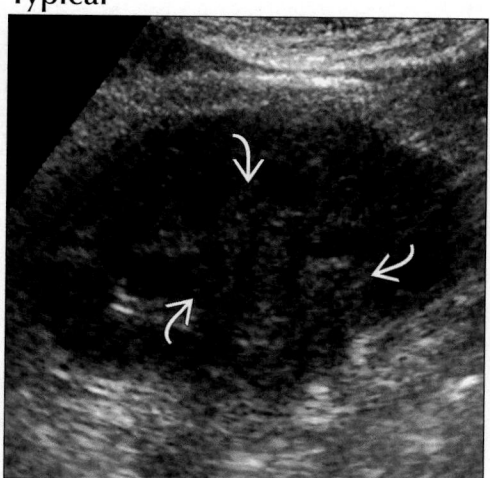 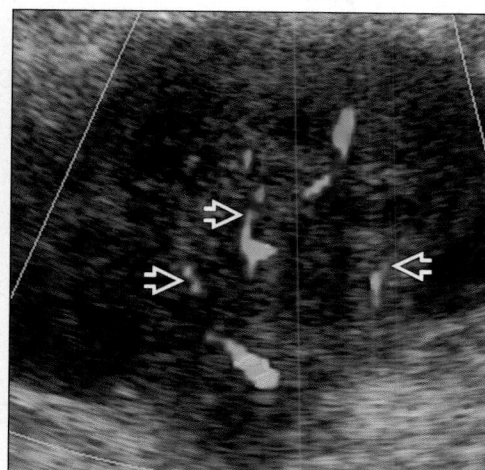

(Left) Longitudinal transabdominal ultrasound shows a hypoechoic renal sinus TCC ➡, with associated caliectasis. Note blood clots and pus may show a similar appearance. *(Right)* Longitudinal color Doppler ultrasound shows the same TCC as in the previous image with vascularity ➡. Detection of internal vascularity rules out clots and pus but avascularity does not exclude tumor.

Typical

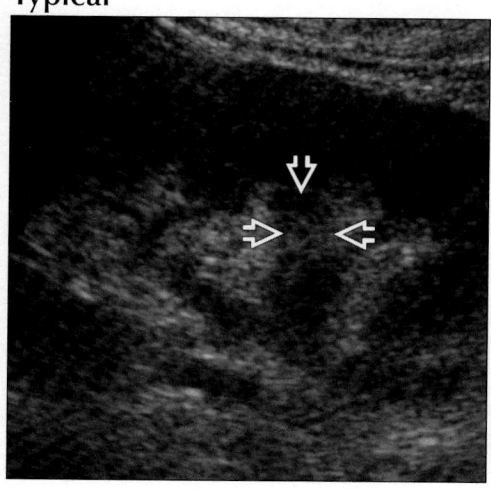 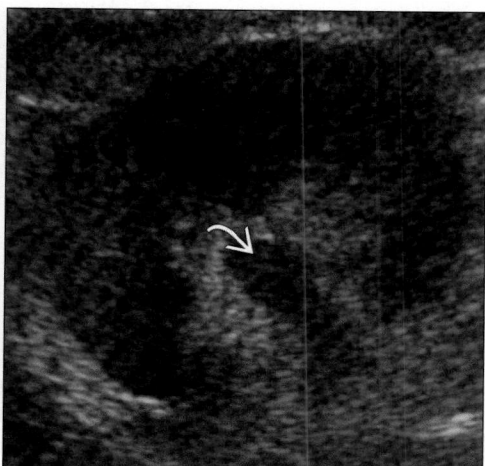

(Left) Longitudinal transabdominal ultrasound shows a small papillary TCC ➡ in the mid-pole of the kidney with mild hydrocalices, confirmed by CT. Ultrasound is insensitive in detecting small TCC. *(Right)* Transverse transabdominal ultrasound shows the previous TCC ➡ within the collecting system. Depiction of a small TCC is difficult and it can be mistaken for debris, urothelial thickening or clot.

Typical

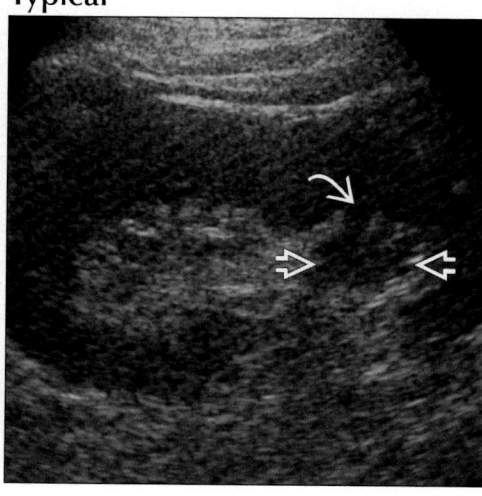 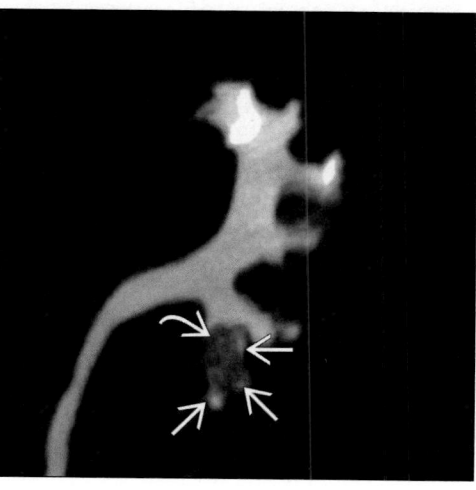

(Left) Longitudinal transabdominal ultrasound shows a small hypoechoic mass ➡ in the lower pole extending into adjacent renal parenchyma ➡. Features are typical of infiltrative TCC. *(Right)* CT urography of the same patient shows an irregular filling defect ➡ within the lower pole calices. Contrast is noted in the curvilinear calyceal spaces (crust-like rims) ➡ around the periphery of tumor.

Typical

(Left) Longitudinal transabdominal ultrasound shows an infiltrative TCC ➡ in the upper pole of kidney. Note that the tumor destroys upper calyces ➡ and infiltrates into the posterior renal cortex ➡. **(Right)** Longitudinal color Doppler ultrasound shows a TCC ➡ in the same patient as previous image with scarce rim vascularity ➡. Tumor vascularity is the only diagnostic sign for malignancy.

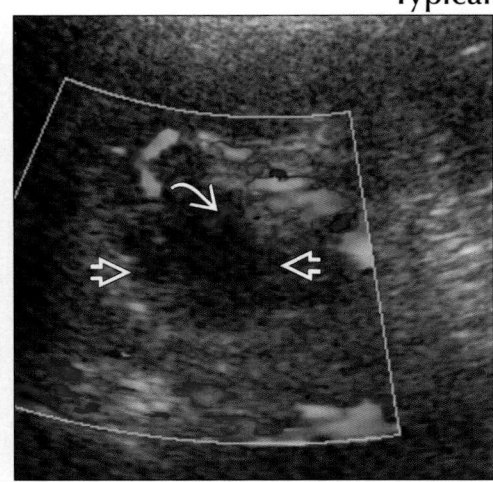

5

102

Typical

(Left) Longitudinal transabdominal ultrasound shows an echogenic TCC ➡ occupying the entire collecting system. High grade TCC is echogenic with no shadowing and can mimic a calculus and a fungus ball. **(Right)** Transverse color Doppler ultrasound shows a TCC ➡ in previous image. It is important not to confuse a high grade TCC with echogenic pus in pyonephrosis by identifying tumor vascularity ➡.

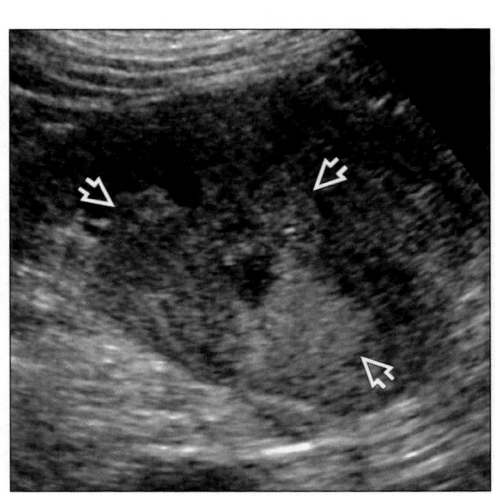
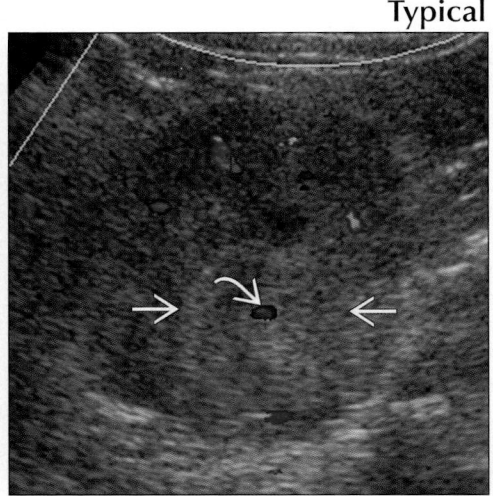

Typical

(Left) Longitudinal color Doppler ultrasound shows a high grade infiltrative TCC ➡ involving the lower pole calyceal system with complete tumor replacement. In such cases hydronephrosis may not be seen. **(Right)** Transverse transabdominal ultrasound shows the same infiltrative TCC ➡ as previous image. Echogenicity may be increased in a high-grade tumor due to formation of keratin pearls in squamous metaplasia.

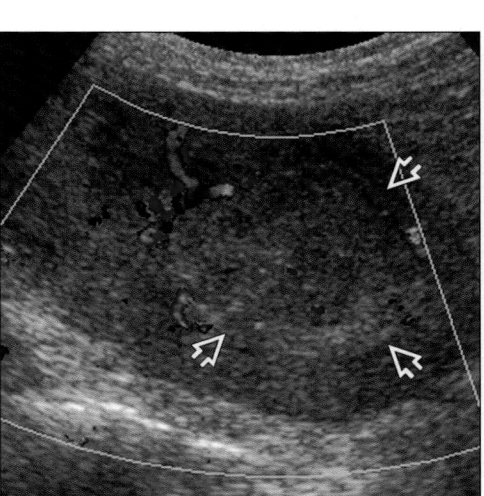
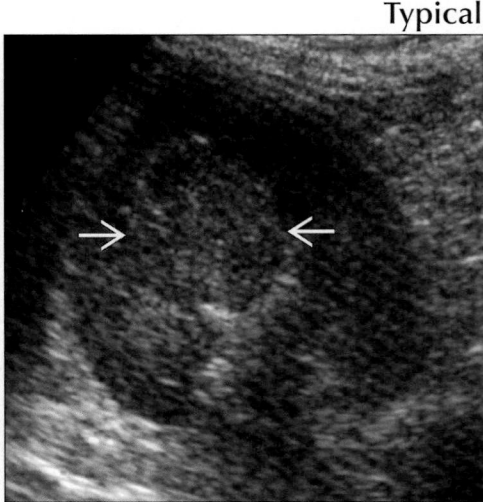

TRANSITIONAL CELL CARCINOMA

Typical

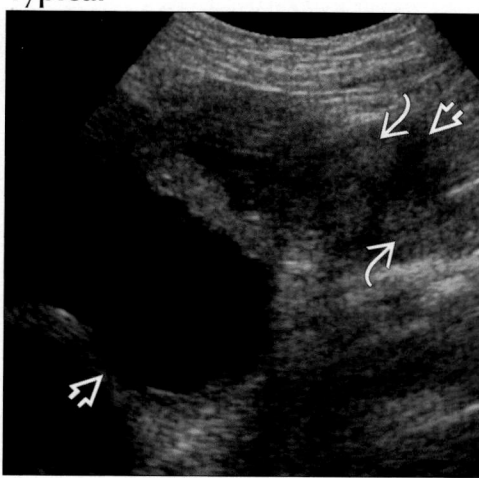

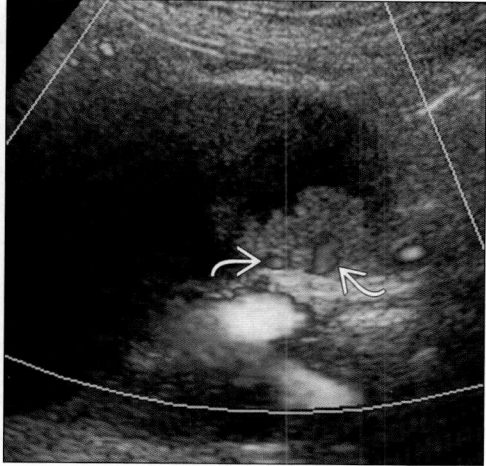

(Left) Longitudinal transabdominal ultrasound shows a severe hydronephrotic kidney ➡ with hypoechoic solid material ➡ in the lower pole calices. Features may represent blood clots, pus or a neoplasm. *(Right)* Oblique power Doppler ultrasound of a kidney in the previous image shows tumor vascularity ➡, compatible with a renal TCC. Synchronous TCC must be excluded by IVP or CT urography.

Typical

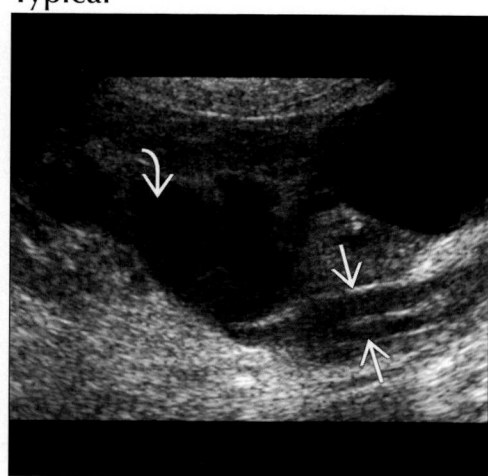

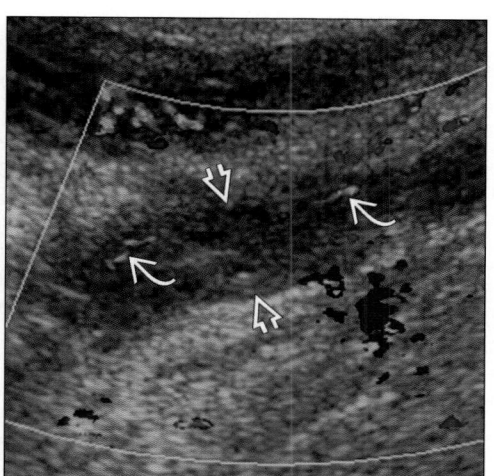

(Left) Longitudinal transabdominal ultrasound shows a dilated ureter ➡ with advanced TCC and associated hydronephrosis ➡. Ultrasound is insensitive in detecting small non-obstructing TCC. *(Right)* Oblique color Doppler ultrasound shows a ureteral TCC ➡ in the previous image with tumor vascularity ➡. Incidence of ureteral TCC is low and accounts for about 2% of all TCC.

Typical

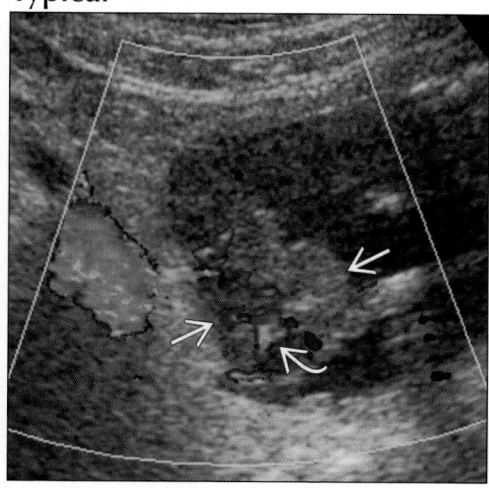

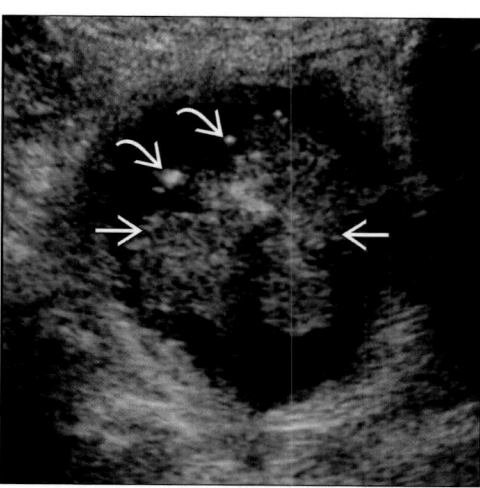

(Left) Oblique color Doppler ultrasound shows a classical lobulated bladder TCC ➡ arising from the right lateral wall. Tumor is highly vascular ➡ and was immobile with a change in patient position. *(Right)* Oblique transabdominal ultrasound shows a bladder TCC in the same patient as previous image with frond-like projections into the bladder resembling "cauliflower" ➡. Surface punctate calcifications ➡ are noted.

RENAL LYMPHOMA

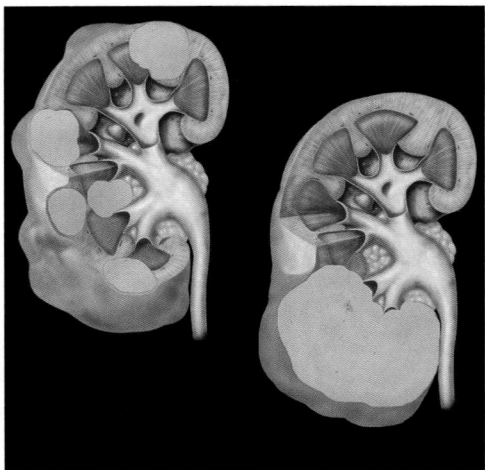

Graphic shows different manifestations of renal lymphoma. Multiple masses are depicted in variable locations in renal parenchyma (left) whereas a solitary mass replaces a lobar segment (right).

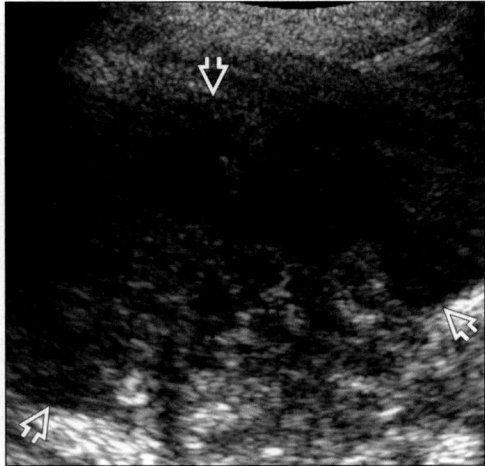

Longitudinal transabdominal ultrasound shows a biopsy proven primary renal B-cell lymphoma ➡. The kidney is heterogeneous and grossly abnormal with complete destruction of renal architecture.

TERMINOLOGY

Abbreviations and Synonyms
- Primary renal lymphoma; secondary renal lymphoma; metastatic renal involvement by lymphoma

Definitions
- Lymphoma: Malignant tumor of B lymphocytes
- Non-Hodgkin > Hodgkin; often bilateral
- Primary: When initial manifestation involves kidney or tumor is confined to it, rare accounting for 3% of cases
- Secondary: Dissemination of extrarenal lymphoma by hematogenous spread (90%) or direct extension via retroperitoneal lymphatic channels

IMAGING FINDINGS

General Features
- Best diagnostic clue: Unilateral or bilateral renal enlargement + altered renal echogenicity ± distortion of renal contour or architecture

Ultrasonographic Findings
- Grayscale Ultrasound
  - Variable manifestations: Solitary, multiple, direct invasion, diffuse infiltration and perirenal involvement; often hypoechoic or near-anechoic
  - Solitary: Focal hypoechoic renal mass indistinct from renal cell carcinoma (RCC)
  - Multiple: Usually bilateral, hypoechoic renal masses
  - Small lesions may be confused with medullary pyramids, renal cysts or abscesses
  - May show posterior acoustic enhancement
  - Direct invasion: Hypoechoic mass extending from retroperitoneum or perirenal space into renal parenchyma or sinus; may simulate transitional cell carcinoma (TCC) or perinephric fluid collection
  - Perirenal lymphoma characterized by hypoechoic "collar" surrounding kidney
  - Early diffuse infiltration: Renal enlargement + preservation of renal architecture and contour + ↓ echogenicity
  - Late diffuse infiltration: Expansile heterogeneous renal mass & loss of normal renal architecture

DDx: Renal Lymphoma Mimics

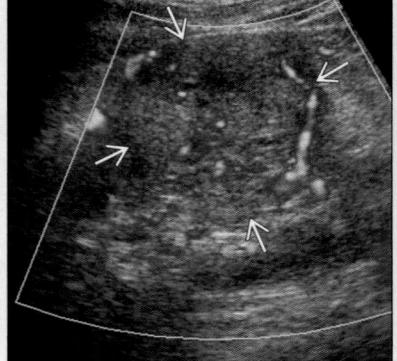

Renal Cell Carcinoma

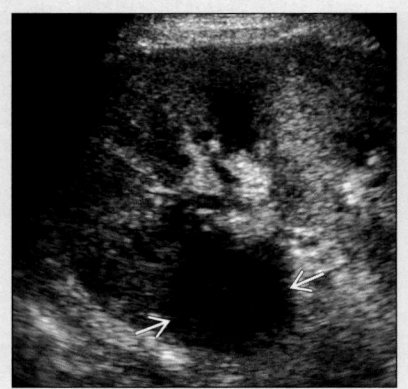

Renal Abscess

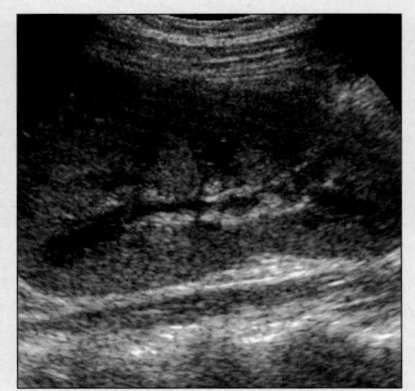

Renal Parenchymal Disease

RENAL LYMPHOMA

Key Facts

Imaging Findings
- Variable manifestations: Solitary, multiple, direct invasion, diffuse infiltration and perirenal involvement; often hypoechoic or near-anechoic
- Solitary: Focal hypoechoic renal mass indistinct from renal cell carcinoma (RCC)
- Multiple: Usually bilateral, hypoechoic renal masses
- Small lesions may be confused with medullary pyramids, renal cysts or abscesses
- May show posterior acoustic enhancement
- Direct invasion: Hypoechoic mass extending from retroperitoneum or perirenal space into renal parenchyma or sinus; may simulate transitional cell carcinoma (TCC) or perinephric fluid collection
- Perirenal lymphoma characterized by hypoechoic "collar" surrounding kidney

- Early diffuse infiltration: Renal enlargement + preservation of renal architecture and contour + ↓ echogenicity
- Late diffuse infiltration: Expansile heterogeneous renal mass & loss of normal renal architecture
- Renal echogenicity uniformly ↑ (similar to liver) may simulate renal parenchymal disease
- Renal vein & inferior vena cava (IVC) tumor thrombosis: Infrequent
- Lymphadenopathy and splenomegaly
- Tumor is typically hypo- or avascular but rarely may show hypervascularity and neovascularity

Top Differential Diagnoses
- Primary Renal Neoplasm: RCC or TCC
- Renal Infection
- Renal Parenchymal Disease

- o Renal echogenicity uniformly ↑ (similar to liver) may simulate renal parenchymal disease
- o Renal vein & inferior vena cava (IVC) tumor thrombosis: Infrequent
- o Lymphadenopathy and splenomegaly
- Color Doppler
  - o Useful to check renal vein and IVC patency
  - o Tumor is typically hypo- or avascular but rarely may show hypervascularity and neovascularity

CT Findings
- CECT is sensitive for evaluation of renal involvement and staging of disease
- Renal masses are homogeneous with minimal contrast-enhancement (10-20 HU)
- Attenuated and poorly opacified collecting systems with variable degree of ↓ enhancement on CECT
- Retroperitoneal adenopathy, splenomegaly or lymphadenopathy at other sites
- Extranodal involvement of gastrointestinal tract, brain, liver and bone marrow, especially in acquired immunodeficiency syndrome (AIDS)

MR Findings
- T1WI: Iso- to slightly hypointense
- T2WI: Hypointense
- T1 C+: Minimal enhancement

Angiographic Findings
- Conventional
  - o Marked attenuation of segmental and interlobar arteries
  - o Masses are usually hypovascular or avascular
  - o Masses rarely demonstrate neovascularity or hypervascularity with arterial venous shunting
  - o Multiple low density cortical defects (nephrogram phase)

Imaging Recommendations
- Best imaging tool
  - o CECT is method of choice for renal involvement and disease staging

- o Ultrasound is ideal for initial investigation and guided percutaneous needle biopsy and follow-up

---

DIFFERENTIAL DIAGNOSIS

Primary Renal Neoplasm: RCC or TCC
- RCC: Round or oval renal cortical mass with central necrosis and grows by expansion; hypervascular
- TCC: Urothelial tumor in collecting system; may be infiltrative extending into renal cortex

Renal Infection
- Pyelonephritis, focal pyelonephritis, renal abscess
- Differentiated by clinical history and urinalysis

Renal Parenchymal Disease
- Due to glomerulonephritis, renal artery stenosis, diabetes, hypertension
- Increase in cortical echogenicity and loss of corticomedullary differentiation
- Reduction in renal volume in chronic disease

Perinephric Fluid Collection
- Retroperitoneal and perirenal lymphoma with direct invasion into renal parenchyma or sinus may simulate perinephric fluid collection
- Color Doppler imaging is not helpful to differentiate it from renal lymphoma because both are avascular

---

PATHOLOGY

General Features
- General path comments
  - o Renal lymphoma
    - 6% of patients with lymphoma at presentation
    - 33-63% of patients dying from malignant lymphoma
    - Renal involvement of non-Hodgkin lymphoma to Hodgkin lymphoma ratio: 10:1
- Etiology

RENAL LYMPHOMA

- o Immunosuppression: Iatrogenic post-organ transplantation or acquired due to AIDS
- o Prior treatment for malignancy
- o Autoimmune disorders
- o Infectious agents e.g., Epstein-Barr virus
- o Secondary renal lymphoma is due to dissemination of advanced disease
- Epidemiology
  - o Primary renal lymphoma (3%)
  - o Secondary renal lymphoma: By hematogenous spread (90%) & via direct spread (7%)
  - o Solitary (10-20%)
  - o Multiple, usually bilateral (60%)
  - o Diffuse infiltration (20%)
  - o Perirenal involvement (10%)

Gross Pathologic & Surgical Features

- Enlarged kidney ± distortion of renal contour
- Expansion of fat caused by homogeneous yellowish tumor infiltration

Microscopic Features

- AIDS: Small cell lymphoma is most common
- Non-Hodgkin lymphoma: Large cell lymphoma is most common
- Tumor foci in renal interstitium, nephrons, collecting system or blood vessels depending on stages of disease

CLINICAL ISSUES

Presentation

- Most common signs/symptoms
  - o Majority are asymptomatic and renal function unaffected
  - o Hematuria, flank pain, palpable mass or renal insufficiency
- Other signs/symptoms
  - o Fever, weight loss
  - o ↑ Serum lactate dehydrogenase
  - o Lymphopenia
- Diagnosis
  - o CT or US-guided percutaneous biopsy

Demographics

- Age: Any (middle-age to elderly more common)
- Gender: Prevalence equal in both sexes

Natural History & Prognosis

- Complications
  - o Renal or perinephric hemorrhage, renal obstruction, renovascular hypertension, acute renal failure
- Prognosis
  - o Renal lymphoma: 57% have complete remission after treatment
    - ■ 4 year survival rate: ~ 40%

Treatment

- Chemotherapy ± radiation therapy
- Nephrectomy if lymphoma is small and isolated to one kidney or have other extenuating circumstances (i.e., severe renal hemorrhage)

DIAGNOSTIC CHECKLIST

Consider

- Clinical history of patient
- Etiology of asymptomatic renal enlargement
- Overlapping sonographic features of renal metastases, renal lymphoma and primary renal carcinoma
- Ultrasound guided renal biopsy in equivocal cases

Image Interpretation Pearls

- Hypoechoic or anechoic renal mass with minimal acoustic enhancement
- Always look for evidence of multisystem involvement in liver, lung, CNS, bone marrow and gastrointestinal tract

SELECTED REFERENCES

1. Barreto F et al: Renal lymphoma. Atypical presentation of a renal tumor. Int Braz J Urol. 32(2):190-2, 2006
2. Bozas G et al: Non-Hodgkin's lymphoma of the renal pelvis. Clin Lymphoma Myeloma. 6(5):404-6, 2006
3. Kunthur A et al: Renal parenchymal tumors and lymphoma in the same patient: case series and review of the literature. Am J Hematol. 81(4):271-80, 2006
4. Porcaro AB et al: Primary lymphoma of the kidney. Report of a case and update of the literature. Arch Ital Urol Androl. 74(1):44-7, 2002
5. Rendon RA et al: The natural history of small renal masses. J Urol. 164(4):1143-7, 2000
6. Urban BA et al: Renal lymphoma: CT patterns with emphasis on helical CT. Radiographics. 20(1):197-212, 2000
7. Sheeran SR et al: Renal lymphoma: spectrum of CT findings and potential mimics. AJR Am J Roentgenol. 171(4):1067-72, 1998
8. Smith PA et al: Spiral computed tomography evaluation of the kidneys: state of the art. Urology. 51(1):3-11, 1998
9. Wyatt SH et al: Spiral CT of the kidneys: role in characterization of renal disease. Part II: Neoplastic disease. Crit Rev Diagn Imaging. 36(1):39-72, 1995
10. Volpe JP et al: The radiologic evaluation of renal metastases. Crit Rev Diagn Imaging. 30(3):219-46, 1990
11. Levine E et al: Small renal neoplasms: clinical, pathologic, and imaging features. AJR Am J Roentgenol. 153(1):69-73, 1989
12. Pollack HM et al: Other malignant neoplasms of the renal parenchyma. Semin Roentgenol. 22(4):260-74, 1987
13. Curry NS et al: Small renal neoplasms: diagnostic imaging, pathologic features, and clinical course. Radiology. 158(1):113-7, 1986
14. Heiken JP et al: Computed tomography of renal lymphoma with ultrasound correlation. J Comput Assist Tomogr. 7(2):245-50, 1983
15. Hartman DS et al: Renal lymphoma: radiologic-pathologic correlation of 21 cases. Radiology. 144(4):759-66, 1982
16. Jafri SZ et al: CT of renal and perirenal non-Hodgkin lymphoma. AJR Am J Roentgenol. 138(6):1101-5, 1982
17. Rubin BE: Computed tomography in the evaluation of renal lymphoma. J Comput Assist Tomogr. 3(6):759-64, 1979

RENAL LYMPHOMA

IMAGE GALLERY

Typical

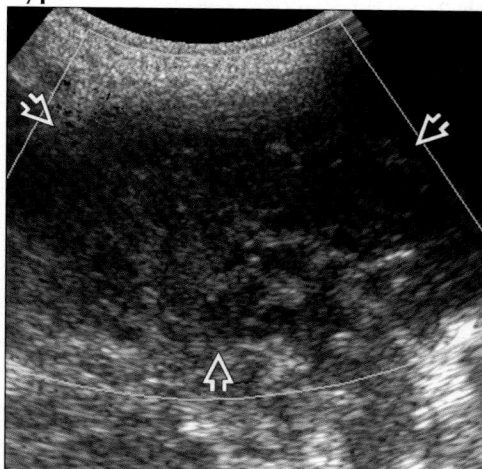
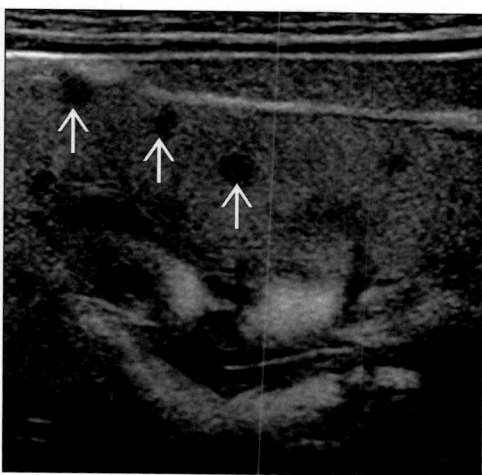

(Left) Longitudinal color Doppler ultrasound in a renal lymphoma ➡ shows an absence of vascularity. Renal lymphoma is typically avascular likely due to vessel occlusion by tumor foci. *(Right)* Longitudinal contrast-enhanced ultrasound shows a renal lymphoma seen as multiple small hypoechoic masses ➡ in an AIDS patient. Note cysts and abscesses have a similar appearance.

Typical

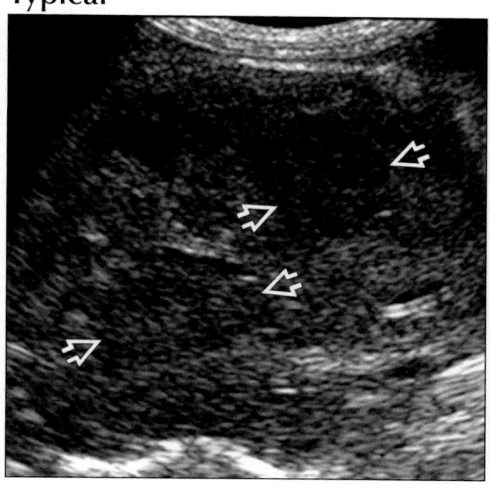
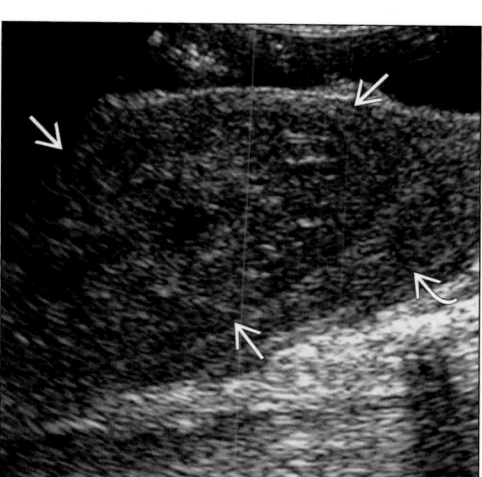

(Left) Longitudinal transabdominal ultrasound shows renal involvement by lymphoma seen as focal hypoechoic masses ➡. This is the most common presentation representing advanced disease. *(Right)* Longitudinal transabdominal ultrasound shows the "hepatization" of renal lymphoma. Note that the kidney is echogenic ➡ simulating renal parenchymal disease. There is also perirenal involvement ➡.

Typical

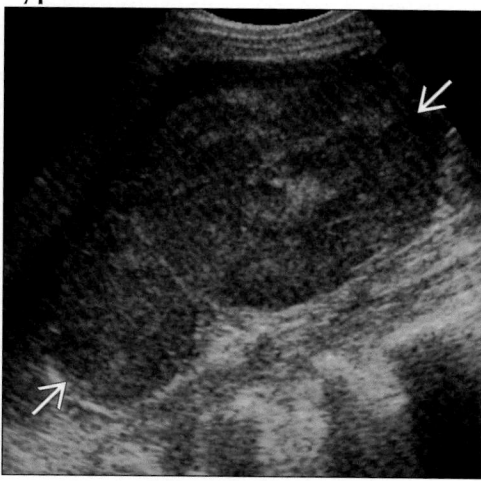
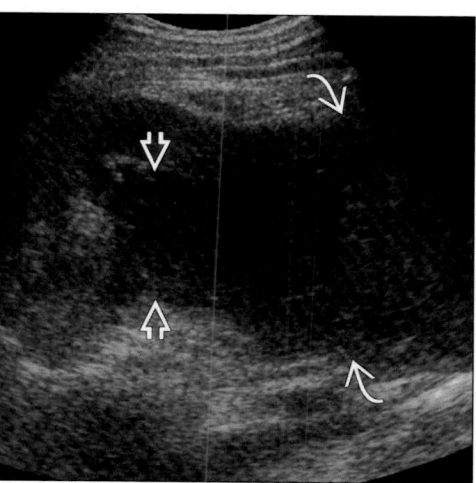

(Left) Longitudinal transabdominal ultrasound shows an advanced diffuse renal infiltration by lymphoma ➡. Note complete loss of normal renal architecture. *(Right)* Transverse transabdominal ultrasound shows lymphoma with direct retroperitoneal extension ➡ into the renal sinus ➡. The mass is large and hypoechoic mimicking perinephric fluid.

RENAL ARTERY STENOSIS

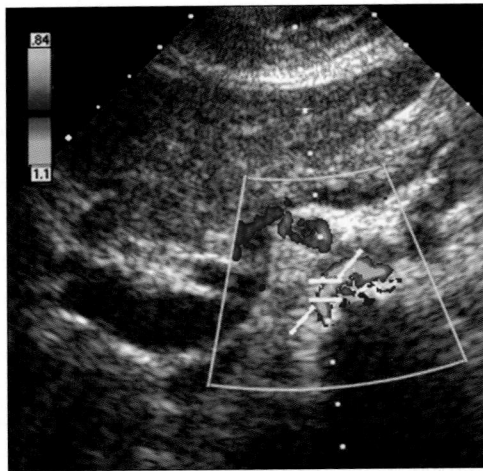

Transverse color Doppler ultrasound in an elderly woman with recurrent hypertension. 8 months post angioplasty shows color aliasing in the proximal right renal artery (sample volume).

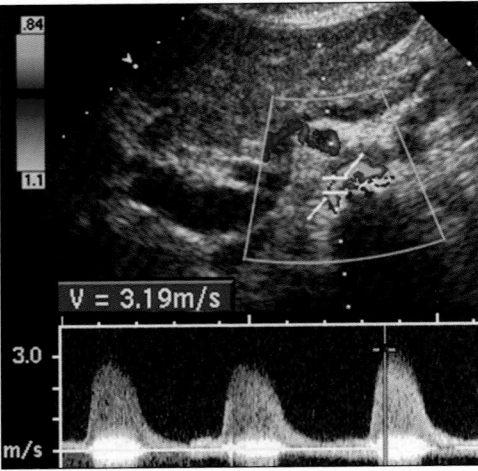

Pulsed Doppler ultrasound shows a peak systolic velocity of 319 cm/sec at location of aliasing, consistent with high grade stenosis. The renal aortic ratio was 4.0.

TERMINOLOGY

Abbreviations and Synonyms
- Renal artery stenosis (RAS)

Definitions
- Narrowing of renal arterial lumen

IMAGING FINDINGS

General Features
- Best diagnostic clue
  - Focal high velocity flow with adjacent post-stenotic turbulence on color Doppler US
  - Documented high peak systolic velocity with spectral Doppler
- Location
  - Ostium/intramural: Primary aortic disease
  - Atherosclerosis: Proximal 2 cm
  - Fibromuscular dysplasia (FMD): Distal renal artery (RA), hilar branches

Ultrasonographic Findings
- Grayscale Ultrasound
  - Possible reduced kidney size (length < 8 cm)
  - Possible increased parenchymal echogenicity (chronic, severe ischemia)
  - Possible FMD "string of beads" appearance of arterial wall (requires excellent visualization)
- Pulsed Doppler
  - Normal RA peak systolic velocity 75-125 cm/sec
  - Doppler criteria ≥ 50-60% diameter stenosis
    - Peak systolic velocity in stenosis ≥ 180-200 cm/sec
    - Renal/aortic ratio > 3.5 (peak systole in RAS/peak systole in aorta at level of RAs)
    - Post-stenotic Doppler spectral broadening
  - Intrarenal Doppler waveform signs of significant RAS
    - Damped Doppler waveforms in lobar/interlobar arteries in RAS
    - Damped: "Pulsus parvus/tardis" waveform shape; parvus = low velocity, tardis = delayed acceleration
    - Acceleration to peak systole > 0.07 sec in RAS
    - Low resistive index < 0.5 (compare with other kidney) in RAS

DDx: Renal Artery Stenosis

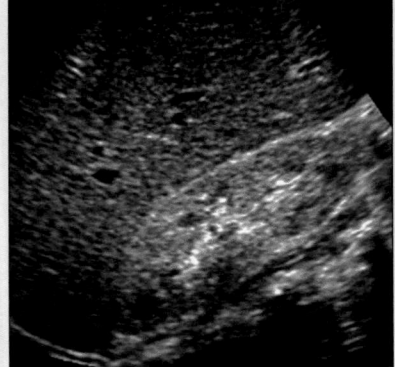

Medical Renal Disease

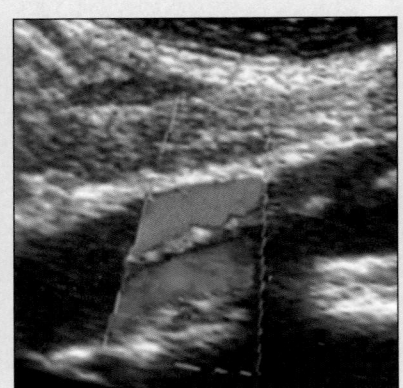

Aortic Dissection

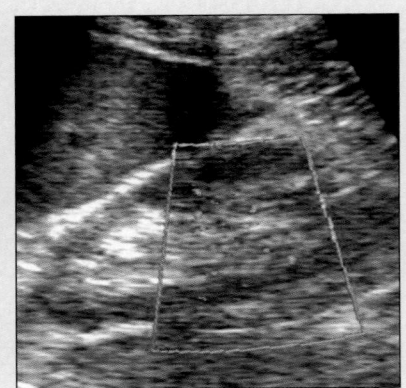

Renal Artery Occlusion

RENAL ARTERY STENOSIS

Key Facts

Imaging Findings

- Focal high velocity flow with adjacent post-stenotic turbulence on color Doppler US
- Normal RA peak systolic velocity 75-125 cm/sec
- Peak systolic velocity in stenosis ≥ 180-200 cm/sec
- Renal/aortic ratio > 3.5 (peak systole in RAS/peak systole in aorta at level of RAs)
- Post-stenotic Doppler spectral broadening
- Damped Doppler waveforms in lobar/interlobar arteries in RAS
- Damped: "Pulsus parvus/tardis" waveform shape; parvus = low velocity, tardis = delayed acceleration
- Acceleration to peak systole > 0.07 sec in RAS
- Low resistive index < 0.5 (compare with other kidney) in RAS

- Color shift/color aliasing in RA at site of stenosis = high velocity flow
- Imaging goal: Accurately diagnose ≥ 50-60% diameter RAS
- Protocol advice: **Imaging for RAS (regardless of modality) is indicated only after appropriate clinical screening**

Top Differential Diagnoses

- Chronic Parenchymal Renal Disease Unrelated to RAS
- Aortic Dissection
- Renal Artery Occlusion

Diagnostic Checklist

- Atherosclerotic RAS: Proximal 2 cm of RA
- FMD-RAS: Mid or distal RA ± intrarenal branches & "string-of-beads" appearance

---

- Cannot accurately diagnose RAS **solely** by intra-renal arterial waveform analysis
  - Accurate Doppler angle ≤ 60° essential
- Color Doppler
  - Color shift/color aliasing in RA at site of stenosis = high velocity flow
  - Post-stenotic turbulence, possibly with soft tissue vibrations

Angiographic Findings

- Contrast enhanced MRA, CTA, or DSA
  - Atherosclerotic lesions: Focal eccentric/concentric stenosis
  - FMD: Most commonly serial ridges or "string-of-beads" pattern

Imaging Recommendations

- Best imaging tool
  - Imaging goal: Accurately diagnose ≥ 50-60% diameter RAS
  - Contrast-enhanced MRA or CTA
  - DSA may be needed for accurate FMD diagnosis in distal RA, hilar branches
  - Duplex ultrasound problems
    - Technically difficult/high exam failure rate
    - Failure to recognize duplicate RAs
    - Inadequate visualization for distal/hilar RAS
    - Wide reported accuracy range; best results for proximal (atherosclerosis-related) RAS
- Protocol advice: **Imaging for RAS (regardless of modality) is indicated only after appropriate clinical screening**

DIFFERENTIAL DIAGNOSIS

Primary Hypertension

- Renal arteries normal

Chronic Parenchymal Renal Disease Unrelated to RAS

- Increased parenchymal echogenicity from interstitial fibrosis

- Increased resistivity index (> 0.7) interlobar/arcuate arteries
- Decreased kidney size from parenchymal destruction (length < 8 cm)

Aortic Dissection

- Possible ostial/intramural obstruction
- Dissection may extend into RA
- US findings: Dissection plane/two lumens seen on color Doppler US

Renal Artery Occlusion

- Etiology
  - Subsequent to RAS
  - Embolic
  - Primary aortic disease
- US findings
  - Absent RA on color Doppler US
  - No or very weak/damped arterial signals in kidney if acute
  - Intrarenal Doppler signals may be normal if chronic (collateralized)
  - Decreased kidney size (length < 8 cm) if chronic

PATHOLOGY

General Features

- Etiology
  - Atherosclerosis
    - Atherosclerotic plaque reducing lumen caliber
    - Ostium (aortic plaque) or proximal 2 cm of renal artery
    - RAS bilateral in 30-40% of atherosclerosis cases
  - FMD
    - Medial fibroplasia 70-80% FMD; intimal hyperplasia: 10-15%; subadventitial fibroplasia 10-15%
    - Most common mid or distal main renal artery ± hilar branches
    - Right RA > left; bilateral 2/3 of cases
  - Aortic dissection
  - Aortic aneurysm (RA compression)

- o Thromboembolism (more likely leads to occlusion than RAS)
- o Arteritis (e.g., Takayasu, polyarteritis nodosa)
- o Retroperitoneal fibrosis
- o Congenital RAS = intimal fibroplasia distal 2/3 RA + branches
- Epidemiology
  - o RAS most common cause of secondary hypertension
    - Called "renovascular hypertension"
    - Accounts for 1-4% of all hypertension cases (higher in some series)
  - o Atherosclerosis
    - Most common cause of RAS (60-90% of cases)
    - Majority > 50 years
    - Males > females
  - o FMD
    - Second most common cause of RAS overall (10-30% cases)
    - Most common cause of renovascular hypertension in children & young adults
    - Male << female (< 2/3 of RAS FMD cases)

Gross Pathologic & Surgical Features
- Atherosclerosis
  - o Eccentric or circumferential plaque in proximal RA
  - o Possible turbulence-related post-stenotic dilatation
- Medial fibroplasia FMD
  - o "String-of-beads" appearance
- Renal parenchymal atrophy (renal length ≤ 8 cm) moderate/severe RAS

Microscopic Features
- Atherosclerotic plaque: Subintimal fibro-fatty plaque, possibly calcified
- Medial fibroplasia FMD: Fibrous ridges with intervening media thinning/aneurysmal dilatation

Staging, Grading or Classification Criteria
- Hemodynamically significant arterial stenosis = pressure/flow reducing lesion
- Hemodynamically significant RAS: ≥ 50-60% diameter reduction

CLINICAL ISSUES

Presentation
- Most common signs/symptoms
  - o No signs or symptoms specific for RA hypertension
  - o Clinical scenarios suggesting RA hypertension & **justifying RA imaging**
    - Hypertension in a child or young adult
    - Hypertension uncontrolled with three or more drugs
    - Previously controlled hypertension newly uncontrollable
    - Rapidly worsening (malignant) hypertension
    - Hypertension with deteriorating renal function
- Other signs/symptoms: Unilateral small kidney

Demographics
- Age
  - o Atherosclerosis: > Age 50 years
  - o FMD: Usually young adulthood

- Gender
  - o Atherosclerosis: Male predominance
  - o FMD: Female predominance

Natural History & Prognosis
- Atherosclerosis: Poor prognosis after RAS angioplasty/surgery
  - o Mixed results for hypertension control
  - o Impossible to predict who is likely to respond
  - o Very poor results for arresting renal function decline
- FMD: Good prognosis after RAS angioplasty
  - o Hypertension ameliorated or medically controlled
  - o Recurrent stenosis possible

Treatment
- Angiotensin converting enzyme (ACE) inhibitors
- Transluminal angioplasty: 80% RAS correction rate for non-ostial lesions; 25-30% ostial
- Surgical revascularization: 80-90% success rate (bypass stenosis)
- Successful stenosis treatment not consistently = clinical improvement

DIAGNOSTIC CHECKLIST

Consider
- RAS/RA occlusion with unilateral small kidney

Image Interpretation Pearls
- Atherosclerotic RAS: Proximal 2 cm of RA
- FMD-RAS: Mid or distal RA ± intrarenal branches & "string-of-beads" appearance

SELECTED REFERENCES

1. Pellerito JS et al: Ultrasound assessment of native renal vessels and renal allografts. In, Zwiebel WJ: Introduction to Vascular Ultrasonography. Ed 5. Philadelphia, Saunders/Elsevier. 611-636, 2005
2. Urban BA et al: Three-dimensional volume-rendered CT angiography of the renal arteries and veins: normal anatomy, variants, and clinical applications. Radiographics. 21(2):373-86; questionnaire 549-55, 2001
3. Gilfeather M et al: Renal artery stenosis: evaluation with conventional angiography versus gadolinium-enhanced MR angiography. Radiology. 210(2):367-72, 1999
4. Isaacson JA et al: Direct and indirect renal arterial duplex and Doppler color flow evaluation. J Vasc Technol. 19:105-10, 1995
5. Taylor DC et al: Duplex ultrasound scanning in the diagnosis of renal artery stenosis: a prospective evaluation. J Vasc Surg. 7(2):363-9, 1988
6. Dubbins PA: Renal artery stenosis: duplex Doppler evaluation. Br J Radiol. 59(699):225-9, 1986
7. Kohler TR et al: Noninvasive diagnosis of renal artery stenosis by ultrasonic duplex scanning. J Vasc Surg. 4(5):450-6, 1986
8. Norris CS et al: Noninvasive evaluation of renal artery stenosis and renovascular resistance. Experimental and clinical studies. J Vasc Surg. 1(1):192-201, 1984

IMAGE GALLERY

Typical

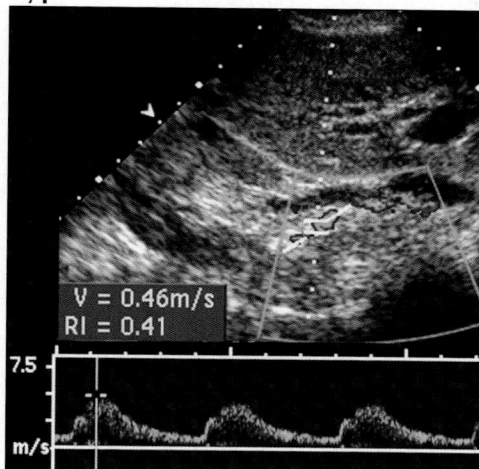

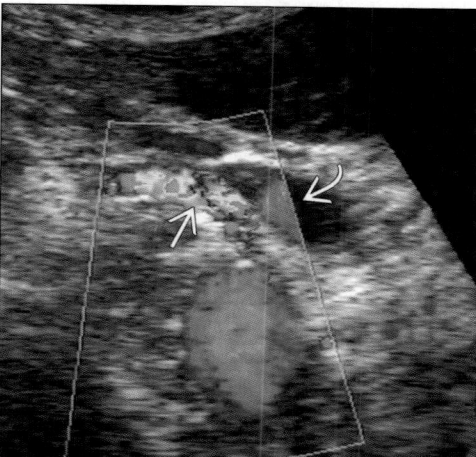

(Left) Transverse pulsed Doppler ultrasound in the same patient as previous image, shows damped Doppler waveforms distal to the right RAS. *(Right)* Oblique color Doppler ultrasound from a right lateral transducer position, shows marked turbulence ➡ in the right renal artery just distal to high-grade proximal stenosis (➡ = IVC).

Typical

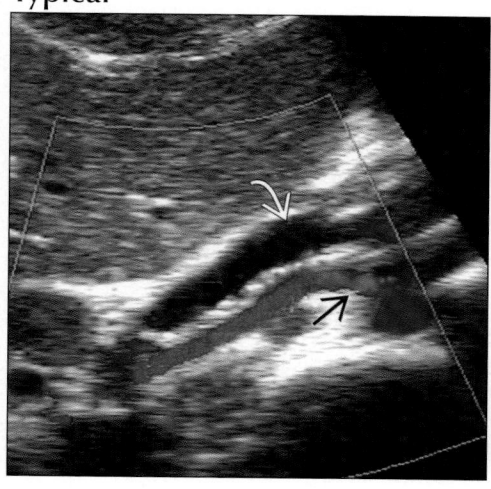

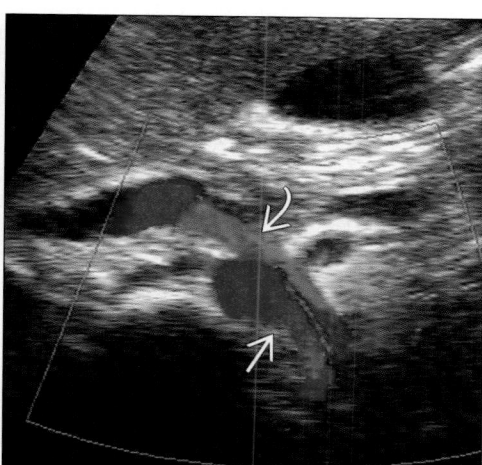

(Left) Oblique color Doppler ultrasound shows a normal right renal artery, which consistently arises from the anterolateral aspect of the aorta ➡ and travels posterior to the IVC ➡. *(Right)* Oblique color Doppler ultrasound shows the origin of the left renal artery ➡, which varies from anterolateral to posterolateral, but always lies posterior to the left renal vein ➡.

Typical

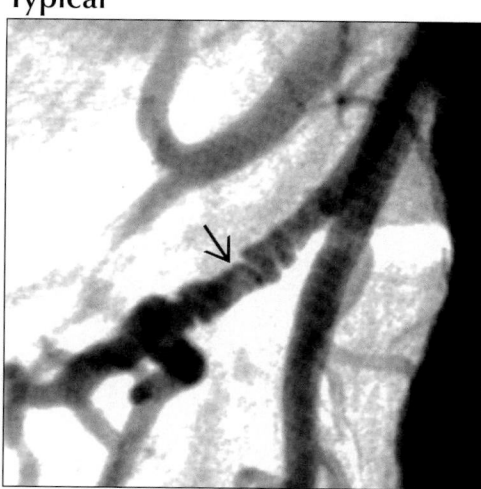

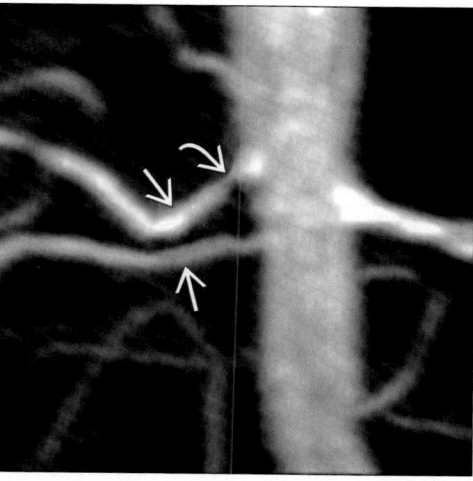

(Left) Oblique DSA shows a series of ridges in the distal right renal artery ➡, typical of FMD, in a middle-aged woman with poorly controlled hypertension. *(Right)* Oblique MRA shows duplicated right renal arteries ➡, with the upper one having a significant stenosis ➡. It is easy to envision why renal artery duplication is often missed with US.

RENAL VEIN THROMBOSIS

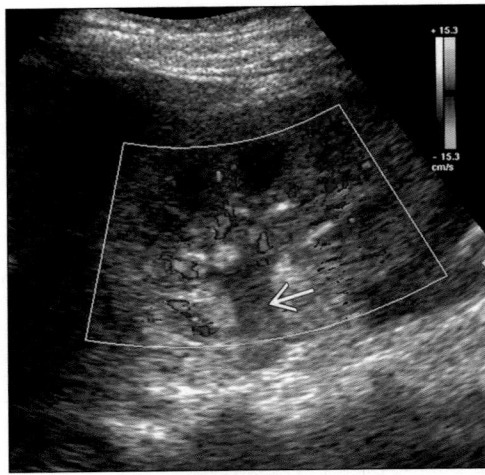

Longitudinal color Doppler ultrasound shows echogenic material distending the renal vein ➡ and absence of venous blood flow.

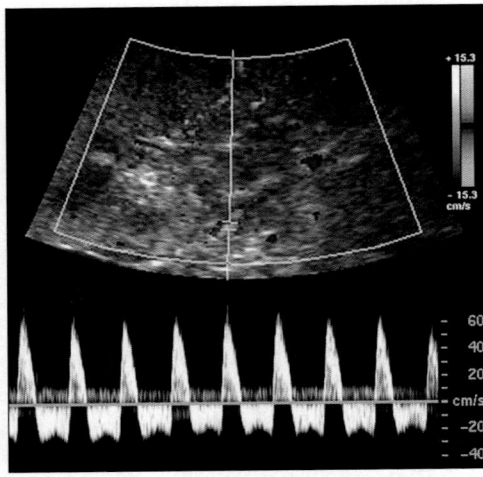

Corresponding oblique pulsed Doppler ultrasound shows striking diastolic flow reversal in the renal artery, characteristic of renal vein thrombosis.

TERMINOLOGY

Abbreviations and Synonyms
- Renal vein thrombosis (RVT)
- Renal vein (RV)

Definitions
- Obstruction of renal vein by thrombus

IMAGING FINDINGS

General Features
- Best diagnostic clue: Echogenic material in renal vein with absence of flow on color Doppler US
- Location
  - Unilateral > bilateral
  - Left renal vein > right renal vein
  - Possible inferior vena cava (IVC) thrombus extension
- Size
  - Kidney enlarged acutely in 75% cases
  - Renal vein dilated acutely
  - Possible shrunken, scarred kidney chronically

Ultrasonographic Findings
- Grayscale Ultrasound
  - **Acute thrombosis**
  - Kidney enlargement most noticeable feature
    - Venous congestion → edema → renal enlargement
    - Enlargement varies & depends on degree of RV obstruction
  - Altered parenchymal echogenicity (3 patterns)
    - Diffusely hypoechoic, no corticomedullary differentiation
    - Diffusely heterogeneous (if extensive hemorrhage and necrosis)
    - Linear echogenic "streaks" radiating from hilum (thrombosed parenchymal veins)
  - Renal vein distended (faintly echogenic material)
  - IVC thrombus extension (uncommon)
  - **Subacute thrombosis**
  - ↑ Cortical echogenicity, ↑ corticomedullary contrast (after 10-14 days)
  - Reduced RV size, increased thrombus echogenicity
  - **Chronic thrombosis**
  - Appearance depends on amount of renal damage, degree of RV flow restoration

DDx: Renal Vein Thrombosis

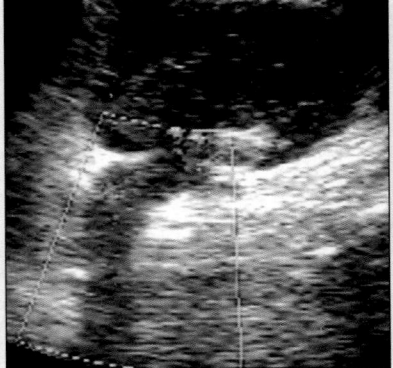

Renal Vein Tumor

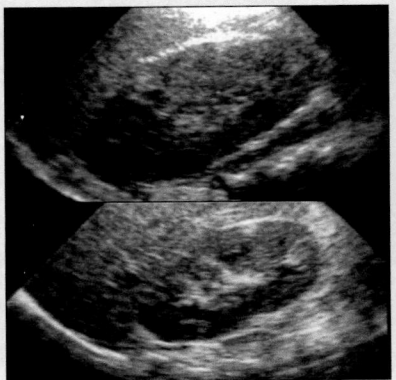

Acute Pyelonephritis

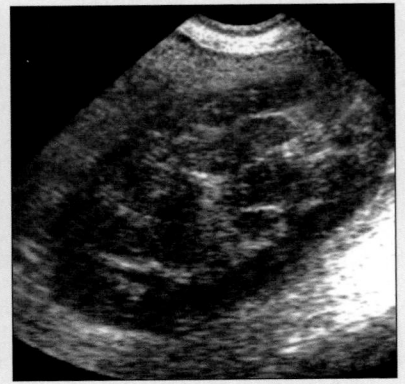

Infiltrative Disorders

RENAL VEIN THROMBOSIS

Key Facts

Imaging Findings
- **Acute thrombosis**
- Kidney enlargement most noticeable feature
- Venous congestion → edema → renal enlargement
- Altered parenchymal echogenicity (3 patterns)
- Diffusely hypoechoic, no corticomedullary differentiation
- Diffusely heterogeneous (if extensive hemorrhage and necrosis)
- Linear echogenic "streaks" radiating from hilum (thrombosed parenchymal veins)
- Renal vein distended (faintly echogenic material)
- IVC thrombus extension (uncommon)
- **Subacute thrombosis**
- ↑ Cortical echogenicity, ↑ corticomedullary contrast (after 10-14 days)

- Reduced RV size, increased thrombus echogenicity
- **Chronic thrombosis**
- Appearance depends on amount of renal damage, degree of RV flow restoration
- Normal grayscale appearance
- ↑ Parenchymal echogenicity
- ↓ Kidney size (scar)
- **Altered renal artery spectral waveforms**
- ↑ Systolic pulsatility (narrow, sharp systolic peaks)
- Persistent retrograde diastolic flow
- **Acute occlusive thrombus**
- Absent RV blood flow
- **Acute non-occlusive thrombus**
- Thrombus "filling defect" in RV flow column
- Do not mistake splenic vein for RV
- Splenic vein **anterior** to superior mesenteric artery
- RV **posterior** to superior mesenteric artery

5

113

- ▪ Normal grayscale appearance
- ▪ ↑ Parenchymal echogenicity
- ▪ ↑ Corticomedullary contrast
- ▪ ↓ Kidney size (scar)
- Pulsed Doppler
  - ○ **Altered renal artery spectral waveforms**
    - ▪ ↑ Systolic pulsatility (narrow, sharp systolic peaks)
    - ▪ Persistent retrograde diastolic flow
  - ○ Focal ↑ flow velocity around thrombus if non-occlusive
- Color Doppler
  - ○ **Acute occlusive thrombus**
    - ▪ Absent RV blood flow
    - ▪ Possible "tram-track" (small flow channels around thrombus)
  - ○ **Acute non-occlusive thrombus**
    - ▪ Thrombus "filling defect" in RV flow column
    - ▪ Possible color shift from ↑ flow velocity around thrombus
  - ○ **Subacute/chronic**
    - ▪ Variable restoration of flow, depending on degree of lysis
    - ▪ Possible collateral veins (hilar, capsular-retroperitoneal, renal-splenic)

Other Modality Findings
- CT/MR
  - ○ Morphologic and vascular findings analogous to US
    - ▪ ↓ Kidney perfusion/excretion acutely
    - ▪ May persist → chronic phase

Imaging Recommendations
- Best imaging tool
  - ○ Color Doppler US for initial diagnosis
  - ○ CT/MRI for comprehensive assessment, follow-up
- Protocol advice
  - ○ Do not mistake splenic vein for RV
    - ▪ Splenic vein **anterior** to superior mesenteric artery
    - ▪ RV **posterior** to superior mesenteric artery
  - ○ Doppler angle, pulse repetition frequency, and gain must be appropriate for low velocity flow

DIFFERENTIAL DIAGNOSIS

Renal Vein Tumor Invasion
- RV distended by faintly echogenic tumor (looks like thrombus)
- May see tumor vessels in RV with color Doppler
- Kidney may be infiltrated, enlarged
- Renal cell carcinoma, transitional cell carcinoma, Wilms tumor

Renal Parenchymal Infiltration
- Diffusely enlarged, hypoechoic kidney, loss of corticomedullary differentiation
- Appearance identical to RVT
- Lymphoma, renal cell carcinoma, transitional cell carcinoma, amyloid

Pyelonephritis
- Enlarged, hypoechoic kidney, loss of corticomedullary differentiation
- Appearance identical to RVT, but RV patent

Urinary Tract Obstruction
- Possible kidney enlargement
- Normal echogenicity maintained acutely
- Dilated pelvis/calyces almost always seen

PATHOLOGY

General Features
- General path comments
  - ○ Nephrotic syndrome is most common cause of RVT in adults
  - ○ Dehydration/sepsis is most common cause of RVT in children
- Genetics: Inherited hypercoagulable states possible cause
- Etiology
  - ○ Nephrotic syndrome
    - ▪ Especially membranous glomerulonephritis
  - ○ Hypovolemia/renal hypoperfusion

- Dehydration, sepsis, hemorrhage, pericarditis, CHF
  - Hypercoagulable states (malignancy-related, pregnancy, genetic)
  - Abdominal/renal trauma
  - Mechanical RV compression
  - Drugs (e.g., oral contraceptives, steroids)
  - Systemic diseases (e.g., sickle cell, systemic lupus)
  - Post-operative renal transplantation
- Epidemiology
  - Nephrotic syndrome underlying cause 16-42% RVT
  - Dehydration/sepsis most commonly → RVT in children < 2 years of age

Gross Pathologic & Surgical Features

- Congested, enlarged kidney acutely → scarred, small kidney chronically

Microscopic Features

- Acute: Vascular congestion, edema → tissue necrosis, hemorrhage
- Chronic: Fibrosis, dystrophic calcification

CLINICAL ISSUES

Presentation

- Most common signs/symptoms
  - Acute
    - Flank/abdominal pain, nausea, vomiting
    - Mass (enlarged kidney)
    - Proteinuria, hematuria. acute renal failure
  - Chronic
    - Asymptomatic (if RVT unilateral or with complete recovery)
    - Renal failure/hypertension
- Other signs/symptoms: Related to acute pulmonary embolization (most common RVT complication)

Demographics

- Age: Adults (most common) or < 2 years of age

Natural History & Prognosis

- Sparse data, small anecdotal clinical series
- Outcome depends on time to occlusion, duration of occlusion, recanalization, collateralization
- Prognosis seems good; frequent spontaneous recovery

Treatment

- Anticoagulation: Heparin then Coumadin
- Thrombolysis/surgical thrombectomy: Heroic measure for life-threatening situations
- Suprarenal caval filter (IVC thrombus)

DIAGNOSTIC CHECKLIST

Consider

- RVT with diffusely enlarged, hypoechoic/heterogeneous kidney

Image Interpretation Pearls

- Persistent diastolic flow reversal in renal artery suggests RVT

SELECTED REFERENCES

1. Urban BA et al: Three-dimensional volume-rendered CT angiography of the renal arteries and veins: normal anatomy, variants, and clinical applications. Radiographics. 21(2):373-86; questionnaire 549-55, 2001
2. Heiss SG et al: Contrast-enhanced three-dimensional fast spoiled gradient-echo renal MR imaging: evaluation of vascular and nonvascular disease. Radiographics. 20(5):1341-52; discussion 1353-4, 2000
3. Kawashima A et al: CT evaluation of renovascular disease. Radiographics. 20(5):1321-40, 2000
4. Zigman A et al: Renal vein thrombosis: a 10-year review. J Pediatr Surg. 35(11):1540-2, 2000
5. Helenon O et al: Renovascular disease: Doppler ultrasound. Semin Ultrasound CT MR. 18(2):136-46, 1997
6. Tempany CM et al: MRI of the renal veins: assessment of nonneoplastic venous thrombosis. J Comput Assist Tomogr. 16(6):929-34, 1992
7. Gatewood OM et al: Renal vein thrombosis in patients with nephrotic syndrome: CT diagnosis. Radiology. 159(1):117-22, 1986
8. Glazer GM et al: Computed tomography of renal vein thrombosis. J Comput Assist Tomogr. 8(2):288-93, 1984
9. Jeffrey RB et al: CT and ultrasonography of acute renal abnormalities. Radiol Clin North Am. 21(3):515-25, 1983
10. Bradley WG Jr et al: Renal vein thrombosis: occurrence in membranous glomerulonephropathy and lupus nephritis. Radiology. 139(3):571-6, 1981
11. Cade R et al: Chronic renal vein thrombosis. Am J Med. 63(3):387-97, 1977
12. Chait A et al: Renal vein thrombosis. Radiology. 90(5):886-96, 1968

RENAL VEIN THROMBOSIS

IMAGE GALLERY

Typical

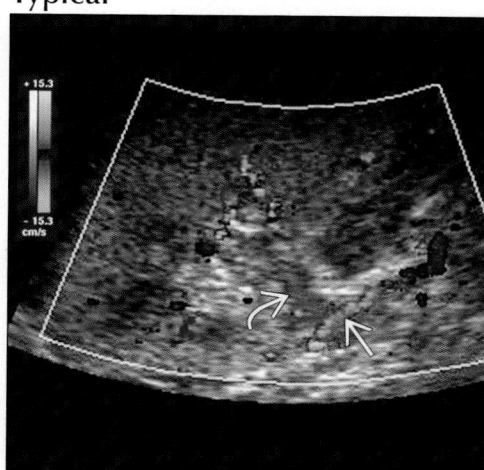 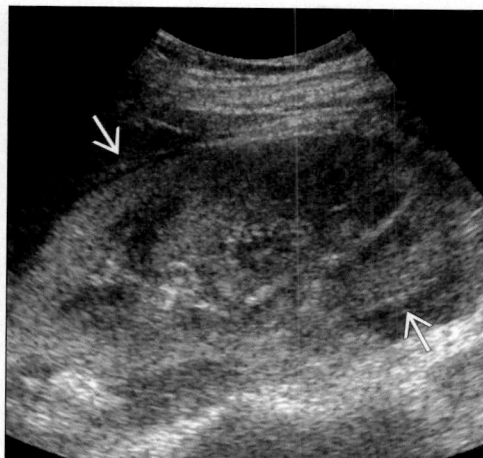

(Left) Longitudinal color Doppler ultrasound in case shown on first page, shows renal artery blood flow ➡ but absence of flow in the renal vein ➡. *(Right)* Longitudinal ultrasound in the same patient as the previous image, shows perinephric fluid ➡, due to congestion, and increased cortical echogenicity.

Typical

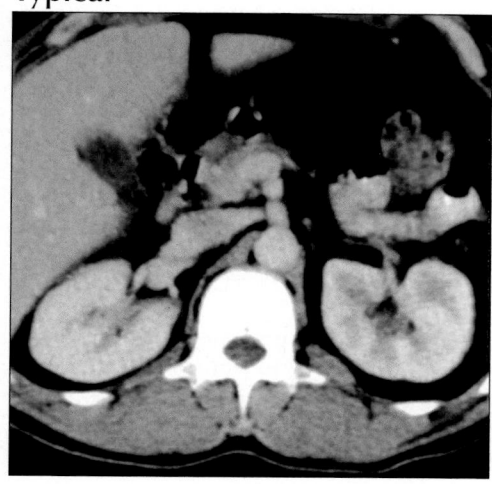 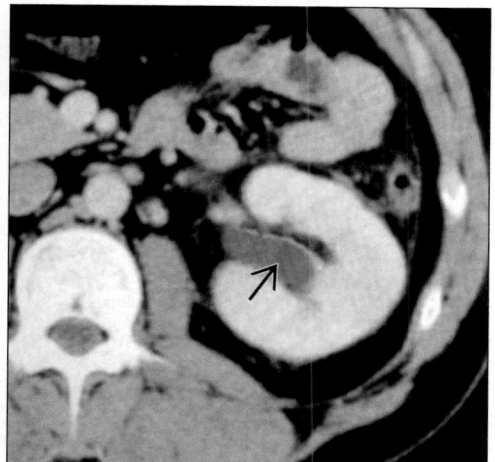

(Left) Transverse CECT in an adult with left flank pain and hematuria 2 days after a fall, shows delayed contrast equilibration in the left kidney, as compared to the right. *(Right)* Transverse CECT shows a thrombus filling the left renal vein ➡, accounting for circulatory delay seen in the prior image.

Typical

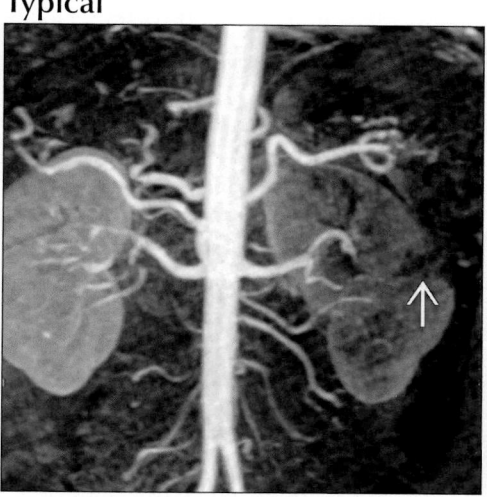 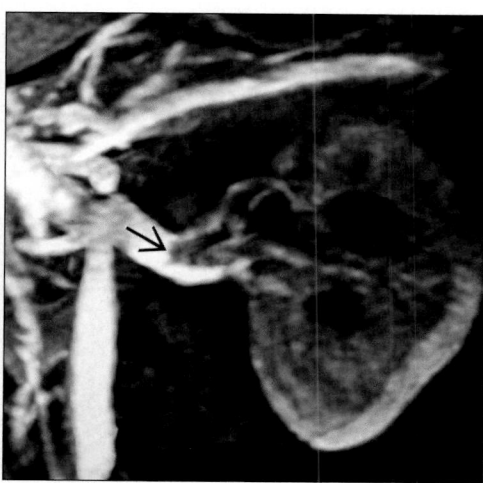

(Left) T1 C+ MR in the arterial phase shows hypoperfusion of the left kidney in the same patient as the previous images. Note parenchymal laceration ➡. *(Right)* T1 C+ MR in the venous phase, shows thrombus ➡ within the proximal left renal vein.

PROSTATIC HYPERTROPHY

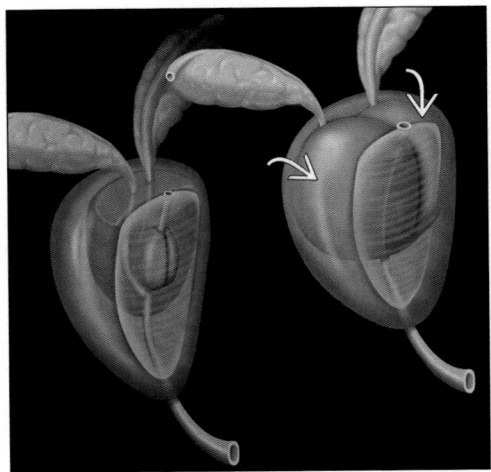

Graphic shows a normal (left) and hypertrophic (right) prostatic gland. Note uniform enlargement of the transitional zone (blue ➡️) compressing on the urethra, as is typical of BPH.

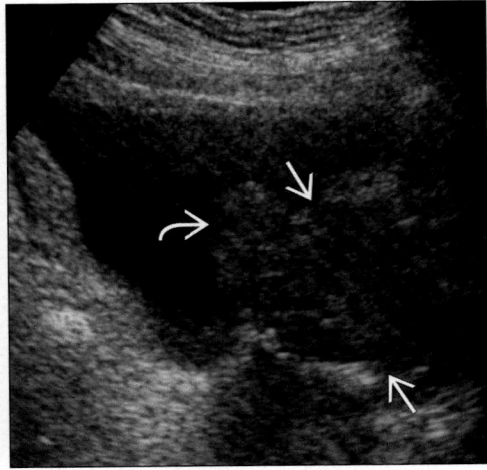

Longitudinal transabdominal ultrasound shows BPH with enlargement of the median lobe ➡️ protruding into the bladder lumen ➡️. Appearance simulates polypoid bladder CA arising from bladder base.

TERMINOLOGY

Abbreviations and Synonyms
- Benign prostatic hypertrophy (BPH), nodular hyperplasia, prostatism

Definitions
- Enlargement of prostate from benign hyperplastic nodule (fibromyoadenomatous nodule)
- Prostate is divided into four glandular zones surrounding the urethra: Peripheral, central, transitional and periurethral glandular
- Peripheral zone is the largest in normal gland
  - Occupies about 70% of prostatic tissue
  - Common site for prostate cancer, accounting for about 70% of cases
  - Is located posteriorly and laterally and becomes thicker in apical (inferior) region
- Central zone is the second largest zone
  - Situated deep to the gland between peripheral and transitional zones
  - Located predominantly in the base (superior) region
  - About 5% prostate cancer found in central zone
- Transitional zone is the site where BPH arises
  - Located in periurethral region between the base and apex
  - Cannot be depicted on sonography unless enlarged
  - About 20% of prostate cancer occur in transitional zone
- Periurethral zone, also known as internal prostatic sphincter

IMAGING FINDINGS

General Features
- Best diagnostic clue: Enlarged prostate on CT, US or MR with nodular hypertrophy in transitional or periurethral zone
- Location: Transition zone and periurethral zone proximal to verumontanum; "lateral lobe" = 82%, median lobe = 12%
- Size: Variable; may be up to 10-12 cm
- Morphology: Rounded or lobulated soft tissue hypertrophy; nodules typically 60-100 gm

Ultrasonographic Findings
- Grayscale Ultrasound

DDx: Benign Prostatic Hypertrophy Mimics

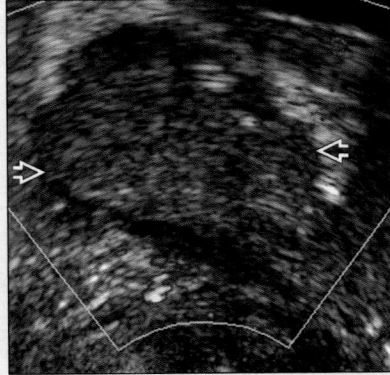

Diffuse Prostate CA

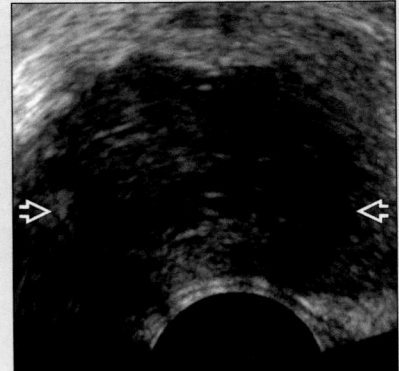

Prostatic Abscess

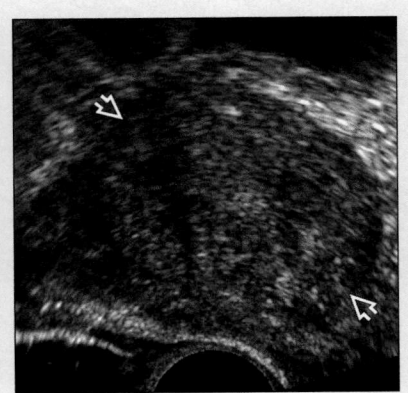

Chronic Prostatitis

PROSTATIC HYPERTROPHY

Key Facts

Terminology
- Enlargement of prostate from benign hyperplastic nodule (fibromyoadenomatous nodule)
- Transitional zone is the site where BPH arises

Imaging Findings
- Role of ultrasound is to distinguish BPH from malignant or inflammatory prostatic disease
- In BPH, secondary alteration of bladder and upper urinary tract should be evaluated
- Investigation of BPH is best done transvesically to assess associated urinary tract abnormalities
- Sonographic appearance of BPH variable, depending on histopathologic changes
- Diffusely enlarged transitional zone; inhomogeneous nodular echotexture; occasional finding of calcification and cystic change (80%)

- Isoechoic hyperplastic nodules with halo may appear in peripheral zone mimicking carcinoma (20%)
- Cysts seen in midline of prostatic base include utricle cysts, müllerian duct cysts and ejaculatory duct cysts
- Sites of degenerative or retention cysts varied
- Vascularity usually is higher in malignancy and prostatitis than in BPH
- Neovascularization is absent in hyperplastic nodules
- Transabdominal ultrasound is preferred to evaluate BPH for prostatic size and associated urinary tract abnormalities

Top Differential Diagnoses
- Prostate Carcinoma
- Bladder Carcinoma
- Prostatitis
- Prostatic Abscess

- Role of ultrasound is to distinguish BPH from malignant or inflammatory prostatic disease
- In BPH, secondary alteration of bladder and upper urinary tract should be evaluated
- Investigation of BPH is best done transvesically to assess associated urinary tract abnormalities
  - To evaluate prostatic size, median lobe enlargement, postvoid bladder volume, associated urinary tract abnormalities such as trabeculation, diverticula, calculi, hydronephrosis
- On transrectal ultrasound (TRUS), normal prostate is homogeneous with peripheral zone slightly more echogenic than central zone
- Sonographic appearance of BPH variable, depending on histopathologic changes
  - Diffusely enlarged transitional zone; inhomogeneous nodular echotexture; occasional finding of calcification and cystic change (80%)
  - Isoechoic hyperplastic nodules with halo may appear in peripheral zone mimicking carcinoma (20%)
  - Delineation between peripheral zone and central zone becomes more obvious, sometimes outlined by corpora amylacea along surgical capsule
  - Hyperplastic nodules may undergo cystic degeneration forming ragged cystic masses
  - Cyst aspiration under TRUS guidance is required to differentiate between these cysts from cystic prostate carcinoma (CA)
- Prostatic volume can be measured with either transvesical or transrectal approach using formula: 0.523 (length x width x thickness) of gland
- Cysts seen in midline of prostatic base include utricle cysts, müllerian duct cysts and ejaculatory duct cysts
  - Utricle cysts, typically "teardrop" in shape pointing toward verumontanum
- Sites of degenerative or retention cysts varied
- Color Doppler
  - Normal prostate is moderately vascular
  - Vascularity increases in dependent lobe

- Vascularity usually is higher in malignancy and prostatitis than in BPH
- Power Doppler
  - Neovascularization is absent in hyperplastic nodules
  - Is not sensitive enough to differentiate BPH from prostatic cancer

Radiographic Findings
- IVP: Extrinsic impression on base of bladder with "J hooking" or "fish hooking" of distal ureters

CT Findings
- NECT: Enlarged prostate; calcification may be seen in enlarged gland
- CECT: Enlarged prostate with extrinsic compression on base of bladder

MR Findings
- T1WI: Enlarged prostate
- T2WI
  - Low or heterogeneous signal nodular adenoma involving transition or periurethral zone
  - Cannot distinguish BPH from carcinoma
- T1 C+
  - Data mixed on whether dynamic contrast-enhancement may aid in differentiating BPH from carcinoma
  - Carcinoma in general has more rapid uptake of gadolinium on dynamic MR

Imaging Recommendations
- Best imaging tool
  - Transabdominal ultrasound is preferred to evaluate BPH for prostatic size and associated urinary tract abnormalities
  - TRUS ± biopsy is not necessary if index of suspicion of malignancy is low

DIFFERENTIAL DIAGNOSIS

Prostate Carcinoma
- Typically involves peripheral zone (70%)
- No specific sonographic appearance

PROSTATIC HYPERTROPHY

- Classical appearance: Hypoechoic nodule in peripheral zone with increased vascularity
- Mimickers: Prostatitis, atrophy, fibrosis, infarct, BPH

Bladder Carcinoma
- Majority of bladder CA along posterior wall
- Sonographically, depicted as polypoid mass protruding into bladder lumen
- Enlarged median lobe in BPH simulates bladder CA arising from bladder base

Prostatitis
- On sonography, mostly normal in appearance
- Patients manifest with variable symptoms
- Acute prostatitis, usually clinically evident with tender prostate and rectum
  - Sonographic appearance may simulate carcinoma
  - Ultrasound features include hypoechoic swollen gland with increase in vascularity ± cystic areas suggestive of abscesses
- Chronic prostatitis: Sonographic findings include focal masses of varying echogenicity, ejaculatory duct calcification, thickened and irregular capsule, irregular periurethral glandular area, dilated periprostatic veins and distended seminal vesicles

Prostatic Abscess
- Develops as complication of prostatitis or is due to hematogenous spread
- TRUS is preferred method of evaluation
- Appears as low attenuation fluid collection with thick septae bulging capsule
- Ultrasound guided aspiration required for diagnosis and therapy

PATHOLOGY

General Features
- General path comments: Firm hypertrophied tissue
- Etiology: Stromal hyperplasia stimulated by normal action of dehydrotestosterone and growth factors (fibroblast growth factor, insulin-like growth factor)
- Epidemiology: 70% of men have BPH by age 70; 80% of men have BPH by age 80
- Associated abnormalities
  - Bladder wall hypertrophy with trabeculation and diverticula
  - Hydronephrosis

Gross Pathologic & Surgical Features
- Enlarged, firm gland at prostatectomy

Microscopic Features
- Hyperplastic nodules due to glandular proliferation and/or fibrous or muscular proliferation of stroma
- Nodules may be fibroblastic, fibromuscular, muscular, hyperadenomatous, or fibroadenomatous

CLINICAL ISSUES

Presentation
- Most common signs/symptoms

- Urinary hesitancy, retention and frequency; nocturnal dribbling; poor urethral stream
- Symptom severity does not correlate strongly with size of gland on imaging
- Other signs/symptoms: Hydronephrosis
- Clinical Profile: Acute retention with bladder outlet obstruction (BOO); enlarged prostate on rectal exam; may have elevated prostate-specific antigen

Demographics
- Gender: Male

Natural History & Prognosis
- May progress to BOO, hydronephrosis if severe
- May lead to urinary infection, gross hematuria

Treatment
- Options, risks, complications
  - Open surgery for gland > 80 gm
  - Transurethral resection for smaller glands
  - Medical therapy with alpha-adrengeric blockers, finasteride for mild symptoms

DIAGNOSTIC CHECKLIST

Consider
- Prostate carcinoma
- Prostatitis

Image Interpretation Pearls
- Median lobe hypertrophy may simulate bladder mass

SELECTED REFERENCES
1. Trabulsi EJ et al: New imaging techniques in prostate cancer. Curr Urol Rep. 7(3):175-80, 2006
2. Tubaro A et al: Investigation of benign prostatic hyperplasia. Curr Opin Urol. 13(1):17-22, 2003
3. Grossfeld GD et al: Benign prostatic hyperplasia: clinical overview and value of diagnostic imaging. Radiol Clin North Am. 38(1):31-47, 2000
4. Aarnink RG et al: Aspects of imaging in the assessment and follow up of benign prostatic hyperplasia. Curr Opin Urol. 9(1):21-9, 1999
5. Geboers AD et al: Imaging in BPH patients. Arch Esp Urol. 47(9):857-64; discussion 864-5, 1994
6. Oyen RH et al: Benign hyperplastic nodules that originate in the peripheral zone of the prostate gland. Radiology. 189(3):707-11, 1993
7. Rifkin MD: MRI of the prostate. Crit Rev Diagn Imaging. 31(2):223-62, 1990
8. Shabsigh R et al: The role of transrectal ultrasonography in the diagnosis and management of prostatic and seminal vesicle cysts. J Urol. 141(5):1206-9, 1989
9. Cytron S et al: Value of transrectal ultrasonography for diagnosis and treatment of prostatic abscess. Urology. 32(5):454-8, 1988
10. Burks DD et al: Transrectal sonography of benign and malignant prostatic lesions. AJR Am J Roentgenol. 146(6):1187-91, 1986

PROSTATIC HYPERTROPHY

IMAGE GALLERY

Typical

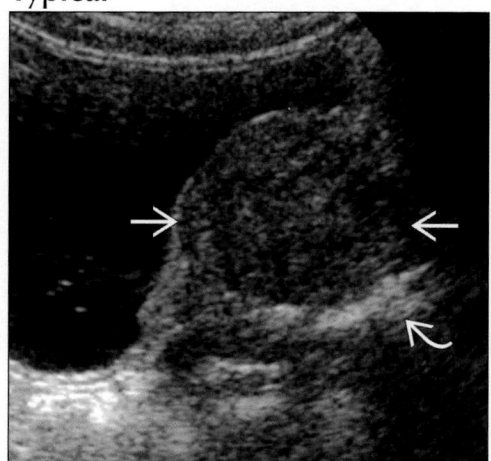
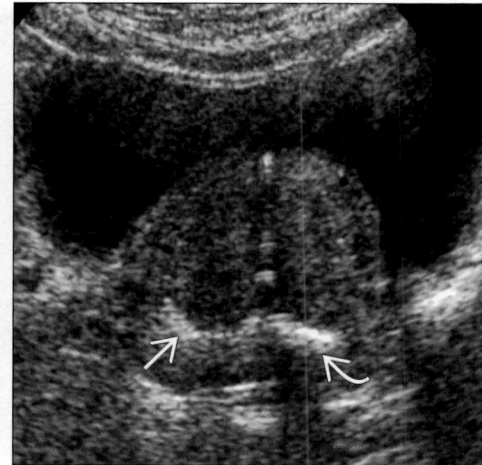

(Left) Longitudinal transabdominal ultrasound shows BPH ➡ abutting the bladder base without protrusion into the bladder. Note calcifications and corpora amylacea ➡ along the surgical capsule. *(Right)* Transverse transabdominal ultrasound shows BPH. Note clear delineation between the central and peripheral zones by echogenic corpora amylacea ➡ and calcification ➡.

Typical

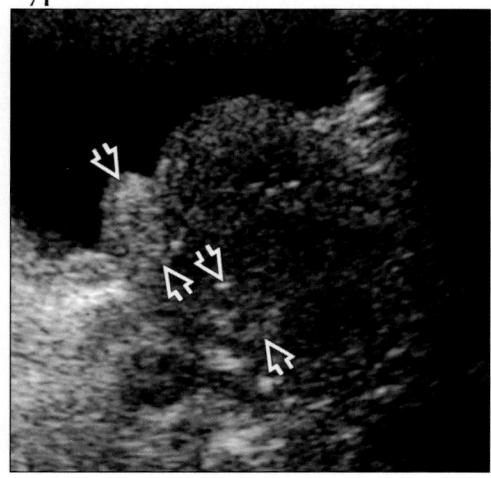
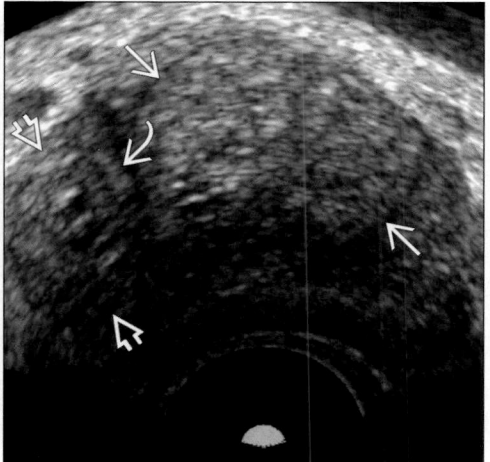

(Left) Longitudinal transabdominal ultrasound shows typical BPH with hyperechoic nodules ➡ seen in the peripheral lobe. Findings warrant TRUS ± biopsy and PSA correlation to exclude malignancy. *(Right)* Transverse TRUS shows asymmetric BPH with markedly enlarged left transition zone ➡ compared to the right ➡. Note the urethra ➡ is displaced to the right side by an enlarged left lobe.

Typical

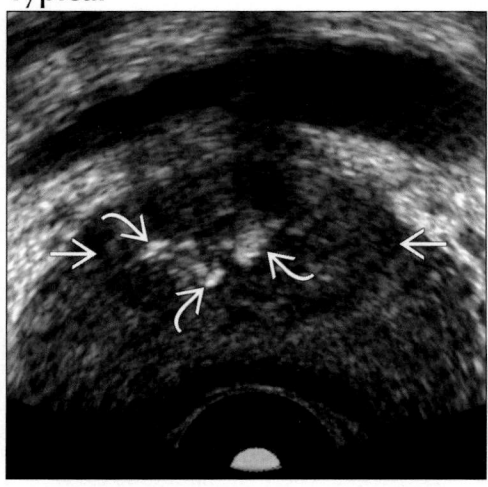
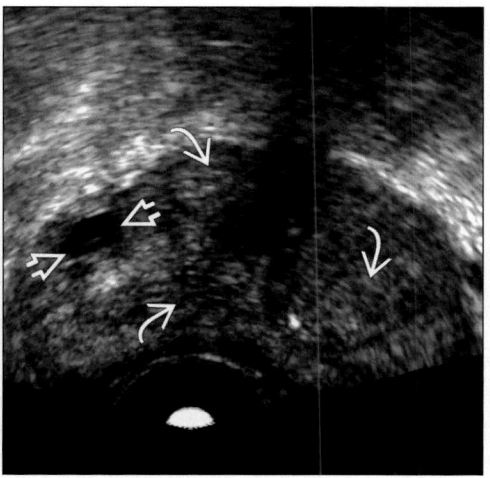

(Left) Transverse TRUS shows typical features of BPH with enlargement of the transition zone ➡ and calcifications ➡. Note the inner gland is relatively hypoechoic compared to the peripheral zone. *(Right)* Transverse TRUS shows BPH with a nodular echo pattern ➡. The small cyst ➡ in the right lobe probably represents a retention or degenerative cyst. The diagnosis is made by guided aspiration.

PROSTATIC CARCINOMA

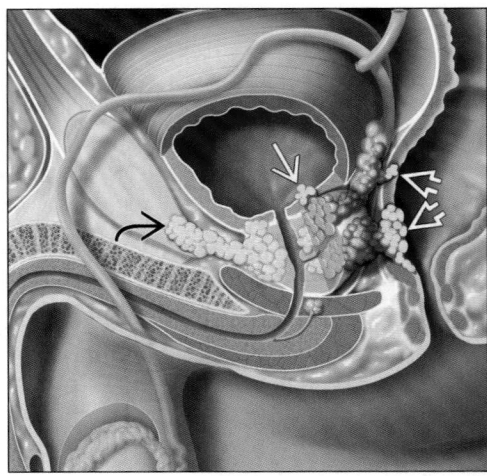

Longitudinal graphic shows advanced prostatic Ca with extracapsular spread to the adjacent pelvic structures such as the bladder ➡, rectal wall ➡ and symphysis pubis ➡.

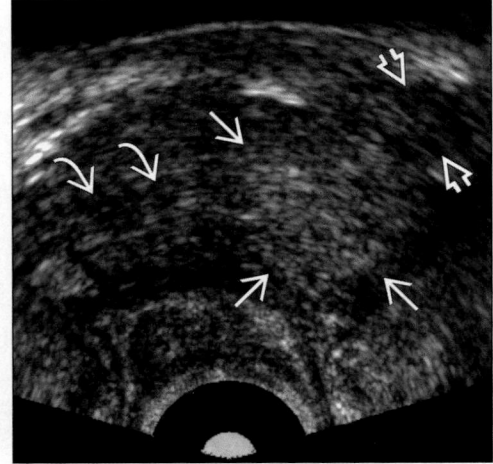

Transverse TRUS shows advanced prostatic Ca. A large, hyperechoic, lobulated mass ➡ arises from the left lobe with extracapsular extension ➡. Satellite lesions ➡ are noted in the right lobe.

TERMINOLOGY

Abbreviations and Synonyms
- Prostatic adenocarcinoma; prostatic glandular cancer

IMAGING FINDINGS

General Features
- Best diagnostic clue: Areas of increased vascularity shown by contrast enhanced imaging modalities
- Location
  - Peripheral zone (70%): Posterior region (most common)
  - Transition zone (20%), central (5%)
  - Typical bony metastases (pelvis & lower vertebrae)
- Other general features
  - Diagnosis of prostate cancer is suggested on basis of
    - Abnormal digital rectal examination (DRE), prostate specific antigen (PSA) level and transrectal ultrasonography (TRUS)
    - Confirmed at biopsy
  - Key factor affecting prognosis & treatment choice is whether there is extracapsular spread (ECS)

- Role of diagnostic imaging in prostate cancer remains unclear
- Prostatic Ca arises in prostatic peripheral zone in most patients and urinary obstruction is seen in advanced stage
- Imaging accuracy for local staging suboptimal
  - Better for advanced disease & metastases
- Spread: Hematogenous and lymphatic

Ultrasonographic Findings
- Grayscale Ultrasound
  - Transrectal approach is preferred to transabdominal approach for evaluation of prostatic carcinoma (Ca)
  - Primary role of ultrasound is for guidance of biopsy and therapy
  - Prostatic Ca can appear as hypoechoic (60-70%), hyperechoic (1-5%), isoechoic (30-40%) or diffuse lesions
  - Echogenicity of prostatic Ca depends on amount of stromal fibrosis
  - Most peripheral isoechoic lesions close to capsule cause asymmetric contour and bulging of lateral border

DDx: Mimics of Prostatic Ca

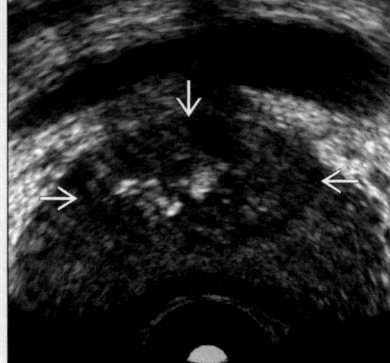

Benign Prostatic Hypertrophy

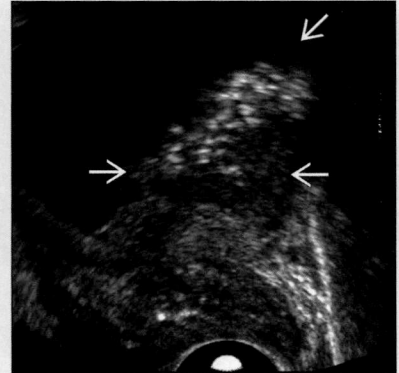

Bladder Ca

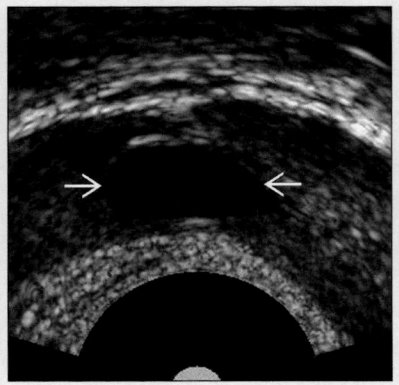

Prostatic Cyst

PROSTATIC CARCINOMA

Key Facts

Imaging Findings

- Peripheral zone (70%): Posterior region (most common)
- Transrectal approach is preferred to transabdominal approach for evaluation of prostatic carcinoma (Ca)
- Primary role of ultrasound is for guidance of biopsy and therapy
- Prostatic Ca can appear as hypoechoic (60-70%), hyperechoic (1-5%), isoechoic (30-40%) or diffuse lesions
- Echogenicity of prostatic Ca depends on amount of stromal fibrosis
- About 30% of prostatic Ca, not evident on ultrasound
- Isoechoic tumors identified by indirect signs: Areas of attenuation, glandular asymmetry, capsular distortion

- Benign prostatic cyst cannot be differentiated from cystic prostatic Ca on ultrasound, need biopsy for diagnosis
- Benign nodules related to prostatitis, BPH, atrophy and infarction can mimic prostatic Ca
- Prostatic Ca usually appears as hypervascular lesions, however, avascular lesions do not exclude Ca
- Color Doppler can be used to detect neovascularization around prostatic Ca, but is insensitive

Top Differential Diagnoses

- Benign Prostatic Hypertrophy (BPH)
- Bladder Carcinoma
- Prostatic Cysts
- Prostatitis

- About 30% of prostatic Ca, not evident on ultrasound
- Isoechoic tumors identified by indirect signs: Areas of attenuation, glandular asymmetry, capsular distortion
- Large, diffuse tumors tend to be more echogenic
- Benign prostatic cyst cannot be differentiated from cystic prostatic Ca on ultrasound, need biopsy for diagnosis
- Benign nodules related to prostatitis, BPH, atrophy and infarction can mimic prostatic Ca
- Color Doppler
  - Prostatic Ca usually appears as hypervascular lesions, however, avascular lesions do not exclude Ca
  - Prostatic vascularity is position-dependent
  - Color Doppler can be used to detect neovascularization around prostatic Ca, but is insensitive
  - Contrast-enhanced TRUS improves sensitivity but is of low specificity
- Power Doppler: No significant improvement to detect prostatic Ca compared to color Doppler imaging

CT Findings

- Not accurate in detection of cancer within prostate
- Signs of ECS
  - Obliteration of periprostatic fat plane
  - Abnormal enhancement of contiguous neurovascular bundle
  - Urinary bladder, rectal invasion
  - Lymphadenopathy

MR Findings

- Endorectal MR is complementary to TRUS and DRE for prostatic Ca localization
- Prostatic Ca is best seen on T2WI
  - Abnormal low signal in normally high signal peripheral zone
  - Signs of ECS
    - Obliteration of rectoprostatic angle & neurovascular bundle
    - Urinary bladder, rectal invasion well depicted
  - Osteoblastic bone metastases

- Low signal intensity on both T1WI & T2WI
- 3D MR spectroscopy (↑ choline & ↓ citrate levels) + endorectal MR imaging ↑ accuracy in detecting & staging of local + ECS of prostatic Ca
- T1 contrast-enhanced scan: Tumor foci & ECS are well depicted

Nuclear Medicine Findings

- PET: Increased uptake of FDG: Early detection of metastatic foci
- Bone Scan: Tc-99m methylene diphosphonate (MDP) bone scan detects osteoblastic metastases by ↑ uptake

Imaging Recommendations

- Best imaging tool
  - TRUS is method of choice for prostatic Ca evaluation and guided biopsy
  - Role of transabdominal ultrasound is limited to detecting abnormal prostatic echo pattern raising possibility of prostatic Ca
  - In patients with known prostatic Ca, it is useful in delineating extent and presence of local and regional metastases

---

DIFFERENTIAL DIAGNOSIS

Benign Prostatic Hypertrophy (BPH)

- Involves transition zone with enlargement
- Typical appearance is enlargement of inner gland which is hypoechoic relative to peripheral zone
- Cysts and calcifications may be found

Bladder Carcinoma

- Patients usually present with hematuria
- 90% are transitional cell carcinoma
- Bladder Ca in posterior wall near trigone may mimic BPH with enlarged median lobe or prostatic Ca with local invasion of bladder

Prostatic Cysts

- Cystic prostatic Ca though rare, can be confused with benign prostatic cysts on ultrasound
- Diagnosis made by biopsy

PROSTATIC CARCINOMA

Prostatitis
- Foci of infection in acute prostatitis can mimic prostatic Ca
- Chronic granulomatous prostatitis with diffuse large and small hypoechoic areas simulate prostatic Ca
- Increase glandular vascularity in prostatitis often produces confusing images suggestive of Ca

PATHOLOGY

General Features
- Etiology
  - Unknown
  - Advancing age, hormonal influence, environmental & genetic factors play a role in development
- Epidemiology
  - Second leading cause of non-skin cancer deaths in men following lung Ca
  - High risk in African-Americans, common in Caucasian and rare in Asians

Gross Pathologic & Surgical Features
- Growth: Usually more common in peripheral zone
  - Localized, diffuse or ECS
  - Firm or "gritty" as a result of fibrosis

Microscopic Features
- 95% of tumors are adenocarcinoma

Staging, Grading or Classification Criteria
- Jewett-Whitmore & TNM staging
  - A & T1: Clinically localized (tumor not palpable on digital rectal exam)
  - B & T2: Clinically localized (tumor palpable)
  - C & T3: Locally invasive beyond prostatic capsule (tumor palpable)
  - D & N/M: Lymph node & distant metastases (bones, lung, liver & brain)
- Gleason score (2-10) used to grade prostate tumors, score 10 being most abnormal

CLINICAL ISSUES

Presentation
- Most common signs/symptoms
  - Early: Asymptomatic, elevated PSA noticed incidentally
  - Urination: Hesitancy, urgency, increased frequency, pain and burning
  - Sexual dysfunction: Difficulty in erection, painful ejaculation, hematospermia
- Other signs/symptoms
  - Bone pain: Spine, pelvis, ribs due to metastasis
  - Limb weakness, urinary and fecal incontinence due to cord compression
  - Hydronephrosis due to outflow tract tumor obstruction
- Lab data
  - Increased PSA level > 4 ng/mL
    - Values 4-10 ng/ml also seen in BPH
- Diagnosis: Imaging findings & biopsy

Demographics
- Age: Adults above 40 years (risk ↑ with age)
- Gender: Male
- Ethnicity: African-Americans > Caucasians > Asians

Natural History & Prognosis
- Prognosis
  - After radical prostatectomy (for local cancer), life expectancy > 15 years
  - Radiation & hormonal therapy without surgery, life expectancy < 5 years
- Complications
  - Bladder outlet & rarely rectal obstruction
  - Obstructive uropathy, uremia, pathological fractures

Treatment
- Radical resection (for cancer confined to capsule)
- Radiation therapy (for cancer confined to capsule + outside capsule & localized spread)
- Hormonal therapy for metastases: Diethylstilbestrol & leuprolide; surgical orchiectomy
- Chemotherapy & cryosurgery

DIAGNOSTIC CHECKLIST

Consider
- Annual screening: PSA levels + DRE
- Findings abnormal: TRUS ± biopsy

Image Interpretation Pearls
- Areas of hypervascularity in prostate despite no discrete nodule seen on grayscale TRUS, suggestive of malignancy

SELECTED REFERENCES

1. Halpern EJ et al: Detection of prostate carcinoma with contrast-enhanced sonography using intermittent harmonic imaging. Cancer. 104(11):2373-83, 2005
2. Mullerad M et al: Comparison of endorectal magnetic resonance imaging, guided prostate biopsy and digital rectal examination in the preoperative anatomical localization of prostate cancer. J Urol. 174(6):2158-63, 2005
3. Pepe P et al: Does the adjunct of ecographic contrast medium Levovist improve the detection rate of prostate cancer? Prostate Cancer Prostatic Dis. 6(2):159-62, 2003
4. Halpern EJ et al: Prostate: high-frequency Doppler US imaging for cancer detection. Radiology. 225(1):71-7, 2002
5. Kurhanewicz J et al: The prostate: MR imaging and spectroscopy. Present and future. Radiol Clin North Am. 38(1):115-38, viii-ix, 2000
6. Presti JC Jr et al: Local staging of prostatic carcinoma: comparison of transrectal sonography and endorectal MR imaging. AJR Am J Roentgenol. 166(1):103-8, 1996
7. Mirowitz SA et al: Evaluation of the prostate and prostatic carcinoma with gadolinium-enhanced endorectal coil MR imaging. Radiology. 186(1):153-7, 1993
8. Hricak H et al: Prostatic carcinoma: staging by clinical assessment, CT, and MR imaging. Radiology. 162(2):331-6, 1987

PROSTATIC CARCINOMA

IMAGE GALLERY

Typical

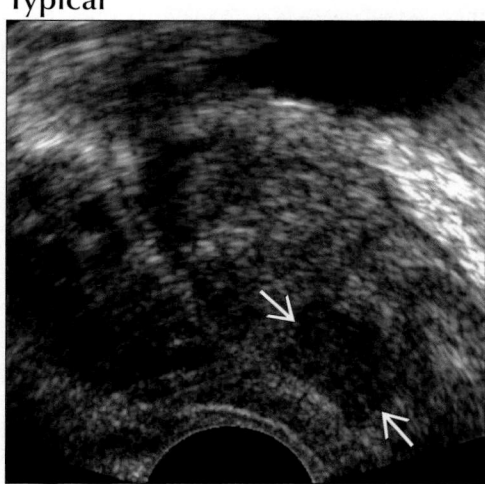 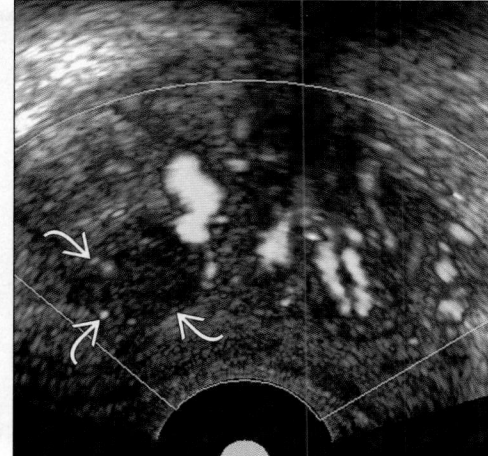

(Left) Longitudinal TRUS shows a hypoechoic lesion in the right peripheral zone typical of prostatic Ca ➡. About 70% of prostatic Ca occur in the peripheral zone. *(Right)* Transverse power Doppler ultrasound TRUS (same patient as in previous image) shows neovascularization ➡ around the mass. Increased vascularity of the left lobe may be due to its dependent position.

Typical

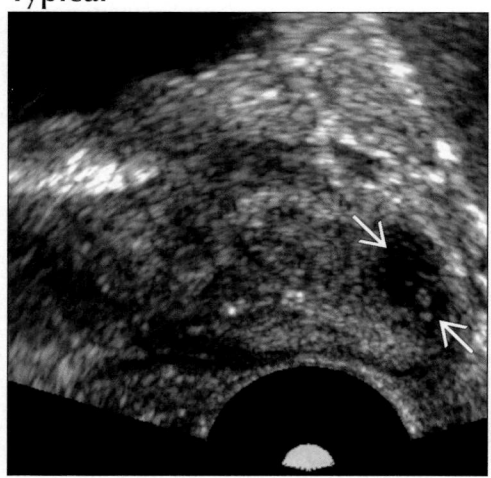 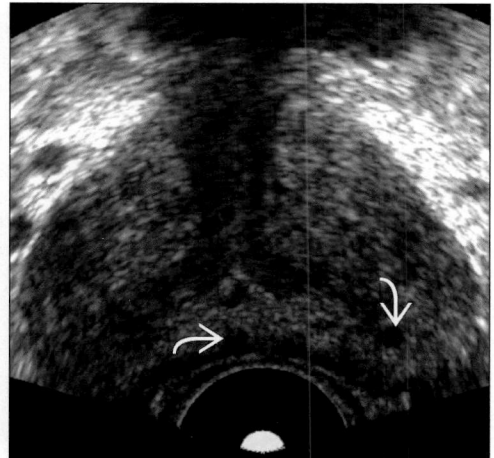

(Left) Longitudinal TRUS shows a small, hypoechoic lesion ➡ in the peripheral zone. Biopsy showed Ca. Note benign nodules related to prostatitis, BPH, atrophy and infarction may mimic prostatic Ca. *(Right)* Transverse TRUS shows a mildly enlarged prostate with small, hypoechoic lesions ➡ in the peripheral zone. The PSA level was elevated (14.2 ng/mL). Biopsy of lesions confirmed Ca.

Typical

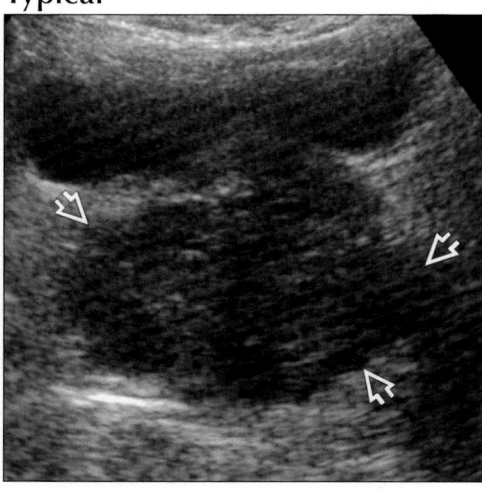 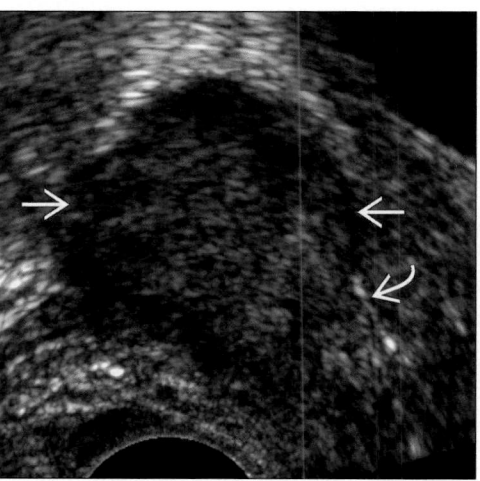

(Left) Transverse transabdominal ultrasound shows a irregularly enlarged prostate in a patient with an elevated PSA level. Findings are suspicious for prostate Ca with ECS. Note lobulated margin of the gland ➡. *(Right)* Longitudinal TRUS shows an irregular, heterogeneous prostatic Ca ➡ compressing the proximal urethra ➡. Compression causes dysuria which is a common complication of prostatic Ca.

DIFFUSE BLADDER WALL THICKENING

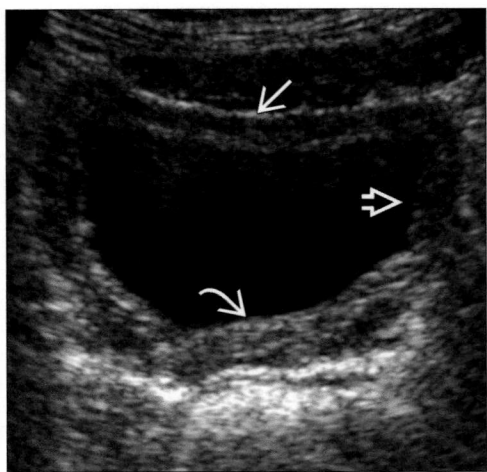

Transverse ultrasound shows diffuse, smooth thickening of the anterior ➡, lateral ⇨ and posterior ↪ walls of the urinary bladder.

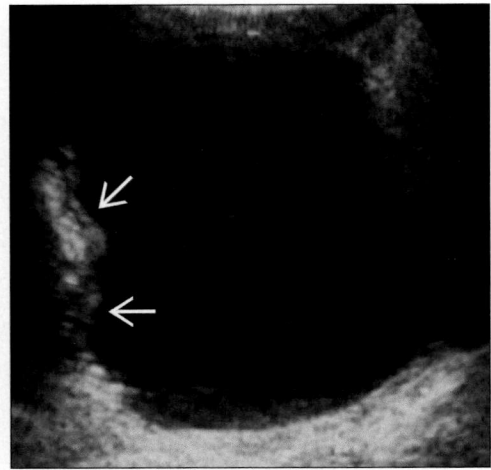

Transverse transabdominal ultrasound shows wall thickening and an irregular inner bladder surface (trabeculations) ➡ in a neurogenic bladder.

TERMINOLOGY

Definitions
- Abnormal thickening of the bladder wall

IMAGING FINDINGS

General Features
- Location: Usually involves entire bladder wall, but may be focal
- Morphology: Contracted and small volume bladder in chronic disease

Ultrasonographic Findings
- Grayscale Ultrasound
  - Diffuse bladder wall thickening
  - Trabeculation: Irregular outline of inner bladder wall
  - +/- Focal pseudopolyp which are indistinguishable from tumor
  - Intraluminal gas and intramural gas in emphysematous cystitis
    - Echogenic foci with ring-down artifact within bladder wall
  - Cysts or solid papillary mass in chronic cystitis indistinguishable from tumor
  - Non-dependent linear echogenic focus with distal shadowing if complicated with fistula
  - Echogenic mobile blood clots if hemorrhagic cystitis
- Color Doppler
  - Neoplastic cause: Vascularity of tumor may be demonstrated
  - Infectious/inflammatory: Vascularity seen in adjacent soft tissues

Radiographic Findings
- Radiography
  - TB, schistosomiasis: Bladder wall calcifications
  - +/- Bladder stone
  - Emphysematous cystitis: Translucent ring of air bubbles in bladder wall
- IVP
  - Acute cystitis: Usually normal bladder, therefore insensitive for detection
  - Acute: Thickened, coarse mucosal folds with cobblestone appearance
  - Chronic: Contracted, irregular thick-walled bladder
  - Neurogenic bladder: Christmas tree shaped bladder

DDx: Bladder Wall Thickening

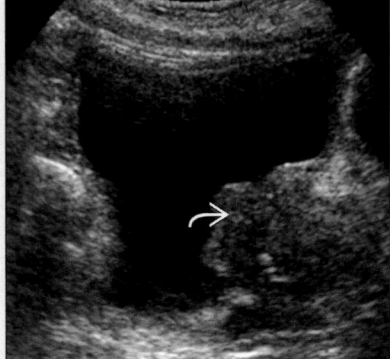

Benign Prostatic Hypertrophy

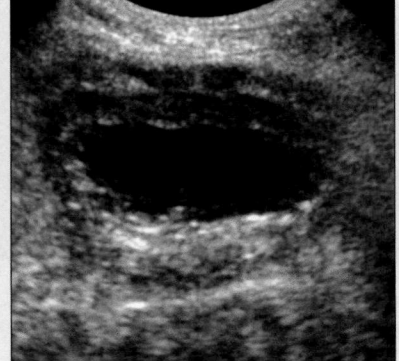

Under-Filled Bladder

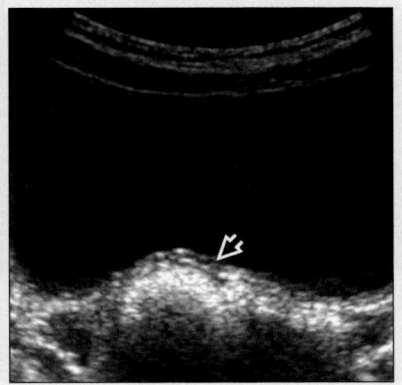

Normal Trigone

DIFFUSE BLADDER WALL THICKENING

Key Facts

Imaging Findings
- Diffuse bladder wall thickening
- Trabeculation: Irregular outline of inner bladder wall
- +/- Focal pseudopolyp which are indistinguishable from tumor
- Intraluminal gas and intramural gas in emphysematous cystitis
- Echogenic foci with ring-down artifact within bladder wall
- Cysts or solid papillary mass in chronic cystitis indistinguishable from tumor
- Non-dependent linear echogenic focus with distal shadowing if complicated with fistula
- Echogenic mobile blood clots if hemorrhagic cystitis
- Neoplastic cause: Vascularity of tumor may be demonstrated

- Infectious/inflammatory: Vascularity seen in adjacent soft tissues

Top Differential Diagnoses
- Benign Prostatic Hypertrophy (BPH)
- Under-Filled Bladder
- Bladder Trigone

Diagnostic Checklist
- Primary bladder tumor if predominantly focal bladder wall thickening
- Tuberculosis if bladder of small volume and thick-walled but patient has subjective feeling of full bladder
- Malignant change in schistosomiasis if irregularity of surface
- Gas in bladder wall always secondary to infection

CT Findings
- CECT
  - Bladder wall thickening +/- hypodense wall
  - Emphysematous cystitis: Gas in bladder wall +/- lumen
  - Infiltrating tumor: Enhancing soft tissue mass, extending to extravesical fat; lack of tissue plane with adjacent structures, such as rectum, uterus/cervix

DIFFERENTIAL DIAGNOSIS

Benign Prostatic Hypertrophy (BPH)
- Simulates tumor at bladder base
- Differentiate by transrectal US

Under-Filled Bladder
- Bladder wall thickness returns to normal when bladder distends

Bladder Trigone
- Normal structure of bladder, focal thickening between the inter-ureteric ridge

PATHOLOGY

General Features
- Etiology
  - Infectious/Inflammatory: Usually smooth thickening
    - Bacterial: Transurethral invasion of bladder by perineal flora in sexually active women
    - Bacterial: Bladder outlet obstruction and urinary stasis in men
    - Tuberculosis: Descending infection from kidney
    - Schistosomiasis: Inflammatory response to ova deposited in bladder
    - Emphysematous: E. coli, aerobacter aerogenes or candida infection, related to hyperglycemia
    - Other infectious agent: Viral, fungal (candida)
    - Alkaline encrustation: Infection by urea-splitting organism → alkaline urine and focal necrosis → dystrophic calcification
    - Mechanical: Local irritation from prolonged catheterization, stone, foreign body, etc.
    - Drug induced: Cyclophosphamide, in 15% patients within first year treatment; caused by breakdown products
    - Radiation-induced
  - Medical disease
    - Intersitial cystitis = pancystitis causing urgency and frequency; post-menopausal female
    - Amyloidosis
    - Systemic lupus erythematosus
  - Neurogenic bladder: Typical "Christmas tree" shape
    - Detrusor hyperreflexia: Gross trabeculation and abnormal shape
  - Chronic bladder outlet obstruction: Trabeculated bladder
    - Muscular hypertrophy leading to irregular outline of inner bladder wall (trabeculation)
  - Neoplasm: More common focal bladder wall thickening, frondlike projection, polypoidal or broad based
    - Transitional cell carcinoma 95%
    - Squamous cell carcinoma
    - Adenocarcinoma
  - Invasion by adjacent tumors and disease
    - Common tumors: Rectal CA, prostatic CA in male, uterus/cervical CA in female
    - Crohn disease: Inflamed bowel or fistula formation
    - Endometriosis
- Associated abnormalities
  - Chronic cystitis: Decreased bladder capacity and vesicoureteric reflux
  - Chronic cystitis: Other complications
    - Hyperplastic uroepithelial cell clusters (Brunn nests) form in bladder submucosa
    - Fluid accumulation → pseudocysts = cystitis cystica, potentially malignant
    - Transformation into gland: Cystitis glandularis

- Recurrent bacterial infection: Malakoplakia
  - Associated with E. coli infection
  - Granulomatous inflammatory process
  - Caused by deficient function of lysosomes in macrophages
- Schistosomiasis: Squamous cell carcinoma of bladder

Gross Pathologic & Surgical Features

- Cystitis: Smooth thickening of bladder wall = erythema of bladder mucosa; small excrescences in severe case = ulceration, petechiae
- Chronic tuberculosis: Small bladder volume, +/- mid ureteric stricture, isolated calyceal dilatation and calcification
- Chronic schistosomiasis: Polypoidal extension into bladder +/- ureteric stricture
- Emphysematous: Gas within bladder mucosa or in bladder lumen
- Interstitial cystitis: Pink pseudoulceration of bladder mucosa, characteristically at vertex of bladder = Hunner ulcer
- Squamous metaplasia: Transformation of urothelium into keratin producing squamous cells
  - May see white patches (leukoplakia) on foci of squamous metaplasia

CLINICAL ISSUES

Presentation

- Most common signs/symptoms: Dysuria, frequency, urgency
- Other signs/symptoms
  - Gross hematuria, pyuria, bacteriuria
  - Infiltrating tumor: Symptoms of primary site, such as change of bowel habit, weight loss in rectal CA

Demographics

- Gender: Bacterial cystitis: M < F due to short urethra

Natural History & Prognosis

- Bladder wall appears normal in early stages of inflammatory disease
- Bladder wall becomes diffusely or non-diffusely hypoechoic, thickened as inflammation duration increases
- Bladder wall becomes fibrotic and scarred as inflammatory process progresses

Treatment

- Infectious cystitis: Usually respond to antibiotics or corresponding anti-organism agent

DIAGNOSTIC CHECKLIST

Consider

- Invasion by adjacent tumors or inflammatory disease if abnormal area of bladder continues with primary tumor or disease process
- Primary bladder tumor if predominantly focal bladder wall thickening
- Nodular bladder wall thickening in cystitis may mimic bladder carcinoma

- Tuberculosis if bladder of small volume and thick-walled but patient has subjective feeling of full bladder
- Malignant change in schistosomiasis if irregularity of surface

Image Interpretation Pearls

- Schistosomiasis progresses proximally; TB progresses distally
- Gas in bladder wall always secondary to infection

SELECTED REFERENCES

1. Lee G et al: Case report: cystitis glandularis mimics bladder tumour: a case report and diagnostic characteristics. Int Urol Nephrol. 37(4):713-5, 2005
2. Barese CN et al: Recurrent eosinophilic cystitis in a child with chronic granulomatous disease. J Pediatr Hematol Oncol. 26(3):209-12, 2004
3. Pavlica P et al: Sonography of the bladder. World J Urol. 22(5):328-34, 2004
4. Choong KK: Sonographic detection of emphysematous cystitis. J Ultrasound Med. 22(8):847-9, 2003
5. Huang WC et al: Sonographic findings in a case of postradiation hemorrhagic cystitis resolved by hyperbaric oxygen therapy. J Ultrasound Med. 22(9):967-71, 2003
6. Wise GJ et al: Genitourinary manifestations of tuberculosis. Urol Clin North Am. 30(1):111-21, 2003
7. Thoumas D et al: Imaging characteristics of alkaline-encrusted cystitis and pyelitis. AJR Am J Roentgenol. 178(2):389-92, 2002
8. Gomes CM et al: Significance of hematuria in patients with interstitial cystitis: review of radiographic and endoscopic findings. Urology. 57(2):262-5, 2001
9. Goodman TR et al: Eosinophilic cystitis following an infected urachal remnant. Pediatr Radiol. 29(6):487-8, 1999
10. Eschwege P et al: Imaging analysis of encrusted cystitis and pyelitis in renal transplantation. Transplant Proc. 27(4):2444-5, 1995
11. Roy C et al: Alkaline-encrusted cystitis: imaging findings. AJR Am J Roentgenol. 164(3):769, 1995
12. Djavan B et al: Bladder ultrasonography. Semin Urol. 12(4):306-19, 1994
13. Leibovitch I et al: Ultrasonographic detection and control of eosinophilic cystitis. Abdom Imaging. 19(3):270-1, 1994
14. Rosenberg HK et al: Benign cystitis in children mimicking rhabdomyosarcoma. J Ultrasound Med. 13(12):921-32, 1994
15. Cartoni C et al: Role of ultrasonography in the diagnosis and follow-up of hemorrhagic cystitis after bone marrow transplantation. Bone Marrow Transplant. 12(5):463-7, 1993
16. Friedman EP et al: Pseudotumoral cystitis in children: a review of the ultrasound features in four cases. Br J Radiol. 66(787):605-8, 1993
17. Kumar A et al: The sonographic appearance of cyclophosphamide-induced acute haemorrhagic cystitis. Clin Radiol. 41(4):289-90, 1990
18. Hassel DR et al: Granulomatous cystitis in chronic granulomatous disease: ultrasound diagnosis. Pediatr Radiol. 17(3):254-5, 1987
19. Doehring E et al: Reversibility of urinary tract abnormalities due to Schistosoma haematobium infection. Kidney Int. 30(4):582-5, 1986
20. Gooding GA: Varied sonographic manifestations of cystitis. J Ultrasound Med. 5(2):61-3, 1986
21. Manco LG: Cystitis cystica simulating bladder tumor at sonography. J Clin Ultrasound. 13(1):52-4, 1985

DIFFUSE BLADDER WALL THICKENING

Typical

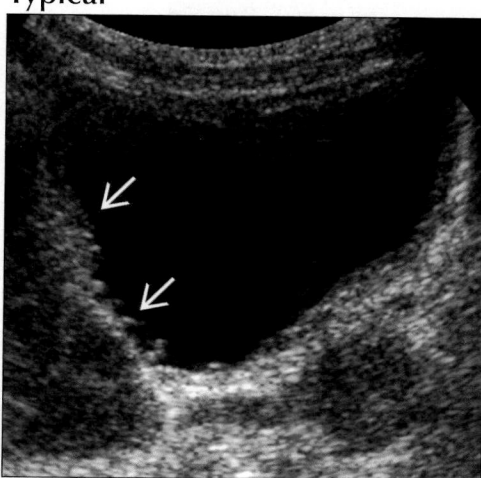
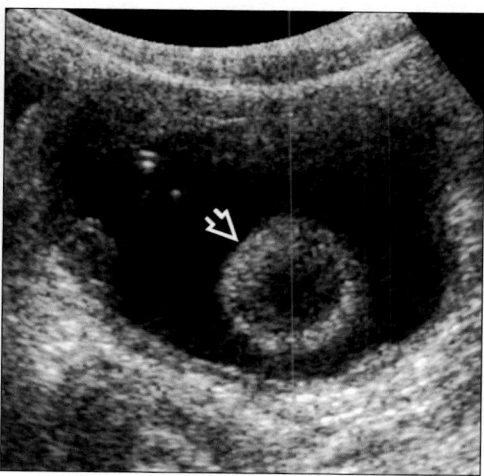

(Left) Transverse transabdominal ultrasound shows an irregular inner bladder outline compatible with trabeculations ➡ in a patient with chronic outflow obstruction. *(Right)* Transverse transabdominal ultrasound shows a diffuse bladder wall thickening and fungal ball ➡ within the bladder of a patient with fungal cystitis.

Typical

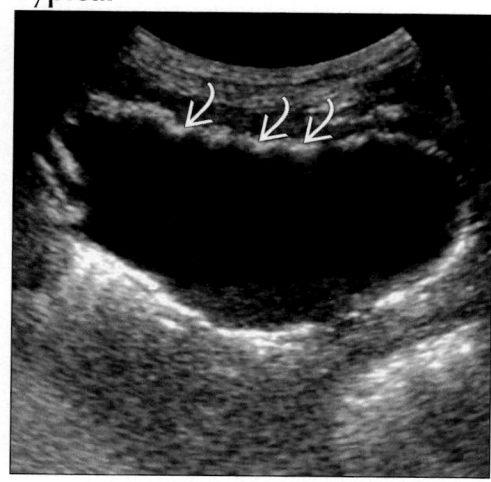
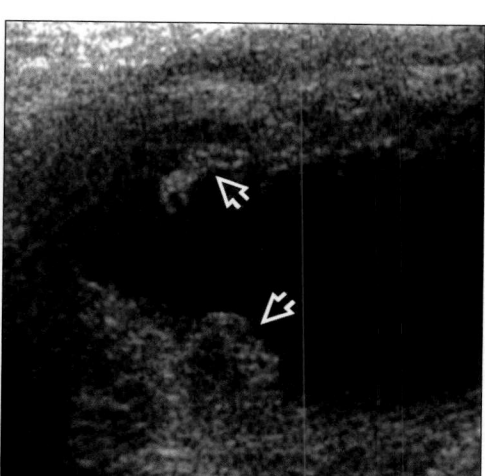

(Left) Longitudinal transabdominal ultrasound in a patient with emphysematous cystitis shows intramural gas as echogenic foci ➡ with ring-down artifact. Also note markedly thickened bladder wall. *(Right)* Oblique transabdominal ultrasound shows small excrescences ➡ in a patient with severe cystitis.

Typical

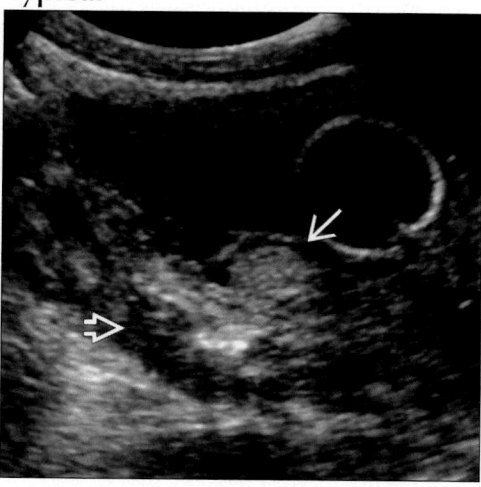
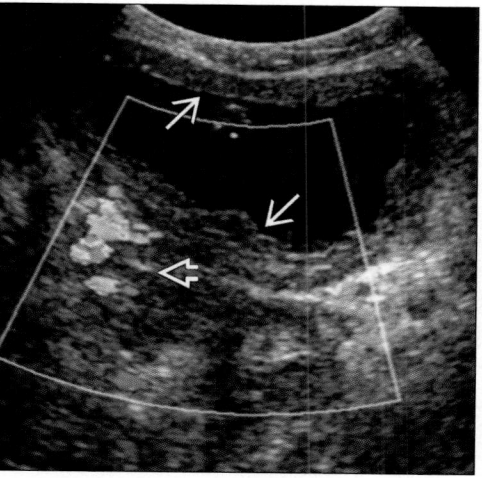

(Left) Oblique transabdominal ultrasound shows bladder wall thickening ➡ due to invasion by adjacent rectal cancer ➡. *(Right)* Longitudinal color Doppler ultrasound shows diffuse bladder wall thickening ➡ due to uterine cancer. Increased vascularity is present in the tumor tissue ➡.

5

127

BLADDER CARCINOMA

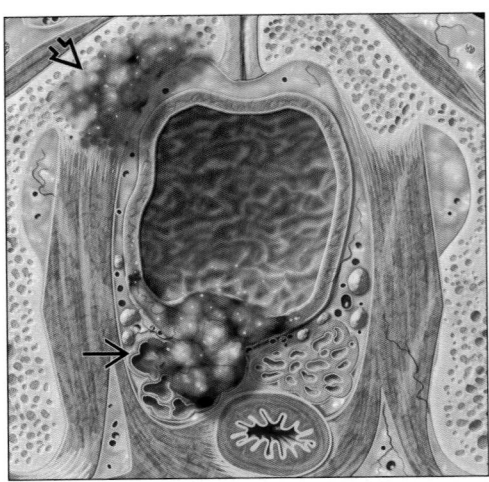

Graphic shows an irregular bladder tumor infiltrating beyond the muscular layer of the bladder wall into the right seminal vesicle ➡. There is a hematogenous metastasis to the right pubic symphysis ▷.

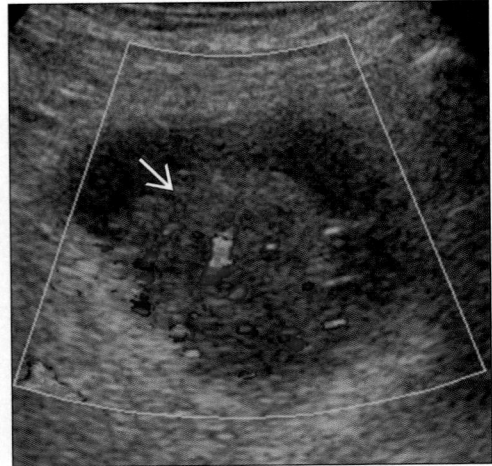

Transverse color Doppler ultrasound shows a large, immobile soft tissue tumor ➡ at the base of the urinary bladder with characteristic intralesional vascularity.

TERMINOLOGY

Definitions
- Malignant tumor growth within bladder

IMAGING FINDINGS

General Features
- Best diagnostic clue: Bladder wall invasion by intraluminal soft tissue mass on CT or MR

Ultrasonographic Findings
- Focal non-mobile mass in bladder, of mixed echogenicity, without acoustic shadowing
- May present as focal bladder wall thickening
- Diverticular tumor appears as moderately echogenic non-shadowing mass
- Color Doppler shows increased vascularity in large tumor
- Reported sensitivities range from 50-95%
- US plays an important role in detection of tumor arising from bladder diverticulum
  - Tumor inaccessible by cystoscopy due to narrow neck of diverticulum
  - Periureteric and posterolateral wall location of most bladder diverticula allow for adequate sonographic visualization
- Tumors near bladder base in male may be confused with prostatic enlargement
  - Transrectal ultrasound differentiates bladder tumors from prostatic lesion
  - Bladder tumors and prostatic enlargement often co-exist and bladder tumors may invade prostate
- Transvaginal or transrectal US: To assess a bladder wall mass if suprapubic visualization is poor
  - Poor transabdominal visualization may be due to obesity, scars on wall and poor bladder distension
- Transurethral US: To stage tumor confined to bladder wall and detect tumors in diverticulum
  - Monitoring distensibility of bladder wall and transurethral resection of disease
  - Disadvantages: Invasive, requires anesthesia
  - Limitations: Unable to discriminate between tumor stages and to detect involvement of pelvic lymph nodes

DDx: Bladder Carcinoma

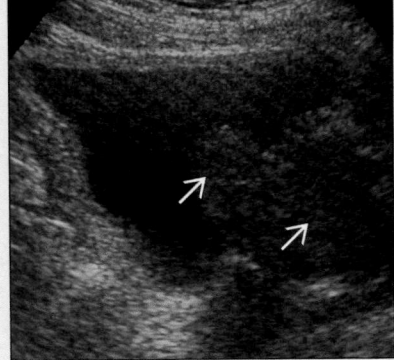

Benign Prostate Hypertrophy

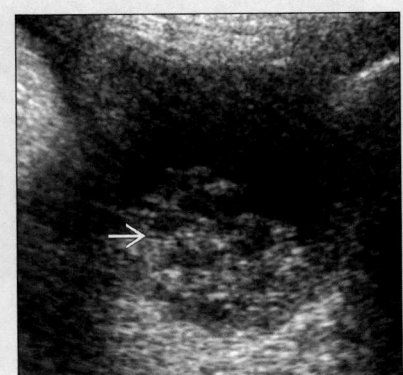

Bladder Sludge

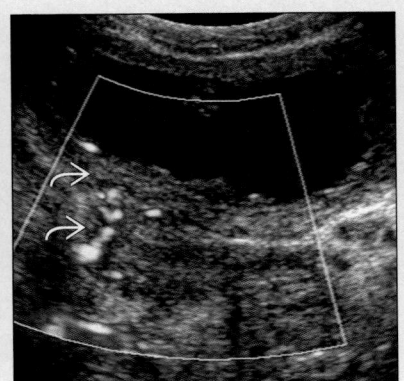

Extrinsic Tumor

BLADDER CARCINOMA

Key Facts

Imaging Findings
- Focal non-mobile mass in bladder, of mixed echogenicity, without acoustic shadowing
- Diverticular tumor appears as moderately echogenic non-shadowing mass
- Color Doppler shows increased vascularity in large tumor
- US plays an important role in detection of tumor arising from bladder diverticulum
- Transrectal ultrasound differentiates bladder tumors from prostatic lesion
- Bladder tumors and prostatic enlargement often co-exist and bladder tumors may invade prostate
- Transurethral US: To stage tumor confined to bladder wall and detect tumors in diverticulum

- Recent advances: 3D US rendering may help to discriminate between superficial stages < pT1 and muscle invasive carcinoma > pT1

Top Differential Diagnoses
- Benign Prostatic Hypertrophy (BPH)
- Bladder Sludge/Blood Clot
- Extrinsic Tumor

Diagnostic Checklist
- US detected immobile soft tissue mass in bladder
- Distinction of benign from malignant tumor by cystoscopy ± biopsy
- CT/MR used for staging for treatment and prognosis
- Check kidneys, ureters for synchronous and metachronous tumors

- Recent advances: 3D US rendering may help to discriminate between superficial stages < pT1 and muscle invasive carcinoma > pT1

Radiographic Findings
- IVP
  - Multifocal (2-3% of urothelial cancers)
  - Punctate or speckled calcification on fronds of villous, papillary tumors (en face view)
  - Linear or curvilinear calcification on surface of sessile tumors
  - Central calcification (necrosis)
  - Nonspecific filling defects within bladder
- Cystography
  - ± Bladder diverticulum (2-10% contain neoplasm)

CT Findings
- Sessile or pedunculated soft tissue mass projecting into lumen; similar density to bladder wall
- ± Enlarged (> 10 mm) metastatic lymph nodes; extravesical tumor extension
- Fine punctate calcification in tumor; may suggest mucinous adenocarcinoma
- Ring pattern of calcification; may suggest pheochromocytoma
- Inability to distinguish tumors from bladder wall hypertrophy, local inflammation and fibrosis
- Unable to differentiate Ta-T3a, invasion of dome/base of bladder or local organ (due to partial volume effect), non enlarged lymph nodes
- Urachal adenocarcinoma
  - Midline abdominal mass ± calcification
  - Solitary lobulated tumor arising from dome of bladder on ventral surface

MR Findings
- T1WI
  - Tumor has intermediate signal intensity, equal to muscle layer of bladder wall
  - Infiltration of perivesical fat (high signal intensity)
  - Endoluminal tumor in urine filled bladder (low signal intensity)

  - Bone marrow metastases; similar signal intensity as primary tumor
- T2WI
  - Tumor has intermediate signal intensity, higher than bladder wall or fibrosis, lower than urine
  - Determine tumor infiltration of perivesical fat (either low or high signal intensity)
  - Invasion of prostate, rectum, uterus, vagina ⇒ ↑ signal intensity
  - Direct invasion of seminal vesicles (sagittal plane) ⇒ ↑ size, ↓ signal intensity & obliteration of angle between seminal vesicle & posterior bladder wall
  - Confirm bone marrow metastases
- T1 C+
  - Mild enhancement in primary, perivesical, nodal or bone invasion
  - Tumor shows earlier than & ↑ enhancement than bladder wall or other benign tissues; assess infiltration
  - Earlier enhancement than edema and granulation tissue
- ± Enlarged (> 10 mm) metastatic lymph nodes
- Unable to differentiate stage T1 from stage T2, acute edema or hyperemia from first week post-biopsy or non enlarged lymph nodes
- Urachal adenocarcinoma
  - Varied appearance
  - T2WI: Increased signal intensity

Imaging Recommendations
- Best imaging tool
  - US: Useful for bladder tumor screening in patients with schistosomiasis, tumor within diverticulum
  - IVP: Screening upper urinary tract
  - MR: Staging bladder carcinoma
    - Accuracy 73-96% (10-33% more accurate than CT)

DIFFERENTIAL DIAGNOSIS

Benign Prostatic Hypertrophy (BPH)
- Enlarged median lobe of prostate may appear as an irregular mass lying free within bladder in some planes

BLADDER CARCINOMA

- On angling transducer caudad, enlarged prostatic median lobe can be shown to be part of prostate gland

Bladder Sludge/Blood Clot
- Mobile mass, does not cast acoustic shadow

Extrinsic Tumor
- Rectal, ovarian, vaginal tumor or fibroids overlying bladder; may simulate bladder carcinoma

Bladder Inflammation
- Cystitis may cause mural thickening and hemorrhage

PATHOLOGY

General Features
- General path comments
  - 95% of bladder neoplasms are malignant
  - Types of epithelial bladder carcinoma
    - Transitional cell carcinoma (90-95%)
    - Squamous cell carcinoma (5%)
    - Adenocarcinoma (2%): Urachal origin, secondary to cystitis glandularis, secondary to extrophy
    - Carcinosarcoma
    - Other rare tumors: Carcinoid, rhabdoid, villous, small cell
    - Metastasis: Gastrointestinal tract, melanoma
  - Types of nonepithelial bladder carcinoma
    - Pheochromocytoma
    - Leiomyosarcoma
    - Embryonal rhabdomyosarcoma (most common bladder neoplasm in children)
    - Lymphoma
    - Plasmacytoma
- Etiology
  - Aromatic amines, nitrosamines, aldehydes (e.g., acrolein)
  - Risk factors
    - Environment: Smoking
    - Infection: Schistosomiasis, chronic cystitis
    - Iatrogenic: Cyclophosphamide, radiation therapy
    - Occupation: Chemical, dye (e.g., aniline dye), rubber and textile industries

Gross Pathologic & Surgical Features
- Superficial and are usually papillary (66%)
- Infiltrating in/beyond muscular layer of wall (33%)

Staging, Grading or Classification Criteria
- TNM classification of bladder carcinoma
  - T0: No tumor
  - Tis: Carcinoma in situ
  - Ta: Papillary tumor confined to mucosa (epithelium)
  - T1: Invasion of lamina propria (subepithelial connective tissue)
  - T2: Invasion of inner half of muscle (detrusor)
  - T2b: Invasion of outer half of muscle
  - T3a: Microscopic invasion of perivesical fat
  - T3b: Macroscopic invasion of perivesical fat
  - T4a: Invasion of surrounding organs
  - T4b: Invasion of pelvic or abdominal wall
  - N1-3: Pelvic lymph node metastases
  - N4: Lymph node metastases above bifurcation

  - M1: Distant metastases

CLINICAL ISSUES

Presentation
- Most common signs/symptoms: Painless hematuria

Demographics
- Age
  - 50-60 years of age
  - Increasing incidence in patients < 30 years of age
- Gender: M:F = 4:1
- Ethnicity: Caucasian-to-African-American ratio: 1.5:1

Natural History & Prognosis
- Complications
  - Hydronephrosis, incontinence & urethral stricture
- Prognosis
  - 5 year survival rate: 82% in all stages combined
    - 94% in localized stages
    - 48% in regional stages
    - 6% in distant stages

Treatment
- < T2: Local endoscopic resection ± intravesical instillation or bacille Calmette-Guérin therapy
- T2 to T4a: Radical cystectomy or radiotherapy (cure)
- > T4b: Chemotherapy or radiotherapy ± adjuvant surgery (palliative)

DIAGNOSTIC CHECKLIST

Consider
- US detected immobile soft tissue mass in bladder
- Distinction of benign from malignant tumor by cystoscopy ± biopsy
- CT/MR used for staging for treatment and prognosis
- Check kidneys, ureters for synchronous and metachronous tumors

Image Interpretation Pearls
- Transrectal ultrasound may differentiate bladder tumors from prostatic lesion
- MR is superior in staging and used in patients with high grade stage T1 or > stage T2

SELECTED REFERENCES

1. Tekes A et al: Dynamic MRI of bladder cancer: evaluation of staging accuracy. AJR Am J Roentgenol. 184(1):121-7, 2005
2. Wagner B et al: Staging bladder carcinoma by three-dimensional ultrasound rendering. Ultrasound Med Biol. 31(3):301-5, 2005
3. Koraitim M et al: Transurethral ultrasonographic assessment of bladder carcinoma: its value and limitation. J Urol. 154(2 Pt 1):375-8, 1995
4. Kim B et al: Bladder tumor staging: comparison of contrast-enhanced CT, T1- and T2-weighted MR imaging, dynamic gadolinium-enhanced imaging, and late gadolinium-enhanced imaging. Radiology. 193(1):239-45, 1994

IMAGE GALLERY

Typical

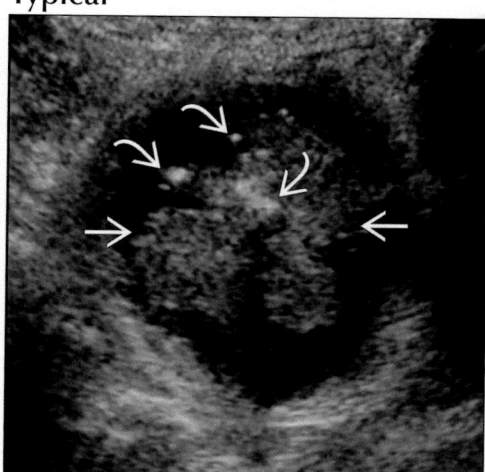
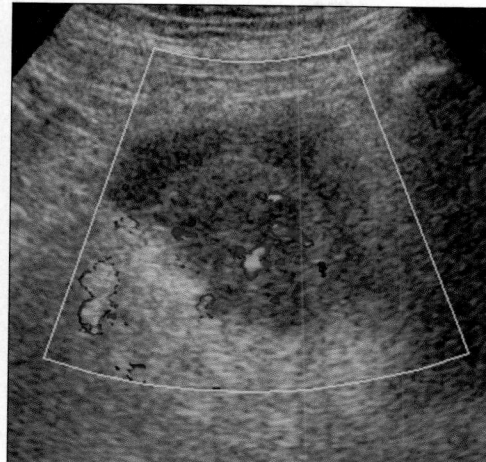

(Left) Longitudinal transabdominal ultrasound shows an irregular, intravesicular polypoid mass ➡ resembling a "cauliflower" arising from the right lateral bladder wall. Punctate calcifications are present within the tumor ➡. (Right) Transverse color Doppler ultrasound shows increased vascularity within this tumor.

Typical

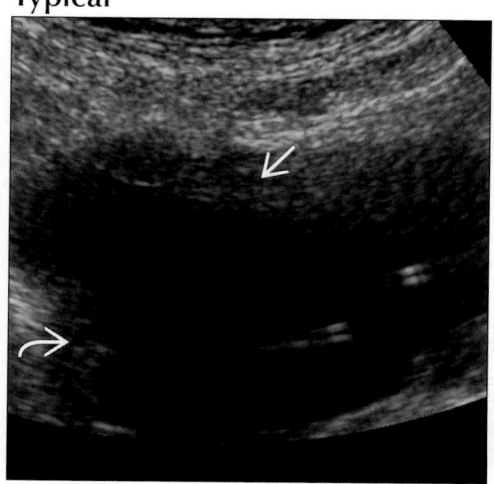
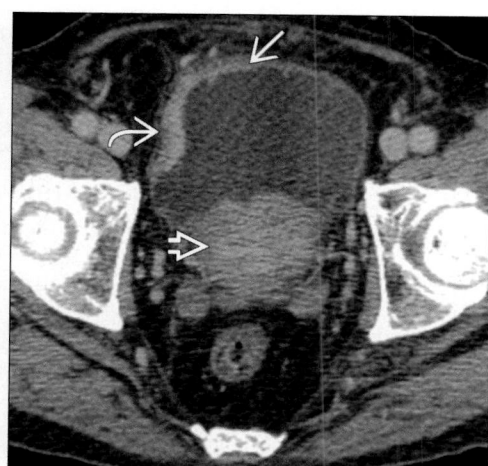

(Left) Transverse transabdominal ultrasound shows biopsy proven bladder cancer seen as focal areas of wall thickening over the lateral ➡ and anterior wall ➡ of the urinary bladder. (Right) Transverse CECT corresponding to previous image shows the lateral ➡ and anterior wall ➡ thickening of the bladder. Note benign hypertrophy of the prostate ➡ at the base of the urinary bladder.

Typical

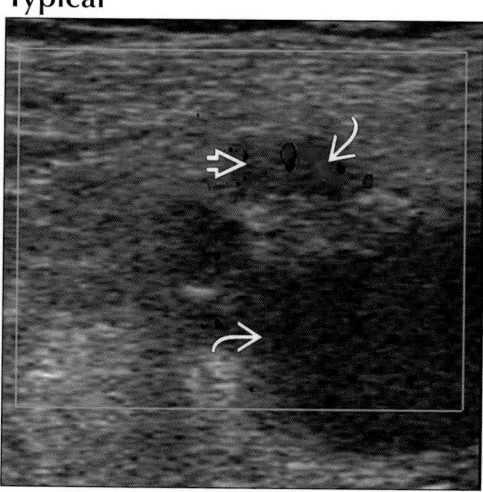
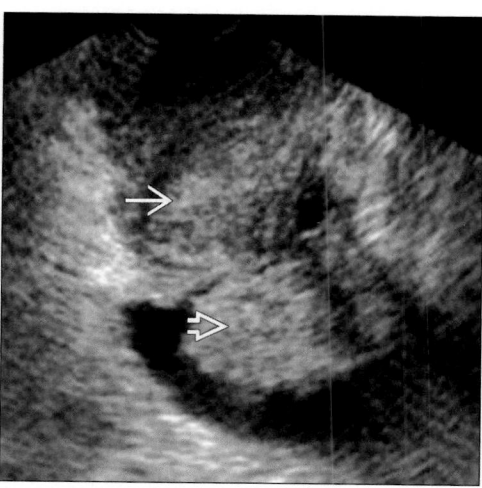

(Left) Transverse color Doppler ultrasound shows a vascular soft tissue mass ➡ within a diverticulum ➡, confirmed to be cancer on histology. (Right) Transrectal US shows a fungating tumor ➡ arising from the bladder base. Note its relationship to the adjacent prostate gland ➡.

URETEROCELE

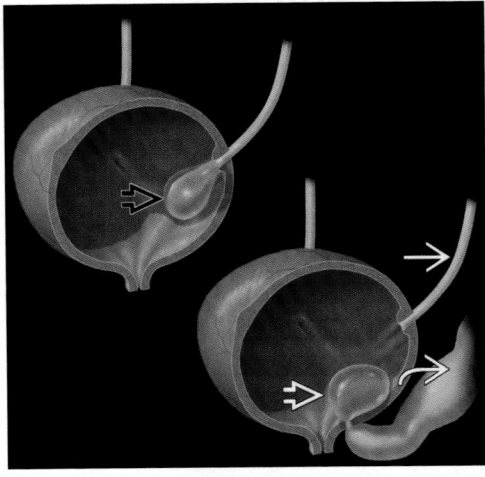

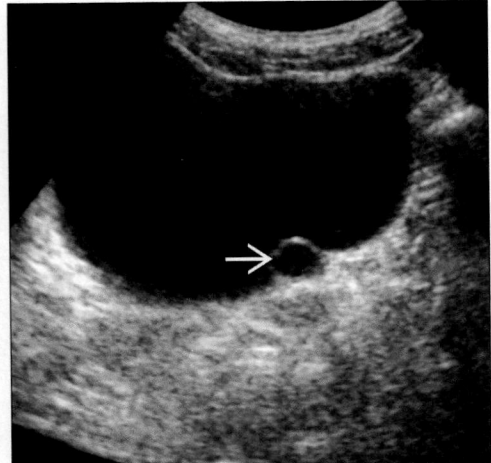

Graphic (upper) orthotopic ureterocele ⇨ at trigone in single system. (Lower) ectopic ureterocele ⇨ with hydroureter ⇉ of the upper moiety, inserting inferior & medial to the lower moiety ureter ➡ in duplex system.

Oblique transabdominal ultrasound shows typical ureterocele ➡ as a thin-walled sac within the urinary bladder.

TERMINOLOGY

Abbreviations and Synonyms
- Simple: Orthotopic or adult-type ureteroceles

Definitions
- Balloon-like dilatation of the intramural portion of ureter bulging into bladder
- **Orthotopic ureterocele**: Normal insertion at trigone and otherwise normal ureter
  ○ Single ureter system
  ○ Bilateral in 33%
- **Ectopic ureterocele**: Inserts below trigone
  ○ Duplicated collecting systems in 80%
    ▪ Upper moiety ureter often distal to proximal sphincter
    ▪ Male: Low in bladder, bladder neck, prostatic urethra, vas deferens, seminal vesicle
    ▪ No wetting in males as insertion always above external sphincter
    ▪ Female: Distal urethra, vaginal vestibule, vagina, cervix, uterus, fallopian tube
    ▪ Wetting in females only if insertion below external sphincter

  ○ Single nonduplicated system in 20%
    ▪ Small/poorly functioning kidney, may be invisible on imaging

IMAGING FINDINGS

General Features
- Best diagnostic clue
  ○ Orthotopic: Thin-walled saclike structure continuous with distal ureter
  ○ Ectopic: Continuous with hydronephrotic obstructive (usually upper) moiety and hydroureter
- Location
  ○ Ectopic: 50% in bladder and 50% in posterior urethra; 10% bilateral
    ▪ Males: Insertion always above external sphincter
- Size: Up to several cm in diameter
- Morphology: Smooth, round, or ovoid

Ultrasonographic Findings
- Grayscale Ultrasound
  ○ Thin walled, cystic intravesical mass near ipsilateral ureter
  ○ Fluctuates in size with ureteric peristalsis

DDx: Ureterocele

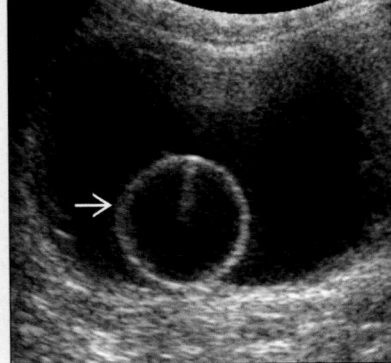

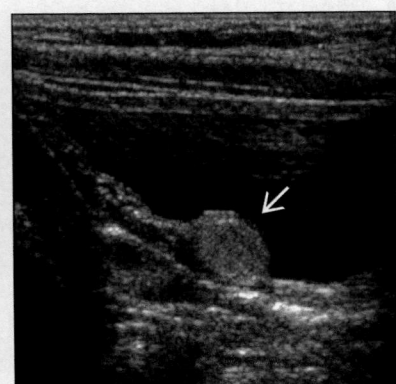

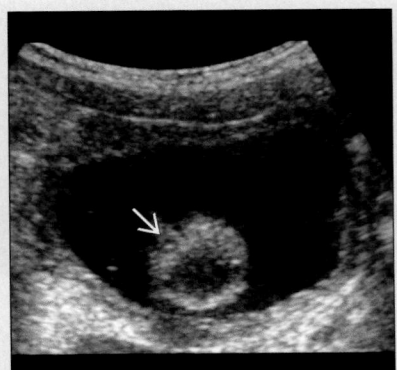

Foley Catheter

Deflux Injection

Fungus Ball

URETEROCELE

Key Facts

Terminology
- Balloon-like dilatation of the intramural portion of ureter bulging into bladder
- **Orthotopic ureterocele**: Normal insertion at trigone and otherwise normal ureter
- Single ureter system
- **Ectopic ureterocele**: Inserts below trigone
- Duplicated collecting systems in 80%

Imaging Findings
- Fluctuates in size with ureteric peristalsis
- Occasionally, in full bladder, ureteroceles may invert, giving an appearance similar to diverticulum
- Inverted ureterocele reverts to its usual appearance upon partial emptying of bladder
- Ectopic ureteroceles inserting outside bladder mimic pelvic cyst

- Pulsed Doppler: In obstructive ureterocele, there is significant difference in frequency, duration & velocity of ureteric jet compared with normal contralateral side
- Color Doppler: Demonstrates ureteric jet from tip of ureterocele

Top Differential Diagnoses
- Foley Catheter
- Pseudoureterocele
- Fungal Ball

Diagnostic Checklist
- Big ureterocele may occupy the entire bladder mimicking bladder itself, especially if bladder is empty

---

- ○ Midline echogenic tubular structure may be seen, leading to outlet obstruction
- ○ Occasionally, in full bladder, ureteroceles may invert, giving an appearance similar to diverticulum
  - ▪ Inverted ureterocele reverts to its usual appearance upon partial emptying of bladder
- ○ Wall thickening secondary to edema from impacted stone/infection
- ○ Ectopic ureteroceles inserting outside bladder mimic pelvic cyst
- Pulsed Doppler: In obstructive ureterocele, there is significant difference in frequency, duration & velocity of ureteric jet compared with normal contralateral side
- Color Doppler: Demonstrates ureteric jet from tip of ureterocele

Radiographic Findings
- IVP/cystography
  - ○ Orthotopic ureterocele: Cobra-head deformity
    - ▪ Dilated distal ureter projecting into lumen of bladder with surrounding radiolucent halo
  - ○ Ectopic ureterocele: Smooth, radiolucent intravesicular mass near bladder base
    - ▪ May evert during voiding and mimic diverticulum
    - ▪ Lumen opacification depends on function of upper pole moiety
    - ▪ Drooping lily sign: Displacement of lower pole collecting system by obstructed upper pole moiety

CT Findings
- CECT: Intravesicular mass at ureterovesical junction (UVJ)

MR Findings
- T2WI
  - ○ Intravesicular mass at UVJ
    - ▪ Ectopic: May see ectopic insertion into urethra, vagina, etc.
  - ○ Maximum intensity projection (MIP) image demonstrates relative positions of upper and lower moiety ureters in duplex system

- ▪ Superior to demonstrate ectopic ureter extending from poorly functioning moiety invisible on other imaging
- ▪ Ureterocele may be masked by fluid within urinary bladder
- Contrast-enhanced MR urography
  - ○ Best for detection of ureterocele in duplex system
  - ○ Intravesicular cyst filled by contrast with surrounding halo within bladder during early filling phase
  - ○ Continuous with hydronephrotic upper moiety & hydroureter if function of upper pole moiety preserved
  - ○ Poor or no excretion by upper pole of duplex kidney if dysplastic

Imaging Recommendations
- Best imaging tool: US and IVP
- Protocol advice
  - ○ US: Get images when bladder is reasonably full
  - ○ Cystogram: Get early images of bladder filling; overfilling may collapse/invert low-pressure ureterocele

DIFFERENTIAL DIAGNOSIS

Foley Catheter
- Characteristic shape
- Midline echogenic tubular structure may be seen

Pseudoureterocele
- Focal mucosal bulging after deflux injection in treatment of vesicoureteric reflux

Fungal Ball
- Mobile mass within bladder

Prolapsing Ureterocele: Vaginal Mass In Girls
- Bladder diverticulum: Indistinguishable with everted ureterocele
  - ○ Sac formed by herniation of bladder mucosa, connects to bladder cavity via neck

URETEROCELE

○ Does not return to intravesicle position after micturition
• Gartner duct cyst: Cyst in vaginal wall
○ Transvaginal US defines origin

PATHOLOGY

General Features
• Etiology: Congenital anomaly
• Epidemiology: US: 1:12,000-1:5,000
• Associated abnormalities
○ Single system ectopic ureteroceles: Cardiac and genital anomalies
○ Duplex system: Commonly upper moiety ureter associated with ureterocele
▪ Obstruction leading to hydronephrosis and hydroureter
▪ Occasional dysplastic small upper pole moiety with hydroureter
▪ Lower pole moiety can be hydronephrotic due to reflux

Gross Pathologic & Surgical Features
• Simple ureteroceles: Pin-point orifices but no significant obstruction
• Ectopic ureteroceles: Often obstructed, with dysplasia of upper pole kidney
• Ureteric orifice, which is narrowed, usually opens at tip, occasionally at base
• Sometimes portion of ureter extends distal to ureterocele to open in an ectopic position in bladder or urethra

Microscopic Features
• Thin wall: Covered by bladder mucosa and lined by ureteral mucosa
• Sometimes with only mucosal layer, sometimes with mucosal and thin muscularis layer

Staging, Grading or Classification Criteria
• Orifice type: Stenotic, sphincteric, sphincterostenotic, cecoureterocele
○ Sphincteric: Orifice distal to bladder neck
○ Cecoureterocele: Intravesical orifice; submucosal extension to urethra

CLINICAL ISSUES

Presentation
• Most common signs/symptoms
○ Orthotopic: Usually asymptomatic; incidental finding
○ Ectopic ureteroceles: Urinary tract infection (UTI), incontinence, vaginal mass
• Other signs/symptoms: Rarely, prolapse into bladder neck/urethra, causing obstruction
• Clinical Profile: Ectopic: Infant or child with UTI or sepsis

Demographics
• Age
○ Ectopic: Median age 3 months at diagnosis

▪ Often diagnosed with prenatal ultrasound
• Gender: Ectopic ureterocele with duplicated system M:F = 1:4

Natural History & Prognosis
• Severe obstruction: Primarily ectopic ureteroceles
○ Dysplasia of obstructed upper pole moiety

Treatment
• Options, risks, complications: Obstructed ureteroceles may cause stasis and stone formation

DIAGNOSTIC CHECKLIST

Consider
• Look for ureterocele in reasonably full bladder if duplex renal system detected
• Big ureterocele may occupy the entire bladder mimicking bladder itself, especially if bladder is empty

Image Interpretation Pearls
• Long axis of ectopic ureterocele points to side of origin

SELECTED REFERENCES

1. Zougkas K et al: Assessment of obstruction in adult ureterocele by means of color Doppler duplex sonography. Urol Int. 75(3):239-46, 2005
2. Bolduc S et al: The predictive value of diagnostic imaging for histological lesions of the upper poles in duplex systems with ureteroceles. BJU Int. 91(7):678-82, 2003
3. do Nascimento H et al: Magnetic resonance in diagnosis of ureterocele. Int Braz J Urol. 29(3):248-50, 2003
4. Sepulveda W et al: Prenatal sonographic diagnosis of bilateral ureteroceles: the pseudoseptated fetal bladder. J Ultrasound Med. 22(8):841-4; quiz 845-6, 2003
5. Shimoya K et al: Diagnosis of ureterocele with transvaginal sonography. Gynecol Obstet Invest. 54(1):58-60, 2002
6. Shokeir AA et al: Ureterocele: an ongoing challenge in infancy and childhood. BJU Int. 90(8):777-83, 2002
7. Walsh PC et al: Campbell's Urology. 8th ed. Philadelphia, Saunders. 2007-52, 2002
8. Gilbert WB et al: Development of small calculi in an infant with bilateral single system ureteroceles. J Urol. 166(5):1860-1, 2001
9. Ogunyemi D: Prenatal sonographic diagnosis of bladder outlet obstruction caused by a ureterocele associated with hydrocolpos and imperforate hymen. Am J Perinatol. 18(1):15-21, 2001
10. Shankar KR et al: Outcome of patients with prenatally detected duplex system ureterocele; natural history of those managed expectantly. J Urol. 165(4):1226-8, 2001
11. Madeb R et al: Evaluation of ureterocele with Doppler sonography. J Clin Ultrasound. 28(8):425-9, 2000
12. Zerin JM et al: Single-system ureteroceles in infants and children: imaging features. Pediatr Radiol. 30(3):139-46, 2000
13. Davidson AJ et al: Radiology of the kidney and genitourinary tract. 3rd ed. Philadelphia, W.B. Saunders. 213-6, 1999
14. Abrahamsson K et al: Bladder dysfunction: an integral part of the ectopic ureterocele complex. J Urol. 160(4):1468-70, 1998
15. Austin PF et al: Prenatal bladder outlet obstruction secondary to ureterocele. Urology. 52(6):1132-5, 1998
16. Glazier DB et al: Infected obstructive ureterocele. Urology. 50(6):972-3, 1997

URETEROCELE

IMAGE GALLERY

Typical

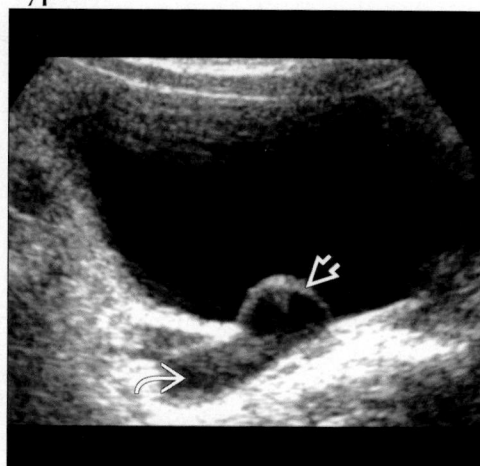
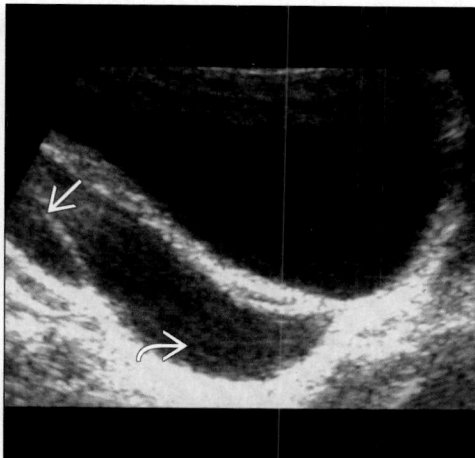

(Left) Longitudinal transabdominal ultrasound shows a typical ureteric duplex system associated with a small ureterocele ➡ at the distal end of the upper pole moiety ureter. The ureter is dilated ➡. (Right) Oblique transabdominal ultrasound shows the lower moiety ureter ➡ is mildly dilated due to reflux. It has a higher bladder insertion than the obstructed upper moiety ureter ➡ (same patient as in previous image).

Typical

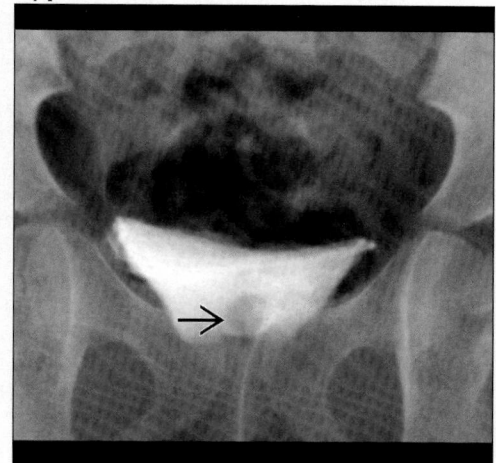
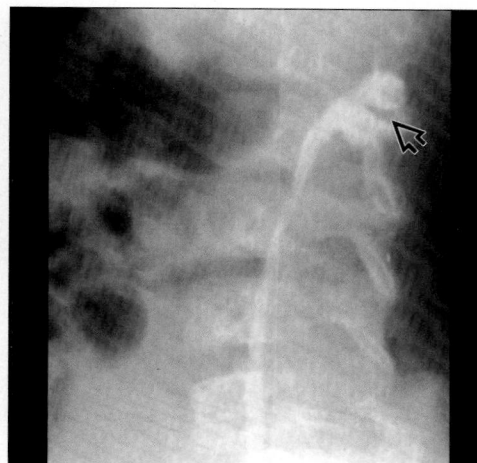

(Left) Transverse contrast cystogram shows a round filling defect ➡ within the urinary bladder compatible with a ureterocele. (Right) Longitudinal contrast cystogram shows a "drooping-lily" appearance of a refluxing lower moiety ➡, which is displaced inferolaterally by a non-refluxing hydronephrotic upper moiety (not visualized).

Typical

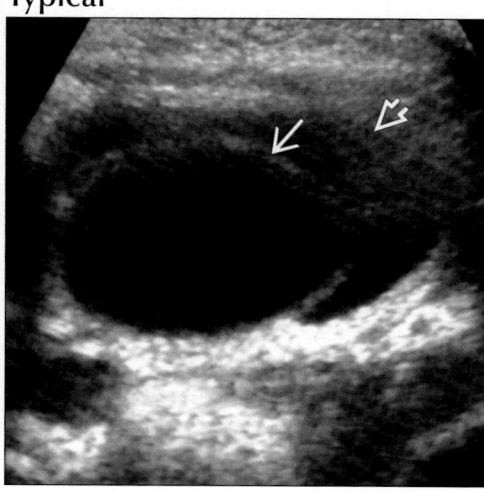
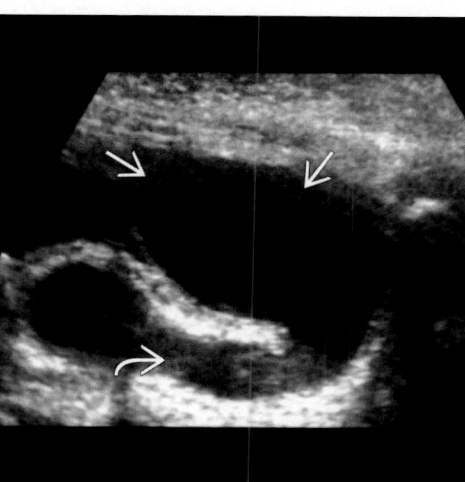

(Left) Transverse ultrasound shows presence of a large ureterocele ➡, almost occupying the whole urinary bladder ➡. These can be easily missed if the bladder is decompressed. (Right) Oblique transabdominal ultrasound shows a large ureterocele ➡ obstructing a dilated ureter ➡.

(Left) Transverse transabdominal ultrasound shows a small orthotopic ureterocele ➡ at the normal position in the trigone of bladder. Distal ureter connecting to the ureterocele is mildly dilated ➡. *(Right)* Longitudinal transabdominal ultrasound shows a typical orthotopic ureterocele ➡ in a single system, at the normal position of the bladder trigone, without ureteric dilatation.

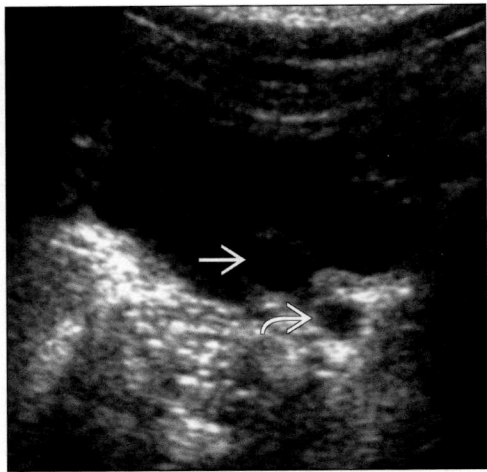
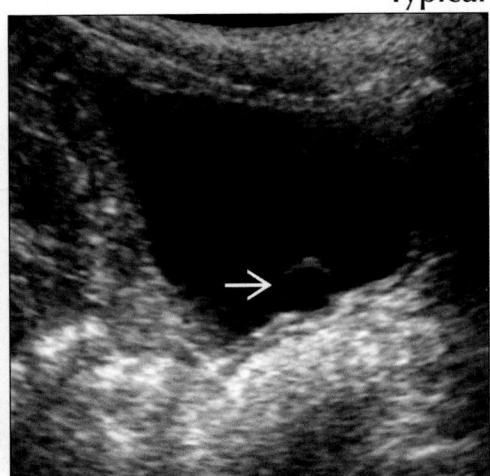

(Left) Transverse transabdominal ultrasound shows bilateral, thin-walled ureteroceles ➡ present in the bladder trigone. There was no evidence of obstructive hydronephrosis. *(Right)* Maximum intensity projection heavily T2-weighted MR urography cannot detect presence of a ureterocele within the urinary bladder.

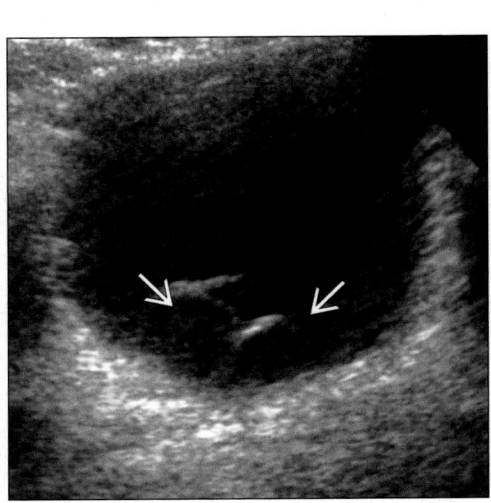
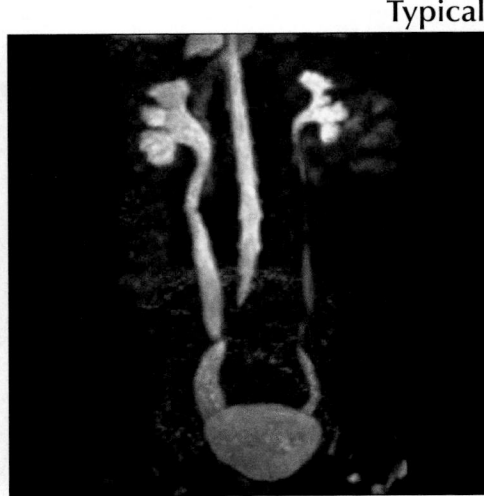

(Left) Maximum intensity projection contrast enhanced MR urography shows a right ureterocele ➡ is not yet filled with contrast and appears as a filling defect during the early dynamic phase. *(Right)* Maximum intensity projection contrast enhanced MR urography shows contrast filling the ureterocele ➡ during the delayed phase.

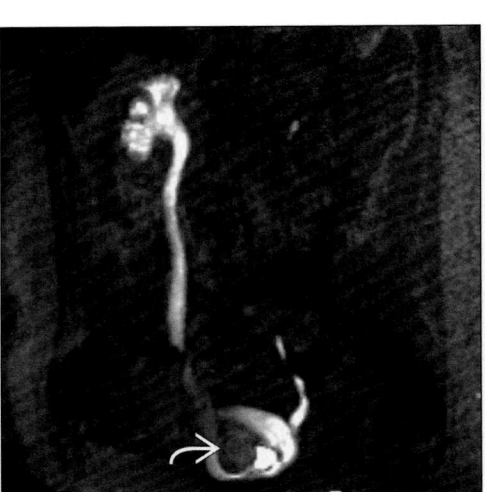
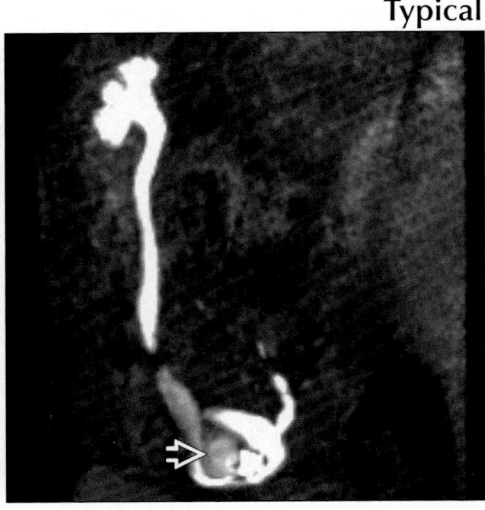

Typical

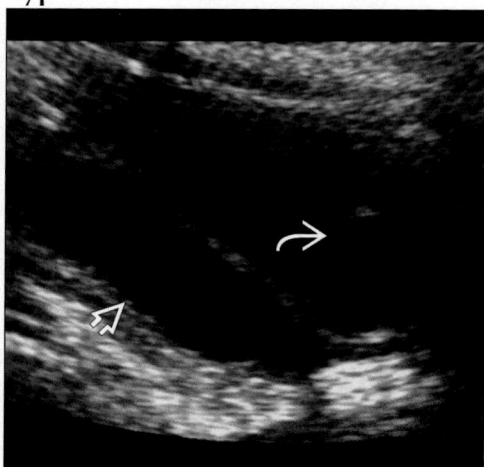
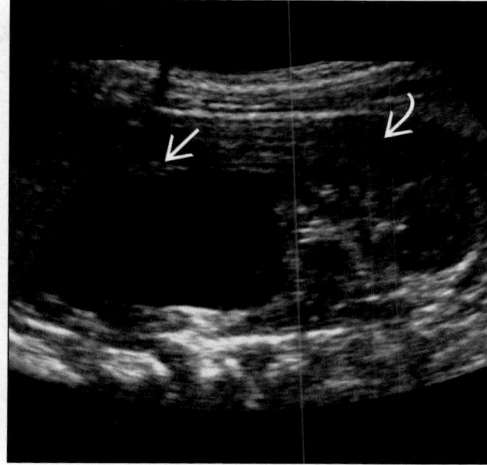

(Left) Oblique transabdominal ultrasound shows a ureterocele ⇒ at the vesicoureteric junction resulting in obstruction of the upper moiety ureter ⇒ of a duplex system. (Right) Longitudinal transabdominal ultrasound shows a dilated upper pole collecting system ⇒ associated with cortical thinning. Lower moiety ⇒ is unremarkable.

Typical

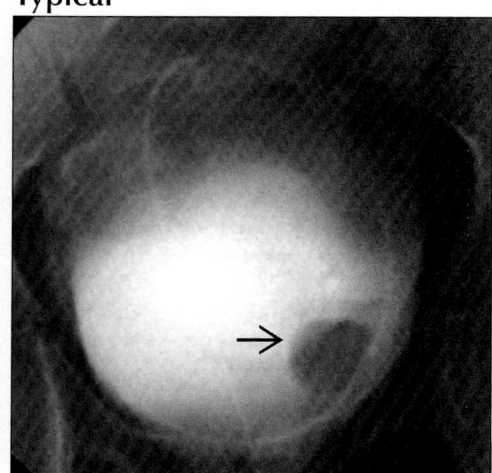
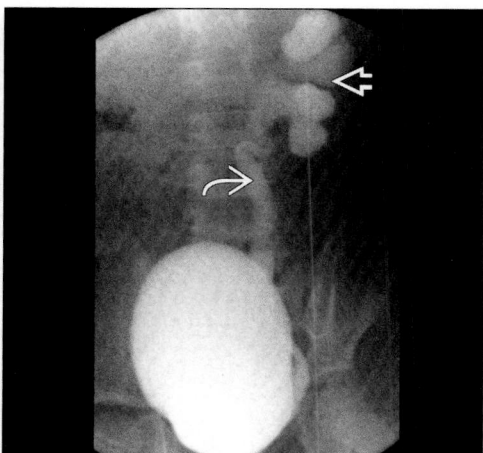

(Left) Contrast micturition cystogram shows a round filling defect ⇒ within the urinary bladder, compatible with a ureterocele. (Right) Voiding cystogram shows high grade reflux into the lower moiety ureter ⇒ in a duplex system. There is gross hydronephrosis of the lower moiety ⇒. Upper moiety is dysplastic.

Typical

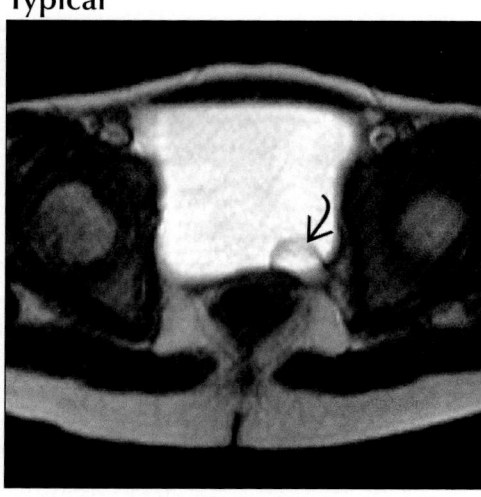
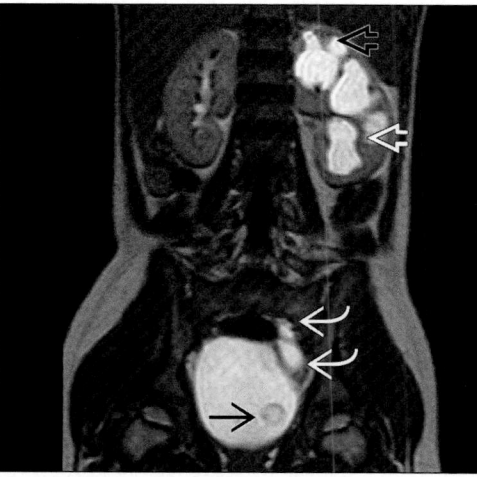

(Left) Axial post-contrast delayed T1-weighted MR shows a ureterocele ⇒ as a lucent halo within a contrast filled urinary bladder. (Right) Coronal post-contrast T1-weighted MR shows the ureterocele ⇒ obstructing a dysplastic upper moiety ⇒. The lower moiety ⇒ is dilated due to reflux. Two ureters ⇒ are noted.

BLADDER DIVERTICULUM

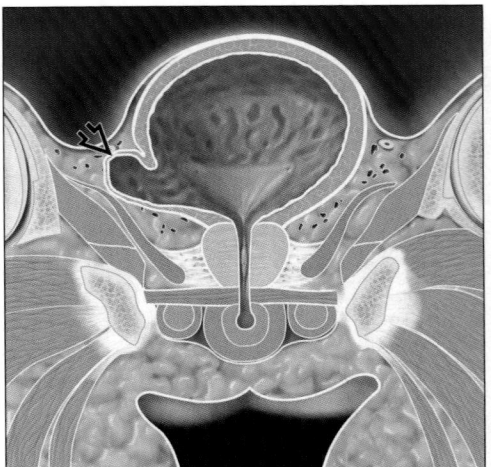

Graphic shows a diverticulum ⟹ arising from the lateral bladder wall, due to herniation of the mucosa and submucosa through the muscular wall.

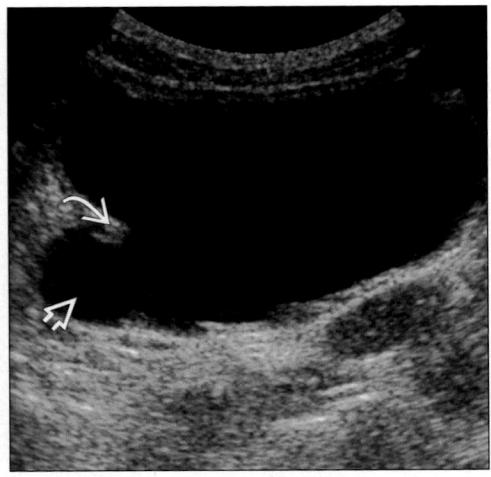

Transverse transabdominal ultrasound shows a typical diverticulum ⟹ arising from the posterolateral wall of the urinary bladder. Note its wide neck ⟹.

TERMINOLOGY

Abbreviations and Synonyms
- Bladder diverticulum/diverticula

Definitions
- Sac formed by herniation of bladder mucosa and submucosa through muscular wall
- Joined to bladder cavity by a constricted neck

IMAGING FINDINGS

General Features
- Best diagnostic clue: Perivesical cystic mass with connection to bladder lumen
- Location
  - Near ureterovesical junction (UVJ)
  - Bladder dome: Likely urachal if solitary
- Size: Small to very large; can exceed size of bladder
- Morphology: Single or multiple; smooth wall

Ultrasonographic Findings
- Grayscale Ultrasound

- Anechoic outpouching from bladder
- Internal echogenicity of diverticulum varies depending on its contents
- Narrow or wide neck; easily appreciated on US
- May contain calculi, hematoma or tumor
- Empty with micturition
- Color Doppler
  - Urine may be seen flowing into and out of diverticulum
    - Color jet connecting to bladder very useful to distinguish diverticulum from other paravesical masses
- Sonographic air/CO_2 contrast
  - Differentiate bladder diverticula (filled by air/contrast) from other lesions that do not communicate with bladder (cysts of ovarian/enteric origin)

Radiographic Findings
- IVP
  - Medial deviation of ipsilateral ureter
  - Usually fills with contrast unless obstructed
  - Diverticulum may contain stones, debris, or tumor

DDx: Bladder Diverticulum

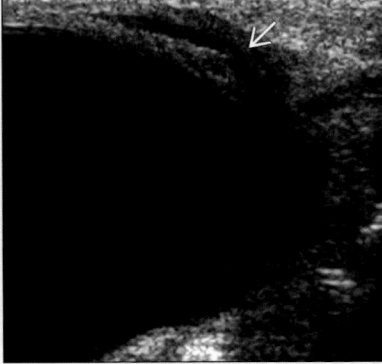

Patent Urachus

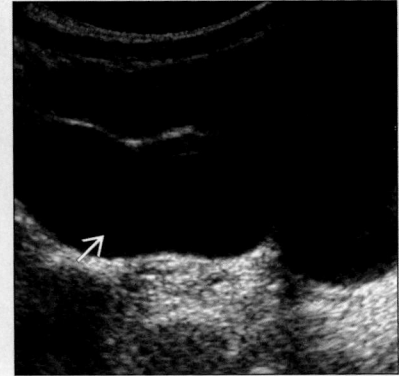

Everted Ureterocele

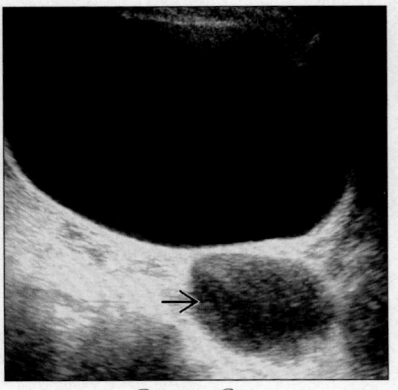

Gartner Cyst

BLADDER DIVERTICULUM

Key Facts

Terminology
- Sac formed by herniation of bladder mucosa and submucosa through muscular wall

Imaging Findings
- Best diagnostic clue: Perivesical cystic mass with connection to bladder lumen
- Near ureterovesical junction (UVJ)
- Narrow or wide neck; easily appreciated on US
- May contain calculi, hematoma or tumor
- Color jet connecting to bladder very useful to distinguish diverticulum from other paravesical masses
- Differentiate bladder diverticula (filled by air/contrast) from other lesions that do not communicate with bladder (cysts of ovarian/enteric origin)

- Best imaging tool: Ultrasound, cystogram
- Protocol advice: Check emptying of diverticulum on post-void studies

Top Differential Diagnoses
- Urachus
- Everted Ureterocele
- Paraovarian Cysts in Female (e.g. Gartner Cyst)

Clinical Issues
- Secondary inflammation predisposes to development of carcinoma within diverticulum
- Tumors in diverticula have worse prognosis; poorly formed wall leads to more rapid local invasion into surrounding perivesical fat

- Cystogram: Oblique films may show configuration of diverticulum neck

CT Findings
- CECT
  - Fluid attenuation outpouching from bladder
  - Usually fills with contrast on delayed images

MR Findings
- T1WI: Low signal mass contiguous with bladder
- T2WI
  - High signal mass contiguous with bladder
  - May see dephasing with motion of urine between it and bladder lumen

Fluoroscopic Findings
- Voiding Cystourethrogram: Evaluates diverticulum if US cannot differentiate it from pelvic cyst

Imaging Recommendations
- Best imaging tool: Ultrasound, cystogram
- Protocol advice: Check emptying of diverticulum on post-void studies

DIFFERENTIAL DIAGNOSIS

Urachus
- Cord-like embryonic remnant that connects bladder apex with umbilicus
- Characteristic midline position

Everted Ureterocele
- Continuous with ureter
- Assumes its more usual appearance of bulging into bladder upon partial bladder emptying

Paraovarian Cysts in Female (e.g. Gartner Cyst)
- Vestigial remnant of Wolffian duct in mesosalpinx
- Gartner cyst: Inclusion cyst, lateral to vagina and uterine wall
- No communication with bladder
- Do not empty with micturition

- Transvaginal US accurately defines spatial relationship to urethra and bladder

Pelvic Cysts in Male
- Prostatic utricle cyst: Dilatation of prostatic utricle, in midline
- Müllerian cyst: Arise from remnants of müllerian duct, may extend lateral to midline
- Ejaculatory duct cyst: Cystic dilatation of ejaculatory duct, usually small
- Seminal vesicle cysts: Wolffian duct anomaly, usually large and solitary
- Transrectal US defines their origins and shows no communication with bladder

PATHOLOGY

General Features
- Etiology
  - Acquired: Most common secondary to bladder outlet obstruction (60%)
    - Associated with weakening of muscle layers from long-standing bladder outlet obstruction
    - In children: Posterior urethral valves, large ureterocele, neurogenic bladder, bladder neck stenosis
    - In adult: Secondary to prostatic enlargement, post traumatic urethral stricture
    - May occur anywhere, most common near ureteric orifices
    - Associated with syndromes: Prune-belly syndrome, Ehlers-Danlos, Menkes kinky-hair syndrome, Diamond-Blackfan syndrome
  - Congenital: Hutch diverticulum (40%)
    - Weakness in detrusor muscle adjacent to ureteral orifice
    - With or without vesicoureteral reflux
    - Typically in paraureteral region
- Epidemiology
  - Prevalence 1.7% in children

BLADDER DIVERTICULUM

○ Multiple diverticula in children: Neurogenic dysfunction, posterior urethral valves, prune belly syndrome
• Associated abnormalities: Ureteral reflux

Gross Pathologic & Surgical Features
• Bladder mucosa herniates through weak areas in wall
• Composed only of mucosa and submucosa without muscularis layer present
• Typically located at areas of congenital weakness of muscular wall at ureteral meatus or posterolateral wall (= paraureteral)

Microscopic Features
• Uroepithelial lining

CLINICAL ISSUES

Presentation
• Most common signs/symptoms: Usually asymptomatic
• Other signs/symptoms
  ○ Hematuria due to complications: Calculi or vesical carcinoma due to chronic inflammation (in older patients)
  ○ May present as abdominal mass and acute urinary retention in infant
  ○ Voiding difficulty in case of big diverticulum with bladder outlet obstruction
• Clinical Profile: Older male with benign prostatic hyperplasia (BPH); spinal cord injury patient

Demographics
• Age: 6th and 7th decade
• Gender: M:F = 9:1

Natural History & Prognosis
• Wide-neck diverticula: Empty readily with the bladder
• Narrow-neck diverticula: Urinary stasis → complications such as infection, stone and ureteral obstruction
• Secondary inflammation predisposes to development of carcinoma within diverticulum
• Tumors in diverticula have worse prognosis; poorly formed wall leads to more rapid local invasion into surrounding perivesical fat
• Rarely, spontaneous rupture

Treatment
• Options, risks, complications
  ○ Complications: Carcinoma, vesico-ureteral reflux, ureteral obstruction
  ○ Surgery may be indicated for persistent infection, stone formation, or ureteral obstruction

DIAGNOSTIC CHECKLIST

Consider
• Large diverticulum may be confused with bladder especially if bladder is contracted
• Look for filling defects, which may be calculi, hematoma or tumor

Image Interpretation Pearls
• Continuity with urethra distinguishes bladder from diverticulum
• Differentiated from pelvic cysts by demonstration of diverticulum neck connecting to bladder in appropriate plane

SELECTED REFERENCES

1. Aslam F et al: Acute urinary retention as a result of a bladder diverticulum. Int J Urol. 13(5):628-30, 2006
2. Pace AM et al: Congenital vesical diverticulum in a 38-year-old female. Int Urol Nephrol. 37(3):473-5, 2005
3. Yang JM et al: Transvaginal sonography in the diagnosis, management and follow-up of complex paraurethral abnormalities. Ultrasound Obstet Gynecol. 25(3):302-6, 2005
4. Shukla AR et al: Giant bladder diverticula causing bladder outlet obstruction in children. J Urol. 172(5 Pt 1):1977-9, 2004
5. Wang CW et al: Pitfalls in the differential diagnosis of a pelvic cyst: lessons from a post-menopausal woman with bladder diverticulum. Int J Clin Pract. 58(9):894-6, 2004
6. Cappele O et al: A study of the anatomic features of the duct of the urachus. Surg Radiol Anat. 23(4):229-35, 2001
7. Yu JS et al: Urachal remnant diseases: spectrum of CT and US findings. Radiographics. 21(2):451-61, 2001
8. Khati NJ et al: Imaging of the umbilicus and periumbilical region. Radiographics. 18(2):413-31, 1998
9. Sharma R et al: Giant diverticulum of urinary bladder causing bilateral hydronephrosis in an adult. Diagnostic features on radionuclide scintigraphy. Clin Nucl Med. 22(6):385-7, 1997
10. Maynor CH et al: Urinary bladder diverticula: sonographic diagnosis and interpretive pitfalls. J Ultrasound Med. 15(3):189-94, 1996
11. Bellah RD et al: Ureterocele eversion with vesicoureteral reflux in duplex kidneys: findings at voiding cystourethrography. AJR Am J Roentgenol. 165(2):409-13, 1995
12. Itoh N et al: Spontaneous rupture of a bladder diverticulum: ultrasonographic diagnosis. J Urol. 152(4):1206-7, 1994
13. Levine D et al: Using color Doppler jets to differentiate a pelvic cyst from a bladder diverticulum. J Ultrasound Med. 13(7):575-7, 1994
14. Weingardt JP et al: The diverticular jet effect: color Doppler differentiation of bladder diverticula from other pelvic fluid collections. J Clin Ultrasound. 22(6):397-400, 1994
15. Dondalski M et al: Carcinoma arising in urinary bladder diverticula: imaging findings in six patients. AJR Am J Roentgenol. 161(4):817-20, 1993
16. Farhi J et al: Giant diverticulum of the bladder simulating ovarian cyst. Int J Gynaecol Obstet. 36(1):55-7, 1991
17. Walz PH et al: Ultrasound examination of bladder and prostate. Urol Int. 45(4):217-30, 1990
18. Patel PJ et al: Vesicourachal diverticulum in association with other urological anomalies. Eur Urol. 13(6):417-8, 1987
19. Schneider K et al: Differential diagnosis of intra- and perivesical abnormalities using bladder air/CO2 contrast sonography. Pediatr Radiol. 16(4):309-12, 1986
20. Bellinger MF et al: Bladder diverticulum associated with ureteral obstruction. Pediatr Radiol. 15(3):207-8, 1985
21. Dragsted J et al: Urothelial carcinoma in a bladder diverticulum evaluated by transurethral ultrasonography. Scand J Urol Nephrol. 19(2):153-4, 1985
22. Saez F et al: Carcinomas in vesical diverticula: the role of ultrasound. J Clin Ultrasound. 13(1):45-8, 1985

BLADDER DIVERTICULUM

IMAGE GALLERY

Typical

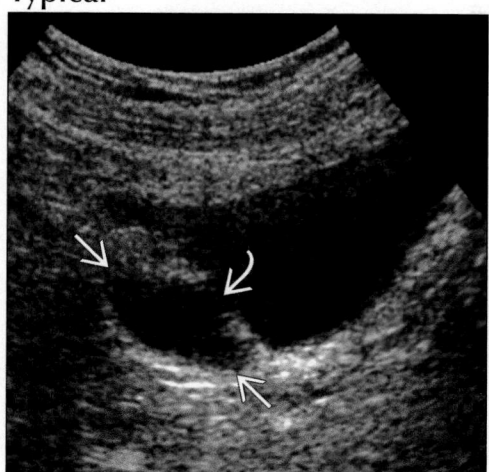
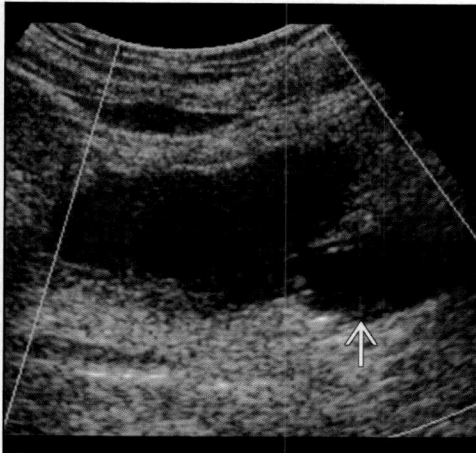

(Left) Longitudinal transabdominal ultrasound shows a small pouch ➡ arising from the supero-posterior aspect of the bladder wall. Note communication between the diverticulum and bladder through narrow neck ➡. *(Right)* Transverse color Doppler ultrasound shows no color signals within the diverticulum ➡, confirming its avascular nature.

Typical

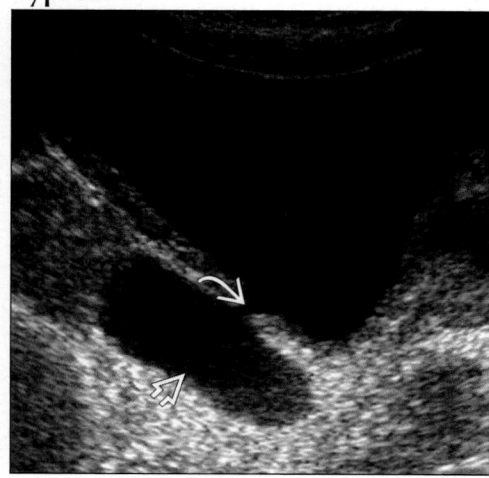
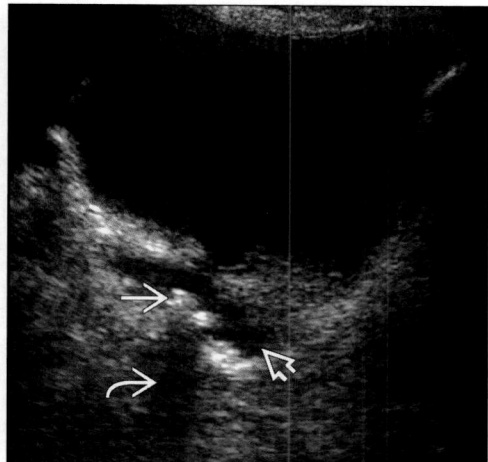

(Left) Longitudinal transabdominal ultrasound shows Hutch diverticulum ➡ arising from the posterolateral wall with a narrow neck ➡. *(Right)* Oblique transabdominal ultrasound shows multiple, small, echogenic calculi ➡ within the bladder diverticulum ➡. Note posterior acoustic shadowing ➡.

Typical

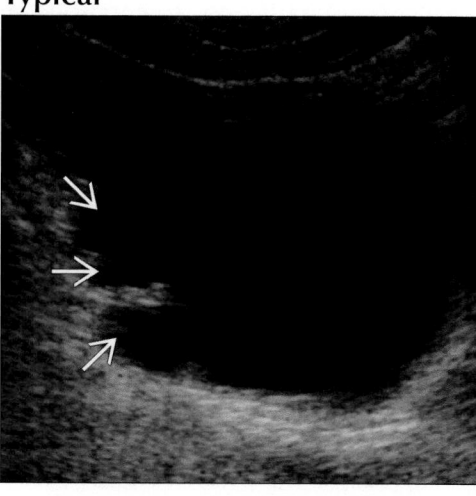
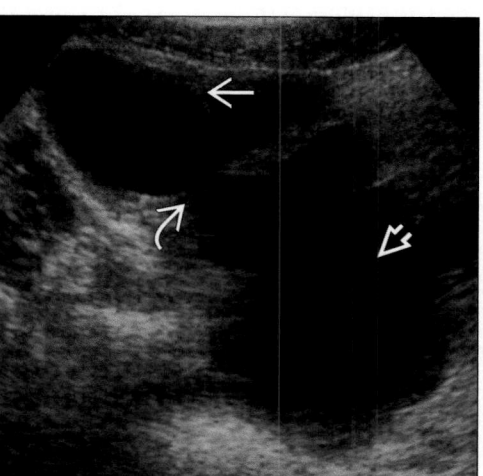

(Left) Transverse transabdominal ultrasound shows multiple, wide-neck diverticula ➡ arising from the lateral wall of the urinary bladder in a patient with urine retention. *(Right)* Oblique transabdominal ultrasound shows a large diverticulum ➡ with a wide neck ➡, arising from the urinary bladder ➡. Note, diverticulum is larger than the bladder.

BLADDER CALCULI

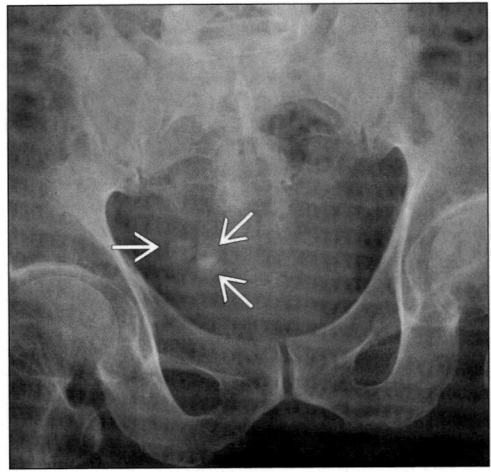

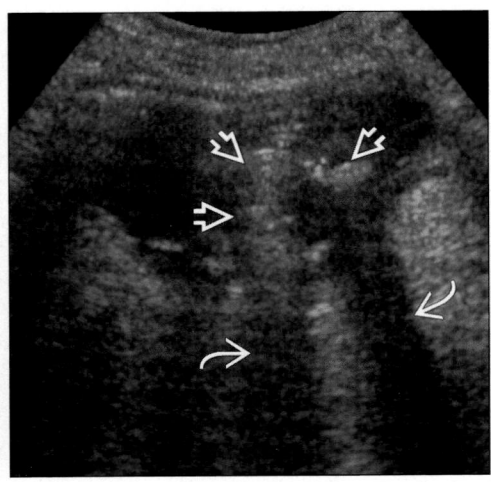

Pelvic radiograph shows three smooth, round, lamellated calcifications ➡ in the lower pelvis, typical of bladder calculi.

Transverse transabdominal ultrasound shows three echogenic foci ➡ with posterior acoustic shadowing ➡ within the urinary bladder.

TERMINOLOGY

Abbreviations and Synonyms
- Bladder stones, vesical calculi, cystolithiasis

Definitions
- Concretions of mineral salts within bladder lumen

IMAGING FINDINGS

General Features
- Best diagnostic clue
  - Mobile echogenic focus in bladder with acoustic shadowing on US
  - Smooth round or ovoid laminated calcification in bladder on plain radiograph
- Location
  - Bladder lumen: Usually midline with patient supine
    - Eccentric if within bladder augmentation or diverticulum
- Size: Variable
- Morphology: Round, oval, spiculated, laminated, faceted

Ultrasonographic Findings
- Grayscale Ultrasound
  - Crescentic echogenic focus with sharp acoustic shadowing
  - Mobile, changes position on decubitus scans
  - Occasional stone adheres to bladder wall due to inflammation
  - Associated with edema of ureteral orifices and thickening of bladder wall if large calculus

Radiographic Findings
- Radiography
  - Solitary or multiple calcifications overlying bladder
  - Most are radiopaque but opacity variable
- IVP: Filling defect or radiopacity, depending on relative density of stone vs. contrast material

CT Findings
- NECT: All bladder calculi are radiopaque on CT

MR Findings
- All pulse sequences: Signal void(s) in bladder

DDx: Bladder Calculus

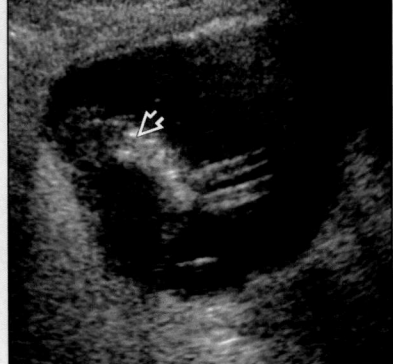

Bladder Carcinoma

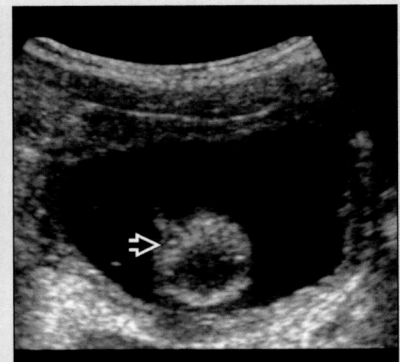

Fungal Ball

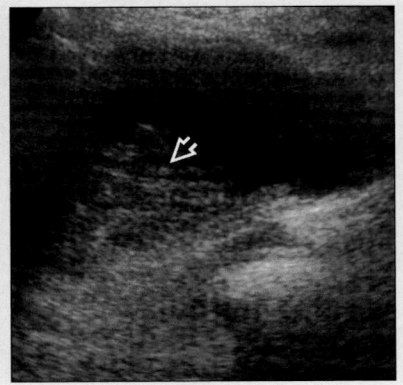

Blood Clot

BLADDER CALCULI

Key Facts

Imaging Findings
- Bladder lumen: Usually midline with patient supine
- Crescentic echogenic focus with sharp acoustic shadowing
- Mobile, changes position on decubitus scans
- Occasional stone adheres to bladder wall due to inflammation
- Associated with edema of ureteral orifices and thickening of bladder wall if large calculus

Top Differential Diagnoses
- Bladder Neoplasm
- Fungal Ball
- Blood Clot

Diagnostic Checklist
- Carcinoma resulting from chronic bladder irritation may co-exist with bladder stone

DIFFERENTIAL DIAGNOSIS

Bladder Neoplasm
- Focal non-mobile mass in bladder
- May show increased vascularity on color Doppler

Fungal Ball
- Rare entities occurring in diabetics or immunocompromised patients
- Medium echogenicity, non-shadowing, rounded mobile lesions within bladder

Blood Clot
- Medium slightly speckled echodensity, without acoustic shadowing
- Diagnosis suggested if history of hematuria

PATHOLOGY

General Features
- General path comments
  - Most are mixture of calcium oxalate and calcium phosphate
  - Infection stones: Magnesium ammonium phosphate ("struvite")
- Etiology
  - Stasis: Bladder outlet obstruction, neurogenic bladder, bladder diverticula
  - Infection, especially proteus mirabilis
  - Foreign bodies: Nidus for crystal growth
  - Bladder augmentation: Local metabolic derangement

CLINICAL ISSUES

Presentation
- Most common signs/symptoms
  - Most asymptomatic
  - Other signs/symptoms
    - Suprapubic pain, foul smelling urine
    - Microscopic hematuria, gross hematuria is rare

Demographics
- Gender: M > F

Natural History & Prognosis
- Complication: Malignant bladder tumors in patients with stones from indwelling Foley catheters

DIAGNOSTIC CHECKLIST

Image Interpretation Pearls
- Carcinoma resulting from chronic bladder irritation may co-exist with bladder stone

SELECTED REFERENCES
1. Schwartz BF et al: The vesical calculus. Urol Clin North Am. 27(2):333-46, 2000

IMAGE GALLERY

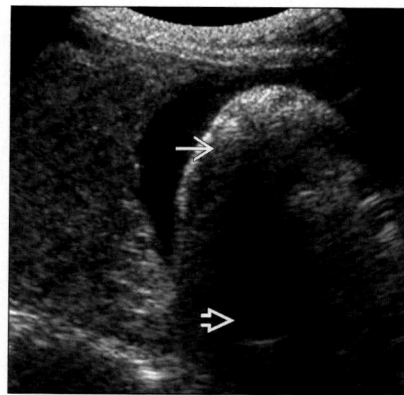 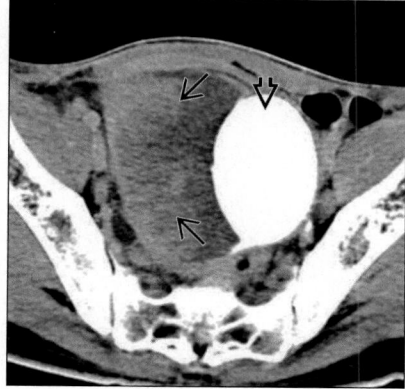 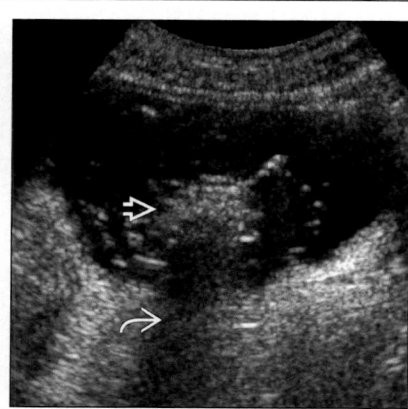

(Left) Longitudinal transabdominal US shows a large, smooth, echogenic bladder calculus ➡ with posterior acoustic shadowing ⤑. It was mobile on real-time US. *(Center)* Transverse NECT shows a large bladder calculus ▷ located towards the left side of the bladder, as the patient was in a slight left decubitus position during scanning. Note associated Carcinoma ➔. *(Right)* Transverse transabdominal US shows a large echogenic stone ⇒ within the urinary bladder. It is lobulated in contour and associated with posterior acoustic shadowing ⤑.

SCHISTOSOMIASIS, BLADDER

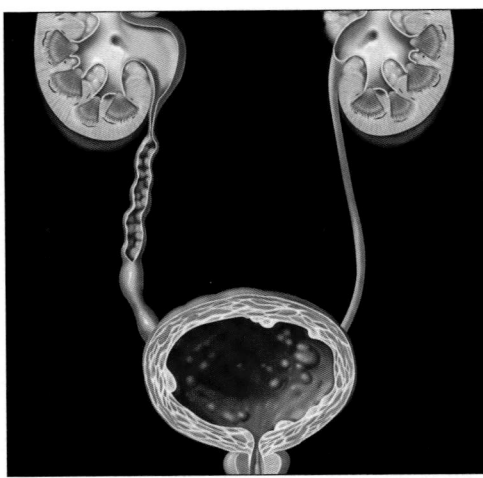

Graphic shows a markedly thickened urinary bladder wall with inflammatory polyps and calcifications. Urteritis cystica changes are present in the dilated right ureter.

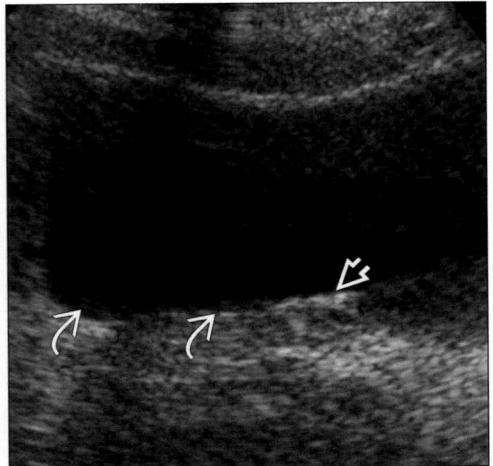

Transverse transabdominal ultrasound shows a linear echogenic calcification ➤ and irregular thickening ➤ over the posterior bladder wall in a patient with schistosomiasis.

TERMINOLOGY

Abbreviations and Synonyms
- Bilharziasis, parasitic infection

Definitions
- Infection of urinary system by parasite Schistosoma hematobium

IMAGING FINDINGS

General Features
- Best diagnostic clue: Curvilinear calcification of bladder wall on plain radiograph

Ultrasonographic Findings
- Thick-walled fibrotic bladder
- Echogenic calcification within bladder wall
- Small capacity bladder with significant postvoid residue
- Hydronephrosis and hydroureter due to distal ureteric stricture

Radiographic Findings
- Calcifications of bladder wall (4-56%)
- ± Calcification of ureter (34%), seminal vesicle (late)

CT Findings
- NECT: Better delineates extent of bladder calcification, compared to plain radiograph

Fluoroscopic Findings
- Mucosal irregularity, inflammatory pseudopolyps of bladder
- Ureteritis cystica, distal ureteric stricture
- Vesicoureteric reflux

Imaging Recommendations
- Best imaging tool: US for screening of bladder mass as late complication

DIFFERENTIAL DIAGNOSIS

Bladder Calculus
- Mobile echogenic focus within bladder

DDx: Bladder Schistosomiasis

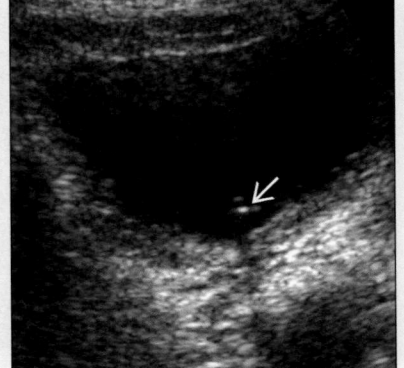

Bladder Calculus

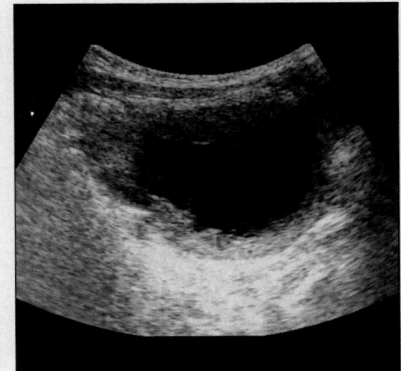

Cystitis

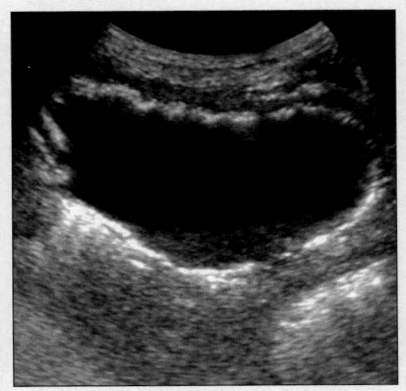

Emphysematous Cystitis

SCHISTOSOMIASIS, BLADDER

Key Facts

Imaging Findings
- Thick-walled fibrotic bladder
- Echogenic calcification within bladder wall
- Small capacity bladder with significant postvoid residue
- Hydronephrosis and hydroureter due to distal ureteric stricture
- Best imaging tool: US for screening of bladder mass as late complication

Top Differential Diagnoses
- Bladder Calculus
- Bladder Cystitis
- Emphysematous Cystitis

Diagnostic Checklist
- Degree of hydronephrosis & irregularity of bladder wall seen on US correlates strongly with prevalence & intensity of S. hematobium infection, microhematuria & proteinuria

---

Bladder Cystitis
- Diffuse/non-diffuse hypoechoic thickening of bladder wall; no wall calcification

Emphysematous Cystitis
- Infection by gas-forming organism
- Echogenic foci within area of bladder wall thickening with ring-down shadowing

PATHOLOGY

General Features
- Epidemiology: Endemic in Middle East, India, Africa, Central America and South America

Gross Pathologic & Surgical Features
- Thickened and ulcerated bladder mucosa; progresses to scarring and muscular hypertrophy

Microscopic Features
- Encapsulated eggs in vesicle tissue cause inflammatory granulomatous reaction
- Fibrosis traps ova in tunica propria of bladder wall where ova die and calcify

CLINICAL ISSUES

Presentation
- Most common signs/symptoms: Frequency, urgency, dysuria, hematuria

- Other signs/symptoms
  - Ureteric stricture, causing hydronephrosis
  - Squamous cell carcinoma of bladder as late complication

Natural History & Prognosis
- Female parasite discharges eggs into urine & feces
- Ova hatch into miracidia infecting fresh water snails (intermediate host)
- Cercaria pass from snail to water & penetrate human skin
- Pass into lymphatics and migrate to pelvic venous plexus
- Ultimately eggs deposited and erode bladder mucosa

Treatment
- Drug: Praziquantel, metrifonate

DIAGNOSTIC CHECKLIST

Image Interpretation Pearls
- Degree of hydronephrosis & irregularity of bladder wall seen on US correlates strongly with prevalence & intensity of S. hematobium infection, microhematuria & proteinuria

SELECTED REFERENCES
1. Degremont A et al: Value of ultrasonography in investigating morbidity due to Schistosoma haematobium infection. Lancet. 1(8430):662-5, 1985

IMAGE GALLERY

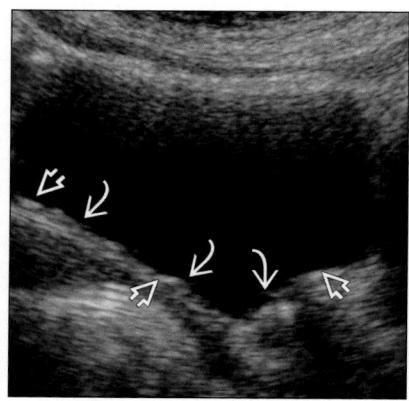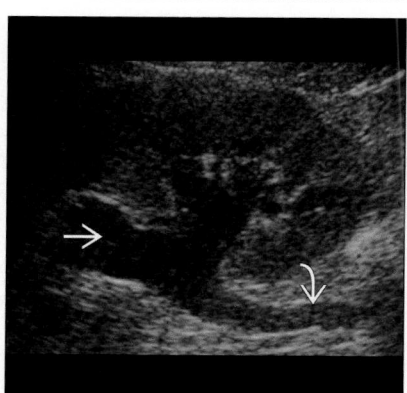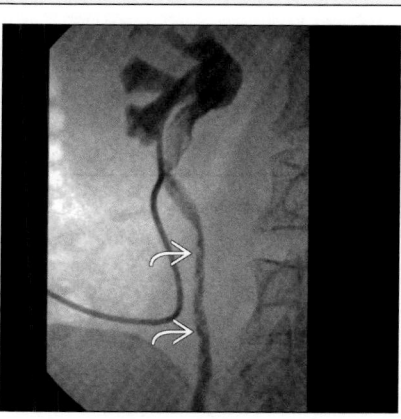

(Left) Longitudinal transabdominal ultrasound shows multiple echogenic foci of calcifications ➡ and mucosal irregularity ➡ of the posterior bladder wall. Bladder volume is reduced. *(Center)* Oblique transabdominal ultrasound shows moderate hydronephrosis ➡ and hydroureter ➡ due to distal ureteral stricture caused by infection with S. hematobium. *(Right)* Percutaneous contrast pyelogram shows typical appearance of ureteritis cystica ➡ caused by infection with S. hematobium.

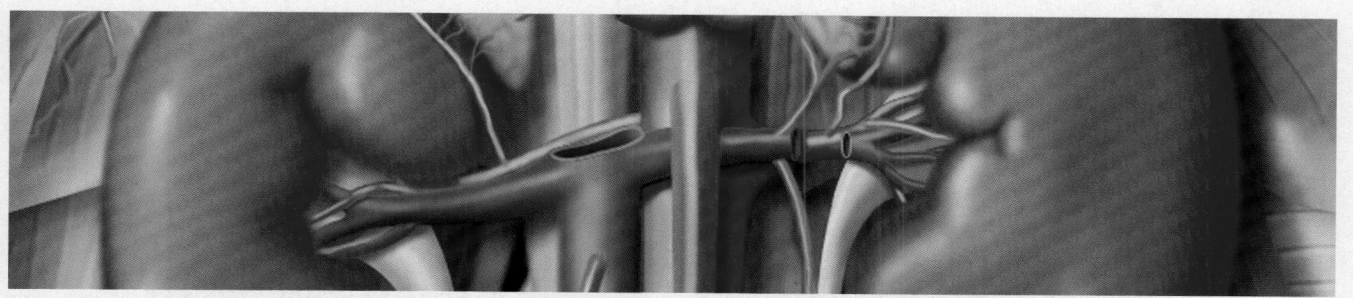

SECTION 6: Renal Transplants

Introduction and Overview

SONOGRAPHIC FEATURES OF RENAL ALLOGRAFTS

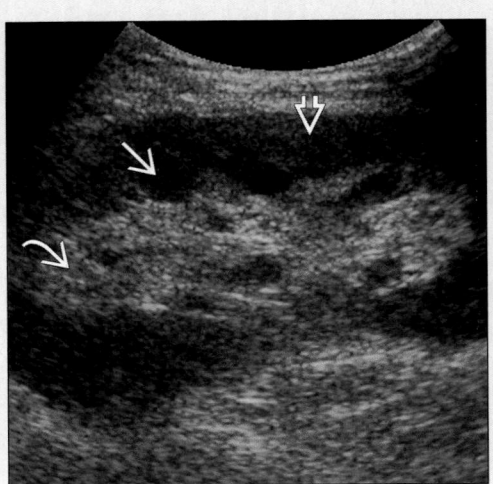

Oblique transabdominal ultrasound shows a normal renal allograft with smooth contour, echogenic central sinus ➡, relatively hypoechoic cortex ➡ and echo-poor medullary pyramids ➡.

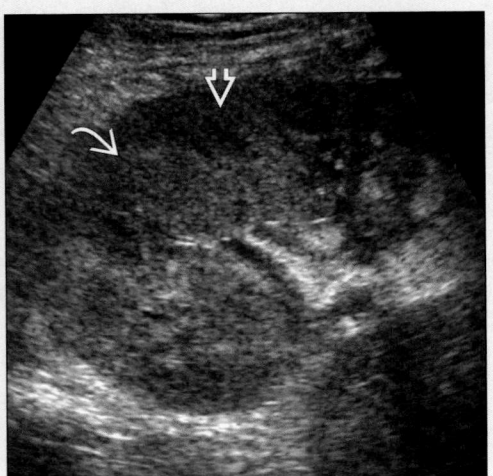

Oblique transabdominal ultrasound shows a swollen renal allograft with an abnormal parenchymal echo pattern, echogenic cortex ➡, ↓ CM differentiation ➡ and effaced central sinus.

TERMINOLOGY

Synonyms
- Kidney/renal transplant

Definitions
- Kidney transplanted from either living or cadaveric donor

IMAGING ANATOMY

General Anatomic Considerations
- Vessel anastomosis
  - Typical: End-to-side anastomosis of donor renal artery (RA) and vein (RV) to recipient external iliac artery (EIA) and vein (EIV)
  - Living kidney: End-to-side anastomosis of donor main RA to recipient internal iliac artery (IIA)
  - Small children: Anastomosis of donor main RA to distal aorta and RV to inferior vena cava
- Ureteric anastomosis
  - Ureterovesical (most common)
  - Ureteropelvic or ureteroureter less frequent because of higher incidence of associated urinomas
- Normal renal parenchyma
  - Similar to that of native kidney
  - Smooth renal contour
  - Echogenicity: Central sinus > cortex > pyramids
  - Medullary pyramids > overlying renal cortical thickness ⇒ swollen pyramids
- Renal size
  - Tends to be larger than native kidneys
  - Probably secondary to hypertrophy after transplantation
- Collecting system
  - Mild pelvicaliectasis is common; possibly related to bladder distension
- Urothelial wall
  - Normal wall thickness ⇒ barely visible
  - Perceptible urothelial wall ⇒ wall thickening

Critical Anatomic Structures
- Bladder in the vicinity of renal allograft must not be mistaken as perinephric fluid collection
- Iliac and graft vessels confused with dilated ureter

Anatomic Relationships
- Superficially located in either iliac fossa of recipient
- Usually extraperitoneal, anterior to iliacus muscle and lateral to iliac vessels
- Cephalad and lateral to bladder, close to but separated from it
- In small children, it is transplanted intraperitoneally

ANATOMY-BASED IMAGING ISSUES

Key Concepts or Questions
- Renal axis is variable dependent on surgical procedure
- Renal parenchymal changes
  - Acute rejection: Hypoechoic renal cortex; swollen medullary pyramids and effacement of central echo complex
  - Differentials include acute tubular necrosis (ATN), glomerulonephritis, nephrocalcinosis, cyclosporine nephrotoxicity
- Renal enlargement
  - Occurs in ATN, acute rejection, obstruction, infection and renal vein thrombosis
  - Renal volume is best parameter for assessing renal enlargement
- Pelviectasis
  - Best demonstrated by ultrasound
  - May be related to degree of bladder distension
  - Post-voiding scan is recommended to exclude obstruction
  - Ureter may be large post-operatively secondary to denervation and possibly mild ischemia mimicking hydroureter
- Urothelial wall thickening
  - Non-specific finding
  - Seen as hypoechoic rim along the inner wall

SONOGRAPHIC FEATURES OF RENAL ALLOGRAFTS

Key Facts

Imaging Issues

- Common complications include ATN, rejection, perinephric fluid collections, obstructive uropathy and vascular abnormalities
- Renal enlargement may occur in ATN, acute rejection, obstruction, infection and renal vein thrombosis
- Renal parenchymal changes may reflect ATN, rejection, glomerulonephritis, nephrocalcinosis, cyclosporine nephrotoxicity
- ATN and rejection may have overlapping sonographic features
- Mild pelvicaliectasis is common; may be related to bladder distension
- Normal urothelial wall is barely visible, if perceptible ⇒ thickening

- Focal color aliasing, high-velocity post-stenotic turbulence ⇒ severe RA stenosis
- High-velocity, low resistance flow in feeding artery; arterialization of venous signals ⇒ AVF
- Pulsatile hypoechoic mass with high-velocity jet or to-and-fro flow at aneurysm neck ⇒ pseudoaneurysm

Pitfalls

- Pelvicaliectasis due to bladder distension or ↓ ureteral tone mimics obstructive uropathy
- Bladder confused with urinoma or lymphocele
- Iliac vessels and allograft hilar vessels confused with dilated ureter
- Normal post-operative renal hypertrophy may mimic those caused by ATN or rejection
- Vessel kinking and tortuosity may simulate significant RA stenosis

- ○ Caused by acute rejection, inflammatory cell infiltrate, fibrosis, muscular hypertrophy, or hemorrhage
- ○ Wall thickening > 2 mm associated with rejection
- RA stenosis
  - ○ Ideally assessed by color Doppler imaging
  - ○ Usually occurs at anastomosis or at proximal donor artery; related to surgical procedure
  - ○ Kinks and tortuosity of main allograft RA may be confused with arterial stenosis

Imaging Approaches

- Knowledge of technique of anastomosis before exam
- High frequency transducer ≥ 5 MHz used to evaluate parenchymal detail
- Supine, transabdominal anterior approach
- Morphologic evaluation by gray scale imaging
  - ○ Assess cortical echogenicity and corticomedullary (CM) differentiation
  - ○ Measure maximum length of renal axis and anteroposterior & transverse diameters relative to renal axis
- Vascular evaluation by color Doppler imaging
  - ○ Evaluate patency of renal vessels and graft vascularity

Imaging Pitfalls

- Bladder confused with urinoma or lymphocele
- Iliac vessels and allograft hilar vessels confused with dilated ureter

Normal Measurements

- Grayscale imaging
  - ○ On average 11 ± 2 cm in length
  - ○ 7-25% volume ↑ by end of 2nd week post-transplantation
  - ○ 24% volume ↑ in follow-up versus baseline scan
- Doppler parameters
  - ○ Normally peak systolic velocity (PSV) < 180 cm/s, if > 250 cm/s ⇒ 60% RA stenosis (highly specific)
  - ○ Systolic velocity ratio [PSV at stenosis/PSV in renal artery (RA) at external iliac artery] > 3.0 ⇒ 60% RA stenosis

PATHOLOGIC ISSUES

General Pathologic Considerations

- Frequent complications: ATN, rejection, perinephric fluid collections, obstructive uropathy and vascular abnormalities
- ATN
  - ○ Most common cause of acute post-transplant renal failure
  - ○ Seen in 50% cadaver kidneys
  - ○ Uncomplicated ATN is reversible
- Rejection
  - ○ Most common cause of renal failure after 1st week post-transplantation
  - ○ Divided into acute and chronic based on nature of microscopic inflammatory lesion
  - ○ Cortical ischemia may result in parenchymal foci of edema, hemorrhage or infarction
  - ○ Both ATN and acute rejection are characterized by diminished perfusion
- Perinephric fluid collections
  - ○ Hematomas and seromas: Sequela of surgery
  - ○ Urinomas: Urine leaks at ureterovesical anastomosis related to surgical technique or distal ureteral necrosis
  - ○ Lymphoceles: Due to surgical disruption of lymphatic drainage
  - ○ Abscesses: Due to infection
- Obstructive uropathy
  - ○ Obstructive causes: Ureteral strictures, torsion, ureteral necrosis (most common), blood clots, calculi, ureteral kinking and extrinsic compression by perinephric fluid collection
  - ○ Non-obstructive causes: Diminished ureteral tone, bladder distension
- Vascular complications
  - ○ RA stenosis, vascular occlusion, AVF and pseudoaneurysm
  - ○ Causes of RA stenosis: Type of anastomosis, surgical procedure, arterial trauma during harvesting and chronic rejection

SONOGRAPHIC FEATURES OF RENAL ALLOGRAFTS

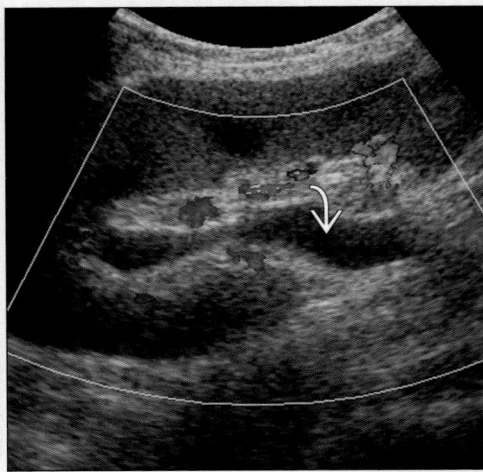

Oblique color Doppler ultrasound shows pelvicaliectasis 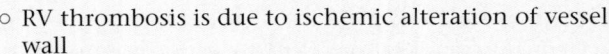 *in a renal allograft due to bladder distension. The degree of dilatation is affected by amount of bladder distension.*

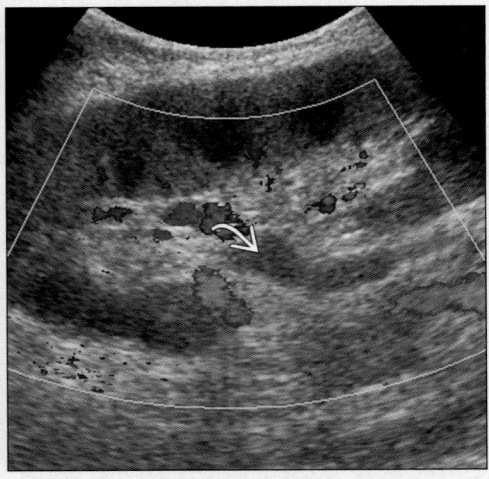

Oblique color Doppler ultrasound shows previous allograft after micturition. The collecting system is decompressed ➡ *and obstructive uropathy is excluded.*

- ○ RV thrombosis is due to ischemic alteration of vessel wall
- ○ AVF and pseudoaneurysm are uncommon complications of renal biopsies

PATHOLOGY-BASED IMAGING ISSUES

Key Concepts or Questions

- Rejection
  - ○ Renal enlargement, swollen medullary pyramids and high RI > 0.9 (highly specific)
  - ○ Renal volume ↑ (rejection > ATN: 73% versus 27%) compared to early post-operative baseline scan
  - ○ ATN and rejection may have overlapping sonographic features
  - ○ Parenchymal changes determined by severity of impaired cortical perfusion and vascular occlusion
- Perinephric fluid collection
  - ○ Small amount of perigraft fluid may be normal post-operatively
  - ○ Characterization of fluid collections is insensitive by ultrasound and must be diagnosed by aspiration
- Hydronephrosis
  - ○ Intrarenal spectral Doppler may be useful in diagnosis of obstruction
  - ○ Obstruction: High resistivity index (RI > 0.75), but is non-specific
- Vascular complications
  - ○ RA stenosis: Focal color aliasing, high-velocity post-stenotic turbulence
  - ○ AVF: High-velocity, low resistance flow in feeding artery; arterialization of venous signals
  - ○ Pseudoaneurysm: Pulsatile hypoechoic mass with characteristic high-velocity jet or to-and-fro flow at aneurysm neck

Imaging Approaches

- Check for urothelial wall thickening, pelvicaliceal distension and calculus formation
- Look for perirenal and pelvic fluid collection

- Suspected perinephric fluid collections or hydronephrosis should be rescanned following patient voiding
- Scrutinize for presence of arteriovenous fistula (AVF) or pseudoaneurysm after renal biopsy
- Native kidneys and renal allograft should be scanned for neoplasms in routine follow-up scan

Imaging Protocols

- Baseline ultrasound performed in early post-operative period; 2nd scan in 2 weeks and 3rd scan in 3 months
- Equivocal RA stenosis should be re-scanned by ultrasound or excluded by angiography or MRA
- Annual follow-up of both native kidneys and renal allograft for neoplasms is recommended

Imaging Pitfalls

- Normal post-operative renal hypertrophy may mimic those caused by ATN or rejection
- Pelvicaliectasis due to bladder distension or ↓ ureteral tone mimics obstructive uropathy
- Vessel kinking simulates significant RA stenosis

CLINICAL IMPLICATIONS

Clinical Importance

- Early detection and diagnosis of allograft complications guides proper therapy and prolongs life of allograft

RELATED REFERENCES

1. Baxter GM: Ultrasound of renal transplantation. Clin Radiol. 56(10):802-18, 2001
2. Baxter GM et al: Colour Doppler ultrasound in renal transplant artery stenosis: which Doppler index? Clin Radiol. 50(9):618-22, 1995
3. Dodd GD 3rd et al: Imaging of vascular complications associated with renal transplants. AJR Am J Roentgenol. 157(3):449-59, 1991
4. Raiss GJ et al: Further observations in the ultrasound evaluation of renal allograft rejection. J Ultrasound Med. 5(8):439-44, 1986

IMAGE GALLERY

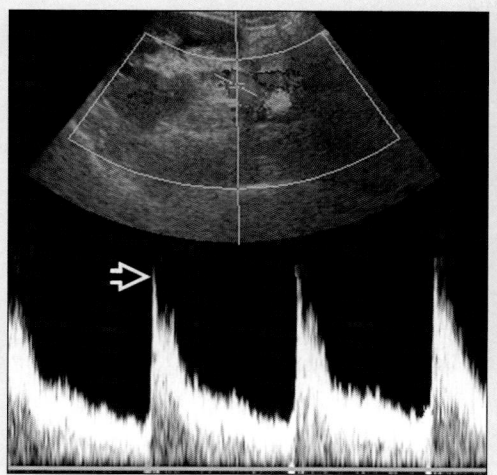

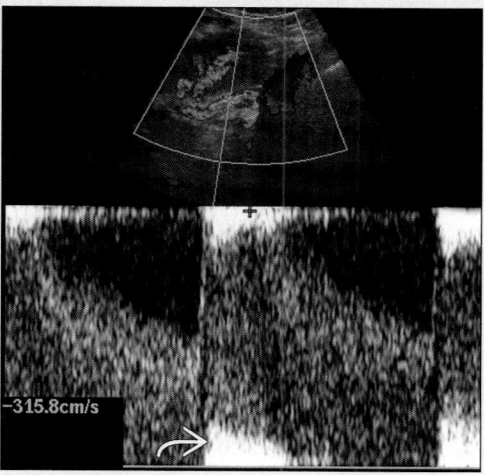

(Left) Transverse color Doppler ultrasound shows a normal allograft RA waveform. There is a low resistance waveform with a rapid systolic upstroke ➡ and PSV < 180 cm/s. (Right) Transverse color Doppler ultrasound shows high-velocity (> 300 cm/s) turbulent flow with aliasing ➡ at the origin of the allograft RA. Findings are consistent with severe stenosis > 60%.

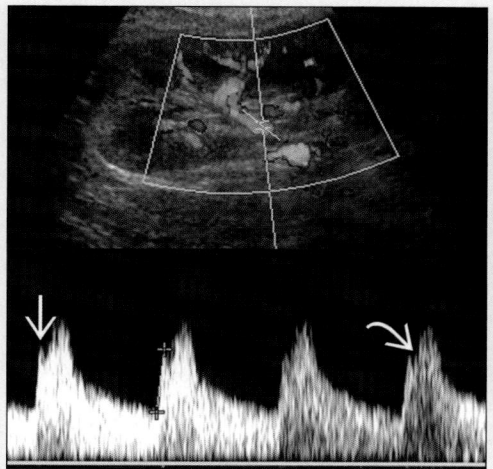

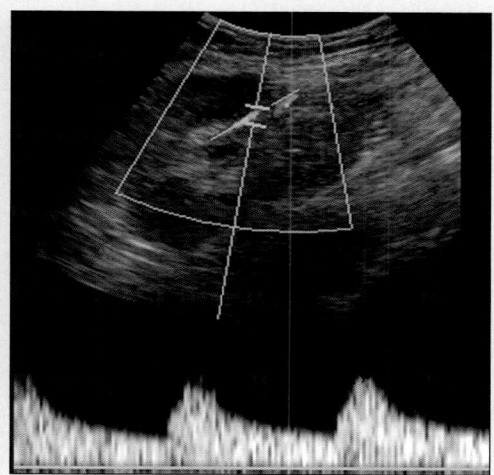

(Left) Oblique color Doppler ultrasound shows a normal allograft intra-RA waveform with a sharp systolic stroke, early systolic peak ➡, dicrotic notch ➡ and acceleration time (AT) < 100 ms. (Right) Transverse color Doppler ultrasound shows a "tardus parvus" waveform in allograft intra-RA. Note the delayed systolic upstroke, lost dicrotic notch and prolonged AT > 100 ms.

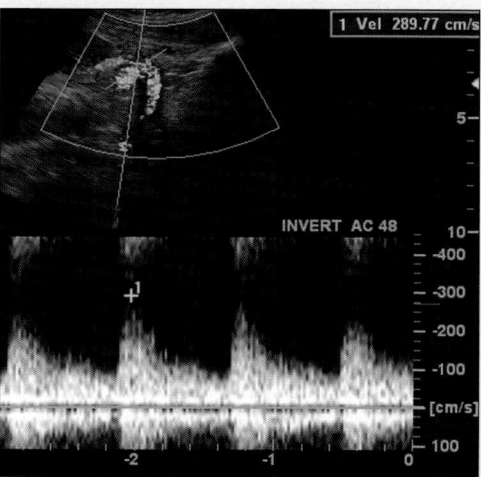

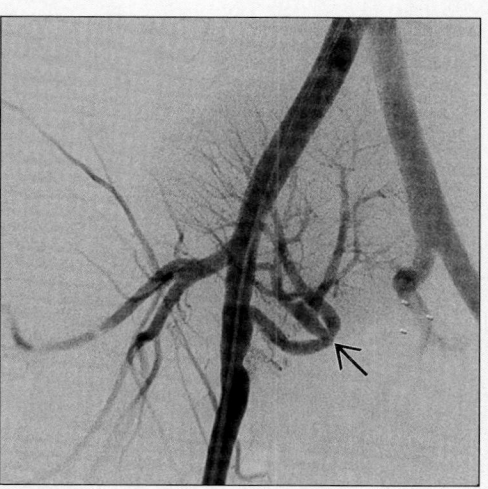

(Left) Transverse color Doppler ultrasound shows a vessel kink mimicking stenosis in an allograft RA. Note high-velocity turbulent flow present at one hilar artery; suspicious of severe stenosis. (Right) DSA shows previous allograft RA ➡. There is no delay in contrast opacification of both hilar arteries nor intra-RA pressure drop, which is more suggestive of a vessel kink rather than stenosis.

ALLOGRAFT HYDRONEPHROSIS

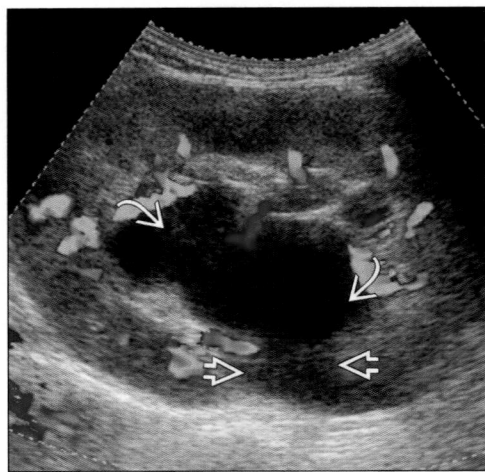

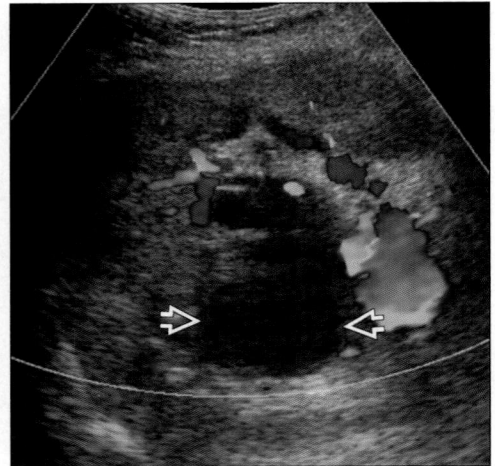

Longitudinal color Doppler ultrasound shows severe graft hydronephrosis secondary to ureteric stricture. Note both calyces ⇶ and renal pelvis ➤ are dilated.

Transverse color Doppler ultrasound of the dilated renal pelvis ➤ of the same graft as the previous image.

TERMINOLOGY

Abbreviations and Synonyms
- Obstructive pyelocaliectasis

Definitions
- Pelvicaliceal dilatation with or without hydroureter

IMAGING FINDINGS

General Features
- Best diagnostic clue: Splitting of central calyceal system with dilated renal pelvis
- Location: Approximately 90% of obstructions occur at ureterovesical junction as a result of ureteric stricture or ischemia
- Morphology
  - True obstruction results from ureteral stricture, blood clot, fungal ball or calculus
  - Very rarely a sloughed papilla may cause ureteral obstruction
  - Obstruction may be secondary to ureteric compression by perigraft fluid collections
  - Non-obstructive causes: Ureteral edema, rejection, reflux, decreased ureteral tone or ureteral kinking
  - Hydronephrosis may be transient in immediate posttransplantation due to edema at ureteric anastomosis
  - Pelviectasis rarely associated with obstruction unless occurring within a month posttransplantation
  - Calculus is rare, present in < 2% of renal allograft

Ultrasonographic Findings
- Grayscale Ultrasound
  - Ultrasound: Sensitive and specific for hydronephrosis
  - Harmonic imaging is better than fundamental gray scale imaging for evaluating subtle calyceal dilatation and small calculi (less side lobe, scatter artifact)
  - Has limitation to locate site of obstruction
  - Dilatation of renal pelvis and calyceal system which appears as a hypoechoic branching structure
  - Hydroureter depicted as avascular tubular structure arising from renal hilum
  - Echoes within calyceal system, suggestive of pyo- or hemonephrosis

DDx: Allograft Hydronephrosis

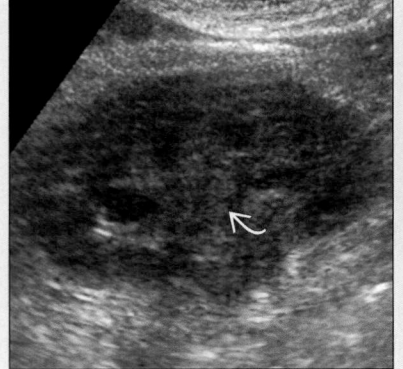

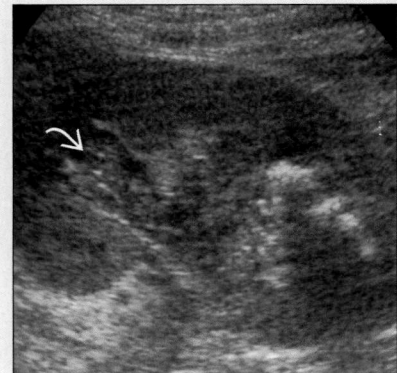

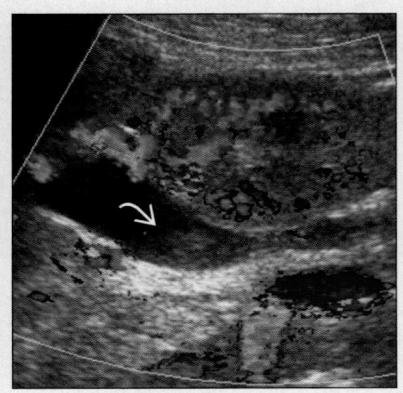

Transitional Cell Carcinoma

Pyonephrosis

Hemonephrosis

ALLOGRAFT HYDRONEPHROSIS

Key Facts

Imaging Findings
- Best diagnostic clue: Splitting of central calyceal system with dilated renal pelvis
- True obstruction results from ureteral stricture, blood clot, fungal ball or calculus
- Very rarely a sloughed papilla may cause ureteral obstruction
- Obstruction may be secondary to ureteric compression by perigraft fluid collections
- Ultrasound: Sensitive and specific for hydronephrosis
- Harmonic imaging is better than fundamental gray scale imaging for evaluating subtle calyceal dilatation and small calculi (less side lobe, scatter artifact)
- Echoes within calyceal system, suggestive of pyo- or hemonephrosis
- Highly echogenic, weakly shadowing masses, suggestive of fungal balls
- Avascular hypoechoic material in dilated ureter, indicative of blood clot
- Graft calculi if small may not show shadowing
- "Twinkling" artifact: Color "comet-tail" is typical of renal calculus
- Color Doppler: Useful to demonstrate tiny vessels within urothelial tumors
- Ultrasound, offered as initial investigation during post-operative period

Top Differential Diagnoses
- Transitional Cell Carcinoma (TCC)
- Pyo- or Hemonephrosis
- Renal Cysts
- Prominent Hilar Vessels

- Highly echogenic, weakly shadowing masses, suggestive of fungal balls
- Avascular hypoechoic material in dilated ureter, indicative of blood clot
- Graft calculi if small may not show shadowing
- Dilatation of renal pelvis and ureter may be associated with full bladder
- Unable to provide functional assessment
- Color Doppler
  - Useful to distinguish hilar vessels from dilated ureter
  - RI > 0.7 is suggestive of obstructive uropathy, but this finding is nonspecific and of little diagnostic value
  - Normal RI is strongly against obstruction unless a ureteral leak is present
  - "Twinkling" artifact: Color "comet-tail" is typical of renal calculus
  - Color Doppler: Useful to demonstrate tiny vessels within urothelial tumors
- Power Doppler
  - Has limited role in diagnosing hydronephrosis except for differentiating hilar vessels from dilated ureter
  - "Twinkling" artifact may appear distal to calculus
  - Useful to demonstrate tiny vessels within urothelial tumors

MR Findings
- T2WI FS
  - Highly sensitive for fluid collection and allows differentiation between hydronephrosis and renal cysts
  - Short acquisition time (1 second/slice) ideal for uncooperative patients
  - Provides high-resolution display of urinary tract (UT)
  - MR: Localization of obstruction is superior to Intravenous pyelogram and ultrasound
  - Can demonstrate UT distal to obstruction
  - MR can provide renal functional assessment
  - Advantage: Avoids potential side effects of iodinated contrast medium administration

Fluoroscopic Findings
- Antegrade pyelography (AP) is invasive
- Antegrade pyelography is gold standard in differentiating true from transient obstruction
- Provides valuable anatomic and physiologic information about site and significance of obstruction
- Disadvantage is the administration of iodinated contrast medium
- For interventional procedures, it is performed under ultrasound guidance

Imaging Recommendations
- Best imaging tool
  - Ultrasound, offered as initial investigation during post-operative period
  - Harmonic imaging is better than fundamental gray scale imaging
- Protocol advice
  - If ultrasound fails to delineate cause/site of obstruction, MRU may be considered
  - AP should be solely reserved for interventional procedure under ultrasound guidance for decompressing obstruction

DIFFERENTIAL DIAGNOSIS

Transitional Cell Carcinoma (TCC)
- Patients usually present with painless hematuria
- Coexists with hydronephrosis
- Hypoechoic urothelial tumor mimics hydronephrosis, unless demonstrated by color Doppler imaging

Pyo- or Hemonephrosis
- Dilated calyceal system filled with low level echoes
- Patient's clinical symptoms provide important clues to diagnosis

Renal Cysts
- To rule out cysts, important to show communication between cystic lesion and collecting system

ALLOGRAPH HYDRONEPHROSIS

Urothelial Thickening
- Secondary to acute rejection, and infection
- Appears as hypoechoic lining within collecting system; if grossly thickened, can mimic hydronephrosis

Prominent Hilar Vessels
- Mimicking dilated ureter
- Easily differentiated from dilated ureter with the aid of color Doppler imaging

PATHOLOGY

General Features
- Epidemiology
  - Incidence of obstructive hydronephrosis accounts for about 9% of cases
  - Ureteral obstruction occurs in 3-6% of renal allografts
- Associated abnormalities
  - Acute or chronic rejection
  - Nephrolithiasis
  - Infection
  - Urothelial tumors

Gross Pathologic & Surgical Features
- Fibrosis due to ureteral ischemia or rejection
- Ureteral edema or intraluminal blood clot
- Cortical thinning if hydronephrosis is long-standing and severe

CLINICAL ISSUES

Presentation
- Most common signs/symptoms
  - Rising creatinine level
  - Typically asymptomatic
    - Because allograft is denervated, collecting system dilates without causing pain or discomfort
  - Diagnosis is usually made as incidental finding or work-up in transplant patient with asymptomatic deterioration of renal function
- Other signs/symptoms: Tender graft

Natural History & Prognosis
- For non-obstructive causes, hydronephrosis usually is mild and transient and requires no intervention
- For obstructive causes if detected early, it is mostly correctable with good prognosis

Treatment
- Stent placement
- Balloon dilatation
- Removal of intrinsic obstruction such as clot, calculus
- Correction of extrinsic compression (e.g., percutaneous aspiration of perigraft fluid collection)
- Surgical reconstruction required for long or recurrent strictures

DIAGNOSTIC CHECKLIST

Consider
- Ultrasound offers as initial investigation in immediate post-operative period and in follow-up
- MRU is complementary to ultrasound to evaluate causes of obstruction and renal function assessment
- Ultrasound guided AP for interventional procedures if required

Image Interpretation Pearls
- Splitting of calyceal system
- Use of harmonic imaging for evaluating subtle calyceal dilatation and small calculi as with harmonic imaging there is less side lobe and scatter artifact

SELECTED REFERENCES

1. Browne RF et al: Imaging of the renal transplant: comparison of MRI with duplex sonography. Abdom Imaging. 2006
2. Kamath S et al: Papillary necrosis causing hydronephrosis in renal allograft treated by percutaneous retrieval of sloughed papilla. Br J Radiol. 78(928):346-8, 2005
3. Pepe P et al: Functional evaluation of the urinary tract by color-Doppler ultrasonography (CDU) in 100 patients with renal colic. Eur J Radiol. 53(1):131-5, 2005
4. Sandhu C et al: Renal transplantation dysfunction: the role of interventional radiology. Clin Radiol. 57(9):772-83, 2002
5. Lee JY et al: Color and power Doppler twinkling artifacts from urinary stones: clinical observations and phantom studies. AJR Am J Roentgenol. 176(6):1441-5, 2001
6. Brown ED et al: Complications of renal transplantation: evaluation with US and radionuclide imaging. Radiographics. 20(3):607-22, 2000
7. Shapeero LG et al: Papillary necrosis causing hydronephrosis in the renal allograft. Sonographic findings. J Ultrasound Med. 8(10):579-81, 1989
8. Straiton JA et al: Ultrasound in suspected obstruction complicating renal transplantation. Br J Radiol. 62(741):803-6, 1989

ALLOGRAFT HYDRONEPHROSIS

IMAGE GALLERY

Typical

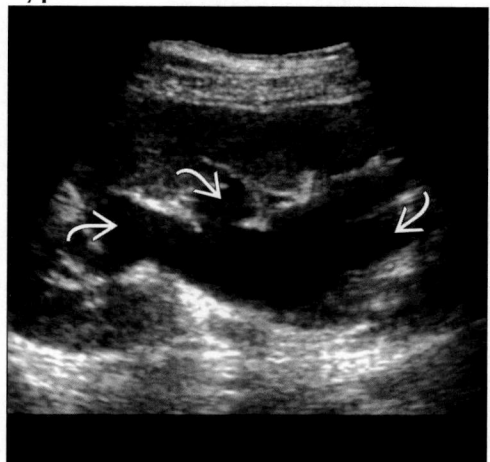

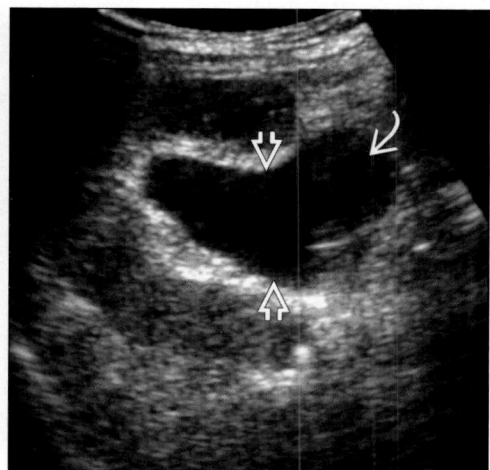

(Left) Longitudinal transabdominal ultrasound shows a renal transplant allograft with severe hydronephrosis and calyceal clubbing ➡. *(Right)* Transverse transabdominal ultrasound shows a distended renal pelvis ➡ & proximal ureter ➡, in the same graft as the previous image. Often distal obstruction cannot be identified on US. MRU may help delineate the point of obstruction.

Typical

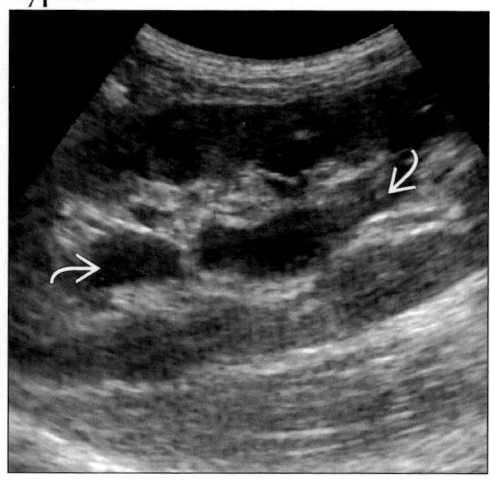

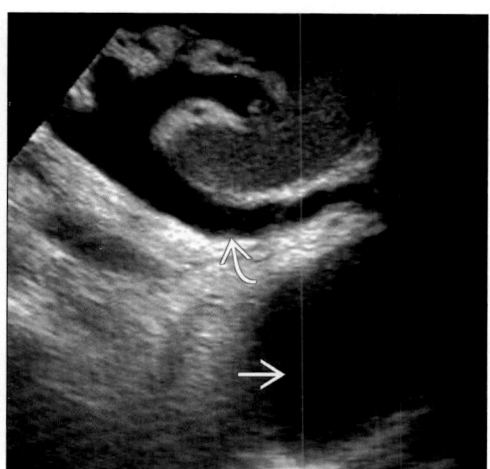

(Left) Longitudinal transabdominal ultrasound shows a mildly hydronephrotic graft with splitting of the calyceal system ➡. The site of obstruction was not identified on ultrasound. *(Right)* Longitudinal transabdominal ultrasound shows graft hydronephrosis with ureteral dilatation ➡ seen down to the bladder ➡. The ureter is denervated so dilatation does not cause pain or discomfort.

Typical

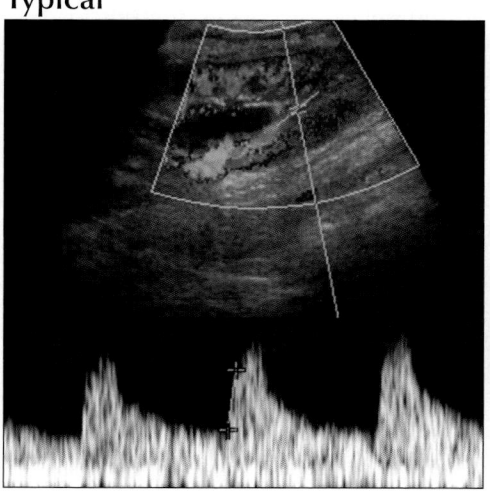

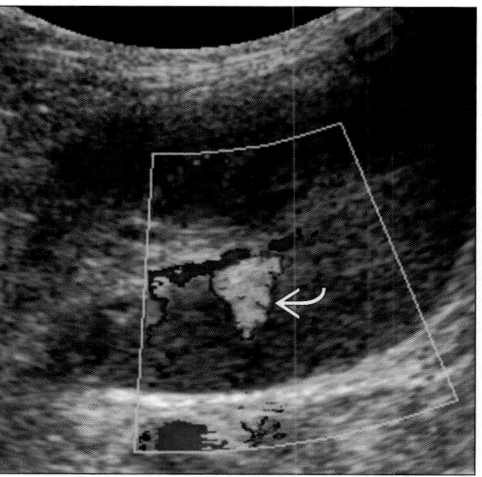

(Left) Longitudinal color Doppler ultrasound shows a low RI spectral waveform of a hydronephrotic graft. A high RI > 0.7 is suspicious of urinary obstruction but is nonspecific. *(Right)* Transverse color Doppler ultrasound shows a "twinkling" artifact with a classical color "comet-tail" ➡ arising from an echogenic focus in the graft kidney. This finding is typical of a renal calculus.

PERIGRAFT FLUID COLLECTIONS

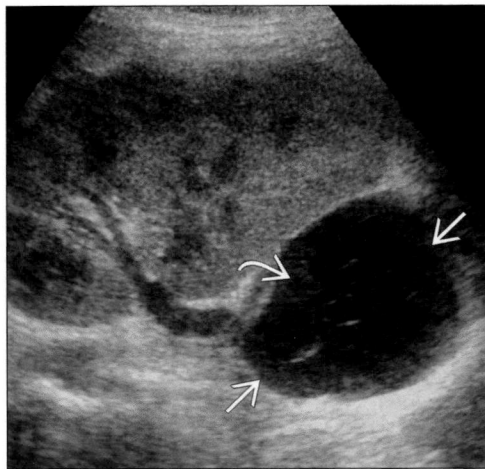

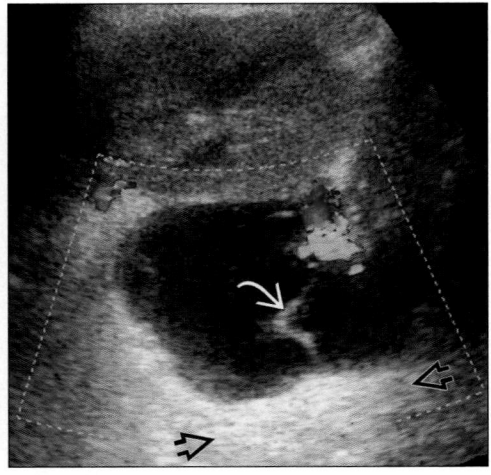

Longitudinal transabdominal ultrasound shows PFC ➡ containing internal echoes ➡ and abutting graft lower pole in a febrile patient. Aspiration confirmed an abscess.

Transverse color Doppler ultrasound shows same abscess as in previous image with thick internal septa ➡. Note characteristic posterior enhancement ➡.

TERMINOLOGY

Abbreviations and Synonyms
- Perigraft fluid collections (PFC)

Definitions
- Occur in approx 14% in early post-operative period
- Includes hematomas, seromas, urinomas, lymphoceles and abscesses
- May cause graft hydronephrosis
- Lymphoceles, most common PFC, occur in 5-15% patients
  - Most frequently associated with graft hydronephrosis due to extrinsic ureteral compression
- Urinomas occur in 2-5% of patients secondary to anastomotic leak or ureteric ischemia
- Hematomas/seromas: Normal sequela of surgery often small and seen immediately after transplantation
- Abscesses are found later in the post-operative period with clinical evidence of infection
  - Bacterial or fungal infection is not uncommon in renal transplant patients due to immunosuppression

IMAGING FINDINGS

General Features
- Best diagnostic clue
  - Perigraft space occupying cystic structures, either localized or free
  - Appearance and complications of PFC depend on its composition and location
  - Definitive diagnosis established by ultrasound-guided needle aspiration
- Location: Variable
- Size: Variable
- Morphology: Depends on composition of PFC

Ultrasonographic Findings
- Grayscale Ultrasound
  - PFC possess sonographic characteristics of cystic structures: Anechoic or hypoechoic with posterior enhancement
  - Lymphoceles are well-defined, large anechoic or heavily septated
  - Urinomas usually manifest as localized or free anechoic collections without septations
    - May be undetectable when small

DDx: Differentials of Allograft Perinephric Collections

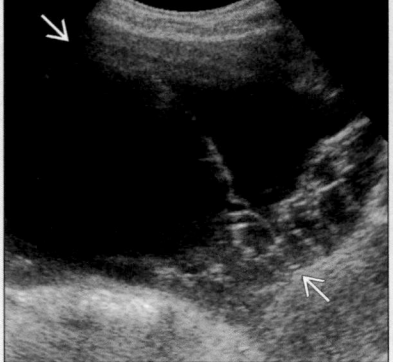

Mucinous Cystadenoma

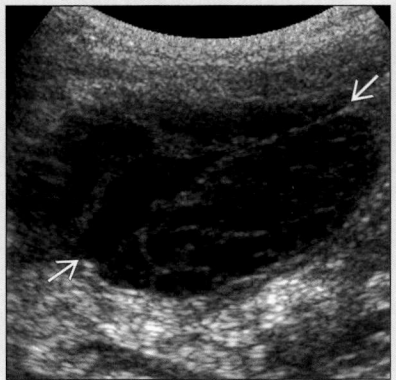

Pancreatic Pseudocyst

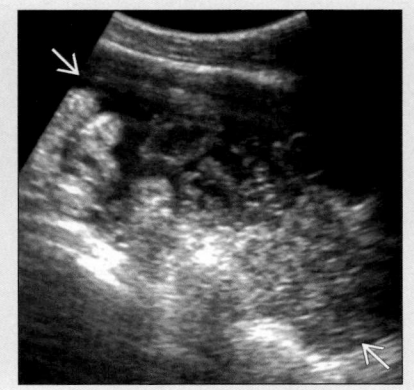

Pseudomyxoma Peritonei

ALLOGRAFT REJECTION

Key Facts

Terminology
- Common complication posttransplantation
- Occurs in acute/active form acute rejection (AR) and/or as chronic/fibrosing process chronic rejection (CR)
- Classification: Antibody (humoral) or cellular

Imaging Findings
- AR: Edematous renal allograft, swollen medullary pyramids, effacement of central sinus echo complex
- CR: Small and echogenic graft, cortical thinning, sparing of medullary pyramids, mild hydronephrosis
- AR: Resistivity index (RI) lacks sensitivity and specificity, RI 0.8-0.9 suspicious, abnormal > 0.9
- AR: Abnormal parenchymal vascularity (blush) may or may not be present
- CR: Scarce parenchymal vascularity

- Best imaging tool: Ultrasound, easily available and radiation-free, is ideal for immediate posttransplantation and follow-up
- Equivocal ultrasound findings, prompt for renal scintigraphy or MR
- If inconclusive, must perform renal biopsy for definitive diagnosis

Top Differential Diagnoses
- Acute Tubular Necrosis (ATN)
- Glomerulonephritis
- Nephrocalcinosis
- Renal Artery Stenosis
- Cyclosporine Nephrotoxicity

- Focal area of hypoechogenicity suggestive of infarction
- Perinephric fluid due to necrosis or hemorrhage may be present
- CR: Small and echogenic graft, cortical thinning, sparing of medullary pyramids, mild hydronephrosis
- Color Doppler
  - AR: Resistivity index (RI) lacks sensitivity and specificity, RI 0.8-0.9 suspicious, abnormal > 0.9
  - Early rejection, RI may be normal (0.6-0.8)
  - If abnormal RI (> 0.9), increases with increasing severity of rejection
  - Diastolic flow may be reversed
  - Values overlap with that of acute tubular necrosis (ATN)
  - CR: RI may be normal or slightly raised with reduced vascularity
  - CR: May have vascular pruning
- Power Doppler
  - AR: Abnormal parenchymal vascularity (blush) may or may not be present
  - If abnormal, highly predictive
  - CR: Scarce parenchymal vascularity

MR Findings
- T1WI
  - Post-gadolinium, renal cortex, medulla and collecting system depicted clearly
  - Abnormal nephrogram seen with rejection, ATN and vascular insult
  - Early cortical enhancement on MR: Diminished CM differentiation, suggestive of AR

Nuclear Medicine Findings
- Tc-99m DPTA renal scintigraphy
  - Useful in evaluating renal allograft function but is nonspecific
  - AR characterized by poor perfusion with decrease uptake and minimal excretion
  - Progressive impaired renal function on serial scintigraphy, suggestive of AR

- On single scan: Raised perfusion to uptake ratio, flat uptake curve and preserved peak/plateau pattern, specific for low grade AR
  - Flat uptake curve with loss of peak/plateau, indicative of high grade AR

Imaging Recommendations
- Best imaging tool: Ultrasound, easily available and radiation-free, is ideal for immediate posttransplantation and follow-up
- Protocol advice
  - Equivocal ultrasound findings, prompt for renal scintigraphy or MR
  - If inconclusive, must perform renal biopsy for definitive diagnosis

DIFFERENTIAL DIAGNOSIS

Acute Tubular Necrosis (ATN)
- Most common cause of delayed graft dysfunction in cadaveric transplants
- Generally self-limiting, renal function recovers within days to weeks
- Ultrasound features are variable and overlap with that of AR: Baseline transient renal enlargement and transient increase in RI

Glomerulonephritis
- Enlarged allograft with diminished parenchymal perfusion
- Echo-poor areas may be seen in CM region
- Spectral Doppler findings are nonspecific

Nephrocalcinosis
- Occurs in transplant kidneys involving renal cortex
- Results from chronic renal tubular acidosis

Renal Artery Stenosis
- Treatable if detected early
- Angiography being gold standard
- On Doppler ultrasound, peak systolic velocity (PSV) > 250 cm/s, predictive of stenosis > 60%

ALLOGRAFT REJECTION

- Post-stenotic turbulence, dampened signal distal to stenosis (tardus-parvus waveform)

Cyclosporine Nephrotoxicity
- Vasoconstrictive effect on afferent glomerular arterioles
- Decreased effective renal plasma flow
- No change in renal size
- No change or increase of RI

PATHOLOGY

General Features
- Etiology
  - ACR: Mediated by alloreactive T-lymphocytes that infiltrate allograft through endothelium with subsequent graft destruction by inflammatory and cytotoxic effects
  - AMR: Mediated by complex interaction of immunoglobulin antibodies that bind to antigens on vascular endothelium with formation of membrane attack complex and chemotactic factors, resulting in endothelial injury and graft damage
  - CR: Fibrotic changes in arteries and capillaries due to autoimmune mechanisms
- Epidemiology
  - AMR: Incidence varies between 0-9% and up to 30-35% of AR episodes
    - Risk factors: Previous transplant, female gender, pregnancy, positive cross-match, increased positive reactive antibody
- Associated abnormalities
  - Glomerulitis; capillaritis; severe necrotizing arteritis
  - Capillary leak with interstitial edema and/or hemorrhage
  - Thrombosis or infarction

Gross Pathologic & Surgical Features
- Acute: Swollen and hemorrhagic
- Chronic: Small, may have focal hemorrhage

Microscopic Features
- ACR: Lymphocytic tubulitis as classical feature
- AMR: Tubulitis and intimal arteritis as cardinal features where tubulitis > ACR
  - Early: Edema, tubular injury, little inflammation
  - Moderate: Capillaritis or glomerulitis
  - Severe: Arteritis
- CR: Thickened arteries with intimal fibrosis and chronic inflammation
  - Capillary basement membrane multilayering in glomeruli and peritubular capillaries

CLINICAL ISSUES

Presentation
- Most common signs/symptoms
  - Acute: Often asymptomatic apart from deranged renal function, allograft may be swollen and tender
  - Chronic: Hypertension, proteinuria, progressive deranged renal function
- Other signs/symptoms

- Fever
- Malaise
- Edema and weight gain
- Symptomatic azotemia

Natural History & Prognosis
- Generally good, if renal allograft is salvaged by antirejection therapy at early and mild stage
- Prognosis of ACR is generally better than AMR
- AMR is frequently associated with chronic allograft nephropathy or graft loss due to on-going immune injury

Treatment
- Multi-drug immunosuppression

DIAGNOSTIC CHECKLIST

Consider
- Ultrasound remains method of choice in immediate post-operative period and long term follow-up
- Renal scintigraphy and MR as second line investigations
- Renal biopsy if these investigations are inconclusive

Image Interpretation Pearls
- Ultrasound findings: Enlarged allograft with decreased parenchymal vascularity and high RI > 0.9

SELECTED REFERENCES

1. Aktas A et al: Indicators of Acute Rejection on Tc-99m DTPA Renal Scintigraphy. Transplant Proc. 38(2):443-8, 2006
2. Browne RF et al: Imaging of the renal transplant: comparison of MRI with duplex sonography. Abdom Imaging. 2006
3. Johnson HJ et al: Solid-Organ Transplant. In: Pharmacotherapy: A Pathophysiologic Approach. 6th ed. New York, McGrawHill. 1613-43, 2005
4. Racusen LC et al: Banff 2003 meeting report: new diagnostic insights and standards. Am J Transplant. 4(10):1562-6, 2004
5. Racusen LC: Antibody-mediated rejection in the kidney. Transplant Proc. 36(3):768-9, 2004
6. Dupont PJ et al: Role of duplex Doppler sonography in diagnosis of acute allograft dysfunction-time to stop measuring the resistive index? Transpl Int. 16(9):648-52, 2003
7. Chow L et al: Power Doppler imaging and resistance index measurement in the evaluation of acute renal transplant rejection. J Clin Ultrasound. 29(9):483-90, 2001
8. Brown ED et al: Complications of renal transplantation: evaluation with US and radionuclide imaging. Radiographics. 20(3):607-22, 2000
9. Heering P et al: Tubular dysfunction following kidney transplantation. Nephron. 74(3):501-11, 1996
10. Genkins SM et al: Duplex Doppler sonography of renal transplants: lack of sensitivity and specificity in establishing pathologic diagnosis. AJR Am J Roentgenol. 152(3):535-9, 1989

ALLOGRAFT REJECTION

Typical

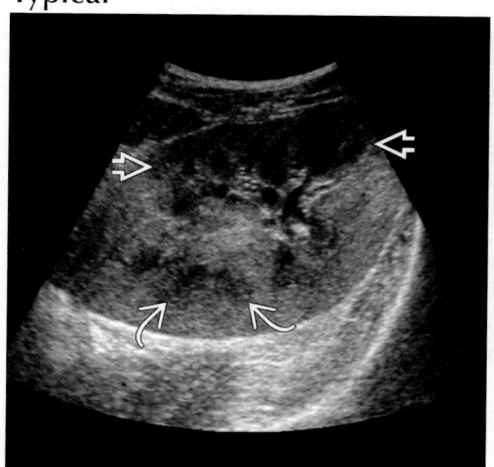
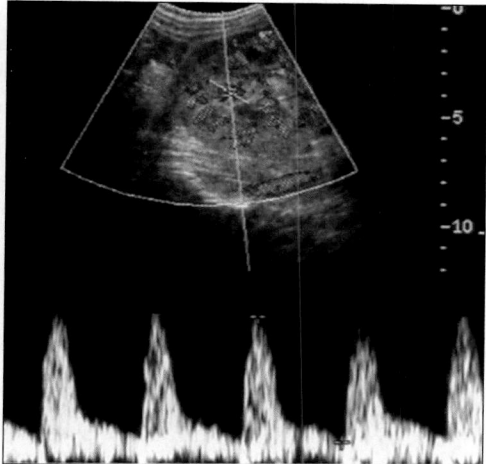

(Left) Longitudinal transabdominal ultrasound shows a swollen graft with AR. Note loss of CM differentiation ➜ and focal hypoechoic area ➡ probably representing focal infarction or phlegmon. (Right) Transverse color Doppler ultrasound of same graft as previous image shows intrarenal flow of high RI with low end-diastolic flow.

Typical

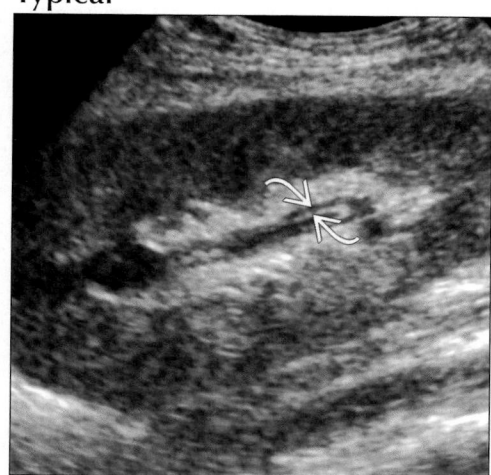
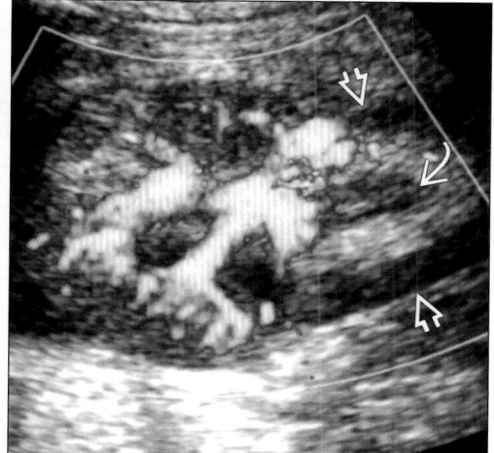

(Left) Longitudinal transabdominal ultrasound shows a renal allograft with AR. Urothelium ➜ is diffusely thickened indicative of collecting system edema. (Right) Longitudinal power Doppler ultrasound shows severe CR in cadaveric graft complicated by lobar infarction. Note absent Doppler signal and thick urothelium ➜ in atrophic lower pole ➡.

Typical

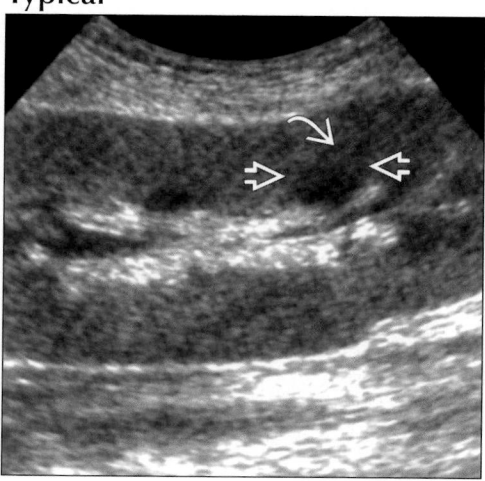
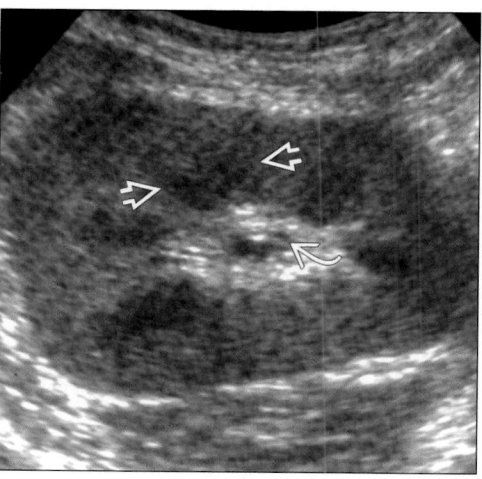

(Left) Longitudinal transabdominal ultrasound shows AR in cadaveric graft. Note swollen graft with prominent pyramids ➡ and diminished CM differentiation ➜. (Right) Transverse transabdominal ultrasound shows same renal graft as previous image. Medullary pyramids are swollen ➡ and urothelium is thickened ➜. Appearances are due to diffuse graft edema secondary to AR.

RENAL TRANSPLANT VASCULAR DISORDERS

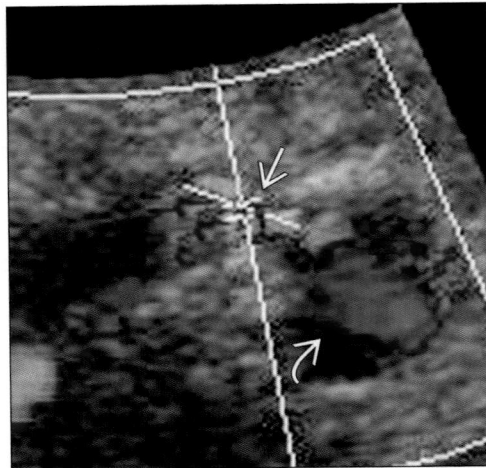

Oblique color Doppler ultrasound shows TRAS ➡ and post-stenotic turbulence, near the anastomosis with the iliac artery ➡.

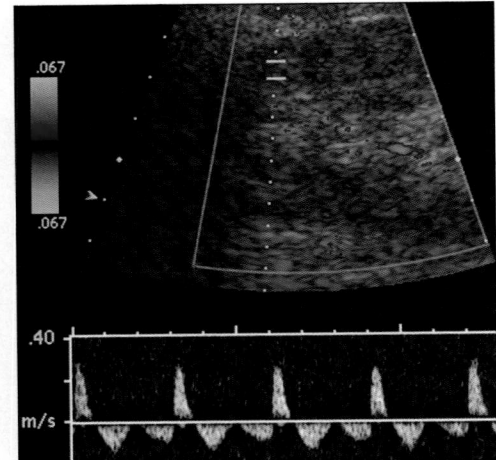

Longitudinal pulsed Doppler ultrasound shows high resistance intrarenal arterial Doppler waveforms with reversed diastolic flow in an inverted "M" pattern, due to renal vein thrombosis.

TERMINOLOGY

Abbreviations and Synonyms
- Transplant renal artery stenosis (TRAS)
- Transplant renal artery thrombosis (TRAT)
- Transplant renal vein thrombosis (TRVT)

Definitions
- TRAS: Narrowing of the transplant renal artery (TRA)
- TRAT: Complete obstruction of the transplant renal artery due to thrombus formation
- TRVT: Blockage of transplant renal vein due to thrombus formation

IMAGING FINDINGS

General Features
- Best diagnostic clue
  - TRAS: Focal elevation of TRA blood flow velocity with post-stenotic turbulence
  - TRAT: Absence of blood flow in TRA; absent arterial flow in kidney
  - TRVT: Absence of blood flow in TRV and persistent diastolic flow reversal in the TRA
- Location
  - TRAS: At artery origin or distally, near/in hilum
  - TRA and TRV thrombosis: Entire vessel
- Surgical anatomy
  - End of graft artery-to-side of external iliac artery
    - Performed in living donor and some cadaveric grafts
    - Common
  - End of graft artery-to-end of internal iliac artery or branch
    - Living donor or cadaveric graft
    - Uncommon
  - Patch of donor aorta (with renal artery attached)-to-side of external iliac artery
    - Cadaveric graft only
    - Common

Ultrasonographic Findings
- Grayscale Ultrasound
  - TRAS: Relevant grayscale findings unlikely
    - Appearance usually normal
  - TRAT: Kidney length < 8.5 cm

DDx: Transplant Vascular Disorders

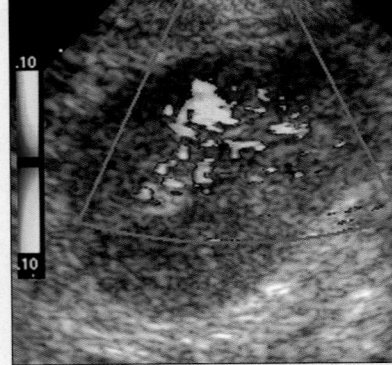

AV Fistula/Pseudoaneurysm

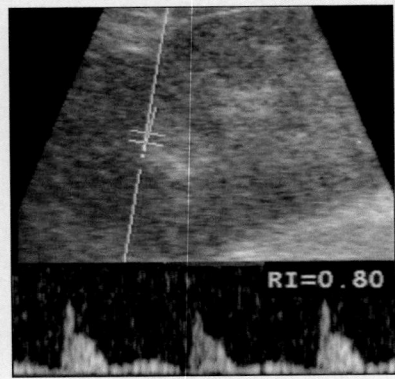

Acute Severe Rejection

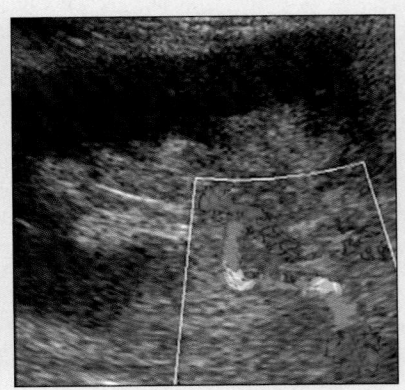

Tortuous Renal Artery

RENAL TRANSPLANT VASCULAR DISORDERS

Key Facts

Terminology
- Transplant renal artery stenosis (TRAS)
- Transplant renal artery thrombosis (TRAT)
- Transplant renal vein thrombosis (TRVT)

Imaging Findings
- TRAS: Focal elevation of TRA blood flow velocity with post-stenotic turbulence
- TRAT: Absence of blood flow in TRA; absent arterial flow in kidney
- TRVT: Absence of blood flow in TRV and persistent diastolic flow reversal in the TRA
- TRAS: Focal color shift or aliasing indicating elevated flow velocity
- TRAS: Post-stenotic turbulence
- TRAT: TRA visualized but without blood flow

- TRAT: Absent arterial flow in kidney hilum and parenchyma
- TRVT: TRV visualized, distended, and without blood flow
- TRVT: Absent venous flow in kidney hilum and parenchyma
- TRAS: PSV > 200 or 300 cm/sec (> 50-60%d) to > 400 cm/sec (> 70%d) (d = diameter reduction)
- TRAT: Absent or severely damped (collateralized) spectral Doppler signals in kidney
- TRVT: Sustained flow reversal in TRA, with shelf-like or inverted "M" shape

Top Differential Diagnoses
- Abrupt TRA Curves & Kinks: Mimic TRAS
- Acute, Severe Rejection or Tubular Necrosis: Mimic TRA & TRVT

- TRVT
  - TRV distended by low echogenicity thrombus
  - Kidney markedly enlarged and hypoechoic due to edema (congestion)
- Color Doppler
  - TRAS
    - TRAS: Focal color shift or aliasing indicating elevated flow velocity
    - TRAS: Post-stenotic turbulence
    - Possible soft tissue vibration adjacent to stenosis
  - TRAT
    - TRAT: TRA visualized but without blood flow
    - TRA not visualized
    - TRAT: Absent arterial flow in kidney hilum and parenchyma
  - TRVT
    - TRVT: TRV visualized, distended, and without blood flow
    - TRV not visualized
    - TRVT: Absent venous flow in kidney hilum and parenchyma
- Spectral Doppler
  - TRAS
    - Elevated flow velocity in stenotic area
    - Moderate-to-severe post-stenotic turbulence
    - Note: Wide range of peak systolic velocities (PSVs) in normal graft arteries: 60-200 cm/sec
    - Note: Doppler stenosis criteria not well established; following criteria reported
    - TRAS: PSV > 200 or 300 cm/sec (> 50-60%d) to > 400 cm/sec (> 70%d) (d = diameter reduction)
    - Damped arterial waveforms hilar/interlobar arteries with prolonged systolic acceleration > 0.07, > 0.08, and > 0.10 sec (range > 50-70%d)
    - PSV stenosis/PSV interlobar arteries > 13 (> 70%d)
    - PSV stenosis/PSV aorta > 3.0 to 3.5 (> 60%d)
    - PSV stenosis/PSV iliac artery > 2 (> 50-60%d), to > 5 (> 70%d)
  - TRAT
    - Absent spectral Doppler signals in TRA
    - TRAT: Absent or severely damped (collateralized) spectral Doppler signals in kidney

- TRVT
  - TRVT: Sustained flow reversal in TRA, with shelf-like or inverted "M" shape
  - Absent spectral Doppler signals in TRV and kidney hilum

Imaging Recommendations
- Best imaging tool: Color, power, spectral Doppler US
- Protocol advice: Correct adjustment of pulse repetition frequency, gain, other Doppler controls is essential

DIFFERENTIAL DIAGNOSIS

Abrupt TRA Curves & Kinks: Mimic TRAS
- Curves and kinks elevate flow velocity without stenosis
- Do not try to diagnose stenosis when curves or kinks are present
- Be wary of diagnosing flow-limiting stenoses in absence of post-stenotic flow disturbance

Transplant Arteriovenous Fistula
- Another cause of hypertension

Acute, Severe Rejection or Tubular Necrosis: Mimic TRA & TRVT
- Flow resistance in renal parenchyma markedly elevated, causing
  - Diminished or absent arterial flow in kidney hilum/interlobar arteries
  - Persistent diastolic flow reversal in TRA

PATHOLOGY

General Features
- Etiology
  - TRAS and TRAT
    - Surgical injury (harvesting or transplantation)
    - Anastomotic technical problems
    - Neointimal hyperplasia
    - Rejection > scarring

RENAL TRANSPLANT VASCULAR DISORDERS

- ○ TRVT
  - Usual: Surgical injury or technical problem
  - Less commonly: Thrombus propagation from common femoral/external iliac vein
  - Less common: Vein compression by confined fluid collection (e.g., hematoma, lymphocele)
  - Hypovolemia = possible contributing factor
- Epidemiology
  - ○ TRAS
    - Most common graft vascular problem
    - 3-10% of transplants
  - ○ TRAT: < 1% of transplants
  - ○ TRVT: ≤ 4% of transplants
- Associated abnormalities
  - ○ Marked graft congestion/edema with TRV occlusion
  - ○ Confined fluid collections > TRV occlusion

Gross Pathologic & Surgical Features
- TRAS: Arterial wall fibrosis → luminal narrowing
- TRAT: Stenosis → thrombosis
- TRVT: Intraluminal thrombus formation

Microscopic Features
- Surgical injury, inflammation, arterial wall fibrosis, thrombus

CLINICAL ISSUES

Presentation
- Most common signs/symptoms
  - ○ TRAS
    - Post-op complication or later; usually first 3 years
    - Hypertension = principal symptom; newly developed, progressive, or resistant to therapy
    - Transplant dysfunction
    - Bruit in vicinity of transplant/iliac artery
  - ○ TRAT
    - Usually 1st post-operative month
    - Abrupt onset of oliguria, decreased function
    - Almost always → loss of graft
  - ○ TRVT
    - Usually within 48 hours post-op
    - Abrupt onset of graft tenderness and swelling, oliguria, proteinuria, decreased function

Natural History & Prognosis
- TRAS: Excellent prognosis with successful treatment of stenosis/surgical revision
- TRAT: Poor prognosis, graft loss typical
- TRAT: Good prognosis with prompt thrombectomy/surgical revision

Treatment
- TRAS: Angioplasty or surgical revision of TRA
- TRAT: Thrombectomy, surgical TRA revision
- TRVT: Thrombectomy, surgical TRV revision

DIAGNOSTIC CHECKLIST

Consider
- Curves and kinks mimicking TRAS
- Transplant arteriovenous fistula causing hypertension

- Severe acute rejection or tubular necrosis mimicking TRA or TRV occlusion

Image Interpretation Pearls
- TRAS: Look for focal, high TRA velocity **and** turbulence
- TRVT: Marked graft swelling, persistent TRA diastolic flow reversal

SELECTED REFERENCES

1. Li JC et al: Evaluation of severe transplant renal artery stenosis with Doppler sonography. J Clin Ultrasound. 33(6):261-9, 2005
2. de Morais RH et al: Duplex Doppler sonography of transplant renal artery stenosis. J Clin Ultrasound. 31(3):135-41, 2003
3. Osman Y et al: Vascular complications after live donor renal transplantation: study of risk factors and effects on graft and patient survival. J Urol. 169(3):859-62, 2003
4. Patel U et al: Doppler ultrasound for detection of renal transplant artery stenosis-threshold peak systolic velocity needs to be higher in a low-risk or surveillance population. Clin Radiol. 58(10):772-7, 2003
5. Patel NH et al: Renal arterial stenosis in renal allografts: retrospective study of predisposing factors and outcome after percutaneous transluminal angioplasty. Radiology. 219(3):663-7, 2001
6. Souza de Oliveira IR et al: Colour Doppler ultrasound: a new index improves the diagnosis of renal artery stenosis. Ultrasound Med Biol. 26(1):41-7, 2000
7. Loubeyre P et al: Transplanted renal artery: detection of stenosis with color Doppler US. Radiology. 203(3):661-5, 1997
8. Miralles M et al: Value of Doppler parameters in the diagnosis of renal artery stenosis. J Vasc Surg. 23(3):428-35, 1996
9. Baxter GM et al: Colour Doppler ultrasound in renal transplant artery stenosis: which Doppler index? Clin Radiol. 50(9):618-22, 1995
10. Gottlieb RH et al: Diagnosis of renal artery stenosis in transplanted kidneys: value of Doppler waveform analysis of the intrarenal arteries. AJR Am J Roentgenol. 165(6):1441-6, 1995
11. Kribs SW et al: Doppler ultrasonography after renal transplantation: value of reversed diastolic flow in diagnosing renal vein obstruction. Can Assoc Radiol J. 44(6):434-8, 1993
12. Baxter GM et al: Acute renal vein thrombosis in renal allografts: new Doppler ultrasonic findings. Clin Radiol. 43(2):125-7, 1991
13. Dodd GD 3rd et al: Imaging of vascular complications associated with renal transplants. AJR Am J Roentgenol. 157(3):449-59, 1991
14. Pozniak MA et al: Renal transplant ultrasound: imaging and Doppler. Semin Ultrasound CT MR. 12(4):319-34, 1991
15. Kaveggia LP et al: Duplex Doppler sonography in renal allografts: the significance of reversed flow in diastole. AJR Am J Roentgenol. 155(2):295-8, 1990

IMAGE GALLERY

Typical

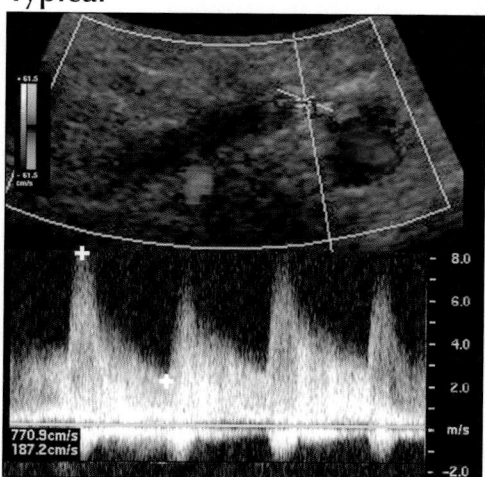 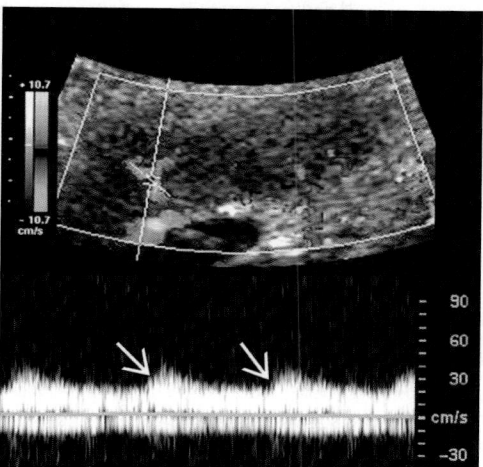

(Left) Oblique color Doppler ultrasound shows a very high peak systolic velocity of 771 cm/sec and end diastolic velocity of 187 in a patient with TRAS. *(Right)* Oblique color Doppler ultrasound shows markedly damped segmental arterial waveforms, as indicated by a sloped early systolic waveform ➡. This is another finding seen in TRAS.

Typical

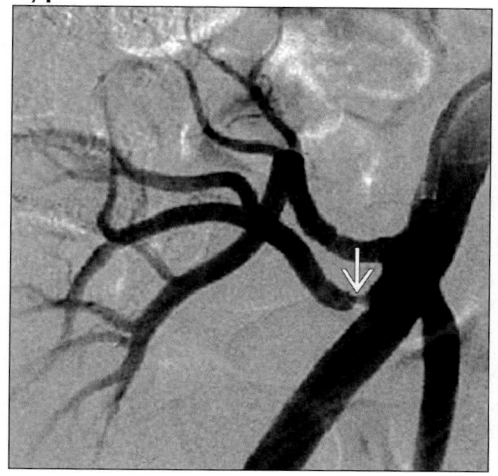 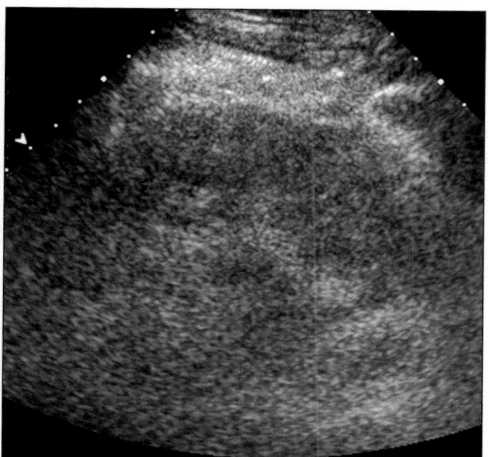

(Left) Oblique DSA on the same patient as the previous image shows two renal arteries, with severe stenosis ➡ on the one with the abnormal Doppler. *(Right)* Longitudinal ultrasound (same case as previous image) performed at 48 hrs post-transplant shows an indistinct, hypoechoic, edematous kidney that had increased in length from 12 cm at 24 hrs to almost 15 cm.

Typical

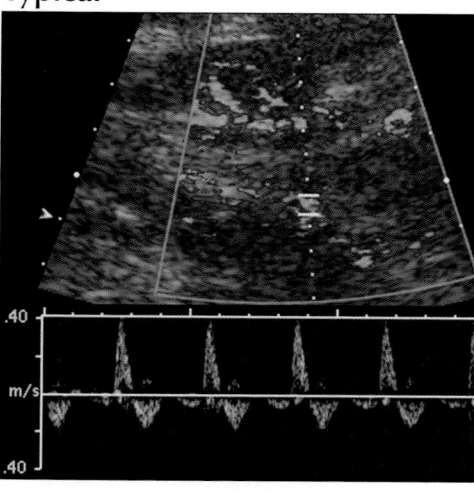 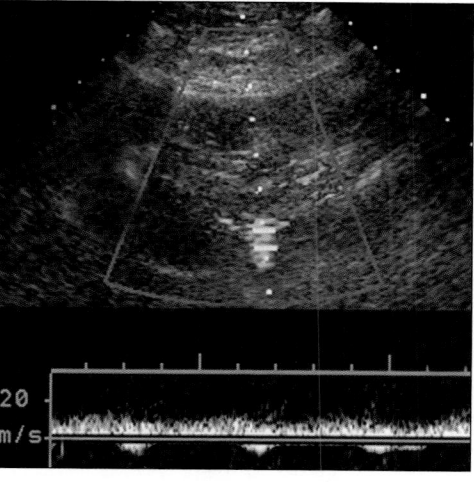

(Left) Longitudinal pulsed Doppler ultrasound in a patient with renal vein thrombosis shows only arterial flow in the renal hilum. Renal vein could not be identified. *(Right)* Longitudinal color Doppler ultrasound 24 hours after thrombectomy shows renal vein flow in the kidney hilum. No further complications occurred and kidney resumed normal function.

RENAL TRANSPLANT FISTULA/PSEUDOANEURYSM

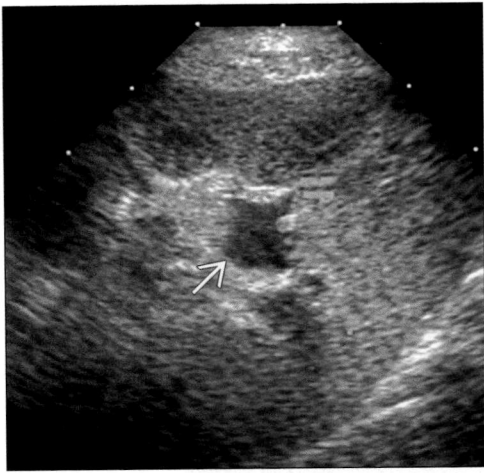

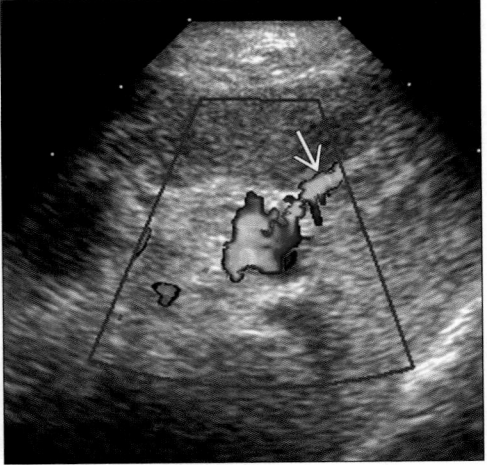

Oblique ultrasound shows cyst-like structure ➔ in renal sinus of this transplanted kidney approximately 1 month after percutaneous biopsy. Patient was asymptomatic.

Oblique color Doppler ultrasound shows blood flow in the structure shown on left indicating that it is pseudoaneurysm, not cyst. Note vessel ➔ extending from pseudoaneurysm.

TERMINOLOGY

Definitions
- Arteriovenous fistula (AVF): Abnormal, direct communication between an artery and a vein
- Pseudoaneurysm (PA): Saccular chamber into which blood circulates from a rent in an adjacent artery

IMAGING FINDINGS

General Features
- Best diagnostic clue
  - AVF: Focal soft tissue vibrations in transplant parenchyma on color Doppler US
  - PA: Focal vascular "lake" with turbulent blood flow
- Location: Usually in renal parenchyma, may be extrarenal
- Size: Parenchymal PA: Usually ≤ 1 cm, extrarenal PA may be larger
- Morphology: PAs are saccular, round or ovoid

Ultrasonographic Findings
- Pulsed Doppler

- AVF: Elevated velocity in feeding artery; turbulent/pulsatile flow draining vein
  - PA: Turbulent/pulsatile/to-and-fro waveforms
- Color Doppler
  - AVF
    - AVF: Focal montage of color in adjacent tissues
    - AVF: Prominent draining vein with turbulent flow
  - PA: Vascular "lake" with turbulent/swirling flow

Imaging Recommendations
- Best imaging tool: Color Doppler sonography
- Protocol advice: Proper Doppler adjustment is essential

DIFFERENTIAL DIAGNOSIS

Hydronephrosis Unrelated to AVF/PA
- Dilated renal pelvis, anechoic ± dilated calyx, ± dilated ureter
- If internal debris, echoes consider pyonephrosis

Renal Artery Stenosis
- Narrowing, increased peak systolic velocity
- Post-stenotic spectral broadening ± flow reversal
- Significant hypertension

DDx: Renal Transplant Arteriovenous Fistula/Pseudoaneurysm

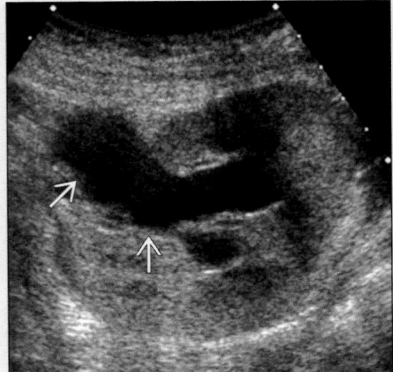

Hydronephrosis

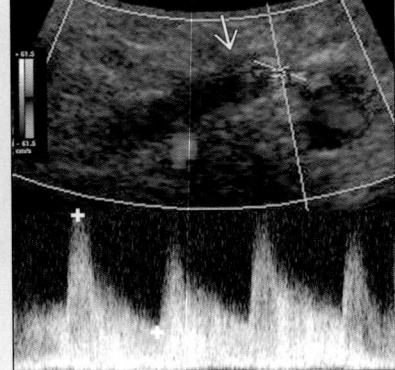

Transplant Renal Artery Stenosis

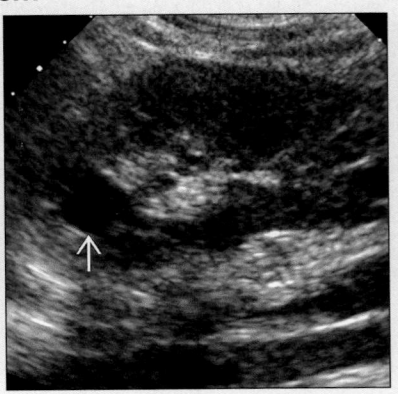

Renal Cyst

RENAL TRANSPLANT FISTULA/PSEUDOANEURYSM

Terminology
- Arteriovenous fistula (AVF): Abnormal, direct communication between an artery and a vein
- Pseudoaneurysm (PA): Saccular chamber into which blood circulates from a rent in an adjacent artery

Imaging Findings
- AVF: Elevated velocity in feeding artery; turbulent/pulsatile flow draining vein
- PA: Turbulent/pulsatile/to-and-fro waveforms

Key Facts
- AVF: Focal montage of color in adjacent tissues
- PA: Vascular "lake" with turbulent/swirling flow

Clinical Issues
- 50% of parenchymal AVFs disappear in 48 hours; 75% within 4 months; 3% of AVFs persist > 1 year

Diagnostic Checklist
- Focal, strong parenchymal color focus = AVF or PA
- Cyst-like lesion on grayscale; think of PA

Cysts or Fluid Collections
- Anechoic, thin walled with posterior enhancement
- No flow on color Doppler

PATHOLOGY

General Features
- Etiology
  - Percutaneous biopsy/nephrostomy complication
  - Surgical complication, usually anastomotic
- Epidemiology: Post-biopsy incidence: AVF 17%, PA 6%
- Associated abnormalities: AVF and PA often coexist

Microscopic Features
- PA: Confined by organized thrombus or fibrous tissue

CLINICAL ISSUES

Presentation
- Most common signs/symptoms: Most PAs/AVFs are asymptomatic
- Other signs/symptoms
  - Hypertension/renal dysfunction from large AVF
  - Hematuria/urinary tract obstruction from clots
  - Pain/other symptoms of PA rupture

Natural History & Prognosis
- AVFs and PAs
  - 50% of parenchymal AVFs disappear in 48 hours; 75% within 4 months; 3% of AVFs persist > 1 year
  - Extrarenal/sinus AVFs/PAs larger, more dangerous

Treatment
- Embolization, covered stents, surgery

DIAGNOSTIC CHECKLIST

Image Interpretation Pearls
- Focal, strong parenchymal color focus = AVF or PA
- Cyst-like lesion on grayscale; think of PA

SELECTED REFERENCES
1. Brandenburg VM et al: Color-coded duplex sonography study of arteriovenous fistulae and pseudoaneurysms complicating percutaneous renal allograft biopsy. Clin Nephrol. 58(6):398-404, 2002
2. Dodd GD 3rd et al: Imaging of vascular complications associated with renal transplants. AJR Am J Roentgenol. 157(3):449-59, 1991
3. Hubsch PJ et al: Evaluation of arteriovenous fistulas and pseudoaneurysms in renal allografts following percutaneous needle biopsy. Color-coded Doppler sonography versus duplex Doppler sonography. J Ultrasound Med. 9(2):95-100, 1990

IMAGE GALLERY

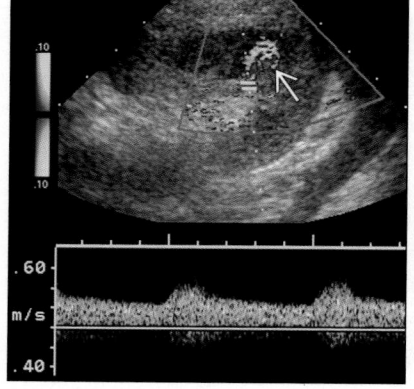 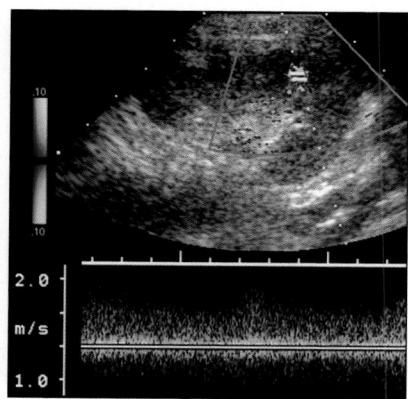 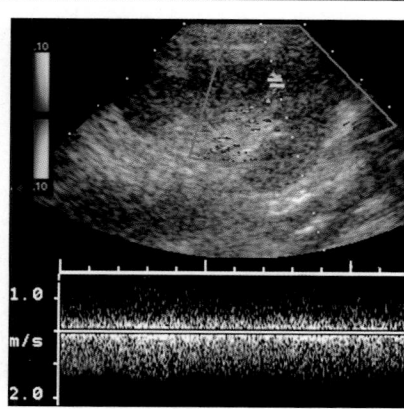

(Left) Longitudinal color Doppler ultrasound of a post-biopsy renal transplant shows high velocity blood flow in an artery feeding an arteriovenous fistula ➡. *(Center)* Oblique color Doppler ultrasound shows turbulent blood flow in the fistula. *(Right)* Oblique color Doppler ultrasound shows turbulent blood flow in the vein draining the fistula.

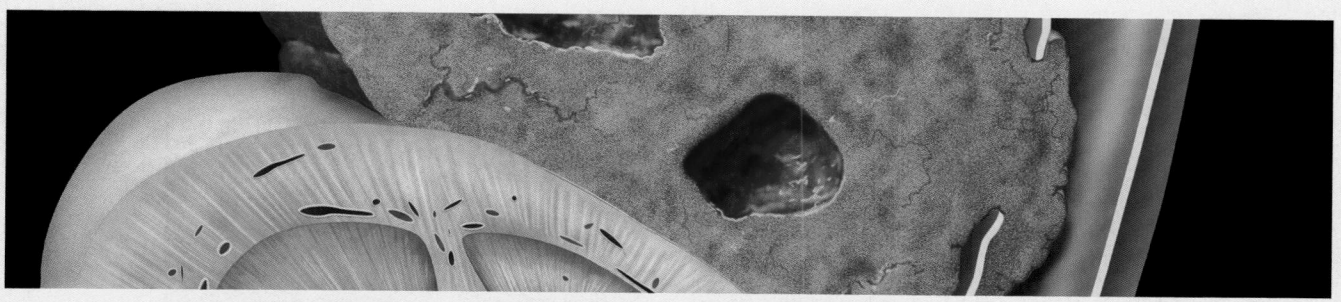

SECTION 7: Adrenal Gland

ADRENAL HEMORRHAGE

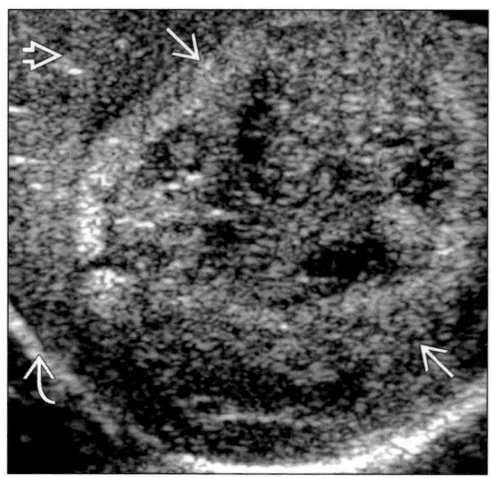

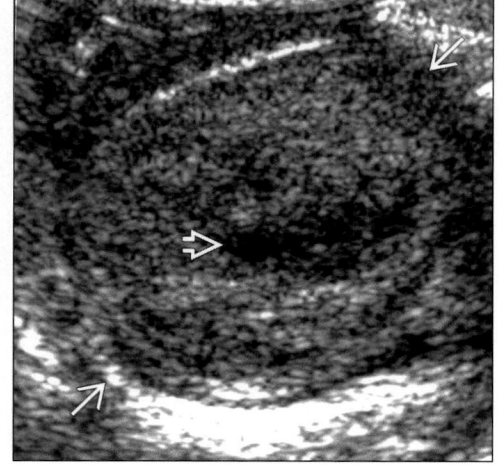

Longitudinal transabdominal ultrasound in a neonate shows a large, hyperechoic, acute right adrenal hemorrhage ➡. Note liver ➡ & diaphragm ➡.

Transverse transabdominal ultrasound (same patient as in previous image) shows hyperechoic acute adrenal hemorrhage ➡. Note central hypoechoic area ➡ representing liquefaction.

TERMINOLOGY

Abbreviations and Synonyms
- Adrenal hemorrhage, adrenal hematoma (AH)

Definitions
- Hemorrhage either within adrenal gland or an adrenal tumor

IMAGING FINDINGS

General Features
- Best diagnostic clue: Hyperechoic well-defined lesion within adrenal gland
- Key concepts
  - Relatively uncommon condition but potentially catastrophic event
    - More common in neonates than children & adults
  - Secondary to traumatic & nontraumatic causes
    - Traumatic more common than nontraumatic
    - May be unilateral or bilateral
  - Traumatic hemorrhage: Blunt abdominal trauma

- 25% of patients with blunt abdominal trauma have adrenal hemorrhage
- Unilateral in 80% of cases: Right (85%), left (15%)
  - Nontraumatic hemorrhage (often bilateral)
    - Stress, bleeding disorders, adrenal tumors
    - Neonatal stress (birth asphyxia), idiopathic
  - Bilateral AH in 15% of individuals who die of shock
  - Adrenal insufficiency occurs when 90% of adrenal tissue is destroyed
  - Neonatal adrenal hemorrhage
    - Most common cause of adrenal mass in infancy
    - Usually seen during first week of life
    - Incidence ranges from 1.7-3% per 1,000 births
    - Gland is hypervascular & weighs twice that of adults

Ultrasonographic Findings
- Grayscale Ultrasound
  - Unilateral or bilateral adrenal hematomas
  - AH appears as round or oval, well-defined adrenal mass with variable echogenicity depending on the stage of hemorrhage
  - Acute hematoma: Hyperechoic

DDx: Adrenal Hemorrhage

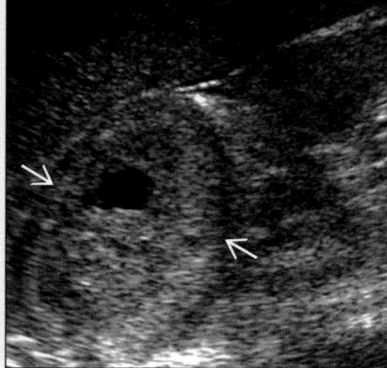

Pheochromocytoma

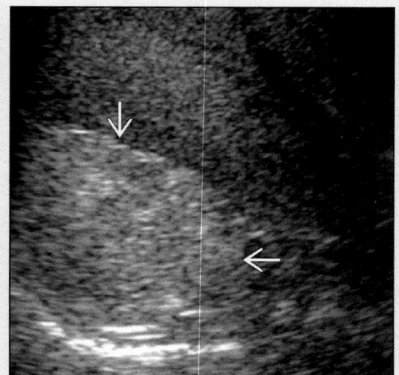

Myelolipoma

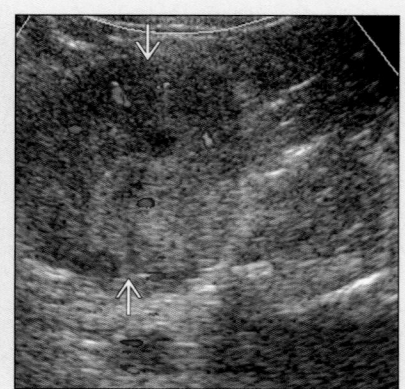

Renal Cell Carcinoma

ADRENAL HEMORRHAGE

Key Facts

Imaging Findings

- Best diagnostic clue: Hyperechoic well-defined lesion within adrenal gland
- Unilateral or bilateral adrenal hematomas
- AH appears as round or oval, well-defined adrenal mass with variable echogenicity depending on the stage of hemorrhage
- Acute hematoma: Hyperechoic
- Subacute hematoma: Mixed echogenicity ± central hypoechoic area
- Chronic hematoma: Anechoic & cyst-like lesion; ± curvilinear/eggshell calcification
- Asymmetric enlargement of adrenal glands
- ± Peri-adrenal hemorrhage ± perinephric extension
- Displacement & mass effect on kidney & IVC

- Hyperechoic hemorrhage within pre-existing adrenal mass
- Avascular hematoma on color Doppler
- ± Associated renal vein thrombosis
- ± Extension of thrombus into IVC
- Secondary adrenal hemorrhage; variable vascularity of underlying adrenal tumor
- US for initial screening & detection followed by CT/MR for further characterization
- Left adrenal gland can be difficult to see on US & small lesions may be obscured

Top Differential Diagnoses

- Pheochromocytoma
- Myelolipoma
- Adjacent Neoplasm

- o Subacute hematoma: Mixed echogenicity ± central hypoechoic area
- o Chronic hematoma: Anechoic & cyst-like lesion; ± curvilinear/eggshell calcification
- o Asymmetric enlargement of adrenal glands
- o ± Peri-adrenal hemorrhage ± perinephric extension
- o Displacement & mass effect on kidney & IVC
- o Hyperechoic hemorrhage within pre-existing adrenal mass
  - ▪ Adrenal carcinoma/pheochromocytoma; usually large heterogeneous adrenal mass
  - ▪ Myelolipoma; variable size echogenic adrenal mass
  - ▪ Adrenal cyst; anechoic well-defined lesion with internal debris & echoes due to hemorrhage
- Color Doppler
  - o Avascular hematoma on color Doppler
  - o ± Associated renal vein thrombosis
  - o ± Extension of thrombus into IVC
  - o Secondary adrenal hemorrhage; variable vascularity of underlying adrenal tumor
    - ▪ Adrenal carcinoma/pheochromocytoma; usually hypervascular
    - ▪ Myelolipoma/adrenal cyst; hypo to avascular

CT Findings

- Acute or subacute hematoma
  - o Round or oval mass of high attenuation (50-90 HU)
  - o Homogeneous & no enhancement with contrast
  - o Inflammatory stranding of peri-adrenal fat
  - o Thickening of adjacent diaphragmatic crura
  - o ± Associated upper abdominal trauma findings
    - ▪ Pneumothorax, hydropneumothorax, rib fracture
    - ▪ Contusion of lung, liver, spleen or pancreas
- Chronic hematoma
  - o Mass with hypoattenuating center (pseudocyst)
  - o Lack of enhancement
  - o Calcification (usually seen after 1 year in adults)
    - ▪ Neonates: Seen within 1-2 weeks after trauma
- Hematomas ↓ in size & attenuation over a period of time
- ± Underlying large adrenal mass (adrenal carcinoma, pheochromocytoma, cyst, myelolipoma)

- o Intracystic or intratumoral hemorrhage

MR Findings

- T1 & T2WI: Varied signal based on age of hematoma
- Acute hematoma (less than 7 days after onset)
  - o T1WI: Isointense or slightly hypointense
  - o T2WI: Markedly hypointense
- Subacute hematoma (7 days to 7 weeks after onset)
  - o T1WI: Hyperintense; due to free methemoglobin
  - o T2WI: Markedly hyperintense; due to serum & clot
  - o Large hematoma: Irregular clot lysis; multilocular, fluid-fluid levels
- Chronic hematoma (beyond 7 weeks after onset)
  - o T1 & T2WI: Hyperintense hematoma; due to persistence of free methemoglobin
  - o T1 & T2WI: Hypointense rim; due to hemosiderin deposition in fibrous capsule
- Gradient-echo imaging
  - o Demonstrates "blooming" effect (magnetic susceptibility) due to hemosiderin deposition

Nuclear Medicine Findings

- Tc-99m dimercaptosuccinic acid study (DMSA)
  - o Adrenal hematoma: Photopenic suprarenal mass with inferior displacement of kidney

Angiographic Findings

- Conventional
  - o Usually not recommended in adrenal hemorrhage
  - o Adrenal hemorrhage & pseudocyst: Avascular
  - o Adrenal mass: Neovascularity seen

Imaging Recommendations

- Best imaging tool
  - o US for initial screening & detection followed by CT/MR for further characterization
    - ▪ Left adrenal gland can be difficult to see on US & small lesions may be obscured
- Protocol advice
  - o CT: 3 mm thick section at 3 mm intervals or less
  - o MR: Spin-echo & gradient-echo imaging

ADRENAL HEMORRHAGE

DIFFERENTIAL DIAGNOSIS

Pheochromocytoma
- Variable appearance; purely solid (68%), complex (16%) & cystic tumor (16%)
- Large tumors may appear purely solid with a homogeneous (46%) or heterogeneous (54%) echo pattern
- Predominantly cystic lesions are due to chronic hemorrhage & necrotic debris (± fluid-fluid levels)

Myelolipoma
- Well-defined homogeneous echogenic mass (when fat cells predominate)
- Heterogeneous mass (when myeloid cells predominate)

Adjacent Neoplasm
- Renal cell carcinoma, angiomyolipoma
- Large exophytic liver tumor; hepatocellular carcinoma, atypical hepatic hemangioma

Adrenal Metastases
- Malignant melanoma: Hypervascular metastases
- Lung cancer: Hemorrhagic; enhancing adrenal mass

PATHOLOGY

General Features
- Etiology
  - Bilateral adrenal hemorrhage
    - Anticoagulation therapy (most common)
    - Antiphospholipid antibody syndrome & disseminated intravascular coagulopathy
    - Stress: Surgery, sepsis, burns, hypotension, steroids
    - Pheochromocytoma, adrenal hyperplasia, myelolipoma
    - Metastases: Lung cancer & malignant melanoma
  - Unilateral adrenal hemorrhage
    - Blunt abdominal trauma (right gland > left gland)
    - Adrenal vein thrombosis; adrenal tumor
    - Adrenal neoplasm; adrenal carcinoma, unilateral pheochromocytoma
  - Neonates
    - Difficult labor or delivery; renal vein thrombosis
    - Asphyxia or hypoxia; hemorrhagic disorders
    - Meningococcal septicemia (Waterhouse-Friderichsen syndrome)
  - Pathogenesis (nontraumatic)
    - Stress or adrenal tumor → ↑ adrenocorticotrophic hormone → ↑ arterial blood flow + limited venous drainage → hemorrhage
    - Stress or tumor → ↑ catecholamines → adrenal vein spasm → stasis → thrombosis → hemorrhage
    - Coagulopathies → ↑ venous stasis → thrombosis → hemorrhage
- Epidemiology
  - Autopsy studies: 0.3-1.8% of unselected cases
  - 15% of individuals who die of shock
  - 2% of orthotopic liver transplantations

Gross Pathologic & Surgical Features
- Hematoma, enlarged gland, peri-adrenal stranding

Microscopic Features
- Necrosis of all 3 cortical layers + medullary cells

CLINICAL ISSUES

Presentation
- Most common signs/symptoms
  - Nonspecific: Abdominal, lumbar, thoracic pain
  - Fever, tachycardia, hypotension
  - Acute abdomen
    - Guarding, rigidity, rebound tenderness
  - Confusion, disorientation, shock in late phase
  - Acute adrenal insufficiency
    - Fatigue, anorexia, nausea & vomiting
  - ± Symptoms of associated underlying condition
  - Rarely, asymptomatic; incidental finding (imaging)
  - Waterhouse-Friderichsen syndrome: Skin rash, cough, headache, dizziness, arthralgia & myalgia

Demographics
- Age
  - Any age group
    - More common in neonates than children & adults
  - Nontraumatic (40-80 years); traumatic (20-30 years)
- Gender: M:F = 2:1

Natural History & Prognosis
- Complications
  - Adults: Adrenal crisis; neonate: Death (> blood loss)
  - Prerenal azotemia, adrenal abscess, shock
- Prognosis
  - Prognosis depends on etiology rather than extent of adrenal hemorrhage
  - Overall, AH is associated with a 15% mortality rate
    - Waterhouse-Friderichsen syndrome: 55-60%

Treatment
- Medical
  - Correct fluid, electrolytes & treat underlying cause
- Surgical: Adrenalectomy (open or laparoscopic)
  - Surgery not required, except in adrenal tumors

DIAGNOSTIC CHECKLIST

Consider
- Check for history of trauma, anticoagulant therapy, coagulopathies, malignancies, stress, adrenal tumor

Image Interpretation Pearls
- US; hyperechoic avascular lesion within adrenal gland with relevant clinical features
- MR: Signal intensity varies with age of hematoma

SELECTED REFERENCES
1. Dunnick NR et al: Imaging of adrenal incidentalomas: Current status. AJR. 179:559-68, 2002
2. Mayo-Smith WW et al: State-of-the-art adrenal imaging. Radiographics. 21(4):995-1012, 2001
3. Vella A et al: Adrenal hemorrhage: a 25-year experience at the Mayo Clinic. Mayo Clin Proc. 76(2):161-8, 2001

ADRENAL HEMORRHAGE

Typical

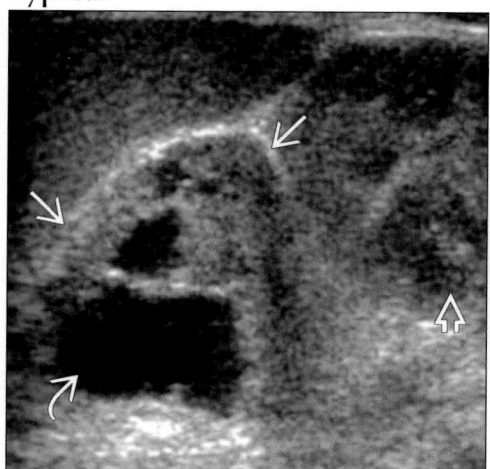 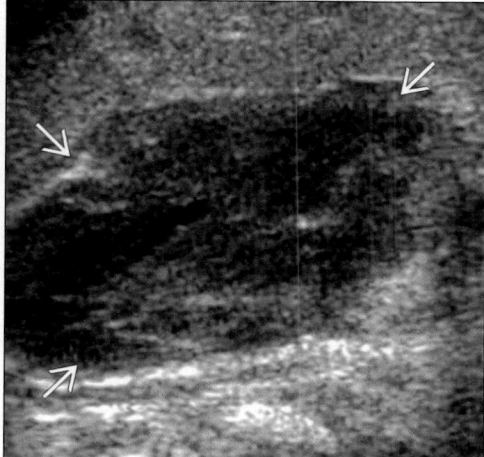

(Left) Transverse transabdominal ultrasound shows a large, well-defined, sub-acute left adrenal hematoma ➡. Note the central anechoic areas representing liquefaction ➡ (left kidney ➡). (Right) Longitudinal transabdominal ultrasound shows a hypoechoic, subacute adrenal hemorrhage ➡. Note the heterogeneous echo pattern of the hematoma.

Typical

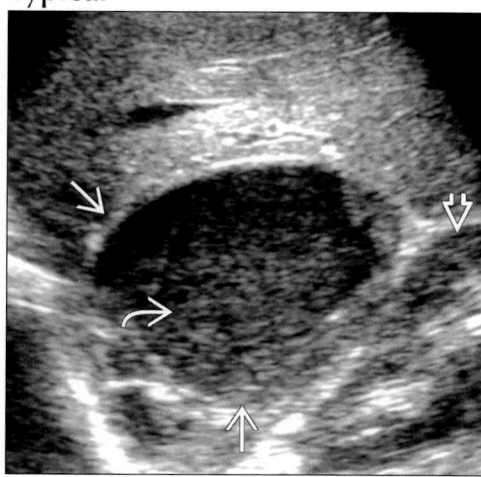 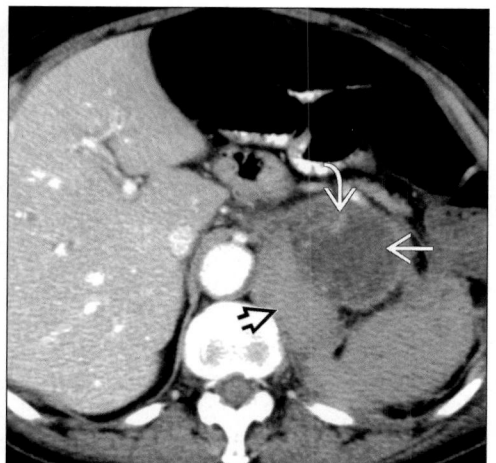

(Left) Longitudinal transabdominal ultrasound shows chronic changes in an old right adrenal hematoma ➡, with cystic degeneration/pseudocyst formation. Note the fine internal echoes ➡ (right kidney ➡). (Right) Transverse CECT shows a large, hypodense, nonenhancing subacute hemorrhage ➡ in a left adrenal gland metastasis ➡. Note an area of hyperdense acute blood ➡.

Typical

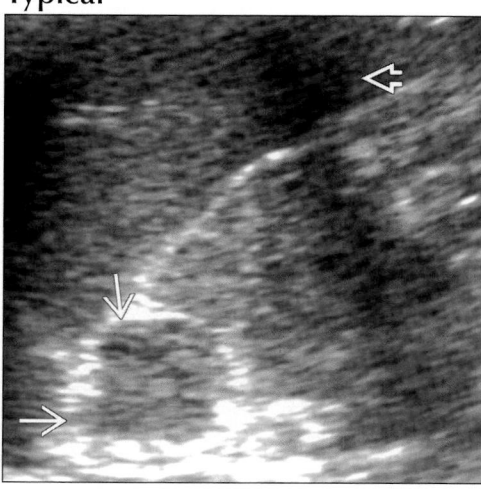 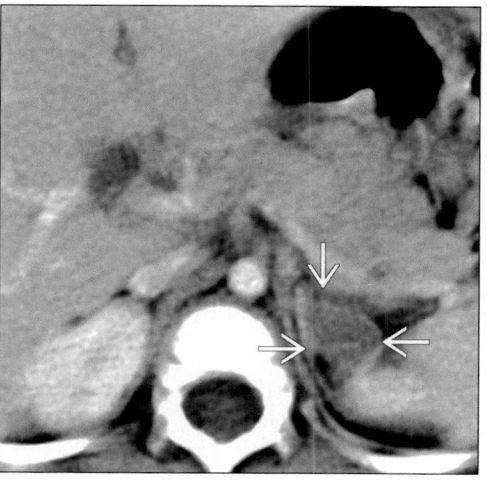

(Left) Oblique transabdominal ultrasound shows a small left adrenal hemorrhage ➡. Note its relationship to the spleen ➡. (Right) Transverse CECT (same patient as previous image) shows a well-defined, hypodense, nonenhancing left adrenal subacute hemorrhage ➡.

MYELOLIPOMA

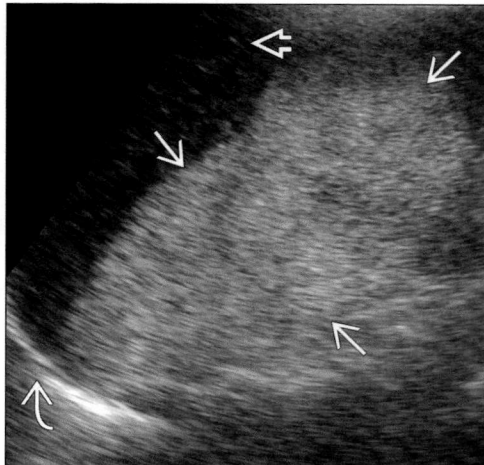

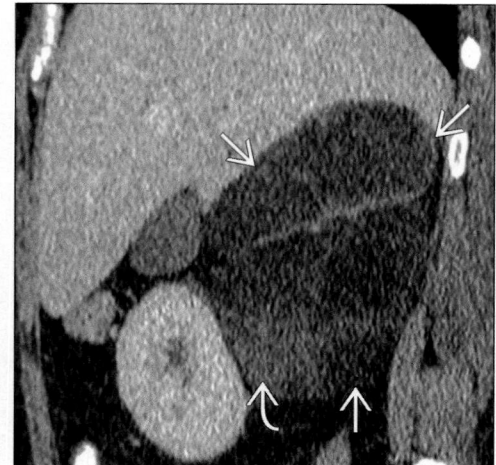

Longitudinal transabdominal ultrasound shows a large lobulated hyperechoic right adrenal myelolipoma ➡ with artifactual step defect in echogenic diaphragm ➡. Note adjacent liver ➡ echogenicity.

CECT sagittal reconstruction (same patient as previous image) shows the large, hypodense right adrenal myelolipoma ➡. The faintly enhancing area represents the myeloid component ➡.

TERMINOLOGY

Definitions
- Rare benign tumor composed of mature fat tissue & hematopoietic elements (myeloid & erythroid cells)

IMAGING FINDINGS

General Features
- Best diagnostic clue: Heterogeneous fatty adrenal mass
- Location
  - Adrenal gland (85%): Thought to arise in the zona fasciculata of the adrenal cortex
  - Typically unilateral & very rarely bilateral: 10:1
  - Extra-adrenal (15%): Retroperitoneal (12%) & intrathoracic (3%)
- Size: Usually 2-10 cm, rarely 10-20 cm
- Key concepts
  - Rare, benign neoplasm of adrenal gland
  - Seen in 0.2-0.4% of cases based on autopsy series
  - Frequency among all incidentaloma is 7-15%
  - Composed of myeloid and fatty tissue similar to bone marrow
  - Large tumor can bleed spontaneously or undergo necrosis
  - Non-functioning (do not secrete hormones)
  - Large myelolipoma can mimic retroperitoneal lipoma or liposarcoma
  - Malignant transformation is not known to occur

Ultrasonographic Findings
- Grayscale Ultrasound
  - Well-defined, homogeneous, echogenic mass (when predominantly composed of fatty tissue)
  - When small difficult to distinguish from the echogenic retro-peritoneal fat
  - "Apparent diaphragm disruption": Propagation speed artifact; decreased sound velocity through a fatty mass leads to this appearance, usually seen when tumor > 4 cm
  - Heterogeneous mass (when myeloid cells predominate), may be isoechoic or hypoechoic
  - Heterogeneous echo pattern may also be due to internal hemorrhage (common), ± calcification
  - When large & atypical: Ultrasound-guided FNAC can be performed to confirm diagnosis

DDx: Adrenal Myelolipoma

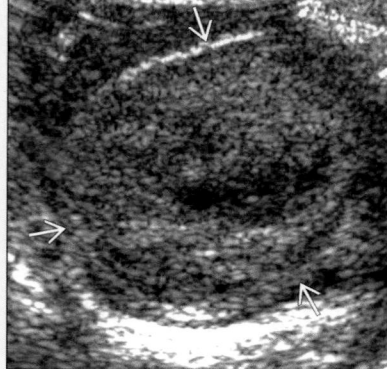

Adrenal Hemorrhage - Acute

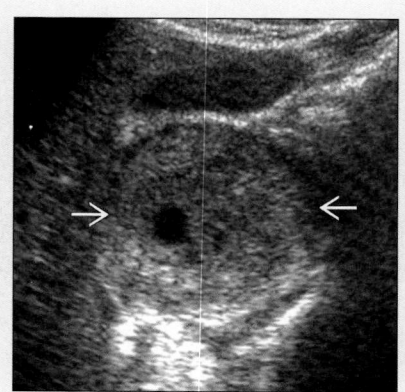

Pheochromocytoma

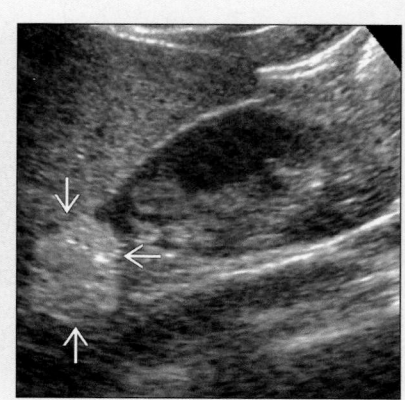

Renal Cell Carcinoma

MYELOLIPOMA

Key Facts

Terminology
- Rare benign tumor composed of mature fat tissue & hematopoietic elements (myeloid & erythroid cells)

Imaging Findings
- Best diagnostic clue: Heterogeneous fatty adrenal mass
- Well-defined, homogeneous, echogenic mass (when predominantly composed of fatty tissue)
- When small difficult to distinguish from the echogenic retro-peritoneal fat
- "Apparent diaphragm disruption": Propagation speed artifact; decreased sound velocity through a fatty mass leads to this appearance, usually seen when tumor > 4 cm
- Heterogeneous mass (when myeloid cells predominate), may be isoechoic or hypoechoic

- Heterogeneous echo pattern may also be due to internal hemorrhage (common), ± calcification
- When large & atypical: Ultrasound-guided FNAC can be performed to confirm diagnosis
- Color Doppler: Avascular to hypovascular adrenal mass

Top Differential Diagnoses
- Adrenal Hemorrhage
- Pheochromocytoma
- Renal cell carcinoma (RCC)

Diagnostic Checklist
- Ultrasound is useful in the diagnosis of large masses, CT is better for detection of smaller lesions
- Presence of tumoral fat confirming benign nature, further work-up for incidental mass may be avoided

---

- Color Doppler: Avascular to hypovascular adrenal mass

Radiographic Findings
- Radiography
  - Lucent mass with rim of residual normal adrenal cortex
  - Calcification present (due to previous hemorrhage in up to 22%)

CT Findings
- CT appearance depends on histologic composition
  - Most tumors are heterogeneous fatty adrenal masses
    - Presence of pure fat within tumor is diagnostic
    - Low-attenuation of fat density (-30 to -90 HU)
    - Amount of fat is widely variable; completely fat, to more than half fat (50%), to only a few tiny foci of fat in a soft tissue mass (10%)
- Usually well-defined mass with recognizable capsule
- Interspersed "smoky" areas of higher CT values than those of retroperitoneal fat because of the presence of hematopoietic tissue in myelolipoma
- Mass may have attenuation values between fat & water due to diffusely mixed fat and myeloid elements
- With hemorrhage: High density areas may be seen
- Punctate calcification seen (20% of cases)
- Occasionally the mass may appear to extend into the retroperitoneum
- Thin-sections are recommended (to avoid volume averaging) if the fatty tissue is not predominant

MR Findings
- MR appearance depends on histologic composition
  - Tumor with major fat component
    - T1WI in phase: Typically hyperintense
    - Fat suppression/opposed phase sequences: Loss of signal
    - If mass is completely composed of mature fat cells: No loss of signal on opposed phase sequence
  - Tumor with major bone marrow elements (myeloid & erythroid cells)
    - Low signal on T1WI; moderate signal on T2WI

  - Enhance brightly after intravenous administration of gadolinium

Angiographic Findings
- Conventional: Differentiate myelolipoma from retroperitoneal liposarcoma by determining origin of blood supply & vascularity of tumors

Imaging Recommendations
- Protocol advice: Ultrasonography is useful in the diagnosis of large tumors, CT is better in detecting smaller mass
- NECT or MR with fat suppression sequence

DIFFERENTIAL DIAGNOSIS

Adrenal Hemorrhage
- Usually well-defined & round in shape
- Acute: Echogenic or heterogeneous echo pattern in adrenal mass
- Chronic: Large, well-defined, hypoechoic adrenal mass

Pheochromocytoma
- Variable appearance; purely solid (68%), complex (16%) & cystic tumor (16%)
- Small tumor: Round solid, well-circumscribed mass with uniform echogenicity
- Large tumor may appear as purely solid mass of homogeneous (46%) or heterogeneous (54%) echo pattern
- Highly vascular; prone to hemorrhage & necrosis

Adjacent Neoplasm
- Renal cell carcinoma (RCC)
  - Exophytic upper pole RCC in the adjacent kidney may simulate a myelolipoma
  - Variable echogenicity; usually an echogenic, well-defined mass
  - When large may appear heterogeneous due to areas of necrosis & hemorrhage
- Angiomyolipoma
  - Upper pole renal cortical angiomyolipoma may simulate myelolipoma

MYELOLIPOMA

- ○ Hyperechoic well-defined renal parenchymal neoplasm
- Exophytic atypical hepatic hemangioma/hepatocellular carcinoma: Arising from the inferior margin of liver
  - ○ May appear as a large echogenic mass extending into the suprarenal space
  - ○ Displacement of retroperitoneal fat reflection posteriorly by hepatic masses

Liposarcoma
- Retroperitoneal primary sarcoma involving perirenal space may simulate adrenal (or renal) fatty tumor

Adrenal Adenoma
- Most common benign tumor of adrenal gland (cortex)
- Well-defined, small, solid, round, soft tissue adrenal mass

Adrenal Metastases & Lymphoma
- Adrenal metastases
  - ○ Unilateral or bilateral hypoechoic masses ± necrosis or hemorrhage
  - ○ Size: Usually < 5 cm, may be larger in melanoma
  - ○ Hypervascular on color Doppler
  - ○ Usually known to have a primary malignancy elsewhere
- Adrenal lymphoma
  - ○ Primary (rare); secondary (non-Hodgkin common)
  - ○ Often bilateral; retroperitoneal disease usually seen
  - ○ Discrete or diffuse mass, shape is maintained
  - ○ Extensive retroperitoneal tumor engulfing adrenal

Adrenal Carcinoma
- Rare, unilateral, solid mass with mixed heterogeneous echo pattern
- Areas of necrosis & hemorrhage ± calcification (30%)
- Local spread; renal vein or inferior vena cava (IVC) extension
- Metastases to lung, liver lymph nodes & bones

PATHOLOGY

General Features
- Etiology
  - ○ Unknown
  - ○ Best hypothesis: Reticuloendothelial cell metaplasia of capillaries in adrenal (stress/infection/necrosis)
  - ○ Secondary hypothesis: Myelolipoma represents a site of extramedullary hematopoiesis
- Epidemiology: Autopsy incidence 0.2-0.4%
- Associated abnormalities
  - ○ Adrenal collision tumors: Independently coexisting neoplasms without significant tissue admixture e.g., adrenal adenoma & myelolipoma
  - ○ Endocrine disorders in 7%; Cushing syndrome, congenital adrenal hyperplasia (21-hydroxylase deficiency) and Conn syndrome
  - ○ Non-hyperfunctioning adenoma 15%

Gross Pathologic & Surgical Features
- Cut section: Fat & soft tissue components; fatty tissue interspersed with hematopoietic elements resembling bone marrow + pseudocapsule

Microscopic Features
- Mature fat cells with variable mixture of myeloid cells, erythroid cells, lymphocytes & megakaryocytes; no malignant cells

CLINICAL ISSUES

Presentation
- Most common signs/symptoms
  - ○ Asymptomatic
  - ○ Usually an incidental finding on CT, MR or US
  - ○ "Acute abdomen": Rupture with hemorrhage (rare)
- Other signs/symptoms: Other symptoms may occur if these tumors undergo necrosis, hemorrhage or compress surrounding structures
- Diagnosis: CT or MR; biopsy prone to sampling error

Demographics
- Age: Usually elderly age group: 50-70 years
- Gender: Equally seen in men & women

Natural History & Prognosis
- Complication: Rupture with hemorrhage (rare)
- Prognosis: Excellent

Treatment
- When diagnosis is certain, surgery not needed

DIAGNOSTIC CHECKLIST

Consider
- Differentiate from other tumors (lipid-rich adenoma)

Image Interpretation Pearls
- Ultrasound is useful in the diagnosis of large masses, CT is better for detection of smaller lesions
- Well-defined heterogeneous fat density tumor on CT
- Presence of tumoral fat confirming benign nature, further work-up for incidental mass may be avoided

SELECTED REFERENCES

1. Cobanoglu U et al: Adrenal myelolipoma in a child. Pediatr Surg Int. 2005
2. Schaeffer EM et al: Adrenal myelolipoma. J Urol. 173(5):1760, 2005
3. Cristofaro MG et al: [Giant adrenal myelolipoma: a case report and review of the literature] Ann Ital Chir. 2004
4. Dunnick NR et al: Imaging of adrenal incidentalomas: current status. AJR Am J Roentgenol. 179(3): 559-68, 2002
5. Mayo-Smith WW et al: State-of-the-Art adrenal imaging. Radiographics. 21(4): 995-1012, 2001
6. West DJ et al: Giant myelipoma of the adrenal gland. Clin Radiol. 2001
7. White PC et al: Congenital adrenal hyperplasia due to 21-hydroxylase deficiency. Endocr Rev. 21(3):245-91, 2000
8. Rao P et al: Imaging and pathologic features of myelolipoma. Radiographics. 17: 1373-85, 1997

MYELOLIPOMA

IMAGE GALLERY

Typical

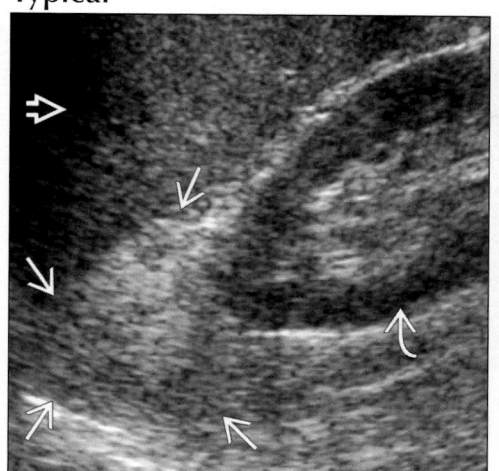
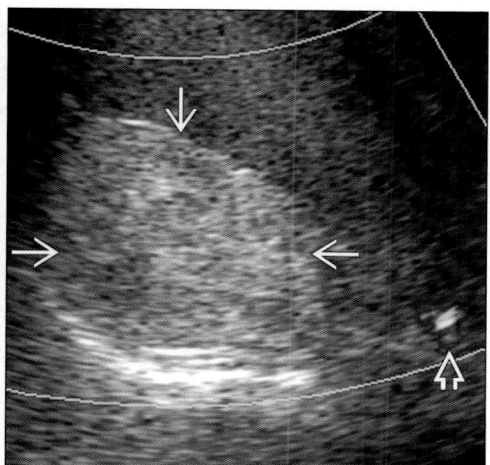

(Left) Longitudinal transabdominal ultrasound shows a right adrenal myelolipoma ➡. Note its relation to the right kidney ➡ and liver ➡. *(Right)* Transverse power Doppler ultrasound (same patient as previous image) shows avascular nature of myelolipoma ➡. Note flow in adjacent IVC ➡.

Typical

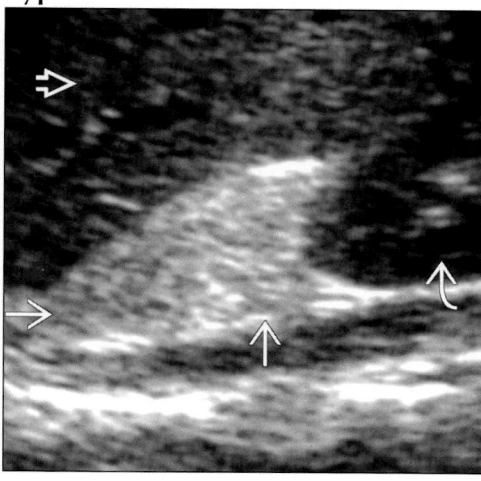
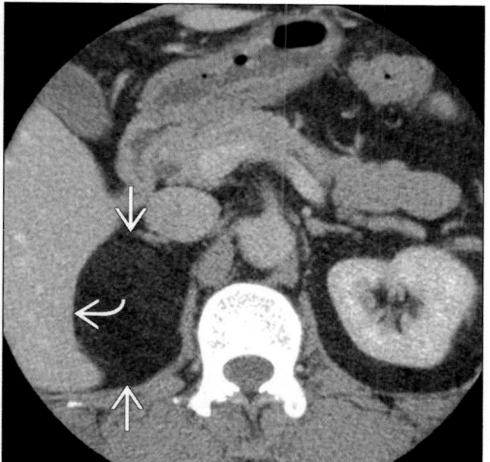

(Left) Longitudinal transabdominal ultrasound shows a right adrenal myelolipoma ➡ with uniform echogenicity. Note adjacent right kidney ➡ and liver ➡. *(Right)* Transverse CECT shows a large, hypodense, nonenhancing right adrenal myelolipoma ➡. Note slight mass effect of adjacent liver ➡. (Courtesy of AD. King, MD).

Variant

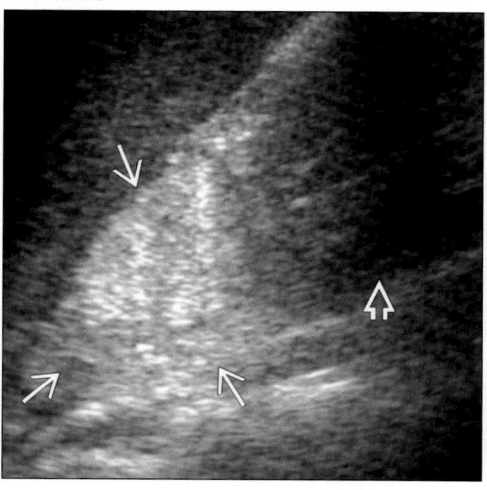
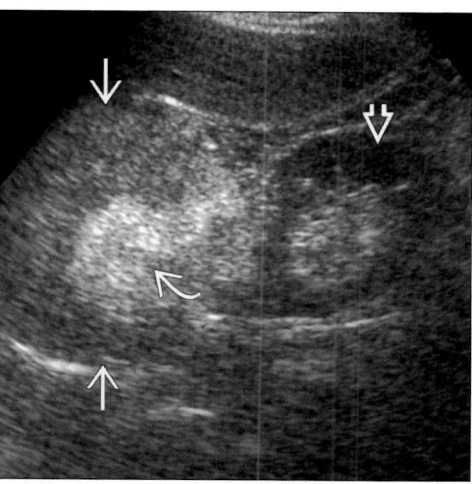

(Left) Longitudinal transabdominal ultrasound in a patient with congenital adrenal hyperplasia shows a well-defined echogenic myelolipoma ➡. Note adjacent kidney ➡. *(Right)* Transverse transabdominal ultrasound shows a large left adrenal myelolipoma ➡ of mixed echogenicity. Note central hyperechoic area ➡ composed predominantly of fatty tissue. Left kidney ➡.

ADRENAL CYSTS

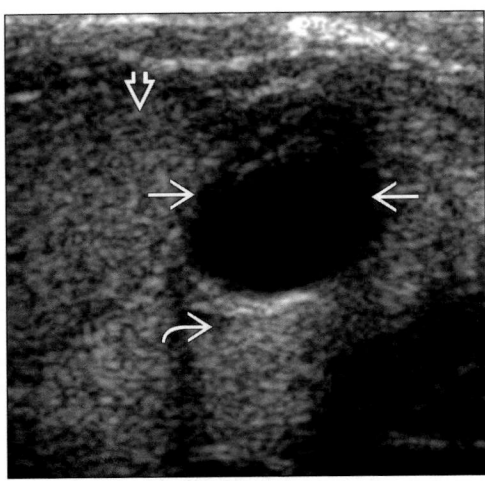
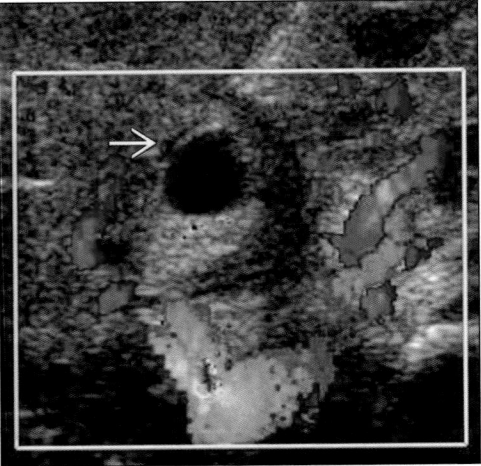

Longitudinal transabdominal ultrasound shows a well-defined left adrenal cyst ➡. Note good posterior sound transmission ⇗, adjacent spleen ⇒.

Longitudinal color Doppler ultrasound (same patient as previous image) confirms avascular nature of the adrenal cyst ➡.

TERMINOLOGY

Definitions
- Cystic mass within the adrenal gland

IMAGING FINDINGS

General Features
- Best diagnostic clue: Well-defined, hypo or anechoic adrenal mass ± calcification
- Location: Unilateral > bilateral (8-10%)
- Size: < 5 cm (50%), up to 20 cm

Ultrasonographic Findings
- Grayscale Ultrasound
  - Unilocular/multilocular, well-defined, adrenal mass
  - Round or oval with thin smooth wall
  - Posterior acoustic enhancement
  - Occasionally with internal debris (hemorrhage) and septation
  - Calcification (15%); variable in shape and location

- Calcification rim-like or nodular (51-69%), centrally along the septation (19%), punctate within intracystic hemorrhage (5%)
  - Complicated cyst; ≥ 5 cm size, internal echoes with septation or thick wall (≥ 3 mm), ↑ malignant potential
  - Ultrasound-guided percutaneous cyst aspiration; ± injection of sclerosing agent
    - Cyst fluid analysis may yield adrenal steroids or cholesterol: Diagnostic of adrenal cyst
    - Therapeutic for cyst without malignant features

CT Findings
- NECT
  - Well-defined, round to oval, homogeneous mass with water (0 HU) or near water density
  - Higher or mixed attenuation cyst contents (hemorrhage, intracystic debris, crystals)
  - ± Calcification (15%)
- CECT: No central enhancement ± wall enhancement

MR Findings
- T1WI: Homogeneous, hypointense mass
- T2WI: Hyperintense mass

DDx: Cystic Adrenal Lesions

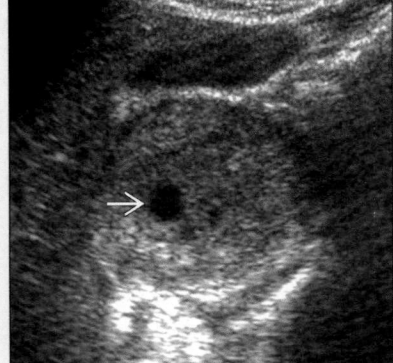
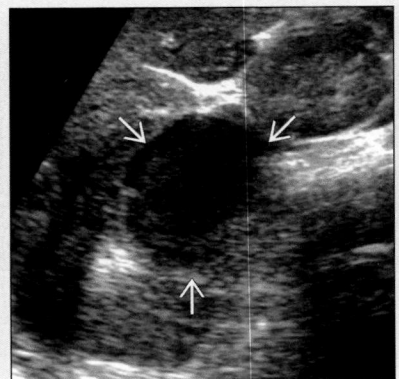
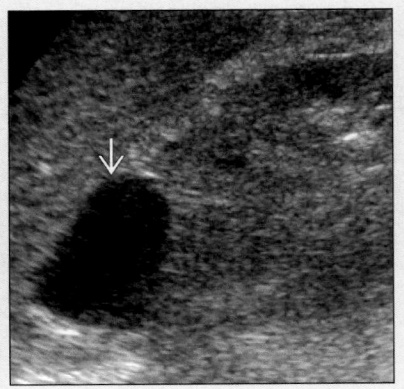

Pheochromocytoma Cystic Necrosis *Cystic Adrenal Metastasis* *Renal Cyst*

ADRENAL CYSTS

Key Facts

Imaging Findings
- Best diagnostic clue: Well-defined, hypo or anechoic adrenal mass ± calcification
- Unilocular/multilocular, well-defined, adrenal mass
- Round or oval with thin smooth wall
- Posterior acoustic enhancement
- Occasionally with internal debris (hemorrhage) and septation
- Calcification (15%); variable in shape and location

- Complicated cyst; ≥ 5 cm size, internal echoes with septation or thick wall (≥ 3 mm), ↑ malignant potential
- Ultrasound-guided percutaneous cyst aspiration; ± injection of sclerosing agent

Top Differential Diagnoses
- Necrotic Adrenal Tumor
- Adjacent Cystic Lesions
- Adrenal Myelolipoma

Imaging Recommendations
- Best imaging tool: US for initial screening and diagnosis followed by CT for further characterization; US for follow-up

DIFFERENTIAL DIAGNOSIS

Necrotic Adrenal Tumor
- Primary or metastatic tumor e.g., pheochromocytoma, adrenal carcinoma, melanoma metastases
- Cystic neuroblastoma in appropriate age group (rare)

Adjacent Cystic Lesions
- Hepatic cyst: Along inferior liver margin
- Renal cyst: Exophytic upper pole renal cyst
- Pancreatic tail pseudocyst, splenic artery pseudoaneurysm, splenic varices

Adrenal Myelolipoma
- Bright echogenic adrenal mass of variable size
- Large tumor: May show areas of cystic necrosis

PATHOLOGY

General Features
- Etiology
  - Endothelial lining (45-48%)
    - Lymphangioma
    - Hemangioma
  - Pseudocyst (39-42%)
    - Prior hemorrhage (e.g., vascular neoplasm, primary adrenal mass) or infarction
  - Epithelial lining: True cyst (9-10%)
    - Glandular or retention cyst
    - Embryonal cyst
    - Cystic adenoma
    - Mesothelial inclusion cyst
  - Parasitic cyst (7%)
    - Hydatid or echinococcal cyst

CLINICAL ISSUES

Natural History & Prognosis
- Complications: Hypertension, infection, rupture with retroperitoneal hemorrhage, intracystic hemorrhage
- Prognosis: Good

Treatment
- Conservative; usually
- Surgical resection; laparoscopic approach
  - Cyst with clear malignant features > 5 cm
  - Patients with symptoms, endocrine abnormalities, complications

SELECTED REFERENCES

1. Kawashima A et al: Imaging of nontraumatic hemorrhage of the adrenal gland. Radiographics. 19(4):949-63, 1999
2. Neri LM et al: Management of adrenal cysts. Am Surg. 65(2):151-63, 1999

IMAGE GALLERY

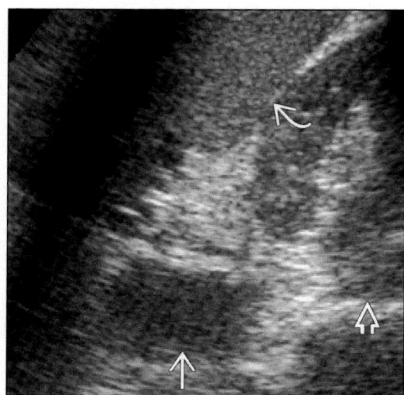 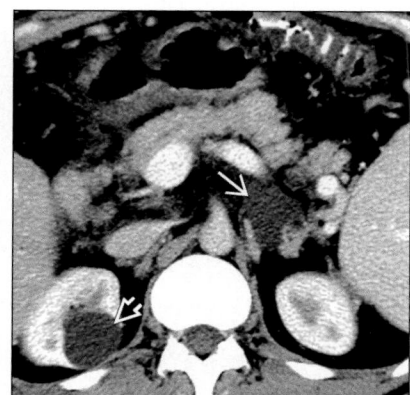 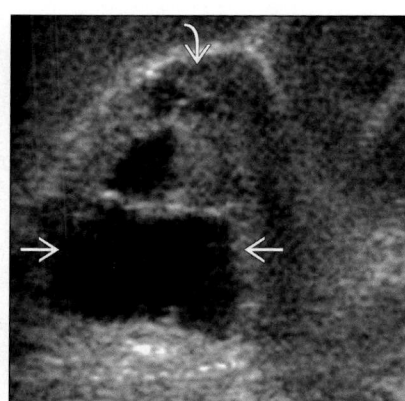

(Left) Transverse transabdominal ultrasound shows an incidental, well-defined left adrenal cyst ➡. Note adjacent spleen ➢, left kidney ➡. *(Center)* Transverse CECT (same patient as previous image) shows well-defined, hypodense, nonenhancing left adrenal cyst ➡, isodense to the right cortical renal cyst ➡. *(Right)* Longitudinal transabdominal ultrasound shows a large adrenal hemorrhage ➢ with cystic liquefaction ➡.

PHEOCHROMOCYTOMA

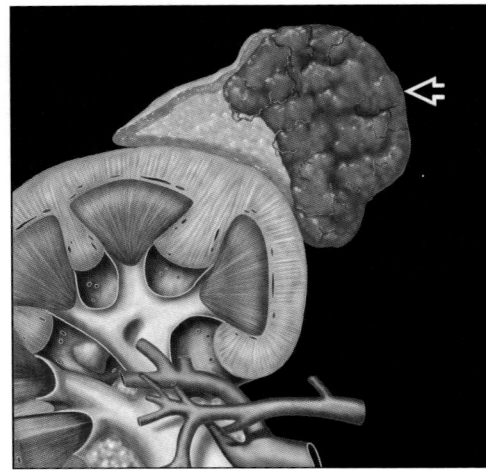

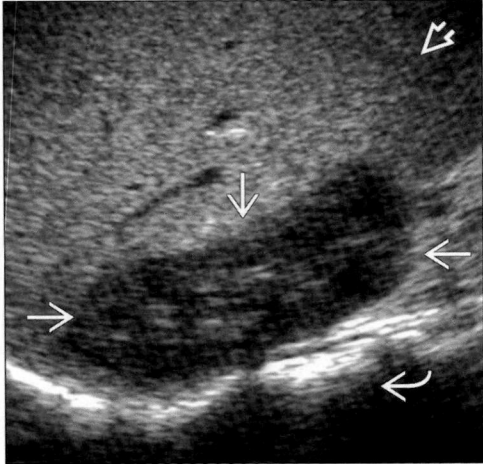

Graphic shows a right adrenal pheochromocytoma ➡. Note its relationship to kidney and hilar vessels. The IVC and renal vein may be compressed/invaded by large pheochromocytomas.

Longitudinal transabdominal ultrasound shows a homogeneous, hypoechoic right adrenal pheochromocytoma ➡. Note its relationship to liver ➡ & spine ➡.

TERMINOLOGY

Abbreviations and Synonyms
- Pheochromocytoma (adrenal) or paraganglioma (extra-adrenal)

Definitions
- Tumor arising from chromaffin cells of adrenal medulla or extra-adrenal ectopic tissue

IMAGING FINDINGS

General Features
- Location
  - Along sympathetic chain: Neck to urinary bladder
  - Subdiaphragmatic (98%); thorax (1-2%)
    - Adrenal medulla (90%); extra-adrenal (10%)
- Size
  - Usually more than 3 cm
  - Weight ranges from 1 gm to over 4 kg
- Morphology
  - Well-circumscribed, encapsulated tumor
    - Solitary (sporadic); multiple (familial)

- Key concepts
  - Remembered as "10% tumors" or "rule of 10s"
  - 10% extra-adrenal: Paragangliomas/chemodectomas
  - 10% bilateral
  - 10% malignant
  - 10% familial, pediatric, silent
  - 10% have autosomal dominant transmission & associated with various other dominant conditions
  - Extra-adrenal tumors arise from sympathetic ganglia
    - Neck, mediastinum, pelvis or urinary bladder
    - Urinary bladder pheochromocytoma (1%), arises from paraganglia of bladder wall
    - Aortic bifurcation (organ of Zuckerkandl, 2.5%): Ganglia at origin of inferior mesenteric artery (IMA)
  - 90% of patients present with hypertension secondary to release of catecholamines
  - Term pheochromocytoma refers to the dusky color it "stains" when treated with chromium salts
  - Imaging: Difficult to distinguish benign, malignant
    - Benign lesions can be locally invasive: Involving inferior vena cava (IVC) & renal capsule
    - Distant metastases indicate malignancy

DDx: Pheochromocytoma Mimics

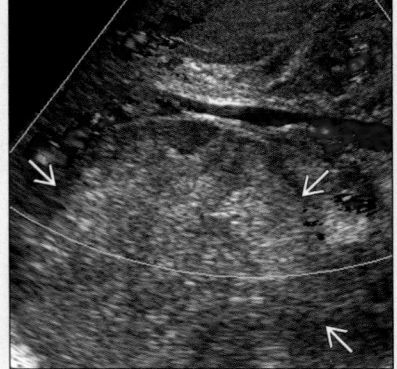

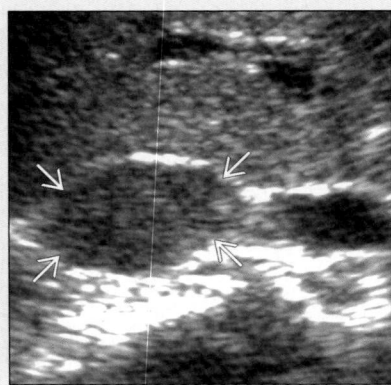

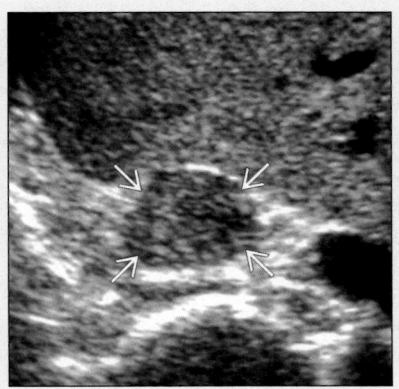

Adrenal Carcinoma

Adrenal Metastasis

Adrenal Adenoma

PHEOCHROMOCYTOMA

Key Facts

Terminology
- Pheochromocytoma (adrenal) or paraganglioma (extra-adrenal)

Imaging Findings
- Remembered as "10% tumors" or "rule of 10s"
- 10% extra-adrenal: Paragangliomas/chemodectomas
- 10% bilateral
- 10% malignant
- 10% familial, pediatric, silent
- 10% have autosomal dominant transmission & associated with various other dominant conditions
- Variable appearance; purely solid (68%), complex (16%) & cystic tumor (16%)
- Small tumors typically solid, round & well-circumscribed masses, with uniform echogenicity

- Large tumors may appear as purely solid masses with homogeneous (46%) or heterogeneous (54%) echo pattern
- Calcification is seen in 10% of pheochromocytomas
- Always evaluate bladder wall, renal hilum & organ of Zuckerkandl at origin of IMA
- Hypervascular on color Doppler

Top Differential Diagnoses
- Adrenocortical Carcinoma
- Adrenal Metastases & Lymphoma
- Adrenal Adenoma

Diagnostic Checklist
- FNAC to be avoided as it may precipitate a hypertensive crisis

Ultrasonographic Findings
- Grayscale Ultrasound
  - Variable appearance; purely solid (68%), complex (16%) & cystic tumor (16%)
  - May present as small (< 2 cm) or large mass
  - Small tumors typically solid, round & well-circumscribed masses, with uniform echogenicity
  - Large tumors may appear as purely solid masses with homogeneous (46%) or heterogeneous (54%) echo pattern
  - Heterogeneous/complex echo pattern in large lesions is due to necrosis (hypoechoic areas) & hemorrhage (hyperechoic areas)
  - Iso/hypoechoic (77%) & hyperechoic (23%) as compared to normal renal cortical parenchyma
  - Predominantly cystic lesions are due to chronic hemorrhage & necrotic debris (sometimes fluid-fluid level seen)
  - Associated retroperitoneal hematoma may be present
  - Calcification is seen in 10% of pheochromocytomas
  - Extra-adrenal pheochromocytoma more difficult to detect due to overlying bowel gas
  - Always evaluate bladder wall, renal hilum & organ of Zuckerkandl at origin of IMA
- Color Doppler
  - Hypervascular on color Doppler
  - Compression/invasion of IVC or renal vein

CT Findings
- NECT
  - Well-defined, round, homogeneous (muscle density)
  - ± Areas of: ↑ Density (hemorrhage), ↓ density (cystic degeneration, necrosis), curvilinear or mural calcification (rarely)
- CECT
  - Shows marked homogeneous enhancement
  - Heterogeneous enhancement: Tissue necrosis & hemorrhage
  - Peripheral enhancement with fluid-levels

  - IV injection of iodinated contrast may precipitate hypertensive crisis in patients not on alpha-adrenergic blockers

MR Findings
- T1WI
  - Isointense to muscle & hypointense to liver
  - Heterogeneous signal intensity: Necrosis & hemorrhage (acute & subacute blood: ↑ Signal intensity)
- T2WI
  - Markedly hyperintense on T2WI (characteristic); ↑ water content due to necrosis
  - Heterogeneous signal intensity (in 33% of cases): Hemorrhage & necrosis with fluid levels
- T1 C+
  - Characteristic "salt & pepper" pattern (due to increased tumor vascularity)
    - Salt: Represents enhancing parenchyma
    - Pepper: Represents flow void of vessels

Nuclear Medicine Findings
- I-131 or 123 Metaiodobenzylguanidine (MIBG)
  - After 24-72 hours: ↑ Uptake of I-131 MIBG in tumor
  - Particularly useful for detecting extra-adrenal tumors
    - Metastatic disease in malignant condition
    - Recurrent & extra-abdominal tumors
  - Sensitivity (80-90%); specificity (90-100%)

Angiographic Findings
- Conventional: Hypervascular tumor with enlarged feeding arteries

Imaging Recommendations
- Protocol advice: US sensitivity similar to CT for detecting adrenal lesions, but poor in detecting extra-adrenal pheochromocytoma
- Helical NE + CECT
  - 93-100% sensitive; localization accurate in 91% with tumor size > 2 cm, up to 40% extra-adrenal lesions may be missed on CT
- T1 C + MR
- MIBG: For ectopic, recurrent & metastatic tumors

PHEOCHROMOCYTOMA

DIFFERENTIAL DIAGNOSIS

Adrenocortical Carcinoma
- Rare; usually unilateral; rarely bilateral (up to 10%)
- Functioning tumors (small); nonfunctioning (large)
- Large unilateral solid adrenal mass with invasive margins, areas of necrosis, hemorrhage ± calcification (30% cases)
- Local spread: Renal vein or IVC extension
- Metastatic tumor spread: Lungs, liver, nodes & bone

Adrenal Metastases & Lymphoma
- Adrenal metastases
  - In a patient with known primary malignancy: Unilateral or bilateral adrenal mass; central necrosis ± hemorrhage
  - e.g., Lung (35-38%, usually solid), breast (50%), renal cell carcinoma (18-25%) & melanoma (50%)
  - Renal cell carcinoma: Adrenal metastases usually ipsilateral & hypervascular
  - Malignant melanoma: Adrenal metastases usually bilateral, solid or cystic component, ± rim calcification
- Adrenal lymphoma
  - Primary (rare); 25% cases of secondary lymphoma (non-Hodgkin common)
  - Often bilateral, discrete or diffuse mass, shape is maintained, extensive retroperitoneal tumor engulfing adrenal
  - Diagnosis by percutaneous aspiration biopsy

Adrenal Adenoma
- Most common benign tumor of adrenal gland (cortex)
- US: Well-defined, small, solid, round, homogeneous, soft tissue adrenal mass

Granulomatous Infection
- e.g., Tuberculosis, histoplasmosis, other fungal diseases
- Usually bilateral, hypoechoic (acute)
- Chronic: Small & calcified adrenals

PATHOLOGY

General Features
- Etiology
  - Chromaffin cells of sympathetic nervous system
    - Adrenal medulla: Pheochromocytoma
    - Extra-adrenal: Paraganglioma
- Epidemiology
  - Incidence
    - 0.13% in autopsy series; 0.1-0.5% of HTN cases
- Associated abnormalities
  - With 10% autosomal dominant variety
    - Multiple endocrine neoplasia syndromes (MEN) type IIA/IIB: Pheochromocytoma, medullary thyroid carcinoma, parathyroid hyperplasia
    - Neurocutaneous syndromes: von Hippel-Lindau syndrome, type 1 neurofibromatosis, tuberous sclerosis, Sturge-Weber syndrome
    - Carney syndrome: Pulmonary chondroma, gastric leiomyosarcoma, pheochromocytoma

Gross Pathologic & Surgical Features
- Round, tan-pink to violaceous, encapsulated mass

Microscopic Features
- Large cells: Granular cytoplasm & pleomorphic nuclei
- Chromaffin reaction: Cells stained with chromium salt

CLINICAL ISSUES

Presentation
- Most common signs/symptoms
  - Symptoms may be episodic or paroxysmal
  - Crisis: Headaches, hypertension (HTN), palpitations, sweating, tremors, arrhythmias, pain
  - Classic: Paroxysmal HTN ± visual changes
  - Atypical: Labile HTN, myocardial infarction, CVA
  - Urinary bladder pheochromocytoma: Adrenergic attacks at micturition or bladder filling, intermittent hypertension
- Clinical Profile: Young patient with paroxysmal attacks of headache, palpitations, sweating & tremors
- Lab data
  - ↑ Levels of vanillylmandelic acid (VMA) 24 hr urine

Demographics
- Age: 3rd & 4th decades; ↑ familial incidence

Natural History & Prognosis
- Complications: During hypertensive crisis
  - Cerebrovascular accidents (CVA)
  - Pregnancy + pheochromocytoma: Mortality (48%)
  - Malignancy in 2-14% cases; distant metastases
- Prognosis
  - Noninvasive & nonmetastatic: Good prognosis
  - Malignant & metastatic: Poor prognosis

Treatment
- Medical therapy: Before, during, after surgery
  - Alpha-adrenergic blockers: Phenoxybenzamine
  - Beta-adrenergic blocker: Propranolol
- Surgical resection: Benign & malignant
- Chemotherapy: Cyclophosphamide + vincristine + dacarbazine

DIAGNOSTIC CHECKLIST

Consider
- Imaging findings + history & labs (usually diagnostic)
- FNAC to be avoided as it may precipitate a hypertensive crisis

Image Interpretation Pearls
- Spherical, usually solid, suprarenal mass, of 3-5 cm size with areas of necrosis & hemorrhage, ± invasion of IVC & renal vein, ± lymph node involvement

SELECTED REFERENCES
1. Dunnick NR et al: Imaging of adrenal incidentalomas: current status. AJR Am J Roentgenol. 179(3):559-68, 2002
2. Mayo-Smith WW et al: State-of-the-art adrenal imaging. Radiographics. 21(4):995-1012, 2001

7

14

PHEOCHROMOCYTOMA

IMAGE GALLERY

Typical

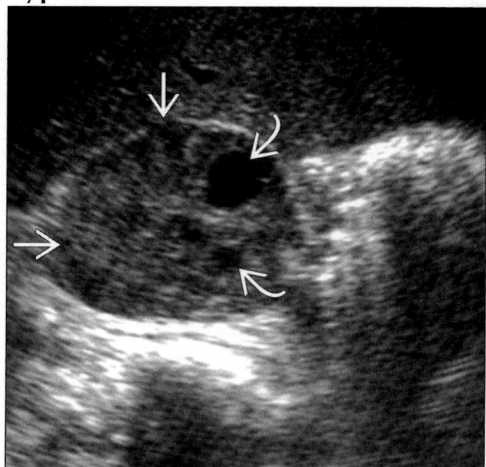 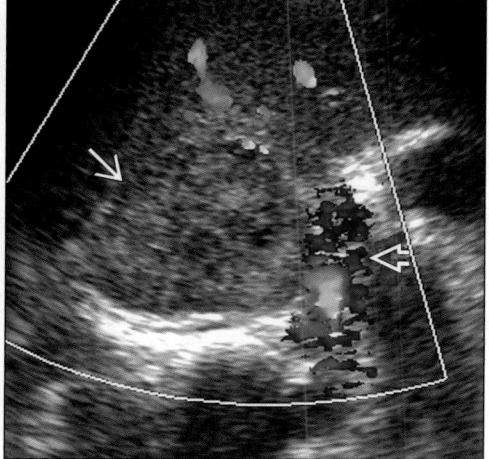

(Left) Transverse transabdominal ultrasound shows a large, well-defined right adrenal pheochromocytoma ➡ with anechoic cystic areas representing necrosis ➡. *(Right)* Transverse color Doppler ultrasound (same patient as previous image) shows the right adrenal pheochromocytoma ➡ displacing & compressing the IVC ➡.

Typical

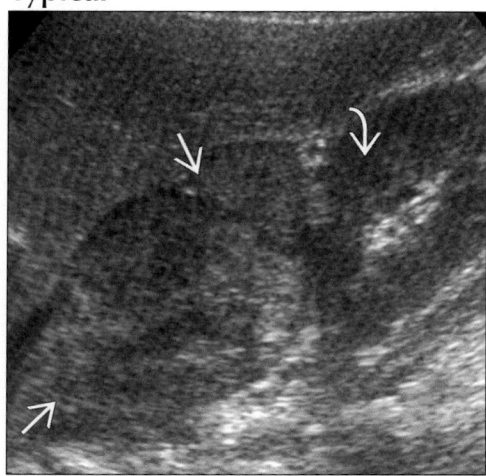 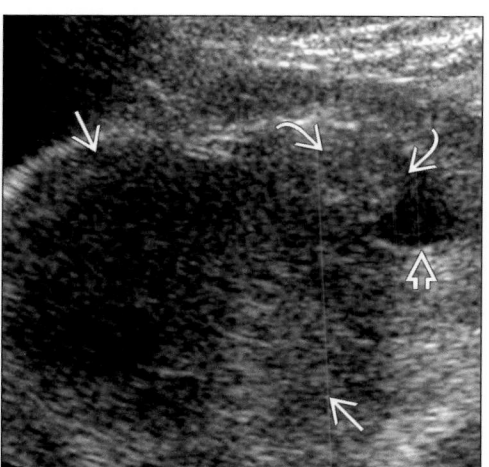

(Left) Longitudinal transabdominal ultrasound shows a large, lobulated right adrenal pheochromocytoma ➡, isoechoic to the adjacent right renal cortex ➡, with a clear plane between them. *(Right)* Transverse transabdominal ultrasound shows a large right adrenal pheochromocytoma ➡ with extension of echogenic tumor thrombus ➡ into the IVC ➡.

Typical

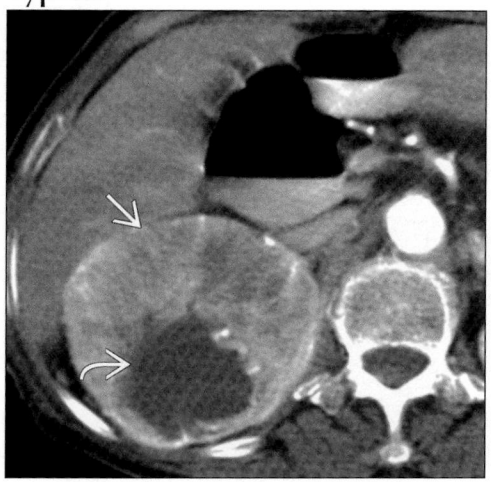 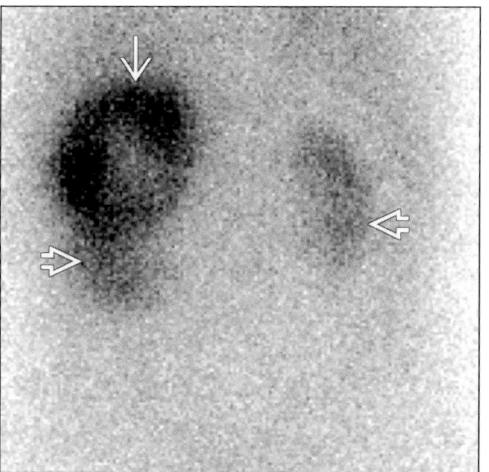

(Left) Transverse CECT shows a large, well-circumscribed, moderately enhancing right adrenal pheochromocytoma ➡ with hypodense area of necrosis ➡. *(Right)* DTPA - MIBG scan (same patient as previous image) shows uptake within the pheochromocytoma ➡. Note DTPA uptake in kidneys ➡. MIBG is useful to detect extra-adrenal tumors.

ADRENAL CARCINOMA

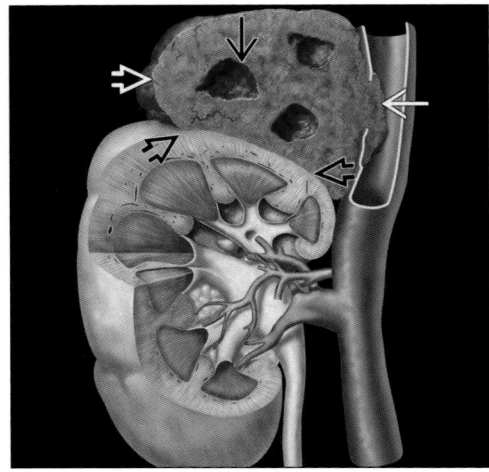

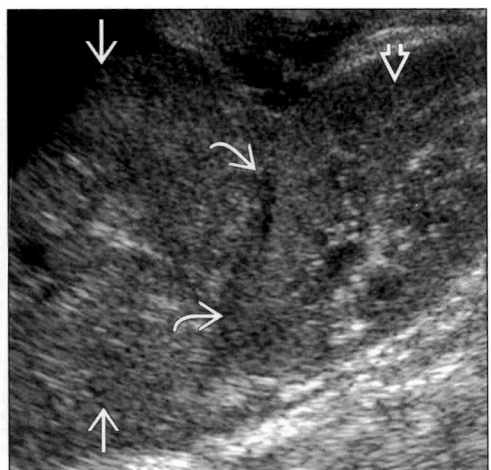

Longitudinal graphic shows a large right adrenal carcinoma ➡ with areas of necrosis ➡, tumor invasion into the IVC ➡ & compression of right renal upper pole ➡.

Longitudinal transabdominal ultrasound shows a large right adrenal carcinoma ➡ causing indentation ➡ of the right renal upper pole ➡.

TERMINOLOGY

Abbreviations and Synonyms
- Adrenocortical carcinoma, adrenal cancer

Definitions
- Malignant growth from one of the adrenal cell lines

IMAGING FINDINGS

General Features
- Best diagnostic clue: Large, solid, unilateral adrenal mass with invasive margins (bilateral in 10%)
- Location: Suprarenal, usually unilateral (left > right)
- Size
  - Functioning tumors: Usually ≤ 5 cm at presentation
  - Nonfunctioning tumors: 10 cm or more
- Morphology
  - Large suprarenal invasive lesion
  - Usually contain hemorrhagic, cystic & calcific areas
- Key concepts
  - Rare & highly malignant neoplasm of adrenal cortex
  - Mostly unilateral, but bilateral in up to 10% of cases
  - Local spread: Renal vein, inferior vena cava (IVC)
  - Metastatic spread: Lungs, liver, nodes, bone; 20% with metastasis at presentation
  - Most patients are at stage 3 or 4 at time of diagnosis
  - Functioning (< 50%); nonfunctioning (> 50%)
  - Accounts for only 0.002% of all childhood cancers
    - Mostly functional, virilization seen in 95% cases

Ultrasonographic Findings
- Grayscale Ultrasound
  - Variable appearance depending on size & contents, ± calcification
  - Small tumors: Echo pattern similar to renal cortex
  - Large tumors: Mixed heterogeneous echo pattern with hypoechoic/anechoic areas (due to necrosis & hemorrhage)
  - "Scar sign": Complex, predominantly echogenic, pattern with radiating linear echoes; when seen in a large adrenal mass suggests adrenal carcinoma
  - Metastasis to regional & periaortic lymph nodes (reliable sign of malignancy)
  - Large tumor may cause compression/indentation of upper pole and anterior surface of the adjacent kidney

DDx: Adrenal Carcinoma Mimics

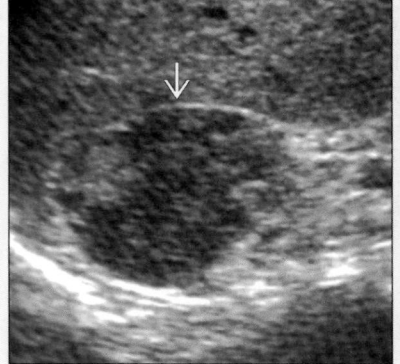

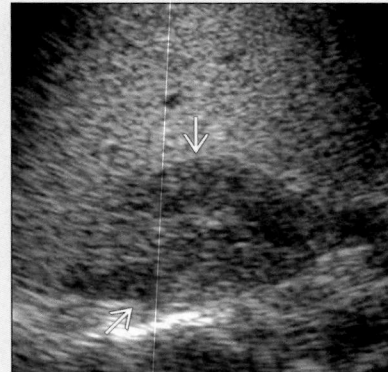

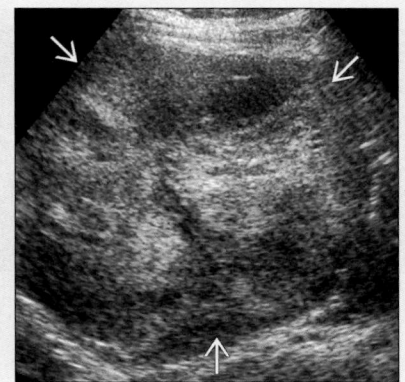

Adrenal Metastasis

Pheochromocytoma

Large HCC

ADRENAL CARCINOMA

Key Facts

Imaging Findings
- Best diagnostic clue: Large, solid, unilateral adrenal mass with invasive margins (bilateral in 10%)
- Functioning tumors: Usually ≤ 5 cm at presentation
- Nonfunctioning tumors: 10 cm or more
- Variable appearance depending on size & contents, ± calcification
- Small tumors: Echo pattern similar to renal cortex
- Large tumors: Mixed heterogeneous echo pattern with hypoechoic/anechoic areas (due to necrosis & hemorrhage)
- Metastasis to regional & periaortic lymph nodes (reliable sign of malignancy)
- Differentiation between adrenal carcinoma, adrenal adenoma & neuroblastoma may not be possible by ultrasound

- Color Doppler: Invasion/occlusion of adrenal vein, renal vein & IVC; visualization of intraluminal tumor thrombus ± vascularity
- Best imaging tool: US for initial screening followed by CT/MR for further characterization, evaluating the tumor extent, vascular invasion & distant metastasis

Top Differential Diagnoses
- Adrenal Metastases & Lymphoma
- Adrenal Hemorrhage
- Adrenal Adenoma

Diagnostic Checklist
- Large to medium sized, unilateral adrenal mass with calcification & invasive margins + venous + nodal or distant metastases: Highly suggestive of adrenal carcinoma

---

  - ○ Differentiation between adrenal carcinoma, adrenal adenoma & neuroblastoma may not be possible by ultrasound
  - ○ Large tumor with calcification: Suggests malignancy
- Color Doppler: Invasion/occlusion of adrenal vein, renal vein & IVC; visualization of intraluminal tumor thrombus ± vascularity

CT Findings
- Solid, well-defined suprarenal mass with invasive margins
- Usually unilateral; may be bilateral in 10% of cases
- Areas of necrosis, hemorrhage, fat, calcification within tumor (30% of cases)
- Variable enhancement (necrosis & hemorrhage), peripheral nodular enhancement (88%)
- ± Renal vein, IVC, adjacent renal extension
- Metastases to lungs, liver or nodes

MR Findings
- T1WI: Hypointense adrenal mass compared to liver
- T2WI: Hyperintense adrenal mass compared to liver
- T1 C+: Heterogeneous nodular enhancement (tumor necrosis) + central hypoperfusion + delayed washout
- Multiplanar contrast-enhanced imaging better depiction & delineation of tumor invasion into the renal vein, IVC (coronal images), adjacent kidney & tumor-liver interface

Nuclear Medicine Findings
- FDG PET
  - ○ Adrenal carcinoma: Increased uptake of FDG
    - ■ Differentiates from adenoma (lack of ↑ uptake)
- Adrenocortical scintigraphy by using NP-59
  - ○ No uptake in either gland with large tumor
    - ■ Carcinoma side: The gland is largely destroyed
    - ■ Contralateral side: Carcinoma ↑ hormone release → pituitary feedback shutdown of normal gland

Angiographic Findings
- Conventional
  - ○ Selective catheterization

  - ■ Inferior phrenic artery opacifies superior adrenal artery, which is often predominant arterial supply
  - ■ Renal artery opacifies inferior adrenal artery
  - ■ Middle adrenal artery arises from aorta
  - ○ Enlarged adrenal arteries, arterio-venous shunting & multiple draining veins; minimal neovascularity
  - ○ Inferior venacavography: Confirms tumor invasion

Imaging Recommendations
- Best imaging tool: US for initial screening followed by CT/MR for further characterization, evaluating the tumor extent, vascular invasion & distant metastasis
- NE + CECT: Study of choice to exclude adenoma

DIFFERENTIAL DIAGNOSIS

Adrenal Metastases & Lymphoma
- Adrenal metastases
  - ○ Unilateral or bilateral hypoechoic masses ± necrosis, hemorrhage
  - ○ Size: Usually < 5 cm, may be larger in melanoma
  - ○ Hypervascular on color Doppler
  - ○ Usually known to have malignancy elsewhere
- Adrenal lymphoma
  - ○ Primary (rare); secondary (non-Hodgkin common)
  - ○ Often bilateral; associated retroperitoneal disease usually seen
  - ○ Discrete or diffuse mass, shape is maintained
  - ○ Extensive retroperitoneal tumor engulfing adrenal

Pheochromocytoma
- Tumor > 3 cm in most cases
- Highly vascular with hemorrhage & necrosis
- Bilateral adrenal tumors in multiple endocrine neoplasia (MEN) IIA & IIB syndromes
- Clinical presentation & lab data may be helpful

Adjacent Malignancy
- Hepatocellular carcinoma: Arising from inferior aspect of right liver lobe
  - ○ Displacement of retroperitoneal fat reflection posteriorly by hepatic & subhepatic masses

ADRENAL CARCINOMA

- Renal cell carcinoma (RCC) upper pole
  - Large upper pole RCC mimics large adrenal carcinoma
- Other: Pancreatic tail neoplasm, lymph nodes, enlarged caudate lobe

Adrenal Hemorrhage
- Adrenal hematoma usually appear round in shape
- Acute: Echogenic or heterogeneous echo pattern adrenal mass
- Chronic: Large, well-defined, hypoechoic adrenal lesion

Adrenal Adenoma
- Well-defined, small, solid, round, soft tissue adrenal mass

PATHOLOGY

General Features
- Genetics
  - More likely to be aneuploid or tetraploid
  - Genetic syndromes may ↑ incidence of tumor
- Etiology: Unknown for sporadic adrenal carcinoma
- Epidemiology
  - 0.05-0.2% of all cancers
  - 1 per 1,500 adrenal tumors are malignant
- Associated abnormalities
  - May be associated with genetic syndromes
    - Beckwith-Wiedemann, Li-Fraumeni, Carney & MEN type 1

Gross Pathologic & Surgical Features
- Usually large & predominantly yellow on cut surface
- Necrotic, hemorrhagic, calcific, lipoid & cystic areas

Staging, Grading or Classification Criteria
- Staging of adrenal carcinoma
  - T1: Diameter ≤ 5 cm without local invasion
  - T2: Diameter > 5 cm without local invasion
  - T3: Any size tumor with local invasion but not involving adjacent organs
  - T4: Any size tumor with local invasion & extension into adjacent organs, nodes & distant metastases

CLINICAL ISSUES

Presentation
- Most common signs/symptoms
  - Presentation with non-hormonally active malignancy
    - Abdominal pain, fullness or palpable mass
    - Incidentally discovered mass on imaging exam
    - Metastatic disease in lung, liver ± bone (20% at presentation)
    - 54% of cases nonfunctioning at presentation
- Presentation with hormonally active malignancy
  - Cushing syndrome (30-40%): ↑ Cortisol
    - Moon facies, truncal obesity, purple striae & buffalo hump
  - Virilization in females (20-30%): ↑ Androgens

- 95% of children with functioning adrenal carcinoma present with virilization
  - Conn syndrome (primary hyperaldosteronism)
    - Hypertension & weakness
  - Feminization in males: ↑ Androgens
- Other clinical syndromes at presentation
  - Hypoglycemia, polycythemia & nonglucocorticoid-related insulin resistance

Demographics
- Age
  - Bimodal distribution
    - 1st peak below age 5
    - 2nd peak in 4-5th decades of life
- Gender
  - Overall, females more than males, females account for (65-90%) of all cases
  - Functioning tumors: More common in females
  - Nonfunctioning tumors: More common in males

Natural History & Prognosis
- Rapid growth with local invasion & distant metastases
- Tumor thrombus: IVC & renal vein
- Mean survival 18 months; children better than adults
- 5 year survival for stage 3 disease is under 30%
- Stage 1 & 2: Good prognosis after surgical removal
- Stage 3 & 4: Poor prognosis with or without treatment

Treatment
- Small lesions: Laparoscopic adrenalectomy
- Large lesions with extension: Radical resection of ipsilateral kidney, adrenal gland, adjacent structures
- Metastatic sites also resected if possible
- Chemotherapy: Mitotane, cisplatin, 5-FU & suramin

DIAGNOSTIC CHECKLIST

Consider
- Rule out other adrenal tumors especially adenoma

Image Interpretation Pearls
- Large to medium sized, unilateral adrenal mass with calcification & invasive margins + venous + nodal or distant metastases: Highly suggestive of adrenal carcinoma

SELECTED REFERENCES

1. Leboulleux S et al: Diagnostic and prognostic value of 18-fluorodeoxyglucose positron emission tomography in adrenocortical carcinoma: a prospective comparison with computed tomography. J Clin Endocrinol Metab. 91(3):920-5, 2006
2. Caoili EM et al: Adrenal masses: characterization with combined unenhanced and delayed enhanced CT. Radiology. 222(3):629-33, 2002
3. Mittelstaedt CA. Retroperitoneum. In: General Ultrasound. Churchill Livingstone. p 791-2, 1992

ADRENAL CARCINOMA

IMAGE GALLERY

Typical

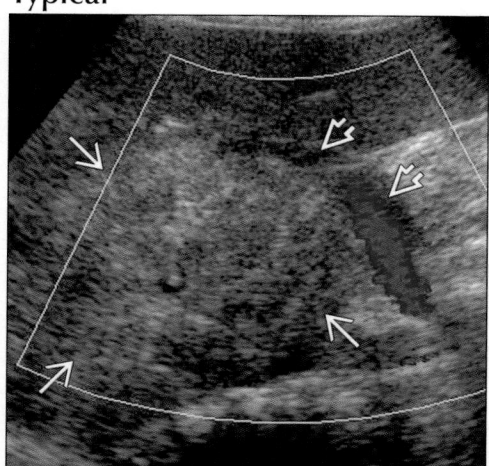

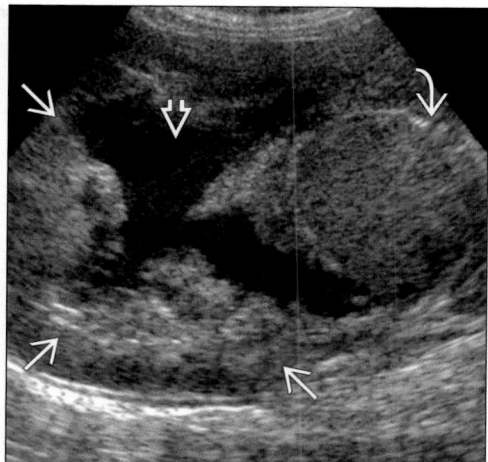

(Left) Longitudinal color Doppler ultrasound shows a large right adrenal carcinoma ➡ with invasion/compression of the IVC ➡. *(Right)* Oblique transabdominal ultrasound shows a large right adrenal carcinoma ➡ with necrosis ➡. There was an associated well-defined hepatic metastasis ➡ next to the adrenal carcinoma.

Typical

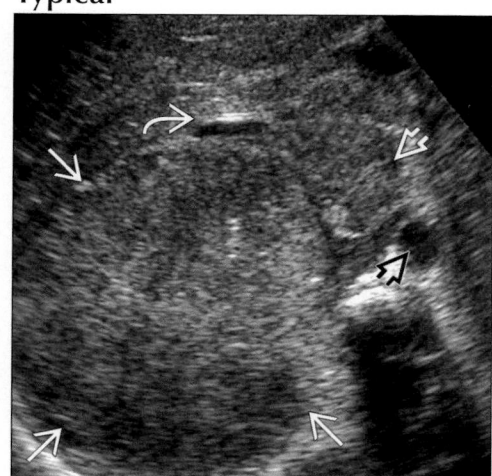

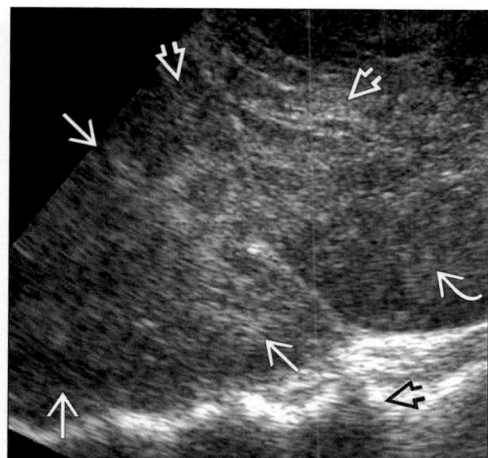

(Left) Transverse transabdominal ultrasound shows a large right adrenal carcinoma ➡ compressing the IVC ➡. Note para-aortic metastatic lymph nodes ➡ around the aorta ➡. *(Right)* Longitudinal transabdominal ultrasound shows a left adrenal carcinoma ➡ with invasion ➡ of the upper pole of left kidney ➡. Note its proximity to the spine posteriorly ➡.

Typical

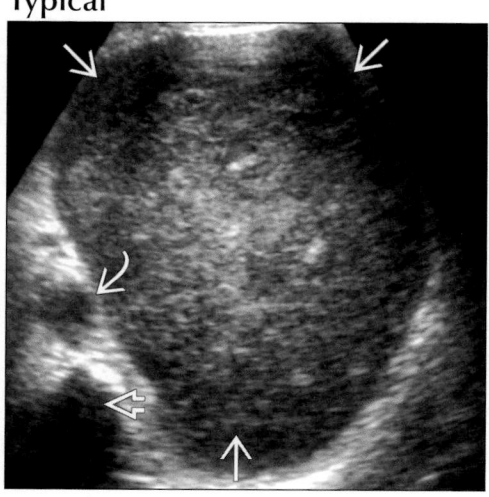

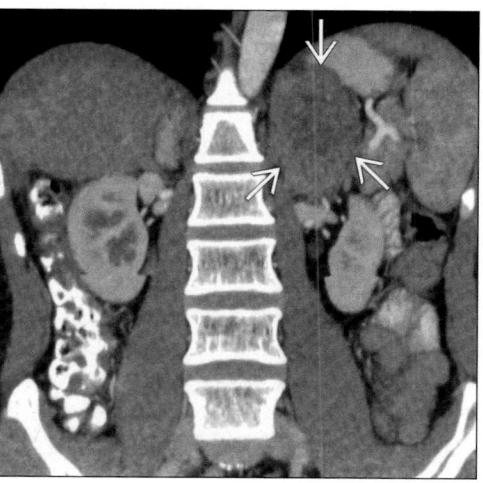

(Left) Transverse transabdominal ultrasound shows a huge, solid left adrenal carcinoma ➡, note aorta ➡ and spine ➡. *(Right)* CECT with coronal reformat shows a large, heterogeneous left adrenal mass ➡. Note how CT provides a better overview of adrenal mass.

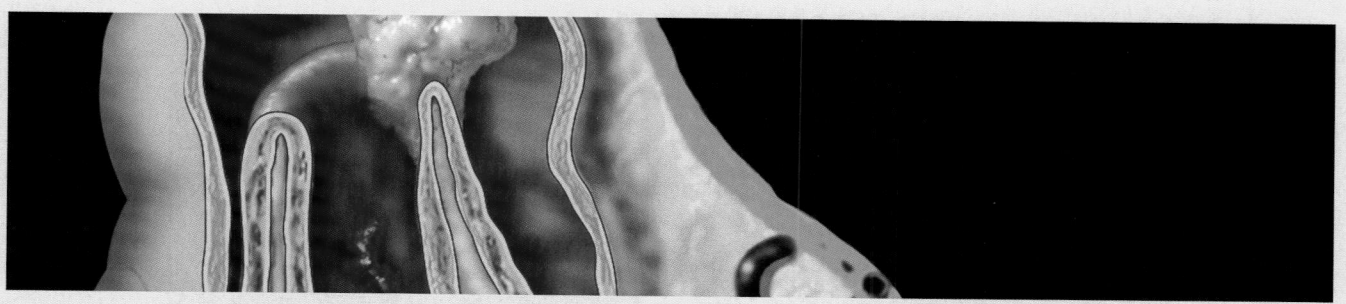

SECTION 8: Abdominal Wall/Peritoneal Cavity

ABDOMINAL WALL HERNIA

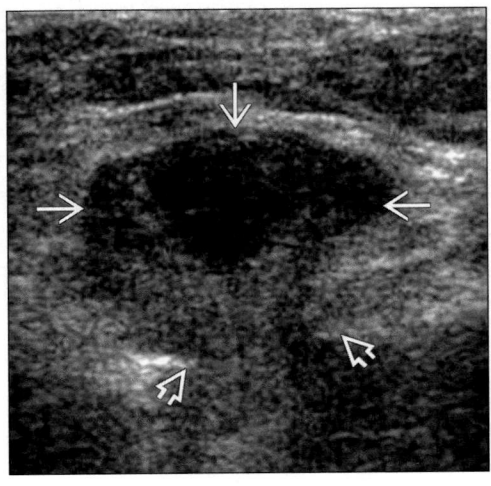

Transverse transabdominal ultrasound shows herniation of small bowel ➡ through an anterior abdominal wall defect ⊵.

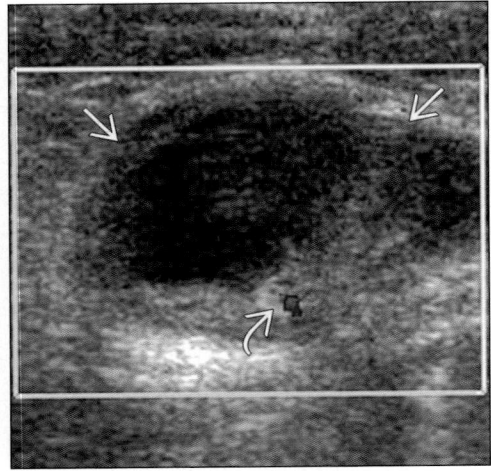

Transverse color Doppler ultrasound (same patient as previous image) shows faint mesenteric vascularity ➡ within the herniated small bowel loop ➡.

TERMINOLOGY

Abbreviations and Synonyms
- Abdominal wall hernia, Spigelian hernia, lumbar hernia

Definitions
- Abnormal protrusion of an organ or part of an organ out of the cavity in which it is normally contained

IMAGING FINDINGS

General Features
- Best diagnostic clue
  - Abdominal wall lump increasing in size with increased intra-abdominal pressure
  - Recent history of trauma, straining activity or surgery
- Location
  - Focal: Midline or lateral to rectus sheath
    - Usually detected incidentally, unless obstructed or strangulated (more common in focal hernias due to small neck)
  - Diffuse: Abdominal wall defects, iliac crest region (seat belt injury), retroperitoneal rent
    - Less likely to strangulate or obstruct due to wider neck
- Size: Fascial or muscle defects vary from small to large tears
- Morphology
  - Abdominal wall; anatomy
    - Layers: Skin, superficial fascia, subcutaneous fat, musculofascial layer, transversalis fascia & extraperitoneal fat
    - Musculofascial layer: Composed of different muscles
    - Anterior wall: Paired rectus muscle, enclosed by rectus sheath (aponeurosis of internal oblique, external oblique & transversus abdominis muscles), which laterally forms the linea semilunaris & centrally fuses to form linea alba
    - Antero-lateral wall: External oblique, internal oblique & transversus abdominis
    - Posterior wall: Quadratus lumborum & erector spinae muscles

DDx: Anterior Abdominal Wall Mass

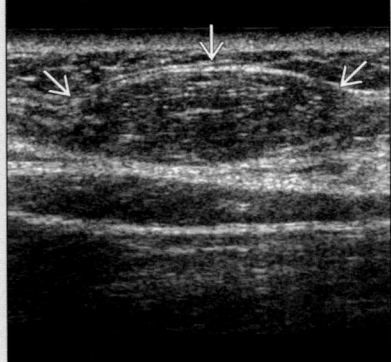

Lipoma

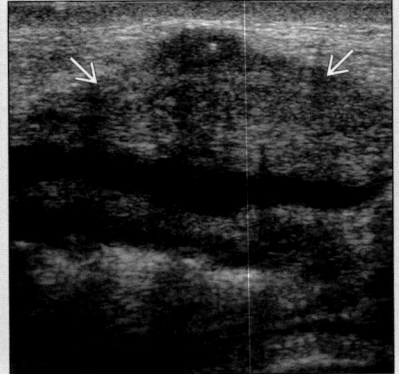

Scar Metastasis

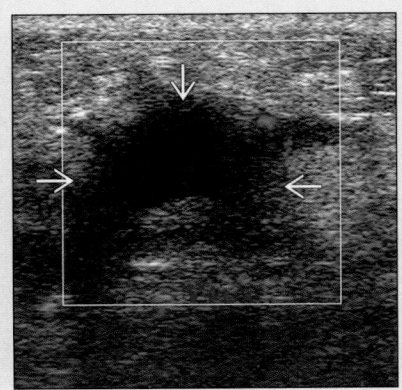

Abdominal Wall Abscess

ABDOMINAL WALL HERNIA

Key Facts

Terminology
- Abnormal protrusion of an organ or part of an organ out of the cavity in which it is normally contained

Imaging Findings
- Abdominal wall lump increasing in size with increased intra-abdominal pressure
- US identifies nature of herniated contents (bowel/omentum) & site of muscle/facial defect
- Omental fat: Echogenic/hypoechoic tissue without peristalsis on ultrasound
- Intestinal loops on ultrasound: "Target" echo pattern with strong central echoes representing air in lumen ± peristalsis

- Obstructed hernia: Tubular fluid-filled structure with valvulae conniventes (small bowel) or fecal material (colon) & dilated fluid-filled intra-peritoneal bowel loops ± free fluid on ultrasound
- Color Doppler: Strangulated hernia; absence of vascularity within bowel wall & mesentery
- Identify anatomical layers, localize focal abdominal wall defect, compare with opposite side & identify contents
- If bowel herniation, check for complications (irreducible/obstruction/strangulation)

Top Differential Diagnoses
- Abdominal Wall Tumor
- Abdominal Wall Abscess/Collection
- Abdominal Wall/Rectus Hematoma

- Arcuate line: Caudal aspect of posterior rectus sheath ends at arcuate line, midway between umbilicus & pubic symphysis
- Distal to arcuate line rectus muscle is separated from peritoneum only by fascia transversalis, as aponeuroses of internal oblique, external oblique & transversus abdominis pass anterior to rectus muscle
  - Ventral hernia
    - Congenital: Gastroschisis (close to cord insertion, not covered by membrane, contains small bowel) & omphalocele (at umbilicus, liver &/or bowel, & other major malformations)
    - Acquired: Weak abdominal wall musculature due to obesity, old age, post-operative
    - Incisional: Previous surgery or laparoscopy, in 0.5-14% of post-operative patients
    - Sites: Midline (linea alba), paramedian (along linea semilunaris)
  - Spigelian hernia
    - Defect in aponeurosis of transversus abdominis muscle lateral to rectus sheath
    - Most commonly located near junction of linea semilunaris & arcuate line
    - Hernia sac dissects laterally to rectus abdominis muscle through a fibrous groove (Spigelian line)
    - Hernia sac may dissect between muscle layers or subcutaneous tissue to expand laterally
    - Only spontaneous hernia of lateral abdominal wall
    - Traumatic hernia may sometimes occur at typical Spigelian hernia site
  - Lumbar hernia
    - Spontaneous lumbar hernia occur in two areas of potential weakness in flank; the superior lumbar triangle (Grynfelt hernia) & inferior lumbar triangle (Petit hernia)
    - Usually asymptomatic due to wide hernia neck, strangulation uncommon (10%)
  - Traumatic abdominal wall hernia

- Variable degree of musculofascial disruption depending on type of force & tensile property of abdominal wall (muscles & fascia) at site of impact
- Skin usually remains intact
- Associated abdominal wall hematoma ± intra-abdominal injury

Ultrasonographic Findings
- Grayscale Ultrasound
  - US identifies nature of herniated contents (bowel/omentum) & site of muscle/facial defect
  - Omental fat: Echogenic/hypoechoic tissue without peristalsis on ultrasound
  - Intestinal loops on ultrasound: "Target" echo pattern with strong central echoes representing air in lumen ± peristalsis
    - Non obstructed hernia: Active peristalsis ± movement of intestinal contents
    - Obstructed hernia: Tubular fluid-filled structure with valvulae conniventes (small bowel) or fecal material (colon) & dilated fluid-filled intra-peritoneal bowel loops ± free fluid on ultrasound
  - US reveals reducible/irreducible nature of hernia
    - Decrease in hernia size with decrease in intra-abdominal pressure or application of external pressure on hernial sac with transducer
    - Increase in hernia size with cough or Valsalva maneuver
- Color Doppler: Strangulated hernia; absence of vascularity within bowel wall & mesentery

Radiographic Findings
- Herniography: Injection of soluble low osmolar contrast medium into peritoneal cavity
  - Frontal (prone, supine, standing), lateral decubitus, oblique and tangential radiographs ± post-exercise radiographs
  - Inguinal and femoral hernias best shown and classified with herniography
  - Useful for detection of small or occult post-surgical hernia
  - Can be followed by CT

ABDOMINAL WALL HERNIA

CT Findings
- Assessment: Size & site of fascial or muscular defect
- Identify nature of herniated contents
- Avulsion of abdominal wall musculature; all layers of abdominal wall may be disrupted
- Associated visceral injury (blunt abdominal trauma)

Fluoroscopic Findings
- Barium study
  - Abdominal wall hernias containing bowel are well visualized in profile on lateral/oblique spot images

Imaging Recommendations
- Best imaging tool
  - US for initial screening & dynamic evaluation of herniated contents
    - CT ± herniography if ultrasound is negative or equivocal
- Protocol advice
  - Identify anatomical layers, localize focal abdominal wall defect, compare with opposite side & identify contents
    - If bowel herniation, check for complications (irreducible/obstruction/strangulation)

DIFFERENTIAL DIAGNOSIS

Abdominal Wall Tumor
- Primary tumor: Desmoid tumor, lipoma, rhabdomyoma, rhabdomyosarcoma
- Secondary tumor: Scar metastasis, metastasis (melanoma, Sister Mary Joseph nodule)

Abdominal Wall Abscess/Collection
- Post-operative abdominal wall abscess
- Suture/scar granuloma
- Subcutaneous collections or cysts

Abdominal Wall/Rectus Hematoma
- Post-traumatic or spontaneous: Bleeding of epigastric artery/vein or primary tear of muscle fibers
- May be associated with endometrioma in women

PATHOLOGY

General Features
- Etiology
  - Chronic increased intra-abdominal pressure, abdominal distension (ascites) ± muscle laxity (obesity, old age)
    - Weak abdominal wall musculature
    - Chronic cough ("internal trauma")
    - Prostatism, constipation, manual labour
  - Trauma: Blunt force or hyperextension strain
    - Insufficient to penetrate skin but strong enough to disrupt muscle & fascia
    - Sudden ↑ in intra-abdominal pressure
    - Shearing force applied across bony prominences
    - Low energy injuries: Impact on small blunt object, blow to abdominal wall
    - High energy injuries: Motor vehicle accidents (steering wheel injury, seat belt injury)
  - Post-operative abdominal wall weakness, surgical scar, suture dehiscence

CLINICAL ISSUES

Presentation
- Most common signs/symptoms
  - Abdominal lump increasing in size with ↑ in intra-abdominal pressure
  - Reducible swelling with a positive cough impulse
  - Intermittent intestinal obstruction

Natural History & Prognosis
- May not be diagnosed initially; delayed presentation ± complications
- Complication: Intestinal obstruction, strangulation ± bowel ischemia

Treatment
- Repair of muscle/fascial defect: Open or laparoscopic technique, meshplasty
- Intestinal obstruction/strangulated hernia; urgent exploratory laparotomy

DIAGNOSTIC CHECKLIST

Consider
- Abdominal wall hernia, if posterior margin of any abdominal wall mass cannot be seen on US

Image Interpretation Pearls
- Check for abdominal wall defect, hernial sac contents, peristaltic movement & vascularity (if bowel)

SELECTED REFERENCES
1. Zafar HM et al: Anterior abdominal wall hernias: findings in barium studies. Radiographics. 26(3):691-9, 2006
2. Aguirre DA et al: Abdominal wall hernias: imaging features, complications, and diagnostic pitfalls at multi-detector row CT. Radiographics. 2005
3. Allewaert S et al: Spigelian hernia with unusual content. Abdom Imaging. 30(6):677-8, 2005
4. Emby DJ et al: Valsalva's maneuver in abdominal wall hernia imaging. AJR Am J Roentgenol. 2005
5. Crespi G et al: Imaging of early postoperative complications after polypropylene mesh repair of inguinal hernia. Radiol Med (Torino). 2004
6. Losanoff JE et al: Handlebar hernia: ultrasonography-aided diagnosis. Hernia. 6(1):36-8, 2002
7. Vasquez JC et al: Traumatic abdominal wall hernia caused by persistent cough. South Med J. 92(9): 907-8, 1999
8. Furtschegger A et al: Sonography in the postoperative evaluation of laparoscopic inguinal hernia repair. J Ultrasound Med. 14(9):679-84, 1995
9. Damschen DD et al: Acute traumatic abdominal hernia: case reports. J Trauma. 36(2): 273-6, 1994
10. Yeh HC et al: Ultrasonography and CT of abdominal and inguinal hernias. J Clin Ultrasound. 12(8):479-86, 1984

ABDOMINAL WALL HERNIA

IMAGE GALLERY

Typical

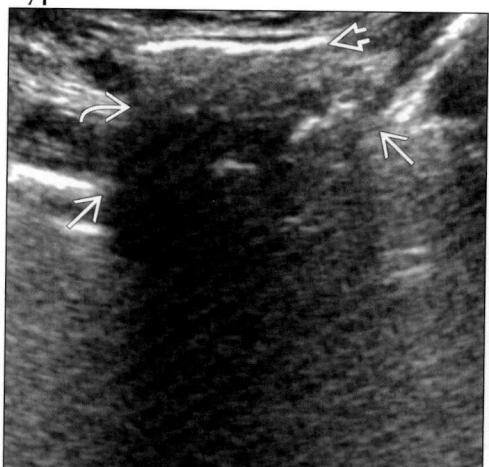

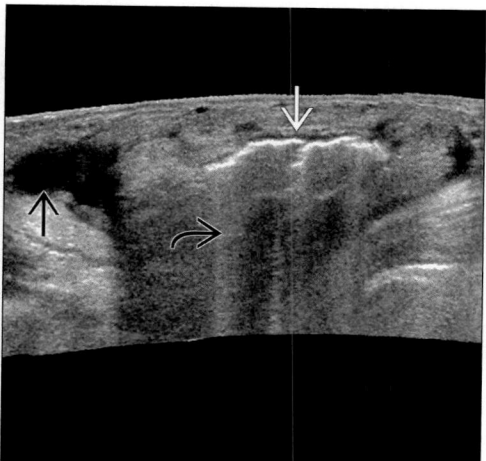

(Left) Transverse transabdominal ultrasound shows an anterior abdominal wall incisional hernia with a wide neck ➡. It contains a bowel loop ⮕, which is causing posterior shadowing ⮞. (Right) Longitudinal transabdominal ultrasound shows an umbilical hernia in patient with portal hypertension. Note herniated bowel loops ➡ with characteristic shadowing ➔ & minimal ascites ➔.

Typical

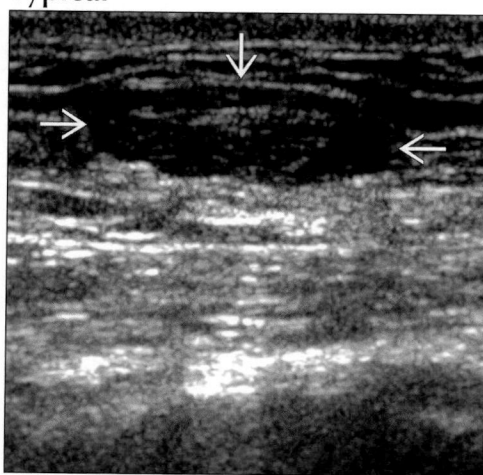

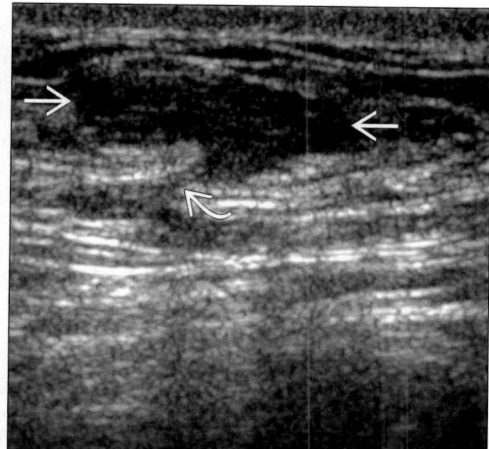

(Left) Transverse transabdominal ultrasound shows a well-defined, ovoid, hypoechoic anterior abdominal wall nodule ➡. (Right) Transverse transabdominal ultrasound (same patient as previous image) with Valsalva maneuver shows a fascial defect ➡ in the abdominal wall with omental herniation ➡. Dynamic maneuvers such as Valsalva can accentuate a hernia, improving detection and diagnosis.

Typical

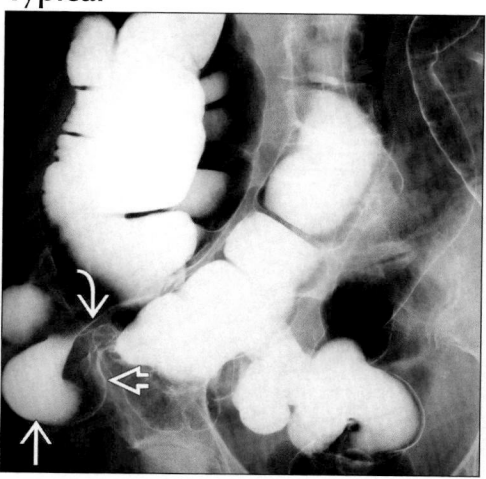

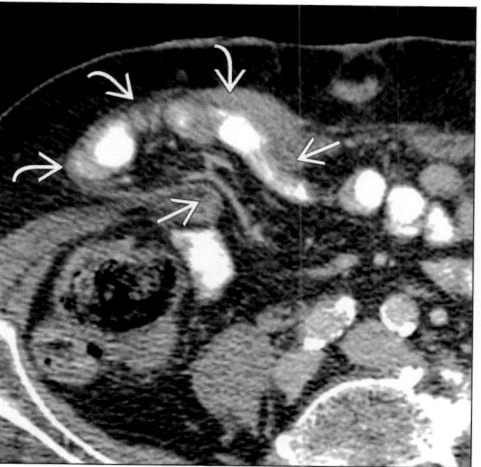

(Left) Barium enema shows large bowel herniation through the lateral abdominal wall ⮕. Note the narrow neck of the hernial sac ⮞ & barium filled bowel loops ➡ herniating through the defect. (Right) Transverse CECT shows a right, paramedial, anterior abdominal wall hernia ➡. Note the wide neck of the hernial sac ➡.

GROIN HERNIAS

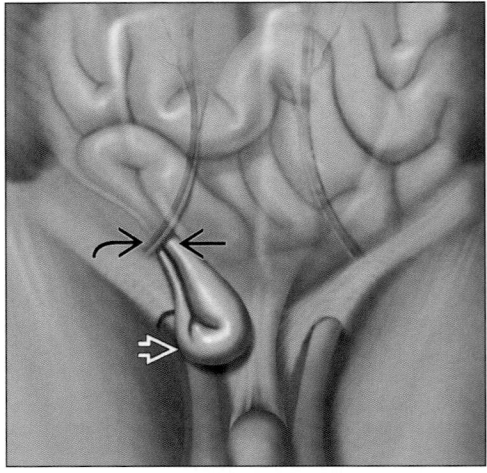

Graphic shows a direct inguinal hernia ⮕. Note the neck ➡ of a direct inguinal hernia is medial to the inferior epigastric vessels ➡.

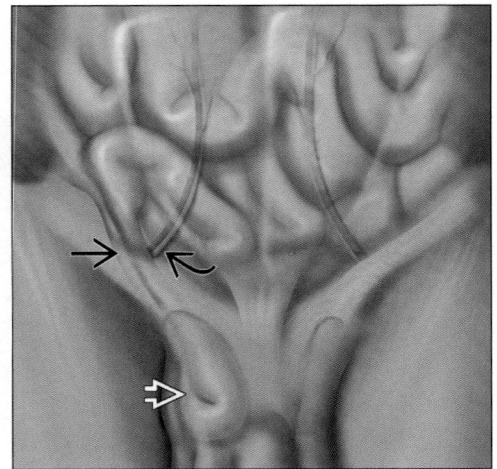

Graphic shows an indirect inguinal hernia ⮕ entering into the right scrotal sac. Note the neck ➡ of an indirect inguinal hernia is lateral to the inferior epigastric vessels ➡.

TERMINOLOGY

Abbreviations and Synonyms
- Inguinal hernia (IH)
- Pelvic & groin hernia

Definitions
- Abnormal protrusion of an organ or part of organ out of the cavity in which it is normally contained
- IH: Inguinal location of hernia orifice

IMAGING FINDINGS

General Features
- Location
  - Indirect IH: Passes through internal inguinal ring, down the inguinal canal & emerges at external ring
    - Can extend along spermatic cord into scrotum; complete hernia
    - In females, hernia follows course of round ligament of uterus into labium majus
    - Passes lateral to epigastric vessels (lateral umbilical fold) & is also known as lateral IH
    - Juxtafunicular: Indirect hernia passes outside spermatic cord
  - Direct IH: Occurs in floor of inguinal canal, through Hesselbach triangle
    - Protrudes medial to inferior epigastric vessels (IEV)
    - Not contained in spermatic cord & generally does not pass into scrotum
    - Medial umbilical fold divides Hesselbach triangle into medial & lateral parts
    - Medial & lateral direct IH
- Morphology
  - Indirect IH in males within spermatic cord has smooth contour & elongated oblique course
    - Juxtafunicular hernias: Irregular contour; do not protrude into a preformed sac
    - Dissect through subcutaneous fat & fibrous tissue
  - Direct IH: Broad & dome-shaped; appears as a small bulge in groin; short & blunt aperture

Ultrasonographic Findings
- Grayscale Ultrasound
  - US: Identifies the nature of herniated contents; bowel (enterocele) or omentum (omentocele) or both

---

DDx: Groin Swelling

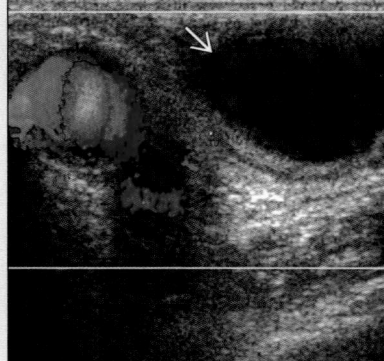

Femoral Hernia

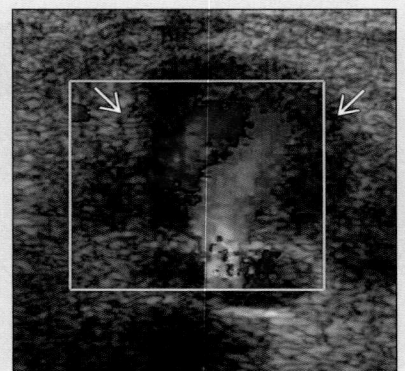

Pseudoaneurysm

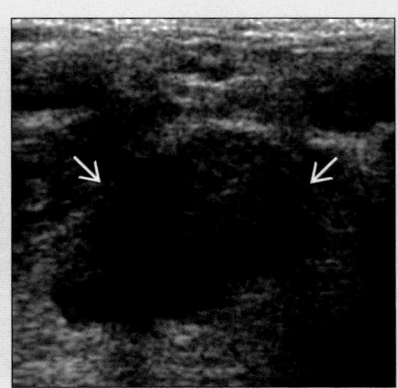

Lymphadenopathy

GROIN HERNIAS

Key Facts

Imaging Findings
- Indirect IH: Passes through internal inguinal ring, down the inguinal canal & emerges at external ring
- Direct IH: Occurs in floor of inguinal canal, through Hesselbach triangle
- US: Identifies the nature of herniated contents; bowel (enterocele) or omentum (omentocele) or both
- Omental fat: Echogenic tissue without peristalsis
- US: Intestinal loops; "target" echo pattern with strong central echoes representing air or fluid in lumen ± peristalsis
- Nonobstructed hernia; active peristalsis ± movement of intestinal contents
- US can reveal reducible/irreducible nature of hernia
- Increase in hernia size during cough or Valsalva maneuver

- Valsalva maneuver may help differentiate type of hernia
- Direct hernia: Distended pampiniform plexus is displaced by hernia sac
- Indirect hernia: Impaired swelling of pampiniform plexus seen

Top Differential Diagnoses
- Femoral Hernia
- Vascular Lesions (Iatrogenic)
- Lymphadenopathy

Pathology
- Inguinal hernia in children is always a result of patent processus vaginalis (indirect hernia); extending into the scrotal sac

---

- ○ Omental fat: Echogenic tissue without peristalsis
- ○ US: Intestinal loops; "target" echo pattern with strong central echoes representing air or fluid in lumen ± peristalsis
  - Nonobstructed hernia; active peristalsis ± movement of intestinal contents
  - Obstructed hernia: Tubular fluid-filled structures with valvulae conniventes (small bowel) or fecal material with haustral pattern (colon); without active peristalsis
- ○ Useful when patient presents non-urgently with history suggesting reducible hernia
  - Real time US examination allows patient to stand upright & perform Valsalva maneuver
- ○ US can reveal reducible/irreducible nature of hernia
  - Decrease in hernia size with decrease in intra-abdominal pressure or application of external pressure to hernial sac with transducer
  - Increase in hernia size during cough or Valsalva maneuver
- ○ Valsalva maneuver may help differentiate type of hernia
  - Direct hernia: Distended pampiniform plexus is displaced by hernia sac
  - Indirect hernia: Impaired swelling of pampiniform plexus seen
- Color Doppler
  - ○ Distinguishes among types of groin hernias; direct or indirect
    - Demonstrate inferior epigastric artery (origin &/or trunk segment) & its relationship with hernia sac
  - ○ Strangulated hernia; absence of vascularity within bowel wall & mesentery

Radiographic Findings
- Radiography
  - ○ Films of abdomen with patient supine may indicate incarceration or strangulation
    - Convergence of distended intestinal loops toward inguinal region
    - Soft tissue density or gas-containing mass overlying obturator foramen on affected side
  - ○ Barium examination of small or large bowel

- Tapered narrowing or obstruction of intestinal segments as it enters hernia orifice
- Herniography: Injection of soluble low osmolar contrast medium into peritoneal cavity
  - ○ Indirect IH: Emerges from lateral inguinal fossa & protrudes medially
    - Roughly parallel to superior pubic ramus
  - ○ Persistent processus vaginalis has a width of 1-2 mm; may extend into scrotum
    - Communicating hydrocele
  - ○ Open Nuck canal in women: Same herniographic appearance as patent processus vaginalis in men
  - ○ Direct hernia: Usually dome-shaped with wide neck
    - More lateral direct IH: Protrudes from medial inguinal fossa
    - More medial direct IH: Protrudes from supravesical fossa & are usually smaller

CT Findings
- Indirect IH: Seen as well-defined ovoid mass in groin
  - ○ Bowel loops & mesenteric fat in hernia sac
- Neck of indirect IH can be demonstrated at deep inguinal ring lateral to IEV
  - ○ Whereas direct IH remain medial to IEV throughout

Imaging Recommendations
- Best imaging tool
  - ○ US/CT for demonstrating acutely strangulated hernia in obese patients
    - In clinical situations where there is diagnostic uncertainty
- Protocol advice
  - ○ US: Examine both inguinal canals & scrotum; during resting phase & with Valsalva maneuver
  - ○ CT: Oral & intravenous CECT; axial plane; thinner slice collimation

DIFFERENTIAL DIAGNOSIS

Femoral Hernia
- Medial position within femoral canal posterior to line of inguinal ligament; caudal & posterior to IH

GROIN HERNIAS

- Frequently has a narrow neck; neck remains below inguinal ligament & lateral to pubic tubercle
- More common in women

Vascular Lesions (Iatrogenic)

- Arterial puncture following arteriography; needle biopsy or aspiration
  - Hematoma formed may extend into rectus muscle or lateral abdominal wall muscles
  - Blood can track directly from groin, along transversalis fascia & transversus abdominis muscle
  - Pseudoaneurysm: Perivascular, rounded mass; neck & track connecting it with injured artery

Lymphadenopathy

- Appears as mass near inguinal ligament
- May be multiple, well defined, hypoechoic or matted conglomerate mass ± central necrosis
- On color Doppler may show hilar or capsular vascularity

PATHOLOGY

General Features

- Etiology
  - Chronic increased intra-abdominal pressure, abdominal distension (ascites) ± muscle laxity
    - Weak abdominal musculature, chronic cough, prostatism, constipation, manual labor
  - Indirect IH considered to be a congenital defect
    - Patency of processus vaginalis; weakness of crus lateralis at lateral aspect of inguinal canal
  - Direct IH considered acquired lesion
    - Weakness in transversalis fascia of posterior wall of inguinal canal in Hesselbach triangle
- Epidemiology
  - 75-80% of all hernias occur in inguinal region
  - Indirect IH are 5 times more common than direct IH
  - Inguinal hernia in children is always a result of patent processus vaginalis (indirect hernia); extending into the scrotal sac
    - Incidence: IH occurs in 1-3% of all children
    - In premature infants, incidence is one-half to two times greater
  - Bilateral patent processus vaginalis occurs in up to 10% of patients with indirect IH
  - Approximately 5% of men develop IH during their lifetime & require an operation

Gross Pathologic & Surgical Features

- Contents: Include small bowel loops or mobile colon segments such as sigmoid, cecum & appendix
- Sliding IH: Partially retroperitoneal organs
  - Urinary bladder, distal ureters or ascending/descending colon, included in herniation
- Littre hernia: Meckel diverticulum in hernia sac
- Richter hernia: Only portion of bowel circumference in sac (antimesenteric)
- Potential indirect hernias are associated with an undescended inguinal testis

CLINICAL ISSUES

Presentation

- Asymptomatic; sudden appearance of lump in groin; intermittently present; ± groin pain; palpable bulge
- Incarcerated or strangulated hernia: Bowel distension; painful & often tense swelling in groin or scrotum
- Physical examination: Recumbent & upright position; may be reducible; bowel sounds audible; ± tenderness
  - Examining finger placed along spermatic cord at scrotum & passed into external ring along canal with ↑ intra-abdominal pressure
    - Indirect hernia touches tip of finger
    - Direct hernia causes bulge forward low in canal

Demographics

- Age
  - Indirect IH may occur from infancy to old age but generally occur by 5th decade of life
  - Direct IH increases in occurrence with age
- Gender
  - Indirect IH five to ten times more common in men
  - Direct IH occurs mostly in men & seldom in women

Natural History & Prognosis

- Pediatric IH: Almost always indirect; higher risk of incarceration
  - Usually on right (60-75%); often bilateral (10-15%)
- Recurrent hernia: Groin hernias recur after herniorrhaphy in up to 20% of patients
  - Direct IH may develop after repair of an indirect hernia
- Multiple hernias: Often one is of direct type
- Saddlebag, pantaloon, combined IH: Simultaneous occurrence of direct & indirect IH in same groin
- Indirect IH accounts for 15% of intestinal obstructions
- Diverticulitis; appendicitis; primary or metastatic tumor may occur within hernia sac
- Complications: Incarceration; strangulation
  - Direct IH rarely undergoes incarceration or strangulation

Treatment

- Laparoscopic or open hernia repair

DIAGNOSTIC CHECKLIST

Consider

- Hernias that protrude from lateral inguinal fossa are indirect IH
- Hernias that protrude from medial & supravesical fossae are direct IH

SELECTED REFERENCES

1. van den Berg JC: Inguinal hernias: MRI and ultrasound. Semin Ultrasound CT MR. 23(2): 156-73, 2002
2. Shadbolt CL et al: Imaging of groin masses: inguinal anatomy and pathologic conditions revisited. Radiographics. 21 Spec No: S261-71, 2001
3. Zhang GQ et al: Groin hernias in adults: value of color Doppler sonography in their classification. J Clin Ultrasound. 29(8): 429-34, 2001

8
8

IMAGE GALLERY

Typical

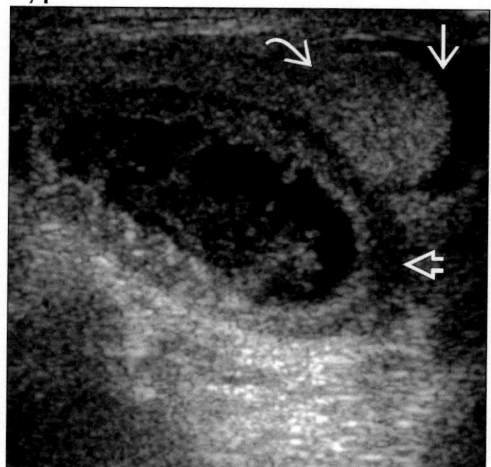
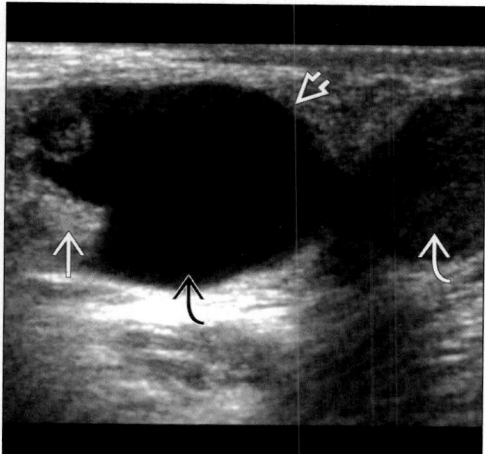

(Left) Longitudinal ultrasound along the inguinal canal shows an indirect, bowel-containing inguinal hernia ➡ entering the scrotal sac & displacing the testis ➡. Note minimal hydrocele ➡. *(Right)* Oblique ultrasound shows an inguinal hernia ➡ containing omentum ➡ & free fluid ➡. Note the relationship of the hernial sac to the testis ➡.

Typical

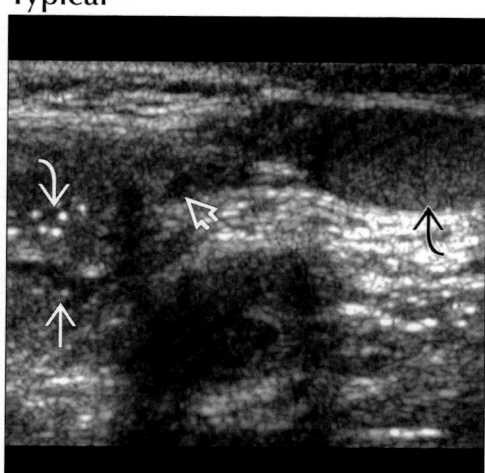
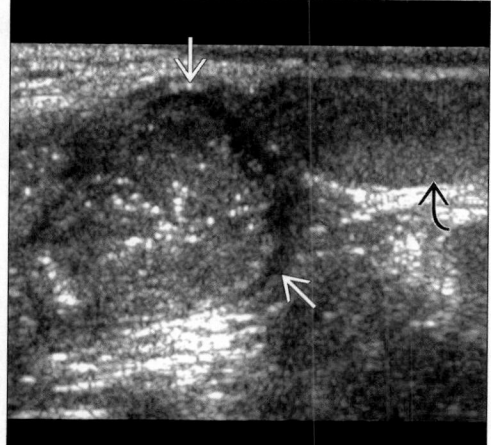

(Left) Oblique transabdominal ultrasound along the inguinal canal ➡ shows a herniating bowel loop ➡ with echogenic contents ➡. Note its relationship to the upper pole of the testis ➡. *(Right)* Oblique transabdominal ultrasound (same patient as previous image), with increased intra-abdominal pressure, shows increased herniation of small bowel loops ➡ into the scrotum. Note the relationship to testis ➡.

Typical

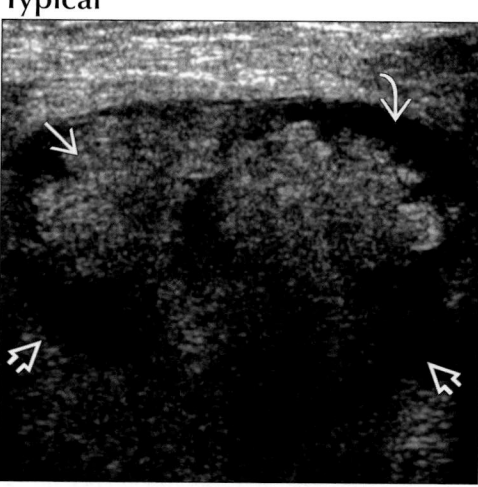
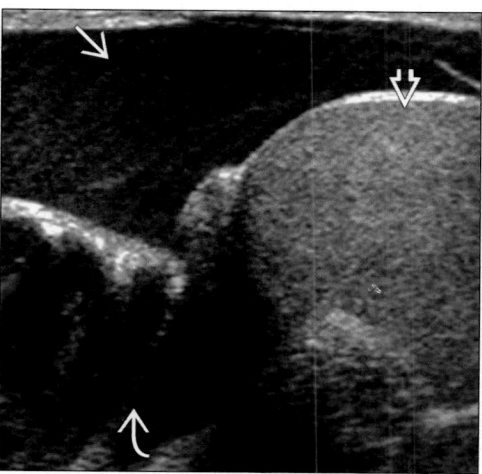

(Left) Transverse ultrasound shows a direct hernia ➡ containing echogenic omentum ➡ surrounded by anechoic peritoneal fluid ➡. *(Right)* Oblique ultrasound shows an indirect inguinal hernia in an infant. There is a patent processus vaginalis with a communicating hydrocele ➡. Note small bowel with valvulae conniventes ➡ & its relationship to the testis ➡.

ASCITES

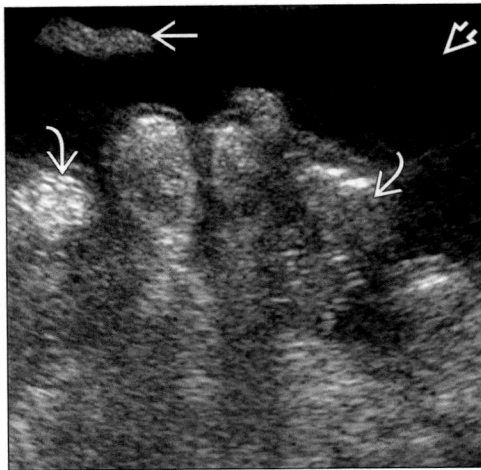 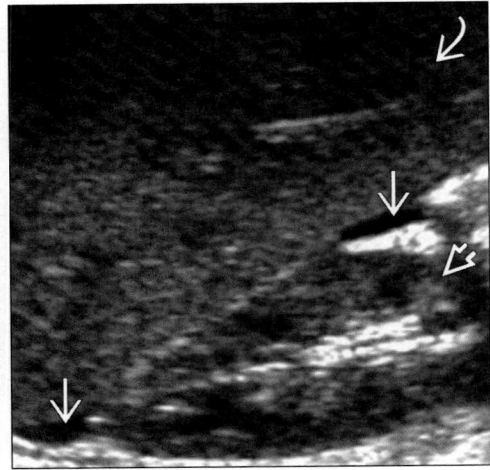

Transverse transabdominal ultrasound shows massive ascites ➡ with floating bowel loops ➡ & echogenic omentum ➡.

Longitudinal transabdominal ultrasound shows minimal ascites in the hepatorenal (Morrison) pouch ➡. Note right kidney ➡ & liver ➡.

TERMINOLOGY

Abbreviations and Synonyms
- Intraperitoneal fluid collection

Definitions
- Pathologic accumulation of fluid within peritoneal cavity

IMAGING FINDINGS

General Features
- Best diagnostic clue: Diagnostic paracentesis
- Location
  - In uncomplicated cases, fluid flows to most dependent position
  - Morrison pouch (hepatorenal fossa): Most dependent upper abdominal recess
  - Pelvis: Most dependent space, pouch of Douglas
  - Paracolic gutters: Along ascending & descending colon
  - Subphrenic spaces
    - Not dependent, but fill due to suction effect of diaphragmatic motion
  - Lesser sac
    - Usually does not fill with ascites
    - Exceptions: Tense ascites, local source (gastric ulcer or pancreatitis)
    - Otherwise, usually due to carcinomatosis or infected ascites
- Morphology
  - Free-flowing: Shaped by surrounding structures & does not deform normal shape of adjacent organs
    - Fluid insinuates itself between organs
  - Loculated: Rounded, bulging contour, encapsulated
    - Does not conform to organ margins
    - Mass effect on adjacent organs
  - Transudative or exudative ascites
  - Chylous, hemorrhagic, bile, pancreatic, urine, cerebrospinal fluid
  - Pseudomyxoma peritonei, malignant ascites

Ultrasonographic Findings
- Grayscale Ultrasound
  - US accurate at quantifying & localizing ascites

DDx: Peritoneal Fluid

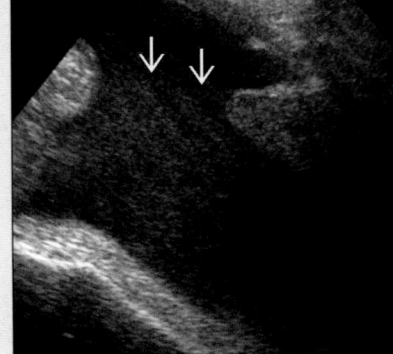 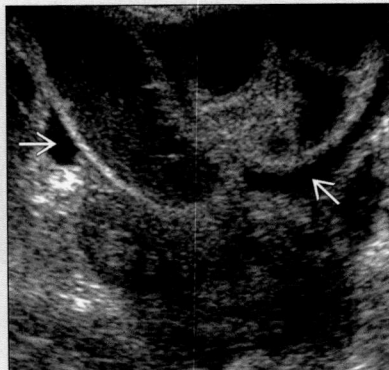 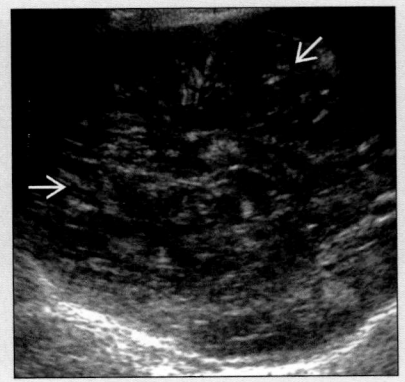

Hemoperitoneum   *Peritoneal Tuberculosis*   *Malignant Ascites*

ASCITES

Key Facts

Imaging Findings

- US accurate at quantifying & localizing ascites
- US: Uncomplicated ascites; homogeneous, freely mobile, anechoic; deep acoustic enhancement
- Free fluid: Acute angles where fluid borders organs
- Free fluid shifts with change in patient position
- Complicated ascites: With coarse or fine internal echoes on US
- Loculated ascites: Adhesions, chronic ascites, malignancy, infection, immobile
- Sonolucent band; small amounts of fluid (5-10 mL) in Morrison pouch, around liver
- Triangular fluid cap; distended bladder displaces fluid to peritoneal reflection adjacent to uterine fundus
- Small free fluid in cul-de-sac; physiologic in women

- Transvaginal US: Excellent for detection of even minimal fluid (0.8 mL) in pelvis
- Thickening of gallbladder wall; more than 3 mm in benign ascites; in carcinomatosis less than 3 mm thick
- Cerebrospinal fluid ascites: Small amounts of free fluid normal with ventriculoperitoneal shunt
- Pancreatic ascites: Peripancreatic, lesser sac, anterior pararenal space
- Bedside US to screen for ascites in critically ill or post-operative patients ± drainage

Top Differential Diagnoses

- Hemoperitoneum
- Infectious Ascites
- Malignant Ascites

- Characterization of ascites: Anechoic or echogenic (debris or particulate)
  - Anechoic (uncomplicated ascites): Usually transudative due to liver disease, congestive cardiac failure, renal failure
  - Echogenic ascites (complicated ascites): Exudative ascites due to infection, inflammation, blood or neoplastic cells
- US: Uncomplicated ascites; homogeneous, freely mobile, anechoic; deep acoustic enhancement
  - Free fluid: Acute angles where fluid borders organs
    - Free fluid shifts with change in patient position
    - Compresses with increased transducer pressure
- Complicated ascites: With coarse or fine internal echoes on US
  - Loculation, atypical fluid distribution, multiple septa on US
  - Matted or clumped; infiltrated bowel loops (tuberculous peritonitis, pseudomyxoma peritonei)
  - Thickened interfaces between fluid & adjacent structures; peritoneal lining, omental thickening
- Loculated ascites: Adhesions, chronic ascites, malignancy, infection, immobile
  - Non compressible
  - Rounded margins with mass effect, frequently displacing adjacent structures
- Sonolucent band; small amounts of fluid (5-10 mL) in Morrison pouch, around liver
- Polycyclic, "lollipop," arcuate appearance
  - Small bowel loops arrayed on either side of vertically floating mesentry; seen with massive ascites
- Transverse & sigmoid colon usually float on top of fluid (nondependent gas content when patient supine)
- Triangular fluid cap; distended bladder displaces fluid to peritoneal reflection adjacent to uterine fundus
- Small free fluid in cul-de-sac; physiologic in women
  - Transvaginal US: Excellent for detection of even minimal fluid (0.8 mL) in pelvis
- Thickening of gallbladder wall; more than 3 mm in benign ascites; in carcinomatosis less than 3 mm thick
- Cerebrospinal fluid ascites: Small amounts of free fluid normal with ventriculoperitoneal shunt

- Localized/loculated collection around tip of shunt tube; pathologic, implies malfunction
- Pancreatic ascites: Peripancreatic, lesser sac, anterior pararenal space
  - Disruption of pancreatic duct or severe pancreatitis

Radiographic Findings

- Plain abdominal film: Insensitive for diagnosis
  - "Hellmer sign", lateral edge of liver medially displaced from adjacent thoracoabdominal wall
  - Obliteration of hepatic & splenic angle
  - Symmetric densities on sides of bladder ("dog's ear")
  - Medial displacement of ascending & descending colon; lateral displacement of properitoneal fat line
  - Indirect signs: Diffuse abdominal haziness; bulging of flanks; poor visualization of psoas & renal outline
    - Separation of small bowel loops; centralization of floating gas-containing small bowel
  - Chest film: Elevation of diaphragm, sympathetic pleural effusion; with massive ascites

CT Findings

- Simple ascites: Low density free fluid collection
  - Transudate: 0-30 Hounsfield units
  - Small amounts in right perihepatic space, Morrison pouch, pouch of Douglas
  - Larger amounts of fluid in paracolic gutters
    - Centralization of bowel loops; triangular configuration within leaves of mesentery
  - Massive ascites; distends peritoneal spaces
- CT findings in other intraperitoneal collections
  - Exudates: Density of ascitic fluid increases with increasing protein content
  - Chylous ascites: Less than 0 HU; intraperitoneal & extraperitoneal water density fluid (in trauma)
  - Bile ascites: Less than 20 HU; typically in right or left supramesocolic spaces
  - Urine ascites: Nonspecific NECT appearance, may be opacified in CECT

Non-Vascular Interventions

- US guided therapeutic & diagnostic paracentesis

ASCITES

Imaging Recommendations
- Best imaging tool
  - US for quantification & characterization (localized or generalized) of peritoneal fluid collections
  - US: Easily available, sensitive (detection of small volume ascites), cost-effective
    - Bedside US to screen for ascites in critically ill or post-operative patients ± drainage
- Protocol advice: US for screening followed by detailed evaluation of peritoneum & abdomen by US/CT/MR

DIFFERENTIAL DIAGNOSIS

Hemoperitoneum
- Trauma, ruptured aneurysm, ruptured ectopic pregnancy, ruptured liver mass, post-surgical bleeding, anticoagulant therapy
- Fluid debris level may develop; patients in supine position for long time
- Massive hemorrhage: Large echogenic mass (clots), later become heterogeneous (lysis)

Infectious Ascites
- Fluid with internal echoes, debris
- Partial loculations; multiple septae
- Peritoneal thickening, matted bowel loops, abscess
- Tuberculosis, acquired immunodeficiency syndrome, fungal infections

Malignant Ascites
- Loculated collections; fluid in greater & lesser sac
- Bowel loops tethered along posterior abdominal wall
- Thickening of peritoneum; peritoneal seeding
- Hepatic, splenic, lymph node lesions; mass arising from ovary, gut, pancreas

PATHOLOGY

General Features
- General path comments: Diminished effective volume (hydrostatic vs. colloid osmotic pressure); overflow
- Etiology
  - Hepatic: Cirrhosis, portal hypertension
    - Budd-Chiari syndrome, portal vein thrombosis, alcoholic hepatitis, fulminant hepatic failure
  - Cardiac: Congestive heart failure, constrictive pericarditis, cardiac tamponade
  - Renal: Nephrotic syndrome, chronic renal failure
  - Neoplasm: Colon, gastric, pancreatic, hepatic, ovarian; metastatic disease (breast/lung etc.)
    - Meigs syndrome, mesothelioma
  - Infections: Bacterial, fungal or parasitic
    - Tuberculosis; acquired immunodeficiency syndrome
  - Trauma: Blunt, penetrating or iatrogenic
    - Diagnostic/therapeutic peritoneal lavage
    - Bile ascites: Trauma, cholecystectomy, biliary or hepatic surgery, biopsy, percutaneous drainage
    - Urine ascites: Trauma to bladder or collecting system, instrumentation
    - Cerebrospinal fluid: Ventriculoperitoneal shunts
  - Chylous: Trauma (blunt, penetrating, surgical), inflammatory, idiopathic
  - Hypoalbuminemia; protein-losing enteropathy
  - Miscellaneous: Myxedema, marked fluid overload

Gross Pathologic & Surgical Features
- Transudate: Clear or straw colored (proteins < 2.5 g/dl)
- Exudate: Yellowish/hemorrhagic (proteins > 2.5 g/dl)
- Neoplasm: Hemorrhagic, clear or chylous (yellowish-white, milky)
- Pyogenic: Turbid (polymorphonuclear leukocyte count > 500/cu mm)
- Pseudomyxoma peritonei: Gelatinous, mucinous

Microscopic Features
- Ascitic fluid may contain blood cells, colloids, protein molecules, or crystalloids (such as glucose) & water

CLINICAL ISSUES

Presentation
- Most common signs/symptoms: Asymptomatic, abdominal discomfort & distension, weight gain
- Physical examination: Bulging flanks, flank dullness, fluid thrill, umbilical hernia, penile or scrotal edema
- Diagnosis: Paracentesis (US guidance or blind tap)
  - Indications: All patients with new onset ascites
    - Chronic ascites with fever, abdominal pain, renal insufficiency, or encephalopathy
  - Fluid analysis: Protein, lactate dehydrogenase, amylase, cytology, pH, triglycerides

Natural History & Prognosis
- Complication: Spontaneous bacterial peritonitis, respiratory compromise, anorexia

Treatment
- Sodium restriction & diuretics
- Refractory cases: Large volume paracentesis
  - Peritoneovenous shunting; LeVeen, Denver
  - Liver transplantation, transjugular intrahepatic portosystemic shunting (TIPSS), IVC or hepatic vein stenting (Budd-Chiari syndrome)

DIAGNOSTIC CHECKLIST

Consider
- Often difficult to characterize nature & underlying cause of peritoneal fluid collections on basis of imaging alone

SELECTED REFERENCES
1. Witte MH et al: Chylothorax and chyloperitoneum. N Engl J Med. 2006
2. Hanbidge AE et al: US of the peritoneum. Radiographics. 23(3):663-84; discussion 684-5, 2003
3. Habeeb KS et al: Management of ascites. Paracentesis as a guide. Postgrad Med. 101(1): 191-2, 195-200, 1997

ASCITES

IMAGE GALLERY

Typical

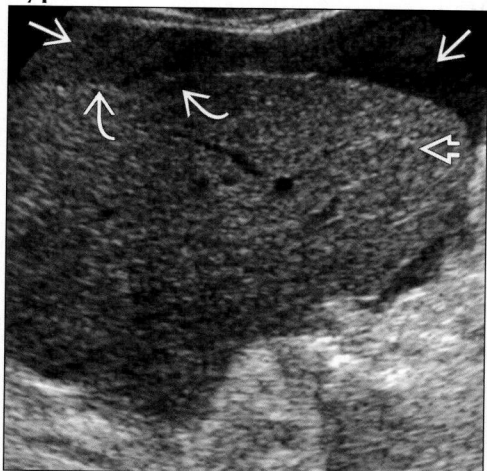
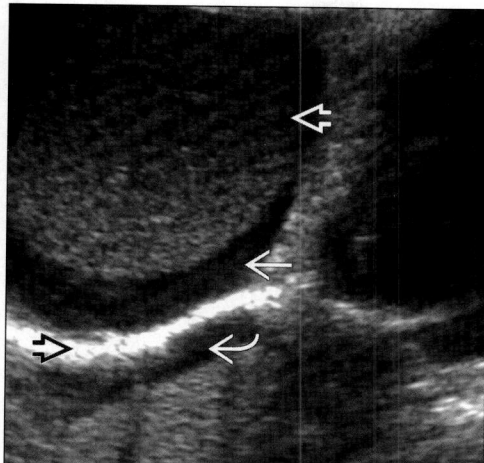

(Left) Oblique transabdominal ultrasound shows ascites ➡ due to liver cirrhosis. Note liver with coarse parenchyma ➡ & surface nodularity ➡. (Right) Transverse transabdominal ultrasound through the epigastric region shows ascites ➡ between the liver ➡ and the echogenic diaphragm ➡. A right pleural effusion ➡ is seen posterior to the diaphragm.

Typical

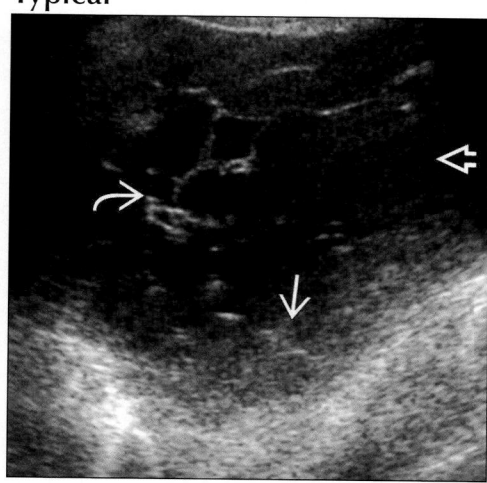
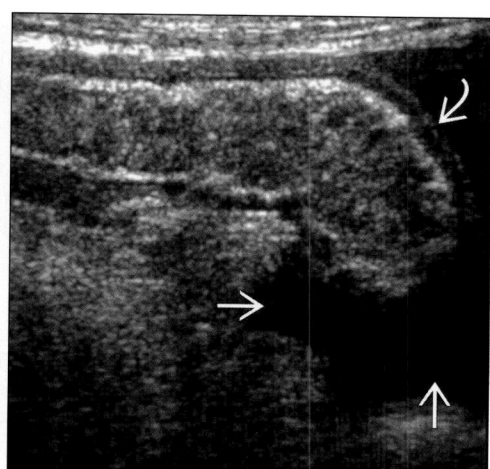

(Left) Transverse transabdominal ultrasound shows chronic, loculated ascites ➡ in the flank. It has internal septations ➡ & debris ➡. (Right) Longitudinal transabdominal ultrasound shows moderate ascites ➡. Note a small bowel loop with thickened serosa ➡.

Typical

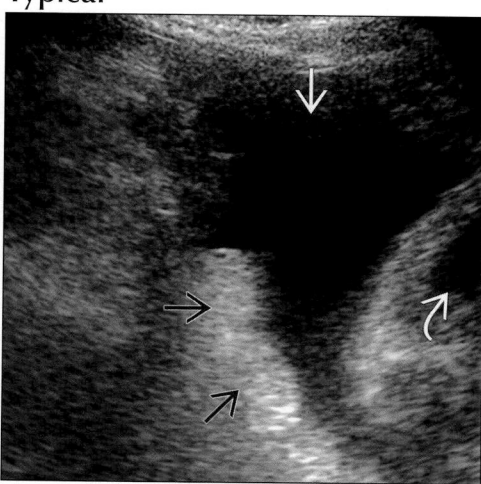
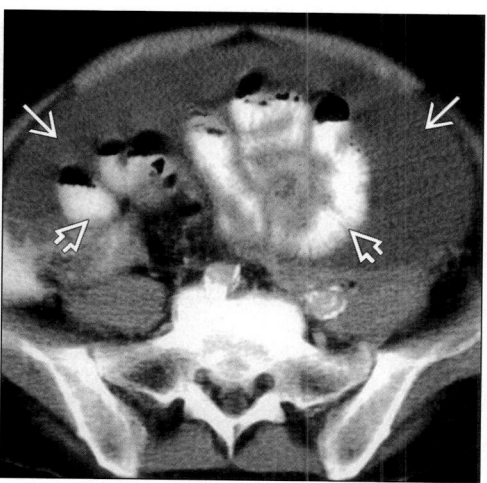

(Left) Longitudinal transabdominal ultrasound shows moderate ascites ➡ in the pelvis (dependent part). Note the empty bladder ➡ & air filled, echogenic bowel loops ➡. (Right) Transverse CECT shows marked ascites ➡, causing central displacement of small bowel loops ➡.

PERITONEAL CARCINOMATOSIS

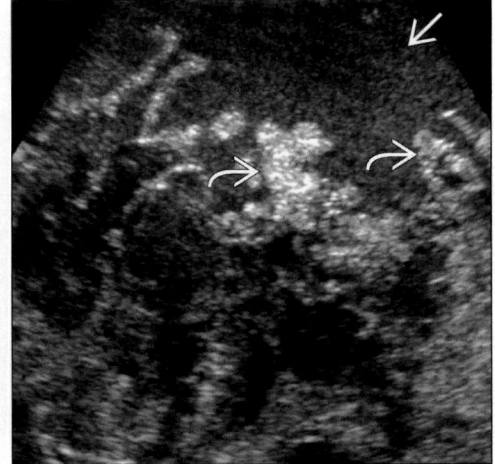

Transverse transabdominal ultrasound shows echogenic small bowel loops ➡. Note markedly thickened & echogenic mesenteric leaves ➡ with classic sunburst appearance ➡.

Longitudinal transabdominal ultrasound shows ascites with echogenic debris ➡. Note thick, nodular mesenteric deposits ➡.

TERMINOLOGY

Abbreviations and Synonyms
- Peritoneal carcinomatosis, peritoneal implants, omental caking

Definitions
- Metastatic disease to the omentum, peritoneal surface, peritoneal ligaments and/or mesentery

IMAGING FINDINGS

General Features
- Best diagnostic clue
  - Omental cake, soft tissue implants on peritoneal surface
  - Cystic peritoneal masses in ovarian carcinoma
  - Ascites, mesenteric stranding, bowel obstruction
- Location: Peritoneum, mesentery, peritoneal ligaments
- Size: Variable; 5 mm nodules to large confluent omental masses (omental cake)
- Morphology: Nodular, plaque-like or large omental mass

Ultrasonographic Findings
- Grayscale Ultrasound
  - Omental deposits: Hypoechoic omental masses, nodular echogenic mass seen against anechoic ascites
  - Thickening of mesenteric leaves due to desmoplastic reaction; typically mesenteric side of terminal ileum
    - May give "sunburst" appearance
  - Peritoneal implants: Nodular masses along the parietal & visceral peritoneum or hypoechoic rind-like thickening of peritoneum
    - Parietal peritoneal line preserved with small implants; often lost as implants grow in size
    - Usually grow inward towards peritoneal cavity; may grow outwards & invade abdominal wall
    - Pouch of Douglas, Morrison pouch & right subphrenic space commonly involved
    - Transvaginal US: Lobulated mass in pouch of Douglas
    - Psammomatous calcification in peritoneal implants seen in ovarian serous cystadenoma (up to 40% with stage III/IV disease)

DDx: Peritoneal Pathologies

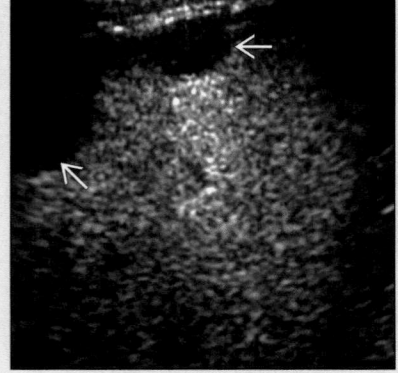

Pseudomyxoma Peritonei

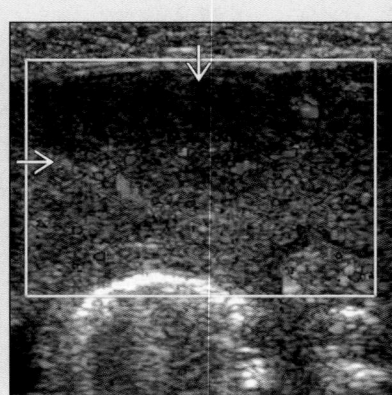

Mesothelioma

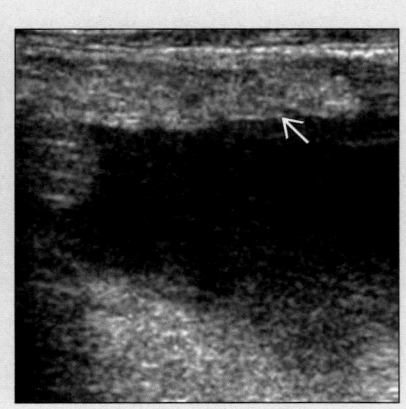

Peritoneal Tuberculosis

PERITONEAL CARCINOMATOSIS

Key Facts

Imaging Findings

- Omental cake, soft tissue implants on peritoneal surface
- Omental deposits: Hypoechoic omental masses, nodular echogenic mass seen against anechoic ascites
- Thickening of mesenteric leaves due to desmoplastic reaction; typically mesenteric side of terminal ileum
- Peritoneal implants: Nodular masses along the parietal & visceral peritoneum or hypoechoic rind-like thickening of peritoneum
- Transvaginal US: Lobulated mass in pouch of Douglas
- Psammomatous calcification in peritoneal implants seen in ovarian serous cystadenoma (up to 40% with stage III/IV disease)
- Ascites: Complex ascites with septation, hyperechoic nodular debris

- In absence of ascites it may be difficult to detect peritoneal implants < 3 mm in size
- ± Enlarged hypoechoic retro-peritoneal & mesenteric lymph nodes
- Bilateral cystic adnexal masses due to peritoneal metastasis from GI malignancies; "Krukenberg" tumor
- Color Doppler: May detect vascularity in omental/peritoneal deposits
- US excellent for initial screening, followed by CT/MR for further evaluation

Top Differential Diagnoses

- Pseudomyxoma Peritonei
- Peritoneal Mesothelioma
- Peritoneal Tuberculosis

- Ascites: Complex ascites with septation, hyperechoic nodular debris
  - May be the only finding
  - Facilitates detection of peritoneal implants
- In absence of ascites it may be difficult to detect peritoneal implants < 3 mm in size
- ± Enlarged hypoechoic retro-peritoneal & mesenteric lymph nodes
- Bilateral cystic adnexal masses due to peritoneal metastasis from GI malignancies; "Krukenberg" tumor
- Color Doppler: May detect vascularity in omental/peritoneal deposits

Radiographic Findings

- Radiography
  - Plain film findings of ascites
    - Medial displacement of cecum in 90% of patients with significant ascites
    - Pelvic "dog's ear" in 90% of patients with significant ascites
    - Medial displacement of lateral liver edge (Hellmer sign) in 80% of patients with significant ascites
    - Bulging of flanks, central displacement of bowel loops, indistinct psoas margin
  - Plain film findings of small bowel obstruction
    - Dilated small bowel > 3 cm
    - Fluid-fluid levels in small bowel on upright film
    - "String of pearls" sign
    - Collapsed gasless colon

CT Findings

- NECT: Ascites
- CECT
  - Ascites, nodular thickening/enhancement of peritoneum, hypovascular omental masses
  - Spiculated mesentery
  - Evidence of bowel obstruction with delineation of transition zone from dilated to non-dilated bowel

Non-Vascular Interventions

- US guided diagnostic & therapeutic aspiration

MR Findings

- T1WI: Low signal ascites, medium signal omental cake
- T2WI: Intermediate signal peritoneal mass and high signal ascites
- T1 C+: Abnormal enhancement of peritoneum with gadolinium, hypointense nodules and masses

Fluoroscopic Findings

- Barium studies
  - Small bowel follow through (SBFT): Dilated bowel with transition zone; partial small bowel obstruction
  - Mural extrinsic filling defects due to serosal implants on small bowel
  - Spiculated extrinsic impression due to tethering of rectosigmoid from intraperitoneal metastases to pouch of Douglas
  - Scalloping of cecum from peritoneal implants
  - "Omental cake" may cause invasion of transverse mesocolon with nodularity & spiculation of superior contour

Imaging Recommendations

- Best imaging tool: CECT
- Protocol advice
  - US excellent for initial screening, followed by CT/MR for further evaluation
    - Detailed search for primary tumor involving, ovaries, stomach, colon, gallbladder & bile ducts
  - US ideal for guiding diagnostic & therapeutic aspiration

DIFFERENTIAL DIAGNOSIS

Pseudomyxoma Peritonei

- Complex ascites; reflecting gelatinous nature of fluid within peritoneum
- Scalloping of lateral contour of liver and spleen
- Etiology related to perforation of mucinous epithelial neoplasm of appendix or ovaries

PERITONEAL CARCINOMATOSIS

Peritoneal Mesothelioma
- 33% of mesotheliomas are peritoneal, most common in middle aged men, association with asbestos exposure
- Thick nodular masses involving anterior parietal peritoneum, becoming confluent, "cake-like"
- Large solid omental and mesenteric masses often infiltrating bowel and mesentery
- Ascites: Seen in 90% of cases, but may be much less in quantity

Peritoneal Tuberculosis
- Nodular or symmetric thickening of peritoneum and mesentery, ± calcification (14%)
- Ascites, ± mesenteric nodes
- Ileo-cecal mural thickening, matted, clumped hypoperistaltic small bowel loops

PATHOLOGY

General Features
- Genetics
  - Colorectal and ovarian CA related to Lynch syndrome (I & II) of hereditary nonpolyposis colorectal cancer
  - GI cancers related to polyposis syndrome
- Etiology
  - Metastatic disease to peritoneal surfaces, omentum and mesentery
  - Ovarian and GI tract adenocarcinomas most common etiologies
  - Krukenberg tumor: Peritoneal spread of GI tract malignancies (usually stomach or colon) to both ovaries
  - Less common causes
    - Metastatic lung, breast and renal CA
    - Sarcoma, lymphoma less common causes

Gross Pathologic & Surgical Features
- Infiltrating masses of peritoneal surfaces, omentum and mesentery
- Omental cake & nodular implants on peritoneal surface
- Ascites: Clear or turbid & thick (viscous)

Microscopic Features
- Varies according to primary tumor
  - Most commonly adenocarcinoma

Staging, Grading or Classification Criteria
- Peritoneal metastases indicate stage IV disease

CLINICAL ISSUES

Presentation
- Most common signs/symptoms: Abdominal distension and pain, weight loss; ascites may or may not be present
- Clinical Profile
  - No reliable lab data
  - Positive cytology on paracentesis
  - Positive FNA of omental mass

Demographics
- Age
  - Adults generally > 40 yrs
  - Younger patients with hereditary syndromes (i.e., Lynch II)
- Gender: More common in females than males, due to ovarian CA

Natural History & Prognosis
- Variable depending on primary tumor; poor prognosis in general
- Progressive if untreated
- Pattern of peritoneal spread
  - Direct seeding along mesentery and ligaments
  - Intraperitoneal seeding along distribution of ascites
  - Lymphatic or hematogenous
- Complication: Bowel obstruction

Treatment
- Cytoreductive surgery for ovarian metastases
- All others combination of systemic and intraperitoneal chemotherapy

DIAGNOSTIC CHECKLIST

Consider
- TB peritonitis
  - Causes symmetric thickening of peritoneum, ileo-cecal thickening, ascites, hypoechoic mesenteric lymph nodes & calcification

Image Interpretation Pearls
- Omental cake
- Peritoneal and mesenteric implants
- Ascites

SELECTED REFERENCES

1. Jayne DG: The molecular biology of peritoneal carcinomatosis from gastrointestinal cancer. Ann Acad Med Singapore. 32(2):219-25, 2003
2. Park CM et al: Recurrent ovarian malignancy: patterns and spectrum of imaging findings. Abdom Imaging. 28(3):404-15, 2003
3. Pavlidis N et al: Diagnostic and therapeutic management of cancer of an unknown primary. Eur J Cancer. 39(14):1990-2005, 2003
4. Canis M et al: Risk of spread of ovarian cancer after laparoscopic surgery. Curr Opin Obstet Gynecol. 13(1):9-14, 2001
5. Chorost MI et al: The management of the unknown primary. J Am Coll Surg. 193(6):666-77, 2001
6. Raptopoulos V et al: Peritoneal carcinomatosis. Eur Radiol. 11(11):2195-206, 2001
7. Sugarbaker PH: Review of a personal experience in the management of carcinomatosis and sarcomatosis. Jpn J Clin Oncol. 31(12):573-83, 2001
8. Tamsma JT et al: Pathogenesis of malignant ascites: Starling's law of capillary hemodynamics revisited. Ann Oncol. 12(10):1353-7, 2001
9. Canis M et al: Cancer and laparoscopy, experimental studies: a review. Eur J Obstet Gynecol Reprod Biol. 91(1):1-9, 2000
10. Leblanc E et al: Surgical staging of early invasive epithelial ovarian tumors. Semin Surg Oncol. 19(1):36-41, 2000

PERITONEAL CARCINOMATOSIS

IMAGE GALLERY

Typical

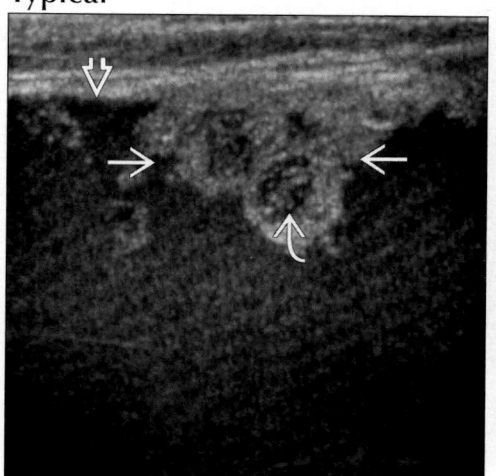

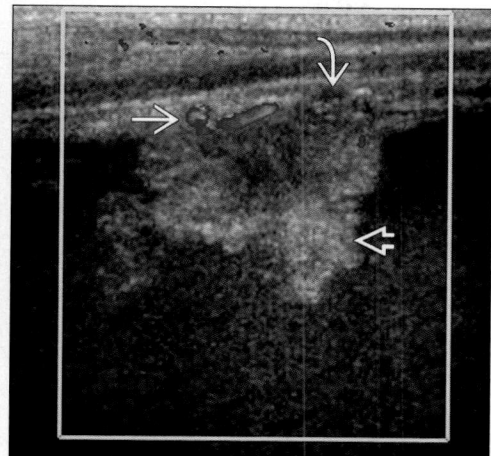

(Left) Transverse transabdominal ultrasound shows a nodular peritoneal deposit ➡️ along the parietal peritoneum ➡️, better seen due to ascites. Note cystic areas within peritoneal deposits ➡️. *(Right)* Transverse color Doppler ultrasound shows minimal vascularity ➡️ within the peritoneal deposit ➡️. Note focal invasion of abdominal wall ➡️.

Typical

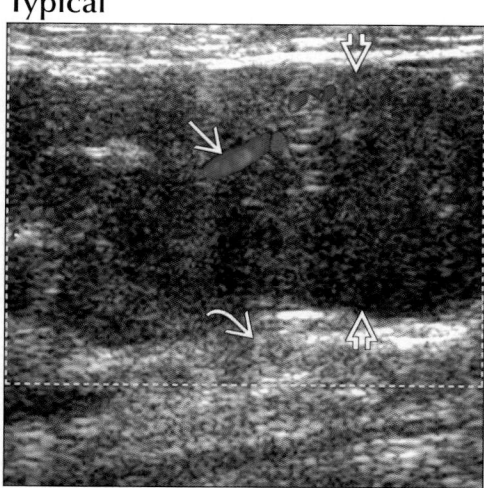

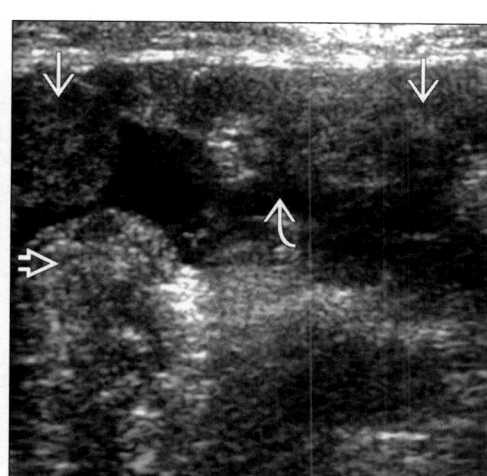

(Left) Longitudinal color Doppler ultrasound shows hypoechoic omental cake (thickening) ➡️ with vascularity ➡️. Note displacement of bowel loops ➡️ by thickened omentum. *(Right)* Longitudinal transabdominal ultrasound shows nodular hypoechoic peritoneal deposits ➡️. They are well delineated due to presence of anechoic ascites ➡️. Note adjacent bowel ➡️.

Typical

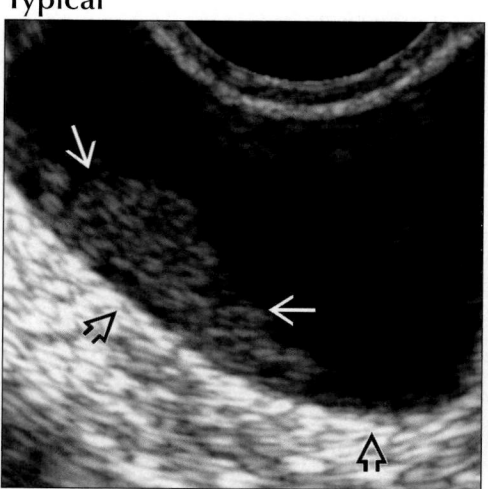

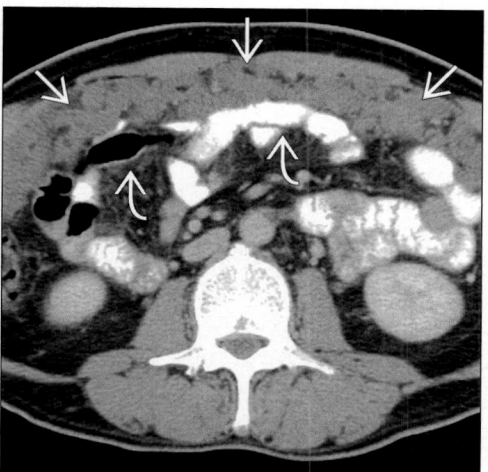

(Left) Longitudinal transvaginal ultrasound shows small nodular peritoneal deposits ➡️ in the pouch of Douglas ➡️. *(Right)* Transverse CECT shows enhancing "cake-like" nodular parietal peritoneal thickening ➡️ due to metastasis. Note displacement of bowel loops ➡️ away from anterior abdominal wall.

PERITONEAL SPACE ABSCESS

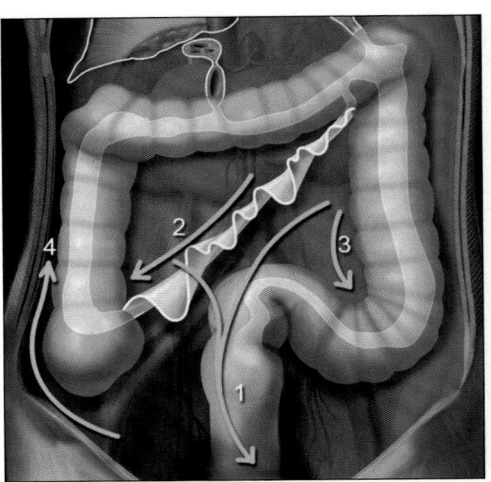

Graphic shows preferential sites of peritoneal collections in the abdomen and pelvis.

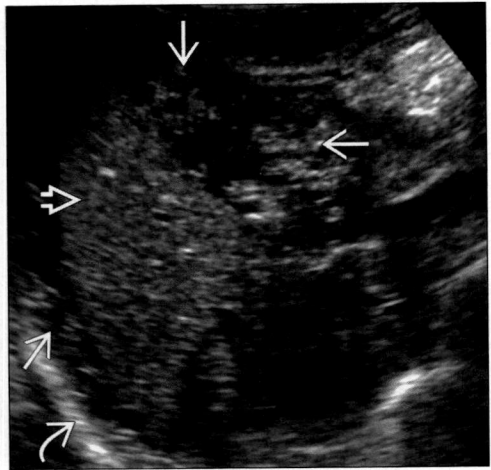

Oblique transabdominal ultrasound shows a perihepatic ➡ collection due to ruptured liver abscess. Note echogenic diaphragm ⮞ & liver ⮞.

TERMINOLOGY

Definitions
- Localized abdominal collection of pus

IMAGING FINDINGS

General Features
- Best diagnostic clue: Fluid collection with mass effect ± gas bubbles or air-fluid level
- Location: Anywhere within abdominal cavity; within intra- or extraperitoneal spaces
- Size: Highly variable; 2-15 cm in diameter or diffuse peritoneal collection
- Morphology: Hypoechoic or anechoic fluid collection ± septations & debris

Ultrasonographic Findings
- Grayscale Ultrasound
  - Complex fluid collection with internal low level echoes, membranes or septations
  - Dependent echoes representing debris; seen as fluid-fluid level
  - Bright linear echoes with reverberation artifacts representing gas bubbles; diagnostic of infection
  - Inflamed fat adjacent to abscess: Echogenic mass
    - Usually seen with abscesses due to appendicitis, diverticulitis, complicated acute cholecystitis, inflammatory bowel disease & pancreatitis
  - Peritonitis (infective): Diffuse inflammation of parietal or visceral peritoneum
    - Ascites: Particulate, loculated or with internal septations, debris or gas (perforation)
    - Diffuse thickening of peritoneum (parietal & visceral), mesentry & omentum
  - Tuberculous peritonitis: Matted bowel loops with heterogeneous inter-bowel exudate
    - ± Necrotic lymphadenopathy (mesenteric & retroperitoneal), may progress to liquefaction & abscess formation
  - Sclerosing peritonitis: Major complication of continuous ambulatory peritoneal dialysis (CAPD) with secondary infection
    - Hyperperistaltic bowel loops with both free & loculated ascites (earlier sign)

DDx: Abdominal Collections

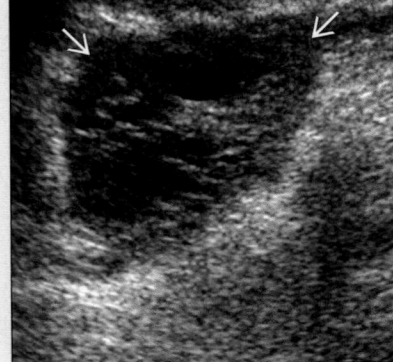

Chronic Loculated Ascites

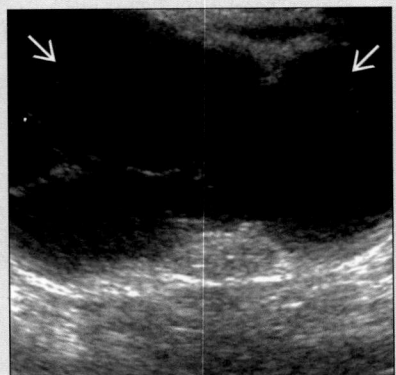

Lymphocele

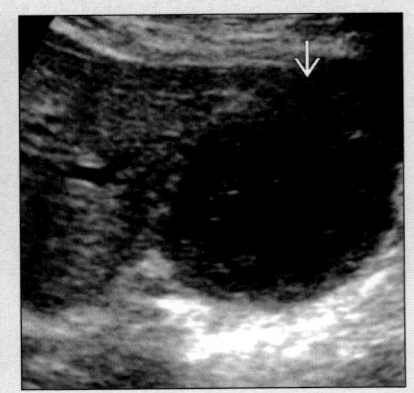

Biloma

PERITONEAL SPACE ABSCESS

Key Facts

Imaging Findings

- Best diagnostic clue: Fluid collection with mass effect ± gas bubbles or air-fluid level
- Complex fluid collection with internal low level echoes, membranes or septations
- Dependent echoes representing debris; seen as fluid-fluid level
- Bright linear echoes with reverberation artifacts representing gas bubbles; diagnostic of infection
- Inflamed fat adjacent to abscess: Echogenic mass
- Peritonitis (infective): Diffuse inflammation of parietal or visceral peritoneum
- Tuberculous peritonitis: Matted bowel loops with heterogeneous inter-bowel exudate
- Color Doppler: Hypervascular periphery, avascular center of abscess & hyperemic (inflamed) adjacent fat

- US-guided: Diagnostic or therapeutic aspiration & percutaneous abscess drainage (PAD)
- US: Very effective screening tool to localize intraperitoneal abscess or collections
- Bedside US: For critically ill or post-operative patients
- US: Evaluation of dependent portion of peritoneal cavity or area surrounding the operative site

Top Differential Diagnoses

- Loculated Ascites
- Lymphocele
- Biloma

Diagnostic Checklist

- Loculated collections with internal debris or septations with appropriate clinical features

---

- Later: Matted, clumped bowel loops tethered to posterior abdominal wall by uniformly echogenic enveloping membrane (1-4 mm thick)
- Post-operative peritoneal abscess
  - Well-defined & irregular wall collection containing clear fluid or complex echogenic collection with debris ± septations
  - Close to site of surgery, around the tip of drainage catheter (if blocked), dependent parts of peritoneal cavity (supine patients)
  - US exam may be suboptimal due to limited patient mobility, open wounds, dressings, drainage tubes, paralytic ileus
  - Probe tenderness: On deep compression with US transducer due to inflammation
- Color Doppler: Hypervascular periphery, avascular center of abscess & hyperemic (inflamed) adjacent fat

Radiographic Findings

- Radiography
  - Ectopic gas (50% of cases)
  - Air-fluid level
  - Soft tissue "mass"
  - Focal ileus
  - Loss of soft tissue-fat interface
  - Subphrenic abscess: Pleural effusion and lower lobe atelectasis

CT Findings

- NECT: Low attenuation fluid collection, mass effect, gas in 50% of cases
- CECT: Peripheral rim-enhancement

Non-Vascular Interventions

- US-guided: Diagnostic or therapeutic aspiration & percutaneous abscess drainage (PAD)

MR Findings

- T1WI: Low signal
- T2WI: Intermediate to high signal fluid collection
- T1 C+: Low signal fluid collection with enhancing rim

Fluoroscopic Findings

- Abscess sinogram

- Useful after percutaneous drainage
- Defines catheter position in dependent portion of abscess
- Detection of fistulas to bowel, pancreas or biliary duct

Nuclear Medicine Findings

- Gallium scan
  - Useful for fever of unknown origin
  - Nonspecific: Positive with tumor such as lymphoma and granulomatous lesions
- WBC scan
  - 73-83% sensitivity
  - False positives with bowel infarct or hematoma
- Newer agents
  - Indium-labeled polyclonal IgG
  - Tc-99m-labeled monoclonal antibody

Imaging Recommendations

- Best imaging tool
  - US: Very effective screening tool to localize intraperitoneal abscess or collections
    - Bedside US: For critically ill or post-operative patients
  - CECT
- Protocol advice
  - CECT: Oral & IV contrast, 150 mL IV contrast at 2.5 mL/sec
  - US: Evaluation of dependent portion of peritoneal cavity or area surrounding the operative site

DIFFERENTIAL DIAGNOSIS

Loculated Ascites

- Evidence for cirrhosis or chronic liver disease
- Minimal or no mass effect
- Often passively conforms to peritoneal space
- May contain septation on US

Lymphocele

- History of lymph node dissection & found adjacent to transplant kidneys

PERITONEAL SPACE ABSCESS

- Fluid collections along lymphatic drainage, may occur lateral to bladder
- Often anechoic & resemble simple cysts

Biloma
- History of biliary or hepatic surgery
- Perihepatic fluid collection commonly in gallbladder fossa or Morrison pouch
- Hypoechoic, rounded collections or complex cystic collections

PATHOLOGY

General Features
- General path comments: Pus collection; peripheral fibrocapillary "capsule"; often polymicrobial from enteric organisms
- Genetics
  - Increased risk if genetically altered immune response
  - Diabetics have increased incidence of gas-forming abscesses
- Etiology
  - Enteric perforation
    - Appendicitis, diverticulitis, Crohn disease
  - Post-operative
    - Typically intraperitoneal spaces such as cul-de-sac, Morrison pouch and subphrenic spaces
  - Bacteremia
  - Trauma
  - CAPD with secondary infection
- Epidemiology
  - Most commonly due to post-operative complication
  - Microabscesses due to fungal infections in immunocompromised patients
  - Higher incidence in diabetics, immunocompromised patients and post-operative patients

Gross Pathologic & Surgical Features
- Often adherent omentum or bowel loops; pus collection
- May or may not have "capsule"

Microscopic Features
- PMN and white cell debris
- Bacteria, fungi detected

Staging, Grading or Classification Criteria
- Organism: Bacterial, fungal, amebic
- Related to organ of origin (i.e., liver abscess)
- Intraperitoneal or extraperitoneal
- Communicating
  - Underlying fistula to GI tract
  - Connection to biliary tract or pancreatic duct

CLINICAL ISSUES

Presentation
- Most common signs/symptoms: Fever, chills, abdomen pain, tachycardia, decreased blood pressure if septic
- Clinical Profile: Leukocytosis, + blood cultures and elevated ESR

Natural History & Prognosis
- Variable depending on extent of abscess, patient's immune system status; often good prognosis

Treatment
- Options, risks, complications
  - Percutaneous abscess drainage (PAD)
    - 80% success rate of percutaneous drainage
    - Patient selection critical for success
    - Best candidates for PAD have well-localized, fluid-filled abscesses > 3 cm with safe catheter access route
  - Contraindications for PAD related to patient
    - Coagulopathy with prothrombin time > 3 sec
    - International normalized ratio > 1.5
    - Platelets < 50,000 μL
  - Contraindications for PAD related to abscess
    - Infected necrosis (i.e., pancreatic abscess)
    - Gas-forming infection such as emphysematous pancreatitis
    - Soft tissue infection (i.e., phlegmon)
    - No safe access route for catheter insertion
  - Surgery indications
    - Extensive intraperitoneal abscesses
    - Debridement of necrotic infected tissue
    - Failed PAD
  - Antibiotic therapy; abscesses < 3 cm

DIAGNOSTIC CHECKLIST

Consider
- Diagnostic mimics: Biloma, lymphocele, loculated ascites or pseudocyst

Image Interpretation Pearls
- Loculated collections with internal debris or septations with appropriate clinical features

SELECTED REFERENCES

1. Benoist S et al: Can failure of percutaneous drainage of postoperative abdominal abscesses be predicted? Am J Surg. 184(2):148-53, 2002
2. Betsch A et al: CT-guided percutaneous drainage of intra-abdominal abscesses: APACHE III score stratification of 1-year results. Acute Physiology, Age, Chronic Health Evaluation. Eur Radiol. 12(12):2883-9, 2002
3. Cinat ME et al: Determinants for successful percutaneous image-guided drainage of intra-abdominal abscess. Arch Surg. 137(7):845-9, 2002
4. Harisinghani MG et al: CT-guided transgluteal drainage of deep pelvic abscesses: indications, technique, procedure-related complications, and clinical outcome. Radiographics. 22(6):1353-67, 2002
5. Lohela P: Ultrasound-guided drainages and sclerotherapy. Eur Radiol. 12(2):288-95, 2002
6. Men S et al: Percutaneous drainage of abdominal abscess. Eur J Radiol. 43(3):204-18, 2002
7. Ralls PW: Inflammatory disease of the liver. Clin Liver Dis. 6(1):203-25, 2002
8. Deck AJ et al: Perinephric abscesses in the neurologically impaired. Spinal Cord. 39(9):477-81, 2001

PERITONEAL SPACE ABSCESS

IMAGE GALLERY

Typical

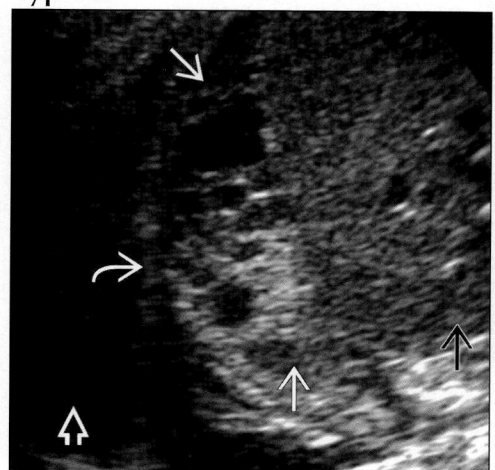

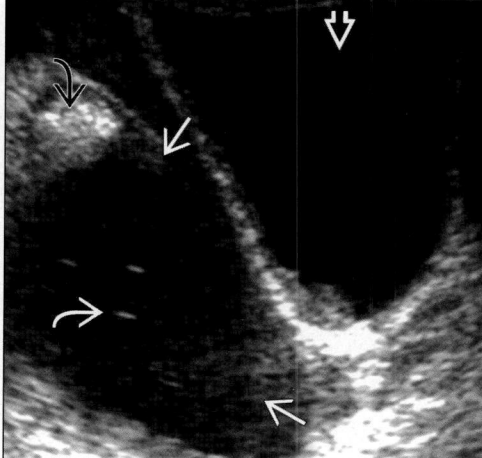

(Left) Longitudinal transabdominal ultrasound shows a right subphrenic abscess ➡ with an associated reactive right pleural effusion ➡. Note adjacent liver ➡ & diaphragm ➡. *(Right)* Longitudinal transabdominal ultrasound shows a post-operative infected collection ➡ in the pelvis, posterior to the bladder ➡. Note air ➡ in the non-dependent portion & fine internal echoes within the collection ➡.

Typical

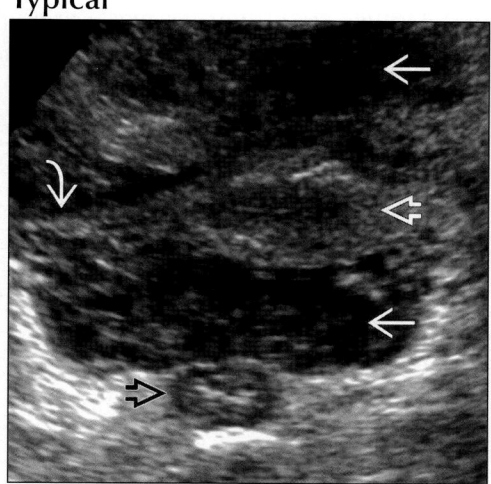

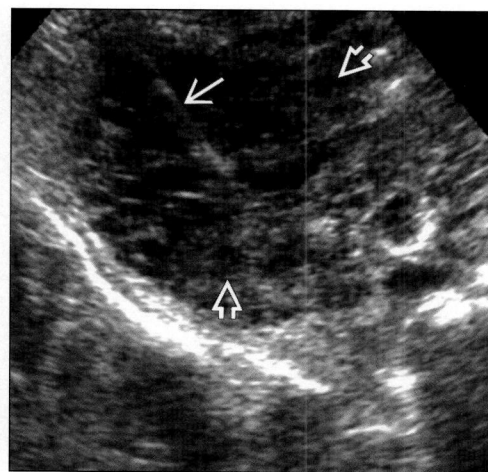

(Left) Transverse transabdominal ultrasound shows a pelvic abscess ➡ in a case of ileal perforation. Note echogenic fluid around the uterus ➡, broad ligament ➡ & rectum ➡. *(Right)* Transverse transabdominal ultrasound shows an US-guided aspiration of an appendicular abscess ➡. Note the linear echogenic aspiration needle ➡.

Typical

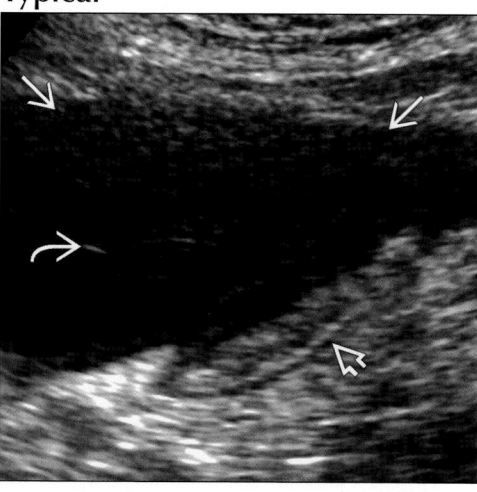

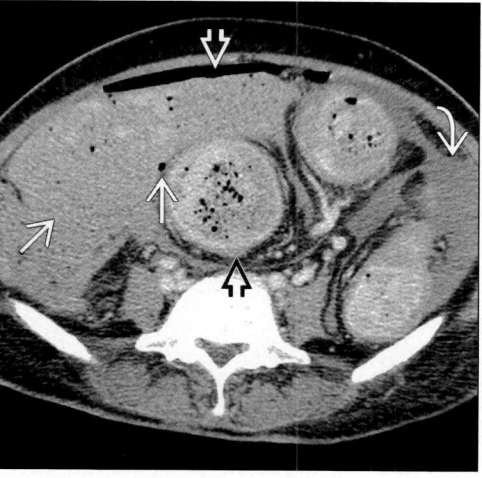

(Left) Oblique transabdominal ultrasound shows an anechoic diverticular abscess ➡, with a few scattered internal echoes ➡ along the sigmoid colon ➡. *(Right)* Transverse CECT shows peritonitis and a pneumoperitoneum ➡, secondary to a bowel perforation ➡. There is a hyperdense fluid collection in the right paracolic region with air loculi ➡. Compare to the hypodense simple ascites in the left paracolic region ➡.

APPENDICITIS

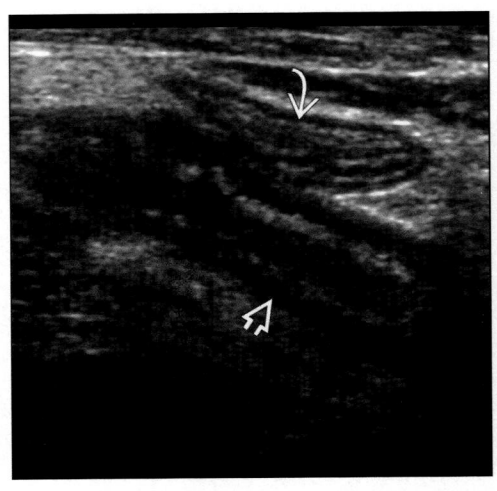 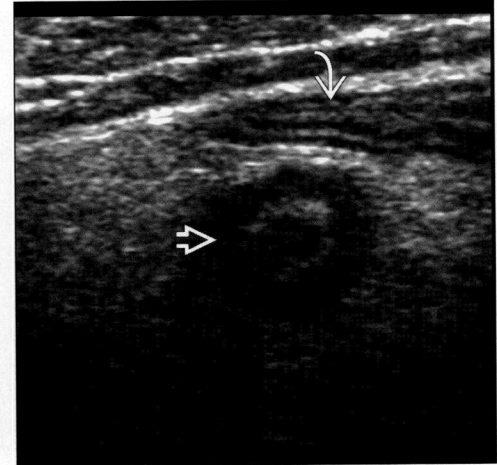

Oblique transabdominal ultrasound shows a blind-ending tubular, dilated and noncompressible acutely inflamed appendix ➤. Adjacent small bowel is compressible ➤.

Transverse transabdominal ultrasound shows cross section of a dilated, non-compressible inflamed appendix ➤, adjacent to a compressible segment of normal small bowel ➤.

TERMINOLOGY

Definitions
- Acute appendiceal inflammation due to luminal obstruction and superimposed infection

IMAGING FINDINGS

General Features
- Best diagnostic clue
  - Distended non-compressible appendix (≥ 7 mm) on ultrasound (US) or CT
  - Periappendiceal fluid collection or edema & abnormal mural vascularity on power Doppler
  - Fat stranding & mural enhancement of appendix on CECT
- Location: Cecal tip
- Size
  - Noncompressible appendix > 6 mm has sensitivity of 100%, but specificity of only 64%
  - Noncompressible appendix > 7 mm has sensitivity of 94% and specificity of 88%
  - Noncompressible appendix 6-7 mm equivocal size; increased flow on color Doppler in appendix suggests appendicitis
- Morphology: Tip of appendix is often first site of inflammation and appendiceal perforation

Ultrasonographic Findings
- Grayscale Ultrasound
  - Non-compressible appendix ≥ 7 mm in diameter, laminated wall with target appearance, mural wall thickness ≥ 2 mm
  - Blind ended, aperistaltic tubular structure, gut signature, close to cecum
  - Sonographic "McBurney sign" with focal pain/tenderness over inflamed appendix: "Graded compression sonography"
  - Gangrenous appendicitis: "Loss of differentiation" of wall layers
  - Increased periappendiceal echogenicity (mesoappendix & pericecal fat infiltration), phlegmonous appendicitis (hypoechoic areas with ill-defined margins within inflamed fat)

DDx: Pathologies Mimicking Appendicitis

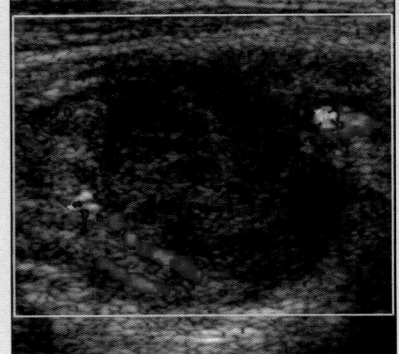 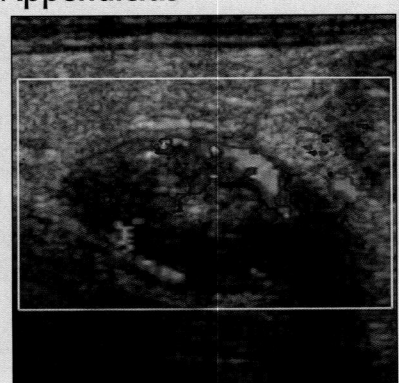 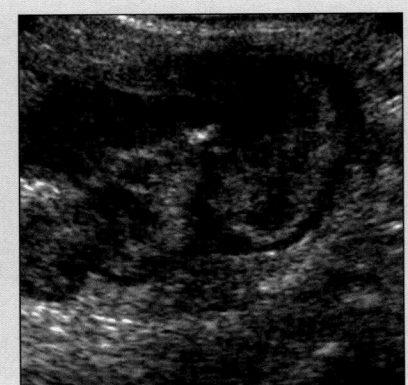

Lymphadenitis   *Ileo-Cecal Tuberculosis*   *Crohn Disease*

INTUSSUSCEPTION

Key Facts

Terminology
- Invagination or telescoping of a proximal segment of bowel (intussusceptum) into lumen of a distal segment (intussuscipiens)

Imaging Findings
- Intussusception can be diagnosed using US with high sensitivity (98-100%) & specificity (88%)
- Transverse US: "Target " sign; peripheral hypoechoic halo: Edematous wall of intussuscipiens
- Intermediate hyperechoic area: Space between intussuscipiens & intussusceptum
- Internal hypoechoic ring: Due to intussusceptum
- Inner ring may also show lymph nodes or lead point/mass that is drawn into intussusception
- Longitudinal US: "Pseudokidney" sign; multiple, thin, parallel, hypoechoic & echogenic stripes

- Free fluid: Small quantity (commonly seen with intussusception)
- Perforation: Large ascites ± internal echoes/debris ± free peritoneal air
- Absent mural vascularity of intussusceptum suggestive of ischemia/infarction, thus high risk of perforation
- Presence of vascularity in intussusceptum is good predictor of reducibility
- US for localization of the intussusception, followed by barium/water/air enema for reduction

Top Differential Diagnoses
- Primary Bowel Tumor
- Appendicular Lump
- Intestinal Helminthiasis

- Internal hypoechoic ring: Due to intussusceptum
- Inner ring may also show lymph nodes or lead point/mass that is drawn into intussusception
  - Longitudinal US: "Pseudokidney" sign; multiple, thin, parallel, hypoechoic & echogenic stripes
  - Trapped fluid seen as anechoic component between compressed bowel segments of intussusception
  - Free fluid: Small quantity (commonly seen with intussusception)
  - Perforation: Large ascites ± internal echoes/debris ± free peritoneal air
  - US: Detects ileo-ileal component of intussusception that may persist, even after successful reduction of ileo-colic intussusception
  - "Transient small bowel intussusception"; very common in hyperperistalsis
    - Not associated with significant bowel edema; peripheral rim is thinner & more echogenic on US
    - Occasionally spontaneous resolution can be observed at US with a little patience
  - Repeat US exam: To check for spontaneous reduction & for follow up of recurrent intussusceptions (4-10%)
  - US features suggesting decreased success of non-surgical reduction (NSR)
    - Peripheral rim thickness greater than 1 cm, lymph nodes size > 1 cm within intussusception & large amounts of internal trapped fluid
  - US guided hydrostatic NSR: Avoids ionizing radiation
- Color Doppler
  - Shows mesenteric vessels dragged between entering and returning wall of intussusceptum
  - Absent mural vascularity of intussusceptum suggestive of ischemia/infarction, thus high risk of perforation
  - Presence of vascularity in intussusceptum is good predictor of reducibility

Radiographic Findings
- Radiography
  - Soft tissue mass
  - Findings of bowel obstruction may be seen (50-60%)

- Nipple-like termination of gas shadow, absence of gas in distal collapsed bowel
- Air-fluid levels; proximal bowel dilatation

CT Findings
- Seen as three different patterns on axial CT scans
  - "Target" sign: Earliest stage of intussusception
    - Outer layer (intussuscipiens) & inner layer (intussusceptum)
  - Sausage-shaped mass: Layering pattern (later)
    - Alternating layers of low-attenuation (mesenteric fat) & high-attenuation areas (bowel wall) with enhancing mesenteric vessels
  - Reniform mass: Due to edema or mural thickening leading to vascular compromise
    - Thick bowel wall with hypodense areas within & crescent-shaped fluid or gas collections
- Intestinal obstruction: Air-fluid levels, proximal bowel distension

Fluoroscopic Findings
- Fluoroscopic guided barium study
  - Antegrade barium study: "Coil spring" appearance
  - Retrograde barium study: Convex intracolic mass with "claw" sign
    - Due to trapping of contrast between folds of intussusceptum & intussuscipiens
  - Beak-like narrowing of barium column demonstrating central channel
  - Not helpful for diagnosis or treatment of intussusceptions restricted to small bowel
- Fluoroscopic guided hydrostatic/contrast (Gastrografin or barium)/pneumatic NSR
  - < 1% mortality if reduction occurs < 24 hr after onset, overall success rate of 18-90%
  - Contraindications; pneumoperitoneum, peritonitis, hypovolemic shock
  - "Rule of three": (1) Enema container 3 feet above table (2) no more than 3 attempts (3) 3 minutes per attempt (4) 3 minutes between attempts

Imaging Recommendations
- Best imaging tool

○ US for localization of the intussusception, followed by barium/water/air enema for reduction
  ▪ CT: For evaluation of lead point/mass

DIFFERENTIAL DIAGNOSIS

Primary Bowel Tumor
• Lymphoma, carcinoid tumor, adenocarcinoma, stromal tumor, lipoma & adenoma

Appendicular Lump
• Right iliac fossa mass
• Visualization of inflamed appendix ± appendicolith
• Inflamed & thickened cecum ± hyperechoic inflamed periappendiceal fat ± fluid

Intestinal Helminthiasis
• Long tubular worms within bowel lumen
• Intestinal obstruction (38-88%): Due to clumped (coiled, tubular) mass of worms; may mimic intussusception in children

Metastases
• Common in small bowel
• From malignant melanoma, lung & breast cancer
• Location: Antimesenteric border

PATHOLOGY

General Features
• Etiology
  ○ Children
    ▪ Idiopathic (95%): Abnormal motility, early weaning, prematurity, hyperperistalsis, hypertrophied payers patches, gastrojejunal feeding tubes
    ▪ Lead point (5%): Meckel diverticulum, polyp, enteric duplication cyst, appendicitis, Henoch-Schönlein purpura, inspissated meconium
  ○ Adults: Long segment (obstructing) & short segment (non obstructing) intussusception
  ○ Long-segment, obstructing intussusception; leading mass, benign tumor (1/3) or malignant tumor (1/5)
    ▪ Benign (more common-small bowel): Polyp, leiomyoma, lipoma, adenoma of appendix, appendiceal stump granuloma
    ▪ Malignant: Primary (more common-colon) polypoid adenocarcinoma, metastases & lymphoma (more common-small bowel)
  ○ Short-segment, non-obstructing intussusception: Without a lead mass, usually self-limited, due to other predisposing conditions
    ▪ Post-operative: Suture lines, ostomy closure sites, adhesions, submucosal edema, abnormal bowel motility, electrolyte imbalance, fasting, chronic dilated loop, long intestinal tubes
    ▪ Miscellaneous: Meckel diverticulum, scleroderma, celiac & Whipple disease, colitis, chronic ulcers, epiploic appendagitis
    ▪ Idiopathic, anxiety & agonal state

Gross Pathologic & Surgical Features
• Three layers are seen
  ○ Intussusceptum: Entering/inner tube + returning/middle tube (intestine)
  ○ Intussuscipiens: Sheath or outer tube (intestine)

CLINICAL ISSUES

Presentation
• Most common signs/symptoms
  ○ Adults: Intermittent pain, vomiting, red blood in stool
  ○ Children: Acute pain, palpable mass, "red currant jelly" stools

Natural History & Prognosis
• Complications: Obstruction, bowel ischemia (infarction & necrosis), perforation & peritonitis
• Prognosis
  ○ Early: Good, (post reduction or surgical resection) recurrence rare
  ○ Late: Poor if severe vascular compromise (gangrene & perforation)

Treatment
• Children: Hydrostatic or pneumatic reduction
  ○ Non reducible; surgical reduction or resection
• Adults: None for transient, non-obstructing
  ○ Non-reducible with lead mass; resection

DIAGNOSTIC CHECKLIST

Consider
• Intussusception: When classical "target" or "doughnut" sign seen (on US/CT) with appropriate clinical features
• Identify bowel segments (forming intussusceptum & intussuscipiens), leading point/mass
• Check for bowel vascularity & complications

SELECTED REFERENCES

1. El Fortia M et al: Tetra-layered sign of adult intussusception (new ultrasound approach). Ultrasound Med Biol. 2006
2. Krishnakumar et al: Ultrasound guided hydrostatic reduction in the management of intussusception. Indian J Pediatr. 73(3):217-20, 2006
3. Applegate KE. Related Articles et al: Clinically suspected intussusception in children: evidence-based review and self-assessment module. AJR Am J Roentgenol. 2005
4. Grunshaw ND. Related Articles et al: The imaging of intussusception. Clin Radiol. 2005
5. Huang BY et al: Adult intussusception: diagnosis and clinical relevance. Radiol Clin North Am. 41(6):1137-51, 2003
6. Lvoff N et al: Distinguishing features of self-limiting adult small-bowel intussusception identified at CT. Radiology. 227(1):68-72, 2003

INTUSSUSCEPTION

IMAGE GALLERY

Typical

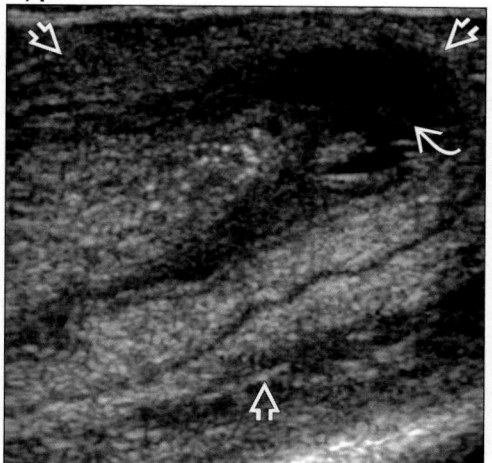

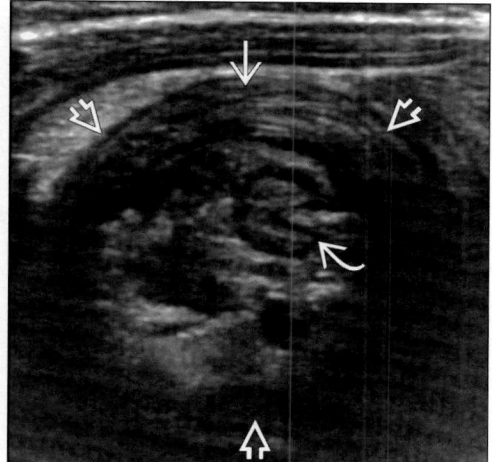

(Left) Longitudinal transabdominal ultrasound shows multilayered appearance of intussusception ⇉ giving rise to "pseudokidney" sign. Note minimal fluid trapped between layers ➡. *(Right)* Transverse transabdominal ultrasound shows classical "target" or "doughnut" sign of intestinal intussusception ⇉. Note ring in ring appearance formed by different layers ➡ of intestine & central lymph node ➡ acting as lead point.

Typical

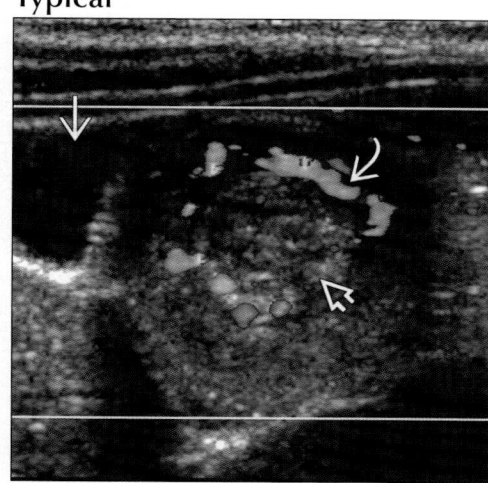

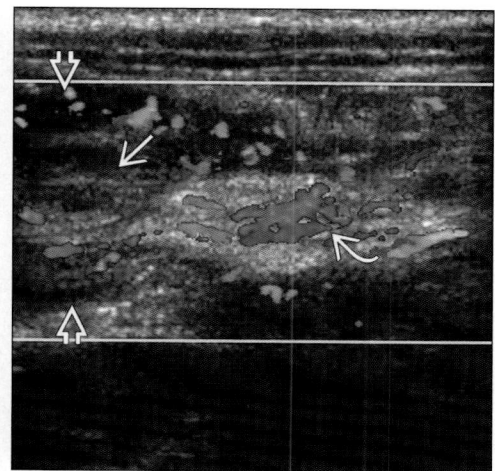

(Left) Transverse color Doppler ultrasound shows mural vascularity ➡ in central intussusceptum ⇉. Note minimal fluid around the intussusception ➡. *(Right)* Longitudinal color Doppler ultrasound of intussusception shows central leash of mesenteric vessels ➡ that are pulled along with intussusceptum ⇉ into outer intussuscipiens ⇉. Presence of vascularity predicts reducibility.

Typical

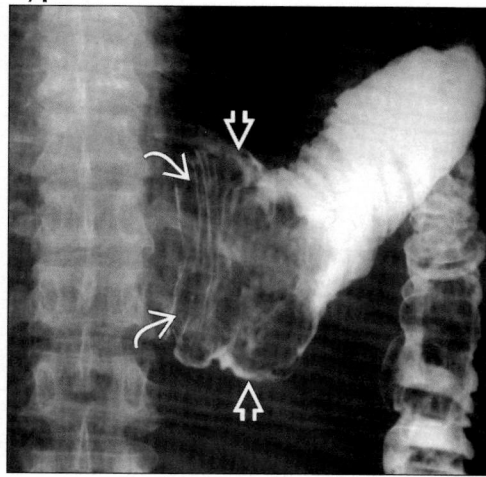

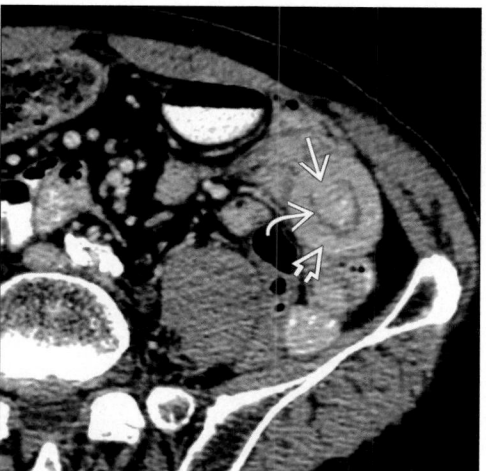

(Left) Barium enema shows colo-colic intussusception involving transverse colon. Note proximal intussusceptum ➡ invaginating into distal intussuscipiens ⇉, with classical "claw sign". *(Right)* Transverse CECT shows ileo-ileal intussusception ⇉ with "target" sign. Note proximal segment ➡ of ileum telescoping into distal segment separated by hypodense rim ➡.

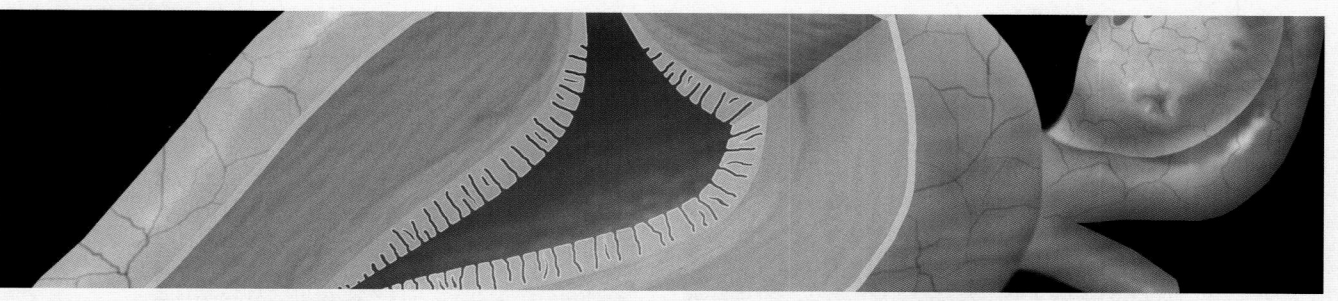

SECTION 9: Female Pelvis

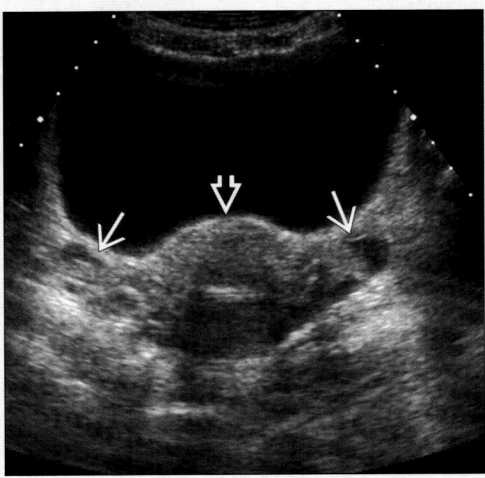

Transabdominal ultrasound shows the uterus ➡ and both ovaries ➡. This gives the "big picture" and provides better evaluation of large masses, which may be incompletely evaluated by transvaginal scanning.

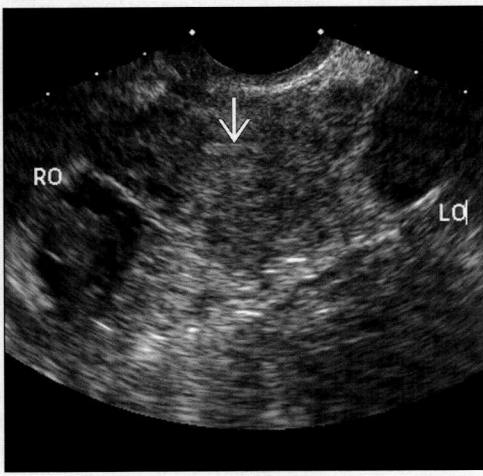

Transvaginal ultrasound gives a more detailed evaluation of both the ovaries and the uterus, and should be performed unless there is a contraindication. (RO - right ovary, LO - left ovary, ➡ - endometrium).

IMAGING ANATOMY

General Anatomic Considerations
- Contents of female pelvis
  - Reproductive organs: Uterus, cervix, fallopian tubes, ovaries, vagina
  - Other organs: Distal ureters, bladder, urethra, rectum
- Reproductive organs are supported by group of visceral ligaments
  - Broad ligament created by two sheets of peritoneum
    - Peritoneum passes over bladder dome to anterior uterus creating **anterior cul-de-sac** (vesico-uterine pouch)
    - Posteriorly, peritoneum extends more inferiorly to to upper portion of vagina creating **posterior cul-de-sac** (pouch of Douglas, recto-uterine pouch)
    - Posterior cul-de-sac most dependent portion in female pelvis
  - Other ligaments include: Round ligaments, cardinal ligaments, uterosacral ligaments, vesicouterine ligaments, suspensory ligaments of ovary, mesosalpinx, and proper ovarian ligaments
- **Ovaries and uterus have dual blood supply**
  - Ovarian arteries arise from aorta below renal arteries
    - Descend to pelvis and enter suspensory ligaments of ovary
    - Continue medially to anastomose with respective uterine arteries
  - Uterine artery arises from internal iliac artery
    - Passes over ureter at level of cervix ("water under the bridge")
    - Courses superiorly over lateral margin of uterus to anastomose with ovarian artery
    - Uterine arteries give rise to **arcuate arteries**, which run in outer third of myometrium
    - Arcuate arteries then give rise to **radial arteries**, which extend through myometrium terminating as **spiral arteries** in endometrium
  - Venous drainage via complex, collateral network in parametrium

- Eventually drain to either ovarian or uterine veins

Menstrual Cycle
- ~ 400,000 follicles present at birth but only 0.1% (400) mature to ovulation
- Terminology based on changes seen in ovary (follicular, luteal phases) or uterus (proliferative, secretory phases)
- **Days 0-14**
  - **Ovary: Follicular phase**
    - Follicle stimulating hormone (FSH) induces several follicles (range 1-11, mean 5) to develop
    - By days 8-12 a dominant follicle develops, while remainder start to regress
  - **Uterus:** Menstruation followed by **proliferative phase**
    - Estrogen induces proliferation of functionalis layer of endometrium
- **Day 14: Ovulation**
  - Egg extruded from ovary
  - Dominant follicle typically 2.0-2.5 cm at ovulation
- **Days 14-28**
  - **Ovary: Luteal phase**
    - Luteinizing hormone (LH) induces formation of a corpus luteum
    - If fertilization does not occur, corpus luteum degenerates to corpus albicans
  - **Uterus: Secretory phase**
    - Progesterone induces endometrium to secrete glycogen, mucus and other substances
    - Endometrial glands become enlarged and tortuous

Uterine/Cervical Ultrasound
- Appearance, size, shape and weight vary with estrogen stimulation and parturition
  - **Premenarche**
    - Cervix is larger than corpus (~ 2/3 of uterine mass)
  - **Menarche**
    - Preferential growth of corpus in response to hormonal stimulation
    - Nulliparous women, corpus and cervix roughly same length

PELVIC ANATOMY & IMAGING ISSUES

Key Facts

Anatomy and Physiology

- Ovaries and uterus have dual blood supply
- Cervix is larger than corpus (~ 2/3 of uterine mass) before menarche, proportions reversed after menarche
- Posterior cul-de-sac most dependent portion of female pelvis
  - Important area to evaluate for fluid and masses (drop metastases, endometriosis, etc.)
- Terminology of menstrual cycle based on changes seen in ovary (follicular, luteal phases) or uterus (proliferative, secretory phases)
- Endometrial appearance varies with phase of menstrual cycle
  - Proliferative phase: Progressive, hypoechoic thickening (4-8 mm)
  - Layered ("sandwich") appearance near ovulation
  - Secretory phase: Becomes thicker (7-14 mm) and more echogenic
- Ovarian cysts up to 3 cm reported in 15% of postmenopausal women and should not be confused with malignancy

Clinical Presentation is Critically Important

- Many pelvic pathologies have similar sonographic appearances
- Narrowing the differential diagnosis requires knowledge of the clinical circumstances
  - Where is the mass?
  - What is the patient's age/hormonal status?
  - What are the symptoms?

- Parous, non-pregnant women corpus is ~ 2/3 of uterine mass
  - **Postmenopausal**
    - Corpus decreases back to premenopausal size
- **Uterine position**
  - **Flexion** is axis of uterine body relative to cervix
  - **Version** is axis of cervix relative to vagina
  - Most uteri are anteverted and anteflexed
- **Myometrium:** 3 layers usually discernible
  - Compacted, thin, hypoechoic inner layer forms **subendometrial halo**
  - Thicker, homogeneous, moderately echogenic middle layer
  - Thinner, hypoechoic outer layer
    - Portion of myometrium peripheral to arcuate vessels
- **Endometrial appearance varies** with phase of menstrual cycle
  - Thin, echogenic line early in menstrual phase
  - Progressive, hypoechoic thickening (4-8 mm) as proliferative phase progresses
  - Layered ("sandwich") appearance near ovulation
    - Thin, outer echogenic stratum basalis (deep layer of endometrium densely adherent to myometrium)
    - Hypoechoic stratum functionalis (superficial layer that grows under hormonal stimulation and sloughs with menstruation)
    - Echogenic central line created where the 2 hypoechoic endometrial walls coapt
  - After ovulation (secretory phase), endometrium becomes thicker (7-14 mm) and more echogenic

Ovarian Ultrasound

- Scan between uterus and pelvic sidewall, following broad ligament
  - Often seen by internal iliac vessels
- Medulla mildly hyperechoic in comparison to hypoechoic cortex
- Developing follicles anechoic
  - Cysts up to 3 cm reported in 15% of postmenopausal women and should not be confused with malignancy

- Corpus luteum may have thick, echogenic wall
  - Hemorrhage common
    - Variable appearances: Lace-like septations, fluid-fluid level, retracting clot
    - Marked flow within wall of corpus luteum cyst
- Normal ovarian pulsed Doppler shows a low-velocity, low-resistance arterial waveform
- **Echogenic foci** common
  - 1-3 mm, non-shadowing, more common in periphery
  - Represent specular reflectors from walls of tiny unresolved cysts
- Volume (.523 x length x width x height) more accurate than individual measurement
  - Premenopausal: Mean ~ 10 +/- 6 cc, max 22 cc
  - Postmenopausal: Mean ~ 4 +/- 2 cc, max 8 cc

ANATOMY-BASED IMAGING ISSUES

Imaging Protocols

- Always use highest frequency transducer possible that gives adequate penetration
- Transabdominal sonogram
  - Gives "big picture"
    - Large masses (fibroids, dermoids, fluid collections, etc.) may be better evaluated transabdominally
  - Should be performed through full urinary bladder
    - Creates acoustic window and pushes bowel out of pelvis
- Transvaginal sonogram
  - Much more detailed evaluation of uterus and ovaries
  - Unless there is a contraindication, should be used in most cases
- Sonohysterography
  - Study of choice for evaluating endometrial pathology
  - Balloon catheter inserted into cervix
  - Sterile saline infused while scanning
    - Separates endometrial walls, allowing for complete evaluation of endometrium
- 3D ultrasound

PELVIC ANATOMY & IMAGING ISSUES

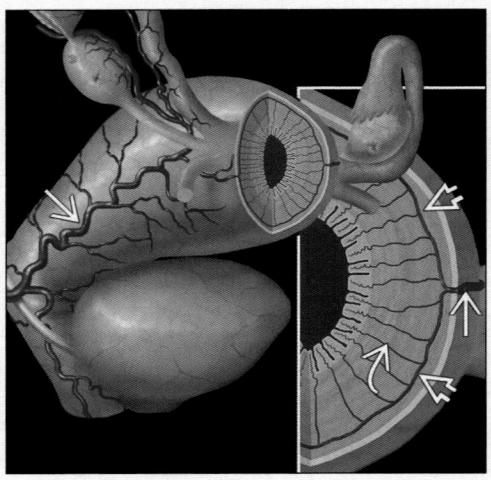

Graphic shows the uterine artery ➡ ascending along the lateral uterine wall. It gives rise to the the arcuate arteries ➡, which course circumferentially in the outer third of the myometrium. (➡ - radial artery).

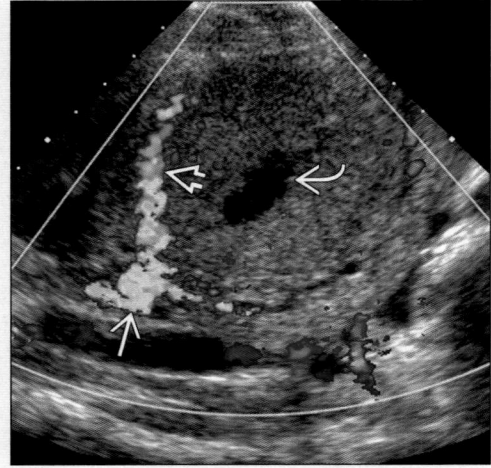

Color Doppler ultrasound of a patient who has just undergone a dilatation and curettage shows prominent uterine ➡ and arcuate ➡ arteries. (➡ - fluid in endometrial cavity).

- o Allows multiple views to be reconstructed from single sweep through uterus
- o Decrease in scan time and potential for increased patient throughput
- **American Institute of Ultrasound in Medicine (AIUM) practice guidelines for female pelvis**
  - o Requires documentation of uterus, adnexa and cul-de-sac
    - ▪ All masses should be measured in at least 2 dimensions and location recorded
  - o Uterus
    - ▪ Size, shape and orientation (longitudinal and axial views)
    - ▪ Endometrial thickness (double layer thickness, exclude fluid in endometrial cavity from measurements)
    - ▪ Myometrium
    - ▪ Cervix
  - o Adnexa
    - ▪ Ovaries should be measured in 3 dimensions using 2 orthogonal planes

PATHOLOGY-BASED IMAGING ISSUES

Key Concepts or Questions
- Many pelvic pathologies have similar sonographic appearances
  - o Narrowing differential diagnosis requires knowledge of clinical circumstances
- Where is the mass?
  - o Uterine mass: Myometrial vs. endometrial
  - o Adnexal mass: Intraovarian vs. extraovarian
- What is the patient's age/hormonal status?
  - o Differential diagnosis can be refined and appropriately ordered knowing if patient is premenarchal, premenopausal or postmenopausal
  - o Findings may be normal in one age group or phase of menstrual cycle, but not in another
- What are the symptoms?

- o Acute pain, chronic pain, incidental finding, hormonal abnormality

EMBRYOLOGY

Embryologic Events
- Uterus if formed from paired paramesonephric (Müllerian) ducts
- These paired ducts meet in midline and fuse
  - o Fusion forms uterovaginal canal (uterus and upper vagina)
  - o Unfused portions remain as fallopian tubes
- Lower vagina formed from urogenital sinus
- Ovaries develop separately by incorporation of germ cells into genital ridges

Practical Implications
- Failure of Müllerian duct development/fusion leads to spectrum of congenital uterine anomalies

RELATED REFERENCES

1. AIUM practice guideline for the performance of the ultrasound examination of the female pelvis. AIUM Clinical Guidelines. 1-4, 2006
2. Benacerraf BR et al: Improving the efficiency of gynecologic sonography with 3-dimensional volumes: a pilot study. J Ultrasound Med. 25(2):165-71, 2006
3. American Institute of Ultrasound in Medicine; American College of Obstetricians and Gynecologists; American College of Radiology: AIUM standard for the performance of saline infusion sonohysterography. J Ultrasound Med. 22(1):121-6, 2003
4. Funt SA et al: Detection and characterization of adnexal masses. Radiol Clin North Am. 40(3):591-608, 2002
5. Laing FC et al: Gynecologic ultrasound. Radiol Clin North Am. 39(3):523-40, 2001
6. Nalaboff KM et al: Imaging the endometrium: disease and normal variants. Radiographics. 21(6):1409-24, 2001
7. Benacerraf BR et al: Is a full bladder still necessary for pelvic sonography? J Ultrasound Med. 19(4):237-41, 2000
8. Kinkel K et al: US characterization of ovarian masses: a meta-analysis. Radiology. 217(3):803-11, 2000

CERVICAL CARCINOMA

IMAGE GALLERY

Typical

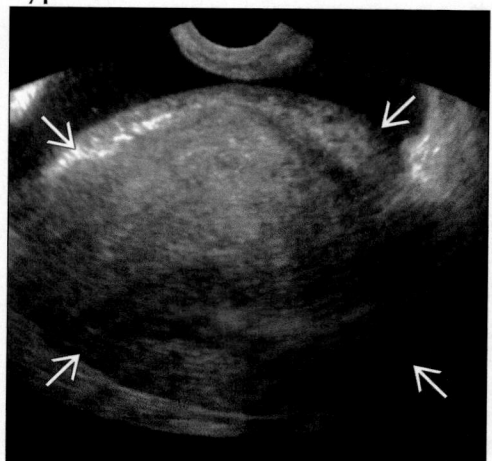 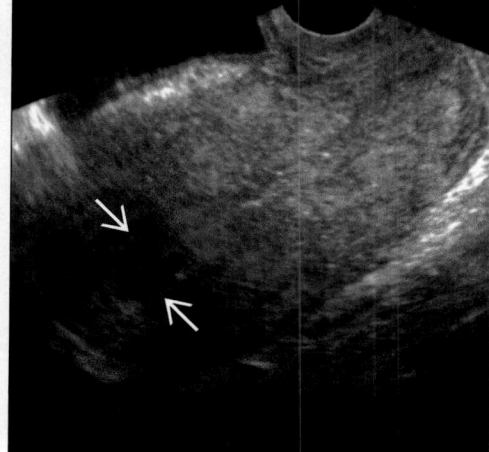

(Left) Transverse transvaginal ultrasound shows a large inhomogeneous mass ➡ replacing the cervix in a patient who presented with intermenstrual bleeding. *(Right)* Longitudinal transvaginal ultrasound in the same patient shows a small amount of fluid ➡ in the endometrial canal. Note that the eccentric, exophytic cervical mass is not apparent on this midline section.

Typical

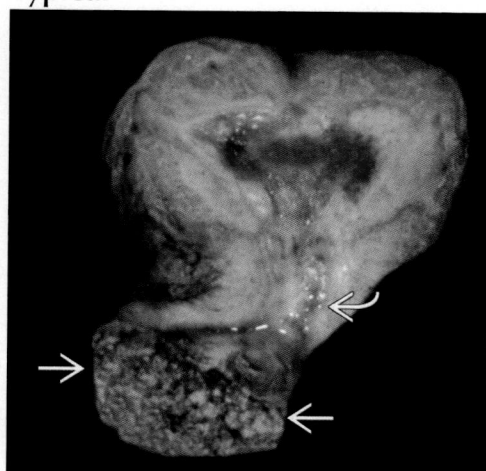 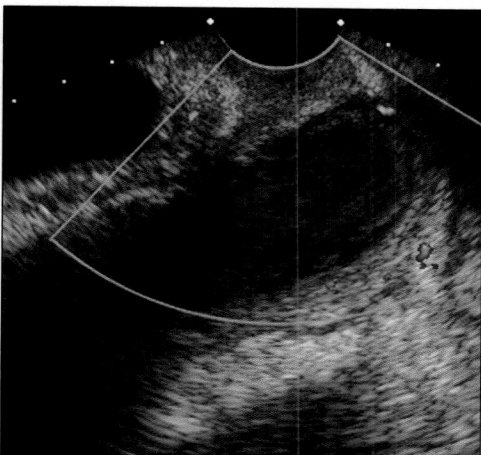

(Left) Gross pathology shows a primarily exophytic tumor ➡ extending from the cervix ➡. This growth pattern is commonly seen in younger patients. *(Right)* Longitudinal transvaginal ultrasound shows hematometra secondary to cervical stenosis. The patient had cervical cancer treated by radiation therapy. Cervical and vaginal stenosis are recognized side effects.

9

13

Typical

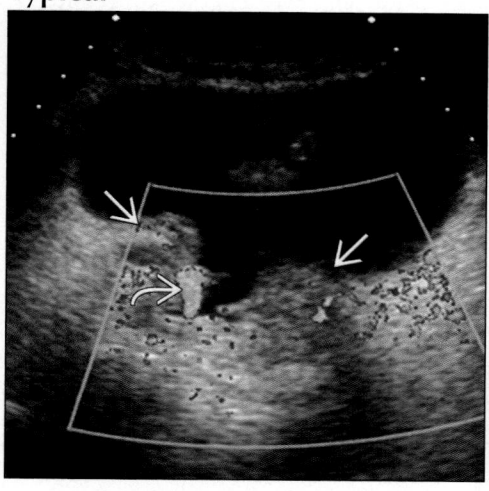 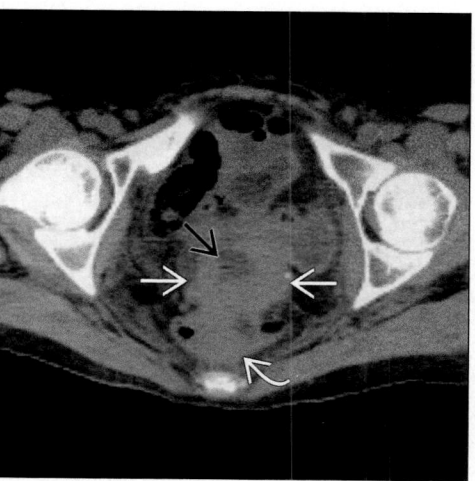

(Left) Transverse color Doppler ultrasound shows an irregular mass ➡ in the posterior bladder with abnormal vessels ➡. She complained of "being wet all the time" and had a vesicovaginal fistula due to an advanced CxCA. *(Right)* Axial NECT shows tumor involvement of the rectum ➡ and vagina ➡. Urine ➡ is present in the vagina despite the presence of urinary catheter.

UTERINE ADENOMYOSIS

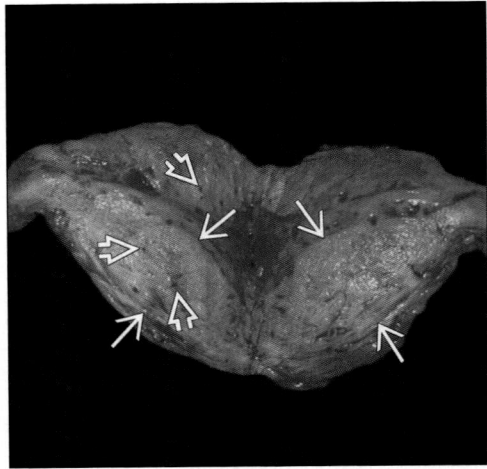

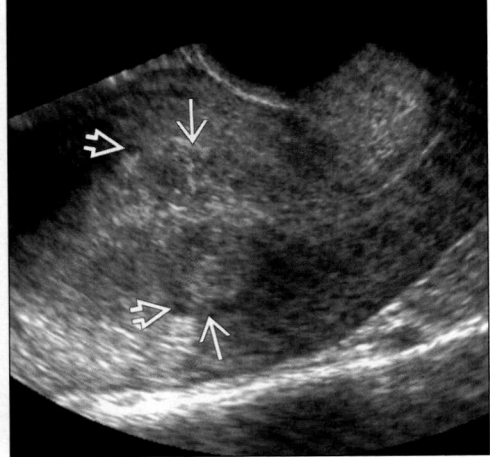

Gross pathology of a coronally sectioned uterus with adenomyosis. The myometrium is diffusely thickened ➡ and contains foci of hemorrhage ⮞ from ectopic endometrial glands.

Longitudinal transvaginal ultrasound shows a diffusely enlarged uterus. The endometrial/myometrial junction is indistinct and thickened ➡. Tiny myometrial cysts are also seen ⮞.

TERMINOLOGY

Abbreviations and Synonyms
- Diffuse adenomyosis
- Focal adenomyoma
- Uterine endometriosis

Definitions
- Endometrial gland migration into myometrium
- Associated smooth muscle hyperplasia

IMAGING FINDINGS

General Features
- Best diagnostic clue
  - Adenomyosis
    - Diffuse uterine enlargement
    - Loss of endometrial/myometrial interface
  - Adenomyoma
    - Focal heterogeneous mass
- Location
  - Adenomyosis can be asymmetric
    - Posterior wall more likely thickened
  - Adenomyoma can occur anywhere in myometrium
    - Often near endometrial/myometrial junction
- Size: Variable
- Morphology
  - Diffuse adenomyosis
    - Globular enlarged uterus
  - Adenomyoma
    - Elliptical more often than round

Ultrasonographic Findings
- Diffuse adenomyosis
  - Globular shaped uterus
    - Enlarged uterus without fibroids
  - Loss of endometrial/myometrial junction
    - Difficult to measure endometrium
    - Equivalent to thickened junctional zone by MR
  - Ill-defined echogenic areas in myometrium
    - Hyperechoic foci are endometrial glands
    - 2° focal smooth muscle hypertrophy
  - Myometrial cysts (50%), "Swiss cheese" appearance of myometrium
    - 1-5 mm
    - Often subendometrial

DDx: Thickened Endometrium

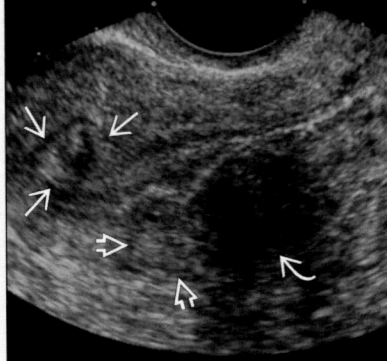

Myoma

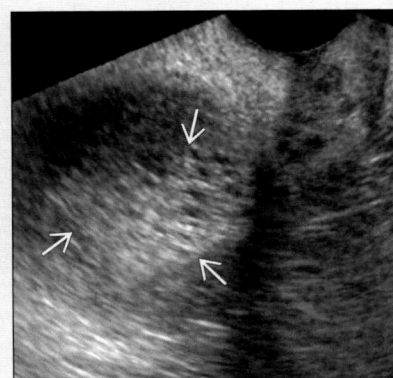

Hyperplasia

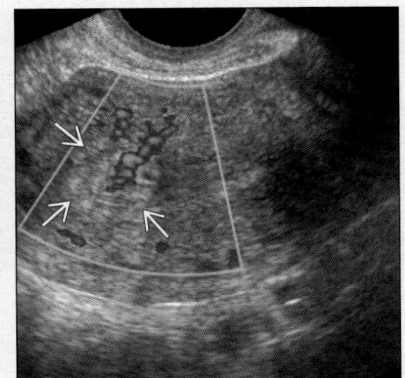

Polyp

UTERINE ADENOMYOSIS

Key Facts

Terminology
- Diffuse adenomyosis
- Focal adenomyoma
- Endometrial gland migration into myometrium

Imaging Findings
- Enlarged uterus without fibroids
- Loss of endometrial/myometrial junction
- Ill-defined echogenic areas in myometrium
- Myometrial cysts (50%), "Swiss cheese" appearance of myometrium
- Echogenic striations from endometrium
- Sawtooth shadowing from myometrium
- Anterior or posterior wall thickening
- Adenomyoma features overlap with myoma
- No mass effect on vessels

Top Differential Diagnoses
- Fibroids
- Endometrial Hyperplasia
- Endometrial Polyp

Clinical Issues
- Menorrhagia (50%)
- Dysmenorrhea (20%)
- Uterine artery embolization is possible emerging treatment

Diagnostic Checklist
- Look at endometrial myometrial junctional zone with ultrasound
- Look carefully for small myometrial cysts
- Recommend MR if findings are equivocal

- Appearance waxes and wanes with menstrual cycle
- Color Doppler differentiates from vessels
  - Echogenic striations from endometrium
    - Nodular or linear extension into myometrium
  - Hypoechoic striations from myometrium
    - Edge shadows
    - Sawtooth shadowing from myometrium
    - From whorls of smooth muscle hypertrophy
  - Asymmetric uterine enlargement possible
    - Anterior or posterior wall thickening
    - No contour abnormality
    - No mass effect
- Adenomyoma
  - Echogenic mass
    - Poorly defined
  - Can be located anywhere in uterus
    - Often near junctional zone
    - Rarely endometrial polypoid mass
  - Adenomyoma features overlap with myoma
    - MR helpful
- Color Doppler characteristics
  - No mass effect on vessels
    - Penetrating vessels
    - No circular vascularization as seen with fibroids
  - Helps differentiate cysts from uterine veins
    - Cysts more likely scattered or near endometrium
    - Uterine veins at periphery

MR Findings
- Thickening of junctional zone on T2WI
  - Low signal zone represents inner layer of myometrium
  - > 12 mm is diagnostic
  - 8-12 mm is suggestive
  - < 8 mm is normal
  - Junctional zone to myometrial thickness > 40%
- Focal areas of bright T2 signal
  - Dilated endometrial glands
- Focal areas of bright T1 signal
  - Foci of hemorrhage
- Adenomyoma
  - Oval ill-defined mass

- Often within junctional zone
  - Low signal intensity on T2
    - From smooth muscle hypertrophy
- Gadolinium not helpful
  - Adenomyomas and fibroids both enhance

Imaging Recommendations
- Best imaging tool
  - Ultrasound is initial study in patients with pelvic symptoms
    - Sensitivity 80-86%
    - Specificity 50-96%
    - Accuracy 68-86%
  - MR best tool for diagnosis but expensive
- Protocol advice
  - Use transvaginal ultrasound to look for subtle findings
    - Concentrate at endometrial/myometrial junction
  - MR for equivocal cases
    - Adenomyoma
    - Fibroids also present

DIFFERENTIAL DIAGNOSIS

Fibroids
- More often present with bleeding or mass
- Fibroids painful if complication
  - Torsion
  - Degeneration
- Ultrasound features
  - Well-defined mass
    - Submucosal
    - Mural
    - Subserosal
  - Often diffusely hypoechoic
  - Can be heterogeneous
    - Calcifications
    - Cystic degeneration
  - Poor posterior transmission of sound
  - Peripheral vascularity
    - Circular spoke-wheel pattern
- MR

UTERINE ADENOMYOSIS

○ Low signal on T1 and T2
○ Normal junctional zone

Endometrial Hyperplasia
• Thickened endometrium
  ○ Often cystic
  ○ Swiss cheese appearance
• Increased incidence in women on tamoxifen
• Considered precancerous especially if pathology shows atypia

Endometrial Polyp
• Focal endometrial thickening
• May contain cysts
• Pedunculated
  ○ Identifiable stalk
    ▪ Color Doppler shows flow in stalk
• Sessile
  ○ Broad based
• Sonohysterography is best imaging test

Endometrial Cancer
• Irregularly thickened endometrium
  ○ Often diffuse
• Invasion into myometrium
  ○ Focal obliteration of junctional zone

PATHOLOGY

General Features
• Etiology
  ○ Endometrial gland migration
    ▪ From basal layer into myometrium
  ○ Subendometrial cysts
    ▪ Continued cyclic function of endometrial glands
• Epidemiology
  ○ 1% of all women
    ▪ More common in multiparous
  ○ Pre-operatively diagnosed in 2.6-26%
• Associated abnormalities: Endometriosis

Gross Pathologic & Surgical Features
• Diffusely thickened myometrium
  ○ Foci of hemorrhage

Microscopic Features
• Endometrial glands in myometrium
  ○ > 2.5 mm beyond basal layer
• Smooth muscle hyperplasia
  ○ Myometrium response to ectopic glands

CLINICAL ISSUES

Presentation
• Most common signs/symptoms
  ○ Soft tender diffusely enlarged uterus
    ▪ Most painful 1 week before onset of menses
  ○ Menorrhagia (50%)
  ○ Dysmenorrhea (20%)
  ○ Metrorrhagia (10%)
  ○ Infertility
• Other signs/symptoms
  ○ Endometriosis

▪ 79% of women with endometriosis also have adenomyosis

Demographics
• Age: 4th and 5th decades

Treatment
• Hormonal control of menstrual cycle
  ○ Oral contraceptives
• Uterine artery embolization is possible emerging treatment
  ○ Adenomyomas noted to embolize along with coexistent fibroids
    ▪ Decrease in size on follow-up MR
  ○ Current studies
    ▪ 44% need additional treatment
    ▪ 28% require hysterectomy
• Hysterectomy is definitive treatment

DIAGNOSTIC CHECKLIST

Consider
• Adenomyosis in patients with enlarged painful uterus
  ○ Fibroids are less likely to be painful

Image Interpretation Pearls
• Look at endometrial myometrial junctional zone with ultrasound
  ○ May see endometrial invasion
• Look carefully for small myometrial cysts
• Asymmetric thickening of uterine wall may be only clue to diagnosis
• Recommend MR if findings are equivocal
• MR most helpful for adenomyoma

SELECTED REFERENCES

1. Bazot M et al: Adenomyosis in endometriosis--prevalence and impact on fertility. Evidence from magnetic resonance imaging. Hum Reprod. 21(4):1101-2; author reply 1102-3, 2006
2. Chopra S et al: Adenomyosis:common and uncommon manifestations on sonography and magnetic resonance imaging. J Ultrasound Med. 25(5):617-27; quiz 629, 2006
3. Ghai S et al: Uterine artery embolization for leiomyomas: pre- and postprocedural evaluation with US. Radiographics. 25(5):1159-72; discussion 1173-6, 2005
4. Kuligowska E et al: Pelvic pain: overlooked and underdiagnosed gynecologic conditions. Radiographics. 25(1):3-20, 2005
5. Pelage JP et al: Midterm results of uterine artery embolization for symptomatic adenomyosis: initial experience. Radiology. 234(3):948-53, 2005
6. Bazot M et al: Ultrasonography compared with magnetic resonance imaging for the diagnosis of adenomyosis: correlation with histopathology. Hum Reprod. 16(11):2427-33, 2001
7. Atri M et al: Adenomyosis: US features with histologic correlation in an in-vitro study. Radiology. 215(3):783-90, 2000
8. Reinhold C et al: Uterine adenomyosis: endovaginal US and MR imaging features with histopathologic correlation. Radiographics. 19 Spec No:S147-60, 1999

9

16

UTERINE ADENOMYOSIS

IMAGE GALLERY

Typical

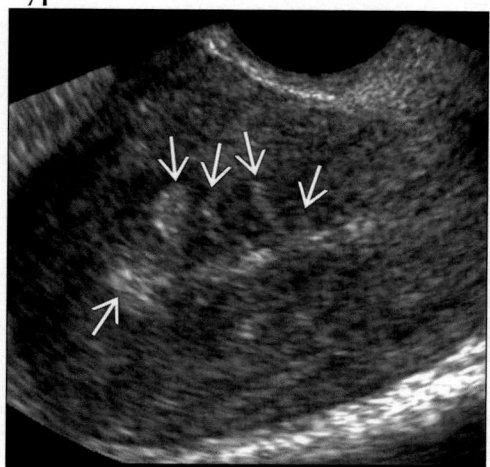
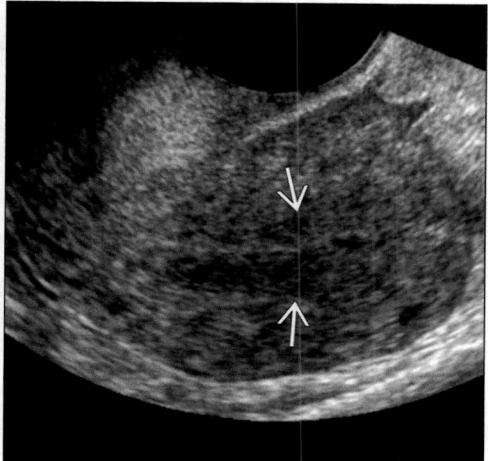

(Left) Longitudinal transvaginal ultrasound shows subtle findings of adenomyosis. Nodular and linear echogenic striations ➡ from the endometrium into the myometrium are due to endometrial gland migration. *(Right)* Longitudinal transvaginal ultrasound shows thickening of the junctional zone ➡. The borders of the endometrium are obliterated. MR confirmed adenomyosis in both cases.

Typical

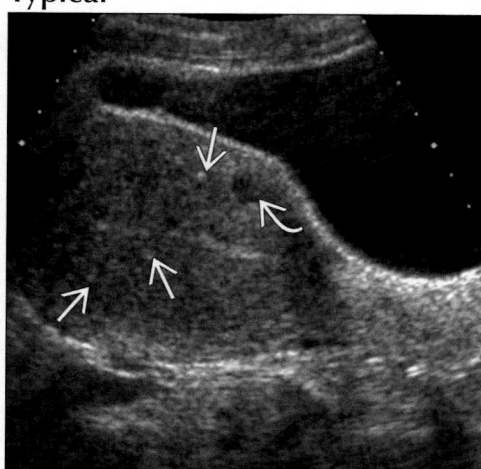
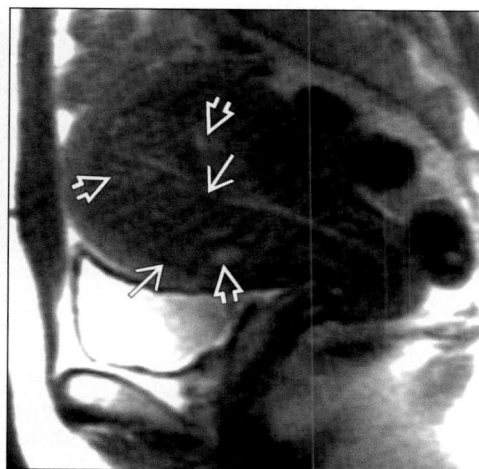

(Left) Longitudinal transabdominal ultrasound shows enlarged globular uterus with multiple myometrial echogenic foci ➡, indistinct endometrium, and myometrial cyst ➡. *(Right)* Longitudinal T2WI MR of the same uterus as previous image, shows markedly thickened junctional zone ➡ and multiple foci of ↑ signal ➡. The hyperintense foci are from myometrial cysts and focal hemorrhage.

Typical

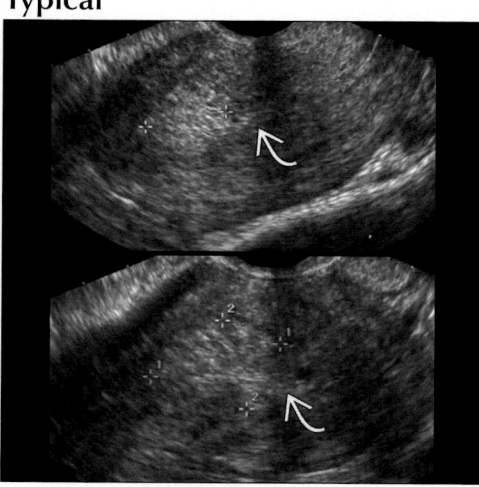
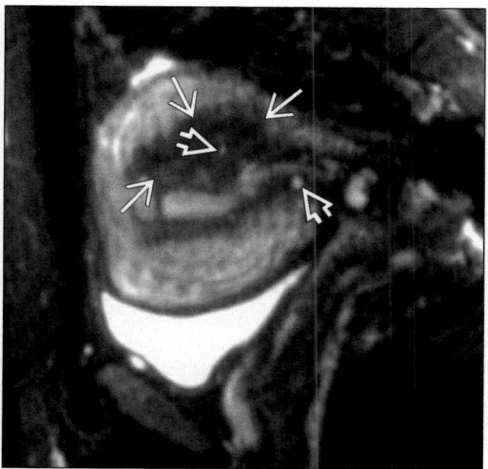

(Left) Transvaginal ultrasound of an adenomyoma in longitudinal (above) and axial planes (below) shows a poorly defined elliptical echogenic mass (calipers) near the endometrium ➡. *(Right)* Longitudinal T2WI MR of another adenomyoma shows a poorly defined elliptical mass ➡ associated with the posterior junctional zone. Several small myometrial cysts are also seen ➡.

UTERINE LEIOMYOMA

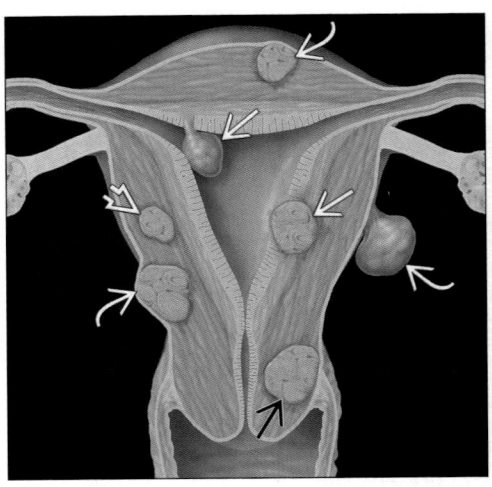

Coronal graphic shows various fibroid locations including submucosal and endocavitary ➡, subserosal and pedunculated ⟹, mural ⬌ and cervical ➡.

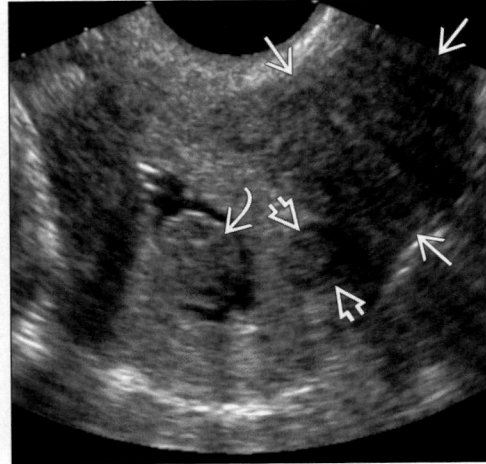

Longitudinal transvaginal ultrasound at time of sonohysterography shows an endocavitary myoma ➡ surrounded by saline. Mural ⬌ and subserosal myomas ➡ are also seen.

TERMINOLOGY

Abbreviations and Synonyms
- Myoma
- Fibroid

Definitions
- Benign uterine smooth muscle proliferation

IMAGING FINDINGS

General Features
- Best diagnostic clue: Focal uterine wall mass
- Location
  - Submucosal
    - In close contact with endometrium
    - Variant is intracavitary
  - Mural
    - Within uterine muscle wall
  - Subserosal
    - Beneath serosa
  - Pedunculated
    - Extrauterine on a stalk
- Size: Extremely variable
- Morphology
  - Often distort uterine contour
  - May exert mass effect upon endometrium

Ultrasonographic Findings
- Well-defined focal mass
  - Hypoechoic to myometrium
  - Poorly reflective
    - Poor through transmission
    - Acoustic shadowing even without calcification
  - Heterogeneous echotexture
    - Foci of hemorrhage
    - Foci of cystic degeneration
    - Calcifications
- Uterine enlargement
  - Normal contour often lost
  - Multiple myomas
    - Difficult to see endometrium
  - Single giant myoma sometimes seen
- Myoma location
  - Submucosal
    - Mass effect on endometrium

DDx: Uterine Enlargement

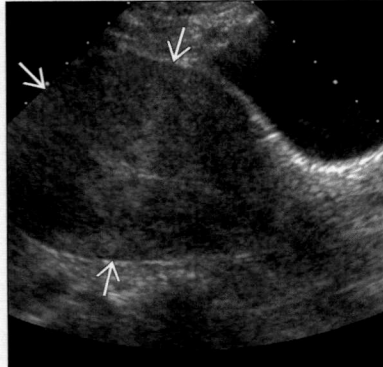

Adenomyosis

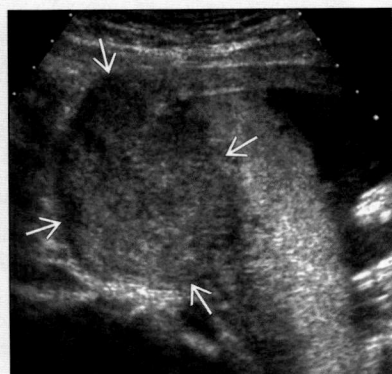

Focal Myometrial Contraction

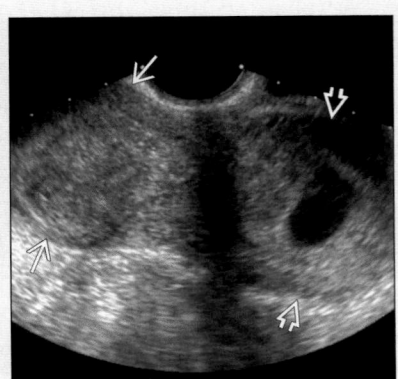

Duplication

UTERINE LEIOMYOMA

Key Facts

Imaging Findings
- Well-defined focal mass
- Hypoechoic to myometrium
- Poorly reflective
- Acoustic shadowing even without calcification
- Heterogeneous echotexture
- Uterine enlargement
- Blood flow from periphery to center
- Low lying fibroids may block birth canal
- MR for complicated cases
- Use both transabdominal and transvaginal ultrasound (TVUS)
- Determine size and location of myomas
- At least largest three myomas should be "mapped"
- Sonohysterography best to determine submucosal component

Top Differential Diagnoses
- Leiomyosarcoma
- Adenomyosis
- Focal Myometrial Contraction (FMC)

Clinical Issues
- Submucosal fibroids cause bleeding
- Pedunculated fibroids can undergo torsion
- Degenerating fibroids cause pain
- Uterine artery embolization popularity growing

Diagnostic Checklist
- Recommend sonohysterography to better evaluate submucosal myomas
- MR may be necessary to better show myoma relationship to adnexal structures
- Suspect malignancy if rapidly growing myoma seen

- May extend into endometrial cavity as pedunculated mass
  - Intramural
    - Surrounded by normal myometrium
    - No mass effect on endometrium
    - May effect external contour if large
  - Subserosal
    - Beneath serosal surface
    - Always effects uterine contour
    - Far from endometrium
  - Pedunculated
    - Extrinsic myoma attached to uterus by a stalk
    - Vascular connection to uterus seen by Doppler
    - At risk for torsion
    - Must differentiate from ovarian mass
  - Broad ligament myoma
    - Arises within broad ligament
    - May mimic solid ovarian mass
  - Cervical myoma
    - Focal hypoechoic mass in cervix
    - Internal blood flow differentiates from nabothian cyst
    - More focal than cervical cancer
- Sonohysterography helpful in characterizing submucosal fibroids
  - Fibroids more hypoechoic than polyps
  - Echogenic endometrial lining covers myoma
  - Hysteroscopic resection if > 50% of myoma is intracavitary
- Color Doppler findings
  - Blood flow from periphery to center
  - Spoke wheel pattern
- Pulse Doppler Characteristics
  - Low resistive flow
- Fibroids and pregnancy
  - 50% grow during the first 20 weeks
    - Cystic change from degeneration common
    - May be painful
  - Low lying fibroids may block birth canal
    - "Myoma previa"
    - Obligatory cesarian section
  - Placental implantation upon fibroids

- Increased risk for abruption
- Lipoleiomyoma variant
  - Myoma with variable amount of fat
    - Echogenic mass if mostly fat
  - Can mimic dermoid if exophytic

CT Findings
- Enlarged homogeneous uterus
  - Fibroid attenuation similar to uterus
- Heterogeneous attenuation if myoma has focal hemorrhage, cystic degeneration, calcification, necrosis

MR Findings
- T1WI
  - Myoma is isointense to myometrium
  - High signal if blood products present
- T2WI
  - Low signal
  - High signal if cystic degeneration
- Myomas enhance with gadolinium
- Appearance after uterine artery embolization
  - Volume reduction of uterus and fibroids
  - Decreased enhancement
  - Internal focal findings
    - Hemorrhage
    - Necrosis
    - Gas from infection or necrosis
  - Myoma may be expelled vaginally

Imaging Recommendations
- Best imaging tool
  - Ultrasound is initial study of choice
  - Sonohysterography for submucosal myomas
  - MR for complicated cases
    - Embolization cases
    - Multiple myomas
- Protocol advice
  - Use both transabdominal and transvaginal ultrasound (TVUS)
    - May miss pedunculated or subserosal myoma with TVUS alone
  - Measure uterus in 3 orthogonal planes

UTERINE LEIOMYOMA

■ Can follow treatment plans
○ Determine size and location of myomas
■ At least largest three myomas should be "mapped"
○ Sonohysterography best to determine submucosal component

DIFFERENTIAL DIAGNOSIS

Leiomyosarcoma
• Cancer of smooth muscle cells
  ○ 1:7,000,000 incidence
  ○ Rarely arises from preexisting myoma
• Rapidly growing uterine mass
  ○ Appearance otherwise identical to myoma
• Invasion of pelvic structures
• Highly vascular
  ○ Many fibroids also show ↑ flow

Adenomyosis
• Endometrial gland migration into myometrium
• Diffuse adenomyosis
  ○ Enlarged globular uterus
    ■ No distinct masses
  ○ Heterogeneous endometrial/myometrial junction
  ○ Myometrial cysts
• Focal adenomyosis can mimic myoma
  ○ Elliptical more than round
  ○ Heterogeneously echogenic
    ■ Myoma more likely hypoechoic
  ○ Often near endometrium
  ○ MR may be necessary to differentiate from fibroid

Focal Myometrial Contraction (FMC)
• Normal finding in pregnancy
• Focal bulge of myometrium
• Distorts internal contour more than external
• Isoechoic to myometrium
• Resolves with time

Uterine Duplication
• Bicornuate uterus
  ○ 2 fundi with midline contour defect
  ○ 1 fundus can mimic myoma
• Empty horn in pregnancy can mimic myoma
• Look for central endometrial echogenicity
  ○ Longitudinal images helpful

PATHOLOGY

General Features
• Epidemiology
  ○ 25-30% incidence in US
  ○ Higher incidence in African American women
  ○ 77% incidence in hysterectomy specimens

Microscopic Features
• Spindle shaped smooth muscle cells
• Variable amounts of fibrin, collagen and extra-cellular matrix

CLINICAL ISSUES

Presentation
• Most common signs/symptoms
  ○ Symptoms related to myoma location
    ■ Submucosal fibroids cause bleeding
    ■ Pedunculated fibroids can undergo torsion
    ■ Cornual fibroids can cause tubal obstruction
  ○ Symptoms related to myoma size and growth
    ■ Degenerating fibroids cause pain
    ■ Urinary urgency
    ■ Constipation
  ○ Symptoms related to pregnancy
    ■ Pregnancy loss
    ■ Premature labor
    ■ Fetal malpresentation
    ■ Myoma previa

Demographics
• Age: Increase in size and frequency with age

Natural History & Prognosis
• Tend to involute after menopause

Treatment
• Hormonal therapy
• Uterine artery embolization popularity growing
• Myomectomy
• Hysterectomy

DIAGNOSTIC CHECKLIST

Image Interpretation Pearls
• Recommend sonohysterography to better evaluate submucosal myomas
• MR may be necessary to better show myoma relationship to adnexal structures
• Suspect malignancy if rapidly growing myoma seen

SELECTED REFERENCES

1. Dixon D et al: The second National Institutes of Health International Congress on advances in uterine leiomyoma research: conference summary and future recommendations. Fertil Steril. 86(4):800-6, 2006
2. Spielmann AL et al: Comparison of MRI and sonography in the preliminary evaluation for fibroid embolization. AJR Am J Roentgenol. 187(6):1499-504, 2006
3. Ghai S et al: Uterine artery embolization for leiomyomas: pre- and postprocedural evaluation with US. Radiographics. 25(5):1159-72; discussion 1173-6, 2005
4. Davis PC et al: Sonohysterographic findings of endometrial and subendometrial conditions. Radiographics. 22(4):803-16, 2002
5. Nalaboff KM et al: Imaging the endometrium: disease and normal variants. Radiographics. 21(6):1409-24, 2001
6. Kliewer MA et al: Acoustic shadowing from uterine leiomyomas: sonographic-pathologic correlation. Radiology. 196(1):99-102, 1995

9

20

UTERINE LEIOMYOMA

IMAGE GALLERY

Typical

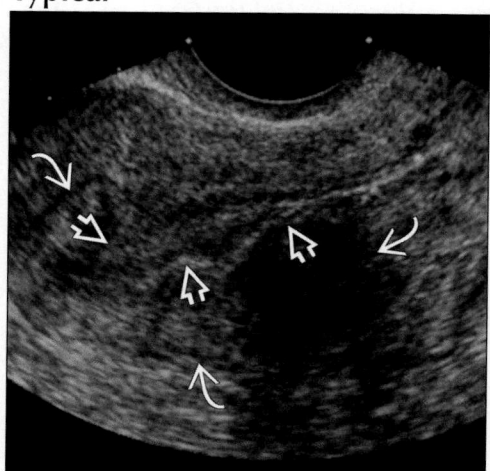

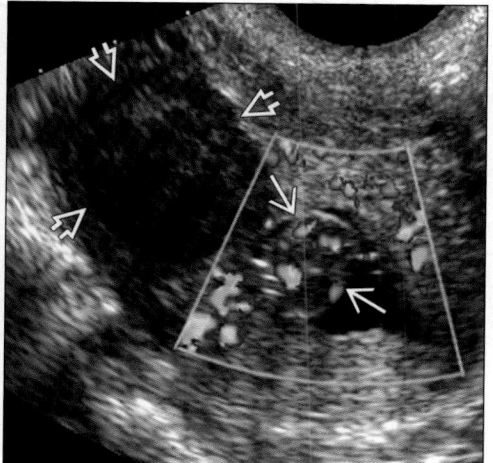

(Left) Longitudinal transvaginal ultrasound shows 3 fibroids ➡ with mass effect on endometrium ⇨. These submucosal fibroids were the cause of the patient's bleeding. Note shadowing from the largest fibroid. *(Right)* Transverse color Doppler ultrasound shows circular peripheral blood flow in another submucosal intracavitary myoma ➡. An adjacent mural myoma is also seen ⇨.

Typical

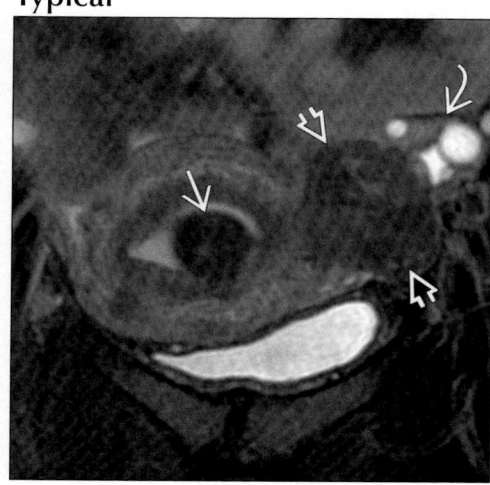

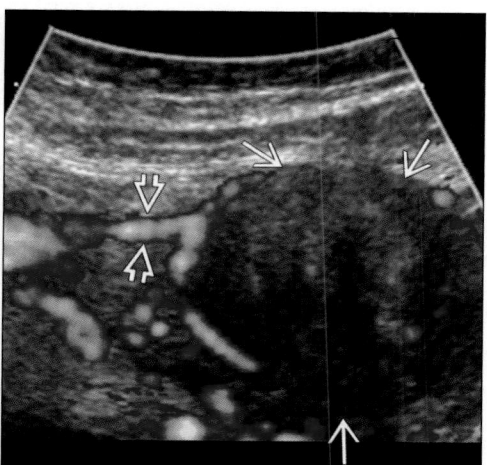

(Left) Transverse T2WI MR shows an intracavitary ➡ and left pedunculated ⇨ myoma. Normal and separate left ovary ➡ is easily identified with MR. *(Right)* Transverse power Doppler ultrasound shows pedunculated myoma ➡ attached to the uterus by a vascular stalk ⇨. Doppler and MR help differentiate exophytic myomas from ovarian masses.

Variant

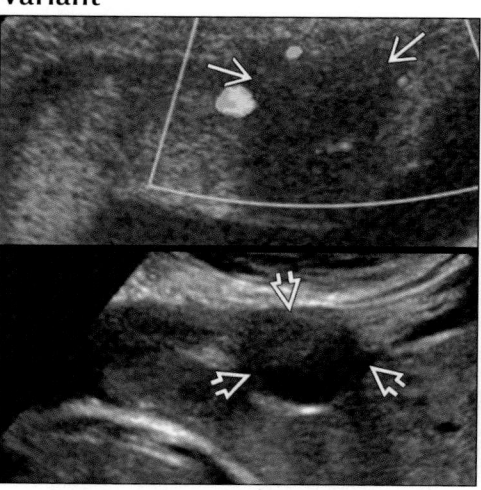

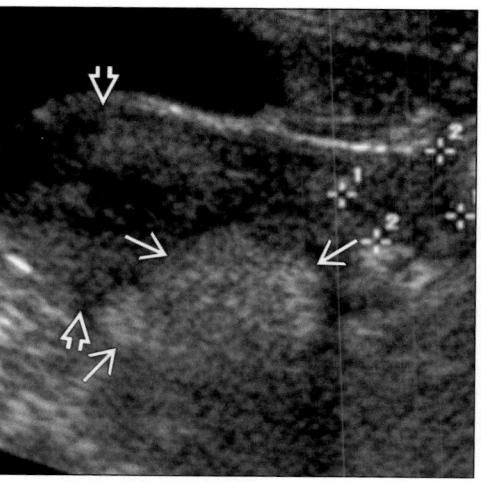

(Left) Transverse ultrasound during pregnancy shows subplacental myoma ➡ in 2nd trimester (upper) with peripheral flow and shadowing. Follow-up (lower), in 3rd trimester, shows cystic degeneration ⇨. *(Right)* Transverse transabdominal ultrasound shows an echogenic mass ➡ arising from the uterus ⇨, separate from the left ovary (calipers). MR confirmed the diagnosis of lipoleiomyoma.

HEMATOMETROCOLPOS

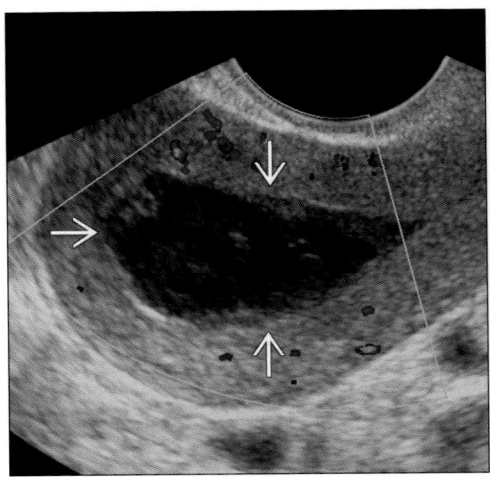

Longitudinal color Doppler ultrasound during a transvaginal study shows the uterine cavity ➡ distended by blood clot. As expected there is no flow in the endocavitary blood clot.

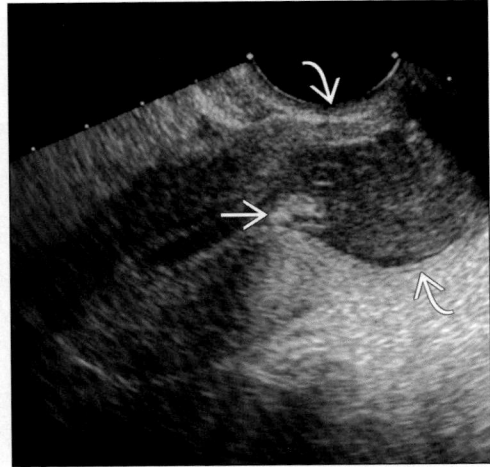

Longitudinal transvaginal ultrasound shows active bleeding ➡ within a collection of older blood products distending the cervix ➡. Cervical stenosis was due to radiation therapy for cervical cancer.

TERMINOLOGY

Abbreviations and Synonyms
- Hematometra (HM)
- Hematocolpos (HC)
- Müllerian duct anomaly (MDA)
- Cloacal malformation (CM)

Definitions
- HM: Distension of uterine cavity by blood products
- HC: Distension of vagina by blood products
- Hematometrocolpos: Distension of uterus and vagina by accumulated blood
- MDA: Series of uterine malformations as result of abnormal fusion of Müllerian ducts
  - Unicornuate, bicornuate, didelphys uterus ± cervical/vaginal malformation
- CM: Confluence of rectum vagina and urethra into a single common channel

IMAGING FINDINGS

General Features
- Best diagnostic clue: Echogenic fluid within distended uterus ± vagina

Ultrasonographic Findings
- Grayscale Ultrasound
  - Mass arising from pelvis
    - HM appears thick-walled due to myometrium
    - HC lower in pelvis and thin-walled compared to HM
  - Fetal diagnosis reported
    - Thin bulging membrane separating labia
    - Distended vagina
    - May be associated with ascites attributed to uterine reflux via fallopian tubes versus associated distal urinary obstruction
- Color Doppler: No flow
- 3D
  - 3D allows better sonographic evaluation of uterine fundal contour
    - Vital for diagnosis of MDA

DDx: Uterine Distension

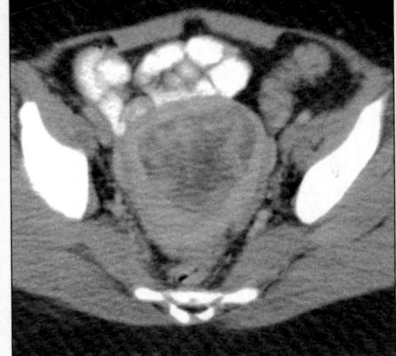

Molar Pregnancy

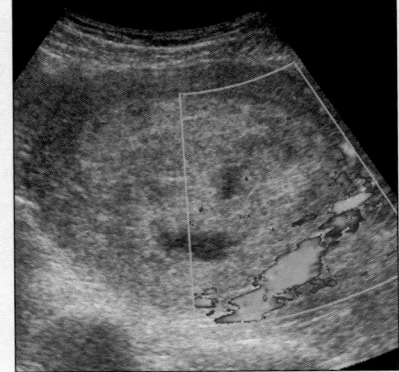

Retained Products of Conception

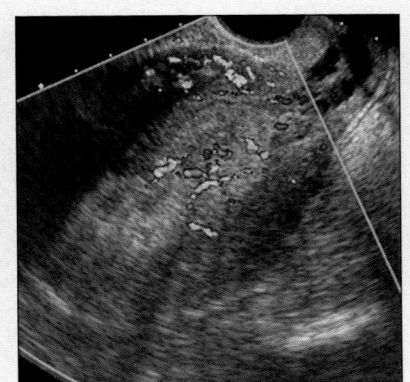

Endometrial Cancer

HEMATOMETROCOLPOS

Key Facts

Imaging Findings
- Best diagnostic clue: Echogenic fluid within distended uterus ± vagina
- Mass arising from pelvis
- HM appears thick-walled due to myometrium
- HC lower in pelvis and thin-walled compared to HM
- Color Doppler: No flow
- 3D allows better sonographic evaluation of uterine fundal contour
- MR best to confirm blood products
- MR very helpful to clarify anatomy, relationship of pelvic organs
- Consider use of translabial scans

Top Differential Diagnoses
- Pyometra
- Muco/Hydrometrocolpos
- Endometritis
- Gestational Trophoblastic Disease
- Retained Products of Conception

Clinical Issues
- Present at puberty if associated with MDA/CM
- Present later if associated with cervical cancer
- If clinical or sonographic diagnosis avoid aspiration as risk of infection → pyocolpos/pyometra
- Schedule MR to verify diagnosis and assess extent of associated malformation

Diagnostic Checklist
- HM/HC should be excluded in any young female with cyclical pelvic pain
- Female fetus/infant with pelvic mass + urinary obstruction → strongly suggests CM

Imaging Recommendations
- Best imaging tool
  - MR best to confirm blood products
  - MR very helpful to clarify anatomy, relationship of pelvic organs
- Protocol advice
  - Ultrasound
    - Consider use of translabial scans
    - Some reports of transrectal sonography
  - MR
    - Include renal images on coronal scout views
    - True coronal images of uterus to evaluate fundal contour
    - Distend vagina with Surgilube if possible, helpful to inject even if tiny perineal orifice

DIFFERENTIAL DIAGNOSIS

Pyometra
- Associated with fever, elevated white cell count
- Clinical diagnosis as complex fluid on imaging may be pus or blood
- Does not involve vagina

Muco/Hydrometrocolpos
- Uterus/vagina distended with mucous secretions not blood
- Most commonly associated with imperforate hymen
- Hymenal membrane appears white
  - HC/HM hymenal membrane appears bluish due to accumulated blood products

Endometritis
- Seen after childbirth, uterine instrumentation
- Look for gas bubbles within endometrial cavity
- Not associated with amenorrhea
- Does not involve vagina

Gestational Trophoblastic Disease
- Uterus distended by complete mole has typical "snowstorm" appearance, not echogenic fluid
- Invasive mole typically hypervascular mass invading myometrium
  - Myometrium may be thinned in HM but is intact
- Does not involve vagina

Retained Products of Conception
- History of recent delivery
- Solid perfused tissue
- Retained clot is hypoechoic, non vascular, smaller in volume than that seen with HM
- Does not involve vagina

Complex Adnexal Mass
- Always identify organ of origin of adnexal mass
  - Most are ovarian: Normal uterus can be identified separately
  - Pedunculated fibroids with cystic degeneration can be confusing
    - Not associated with amenorrhea
    - Look for vessels from myometrium to mass
    - Often other fibroids in uterine corpus in addition to pedunculated
- If normal uterus not identified could "mass" be abnormal uterus?
- May require MR to visualize normal ovaries
  - If large complex pelvic mass
  - If vaginal sonography not possible

PATHOLOGY

General Features
- Etiology
  - Imperforate hymen
    - Most frequent cause of vaginal outflow obstruction
  - Mullerian duct anomaly
    - Vaginal septum: Transverse or vertical
    - Vaginal agenesis
    - Cervical agenesis
    - Uterus didelphys with obstructed hemivagina is most confusing as normal menstruation occurs through non-obstructed side

- ○ Cloacal malformation
  - One series 68% uterine function
  - 32% normal menstruation
  - 36% presented with hematometra/hematocolpos
  - 20% primary amenorrhea
  - 36% uterine obstruction requiring surgery (hysterectomy, partial hysterectomy with vaginoplasty, vaginoplasty alone)
  - Obstruction due to vaginal stenosis after reconstruction, stenosis of persistent urogenital sinus (no previous reconstruction) or cervical stenosis
  - ○ Cervical/vaginal stenosis
    - Post radiation therapy for gynecologic/colorectal malignancies
    - Post reconstructive surgery
    - Vaginal stenosis described in chronic graft versus host disease
- Epidemiology
  - ○ Imperforate hymen 1:1,000
  - ○ Vaginal agenesis 1:5,000
  - ○ CM occurs exclusively in females, 1:20,000 live births
  - ○ Vaginal stenosis occurs in up to 88% of cervical cancer patients treated with radiation therapy
- Associated abnormalities
  - ○ Renal anomalies
  - ○ Endometriosis

CLINICAL ISSUES

Presentation

- Most common signs/symptoms: Primary amenorrhea
- Other signs/symptoms
  - ○ Cyclical pelvic pain
  - ○ Low back pain
  - ○ Present at puberty if associated with MDA/CM
    - Primary amenorrhea if obstructed single vagina
    - Uterus didelphys → duplicated vagina → normal menses through unobstructed side with progressive distension of obstructed side
    - Pelvic pressure
    - Distended uterus/vagina → mass effect → acute urinary retention
  - ○ Present later if associated with cervical cancer
    - Average age at diagnosis of CxCA is 50 yrs
    - Radiation therapy induced cervical/vaginal stenosis develops within a year of therapy

Natural History & Prognosis

- Depends on underlying etiology
  - ○ Imperforate hymen easily corrected
  - ○ CM requires complex repair with multiple surgeries
  - ○ MDA repair varies with malformation: Simple septal resection to more complex vaginal reconstruction
- Associated with endometriosis
  - ○ Increased incidence of infertility/ectopic pregnancy
  - ○ Endometriosis causes chronic pelvic pain

Treatment

- If clinical or sonographic diagnosis avoid aspiration as risk of infection → pyocolpos/pyometra

- Schedule MR to verify diagnosis and assess extent of associated malformation
  - ○ Assist with surgical planning
- Imperforate hymen
  - ○ Cruciate incision with marsupialization of edges to vaginal wall
  - ○ Simple incision inadequate → does not guarantee complete drainage → risk of infection
- MDA
  - ○ Incision/removal of vaginal septum
  - ○ Creation of perineal opening/vaginoplasty
  - ○ Uterine surgery may also be required to improve chances of successful pregnancy
- Radiation therapy related
  - ○ Topical estrogen, anti-inflammatory ointment
  - ○ Serial vaginal dilators
- CM
  - ○ Surgical challenge is to create three perineal openings with functional vagina, bladder/bowel control
  - ○ Individual anatomy will direct reconstructive approach

DIAGNOSTIC CHECKLIST

Consider

- HM/HC should be excluded in any young female with cyclical pelvic pain

Image Interpretation Pearls

- Female fetus/infant with pelvic mass + urinary obstruction → strongly suggests CM
  - ○ 50% have hydrocolpos → pressure on bladder trigone → urinary tract obstruction

SELECTED REFERENCES

1. Prada Arias M et al: Uterus didelphys with obstructed hemivagina and multicystic dysplastic kidney. Eur J Pediatr Surg. 15(6):441-5, 2005
2. Ballesio L et al: Hematocolpos in double vagina associated with uterus didelphus: US and MR findings. Eur J Radiol. 45(2):150-3, 2003
3. Chircop R: A case of retention of urine and haematocolpometra. Eur J Emerg Med. 10(3):244-5, 2003
4. Warne SA et al: Long-term gynecological outcome of patients with persistent cloaca. J Urol. 170(4 Pt 2):1493-6, 2003
5. Anguenot JL et al: Vaginal stenosis with hematocolpometra, complicating chronic graft versus host disease. Eur J Obstet Gynecol Reprod Biol. 103(2):185-7, 2002
6. Anguenot JL et al: Hematocolpos secondary to imperforate hymen, contribution of transrectal echography. Acta Obstet Gynecol Scand. 79(7):614-5, 2000
7. Ahmed S et al: Distal mucocolpos and proximal hematocolpos secondary to concurrent imperforate hymen and transverse vaginal septum. J Pediatr Surg. 34(10):1555-6, 1999
8. Fliegner JR et al: Management of vaginal agenesis with a functioning uterus. Is hysterectomy advisable? Aust N Z J Obstet Gynaecol. 34(4):467-70, 1994
9. Agrawal PK et al: Ultrasonographic diagnosis of haematometrocolpos in patients refusing vaginal examination. J Indian Med Assoc. 90(5):127-8, 1992

HEMATOMETROCOLPOS

IMAGE GALLERY

Typical

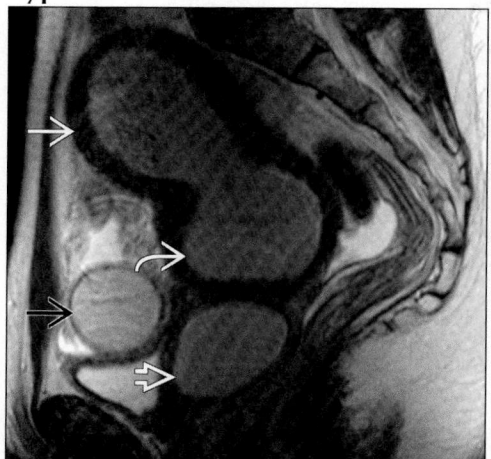

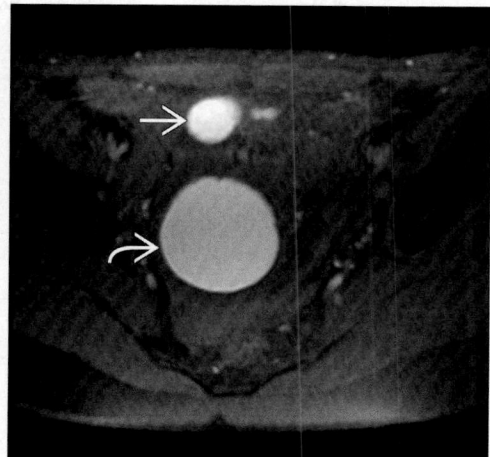

(Left) Longitudinal T2WI MR shows hematometrocolpos with blood distending uterus ➡, cervix ➡ and vagina ➡. Note the intermediate signal structure ➡ superior to the bladder. (Right) T1+ FS MR in true axial plane to uterus shows high signal material i.e., blood products in the cervix ➡ and the structure ➡ superior to bladder indicating that it is an endometrioma. Endometriosis is a common complication of obstructed MDA.

Typical

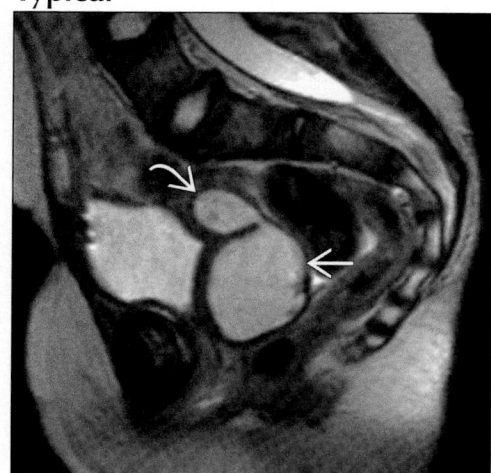

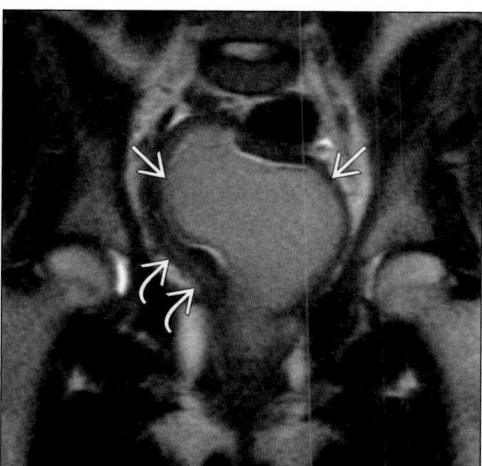

(Left) Longitudinal T2WI MR shows another hematometrocolpos with marked distension of the vagina ➡ and less significant distension of the uterus ➡ which remains intrapelvic in this case. In the previous case the fundus reached the umbilicus. (Right) Coronal T2WI MR shows hematocolpos ➡ in the left hemivagina of a patient with a uterus didelphys and a duplicated vagina. The right hemivagina ➡ is displaced but not obstructed.

Typical

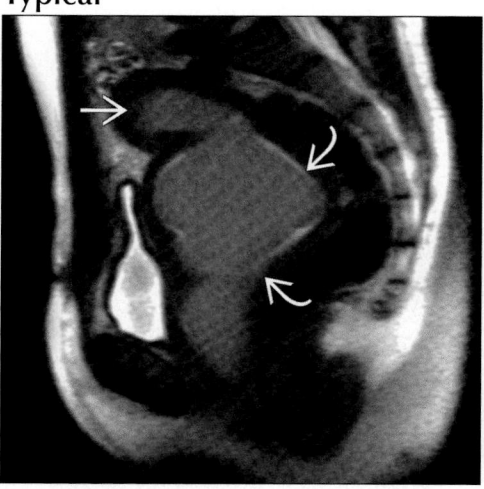

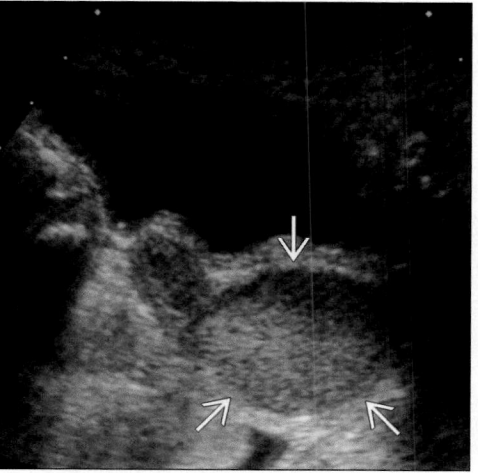

(Left) Longitudinal T2WI MR in the same patient as the previous image shows hematometra ➡ as well as hematocolpos ➡ in the left uterus of the didelphys. (Right) Longitudinal transabdominal ultrasound in a different case shows hematocolpos ➡ without associated hematometra. The patient had distal vaginal stenosis secondary to pelvic irradiation.

ENDOMETRIAL POLYP

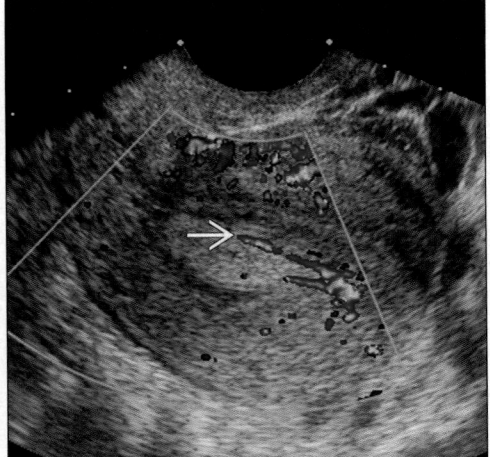

Transverse transvaginal ultrasound shows a focal oval thickening ➡ in the endometrial cavity. This is the typical appearance of an endometrial polyp.

Transverse color Doppler ultrasound shows a feeding vessel ➡ entering the polyp. The vessel is a good indicator of the site of the stalk attachment to the uterus.

TERMINOLOGY

Abbreviations and Synonyms
- Endometrial polyp (EP)

Definitions
- EP: Focal overgrowth of endometrial tissue
- SHSG: Ultrasound of the uterus after distension of the cavity with sterile saline

IMAGING FINDINGS

General Features
- Best diagnostic clue: Focal echogenic endometrial thickening or mass with feeding vessel
- Size: Variable: May be tiny or may be large enough to fill entire uterine cavity
- Morphology
  - Oval or fusiform thickening rather than round
    - Round mass more likely to be submucosal fibroid

Ultrasonographic Findings
- Grayscale Ultrasound
  - Echogenic area in endometrium during proliferative phase of menstrual cycle
    - Proliferative endometrium is normally hypoechoic
    - Secretory endometrium is echogenic, may obscure small polyp
  - Pedunculated or sessile, solitary or multiple
  - Small "cystic" areas within polyp due to dilated endometrial glands
    - Strong correlation with benignity
  - **Hyperechoic line sign**
    - Full/partial echogenic rim around area of endometrial thickening highly specific for endocavitary mass
    - Thought to be compressed endometrium vs. interface of mass with cavity
    - Does not differentiate between masses (polyp vs. fibroid)
- Pulsed Doppler
  - Single feeding vessel in stalk may be evident
    - Divides into smaller vessels within polyp
- 3D
  - Useful for "global view"
  - 3D shows multiple polyps better than 2D

DDx: Mass in Endometrial Cavity

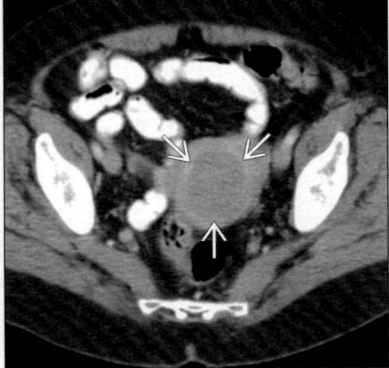

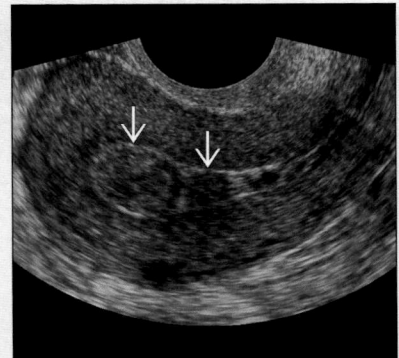

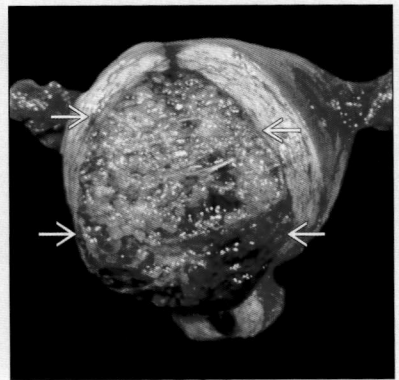

Endometrial Cancer

Fibroids

Complete Mole

ENDOMETRIAL POLYP

Key Facts

Imaging Findings
- Best diagnostic clue: Focal echogenic endometrial thickening or mass with feeding vessel
- Oval or fusiform thickening rather than round
- Echogenic area in endometrium during proliferative phase of menstrual cycle
- Pedunculated or sessile, solitary or multiple
- Small "cystic" areas within polyp due to dilated endometrial glands
- **Hyperechoic line sign**
- Full/partial echogenic rim around area of endometrial thickening highly specific for endocavitary mass
- Does not differentiate between masses (polyp vs. fibroid)
- Single feeding vessel in stalk may be evident
- 3D shows multiple polyps better than 2D

- SHSG best technique to differentiate focal from diffuse endometrial thickening

Top Differential Diagnoses
- Endometrial cancer
- Endometrial hyperplasia
- Submucosal fibroid
- Gestational trophoblastic disease

Diagnostic Checklist
- Benign polyps cannot be differentiated from polyps with atypical hyperplasia
- MR/TV sonography/color Doppler may help to distinguish polyp from carcinoma but biopsy still required
- Cancer may coexist with benign disease

- o Useful during sonohysterography (SHSG) especially if multiple lesions
- Sonohysterography
  - o SHSG best technique to differentiate focal from diffuse endometrial thickening
  - o Focal
    - Polypoid with thin stalk
    - Sessile: If broad based resection is more complex than simple snare
  - o Diffuse
    - Symmetric thickening: "Blind" office biopsy with Pipelle or similar implement
    - Asymmetric: Requires visually directed biopsy of thickest area

MR Findings
- T2WI
  - o Polyp lower signal than normal endometrium
    - Central fibrous core (low signal intensity) within endometrial cavity
    - Intratumoral cysts (high signal intensity) seen more frequently in polyps than carcinomas

Imaging Recommendations
- Best imaging tool: SHSG
- Protocol advice
  - o Schedule scans for abnormal bleeding early in menstrual cycle if possible
  - o Use TV sonography → better resolution
  - o If thick echogenic endometrium seen in premenopausal female
    - > 15 mm → abnormal → SHSG to determine type of biopsy
    - 11-15 mm is indeterminate → follow-up after menstrual period
    - Normal endometrium will slough post menstrually
    - Persistent thickening of increased echogenicity → SHSG
  - o SHSG
    - Schedule within first 10 days of menstrual cycle in menstruating females

- If postmenopausal on hormone replacement therapy (HRT) schedule immediately after withdrawal bleed
- If postmenopausal not on HRT schedule at any time
- Suggest patient take analgesic (non steroidal anti-inflammatory) one hour prior to procedure to minimize discomfort

DIFFERENTIAL DIAGNOSIS

Thickened Endometrium
- Endometrial cancer
  - o Irregular thickening
  - o Often mixed hyper/hypoechoic areas
  - o Irregular endometrial-myometrial interface
  - o May spread to involve cervix/invade through myometrium
    - Polyp may prolapse but will not invade
- Endometrial hyperplasia
  - o More likely diffuse than focal process
  - o Often asymptomatic

Intracavitary Mass
- Submucosal fibroid
  - o Myometrial echogenicity i.e., less echogenic than endometrial stripe
  - o Spherical rather than oval/fusiform
  - o Disrupts endometrial-myometrial interface
  - o Layer of endometrium covers surface of fibroid
  - o Feeding vessel branches over surface of fibroid
    - Often multiple feeding vessels arise from inner myometrium
- Gestational trophoblastic disease
  - o Positive pregnancy test
  - o Often associated with hyperemesis
  - o Beta human chorionic gonadotrophin levels may be ↑ ↑
  - o 25% association with theca lutein cysts
- Retained products of conception
  - o Associated with history of recent gestation

ENDOMETRIAL POLYP

○ Often prominent feeding vessels from myometrium to "mass"
○ May have positive pregnancy test

PATHOLOGY

General Features
- Etiology
  ○ Associated with Tamoxifen treatment in postmenopausal women
    ▪ Premenopausal women taking Tamoxifen for breast cancer are not at increased risk for endometrial cancer
  ○ Lynch syndrome (hereditary nonpolyposis colon cancer) case report of EP containing cancer
- Epidemiology: EP → 30% PMB

Gross Pathologic & Surgical Features
- Circumscribed overgrowth of endometrial mucosa ± stromal tissue
- Protrudes into cavity on fibrovascular stalk

Microscopic Features
- Foci of atypical hyperplasia may be seen within polyps

CLINICAL ISSUES

Presentation
- Most common signs/symptoms
  ○ Abnormal bleeding
    ▪ Intermenstrual
    ▪ Postcoital
    ▪ Postmenopausal
- Other signs/symptoms
  ○ Atypical glandular cells of endometrial origin on Papanicolaou smear
    ▪ Indication for endometrial biopsy as 40% incidence of significant pathology

Natural History & Prognosis
- Polyp site/number/diameter do not correlate with symptomatology
- Often asymptomatic
  ○ 36.1% of postmenopausal women
  ○ 44.4% of reproductive-aged women
- Frequent finding in infertile patients
  ○ Controversial if etiologic factor or if resection improves outcome
  ○ Endometrial polyps < 1.5 cm diameter discovered during ovarian stimulation do not negatively affect pregnancy/implantation outcomes in ICSI (intracytoplasmic sperm injection) cycles

Treatment
- Polypectomy
  ○ Outpatient procedure is safe and better tolerated than operating room hysteroscopic resection
    ▪ Less time away from home
    ▪ Less per/post procedural pain
    ▪ Shorter recovery time

DIAGNOSTIC CHECKLIST

Consider
- Benign polyps cannot be differentiated from polyps with atypical hyperplasia
- MR/TV sonography/color Doppler may help to distinguish polyp from carcinoma but biopsy still required
  ○ Cancer may coexist with benign disease

Image Interpretation Pearls
- Beware of endometrial "wrinkles"
  ○ SHSG should be performed in early proliferative phase
  ○ Endometrium thin and hypoechoic
  ○ Avoids risk of displacing an early pregnancy
  ○ If performed in proliferative phase
    ▪ Endometrium thick and echogenic
    ▪ Uterine contraction is response to cavitary distention → "wrinkles"
    ▪ Wrinkles may be mistaken for sessile polyps

SELECTED REFERENCES

1. American College of Obstetricians and Gynecologists Committee on Gynecologic Practice: ACOG committee opinion. No. 336: Tamoxifen and uterine cancer. Obstet Gynecol. 107(6):1475-8, 2006
2. Hassa H et al: Are the site, diameter, and number of endometrial polyps related with symptomatology? Am J Obstet Gynecol. 194(3):718-21, 2006
3. Isikoglu M et al: Endometrial polyps smaller than 1.5 cm do not affect ICSI outcome. Reprod Biomed Online. 12(2):199-204, 2006
4. Marsh FA et al: A randomised controlled trial comparing outpatient versus daycase endometrial polypectomy. BJOG. 113(8):896-901, 2006
5. Silberstein T et al: Endometrial polyps in reproductive-age fertile and infertile women. Isr Med Assoc J. 8(3):192-5, 2006
6. Sparac V et al: Successful pregnancy after hysteroscopic removal of grade I endometrial carcinoma in a young woman with Lynch syndrome. Int J Gynecol Cancer. 16 Suppl 1:442-5, 2006
7. Jakab A et al: Detection of feeding artery improves the ultrasound diagnosis of endometrial polyps in asymptomatic patients. Eur J Obstet Gynecol Reprod Biol. 119(1):103-7, 2005
8. Le Donne M et al: Uterine pathologies in patients undergoing tamoxifen therapy for breast cancer: ultrasonographic, hysteroscopic and histological findings. Eur J Gynaecol Oncol. 26(6):623-6, 2005
9. Fong K et al: Transvaginal US and hysterosonography in postmenopausal women with breast cancer receiving tamoxifen: correlation with hysteroscopy and pathologic study. Radiographics. 23(1):137-50; discussion 151-5, 2003
10. Grasel RP et al: Endometrial polyps: MR imaging features and distinction from endometrial carcinoma. Radiology. 214(1):47-52, 2000

ENDOMETRIAL POLYP

Typical

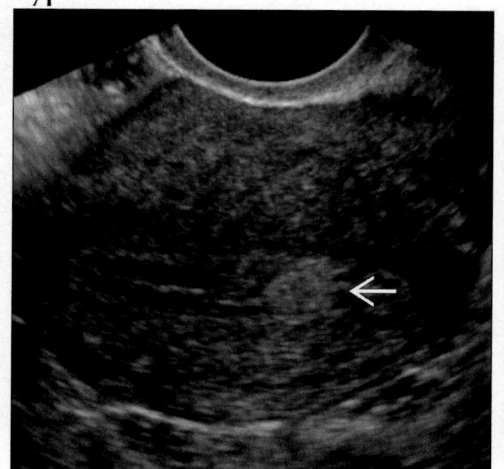 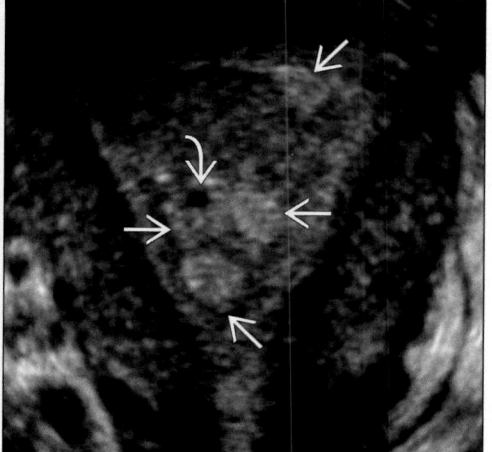

(Left) Transverse transvaginal ultrasound shows a small focal echogenic mass ➡ within the uterine cavity. Note the hypoechoic appearance of the rest of the endometrium. The patient is in the proliferative phase of her menstrual cycle. (Right) 3D ultrasound in same patient as previous image shows multiple polyps ➡, one of which has some internal cysts ➡. Cysts correlate strongly with benignity.

Typical

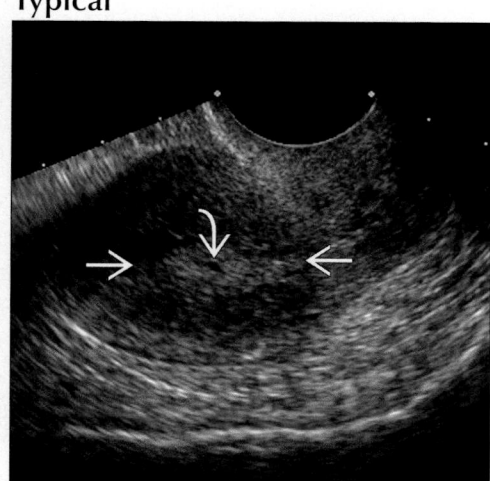 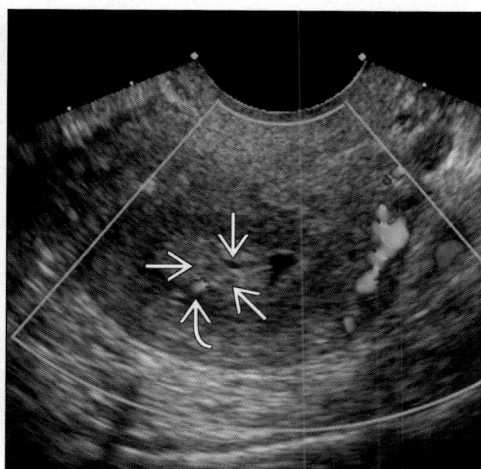

(Left) Longitudinal transvaginal ultrasound shows irregular endometrial thickening ➡ in a patient with postmenopausal bleeding. Note the cystic area ➡. (Right) Transverse color Doppler ultrasound in same patient as previous image shows a feeding vessel ➡ entering the area of focal thickening. Multiple cysts ➡ are visible. Hysteroscopic biopsy showed broad-based sessile polyp.

Typical

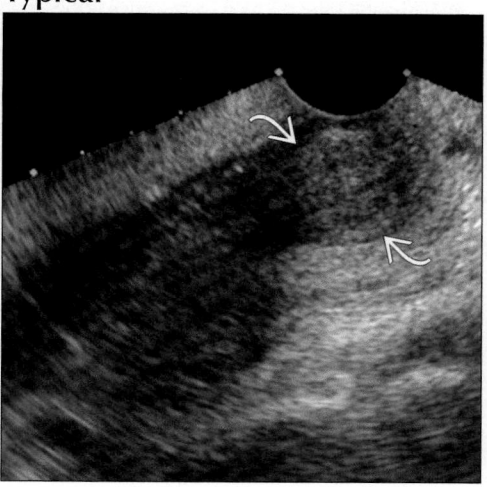 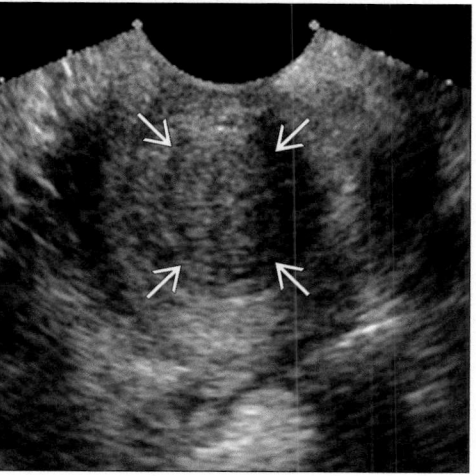

(Left) Longitudinal transvaginal ultrasound shows a large polyp ➡ prolapsing into the cervix. (Right) Transverse transvaginal ultrasound in the same patient as the previous image confirms a well-circumscribed mass ➡ within the cervix. This is difficult to differentiate from a prolapsed fibroid but the well-defined margin decreases suspicion for malignancy.

ENDOMETRIAL POLYP

(Left) Oblique transvaginal ultrasound shows a polyp ➡ outlined by a small amount of endocavitary fluid ⇨ in a patient with cervical stenosis. *(Right)* Longitudinal transvaginal ultrasound shows mildly thickened endometrium to 15 mm in a patient with menorrhagia. There are hypoechoic and hyperechoic areas but no discernible mass.

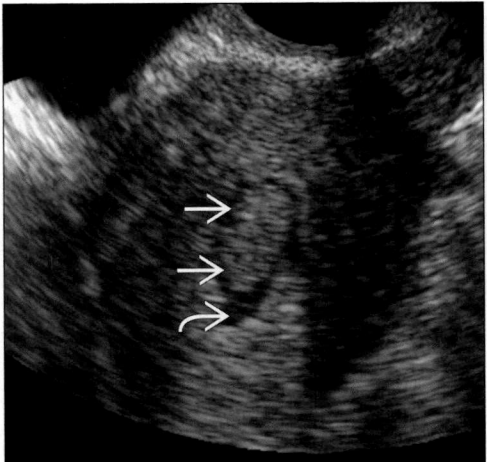
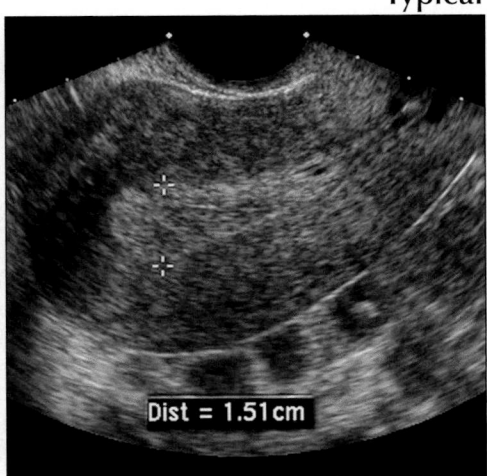

(Left) Longitudinal color Doppler ultrasound in same patient as previous image shows no feeding vessels entering endometrium. *(Right)* Longitudinal transvaginal ultrasound in same patient as previous image shows an early filling view during SHSG. Note how diffuse the irregular thickening of the endometrium is.

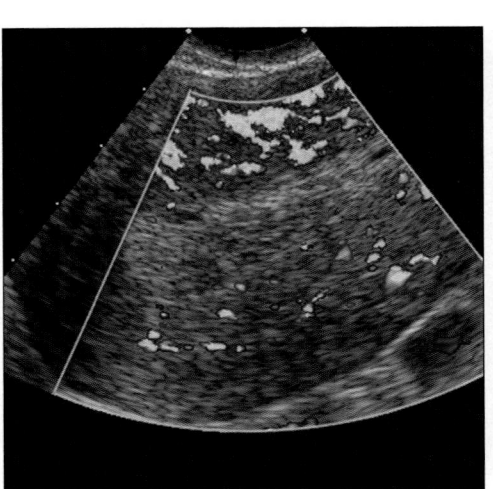
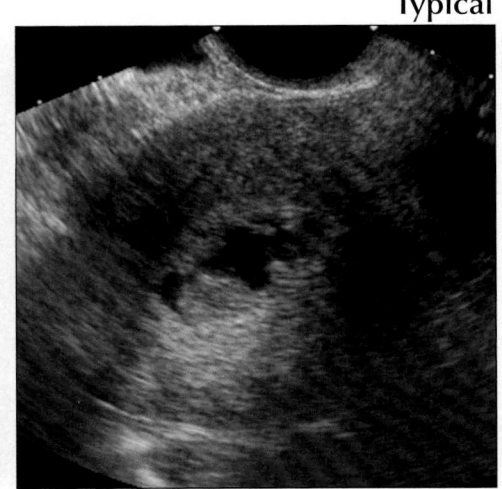

(Left) Longitudinal transvaginal ultrasound during SHSG shows catheter ➡ in place and good uterine distension with saline ➡. *(Right)* Longitudinal transvaginal ultrasound during SHSG shows innumerable polyps ➡ "carpeting" the endometrial cavity. Pathology on D&C curettings showed benign polyps with no atypia.

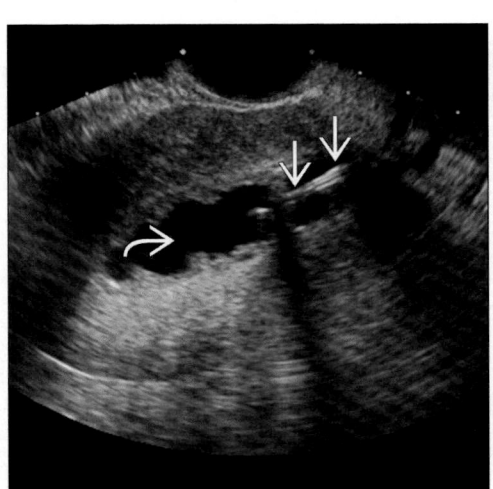
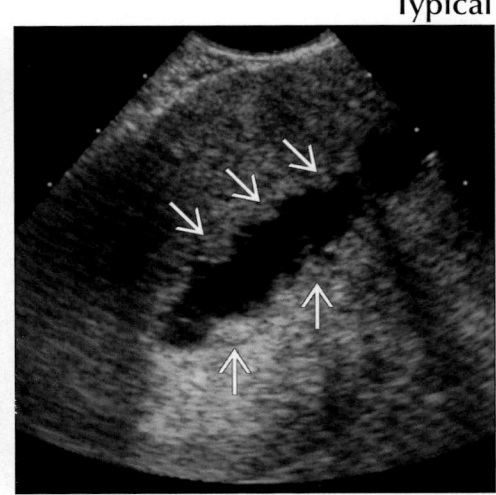

ENDOMETRIAL POLYP

Typical

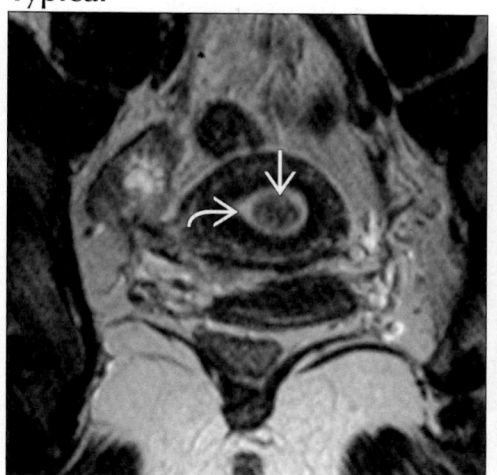
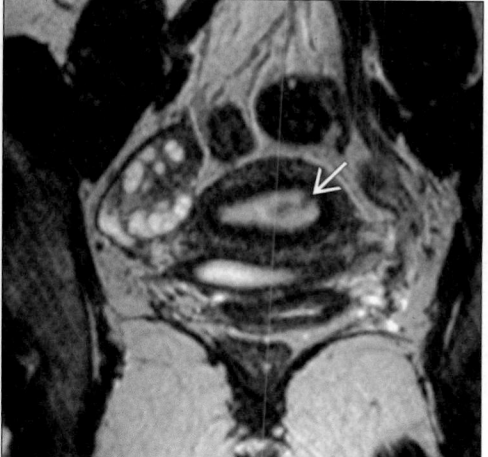

(Left) Coronal T2WI MR shows a mass ➡ in the endometrial cavity of lower signal than the normal endometrium ➡. (Right) T2WI MR image slightly more anterior shows the typical appearance of the fibrovascular stalk as a serpiginous low signal structure ➡ within the endometrial cavity.

Variant

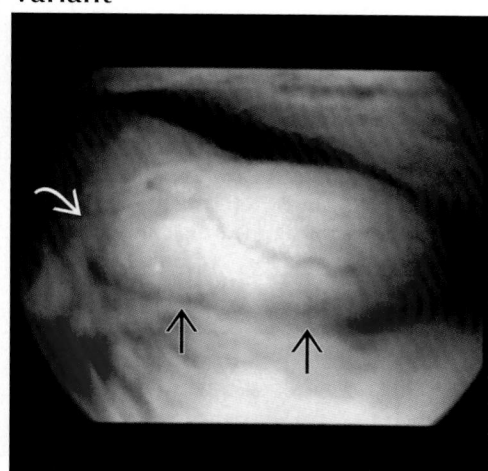
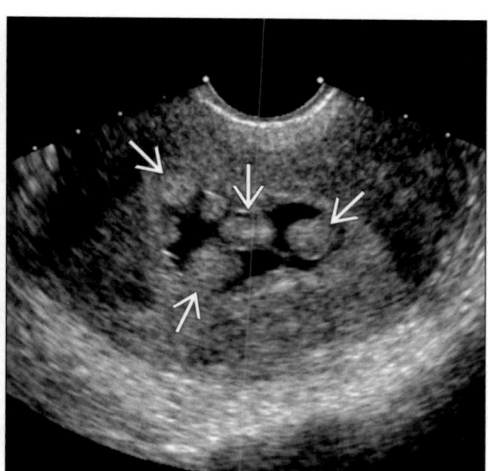

(Left) Clinical photograph through a hysteroscope shows the typical appearance of an oval ➡ endometrial polyp protruding into the uterine cavity. There is a broad-based attachment ➡ to the uterus. (Right) Transverse transvaginal ultrasound during sonohysterography shows multiple polyps ➡ throughout the cavity. Six can be seen in a single scan plane.

Typical

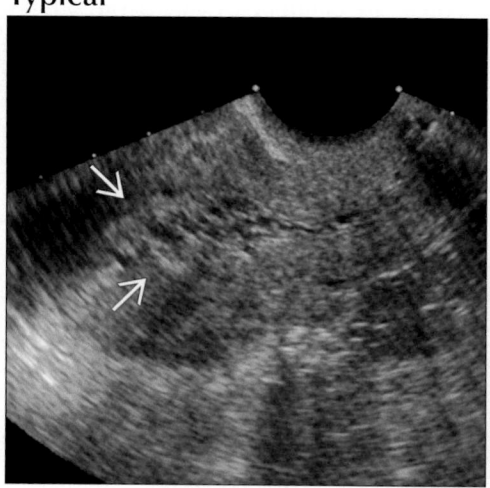
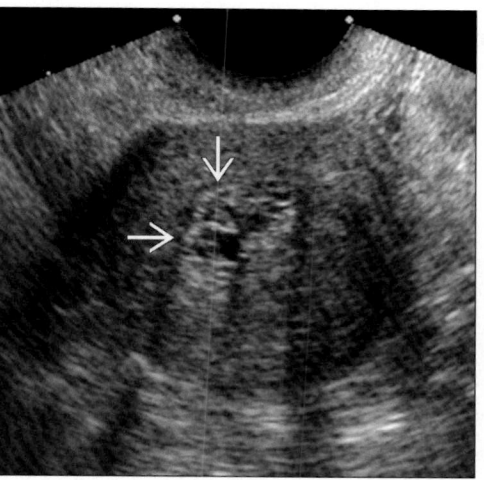

(Left) Longitudinal transvaginal ultrasound shows an area of irregular endometrial thickening ➡ with cystic changes in a postmenopausal patient on Tamoxifen for breast cancer. (Right) Transverse transvaginal ultrasound shows the echogenic line sign ➡ surrounding part of an endometrial mass. Hysteroscopic biopsy showed a benign endometrial polyp. Biopsy is mandatory as carcinoma cannot be excluded by imaging alone.

ENDOMETRIAL HYPERPLASIA

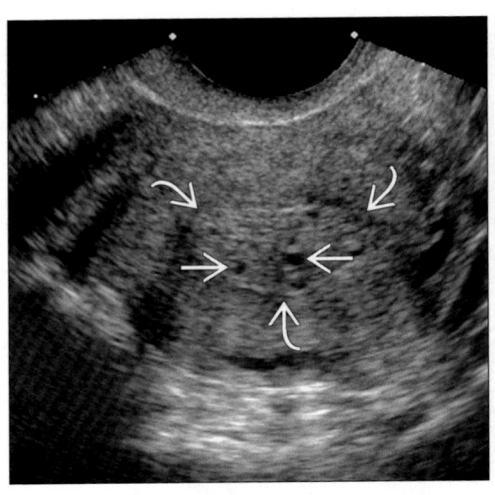

Transverse ultrasound shows cystic areas ➡ within thickened endometrium ➡. Imaging alone cannot always differentiate between hyperplasia, polyp and carcinoma.

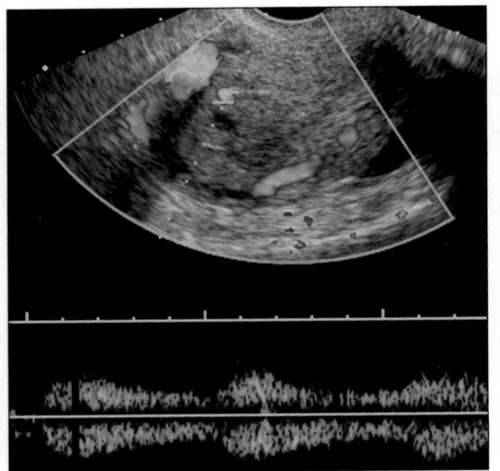

Color Doppler ultrasound (same case as previous image) shows low resistance arterial flow at endometrial myometrial interface but no "stalk". D&C revealed endometrial hyperplasia without atypia.

TERMINOLOGY

Definitions
- Proliferation of endometrial glands

IMAGING FINDINGS

General Features
- Best diagnostic clue: Thickened endometrial echo complex

Imaging Recommendations
- Best imaging tool: Transvaginal sonography: If inadequate consider sonohysterography (SHSG)

DIFFERENTIAL DIAGNOSIS

Endometrial Carcinoma
- Cannot differentiate carcinoma/hyperplasia on basis of imaging findings alone

Endometrial Polyps
- More likely circumscribed oval mass with feeding vessel in stalk

Cystic Endometrial Atrophy
- Pathologic diagnosis: Cannot differentiate from hyperplasia on basis of imaging findings alone

PATHOLOGY

General Features
- Etiology
  - Unopposed estrogen exposure e.g., hormone replacement therapy (HRT)
    - Addition of progestins ↓ decreases risk, most effective as monthly sequential regimen
  - Tamoxifen: Polyps are commonest side effect, often associated with malignancy

Microscopic Features
- Irregular non invasive proliferation of glands with variable amount of stroma

---

DDx: Endometrial Thickening

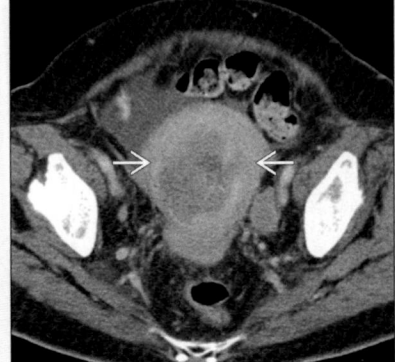

Endometrial Cancer

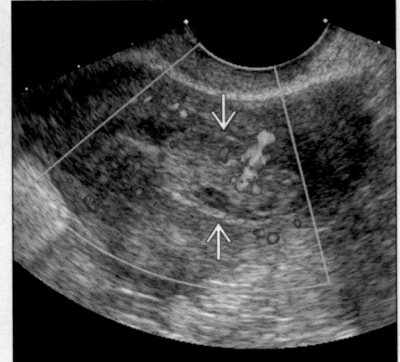

Endometrial Cancer

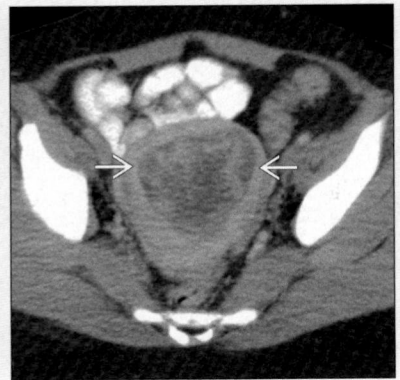

Invasive Mole

ENDOMETRIAL HYPERPLASIA

Key Facts

Top Differential Diagnoses
- Endometrial Carcinoma
- Endometrial Polyps
- Cystic Endometrial Atrophy

Clinical Issues
- Most common signs/symptoms: Menorrhagia or postmenopausal bleeding or unscheduled bleeding on hormone replacement therapy

- Without atypia: > 80% respond to Progestin therapy, < 2% risk of endometrial cancer
- With atypia: < 50% respond to Progestin therapy, 25% risk of endometrial cancer
- Thick endometrium requires biopsy to establish tissue diagnosis

Diagnostic Checklist
- Measure endometrial thickness on sagittal section of uterus

---

- If glandular atypia present ⇒ ↑ risk of developing endometrial cancer ⇒ hysterectomy recommended

CLINICAL ISSUES

Presentation
- Most common signs/symptoms: Menorrhagia or postmenopausal bleeding or unscheduled bleeding on hormone replacement therapy

Natural History & Prognosis
- Without atypia: > 80% respond to Progestin therapy, < 2% risk of endometrial cancer
- With atypia: < 50% respond to Progestin therapy, 25% risk of endometrial cancer

Treatment
- Thick endometrium requires biopsy to establish tissue diagnosis
  - With atypia → hysterectomy
    - If younger patients refuse/wish to preserve fertility → progestin therapy with endometrial biopsy every 3 months
    - Once child bearing complete consider hysterectomy
  - Without atypia → progestin therapy with biopsy every 3-6 months
    - Continue for 12 months after normal biopsy with annual biopsies thereafter
    - If patient > 50 yrs may consider hysterectomy as definitive therapy

DIAGNOSTIC CHECKLIST

Consider
- Women taking Tamoxifen are at increased risk for endometrial hyperplasia/cancer
  - Any abnormal bleeding in this population merits aggressive evaluation
- Presence of endometrial cells on Papanicolaou smear in postmenopausal women not on HRT merits biopsy
  - 19% incidence of hyperplasia or cancer in one study

Image Interpretation Pearls
- Endometrial cancer/hyperplasia occur with unopposed estrogen exposure
  - Unexpected ovarian neoplasm e.g., granulosa cell tumor may be source of excess estrogen
- Measure endometrial thickness on sagittal section of uterus
  - Calipers perpendicular to long axis of cavity, do not include subendometrial hypoechoic zone

SELECTED REFERENCES

1. Mazur MT: Endometrial hyperplasia/adenocarcinoma. a conventional approach. Ann Diagn Pathol. 9(3):174-81, 2005
2. Cohen I: Endometrial pathologies associated with postmenopausal tamoxifen treatment. Gynecol Oncol. 94(2):256-66, 2004
3. Montgomery BE et al: Endometrial hyperplasia: a review. Obstet Gynecol Surv. 59(5):368-78, 2004

IMAGE GALLERY

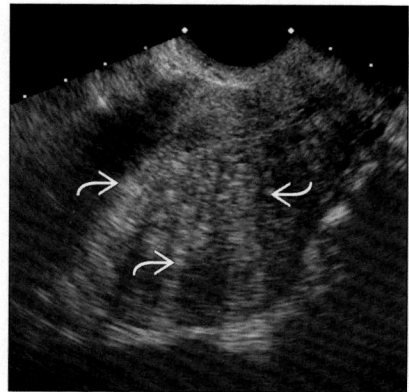 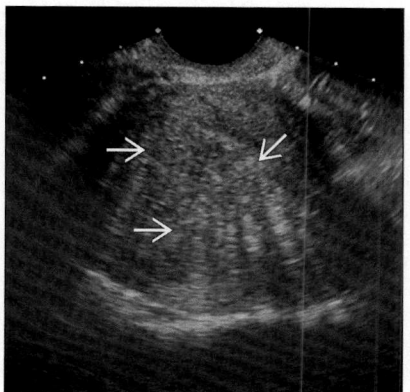 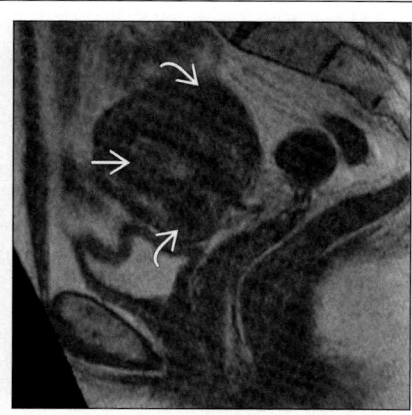

(Left) Longitudinal transvaginal ultrasound shows irregular endometrial thickening ➡. *(Center)* Transverse transvaginal ultrasound (same case as previous image) shows marked heterogeneity of the endometrium ➡. Measurement of the endometrial stripe fails in 5-10% of patients. Biopsy showed only benign hyperplasia. *(Right)* Longitudinal T2WI MR shows endometrial thickening ➡ and fibroids ➡. Fibroids prevented adequate sonographic evaluation of the endometrium and the patient refused SHSG therefore MR was performed. Biopsy: Hyperplasia, no atypia.

ENDOMETRIAL CARCINOMA

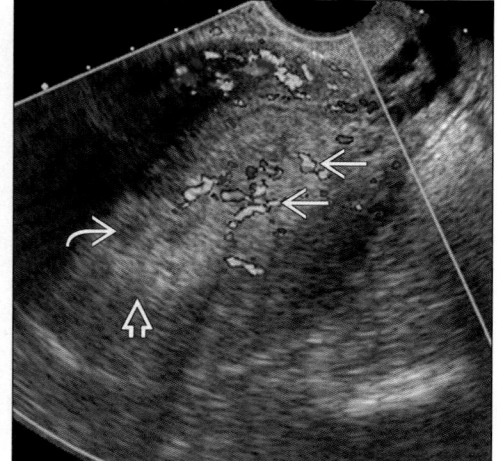

Longitudinal ultrasound shows thick echogenic endometrium ➤ with an irregular endometrial myometrial interface ➤. The patient presented with severe menorrhagia and had two benign biopsies.

Corresponding color Doppler shows abnormal vascularity ➤, hypoechoic endometrial areas ➤ and irregular endometrial myometrial interface ➤ all suspicious for cancer (surgically confirmed).

TERMINOLOGY

Abbreviations and Synonyms
- Endometrial cancer (EC)

Definitions
- Malignant proliferation of abnormal endometrial glands with abnormal gland to gland relationship
  - Atypical irregular glands with multiple lumens
  - Reduced stroma → "back to back" appearance of glands

IMAGING FINDINGS

General Features
- Best diagnostic clue
  - Irregularly thickened endometrial echo complex
    - > 5 mm bilayer thickness in postmenopausal patient → biopsy

Ultrasonographic Findings
- Grayscale Ultrasound
  - Thickened endometrium

- Focal thickening more concerning than diffuse
  - Areas of mixed echogenicity within endometrial thickening more suspicious than homogeneous hyperechogenicity
  - Irregular endometrial myometrial interface
- Power Doppler
  - Increased vascularity within endometrium
  - Irregularly branching vessels
    - Single vessel more likely in fibrovascular stalk of polyp
  - Pulsatility index < 1.5, resistive index < 0.7

Imaging Recommendations
- Best imaging tool
  - Transvaginal ultrasound for detection
  - Contrast-enhanced MR for staging/local extent
- Protocol advice
  - Must see entire endometrial stripe
    - Measure on sagittal section of uterus at widest point
    - Do not include hypoechoic inner myometrium in measurement

DDx: Imaging Findings Associated with Abnormal Bleeding

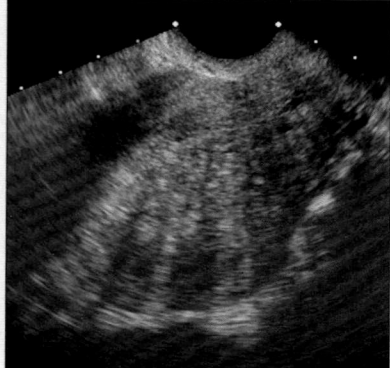

Endometrial Hyperplasia

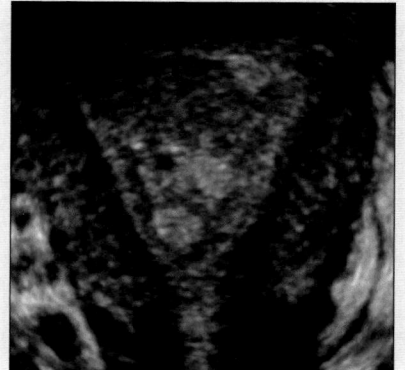

Endometrial Polyps

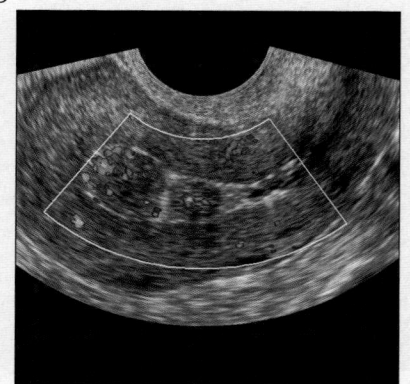

Submucosal Fibroids

ENDOMETRIAL CARCINOMA

Key Facts

Imaging Findings
- Irregularly thickened endometrial echo complex
- Focal thickening more concerning than diffuse
- Areas of mixed echogenicity within endometrial thickening more suspicious than homogeneous hyperechogenicity
- Irregular endometrial myometrial interface
- Increased vascularity within endometrium
- Transvaginal ultrasound for detection
- Contrast-enhanced MR for staging/local extent
- Must see entire endometrial stripe
- Measure on sagittal section of uterus at widest point
- Do not include hypoechoic inner myometrium in measurement
- If inadequate TV US → additional evaluation with sonohysterography (SHSG) or MR

- SHSG distends cavity → shows whether endometrial thickening is focal or diffuse
- In premenopausal women with thick echogenic endometrial stripe
- > 15 mm → SHSG to determine most appropriate type of biopsy
- 11-15 mm → re-image after menstrual period, if persistent abnormal thickness > 15 mm → SHSG/biopsy
- In postmenopausal women bilayer thickness > 5 mm merits biopsy

Top Differential Diagnoses
- Endometrial Hyperplasia
- Endometrial Polyp
- Adenomyosis

- If fluid in endometrial cavity measure each layer separately and report sum, do not include fluid component
- If inadequate TV US → additional evaluation with sonohysterography (SHSG) or MR
  - 5-10% studies are inadequate
- SHSG distends cavity → shows whether endometrial thickening is focal or diffuse
  - Diffuse thickening: "Blind" office biopsy or D&C
  - Focal thickening: Hysteroscopic biopsy necessary to ensure sampling of abnormal area
- In premenopausal women with thick echogenic endometrial stripe
  - > 15 mm → SHSG to determine most appropriate type of biopsy
  - 11-15 mm → re-image after menstrual period, if persistent abnormal thickness > 15 mm → SHSG/biopsy
- In postmenopausal women bilayer thickness > 5 mm merits biopsy
  - SHSG again useful in triage: Blind office biopsy versus hysteroscopic biopsy in operating room

DIFFERENTIAL DIAGNOSIS

Endometrial Hyperplasia
- Imaging cannot differentiate hyperplasia from cancer
- More likely homogeneous thickening than mixed echogenicity

Endometrial Polyp
- More likely to be oval or fusiform mass than diffuse thickening
- Look for single feeding vessel in fibrovascular stalk

Submucosal Fibroids
- Hypoechoic mass/masses in cavity
- Masses arise from myometrium
- SHSG: "Rind" of endometrium covers fibroid surface

Adenomyosis
- Process based in myometrium

- Bulky uterus with areas of acoustic shadowing
- Myometrial/subendometrial cysts

PATHOLOGY

General Features
- Genetics
  - p53 suppressor gene associated with recurrent disease
    - More common in African-American women, may partly explain poorer outcome
  - PTEN mutation more common in Caucasian women, associated with better outcomes
- Etiology
  - Risk factors
    - Nulliparity/low parity
    - Obesity
    - Hypertension
    - Diabetes
    - Polycystic ovarian syndrome: Controversial causative association versus occurrence of two diseases with similar risk factors
    - Hereditary nonpolyposis colorectal cancer syndrome (HNPCC)
    - Prior pelvic radiation
  - Atypical hyperplasia
    - Confers 25% risk of developing endometrial cancer
    - Hyperplasia without atypia → 2% risk
  - Unopposed estrogen exposure
    - Tamoxifen
    - Estrogen secreting tumors
    - Hormone replacement therapy with estrogen without progestins
- Epidemiology
  - Most common gynecologic malignancy
    - 75% postmenopausal
    - 25% premenopausal
  - 4th most common cancer in women
  - Western affluent societies, least common in India/southeast Asia

ENDOMETRIAL CARCINOMA

Microscopic Features
- Majority are adenocarcinoma
- Serous (papillary serous), clear cell types also occur
  - Tend to be in older patients
  - More aggressive behavior
  - Serous type invades lymphovascular spaces →
    metastasizes without invasion of deep myometrium

Staging, Grading or Classification Criteria
- Stage I: Confined to uterus
- Stage II: Spread to involve cervix but not beyond
  uterus
- Stage III: Spread beyond uterus confined to true pelvis
- Stage IV: Disseminated metastases or bladder/bowel
  involvement

CLINICAL ISSUES

Presentation
- Most common signs/symptoms
  - Abnormal bleeding in 90%
    - Postmenopausal bleeding
    - Menometrorrhagia
- Other signs/symptoms: Endometrial cells on
  Papanicolaou smear

Demographics
- Age: Most common in 50-65 yr old age group

Natural History & Prognosis
- Depends on stage at diagnosis
  - Stage I or II: 5 yr survival 96%
  - Stage III: 5 yr survival 63%
  - Stage IV: 5 yr survival 8%
- African-American woman tend to have worse outcome
  than Caucasian women
  - Mortality rates 1.8 times greater
  - Tend to be higher stage at diagnosis
  - Tend to have more aggressive types (papillary
    serous, clear cell)
  - p53 suppressor gene in 34% African-American versus
    11% Caucasian women with stage I EC in one series
    - p53 confers worse prognosis/increased recurrence
      risk

Treatment
- Stage dependent
  - Stage I or II: Surgical ± radiation therapy (XRT)
  - Stage III: Customized to patient/extent of
    parametrial disease
    - Usually combined surgery, XRT
  - Stage IV: Customized to patient
    - Combination of surgery, chemotherapy, XRT
- Surgery
  - Hysterectomy, bilateral salpingo-oophorectomy,
    lymphadenectomy
  - Surgical staging vital as imaging misses microscopic
    disease

DIAGNOSTIC CHECKLIST

Consider
- Endometrial cancer is the most serious cause of PMB
  - 10% of women with PMB will have endometrial
    cancer
  - Other etiologies include hyperplasia, polyps,
    atrophy or fibroids
- TV US is a good test to detect EC
  - Use of 5 mm bilayer thickness as threshold for
    intervention will detect 96% of EC
  - Safe to use TV US as initial diagnostic test
    - Better tolerated than endometrial biopsy
  - Normal appearing endometrium with bilayer
    thickness < 5 mm
    - Negative test for endometrial cancer
    - Obviates need for additional testing in patient
      with PMB and non-diagnostic office biopsy

Image Interpretation Pearls
- Imaging alone cannot differentiate hyperplasia from
  carcinoma
- Cancer may arise within an endometrial polyp

SELECTED REFERENCES

1. Barwick TD et al: Imaging of endometrial adenocarcinoma.
   Clin Radiol. 61(7):545-55, 2006
2. Kirby TO et al: Surgical staging in endometrial cancer.
   Oncology (Williston Park). 20(1):45-50; discussion 50,
   53-4, 63, 2006
3. Kumar R et al: Positron emission tomography in
   gynecological malignancies. Expert Rev Anticancer Ther.
   6(7):1033-44, 2006
4. Messiou C et al: MR staging of endometrial carcinoma.
   Clin Radiol. 61(10):822-32, 2006
5. Rackow BW et al: Endometrial cancer and fertility. Curr
   Opin Obstet Gynecol. 18(3):245-52, 2006
6. Takeuchi M et al: Malignant transformation of pelvic
   endometriosis: MR imaging findings and pathologic
   correlation. Radiographics. 26(2):407-17, 2006
7. Barranger E et al: Lymphatic mapping for gynecologic
   malignancies. Semin Oncol. 31(3):394-402, 2004
8. Moodley M et al: Clinical pathway for the evaluation of
   postmenopausal bleeding with an emphasis on
   endometrial cancer detection. J Obstet Gynaecol.
   24(7):736-41, 2004
9. Tjalma WA et al: The clinical value and the
   cost-effectiveness of follow-up in endometrial cancer
   patients. Int J Gynecol Cancer. 14(5):931-7, 2004
10. McMeekin DS et al: Endometrial cancer: treatment of nodal
    metastases. Curr Treat Options Oncol. 4(2):121-30, 2003
11. Ascher SM et al: Imaging of cancer of the endometrium.
    Radiol Clin North Am. 40(3):563-76, 2002
12. Sugimura K et al: Postsurgical pelvis: treatment follow-up.
    Radiol Clin North Am. 40(3):659-80, viii, 2002

ENDOMETRIAL CARCINOMA

IMAGE GALLERY

Typical

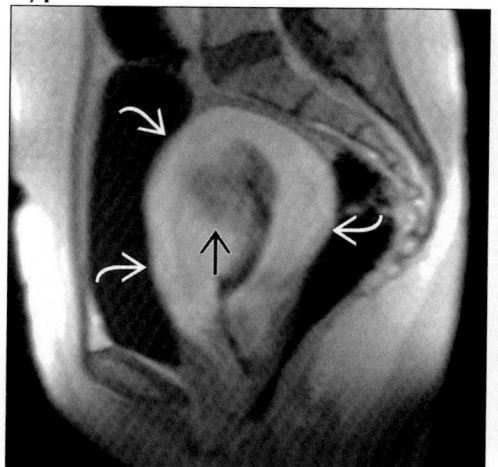

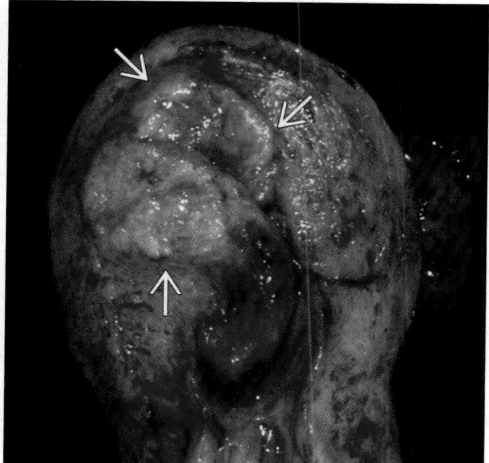

(Left) Longitudinal T1 C+ MR shows endometrial cancer ⇨ invading the myometrium. The tumor enhances less than the surrounding myometrium ⇨. *(Right)* Gross pathology (same patient as previous case) shows endometrial cancer ⇨ invading through more than 50% of the myometrium i.e., stage 1c disease.

Typical

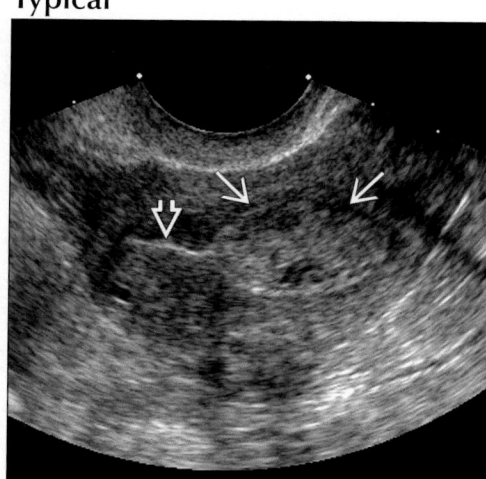

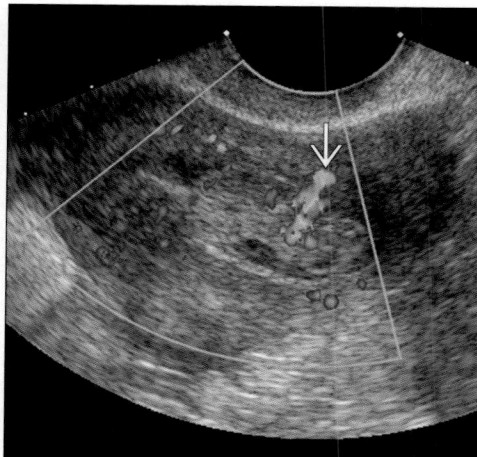

(Left) Transverse transvaginal ultrasound shows an inhomogeneous polypoid mass ⇨ within the endometrial cavity. The normal line of endometrial apposition ⇨ is displaced by the mass indicating that it is within the endometrial cavity. *(Right)* Oblique color Doppler ultrasound shows a prominent vessel ⇨ within the thick area of endometrium. This was thought to be an endometrial polyp but cancer was found at hysteroscopic biopsy.

Typical

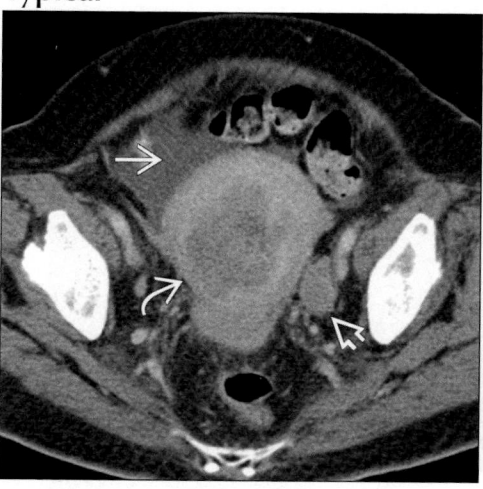

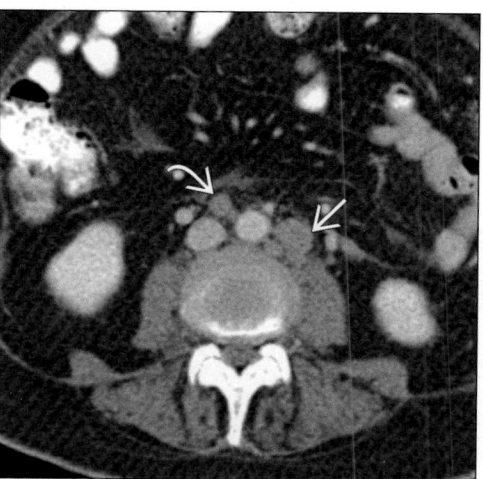

(Left) Transverse CECT shows ascites ⇨, iliac adenopathy ⇨ and an irregular mass ⇨ in the endometrium which invades the myometrium. *(Right)* Transverse CECT in the same patient as previous image shows para-aortic ⇨ and inter-aortocaval ⇨ adenopathy consistent with stage 4 endometrial carcinoma.

ENDOMETRITIS

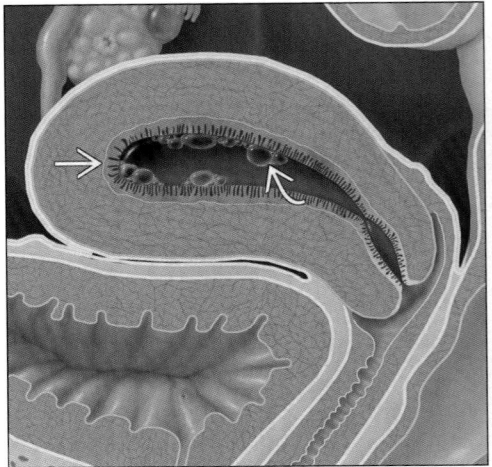

Graphic shows findings in endometritis including hyperemia of the endometrium ➡, with associated fluid and gas bubbles ➡ in the endometrial cavity.

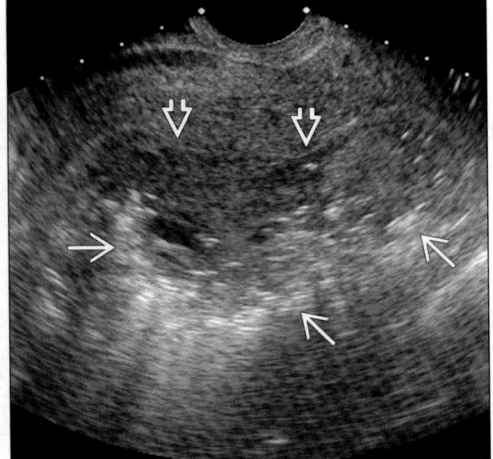

Transverse transvaginal ultrasound shows severe endometritis with pyometrium. The endometrial cavity is distended with echogenic fluid/debris ➡. Multiple echogenic gas bubbles ➡ are seen within this fluid.

TERMINOLOGY

Definitions
- Infection of endometrium is generally caused by ascending infection of organisms through cervix or incision site into uterus
  - May extend to involve myometrium and parametrium
- Endometritis occurs in two clinical settings
  - Fever and pain in postpartum period (most common)
  - Associated with pelvic inflammatory disease (PID) in nonobstetric patient

IMAGING FINDINGS

General Features
- Best diagnostic clue: Endometrial gas and fluid in a patient with postpartum fever and pelvic pain
- Primarily a clinical diagnosis
  - Often no imaging findings in uncomplicated endometritis
  - Primary role of imaging is to evaluate for complications

Ultrasonographic Findings
- Pain may limit ability to perform transvaginal examination
- Endometrium may appear normal
- Findings often nonspecific
  - Thickened, heterogeneous endometrium
  - Endometrial fluid
  - Fluid in cul-de-sac
- Hyperechoic foci within endometrial cavity ± shadowing
  - Intracavitary gas, inflammatory debris
    - Gas bubbles alone are not diagnostic
    - Endometrial gas is seen in up to 21% of healthy patients in postpartum period
  - Large amount of echogenic fluid suspicious for pyometra
- Color Doppler
  - May see increased flow, but not always present
  - Lack of ↑ flow does not rule out endometritis
- Findings overlap with retained products of conception (RPOC)

DDx: Endometritis

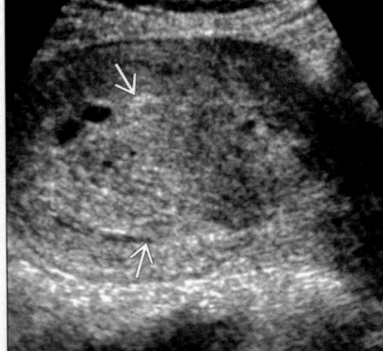

Retained Products of Conception

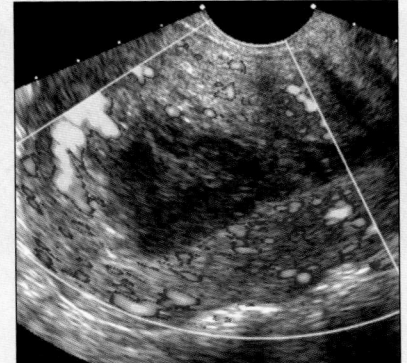

Blood Clot

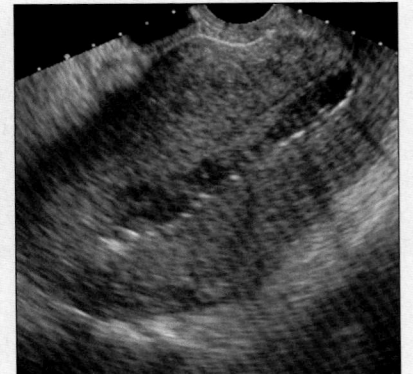

Postpartum Gas

ENDOMETRITIS

Key Facts

Imaging Findings

- Often no imaging findings in uncomplicated endometritis
- Pain may limit ability to perform transvaginal examination
- Gas bubbles alone are not diagnostic
- Endometrial gas is seen in up to 21% of healthy patients in postpartum period
- May see increased flow, but not always present
- Findings overlap with retained products of conception (RPOC)
- Patients may have both RPOC and endometritis

Top Differential Diagnoses

- Retained Products of Conception
- Intrauterine Blood/Clot
- Asymptomatic Postpartum Endometrial Gas

Pathology

- Most common cause of postpartum fever
- Occurs in 1-3% of vaginal deliveries
- Much more common following cesarian section (15-20%)
- 70-90% of patients with PID have coexistent endometritis
- Both infectious and non-infectious endometritis reported in 0.5% of cases after uterine artery embolization

Diagnostic Checklist

- Endometritis is predominantly a clinical diagnosis
- In the appropriate clinical setting (postpartum fever and pain), presence of endometrial fluid and bubbles is highly suggestive of endometritis

---

  - ○ RPOC is a risk factor for developing endometritis
  - ○ Patients may have both RPOC and endometritis
- If associated with PID, may see tubo-ovarian abscess

CT Findings

- Nonspecific, most useful for complications (abscess) or alternative diagnosis
- Uterine enlargement, heterogeneous density
- Distended endometrial cavity
  - ○ May see air-fluid or fluid-fluid level (pus, hematoma)
- Inflammatory changes around uterus better seen than with ultrasound

MR Findings

- T1WI: Low signal uterus and endometrial fluid
- T2WI: Myometrium increased in signal intensity with loss of junctional zone
- Intense enhancement with gadolinium

Imaging Recommendations

- Best imaging tool: Transvaginal ultrasound
- Protocol advice
  - ○ Always use color Doppler to evaluate for possible RPOC
  - ○ Thorough scan of adnexa to look for parametrial or tubo-ovarian abscess

DIFFERENTIAL DIAGNOSIS

Retained Products of Conception

- Echogenic endometrial mass
- Significant overlap in findings with endometritis
- High-velocity, low-resistance flow
  - ○ Not always present
- Presents with postpartum bleeding
  - ○ Simple RPOC should not have fever, ↑ white count
- May have RPOC with superimposed infection

Intrauterine Blood/Clot

- Seen in up to 24% of asymptomatic postpartum patients
- May also be seen with endometritis
- Should not have fever, ↑ white count

- Changes rapidly with resolution on follow-up scans

Asymptomatic Postpartum Endometrial Gas

- Seen in up to 21% of healthy patients in postpartum period
- May be present up to 3 weeks postpartum
- Should not have fever, ↑ white count

Endometrial Calcifications

- Incidental finding in asymptomatic patient
- Curvilinear calcifications along endometrium
- Often history of prior instrumentation (dilatation and curettage)

Other Causes of Postpartum Fever

- Ovarian vein thrombosis
- Atelectasis
- Pneumonia
- Pyelonephritis
- Appendicitis

PATHOLOGY

General Features

- Etiology
  - ○ Ascending infection of vaginal/cervical flora
  - ○ May progress from chorioamnionitis
  - ○ Monomicrobial infection, group B Streptococcus
    - ■ Occurs in first 24-36 hrs
  - ○ Polymicrobial, both aerobic and anaerobic
    - ■ Occurs in first 48 hrs
  - ○ Most infections are polymicrobial
    - ■ Etiologic agent(s) often never identified
  - ○ Common causative agents
    - ■ Vaginal flora including those associated with bacterial vaginosis
    - ■ Neisseria gonorrhoeae
    - ■ Enterococcus
    - ■ Chlamydia and tuberculosis often seen in chronic endometritis
- Epidemiology
  - ○ Most common cause of postpartum fever

ENDOMETRITIS

- ○ Occurs in 1-3% of vaginal deliveries
- ○ Much more common following cesarian section (15-20%)
  - ▪ Prophylactic antibiotics highly effective in reducing risk of endometritis after cesarian section
  - ▪ 50-60% of women undergoing cesarian section without antibiotics will develop endometritis
- ○ Risk factors in obstetric patients
  - ▪ Cesarian section
  - ▪ Preexisting lower genital tract infection
  - ▪ Prolonged labor
  - ▪ Prolonged rupture of membranes
  - ▪ RPOC
  - ▪ Retained clots
- ○ Risk factors in nonobstetric patients
  - ▪ 70-90% of patients with PID have coexistent endometritis
  - ▪ May also occur after invasive gynecologic procedure
  - ▪ Intrauterine device
- ○ Uterine artery embolization
  - ▪ Both infectious and non-infectious endometritis reported in 0.5% of cases after uterine artery embolization
- ○ Chronic endometritis may occur
  - ▪ Associated with RPOC in obstetric population
  - ▪ In nonobstetric population associated with intrauterine device

CLINICAL ISSUES

Presentation

- • Most common signs/symptoms
  - ○ Fever (> 100.4° F) within 36 hours following delivery
  - ○ Pelvic/abdominal pain
  - ○ Uterine tenderness on physical exam and during ultrasound
  - ○ ↑ White blood cell count
- • Other signs/symptoms
  - ○ Malodorous lochia
  - ○ Vaginal bleeding
  - ○ Vaginal discharge
  - ○ Tachycardia

Natural History & Prognosis

- • Cure rates approach 95% with appropriate therapy
- • May extend to myometrium/parametrium if untreated or if caused by drug-resistant organisms
  - ○ Potential complications include pyometrium and pelvic abscess

Treatment

- • Parenteral broad spectrum antibiotics
  - ○ 90-95% defervesce with 48-72 hrs
  - ○ Therapy continued until patient afebrile for 24-48 hrs and white blood cell count returns to normal
- • Persistent fever
  - ○ Resistant organism ⇒ triple antibiotic therapy
  - ○ Abscess ⇒ surgical or percutaneous drainage

DIAGNOSTIC CHECKLIST

Consider

- • Endometritis is predominantly a clinical diagnosis
  - ○ Imaging findings frequently normal in uncomplicated endometritis
- • Imaging usually ordered to look for complications
  - ○ Pyometrium
  - ○ Abscess
  - ○ RPOC

Image Interpretation Pearls

- • In the appropriate clinical setting (postpartum fever and pain), presence of endometrial fluid and bubbles is highly suggestive of endometritis
- • Conversely, endometrial gas in an asymptomatic postpartum patient is likely normal

SELECTED REFERENCES

1. Faro S: Postpartum endometritis. Clin Perinatol. 32(3):803-14, 2005
2. Kitamura Y et al: Imaging manifestations of complications associated with uterine artery embolization. Radiographics. 25 Suppl 1:S119-32, 2005
3. Gibbs RS et al: Maternal and fetal infectious disorders. In: Maternal-Fetal Medicine Principles and Practice, 9th ed. Saunders, Philadelphia. 749-50, 2004
4. Ledger WJ: Post-partum endomyometritis diagnosis and treatment: a review. J Obstet Gynaecol Res. 29(6):364-73, 2003
5. Savelli L et al: Transvaginal sonographic appearance of anaerobic endometritis. Ultrasound Obstet Gynecol. 21(6):624-5, 2003
6. Eckert LO et al: Endometritis: the clinical-pathologic syndrome. Am J Obstet Gynecol. 186(4):690-5, 2002
7. Nalaboff KM et al: Imaging the endometrium: disease and normal variants. Radiographics. 21(6):1409-24, 2001
8. Wachsberg RH et al: Real-time ultrasonographic analysis of the normal postpartum uterus: technique, variability, and measurements. J Ultrasound Med. 13(3):215-21, 1994
9. Lev-Toaff AS et al: Diagnostic imaging in puerperal febrile morbidity. Obstet Gynecol. 78(1):50-5, 1991

SYNECHIAE

Key Facts

Terminology
- Asherman syndrome: More severe form of adhesions with partial or complete obliteration of endometrial cavity
- Clinical symptoms include hypo- or amenorrhea, infertility and recurrent pregnancy loss

Imaging Findings
- Best diagnostic clue: Fixed fibrous strands or nondistensible endometrial cavity during sonohysterography (SHG)
- Difficult diagnosis to make unless endometrial cavity distended by fluid
- Adhesions have variable appearance based on severity
- Thin, undulating membranes
- Thick, adhesive bands which may obliterate large areas of endometrial cavity and prevent distention

- Patients may experience pain during saline injection due to poor distensibility of cavity

Top Differential Diagnoses
- Uterine Septum
- Endometrial Polyp

Pathology
- Most often from prior dilatation and curettage (D&C)
- Present in 68% of women with infertility who have had two or more D&Cs
- Seen in 0.5% of routine pregnancies

Clinical Issues
- After hysteroscopic treatment of severe Asherman syndrome, half of patients will become pregnant and a third have live births

---

- Straight, bulbous free edge with thinner sheet extending to endometrial surface
  - Hypoechoic central area (synechiae) between more hyperechoic layers (fetal membranes)
- Y-shaped notch at endometrial base, created by membranes separating at endometrial margin
- Placenta can abut or even wrap around synechia
  - May be seen in up to 2/3 of cases
- Fetus moves freely around sheet
- Color Doppler may demonstrate flow in membranes around synechiae
  - Differentiates from amniotic band, which has no flow

MR Findings
- T2WI best sequence
  - Low signal intensity band bridging normal, high signal endometrium
  - Loss of normal, high signal endometrium in severe cases

Fluoroscopic Findings
- Hysterosalpingography
  - Injection of endometrial cavity with iodinated contrast
  - Adhesions appear as irregular, intracavitary filling defects
  - Better evaluation of tubal patency than SHG

Imaging Recommendations
- Best imaging tool: SHG
- Protocol advice
  - Purge all bubbles from system before injection
    - May cause confusing filling defects
  - Make sure balloon is well positioned before injection
    - An incomplete seal may allow leaking with non-distention of endometrial cavity
  - Patients may experience pain during saline injection due to poor distensibility of cavity

---

DIFFERENTIAL DIAGNOSIS

Uterine Septum
- Midline, fundal
- May be fibrous or composed of myometrium
- Thicker than synechiae
- Two distinct endometrial cavities

Endometrial Polyp
- Polypoid mass protrudes into endometrial cavity
- Does not extend between uterine walls
- More hyperechoic than synechiae
- Feeding vessel on color Doppler

Endometrial Blood Clot
- Variable morphology
- Appearance changes during SHG

Intrauterine Bands in Pregnancy
- **Amniotic bands**
  - Disruption of amnion
  - Fetus becomes entrapped ⇒ constrictions, amputations, "slash" defects
  - Bands are thinner than synechiae
    - Often difficult to see
  - Do not attach to both uterine walls
- **Circumvallate placenta**
  - Margin of placenta is elevated off uterine wall
  - Creates a "marginal shelf" when scanning parallel to edge
    - Scanning perpendicularly shows "curled lip" of placental margin
- **Chorioamnionic separation**
  - Amnion forms sac around fetus
    - Does not go wall-to-wall
  - Normally fuses 12-14 weeks
  - Delayed fusion associated with aneuploidy
    - Trisomy 21 most common
- **Twins**
  - 2 fetuses
  - Dichorionic, diamniotic ⇒ thick membrane
  - Monochorionic, diamniotic ⇒ thin membrane

SYNECHIAE

PATHOLOGY

General Features
- Etiology
  - Instrumentation, trauma or infection causing destruction of basalis layer of endometrium
    - Adhesions form between opposing uterine walls
  - Most often from prior dilatation and curettage (D&C)
    - Curettage denudes basalis layer
  - Retained placental/villous elements increase risk of forming adhesions (abortion or postpartum)
    - Promotes fibroblastic proliferation before endometrial regeneration can occur
  - Postpartum uterus predisposed to form adhesions
    - Related to temporary hypoestrogenic state
    - Higher risk if breast feeding (prolonged hypoestrogenic state and delayed endometrial proliferation)
- Epidemiology
  - Present in 5-39% of women with recurrent miscarriages
  - Present in 68% of women with infertility who have had two or more D&Cs
  - Seen in 0.5% of routine pregnancies
- Associated abnormalities
  - Rarely associated with deeply invasive adenomyosis
  - In pregnancy may cause abnormal fetal lie
    - Adhesions oriented perpendicular to placental surface more likely to have abnormal fetal lie

Gross Pathologic & Surgical Features
- Fibrous adhesions and endometrial sclerosis
- Most commonly multiple but may be single
- Variable morphology from thin endometrial strands to thick fibrous bands

CLINICAL ISSUES

Presentation
- Most common signs/symptoms
  - Hypo- or amenorrhea
  - Infertility
  - Recurrent spontaneous abortions
- Other signs/symptoms
  - Dyspareunia
  - Abdominal pain
  - Incidental finding in 2nd trimester ultrasound
    - May no longer be visible in 3rd trimester (compression or rupture of adhesion)

Natural History & Prognosis
- Variable outcomes depending on severity
  - May be asymptomatic and have normal pregnancy
    - Higher incidence of cesarian section for abnormal fetal lie
  - Myometrial adhesions have poor prognosis
    - Need basalis layer for new endometrium to proliferate following adhesiolysis
  - Patient with atrophic endometrium have extremely poor prognosis

- After hysteroscopic treatment of severe Asherman syndrome, half of patients will become pregnant and a third have live births
  - Up to 50% have preterm labor
  - Increased risk of placenta previa and adhesions

Treatment
- Lysis of adhesions for those with infertility
  - Hysteroscopy preferred approach
- Treatment following adhesiolysis
  - Loop intrauterine device placed in uterine cavity
    - Reduces chance of re-adherence of endometrial walls
    - High dose sequential estrogen-progestin treatment to promote re-epithelization of endometrium

DIAGNOSTIC CHECKLIST

Consider
- Suspect diagnosis in patient with secondary hypo- or amenorrhea with prior history of D&C
- Synechiae do not cause fetal structural defects
  - Important to differentiate from other more serious entities such as amniotic bands

SELECTED REFERENCES

1. Fedele L et al: Septums and synechiae: approaches to surgical correction. Clin Obstet Gynecol. 49(4):767-88, 2006
2. Davis PC et al: Sonohysterographic findings of endometrial and subendometrial conditions. Radiographics. 22(4):803-16, 2002
3. Salle B et al: Transvaginal sonohysterographic evaluation of intrauterine adhesions. J Clin Ultrasound. 27(3):131-4, 1999
4. Korbin CD et al: Placental implantation on the amniotic sheet: effect on pregnancy outcome. Radiology. 206(3):773-5, 1998
5. Ball RH et al: Clinical significance of sonographically detected uterine synechiae in pregnant patients. J Ultrasound Med. 16(7):465-9, 1997
6. Fedele L et al: Intrauterine adhesions: detection with transvaginal US. Radiology. 199(3):757-9, 1996
7. Lazebnik N et al: The effect of amniotic sheet orientation on subsequent maternal and fetal complications. Ultrasound Obstet Gynecol. 8(4):267-71, 1996
8. Cullinan JA et al: Sonohysterography: a technique for endometrial evaluation. Radiographics. 15(3):501-14; discussion 515-6, 1995
9. Finberg HJ: Uterine synechiae in pregnancy: expanded criteria for recognition and clinical significance in 28 cases. J Ultrasound Med. 10(10):547-55, 1991

SYNECHIAE

IMAGE GALLERY

Typical

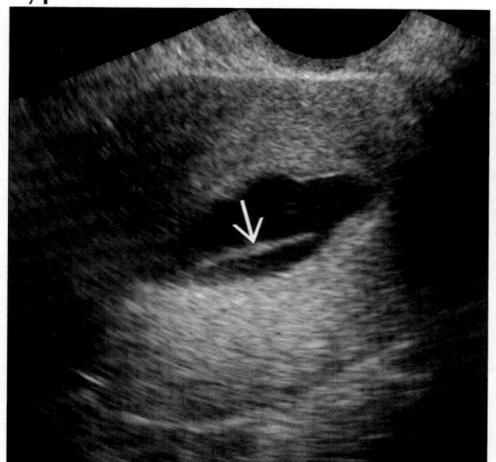 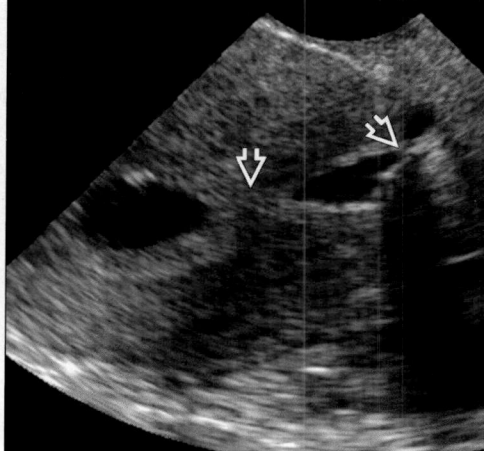

(Left) Longitudinal transvaginal ultrasound during SHG shows a single, undulating adhesion ➡ within the endometrial cavity. Cavity is otherwise normal with good distention. (Right) Longitudinal transvaginal ultrasound from SHG in a patient with severe adhesions shows extensive adherence of uterine walls ⇒. Synechiae can be quite variable in severity.

Typical

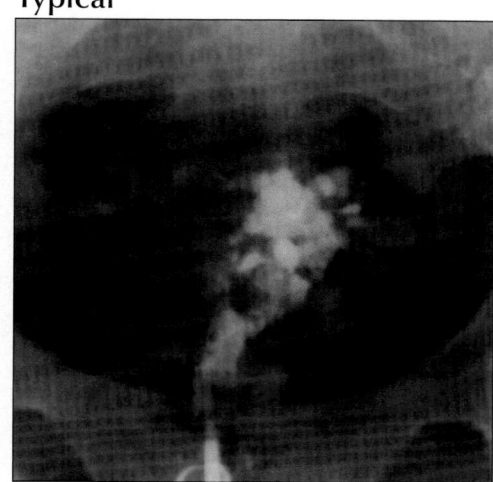 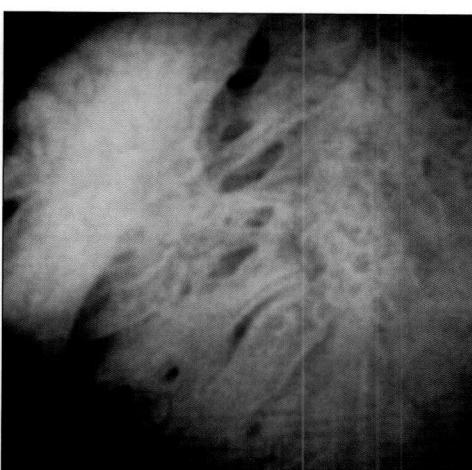

(Left) Spot film from hysterosalpingogram shows multiple irregular filling defects within the endometrial cavity, as well as occlusion of the fallopian tubes. This patient had hypomenorrhea and infertility, classic features of Asherman syndrome. (Right) Hysteroscopic view of uterine synechiae shows fibrous bands extending across the endometrium.

Typical

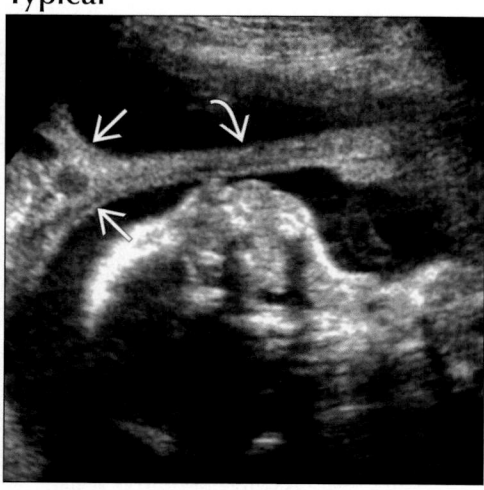 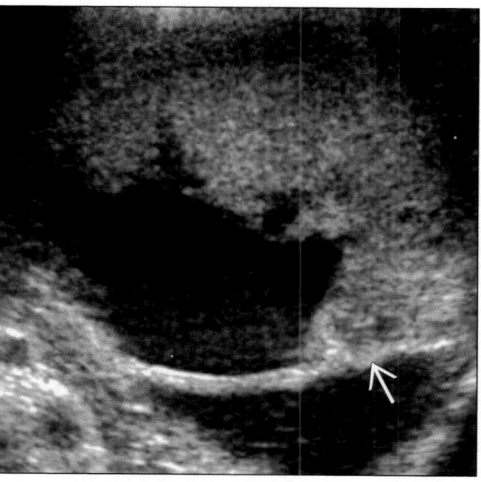

(Left) Ultrasound shows an amniotic sheet ➡, which is caused by fetal membranes wrapping around a synechium. The membranes split at the endometrium, creating a Y-shaped notch ➡. (Right) Ultrasound shows partial implantation of the placenta on a synechium ➡. Synechiae such as these generally have no adverse effect on pregnancy outcome and should not be confused with something more ominous, such as an amniotic band.

ECTOPIC PREGNANCY

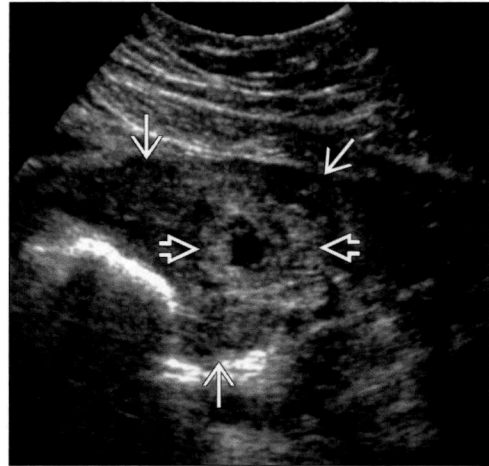

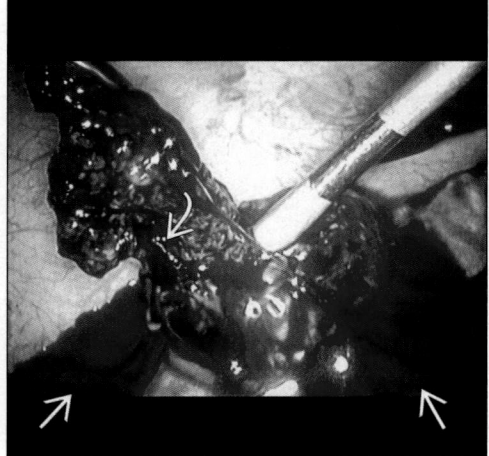

Transverse transvaginal ultrasound shows echogenic blood ⇒ surrounding the echogenic ring ⇒ of an ectopic pregnancy. The presence of a large amount of blood suggests a ruptured tube.

Clinical photograph at the time of laparoscopy shows a ruptured right fallopian tube ⇒ and blood in the peritoneal cavity ➡.

TERMINOLOGY

Abbreviations and Synonyms
- Ectopic pregnancy (EP)
- Tubal pregnancy

Definitions
- Gestation occurring outside of uterus

IMAGING FINDINGS

General Features
- Best diagnostic clue
  - No intrauterine pregnancy (IUP)
  - Tubal mass
  - Echogenic fluid in cul-de-sac (blood)
- Location
  - 95% are tubal
  - 5% are cervical, interstitial, ovarian, abdominal

Ultrasonographic Findings
- Uterine findings
  - Thick echogenic endometrium
    - Decidual reaction
    - Endometrial cysts
  - "Pseudogestational sac" sign
    - Decidual cast of blood
    - No double-decidual sac sign of IUP
  - Heterotopic pregnancy is rare
    - IUP + EP
- Tubal findings in 80-95%
  - Tubal hematoma (40-60%)
    - Heterogeneous mass
  - Tubal ring (50%): Echogenic ring separate from ovary
    - ± Yolk sac ± embryo
  - Tubal ring "lights up" with color Doppler
    - "Ring of fire"
    - May show small EP missed otherwise
  - Pulsed Doppler findings
    - High-velocity, low-resistance flow
    - Systolic velocity > 2-4 kHz frequency shift common for trophoblastic flow
- Ovary findings with tubal ectopic
  - 85% tubal EP on same side as corpus luteum
  - Corpus luteum (CL) appearance is variable
    - Anechoic cyst → complex hemorrhagic cyst

DDx: Adnexal Mass in Pregnancy

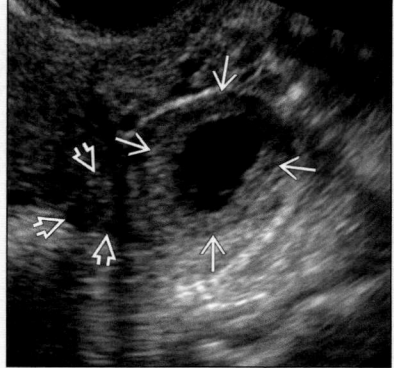

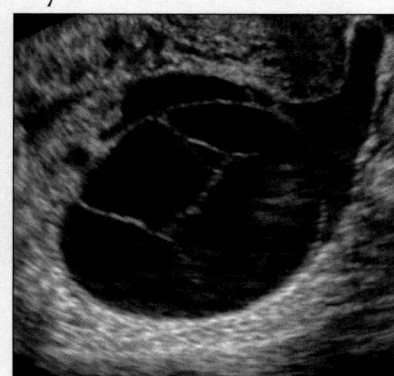

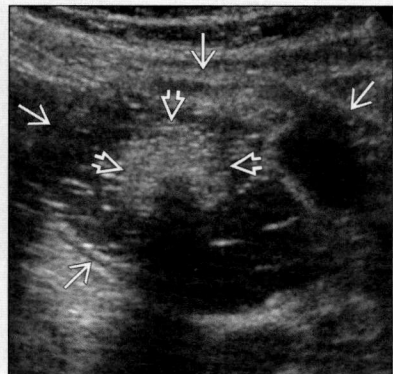

Corpus Luteum

Hemorrhagic Cyst

Dermoid

ECTOPIC PREGNANCY

Key Facts

Terminology
- Gestation occurring outside of uterus

Imaging Findings
- No intrauterine pregnancy (IUP)
- Tubal mass
- Echogenic fluid in cul-de-sac (blood)
- "Pseudogestational sac" sign
- Tubal hematoma (40-60%)
- Tubal ring (50%): Echogenic ring separate from ovary
- Tubal ring "lights up" with color Doppler
- 85% tubal EP on same side as corpus luteum
- Ultrasound completely negative in 5-10% of cases
- 91% of EP accurately diagnosed
- Use endovaginal probe as a palpation tool

Top Differential Diagnoses
- Corpus Luteum of Pregnancy
- Incidental Adnexal Mass
- Intrauterine Pregnancy

Pathology
- 1.4% of all pregnancies are ectopic
- 95% of all ectopics are tubal

Clinical Issues
- Medical treatment with methotrexate

Diagnostic Checklist
- Presence of IUP is best negative predictor of EP
- Can often find EP with hCG levels < 2,000 mIU/mL
- Look for "ring of fire" in adnexa with color Doppler
- Corpus luteum can mimic EP

- Corpus luteum can mimic EP
  - Corpus luteum Doppler findings
    - Similar to "ring of fire" but in ovary
    - CL flow velocity < trophoblastic tissue velocity
- Echogenic fluid in cul-de-sac
  - Blood in peritoneal space
  - May need ↑ gain settings to see echoes
    - Anechoic fluid considered physiologic
  - Clotted blood often mass-like
  - Blood may be isolated finding
    - 73% will have EP if ↑ echogenic fluid seen
- Ultrasound completely negative in 5-10% of cases
  - No IUP, normal adnexa, no cul-de-sac fluid
- Non-tubal EP
  - Cervical EP
    - Implantation in cervical stroma
    - Hourglass shaped uterus
    - Marked peritrophoblastic flow
    - Differentiate from abortion in progress
  - Cornual ectopic
    - Implantation in interstitial portion of fallopian tube
    - < 5 mm surrounding myometrium
    - Intersitial line sign: Echogenic line from endometrium to sac
  - Ovarian ectopic
    - Implantation within ovary
    - Mimics corpus luteum
    - Look for yolk sac and embryo
  - Abdominal pregnancy
    - Implantation in peritoneal space
    - Lack of myometrium
    - Most often in pouch of Douglas
  - Cesarean section EP
    - Implantation in lower myometrium near cervical junction

Imaging Recommendations
- Best imaging tool
  - Transvaginal ultrasound + color Doppler
    - 91% of EP accurately diagnosed
- Protocol advice

- Correlate findings with human chorionic gonadotropin (hCG) levels
  - Should see IUP when hCG levels are > 2,000 mIU/mL IRP (international reference preparation)
- Lack of IUP at low hCG levels does not rule out EP
- Obtain sagittal cul-de-sac view in every case
  - Look for echogenic blood
- Look for CL
  - EP often on same side as CL
  - CL hemorrhage or rupture may be cause of pain
  - Do not confuse CL for EP
- Use color Doppler
  - Look for small EP
- Use endovaginal probe as a palpation tool
  - Gently wedge probe between mass and ovary
  - Free hand on abdomen palpates same area
  - EP moves independent of ovary
  - CL moves with ovary

DIFFERENTIAL DIAGNOSIS

Corpus Luteum of Pregnancy
- Variable appearance
  - Anechoic
  - Diffusely hypoechoic
  - Hemorrhagic
    - Fibrin strands
- Often with echogenic thick wall
  - ↑ Blood flow in wall only
  - Low resistance flow

Incidental Adnexal Mass
- Teratoma (dermoid)
  - Complex mass with fat, fluid, calcification
- Neoplasm
  - Complex mass with nodularity and thick septations
- Paraovarian cyst

Intrauterine Pregnancy
- Double decidual sac sign
- Perigestational hemorrhage common
  - Resembles pseudosac

ECTOPIC PREGNANCY

- Presence of IUP makes EP less likely
- Anechoic cul-de-sac fluid

PATHOLOGY

General Features
- Etiology
  - Abnormal blastocyst implantation
    - Normally in utero on day 7
  - Abnormal tube is a risk factor for tubal ectopic
    - Chronic salpingitis
    - Salpingitis isthmica nodosa
    - Tubal surgery
    - Prior EP
  - Endometrial injury is a risk factor for cervical ectopic
- Epidemiology
  - 1.4% of all pregnancies are ectopic
  - 95% of all ectopics are tubal
  - 10-40% risk in fertility patients
  - 5-20% incidence if patient presents with pain/bleeding

CLINICAL ISSUES

Presentation
- Most common signs/symptoms
  - Pelvic pain
  - Vaginal bleeding
  - Palpable mass
  - Cardiovascular shock
- Other signs/symptoms
  - No IUP when hCG > 2,000 mIU/mL IRP
    - Differential is EP vs. failing IUP
  - Low hCG level and negative ultrasound
    - EP vs. early IUP vs. failed IUP
  - Maternal serum progesterone levels
    - Helps predict normal IUP vs. EP/failing IUP
    - Cannot differentiate EP from failed IUP
    - < 5 ng/mL = nonviable pregnancy in 100%
    - Office curettage can rule out failed IUP
    - > 25 ng/mL excludes ectopic with 97.5% sensitivity

Natural History & Prognosis
- Delayed diagnosis ⇒ ↑ morbidity and death
  - Fatality rate has ↓ from 3.5 to 1:1,000
- Prognosis for future pregnancies
  - 80% will have future IUP
  - 15-20% will have future EP
- EP may resolve on own
  - More likely if hCG levels are < 1,000 mIU/mL IRP
  - Must follow dropping hCG levels very carefully
  - 24% of all EP may spontaneously resolve

Treatment
- Medical treatment with methotrexate
  - Patient must be hemodynamically stable
  - No evidence for tube rupture
    - Little or no peritoneal fluid
  - Early, unruptured, small ectopic
    - 90% success rate
    - EP < 4 cm

- HCG levels < 5,000 mIU/mL
- ≤ 8 weeks gestation
  - 70% success rate if living embryo
  - Multiple doses may be necessary
  - Ultrasound after treatment is often confusing
    - ↑ Hemorrhage around EP
    - ↑ Size of EP
    - Use only if suspect tubal rupture
- Surgical therapy
  - Salpingectomy
    - Segment of tube removed
    - Ends reconnected if possible
    - Only choice for ruptured EP
  - Salpingotomy
    - Small lengthwise incision in tube
    - Removal of EP
- Ultrasound guided local injection
  - Methotrexate or potassium chloride (KCl)
    - Injected directly into gestational sac
  - Live ectopic + unruptured tube
    - 30% fail systemic treatment
  - Preferred method for cornual and cervical ectopics

DIAGNOSTIC CHECKLIST

Consider
- Serial hCG levels in indeterminate cases
  - Levels double every 2 days with normal IUP
  - Repeat ultrasound if hCG levels are rising
  - Dropping levels suggest failing pregnancy

Image Interpretation Pearls
- Presence of IUP is best negative predictor of EP
- Can often find EP with hCG levels < 2,000 mIU/mL
  - Do not delay ultrasound
- Look for "ring of fire" in adnexa with color Doppler
  - May detect a small EP when grayscale findings are negative
- Be aware of, and beware of, corpus luteum
  - Corpus luteum can mimic EP
  - Often EP on same side
  - Can be cause of pain

SELECTED REFERENCES

1. Blaivas M et al: Reliability of adnexal mass mobility in distinguishing possible ectopic pregnancy from corpus luteum cysts. J Ultrasound Med. 24(5):599-603; quiz 605, 2005
2. Condous G et al: The accuracy of transvaginal ultrasonography for the diagnosis of ectopic pregnancy prior to surgery. Hum Reprod. 20(5):1404-9, 2005
3. Dogra V et al: First trimester bleeding evaluation. Ultrasound Q. 21(2):69-85; quiz 149-50, 153-4, 2005
4. Monteagudo A et al: Non-surgical management of live ectopic pregnancy with ultrasound-guided local injection: a case series. Ultrasound Obstet Gynecol. 25(3):282-8, 2005
5. Dialani V et al: Ectopic pregnancy: a review. Ultrasound Q. 20(3):105-17, 2004
6. Sowter MC et al: Ectopic pregnancy: an update. Curr Opin Obstet Gynecol. 16(4):289-93, 2004

ECTOPIC PREGNANCY

IMAGE GALLERY

Typical

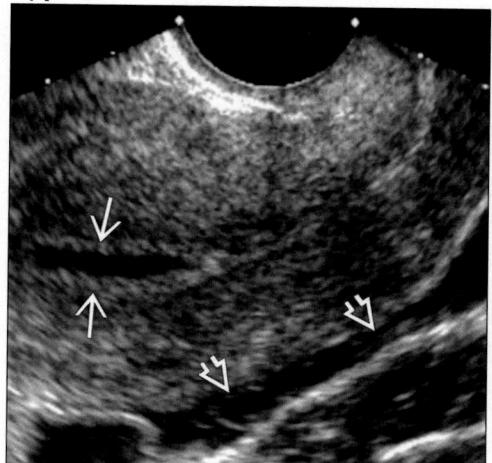

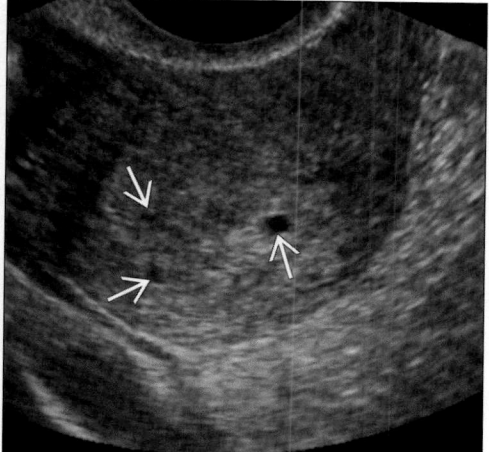

(Left) Longitudinal transvaginal ultrasound shows a pseudogestational sac. The fluid in the endometrial cavity ➡ is blood and can mimic a gestational sac. Note the presence of complex pelvic fluid ➡. (Right) Transverse transvaginal ultrasound shows endometrial cysts ➡ commonly seen with ectopic pregnancy. They should not be confused with a gestational sac.

Typical

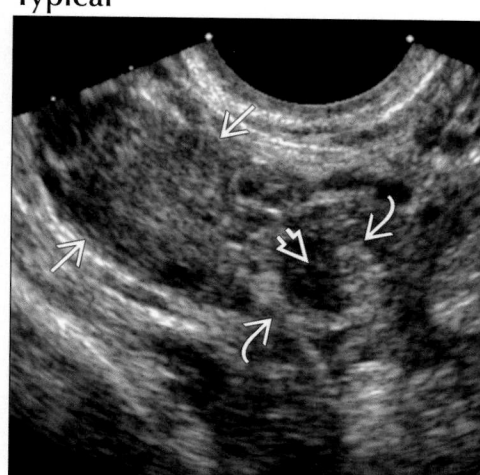

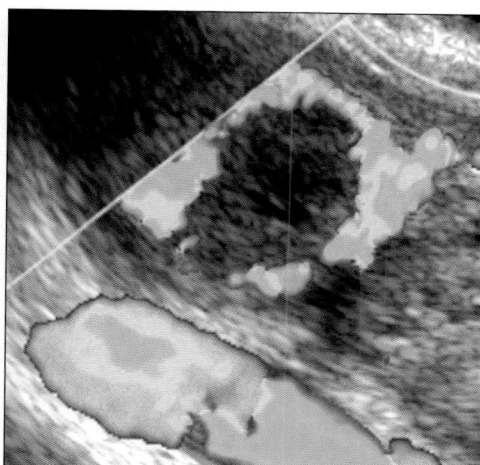

(Left) Transverse transvaginal ultrasound shows a tubal echogenic ring ➡ next to the ovary ➡. The sac contains a faint yolk sac ➡. Lack of peritoneal fluid suggests non-ruptured tubal EP. (Right) Corresponding transverse color Doppler ultrasound shows the classic "ring of fire". A small ectopic pregnancy will light up when color Doppler is used.

Variant

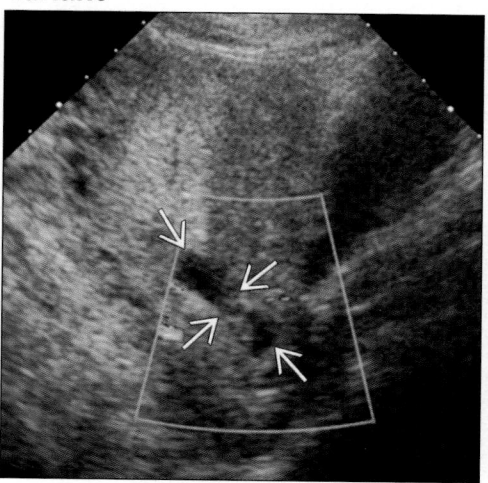

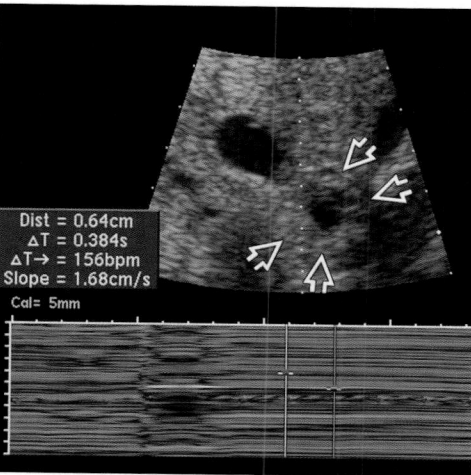

Dist = 0.64cm
ΔT = 0.384s
ΔT→ = 156bpm
Slope = 1.68cm/s
Cal= 5mm

(Left) Longitudinal transabdominal ultrasound shows a cervical ectopic pregnancy ➡. The gestational sac is within the cervix and is misshapen. The appearance mimics an abortion in progress. (Right) Longitudinal transvaginal ultrasound with M-mode technique shows a living embryo within the sac and an echogenic ring around the sac ➡ suggesting implantation within the cervix and not abortion in progress.

INTERSTITIAL ECTOPIC PREGNANCY

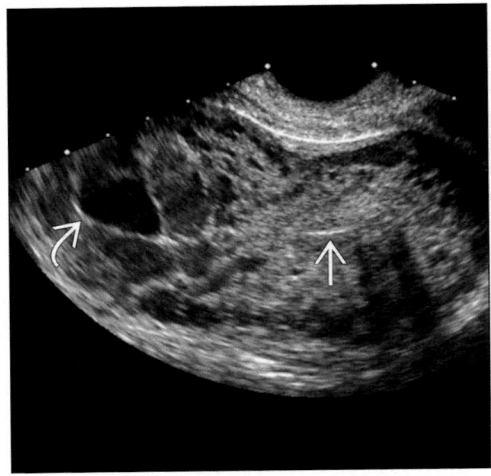

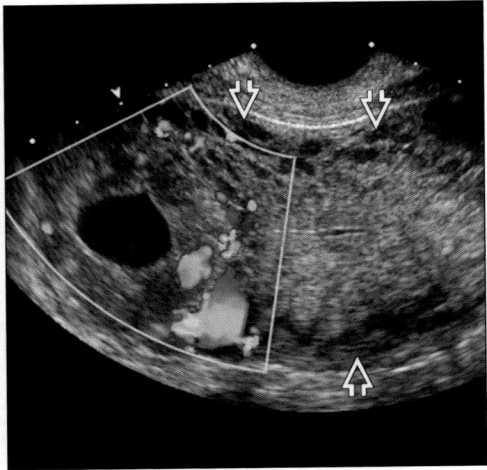

Transverse transvaginal ultrasound shows a large gestational sac ➡ in the uterine cornua. It is eccentrically located with respect to the endometrial cavity ➡.

Color Doppler ultrasound shows significant flow around interstitial ectopic and prominent arcuate vessels ➡ in the outer third of myometrium. Exsanguination may occur if the uterus ruptures.

TERMINOLOGY

Abbreviations and Synonyms
- Interstitial ectopic pregnancy (preferred term)
- Cornual ectopic pregnancy
  - Often used interchangeably
  - More appropriately applied to pregnancies in a rudimentary horn
- Intramural ectopic pregnancy
- Angular pregnancy
  - Pregnancy implanted at lateral angle of uterine cavity by ostium, medial to interstitial portion of tube

Definitions
- Pregnancy occurring in interstitial (intramural) portion of fallopian tube

IMAGING FINDINGS

General Features
- Best diagnostic clue
  - Combination of findings

- Interstitial line sign: Echogenic line from endometrium to ectopic sac
- Myometrium thinned to < 5 mm
- Location
  - Interstitial (intramural) portion of fallopian tube
    - Connects uterine cavity to isthmus (extrauterine portion of tube)
    - 1 cm in length, 1 mm in diameter
- Size: Covered by myometrium so can grow to larger size than tubal ectopics
- Early interstitial pregnancy often difficult to diagnose
  - 42% of cases missed in one large series

Ultrasonographic Findings
- Gestational sac located high in fundus
  - Eccentrically located with respect to endometrial cavity
- Appearance of sac contents quite variable
  - Gestational sac ± yolk sac, embryo
    - Gestational sac and embryo can be quite large
  - May appear as echogenic mass within cornua
    - Combination of trophoblastic tissue, hematoma
    - No definable sac
- Thinned myometrium

DDx: Interstitial Ectopic

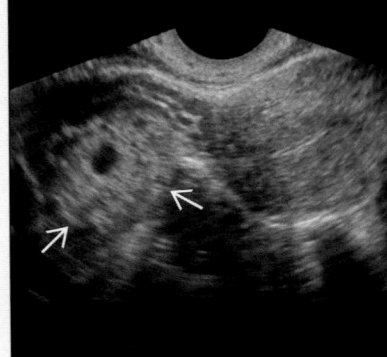

Tubal Ectopic

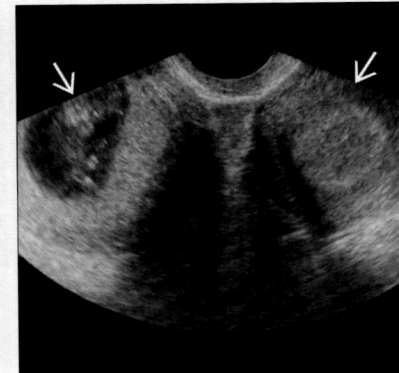

Uterus Didelphys

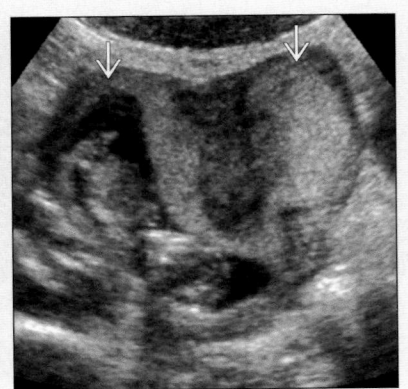

Septate Uterus

INTERSTITIAL ECTOPIC PREGNANCY

Key Facts

Terminology
- Pregnancy occurring in interstitial (intramural) portion of fallopian tube

Imaging Findings
- Interstitial line sign: Echogenic line from endometrium to ectopic sac
- Gestational sac located high in fundus
- Eccentrically located with respect to endometrial cavity
- Gestational sac and embryo can be quite large
- May appear as echogenic mass within cornua
- < 5 mm of surrounding myometrium very suggestive
- Normal myometrium may be seen early and does not exclude an interstitial ectopic
- Interstitial line sign has reported sensitivity of 80% and specificity of 98%

- If diagnosis is unclear, short term follow-up with careful instructions to patient to return immediately if symptoms occur

Top Differential Diagnoses
- Normal Intrauterine Pregnancy
- Uterine Duplications

Pathology
- 2-4% of ectopic pregnancies are interstitial
- Mortality rate 2-2.5%

Clinical Issues
- Hypotension and shock if presenting with rupture
- Significantly greater morbidity and mortality than for tubal ectopics
- Uterine rupture most commonly occurs at 9-12 weeks

  - < 5 mm of surrounding myometrium very suggestive
  - May have areas where no definable myometrium is seen
  - Normal myometrium may be seen early and does not exclude an interstitial ectopic
- Interstitial line sign has reported sensitivity of 80% and specificity of 98%
  - Echogenic line can be followed from endometrium to ectopic sac
- 3D ultrasound
  - Multiple case reports show improved diagnosis
  - Improved spatial orientation of ectopic in relation to uterine cavity
- Doppler findings
  - Trophoblastic tissue is highly vascular
  - Marked flow identified on color and power Doppler
  - Pulsed Doppler shows high-velocity, low-resistance waveform
  - May see prominent arcuate vessels in outer third of myometrium

MR Findings
- Has been shown accurate in diagnosis
  - Eccentric sac separated from endometrium by junctional zone
- Generally not necessary
- Consider when ultrasound findings are equivocal or pre-operative planning for large ectopics
- Generally avoided in first trimester unless clinical situation warrants

Imaging Recommendations
- Always document location of sac with respect to endometrium in both transverse and longitudinal planes
- Measure surrounding myometrium if it appears thin
  - < 5 mm more likely to be an interstitial ectopic
- Look for echogenic line leading to myometrium (interstitial line sign)
- Use 3D ultrasound if available
- If diagnosis is unclear, short term follow-up with careful instructions to patient to return immediately if symptoms occur

- May consider MR if still unclear

DIFFERENTIAL DIAGNOSIS

Normal Intrauterine Pregnancy
- High, eccentric implantation can be confusing
- Should always have normal myometrial coverage
- Follow-up scan shows normal development

Uterine Duplications
- Duplication of endometrial cavity
- Implantation within one horn gives eccentric appearance
- Myometrium will completely surround gestational sac in all types
- May give false appearance of interstitial line sign
  - Can follow an echogenic line to main cavity
    - Close evaluation shows it is curved, rather than straight
- Classification system based on external contour
  - Uterus didelphys
    - Two separate uteri
    - Easiest to distinguish from interstitial ectopic
  - Bicornuate
    - External contour of uterus is concave
    - Must examine uterine fundus to adequately evaluate contour
  - Septate
    - External uterine contour is normal
    - Most likely congenital anomaly to be confused with interstitial ectopic
    - Septum extends for variable lengths (subseptate vs. complete)

Tubal Ectopic
- Can occasionally be confusing if adjacent to uterine cornua
- Use ultrasound probe to gently separate structures

INTERSTITIAL ECTOPIC PREGNANCY

PATHOLOGY

General Features
- Etiology
  - Risk factors
    - History of prior tubal surgery, especially salpingectomy
    - Prior ectopic pregnancy
    - Assisted reproductive technology (ART) pregnancies
    - May see heterotopic pregnancy with ART, with one sac in cornua
  - Intrauterine contraceptive devices (IUD) are not associated with interstitial ectopics
    - Ectopic pregnancies more likely to be in tube when IUD present
- Epidemiology
  - 2-4% of ectopic pregnancies are interstitial
  - Mortality rate 2-2.5%

Microscopic Features
- Interstitial portion of tube composed of multiple layers
  - Endosalpinx (mucosa)
  - Myosalpinx
    - 3 layers of muscle
    - Highly vascularized
  - Serosa is directly contiguous with peritoneum

CLINICAL ISSUES

Presentation
- Most common signs/symptoms
  - Pelvic/abdominal pain
  - Vaginal bleeding
- Other signs/symptoms
  - Hypotension and shock if presenting with rupture
  - May be an incidental finding on routine 1st trimester scan
    - Easy to miss on early scan

Natural History & Prognosis
- Significantly greater morbidity and mortality than for tubal ectopics
  - Surrounding myometrium is distensible, allowing for greater gestational sac size
  - Uterine rupture most commonly occurs at 9-12 weeks
    - May occur earlier
  - Potential exsanguination
    - Large arcuate vessels run in outer third of myometrium
- Good outcome, with preserved future fertility, with appropriate treatment

Treatment
- Systemic methotrexate
  - Follow human chorionic gonadotropin (hCG) after initial dose
  - May require second dose if levels do not fall appropriately
  - Failed treatment goes to surgery
- Sac injection
  - Generally with methotrexate

- Via laparoscopy or ultrasound guidance
  - Potassium chloride, etoposide also used
- Cornuostomy with sac excision
  - May be done with laparoscopy or laparotomy
- Expectant management
  - Considered only if small sac and no living embryo
- Rupture may require hysterectomy
  - May consider uterine artery embolization prior to surgery

DIAGNOSTIC CHECKLIST

Consider
- 3D ultrasound for improved spatial orientation of sac to endometrial cavity

Image Interpretation Pearls
- Despite technical advances, diagnosis of interstitial ectopic pregnancy remains difficult
  - Must have a high degree of suspicion, especially in a high-risk patient
  - Short term follow-up for any sac which appears high and eccentric

SELECTED REFERENCES

1. Deruelle P et al: Management of interstitial pregnancy using selective uterine artery embolization. Obstet Gynecol. 107(2 Pt 1):427-8, 2006
2. Lee GS et al: Diagnosis of early intramural ectopic pregnancy. J Clin Ultrasound. 33(4):190-2, 2005
3. Coric M et al: Laparoscopic approach to interstitial pregnancy. Arch Gynecol Obstet. 270(4):287-9, 2004
4. Jermy K et al: The conservative management of interstitial pregnancy. BJOG. 111(11):1283-8, 2004
5. Tarim E et al: Angular pregnancy. J Obstet Gynaecol Res. 30(5):377-9, 2004
6. Tulandi T et al: Interstitial pregnancy: results generated from the Society of Reproductive Surgeons Registry. Obstet Gynecol. 103(1):47-50, 2004
7. Akrivis Ch et al: Early ultrasonographic diagnosis of unrupted interstitial pregnancy: a case report and review of the literature. Clin Exp Obstet Gynecol. 30(1):60-4, 2003
8. Chan LY et al: Pitfalls in diagnosis of interstitial pregnancy. Acta Obstet Gynecol Scand. 82(9):867-70, 2003
9. Izquierdo LA et al: Three-dimensional transvaginal sonography of interstitial pregnancy. J Clin Ultrasound. 31(9):484-7, 2003
10. Bouyer J et al: Sites of ectopic pregnancy: a 10 year population-based study of 1800 cases. Hum Reprod. 17(12):3224-30, 2002
11. Sagiv R et al: Three conservative approaches to treatment of interstitial pregnancy. J Am Assoc Gynecol Laparosc. 8(1):154-8, 2001
12. Takeuchi K et al: Comparison of magnetic resonance imaging and ultrasonography in the early diagnosis of interstitial pregnancy. J Reprod Med. 44(3):265-8, 1999
13. Ackerman TE et al: Interstitial line: sonographic finding in interstitial (cornual) ectopic pregnancy. Radiology. 189(1):83-7, 1993

IMAGE GALLERY

Typical

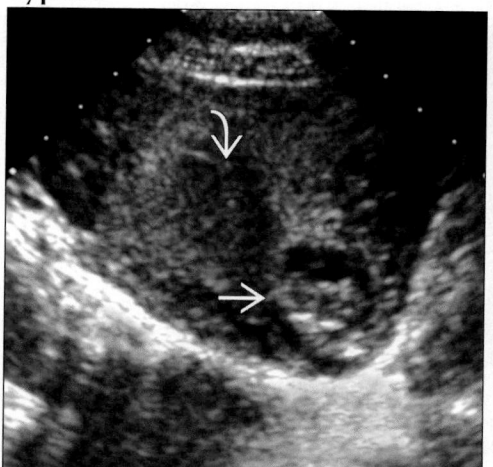

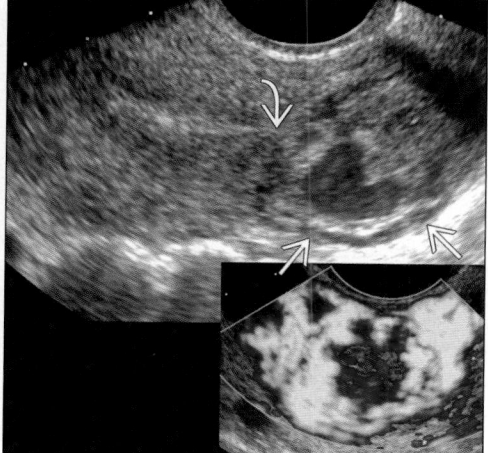

(Left) Transabdominal ultrasound shows gestational sac ➘ bulging uterine contour at left cornua. Note sac is eccentric with respect to the endometrial cavity ➔. (Right) Transverse transvaginal ultrasound shows interstitial line sign ➔, an echogenic line that can be followed from the endometrium to the ectopic sac. There is severe thinning of the myometrium ➔ and marked trophoblastic flow is seen with power Doppler (inset).

Typical

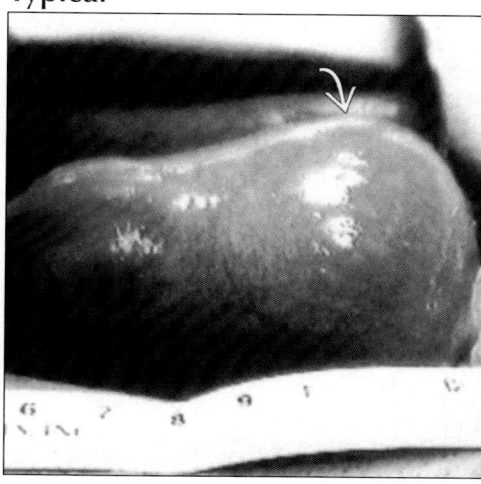

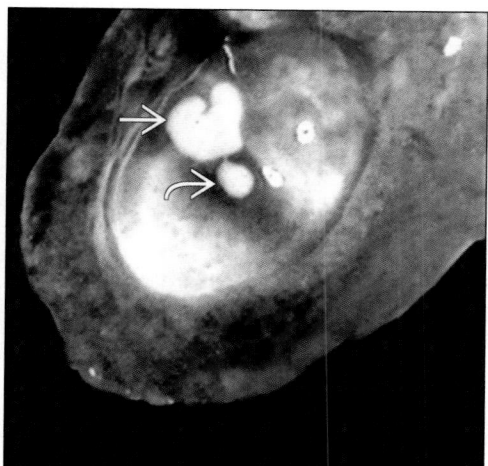

(Left) Intra-operative photograph shows bulging, thinned myometrium at the site of interstitial ectopic ➔. The patient underwent cornuostomy and sac excision. (Right) Gross photograph of the resected gestational sac. Clearly defined embryo ➔ and yolk sac ➘ are seen.

Typical

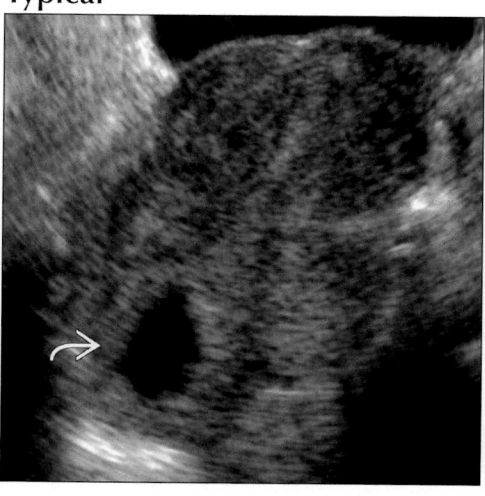

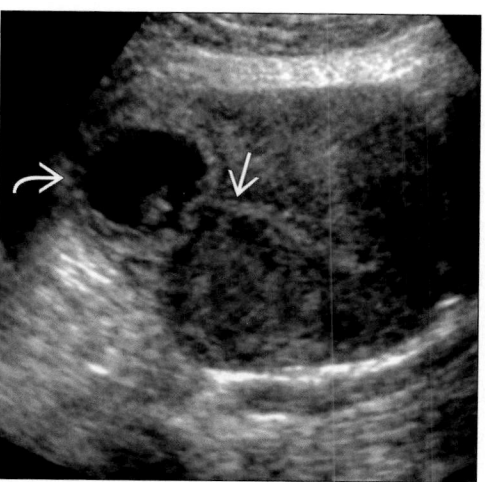

(Left) Longitudinal transvaginal ultrasound of a retroverted uterus shows a gestational sac ➘ higher in the uterine cavity than expected. (Right) Transverse plane shows the interstitial line sign ➘, leading from endometrial cavity to ectopic gestational sac ➘. Note thinned overlying myometrium. The transverse plane is often most helpful for diagnosing an interstitial ectopic.

FAILED FIRST TRIMESTER PREGNANCY

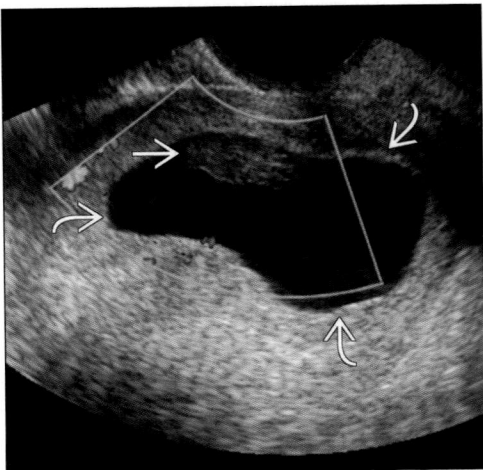

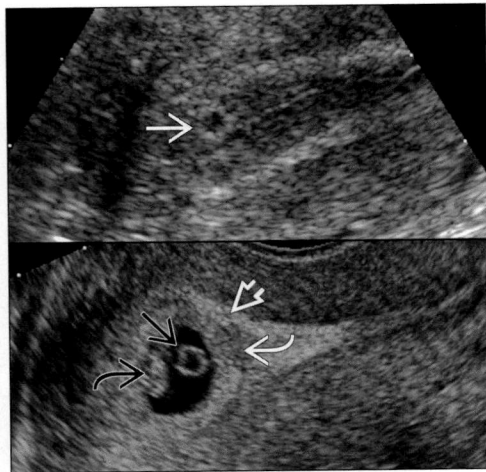

Transvaginal ultrasound with color Doppler shows a dead embryo ➡. Absent cardiac activity in an embryo > 5 mm in size implies demise. Note poor decidual reaction ➡ and irregular sac shape.

Compare with TV scans of normal early pregnancy. Follow the intradecidual sac sign ➡ to confirm development of the double decidual sac sign ➡ ➡. Lower image also shows yolk sac ➡ and embryo ➡.

TERMINOLOGY

Abbreviations and Synonyms
- Anembryonic pregnancy (AP)
- Blighted ovum

Definitions
- Anembryonic pregnancy
  - Gestational sac without visible embryo
    - Failure of embryo to develop versus early demise with resorption of embryonic pole
- Embryonic demise
  - Gestational sac with visible dead embryo
- Consider term "failed first trimester pregnancy"
  - Avoids confusion and simplifies terminology

IMAGING FINDINGS

General Features
- Gestational sac without identifiable embryo
  - Sac size must have reached discriminatory threshold
- Discriminatory criteria for anembryonic pregnancy by transvaginal (TV) ultrasound

- Mean sac diameter > 10 mm without a yolk sac (YS)
  - Some authors use 8 mm
- Mean sac diameter > 18 mm without an embryo
  - Some authors use 16 mm
- Discriminatory criteria for anembryonic pregnancy by transabdominal ultrasound
  - Mean sac diameter > 20 mm without a yolk sac
  - Mean sac diameter > 25 mm without an embryo
- Very few indications for performing transabdominal scan alone: Resolution much better with TV scans
  - Victims of abuse, patients with pelvic/perineal trauma

Ultrasonographic Findings
- Grayscale Ultrasound
  - Empty amnion sign
    - Specific sign of anembryonic gestation
    - Amniotic sac without an embryo
    - YS may be visible: Outside amnion
  - Abnormal yolk sac
    - YS forms after amnion but is easier to see
    - Embryo first seen as focal thickening on YS
    - Amnion becomes visible, enlarges rapidly to envelop embryo

DDx: Abnormal First Trimester Pregnancy

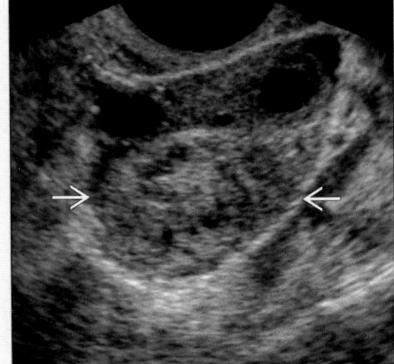

Adnexal Ectopic

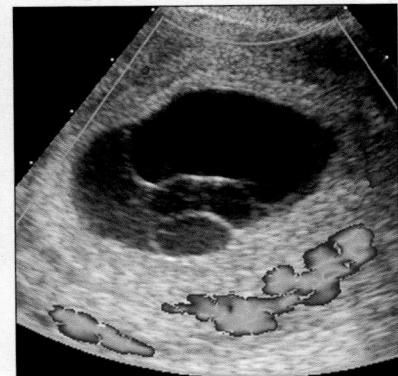

Partial Mole

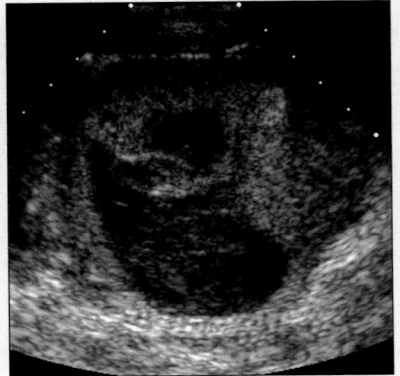

Subchorionic Bleed

FAILED FIRST TRIMESTER PREGNANCY

Key Facts

Terminology
- Gestational sac without visible embryo
- Consider term "failed first trimester pregnancy"

Imaging Findings
- Sac size must have reached discriminatory threshold
- Mean sac diameter > 10 mm without a yolk sac (YS)
- Mean sac diameter > 18 mm without an embryo
- Empty amnion sign
- Poor color Doppler signal around gestation sac

Top Differential Diagnoses
- Normal Early Intrauterine Pregnancy (IUP)
- Retained Products of Conception (RPOC)
- Gestational Trophoblastic Disease (GTD)

Pathology
- 60% of spontaneous abortions < 12 weeks due to abnormal chromosomes

Clinical Issues
- No specific recurrence risk if isolated
- Most will spontaneously abort without treatment

Diagnostic Checklist
- Abnormalities common in early pregnancy
- Diagnosis depends on knowledge of normal early pregnancy milestones
- If in doubt, wait and see
- "Empty amnion sign" is a specific indicator of anembryonic gestation

---

- YS eventually obliterated as amnion fuses with chorion
- Pyknotic (collapsed), calcified or large YS → poor prognosis
  - Signs of abnormal pregnancy
    - Irregular gestation sac shape, may be "tear-drop" or "amoeboid" in shape
    - Poor decidual reaction
    - Gestation sac positioned low in uterus
- Color Doppler
  - Poor color Doppler signal around gestation sac
    - Use with caution to support abnormal diagnosis
    - Doppler delivers greater energy with theoretic risks to developing embryo from heating and cavitation
    - If possibility of normal early gestation, follow-up with grayscale rather than use Doppler

Imaging Recommendations
- Use TV sonography
  - Better resolution → more confidence in diagnosis
- Be sure to scan through entire uterus in longitudinal and transverse planes
  - Must look carefully for yolk sac, embryo
  - Avoids missing multiple gestations
- Measure sac diameter in 3 planes
  - Measurement does not include chorionic reaction
  - Mean sac diameter = average of these three measurements
- Follow-up if possible normal early pregnancy
  - Check menstrual history
    - Verify date of last menstrual period (LMP)
    - Is cycle regular?
    - What is cycle length?
  - Know anatomy and developmental stages
    - "Double bleb": Embryonic disc between amnion and yolk sac
    - Yolk sac and amnion should be visible by 7 weeks post LMP
    - Embryo lies inside amniotic cavity, YS lies outside
    - Normal yolk sac round in shape, ≤ 6 mm diameter

DIFFERENTIAL DIAGNOSIS

Normal Early Intrauterine Pregnancy (IUP)
- Double decidual sac sign (DDSS)
- Thick echogenic decidual reaction
- Yolk sac may not be seen if MSD < 10 mm TV
  - > 10 mm + no yolk sac = failed IUP
- Prominent color flow around sac
- Low-resistance, high-velocity flow on spectral analysis of chorion

Pseudosac of Ectopic Pregnancy
- Sac central in endometrial cavity
- No DDSS
- Doppler: Absent or low velocity flow, peak systolic velocity < 8 cm/sec

Retained Products of Conception (RPOC)
- Disorganized material in uterine cavity
- Echogenic material with flow on color Doppler → most likely RPOC
- Retained clot is usually hypoechoic, non-perfused
- No recognizable gestation sac

Gestational Trophoblastic Disease (GTD)
- Classic hydatidiform mole has "swiss cheese" appearance
- May see abnormal appearing gestational sac
  - Can mimic anembryonic sac
- May see associated ovarian theca lutein cysts

Perigestational Hemorrhage
- Usually crescentic around periphery of gestational sac
- ± Living embryo

PATHOLOGY

General Features
- General path comments
  - 60% of spontaneous abortions < 12 weeks due to abnormal chromosomes
    - Trisomies/triploidy/tetraploidy

FAILED FIRST TRIMESTER PREGNANCY

- 45 XO
- Translocations/mosaics
  - Early US/embryoscopy have shown structural anomalies in karyotypically normal embryos in which pregnancy ended in missed abortion
    - Research into potential role of cytokines in excessive apoptosis as cause of anomalies/demise
- Epidemiology
  - 30-60% documented elevations of beta human chorionic gonadotrophin end as failed pregnancy
  - Up to 20% of confirmed first trimester pregnancies end in spontaneous abortion
  - Pathology series of abnormal early pregnancies
    - 35% anembryonic, 54% early loss (cause not specified), 11% molar (partial or complete)
  - Groups with increased incidence of early pregnancy failure
    - Advanced maternal age
    - Poor diabetic control
    - History recurrent abortions

Microscopic Features
- Chorionic villi present in uterine curettings
  - Significant reduction in number of vessels per chorionic villus when compared to normal pregnancy
  - Vessels abnormally located within chorionic villi: Remain as central cords
    - Vessels marginalize to periphery of villus in normal pregnancy
    - Thought to relate to inadequate vasculogenesis, abnormal development of vasculosyncitial membrane
- Other studies failed to show pivotal role for trophoblast invasion/spiral artery transformation in early miscarriage
  - May be more important in poor outcome/maternal complications
- Nuclear DNA abnormal in up to 40%
  - Suggests that chromosomal aberrations → abnormal embryogenesis → anembryonic gestation

CLINICAL ISSUES

Presentation
- May be asymptomatic with diagnosis made during routine first trimester scan
- If spontaneous miscarriage imminent
  - Vaginal bleeding, pelvic pain, uterine contractions
- Patient perception
  - Diminished breast tenderness, morning sickness
  - "Doesn't feel like other pregnancies"

Natural History & Prognosis
- Random event
- No specific recurrence risk if isolated
  - Patients with recurrent abortion are empirically treated with aspirin, heparin
  - Luteal phase insufficiency treated with progesterone supplementation
- Threatened abortion occurs in 25% first trimester pregnancies

Treatment
- "Wait and see"
  - Most will spontaneously abort without treatment
- Vaginal misoprostol
  - Successful evacuation of uterus in majority of patients
  - Many patients prefer definitive treatment to expectant management
  - Some will require curettage but overall expect 50% reduction in need for surgical management
- Suction curettage
  - Small associated risk of excessive bleeding, uterine rupture, Asherman syndrome

DIAGNOSTIC CHECKLIST

Consider
- Abnormalities common in early pregnancy
- Anembryonic pregnancy often due to chromosomal aberration
- Diagnosis depends on knowledge of normal early pregnancy milestones
- If in doubt, wait and see
  - Normal pregnancies grow in a predictable manner
  - MSD increases by 1 mm per day
  - Schedule follow-up for a time when gestational sac should have reached discriminatory threshold
- With modern equipment many anomalies can be detected in first trimester
  - Scans are not just for "viability" any more
  - Early detection of anomalies → option for early diagnosis of aneuploidy with chorionic villus sampling

Image Interpretation Pearls
- "Empty amnion sign" is a specific indicator of anembryonic gestation
  - Gestational sac with amnion but no visible embryo
  - YS may be visible

SELECTED REFERENCES

1. Ball E et al: Early embryonic demise: no evidence of abnormal spiral artery transformation or trophoblast invasion. J Pathol. 208(4):528-34, 2006
2. Chama CM et al: The value of the secondary yolk sac in predicting pregnancy outcome. J Obstet Gynaecol. 25(3):245-7, 2005
3. Jauniaux E et al: The role of ultrasound imaging in diagnosing and investigating early pregnancy failure. Ultrasound Obstet Gynecol. 25(6):613-24, 2005
4. Carp H: Cytokines in recurrent miscarriage. Lupus. 13(9):630-4, 2004
5. Lisman BA et al: Abnormal development of the vasculosyncytial membrane in early pregnancy failure. Fertil Steril. 82(3):654-60, 2004
6. Sohaey R et al: First-trimester ultrasound: the essentials. Semin Ultrasound CT MR. 17(1):2-14, 1996

IMAGE GALLERY

Typical

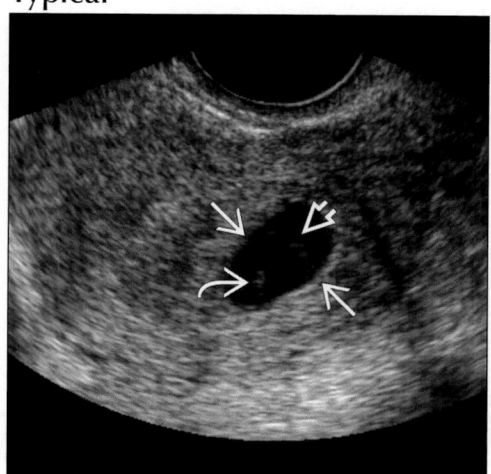 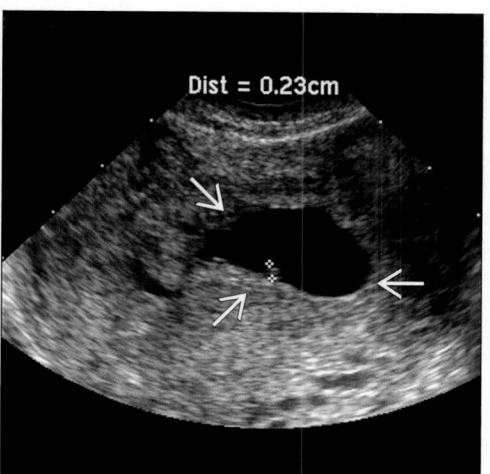

(Left) Transvaginal ultrasound in a patient with recurrent abortions shows an early IUP with appropriate milestones. There is an embryo ➔, amnion ➔ and yolk sac (not shown). However, decidual reaction ➔ is poor. (Right) Repeat TV US one week later shows no interval embryonic growth with a CRL of 2.3 mm and collapse of the gestational sac, which is now irregular in shape ➔ indicating early pregnancy failure.

Typical

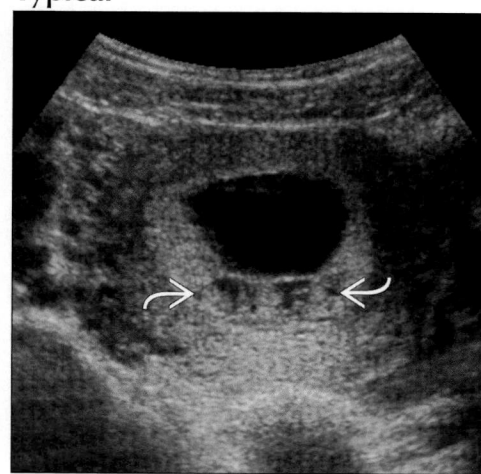 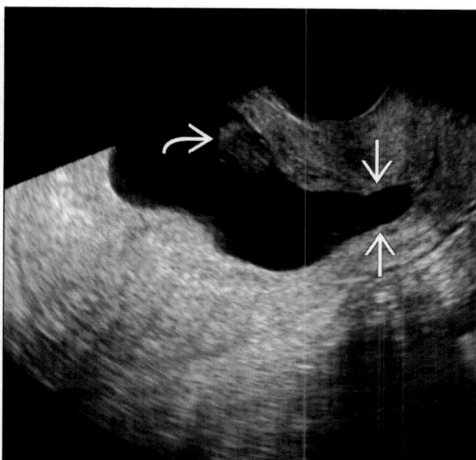

(Left) Transabdominal ultrasound shows hypoechoic areas within the chorion frondosum ➔. This appearance is created by hydropic placental villi. No embryo was visible in this sac with mean diameter of 25 mm. (Right) Transvaginal ultrasound shows a dead embryo ➔ within a large, irregular gestational sac with poor decidual reaction. The cervix has started to dilate ➔, consistent with an impending spontaneous abortion.

Typical

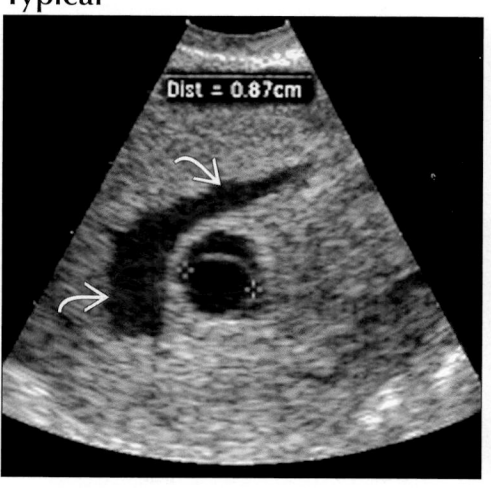 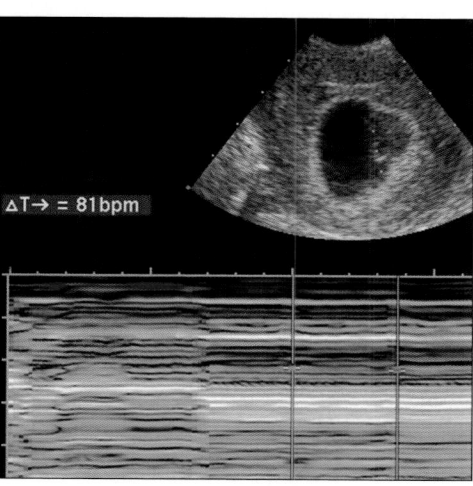

(Left) Transvaginal ultrasound shows an abnormally large yolk sac (calipers) measuring 8.7 mm associated with large perigestational hemorrhage ➔ and poor decidual reaction. Spontaneous abortion occurred. (Right) M-mode Doppler shows an embryonic heart rate of 81 bpm. This is associated with poor outcome, one week later embryonic demise was confirmed.

RETAINED PRODUCTS OF CONCEPTION

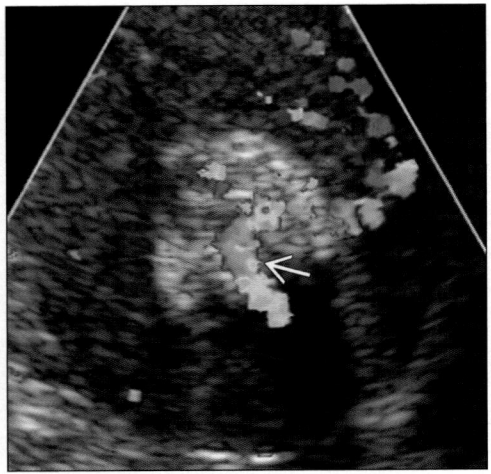

Color Doppler ultrasound of a postpartum woman with bleeding shows a thickened, echogenic endometrial cavity ➡ with a focal area with Doppler flow ➔. D&C showed RPOC.

Color Doppler ultrasound shows flow ➡ within this echogenic endometrial mass, which helps confirm RPOC. Note that color flow is not always seen.

TERMINOLOGY

Abbreviations and Synonyms
- Retained products of conception (RPOC)
- Retained placenta, retained trophoblastic tissue

Definitions
- Incomplete uterine evacuation, with retention of placental tissue within endometrial cavity
  ○ Occurs after delivery or termination

IMAGING FINDINGS

General Features
- Best diagnostic clue: Echogenic endometrial mass with low-resistance, high-velocity flow
- Significant overlap in ultrasound findings between normal postpartum uterus and RPOC
  ○ Overall false positive rate for RPOC is 34%
    - 28.9% after delivery
    - 51.5% after therapeutic abortion

Ultrasonographic Findings
- Solid, heterogeneous, echogenic mass
- Irregular interface between endometrium and myometrium
- Intrauterine fluid common
- Persistent, thickened endometrium
- Doppler shows high-velocity, low-resistance flow
  ○ Peak velocity ≥ 21 cm/sec
  ○ Lack of increased flow does not rule out RPOC

DIFFERENTIAL DIAGNOSIS

Normal Postpartum Uterus
- Highly variable, from smooth to irregular endometrium
- Small echogenic foci and fluid common
- Foci of gas may be seen in up to 21%
- Endometrial thickness < 2 cm initially and should decrease to < 8 mm with uterine involution

Uterine Atony
- Primary differential consideration for immediate postpartum hemorrhage

DDx: Retained Products of Conception

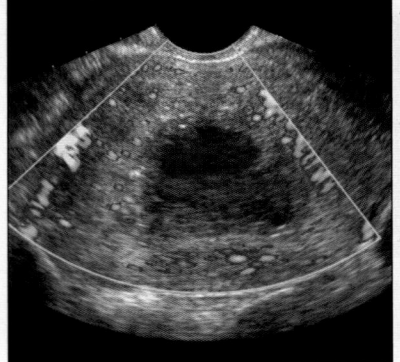

Endometritis

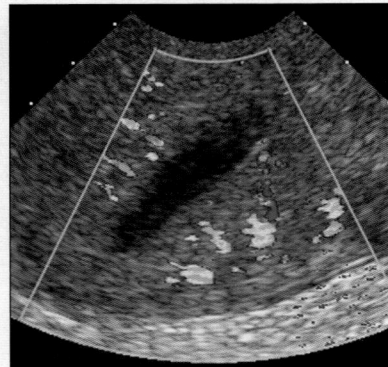

Clot

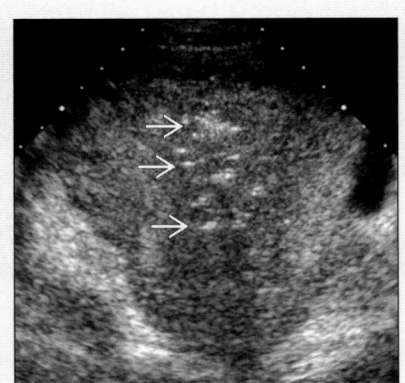

Endometritis

RETAINED PRODUCTS OF CONCEPTION

Key Facts

Imaging Findings
- Significant overlap in ultrasound findings between normal postpartum uterus and RPOC
- Overall false positive rate for RPOC is 34%
- Solid, heterogeneous, echogenic mass
- Irregular interface between endometrium and myometrium
- Lack of increased flow does not rule out RPOC

Top Differential Diagnoses
- Normal Postpartum Uterus
- Intrauterine Blood/Clot

Clinical Issues
- Delayed postpartum bleeding

Diagnostic Checklist
- If no mass or fluid and endometrial thickness < 10 mm, RPOC extremely unlikely

---

- Should not see any retained products within endometrial cavity
  - Blood/clot may potentially be confusing

Intrauterine Blood/Clot
- No flow with Doppler
- Changes/resolves on follow-up scans

Endometritis
- Postpartum fever and pelvic pain
- May see gas in endometrium, nonspecific
- Patient may have both RPOC and endometritis

PATHOLOGY

General Features
- Epidemiology
  - ~ 1% of all pregnancies
  - More frequent following termination
  - ↑ Incidence with placenta accreta

CLINICAL ISSUES

Presentation
- Delayed postpartum bleeding
  - Most present within a few days of delivery or abortion, although some may present in immediate postpartum period
  - May rarely present weeks after delivery with vaginal bleeding or infection

Treatment
- May monitor 24-48 hours, especially if ultrasound findings are equivocal
  - ± Repeat ultrasound to re-evaluate
- Dilatation and curettage (D&C) for persistent bleeding or obvious RPOC
  - Failure to evacuate ⇒ prolonged hemorrhage and infection

DIAGNOSTIC CHECKLIST

Image Interpretation Pearls
- Uterine atony vs. RPOC primary differential for immediate postpartum hemorrhage
  - Atony: Normal appearing cavity
  - RPOC: Echogenic, intracavitary mass
- If no mass or fluid and endometrial thickness < 10 mm, RPOC extremely unlikely

SELECTED REFERENCES

1. Durfee SM et al: The Sonographic and Color Doppler Features of Retained Products of Conception. J Ultrasound Med. 24(9):1181-1186, 2005
2. Sadan O et al: Role of sonography in the diagnosis of retained products of conception. J Ultrasound Med. 23(3):371-4, 2004

9

IMAGE GALLERY

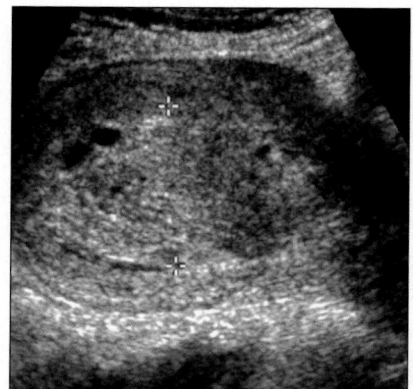 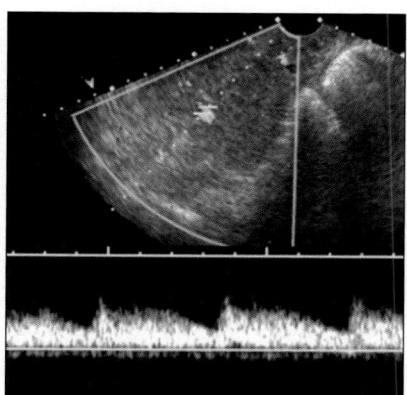 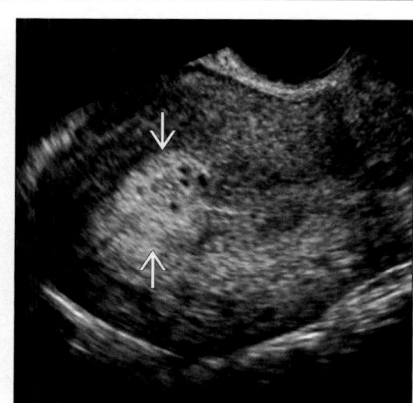

(Left) Longitudinal transabdominal ultrasound of the uterus shows RPOC in a woman presenting with postpartum bleeding. There is a complex, echogenic mass (calipers) distending the endometrial cavity. *(Center)* Pulsed Doppler ultrasound in the same case shows the characteristic high-velocity, low-resistance flow within RPOC. *(Right)* Transvaginal ultrasound shows a focal area of endometrial thickening ➡ near the fundus. This is RPOC in a woman who presented with delayed postpartum bleeding.

GESTATIONAL TROPHOBLASTIC NEOPLASM

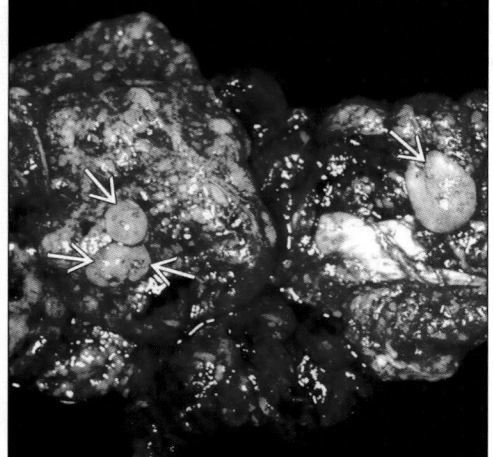

Transverse transabdominal ultrasound shows a molar pregnancy. The uterine cavity is distended by a cystic placental mass. Note that the intact myometrial wall is discernible ➡.

Gross pathology of molar pregnancy shows the typical trophoblastic hydropic villi within the placental mass. This grouping of cysts ➡ has been called the "cluster of grapes" appearance.

TERMINOLOGY

Abbreviations and Synonyms
- Gestational trophoblastic neoplasm (GTN) subtypes
  - Complete hydatidiform mole (CHM)
  - Invasive mole
  - Choriocarcinoma
  - Partial mole (triploidy)

Definitions
- Abnormal proliferation of trophoblastic tissue

IMAGING FINDINGS

General Features
- Best diagnostic clue
  - Placental cysts
  - ± Ovarian theca lutein cysts
- Location
  - CHM confined to endometrium
  - Invasive mole invades myometrium
  - Choriocarcinoma often metastatic

Ultrasonographic Findings
- CHM is most common type of GTN
  - Cystic intrauterine mass
    - Hydropic placenta
  - No embryo or fetus
  - Color Doppler shows marked vascularity
    - High-velocity, low-impedance flow
    - Mean resistive index (RI) of 0.55
  - First trimester CHM has variable appearance
    - Only 56% with endometrial cysts
    - Can look identical to anembryonic gestation
    - Theca lutein cysts rare < 13 weeks
    - HCG not extremely elevated
  - Often associated with hemorrhage
    - Adjacent sonolucent hematoma
    - Hemorrhage within mass
  - Coexistent mole and fetus is variant of CHM
    - Dizygotic twin pregnancy
    - One normal fetus, one CHM
    - Normal fetus has a normal placenta
- **Partial mole with triploid karyotype**
  - Abnormal fetus
    - Profound intrauterine growth restriction

DDx: Placental Cysts

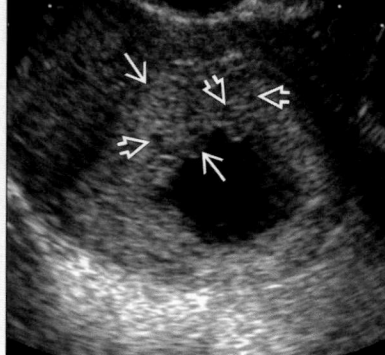

Hydropic Placenta

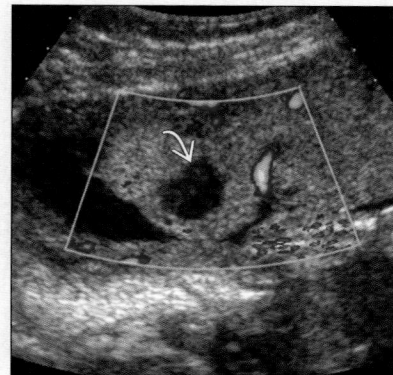

Sonolucencies

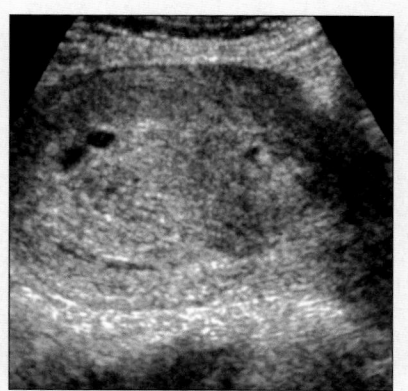

Retained Products of Conception

GESTATIONAL TROPHOBLASTIC NEOPLASM

Key Facts

Imaging Findings
- CHM confined to endometrium
- Invasive mole invades myometrium
- Choriocarcinoma often metastatic
- **CHM is most common type of GTN**
- Cystic intrauterine mass
- Color Doppler shows marked vascularity
- Often associated with hemorrhage
- Coexistent mole and fetus is variant of CHM
- **Theca lutein cysts (TLC): Bilateral multiseptated ovarian cysts**
- 2° to ovarian hyperstimulation
- 50% CHM have associated theca lutein cysts
- 12-15% CHM progress to invasive mole
- 5-8% of CHM progress to choriocarcinoma
- MR helpful in assessing molar invasion

- Transvaginal ultrasound for CHM
- MR with gadolinium for invasive mole
- CT for metastatic choriocarcinoma

Top Differential Diagnoses
- Placental Hydropic Degeneration
- Placental Sonolucencies (Pseudomole)
- Retained Products of Conception (RPOC)

Clinical Issues
- Hyperemesis
- ↑ hCG levels
- Chemotherapy for invasive disease highly effective

Diagnostic Checklist
- Normal hCG levels do not rule out CHM if < 13 wks
- CHM can look identical to anembryonic pregnancy

- ▪ Multiple anomalies
- ○ Variable appearance of placenta
  - ▪ Cystic placenta if extra paternal chromosomes
  - ▪ Small placenta if extra maternal chromosomes
- **Theca lutein cysts (TLC): Bilateral multiseptated ovarian cysts**
  - ○ 2° to ovarian hyperstimulation
    - ▪ ↑ Human chorionic gonadotropin (hCG) hormone
  - ○ 50% CHM have associated theca lutein cysts
- **Malignant GTN**
  - ○ Invasive mole
    - ▪ Invasion of myometrium and beyond
    - ▪ 12-15% CHM progress to invasive mole
    - ▪ Heterogeneous cystic mass in myometrium
    - ▪ ↑ Flow by Doppler
  - ○ Choriocarcinoma
    - ▪ 5-8% of CHM progress to choriocarcinoma
    - ▪ Often present with metastases
    - ▪ Variable uterine findings (often minimal)
  - ○ MR helpful in assessing molar invasion
    - ▪ Myometrial mass
    - ▪ Variable signal intensity
    - ▪ Enhancement with gadolinium
  - ○ Imaging often negative if HCG levels low

Imaging Recommendations
- Best imaging tool
  - ○ Transvaginal ultrasound for CHM
  - ○ MR with gadolinium for invasive mole
  - ○ CT for metastatic choriocarcinoma
- Protocol advice
  - ○ Suspect GTN if hCG levels are atypical
    - ▪ Too high for gestational age
    - ▪ Not resolving normally
  - ○ Look for cystic placenta
  - ○ Anembryonic sac may be CHM
  - ○ Look for signs of invasion
    - ▪ Myometrial vascular cystic spaces

DIFFERENTIAL DIAGNOSIS

Placental Hydropic Degeneration
- Hydropic change without proliferation
- Seen after pregnancy failure
  - ○ Embryonic demise
  - ○ Anembryonic gestation
- Can look identical to CHM
  - ○ Need histologic diagnosis
- Less vascular than CHM
  - ○ ↓ Velocity, ↓ impedance
- Low hCG levels

Placental Sonolucencies (Pseudomole)
- Occasional sonolucencies are normal
  - ○ Placental lakes
  - ○ Intervillous thrombus
  - ○ Often seen > 25 weeks
- "Swiss cheese" variant mimics CHM
  - ○ Pseudomole
  - ○ Often with placentomegaly
  - ○ Associated with maternal/fetal morbidity
    - ▪ Oligohydramnios
    - ▪ Preeclampsia
    - ▪ Intrauterine growth restriction (IUGR)
- Not associated with aneuploidy

Retained Products of Conception (RPOC)
- Incomplete uterine evacuation
  - ○ After normal delivery
  - ○ After abortion or miscarriage
- Complex endometrial mass
  - ○ High-velocity low-resistive blood flow
- Normal to slightly elevated hCG levels

PATHOLOGY

General Features
- General path comments: Abnormal trophoblast proliferation
- Genetics
  - ○ CHM

GESTATIONAL TROPHOBLASTIC NEOPLASM

- 100% paternal genetic makeup
- 46 XX more common than 46 XY
  ○ Triploidy
    - 3 complete sets of chromosomes
    - Diandry = 2 paternal + 1 maternal
    - Digyny = 2 maternal + 1 paternal
- Etiology
  ○ CHM
    - Autonomous trophoblast growth
    - Size of villi ↑ as gestation progresses
  ○ Theca lutein cysts
    - Ovarian hyperstimulation by ↑ hCG
    - Only present in 50%
    - Rare < 13 weeks
- Epidemiology
  ○ CHM
    - 0.5:1,000 in United States
    - 8:1,000 in Asia
    - 12-15% become invasive
  ○ Choriocarcinoma
    - 50% originate from CHM
    - 25% occur after failed pregnancy
    - 25% after normal pregnancy

Gross Pathologic & Surgical Features
- Cystic villi resemble "cluster of grapes"

Microscopic Features
- Trophoblastic hyperplasia
- Hydropic villi

Staging, Grading or Classification Criteria
- Choriocarcinoma
  ○ Stage 1: Confined to uterus
  ○ Stage 2: Limited to pelvis
  ○ Stage 3: Lung metastases
  ○ Stage 4: Other metastases

CLINICAL ISSUES

Presentation
- Most common signs/symptoms
  ○ First trimester CHM
    - Vaginal bleeding
    - Rapid uterine enlargement
    - Hyperemesis
    - HCG levels may be normal
  ○ Second trimester CHM
    - ↑ hCG levels
    - Preeclampsia
  ○ Invasive mole
    - ↑ hCG levels after CHM treatment
  ○ Choriocarcinoma
    - Symptoms of metastatic disease
    - Variable hCG levels
  ○ Triploidy
    - Abnormal fetus
    - Cystic placenta if diandry
    - Small placenta if digyny
- Other signs/symptoms
  ○ Adnexal pain or mass
    - Theca lutein cysts

Demographics
- Age
  ○ ↑ Risk with advanced maternal age
    - ≥ 35 year old at time of delivery
- Ethnicity: ↑ Risk for Asian women

Natural History & Prognosis
- CHM has excellent prognosis
  ○ Evacuation often curative
- Invasive disease
  ○ Near 100% cure with chemotherapy
  ○ 75% remission even if extensive metastases
  ○ Early diagnosis and treatment important

Treatment
- CHM
  ○ Suction evacuation of mass
  ○ Curettage of endometrium
    - Helps determine myometrial invasion
  ○ Serial hCG levels
    - 1 year surveillance
- Chemotherapy for invasive disease highly effective
  ○ Methotrexate
  ○ Actinomycin D
  ○ Etoposide

DIAGNOSTIC CHECKLIST

Consider
- CHM with atypical anembryonic gestation
- Rule out CHM when hCG levels are ↑
- Normal hCG levels do not rule out CHM if < 13 wks
- Careful evaluation for invasive disease
  ○ Color Doppler of myometrium
  ○ MR

Image Interpretation Pearls
- Repeat imaging if hCG levels ↑ after treatment
  ○ Ultrasound to look for myometrial vascular cysts
  ○ MR
- CHM can look identical to anembryonic pregnancy

SELECTED REFERENCES
1. Zhou Q et al: Sonographic and Doppler imaging in the diagnosis and treatment of gestational trophoblastic disease: a 12-year experience. J Ultrasound Med. 24(1):15-24, 2005
2. Garner EI et al: Subsequent pregnancy experience in patients with molar pregnancy and gestational trophoblastic tumor. J Reprod Med. 47(5):380-6, 2002
3. Matsui H et al: Outcome of subsequent pregnancy after treatment for persistent gestational trophoblastic tumour. Hum Reprod. 17(2):469-72, 2002
4. Benson CB et al: Sonographic appearance of first trimester complete hydatidiform moles. Ultrasound Obstet Gynecol. 16(2):188-91, 2000
5. Lazarus E et al: Sonographic appearance of early complete molar pregnancies. J Ultrasound Med. 18(9):589-94; quiz 595-6, 1999
6. Jauniaux E et al: Early ultrasound diagnosis and follow-up of molar pregnancies. Ultrasound Obstet Gynecol. 9(1):17-21, 1997

FUNCTIONAL OVARIAN CYST

Typical

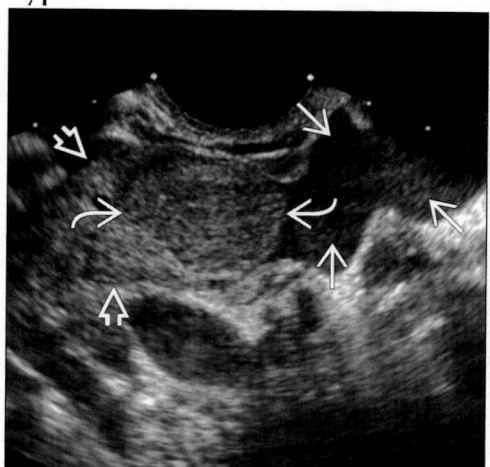
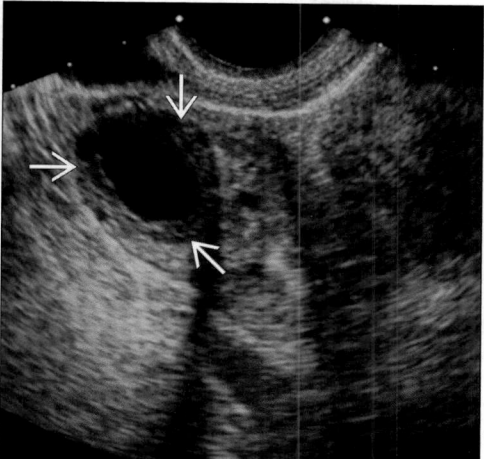

(Left) Transvaginal ultrasound shows significant hemorrhage ⇨ secondary to a rupture of the hemorrhagic CL cyst ⇨ of the right ovary ⇨ in early pregnancy. *(Right)* Transverse transvaginal ultrasound shows the typical thick-wall ⇨ of a corpus luteum cyst. In contrast follicular cysts are thin-walled.

Typical

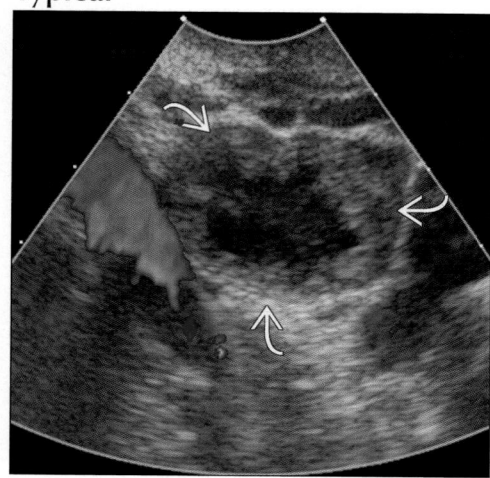
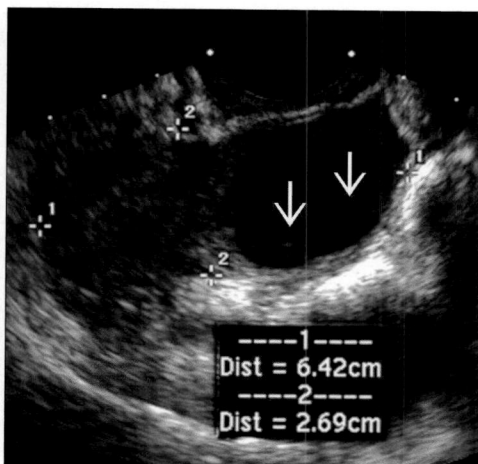

(Left) Oblique transvaginal ultrasound shows another less common appearance of a corpus luteum cyst. The wall ⇨ is thick and echogenic but also irregular or "crenelated". This occurs with collapse of the cyst wall following ovulation. *(Right)* Longitudinal transvaginal ultrasound shows an exophytic corpus luteum cyst with fluid-fluid level ⇨ consistent with hemorrhage. Scan was requested for dating as uterus felt large on bimanual examination.

----1----
Dist = 6.42cm
----2----
Dist = 2.69cm

Typical

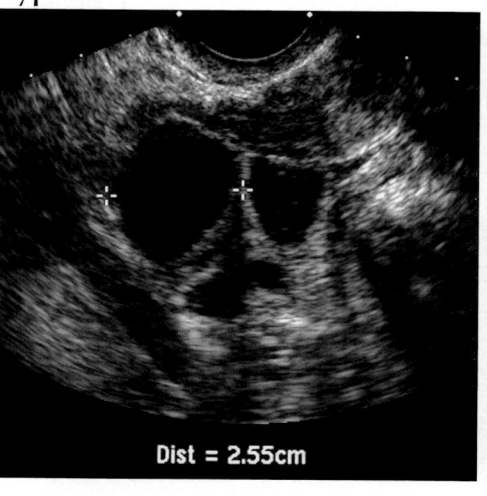
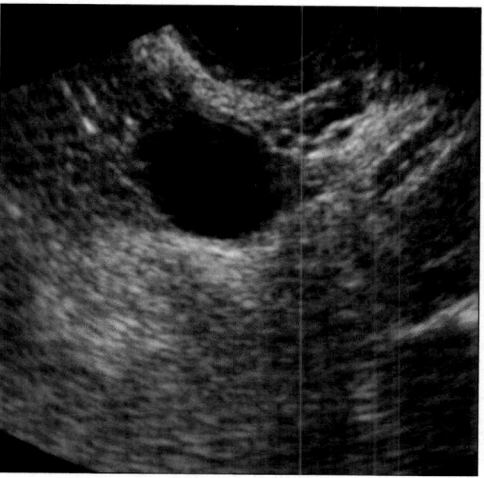

(Left) Longitudinal transvaginal ultrasound shows dominant cystic structure (calipers) measuring 2.55 cm in a patient undergoing ovarian suppression prior to superovulation for assisted reproduction. This is a follicular cyst. *(Right)* Transvaginal ultrasound in her next cycle shows a similar cyst of the opposite ovary. Both were associated with elevated serum estrogen. Superovulation had to be deferred.

Dist = 2.55cm

HEMORRHAGIC CYST

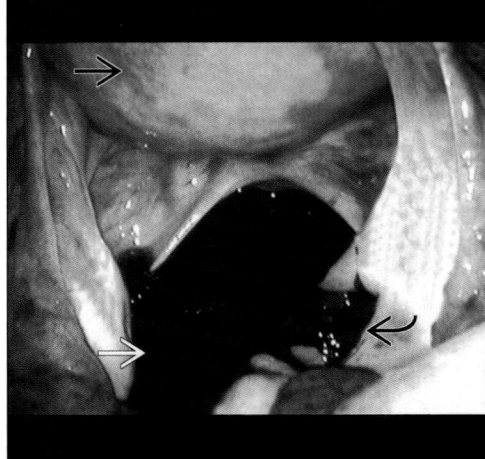

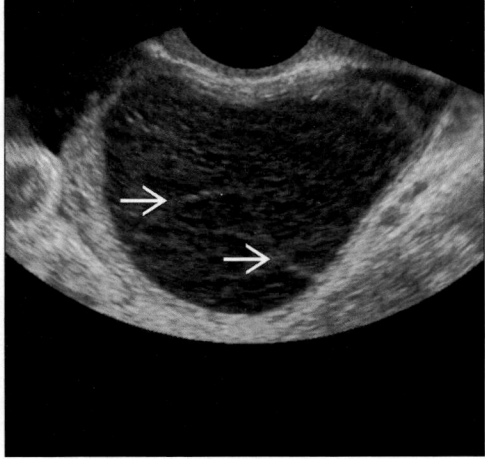

Clinical photograph during laparoscopy shows blood in a cul de sac ➡ behind the uterus ➡ secondary to the ruptured hemorrhagic cyst. Clot ➡ is seen adherent to the ovarian capsule.

Transverse transvaginal ultrasound shows the typical internal architecture of a hemorrhagic cyst, with lacy fibrin strands ➡ within the internal clot. The patient presented with acute pelvic pain.

TERMINOLOGY

Abbreviations and Synonyms
- Hemorrhagic cyst (HC)
- Hemorrhagic corpus luteum (HCL)

Definitions
- Hemorrhage into a cystic space in ovarian parenchyma
  - Commonest at time of ovulation → HCL
  - May occur into follicular cyst
  - Acute hemorrhage may occur into an established endometrioma

IMAGING FINDINGS

General Features
- Best diagnostic clue: Avascular hypoechoic adnexal "mass" with fine lacy interstices
- Location: Intraovarian
- Size: Variable, up to 8 cm diameter

Ultrasonographic Findings
- Grayscale Ultrasound
  - 92% show increased through transmission
    - Indicates "cystic" nature even though initial assessment may suggest solid mass
  - May appear as mixed echogenicity mass
  - Acute clot with fibrin strands → lacy interstices
  - Clot retraction → rim of fluid within cyst surrounding clot
  - Clot fragmentation → angular margins of clot fragments
    - Fragments adhere to cyst wall
    - Float in fluid component
    - "Jelly-like" motion with transducer compression
  - As clot resorbs HC becomes more like a simple cyst
  - Majority resorb quickly and leave no sequela on 6 week follow-up scans
  - HC may rupture
    - Look for echogenic fluid in cul de sac
    - With significant hemorrhage may see hemoperitoneum
    - Remember to check for fluid in hepatorenal fossa/subphrenic spaces
  - Cyst wall often appears thick
- Color Doppler
  - Clot is avascular

DDx: Palpable Adnexal Mass

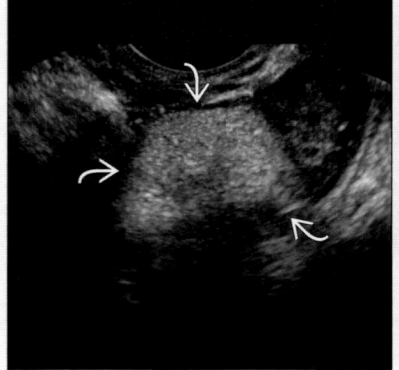

Teratoma

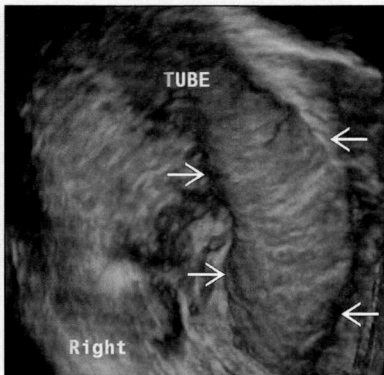

Hydrosalpinx

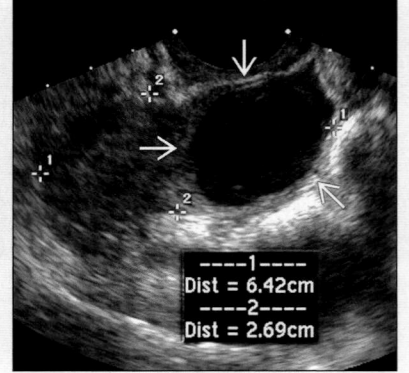

Functional Luteal Cyst

HEMORRHAGIC CYST

Key Facts

Terminology
- Hemorrhage into a cystic space in ovarian parenchyma

Imaging Findings
- Best diagnostic clue: Avascular hypoechoic adnexal "mass" with fine lacy interstices
- 92% show increased through transmission
- May appear as mixed echogenicity mass
- Clot retraction → rim of fluid within cyst surrounding clot
- Clot fragmentation → angular margins of clot fragments
- Majority resorb quickly and leave no sequela on 6 week follow-up scans
- HC may rupture

- May see increased flow at margins of corpus luteum: "Ring of fire" appearance

Top Differential Diagnoses
- Endometrioma
- Ectopic Pregnancy
- Torsion
- Pelvic Abscess

Clinical Issues
- May complicate ovulation induction in assisted reproduction

Diagnostic Checklist
- Hemorrhage can be cause or effect of ovarian torsion
- 90% of hemorrhagic ovarian cysts will exhibit fibrin strands or retracting clot

---

- ○ May see increased flow at margins of corpus luteum: "Ring of fire" appearance
- ○ Look for flow in ovarian parenchyma
  - ▪ HC may → torsion
  - ▪ Any mass → torsion → infarction → hemorrhage

CT Findings
- May appear simple
- May see fluid-fluid level
- May show ring-enhancement
- May see high attenuation material in adnexal mass

MR Findings
- T1WI
  - ○ Typically intermediate to high signal blood products with no loss of signal on FS images but
    - ▪ 64% of 22 confirmed HC were hypointense on T1 weighted images
    - ▪ 18% were also hyperintense on T2 weighted images
  - ○ Hematocrit effect: High signal layering blood akin to sonographic fluid-fluid level
- T2WI: Typically intermediate to low signal

Imaging Recommendations
- Best imaging tool: Transvaginal ultrasound

DIFFERENTIAL DIAGNOSIS

Endometrioma
- More likely to have history of chronic pelvic pain
- Uniform low-level internal echoes from blood breakdown products rather than lacy fibrin strands in clot
- Walls often contain punctate high echogenic foci
- Will not change much on follow-up
  - ○ HC would be expected to resolve or decrease significantly in size
- Occasionally an acute bleed into an endometrioma may produce a confusing picture
  - ○ Follow-up will show resolution of acute clot with persistent background endometrioma

Ectopic Pregnancy
- Positive pregnancy test
- Hemorrhagic adnexal mass rather than intra-ovarian
  - ○ Ovarian ectopics are very uncommon
- Use realtime observation during transducer pressure
  - ○ Ovary will "slide" over an adnexal mass
  - ○ Intra-ovarian mass moves with the ovary
- May see "ring of fire" sign of increased flow in trophoblastic tissue
  - ○ Make sure it is not around a corpus luteum in the ovary
  - ○ Not all ectopics demonstrate this sign

Torsion
- Look for flow in walls of cyst or adjacent parenchyma
  - ○ Venous system low pressure therefore more affected than arterial
  - ○ If no venous flow in an enlarged tender ovary torsion is very likely

Solid Ovarian Mass
- Papillary projections more likely than angular fragments
- Solid masses reflect sound equally with ovarian parenchyma
  - ○ No increased through transmission
- Internal perfusion seen with Doppler interrogation

Pelvic Abscess
- Febrile patient
- May see echogenic fluid in cul de sac due to inflammatory exudate
- Pelvic inflammatory disease → edema → loss of tissue planes → difficulty identifying structures
  - ○ May be associated with purulent discharge
  - ○ Often extremely tender during sonography
- Appendix abscess may form in the pelvis: Remember non-gynecologic causes

HEMORRHAGIC CYST

PATHOLOGY

General Features
- Epidemiology
  - One series 112 patients
    - 71% in nulliparous patients
    - 29% multiparous
    - 77% in luteal phase of menstrual cycle
    - 12% in proliferative phase
    - 11% in early gestation
- Majority occur as result of bleeding into functional ovarian cyst; follicular/corpus luteum

CLINICAL ISSUES

Presentation
- Most common signs/symptoms: Acute pelvic pain
- Other signs/symptoms
  - May be asymptomatic
    - In one series of 112 patients only 38% presented with acute pain
    - Remaining cases detected during sonography for other indications most commonly palpable mass on pelvic examination
  - Mittelschmerz
    - Ovulation pain
  - May complicate ovulation induction in assisted reproduction
    - Rupture may → significant hemorrhage
    - Acute pain can be confusing for torsion of enlarged stimulated ovary
  - Neonatal presentation
    - Fetal ovarian cysts are well described
    - Development of a fluid-fluid level in utero is very suspicious for hemorrhage/torsion
    - Infants are generally asymptomatic at birth
    - Elective surgery recommended to fix the contralateral ovary/prevent future torsion

Natural History & Prognosis
- Majority resolve spontaneously
  - Severe pain resolves within hours in > 90%
  - Mass will disappear in > 90% within 8 weeks
- If large may cause adnexal torsion
- Larger cysts more likely to cause acute pain/presentation with acute abdomen
- May rupture
  - Supportive treatment adequate in most
  - Occasional need for laparoscopy

Treatment
- Symptomatic
- If recurrent consider ovulation suppression

DIAGNOSTIC CHECKLIST

Consider
- Look for rind of ovarian tissue containing follicles: "Claw" sign
  - Confirms intraovarian process

- Increased through transmission suggests cystic entity rather than solid mass
- Hemorrhage can be cause or effect of ovarian torsion

Image Interpretation Pearls
- 90% of hemorrhagic ovarian cysts will exhibit fibrin strands or retracting clot
  - Lacy interstices due to fibrin strands are characteristic of acute clot
  - "Mass" with angular margins suggests fragmented clot rather than papillary projections from neoplasm
- Beware the "ring of fire" sign
  - Frequently around corpus luteum, does not imply ectopic pregnancy
  - Majority of hemorrhagic cysts can be managed conservatively unlike ruptured ectopic pregnancies
- Reported cause or false positive F-18 FDG uptake in PET scans
  - Consider ultrasound for any unexpected ovarian mass on PET scans

SELECTED REFERENCES

1. Kanso HN et al: Variable MR findings in ovarian functional hemorrhagic cysts. J Magn Reson Imaging. 24(2):356-61, 2006
2. Ames J et al: 18F-FDG uptake in an ovary containing a hemorrhagic corpus luteal cyst: false-positive PET/CT in a patient with cervical carcinoma. AJR Am J Roentgenol. 185(4):1057-9, 2005
3. Kurioka H et al: Hemorrhagic ovarian cyst without peritoneal bleeding in a patient with ovarian hyperstimulation syndrome: case report. Chin Med J (Engl). 118(18):1577-81, 2005
4. Patel MD et al: The likelihood ratio of sonographic findings for the diagnosis of hemorrhagic ovarian cysts. J Ultrasound Med. 24(5):607-14; quiz 615, 2005
5. Condous G et al: Should we be examining the ovaries in pregnancy? Prevalence and natural history of adnexal pathology detected at first-trimester sonography. Ultrasound Obstet Gynecol. 24(1):62-6, 2004
6. Kives SL et al: Ruptured hemorrhagic cyst in an undescended ovary. J Pediatr Surg. 39(11):e4-6, 2004
7. Swire MN et al: Various sonographic appearances of the hemorrhagic corpus luteum cyst. Ultrasound Q. 20(2):45-58, 2004
8. Edwards A et al: Acoustic streaming: a new technique for assessing adnexal cysts. Ultrasound Obstet Gynecol. 22(1):74-8, 2003
9. Nemoto Y et al: Ultrasonographic and clinical appearance of hemorrhagic ovarian cyst diagnosed by transvaginal scan. J Nippon Med Sch. 70(3):243-9, 2003
10. Teng SW et al: Comparison of laparoscopy and laparotomy in managing hemodynamically stable patients with ruptured corpus luteum with hemoperitoneum. J Am Assoc Gynecol Laparosc. 10(4):474-7, 2003
11. Jain KA: Sonographic spectrum of hemorrhagic ovarian cysts. J Ultrasound Med. 21(8):879-86, 2002
12. Hertzberg BS et al: Ovarian cyst rupture causing hemoperitoneum: imaging features and the potential for misdiagnosis. Abdom Imaging. 24(3):304-8, 1999
13. O'Brien PM et al: Management of an acute hemorrhagic ovarian cyst in a female patient with hemophilia A. J Pediatr Hematol Oncol. 18(2):233-6, 1996

OVARIAN HYPERSTIMULATION

Key Facts

Imaging Findings

- Bilaterally enlarged, cystic ovaries
- Heterogeneous complex ovarian cysts with debris, septa if hemorrhagic component present
- Ascites
- Pleural effusion

Top Differential Diagnoses

- Theca Lutein Cysts
- Echogenic peritoneal fluid

Pathology

- Exaggerated response to ovulation induction
- Increased permeability of peritoneal and pleural surfaces
- Protein-rich fluid leaks out of intravascular space

Clinical Issues

- Polycystic ovarian syndrome major risk factor
- Early type occurs < 5 days after oocyte retrieval
- Late type occurs ≥ 5 days (range 5-15 days) after oocyte retrieval
- Late type always associated with pregnancy
- Should be self-limiting as long as supportive care started early in process
- More severe in patients who become pregnant
- Severe OHSS potentially life-threatening

Diagnostic Checklist

- Avoid aggressive transvaginal imaging as ovaries can be friable
- Correlate imaging appearance of ovaries with clinical history for diagnosis

DIFFERENTIAL DIAGNOSIS

Theca Lutein Cysts

- Multiple cysts within enlarged ovaries
- Not associated with ascites, pleural effusions or oliguria
- Multiple etiologies
  - Multiple gestation
  - Exogenous hormonal stimulation
  - Gestational trophoblastic disease
  - Triploidy

Hyperreactio Luteinalis

- More mild, indolent course within spectrum of OHSS
- Bilateral ovarian enlargement with multiple theca lutein cysts
- Always associated with pregnancy
- High maternal human chorionic gonadotropin (hCG) serum levels
  - No exogenous hCG administered
  - May be a response to chronic exposure to elevated hCG levels

Cystic Ovarian Neoplasm

- Usually unilateral
- Serous cystadenoma/cystadenocarcinoma
- Mucinous cystadenoma/cystadenocarcinoma
- Cystic germ cell tumors

Polycystic Ovarian Syndrome

- Bilateral enlarged ovaries with hyperechoic central stroma
- Multiple small peripheral follicles ("string-of-pearls")
- Chronic anovulation
- Associated with obesity and insulin resistance

Ectopic and Heterotopic Pregnancy

- Echogenic peritoneal fluid
- Adnexal mass
- Higher risk in women undergoing ovulation induction

PATHOLOGY

General Features

- Epidemiology
  - Moderate OHSS: 3-6% of in vitro fertilization (IVF) cases
  - Severe OHSS: 0.1-2.0% of IVF cases
- Exaggerated response to ovulation induction
  - Almost exclusively associated with exogenous gonadotropin use
  - Numerous potential pathophysiologic mediators
    - Cytokines
    - Growth factors
- Most likely associated with vascular endothelial growth factor (VEGF)
  - Granulosa cells are one site of production
  - hCG and VEGF serum levels correlate with severity of OHSS
- Paradoxical arterial dilation and ↓ peripheral vascular resistance
  - Leads to compensatory release of vasoactive substances
    - Aldosterone
    - Antidiuretic hormone
    - Norepinephrine
    - Renin
  - Increased permeability of peritoneal and pleural surfaces
    - Protein-rich fluid leaks out of intravascular space
    - Leads to ascites and pleural effusions

Gross Pathologic & Surgical Features

- Ovaries appear similar to changes seen with theca lutein cysts
  - Bilaterally enlarged
  - Multiple follicular cysts with prominent luteinization of theca interna layer
- Corpus luteum present
  - May be more than one

OVARIAN HYPERSTIMULATION

CLINICAL ISSUES

Presentation
- Most common signs/symptoms
  - Abdominal pain
  - Nausea/vomiting/diarrhea
  - Weight gain
  - Oliguria
- Other signs/symptoms
  - Abdominal distention from ascites
  - Shortness of breath from pleural effusion
  - Hypotension
  - Electrolyte imbalance
- Typically seen in women undergoing ovulation induction
  - Follicle stimulating hormone (FSH) followed by hCG
- Relative hemoconcentration due to fluid leaking into peritoneal/pleural spaces
  - Increased risk of thromboembolism
  - Oliguria

Demographics
- Risk factors
  - Polycystic ovarian syndrome major risk factor
    - May be related to increased number of follicles/oocytes produced when stimulated
    - Oligomenorrhea itself also a risk factor
  - Younger age
  - Previous OHSS history
- Risk correlates with increasing
  - Ovarian volumes
  - Number of oocytes retrieved
  - Number of baseline follicles
  - Number of developing follicles during FSH stimulation
    - Especially intermediate size (10-15 mm)
  - Serum estradiol concentrations

Natural History & Prognosis
- Occurs after ovulation
  - Early type occurs < 5 days after oocyte retrieval
    - Induced by exogenous hCG administration
  - Late type occurs ≥ 5 days (range 5-15 days) after oocyte retrieval
    - Induced by endogenous hCG from implanted pregnancy
    - Late type always associated with pregnancy
- Should be self-limiting as long as supportive care started early in process
- Usually regresses over 10-14 days unless pregnancy implantation occurs
  - Subsequently can have increase in endogenous hCG
  - May prolong OHSS or initiate late form of OHSS
- More severe in patients who become pregnant
- Severe OHSS potentially life-threatening
  - Mortality estimated at 1:45,000 cases of OHSS

Treatment
- No known therapy to immediately reverse OHSS
- Avoid pelvic trauma to ovaries
  - No intercourse, pelvic exams, strenuous exercise
- Conservative therapy with observation warranted
  - May be monitored as an outpatient

- Frequent vital sign and electrolyte checks
  - Maintain intravascular volume and urine output
    - 24 urine volume measurements
    - Daily weights
  - Consider ultrasound guided paracentesis or thoracentesis for symptoms
    - Serial abdominal girth measurements
  - Prophylactic anticoagulation
    - Useful due to relative hemoconcentration
- Some advocate proactive management to shorten course of symptoms
  - Most often considered if moderate to severe OHSS
  - Actively administer fluids and/or albumin
    - Diuretics considered when adequate intravascular volume achieved
  - Benefits of ultrasound guided paracentesis
    - ↓ Hospitalization
    - ↓ Hemoconcentration
    - ↑ Urine output
    - Ameliorates electrolyte abnormalities
- Hospitalization criteria
  - Intractable pain
  - Intractable nausea/vomiting
  - Respiratory difficulties
  - Suspected infection/hemorrhage
  - Hypotension
  - Electrolyte imbalance
  - Leukocytosis
  - HCT > 45%
  - ↑ Liver function tests
  - Oliguria
  - Creatinine > 1.2 mg/dL or creatinine clearance < 50 mL/min
- Surgical intervention only rarely required
  - Ovarian torsion
  - Cyst rupture with hemoperitoneum
- Partial oophorectomy for severe cases reported

DIAGNOSTIC CHECKLIST

Image Interpretation Pearls
- Avoid aggressive transvaginal imaging as ovaries can be friable
- Correlate imaging appearance of ovaries with clinical history for diagnosis

SELECTED REFERENCES

1. Suzuki S: Comparison between spontaneous ovarian hyperstimulation syndrome and hyperreactio luteinalis. Arch Gynecol Obstet. 269(3):227-9, 2004
2. Aboulghar MA et al: Ovarian hyperstimulation syndrome: classifications and critical analysis of preventive measures. Hum Reprod Update. 9(3):275-89, 2003
3. Delvigne A et al: Review of clinical course and treatment of ovarian hyperstimulation syndrome (OHSS). Hum Reprod Update. 9(1):77-96, 2003
4. Delvigne A et al: Epidemiology and prevention of ovarian hyperstimulation syndrome (OHSS): a review. Hum Reprod Update. 8(6):559-77, 2002
5. Mathur RS et al: Distinction between early and late ovarian hyperstimulation syndrome. Fertil Steril. 73(5):901-7, 2000

OVARIAN HYPERSTIMULATION

Typical

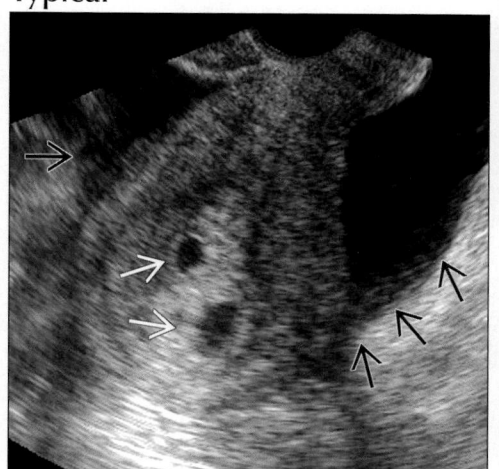
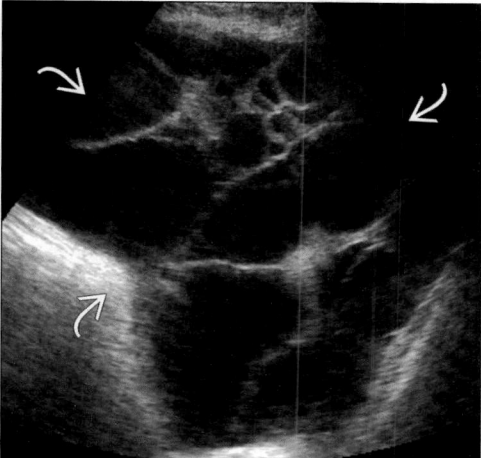

(Left) Transvaginal ultrasound of a patient with late OHSS shows two gestational sacs ➡ present in the uterus, with free fluid in the pelvis ➡. (Right) Transverse ultrasound shows the right ovary ➚, which measures up to 31 cm. The left ovary measured up to 19 cm (not shown). In addition, the patient required thoracentesis for large a right pleural effusion.

Typical

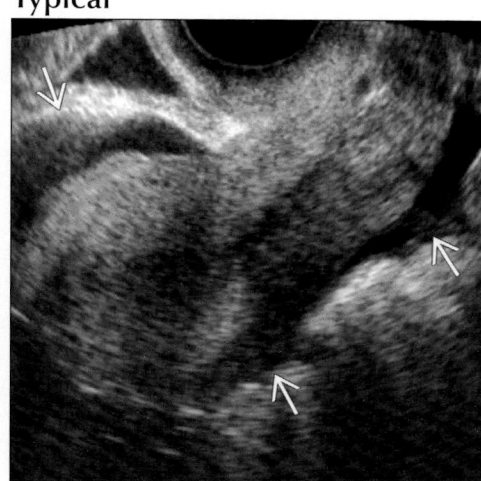
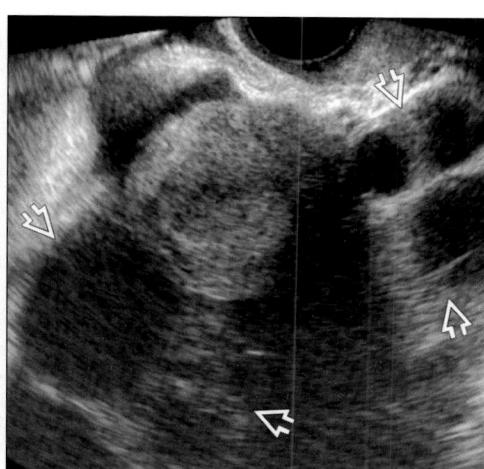

(Left) Transvaginal ultrasound shows initial imaging of the uterus post-oocyte retrieval without a visible gestational sac, however free fluid is present surrounding the uterus ➡. (Right) Transverse transvaginal ultrasound shows bilaterally enlarged cystic ovaries ➡. Early OHSS typically occurs within 5 days after oocyte retrieval, prior to documentation of intrauterine pregnancy.

Typical

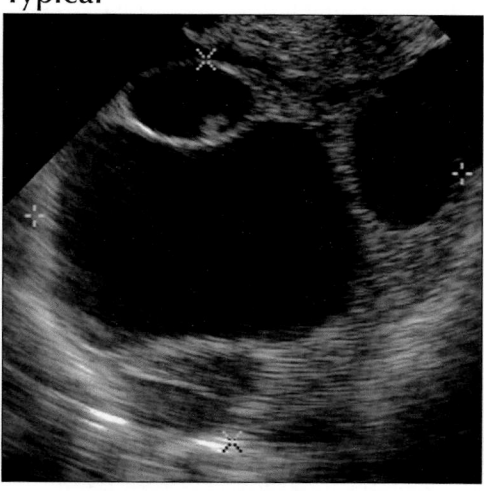
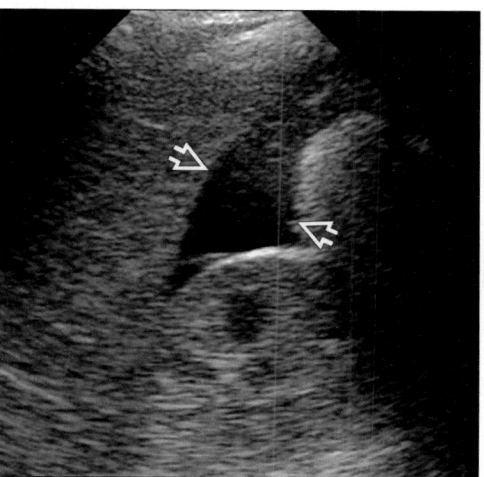

(Left) Longitudinal transabdominal ultrasound shows large cysts in the right ovary (calipers) in a patient with early hyperstimulation syndrome. This ovary measures 7 x 8.5 cm, and the left ovary had a similar appearance. (Right) Transverse transabdominal ultrasound shows free fluid ➡ in the upper abdomen at the margin of liver as well.

SEROUS OVARIAN CYSTADENOMA/CARCINOMA

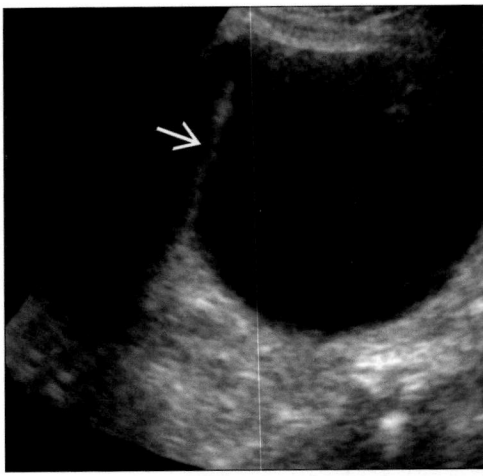

Transabdominal ultrasound shows a cystic ovarian mass with a single, thin septation ➡. There are no papillary projections or solid components. The fluid within the cyst is anechoic.

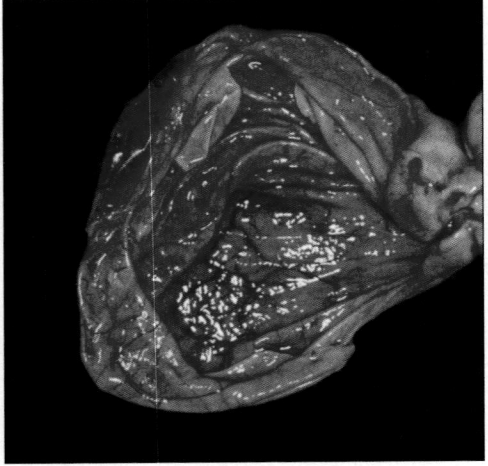

Gross pathology after the fluid has been drained shows the thin wall typical of a serous cystadenoma. They are typically unilocular or have few septations, and can be quite large.

TERMINOLOGY

Abbreviations and Synonyms
- Benign or malignant serous tumor

Definitions
- Serous epithelial neoplasm, which can be benign (serous cystadenoma), borderline (low malignant potential) or malignant (serous cystadenocarcinoma)

IMAGING FINDINGS

General Features
- Best diagnostic clue: Large, thin-walled, unilocular mass with papillary projections
- Location: Bilateral in 25% of benign tumors and 65% of malignant tumors
- Size: Variable but often large

Ultrasonographic Findings
- Grayscale Ultrasound
  - Typically unilocular or few septations even in malignant tumors
  - Cyst fluid clear to mildly echogenic
    - Usually less echogenic than mucinous counterpart
  - Septae often thin but may be thick, especially in malignant tumors
  - Papillary projections common
    - Does not necessarily indicate malignancy
    - Likelihood of malignancy does increase with increased amount of solid components
  - May see ascites and peritoneal implants in metastatic disease
    - Ascites very concerning for metastatic disease (positive predictive value of 72-80% as a sign of peritoneal metastases)
  - ≈ 1/3 have microcalcifications (psammoma bodies) in primary tumor and peritoneal metastases
    - Usually not discernible by ultrasound
- Doppler ultrasound
  - Flow seen in solid components
  - Central flow within a mass is more suggestive of malignancy than peripheral flow
  - Malignant lesions often have increased flow but quantitative parameters, such as pulsatility index and resistive index, are not reliable in differentiating benign from malignant

DDx: Complex Ovarian Mass

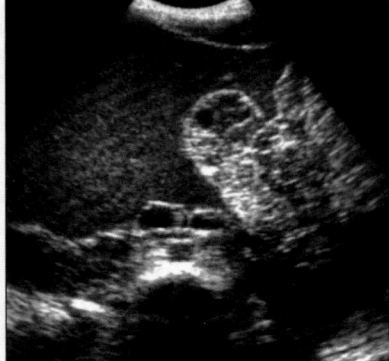

Mucinous Cystadenocarcinoma

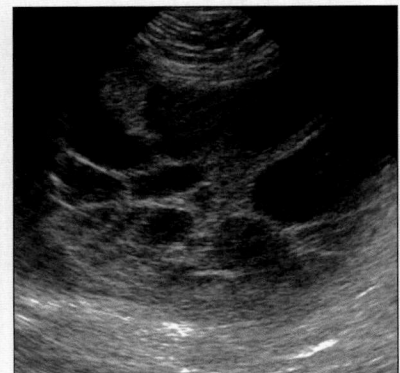

Metastases

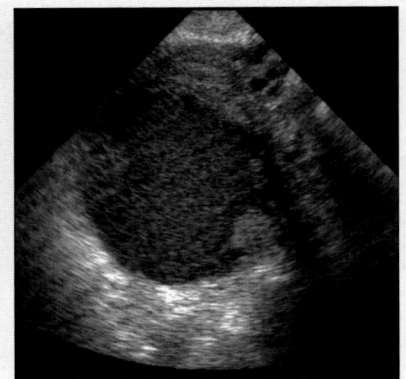

Clear Cell Carcinoma

SEROUS OVARIAN CYSTADENOMA/CARCINOMA

Key Facts

Imaging Findings
- Typically unilocular or few septations even in malignant tumors
- Cyst fluid clear to mildly echogenic
- Usually less echogenic than mucinous counterpart
- Papillary projections common
- Ascites very concerning for metastatic disease (positive predictive value of 72-80% as a sign of peritoneal metastases)
- Malignant lesions often have increased flow but quantitative parameters, such as pulsatility index and resistive index, are not reliable in differentiating benign from malignant

Top Differential Diagnoses
- Other Epithelial Tumors
- Ovarian Metastases

Pathology
- Epithelial tumors 60-70% of all tumors: 85-90% of malignancies
- Serous tumors most common epithelial neoplasm
- Malignant 25%, borderline (low malignant potential) 15%, benign 60%
- Bilateral in 25% of benign tumors, 30% of borderline tumors and 65% of malignant tumors

Clinical Issues
- 70% of patients with malignant tumors have peritoneal involvement at time of diagnosis

Diagnostic Checklist
- Serous cystadenoma is most likely diagnosis for a large, simple-appearing, unilocular cyst in a postmenopausal woman

---

CT Findings
- Calcifications more likely to be identified
- Soft tissue components enhance with contrast
- Study of choice for tumor staging

MR Findings
- T1WI: Low-signal cyst fluid, with intermediate signal solid component
- T2WI: High-signal cyst fluid, with heterogeneous solid components
- T1 C+: Enhancement of solid components

Imaging Recommendations
- Best imaging tool
  - Ultrasound ideal method for lesion detection and characterization
    - Always use Doppler to evaluate for flow
  - CT preferred for tumor staging
- Protocol advice: Evaluate along paracolic gutters and capsule of liver for possible peritoneal implants

DIFFERENTIAL DIAGNOSIS

Mucinous Cystadenoma/Carcinoma
- Multilocular masses with low-level echoes

Other Epithelial Tumors
- Significant overlap in imaging findings
- All less common than serous tumors

Ovarian Metastases
- Look for upper abdominal malignancy

PATHOLOGY

General Features
- General path comments
  - **Ovarian neoplasms**
    - Epithelial tumors 60-70% of all tumors: 85-90% of malignancies

- Germ cell tumors 15-20% of all tumors: 3-5% of malignancies
- Sex cord-stromal tumors 5-10% of all tumors: 2-3% of malignancies
- Metastases and lymphoma 5-10% of all tumors: 5-10% of malignancies
  - **Benign epithelial tumors**
    - Serous cystadenoma 20-25%
    - Mucinous cystadenoma 20-25%
  - **Malignant epithelial tumors**
    - Serous cystadenocarcinoma 40-50%
    - Endometrioid carcinoma 20-25%
    - Mucinous cystadenocarcinoma 5-10%
    - Clear cell carcinoma 5-10%
    - Brenner tumor 1-2%
    - Undifferentiated carcinoma 4-5%
- Genetics: Hereditary causes in 5-10% of ovarian cancers (mutations in BRCA1 and BRCA2 tumor suppressor genes)
- Etiology
  - Not completely understood
  - One theory is "incessant ovulation": Repeated microtrauma with cellular repair to surface epithelium
    - Increased risk: Nulliparity, early menarche, late menopause (more ovulatory cycles)
    - Reduced risk: Multiparity, late menarche, early menopause, oral contraceptive use (fewer ovulatory cycles)
- Epidemiology
  - Serous tumors most common epithelial neoplasm
  - Malignant 25%, borderline (low malignant potential) 15%, benign 60%
  - Bilateral in 25% of benign tumors, 30% of borderline tumors and 65% of malignant tumors
- Associated abnormalities: May occasionally be hormonally active producing estrogen
- Methods of spread
  - Intraperitoneal dissemination most common
    - Greater omentum, right subphrenic region, and pouch of Douglas most common sites found at surgery

SEROUS OVARIAN CYSTADENOMA/CARCINOMA

○ Direct extension into surrounding organs
○ Lymphatic spread to paraaortic and pelvic nodes
○ Hematogenous spread least common
  ▪ Liver and lung most common sites

Staging, Grading or Classification Criteria
• FIGO staging system of ovarian carcinoma
  ○ Stage I: Tumor limited to ovaries
    ▪ IA: Unilateral, no malignant ascites
    ▪ IB: Bilateral, no malignant ascites
    ▪ IC: IA or IB with malignant ascites or positive peritoneal washings
  ○ Stage II: Tumor involves one or both ovaries with pelvic extension
    ▪ IIA: Extension to uterus or fallopian tubes, no malignant ascites
    ▪ IIB: Extension to other pelvic tissues, no malignant ascites
    ▪ IIC: IIA or IIB with malignant ascites or positive peritoneal washings
  ○ Stage III: Peritoneal implants or nodal metastases outside the pelvis
    ▪ IIIA: Microscopic peritoneal implants
    ▪ IIIB: Macroscopic implants < 2 cm
    ▪ IIIC: Implants > 2 cm or lymph node metastases
  ○ Stage IV: Distant metastases (excluding peritoneal implants)

CLINICAL ISSUES

Presentation
• Most common signs/symptoms
  ○ Incidental discovered on physical exam
  ○ Pelvic discomfort/pain from large tumors
  ○ Symptoms from metastatic disease
    ▪ 70% of patients with malignant tumors have peritoneal involvement at time of diagnosis
• Abnormal CA-125: Strongest association with serous cystadenocarcinoma (compared to other histologic types)
  ○ Important to know limitations
    ▪ False negative in 50% of stage I tumors (inadequate as screening tool)
    ▪ False positives occur (especially in premenopausal women) with benign neoplasms, endometriosis
  ○ Most commonly used to follow known disease

Demographics
• Age
  ○ Serous cystadenoma in 30s and 40s
  ○ Serous cystadenocarcinoma in peri- and postmenopausal age group

Natural History & Prognosis
• 95% 5 year survival for low malignant potential tumors
  ○ If metastatic, prognosis is similar to those with frankly malignant histology
• 5 year survival rate for malignant epithelial tumors
  ○ Stage I - 80%
  ○ Stage II - 50%
  ○ Stage III - 30%
  ○ Stage IV - 8%

Treatment
• Primary treatment is surgery
  ○ Should do complete staging laparotomy and tumor debulking (cytoreduction)
    ▪ Staging laparotomy includes hysterectomy with bilateral salpingo-oophorectomy, pelvic and paraaortic node biopsies, omentectomy, peritoneal biopsies and washings
    ▪ More conservative surgery may be done for women with stage I disease in reproductive age group
    ▪ Debulking considered optimal if < 1.5-2.0 cm residual tumor remains
• Chemotherapy after cytoreductive surgery
• Neoadjuvant chemotherapy before cytoreductive surgery in patients with unresectable disease
  ○ Includes bulky disease in difficult to reach areas (porta hepatis, lesser sac, root of mesentery), extensive surrounding organ or sidewall invasion, or stage IV disease

DIAGNOSTIC CHECKLIST

Consider
• In trying to determine benign from malignant ovarian masses must consider multiple parameters
  ○ Morphologic appearance: Septations, papillary projections, solid components
  ○ Doppler: Presence of flow, location and quantitative parameters
  ○ Age and hormonal status
  ○ Clinical history
  ○ Ancillary findings (e.g., ascites)

Image Interpretation Pearls
• Serous cystadenoma is most likely diagnosis for a large, simple-appearing, unilocular cyst in a postmenopausal woman

SELECTED REFERENCES

1. Woodward PJ et al: From the archives of the AFIP: radiologic staging of ovarian carcinoma with pathologic correlation. Radiographics. 24(1):225-46, 2004
2. Hanbidge AE et al: US of the peritoneum. Radiographics. 23(3):663-84; discussion 684-5, 2003
3. Coakley FV et al: Peritoneal metastases: detection with spiral CT in patients with ovarian cancer. Radiology. 223(2):495-9, 2002
4. Sawicki W et al: Preoperative discrimination between malignant and benign adnexal masses with transvaginal ultrasonography and colour blood flow imaging. Eur J Gynaecol Oncol. 22(2):137-42, 2001
5. Holschneider CH et al: Ovarian cancer: epidemiology, biology, and prognostic factors. Semin Surg Oncol. 19(1):3-10, 2000
6. Brown DL et al: Benign and malignant ovarian masses: selection of the most discriminating gray-scale and Doppler sonographic features. Radiology. 208(1):103-10, 1998
7. Wagner BJ et al: From the archives of the AFIP. Ovarian epithelial neoplasms: radiologic-pathologic correlation. Radiographics. 14(6):1351-74; quiz 1375-6, 1994

IMAGE GALLERY

Typical

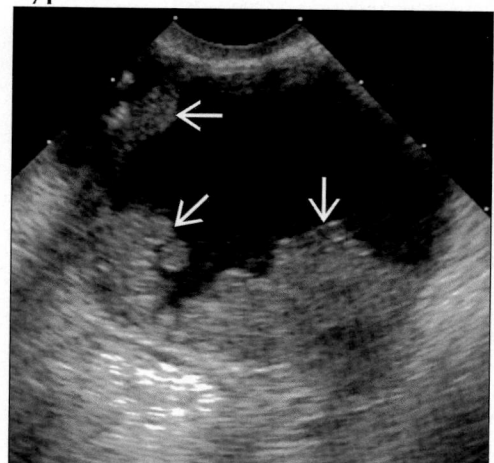 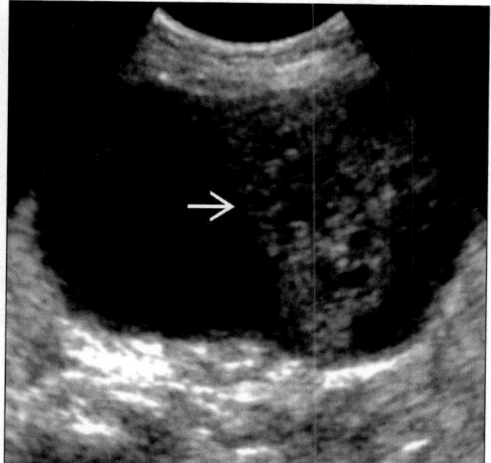

(Left) Transvaginal ultrasound shows a unilocular mass with multiple, solid papillary projections ➡. Despite this very worrisome appearance, histology showed a serous tumor of low malignant potential, which has a much better prognosis than frankly malignant tumors. (Right) Transabdominal ultrasound shows a unilocular cystic mass with a large, solid component ➡. Histology showed a serous cystadenocarcinoma.

Typical

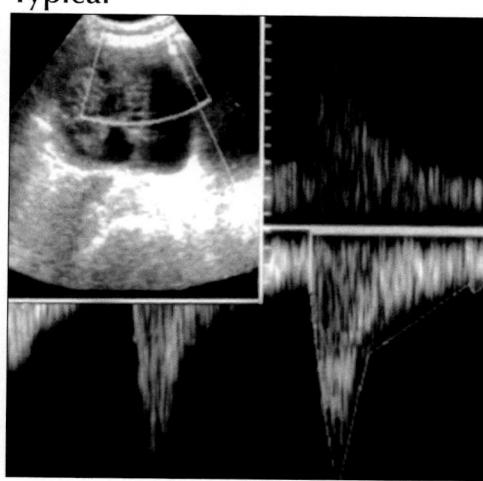 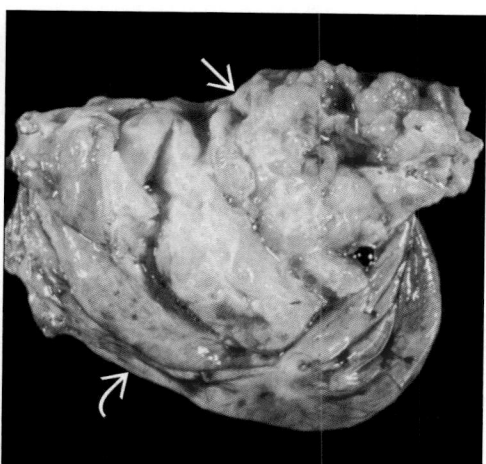

(Left) Pulsed Doppler ultrasound from the prior case shows marked flow within the solid component of the mass. (Right) Gross pathology after the fluid has been drained shows the large solid component ➡, within the otherwise thin sac ➡.

Typical

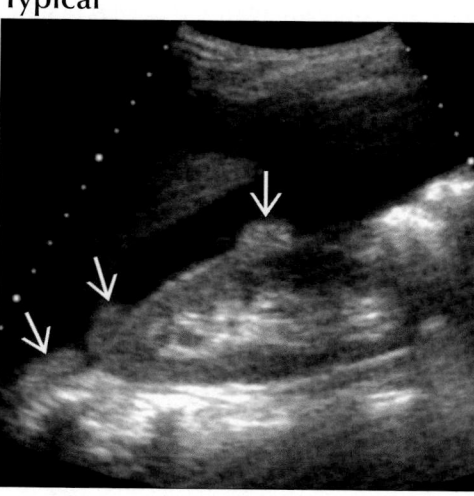 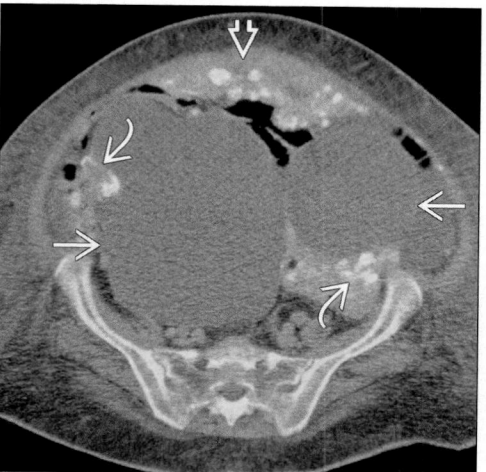

(Left) Longitudinal ultrasound of the right paracolic gutter shows several peritoneal implants ➡ in a case of metastatic serous cystadenocarcinoma. (Right) CECT shows bilateral, serous cystadenocarcinomas ➡ with spread to the omentum ➡. Note the calcifications within the omental metastases and primary tumors ➡. Malignant tumors are bilateral in 65% of cases and calcifications have been reported in 33% of peritoneal metastases.

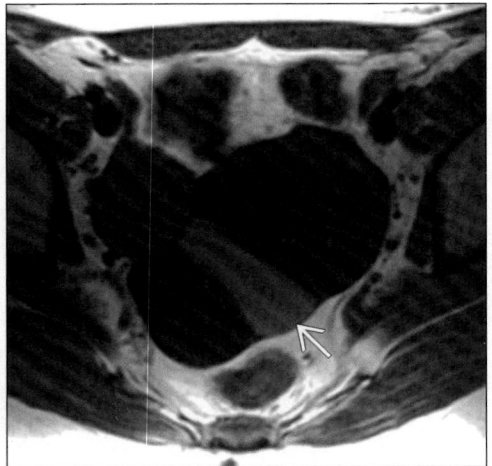

Transvaginal ultrasound shows a multilocular ovarian mass with uniform, low-level echoes, typical of a mucinous cystadenoma. No solid components are seen.

Axial T1WI shows one loculus →has slightly increased signal, while the others are low signal. Signal varies according to the concentration of mucin. This creates what has been called the "stained glass" appearance.

TERMINOLOGY

Abbreviations and Synonyms
- Benign or malignant mucinous tumor

Definitions
- Mucinous epithelial neoplasm, which can be benign (mucinous cystadenoma), borderline (low malignant potential) or malignant (mucinous cystadenocarcinoma)

IMAGING FINDINGS

General Features
- Best diagnostic clue: Multilocular cystic mass with low-level echoes
- Location: Bilateral in 5% of benign and 20% of malignant tumors
- Size
  - Variable but often large, filling entire pelvis and extending into upper abdomen
  - Some of the largest tumors ever reported are mucinous cystadenomas
    - Up to 100 kg

Ultrasonographic Findings
- Grayscale Ultrasound
  - Typically multiloculated
  - Septae often thin
  - Papillary projections much less common than in serous tumors
  - Mucin creates low-level echoes within loculi
    - Echogenicity can be quite variable depending on concentration of mucin
    - Typically have multiple loculi of varying echogenicity
  - Solid components suspicious of malignancy
  - Pseudomyxoma peritonei potential form of peritoneal spread with amorphous, mucoid material insinuating itself around mesentery, bowel, and solid organs
    - More echogenic than simple ascites
    - Has mass effect with scalloping along solid organs (especially liver) and bowel matted posteriorly (rather than free-floating)
    - May have subtle septations
- Color Doppler: Flow seen within solid components

DDx: Echogenic Ovarian Masses

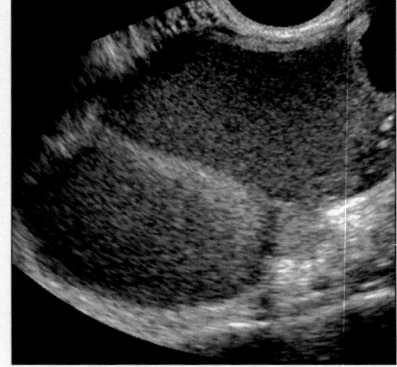

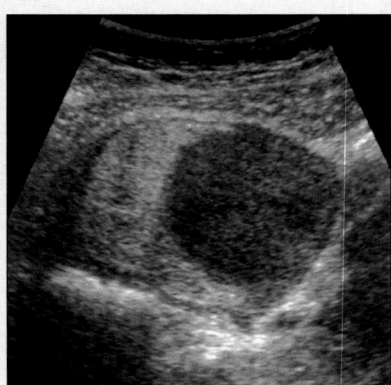

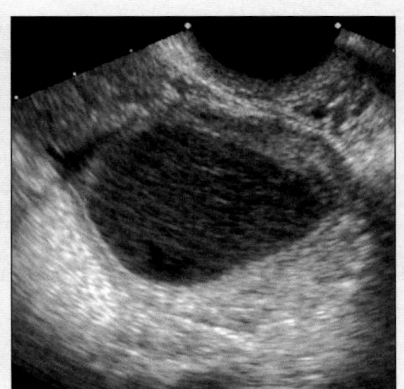

Endometrioma   *Dermoid*   *Hemorrhagic Cyst*

MUCINOUS OVARIAN CYSTADENOMA/CARCINOMA

Key Facts

Imaging Findings
- Some of the largest tumors ever reported are mucinous cystadenomas
- Typically multiloculated
- Papillary projections much less common than in serous tumors
- Mucin creates low-level echoes within loculi
- Echogenicity can be quite variable depending on concentration of mucin
- Pseudomyxoma peritonei potential form of peritoneal spread with amorphous, mucoid material insinuating itself around mesentery, bowel, and solid organs
- Has mass effect with scalloping along solid organs (especially liver) and bowel matted posteriorly (rather than free-floating)

Top Differential Diagnoses
- Endometriomas
- Serous Cystadenoma/Carcinoma

Pathology
- Epithelial tumors 60-70% of all tumors: 85-90% of malignancies
- Mucinous tumors second most common epithelial neoplasm (serous most common)
- Malignant 10%, borderline (low malignant potential) 10%, benign 80%
- Bilateral in 5% of benign tumors, 10% of borderline tumors and 20% of malignant tumors

Clinical Issues
- Gelatinous, insinuating nature of pseudomyxoma peritonei makes complete resection difficult

CT Findings
- Variable attenuation of loculi depending on concentration of mucin
- Peritoneal metastases often low attenuation
  - May be difficult to differentiate from fluid-filled bowel
- Enhancement of solid portions with contrast

MR Findings
- Signal intensity varies depending on degree of mucin concentration
- Loculi with high concentration of mucin will be higher signal on T1WI and lower signal on T2WI than those with lower concentration
  - Creates a "stained glass" appearance

DIFFERENTIAL DIAGNOSIS

Endometriomas
- Also contain low-level echoes
- MRI helpful: Blood high signal on T1WI with T2 shading

Serous Cystadenoma/Carcinoma
- More often unilocular
- Cyst contents not as echogenic
- Papillary projections common

Germ Cell Tumors
- Can have low-level echoes similar to mucin
- Typically more complicated with calcifications, fluid-fluid levels, etc.

Hemorrhagic Cyst
- Smaller and unilocular
- Resolves on follow-up scan

Mucocele
- Dilated appendix filled with mucinous material

PATHOLOGY

General Features
- General path comments
  - **Ovarian neoplasms**
    - Epithelial tumors 60-70% of all tumors: 85-90% of malignancies
    - Germ cell tumors 15-20% of all tumors: 3-5% of malignancies
    - Sex cord-stromal tumors 5-10% of all tumors: 2-3% of malignancies
    - Metastases and lymphoma 5-10% of all tumors: 5-10% of malignancies
  - **Benign epithelial tumors**
    - Serous cystadenoma 20-25%
    - Mucinous cystadenoma 20-25%
  - **Malignant epithelial tumors**
    - Serous cystadenocarcinoma 40-50%
    - Endometrioid carcinoma 20-25%
    - Mucinous cystadenocarcinoma 5-10%
    - Clear cell carcinoma 5-10%
    - Brenner tumor 1-2%
    - Undifferentiated carcinoma 4-5%
- Genetics: Hereditary causes in 5-10% of ovarian cancers (mutations in BRCA1 and BRCA2 tumor suppressor genes)
- Etiology
  - Not completely understood
  - One theory is "incessant ovulation": Repeated microtrauma with cellular repair to surface epithelium
    - Increased risk: Nulliparity, early menarche, late menopause (more ovulatory cycles)
    - Reduced risk: Multiparity, late menarche, early menopause, oral contraceptive use (fewer ovulatory cycles)
- Epidemiology
  - Mucinous tumors second most common epithelial neoplasm (serous most common)
  - Malignant 10%, borderline (low malignant potential) 10%, benign 80%

MUCINOUS OVARIAN CYSTADENOMA/CARCINOMA

○ Bilateral in 5% of benign tumors, 10% of borderline tumors and 20% of malignant tumors
- Associated abnormalities: May occasionally be hormonally active producing estrogen
- Method of spread
  ○ Intraperitoneal dissemination most common
    ■ Greater omentum, right subphrenic region, and pouch of Douglas most common sites found at surgery
  ○ Direct extension to surrounding organs
  ○ Lymphatic spread to paraaortic and pelvic nodes
  ○ Hematogenous spread least common
    ■ Liver and lung most common sites

Microscopic Features
- Ovarian origin of pseudomyxoma peritonei called into question
  ○ Most cases now thought to be appendiceal with metastases to ovary
  ○ Appendix should be thoroughly examined with special tissue staining in every case

Staging, Grading or Classification Criteria
- FIGO staging system of ovarian carcinoma
  ○ Stage I: Tumor limited to ovaries
    ■ IA: Unilateral, no malignant ascites
    ■ IB: Bilateral, no malignant ascites
    ■ IC: IA or IB with malignant ascites or positive peritoneal washings
  ○ Stage II: Tumor involves one or both ovaries with pelvic extension
    ■ IIA: Extension to uterus or fallopian tubes, no malignant ascites
    ■ IIB: Extension to other pelvic tissues, no malignant ascites
    ■ IIC: IIA or IIB with malignant ascites or positive peritoneal washings
  ○ Stage III: Peritoneal implants or nodal metastases outside the pelvis
    ■ IIIA: Microscopic peritoneal implants
    ■ IIIB: Macroscopic implants < 2 cm
    ■ IIIC: Implants > 2 cm or lymph node metastases
  ○ Stage IV: Distant metastases (excluding peritoneal implants)

CLINICAL ISSUES

Presentation
- Most common signs/symptoms
  ○ Incidental mass discovered on exam
  ○ Pelvic discomfort/pain from large tumors
    ■ Massive tumors can actually cause weight gain and a distended abdomen
  ○ Symptoms from metastatic disease
- CA-125 not useful for mucinous tumors: False negative in 30%

Demographics
- Age
  ○ Mucinous cystadenoma 3rd-5th decade
  ○ Mucinous cystadenocarcinoma in peri- and postmenopausal age group

Natural History & Prognosis
- 95% 5 year survival for low malignant potential tumors
  ○ If metastatic, prognosis is similar to those with frankly malignant histology
- 5 year survival for malignant epithelial tumors
  ○ Stage I - 80%
  ○ Stage II - 50%
  ○ Stage III - 30%
  ○ Stage IV - 8%

Treatment
- Primary treatment is surgery
  ○ Should do complete staging laparotomy and tumor debulking (cytoreduction)
    ■ Staging laparotomy includes hysterectomy with bilateral salpingo-oophorectomy, pelvic and paraaortic node biopsies, omentectomy, peritoneal biopsies and washings
    ■ More conservative surgery may be done for women with Stage I disease in reproductive age group
    ■ Debulking considered optimal if < 1.5-2.0 cm residual tumor remains
  ○ Gelatinous, insinuating nature of pseudomyxoma peritonei makes complete resection difficult
    ■ Recurrence common and multiple laparotomies required
  ○ Chemotherapy after cytoreductive surgery
  ○ Neoadjuvant chemotherapy before cytoreductive surgery in patients with unresectable disease
    ■ Includes bulky disease in difficult to reach areas (porta hepatis, lesser sac, root of mesentery), extensive surrounding organ or sidewall invasion, or Stage IV disease

DIAGNOSTIC CHECKLIST

Image Interpretation Pearls
- Mucinous tumors are less commonly malignant than serous tumors

SELECTED REFERENCES

1. Woodward PJ et al: From the archives of the AFIP: radiologic staging of ovarian carcinoma with pathologic correlation. Radiographics. 24(1):225-46, 2004
2. Hanbidge AE et al: US of the peritoneum. Radiographics. 23(3):663-84; discussion 684-5, 2003
3. Holschneider CH et al: Ovarian cancer: epidemiology, biology, and prognostic factors. Semin Surg Oncol. 19(1):3-10, 2000
4. Kawamoto S et al: CT of epithelial ovarian tumors. Radiographics. 19 Spec No:S85-102; quiz S263-4, 1999
5. Wagner BJ et al: From the archives of the AFIP. Ovarian epithelial neoplasms: radiologic-pathologic correlation. Radiographics. 14(6):1351-74; quiz 1375-6, 1994
6. Ronnett BM et al: Disseminated peritoneal adenomucinosis and peritoneal mucinous carcinomatosis. A clinicopathologic analysis of 109 cases with emphasis on distinguishing pathologic features, site of origin, prognosis, and relationship to "pseudomyxoma peritonei".

IMAGE GALLERY

Typical

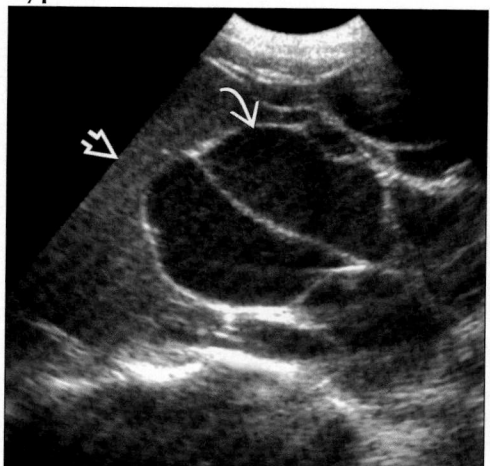 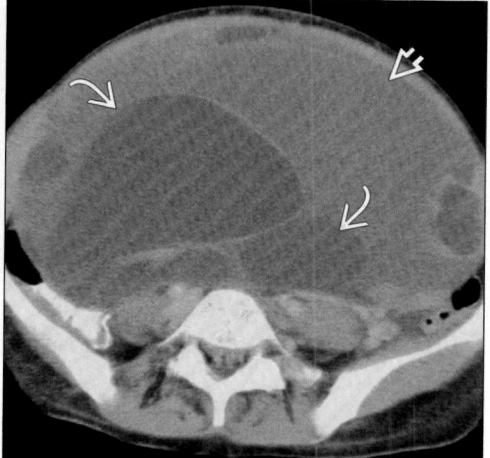

(Left) Transverse ultrasound of a mucinous tumor of low malignant potential shows multiple loculi of varying echogenicity. Some are very echogenic ➡, having the classic appearance, while others have few echoes ➡. *(Right)* CECT shows the corresponding CT appearance with some loculi having increased attenuation ➡, while others have decreased attenuation ➡. This varied appearance is typical for mucinous tumors.

Typical

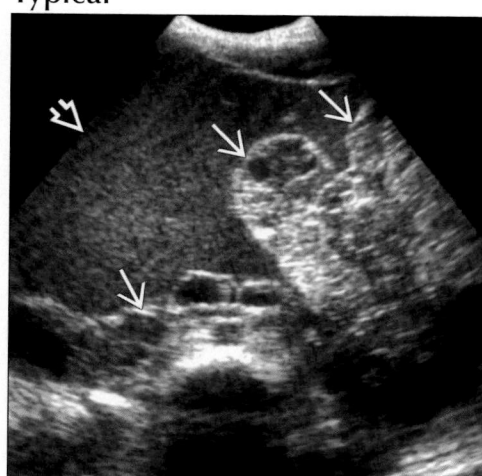 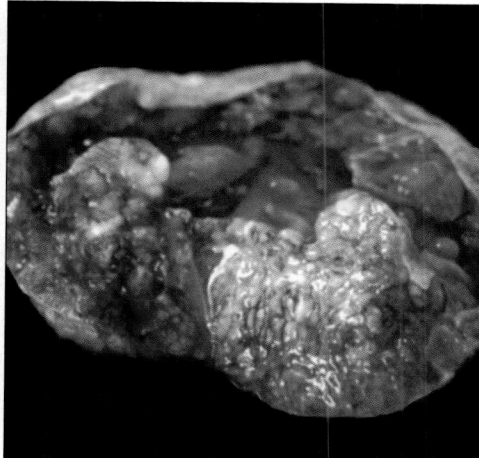

(Left) Transverse ultrasound of a mucinous cystadenocarcinoma shows significant solid components ➡, as well as echogenic fluid ➡, within this large tumor. *(Right)* Gross pathology of the resected mass shows the corresponding solid areas. The greater the amount of solid material, the greater the likelihood of malignancy.

9

87

Typical

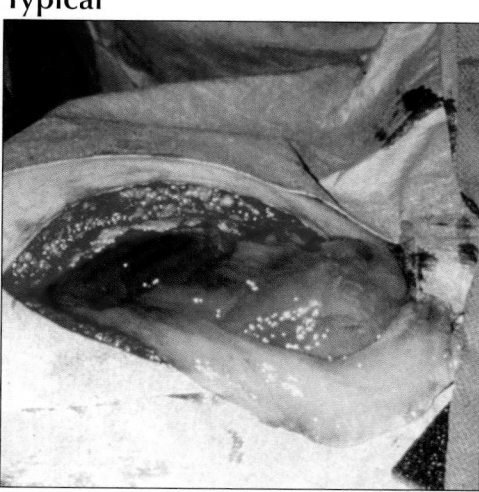 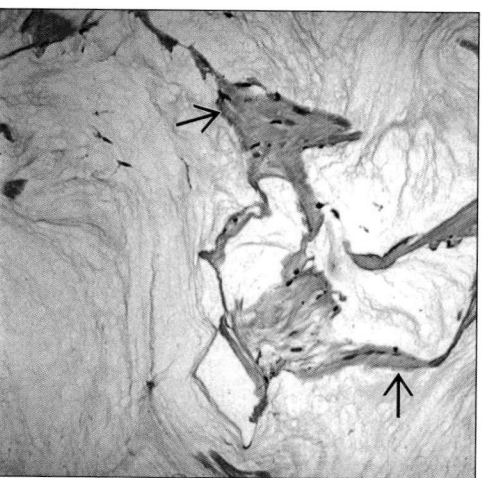

(Left) Intraoperative photograph of a patient with pseudomyxoma peritonei shows thick, gelatinous material exuding from the incision site. *(Right)* Photomicrograph shows pools of acellular mucin dissecting through bands of fibrous tissue ➡. *(Shown in Radiographics, ref 1).*

OVARIAN TERATOMA

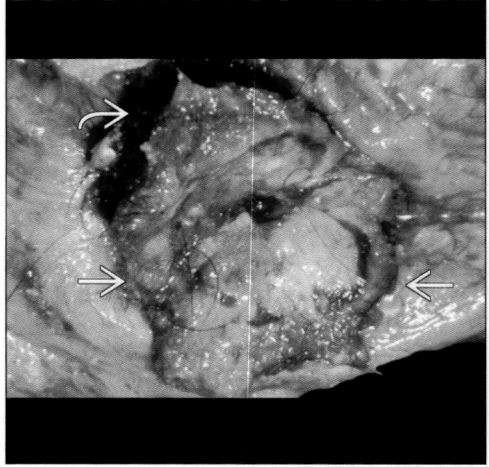

Gross pathology shows the typical appearance of a Rokitansky nodule ➡ within the dissected mature cystic teratoma. Hair ⇒ arises from nodule.

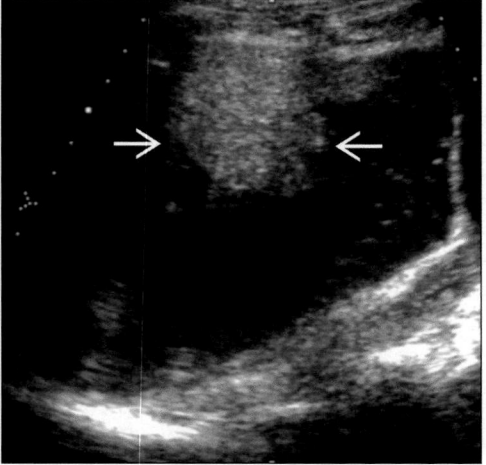

Corresponding transabdominal ultrasound shows the Rokitansky nodule ➡. It is usually echogenic and often causes distal acoustic shadowing.

TERMINOLOGY

Abbreviations and Synonyms
- Dermoid cyst

Definitions
- Ovarian teratoma includes
  - Mature cystic teratoma (MCT) = dermoid cyst
  - Immature teratoma (IT)
  - Monodermal teratoma in which one cell line predominates
    - Struma ovarii
    - Carcinoid tumor

IMAGING FINDINGS

General Features
- Best diagnostic clue: Ovarian mass with echogenic shadowing mural nodule on US

Ultrasonographic Findings
- Grayscale Ultrasound

- Mature cystic teratomas have a variety of appearances
- Heterogeneous mass with echogenic component
- Highly echogenic components due to fat content
- ± Fat fluid level
- Shadowing echogenic mural nodule (sebaceous material)
  - Rokitansky plug
- Hair
  - Punctate echoes in one plane
  - Elongate to become linear echoes in orthogonal plane
  - Hair will move through more fluid component with transducer pressure
- Teeth
  - Highly echogenic focus/foci with distal acoustic shadowing represent teeth
- "Tip of the iceberg sign": Only leading edge of the mass identified
  - Distal acoustic shadowing prevents assessment of deep edge
  - Size cannot be measured
  - Mass may be much larger than suggested by leading edge echoes

DDx: Complex Adnexal Mass

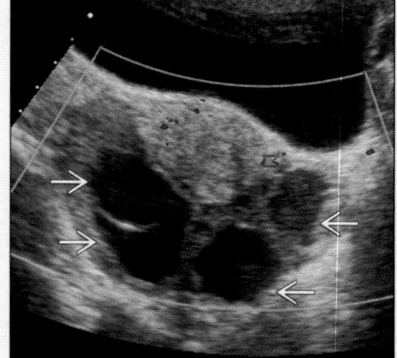

Hemorrhagic Cysts

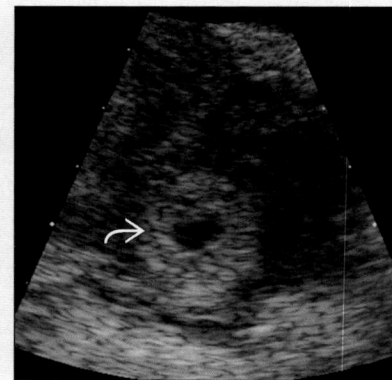

Ruptured Ectopic

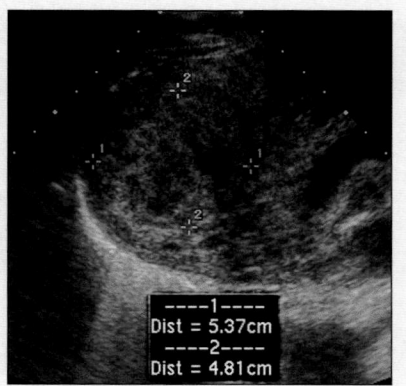

Degenerated Fibroid

OVARIAN TERATOMA

Typical

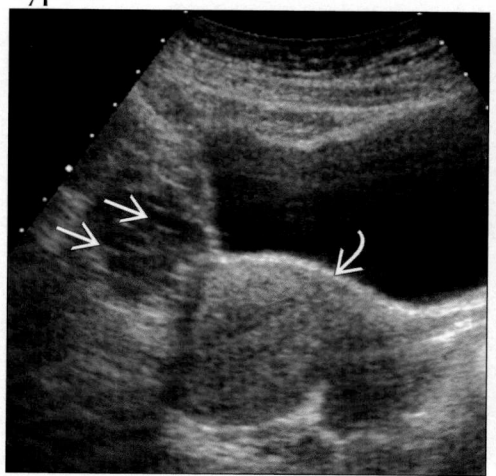 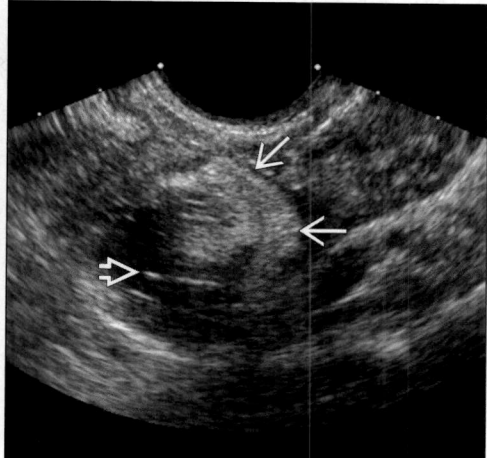

(Left) Longitudinal transabdominal ultrasound shows a mass containing linear echoes ➡ superior to the uterus ➡. Linear echoes are created by hair in mature cystic teratoma. *(Right)* Corresponding transverse transvaginal ultrasound shows the echogenic fatty component ➡ to better advantage than the transabdominal scan. Again note linear echoes ➡ from hair.

Typical

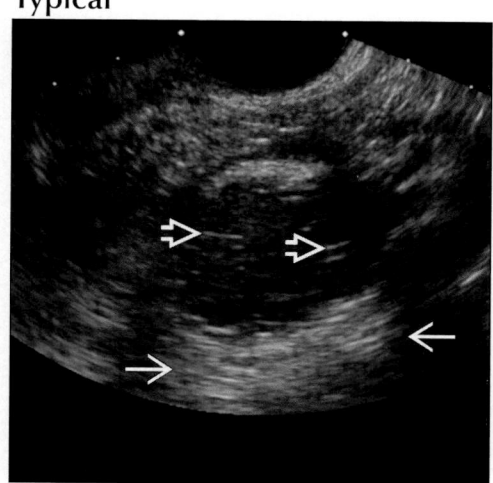 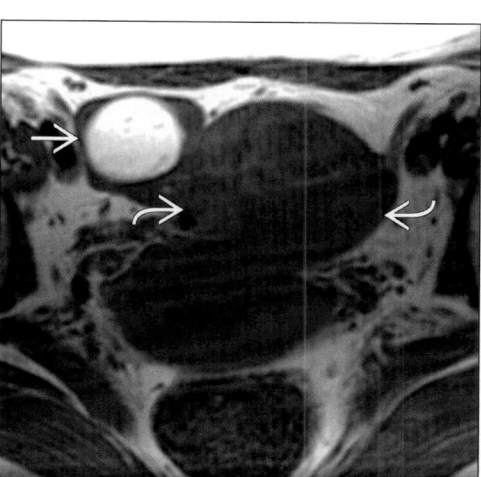

(Left) Longitudinal transvaginal ultrasound shows linear echoes from hair ➡ floating in the cystic component. Note acoustic enhancement ➡ distal to the cystic component. *(Right)* Transverse T1WI MR shows a high signal right adnexal mass ➡. The uterus ➡ is not well evaluated on this sequence.

Typical

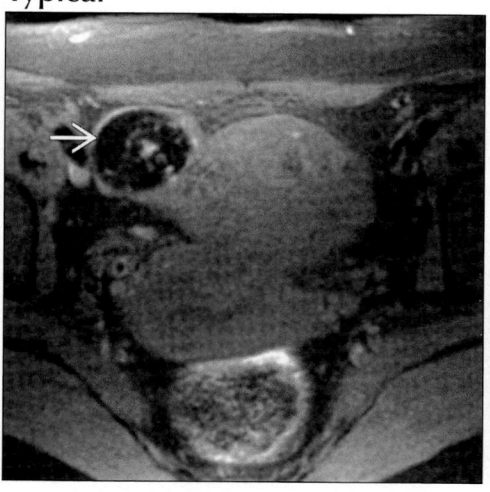 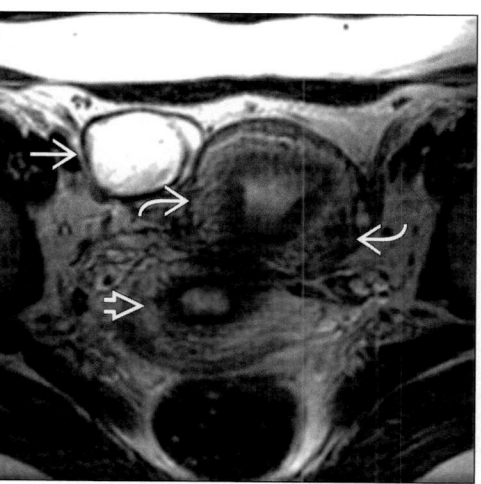

(Left) Transverse T1WI MR with fat-saturation shows loss of signal in the mass ➡ confirming fat content. This is typical of mature cystic teratoma, same case as previous image. *(Right)* Transverse T2WI MR shows high signal in the mass ➡ as well as the normal internal architecture of the uterus ➡ and cervix ➡, same patient as previous two images.

POLYCYSTIC OVARIAN SYNDROME

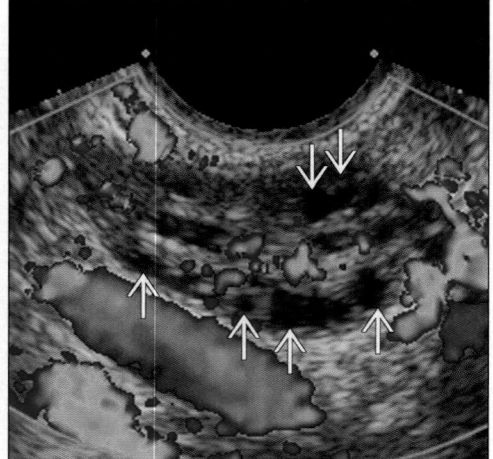

Longitudinal transvaginal ultrasound shows a large left ovary with calculated volume of 18.9 cc. Ovarian enlargement is one of the key findings in polycystic ovarian syndrome.

Longitudinal color Doppler ultrasound shows a large ovary with multiple small follicles ➡ and increased stromal vascularity.

TERMINOLOGY

Abbreviations and Synonyms
- Polycystic ovarian syndrome (PCOS)
- Polycystic ovary (PCO) appearance in asymptomatic women
- Insulin-like growth factor binding protein (IGFBP)
- Insulin-like growth factor (IGF)
- Stein-Leventhal syndrome: Hyperandrogenemia ⇒ polycystic ovaries, hirsutism, menstrual abnormalities, obesity

Definitions
- Refined definition of PCOS developed in 2003: Two of three criteria must be present
  ○ Oligo ± anovulation
  ○ Hyperandrogenism (clinical or biochemical) after exclusion of other causes
  ○ Polycystic ovaries (one or both) after exclusion of other etiologies
- Some authors suggest PCO are more correctly polyfollicular, PCOS should be called "functional hyperandrogenism"

○ Subtypes of functional hyperandrogenism account for variable clinical presentation
  ■ Allow for better individualized treatment
  ■ Decrease bias in future scientific/clinical studies

IMAGING FINDINGS

General Features
- Best diagnostic clue
  ○ Enlarged ovaries with volume > 10 cc or
  ○ ≥ 12 follicles per ovary measuring 2-9 mm in diameter

Ultrasonographic Findings
- Pulsed Doppler
  ○ Stromal arteries
    ■ Resistive index (RI) and pulsatility index (PI) are significantly lower in PCOS than in normals
    ■ Peak systolic velocity (PSV) higher in PCOS than in normals
    ■ Flow evaluation may predict risk for hyperstimulation syndrome during gonadotropin therapy

DDx: Multicystic Ovaries

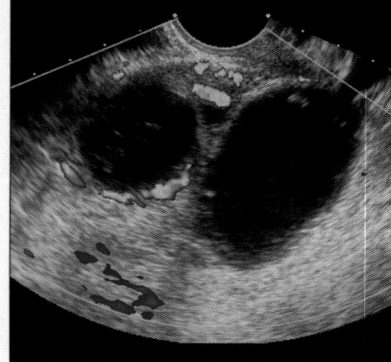

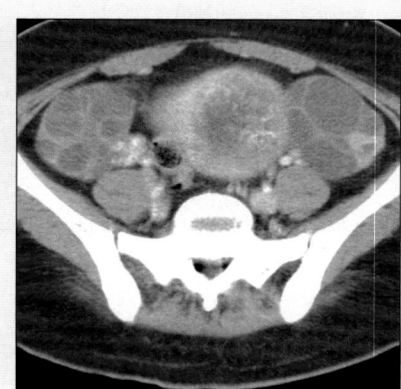

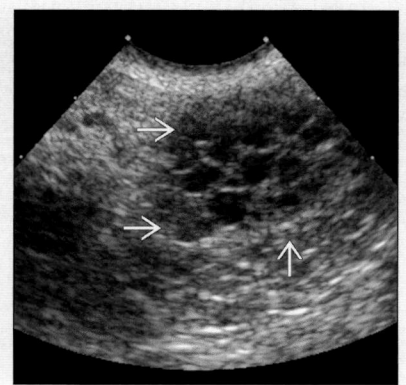

Hemorrhagic Cysts

Theca Lutein Cysts

Polyfollicular Ovary

POLYCYSTIC OVARIAN SYNDROME

Key Facts

Terminology
- Refined definition of PCOS developed in 2003: Two of three criteria must be present
- Oligo ± anovulation
- Hyperandrogenism (clinical or biochemical) after exclusion of other causes
- Polycystic ovaries (one or both) after exclusion of other etiologies

Imaging Findings
- Enlarged ovaries with volume > 10 cc or
- ≥ 12 follicles per ovary measuring 2-9 mm in diameter

Top Differential Diagnoses
- Other Causes of Hyperandrogenism
- Multicystic/multifollicular ovary

Pathology
- Commonest cause of anovulatory infertility in USA

Clinical Issues
- Traditional treatment centers on ovulation induction, treatment of acne/hirsutism, prevention of endometrial cancer

Diagnostic Checklist
- Clinical presentation is highly variable
- Features seen in one ovary are sufficient to diagnose PCOS
- PCO detection in ovulatory infertile women indicates increased risk for ovarian hyperstimulation syndrome
- In virginal, obese patients MR allows accurate characterization of ovarian morphology

---

- 3D: More precise than 2D for measurement of ovarian volume
- Uterus often enlarged due to estrogenization
  - Uterine volume not reliable enough to be used as diagnostic criterion
- Ovarian stromal echogenicity
  - Subjective, influenced by gain settings
  - Although strongly correlated with diagnosis of PCOS it is not one of the consensus criteria due to subjective nature of evaluation
- Ovarian stromal volume
  - Stromal volume is increased in PCOS (main cause of ↑ ovarian volume, follicles do not contribute significantly)
  - Overall ovarian volume easier to measure in routine practice therefore it is selected as a diagnostic criterion

Imaging Recommendations
- Best imaging tool: Transvaginal ultrasound
- Protocol advice
  - Measure ovarian diameters in three planes
  - Calculate volume using formula for prolate ellipsoid (longitudinal x transverse x AP diameter x 0.5233)
    - Normal women 7.94 ± 2.34 cc
    - PCOS patients 10.04 ± 7.36 cc
  - Follicle numbers should be assessed in at least two planes to confirm size and position
  - Follicle diameter should be measured as the mean of three planes
  - If a dominant follicle (> 10 mm diameter) or corpus luteum seen repeat scan during next cycle to avoid false elevation of volume
  - Regularly menstruating women should be scanned day 3-5, oligo/amenorrheic women can be scanned at random or 3-5 days after progestogen-induced bleed

DIFFERENTIAL DIAGNOSIS

Normal
- Ovarian morphology alone is insufficient for diagnosis of PCOS
  - PCO morphology seen in approximately 22% of women, PCOS prevalence is 5-10%

Suppressed Ovary
- Oral contraceptive pills suppress ovulation → multiple small follicles

Other Causes of Hyperandrogenism
- Hyperthecosis, congenital adrenal hyperplasia, 21-hydroxylase deficiency, Cushing syndrome, Androgen producing neoplasm

Other Causes of "Polycystic" Appearance
- Multicystic/multifollicular ovary
  - ≥ 6 follicles 4-10 mm in diameter with normal stromal echogenicity
  - Typically seen at puberty or in women recovering from hypothalamic amenorrhea
    - Follicular growth without consistent recruitment of dominant follicle

PATHOLOGY

General Features
- Etiology: No single etiologic factor identified, no responsible gene as yet isolated
- Epidemiology
  - Commonest cause of anovulatory infertility in USA
  - Affects 6-10% of females in reproductive age group
- Associated abnormalities: Obesity, hirsutism
- Endometrium
  - Androgen receptors/steroid receptor coactivators are overexpressed in PCOS endometrium
  - Markers of bioreceptivity to embryonic implantation are decreased

POLYCYSTIC OVARIAN SYNDROME

○ Endometrium is a target for insulin in addition to steroid hormones (estradiol, progesterone, androgens)
  ▪ Insulin receptors are cyclically regulated in normo-ovulatory women
  ▪ Hyperinsulinemia down regulates hepatic IGFBP-1 → ↑ IGF-1 in circulation
  ▪ In vitro insulin inhibits decidualization of endometrium therefore ↑ IGF likely contributes to endometrial dysfunction

Gross Pathologic & Surgical Features
• Prominent theca, fibrotic thickening of tunica albuginea
• Multiple cystic follicles (vs. pathologic cysts)

Microscopic Features
• Atretic follicles ± degenerating granulosa cells
• Hypertrophy/luteinization inner theca cell layer
• 2-3 fold increased number of follicles

CLINICAL ISSUES

Presentation
• Most common signs/symptoms
  ○ PCOS phenotype has three components
    ▪ Anovulation → oligo/amenorrhea
    ▪ Hyperandrogenism → hirsutism
    ▪ Obesity with associated hyperinsulinemia/insulin resistance
• Metabolic effects of syndrome
  ○ Insulin resistance seen in almost all obese women and > 50% normal weight women with PCOS
  ○ Hyperlipidemia, low serum HDL cholesterol

Natural History & Prognosis
• If conception occurs increased risk of
  ○ Early pregnancy loss
  ○ Gestational diabetes
  ○ Pregnancy induced hypertension/preeclampsia (controversial if true association)
  ○ Delivery of small for gestational age babies
    ▪ Impaired insulin mediated growth/fetal programming
• Associated with dysmetabolic syndrome
  ○ 3-7x ↑ risk maturity onset diabetes, some studies suggest ↑ cardio/cerebrovascular events
• Possible increased risk of endometrial cancer
  ○ Ongoing research to evaluate if causal relationship versus association with obesity/infertility

Treatment
• Traditional treatment centers on ovulation induction, treatment of acne/hirsutism, prevention of endometrial cancer
• Ovulation induction
  ○ Clomiphene citrate followed by FSH
  ○ Gonadotropin (GN) therapy next line if no response to clomiphene
• Metformin/other insulin sensitizing drugs
  ○ Agent for ovulation induction in this group of patients

▪ Use also associated with ↓ androgen/GN levels, improved serum lipids, improved acne and hirsutism
○ Sustained use in pregnancy controversial
  ▪ Hope is to prevent early pregnancy loss/gestational diabetes
  ▪ Concern that it may increase preeclampsia
○ Improves
  ▪ Insulin sensitivity, lipid profiles, plasma glucose concentrations
• Laparoscopic surgery "ovarian drilling" electrocautery
  ○ Lower cost per pregnancy than GN induced ovulation induction
  ○ Better long term reproductive performance & menstrual regularity
• Lifestyle modification with diet and exercise for obese patients
• Comprehensive evaluation for diabetes/other cardiovascular risk factors

DIAGNOSTIC CHECKLIST

Consider
• Consensus criteria selected for ease of performance and reproducibility
  ○ Still some controversy regarding method of follicle count and absolute number of follicles for diagnosis
• Other techniques; e.g., pulse Doppler may be clinically useful to refine diagnosis, predict response to therapy
• Clinical presentation is highly variable
  ○ Ovulatory PCOS
  ○ Non-hirsute anovulatory PCOS

Image Interpretation Pearls
• Features seen in one ovary are sufficient to diagnose PCOS
• Ovarian volume is suppressed in women taking oral contraceptives but appearance may still be polycystic
• Criteria to distinguish PCO from multicystic ovary in adolescents are not yet established
• PCO detection in ovulatory infertile women indicates increased risk for ovarian hyperstimulation syndrome
• In virginal, obese patients MR allows accurate characterization of ovarian morphology

SELECTED REFERENCES

1. Balen A: Surgical treatment of polycystic ovary syndrome. Best Pract Res Clin Endocrinol Metab. 20(2):271-80, 2006
2. Essah PA et al: The metabolic syndrome in polycystic ovary syndrome. J Endocrinol Invest. 29(3):270-80, 2006
3. Giudice LC: Endometrium in PCOS: Implantation and predisposition to endocrine CA. Best Pract Res Clin Endocrinol Metab. 20(2):235-44, 2006
4. Homburg R: Pregnancy complications in PCOS. Best Pract Res Clin Endocrinol Metab. 20(2):281-92, 2006
5. Moran LJ et al: Effects of lifestyle modification in polycystic ovarian syndrome. Reprod Biomed Online. 12(5):569-78, 2006
6. Pasquali R et al: Insulin-sensitizing agents in polycystic ovary syndrome. Eur J Endocrinol. 154(6):763-75, 2006
7. Balen AH et al: Ultrasound assessment of the polycystic ovary: international consensus definitions. Hum Reprod Update. 9(6):505-14, 2003

POLYCYSTIC OVARIAN SYNDROME

IMAGE GALLERY

Typical

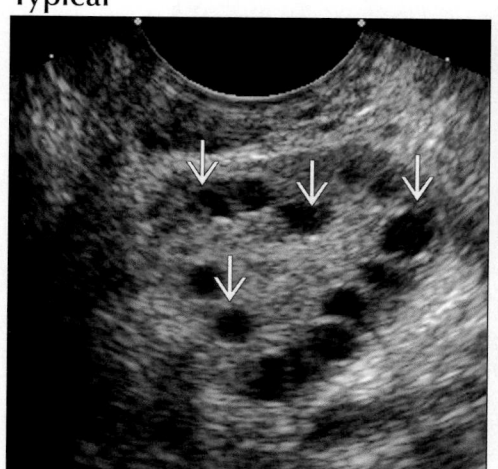 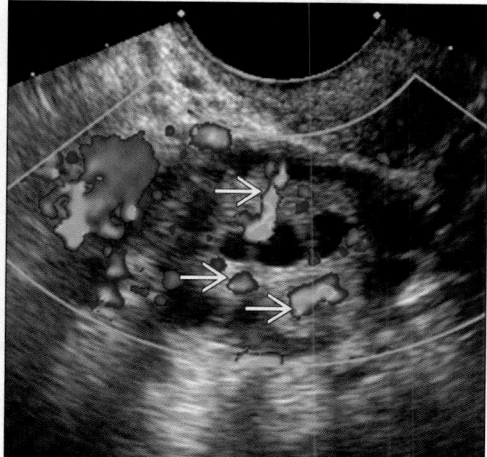

(Left) Transverse transvaginal ultrasound through the right ovary shows thirteen follicles ➡. One criteria for diagnosis is ≥ 12 follicles per ovary. (Right) Transverse color Doppler ultrasound in a different patient shows multiple easily visible stromal arteries ➡. Though not one of the diagnostic criteria increased stromal flow has been observed in PCOS.

Typical

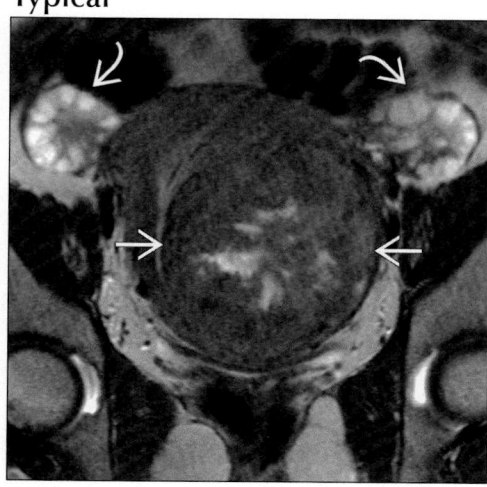 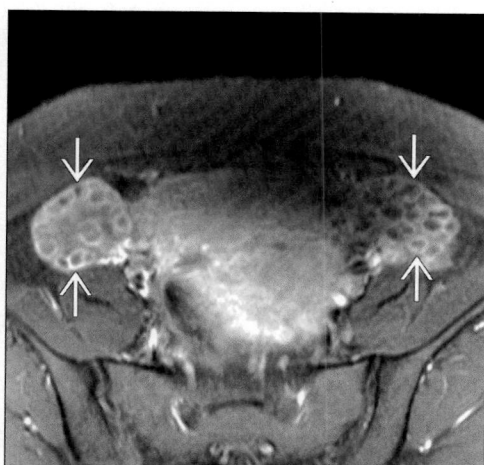

(Left) Coronal T2 weighted MR shows multiple small follicles of similar sizes in enlarged ovaries ➡. There is also a degenerated uterine fibroid ➡. (Right) Axial T1 weighted MR post-gadolinium administration in the same patient as previous image shows innumerable enhancing follicles ➡ within enlarged ovaries. MR may be very helpful to assess ovarian morphology in obese virginal patients.

Other

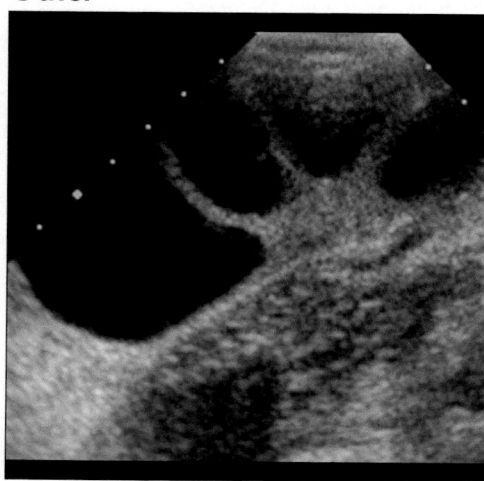 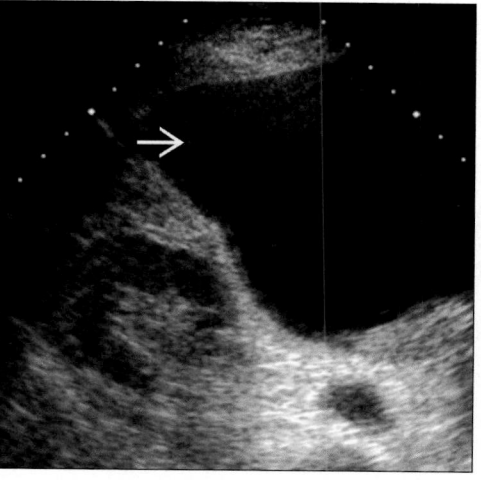

(Left) Longitudinal transabdominal ultrasound shows enlarged ovary with multiple large follicles as a result of ovulation induction. PCOS patients often require assisted reproduction. (Right) Transverse transabdominal ultrasound shows ascites ➡ in association with ovarian hyperstimulation syndrome. Ovulatory patients with PCOS are at increased risk for this complication of assisted reproduction.

HYDROSALPINX

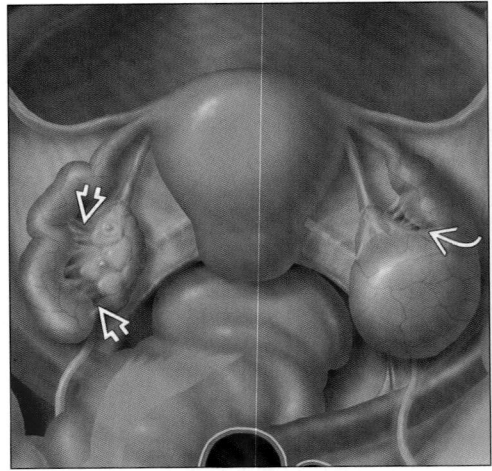

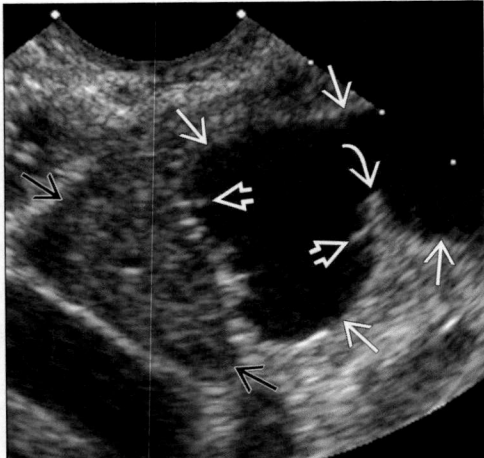

Graphic shows bilateral hydrosalpinx. The left tube folds upon itself ➡ which appears as an incomplete septum on ultrasound. Adhesions ➡ and hydrosalpinx are sequelae of PID.

Oblique transvaginal ultrasound shows a fluid-filled thin-walled fallopian tube ➡ with an incomplete septum ➡ and thin endosalpingeal folds ➡. The ovary ➡ is seen separately.

TERMINOLOGY

Definitions
- Fallopian tube distended with fluid
- Chronic phase of pelvic inflammatory disease (PID)

IMAGING FINDINGS

General Features
- Best diagnostic clue: Thin-walled adnexal tubular structure with anechoic fluid
- Location: Adnexal but separate from ovary
- Morphology
  - Oval
  - Pear-shaped
  - Retort-shaped
    - Tube doubled-up on self
  - Serpiginous

Ultrasonographic Findings
- Thin-walled distended tube, tube wall < 3 mm
- Thin endosalpingeal folds
  - "Beads on a string" appearance

- Incomplete septae
  - Tube folds upon itself
- Fluid in tube and cul-de-sac is anechoic
  - Debris or echoes suggest acute PID
- Separate normal ovary
- Doppler findings
  - High resistive flow in wall of hydrosalpinx
    - Resistive index (RI) ≥ 0.7
    - Higher resistance than acute PID
  - No flow in endosalpingeal folds
- Adnexal torsion is a complication

Imaging Recommendations
- Best imaging tool: Transvaginal ultrasound
- Protocol advice
  - Look for intact separate ovary
  - Use high gain settings to look for echoes in fluid

DIFFERENTIAL DIAGNOSIS

Pyosalpinx (Acute PID)
- Tube distended with echogenic material
- Tube wall > 5 mm and thick endosalpingeal folds
  - "Cogwheel" appearance

DDx: Tubal Lesions

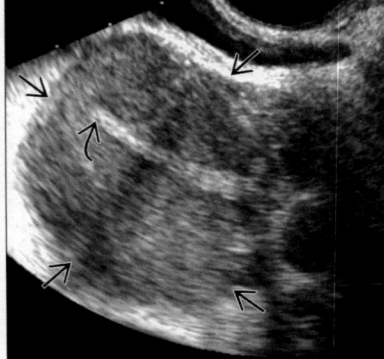

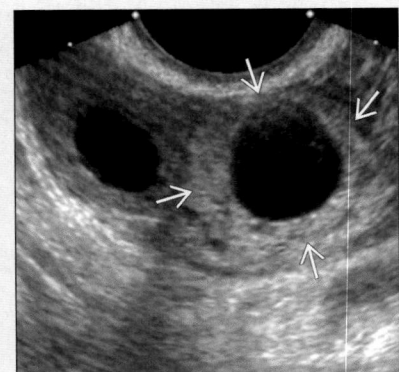

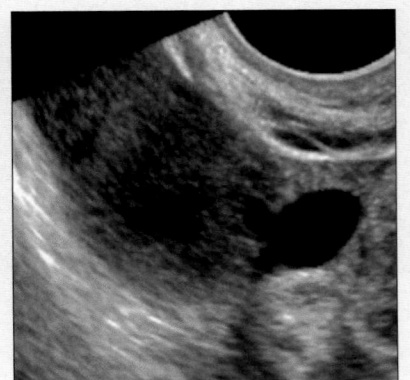

Pyosalpinx (PID) Ectopic Pregnancy Paraovarian Cyst

HYDROSALPINX

Key Facts

Terminology
- Fallopian tube distended with fluid
- Chronic phase of pelvic inflammatory disease (PID)

Imaging Findings
- Thin-walled distended tube, tube wall < 3 mm
- Thin endosalpingeal folds
- Incomplete septae
- Fluid in tube and cul-de-sac is anechoic
- Separate normal ovary

- High resistive flow in wall of hydrosalpinx
- Adnexal torsion is a complication
- Best imaging tool: Transvaginal ultrasound
- Look for intact separate ovary
- Use high gain settings to look for echoes in fluid

Top Differential Diagnoses
- Pyosalpinx (Acute PID)
- Paraovarian Cyst
- Ectopic Tubal Pregnancy

- Low resistive flow in walls and folds (≤ 0.5)

Paraovarian Cyst
- Unilocular anechoic broad ligament cyst
- More round than hydrosalpinx

Ectopic Tubal Pregnancy
- Echogenic ring in adnexa with ↑ flow
- Cul-de-sac fluid contains echoes

PATHOLOGY

General Features
- Etiology: Tube obstruction from PID
- Associated abnormalities
  - Infertility
  - Ectopic pregnancy
  - Chronic pelvic pain

Microscopic Features
- Chronic salpingitis
- Fibrotic endosalpingeal folds

CLINICAL ISSUES

Presentation
- Most common signs/symptoms
  - Asymptomatic
  - History of PID
- Other signs/symptoms: Acute pain if adnexal torsion

Demographics
- Age: Perimenopausal

Treatment
- None necessary if asymptomatic

DIAGNOSTIC CHECKLIST

Image Interpretation Pearls
- Look for signs of acute PID
- Find separate intact ovary (avoid surgery)

SELECTED REFERENCES

1. Patel MD et al: Likelihood ratio of sonographic findings in discriminating hydrosalpinx from other adnexal masses. AJR Am J Roentgenol. 186(4):1033-8, 2006
2. Shukla R: Isolated torsion of the hydrosalpinx: a rare presentation. Br J Radiol. 77(921):784-6, 2004
3. Guerriero S et al: Transvaginal ultrasonography associated with colour Doppler energy in the diagnosis of hydrosalpinx. Hum Reprod. 15(7):1568-72, 2000
4. Zalel Y et al: Contribution of color Doppler flow to the ultrasonographic diagnosis of tubal abnormalities. J Ultrasound Med. 19(9):645-9, 2000
5. Timor-Tritsch IE et al: Transvaginal sonographic markers of tubal inflammatory disease. Ultrasound Obstet Gynecol. 12(1):56-66, 1998

IMAGE GALLERY

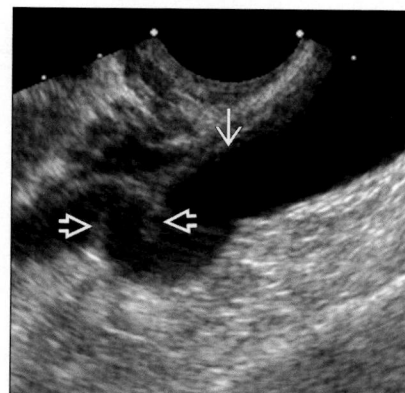 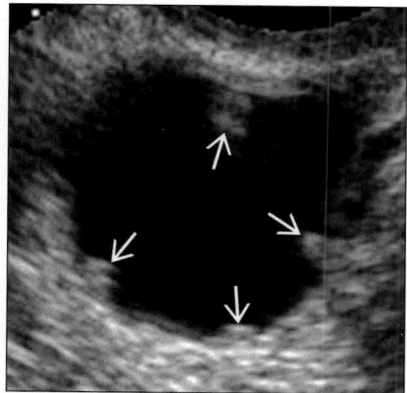 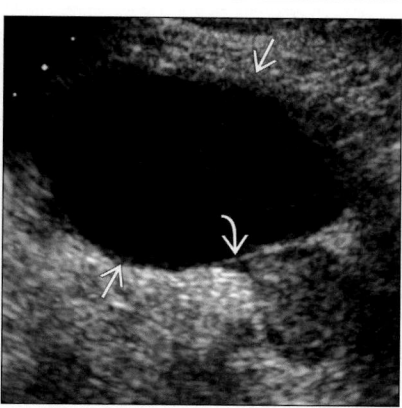

(Left) Longitudinal transvaginal ultrasound shows serpiginous fluid-filled fallopian tube ➡ with incomplete septae ➡. *(Center)* Transverse transvaginal ultrasound shows the tube contains anechoic fluid and thin fibrotic endosalpingeal folds ➡. *(Right)* Longitudinal ultrasound in a patient with acute adnexal pain shows a markedly distended tube ➡ which has lost its fallopian tube features. Notice "twist" of junction with the ovary ➡. This patient had torsion of the hydrosalpinx and her ovary was salvaged.

TUBOVARIAN ABSCESS

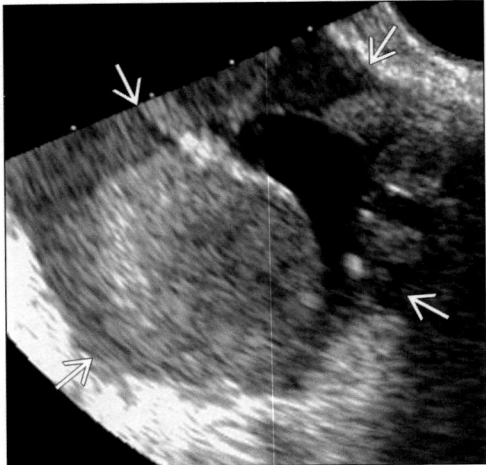

Transverse transvaginal ultrasound shows a complex right adnexal mass ➡ at the distal end of a dilated fallopian tube. A separate ovary is not seen, consistent with a TOA.

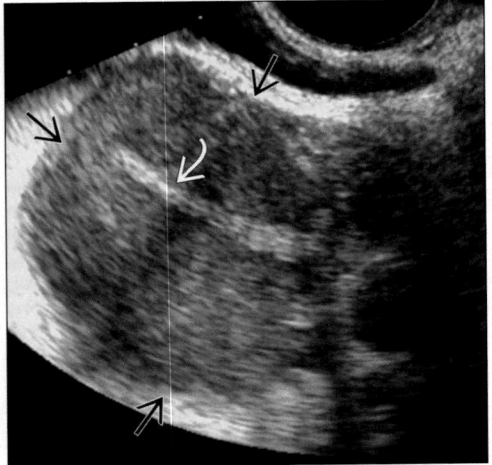

Oblique transvaginal ultrasound shows a distended pus-filled fallopian tube ➡ associated with the TOA. An incomplete septum ➡ is formed by the tube folding upon itself.

TERMINOLOGY

Abbreviations and Synonyms
- Pelvic inflammatory disease (PID)
- Pyosalpinx
- Tubo-ovarian complex (TOC)
- Tubo-ovarian abscess (TOA)

Definitions
- PID
  - Upper genital tract infection
  - Sexually transmitted disease (STD)
- Pyosalpinx
  - Tube distended with pus
- Tubo-ovarian complex
  - Ovary adherent to tube
  - Distinguishable separate ovary
- TOA
  - Abscess involving tube and ovary
  - Separate ovary no longer distinguishable

IMAGING FINDINGS

General Features
- Best diagnostic clue
  - TOA: Painful complex adnexal mass
  - Pyosalpinx: Serpiginous mass with echogenic material
- Location
  - TOA often bilateral, infection spreads from one side to other
    - TOA often in posterior cul-de-sac
  - Early PID is unilateral
- Morphology: Depends on structures involved

Ultrasonographic Findings
- **Fallopian tube distended with echogenic fluid**
  - Distal obstruction causes distention
    - Distended serpiginous, ovoid or pear-shaped tube
  - Tubes extend posteriorly
    - Look in cul-de-sac
  - Complex fluid
    - Layering debris common, ± gas
  - Thickened tube walls
    - Often > 5 mm

DDx: Non-Ovarian Adnexal Cysts

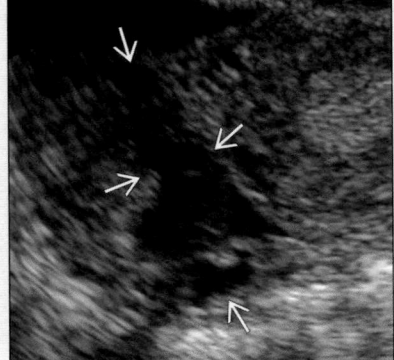

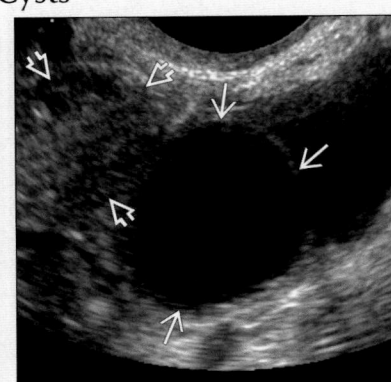

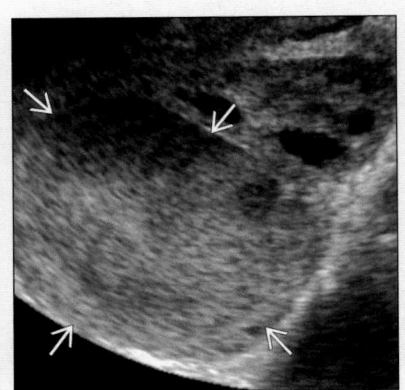

Hydrosalpinx *Paraovarian Cyst* *Endometrioma*

TUBOVARIAN ABSCESS

Key Facts

Imaging Findings
- TOA: Painful complex adnexal mass
- Pyosalpinx: Serpiginous mass with echogenic material
- TOA often bilateral, infection spreads from one side to other
- **Fallopian tube distended with echogenic fluid**
- Distended serpiginous, ovoid or pear-shaped tube
- Layering debris common, ± gas
- Thickened endosalpingeal folds: "Cog wheel sign" in cross-section
- Incomplete septi: Distended tube folds on itself
- As PID progresses ovary appearance varies from enlargement to complex mass
- **Tubo-ovarian complex**
- Enlarged ovary adheres to enlarged tube
- Can recognize both structures separately

- **Tubo-ovarian abscess**
- Complex adnexal mass
- Ovary not recognizable
- Increased color Doppler flow
- Low resistive flow
- Sonographic findings resolve quickly with treatment

Top Differential Diagnoses
- Endometriosis
- Hydrosalpinx
- Paraovarian Cyst

Diagnostic Checklist
- Acute PID may have minimal findings
- Abdominal ultrasound or CT important to assess extent of disease

---

- ○ Thickened endosalpingeal folds: "Cog wheel sign" in cross-section
- ○ Incomplete septi: Distended tube folds on itself
- As PID progresses ovary appearance varies from enlargement to complex mass
  - ○ Early ovarian involvement
    - ▪ Enlarged edematous ovary
    - ▪ ↑ Number and size of follicles
  - ○ Tubo-ovarian complex
    - ▪ Enlarged ovary adheres to enlarged tube
    - ▪ Can recognize both structures separately
  - ○ Tubo-ovarian abscess
    - ▪ Complex adnexal mass
    - ▪ Ovary not recognizable
    - ▪ May still see pyosalpinx
- **Complex pelvic fluid (pus)**
  - ○ High gain settings to see echoes
  - ○ Seen early in course of PID
- **Doppler findings**
  - ○ Increased color Doppler flow
    - ▪ Walls and folds of tube light up
    - ▪ Involved ovary with ↑ flow
  - ○ Pulsed Doppler
    - ▪ Low resistive flow
    - ▪ Resistive index near 0.5
- Sonographic findings resolve quickly with treatment
  - ○ Pyosalpinx → hydrosalpinx → ± resolution
  - ○ Complex pelvic fluid resolution
  - ○ TOA may require drainage/surgery

CT Findings
- CT often ordered 1st if generalized symptoms
  - ○ Rule out appendicitis & diverticulitis
- Similar findings as on ultrasound
  - ○ Enlarged ovaries
  - ○ Dilated tubes
  - ○ Free fluid
- CT is often less specific than ultrasound
  - ○ Difficult to differentiate between pyosalpinx, tubo-ovarian complex and TOA
- Inflammatory changes seen better with CT
  - ○ Thickening of uterosacral ligament
  - ○ Pelvic fat haziness

- ○ Periovarian stranding
- ○ Inflammation beyond pelvis
- Involvement of adjacent structures
  - ○ Ureteral obstruction
    - ▪ Hydronephrosis
  - ○ Secondary inflammation
    - ▪ Appendix
    - ▪ Bowel
- Fitz-Hugh-Curtis syndrome
  - ○ Perihepatic spread of infection
    - ▪ Pouch of Douglas → paracolic gutter → peritoneum
    - ▪ Right upper quadrant pain presentation
  - ○ CT findings
    - ▪ ↑ Enhancement of anterior liver peritoneal surface
    - ▪ Transient hepatic attenuation difference
    - ▪ Gallbladder wall thickening

Imaging Recommendations
- Best imaging tool: Transvaginal ultrasound
- Protocol advice
  - ○ Remember acute PID has subtle, nonspecific findings
    - ▪ Enlarged edematous uterus
    - ▪ Endometrial fluid
    - ▪ Increased pelvic fat echogenicity
    - ▪ Use probe to assess region of pain
  - ○ Use probe to diagnose tuboovarian complex
    - ▪ Do ovary and tube move together or apart?
  - ○ Look in abdomen when pelvic findings are extensive
    - ▪ Consider abdominal ultrasound/CT to evaluate extent of disease
    - ▪ Complex fluid may ascend
    - ▪ Look for hydronephrosis

DIFFERENTIAL DIAGNOSIS

Endometriosis
- Ectopic endometrial glands
  - ○ Functioning cells
  - ○ Cyclic bleeding
- Multiple lesions common

TUBOVARIAN ABSCESS

- Bilateral adnexal masses
- Often ovarian
  - ± Tube involvement
  - ± Other pelvic organ involvement
- Round masses more often than tubular
  - Diffuse low-level echoes
  - Thick wall and nodularity common
  - May have fluid/fluid levels

Hydrosalpinx
- Anechoic fluid distends fallopian tube
  - Thin tube wall
  - Normal endosalpingeal folds
    - "Beads on a string" sign
- Not painful
- Sequelae of PID
  - May resolve or persist

Paraovarian Cyst
- Broad ligament cyst
- Unilocular anechoic cyst
  - Thin wall
  - Ovary displaced peripherally
- No endosalpingeal folds

PATHOLOGY

General Features
- Etiology
  - Bacteria damage endocervical canal and ascend
    - Chlamydia most common organism
    - Neisseria gonorrhoeae
    - Co-existing infections common
    - Actinomycosis israelii (from intrauterine device)
  - Cervical ectopy may play a role
    - Endocervical epithelium extends beyond cervix
    - Larger area susceptible to infection
    - Cervical ectopy more common in teenagers
- Epidemiology
  - 780,000 new cases acute PID annually
  - 4.2% of young adults with chlamydial infection
- Associated abnormalities
  - Ectopic pregnancy
  - Infertility
  - Chronic pelvic pain

CLINICAL ISSUES

Presentation
- Most common signs/symptoms
  - Pelvic pain
    - Cervical motion tenderness
  - Fever
  - Vaginal discharge
- Other signs/symptoms
  - Right upper quadrant pain rare
    - Fitz-Hugh-Curtis syndrome
- Clinical Profile
  - Risk factors related to exposure to STD
    - Multiple partners
    - Sexual intercourse at early age
    - Prior STD

Demographics
- Age: Women < 25 y at ↑ risk

Natural History & Prognosis
- Fallopian tube scarring sequelae
  - Infertility
  - Ectopic pregnancy
  - Salpingitis isthmica nodosa
    - Diverticulae of fallopian tube
    - Mostly at isthmus
- Chronic pelvic pain

Treatment
- Prompt antibiotic therapy
  - 14 days of treatment
  - Polymicrobial coverage
- Pain relief
- 25% need hospitalization
- Nonresolving TOA requires surgery/drainage

DIAGNOSTIC CHECKLIST

Image Interpretation Pearls
- Acute PID may have minimal findings
  - Pain will be disproportionate to findings
  - Look for subtle inflammatory change
  - Look in posterior cul-de-sac for pus
- TOA is nonspecific complex adnexal mass
  - Use color Doppler to show ↑ inflammation
- Abdominal ultrasound or CT important to assess extent of disease

SELECTED REFERENCES

1. Barrett S et al: A review on pelvic inflammatory disease. Int J STD AIDS. 16(11):715-20; quiz 721, 2005
2. Miller WC et al: Epidemiology of chlamydial infection, gonorrhea, and trichomoniasis in the United States--2005. Infect Dis Clin North Am. 19(2):281-96, 2005
3. Piscaglia F et al: Fitz-Hugh-Curtis-syndrome mimicking acute cholecystitis: value of new ultrasound findings in the differential diagnosis. Ultraschall Med. 26(3):227-30, 2005
4. Ghiatas AA: The spectrum of pelvic inflammatory disease. Eur Radiol. 14 Suppl 3:E184-92, 2004
5. Horrow MM: Ultrasound of pelvic inflammatory disease. Ultrasound Q. 20(4):171-9, 2004
6. Lambert MJ et al: Gynecologic ultrasound in emergency medicine. Emerg Med Clin North Am. 22(3):683-96, 2004
7. Ignacio EA et al: Ultrasound of the acute female pelvis. Ultrasound Q. 19(2):86-98; quiz 108-10, 2003
8. Pickhardt PJ et al: Fitz-Hugh-Curtis syndrome: multidetector CT findings of transient hepatic attenuation difference and gallbladder wall thickening. AJR Am J Roentgenol. 180(6):1605-6, 2003

TUBOVARIAN ABSCESS

IMAGE GALLERY

Typical

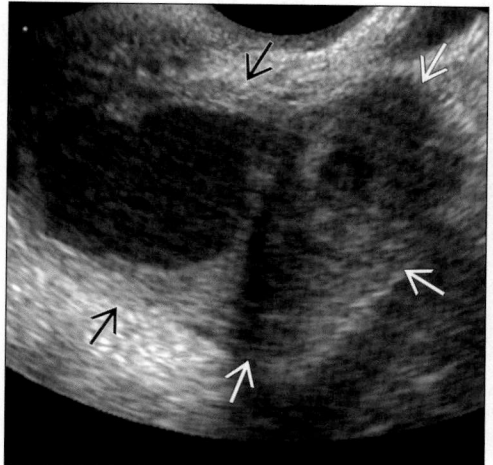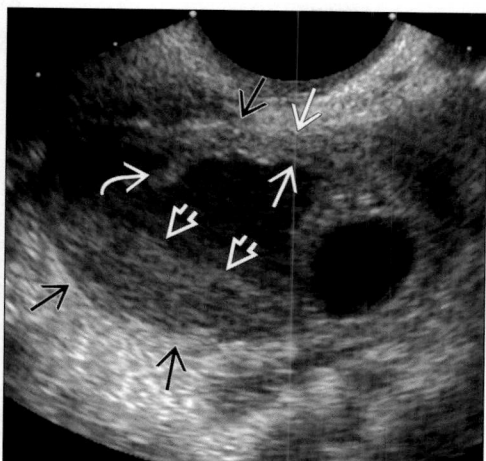

(Left) Transverse transvaginal ultrasound shows a distended thick-walled fallopian tube ➡ adherent to an edematous indistinct ovary ➡ in this case of tubo-ovarian complex. (Right) Longitudinal transvaginal ultrasound of a distended tube ➡ shows layering debris ➡, a thickened endosalpingeal fold ➡ and thickening of the fallopian tube wall ➡.

Typical

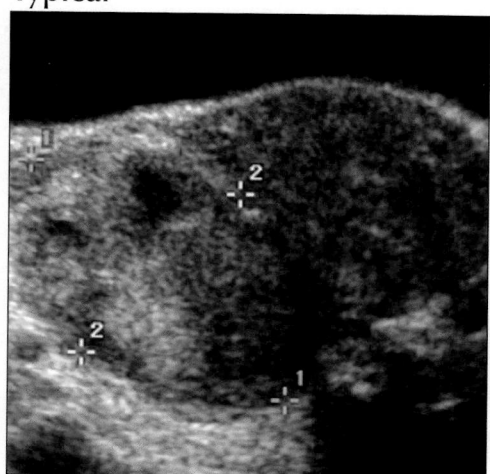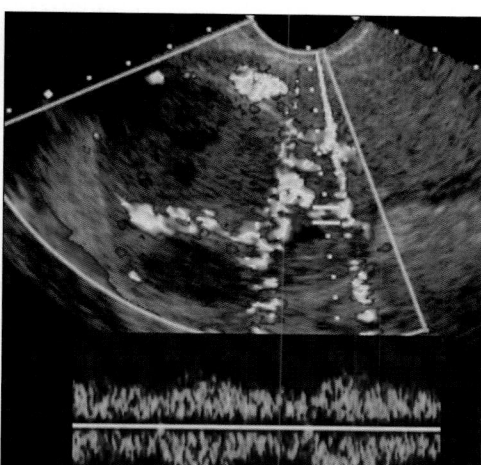

(Left) Transverse transabdominal ultrasound shows an enlarged edematous ovary (calipers) in a patient with early PID. (Right) Transverse color Doppler ultrasound shows increased low resistive blood flow to the ovary. The ultrasound features are nonspecific but correlated with the clinical picture of PID.

Typical

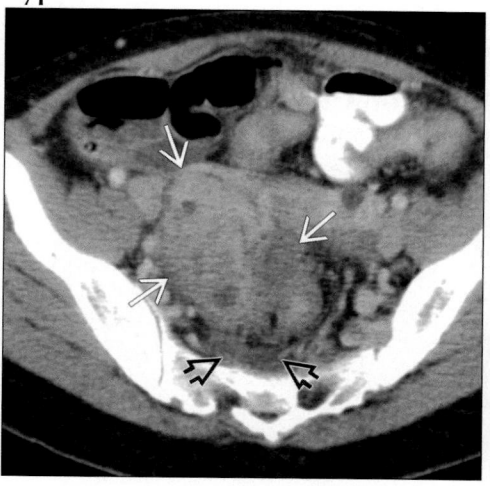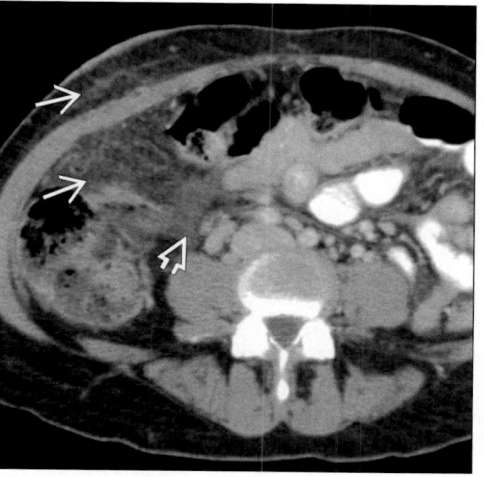

(Left) Transverse CECT shows a TOA ➡. Note that the ovary and tube are not distinguishable and there is inflammatory change in the posterior cul-de-sac ➡. (Right) Transverse CECT shows inflammatory change ➡ and fluid ➡ extending beyond the pelvis in this patient with extensive TOA.

PAROVARIAN CYSTS

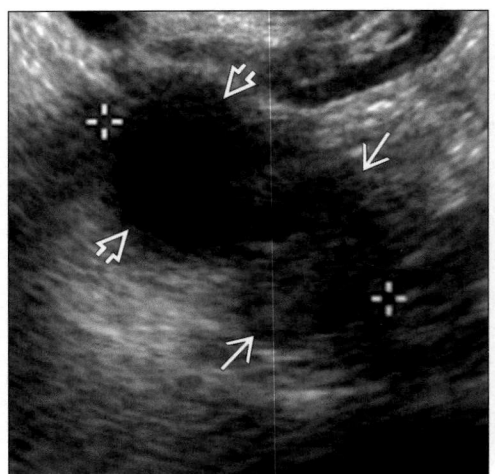

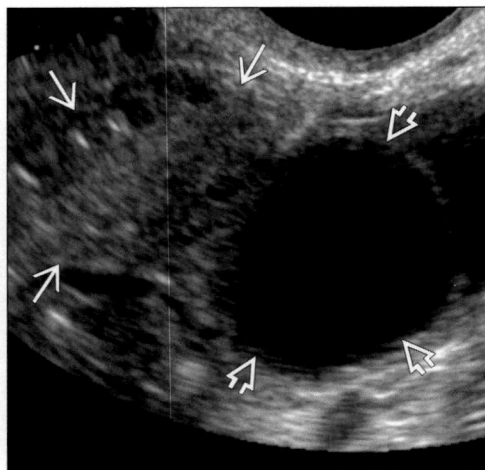

Oblique transabdominal ultrasound shows an adnexal mass (calipers) which initially appears to have solid ➡ & cystic ⬇ components.

Transverse transvaginal ultrasound shows an intact normal ovary ➡ & a unilocular thin-walled paraovarian cyst ⬇ medial to the ovary. Same patient as previous image.

TERMINOLOGY

Abbreviations and Synonyms
- Paratubal cyst

Definitions
- Cyst originating from mesosalpinx or broad ligament

IMAGING FINDINGS

General Features
- Best diagnostic clue: Unilocular cyst near ovary
- Size: Mean diameter is 40 mm (15-120 mm)
- Morphology
  - Well-defined round or oval mass
    - May be pedunculated & those with long pedicles tend to undergo torsion

Ultrasonographic Findings
- Adnexal cyst medial to ovary
  - Lack of follicles distinguishes from ovary
- Unilocular in 95%
- Multilocular in 5%

- Septae are thin, smooth, complete
- May represent multiple cysts
- Fluid is anechoic in 91%
  - 9% with small floating echoes (probably from hemorrhage)
- Thin outer wall (< 3 mm)
  - Some with 2-5 mm papillae

Imaging Recommendations
- Best imaging tool: Transvaginal ultrasound
- Protocol advice
  - Study any adnexal mass from border to border
    - Decide ovarian vs. extraovarian
  - Study cyst characteristics carefully
    - Measure in 3 orthogonal planes
    - Note shape and content
    - Study cyst wall
  - Study cyst mobility with vaginal probe
    - "Split sign" (cyst moves separate from ovary)

DIFFERENTIAL DIAGNOSIS

Peritoneal Inclusion Cyst (PIC)
- Multilocular cyst with undefined walls

DDx: Cystic Adnexal Mass

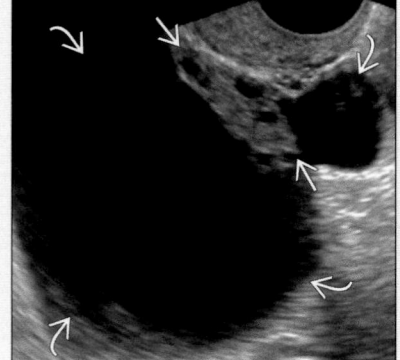

Peritoneal Inclusion Cyst

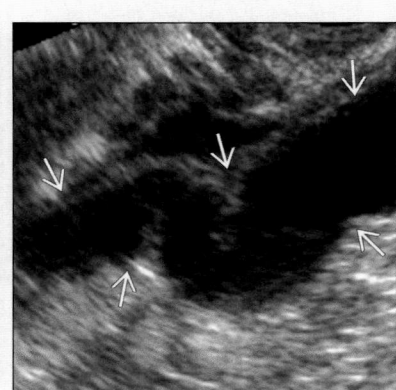

Hydrosalpinx

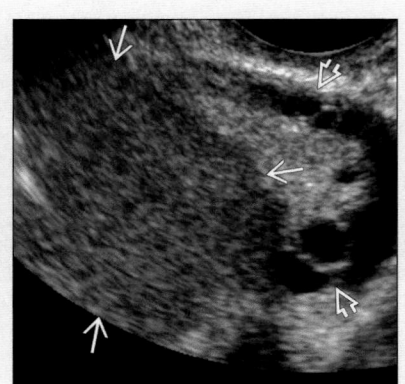

Ovarian Cyst

PAROVARIAN CYSTS

Key Facts

Terminology
- Cyst originating from mesosalpinx or broad ligament

Imaging Findings
- Adnexal cyst medial to ovary
- Unilocular in 95%
- Thin outer wall (< 3 mm)
- "Split sign" (cyst moves separate from ovary)

Pathology
- 98% benign serous cyst

Clinical Issues
- Other signs/symptoms: Torsion, growth, malignancy are rare complications
- Surgery avoided if cyst < 5 cm and no papillae

Diagnostic Checklist
- Do not assume every adnexal mass is ovarian

- Ovary surrounded by fluid and adhesions

Hydrosalpinx
- Tubular morphology with separate ovary
- Hyperechoic mural nodules common

True Ovarian Cyst
- Unilocular or complex
- Look for ovarian tissue at cyst borders

PATHOLOGY

General Features
- Epidemiology: 5-20% of all adnexal masses

Gross Pathologic & Surgical Features
- 98% benign serous cyst
- 2% with malignant features
  - Serous papillary tumors

CLINICAL ISSUES

Presentation
- Most common signs/symptoms
  - Asymptomatic
  - Adnexal mass
- Other signs/symptoms: Torsion, growth, malignancy are rare complications

Treatment
- Surgery avoided if cyst < 5 cm and no papillae

DIAGNOSTIC CHECKLIST

Consider
- Often misdiagnosed as true ovarian cyst

Image Interpretation Pearls
- Do not assume every adnexal mass is ovarian
- Correct diagnosis important to avoid surgery
- MR can help make a more precise diagnosis

SELECTED REFERENCES

1. Puig F et al: Serous cystadenoma of borderline malignancy arising in a parovarian paramesonephric cyst. Eur J Gynaecol Oncol. 27(4):417-8, 2006
2. Savelli L et al: Paraovarian/paratubal cysts: comparison of transvaginal sonographic and pathological findings to establish diagnostic criteria. Ultrasound Obstet Gynecol. 28(3):330-4, 2006
3. Blaivas M et al: Reliability of adnexal mass mobility in distinguishing possible ectopic pregnancy from corpus luteum cysts. J Ultrasound Med. 24(5):599-603; quiz 605, 2005
4. Korbin CD et al: Paraovarian cystadenomas and cystadenofibromas: sonographic characteristics in 14 cases. Radiology. 208(2):459-62, 1998
5. Kim JS et al: Sonographic diagnosis of paraovarian cysts: value of detecting a separate ipsilateral ovary. AJR Am J Roentgenol. 164(6):1441-4, 1995

IMAGE GALLERY

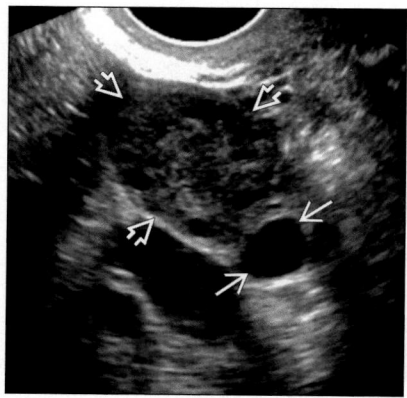 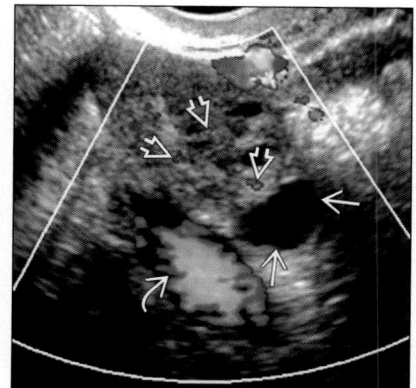 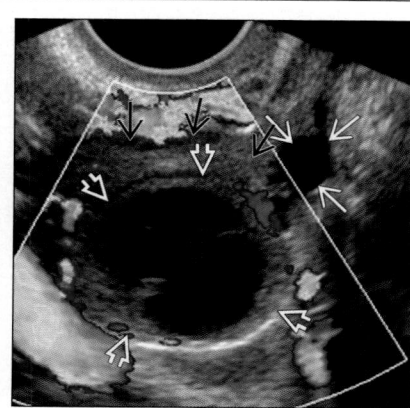

(Left) Oblique transvaginal ultrasound shows small paraovarian cyst ➡ adjacent to the right ovary ➡. *(Center)* Oblique color Doppler ultrasound shows blood flow in the ovary ➡ and iliac artery ➡ but not in the paraovarian cyst ➡. *(Right)* Transverse color Doppler ultrasound of the other ovary shows hemorrhagic corpus luteal cyst ➡ & another small paraovarian cyst ➡. Ovarian tissue ➡ "hugs" the periphery of the intraovarian cyst.

BARTHOLIN CYST

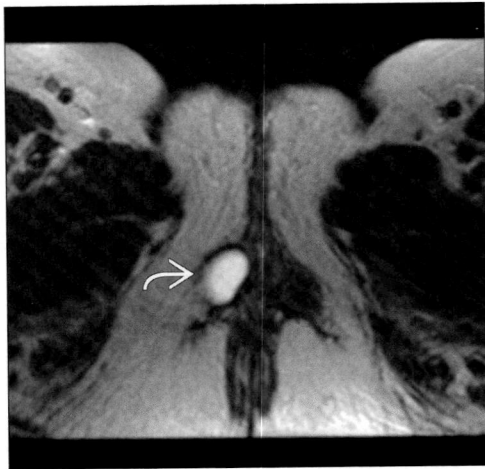

T2WI MR in an axial plane, low in the pelvis shows the typical appearance of a Bartholin cyst as a high signal cyst ➡ in the posterior labia minora.

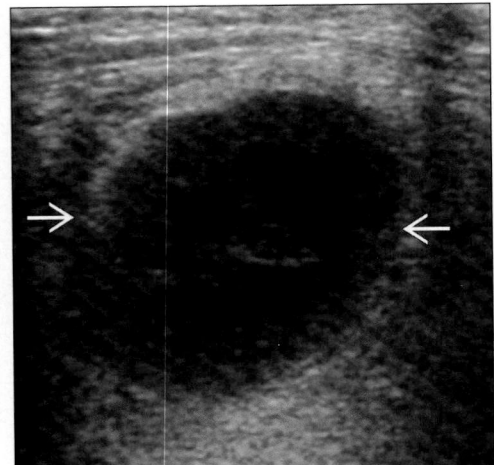

Longitudinal ultrasound shows a complex fluid collection ➡ associated with labial swelling and perineal pain. This is a typical presentation for Bartholin abscess.

TERMINOLOGY

Definitions
- Cystic dilatation of Bartholin gland secondary to duct obstruction

IMAGING FINDINGS

General Features
- Best diagnostic clue: Palpable, visible mass in posterior labia minora
- Location: Bilateral vulvovaginal bodies in labia minora at 4 and 8 o'clock positions, posterolateral vestibule

Ultrasonographic Findings
- Grayscale Ultrasound: Cystic structure: Anechoic to mixed echogenicity if complicated by hemorrhage or infection
- Power Doppler: No internal vascularity, may see reactive hyperemia around Bartholin abscess

MR Findings
- T1WI: Low signal fluid if uncomplicated, signal may ↑ with infection or hemorrhage
- T2WI: High signal fluid if uncomplicated, proteinaceous fluid often lower signal than simple fluid

Imaging Recommendations
- Protocol advice: Clinical diagnosis: Imaging generally not required

DIFFERENTIAL DIAGNOSIS

Other Labial Masses
- Sebaceous cyst: Epidermal inclusion cysts, may become infected, respond well to incision and drainage
- Dysontogenetic cyst: Mucus-containing cysts at introitus/labia minora
- Hematoma: Straddle injury, abuse
- Tumors: Rare, usually clinically obvious

DDx: Vaginal/Perineal Mass

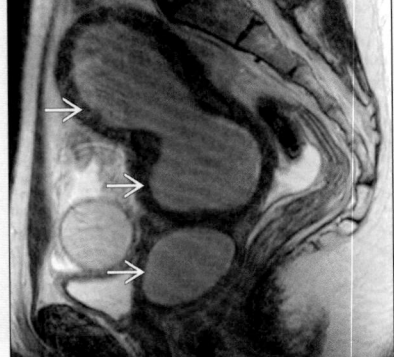

Hematometrocolpos

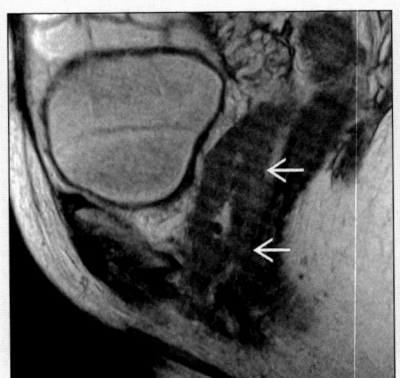

Vaginal Carcinoma

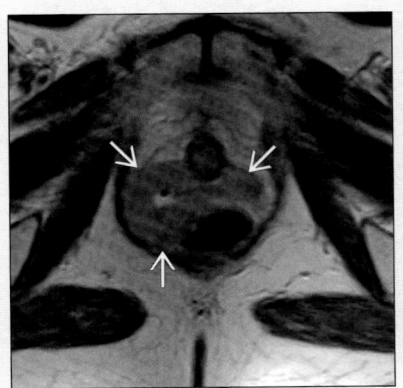

Vaginal Carcinoma

BARTHOLIN CYST

Key Facts

Terminology
- Cystic dilatation of Bartholin gland secondary to duct obstruction

Imaging Findings
- Best diagnostic clue: Palpable, visible mass in posterior labia minora
- Grayscale Ultrasound: Cystic structure: Anechoic to mixed echogenicity if complicated by hemorrhage or infection

Top Differential Diagnoses
- Other Labial Masses
- Vulval Varices

Pathology
- Epidemiology: Approximately 2% of women

Clinical Issues
- May become infected → Bartholin abscess

Vulval Varices
- Associated with pelvic congestion syndrome
- Throughout vulva, not limited to vestibule

PATHOLOGY

General Features
- Etiology: Obstruction of normal Bartholin gland
- Epidemiology: Approximately 2% of women

Microscopic Features
- Squamous or adenocarcinoma can develop in a Bartholin gland
  - Gland lined with cuboidal epithelium, duct lined with squamous epithelium
  - Incidence of cancer is low: 0.114 per 100,000 woman-years

CLINICAL ISSUES

Presentation
- Most common signs/symptoms: Palpable mass posterior labia, 1-3 cm but may become much larger

Natural History & Prognosis
- Most are uncomplicated
- May become infected → Bartholin abscess
  - Perineal pain
  - Tender labial mass
  - Increased size of pre-existing mass

Treatment
- Incision/drainage ± silver nitrate cautery
- Marsupialization or excision for recurrent cases
- Abscess
  - Sitz baths/symptomatic therapy if spontaneous rupture
  - Test for gonococcus/chlamydia
  - Broad spectrum antibiotics after surgical drainage
    - Simple aspiration insufficient for Bartholin abscess
    - Will recur if gland drainage remains obstructed

SELECTED REFERENCES

1. Ergeneli MH: Silver nitrate for Bartholin gland cysts. Eur J Obstet Gynecol Reprod Biol. 82(2):231-2, 1999
2. Hill DA et al: Office management of Bartholin gland cysts and abscesses. Am Fam Physician. 57(7):1611-6, 1619-20, 1998
3. Yuce K et al: Outpatient management of Bartholin gland abscesses and cysts with silver nitrate. Aust N Z J Obstet Gynaecol. 34(1):93-6, 1994
4. Brenner B: Laser vaporisation of Bartholin duct cysts. N Z Med J. 104(906):80-1, 1991
5. Cho JY et al: Window operation: an alternative treatment method for Bartholin gland cysts and abscesses. Obstet Gynecol. 76(5 Pt 1):886-8, 1990

IMAGE GALLERY

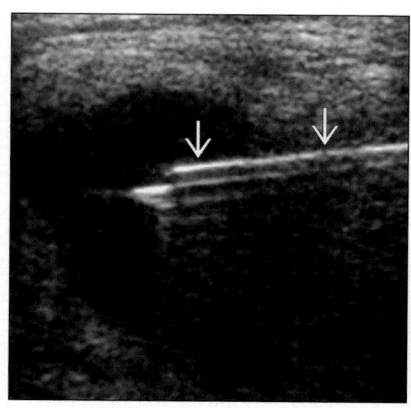 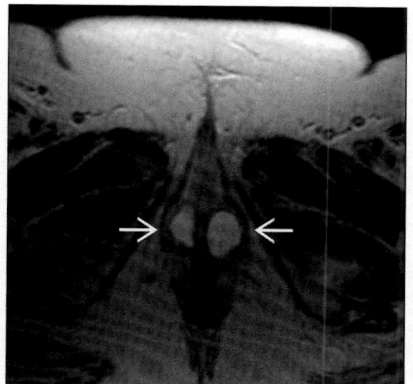 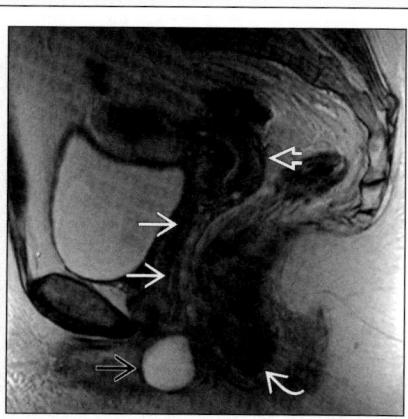

(Left) Longitudinal ultrasound shows needle ➡ in center of collection. Aspiration provides temporary relief and sample for culture but most Bartholin abscesses require more definitive therapy than simple aspiration. *(Center)* Transverse T2 weighted MR shows bilateral Bartholin cysts ➡. They are often an incidental finding. *(Right)* Sagittal T2 weighted MR in same patient as previous image shows typical location ➡ in posterior labia. Cervix ➡, vagina ➡ and rectum ➡ are well seen on MR.

GARTNER DUCT CYST

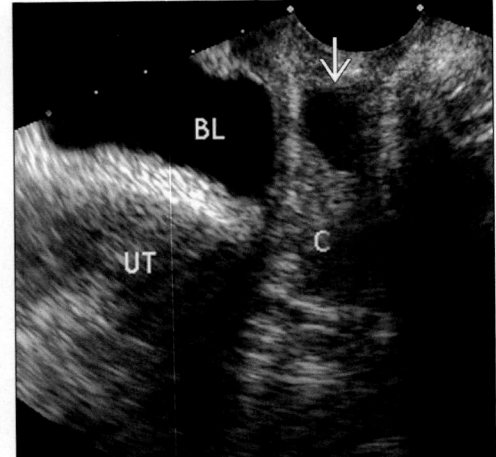

Longitudinal transvaginal ultrasound shows normal appearances of uterus ➡, cervix ➤ and bladder ➡ in patient who was scanned because of history of irregular bleeding.

Oblique transvaginal ultrasound in same case as previous image shows typical Gartner duct cyst in anterior vaginal wall ➡. This is separate from cervix (C) and lateral to uterine (UT) long axis. Bladder (BL).

TERMINOLOGY

Abbreviations and Synonyms
- Gartner duct cyst (GDC)
- Gartner duct (GD)
- Müllerian duct anomalies (MDA)

Definitions
- Cystic dilatation of Gartner duct
  - Remnant of embryonic mesonephric (Wolffian) ducts
  - Cyst can occur anywhere along course of duct, most commonly anterolateral part of proximal 1/3rd of vaginal wall

IMAGING FINDINGS

General Features
- Best diagnostic clue: Fluid-filled structure in anterolateral vaginal wall
- Size: Generally < 2 cm diameter

Ultrasonographic Findings
- Grayscale Ultrasound
  - Cyst characteristics
    - Anechoic to hypoechoic
    - Increased through transmission
    - Well defined wall
  - Infection or hemorrhage → increased echogenicity of fluid component
- Power Doppler
  - No internal flow on Doppler
  - Helps to confirm cystic nature rather than solid mass such as vaginal tumor

Radiographic Findings
- GD may opacify on hysterosalpingography
  - If GDC present it will opacify as a focal ductal dilatation
- GD runs parallel to cervical canal

MR Findings
- T1WI: Intermediate to high signal due to proteinaceous nature of fluid
- T2WI: High signal fluid content
- In anterolateral vaginal wall

DDx: Findings at the Vaginal Vault

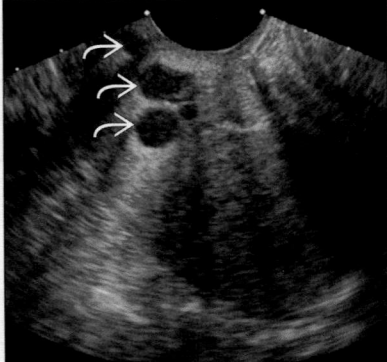

Nabothian Cyst

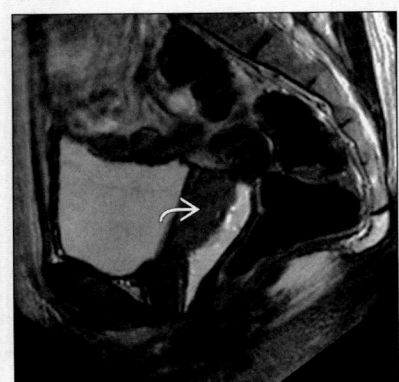

Vaginal Tumor

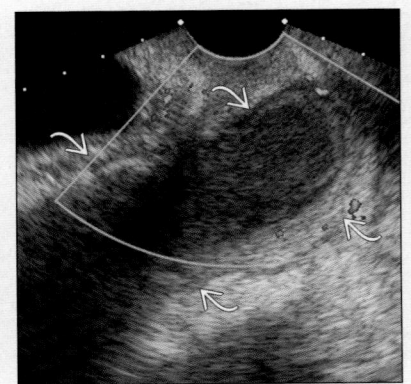

Hematometra

GARTNER DUCT CYST

Key Facts

Terminology
- Cystic dilatation of Gartner duct

Imaging Findings
- Best diagnostic clue: Fluid-filled structure in anterolateral vaginal wall
- Anechoic to hypoechoic
- Infection or hemorrhage → increased echogenicity of fluid component
- No internal flow on Doppler
- Pelvic MR may be helpful to show location within vaginal wall/relationship to surrounding tissues
- In infants consider vaginal distension with saline via catheter

Top Differential Diagnoses
- Nabothian cysts

- Vaginal inclusion cysts
- Endometriosis implant
- Hematometra/hematocolpos
- Vaginal tumor
- Uterine/cervical fibroid

Clinical Issues
- Usually asymptomatic

Diagnostic Checklist
- In girls with ipsilateral renal dysgenesis a ureterocele-like "cyst" without associated ureteric dilatation is highly suspicious for GDC
- In an infant with a pelvic cyst, distension of the vagina with saline allows confirmation that cyst arises in vaginal wall

---

- ○ Vaginal distension with Surgilube → better delineation of vaginal walls
- When large or recurrent may be multiloculated

Imaging Recommendations
- Best imaging tool: Transvaginal sonography
- Protocol advice
  - ○ Pelvic MR may be helpful to show location within vaginal wall/relationship to surrounding tissues
    - Always include kidneys on coronal scout images
    - Have patient inject water soluble gel ("Surgilube") into vagina immediately prior to study: Provides clear delineation of vaginal fornices
  - ○ In infants consider vaginal distension with saline via catheter
    - Will confirm cyst in vaginal wall not in pelvis

DIFFERENTIAL DIAGNOSIS

Cystic Appearance
- Nabothian cysts
  - ○ Within cervix
  - ○ Eccentric to cervical canal
  - ○ GDC is adjacent to but separate from cervix
- Vaginal inclusion cysts
  - ○ Occur as a result of obstetric or gynecologic trauma
  - ○ Usually posterior wall
    - GDC are anterolateral in location
  - ○ Ask patient about prior deliveries/surgeries
- Endometriosis implant
  - ○ More complex architecture
  - ○ Thick wall, low level internal echoes
  - ○ Likely to have other manifestations of endometriosis
  - ○ MR likely to show evidence of blood products
- Hematometra/hematocolpos
  - ○ Echogenic fluid in vag. lumen due to blood products
  - ○ Associated with obstructed vagina
    - Often history of primary amenorrhea/cyclical pain

Solid Appearance
- Vaginal tumor
  - ○ Extremely rare

- ○ Patients are usually symptomatic
- ○ Solid mass; palpable, visible on speculum exam
  - Squamous cell carcinoma may undergo cystic degeneration
  - Vaginal sarcoma
- Uterine/cervical fibroid
  - ○ Prolapsed submucosal fibroid
    - Solid
    - Protrudes though cervix
    - Visible on speculum exam
  - ○ Cervical fibroid
    - Solid
    - Arises from cervical stroma

PATHOLOGY

General Features
- Epidemiology
  - ○ Remnants of GD can be detected in 25% of adult women
  - ○ GDC reported to occur in 1-2% of women
  - ○ More common in Asian patients
- Associated abnormalities
  - ○ Müllerian duct anomalies
    - Unicornuate, bicornuate, didelphys or septate uterus
    - Carry ↑ risk infertility, spontaneous abortion
    - May present with hematocolpos/primary amenorrhea
  - ○ Renal anomalies
    - Ipsilateral renal dysgenesis/agenesis
    - Crossed fused ectopia
    - Ectopic ureter: Reports of ectopic ureter terminating in GDC
  - ○ Diverticulosis of fallopian tubes (salpingitis isthmica nodosa)
    - Associated with increased incidence of infertility/increased risk for ectopic
- Embryology
  - ○ Mesonephric ducts normally resorb in females

GARTNER DUCT CYST

○ Remnants form an interrupted channel along genital tract = GD
○ Dilatation of any portion of mesonephric duct remnants → GDC
  ▪ Commonest in vaginal wall
○ Ureteral bud also develops from mesonephric duct
  ▪ Associated renal/ureteric anomalies are common

CLINICAL ISSUES

Presentation
• Most common signs/symptoms
  ○ Usually asymptomatic
  ○ May be incidental finding on transvaginal ultrasound
  ○ May be incidental finding on pelvic examination
    ▪ Usually soft to palpation
    ▪ Cyst wall has blue tinge on speculum examination
• Other signs/symptoms
  ○ May be symptomatic if large
    ▪ Pelvic pressure symptoms
    ▪ Dyspareunia
    ▪ Obstructed labor
    ▪ Mass at introitus described in neonate
  ○ May present with urologic symptoms
    ▪ Cyst may be seen posterior to bladder or protrude into bladder mimicking a ureterocele
    ▪ May cause ureteric or urethral obstruction
    ▪ Reported cases of recurrent urinary retention in children requiring surgical resection of GDC
    ▪ Urinary incontinence in children

Natural History & Prognosis
• Usually asymptomatic
• No specific treatment required
• Infection/hemorrhage may cause acute pain
• May be associated with
  ○ Müllerian duct anomalies
  ○ Renal anomalies
• Large cysts tend to be symptomatic
• GDC may recur post-operatively
  ○ Recurrences tend to be multilocular
    ▪ May be mistaken for ovarian carcinoma, lymphocele, abscess
  ○ Pelvic MR will show location inferior to levator plate

Treatment
• If symptomatic
  ○ Aspiration
  ○ Sclerotherapy
    ▪ Aspirate fluid
    ▪ Inject with 5% tetracycline solution in volume equal to aspirate
    ▪ Tetracycline solution reaspirated after 24 hrs
  ○ Marsupialization
  ○ Surgical excision
• Check uterine/renal anatomy for possible associated malformations

DIAGNOSTIC CHECKLIST

Consider
• In girls with ipsilateral renal dysgenesis a ureterocele-like "cyst" without associated ureteric dilatation is highly suspicious for GDC
  ○ Strong association with MDA
  ○ 6/10 in one series had obstructing vaginal septum

Image Interpretation Pearls
• In an infant with a pelvic cyst, distension of the vagina with saline allows confirmation that cyst arises in vaginal wall
• Associated with müllerian duct/renal anomalies
  ○ If cyst seen on pelvic imaging check kidneys

SELECTED REFERENCES

1. Lopez C et al: MRI of vaginal conditions. Clin Radiol. 60(6):648-62, 2005
2. Eilber KS et al: Benign cystic lesions of the vagina: a literature review. J Urol. 170(3):717-22, 2003
3. Fan EW et al: Pyonephrosis and urinary retention secondary to a large Gartner's duct cyst associated with single ectopic ureter in a pregnant woman. BJU Int. 89(1):136-7, 2002
4. Ohya T et al: Diagnosis and treatment for persistent Gartner duct cyst in an infant: A case report. J Pediatr Surg. 37(4):E4, 2002
5. Emmons SL et al: Recurrent giant Gartner's duct cysts. A report of two cases. J Reprod Med. 46(8):773-5, 2001
6. Kiechl-Kohlendorfer U et al: Diagnosing neonatal female genital anomalies using saline-enhanced sonography. AJR Am J Roentgenol. 177(5):1041-4, 2001
7. Sherer DM et al: Transvaginal ultrasonographic depiction of a Gartner duct cyst. J Ultrasound Med. 20(11):1253-5, 2001
8. Holmes M et al: Gartner's duct cyst with unilateral renal dysplasia presenting as an introital mass in a new born. Pediatr Surg Int. 15(3-4):277-9, 1999
9. Sheih CP et al: Diagnosing the combination of renal dysgenesis, Gartner's duct cyst and ipsilateral mullerian duct obstruction. J Urol. 159(1):217-21, 1998
10. Sheih CP et al: Duplex kidney, Gartner's duct cyst and ipsilateral Mullerian duct obstruction. J Urol. 159(6):2120-1, 1998
11. Leonovicz PF 3rd et al: Vaginal ectopic ureter with Gartner's duct cyst. J Urol. 158(6):2235, 1997
12. Rosenfeld DL et al: Gartner's duct cyst with a single vaginal ectopic ureter and associated renal dysplasia or agenesis. J Ultrasound Med. 12(12):775-8, 1993
13. Li YW et al: MR imaging and sonography of Gartner's duct cyst and single ectopic ureter with ipsilateral renal dysplasia. Pediatr Radiol. 22(6):472-3, 1992
14. Abd-Rabbo MS et al: Aspiration and tetracycline sclerotherapy: a novel method for management of vaginal and vulval Gartner cysts. Int J Gynaecol Obstet. 35(3):235-7, 1991
15. Pradhan S et al: Vaginal cysts: a clinicopathological study of 41 cases. Int J Gynecol Pathol. 5(1):35-46, 1986

GARTNER DUCT CYST

IMAGE GALLERY

Typical

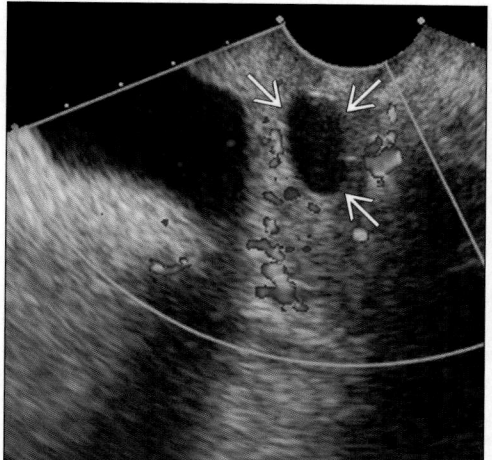

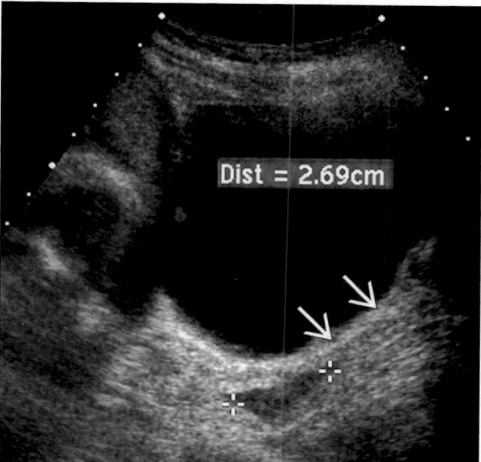

(Left) Oblique color Doppler ultrasound shows no internal flow and well-defined cyst walls ➡. This is an incidental Gartner duct cyst which was asymptomatic. (Right) Longitudinal transabdominal ultrasound shows a hypoechoic "mass" (calipers) aligned with the long axis of the vagina ➡ in a pregnant patient. The cervix was seen separately, adjacent to this "mass".

Typical

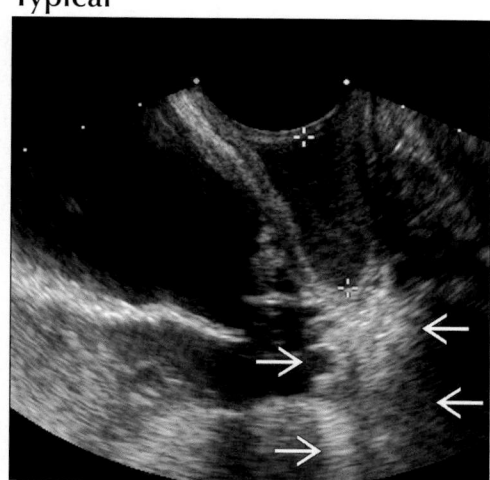

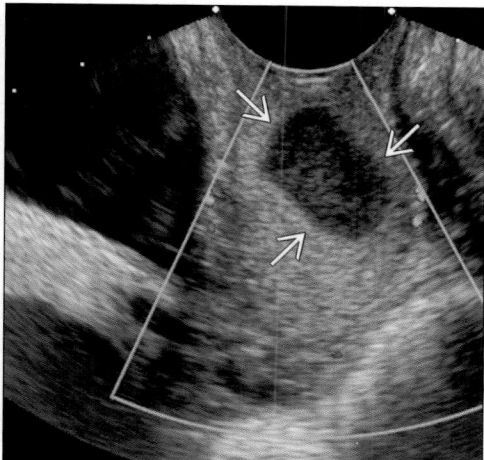

(Left) Oblique transvaginal ultrasound shows that the "mass" (calipers) is cystic and within the walls of the vagina. Note distal acoustic enhancement ➡ confirming its cystic nature. (Right) Transverse color Doppler ultrasound in the same patient as the previous image shows low level internal echoes in the cyst fluid ➡ but no internal vascularity.

Typical

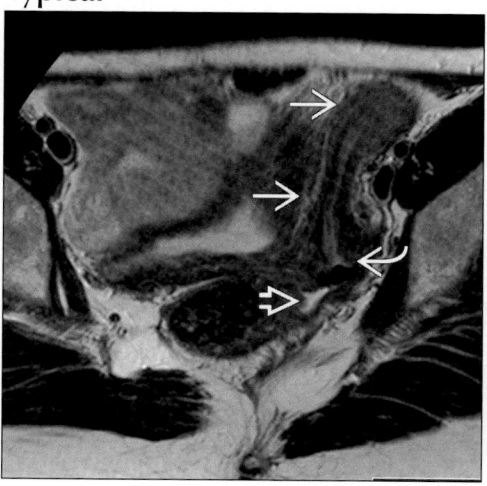

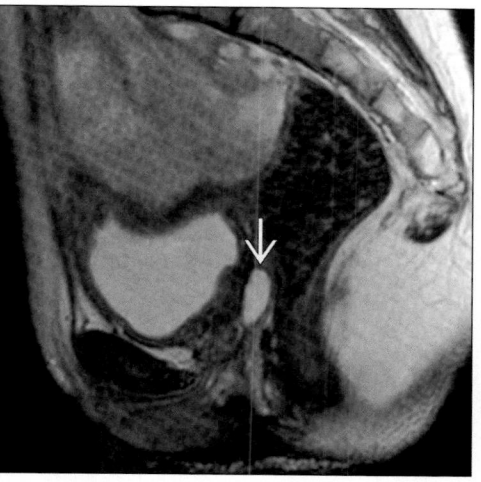

(Left) Axial T2WI MR shows an unicornuate uterus ➡ and fluid signal structure ➡ in the vagina adjacent to the cervix ➡. This is the typical location for a Gartner duct cyst. (Right) Sagittal T2WI MR in the same patient as the previous image confirms location of the cyst ➡ in the vaginal wall. Gartner duct cysts may be associated with Müllerian duct anomalies and renal anomalies.

SEX CORD-STROMAL TUMOR

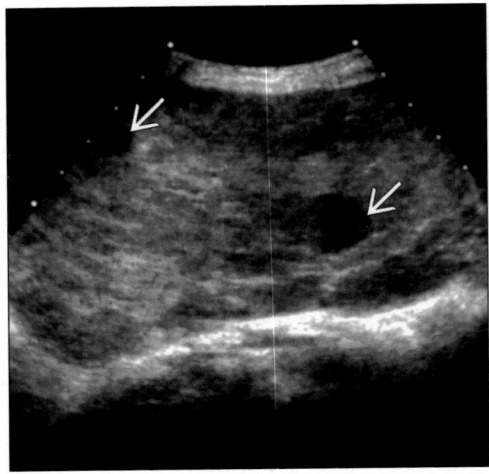

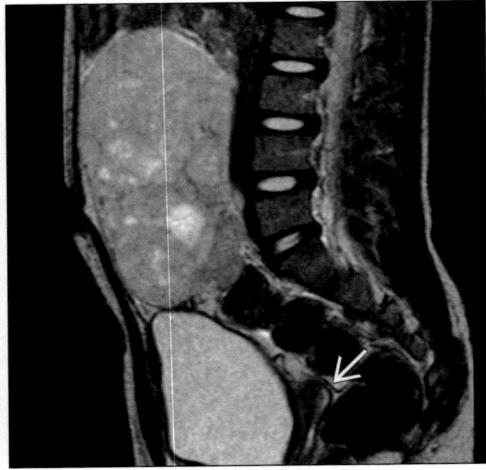

Ultrasound of a 6 yo girl with precocious puberty shows a predominately solid ovarian mass with scattered cysts ➡. With this history and appearance, juvenile granulosa cell tumor is the most likely diagnosis.

Sagittal T2WI shows the mass is intermediate-signal intensity with scattered high-signal areas giving it a "sponge-like" appearance. The mass is clearly separate from the uterus ➡. Histology confirmed the diagnosis.

TERMINOLOGY

Definitions
- Group of ovarian tumors arising from either embryonic sex cords or mesenchyme
  - Fibroma, thecoma, fibrothecoma
  - Granulosa cell tumor: Occurs in both adult and juvenile forms
  - Sertoli-Leydig tumor (androblastoma)
  - Sclerosing stromal tumor, steroid cell tumors, gynandroblastoma and sex cord tumor with annular tubules

IMAGING FINDINGS

General Features
- Sex cord-stromal tumors are generally solid or have significant solid components
- Hormonally active tumors may be small and difficult to find

Ultrasonographic Findings
- Ultrasound findings of sex cord-stromal tumors are diverse and non-specific
  - Range from small, solid tumors to large, multicystic masses
- **Granulosa cell tumors**
  - More often contain cysts, with "sponge-like" appearance
  - Cysts may be complex and contain hemorrhagic fluid
    - May rupture and cause hemoperitoneum
  - Adult and juvenile forms have similar appearance
  - Cysts will be thick-walled
  - Calcifications are rare
  - May be bilateral in 5%
- **Sertoli-Leydig tumors**
  - Significant overlap with granulosa cell tumors
  - Not as frequently cystic as granulosa cell tumors
  - Less likely to have hemorrhage
- **Fibrothecomas**
  - Hypoechoic with posterior acoustic attenuation
    - Similar to uterine leiomyoma
- **Steroid cell tumors**

DDx: Complex Ovarian Mass

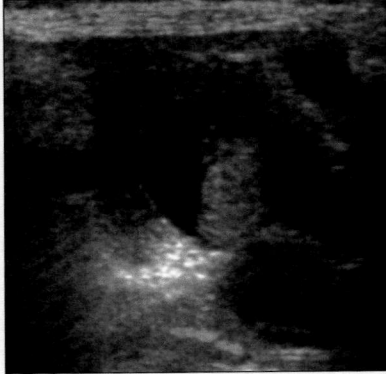

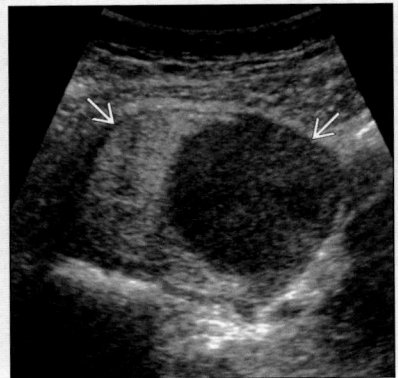

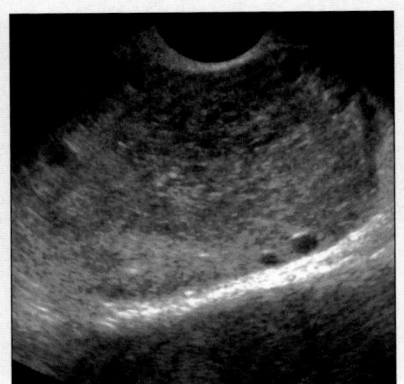

Cystadenocarcinoma

Dermoid

Ovarian Torsion

SEX CORD-STROMAL TUMOR

Key Facts

Terminology
- Group of ovarian tumors arising from either embryonic sex cords or mesenchyme

Imaging Findings
- Sex cord-stromal tumors are generally solid or have significant solid components
- Hormonally active tumors may be small and difficult to find
- **Granulosa cell tumors**
- More often contain cysts, with "sponge-like" appearance
- Cysts may be complex and contain hemorrhagic fluid
- Adult and juvenile forms have similar appearance
- **Sertoli-Leydig tumors**
- Not as frequently cystic as granulosa cell tumors
- Less likely to have hemorrhage

Top Differential Diagnoses
- Ovarian Carcinoma

Pathology
- Sex cord-stromal tumors represent 5-10% of ovarian neoplasms and 2% of ovarian malignancies
- ~ 50% are fibrothecomas
- 10-20% granulosa cell tumors
- 5% Sertoli-Leydig tumors
- Remainder include sclerosing stromal tumor, steroid cell tumors, gynandroblastoma and sex cord tumor with annular tubules

Clinical Issues
- Granulosa cell tumors and thecomas are estrogen producing tumors
- Sertoli-Leydig tumors are androgen producing

- Typically small, without cysts

MR Findings
- T1WI
  - May see high signal from hemorrhage in granulosa cell tumor
  - High lipid content may cause steroid tumors to be high signal
- T2WI
  - Most intermediate signal with cystic area being high signal
    - Granulosa cell tumors may have network of smaller cysts creating a "sponge-like" appearance
- T1 C+: Most enhance except fibrothecomas

Imaging Recommendations
- Protocol advice
  - Evaluate uterus carefully
    - Hormonal stimulation may cause uterine enlargement and endometrial thickening (hyperplasia, polyps or carcinoma)

DIFFERENTIAL DIAGNOSIS

Ovarian Carcinoma
- Most epithelial tumors have dominant cystic component
- Confusion may occur if there is a large solid component

Germ Cell Tumors
- Much more heterogeneous with calcifications, fluid-fluid levels, etc.

Ovarian Torsion
- Edematous, enlarged ovary with peripheral cysts
- Patient is acutely symptomatic

Hormonally Functioning Ovarian Masses
- Patients may present with symptoms related to hormone production rather than mass
- May present with either hyperandrogenism or hyperestrogenism (some may do both)

- **Hyperandrogenism** (virilization with hirsutism, male pattern baldness, loss of female body contour, clitoromegaly)
  - Sertoli-Leydig tumor
  - Sclerosing stromal tumor
  - Gonadoblastoma
  - Brenner tumor
  - Polycystic ovarian disease
  - Stromal hyperplasia
  - Stromal hyperthecosis
  - Hyperreactio luteinalis
  - Non-ovarian causes
    - Pituitary (Cushing disease)
    - Adrenal (Cushing syndrome)
- **Hyperestrogenism** (pseudoprecocious puberty, postmenopausal bleeding)
  - Granulosa cell tumor
  - Thecoma
  - Serous tumors
  - Mucinous tumors
  - Endometrioid tumors

PATHOLOGY

General Features
- Etiology
  - Derive from two embryologically distinct groups of cells
    - Stromal cells: Fibroblasts, theca cells and Leydig cells
    - Sex cords: Granulosa cells and Sertoli cells
  - Most tumors have more than one cell type
- Epidemiology
  - Sex cord-stromal tumors represent 5-10% of ovarian neoplasms and 2% of ovarian malignancies
  - Distribution of sex cord-stromal tumors
    - ~ 50% are fibrothecomas
    - 10-20% granulosa cell tumors
    - 5% Sertoli-Leydig tumors

SEX CORD-STROMAL TUMOR

- Remainder include sclerosing stromal tumor, steroid cell tumors, gynandroblastoma and sex cord tumor with annular tubules
  ○ Granulosa cell tumors occur in two distinct groups (juvenile and adult)
    ▪ 5% are juvenile granulosa cell tumor and present < 30 years
    ▪ Mean age for juvenile granulosa cell tumors is 13 years, with many presenting before puberty
    ▪ 95% are adult granulosa cell tumors and present in perimenopausal and postmenopausal women (mean age, 52 years)
  ○ Sertoli-Leydig tumor, mean age 25 years
- Associated abnormalities
  ○ **Adult granulosa cell tumor**
    ▪ Endometrial hyperplasia, polyps and carcinoma
  ○ **Juvenile granulosa cell tumor**
    ▪ Pseudoprecocious puberty
    ▪ Ollier disease (multiple enchondromas)
    ▪ Maffucci syndrome (multiple enchondromas and hemangiomas)
  ○ **Sertoli-Leydig** most common virilizing tumor
    ▪ Amenorrhea, hirsutism, deepening voice, male pattern baldness
  ○ **Sex cord tumor with annular tubules**
    ▪ Peutz-Jeghers syndrome (autosomal dominant disorder with multiple gastrointestinal hamartomas and mucocutaneous pigmentation); ovarian tumors often bilateral

Microscopic Features
- Granulosa cell tumors are composed of granulosa cells growing in numerous patterns
  ○ Frequently accompanied by theca cells and fibroblasts
- Sertoli-Leydig cell tumors are composed of Sertoli cells, Leydig cells and fibroblasts
  ○ May have tumors from a single cell line
- Steroid cell tumors contain lutein cells, Leydig cells and adrenocortical cells

CLINICAL ISSUES

Presentation
- Smaller masses may be incidental findings
- Pelvic pain/discomfort from larger masses
- Symptoms related to hormone production
- Granulosa cell tumors and thecomas are estrogen producing tumors
  ○ Clinical effects depend on patient age
  ○ Pseudoprecocious puberty in pediatric population
    ▪ Not true precocious puberty because no ovulation or progesterone production
    ▪ Present in 80% of juvenile granulosa cell tumors
    ▪ Juvenile granulosa cell tumors account for 10% of precocious puberty cases
  ○ Uterine bleeding in postmenopausal patient
    ▪ Endometrial stimulation with hyperplasia or carcinoma
    ▪ 30-50% have hyperplasia
    ▪ 3-25% have endometrial carcinoma

○ Women in reproductive age group may have irregular, heavy periods
- Sertoli-Leydig tumors are androgen producing
  ○ Symptoms in 30% of patients

Natural History & Prognosis
- Many are low grade malignancies and surgery is curative
- Juvenile granulosa cell tumors have excellent prognosis
  ○ Most are stage 1
- Adult granulosa cell tumors may act in more aggressive fashion with late recurrences (potentially decades) not uncommon
  ○ > 90% are stage 1
  ○ 90-95% 5 year survival for stage 1
  ○ 25-50% 5 year survival for advanced disease
  ○ Mean survival after recurrence is 5 years
- 80-90% of Sertoli-Leydig cell tumors are stage 1 and are cured with resection
  ○ 10-20% behave in more malignant fashion
  ○ Most recurrences are in first 5 years
- Fibrothecomas are benign

DIAGNOSTIC CHECKLIST

Consider
- Key features differentiating sex cord-stromal tumors from more common epithelial neoplasms
  ○ More likely to present with symptoms from hormone production
  ○ Most are stage 1 with good prognosis
  ○ Affect all age groups, including pediatrics
  ○ More often solid
  ○ Cystic masses less likely to have papillary projections

Image Interpretation Pearls
- Multicystic lesion with hemorrhage in a patient under 30, strongly suggests juvenile granulosa cell tumor
- Granulosa tumors are most common hormonally active tumor and produce estrogen
  ○ Thecomas second most common estrogen producing ovarian tumor
- Sertoli-Leydig cell tumor most common virilizing ovarian tumor

SELECTED REFERENCES
1. Tanaka YO et al: Functioning ovarian tumors: direct and indirect findings at MR imaging. Radiographics. 24 Suppl 1:S147-66, 2004
2. Kim SH et al: Granulosa cell tumor of the ovary: common findings and unusual appearances on CT and MR. J Comput Assist Tomogr. 26(5):756-61, 2002
3. Outwater EK et al: Virilizing tumors of the ovary: imaging features. Ultrasound Obstet Gynecol. 15(5):365-71, 2000
4. Outwater EK et al: Sex cord-stromal and steroid cell tumors of the ovary. Radiographics. 18(6):1523-46, 1998
5. Malmstrom H et al: Granulosa cell tumors of the ovary: prognostic factors and outcome. Gynecol Oncol. 52(1):50-5, 1994

SEX CORD-STROMAL TUMOR

IMAGE GALLERY

Typical

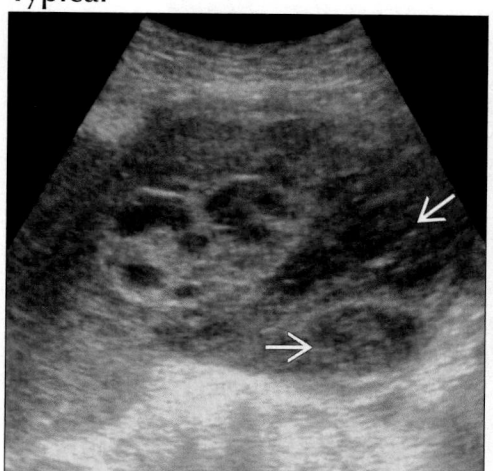

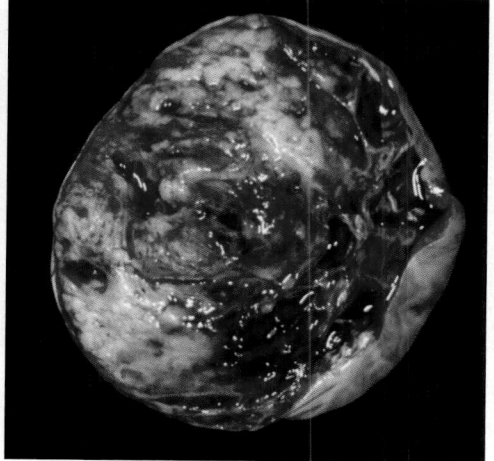

(Left) Transverse ultrasound of an adult granulosa cell tumor shows multiple, complex cysts. Some of these cysts are filled with low level echoes ➡, which proved to be hemorrhage at pathology. *(Right)* Gross pathology shows multiple areas of hemorrhage, corresponding with the ultrasound. Granulosa cell tumors will frequently have hemorrhage.

Typical

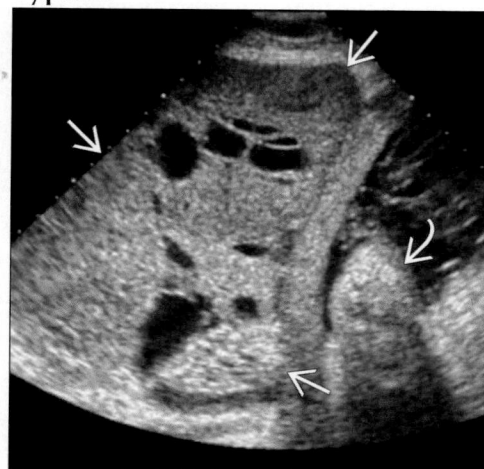

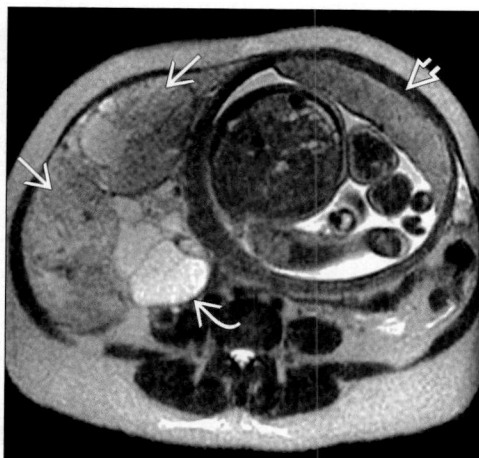

(Left) A third trimester ultrasound shows a predominately solid adnexal mass ➡, with scattered cysts. Fetal leg ➡. *(Right)* T2WI MR shows areas of both intermediate signal ➡ (solid components) and high signal ➡ (cystic components). The gravid uterus ➡ is being displaced laterally. Histology showed an adult granulosa cell tumor.

Typical

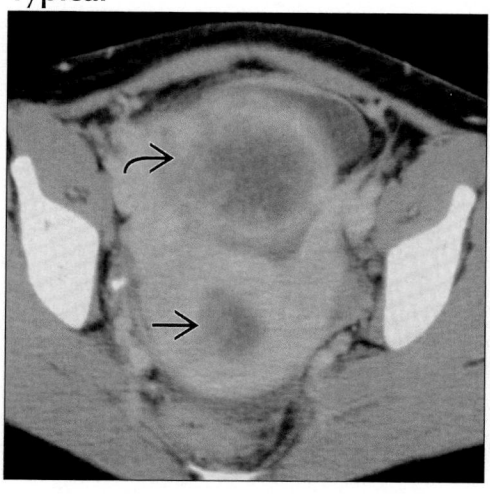

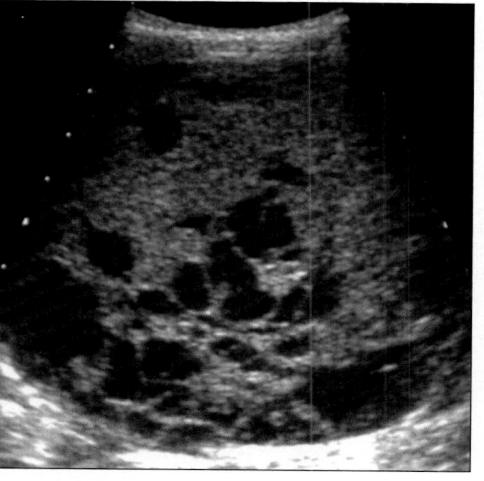

(Left) CECT of an adult granulosa cell tumor shows not only the ovarian mass ➡ but also an irregular, thickened endometrium ➡. Endometrial biopsy was positive for endometrial carcinoma, a common association. *(Right)* Ultrasound of a Sertoli-Leydig cell tumor shows a predominately solid mass, with scattered cysts. The appearance is non-specific and a history of virilization would be necessary to make the diagnosis pre-operatively.

OVARIAN FIBROTHECOMA

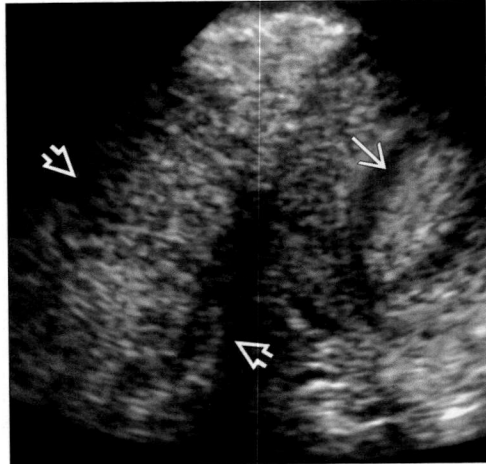

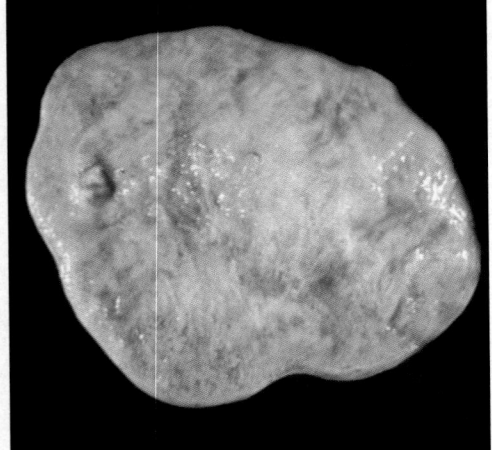

Longitudinal ultrasound shows a solid adnexal mass ➡, very similar in appearance to a pedunculated uterine fibroid. Note thickened endometrium ➡. Biopsy showed endometrial hyperplasia.

Gross pathology confirmed fibrothecoma. The cut surface has a fibrous appearance similar to leiomyoma. These tumors are often estrogen producing & may cause endometrial hyperplasia or carcinoma.

TERMINOLOGY

Abbreviations and Synonyms
- Benign sex cord-stromal tumor
- Fibrotic lesion of the ovary

Definitions
- Thecoma: Tumor of lipid-containing thecal cells
- Fibroma: Mesenchymal tumor consisting of stromal cells
- Fibrothecoma: Composite tumor containing both elements
  - More common than either fibroma or thecoma in pure form

IMAGING FINDINGS

General Features
- Best diagnostic clue: Solid hypoechoic mass with posterior acoustic shadowing
- Location
  - Typically unilateral
  - Rare reports of bilateral tumors
    - Most common association of bilateral tumors is Gorlin syndrome
- Size
  - Variable, but usually large
  - 13 cm mean

Ultrasonographic Findings
- Grayscale Ultrasound
  - Most common presentation is solid, hypoechoic mass
    - Appearance mimics uterine leiomyoma
  - Marked attenuation of ultrasound beam with posterior acoustic attenuation
  - Variations in appearance common
  - May be hyperechoic (more common with thecomas)
  - Occasional calcifications
    - Usually punctate and diffuse but may be more localized
  - Hemorrhage, edema, cystic areas, more common in larger lesions
    - Seen with degeneration (consider infarction or torsion if acutely symptomatic)
  - Intraperitoneal fluid associated with larger lesions
  - Ascites & pleural effusion with Meigs syndrome

DDx: Solid Pelvic Masses

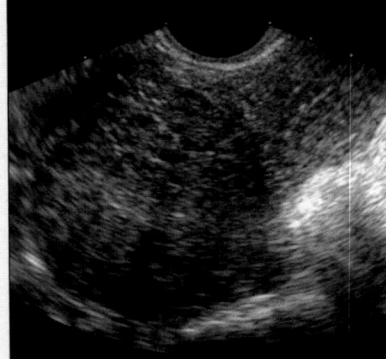

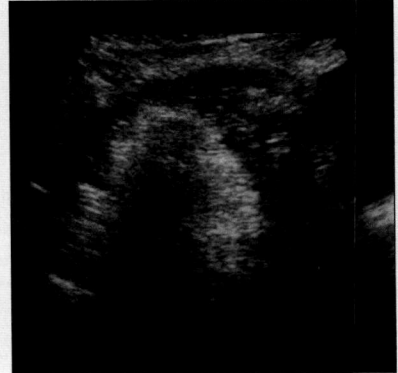

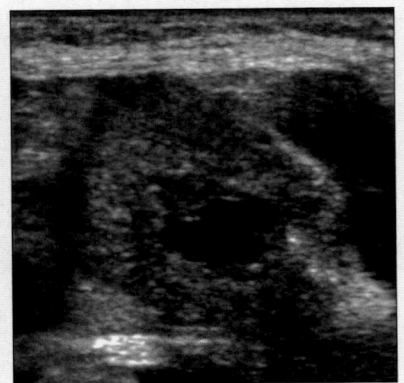

Fibroid

Dermoid

Cystadenocarcinoma

ENDOMETRIOMAS

Key Facts

Imaging Findings
- Best diagnostic clue: Adnexal cyst with diffuse low-level echoes
- Ovarian in 75%, bilateral 50%
- Varies from unilocular cyst to multilocular mass
- Adhesions distort normal pelvic anatomy
- Endometriomas light up with T1 FS
- T2 "shading" is distinguishing feature
- Diffuse low-level internal echoes in 95%
- Tiny bright foci in cyst wall is specific finding (35%)
- Blood of different ages will layer
- Calcifications are rare
- Ultrasound is first imaging tool
- MR has greater specificity
- True nodules and thick septations raise suspicion for malignancy

Top Differential Diagnoses
- Hemorrhagic Cyst
- Dermoid Cyst (Teratoma)
- Cystic Neoplasm

Clinical Issues
- Infertility
- Cyclical or chronic pain
- Palpable mass
- Incidentally noted mass on ultrasound

Diagnostic Checklist
- Endometrioma if unilocular adnexal cyst with diffuse low-level echoes
- Endometriosis can mimic dermoid and neoplasm
- Multiple lesions are common

- Fluid-fluid level in cyst
  - Blood of different ages will layer
    - Echogenic blood is dependent
    - Hypoechoic blood is supernatant
  - Mimics dermoid but echogenicities are flipped
    - Fat-fluid layer
    - Echogenic fat is supernatant
    - Dependent is hypoechoic
- Calcifications are rare
  - Common in dermoids
- Endometrioma may be multilocular
  - Multiple separate cysts
  - Thin or thick septations between loculi
  - Mimics neoplasia
  - Look for other typical endometriomas
- Non-ovarian endometrioma
  - Same appearance as ovarian
    - Unilocular cyst with diffuse low-level echoes
  - Cesarian section endometrioma
    - Between uterus and bladder
    - Subcutaneous at scar
  - Surface of uterus
  - Peritoneal surface of cul de sac
  - Bowel serosa
  - Bladder serosa
  - Ureter
    - Can cause hydronephrosis

MR Findings
- T1WI
  - Homogeneous high signal
    - Similar to or greater than fat
  - Multiple cysts common
- T1WI FS
  - Endometriomas light up with T1 FS
  - Dermoid would lose signal
- T2WI
  - T2 "shading" is distinguishing feature
    - Loss of signal within lesion on T2
    - Variable amounts of shading seen
  - Secondary signs of adhesion
    - Distortion of pelvic anatomy

Imaging Recommendations
- Best imaging tool
  - Ultrasound is first imaging tool
    - Classic appearance is diagnostic
  - MR has greater specificity
- Protocol advice
  - Endometrioma may look anechoic transabdominally
    - Need transvaginal ultrasound and ↑ gain settings to see internal echoes
  - Look carefully at cyst wall for echogenic foci with comet-tail artifact
    - Cholesterol in cyst wall
    - Do not confuse for nodules
  - True nodules and thick septations raise suspicion for malignancy

---

DIFFERENTIAL DIAGNOSIS

Hemorrhagic Cyst
- Functional ovarian cyst
  - Resolves in 4-6 weeks
- Acute hemorrhage can mimic endometrioma
  - Diffuse low/medium-level echoes
- Evolution of hemorrhage into complex cyst
  - Fibrin strands
    - Thinner than septations
  - Clot retraction
    - Surrounding seroma
- Complete resolution rules out endometrioma
- More likely to present with acute pain

Dermoid Cyst (Teratoma)
- Common benign mass
  - Endoderm, ectoderm, mesoderm components
- Unique identifiers
  - Calcification
    - Focal echogenicity with shadowing
  - Hyperechoic areas from solid fat
  - Fat-fluid level
    - Echogenic fluid on top of hypoechoic fluid
- Blood flow in mass rules out endometrioma

ENDOMETRIOMAS

- 20-30% bilateral
- Symptomatic if rupture or torsion

Cystic Neoplasm

- Multilocular mass
- Thick septations
- Wall nodularity
- Blood flow in septations and nodules
- Associated ascites
- More likely to be unilateral mass

PATHOLOGY

General Features

- Etiology
  o Retrograde menstruation (RM)
    ▪ Metastatic implantation
    ▪ 2° hematogenous or lymphatic spread
  o Metaplasia of coelomic epithelium
    ▪ Peritoneal cells become endometrial cells
  o Induction theory
    ▪ Combination of above two theories
    ▪ RM induces metaplasia
  o Abnormal immunity
    ▪ RM occurs in majority of women but implantation of functioning endometrium is rare
    ▪ ↓ Immunity results in implantation
- Epidemiology
  o Overall prevalence 5-10%
    ▪ 4% of all tubal ligation cases
    ▪ 20% of infertility cases
    ▪ 25% of chronic pelvic pain cases
- Associated abnormalities
  o Adhesions
  o Bowel, ureter, bladder involvement
  o Endometriosis can spread outside of pelvis

Gross Pathologic & Surgical Features

- Chocolate cyst
  o Dark brown viscous blood
- Endometriotic implant appearance variable
  o Immature foci are pale yellow or pink
  o Mature foci are dark brown

Microscopic Features

- Endometrial glands and stroma

CLINICAL ISSUES

Presentation

- Most common signs/symptoms
  o Infertility
  o Cyclical or chronic pain
  o Palpable mass
  o Incidentally noted mass on ultrasound
- Other signs/symptoms
  o Unusual symptoms for atypical locations
    ▪ Gastrointestinal bleeding
    ▪ Ureteral obstruction
    ▪ Pneumothorax
    ▪ Seizure

Demographics

- Age
  o Women of childbearing age
  o Mean age at diagnosis is 25-29 y

Natural History & Prognosis

- Burns out with menopause
  o May remerge with estrogen replacement therapy

Treatment

- Medical treatment
  o Hormonal manipulation of menstrual cycle
- Conservative surgery
  o Reproductive function retained
  o 30-40% recurrence rates
- Definitive surgery
  o Hysterectomy and oophorectomy
  o May recur with exogenous estrogen
- Infertility from endometriosis
  o Conservative surgery
  o Assisted reproductive techniques
  o Monthly fecundity rates of 9-18%

DIAGNOSTIC CHECKLIST

Consider

- Endometrioma if unilocular adnexal cyst with diffuse low-level echoes

Image Interpretation Pearls

- Endometriosis can mimic dermoid and neoplasm
- Multiple lesions are common
- MR findings more specific than ultrasound
  o T2 shading is important finding

SELECTED REFERENCES

1. Alborzi S et al: Management of ovarian endometrioma. Clin Obstet Gynecol. 49(3):480-91, 2006
2. Bhatt S et al: Endometriosis: Sonographic Spectrum. Ultrasound Q. 22(4):273-280, 2006
3. Jain KA: Endometrioma with calcification simulating a dermoid on sonography. J Ultrasound Med. 25(9):1237-41, 2006
4. Valentin L: Imaging in gynecology. Best Pract Res Clin Obstet Gynaecol. 20(6):881-906, 2006
5. Giudice LC et al: Endometriosis. Lancet. 364(9447):1789-99, 2004
6. Hart R: Unexplained infertility, endometriosis, and fibroids. BMJ. 327(7417):721-4, 2003
7. Thurmond AS: Imaging of female infertility. Radiol Clin North Am. 41(4):757-67, vi, 2003
8. Woodward PJ et al: Endometriosis: radiologic-pathologic correlation. Radiographics. 21(1):193-216; questionnaire 288-94, 2001
9. Jain S et al: Chocolate cysts from ovarian follicles. Fertil Steril. 72(5):852-6, 1999

ENDOMETRIOMAS

Typical

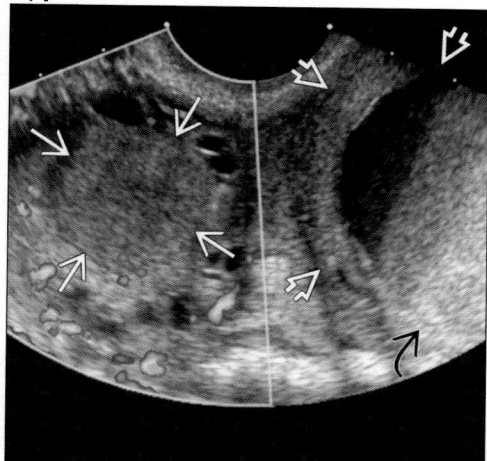

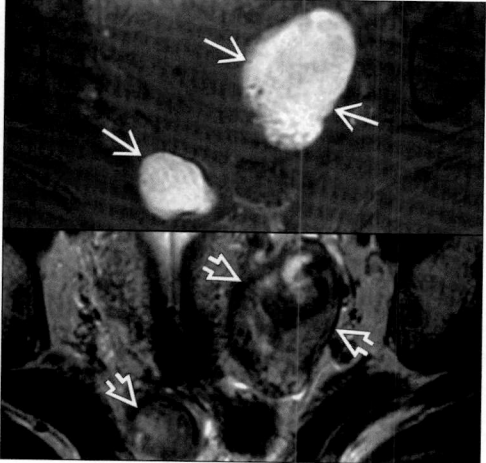

(Left) Transverse transvaginal ultrasound shows a small endometrioma on the right ➡ and layering blood in a large left-sided cyst ➡. Unlike in dermoids, echogenic fluid is dependent ➡. *(Right)* T1WI MR with fat suppression shows bilateral bright signal endometriomas ➡, which drop signal on the T2WI ➡. Amount of T2 shading is variable but specific for endometrioma.

Typical

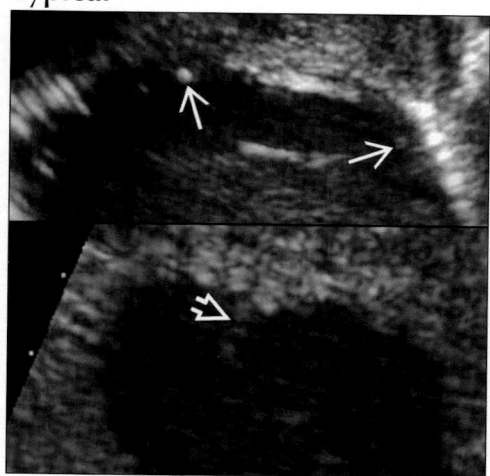

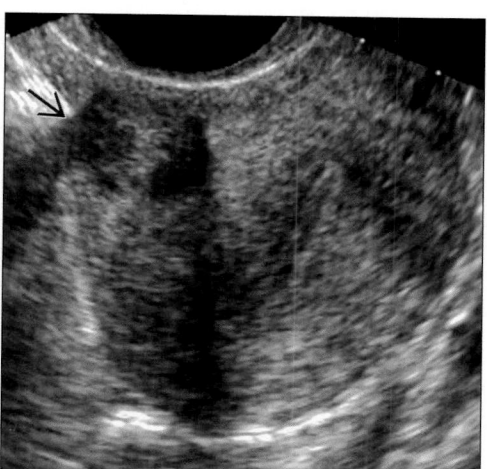

(Left) Transverse ultrasound shows tiny echogenic foci in the wall of an endometrioma ➡. These arise from cholesterol deposits and may produce the comet tail artifact ➡. *(Right)* Longitudinal transvaginal ultrasound shows an endometrioma ➡ arising from the anterior uterine serosa. Multiple other endometriomas, including ovarian, were also present in this patient.

Variant

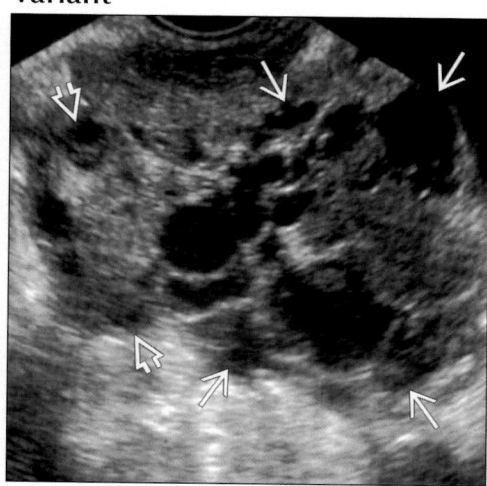

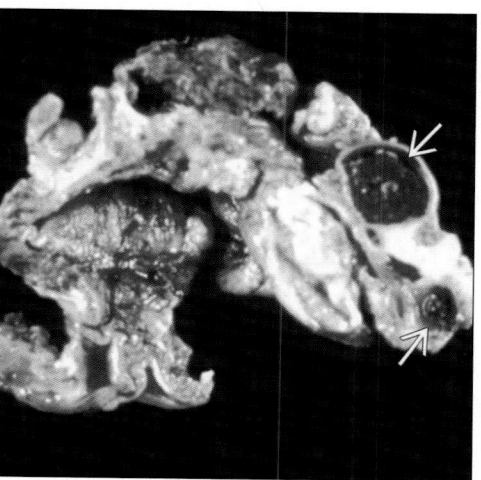

(Left) Transverse transvaginal ultrasound shows a multilocular complex cystic mass ➡ adjacent to the right ovary ➡. *(Right)* Gross pathology of the same mass shows extensive fibrosis and cysts filled with hemorrhage ➡. At surgery, the mass was adherent to the right ovary. Adhesions are common with endometriosis and distort pelvic anatomy.

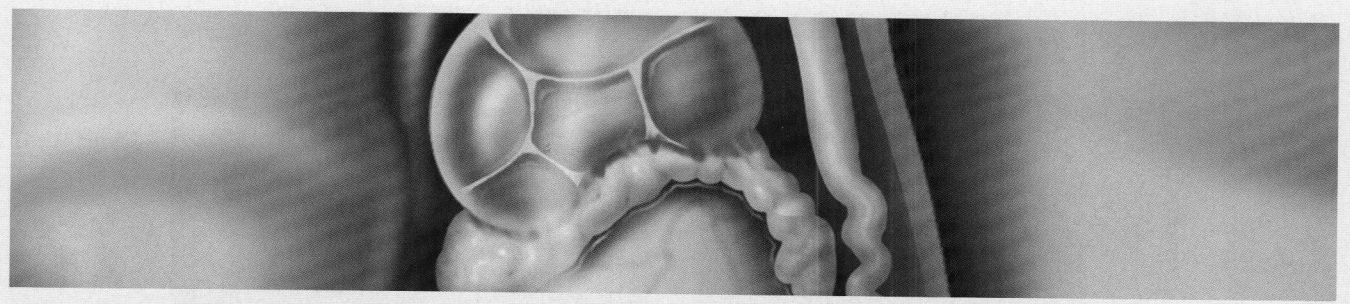

SECTION 10: Scrotum

SCROTAL SONOGRAPHY

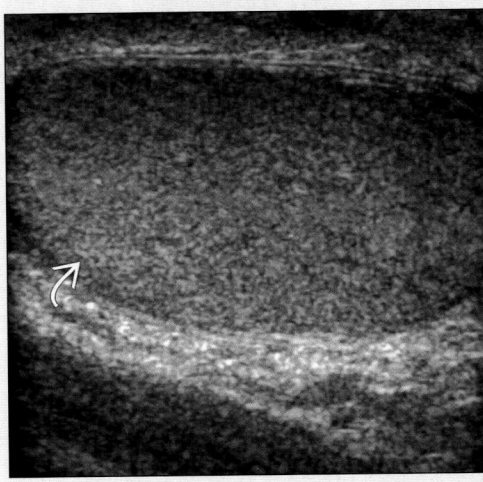

Longitudinal high frequency ultrasound shows a normal shaped testis ➔ with a homogeneous, fine, bright parenchymal echo pattern.

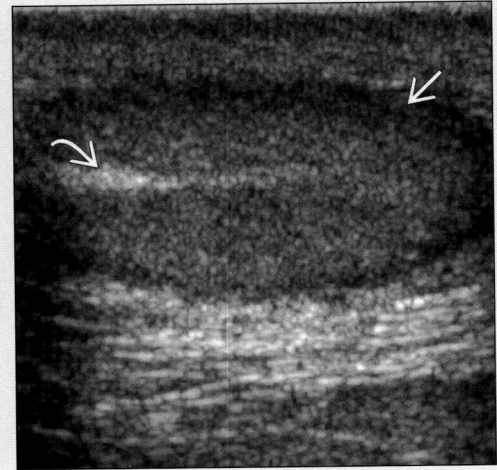

Longitudinal grayscale US shows a normal testis ➔ in young man. Note the normal mediastinum testis seen as an echogenic band ➔ partially bisecting the long axis of the testis.

IMAGING ANATOMY

General Anatomic Considerations

- Ultrasonography (US) must be performed with a high-frequency transducer
- Knowledge of normal scrotal sonographic anatomy is a prerequisite to imaging acute and non-acute diseases of the scrotum
- Scrotum is separated by a midline septum
  - Each half of the scrotum contains testis and associated structures
  - Scrotal wall is composed of six layers, from superficial to deep
    - Rugose skin, superficial fascia, Dartos muscle, external spermatic fascia, cremasteric fascia, and internal spermatic fascia
- Tunica vaginalis consists of visceral and parietal layers normally separated by few milliliters of fluid
  - Layer lining scrotal wall is termed parietal layer, and layer lining testis and epididymis is termed as visceral layer
  - Tunica vaginalis covers testis and epididymis except for small posterior area; bare area
    - Visceral layer covers the tunica albuginea
  - Posterior surface of tunica albuginea projects into interior of testis as incomplete septum, the mediastinum testes
- Spermatic cord consists of vas deferens, three arteries (testicular, cremasteric, deferential), pampiniform plexus and lymphatics
  - Spermatic cord is seen on ultrasound as tubular echogenic structure in subcutaneous tissue of inguinal canal
- Epididymis is best evaluated in longitudinal view when epididymal head (globus major) can be seen as a pyramidal structure 5–12 mm in maximum length lying atop superior pole of testis
  - Narrow body of epididymis (2–4 mm in diameter), is usually indistinguishable from surrounding peri-testicular tissue

- Tail of epididymis (globus minor) is approximately 2–5 mm in diameter and seen as curved structure at inferior pole of testis
- Prepubertal testes are of low to medium echogenicity, whereas pubertal and post-pubertal are of medium homogeneous echogenicity
- Mediastinum testis is seen as an echogenic band of variable thickness and length extending in caudocranial direction
  - Rete testis
    - Seen as a hypoechoic area with a striated configuration adjacent to mediastinum testis
    - Can be identified with high-frequency US in 18% of patients
  - Septula testis
    - Multiple thin septations (septula) arising from the inner aspect of tunica albuginea
    - On US these are seen as linear echogenic or hypoechoic structures in areas away from the mediastinum testis
    - Converge to form rete testis

Critical Anatomic Structures

- Primary vascular supply to testis is through right and left testicular arteries which are branches of abdominal aorta, arising just distal to renal arteries
- Venous drainage is through pampiniform plexus of draining veins
  - Pampiniform plexus is formed around upper half of epididymis in a variable fashion, continuing as testicular vein through deep inguinal ring
  - Right testicular vein empties into inferior vena cava, and left testicular vein empties into left renal vein
- Testicular perfusion can be evaluated with color Doppler, power Doppler, and spectral Doppler US
  - Color Doppler US reliably demonstrates intratesticular arterial and venous flow
  - Power Doppler is valuable in scrotal US because of increased sensitivity to low-flow states and independence of Doppler angle correction
  - Pulsed Doppler US is useful for identifying flow in the testes with use of the time-velocity spectrum to quantify blood flow

SCROTAL SONOGRAPHY

Key Facts

- Ultrasonography (US) must be performed with a high-frequency transducer
  - Knowledge of normal scrotal sonographic anatomy is a prerequisite to imaging acute and non-acute diseases of the scrotum
- Testes and epididymis are examined in at least two planes along longitudinal and transverse axes
  - Size and echogenicity in longitudinal and transverse axes of both testis and epididymis should be routinely compared with contralateral side
  - Prepubertal testes are of low to medium echogenicity, whereas pubertal and post-pubertal are of medium homogeneous echogenicity
- Epididymis is best evaluated in a longitudinal view when epididymal head (globus major) can be seen as pyramidal structure 5-12 mm in maximum length, lying atop superior pole of testis
- Testicular perfusion can be evaluated with color Doppler, power Doppler, and spectral Doppler US
  - Power Doppler is valuable in scrotal US because of increased sensitivity to low-flow states and independence of Doppler angle correction
- High-frequency US in its present state helps to identify certain benign intratesticular lesions, resulting in testis-sparing surgery
  - Familiarity with US characteristics and examination pitfalls of scrotal US is essential for establishing the correct diagnosis and initiating treatment

- Spectral waveform of intratesticular arteries characteristically has low-resistance pattern, with mean resistive index of 0.62 (range: 0.48-0.75)
- Head of epididymis is usually isoechoic to testis, though may have a more coarse echotexture than that of testis
  - Resistive index of normal epididymis ranges from 0.46-0.68
    - Color Doppler US can demonstrate blood flow in a normal epididymis

Anatomic Relationships

- Appendix testis seen as ovoid structure 5 mm in length in groove between testis and epididymis
- Appendix epididymis is of same approximate dimensions as appendix testis but is more often pedunculated
- Normal appendix testis and the appendix epididymis are typically seen only when a hydrocele is present

ANATOMY-BASED IMAGING ISSUES

Imaging Approaches

- Examination is performed most often with transducer in direct contact with skin, but if necessary a stand-off pad can be used for evaluation of superficial structures and lesions
- Scrotal US is performed with patient in supine position & scrotum supported by towel placed between thighs

Imaging Protocols

- Testis and epididymis are examined in at least two planes, along longitudinal and transverse axes
- Size and echogenicity in longitudinal and transverse axes of both testes and epididymi should be routinely compared on contralateral side

Imaging Pitfalls

- Base of penis may be mistaken for contralateral testis while examining from opposite side

Normal Measurements

- Normal scrotal wall thickness is approximately 2-8 mm, depending on state of contraction of cremasteric muscle
- Testicular size depends on age and stage of sexual development
  - At birth, testis measures approximately 1.5 cm in length and 1 cm in width
  - Before age of age 12 years, testicular volume is about 1-2 cm³
  - Testes are symmetric, ovoid structures and measure approximately 5 x 3 x 2 cm in post-puberty

PATHOLOGIC ISSUES

Classification

- Scrotal wall abnormalities
  - Noninflammatory causes: Heart failure, lymphedema, hypoalbuminemia
  - Inflammatory causes: Cellulitis, Fournier gangrene
  - Scrotal wall malignant lesions: Metastases from melanoma, lung and anal carcinoma
- Inguinal and scrotal swelling: Inguinal hernia, hydrocele, pyocele
- Abnormalities of spermatic cord: Varicocele, encysted hydrocele of cord
  - Tumors: Rhabdomyomas and sarcoma
- Epididymis
  - Epididymo-orchitis: Acute/chronic
  - Epididymal masses: Epididymal cyst, spermatocele and sperm granuloma, tumors; adenomatoid tumors, papillary cystadenoma and rare tumors
- Testicular abnormalities
  - Testicular torsion: Extra/intravaginal torsion of spermatic cord leading to vascular occlusion
  - Orchitis: Primary and secondary
  - Benign testicular mass: Intratesticular cysts, epidermoid cyst, intratesticular varicocele
  - Malignant testicular tumors: Germ cell tumors: Seminomatous/non seminomatous

SCROTAL SONOGRAPHY

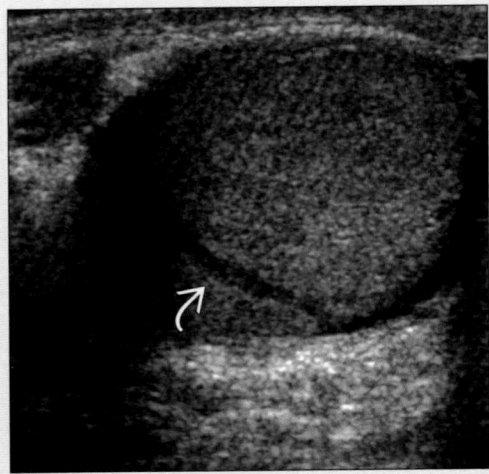

Oblique grayscale ultrasound shows a hypoechoic band created by the transmediastinal artery ➤ running across testicular parenchyma.

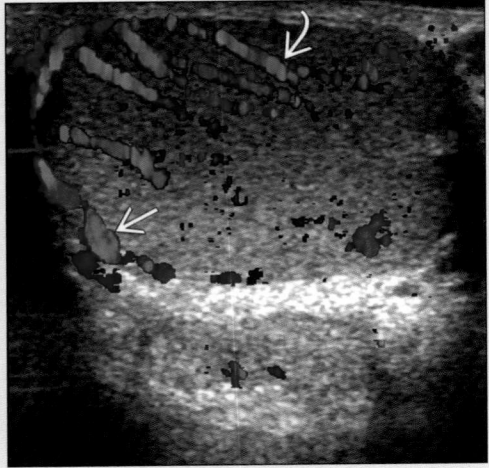

Oblique color Doppler ultrasound shows normal capsular and intratesticular veins ➤ and arteries ➤.

- Non-germ cell tumors: Lymphoma, leukemia, metastases, sex cord-stromal tumors: Sertoli cell and Leydig cell tumor
  - ○ Testicular trauma: Testicular hematoma, hematocele, fracture and rupture of testis

PATHOLOGY-BASED IMAGING ISSUES

Key Concepts or Questions
- Is there an abnormality present?
  - ○ Familiarization with normal ultrasound appearances of scrotum
- Where is the abnormality located?
  - ○ Is it located in testis, in epididymis, in both or none of these structures
  - ○ Does it involve one or both sides of scrotum
- Is it predominantly solid or cystic?
- Is there a malignant tumor present?
  - ○ Vast majority of intrascrotal malignant masses are intratesticular
  - ○ Most testicular masses are malignant and some may have cystic component
  - ○ Familiarization with ultrasound appearances of malignant masses is essential

Imaging Approaches
- High frequency ultrasound helps to reliably identify most intrascrotal pathologies
  - ○ Follow-up ultrasound will usually enable the correct diagnosis to be reached in less common conditions
  - ○ Additional imaging is not routinely needed
- High-frequency US in its present state helps to identify certain benign intratesticular lesions, resulting in testes-sparing surgery

Imaging Pitfalls
- In cases of large hydroceles, both testes should be scanned in at least one single plane, to rule out absent or undescended testis

- In large hydroceles, involved testis can be seen from many scan planes and may be misinterpreted as contralateral testis in cases of absent testis/cryptorchism
  - ○ Similarly, masses in contralateral testis may be overlooked
- Some cystic scrotal masses (e.g., spermatocele) may appear solid
  - ○ Acoustic enhancement is clue to their cystic nature

EMBRYOLOGY

Embryologic Events
- Cryptorchism is defined as complete or partial failure of intra-abdominal testes to descend in scrotum
  - ○ Most common location is in inguinal canal (72%), followed by high scrotal (20%) and abdominal (8%)
- Congenital hydroceles result from a patent processus vaginalis which allows peritoneal fluid to accumulate in scrotal sac
- Testicular microlithiasis is generally bilateral
- Anorchia, a rare condition, presents with absent testis and developed scrotum; testis cannot be located even after detailed investigation

Practical Implications
- Major complications of cryptorchism are malignant degeneration, infertility and torsion
  - ○ Bowel incarceration due to associated indirect inguinal hernia
- Testicular microlithiasis has been associated with testicular neoplasia in 18–75% of cases

CLINICAL IMPLICATIONS

Clinical Importance
- Ultrasound is of vital importance in investigating and follow-up of scrotal disorders
  - ○ Its high sensitivity and specificity allows a correct diagnosis to be made in most conditions

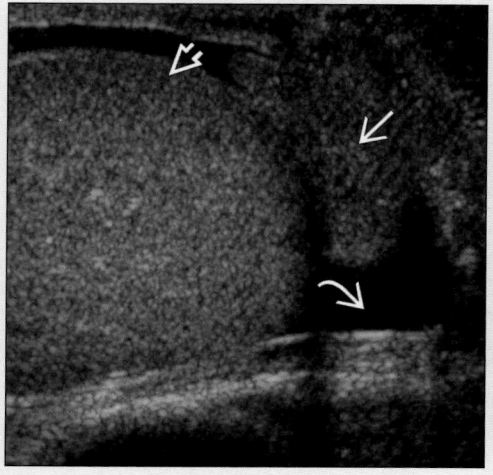

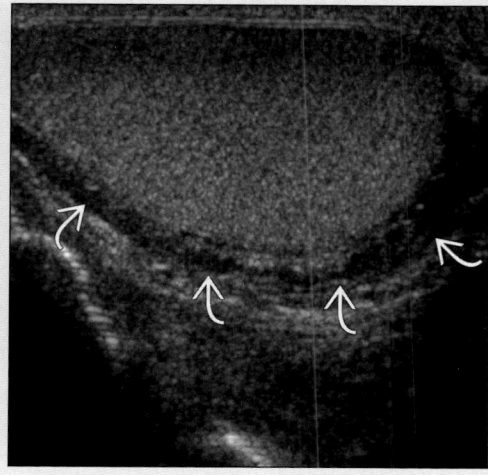

(Left) Oblique grayscale ultrasound shows the hypoechoic head of epididymis ➡ overlying the superior pole of testis ➡. Note minimal fluid in tunica vaginalis ➡. *(Right)* Longitudinal grayscale ultrasound of the scrotum in a young man shows a hypoechoic body and tail of epididymis ➡ coursing along the posterolateral aspect of testis.

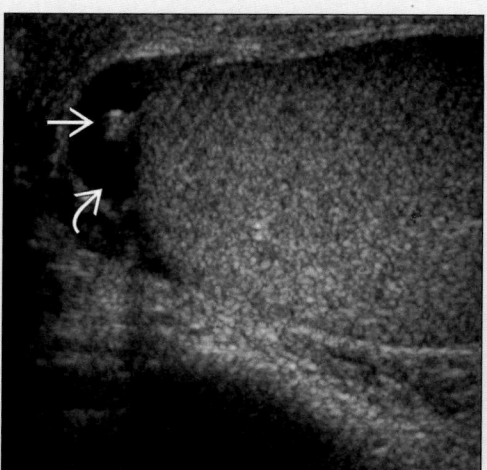

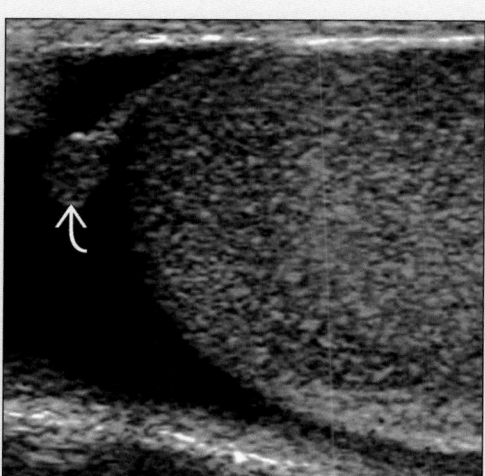

(Left) Longitudinal grayscale ultrasound of a normal scrotum in a young man shows a small sessile hypoechoic appendix testis ➡. Presence of a hydrocele ➡ allows visualization of testicular appendages. *(Right)* Longitudinal grayscale ultrasound of the scrotum in a young man shows a small pedunculated hypoechoic appendix epididymis ➡.

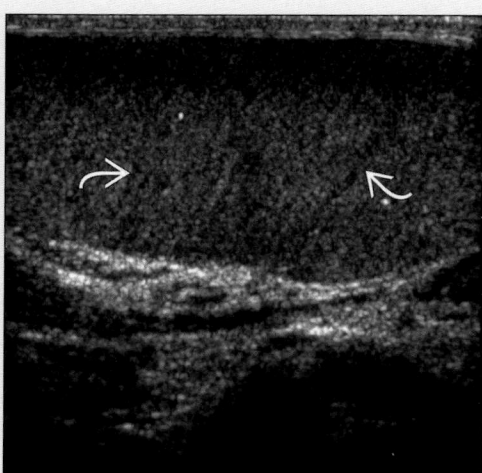

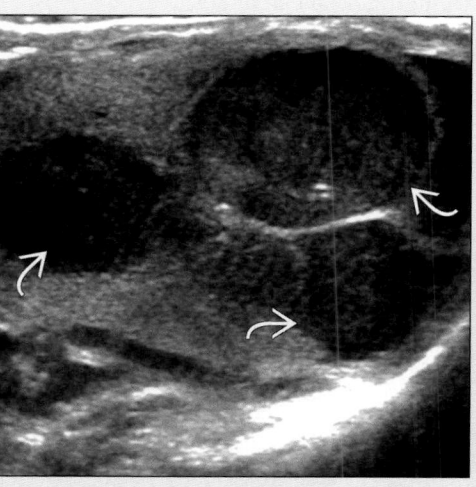

(Left) Longitudinal grayscale ultrasound shows the striated appearance ➡ of the septula testis. *(Right)* Transverse grayscale ultrasound shows multiple, large, well-defined hypoechoic masses ➡ in the testicular substance. Features indicate testicular metastasis.

TESTICULAR ATROPHY

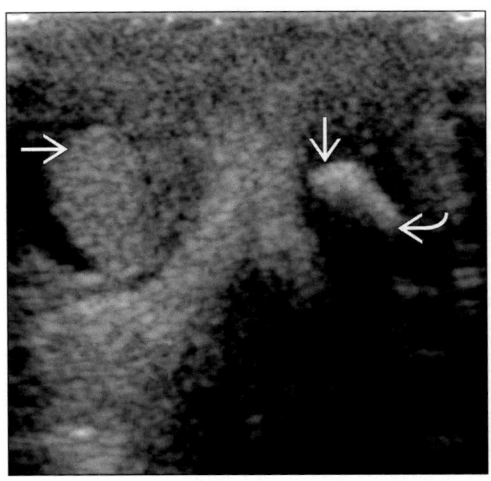

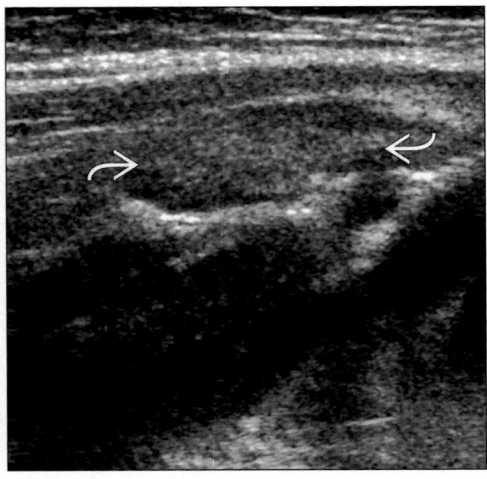

Transverse grayscale ultrasound of the scrotal sac in a young boy shows bilateral, small, shrunken echogenic testes ➡. Note calcified testis ➡ on left side.

Oblique grayscale ultrasound at inguinal region shows a heterogeneous, small, atrophic cryptorchid testis ➡.

TERMINOLOGY

Abbreviations and Synonyms
- "Vanishing testis syndrome", "testicular regression syndrome"

Definitions
- Testicular atrophy is defined as a difference in size and consistency of testes between affected and healthy sides

IMAGING FINDINGS

General Features
- Best diagnostic clue: Testicular atrophy - palpably shrunken, small sized (objective measurements using US), coupled with altered echo pattern
- Location: Intrascrotal in location, inguinal canal, 50% of testis located in abdomen undergo atrophy
- Size: Testicular atrophy is considered to be present if the combined axis measurements of the two sides differ by 10 mm or more, or testicular size less than 4.0 x 2.0 cm

- Morphology: Reduction in size is arbitrarily considered significant only if the volume of affected testis is reduced to 50% of the unaffected side

Ultrasonographic Findings
- Grayscale Ultrasound
  - Shrunken testis displaying increased echogenicity due to fibrosis
    - Foci of calcification may be seen as punctate echoes with posterior acoustic shadowing
  - Uniformly hypoechoic testis may be seen with associated ischemia
    - Reduced echogenicity is a sensitive marker of poor outcome (late atrophy), compared to clinical parameters
  - Focal parenchymal heterogeneity if post-traumatic
- Color Doppler
  - Undescended atrophic testis shows hypoplastic vessels
  - Blind ending vas deferens without evidence of testicular vessels is well demonstrated

Angiographic Findings
- Atrophic testis has diminutive vessels on retrograde venography

---

DDx: Testicular Atrophy

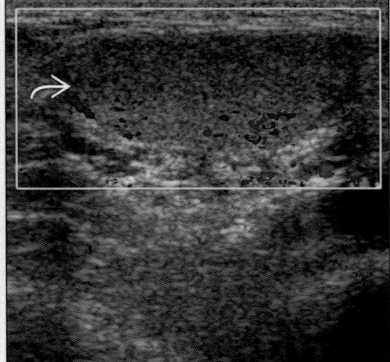

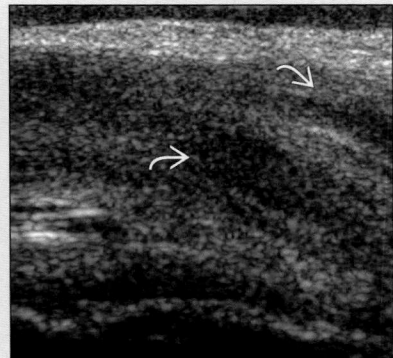

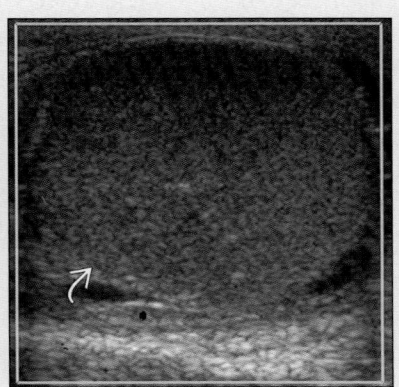

| Undescended Testis | Anorchia | Testicular Torsion |

TESTICULAR ATROPHY

Key Facts

Terminology
- Testicular atrophy is defined as a difference in size and consistency of testes between affected and healthy sides

Imaging Findings
- Size: Testicular atrophy is considered to be present if the combined axis measurements of the two sides differ by 10 mm or more, or testicular size less than 4.0 x 2.0 cm
- Shrunken testis displaying increased echogenicity due to fibrosis
- Uniformly hypoechoic testis may be seen with associated ischemia
- Reduced echogenicity is a sensitive marker of poor outcome (late atrophy), compared to clinical parameters
- Focal parenchymal heterogeneity if post-traumatic
- Undescended atrophic testis shows hypoplastic vessels

DIFFERENTIAL DIAGNOSIS

Undescended Testis
- Testis may be located anywhere along the tract of descent

Anorchia
- Bilateral absent testes

Testicular Torsion
- Vascular compromise of testis due to "torsion knot" of spermatic cord

PATHOLOGY

General Features
- Etiology
  - Secondary to
    - Spermatic cord torsion in utero in 45%
    - Epididymo-orchitis, due to severe degree of inflammation/induration of cord
    - "Missed torsion": Ischemic damage due to compromised blood flow
    - Sequel of scrotal trauma, due to resorption of non-viable testicular tissue & ischemia due to raised pressure within testicular tunics
    - Post inguinal hernioplasty
- Epidemiology: 4-5.5% of cryptorchid testes undergo atrophy
- Associated abnormalities
  - Cryptorchism: Commonly associated with testicular atrophy
  - Kallmann syndrome, hypogonadotrophic hypogonadism

Gross Pathologic & Surgical Features
- Atrophied testis can be identified by presence of atrophic vas deferens and epididymis, with dystrophic calcification, hemosiderin deposits, dominant vein, pampiniform plexus and vascularized fibrous nodule (VFN) formation
  - "Fibrous nubbin" or "atrophic testis" is found at the terminus of spermatic cord

CLINICAL ISSUES

Presentation
- Most common signs/symptoms: Previous history of trauma, epididymo-orchitis, "missed torsion"

Treatment
- It is critical to identify viable testis so that orchiopexy or an orchiectomy if non-viable, can be performed

SELECTED REFERENCES
1. Spires SE et al: Testicular regression syndrome: a clinical and pathologic study of 11 cases. Arch Pathol Lab Med. 124(5):694-8, 2000
2. Cross JJ et al: Scrotal trauma: a cause of testicular atrophy. Clin Radiol. 54(5):317-20, 1999

IMAGE GALLERY

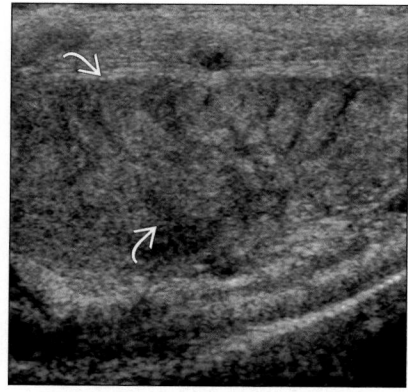 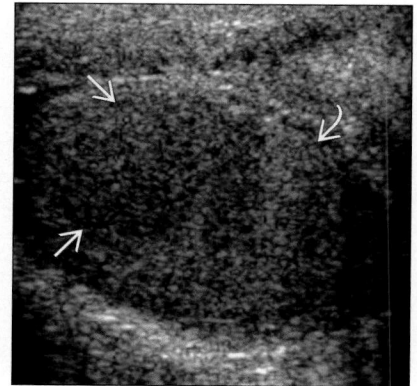 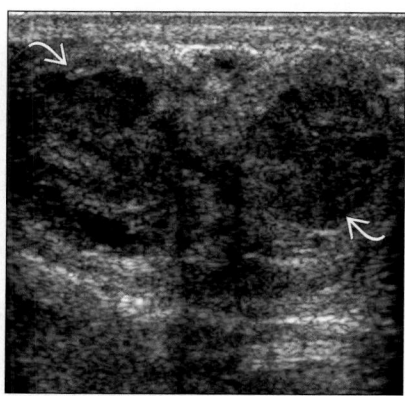

(Left) Longitudinal grayscale ultrasound shows a heterogeneous, shrunken, atrophied testis ⇨ in a patient with chronic testicular torsion. *(Center)* Oblique grayscale ultrasound shows a heterogeneous echo pattern ⇨ of detorted testis with focal area of low reflectivity ⇨ indicative of infarction and early atrophy. *(Right)* Transverse grayscale ultrasound shows a heterogeneous spermatic cord indicative of cord hematoma ⇨ due to thrombosis as complication of inguinal hernioplasty, leading to vascular compromise of testis and subsequent atrophy.

UNDESCENDED TESTIS

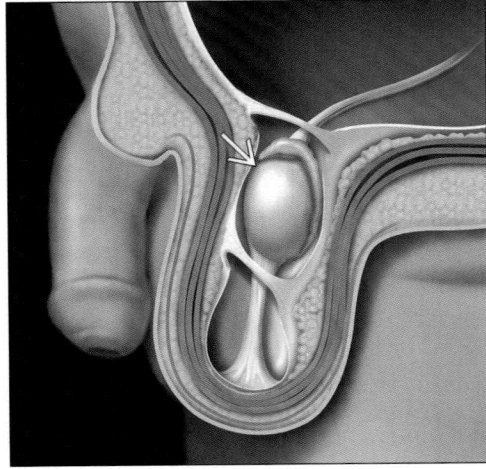

Graphic shows a testis ➡ at a high scrotal location due to incomplete descent. An undescended testis may be located anywhere from the kidney to the inguinal canal.

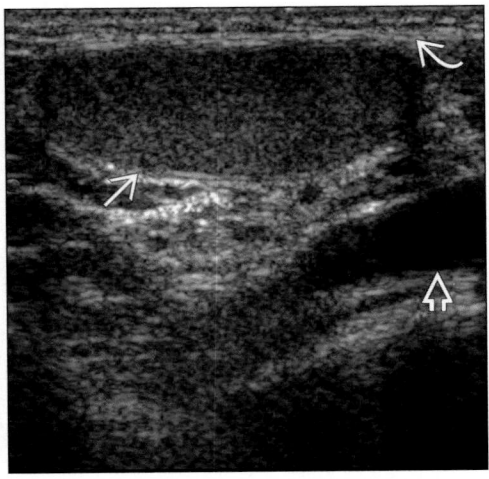

Oblique ultrasound shows an oblong, hypoechoic testis ➡ deep to the subcutaneous tissue & fascia of the inguinal musculature ⇥. Note femoral vessel ⇉ crossing inguinal ligament.

TERMINOLOGY

Abbreviations and Synonyms
- Cryptorchidism, cryptorchism

Definitions
- Incomplete descent of testis into base of scrotum

IMAGING FINDINGS

General Features
- Best diagnostic clue: Unilateral absence of testis in scrotum
- Location
  - Anywhere from kidney to inguinal canal
  - Bilateral in 10%
  - Inguinal canal most common (80%)
- Size
  - Cryptorchid testis smaller than normal testis
  - Adults: Undescended testis exhibit different degrees of atrophy
- Morphology: Ovoid well-circumscribed mass

Ultrasonographic Findings
- Grayscale Ultrasound
  - 20-88% sensitivity to detect inguinal position of testis
  - Lack of surrounding fluid & compression by adjacent structures make the testicular margins less defined than normally located testes
  - Ovoid homogeneous, less echogenic, well-circumscribed structure smaller than normal descended testis
    - Echogenic line of mediastinum testis
  - Spermatic cord not seen in inguinal canal; in 30% of cases epididymis cannot be identified separately
  - Testes less than 1 cm cannot be detected
  - Undescended testis in adults exhibit different degrees of atrophy with altered parenchymal echogenicity
  - Associated with microlithiasis, neoplastic foci if present may be detected

MR Findings
- MR imaging should be used in US negative cases
- T1WI: Low signal intensity ovoid mass; T2WI: High signal intensity ovoid mass

DDx: Undescended Testis

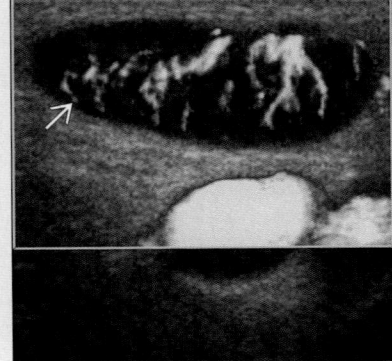

Inguinal Lymphadenopathy

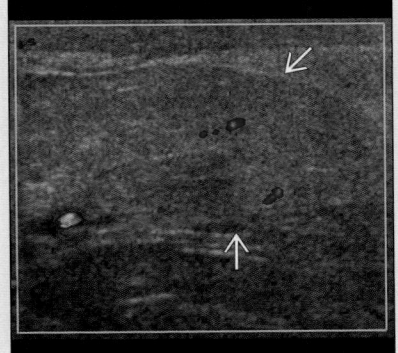

Inguinal Hernia

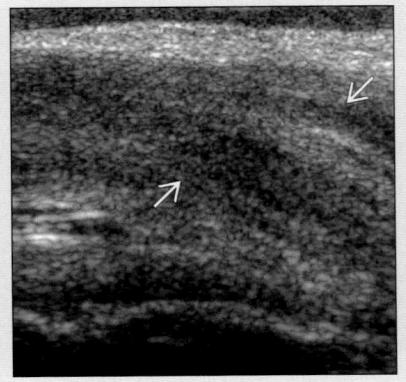

Anorchia

UNDESCENDED TESTIS

Key Facts

Imaging Findings
- Best diagnostic clue: Unilateral absence of testis in scrotum
- Lack of surrounding fluid & compression by adjacent structures make the testicular margins less defined than normally located testes
- Ovoid homogeneous, less echogenic, well-circumscribed structure smaller than normal descended testis
- Spermatic cord not seen in inguinal canal; in 30% of cases epididymis cannot be identified separately
- High-resolution US (≥ 7.5) imaging modality of choice for inguinal testis

Top Differential Diagnoses
- Inguinal Lymphadenopathy
- Inguinal Hernia
- Anorchia: Absent Testis

Imaging Recommendations
- Best imaging tool
  - High-resolution US (≥ 7.5) imaging modality of choice for inguinal testis
  - MR: 90-95% sensitive for intra-abdominal testis

DIFFERENTIAL DIAGNOSIS

Inguinal Lymphadenopathy
- Commonest groin "mass" seen in multiple pathologies

Inguinal Hernia
- Direct/indirect inguinal hernia, bowel/omentum as hernia content

Anorchia: Absent Testis
- Congenital or prior resection

PATHOLOGY

General Features
- Etiology: Interruption of embryologic testicular descent from abdomen into scrotal sac
- Epidemiology
  - Testis may be absent from scrotum in 4% of newborns (spontaneous descent in first few months)
  - Incidence of testis cancer: 1:1,000-1:2,500
- Associated abnormalities: Renal agenesis/ectopia, prune belly syndrome, epispadias

Staging, Grading or Classification Criteria
- Types: Retractile, high scrotal, canalicular (inguinal), abdominal, ectopic (anywhere from kidney to canal)
- Complications: Torsion, infertility, trauma
  - Malignant change, seminoma, embryonal cell CA

CLINICAL ISSUES

Natural History & Prognosis
- 30-50 times ↑ risk of malignant neoplasm in cryptorchid testis; also ↑ risk in contralateral testis

Treatment
- Orchiopexy before age 2 to preserve fertility; surgical removal post-puberty

DIAGNOSTIC CHECKLIST

Image Interpretation Pearls
- Absent spermatic cord on one side → cryptorchidism
- Identify mediastinum of testes to distinguish cryptorchid testis from other inguinal masses on US

SELECTED REFERENCES

1. Zagoria RJ: Genitourinary Radiology. 2nd ed. Philadelphia, Mosby. 327-9, 2004
2. Nguyen HT et al: Cryptorchidism: strategies in detection. Eur Radiol. 9(2):336-43, 1999

IMAGE GALLERY

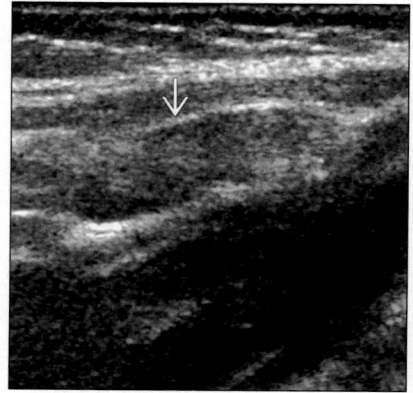 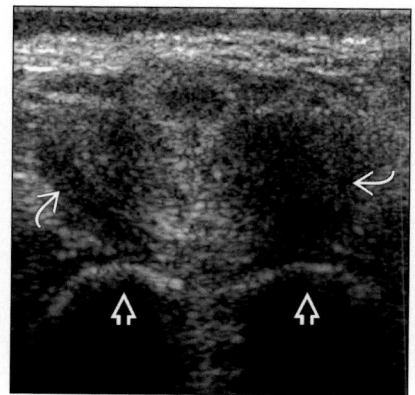 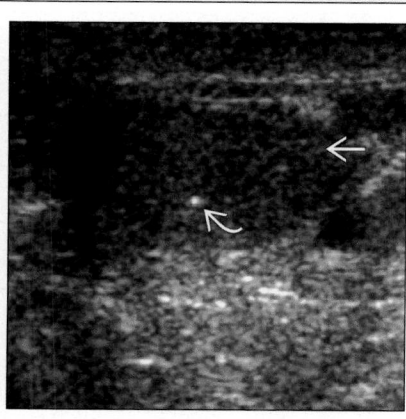

(Left) Oblique ultrasound shows well-defined oblong shaped atrophic testis ➡ in inguinal canal, note heterogeneous echo pattern. *(Center)* Transverse ultrasound shows empty scrotal sac on both sides ➡. The scrotal sac appears crumpled & small in size. Note pubic symphysis ➡. *(Right)* Ultrasound shows hypoechoic testis in the inguinal canal ➡. Note echogenic foci of testicular microlithiasis ➡.

HYDROCELE

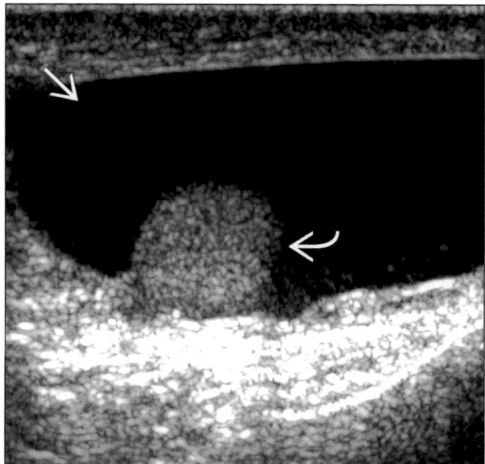

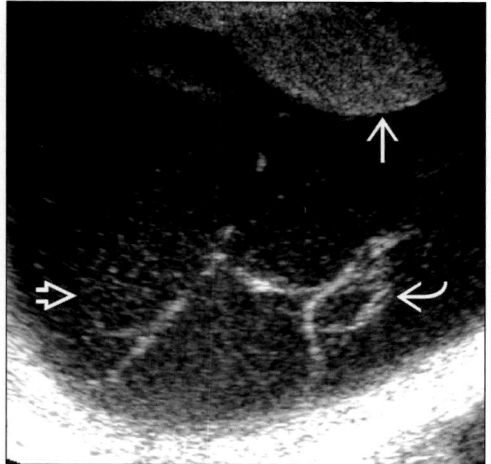

Longitudinal grayscale ultrasound of a scrotum shows anechoic fluid ➡ within the tunica vaginalis indicative of simple hydrocele. Note testis ➡ is attached to tunica vaginalis posteriorly.

Transverse grayscale ultrasound shows moderate fluid in tunica vaginalis, with low-level echoes due to debris ➡ and multiple septae ➡. Note anterolateral displacement of testis ➡.

TERMINOLOGY

Definitions
- Congenital or acquired serous fluid contained within layers of tunica vaginalis

IMAGING FINDINGS

General Features
- Best diagnostic clue: Scrotal fluid surrounding testis, except for "bare area" where tunica vaginalis does not cover testis & is attached to epididymis
- Location: Tunica vaginalis
- Morphology
  - Congenital form of hydrocele is seen in children due to persistent communication with the peritoneal cavity through patent processus vaginalis
  - Types
    - Congenital: Trapped ascites in processus vaginalis
    - Infantile: Fluid in funicular process
    - Primary: Idiopathic
    - Secondary: Post-inflammatory/trauma

Ultrasonographic Findings
- Grayscale Ultrasound
  - Acute hydrocele (AH): Crescentic anechoic fluid collection surrounding anterolateral aspect of testis
    - AH: Usually testis is displaced posteromedially
  - Chronic hydroceles (CH): Low-level, mobile echoes
    - CH: Cholesterol crystals presumed to cause these low-level mobile echoes & cannot be distinguished from inflammatory debris
    - CH: Diffuse scrotal wall thickening, parietal calcifications & scrotoliths
    - CH: Septations are infrequent and mostly due to secondary trauma or infection
- Power Doppler: May demonstrate movement of internal debris in chronic hydrocele

MR Findings
- T1WI: Low signal fluid collection
- T2WI: High signal consistent with serous fluid

Imaging Recommendations
- High resolution US (≥ 7.5 MHz) is modality of choice

DDx: Hydrocele

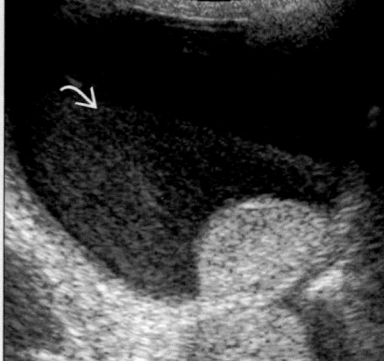

Pyocele

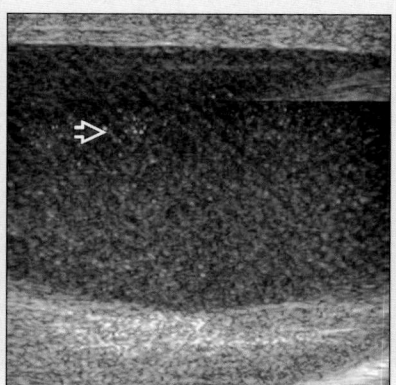

Hematocele

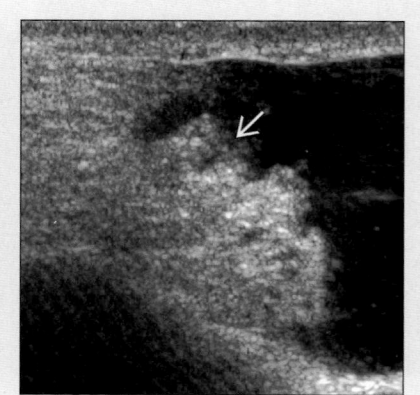

Scrotal Hernia

HYDROCELE

Key Facts

Imaging Findings
- Acute hydrocele (AH): Crescentic anechoic fluid collection surrounding anterolateral aspect of testis
- AH: Usually testis is displaced posteromedially
- Chronic hydroceles (CH): Low-level, mobile echoes
- CH: Diffuse scrotal wall thickening, parietal calcifications & scrotoliths
- Power Doppler: May demonstrate movement of internal debris in chronic hydrocele

- High resolution US (≥ 7.5 MHz) is modality of choice

Top Differential Diagnoses
- Pyocele
- Hematocele
- Scrotal Hernia

Pathology
- Congenital: Incomplete closure of tunica vaginalis
- Acquired: Epididymitis, torsion, trauma; rarely tumor

DIFFERENTIAL DIAGNOSIS

Pyocele
- Septated fluid with low-level internal echoes
- Associated with epididymitis, intrascrotal abscess and clinical signs of inflammation

Hematocele
- Complex echogenic fluid in tunica vaginalis on US
- Associated with trauma, torsion and infarct

Scrotal Hernia
- Bowel or echogenic omentum seen within scrotum due to indirect inguinal hernia

PATHOLOGY

General Features
- General path comments
  - Simple fluid collection within tunica vaginalis
  - Chronic cases show thickened tunica with septation
- Etiology
  - Embryology-anatomy
    - Congenital or communicating hydrocele is due to failure of processus vaginalis to close
    - Secondary occurrence in adults due to epididymitis or surgery for varicocele
- Epidemiology: 10% of testicular tumors have associated hydrocele

Staging, Grading or Classification Criteria
- Congenital: Incomplete closure of tunica vaginalis
- Acquired: Epididymitis, torsion, trauma; rarely tumor

CLINICAL ISSUES

Presentation
- Most common signs/symptoms: Asymptomatic (painless) scrotal mass/enlargement

Treatment
- Surgical resection: Oversewing of hydrocele sac edges

DIAGNOSTIC CHECKLIST

Image Interpretation Pearls
- Anechoic fluid collection in tunica vaginalis along anterolateral aspect of testis

SELECTED REFERENCES

1. Kapur P et al: Pediatric hernias and hydroceles. Pediatr Clin North Am. 45(4):773-89, 1998
2. Fowler RC et al: Scrotal ultrasonography: a clinical evaluation. Br J Radiol. 60(715):649-54, 1987
3. Meizner I et al: In utero diagnosis of congenital hydrocele. J Clin Ultrasound. 1983

IMAGE GALLERY

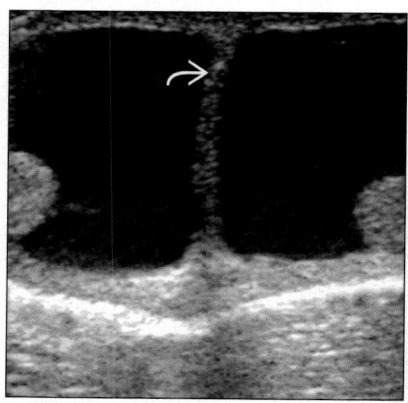 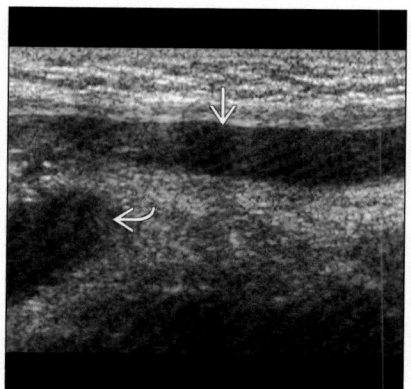 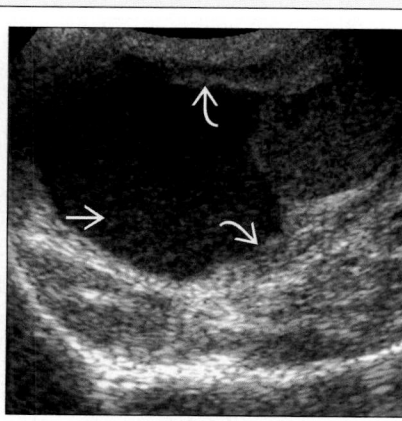

(Left) Transverse ultrasound shows symmetrical hydrocele in both hemiscrotum with clear separation ➦ between right & left scrotal sac characteristic of neonatal hydrocele. *(Center)* Longitudinal ultrasound at inguinal canal shows encysted hydrocele of cord ➦ due to patent processus vaginalis in an infant. Note small amount of associated ascites ➦. *(Right)* Transverse ultrasound shows large, chronic hydrocele with multiple, fine, diffuse echoes ➦ suggestive of cholesterol crystals. Note thickening of tunica vaginalis ➦.

TESTICULAR & EPIDIDYMAL CYSTS

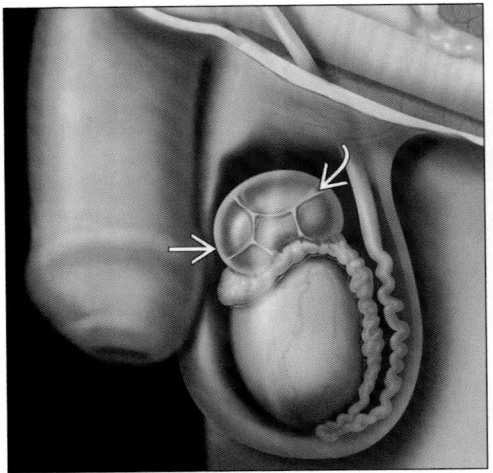

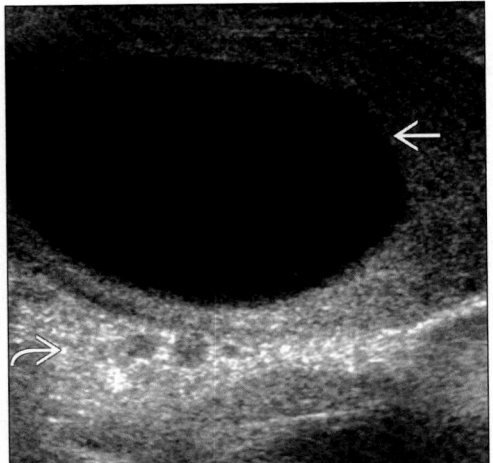

Graphic shows a smooth walled cyst ➡ *at the head of the epididymis. Large cysts may show septations* ➡.

Longitudinal grayscale ultrasound a shows well-defined, intratesticular, anechoic cyst ➡ *with an imperceptible wall and posterior enhancement* ➡; *all features of a simple testicular cyst.*

TERMINOLOGY

Definitions
- Anechoic structures within the substance of testis and epididymis with imperceptible walls and posterior enhancement

IMAGING FINDINGS

General Features
- Best diagnostic clue: Anechoic mass with posterior enhancement and no perceptible wall
- Location
  - Epididymal cyst
    - Simple epididymal cyst: May arise throughout epididymis
    - Spermatocele: Head of epididymis
  - Testicular cyst
    - Tunica albuginea, tunica vaginalis
    - Intraparenchymal: Simple cyst, epidermoid cyst
  - Intratesticular spermatocele is seen in the region of rete testis, and communicates with seminiferous tubules

- Size
  - Epididymal cyst
    - Simple epididymal cyst: ≤ 1 cm
    - Spermatocele: 1-2 cm
  - Testicular cyst
    - Tunica albuginea cyst: 2-5 mm
    - Simple testicular cyst: 2 mm to 2 cm
    - Epidermoid cyst: 1-3 cm
- Morphology
  - Epididymal cyst: 20-40% of individuals, multiple in 29%
    - Simple epididymal cyst: Lined with epithelium, contains clear serous fluid and likely to be lymphatic in origin
    - Spermatocele: Contains thick milky fluid comprising spermatozoa, lymphocytes and cellular debris
    - Cystic degeneration of epididymis: Cannot be differentiated from simple epididymal cyst
    - Larger cysts may have septation and may be confused with hydroceles
  - Testicular cyst: Incidentally detected on sonography in 8-10% of population

DDx: Testicular and Epididymal Cysts

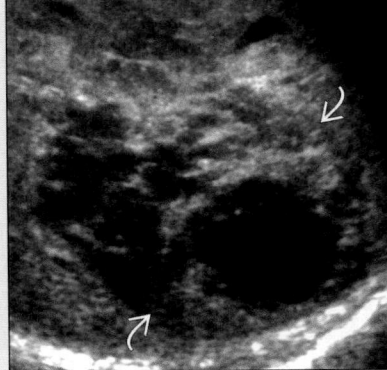

Mature Cystic Teratoma

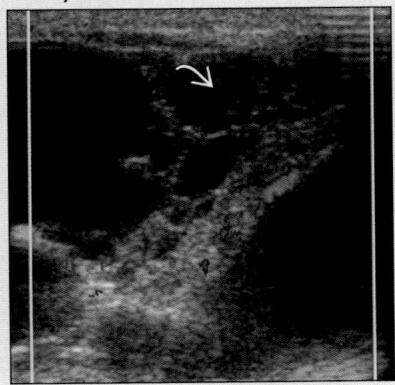

Tubular Ectasia of Rete Testis

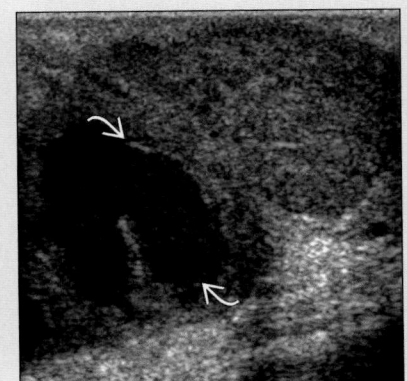

Testicular Abscess

TESTICULAR & EPIDIDYMAL CYSTS

Key Facts

Imaging Findings
- **Simple epididymal cyst:** Well-defined, anechoic
- May be seen throughout epididymis
- Aspiration of fluid is diagnostic of simple cyst but not usually necessary
- **Spermatocele:** Well-defined hypoechoic
- Located at head of epididymis
- Low-level echoes due to proteinaceous fluid and spermatozoa
- Spermatoceles usually displace testis anteriorly
- **Tunica albuginea cyst:** Meets all the characteristics of simple cyst
- Located at upper anterior or lateral aspect of testis
- **Simple testicular cyst:** Located anywhere in the testis, but most commonly near mediastinum testis
- Anechoic center, posterior enhancement
- Commonly associated with extratesticular spermatoceles
- **Epidermoid cyst:** Circumscribed hypoechoic mass
- Target appearance: Hypoechoic halo with central area of increased echogenicity
- "Onion-ring" pattern with alternating hyperechoic and hypoechoic layers
- **Congenital cystic dysplasia:** Appearance similar to acquired cystic dilation of rete testis
- Pressure atrophy of adjacent testicular parenchyma
- Multiple, interconnecting anechoic cysts of various sizes and shapes

Top Differential Diagnoses
- Mature Cystic Teratoma
- Tubular Ectasia of Rete Testis
- Intratesticular Abscess

- Tunica albuginea cyst: Mesothelial in origin, unilocular or multilocular
- Tunica vaginalis cyst: Located between visceral or parietal layer of tunica vaginalis
- Congenital cystic dysplasia of testis is a rare congenital defect characterized by formation of multiple irregular cystic spaces in mediastinum testis

Ultrasonographic Findings
- Grayscale Ultrasound
  - **Simple epididymal cyst:** Well-defined, anechoic
    - May be seen throughout epididymis
    - Contains clear fluid
    - Aspiration of fluid is diagnostic of simple cyst but not usually necessary
  - **Spermatocele:** Well-defined hypoechoic
    - Located at head of epididymis
    - Posterior acoustic enhancement
    - Low-level echoes due to proteinaceous fluid and spermatozoa
    - Spermatoceles usually displace testis anteriorly
  - **Tunica albuginea cyst:** Meets all the characteristics of simple cyst
    - Unilocular or multilocular, eccentrically placed
    - Anechoic center, through transmission, may calcify (posterior acoustic shadowing)
    - Located at upper anterior or lateral aspect of testis
    - Complex tunica albuginea cysts may simulate a testicular neoplasm, scanning in multiple planes helps identify benign nature of these cysts
  - **Simple testicular cyst:** Located anywhere in the testis, but most commonly near mediastinum testis
    - Well-defined, thin, smooth, imperceptible walls
    - Anechoic center, posterior enhancement
    - Commonly associated with extratesticular spermatoceles
    - Careful analysis helps differentiate from cystic neoplasm, especially teratomas; if any solid component, then should be considered malignant
  - **Tunica vaginalis cyst:** Single or multiple
    - Anechoic, may have septation or internal echoes due to hemorrhage
  - **Epidermoid cyst:** Circumscribed hypoechoic mass
    - Target appearance: Hypoechoic halo with central area of increased echogenicity
    - "Onion-ring" pattern with alternating hyperechoic and hypoechoic layers
  - **Congenital cystic dysplasia:** Appearance similar to acquired cystic dilation of rete testis
    - Pressure atrophy of adjacent testicular parenchyma
    - Multiple, interconnecting anechoic cysts of various sizes and shapes
    - Renal agenesis or dysplasia frequently co-exist

MR Findings
- MR imaging useful in evaluating painful scrotal cysts that may be too tender to be examined with ultrasound

Imaging Recommendations
- Best imaging tool: High-resolution US (≥ 7.5 MHz) is imaging modality of choice

DIFFERENTIAL DIAGNOSIS

Mature Cystic Teratoma
- Constitute approximately 5-10% of primary testicular neoplasms
  - Commonest differential of cystic intratesticular mass
- Sonographically teratomas are well-defined, markedly heterogeneous with cystic and solid areas
  - Dense echogenic foci causing acoustic shadowing are common

Tubular Ectasia of Rete Testis
- Partial or complete obliteration of efferent ductules causing ectasia of rete testis
  - Occur in patients ≥ 55 years, frequently bilateral
- Elliptical hypoechoic mass with branching tubular structures
- Associated epididymal cyst is characteristic

Intratesticular Abscess
- Secondary to epididymo-orchitis

TESTICULAR & EPIDIDYMAL CYSTS

○ Other causes are mumps, trauma and testicular infarctions
• Thick irregular walls, low level internal echoes and occasionally hypervascular margins

PATHOLOGY

General Features
• Etiology
  ○ Simple cysts result from previous trauma, surgery and prior inflammation
  ○ Spermatoceles usually result from prior vasectomy
  ○ Tunica albuginea cysts may develop secondary to fluid accumulation within small mesothelial rests or may result from fluid in blind-ending efferent ductules
• Epidemiology
  ○ Epididymal cysts seen in 1/3 of asymptomatic adults
    ■ Increased incidence of epididymal cysts has been reported in boys who are exposed in-utero to diethylstilbestrol
  ○ Testicular cysts are incidentally detected on sonography in 8-10% of population
• Associated abnormalities
  ○ Co-existent genitourinary lesions are commonly associated with congenital cystic dysplasia of testis and include
    ■ Absence of ipsilateral kidney, multicystic dysplastic kidney, duplication anomalies, and cryptorchidism

CLINICAL ISSUES

Presentation
• Most common signs/symptoms
  ○ Painless palpable testicular mass
    ■ Tunica albuginea cysts are firm and are palpable even when small in size
  ○ Simple cysts are incidental findings as they are not easily palpable, usually they are not firm even if large in size

Demographics
• Age
  ○ Epididymal cyst: Any age
    ■ Spermatocele: More common in post-vasectomy individuals
  ○ Testicular cyst: 5th-6th decade

Natural History & Prognosis
• Complex cysts of tunica albuginea may mimic intratesticular neoplasm, thus necessitating orchiectomy
• High-resolution sonography permits unequivocal sonographic differentiation between intratesticular cysts and cystic neoplasms by demonstrating solid components within, however
  ○ Histopathological correlation is needed in suspicious cystic masses
• Surgery for benign intrascrotal pathologies like cysts are frequently undertaken for weak clinical indications and carries significant associated morbidity

○ This could be avoided in many cases by simple reassurance and judicious use of ultrasonography
○ Policy of selective surgical intervention is strongly advocated

Treatment
• Simple cysts of epididymis and testis require no treatment
  ○ Asymptomatic simple cysts can be observed
  ○ Symptomatic simple cysts should be treated ideally with local parenchyma-sparing excision
    ■ Gonadal preservation and enucleation of testicular cysts are possible with a careful surgical approach, and orchiectomy is not necessary
• Spermatocele may be treated with ethanolamine oleate sclerotherapy
  ○ US may be used as the guiding tool
  ○ Cure rate is over 80%

DIAGNOSTIC CHECKLIST

Consider
• Cystic testicular tumors (non seminomatous germ cell tumors) are an important differential
• Combination of clinical and US findings facilitates the differentiation between non-neoplastic and neoplastic testicular cysts

Image Interpretation Pearls
• Anechoic, posterior enhancement, no solid component and no perceptible wall characterizes epididymal and testicular cysts

SELECTED REFERENCES

1. Dogra VS et al: Sonography of the scrotum. Radiology. 227(1):18-36, 2003
2. Woodward PJ et al: From the archives of the AFIP: tumors and tumorlike lesions of the testis: radiologic-pathologic correlation. Radiographics. 22(1):189-216, 2002
3. Munden MM et al: Scrotal pathology in pediatrics with sonographic imaging. Curr Probl Diagn Radiol. 29(6):185-205, 2000
4. Ushida H et al: [Bilateral synchronous multilocular epididymal cysts: a case report] Nippon Hinyokika Gakkai Zasshi. 90(7):692-5, 1999
5. Hobarth K et al: High resolution ultrasonography in the diagnosis of simple intratesticular cysts. Br J Urol. 70(5):546-9, 1992

TESTICULAR & EPIDIDYMAL CYSTS

IMAGE GALLERY

Typical

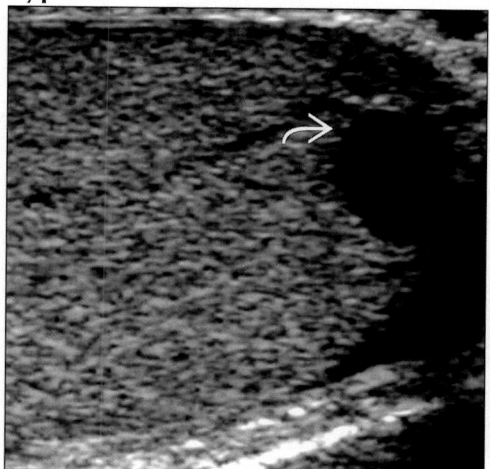
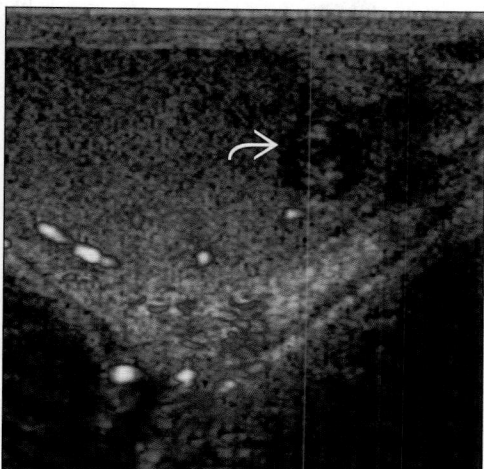

(Left) Oblique grayscale ultrasound shows a well-defined cyst ➥ located in the anterior and upper portion of the testis; a characteristic location for a tunica albuginea cyst. (Courtesy A. Gutte, MD). *(Right)* Oblique power Doppler ultrasound shows a well-circumscribed, avascular, hypoechoic, testicular mass ➔ with a concentric lamellar pattern referred to as an "onion-ring" appearance, characteristic of epidermoid cyst.

Typical

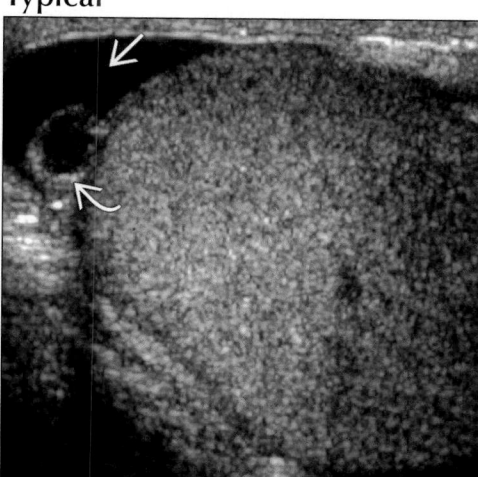
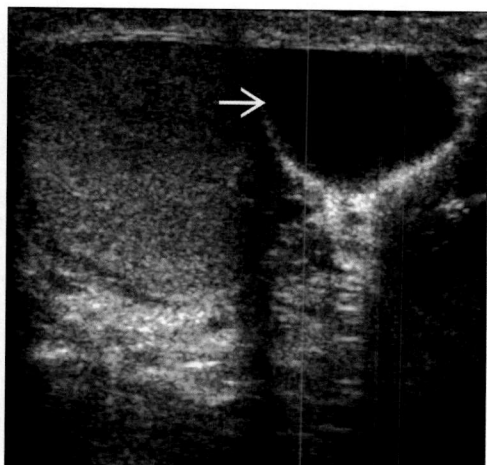

(Left) Oblique grayscale ultrasound shows a small anechoic cyst ➔ in the testicular appendage (appendix testis). A small hydrocele ➔ allows clear visualization of the testicular appendage. *(Right)* Transverse ultrasound shows a well-defined epididymal cyst ➔ in the head of the epididymis. Note contents of the cyst are clear, which differentiates it from a spermatocele. Aspiration of fluid to rule out spermatozoa is diagnostic but seldom necessary.

Typical

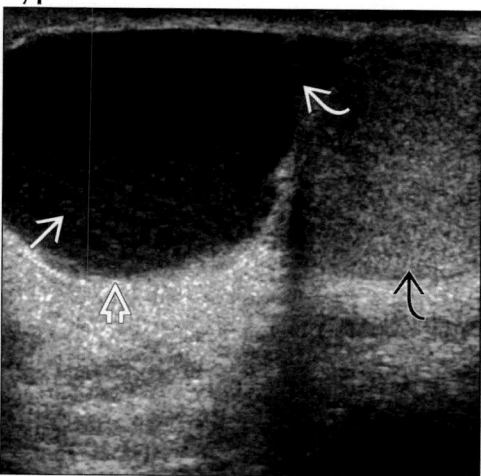
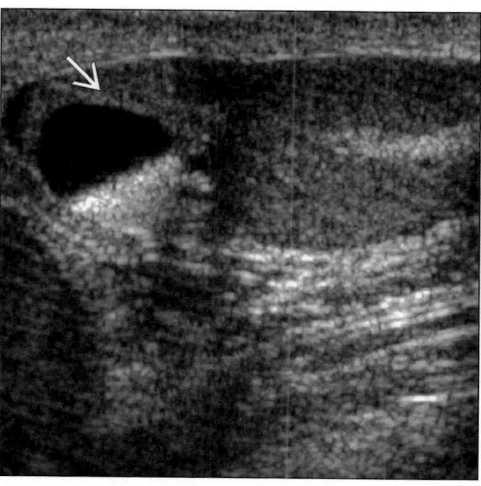

(Left) Oblique grayscale ultrasound shows a large anechoic cyst ➔ with low-level internal echoes ➔ in the head of the epididymis, indicative of a spermatocele. Note the septa ➔ at edge of cyst. Spermatoceles displace the testis ➔ anteriorly. *(Right)* Oblique grayscale ultrasound of a scrotum shows a small spermatocele ➔ in the head of the epididymis, with layered echogenic debris.

EPIDERMOID CYST

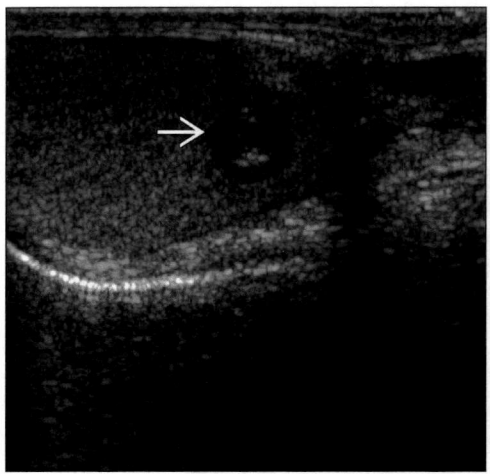

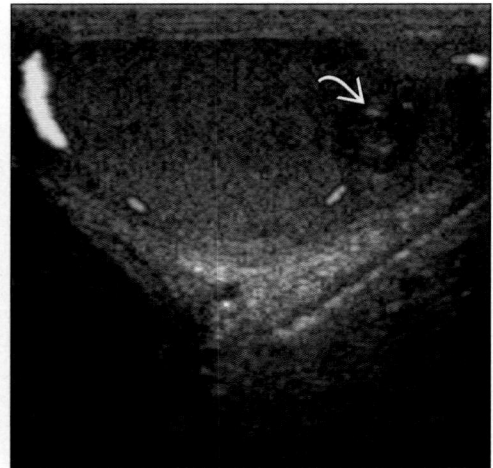

Longitudinal ultrasound shows a well circumscribed, hypoechoic testicular "mass" ➡ with a concentric lamellar pattern referred to as an "onion-ring" appearance. This is characteristic of an epidermoid cyst.

Longitudinal power Doppler ultrasound (same patient as previous image) shows the avascular nature of epidermoid cysts ➡.

TERMINOLOGY

Abbreviations and Synonyms
- "Monodermal dermoid", "keratin/cyst of testis"

Definitions
- Benign teratoma with only ectodermal components/squamous metaplasia of surface mesothelium

IMAGING FINDINGS

General Features
- Best diagnostic clue: "Target/bull's eye" appearance of an avascular testicular "mass"
- Location: Confined to tunica albuginea
- Size: 0.5-10.5 cm in diameter
- Morphology: Cyst contains keratin debris, wall composed of fibrous tissue

Ultrasonographic Findings
- Grayscale Ultrasound
  - Sharply circumscribed encapsulated round "mass"
  - Appearances vary with the maturation, compactness and amount of keratin present
  - "Onion-skin" appearance due to alternating hypo- and hyperechoic rings
    - Hyperechoic fibrous cyst wall ± shadowing from calcifications/ossifications
    - Hypoechoic cyst contents (laminated keratin debris)
  - "Target/bull's eye" appearance due to echogenic center (secondary to compact keratin/calcification)
- Color Doppler: Avascular, no blood flow demonstrable

MR Findings
- Target appearance
- Low intensities on T1WI & T2WI
- Water and lipid contents may give high signals on T1WI & T2WI

Imaging Recommendations
- Best imaging tool: High resolution US (≥ 7.5 MHz) is imaging modality of choice

DDx: Epidermoid Cyst

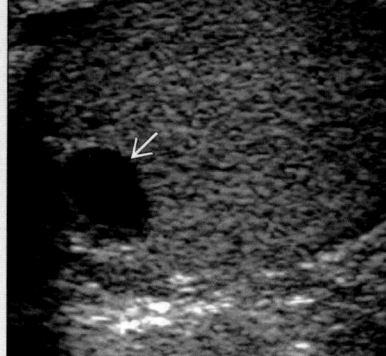

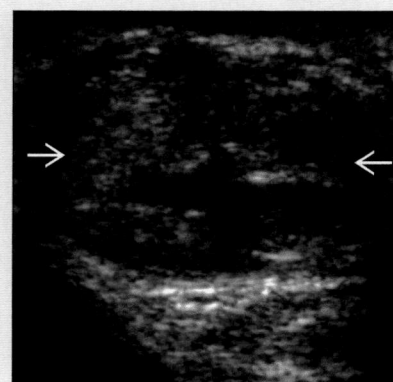

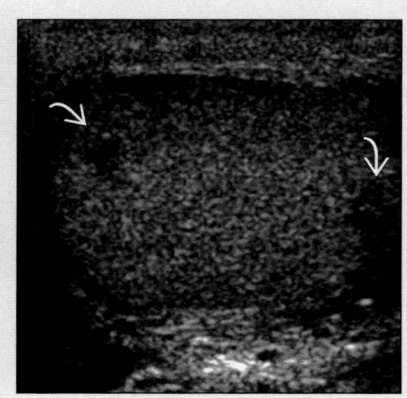

Tunica Albuginea Cyst

Mature Teratoma

Testicular Granuloma

EPIDERMOID CYST

Key Facts

Imaging Findings
- Best diagnostic clue: "Target/bull's eye" appearance of an avascular testicular "mass"
- Sharply circumscribed encapsulated round "mass"
- Appearances vary with the maturation, compactness and amount of keratin present
- "Onion-skin" appearance due to alternating hypo- and hyperechoic rings

- Hyperechoic fibrous cyst wall ± shadowing from calcifications/ossifications
- Hypoechoic cyst contents (laminated keratin debris)
- Color Doppler: Avascular, no blood flow demonstrable

Top Differential Diagnoses
- Tunica Albuginea Cyst
- Germ Cell Tumor
- Testicular Granuloma

DIFFERENTIAL DIAGNOSIS

Tunica Albuginea Cyst
- Located within the tunica, solitary and unilocular

Germ Cell Tumor
- Heterogeneous mass with vascularity seen on Doppler

Testicular Granuloma
- Most probably due to TB, usually multiple

PATHOLOGY

General Features
- Etiology: Monodermal development of teratoma along the line of ectodermal cell differentiation
- Epidemiology: 1% of all testicular tumors

Microscopic Features
- Tumor wall is composed of fibrous tissue and inner lining of squamous epithelium

CLINICAL ISSUES

Presentation
- Most common signs/symptoms: Painless tumor, incidentally noted, may cause diffuse testicular enlargement, negative tumor markers

Demographics
- Age: May occur at any age, 2nd-4th decade most common

Natural History & Prognosis
- No malignant potential

Treatment
- Conservative testicle sparing approach with local excision (enucleation)

DIAGNOSTIC CHECKLIST

Consider
- Germ cell tumor

Image Interpretation Pearls
- "Onion-skin"/ringed appearance in a well circumscribed testicular mass on US
- Avascular benign mass on color Doppler

SELECTED REFERENCES
1. Muttarak M et al: Painless scrotal swelling: ultrasonographical features with pathological correlation. Singapore Med J. 46(4):196-201; quiz 202, 2005
2. Dogra VS et al: Benign intratesticular cystic lesions: US features. Radiographics. 21 Spec No:S273-81, 2001

IMAGE GALLERY

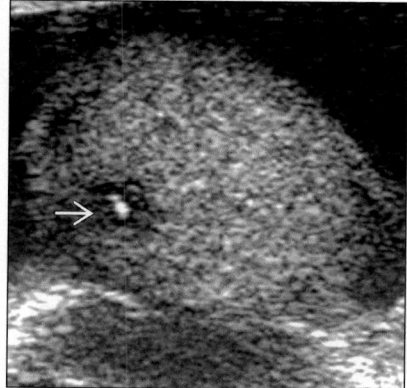 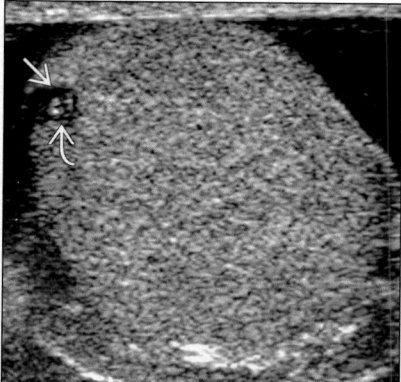 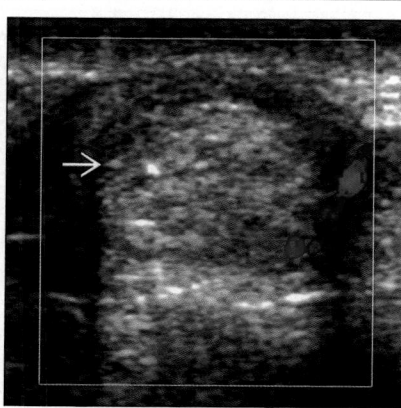

(Left) Transverse grayscale ultrasound shows a well-circumscribed, hypoechoic mass with central calcification ➡. *(Center)* Longitudinal grayscale ultrasound (same patient as previous image) shows its eccentric location, hypoechoic rim ➡, and hyperechoic center ➡. *(Right)* Transverse color Doppler ultrasound shows a large hyperechoic epidermoid cyst with no vascularity ➡. Such appearance may simulate mature teratoma, however absence of vascularity on color Doppler US is characteristic of epidermoid cyst.

TESTICULAR CARCINOMA

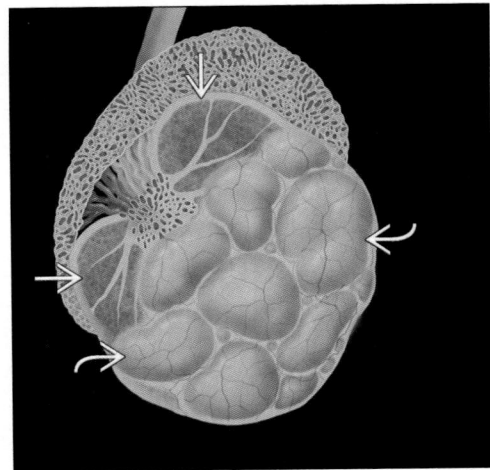

Graphic shows a multilobulated testicular mass →. Note the compressed and near complete replacement of normal testicular parenchyma →.

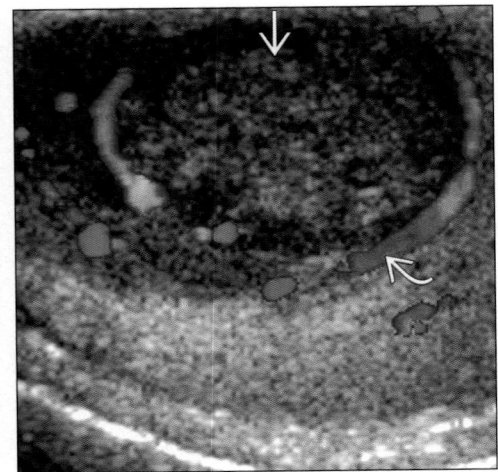

Longitudinal color Doppler ultrasound shows a solid, homogeneous, hypoechoic testicular mass → with increased peripheral vascularity →. Features suggest testicular seminoma.

TERMINOLOGY

Abbreviations and Synonyms
- Germ cell tumor of testis

Definitions
- Malignant germ cell tumor of testis

IMAGING FINDINGS

General Features
- Best diagnostic clue: Discrete hypoechoic or mixed echogenic testicular mass, ± vascularity
- Morphology
  - Most common neoplasm in males between ages 15-34 years
  - Mostly unilateral; contralateral tumor develops eventually in 8%
  - Seminoma is most common pure germ cell tumor of testis
    - Bilateral in 1-3%, almost always asynchronous

Ultrasonographic Findings
- Grayscale Ultrasound
  - Seminoma
    - Seminomas are usually well-defined, hypoechoic, solid without calcification or tunica invasion
    - With high resolution US some lesions show a heterogeneous echo pattern, ± lobulation
    - May very rarely undergo necrosis and appear partly cystic
  - Teratoma/teratocarcinoma
    - Well-defined, anechoic/complex heterogeneous cystic mass
    - Cystic areas, calcification (cartilage, immature bone) ± fibrosis characterize teratoma/teratocarcinoma
  - Embryonal cell carcinoma
    - Heterogeneous, predominantly solid mass, of mixed echogenicity
    - Poorly marginated, 1/3 have cystic necrosis
    - Coarse calcification infrequently seen
    - Embryonal cell carcinoma may invade tunica albuginea and distort testicular contour
  - Choriocarcinoma

DDx: Testicular Carcinoma

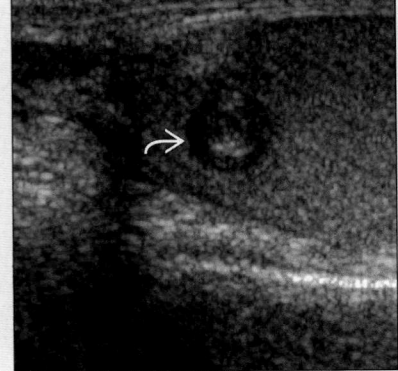

Epidermoid Cyst

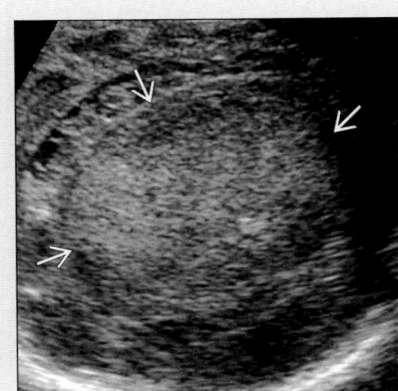

Lymphoma

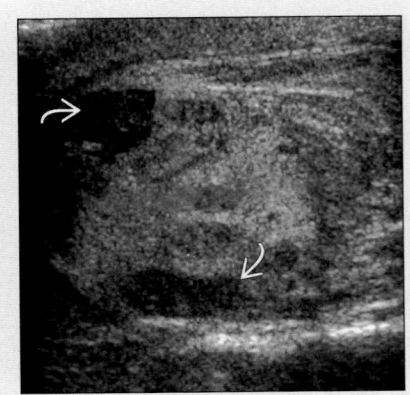

Testicular Hematoma

TESTICULAR CARCINOMA

Key Facts

Terminology
- Malignant germ cell tumor of testis

Imaging Findings
- Best diagnostic clue: Discrete hypoechoic or mixed echogenic testicular mass, ± vascularity
- Seminoma is most common pure germ cell tumor of testis
- Seminomas are usually well-defined, hypoechoic, solid without calcification or tunica invasion
- Cystic areas, calcification (cartilage, immature bone) ± fibrosis characterize teratoma/teratocarcinoma
- Embryonal cell carcinoma may invade tunica albuginea and distort testicular contour
- Hemorrhage with focal necrosis is typical feature of choriocarcinoma

- Tumor < 1.5 cm is commonly hypovascular, and tumors > 1.6 cm are more often hypervascular
- Best imaging tool: US to identify and characterize scrotal mass; CT or MR for metastatic staging; PET to evaluate post-treatment residual masses

Top Differential Diagnoses
- Epidermoid Cyst
- Lymphoma
- Subacute Hematoma

Diagnostic Checklist
- Consider testicular lymphoma if bilateral lesions identified, and particularly if patient is > 50 years
- Presence of discrete mass on grayscale ultrasound with abnormal intrinsic vessels on color Doppler should raise suspicion of testicular carcinoma

---

- Mixed echogenicity, heterogeneous mass
- Cystic areas with calcification common
- Hemorrhage with focal necrosis is typical feature of choriocarcinoma
- Color Doppler
  - Tumor < 1.5 cm is commonly hypovascular, and tumors > 1.6 cm are more often hypervascular
  - Disorganized flow is typical
  - Cystic areas are avascular

CT Findings
- CECT
  - Useful for staging retroperitoneal, nodal and pulmonary metastases
  - Low attenuation nodes
  - Even nodes < 1 cm suspicious if located in typical drainage areas; left renal hilus and right retrocaval in location
  - Helpful to identify retroperitoneal recurrence and/or "growing teratoma" syndrome

MR Findings
- T2WI
  - Useful for identifying nodal metastases
  - Moderate high signal intensity lymphadenopathy in retroperitoneum

Nuclear Medicine Findings
- PET
  - Helpful to reduce false-negative CT study
    - May aid in differentiating residual tumor from scar in treated patients

Imaging Recommendations
- Best imaging tool: US to identify and characterize scrotal mass; CT or MR for metastatic staging; PET to evaluate post-treatment residual masses
- Protocol advice: High frequency (≥ 10 MHz) linear array transducer

DIFFERENTIAL DIAGNOSIS

Epidermoid Cyst
- Cystic cavity lined by stratified squamous epithelium
- "Onion skin" appearance due to alternating layers of keratin and desquamated squamous cells
- May have calcified rim, no enhancement on MR

Lymphoma
- Older age group, most common tumor of testes in men > 60 years
- 50% of cases bilateral, often multiple lesions, associated with lymphadenopathy masses elsewhere
- Hypoechoic and hypervascular on color Doppler

Subacute Hematoma
- History of trauma, associated hematocele
- Hypoechoic on US

Segmental Infarct
- Acute pain, no palpable mass
- Infarct is typically hypoechoic, focal avascular area on color Doppler

Focal Orchitis
- Irregular hypoechoic area within testis, enlarged epididymis
- Increased vascularity on color Doppler without displacement of vessels
- Reactive hydrocele with low level echoes, scrotal wall thickening

PATHOLOGY

General Features
- General path comments
  - 95% of testicular tumors are malignant germ cell tumors
  - Single histologic subtype in 65% of tumors (seminoma most common)
    - 40-50% are seminoma

TESTICULAR CARCINOMA

- 25% have embryonal subtype (often mixed with other subtypes)
- 5-10% are teratomas
- Multiple subtypes in 35%
  - Teratoma and embryonal cell (teratocarcinoma)
  - Seminoma and embryonal cell
  - Seminoma and teratoma
- Genetics: Family history increases risk
- Etiology: Associated with cryptorchidism, previous contralateral cancer; possible association with mumps orchitis, microlithiasis and family history of tumor
- Epidemiology
  - Most common cancer in men aged 15-34
  - 1% of all cancers in men, 4-6% of all male genito urinary tumors, 4th most common cause of death from malignancy between 15-34 years
  - Seminomas most common in men 35-39 years old, most common tumor in undescended testis
  - Seminomas rare before 10 years and after 60 years
  - Lymphoma most common tumor over 50 years
- Associated abnormalities: Gynecomastia, pre-pubescent virilization

Gross Pathologic & Surgical Features
- Solid or solid/cystic intratesticular mass
- 10-15% have epididymis or spermatic cord involvement
- Bilateral in 2-3% of cases

Staging, Grading or Classification Criteria
- Stage I (A): Tumor confined to testis
- Stage II (B): Tumor metastatic to nodes below diaphragm
- Stage IIA (B1): Retroperitoneal node enlargement < 2 cm (5 cm³)
- Stage IIB (B2): Retroperitoneal node enlargement > 2 cm x < 5 cm (10 cm³)
- Stage IIC (B3): Retroperitoneal node enlargement > 5 cm
- Stage III (C): Tumor metastatic to lymph nodes above diaphragm
- Stage IIIA (C1): Metastases confined to lymphatic system
- Stage IIIB or IV: Extranodal metastases

CLINICAL ISSUES

Presentation
- Most common signs/symptoms
  - Palpable mass in testis, painless enlarging mass
  - Dull pain (27%)
  - Acute pain (10%)
- Other signs/symptoms: Gynecomastia, virilization
- Clinical Profile: Young male with palpable testicular mass, elevated tumor markers such as beta-hCG, alfa-feto-protein

Demographics
- Age
  - Seminomatous tumor: Average age 40.5 years
  - Non seminomatous tumor: 20-30 years
  - Endodermal sinus tumor/teratoma: 1st decade

- Ethnicity: Increased incidence in Caucasian and Jewish males

Natural History & Prognosis
- 95% 5 year survival rate overall
- Metastases at presentation is seen in 4-14% of individuals
  - Distant spread occurs along testicular lymphatics
  - Hematogenous dissemination (usually late) to lung, bone, brain
  - Choriocarcinoma has a proclivity for early hematogenous spread especially to brain, death usually within 1 year of diagnosis
- Growing teratoma syndrome: Evolution of mixed germ cell tumor into mature teratoma after chemotherapy (in 40%) followed by interval growth despite maintaining a benign histologic type

Treatment
- Seminoma very sensitive to radiotherapy ± chemotherapy
- Radical orchiectomy; retroperitoneal node dissection for non-seminomatous tumor
- Radiotherapy or chemotherapy for metastatic disease

DIAGNOSTIC CHECKLIST

Consider
- Consider testicular lymphoma if bilateral lesions identified, and particularly if patient is > 50 years

Image Interpretation Pearls
- Presence of discrete mass on grayscale ultrasound with abnormal intrinsic vessels on color Doppler should raise suspicion of testicular carcinoma

SELECTED REFERENCES

1. Bach AM et al: Is there an increased incidence of contralateral testicular cancer in patients with intratesticular microlithiasis? AJR Am J Roentgenol. 180(2):497-500, 2003
2. Hain SF et al: Positron emission tomography for urological tumours. BJU Int. 92(2):159-64, 2003
3. Hussain A et al: The unsuspected nonpalpable testicular mass detected by ultrasound: a management problem. Can J Urol. 10(1):1764-6, 2003
4. Huyghe E et al: Increasing incidence of testicular cancer worldwide: a review. J Urol. 170(1):5-11, 2003
5. Jewett MA et al: Management of recurrence and follow-up strategies for patients with nonseminoma testis cancer. Urol Clin North Am. 30(4):819-30, 2003
6. Jones RH et al: New directions in testicular cancer; molecular determinants of oncogenesis and treatment success. Eur J Cancer. 39(2):147-56, 2003
7. Jones RH et al: Part I: testicular cancer--management of early disease. Lancet Oncol. 4(12):730-7, 2003
8. Patel MI et al: Management of recurrence and follow-up strategies for patients with seminoma and selected high-risk groups. Urol Clin North Am. 30(4):803-17, 2003
9. Woodward PJ et al: From the archives of the AFIP: tumors and tumorlike lesions of the testis: radiologic-pathologic correlation. Radiographics. 22(1):189-216, 2002
10. Albers P et al: Positron emission tomography in the clinical staging of patients with Stage I and II testicular germ cell tumors. Urology. 53(4):808-11, 1999

TESTICULAR CARCINOMA

IMAGE GALLERY

Typical

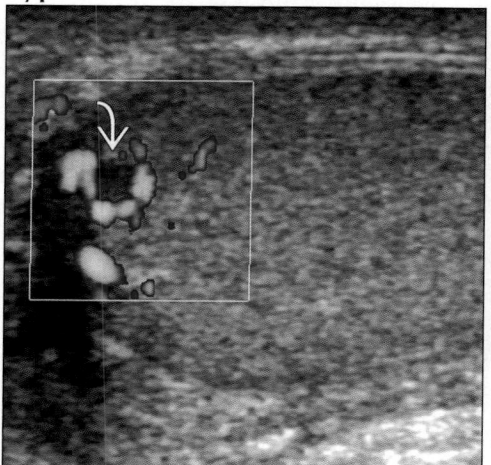

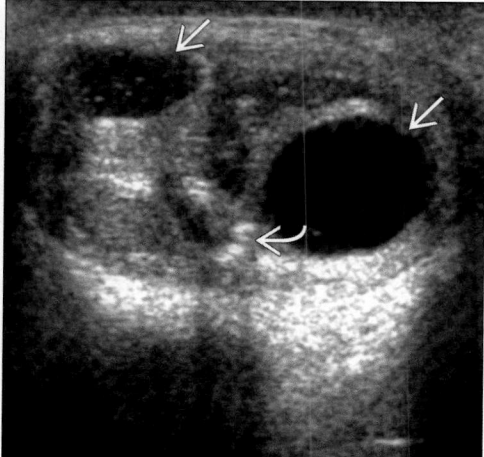

(Left) Longitudinal power Doppler ultrasound shows a small, well-defined, hypoechoic vascular testicular mass ➥ suggestive of small testicular seminoma. *(Right)* Longitudinal ultrasound shows a multilocular cystic ➡ testicular mass, with cysts of varying echogenicity in a cystic teratoma. Note calcific foci ➡ with posterior acoustic shadowing.

Typical

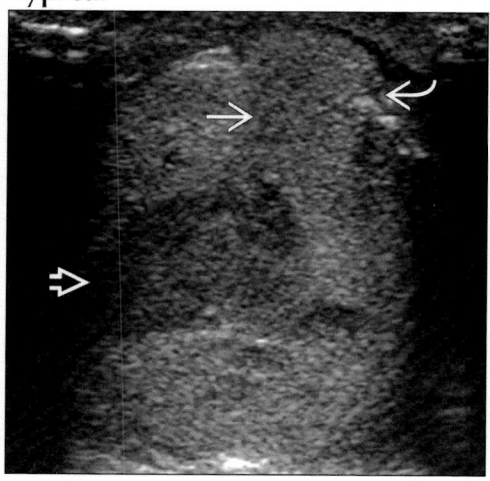

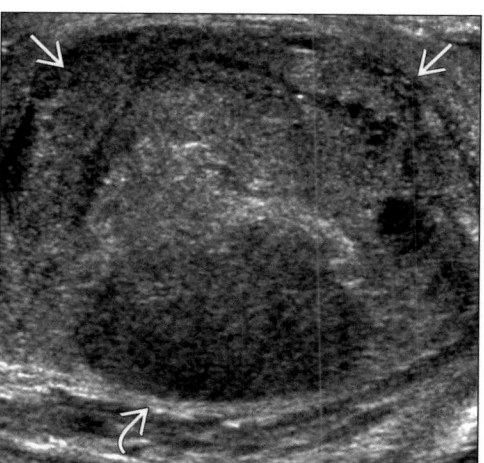

(Left) Transverse ultrasound shows an isoechoic area of choriocarcinoma ➡ invading the tunica albuginea ➡ & adjacent hypoechoic mixed germ cell tumor ➡. *(Right)* Transverse ultrasound of the testis shows a mixed germ cell tumor seen as a large, irregular, heterogeneous mass ➡ invading tunica albuginea ➡.

Typical

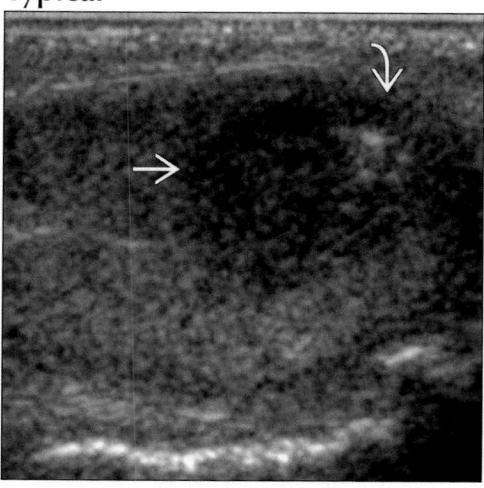

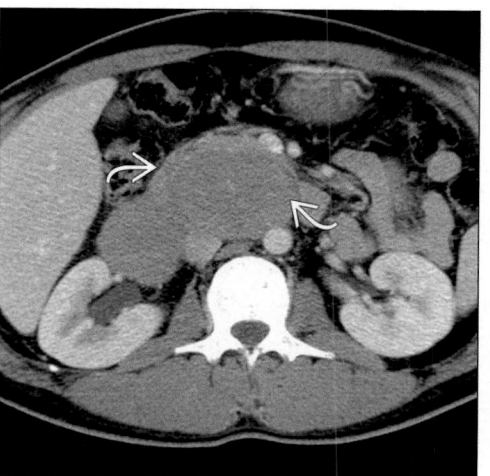

(Left) Oblique ultrasound shows an ill-defined, irregular, hypoechoic, heterogeneous mass ➡ invading the tunica albuginea ➡. Final diagnosis: Embryonal cell carcinoma. *(Right)* Transverse CECT shows a conglomerate of metastatic para-aortic and retroperitoneal lymph nodes ➡ in patient with testicular cancer.

GONADAL STROMAL TUMOR

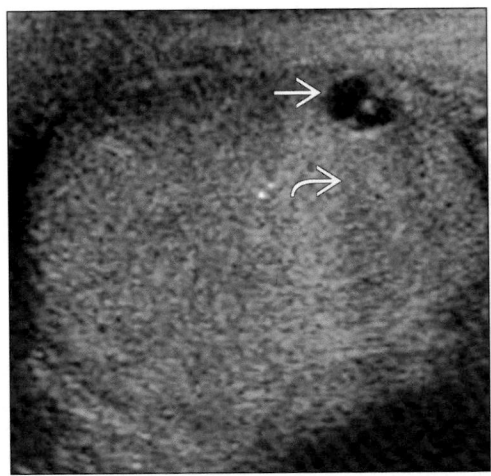
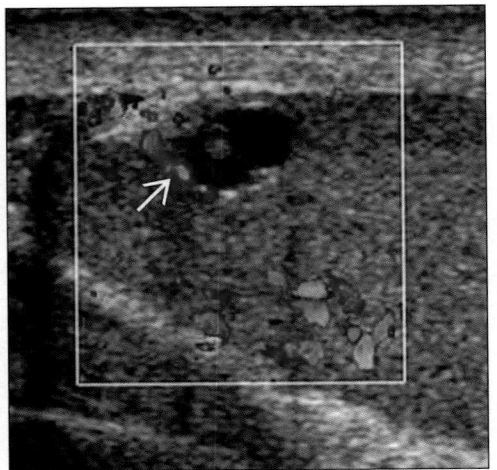

Longitudinal ultrasound shows a well-circumscribed hypoechoic solid mass ➡ in an 8 year old boy. Note areas of shadowing ➡ due to rim calcification. Features suggest gonadal stromal tumor.

Longitudinal color Doppler ultrasound (same patient as previous image) shows peripheral vascularity ➡ in the solid hypoechoic mass.

TERMINOLOGY

Abbreviations and Synonyms
- Gonadal stromal tumors (GST): Also called non-germ cell tumors, interstitial cell tumors, or sex cord tumors

Definitions
- Neoplasm arising from non-germ cell elements
- Leydig cell tumor (LCT): Arise from interstitial cells
- Sertoli cell tumor (SCT): Arise from sustentacular cells lining seminiferous tubules
- Granulosa cell tumor: Rare benign tumor
- Gonadoblastoma: Contains both stromal and germ cell elements

IMAGING FINDINGS

General Features
- Location: Bilateral in 3%
- Size: Benign tumors: Usually < 3 cm; malignant tumors: Usually > 5 cm
- Morphology: Well-circumscribed, round/lobulated

Ultrasonographic Findings
- Grayscale Ultrasound
  - May be indistinguishable from germ cell tumors
  - LCT: Small solid hypoechoic intratesticular mass
    - Larger tumors: Hemorrhage or necrosis leads to heterogeneous echo pattern
    - May occasionally show cystic change
  - SCT: Small hypoechoic mass, hemorrhage may lead to heterogeneity
    - Solid and cystic components
    - ± Punctate calcification; large calcified mass in large-cell calcifying Sertoli cell tumor
  - Gondablastoma: Stromal tumor in conjunction with germ cell tumor, usually mixed sonographic features
- Color Doppler: Internal or perinodular flow

MR Findings
- T2WI: Low signal intratesticular mass ± high signal fibrous capsule rim and high signal intensity foci internally secondary to central scars

Imaging Recommendations
- Best imaging tool: High resolution US (≥ 7.5 MHz)

DDx: Gonadal Stromal Tumor

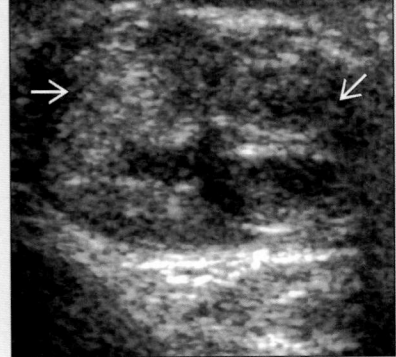
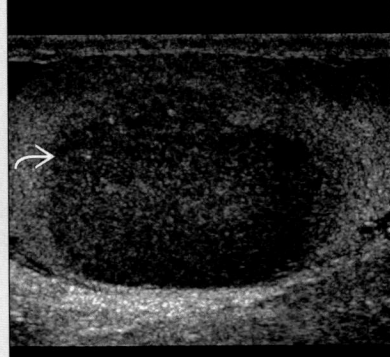
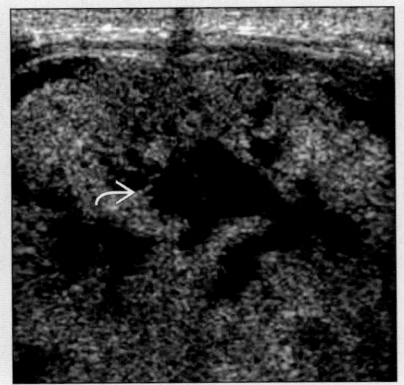

Testicular Teratoma

Testicular Lymphoma

Testicular Hematoma

GONADAL STROMAL TUMOR

Key Facts

Terminology
- Leydig cell tumor (LCT): Arise from interstitial cells
- Sertoli cell tumor (SCT): Arise from sustentacular cells lining seminiferous tubules

Imaging Findings
- May be indistinguishable from germ cell tumors
- LCT: Small solid hypoechoic intratesticular mass
- Larger tumors: Hemorrhage or necrosis leads to heterogeneous echo pattern

- SCT: Small hypoechoic mass, hemorrhage may lead to heterogeneity
- ± Punctate calcification; large calcified mass in large-cell calcifying Sertoli cell tumor
- Best imaging tool: High resolution US (≥ 7.5 MHz)

Diagnostic Checklist
- Consider stromal tumor in any patient with endocrinopathy and testicular mass

DIFFERENTIAL DIAGNOSIS

Testicular Germ Cell Tumors
- May be indistinguishable from stromal tumors on US

Testicular Metastases, Lymphoma, Leukemia
- Often multiple; otherwise indistinguishable

Intratesticular Hematoma
- Scrotal trauma, no internal color flow in hematoma

PATHOLOGY

General Features
- General path comments
  - 3% of all testis tumors; 10-30% occur in childhood
  - Leydig cell tumors: 3% of all testicular tumors
    - 90% benign, 3% bilateral
    - Most common, may produce testosterone
  - Sertoli cell tumors (SCT): 1% of all testis tumors
    - 85-90% benign
    - May produce estrogen/Müllerian inhibiting factor
- Associated abnormalities
  - Leydig cell tumor: Klinefelter syndrome
  - SCT: Peutz-Jeghers syndrome & Carney syndrome

CLINICAL ISSUES

Presentation
- Most common signs/symptoms
  - Painless testicular enlargement
  - 30% of patients have endocrinopathy secondary to testosterone or estrogen production by tumor
    - Precocious virilization in children
    - Gynecomastia, impotence, ↓ libido in adults

Demographics
- Age
  - LCT: 30-60 years; 25% occur before puberty
  - SCT: All age groups; 1/3 < 12 years

Natural History & Prognosis
- Malignant tumors metastasize in same pattern as testicular germ cell tumors

Treatment
- Orchidectomy or testis-sparing surgery

DIAGNOSTIC CHECKLIST

Image Interpretation Pearls
- Consider stromal tumor in any patient with endocrinopathy and testicular mass

SELECTED REFERENCES
1. Dogra VS et al: Sonography of the scrotum. Radiology. 227(1):18-36, 2003
2. Woodward PJ et al: From the archives of the AFIP: tumors and tumorlike lesions of the testis: radiologic-pathologic correlation. Radiographics. 22(1):189-216, 2002

10

23

IMAGE GALLERY

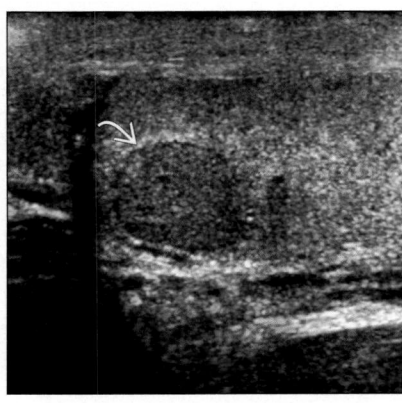 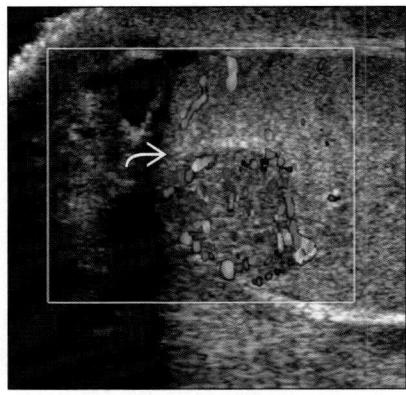 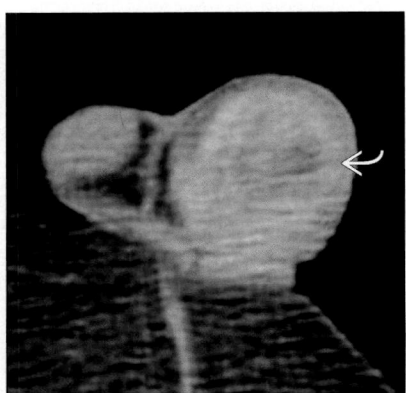

(Left) Transverse ultrasound shows a well-defined, hypoechoic, solid mass ➣ at the upper pole of the testis in a 36 year old adult. *(Center)* Oblique color Doppler ultrasound (same patient as previous image) shows increased vascularity ➣ of the solid mass. Gonadal stromal tumor cannot be differentiated from other testicular tumors. *(Right)* Transverse CECT shows a moderately enhancing, solid testicular tumor ➣ in young boy, surgically proven to be a gonadal stromal tumor.

TESTICULAR MICROLITHIASIS

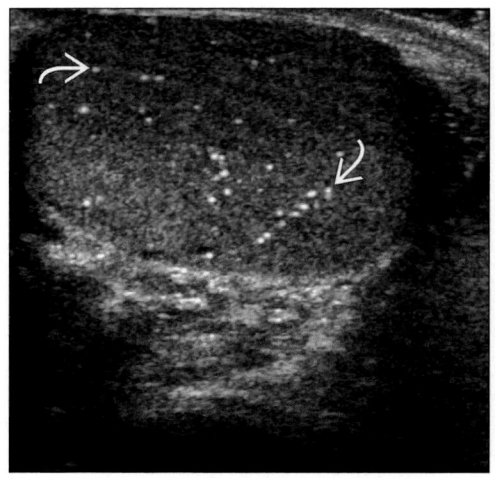
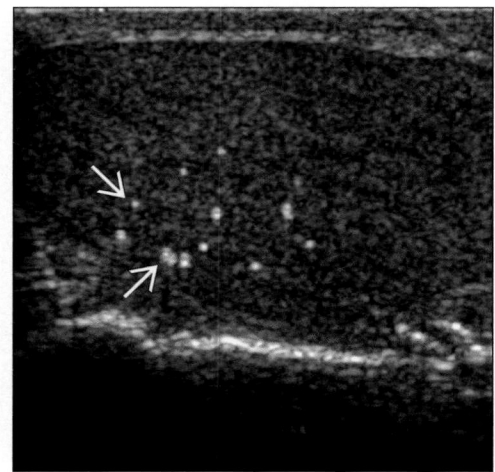

Oblique ultrasound shows multiple, small, hyperechoic non-shadowing foci ➜ diffusely scattered throughout the testicular parenchyma.

Oblique ultrasound shows a few small, non-shadowing echogenic foci ➜ in the testis representing the limited variety of testicular microlithiasis.

TERMINOLOGY

Definitions
- Intratubular calcifications within a multilayered envelope containing organelles, and vesicles surrounded by stratified collagen fibers

IMAGING FINDINGS

General Features
- Best diagnostic clue: Discrete, small, echogenic foci within testicular substance
- Location: Either unilateral or bilateral
- Size: 2-3 mm
- Morphology
  - Asymmetrically distributed, peripheral predominance
  - Multilayered envelope, composed of stratified collagen fibers, is considered to be responsible for absence of acoustic shadowing
  - Majority are idiopathic; previous infection or trauma may also be responsible

Ultrasonographic Findings
- Grayscale Ultrasound
  - Small hyperechoic foci diffusely scattered throughout testicular parenchyma
    - 2-3 mm echogenic foci, no posterior acoustic shadowing
    - May occasionally show a comet tail appearance
    - May have predominant peripheral or segmental distribution
  - Presence of ≥ 5 echogenic foci per transducer field in one testis is abnormal
    - Previously considered insignificant
  - Surrounding hypoechoic foci, if seen, could represent neoplasia
  - Examine abdominal organs to evaluate other concomitant pathology like germ cell tumor, neurofibromatosis and congenital anomalies
- Power Doppler: No role of color/power Doppler ultrasound, except to evaluate concomitant masses if present

Imaging Recommendations
- Best imaging tool: High resolution US (≥ 7.5 MHz) is modality of choice

DDx: Testicular Microlithiasis

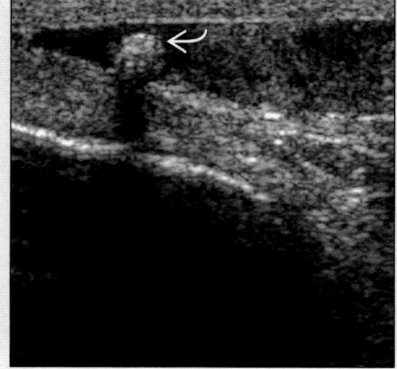
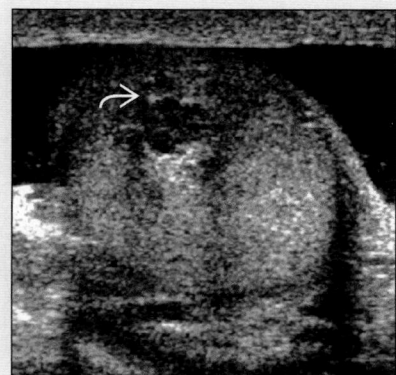
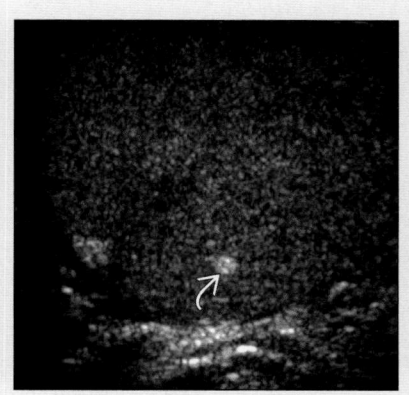

Scrotolith

Sertoli Cell Tumor

Granulomatous Calcification

TESTICULAR MICROLITHIASIS

Key Facts

Imaging Findings
- Best diagnostic clue: Discrete, small, echogenic foci within testicular substance
- Small hyperechoic foci diffusely scattered throughout testicular parenchyma
- 2-3 mm echogenic foci, no posterior acoustic shadowing
- Presence of ≥ 5 echogenic foci per transducer field in one testis is abnormal

- Examine abdominal organs to evaluate other concomitant pathology like germ cell tumor, neurofibromatosis and congenital anomalies
- Best imaging tool: High resolution US (≥ 7.5 MHz) is modality of choice

Top Differential Diagnoses
- Scrotal Pearls (Scrotoliths)
- Large-Cell Calcifying Sertoli Cell Tumor
- Testicular Granuloma

DIFFERENTIAL DIAGNOSIS

Scrotal Pearls (Scrotoliths)
- Extratesticular calcified bodies within scrotum with no clinical significance, result from inflammation of tunica vaginalis or torsion of appendix testis

Large-Cell Calcifying Sertoli Cell Tumor
- Gonadal stromal tumor, often bilateral and multifocal
- Commonest cause of intra-testicular macrolithiasis, mass may be almost completely calcified

Testicular Granuloma
- TB epididymo-orchitis may produce intrascrotal calcifications and scrotal sinus tract

PATHOLOGY

General Features
- Genetics: Associated with Klinefelter syndrome, Down syndrome, male pseudohermaphroditism
- Etiology
  - Defect in phagocytic activity of Sertoli cells leading to degenerated intratubular debris
  - Debris accumulates as glycoprotein and calcium layers and evolves into the histologically and pathologically characteristic form
- Epidemiology: 0.6%, increased detection due to frequent use of high frequency ultrasonography
- Associated abnormalities

  - Testicular neoplasia in 18-75%, intratubular germ cell neoplasia (IGCN), germ cell version of carcinoma in situ
  - Testicular microlithiasis rarely shows association with extratesticular tumors like epididymal or abdominal neoplasms, without testicular tumor

CLINICAL ISSUES

Presentation
- Most common signs/symptoms: Asymptomatic, incidentally seen on US for other scrotal abnormalities

Natural History & Prognosis
- Concurrent germ cell tumor in up to 40%
- Larger population and longer observation periods are required to determine the co-existence of benign and malignant lesions with testicular microlithiasis

Treatment
- No treatment, follow up at 6 month intervals, then yearly/longer intervals ⇒ screen for testicular tumors

SELECTED REFERENCES

1. Kocaoglu M et al: Testicular microlithiasis in pediatric age group: ultrasonography findings and literature review. Diagn Interv Radiol. 11(1):60-5, 2005
2. Dogra VS et al: Sonography of the scrotum. Radiology. 227(1):18-36, 2003

IMAGE GALLERY

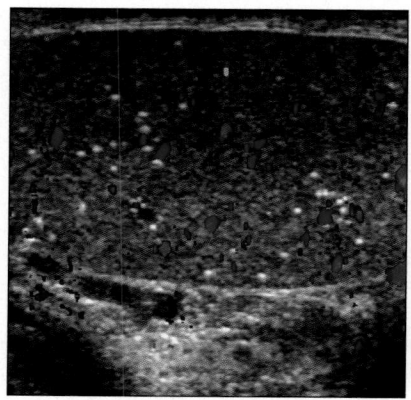 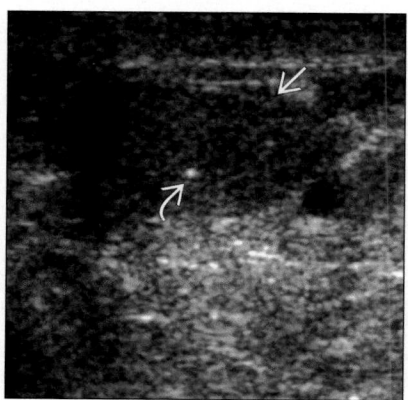 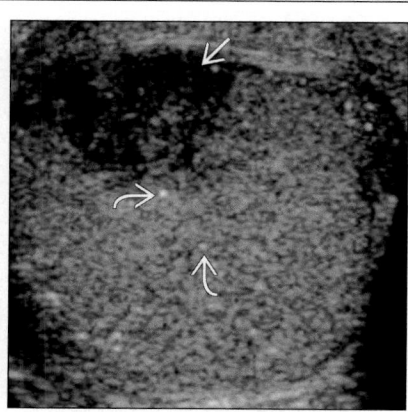

(Left) Oblique color Doppler ultrasound of testicular microlithiasis demonstrates no specific vascularity. *(Center)* Oblique ultrasound shows an undescended testis ➡ within the inguinal canal. Note the echogenic microlith ➡. Such patients have a substantially increased risk of concomitant neoplasm in the future. *(Right)* Transverse ultrasound shows multiple hyperechoic microliths ➡ and hypoechoic focal mass ➡, which was surgically proven to be germ cell tumor.

TUBULAR ECTASIA

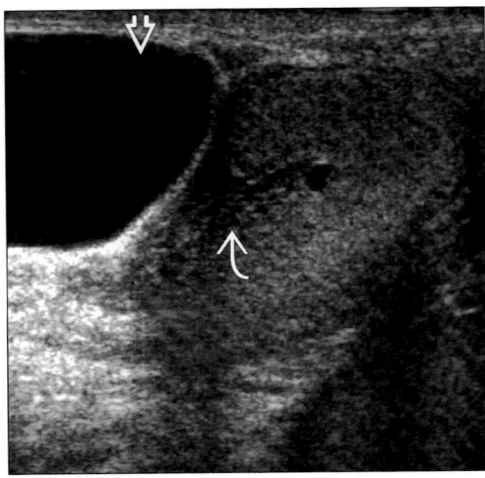

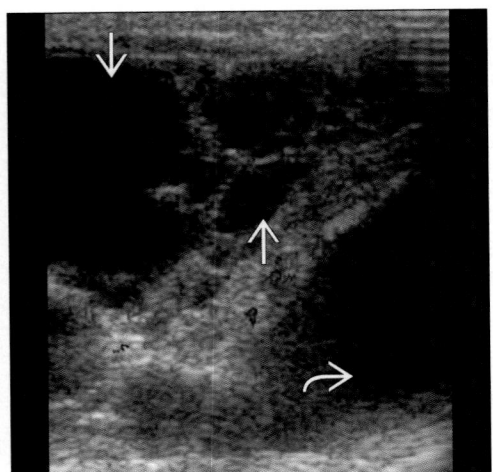

Longitudinal ultrasound shows a hypoechoic "mass" composed of dilated tubules ➔ representing tubular ectasia of rete testis. Note adjacent anechoic epididymal cyst ➔.

Oblique color Doppler image shows multiple, avascular, circular structures ➔ of varying size representing tubular ectasia (cystic transformation) of rete testis. Epididymal cyst (spermatocele) ➔ also seen.

TERMINOLOGY

Definitions
- Dilatation of rete testis, cystic transformation of rete testis

IMAGING FINDINGS

General Features
- Best diagnostic clue: Variable sized cystic masses near mediastinum testis with no associated soft tissue abnormality and no flow on color Doppler
- Location
  - Mediastinum testis
  - Asymmetrical and frequently bilateral
- Size: Variable size cystic spaces
- Morphology
  - Branching tubules converging at mediastinum testis
  - Characteristic appearance and location makes it possible to distinguish this benign condition from malignancy
  - Elongated shaped tubules may completely replace mediastinum testis

Ultrasonographic Findings
- Grayscale Ultrasound
  - Elliptical hypoechoic mass near mediastinum testis with branching tubular structures ± cyst
  - Fluid-filled tubular structures
  - Associated adjacent anechoic epididymal cysts are characteristic
  - Differentiated from cystic malignant masses which have an abnormal rind of parenchyma with increased echogenicity
- Color Doppler: Tubules are avascular and filled with fluid, hence no color flow appreciable

MR Findings
- MR performed for confirmation if a cystic malignant neoplasm cannot be ruled out
- Dilated rete testis appears hypointense on T1WI and iso- hyperintense on T2WI
- Cystic malignant testicular neoplasms show low signal intensity on T2WI

Imaging Recommendations
- Best imaging tool: High resolution US (≥ 7.5 MHz) is imaging modality of choice

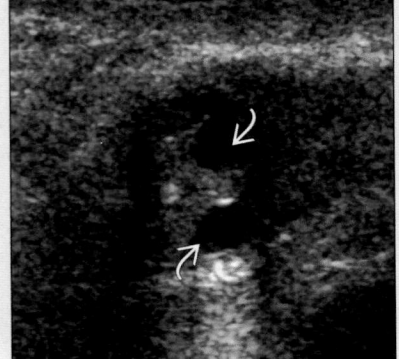

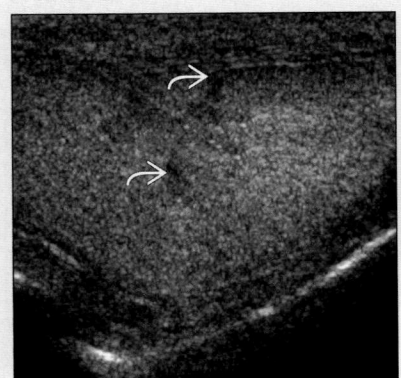

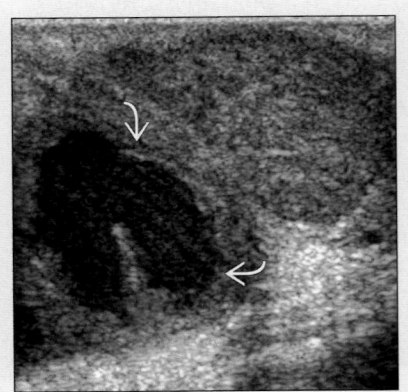

DDx: Tubular Ectasia of Rete Testis

Intratesticular Varicocele

Testicular Infarction

Intratesticular Abscess

TUBULAR ECTASIA

Key Facts

Terminology
- Dilatation of rete testis, cystic transformation of rete testis

Imaging Findings
- Best diagnostic clue: Variable sized cystic masses near mediastinum testis with no associated soft tissue abnormality and no flow on color Doppler
- Elliptical hypoechoic mass near mediastinum testis with branching tubular structures ± cyst

- Color Doppler: Tubules are avascular and filled with fluid, hence no color flow appreciable
- Best imaging tool: High resolution US (≥ 7.5 MHz) is imaging modality of choice

Top Differential Diagnoses
- Intratesticular Varicocele
- Testicular Infarct
- Intratesticular Abscess

DIFFERENTIAL DIAGNOSIS

Intratesticular Varicocele
- Multiple intra-testicular anechoic serpiginous tubules with characteristic color flow on Doppler particularly during Valsalva maneuver
- Pain due to passive congestion

Testicular Infarct
- Avascular hypoechoic mass, as a sequelae of any previous vascular insult

Intratesticular Abscess
- Follows many conditions like epididymo-orchitis, mumps, trauma, infarction
- Collection with irregular thick wall, necrotic center

PATHOLOGY

General Features
- Etiology
  - Partial or complete obliteration of efferent ductules, which cause ectasia and eventually, cystic transformation
  - May be associated with epididymal obstruction due to inflammation or trauma, middle aged to elderly adults are commonly affected
- Associated abnormalities: Spermatocele

CLINICAL ISSUES

Presentation
- Most common signs/symptoms
  - Incidentally noticed, non-palpable
  - Associated spermatocele may become symptomatic

Natural History & Prognosis
- Important to distinguish this condition from malignancy to prevent unnecessary orchiectomy

DIAGNOSTIC CHECKLIST

Consider
- Cystic malignant testicular tumor (teratoma)

Image Interpretation Pearls
- Elongated avascular tubular structures that replace mediastinum testis

SELECTED REFERENCES
1. Dogra VS et al: Benign intratesticular cystic lesions: US features. Radiographics. 21 Spec No:S273-81, 2001
2. Tartar VM et al: Tubular ectasia of the testicle: sonographic and MR imaging appearance. AJR Am J Roentgenol. 160(3):539-42, 1993

IMAGE GALLERY

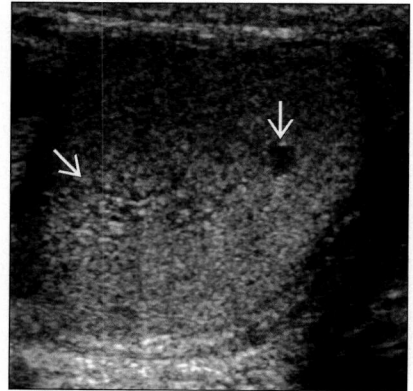 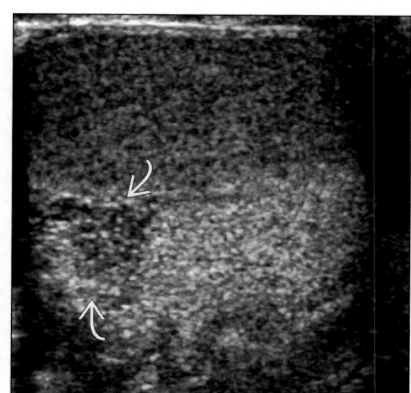 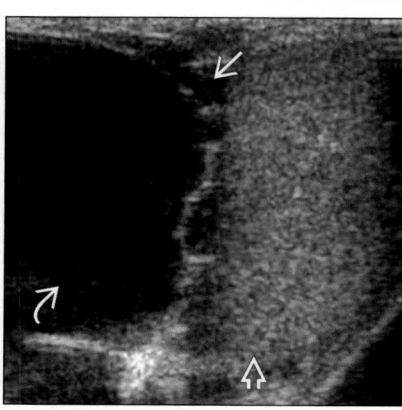

(Left) Transverse ultrasound shows multiple anechoic circular masses ➡ of varying size in postero-lateral aspect of the testis, representing mild tubular ectasia of the rete testis. *(Center)* Transverse grayscale ultrasound of scrotum shows mild to moderate tubular ectasia ➡ of rete testis. *(Right)* Longitudinal ultrasound shows a large anechoic intratesticular cyst ➡ associated with mild dilatation of the rete testis ➡. Note compressed testis due to mass effect ➡.

TESTICULAR TORSION/INFARCTION

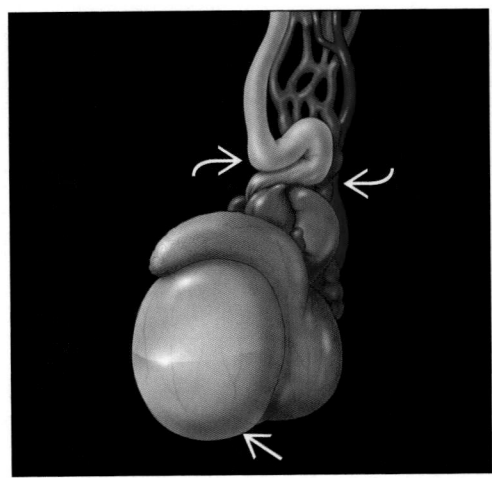

Graphic shows "spiral" twist ➡ of the spermatic cord with torsion, leading to venous congestion and compromised blood supply to the testis ➡.

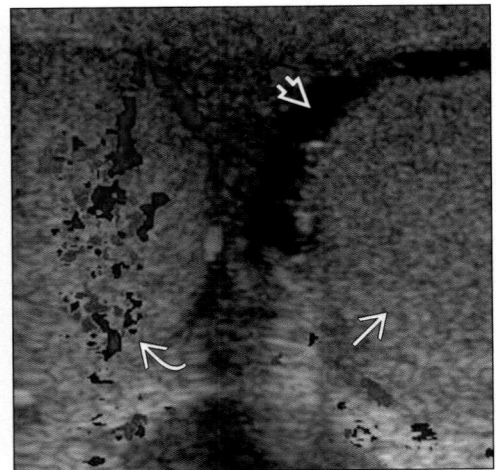

Transverse color Doppler ultrasound shows acute torsion of the left testis ➡. Note absent vascularity in affected testis compared with normal testis ➡. Note small hydrocele ➡ within tunica vaginalis.

TERMINOLOGY

Abbreviations and Synonyms
- Torsion, late or "missed" torsion, acute scrotum
- Spermatic cord torsion

Definitions
- Spontaneous or traumatic twisting of testis & spermatic cord within scrotum, resulting in vascular occlusion/infarction

IMAGING FINDINGS

General Features
- Best diagnostic clue: Decreased or absent testicular blood flow on color Doppler US
- Location: Unilateral in 95% of patients
- Morphology
  - Complete/incomplete torsion
    - Relapsing obstruction to venous outflow ⇒ congestion ⇒ reduced (arterial) inflow
  - Types according to location of "torsion knot"
    - Intravaginal torsion: Torsion knot within tunica vaginalis
    - Extravaginal torsion: Torsion knot outside tunica vaginalis

Ultrasonographic Findings
- Grayscale Ultrasound
  - Testicular torsion
    - Findings vary with duration and degree of rotation of the cord
    - Grayscale appearance during acute phase (critical phase) may be normal
    - "Spiral" twist of spermatic cord cranial to testis and epididymis causing "torsion knot" or "whirlpool" pattern of concentric layers
    - Enlarged testis and epididymis (heterogeneous echotexture, most often decreased echogenicity)
    - Edema of scrotal wall, secondary hydrocele
    - Intratesticular necrosis, hemorrhage or fragmentation if delayed diagnosis
    - At 24 hours after onset, changes like congestion, hemorrhage & infarction seen; condition referred to as "missed torsion"/subacute testicular torsion

DDx: Testicular Torsion

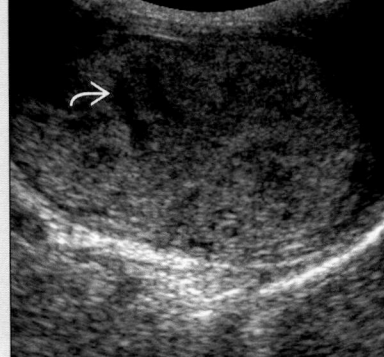

Testicular Trauma

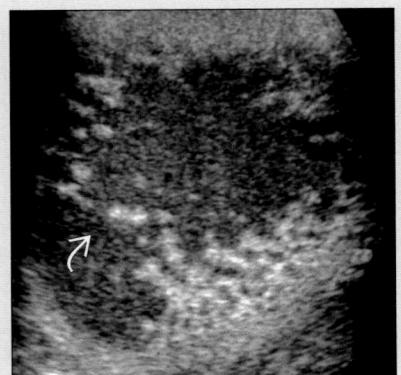

Testicular Abscess

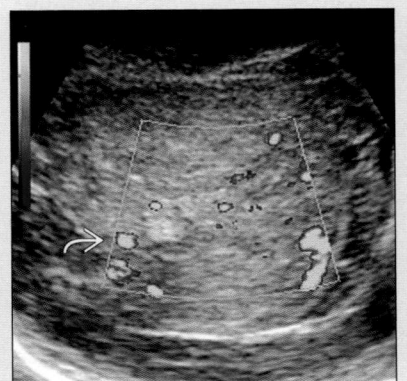

Testicular Lymphoma

TESTICULAR TORSION/INFARCTION

Key Facts

Imaging Findings

- Best diagnostic clue: Decreased or absent testicular blood flow on color Doppler US
- Grayscale appearance during acute phase (critical phase) may be normal
- "Spiral" twist of spermatic cord cranial to testis and epididymis causing "torsion knot" or "whirlpool" pattern of concentric layers
- Enlarged testis and epididymis (heterogeneous echotexture, most often decreased echogenicity)
- Edema of scrotal wall, secondary hydrocele
- Poor testicular echogenicity correlates with prognosis, may indicate non-viability
- Diffusely hypoechoic small testis/focal mass in infarcted testis

- Color Doppler is very useful to establish diagnosis of testicular torsion
- In acute torsion sensitivity, 80-90%; 10% of patients with early or partial torsion have normal exam
- Best imaging tool: US with high-frequency linear transducer & color/power Doppler
- Protocol advice: Compare grayscale, color Doppler appearances to contralateral normal testis

Top Differential Diagnoses

- Testicular Trauma
- Testicular Abscess (Epididymo-Orchitis)
- Testicular Tumor

Diagnostic Checklist

- Normal US (grayscale & Doppler) does not exclude early or partial torsion

---

- Hypoechoic areas associated with testicular infarction may have a linear appearance (due to accentuation of septula testis)
- Poor testicular echogenicity correlates with prognosis, may indicate non-viability
- Subacute phase (1-10 days): Testis echogenicity decreases in initial 4-5 days, then may show focal or diffuse infarction; epididymis may remain echogenic
- Chronic phase: Small atrophied homogeneously hypoechoic testis; enlarged echogenic epididymis
  - Testicular infarction
    - Diffusely hypoechoic small testis/focal mass in infarcted testis
    - Hyperechoic regions (hemorrhage/fibrosis), focal infarctions may have linear appearance
    - Segmental infarction may follow inflammatory process (orchitis)
  - Potential pitfalls are changes due to orchitis, partial torsion, torsion/detorsion
- Color Doppler
  - Color Doppler is very useful to establish diagnosis of testicular torsion
  - In acute torsion sensitivity, 80-90%; 10% of patients with early or partial torsion have normal exam
    - Set-up optimized for detection of slow flow (low pulse repetition frequency, low wall filter, high Doppler gain)
  - Absent or decreased flow
  - Comparison with contralateral spermatic cord and testes is mandatory
  - In subacute or chronic torsion; no flow in testis and increased flow in paratesticular tissues, including epididymis-cord complex and dartos fascia
  - Role of spectral Doppler is limited; in partial torsion of 360° or less, spectral Doppler may show diminished diastolic arterial flow
  - Use of intravascular ultrasound contrast agents may improve sensitivity for detecting blood flow in testes

MR Findings

- Enlarged spermatic cord without increase in vascularity

- Whirlpool pattern (twisting of spermatic cord)
  - "Torsion knot" low signal intensity focus at point of twist (displacement of free water protons from epicenter of twist)

Nuclear Medicine Findings

- Tc-99m pertechnetate: Dynamic flow imaging at 2-5 second intervals for 1 minute (vascular phase); 5 minute intervals for tissue phase; sensitivity 80-90%
  - Can detect reduced or absent testicular flow in 94-99%
  - In testicular torsion, a rounded cold area and a halo of dartos perfusion is seen
    - In "missed" testicular torsion, scrotal scan shows "halo sign" in tissue phase due to intense vascularity in dartos, and "nubbin sign" in perfusion phase due to increased perfusion of spermatic cord vessels

Imaging Recommendations

- Best imaging tool: US with high-frequency linear transducer & color/power Doppler
- Protocol advice: Compare grayscale, color Doppler appearances to contralateral normal testis

---

DIFFERENTIAL DIAGNOSIS

Testicular Trauma

- Hematocele, irregular contours, heterogeneous parenchymal echogenicity
- Avascular fracture plane

Testicular Abscess (Epididymo-Orchitis)

- Thick walled, hypoechoic focus with low level internal echoes, thickened tunica albuginea
- Enlarged hypoechoic epididymis with increased flow on color Doppler

Testicular Tumor

- Focal hypoechoic mass with heterogeneous areas
- Abnormal vascularity within the mass

TESTICULAR TORSION/INFARCTION

PATHOLOGY

General Features
- General path comments
  - Varying degrees of ischemic necrosis & fibrosis depending on duration of symptoms
  - Embryology-anatomy: Deficient testicular fixation related to tunica vaginalis & gubernaculum ("bell clapper" deformity); testicle rotates within scrotum and twists spermatic cord
  - Exocrine and endocrine function is substandard in men with history of unilateral torsion; following three theories explain the contralateral disease noted in torsion
    - Unrecognized or unreported repeated injury to both testes
    - Pre-existing pathologic condition predisposing both testes to abnormal spermatogenesis and torsion of spermatic cord
    - Induction of pathologic changes in the contralateral testis by retention of injured testis
- Etiology: Most occur spontaneously; rarely occurs traumatically
- Epidemiology: Infant & adolescent boys most often affected

Gross Pathologic & Surgical Features
- Purple, edematous, ischemic testicle, may rapidly re-perfuse when manually de-torsed

Microscopic Features
- Hemorrhagic, interstitial edema; necrosis

Staging, Grading or Classification Criteria
- Intravaginal torsion: Common type, most frequently occurs at puberty
  - Results from anomalous suspension of testis by long stalk of spermatic cord, leading to complete investment of testis and epididymis by tunica vaginalis "bell clapper"
  - Anomalous testicular suspension is bilateral in 50-80%
  - 10 fold increase incidence of torsion in undescended testis after orchiopexy
- Extravaginal torsion: Occurs in newborn
  - No "bell clapper" deformity
  - Due to poor or absent attachment of testis to scrotal wall, allowing rotation of testis, epididymis and tunica vaginalis as a unit and causing torsion of the cord at the level of external inguinal ring

CLINICAL ISSUES

Presentation
- Most common signs/symptoms
  - Acute scrotal/inguinal pain; swollen, erythematous hemiscrotum without recognized trauma
  - Other signs/symptoms: Low grade torsion may be tolerated for long periods
- Clinical Profile: > 15 years, male child with acute scrotal pain

Natural History & Prognosis
- Testis usually turns medially up to 1,080°, three full revolutions
  - Diminished blood flow in < 180°, torsion at 1 hour
  - Testicular viability depends on degree of torsion (> 540° worse) and duration of symptoms
  - Absent blood flow occurs with any degree of torsion lasting > 4 hours
- Surgical emergency: Testicular infarction if not treated promptly
- Unilateral testicular loss typically does not lead to infertility

Treatment
- Surgical exploration; de-torsion; bilateral orchidopexy if viable testicle
  - Non-viable testicle usually removed; higher risk of subsequent torsion on contralateral side
- Delaying surgical intervention worsens the intra-operative testicular salvage rate and the extent of subsequent testicular atrophy
- Delay between the onset of symptoms and the time of surgical or manual detorsion is of utmost importance in preserving a viable testis
- Salvage rate of testis versus time interval between onset of pain and surgery
  - 80-100% ⇒ < 6 hours
  - 76% ⇒ 6-12 hours
  - 20% ⇒ 12-24 hours
  - 0% ⇒ > 24 hours

DIAGNOSTIC CHECKLIST

Consider
- Normal US (grayscale & Doppler) does not exclude early or partial torsion
  - Repeat examination at 1-4 hour intervals if conservatively managed

Image Interpretation Pearls
- Decreased or absent flow on Doppler examination

SELECTED REFERENCES

1. Schalamon J et al: Management of acute scrotum in children--the impact of Doppler ultrasound. J Pediatr Surg. 41(8):1377-80, 2006
2. Dogra V et al: Acute painful scrotum. Radiol Clin North Am. 42(2):349-63, 2004
3. Dogra VS et al: Torsion and beyond: new twists in spectral Doppler evaluation of the scrotum. J Ultrasound Med. 23(8):1077-85, 2004
4. Dogra VS et al: Sonography of the scrotum. Radiology. 227(1):18-36, 2003
5. Arce JD et al: Sonographic diagnosis of acute spermatic cord torsion. Rotation of the cord: a key to the diagnosis. Pediatr Radiol. 32(7):485-91, 2002
6. Sidhu PS. Related Articles et al: Clinical and imaging features of testicular torsion: role of ultrasound. Clin Radiol. 54(6):343-52, 1999

IMAGE GALLERY

Typical

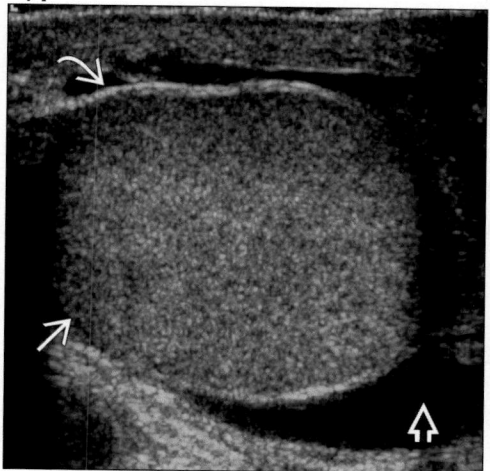
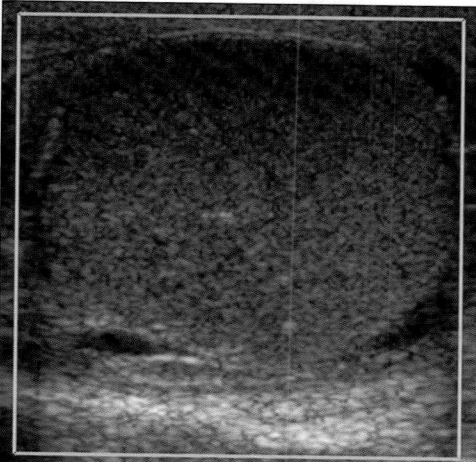

(Left) Longitudinal grayscale ultrasound shows an enlarged hypoechoic testis ➡ in subacute torsion. Note thickened tunica albuginea ➡ and minimal hydrocele ➡. Features may simulate epididymo-orchitis. Doppler helps to differentiate. *(Right)* Longitudinal power Doppler ultrasound shows an enlarged hypoechoic testis in a 20 year old man with no intratesticular blood flow. Surgically proven to be acute torsion.

Typical

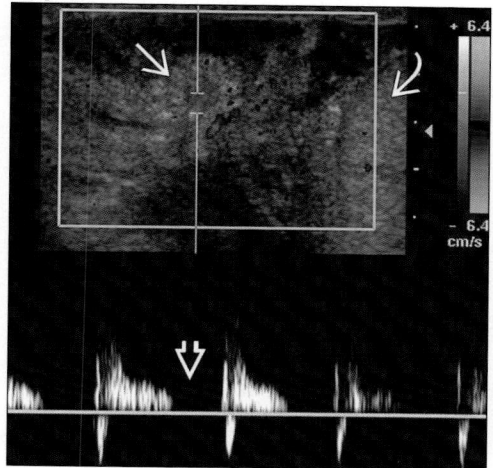
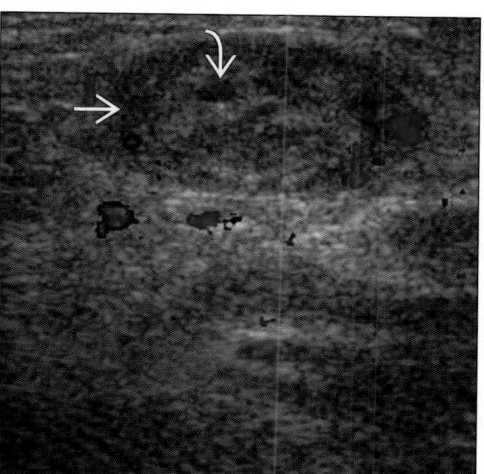

(Left) Longitudinal color Doppler ultrasound shows a "torsion knot" or "whirlpool" pattern ➡ of the spermatic cord immediately cranial to the testis ➡. Spectral waveform shows no diastolic flow ➡. *(Right)* Transverse color Doppler ultrasound (same patient as previous image) shows an enlarged, hypoechoic spermatic cord ➡ immediately proximal to the "torsion knot". Note absent flow in cord vessels ➡.

Typical

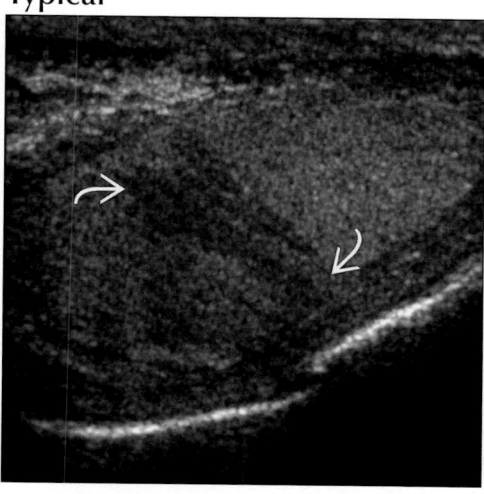
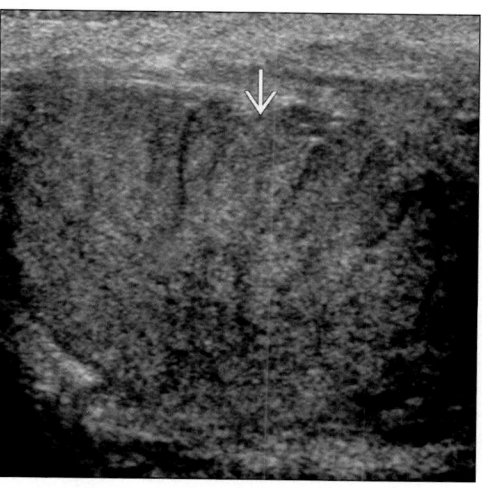

(Left) Oblique ultrasound shows well-demarcated hypoechoic foci ➡ in a testis with previous vascular insult due to partial torsion. Features suggest testicular infarct. *(Right)* Oblique ultrasound shows a moderately shrunken, heterogeneous testis ➡ in a patient with chronic testicular torsion.

SCROTAL TRAUMA

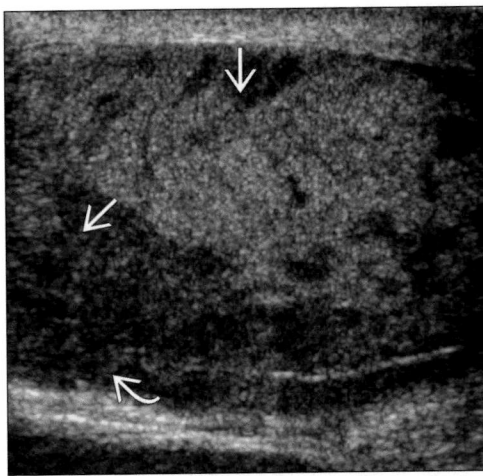
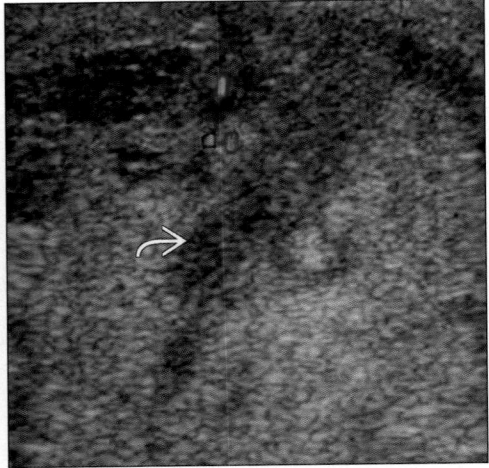

Longitudinal ultrasound shows a heterogeneous testis with irregular, poorly-defined hypoechoic foci ➡. Note interruption of the tunica albuginea ➡ indicating testicular rupture.

Oblique color Doppler ultrasound shows a hypoechoic, avascular, wedge-shaped, testicular fracture ➡.

TERMINOLOGY

Abbreviations and Synonyms
- Testicular rupture, fracture of testis, hematocele

Definitions
- Laceration of tunica albuginea, extrusion of testicular tissue into scrotal sac, collection of blood in tunica vaginalis or scrotal wall

IMAGING FINDINGS

General Features
- Best diagnostic clue: Heterogeneous parenchymal echogenicity of testis on sonography in patients with history of scrotal trauma
- Morphology: Irregularity of testicular contour

Ultrasonographic Findings
- Grayscale Ultrasound
  - Hematocele: Hemorrhage contained within layers of tunica vaginalis
    - Acute hematocele may be echo-lucent
    - Acute echogenic hematocele: Extrusion of disrupted testis most likely
    - Chronic hematocele; linear stranding, septations ± calcification
  - Testicular injury: Testicular rupture, fracture of testis
    - Abnormal testicular parenchymal echogenicity
    - Focal intraparenchymal testicular hematoma
    - Discrete linear or irregular fracture plane within testis (17%)
  - Epididymal injury: Focal epididymal enlargement with reduced echogenicity & abnormal position in relation to testis
- Color Doppler
  - Distorted intratesticular vascularity with interruption of vessels in area of injury
  - Avascular intratesticular hematoma on color Doppler
  - Post-traumatic epididymitis; enlarged epididymis with increased flow

Imaging Recommendations
- Best imaging tool
  - High-resolution US (≥ 7.5 MHz)

DDx: Scrotal Trauma

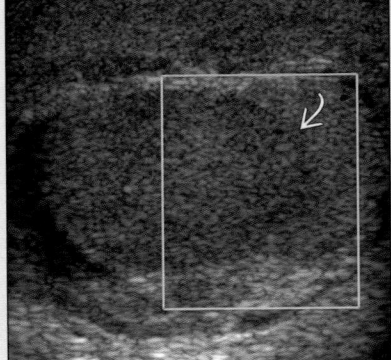
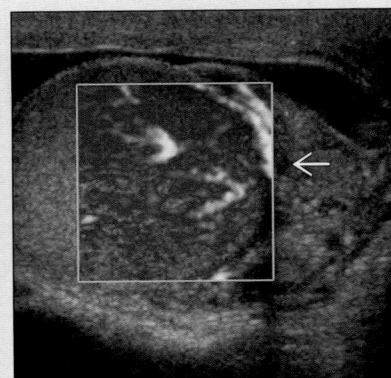
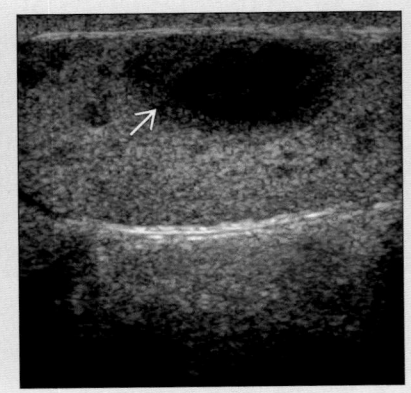

| Testicular Torsion | Epididymo-Orchitis | Testicular Abscess |

SCROTAL TRAUMA

Key Facts

Imaging Findings
- Best diagnostic clue: Heterogeneous parenchymal echogenicity of testis on sonography in patients with history of scrotal trauma
- Hematocele: Hemorrhage contained within layers of tunica vaginalis
- Acute hematocele may be echo-lucent
- Testicular injury: Testicular rupture, fracture of testis
- Abnormal testicular parenchymal echogenicity

- Avascular intratesticular hematoma on color Doppler

Top Differential Diagnoses
- Testicular Torsion
- Epididymo-Orchitis
- Testicular Abscess

Diagnostic Checklist
- Irregularity of testicular contour, heterogeneous parenchyma and echogenic collection

○ Foreign body and air in scrotal collection can be precisely localized

- Intratesticular: Injury to tunica albuginea and testicular parenchyma

DIFFERENTIAL DIAGNOSIS

Testicular Torsion
- ↓ Overall vascularity compared to normal testis

Epididymo-Orchitis
- Acute or chronic pain without history of trauma, enlarged hypoechoic epididymis with increased vascularity in epididymis and testis on color Doppler

Testicular Abscess
- Focal ill defined, thick walled mass & necrotic centre

PATHOLOGY

General Features
- General path comments: Capsular disruption: Hematocele, necrotic testicular parenchyma extrudes into tunica vaginalis
- Etiology
  ○ Sports injuries, vehicular and ballistic trauma
  ○ Blunt trauma impales scrotal contents to symphysis pubis or pubic rami, pelvic fracture

Staging, Grading or Classification Criteria
- Extratesticular: Injury to scrotal wall or tunica vaginalis

CLINICAL ISSUES

Presentation
- Most common signs/symptoms: Acute scrotal hematoma following blunt trauma

Natural History & Prognosis
- Unless repaired within 72 hours, salvage rate only 45%

Treatment
- Drainage: Hematocele
- Orchidectomy: Non viable testis

DIAGNOSTIC CHECKLIST

Image Interpretation Pearls
- Irregularity of testicular contour, heterogeneous parenchyma and echogenic collection

SELECTED REFERENCES
1. Micallef M et al: Ultrasound features of blunt testicular injury. Injury. 32(1):23-6, 2001
2. Simmons MZ: Re: Accuracy of ultrasound diagnosis after blunt testicular trauma. J Urol. 152(3):968-9, 1994

IMAGE GALLERY

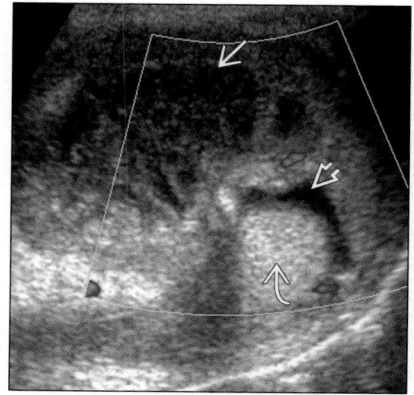 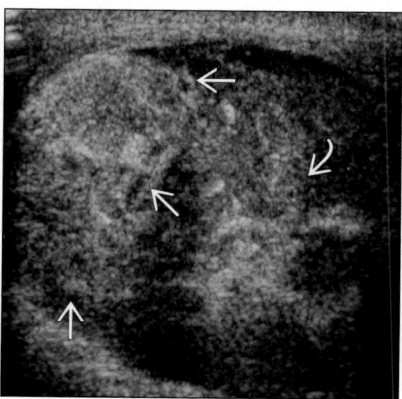 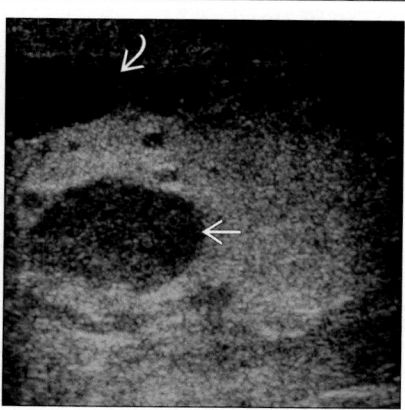

(Left) Transverse power Doppler ultrasound shows a heterogeneous, avascular, organized scrotal wall hematoma ➡. Note compressed ipsilateral testis ➡ and minimal fluid in tunica vaginalis ➡. *(Center)* Oblique ultrasound shows an enlarged, hyperechoic, heterogeneous epididymis ➡ and superior pole of testis ➡ suggesting acute hematoma in a patient with history of scrotal trauma. *(Right)* Oblique ultrasound shows a hypoechoic area within the testis ➡ representing intraparenchymal hematoma. Note surrounding hematocele ➡.

EPIDYMAL MASSES

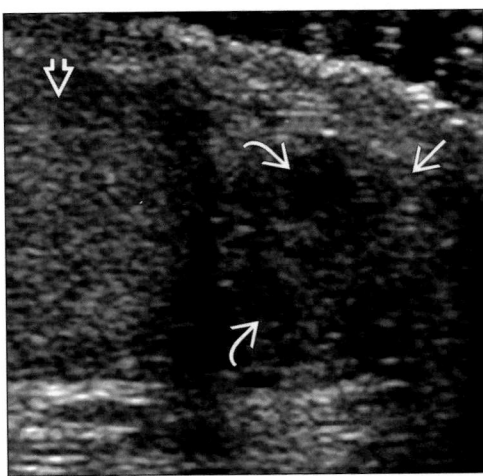

Longitudinal grayscale ultrasound shows an ill-defined, solid, heterogeneous mass ➡, with scattered small cysts ➡, in the epididymal tail. Final diagnosis: Papillary cystadenoma. Normal testis ➡.

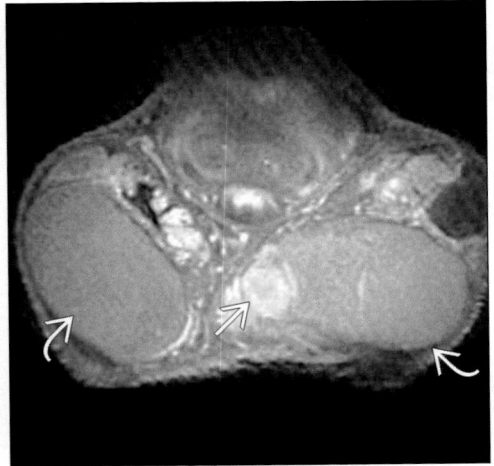

Coronal post-contrast T1WI MR of scrotum (same patient as previous image) shows the enhancing papillary cystadenoma ➡ in left epididymis. Note normal testis ➡ bilaterally.

TERMINOLOGY

Definitions
- Extratesticular neoplasms are rare but clinically significant lesions that affect patients of all ages

IMAGING FINDINGS

General Features
- Location
  - Epididymal cyst: Throughout length of epididymis
  - Spermatocele: Usually head of epididymis
  - Inflammatory mass: Chemical epididymitis involves tail and vas deferens
    - Infective epididymitis involves any part of epididymis
  - Tumors: More frequent in tail of epididymis
- Size
  - Epididymal cyst: 1-4 cm, usually ≤ 1 cm
  - Spermatocele: 1-2 cm
  - Adenomatoid tumor: 3 mm to 5 cm
  - Papillary cystadenoma of epididymis: 1.5-2 cm solid mass

- Morphology
  - Cysts: Most common epididymal mass (20-40%), multiple (29%)
    - Spermatocele: Obstruction and dilatation of efferent ductal system, may show septae, fluid containing spermatozoa and sediment containing lymphocytes, fat globules and cellular debris giving a thick milky appearance to the fluid
    - Epididymal cyst: Lymphatic in origin
  - Inflammatory masses (epididymitis): Focal or diffuse involvement of epididymis
  - Tumor masses
    - Lipoma is the most common extratesticular neoplasm, commonly involves spermatic cord
    - Benign tumors: Solid, well-circumscribed masses
    - Malignant tumors: Sarcoma, metastases, adenocarcinoma

Ultrasonographic Findings
- Grayscale Ultrasound
  - Epididymal cyst: Aspiration of cyst content is diagnostic
    - Simple epididymal cyst: Well-defined, anechoic mass with increased through-transmission

DDx: Epididymal Masses

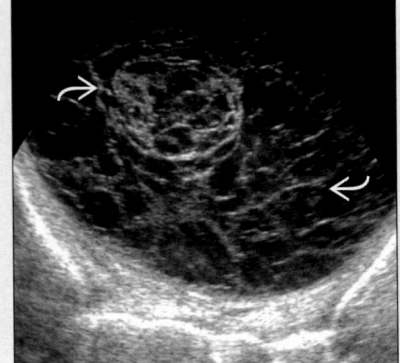

Chronic Hydrocele

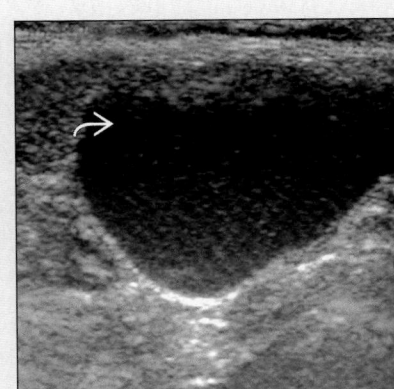

Encysted Hydrocele of Cord

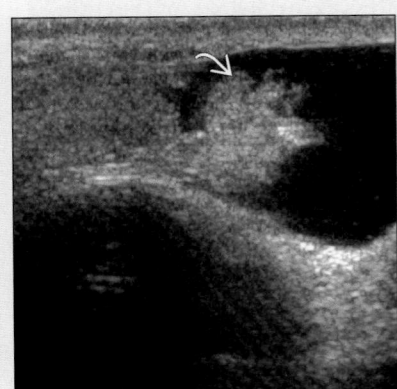

Scrotal Hernia

EPIDIDYMAL MASSES

Key Facts

Imaging Findings
- Lipoma is the most common extratesticular neoplasm, commonly involves spermatic cord
- Benign tumors: Solid well-circumscribed masses
- Leiomyoma, papillary cystadenoma: Large, solid tumors, echogenic, ± cystic spaces
- Adenomatoid tumor: May have variable ultrasound appearances, but typically seen as well-circumscribed, homogeneous, hyperechoic mass
- Lipoma: Homogeneous hyperechoic in appearance, variable size
- In patients with papillary cystadenoma, examine the abdomen to evaluate for concomitant masses, solid organ cysts and other features of von Hippel-Lindau disease

- Malignant tumors: Sarcoma, metastases; nonspecific sonological features
- Sarcoid granuloma: Epididymis is diffusely enlarged, heterogeneous ± solitary hypoechoic mass ± multiple small distinct nodules
- Fibrous pseudotumor: Heterogeneous, paratesticular masses with variable echo pattern
- Inflammatory masses: ↑ Flow on color Doppler (CD)
- Benign/malignant tumors; variable flow on CD
- Best imaging tool: High resolution US (≥ 7.5 MHz) is imaging modality of choice

Top Differential Diagnoses
- Chronic Hydrocele
- Encysted Hydrocele of Cord
- Scrotal Hernia

- Spermatocele: Similar in appearance to epididymal cyst, usually have low level echoes, rarely spermatoceles may be hyperechoic
- Large cysts (either true cysts or spermatocele) may have septations and may be confused with hydrocele; cysts displace the testis, while hydrocele envelopes it
- Inflammatory masses
  - Acute epididymitis: Enlarged, heterogeneous and hypoechoic epididymis; scrotal wall thickening ± hydrocele
  - Chronic epididymitis: Enlarged epididymis with variable appearance, ranging from hypoechoic to hyperechoic, ± calcification
  - Chemical epididymitis: Changes similar to acute epididymitis, limited to tail of epididymis
- Benign tumors: Solid well-circumscribed masses
  - Leiomyoma, papillary cystadenoma: Large, solid tumors, echogenic, ± cystic spaces
  - Adenomatoid tumor: May have variable ultrasound appearances, but typically seen as well-circumscribed, homogeneous, hyperechoic mass
  - Lipoma: Homogeneous hyperechoic in appearance, variable size
- In patients with papillary cystadenoma, examine the abdomen to evaluate for concomitant masses, solid organ cysts and other features of von Hippel-Lindau disease
- Malignant tumors: Sarcoma, metastases; nonspecific sonological features
- Granulomatous disease: Sarcoidosis, tuberculosis
  - Sarcoid granuloma: Epididymis is diffusely enlarged, heterogeneous ± solitary hypoechoic mass ± multiple small distinct nodules
  - Sperm granuloma: Well-demarcated hypoechoic intra epididymal mass ± calcification
- Fibrous pseudotumor: Heterogeneous, paratesticular masses with variable echo pattern
  - Echogenic reactive fibrous tissue may be seen in tunica vaginalis or epididymis
- Color Doppler

- Inflammatory masses: ↑ Flow on color Doppler (CD)
- Benign/malignant tumors; variable flow on CD

MR Findings
- Lipoma: High signal intensity on T1WI
- Sarcoidosis: Both epididymis appear enlarged, heterogeneous and nodular without any signs of testicular involvement; lesion shows mild T2 hyperintensity

Imaging Recommendations
- Best imaging tool: High resolution US (≥ 7.5 MHz) is imaging modality of choice

DIFFERENTIAL DIAGNOSIS

Chronic Hydrocele
- Multiple septations with layering sediment, enveloping testis
- Diffuse thickening of scrotal wall and its lining, tunica vaginalis thickening usually seen
- ± Calcification of wall and contents

Encysted Hydrocele of Cord
- Patent processus vaginalis, seen in infants, associated ascites may be evident
- Elongated fluid collection above the level of testis and epididymis

Scrotal Hernia
- Herniating mesentery ± bowel, mucosal lining of bowel visible, Valsalva maneuver accentuation
- May undergo bowel obstruction ± strangulation

PATHOLOGY

General Features
- Etiology
  - Spermatocele: Obstruction and dilatation of efferent ductal system in post-vasectomy patient
  - Acute infection: N. gonorrhea; chlamydia trachomatis

EPIDIDYMAL MASSES

○ Chronic infection: Tuberculosis, syphilis, parasites
  ▪ Chronic epididymitis usually results from incompletely treated bacterial epididymitis, infections like tuberculosis spread from the adjoining genito-urinary tract
○ Chemical epididymitis due to reflux of sterile urine
○ Sperm granuloma result from extravasation of spermatozoa inducing a necrotizing granulomatous response
• Epidemiology
  ○ Most common mass is cyst; 20-40% of asymptomatic individuals
    ▪ 29% have more than one cyst
  ○ Sarcoidosis most frequently involves epididymis
  ○ Adenomatoid tumor most common epididymal tumor; benign, accounts for 30% of all paratesticular neoplasms
  ○ Genital tract lymphoma; predominantly seen in testis but involves epididymis in 60% and the spermatic cord in 40%
  ○ Malignant tumors; 25% of solid tumors of epididymis are malignant; majority are metastases
• Associated abnormalities
  ○ Papillary cystadenomas have strong association with von Hippel-Lindau disease (VHL)
    ▪ 25% of patients with VHL have epididymal cystadenoma
    ▪ 75% of patients of papillary cystadenoma have VHL
    ▪ Bilateral tumors are virtually pathognomonic for VHL

Gross Pathologic & Surgical Features
• True epididymal cyst lined with epithelium and contains clear serous fluid
  ○ Spermatoceles filled with thicker milky fluid containing spermatozoa, cellular debris
  ○ Differentiation between spermatocele and an epididymal cyst is rarely important clinically
• Lipoma of deeper structures vary much more in shape but also tend to be well delineated from the surrounding tissues by thin capsule
  ○ Uniform greasy surface with an irregular lobulated pattern
• Adenomatoid tumors occur throughout length of epididymis
  ○ Can be seen in spermatic cord and tunica albuginea, may grow intratesticularly, may become indistinguishable from germ cell tumors
• Papillary cystadenoma: Arise from ejaculatory ducts of testes, fibrous capsule surrounds the lesion, composed of multiple cysts lined by papillary fronds

Microscopic Features
• Adenomatoid tumor: Mesothelial in origin
• Papillary cystadenomas have prominent papillae lined by glycogen rich clear cells
• Sperm granuloma forms as a foreign body giant cell reaction to extravasated sperm
• Lipoma is composed of mature fat cells which are slightly larger than the surrounding fat cells
  ○ Admixture of other mesenchymal elements and fibrous connective tissue

○ Lipomas with significant fibrous connective tissue component are classified as fibrolipomas

CLINICAL ISSUES

Presentation
• Most common signs/symptoms
  ○ Most tumors; painless scrotal mass
  ○ Sperm granulomas may occasionally be painful
  ○ Chronic epididymal infection; may present as chronically painful scrotal mass

Demographics
• Age
  ○ Epididymal cyst: Any age
  ○ Adenomatoid tumors: ≥ 20 years
  ○ Papillary cystadenoma: Middle aged

Natural History & Prognosis
• Untreated granulomatous epididymitis will spread to testis in 60-80% of cases
  ○ Focal testicular involvement may simulate a testicular neoplasm
  ○ Tumor marker study will differentiate the two

Treatment
• Conservative management: Antibiotic if infective, analgesics if painful
  ○ Epididymectomy for neoplastic lesion if indicated
• Intrascrotal but extratesticular tumors should to be treated surgically
  ○ If tumor is benign, simple excision suffices
  ○ If malignant, inguinal lymphadenectomy and, as with testicular tumors, lymphography ± retroperitoneal lymphadenectomy
• ± Chemotherapy, ± radiotherapy

DIAGNOSTIC CHECKLIST

Consider
• As opposed to intratesticular masses, most extratesticular masses are benign
• Combination of clinical and US findings facilitates the differentiation between non-neoplastic and neoplastic extratesticular masses

SELECTED REFERENCES

1. Dogra VS et al: Sonography of the scrotum. Radiology. 227(1):18-36, 2003
2. Woodward PJ et al: From the archives of the AFIP: extratesticular scrotal masses: radiologic-pathologic correlation. Radiographics. 23(1):215-40, 2003
3. Ciftci AO et al: Testicular tumors in children. J Pediatr Surg. 36(12):1796-801, 2001
4. Tobias-machado M et al: Fibrous pseudotumor of tunica vaginalis and epididymis. Urology. 56(4):670-2, 2000
5. Frates MC et al: Solid extratesticular masses evaluated with sonography: pathologic correlation. Radiology. 204(1):43-6, 1997
6. Makarainen HP et al: Intrascrotal adenomatoid tumors and their ultrasound findings. J Clin Ultrasound. 21(1):33-7, 1993

EPIDIDYMAL MASSES

IMAGE GALLERY

Typical

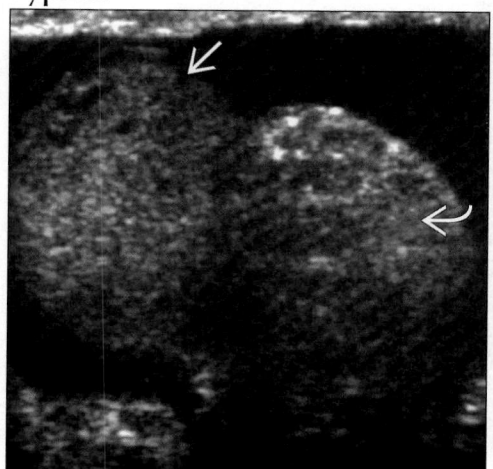
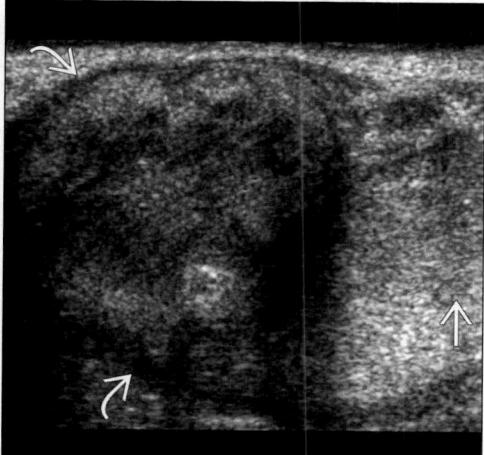

(Left) Oblique ultrasound shows a markedly enlarged, heterogeneous, predominantly hypoechoic epididymis ➔ suggesting granulomatous disease. Final diagnosis: Sarcoidosis. Normal testis ➔. *(Right)* Transverse grayscale ultrasound of the epididymal head shows a lobulated, heterogeneous, hypoechoic mass ➔, suggesting chronic granulomatous inflammatory mass. Final diagnosis: TB. Normal testis ➔.

Typical

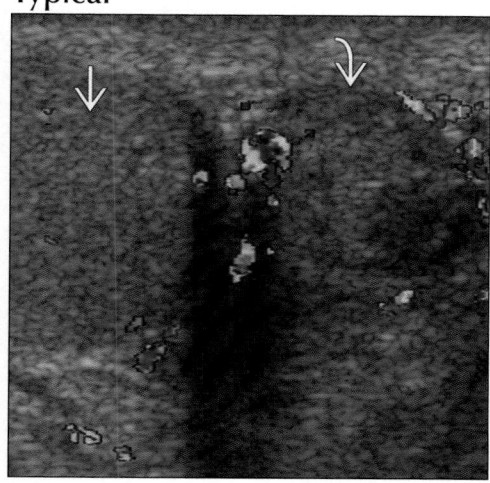
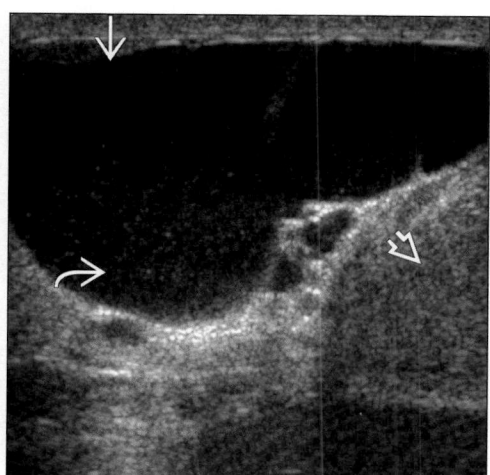

(Left) Longitudinal color Doppler ultrasound shows a well-defined, solid mass ➔ with peripheral vascularity in the head of epididymis. Final diagnosis: Adenomatoid tumor. Normal testis ➔. *(Right)* Longitudinal grayscale ultrasound shows a large, anechoic, septated cyst ➔, with layering of low-level echoes ➔, in the epididymal head, suggesting a spermatocele. Normal testis ➔.

Variant

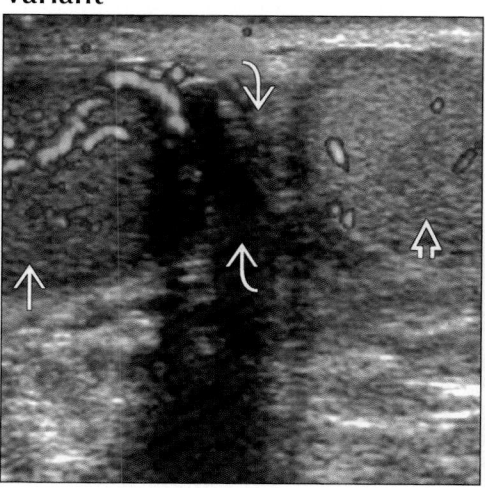
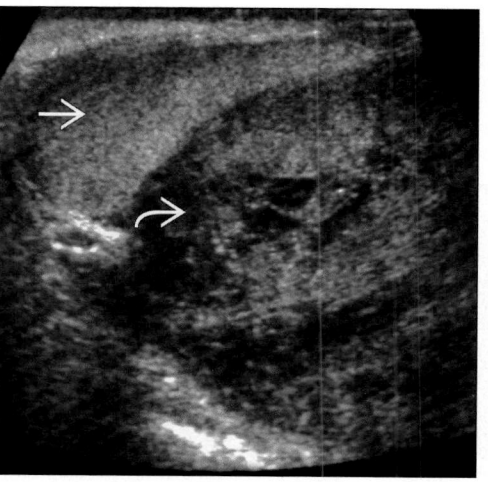

(Left) Longitudinal power Doppler ultrasound shows a well-defined mass ➔ slightly hyperechoic to the testis ➔ arising from the spermatic cord, indicative of lipoma. Note compressed epididymis ➔ between mass and testis ➔. *(Right)* Longitudinal ultrasound shows a large, heterogeneous, paratesticular mass ➔ compressing the testis ➔. The epididymis could not be separately seen. Final diagnosis: Epididymal rhabdomyosarcoma.

EPIDIDYMITIS/ORCHITIS

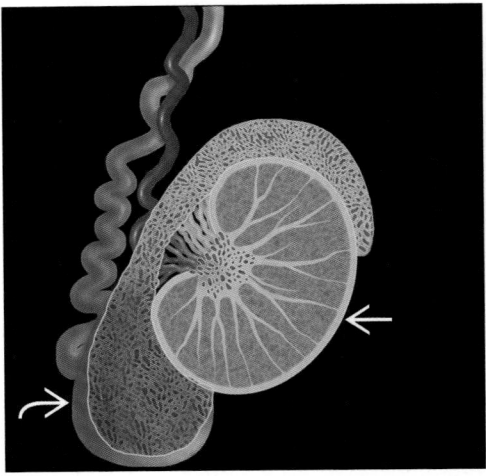

Graphic shows an enlarged and inflamed epididymis ➡ enveloping the testis posteriorly. Note testis ➡ appears normal in size and configuration.

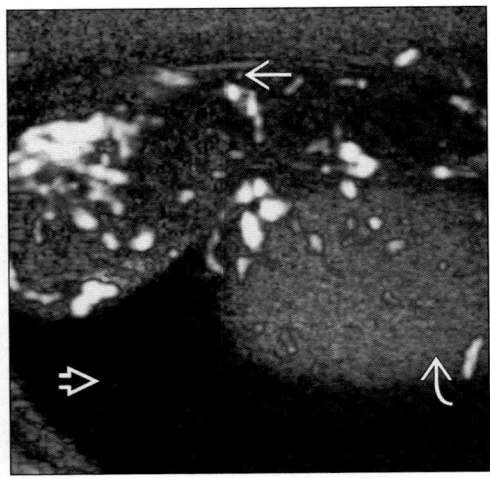

Oblique power Doppler ultrasound shows a markedly enlarged, hypoechoic epididymis, with increased vascularity ➡ suggesting acute epididymitis. Note normal testis ➡ & hydrocele ➡.

TERMINOLOGY

Abbreviations and Synonyms
- Acute scrotum, orchitis, epididymo-orchitis

Definitions
- Infectious inflammation of epididymis and/or testis

IMAGING FINDINGS

General Features
- Best diagnostic clue: Enlarged, hyperemic epididymis and/or testis on color Doppler US
- Location
  - Early epididymitis often involves tail of epididymis
  - Orchitis is usually secondary, occurring in 20-40% of epididymitis due to contiguous spread of infection
    - Primary orchitis is caused by mumps and is usually bilateral
- Size: Epididymis typically 2-3 times larger than normal
- Morphology: Focal enlargement of tail or diffuse enlargement of entire epididymis

Ultrasonographic Findings
- Grayscale Ultrasound
  - Epididymitis: Primarily involved in epididymo-orchitis
    - Acute epididymitis: Enlarged epididymis, decreased echogenicity, coarse heterogeneous echo pattern due to edema & hemorrhage
    - Chronic epididymitis: Enlarged hyperechoic epididymis
  - Orchitis follows in 20-40% of epididymitis due to contiguous spread of infection
    - Orchitis is characterized by edema of the testes contained within a rigid tunica albuginea resulting in heterogeneous parenchymal echogenicity and septal accentuation visible as hypoechoic bands; may be focal or diffuse
    - Focal orchitis: Hypoechoic area adjacent to enlarged portion of epididymis
    - Diffuse orchitis: Testis is diffusely enlarged with inhomogeneous echo pattern, thickening of tunica albuginea (in severe infection)

DDx: Epididymo-Orchitis

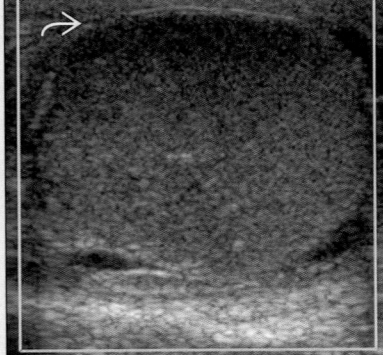

Testicular Torsion

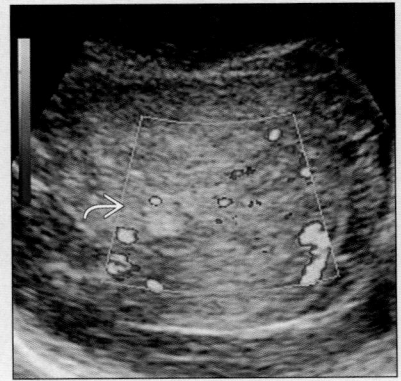

Testicular Lymphoma

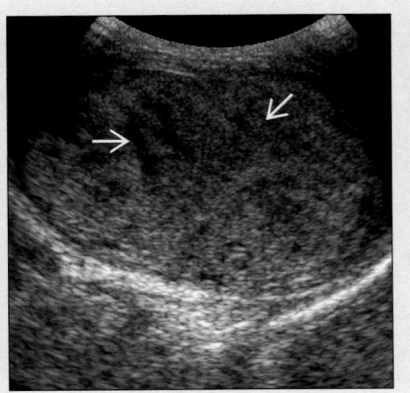

Testicular Trauma

EPIDIDYMITIS/ORCHITIS

Key Facts

Imaging Findings

- Best diagnostic clue: Enlarged, hyperemic epididymis and/or testis on color Doppler US
- Acute epididymitis: Enlarged epididymis, decreased echogenicity, coarse heterogeneous echo pattern due to edema & hemorrhage
- Chronic epididymitis: Enlarged hyperechoic epididymis
- Orchitis follows in 20-40% of epididymitis due to contiguous spread of infection
- Diffuse orchitis: Testis is diffusely enlarged with inhomogeneous echo pattern, thickening of tunica albuginea (in severe infection)
- Spermatic cord may be inflamed, and may appear hypoechoic with associated hyperechoic fat within

- Reactive hydrocele containing low level internal echoes, septae, thickening of tunical layers ± skin edema, all represent changes of periorchitis
- Color Doppler is highly sensitive and specific for epididymo-orchitis
- On color Doppler hyperemia is seen as ↑ number & concentration of vessels in affected region
- Diffuse or focal hyperemia in body and tail of epididymis ± increased vascularity of testis
- In severe epididymo-orchitis, relatively avascular areas within hyperemic testis or epididymis suggests focal infarction

Top Differential Diagnoses

- Testicular Torsion
- Testicular Lymphoma
- Testicular Trauma

- Ischemic changes may result from vascular compromise resulting in testicular infarction with sonographic features indistinguishable from testicular torsion
- Increased intratesticular pressure due to edema and congestion, may lead to venous infarction, may show heterogeneous echo pattern, predominantly hyperechoic initially and hypoechoic later
- Spermatic cord may be inflamed, and may appear hypoechoic with associated hyperechoic fat within
- Reactive hydrocele containing low level internal echoes, septae, thickening of tunical layers ± skin edema, all represent changes of periorchitis
- Color Doppler
  - Color Doppler is highly sensitive and specific for epididymo-orchitis
  - On color Doppler hyperemia is seen as ↑ number & concentration of vessels in affected region
  - Diffuse or focal hyperemia in body and tail of epididymis ± increased vascularity of testis
  - While echogenicity is variable; Doppler flow is invariably increased
  - Increased flow in the tunica vasculosa may be visible as lines of color signal radiating from the mediastinum testis
  - In severe epididymo-orchitis, relatively avascular areas within hyperemic testis or epididymis suggests focal infarction
  - Reversal of arterial diastolic flow of testis (seen due to epididymal edema with obstruction of venous outflow/venous infarction), is an ominous finding associated with testicular infarction in cases with severe epididymo-orchitis
  - Inflammation of epididymis and testis is associated with ↓ vascular resistance compared with healthy individuals
    - Resistive index (RI) less than 0.5 (normal RI in testis ≥ 0.5)

Nuclear Medicine Findings

- Tc-99m: 90% accurate in differentiating torsion from epididymitis

- Increased flow within testicular vessels and vas deferens on flow study
- Markedly increased perfusion through spermatic cord vessels (testicular + deferential arteries)
- Curvilinear increased activity laterally in hemiscrotum on static images (also centrally if testis is involved)

Imaging Recommendations

- Best imaging tool: Color Doppler US; high frequency transducers (≥ 10 MHz)
- Protocol advice: Comparison with contralateral testis is useful when increase in vascularity is subtle

DIFFERENTIAL DIAGNOSIS

Testicular Torsion

- Absent or diminished color Doppler flow, "twist" of spermatic cord in inguinal region
- Epididymis may be enlarged but not hyperemic on color Doppler US
- Clinical differentiation results in 50% false positive rate and unnecessary surgical exploration

Testicular Lymphoma

- Often large in size at the time of diagnosis, commonly occurs in association with disseminated disease
- Heterogeneous echo pattern, often bilateral, involvement of epididymis and spermatic cord is common, hemorrhage and necrosis is rare

Testicular Trauma

- History of trauma; acute pain
- Focal hypoechoic avascular area on color Doppler; rupture of tunica albuginea associated hematocele

PATHOLOGY

General Features

- General path comments: Infectious inflammatory response, can lead to abscess if not treated (6%)

EPIDIDYMITIS/ORCHITIS

- Etiology
  - Bacterial seeding occurs directly in cases with genitourinary (GU) anomaly, and presumably hematogenously in cases without demonstrable anomaly
  - Ascending genito-urinary tract infection: Chlamydia, E. coli, Staphylococcus aureus, M. tuberculosis, mumps virus
    - In prepubertal boys and in men over 35 years of age, the disease is most frequently caused by E. coli, pseudomonas, klebsiella and Proteus mirabilis
  - Primary orchitis is rare and is caused by mumps
  - Drugs such as amiodarone hydrochloride may cause chemical epididymitis
- Epidemiology: Most frequently seen in sexually active young men; also seen in infants and boys

Gross Pathologic & Surgical Features
- Treated surgically only if abscess forms despite antibiotic treatment

Microscopic Features
- Inflammatory infiltrate of testis and epididymis

Staging, Grading or Classification Criteria
- Epididymitis: Isolated epididymitis, focal or diffuse
  - Acute/chronic epididymitis
- Orchitis or combined epididymitis & orchitis
  - Primary: Isolated orchitis (may be seen in boys with mumps)
  - Secondary: Infection spread from adjacent epididymis
  - Acute/chronic orchitis or epididymo-orchitis

CLINICAL ISSUES

Presentation
- Most common signs/symptoms
  - Commonest cause of acute scrotal pain in adolescent boys and adults
  - Scrotal swelling, erythema; fever; dysuria
    - Scrotal pain due to epididymitis is usually relieved after elevation of testes (scrotum) over symphysis pubis (Prehn sign)
    - Prehn sign may help clinically to differentiate epididymo-orchitis from torsion of spermatic cord
  - Associated lower urinary tract infection and its symptoms, urethral discharge
- Other signs/symptoms
  - Pyuria (95%), prostatic tenderness (infrequent)
  - Negative tumor markers like human chorionic gonadotropin (hCG), alpha-fetoprotein (AFP)
- Clinical Profile: Positive urinalysis for WBC and bacteria; may have elevated WBC

Demographics
- Age: Most commonly 15-35 years

Natural History & Prognosis
- Prognosis excellent if treated early with antibiotics
- Complications

- Testicular infarction, intra testicular abscess formation - sequale of epididymo-orchitis
  - Abscess formation (epididymal abscess - 6%, testicular abscess - 6%), microabscesses are usually seen in low grade infection such as tuberculosis and in immunocompromised host
  - Testicular ischemia if thrombosis of main testicular artery or its branches with chronic inflammation
  - Venous infarction: Due to venous outflow obstruction
  - Gangrene is rare but a known complication
  - Late testicular atrophy (21%)
  - Hydropyocele, Fournier gangrene
- Recurrent infection may lead to infertility

Treatment
- Antibiotic therapy; follow-up scans to exclude abscess if no improvement
- Work-up for GU anomalies in younger children and recurrent cases
- Bed rest, scrotal elevation, analgesics

DIAGNOSTIC CHECKLIST

Consider
- Torsion if low or absent flow within testis

Image Interpretation Pearls
- Hyperemic and enlarged epididymis and/or testis

SELECTED REFERENCES

1. Aso C et al: Gray-scale and color Doppler sonography of scrotal disorders in children: an update. Radiographics. 25(5):1197-214, 2005
2. Dogra V et al: Acute painful scrotum. Radiol Clin North Am. 42(2):349-63, 2004
3. Dogra VS et al: Sonography of the scrotum. Radiology. 227(1):18-36, 2003
4. Kraus SJ: Genitourinary imaging in children. Pediatr Clin North Am. 48(6):1381-424, 2001
5. Munden MM et al: Scrotal pathology in pediatrics with sonographic imaging. Curr Probl Diagn Radiol. 29(6):185-205, 2000
6. Dubinsky TJ et al: Color-flow and power Doppler imaging of the testes. World J Urol. 16(1):35-40, 1998
7. Chung JJ et al: Sonographic findings in tuberculous epididymitis and epididymo-orchitis. J Clin Ultrasound. 25(7):390-4, 1997
8. Herbener TE. Related Articles et al: Ultrasound in the assessment of the acute scrotum. J Clin Ultrasound. 24(8):405-21, 1996
9. Bukowski TP et al: Epididymitis in older boys: dysfunctional voiding as an etiology. J Urol. 154(2 Pt 2):762-5, 1995
10. Atkinson GO Jr et al: The normal and abnormal scrotum in children: evaluation with color Doppler sonography. AJR Am J Roentgenol. 158(3):613-7, 1992
11. Deeg KH et al: Colour Doppler imaging--a new method to differentiate torsion of the spermatic cord and epididymo-orchitis. Eur J Pediatr. 149(4):253-5, 1990

EPIDIDYMITIS/ORCHITIS

Typical

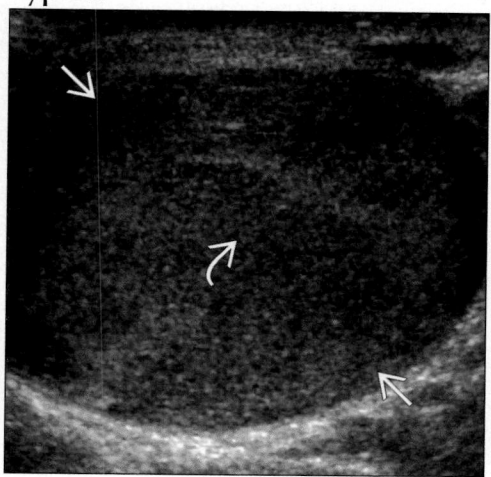
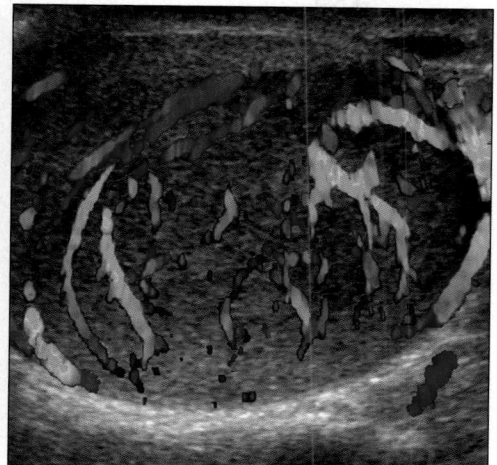

(Left) Transverse grayscale ultrasound shows an enlarged, diffusely hypoechoic testis ➡ more pronounced in the perihilar region ➡, suggesting acute orchitis. *(Right)* Transverse color Doppler ultrasound (same patient as previous image) shows marked increase in vascularity of testis in acute orchitis.

Typical

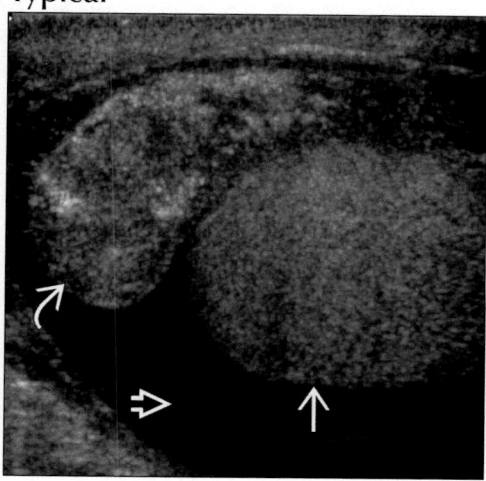
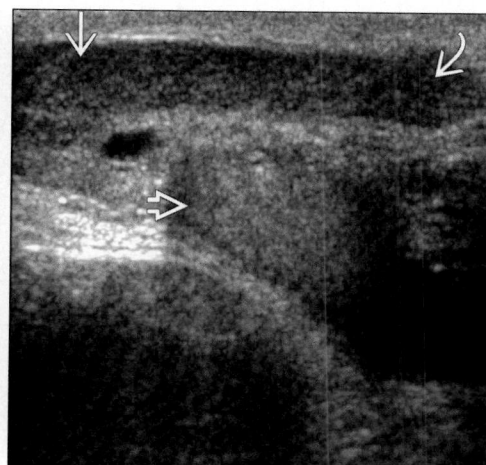

(Left) Longitudinal grayscale ultrasound shows a diffusely enlarged, heterogeneous epididymis ➡ and hypoechoic, heterogeneous adjacent testis ➡ suggesting acute epididymo-orchitis. Note hydrocele ➡. *(Right)* Longitudinal grayscale ultrasound of the scrotum shows an enlarged and hypoechoic body ➡ and tail ➡ of the epididymis. Features suggest epididymitis. Note normal testis ➡.

Typical

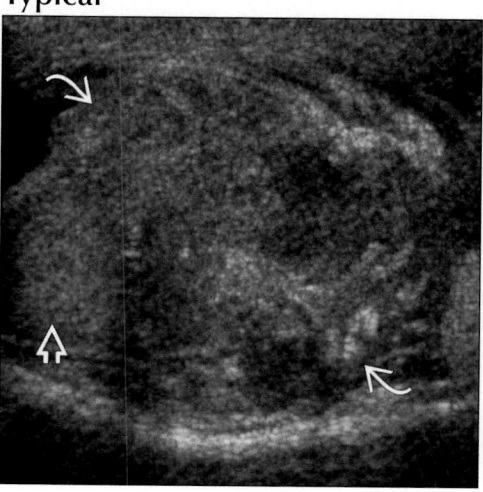
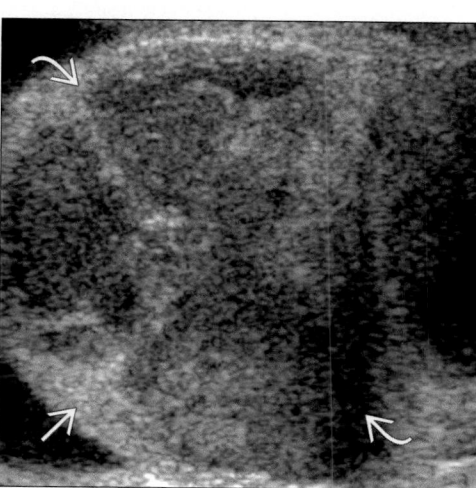

(Left) Oblique grayscale ultrasound of the scrotum shows an irregularly enlarged, hypoechoic, heterogeneous epididymal head ➡. Features of chronic epididymitis. Note normal testis ➡. *(Right)* Transverse grayscale ultrasound shows a hypoechoic, heterogeneous testis ➡ with thick tunica albuginea ➡. Features of chronic orchitis.

(Left) Graphic shows an irregularly enlarged epididymis ➡ with focal cystic areas ➡ indicating early liquefaction and necrosis. *(Right)* Oblique grayscale ultrasound shows an irregularly enlarged, heterogeneous epididymis ➡ with focal hypoechoic areas ➡ within it, indicating necrosis.

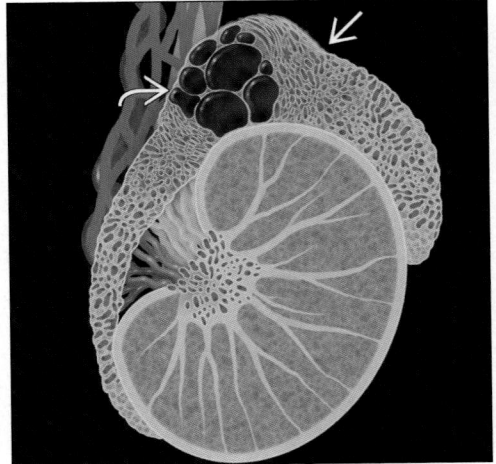
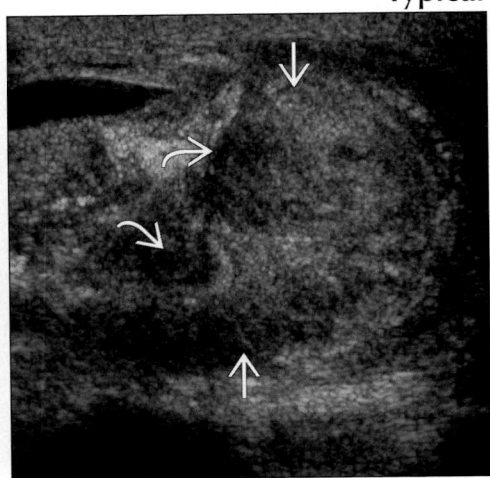

(Left) Oblique grayscale ultrasound shows an enlarged lobulated, predominantly hyperechoic, heterogeneous epididymis ➡ indicating epididymitis. Final diagnosis: Tuberculous epididymitis. *(Right)* Transverse grayscale ultrasound shows an enlarged, lobulated testis ➡ with heterogeneous echo pattern suggesting orchitis. Final diagnosis: Tuberculous orchitis.

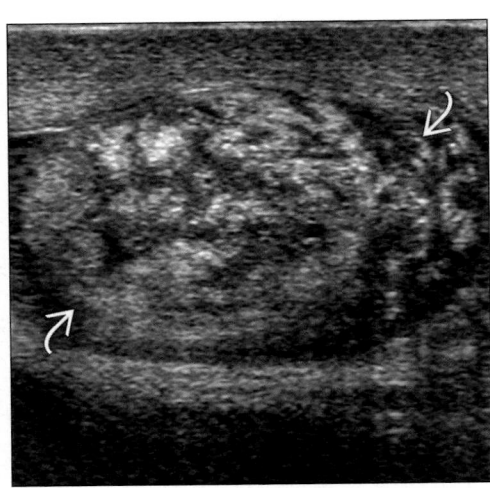
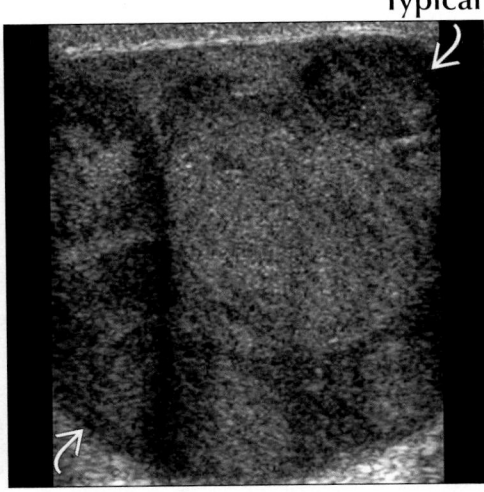

(Left) Longitudinal ultrasound shows an enlarged, heterogeneous, predominantly hypoechoic testis with multiple hypoechoic bands ➡ due to septal accentuation by edema and increased vascularity. *(Right)* Longitudinal grayscale ultrasound of scrotum shows a well-defined, hypoechoic area ➡ within the testicular substance indicative of focal orchitis.

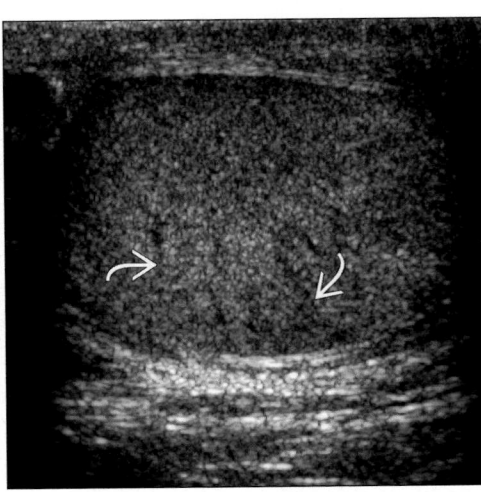
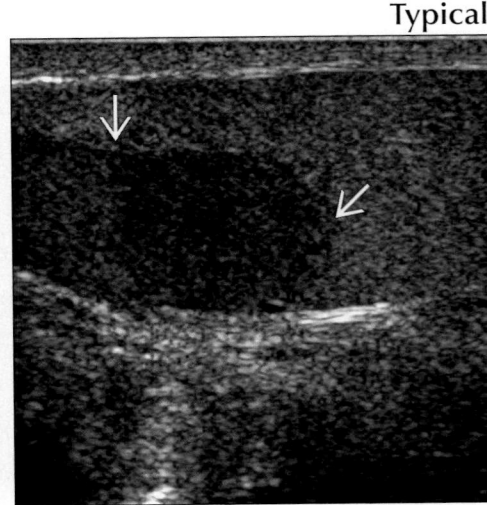

EPIDIDYMITIS/ORCHITIS

Typical

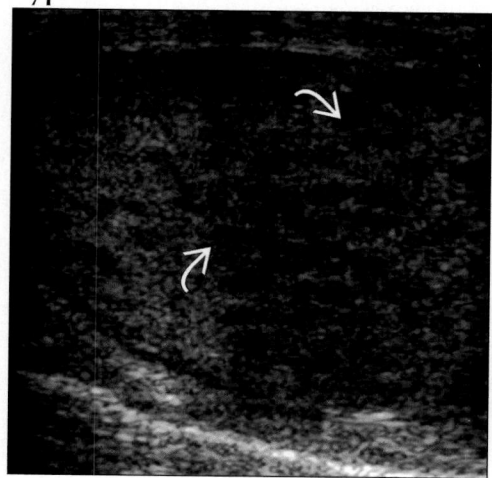

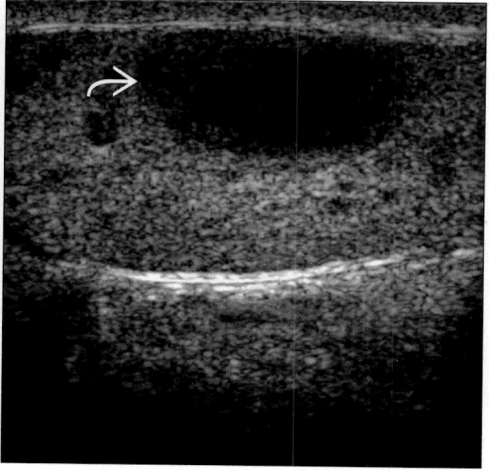

(Left) Longitudinal ultrasound shows multiple hypoechoic foci diffusely spread within the testicular parenchyma representing microabscesses ➡, features of tuberculous infection in immunocompromised host. (Right) Longitudinal ultrasound shows an ill-defined, hypoechoic area ➡ with irregular thick walls, in a patient with epididymo-orchitis. Features suggest testicular abscess.

Typical

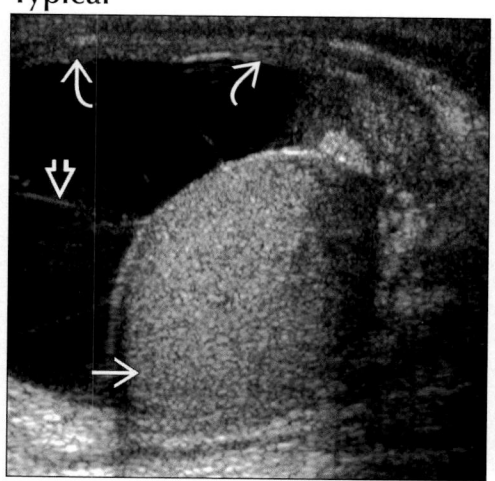

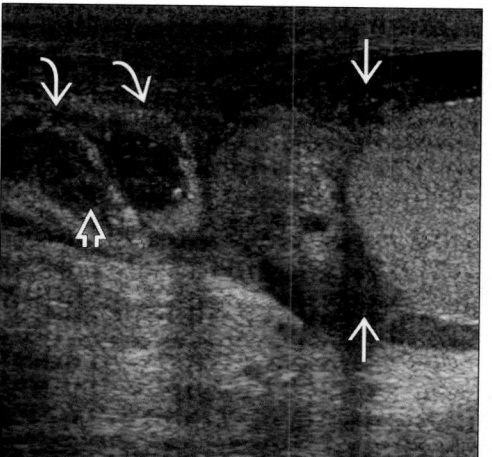

(Left) Transverse grayscale ultrasound shows a hyperechoic testis ➡ with a septate hydrocele ➡ and pachyvaginalitis ➡. Features suggest chronic orchitis and periorchitis. (Right) Longitudinal grayscale ultrasound at the inguinal canal shows an enlarged spermatic cord ➡ with a hypoechoic collection ➡, in a patient with epididymo-orchitis. Features of spermatic cord abscess. Note pyocele in tunica vaginalis ➡.

Typical

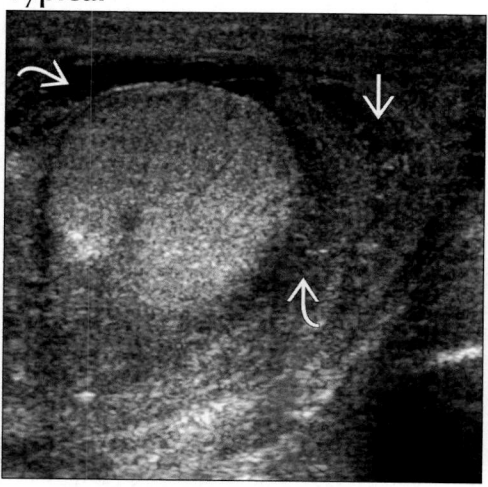

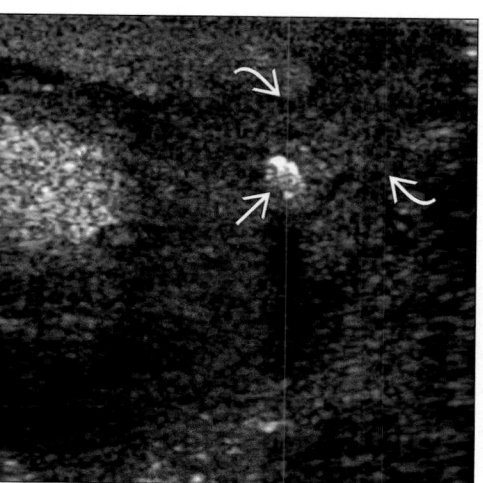

(Left) Oblique grayscale ultrasound of the scrotum shows a pyocele ➡ in the tunica vaginalis and a hypoechoic collection ➡ in the dartos muscle and subdartos planes. Features of scrotal wall abscess. (Right) Oblique grayscale ultrasound shows discharging sinus tract ➡ along tunics and scrotal wall. Note comet tail artifact ➡ due to gas within this collection.

VARICOCELE

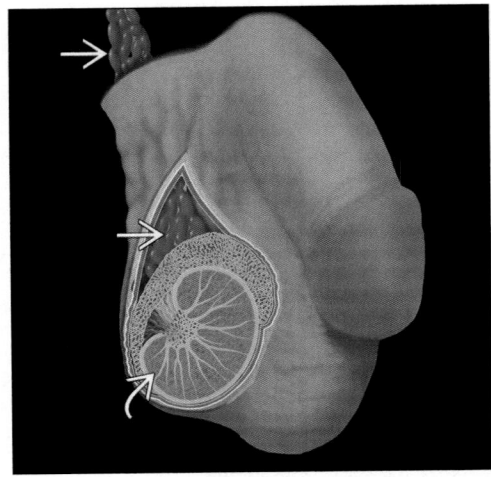

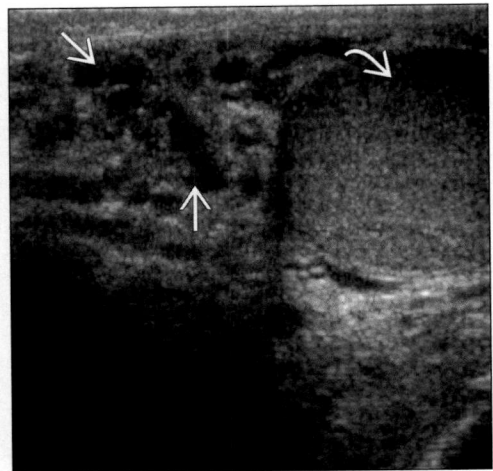

Graphic shows dilated, tortuous varicose veins of the pampiniform plexus ➡ in the spermatic cord and along the postero-superior aspect of testis ➡. Features of varicocele.

Oblique ultrasound of a varicocele seen as multiple serpentine, hypoechoic structures ➡ postero-superior to the testis ➡, representing dilated veins measuring > 2 mm in diameter.

TERMINOLOGY

Definitions
- Dilatation of veins of pampiniform plexus > 2-3 mm in diameter due to retrograde flow in internal spermatic vein

IMAGING FINDINGS

General Features
- Best diagnostic clue
  - Dilated serpiginous veins behind superior pole of testis on color Doppler US
  - Distention, due to retrograde flow, with Valsalva
- Location
  - Left (78%), right (6%), Bilateral (16%)
  - Dilated veins in cremasteric plexus, vein of vas deferens and internal spermatic vein
- Size: Normally veins in pampiniform plexus are ≤ 2 mm; varicocele diagnosed when multiple veins are > 2-3 mm and increase in size with Valsalva
- Morphology: Tortuous vascular channels representing dilated veins

Ultrasonographic Findings
- Grayscale Ultrasound
  - US should be performed in supine and standing positions
    - Multiple, hypoechoic, serpiginous, tubular structures
    - Varying size larger than 2 mm in diameter
  - Best visualized superior and lateral to testis
  - Occasionally low level internal echoes can be detected in dilated veins secondary to slow flow and red cell aggregation
  - Evaluate retroperitoneum and abdomen to exclude secondary varicoceles
- Color Doppler
  - Detection approaches 100% with color Doppler US
  - Doppler parameters are optimized for low flow velocities to confirm the venous flow pattern
  - Bidirectional Doppler sonography (erect with quiet breathing)
  - Secondary varicoceles result from increased pressure on spermatic vein, resulting in non-decompressible veins

---

DDx: Varicocele

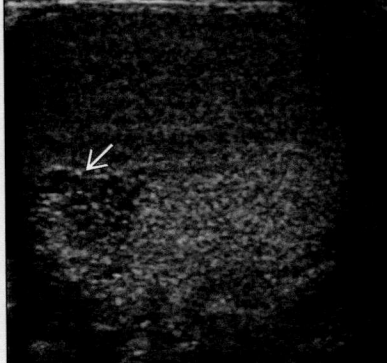

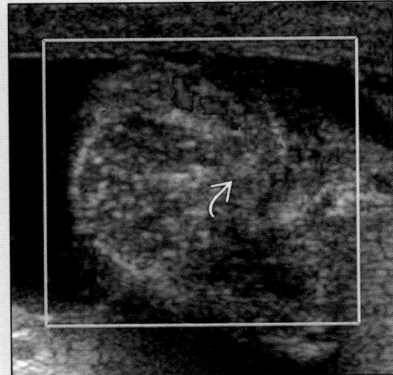

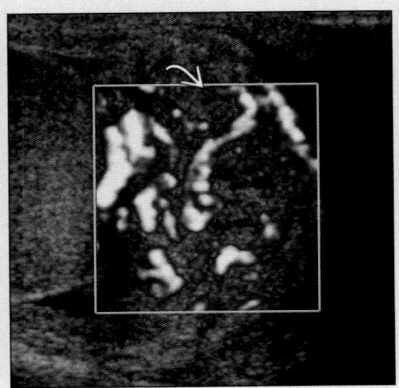

Tubular Ectasia

Testicular Torsion

Epididymitis

VARICOCELE

Key Facts

Terminology
- Dilatation of veins of pampiniform plexus > 2-3 mm in diameter due to retrograde flow in internal spermatic vein

Imaging Findings
- Dilated serpiginous veins behind superior pole of testis on color Doppler US
- Left (78%), right (6%), Bilateral (16%)
- US should be performed in supine and standing positions
- Multiple, hypoechoic, serpiginous, tubular structures
- Evaluate retroperitoneum and abdomen to exclude secondary varicoceles
- Doppler parameters are optimized for low flow velocities to confirm the venous flow pattern

- Bidirectional Doppler sonography (erect with quiet breathing)
- Best imaging tool: US with color Doppler
- Resting and Valsalva color Doppler examination of epididymis

Top Differential Diagnoses
- Tubular Ectasia/Rete Testis
- Testicular Torsion
- Epididymitis

Diagnostic Checklist
- Valsalva essential for diagnosis of small varicoceles
- Varicocele is diagnosed when vessel exceeds 2 mm during quiet respiration in supine position

---

- Shunt-type (86%): Incompetent intrascrotal pampiniform plexus valves allow spontaneous and continuos reflux from internal spermatic vein (retrograde flow) into cremasteric vein and vein of vas deferens (orthograde flow) via collaterals
  - Sperm quality impaired
  - Continuous reflux during Valsalva
  - Clinically plexus type (grade II & III); medium-sized and large varicoceles
- Stop-type/pressure-type (14%): Intact intrascrotal valves allow only brief period of reflux from spermatic vein into pampiniform plexus under Valsalva maneuver
  - Sperm quality normal
  - Short phase of initial retrograde flow during Valsalva
  - Clinically central type (grade 0+ I); subclinical and small varicocele
- Grading of varicoceles
  - Normal: Relaxed state, 2 mm; during Valsalva, 2.7 mm
  - Small varicocele: Relaxed state, 2.5-4 mm; during Valsalva, increase by 1 mm
  - Moderate varicocele: Relaxed state, 4-5 mm; during Valsalva, increase by > 1.2 mm
  - Large varicocele: Relaxed state, > 5 mm; during Valsalva, increase by > 1.5 mm

MR Findings
- Rarely performed, shows similar serpiginous appearance as US
- Signal intensities vary according to blood flow velocity
  - Slow flowing blood: Intermediate signal on T1WI & high signal on T2WI
  - Signal void indicates higher velocity flow
  - Varicoceles show enhancement following gadolinium administration

Other Modality Findings
- Catheter venography via retrograde injection in testicular vein demonstrates dilated venous channels

Imaging Recommendations
- Best imaging tool: US with color Doppler
- Protocol advice
  - Resting and Valsalva color Doppler examination of epididymis
  - Bidirectional Doppler sonography (erect with quiet breathing)

DIFFERENTIAL DIAGNOSIS

Tubular Ectasia/Rete Testis
- Normal variant of dilated seminiferous tubules in mediastinum of testis
- No flow on color Doppler
- May be associated with spermatocele

Testicular Torsion
- Absent or decreased flow to testis on color Doppler
- Hypoechoic testis in late stage

Epididymitis
- Enlarged hypoechoic epididymis with increased flow on color Doppler
- Flow does not show change with Valsalva

PATHOLOGY

General Features
- General path comments
  - Dilated veins within pampiniform plexus
    - Internal spermatic vein (anterior location) draining testis
    - Vein of vas deferens (mediodorsal location) draining epididymis
    - Cremasteric vein (laterodorsal location) draining scrotal wall
  - Varicocele exert their damaging effects by at least three mechanisms

VARICOCELE

- Increased heat: Testes reside in scrotum at 5-7° cooler than body temperature; pooling of blood in varicocele next to testicle causes increase in temperature
  - Oxidative stress: Reactive oxygen species (ROS) creates intratesticular oxidative stress
  - Hemodynamics: Incompetent veins result in high venous pressure compromising arterial inflow
- Etiology
  - Primary: Incompetent/absent venous valve near junction of left renal vein to IVC
    - Left testicular vein is longer
    - Enters left renal vein at right angle
    - Sometimes arches over left renal vein
    - Descending colon distended with feces may compress left testicular vein
  - Secondary: Obstruction or invasion of left renal vein by renal tumor, nodes or adrenal tumor
    - "Nutcracker syndrome": Superior mesenteric artery compressing left renal vein
- Epidemiology
  - 10-15% of men in US have varicoceles
  - Subclinical varicocele in 40-75% of infertile men
  - Most frequent cause of male infertility
- Associated abnormalities: Low sperm count

Gross Pathologic & Surgical Features
- Dilated veins within pampiniform plexus

Staging, Grading or Classification Criteria
- Primary
  - Idiopathic (incompetent valves) 98% on left
  - Most common cause of correctable infertility
- Secondary
  - Obstruction of left renal vein

CLINICAL ISSUES

Presentation
- Most common signs/symptoms
  - Infertility
  - Vague scrotal discomfort or pressure, primarily when standing
- Clinical Profile
  - Majority (78%) left-sided
  - Right sided in 6% of patients
  - Bilateral in 16% of patients
  - Secondary varicocele: Left renal vein occlusion by tumor in elderly male patient presenting with recent onset varicocele

Demographics
- Age
  - Primary: Idiopathic > 15 yrs
  - Secondary: < 40 yrs or elderly

Natural History & Prognosis
- Excellent prognosis in treated cases
- Results for increased fertility have been mixed, may not be as effective as previously thought

Treatment
- No obvious correlation between size of varicocele & degree of testicular damage, hence early detection & treatment of subclinical varicoceles are important
- Catheter embolization if symptomatic or causing low sperm count
- Surgical treatment
  - Ivanissevitch procedure, surgical ligation
  - High ligation: At level of lower pole of kidney; low ligation: At inguinal canal
  - Laparoscopic ligation
- Antegrade sclerotherapy
- After treatment/sclerotherapy blood flow is diverted from pampiniform plexus into other draining veins
  - These alternative pathways can give sonographic evidence of cremasteric plexus & short communicating veins within scrotal wall

DIAGNOSTIC CHECKLIST

Consider
- Left renal vein occlusion by tumor in elderly male patient presenting with recent onset varicocele

Image Interpretation Pearls
- Valsalva essential for diagnosis of small varicoceles
- Varicocele is diagnosed when vessel exceeds 2 mm during quiet respiration in supine position

SELECTED REFERENCES

1. Cimador M et al: The role of Doppler ultrasonography in determining the proper surgical approach to the management of varicocele in children and adolescents. BJU Int. 97(6):1291-7, 2006
2. Cina A et al: Sonographic quantitative evaluation of scrotal veins in healthy subjects: normative values and implications for the diagnosis of varicocele. Eur Urol. 50(2):345-50, 2006
3. Aso C et al: Gray-scale and color Doppler sonography of scrotal disorders in children: an update. Radiographics. 25(5):1197-214, 2005
4. Beddy P et al: Testicular varicoceles. Clin Radiol. 60(12):1248-55, 2005
5. Gat Y et al: Varicocele, hypoxia and male infertility. Fluid Mechanics analysis of the impaired testicular venous drainage system. Hum Reprod. 20(9):2614-9, 2005
6. Kessler A et al: Intratesticular varicocele: gray scale and color Doppler sonographic appearance. J Ultrasound Med. 24(12):1711-6, 2005
7. Muttarak M et al: Painless scrotal swelling: ultrasonographical features with pathological correlation. Singapore Med J. 46(4):196-201; quiz 202, 2005
8. Akcar N et al: Intratesticular arterial resistance and testicular volume in infertile men with subclinical varicocele. J Clin Ultrasound. 32(8):389-93, 2004
9. Park SJ et al: Diagnosis of pelvic congestion syndrome using transabdominal and transvaginal sonography. AJR Am J Roentgenol. 182(3):683-8, 2004
10. Evers JL et al: Assessment of efficacy of varicocele repair for male subfertility: a systematic review. Lancet. 361(9372):1849-52, 2003
11. Kutlu R et al: Intratesticular arteriovenous malformation: color Doppler sonographic findings. J Ultrasound Med. 22(3):295-8, 2003

VARICOCELE

IMAGE GALLERY

Typical

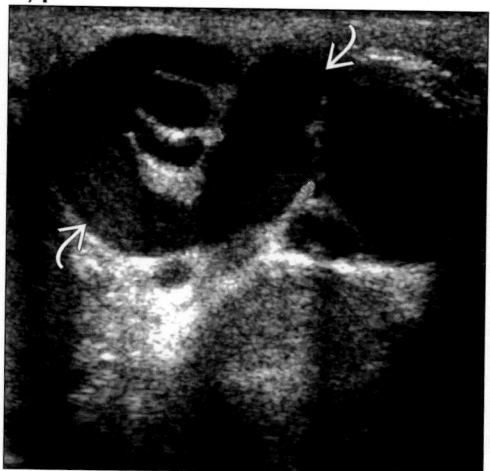
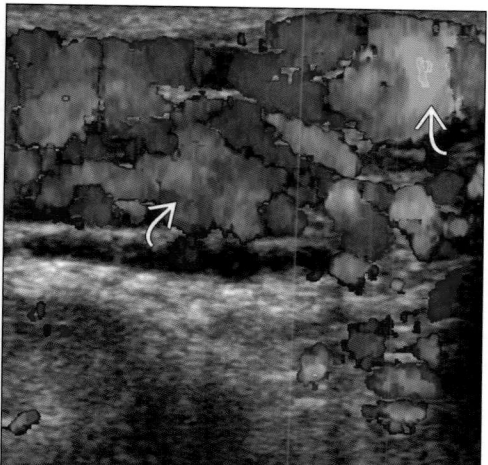

(Left) Oblique grayscale ultrasound through cord, in supine position, with normal respiration shows a dilated tortuous principal vein ➡ in pampiniform plexus measuring 7.5 mm in caliber. *(Right)* Longitudinal color Doppler ultrasound (same patient as previous image) shows blood flow in the principal ➡ and surrounding veins. These features are indicative of large varicocele (grade III).

Typical

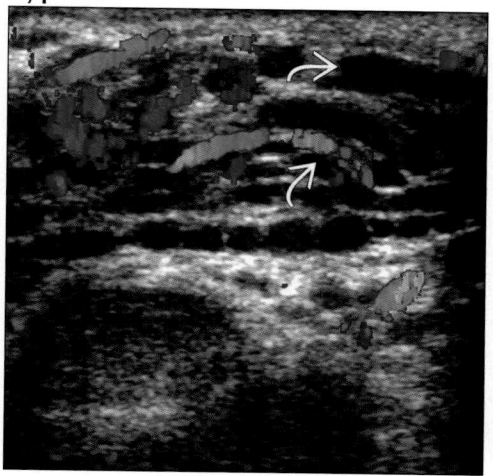
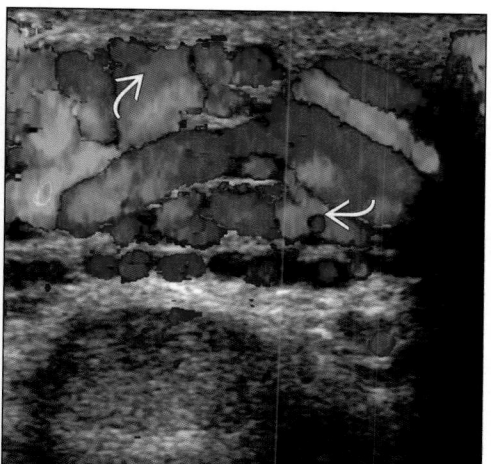

(Left) Longitudinal color Doppler ultrasound shows multiple, serpiginous dilated veins ➡ in pampiniform plexus of cord, along postero-superior aspect of testis in supine position, during normal respiration. *(Right)* Longitudinal color Doppler ultrasound (same patient as previous image) shows flow ➡ in these dilated veins during Valsalva, indicative of moderate varicocele. Blood flow in varicocele is slow and may be detected only with low Doppler settings.

Typical

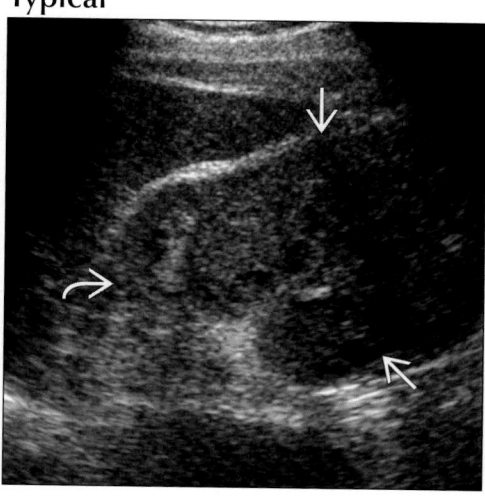
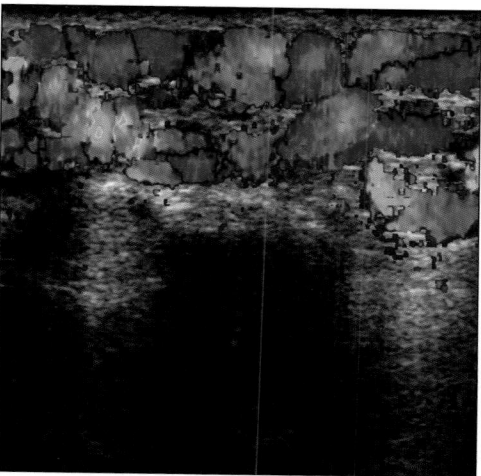

(Left) Longitudinal transabdominal ultrasound shows a large renal cell carcinoma ➡ arising from lower pole of left kidney ➡. *(Right)* Longitudinal color Doppler ultrasound (same patient as previous image) shows serpiginous tubular dilated veins in the pampiniform plexus. Left-sided varicoceles are occasionally seen with left-sided abdominal neoplasms.

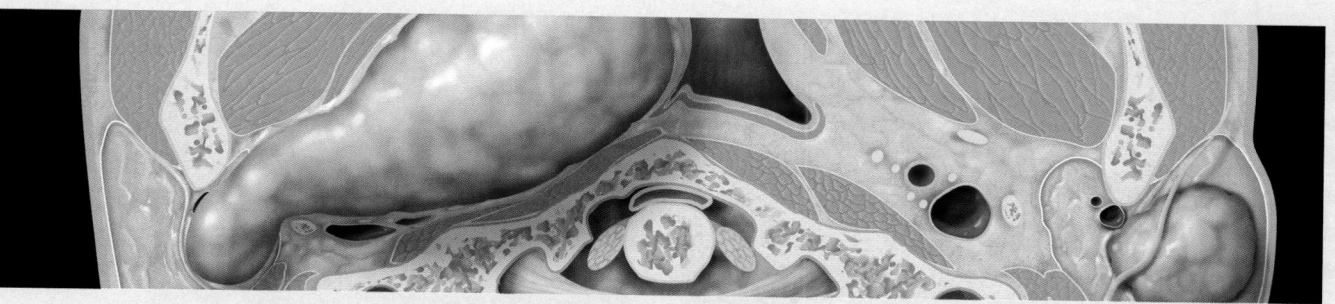

SECTION 11: Head and Neck

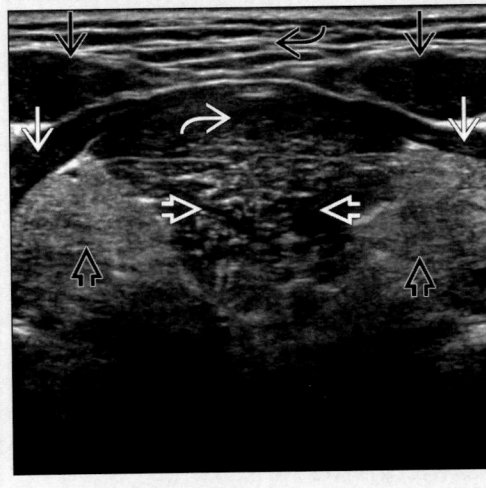

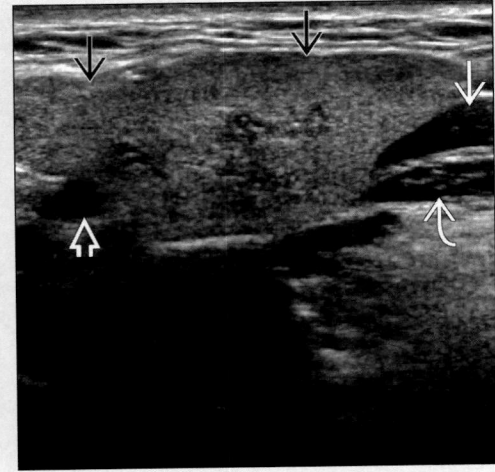

Transverse ultrasound of the submental region shows the platysma ⇗, anterior belly of digastric ⇥, mylohyoid muscle ➡, sublingual glands ⇨, geniohyoid ⇛ & genioglossus muscles ⇻.

Transverse ultrasound shows a fine bright parenchymal pattern of the submandibular gland ⇥, mylohyoid ➡ & hyoglossus ➡ muscles, and facial artery ⇥. Note US readily evaluates the submandibular gland.

IMAGING ANATOMY

Critical Anatomic Structures

- **Submental region**: Key structures to identify are platysma, anterior belly of digastric, mylohyoid, genioglossus & geniohyoid muscles, sublingual glands & lingual artery
  - Lesions deep to mylohyoid are in sublingual space; note posterior border of mylohyoid is free with communication between sublingual & submandibular spaces
  - Small submental lymph nodes are often seen with high-resolution transducers
- **Submandibular region**: Key structures to identify are submandibular gland, lymph nodes, mylohyoid & hyoglossus muscles, anterior & posterior bellies of digastric, facial vein & anterior division of retromandibular vein (RMV)
  - Submandibular duct runs between hyoglossus & mylohyoid muscle; do not mistake it for lingual vein which sits alongside proximal duct; color Doppler helps to identify it
  - Two venous landmarks outline submandibular gland; facial vein courses anteriorly & superiorly and anterior division of RMV (posteriorly)
    - Displacement of these structures helps to identify whether a mass is submandibular or parotid in origin
- **Parotid region**: Extends from external auditory meatus superiorly to angle of mandible inferiorly; key structures to identify are parotid gland, intraparotid duct, RMV, external carotid artery (ECA), intra/periparotid lymph nodes, masseter & buccinator muscles
  - US does not identify course of facial nerve as it runs in parotid; its location can be inferred by identifying ECA, RMV which run alongside facial nerve
  - US only evaluates superficial lobe of parotid gland & does not visualize deep lobe
- **Cervical region**: Commonly divided into upper, mid & lower cervical regions in order to identify relevant groups of jugular cervical lymph nodes

- Upper cervical/internal jugular nodes: Skull base to hyoid bone/carotid bifurcation
- Mid cervical/internal jugular nodes: Hyoid bone/cricoid cartilage
- Lower cervical/internal jugular node: Cricoid cartilage to clavicle
- Key structures in upper cervical region: Jugulodigastric (JD) node resides in close proximity to carotid bifurcation, internal jugular vein (IJV) & posterior belly of digastric muscle
- Key structures in midcervical region: Common carotid artery (CCA), IJV, lymph nodes, omohyoid muscle, esophagus & vagus nerve
- Key structures in lower cervical region: CCA, IJV, vagus nerve, subclavian artery, lymph nodes
- **Posterior triangle**: Bordered anteriorly by sternomastoid & posteriorly by trapezius; floor formed by scalene muscle, levator scapulae and splenius capitis muscle
  - Key structures in posterior triangle: XI nerve, accessory nodal chain, brachial plexus trunks/divisions, fat
- **Supraclavicular fossa**: Key structures include trapezius, sternomastoid, omohyoid, brachial plexus trunks/divisions, transverse cervical chain of nodes
  - Transverse cervical chain of nodes link spinal accessory chain nodal chain laterally with jugular chain medially
- **Midline**: Key structures include hyoid bone, strap muscles, thyroid isthmus, tracheal rings, larynx

ANATOMY-BASED IMAGING ISSUES

Imaging Protocols

- Use of high-resolution transducers is essential (≥ 7.5 MHz)
- For large masses it may not be possible to evaluate all anatomical relations with a high-resolution transducer and one may have to use a 5 MHz transducer and a standoff pad/gel

HEAD & NECK SONOGRAPHY

Key Facts

- **Submental region**: Key structures to identify are platysma, anterior belly of digastric, mylohyoid muscle, genioglossus & geniohyoid muscles, sublingual glands & lingual artery
- **Submandibular region**: Key structures to identify are submandibular gland, lymph nodes, mylohyoid & hyoglossus muscles, anterior & posterior bellies of digastric & facial vein & anterior division of retromandibular vein (RMV)
- **Parotid region**: Key structures to identify are parotid gland, intraparotid duct, RMV, external carotid artery (ECA), intra/periparotid lymph nodes, masseter & buccinator muscles
- **Cervical region**: Commonly divided into upper, mid & lower cervical regions in order to identify relevant groups of jugular cervical lymph nodes

- Key structures in upper cervical region: Jugulodigastric (JD) node is in close proximity to carotid bifurcation, IJV & posterior belly of digastric
- Key structures in midcervical region: CCA, IJV, lymph nodes, omohyoid muscle, esophagus & vagus nerve
- Key structures in lower cervical region: CCA, IJV, vagus nerve, subclavian artery, lymph nodes
- **Posterior triangle**: Key structures in posterior triangle: XI nerve, accessory nodal chain, brachial plexus trunks/divisions, fat
- **Supraclavicular fossa**: Key structures include trapezius, sternomastoid, omohyoid, brachial plexus trunks/divisions, transverse cervical chain of nodes
- **Midline**: Key structures include hyoid bone, strap muscle, thyroid isthmus, tracheal rings, larynx
- US is readily combined with guided FNAC which increases its specificity

---

- Grayscale US and color/power Doppler go hand in hand and in most instances Doppler provides useful, diagnostic supplementary information
- US is readily combined with guided fine needle aspiration cytology (FNAC) or biopsy; this increases its specificity
- In order to perform US of diagnostic quality it is essential to be familiar with sonographic anatomy & meticulous attention to technique (particularly Doppler settings) is necessary
- Be familiar with known nodal draining sites of HN cancers as nodal metastasis from HN cancers are site specific
- Follow a standard scanning protocol as this will prevent missing lesions
- When making images be sure to annotate its exact location and include key identifying landmarks; this helps if second reading is required and in patients who have serial follow-up
- Suggested scanning protocol for neck masses & nodes
  - **Start in the submental region, with transducer held transverse;** most key structures can be identified in transverse plane; Doppler evaluation of abnormal nodes in this region is often better done with transducer held longitudinally
  - **Next proceed to submandibular region which is scanned in transverse & longitudinal/oblique planes** as these best demonstrate floor of submandibular region, hyoglossus & mylohyoid muscles
    - For masses at this site always establish origin of mass, submandibular or extraglandular mass, as this will help to narrow differential diagnosis
    - Remember to evaluate glandular/extraglandular duct dilatation if any and always assess lymph nodes at this site as they are often involved in NHL and adjacent malignancies
  - **Next scan the parotid region in transverse and longitudinal planes**
    - Transverse scans help to define anatomic location of superficial salivary masses in relation to ECA, RMV

- Longitudinal scans help in better evaluating lesions in parotid tail & for Doppler examination
- Always identify origin of mass at angle of mandible as parotid and submandibular salivary masses may be in close proximity; displacement of vessels will help this localization
- US does not evaluate deep lobe masses or deep extension of superficial masses and CECT or MR may be necessary
- In parotid region, 5 MHz transducer with gel block/standoff pad helps to evaluate large masses and probable deep extension
- Evaluate masseter muscle as its lesions will clinically mimic parotid masses
  - **Next move to the upper cervical region with the transducer held transverse;** landmark to identify is carotid bifurcation
    - Always identify and carefully evaluate the JD node (grayscale & Doppler) as it is often involved with HN cancers
    - Color flow imaging helps to identify the major vessels and their anatomic relation to nodes or masses
  - **Now proceed to mid cervical region which is scanned in transverse plane**
    - Always identify CCA, IJV, lymph nodes and vagus nerve in transverse plane
    - Make sure the IJV is compressible and has respiratory phasicity to rule out the presence of a thrombus
  - **Next evaluate lower cervical region in transverse plane**
    - Identify CCA, IJV, subclavian artery & scalenus anterior muscle
    - Note metastatic nodes at this site may be from an infraclavicular primary
  - **Next evaluate the supraclavicular fossa with transducer held in transverse**
    - Identify the brachial plexus and presence of any abnormal nodes
    - Note nodal metastasis from infraclavicular primary may involve this site and brachial plexus

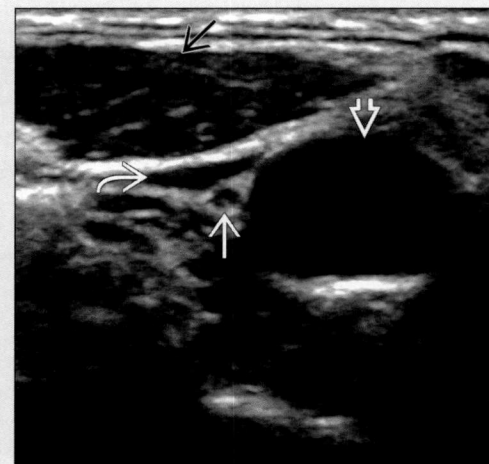

Transverse ultrasound of parotid gland ⇥ at the angle of the mandible. Position of theVII nerve is inferred from its relation to RMV ⇥ & ECA ⇥. Masseter muscle ⇥. Deep lobe obscured by mandible ⇥.

Transverse ultrasound proximal to the carotid bifurcation shows the CCA ⇥, IJV ⇥, sternomastoid muscle ⇥ & vagus nerve ⇥.

- ○ **Now scan posterior triangle transversely along a plane from mastoid process to ipsilateral acromion**
  - ▪ Identify presence of lymph nodes: Evaluate them both longitudinally and in transverse plane
  - ▪ Longitudinal scans facilitate Doppler imaging of nodes at site
  - ▪ Note this is a common site for tuberculous adenitis
- ○ **Now scan thyroid both in longitudinal & transverse planes**
  - ▪ Transverse scans help to locate thyroid nodules, their relationship to trachea, CCA, IJV & evaluate internal architecture & extrathyroid extension
  - ▪ Longitudinal scans help to evaluate internal architecture, vascularity on Doppler & extrathyroid extension if any
  - ▪ Both transverse & longitudinal scans help to differentiate a thyroid nodule from a parathyroid adenoma
- • Above protocol is robust and can be tailored to suit individual clinical conditions
  - ○ One can start with the area of primary lesion (thyroid, salivary, parathyroid etc.) and after that evaluate rest of neck
- • In children it may not be possible to follow protocol as they may be restless; US is usually done without prior sedation
  - ○ It is therefore best to evaluate the primary area of concern first before the child becomes uncooperative

- ○ Sublingual region: Ranula, lesions in sublingual glands
- ○ Submandibular region: Salivary gland masses, abnormal nodes from known draining sites, diving ranula, lymphangioma, extension of 2nd branchial cleft cyst (BCC)
- ○ Parotid region: Salivary masses, nodes in known draining sites, calculus disease, 1st BCC, lesions in masseter muscle (venous vascular malformation, hypertrophy)
- ○ Along internal jugular vein, carotid artery: Lymph nodes, paraganglioma, nerve sheath tumors, 2nd BCC, IJV thrombosis
  - ▪ Thymic cyst, parathyroid lesions, esophageal lesions may be in close proximity
- ○ Posterior triangle: Lymph nodes, cystic hygroma/lymphangioma, lipoma, nerve sheath tumor, venous vascular malformation

RELATED REFERENCES

1. Evans RM et al: Ultrasound. In: Imaging in Head & Neck Cancer: A Practical Approach. London, Greenwich Medical Media. 3-16, 2003
2. Ahuja A et al: An overview of neck sonography. Invest Radiology. 37:333-42, 2002
3. Evans RM: Anatomy & Technique. In: Practical Head & Neck Ultrasound. London, Greenwich Medical Media. 1-16, 2001
4. Hajek PC et al: Lymph nodes of the neck: evaluation with US. Radiology. 158:739-42, 1986

CLINICAL IMPLICATIONS

Clinical Importance

- • Lesions in the neck are often site specific and the knowledge of anatomy, pathology help in narrowing the differential diagnosis at various sites in the neck
- • Common site specific lesions in the neck
  - ○ Submental region: Lymph nodes from known draining sites, dermoid/epidermoid

IMAGE GALLERY

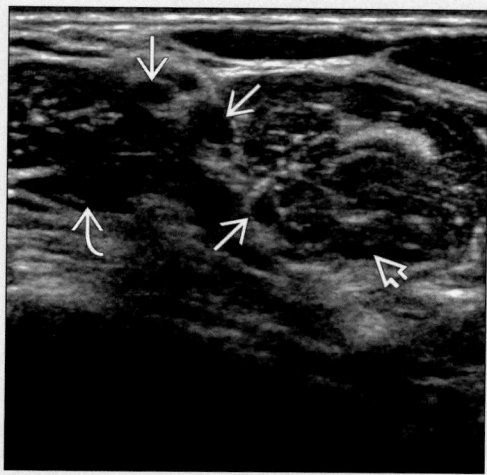
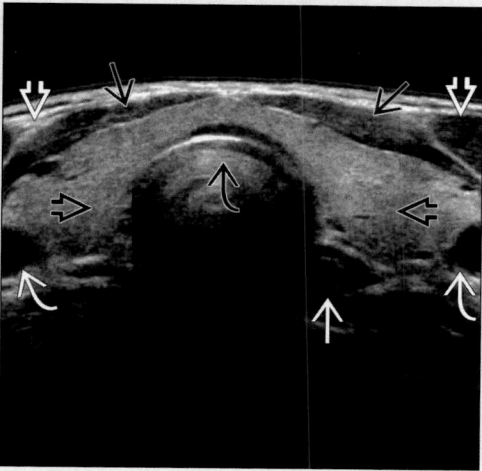

(Left) Transverse ultrasound of the supraclavicular fossa shows the scalenus anterior ➡ & medius ➡ muscles & trunks of the brachial plexus ➡ between them. Do not mistake these for lymph nodes. *(Right)* Transverse ultrasound at the level of the thyroid shows normal, fine, bright thyroid parenchymal echoes ➡. Note esophagus ➡, CCA ➡, strap muscles ➡, sternomastoid ➡ & trachea ➡.

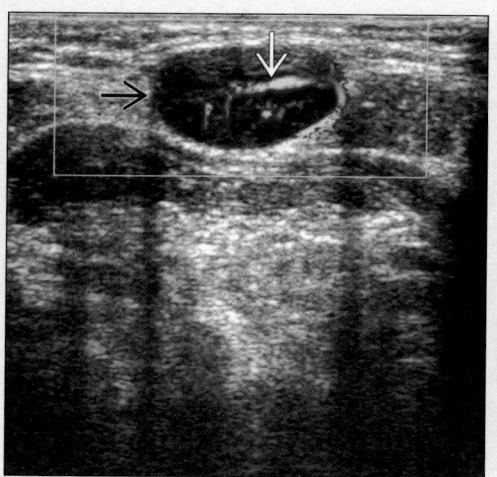
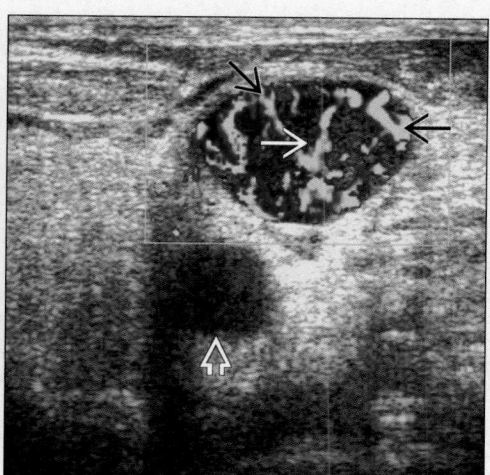

(Left) Transverse power Doppler ultrasound shows a elliptical, solid, hypoechoic reactive lymph node ➡, with normal hilar ➡ vascularity. Note absence of peripheral vessels. *(Right)* Transverse power Doppler ultrasound shows a round, solid, hypoechoic metastatic lymph node with peripheral ➡ & central ➡ vascularity. Peripheral vessels are seen in malignant nodes. CCA ➡.

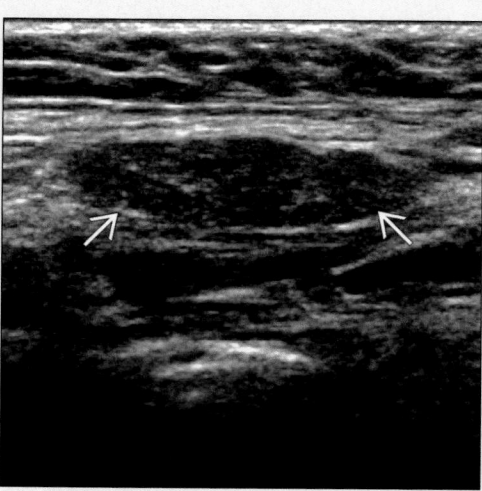
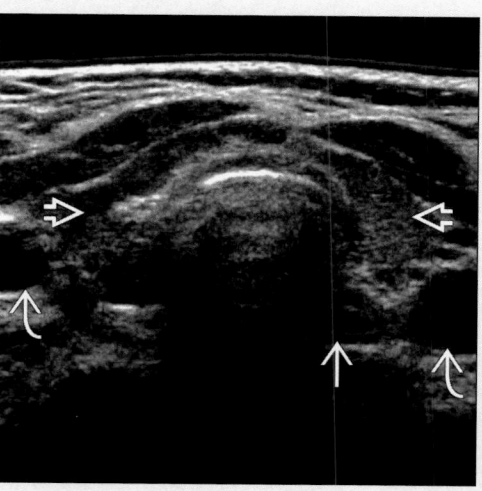

(Left) Transverse ultrasound of the submandibular gland in a patient who received radiotherapy to neck. Note the small, hypoechoic, heterogeneous atrophic submandibular gland ➡. *(Right)* Transverse ultrasound at the level of the thyroid in a patient who received radiotherapy to the neck shows hypoechoic, heterogeneous parenchymal echoes ➡ in an atrophic thyroid gland. CCA ➡, esophagus ➡.

DIFFERENTIATED THYROID CARCINOMA

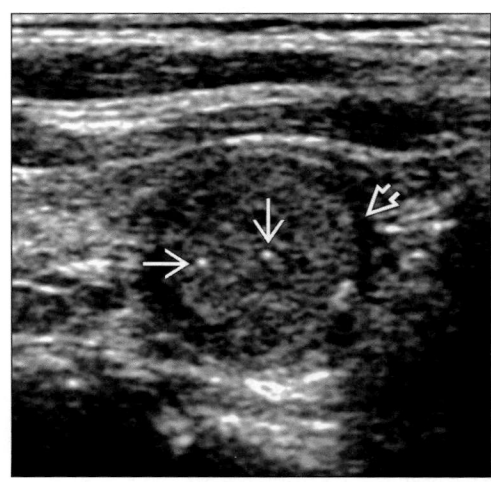

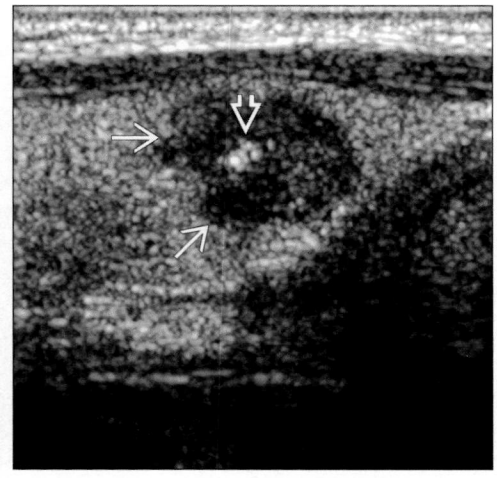

Longitudinal grayscale US shows a partially haloed ➡, hypoechoic, solid nodule with punctate calcifications ➡. FNAC confirmed papillary carcinoma.

Longitudinal grayscale US shows a solid, hypoechoic nodule with microcalcifications ➡. The ill-defined edges ➡ & microcalcifications suggested papillary carcinoma. Confirmed by FNAC.

TERMINOLOGY

Abbreviations and Synonyms
- Differentiated thyroid carcinoma (DTCa)
- Papillary carcinoma (PC), follicular carcinoma (FC), or papillary-follicular carcinoma

Definitions
- DTCa: Thyroid malignancies with well-defined histologies; includes papillary & follicular carcinoma

IMAGING FINDINGS

General Features
- Best diagnostic clue: Focal, intrathyroidal mass ± extracapsular invasion, ± metastatic nodes, ± distant metastases
- Location
  - Primary DTCa: Intrathyroidal
  - Nodal metastases: Most commonly deep cervical, paratracheal & superior mediastinal

Ultrasonographic Findings
- Grayscale Ultrasound
  - Sonographic features of **papillary carcinoma**
    - Solitary or multifocal, on US 10-20% are multifocal, solid (70%) & hypoechoic (77-90%)
    - Predominantly hypoechoic (77-90%) due to sparse colloid & closely packed cellular content
    - Punctate microcalcification is highly specific for papillary carcinoma, typically fine calcification/echogenic foci, ± posterior shadowing
    - Majority are ill-defined with irregular outlines but 15-30% of tumors may show an incomplete halo
    - Large tumors may show signs of invasion to strap muscles, esophagus, trachea, recurrent laryngeal nerve, neck vessels
    - Color Doppler: Multiple, chaotically arranged vessels within the nodule & wall & septa in nodules with cystic change
    - Tumor commonly spreads along rich lymphatic system within & adjacent to thyroid gland; this accounts for multifocal tumors within thyroid & regional nodal spread

DDx: Differentiated Thyroid Carcinoma

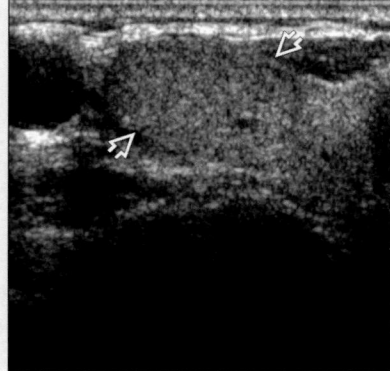

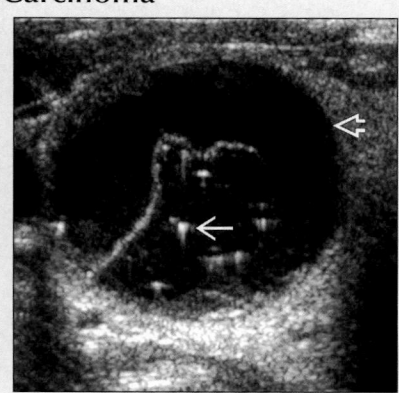

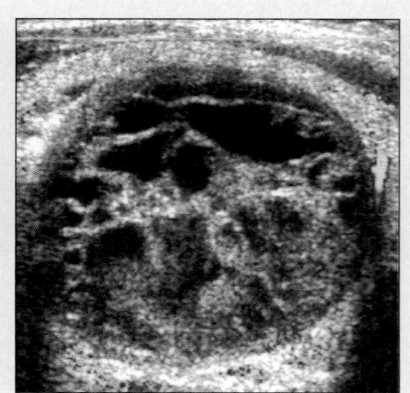

Follicular Adenoma

Hemorrhagic Colloid Cyst

Multinodular Goiter

DIFFERENTIATED THYROID CARCINOMA

Key Facts

Imaging Findings
- Sonographic features of **papillary carcinoma**
- Solitary or multifocal, on US 10-20% are multifocal, solid (70%) & hypoechoic (77-90%)
- Punctate microcalcification is highly specific for papillary carcinoma, typically fine calcification/echogenic foci, ± posterior shadowing
- Majority are ill-defined with irregular outlines but 15-30% of tumors may show an incomplete halo
- Large tumors may show signs of invasion to strap muscles, esophagus, trachea, recurrent laryngeal nerve, neck vessels
- Color Doppler: Multiple, chaotically arranged vessels within the nodule & wall & septa in nodules with cystic change

- Nodes predominantly hyperechoic (80%) compared to muscles with punctate microcalcification (50%)
- Sonographic features of **follicular carcinoma**
- Ill-defined solid tumor with hypoechoic, heterogeneous architecture
- Hypoechoic component to an otherwise iso/hyperechoic solid mass; thick irregular margins/capsule
- Obvious extrathyroid invasion into trachea, esophagus, strap muscles & large vessels
- Color Doppler: Profuse, chaotic perinodular & intranodular vascularity (intranodular > perinodular)

Top Differential Diagnoses
- Follicular Adenoma
- Hemorrhagic Colloid Cyst
- Multinodular Goiter (MNG)

- Lymph node metastasis from papillary carcinoma (PC, LN)
  - Distribution along deep cervical chain, pre & paratracheal nodes
  - Nodes predominantly hyperechoic (80%) compared to muscles with punctate microcalcification (50%)
  - Cystic necrosis (25%) with vascularity within solid portion & septa on color Doppler
- **Follicular carcinoma**
  - Not possible to differentiate benign follicular adenoma from follicular carcinoma by imaging or biopsy; differentiation is made after surgery based on vascular & capsular invasion; they are therefore commonly lumped together as follicular lesions
  - Some cytologists may classify them into microfollicular or macrofollicular types; in 20-25% a microfollicular lesion may be follicular carcinoma; macrofollicular lesions have a low risk of carcinoma
  - In most cases follicular carcinoma develops from a pre-existing adenoma
- Sonographic features of **follicular carcinoma**
  - Ill-defined solid tumor with hypoechoic, heterogeneous architecture
  - Hypoechoic component to an otherwise iso/hyperechoic solid mass; thick irregular margins/capsule
  - Obvious extrathyroid invasion into trachea, esophagus, strap muscles & large vessels
  - Color Doppler: Profuse, chaotic perinodular & intranodular vascularity (intranodular > perinodular)
  - Metastatic disease in bones, lungs, less commonly in lymph nodes; patients often present with bone metastases

CT Findings
- NECT: Cystic change (hypodensity), calcifications (hyperdensity) or well-defined borders to a thyroid mass does not exclude malignancy
- CECT
  - Primary tumor appearance highly variable

- Single vs. multiple nodules vs. diffuse infiltration & extension to surrounding tissues
- Small, well-circumscribed vs. large, ill-defined, heterogeneous mass; solid vs. cystic vs. mixed ± calcification
- Lymph node appearance highly variable
  - Small reactive looking or large heterogeneous, hemorrhagic, cystic nodes with thin walls
  - Solid foci of enhancement, focal calcification may be seen

MR Findings
- T1WI
  - Primary tumor: Intrathyroidal mass, focal, multinodular or diffusely infiltrating
  - Metastatic adenopathy: Areas of high T1 signal caused by hemorrhage ± thyroglobulin possible
- T1 C+: Primary tumor: Mixed signal, heterogeneously enhancing mass nonspecific; invasive margins are key to diagnosis

Nuclear Medicine Findings
- PET: FDG PET (PET/CT) scanning may be useful for detecting de-differentiating recurrent disease
- Tc-99m pertechnetate or I-123 used to assess nodule activity: Cold nodule ~ 20% risk of malignancy
- Diagnostic I-131 scan performed post thyroidectomy to detect local & metastatic disease
  - If positive, therapeutic ablation with I-131

Imaging Recommendations
- Best imaging tool
  - On US solid, hypoechoic, punctate calcification specific for papillary carcinoma & correspond to psammoma bodies on microscopy
    - US identifies malignant nodules, guides needle for fine needle aspiration cytology (FNAC) & helps to follow-up/evaluate post-surgical thyroid bed
    - CT/MR used to stage large tumors as US may not define its entire extent & local infiltration
- Protocol advice: On US in addition to evaluating thyroid gland always look for extracapsular spread, local invasion & nodal metastasis

DIFFERENTIATED THYROID CARCINOMA

DIFFERENTIAL DIAGNOSIS

Follicular Adenoma
- Solitary, well-defined, homogeneous, iso/hyperechoic intrathyroidal mass with perinodular vascularity & no local invasion or adenopathy/metastases

Hemorrhagic Colloid Cyst
- Anechoic nodule with avascular septa, comet tail artifact; solitary vs. multiple; unilateral vs. bilateral

Multinodular Goiter (MNG)
- Multiple nodules, heterogeneous, ± cystic change, ± coarse calcification & perinodular vascularity in thyroid gland

Medullary Carcinoma
- Mimics papillary carcinoma on US; calcification is coarse, shadowing & associated lymph nodes are hypoechoic

Anaplastic Carcinoma
- Rapidly enlarging, invasive thyroid tumor, hypoechoic, ill-defined, ± calcification & profuse chaotic vascularity

PATHOLOGY

General Features
- General path comments
  - Thyroid cancer
    - DTCa: Papillary (80%) & follicular (10%)
    - Medullary carcinoma (5-10%)
    - Anaplastic carcinoma (1-2%)
  - Patterns of spread
    - Local invasion with involvement of recurrent laryngeal nerves, trachea, esophagus
    - Nodal spread: Papillary (50%) > > follicular (10%) microscopic spread at presentation
    - Distant spread: Follicular (20%) > papillary (5-10%), typically occurs to lung, bone & CNS
  - Embryology-anatomy
    - Nodal drainage from thyroid includes paratracheal, deep cervical, spinal accessory, retropharyngeal chains
    - DTCa accesses mediastinum via paratracheal chain
- Etiology: Sporadic, radiation exposure ↑ risk of DTCa
- Epidemiology: Thyroid cancer: 1% of all malignant tumors, DTCa; 90% of all thyroid malignancy

Microscopic Features
- Papillary carcinoma
  - Papillae consisting of neoplastic epithelium overlying fibrovascular stalks
  - Psammoma bodies (50%) = laminated calcific concretions found within tumor stroma
- Follicular carcinoma
  - Neoplastic follicular cells: Solid, trabecular or follicular growth pattern
  - Differentiated from benign follicular adenomas by tumor capsule invasion ± vascular invasion

CLINICAL ISSUES

Presentation
- Most common signs/symptoms: Painless, palpable, solitary thyroid nodule in female
- Other presenting signs/symptoms/history
  - Rapid growth of thyroid mass, extrathyroid hard nodes, hoarseness; history of radiation exposure

Demographics
- Age: Peak incidence in 3rd & 4th decade
- Gender: 3x more common in women

Natural History & Prognosis
- Low mortality malignancy; 20 year survival rate = 90% (papillary), 75% (follicular)

Treatment
- Management of solitary thyroid nodule
  - History & physical, lab evaluation & needle biopsy are key 1st steps
  - Results of needle biopsy determine intervention
- Surgical resection
  - Total thyroidectomy ± regional lymphadenectomy (if nodes present clinically or on imaging)
- I-131scintigraphy
  - DTCa is TSH sensitive (will take up iodine); performed 4-6 weeks after thyroidectomy when patient is hypothyroid (TSH > 50)
  - Diagnostic dose of I-131 1st to assess for any tissue taking up radioiodine; if remnant detected: Ablative dose of I-131 given
- Treatment follow-up
  - Rising serum thyroglobulin indicates recurrence, may occur several decades after 1st treatment
  - US is ideal for evaluating recurrence in thyroid bed, lymph nodes & confirms it by guided FNAC
  - I-131 scintigraphy also identifies site of recurrence; followed by therapeutic dose of I-131

DIAGNOSTIC CHECKLIST

Image Interpretation Pearls
- Consider DTCa in patients with ill-defined, solid, hypoechoic, hypervascular intrathyroid mass, ± extrathyroid extension, ± metastatic nodal/distant metastases

SELECTED REFERENCES

1. Wong KT et al: Ultrasound of thyroid cancer. Cancer Imaging. 5:157-66, 2005
2. Harnsberger HR et al: Diagnostic Imaging: Head & Neck. 1st ed. Salt Lake City, Amisys. III-11-24, 2004

DIFFERENTIATED THYROID CARCINOMA

IMAGE GALLERY

Typical

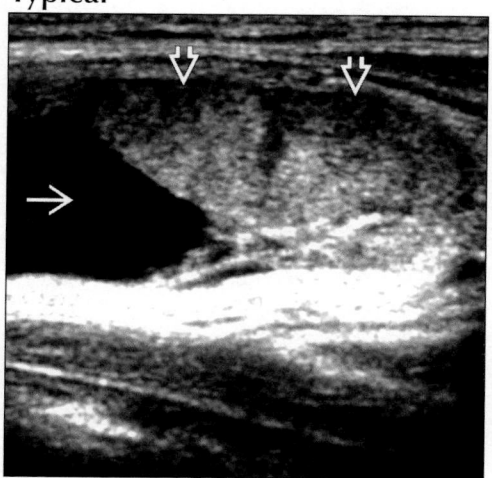
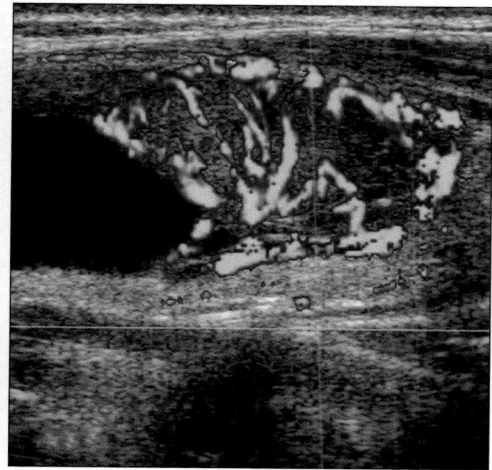

(Left) Longitudinal grayscale US shows cystic ➡ and solid ➡ components in a papillary carcinoma. *(Right)* Corresponding power Doppler shows profuse, chaotic vascularity in the solid component. A FNAC of the solid portion confirmed papillary carcinoma. Benign thyroid nodules show perinodular vascularity.

Typical

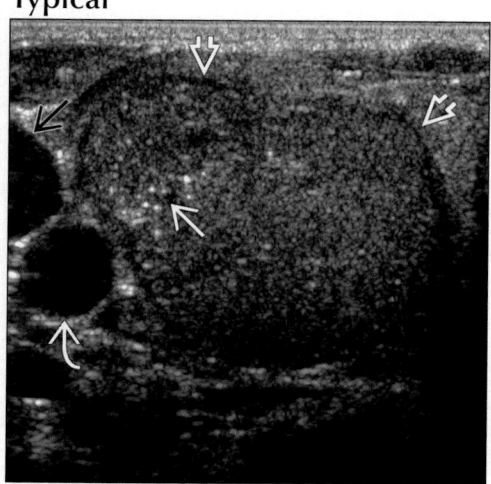
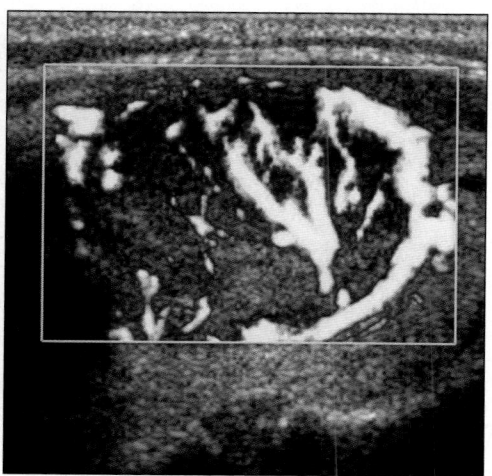

(Left) Transverse grayscale US shows a partially haloed ➡, solid, hypoechoic thyroid nodule, with punctate calcification ➡. Note the relationship to the carotid artery ➡, internal jugular vein ➡. *(Right)* Corresponding power Doppler US shows profuse, chaotic intranodular vascularity. FNAC confirmed papillary carcinoma. The presence of such vascularity should not stop one from safely doing FNAC.

Typical

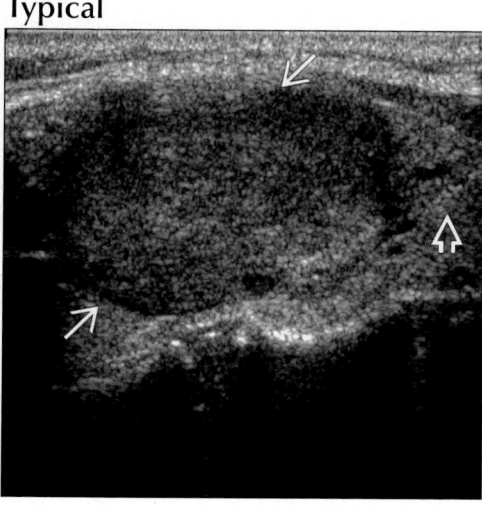
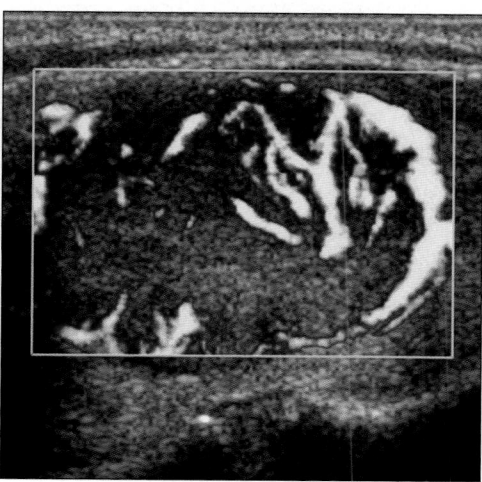

(Left) Longitudinal grayscale US shows an ill-defined, solid, hypoechoic thyroid nodule ➡. Ill-defined edges and hypoechogenicity should raise suspicion of malignancy. Normal thyroid echogenicity ➡. *(Right)* Corresponding power Doppler shows profuse, chaotic intranodular vascularity. FNAC confirmed papillary carcinoma of the thyroid. Such vessels in a thyroid nodule suggest malignancy.

Typical

(Left) Transverse grayscale US shows solid ➡ & cystic ➡ components in a metastatic neck node. Presence of punctate calcifications ➡ suggests metastasis from papillary thyroid cancer. FNAC proven. *(Right)* Corresponding axial T1 C+ MR shows the lymph node ➡ with intense enhancement of the solid portion ➡. Note a focal nodule ➡ in the right lobe of thyroid. FNAC confirmed papillary carcinoma.

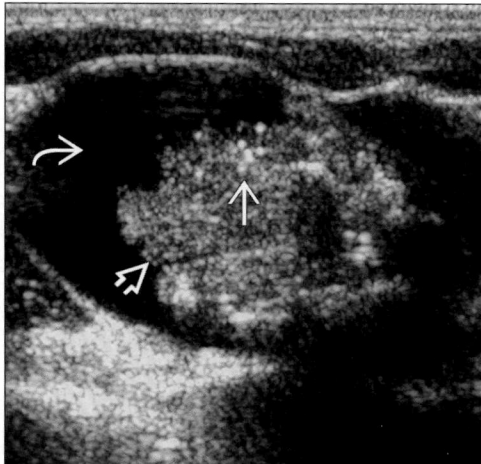

Typical

(Left) Grayscale US shows solid ➡ & cystic components ➡ in a neck lymph node. FNAC of solid portion confirmed metastatic papillary thyroid cancer. Thyroid US detected the primary thyroid tumor. *(Right)* Corresponding color Doppler shows large vessels in the solid component. Blood clots/debris in cystic nodules show no vascularity. Color Doppler helps to guide portion of nodule to be FNAed.

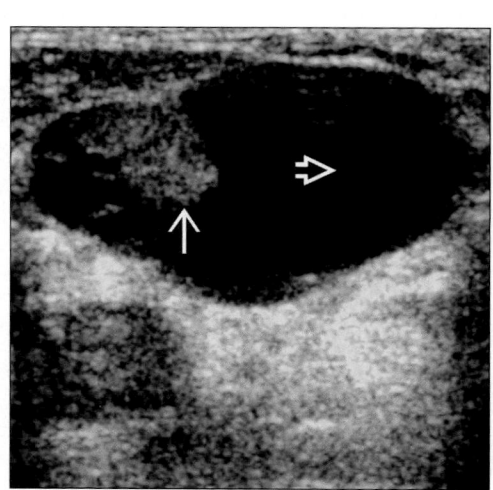
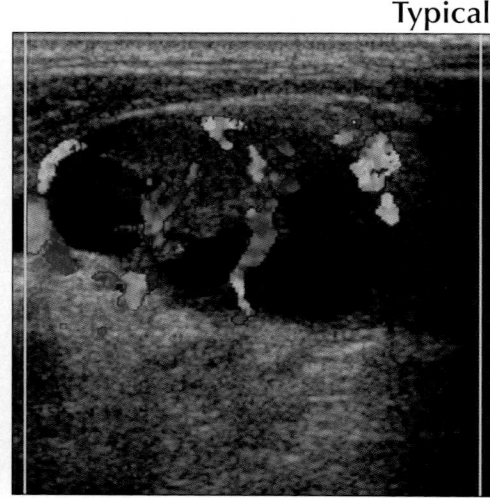

Typical

(Left) Longitudinal grayscale US shows a large, non-calcified, solid hypoechoic thyroid nodule. Note its infiltrative edges ➡. The patient presented with bone metastases. Follicular carcinoma shown at surgery. *(Right)* Corresponding power Doppler clearly demonstrates abnormal chaotic vessels within this thyroid nodule, strongly suggesting malignancy. Benign follicular adenomas show perinodular vascularity.

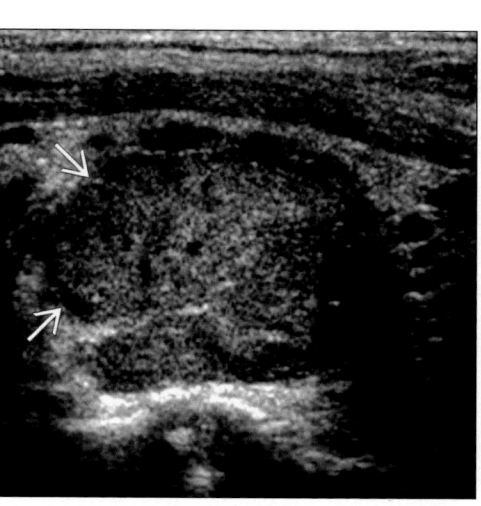
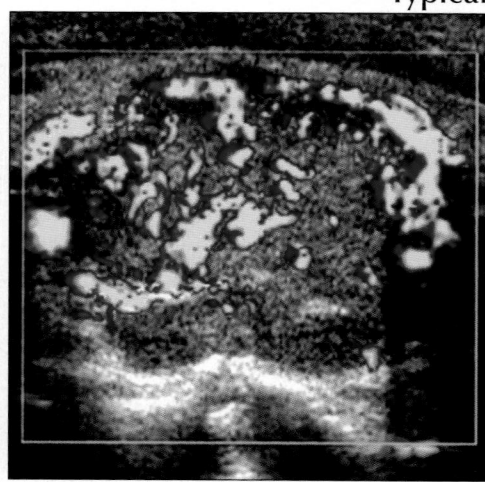

DIFFERENTIATED THYROID CARCINOMA

Typical

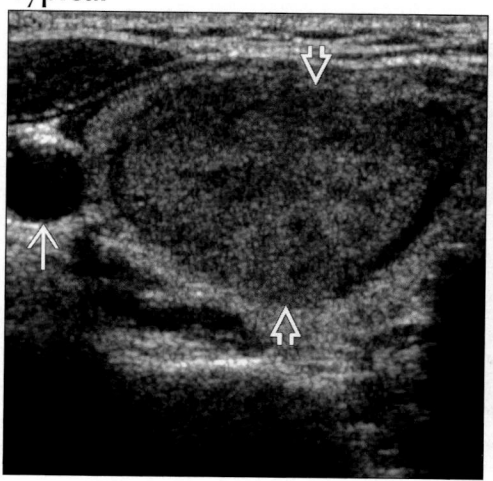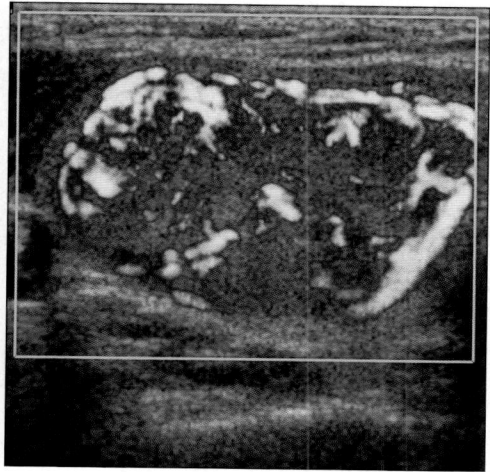

(Left) Transverse grayscale US shows a partially haloed, solid, hypoechoic nodule ⇨ with homogeneous internal echoes. US suggested malignancy; follicular carcinoma confirmed at surgery. Carotid artery ➡. *(Right)* Corresponding power Doppler shows markedly chaotic, large, intranodular vessels suggesting its malignant nature.

Typical

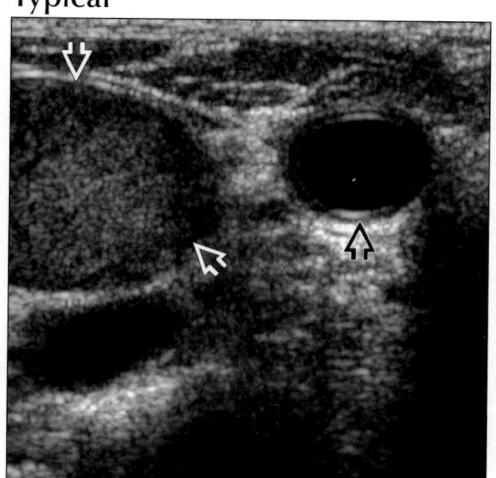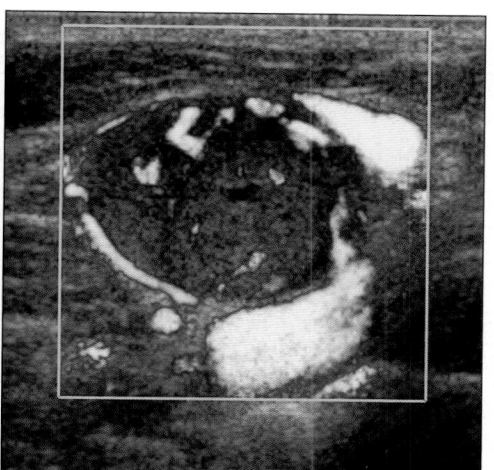

(Left) Transverse grayscale US shows a well-defined, hypoechoic, non-calcified thyroid nodule ⇨ with a homogeneous internal architecture. US suggested a malignant nodule. Carotid artery ➡. *(Right)* Corresponding power Doppler shows abnormal vascularity within this nodule increasing confidence in suggesting a malignant lesion. Follicular carcinoma confirmed at surgery.

Typical

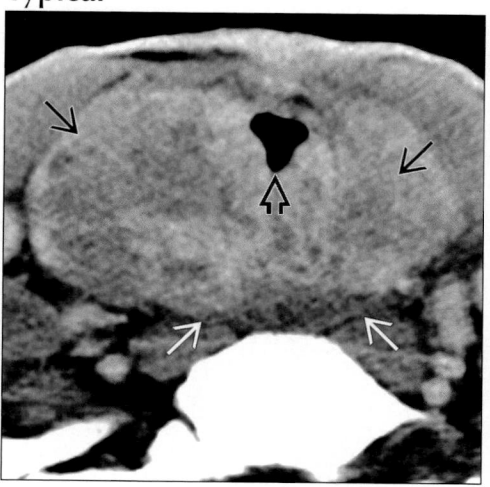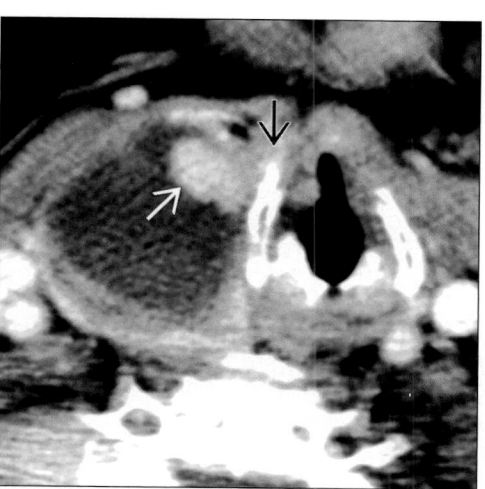

(Left) Axial CECT shows a large follicular carcinoma with diffuse thyroid involvement ➡, compression of the airway ⇨ & extrathyroid spread posteriorly ➡. These features cannot be evaluated by US. *(Right)* Axial CECT of follicular carcinoma shows a cystic & enhancing solid component ➡. Note the infiltration and destruction of the thyroid cartilage anteriorly ➡.

MEDULLARY THYROID CARCINOMA

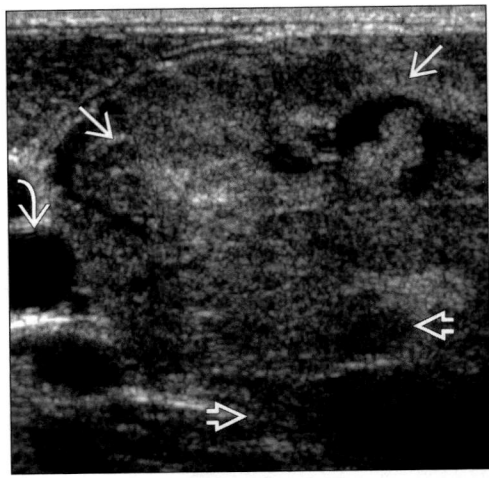

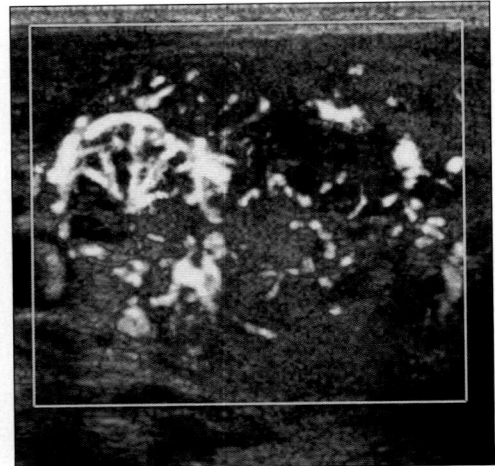

Transverse grayscale US shows a large, heterogeneous thyroid mass ➡ with extracapsular spread posteriorly ➤. US suggested a malignant mass but diagnosis of MTC was only made on FNAC. ➡ Carotid.

Corresponding power Doppler shows the multiple, prominent, chaotically arranged vessels in the tumor. Such vascularity in a thyroid mass is highly suspicious of a malignant nodule & FNAC is indicated.

TERMINOLOGY

Abbreviations and Synonyms
- Abbreviation: Medullary thyroid carcinoma (MTC)

Definitions
- Rare neuroendocrine malignancy arising from thyroid parafollicular "C cells"

IMAGING FINDINGS

General Features
- Best diagnostic clue: Solid lesions in thyroid gland with nodal metastases; ± calcifications
- Location
  - Within thyroid gland, lateral upper 2/3rd of gland (site of maximum C cell concentration)
  - Frequently multifocal, 2/3 of sporadic cases, almost all familial cases
  - Nodal metastases: Level VI & superior mediastinum, retropharyngeal nodes, levels III & IV (mid- & low internal jugular chain)
- Morphology

  - Solid, usually well-circumscribed mass in thyroid gland
  - More infiltrative type seen with familial forms

Ultrasonographic Findings
- Grayscale Ultrasound
  - Medullary carcinoma, primary tumor
    - Solitary or multiple or diffuse involvement of both lobes (especially familial type)
    - Located predominantly in lateral upper 2/3rd of gland in sporadic form
    - Hypoechoic, solid tumor, frequently well-defined but may have infiltrative borders
    - Echogenic foci in 80-90% representing amyloid deposition & associated calcification
    - Echogenic foci are dense & coarse + shadowing compared to papillary carcinoma
  - Lymph node metastases from medullary carcinoma
    - Lymph nodes along mid & low internal jugular chain, superior mediastinum
    - Lymph nodes predominantly hypoechoic with coarse shadowing calcification
- Color Doppler
  - Doppler: Chaotic intratumoral vessels

DDx: Medullary Thyroid Carcinoma

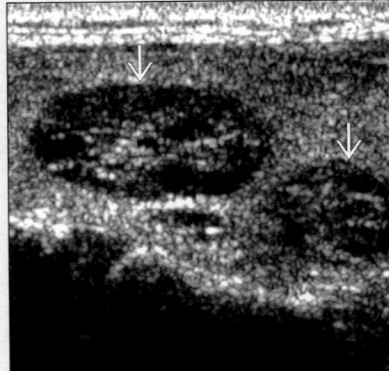

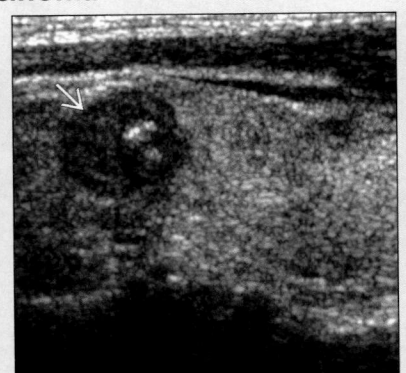

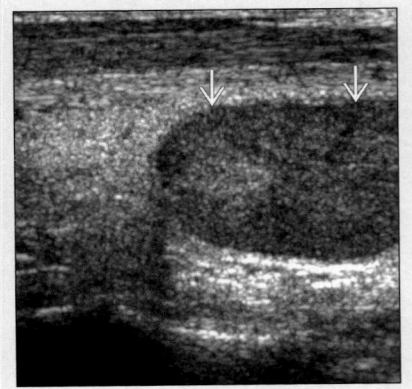

Differentiated Thyroid Carcinoma

Multinodular Goiter

Thyroid Metastases

MEDULLARY THYROID CARCINOMA

Key Facts

Imaging Findings
- Solitary or multiple or diffuse involvement of both lobes (especially familial type)
- Located predominantly in lateral upper 2/3rd of gland in sporadic form
- Hypoechoic, solid tumor, frequently well-defined but may have infiltrative borders
- Echogenic foci in 80-90% representing amyloid deposition & associated calcification
- Echogenic foci are dense & coarse + shadowing compared to papillary carcinoma
- Lymph nodes along mid & low internal jugular chain, superior mediastinum
- Lymph nodes predominantly hypoechoic with coarse shadowing calcification
- Doppler: Chaotic intratumoral vessels

- Doppler: Chaotic intranodal vessels
- On US MTC is invariably mistaken for papillary carcinoma (which is much more common) & diagnosis made only after FNAC
- Sonographic clue to MTC rather than papillary carcinoma is presence of coarse shadowing tumoral calcification (punctate in papillary) & hypoechoic nodes (hyperechoic in papillary) with coarse shadowing
- Evaluate adrenal & parathyroid gland if MTC is part of type 2 multiple endocrine neoplasia (MEN)

Top Differential Diagnoses
- Differentiated Thyroid Carcinoma
- Multinodular Goiter (MNG)
- Thyroid Metastases

- Doppler: Chaotic intranodal vessels

CT Findings
- CECT
  - Solid low density well-circumscribed mass in thyroid; may be multifocal, especially with familial types
  - Fine, punctate calcifications may be found in tumor & in nodal metastases

MR Findings
- MR not routinely used for MTC
- Irregular margins & extraglandular extension may be seen, but MTC frequently well-defined

Nuclear Medicine Findings
- PET
  - Most helpful for suspected recurrence where there is "minimal disease"
    - Elevated tumor markers but no gross disease on cross-sectional imaging
- Octreotide scintigraphy (In-111-pentreotide) or I-13I-MIBG may also be taken up by tumor

Imaging Recommendations
- Best imaging tool
  - Ultrasound (US) is ideal initial tool for evaluation of thyroid nodule when combined with guided fine needle aspiration cytology (FNAC)
    - Sonographically medullary carcinoma closely mimics papillary thyroid carcinoma, both primary tumor & metastatic node
    - On US MTC is invariably mistaken for papillary carcinoma (which is much more common) & diagnosis made only after FNAC
    - Sonographic clue to MTC rather than papillary carcinoma is presence of coarse shadowing tumoral calcification (punctate in papillary) & hypoechoic nodes (hyperechoic in papillary) with coarse shadowing
    - US identifies the malignant nodule, guides needle for FNAC and helps to follow up/evaluate post-surgical thyroid bed and neck

- Cross-sectional imaging is used to stage large tumors as US may not accurately define entire extent, local infiltration & mediastinal nodes
- Protocol advice
  - On US in addition to evaluating thyroid gland always look for extracapsular spread, local invasion and nodal disease
  - Evaluate adrenal & parathyroid gland if MTC is part of type 2 multiple endocrine neoplasia (MEN)

DIFFERENTIAL DIAGNOSIS

Differentiated Thyroid Carcinoma
- Papillary carcinoma has punctate, fine calcifications; nodes are hyperechoic, show cystic change & punctate calcification

Multinodular Goiter (MNG)
- Diffusely enlarged gland with multiple nodules with coarse calcification, ± comet tail artifact

Thyroid Metastases
- Diffuse/focal enlargement of gland, well-defined, solid hypoechoic mass with abnormal vascularity; invariably associated with US evidence of disseminated disease in neck nodes, liver

Follicular Adenoma
- Solitary, well-defined, non-calcified iso/hyperechoic mass with homogeneous internal echogenicity and perinodular vascularity

PATHOLOGY

General Features
- General path comments: Arises from parafollicular "C cells" of thyroid that secrete calcitonin & derived from ultimobranchial body
- Genetics
  - Sporadic (~ 85%) or hereditary, familial forms (15%)

MEDULLARY THYROID CARCINOMA

○ Associated with mutations of RET proto-oncogene on chromosome 10q11.2
  ■ Found in familial (100%) and sporadic (40-60%) cases
  ■ Screening for RET mutations is performed for family members of patients with MTC
• Etiology
  ○ No identified exogenous cause & not related to other thyroid conditions
  ○ Type 2 multiple endocrine neoplasia (MEN) syndromes
    ■ Autosomal dominant
    ■ MEN 2A: Multifocal MTC, pheochromocytoma, parathyroid hyperplasia, hyperparathyroidism
    ■ MEN 2B: Multifocal MTC, pheochromocytoma, mucosal neuromas of lips, tongue, GI tract, conjunctiva; younger patients, more aggressive tumors
  ○ Familial medullary thyroid carcinoma (FMTC)
    ■ Autosomal dominant condition where only neoplasm is MTC
    ■ Later onset, more indolent course than MEN syndromes
• Epidemiology
  ○ 5-10% all thyroid gland malignancies, ≤ 14% thyroid cancer deaths
  ○ 10% pediatric thyroid malignancies (MEN2)

Gross Pathologic & Surgical Features
• Solid, firm, well-circumscribed but non-encapsulated, calcifications may be evident
• Necrosis & hemorrhage only with larger lesions

Microscopic Features
• Stains strongly for calcitonin (80%)
• Also stains for carcinoembryonic antigen (CEA), chromogranin A and neuron-specific enolase

CLINICAL ISSUES

Presentation
• Most common signs/symptoms
  ○ Painless thyroid nodule
  ○ Other signs/symptoms
    ■ Less commonly dysphagia, hoarseness, pain
    ■ Uncommonly presents with paraneoplastic syndromes: Cushing or carcinoid syndromes
    ■ Rarely presents with diarrhea from elevated calcitonin, though often an associated symptom
  ○ Elevated serum calcitonin
    ■ Used as screening tool, for estimation of extent of disease and as baseline for post-operative monitoring
• Clinical Profile: Middle-age patient with lower neck mass or patient with family history of MEN has tumor found on screening exam

Demographics
• Age
  ○ Sporadic form: Mean age = 50 years; familial form: Mean age = 30 years
  ○ Can occur in children, especially with MEN 2B
• Gender: M < F in Caucasians and in children

Natural History & Prognosis
• Familial type almost always multifocal and bilateral
• 2/3 of sporadic cases are bilateral
• Up to 75% have lymphadenopathy at presentation
• Indicators of better prognosis
  ○ Female gender, younger age at surgery
  ○ FMTC and MEN 2A syndromes
  ○ Tumor < 10 cm, no nodes, early stage disease
  ○ Normal pre-operative CEA levels, complete surgical resection
• Overall 5 year survival = 72%; 10 year = 56%

Treatment
• Prophylactic thyroidectomy performed if familial RET mutation detected
  ○ FMTC and MEN 2A perform thyroidectomy at age 5-6
  ○ MEN 2B perform thyroidectomy during infancy
• Mainstay of MTC treatment is complete resection of local and regional disease
  ○ Total thyroidectomy with level VI nodal dissection ± superior mediastinal nodes
  ○ Node levels II-V resected if positive nodes in lateral neck
• Adjuvant radiation therapy
  ○ XRT used if extensive soft tissue invasion or extracapsular nodal spread

DIAGNOSTIC CHECKLIST

Image Interpretation Pearls
• US appearance may exactly mimic papillary thyroid carcinoma
• US readily evaluates post-operative thyroid bed and neck but CT or MR imaging are necessary for detection of nodal metastases in mediastinum as well as distant metastases

SELECTED REFERENCES

1. Wong KT et al: Ultrasound of thyroid cancer. Cancer Imaging. 5:157-66, 2005
2. Harnsberger HR et al: Diagnostic Imaging: Head & Neck. 1st ed. Salt Lake City, Amirsys. III-11-28-31, 2004
3. Ahuja AT et al: Imaging in Head & Neck Cancer: A Practical Approach. London, Greenwich Medical Media. 143-66, 2003
4. Kouvaraki MA et al: Role of preoperative ultrasonography in the surgical management of patients with thyroid cancer. Surgery. 134(6):946-54; discussion 954-5, 2003
5. Ahuja AT et al: Practical Head & Neck Ultrasound. London, Greenwich Medical Media. 35-64, 2000
6. Weber AL et al: The thyroid and parathyroid glands. CT and MR imaging and correlation with pathology and clinical findings. Radiol Clin North Am. 38(5):1105-29, 2000

MEDULLARY THYROID CARCINOMA

IMAGE GALLERY

Typical

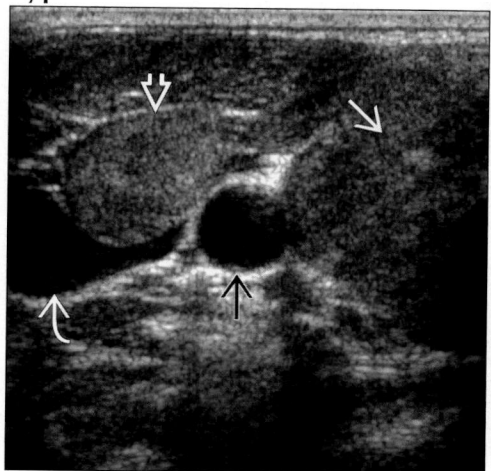
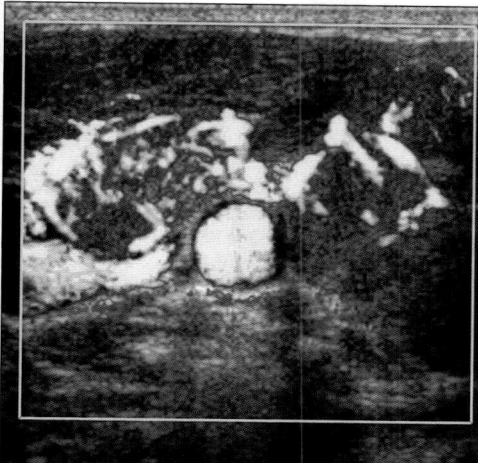

(Left) Transverse grayscale US shows a hypoechoic mass in the thyroid ➡, with an adjacent node ⊞ indenting the internal jugular vein ⊟. Carotid ⊟. FNAC confirmed MTC & MTC LN, commonly mistaken for papillary carcinoma. (Right) Corresponding power Doppler US shows abnormal chaotic vessels in the thyroid mass and adjacent LN. Such prominent vessels should not prevent one from safely doing US-guided FNAC.

Typical

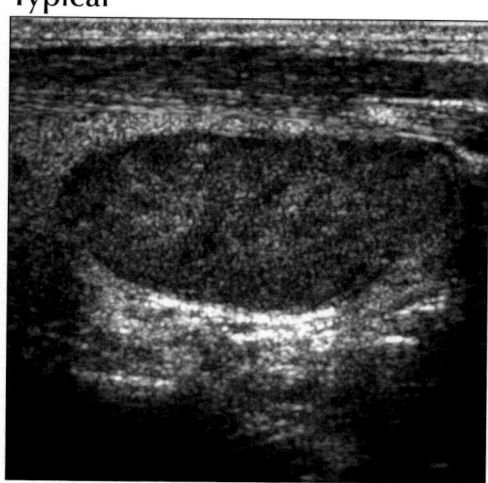
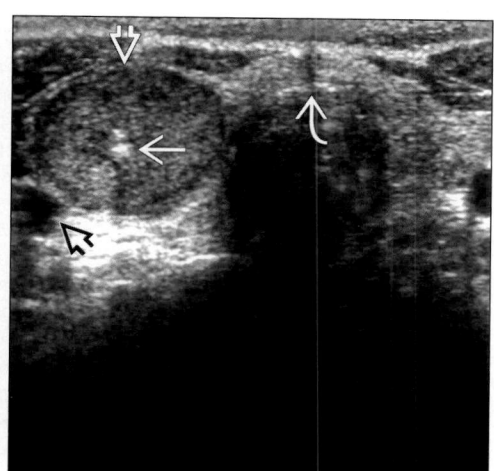

(Left) Longitudinal grayscale US shows a solid, hypoechoic, well-defined thyroid nodule. FNAC confirmed MTC. Malignant masses may have well-defined borders and is a common feature of MTC. (Right) Grayscale US shows a well-defined, solid, hypoechoic MTC ➡ with a densely shadowing echogenic focus ➡ due to amyloid & calcification (unlike punctate calcification in papillary carcinoma). Trachea ⊟, carotid ⊞.

Typical

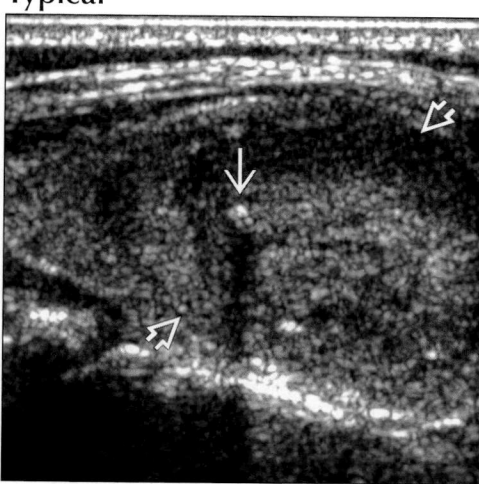
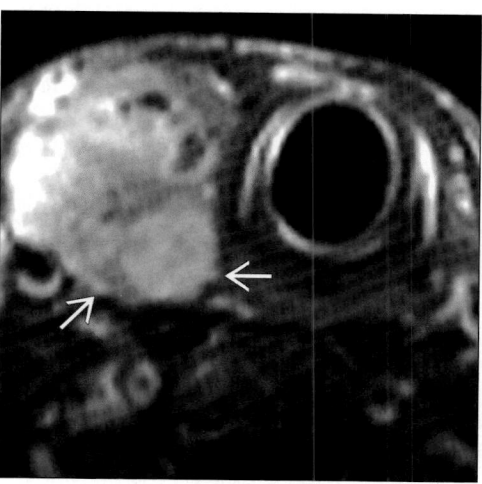

(Left) Grayscale US shows an ill-defined, solid, hypoechoic MTC ⊟ with a densely shadowing focus ➡ due to amyloid & calcification. Papillary carcinoma shows microcalcification ± shadowing. (Right) Axial T2WI MR shows a larger MTC with extracapsular extension posteriorly ➡. US is unable to accurately define extent & spread of large tumors into adjacent structures. CT & MR are better at evaluating invasion into surrounding tissue.

ANAPLASTIC THYROID CARCINOMA

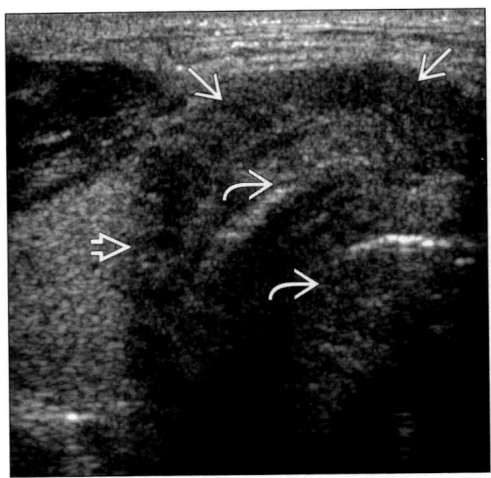

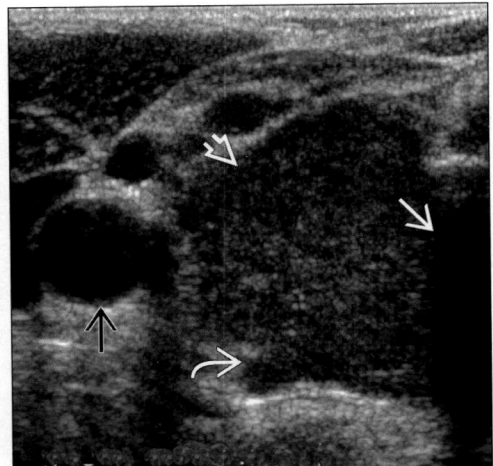

Transverse grayscale US shows a solid, ill-defined hypoechoic thyroid ATCa involving the right lobe ➤ and isthmus ➤ with destruction of tracheal cartilage & tracheal infiltration ➤.

Transverse grayscale US shows an ill-defined, solid, hypoechoic ATCa ➤ with extrathyroid extension posteriorly ➤ & tracheal ➤ involvement medially. Note patent right CCA ➤.

TERMINOLOGY

Abbreviations and Synonyms
- Anaplastic thyroid carcinoma (ATCa)
- Undifferentiated thyroid carcinoma

Definitions
- ATCa: Lethal thyroid malignancy from thyroid-stimulating hormone transformation of either differentiated thyroid carcinoma or multinodular goiter (MNG)

IMAGING FINDINGS

General Features
- Best diagnostic clue: Invasive, hypoechoic thyroid mass, ± focal calcification, ± necrosis against a background of MNG in elderly female
- Size: > 5 cm at presentation typical
- Morphology
  ○ Primary tumor: Large, infiltrating thyroid mass
  ○ Primary tumor + MNG: Diffuse, heterogeneous thyromegaly with infiltrating margins

Ultrasonographic Findings
- Grayscale Ultrasound
  ○ Ill-defined, hypoechoic tumor diffusely involving the entire lobe or gland
  ○ Background of multinodular goiter
  ○ Necrosis (78%), dense amorphous calcification (58%)
    ▪ Dense calcification reflects MNG calcification
  ○ Extracapsular spread with infiltration of trachea, esophagus & perithyroid soft tissues
  ○ Thrombus in IJV and CA causing expansion & occlusion of vessels
  ○ Nodal or distant metastases in 80% of patients
    ▪ Nodes are hypoechoic & necrotic in 50%
  ○ Color Doppler shows prominent, small, chaotic intranodular vessels
    ▪ Necrotic tumor may be avascular/hypovascular (vascular infiltration/occlusion)
    ▪ Abnormal vascularity seen within metastatic nodes
    ▪ Vascularity seen in thrombus in vessels suggesting it to be tumor thrombus & not venous thrombus

11

16

DDx: Anaplastic Thyroid Carcinoma

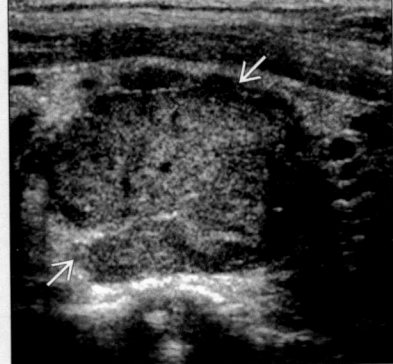

Differentiated Thyroid Carcinoma

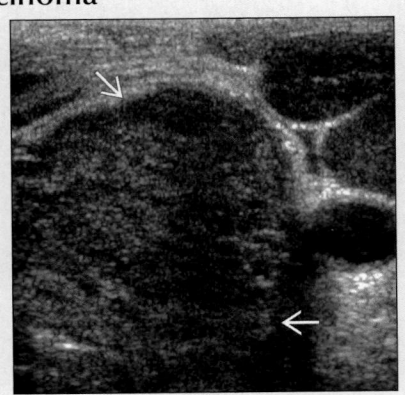

Thyroid Non-Hodgkin Lymphoma

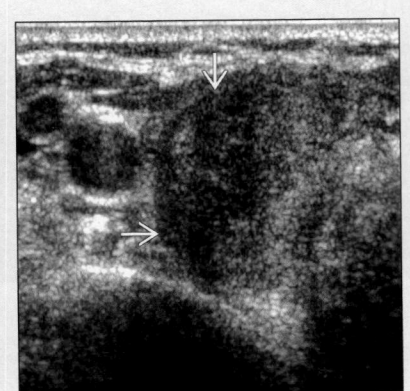

Thyroid Metastases

ANAPLASTIC THYROID CARCINOMA

Key Facts

Imaging Findings
- Best diagnostic clue: Invasive, hypoechoic thyroid mass, ± focal calcification, ± necrosis against a background of MNG in elderly female
- Heterogeneously enhancing lesion, diffusely infiltrating thyroid gland
- Ill-defined, hypoechoic tumor diffusely involving the entire lobe or gland
- Background of multinodular goiter
- Necrosis (78%), dense amorphous calcification (58%)
- Dense calcification reflects MNG calcification
- Extracapsular spread with infiltration of trachea, esophagus & perithyroid soft tissues
- Thrombus in IJV and CA causing expansion & occlusion of vessels
- Nodal or distant metastases in 80% of patients
- Nodes are hypoechoic & necrotic in 50%
- Color Doppler shows prominent, small, chaotic intranodular vessels
- Necrotic tumor may be avascular/hypovascular (vascular infiltration/occlusion)
- Abnormal vascularity seen within metastatic nodes
- Vascularity seen in thrombus in vessels suggesting it to be tumor thrombus & not venous thrombus
- US is ideal bedside imaging tool to evaluate ATCa, its gross extension, nodal disease; it is readily combined with fine needle aspiration cytology (FNAC) to confirm diagnosis

Top Differential Diagnoses
- Differentiated Thyroid Carcinoma (DTCa)
- Non-Hodgkin Lymphoma (NHL)
- Thyroid Metastases

Radiographic Findings
- Radiography: Chest X-ray may demonstrate lung metastases, tracheal narrowing or deviation

CT Findings
- NECT: Calcifications (60%) are typically dense, amorphous, globular (MNG) calcifications
- CECT
  - Primary ATCa tumor
    - Heterogeneously enhancing lesion, diffusely infiltrating thyroid gland
    - Necrosis (75%) & hemorrhage appear as central tumor hypodensity
    - Invades surrounding structures including larynx, trachea, recurrent laryngeal nerve, esophagus, carotid artery (CA), internal jugular vein (IJV) & adjacent infrahyoid neck
  - Metastatic tumor
    - Cervical lymphadenopathy present in 40% & metastatic nodes are necrotic in 50%; CECT shows central hypodensity
    - Distant metastasis present in 50%: Lungs, bones & brain

MR Findings
- T1WI
  - Invasive tumor & adenopathy are diffusely hypointense
  - Hemorrhage, necrosis & calcification may result in heterogeneous mixed signal
- T2WI: Diffuse iso- to hyperintense signal typical, but variable
- T1 C+: Moderate to marked heterogeneous enhancement

Nuclear Medicine Findings
- Bone Scan: Tc-99m MDP scintigraphy used to determine presence of bone metastases
- I-131 scintigraphy
  - ATCa does not concentrate iodine because of highly undifferentiated cells
  - Not used in evaluation or treatment of ATCa
- I-123 scintigraphy
  - Not typically utilized when an invasive thyroid mass is present clinically
  - If performed, ATCa appears as a poorly delineated cold region

Imaging Recommendations
- Best imaging tool
  - Patients with ATCa are often old with poor general condition & present with acute obstructive symptoms such as dyspnea, dysphagia, laryngeal nerve palsy
    - US is ideal bedside imaging tool to evaluate ATCa, its gross extension, nodal disease; it is readily combined with fine needle aspiration cytology (FNAC) to confirm diagnosis
    - US may be unable to evaluate exact infiltration into trachea, larynx, adjacent soft tissues, mediastinal spread & CECT or MR may be necessary
    - CECT is preferable as patients poor condition makes MR imaging suboptimal and CECT is faster
- Protocol advice: Always look for background MNG, extrathyroid & vascular infiltration of ATCa, nodal & distant metastases

DIFFERENTIAL DIAGNOSIS

Differentiated Thyroid Carcinoma (DTCa)
- Ill-defined, solid, hypoechoic, heterogeneous mass with abnormal vascularity, ± punctate calcification, ± adjacent nodal metastases, ± vascular & extrathyroid infiltration

Non-Hodgkin Lymphoma (NHL)
- Focal, hypoechoic, ill-defined areas with abnormal vascularity in thyroid with background evidence of Hashimoto thyroiditis (abnormal architecture, bright fibrotic streaks); rarely calcified or necrotic
- Associated, solid, hypoechoic, reticulated lymphomatous nodes

ANAPLASTIC THYROID CARCINOMA

Thyroid Metastases
- Evidence of a known primary & disseminated disease; solid, hypoechoic mass, ill/well-defined, non-calcified, with abnormal vessels or diffuse hypoechoic enlarged thyroid and nodal metastasis

Medullary Carcinoma
- May exactly mimic morphology of early anaplastic thyroid carcinoma. Solid, hypoechoic, ill-defined with coarse calcification & abnormal adjacent nodes

Multinodular Goiter (MNG)
- Multiple, heterogeneous nodules, ± dense calcification, cystic change, septa, comet tail artifact; no vascular or soft tissue infiltration & no nodal metastasis

PATHOLOGY

General Features
- General path comments
  - ATCa occurs in iodine-deficient areas & setting of pre-existing thyroid pathology
    - Multinodular goiter in 33%: DTCa in 25%
  - Thought to arise from endodermally derived follicular cells
    - ATCa does NOT concentrate iodine or express thyroglobulin
- Etiology
  - Best hypothesis
    - Prolonged stimulation of MNG or DTCa by thyroid-stimulating hormone transforms these conditions into ATCa
- Epidemiology: ATCa is uncommon, representing 1-2% of thyroid malignancy

Gross Pathologic & Surgical Features
- Invasive mass that extends through thyroid gland capsule

Staging, Grading or Classification Criteria
- No generally accepted staging system for ATCa; all ATCa are considered stage IV

CLINICAL ISSUES

Presentation
- Most common signs/symptoms
  - Rapidly growing, large, (> 5 cm) painful mass in thyroid area
  - 50% have associated symptoms from local invasion
    - Larynx or trachea: Dyspnea
    - Recurrent laryngeal nerve: Hoarseness
    - Esophagus: Dysphagia
  - Predisposing factors: Pre-existing MNG
  - Physical exam findings
    - Firm thyroid mass, typically greater than 5 cm, vocal cord paralysis (30%), cervical lymphadenopathy (40%)

Demographics
- Age: ATCa presents at a later age than other thyroid malignancies, most typically 6th or 7th decade

- Gender: Like DTCa, women are more commonly affected than men (M:F = 1:3)

Natural History & Prognosis
- ATCa is one of the most aggressive neoplasms seen in humans & is rapidly fatal with mean survival of 6 months after diagnosis
- Demise is usually secondary to local airway obstruction or complications of pulmonary metastases

Treatment
- Treatment is usually palliative with life expectancy measured in months
- Multimodality with surgery ± radiotherapy & chemotherapy
- Biopsy with tracheostomy followed by combined radio-chemotherapy most commonly employed
- Aggressive surgery probably only warranted when tumor is caught early & has not invaded widely into adjacent spaces

DIAGNOSTIC CHECKLIST

Consider
- Diagnosis is based on clinical evaluation, imaging & biopsy

Image Interpretation Pearls
- Rapidly enlarging thyroid mass suggests DTCa or thyroid NHL

SELECTED REFERENCES

1. Wong KT et al: Ultrasound of thyroid cancer. Cancer Imaging. 5:157-66, 2005
2. Harnsberger HR et al: Diagnostic Imaging: Head & Neck. 1st ed. Salt Lake City, Amirsys. III-11-32-35, 2004
3. Ahuja AT et al: Imaging in Head & Neck Cancer: A Practical Approach. London, Greenwich Medical Media. 143-65, 2003
4. Pasieka JL: Anaplastic thyroid cancer. Curr Opin Oncol. 15(1):78-83, 2003
5. Sherman SI: Thyroid carcinoma. Lancet. 361(9356):501-11, 2003
6. Wiseman SM et al: Anaplastic transformation of thyroid cancer: review of clinical, pathologic, and molecular evidence provides new insights into disease biology and future therapy. Head Neck. 25(8):662-70, 2003
7. Ishikawa H et al: Comparison of primary thyroid lymphoma with anaplastic thyroid carcinoma on computed tomographic imaging. Radiat Med. 20(1):9-15, 2002
8. Stanley MW: Selected problems in fine needle aspiration of head and neck masses. Mod Pathol. 15(3):342-50, 2002
9. Vini L et al: Management of thyroid cancer. Lancet Oncol. 3(7):407-14, 2002
10. Lind P et al: The role of F-18FDG PET in thyroid cancer. Acta Med Austriaca. 27(2):38-41, 2000
11. Takashima S et al: CT evaluation of anaplastic thyroid carcinoma. AJNR Am J Neuroradiol. 11(2):361-7, 1990

ANAPLASTIC THYROID CARCINOMA

Typical

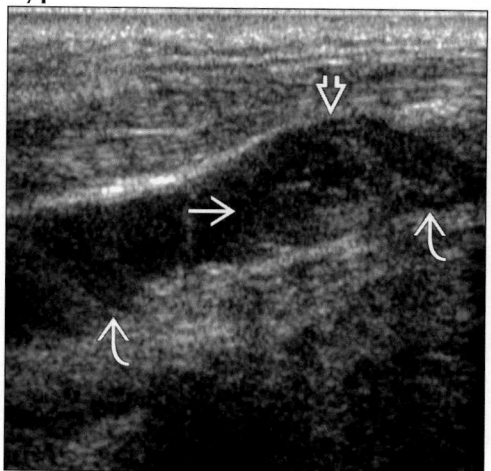
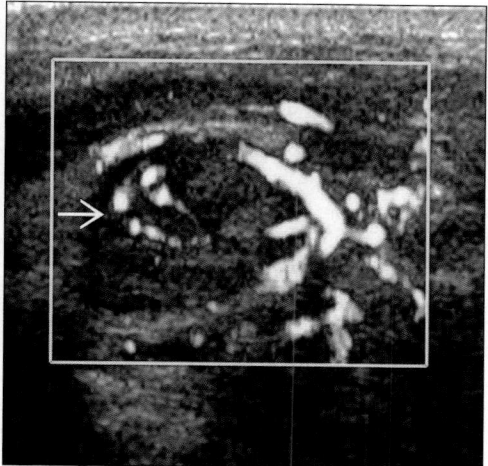

(Left) Longitudinal grayscale US shows a soft tissue thrombus ➡ within the IJV ➡ in a patient with proven ATCa. Note focal expansion of the IJV at the site of the thrombus ➡. *(Right)* Corresponding transverse power Doppler shows vascularity within the thrombus ➡ confirming tumor thrombus (from ATCa) rather than a venous stasis thrombus.

Typical

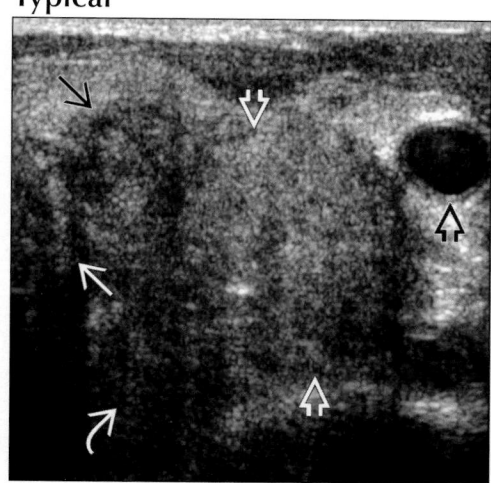
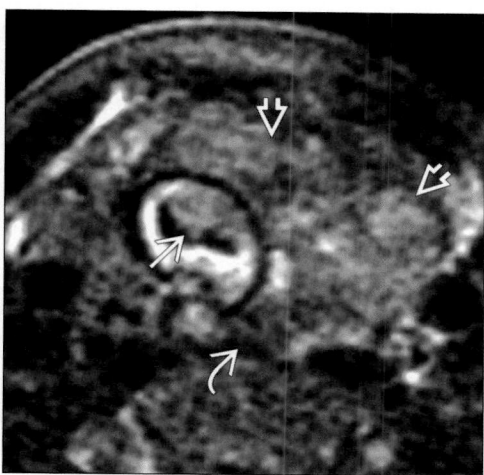

(Left) Transverse grayscale US shows a large, solid, hypoechoic ATCa ➡ with extrathyroid ➡ & tracheal infiltration ➡. Note the adjacent small, heterogeneous nodule ➡ suggestive of background MNG. Note patent left CCA ➡. *(Right)* Axial T2WI FS MR shows an ATCa ➡ with extrathyroid extension ➡ and tracheal infiltration ➡. MR and CECT better demonstrate extrathyroid spread and tracheal involvement.

Typical

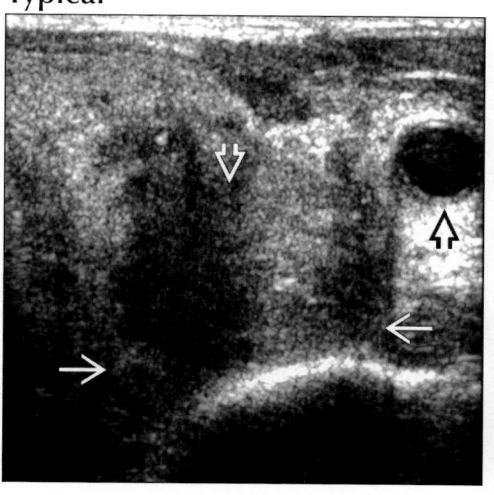
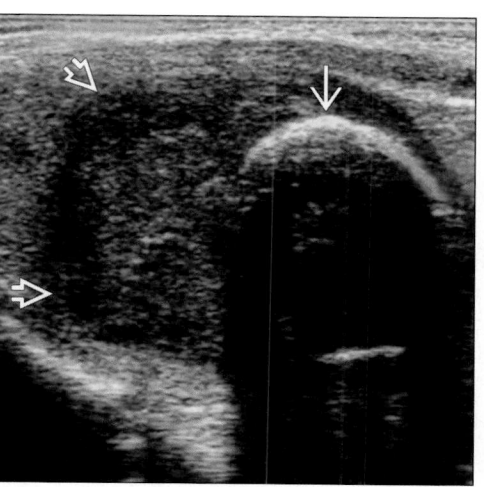

(Left) Transverse grayscale US shows a solid, hypoechoic, ill-defined ATCa ➡ with extrathyroid spread posteriorly ➡. Note patent left CCA ➡. *(Right)* Longitudinal grayscale US shows a solid, ill-defined, hypoechoic ATCa ➡ with dense shadowing calcification ➡. Such dense shadowing is a reflection of MNG calcification.

THYROID NON-HODGKIN LYMPHOMA

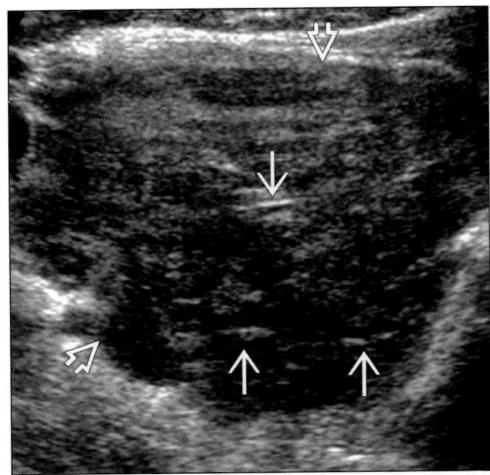

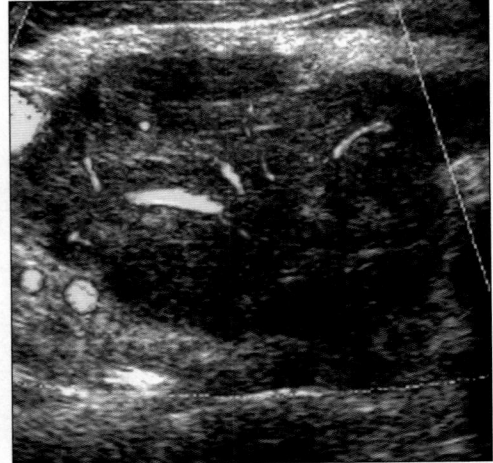

Transverse grayscale US of the thyroid ➡ shows a diffuse, hypoechoic, heterogeneous echo pattern, with fibrotic streaks ➡. History of rapid thyroid enlargement in a patient with HashT. Biopsy showed NHL.

Corresponding power Doppler shows a slight prominence in vascularity but not markedly hypervascular. Color Doppler appearances in thyroid NHL are variable & non-specific.

TERMINOLOGY

Abbreviations and Synonyms
- Thyroid non-Hodgkin lymphoma (NHL)

Definitions
- Primary thyroid NHL is defined as an extranodal, extralymphatic lymphoma that arises from thyroid gland
- Excludes systemic lymphoma that involve thyroid gland secondarily

IMAGING FINDINGS

General Features
- Best diagnostic clue: Rapidly enlarging, solid, non-calcified thyroid mass in elderly female with history of Hashimoto thyroiditis (HashT)
- Size: Often large (5-10 cm)
- Morphology
  - Diffuse, homogeneous thyromegaly if chronic lymphocytic thyroiditis is present, ± lymphomatous neck nodes
  - Primary tumor
    - Rapidly enlarging, homogeneous, solid mass
    - Single mass most common (80%) vs. multiple masses vs. diffusely infiltrated thyroid gland
    - Tendency to compress normal thyroid & surrounding structures without invasion
    - Necrosis, calcification, hemorrhage relatively uncommon (compared to anaplastic thyroid carcinoma)
  - Lymphadenopathy
    - When present, cervical nodes are usually multiple, bilateral & solid/reticulated

Ultrasonographic Findings
- Background evidence of previous HashT: Echogenic fibrous streaks in lobulated, hypoechoic gland
- Focal lymphomatous mass/nodule: "Pseudocystic" appearance with posterior enhancement
- Focal lymphomatous mass/nodule: Well-defined, solid, hypoechoic, heterogeneous, non-calcified
- Diffuse involvement: Hypoechoic, rounded gland with heterogeneous echo pattern
- Diffuse involvement: Simple thyroid enlargement, minimal change in echo pattern (often missed)

DDx: Thyroid Non-Hodgkin Lymphoma

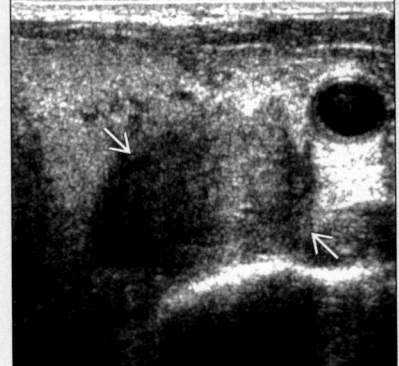

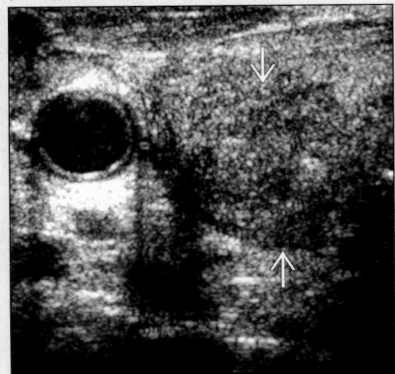

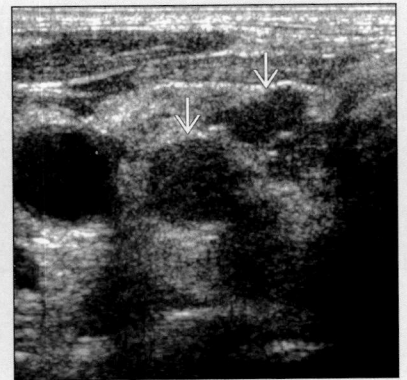

Anaplastic Carcinoma

Papillary Carcinoma

Thyroid Metastasis

THYROID NON-HODGKIN LYMPHOMA

Key Facts

Imaging Findings

- Best diagnostic clue: Rapidly enlarging, solid, non-calcified thyroid mass in elderly female with history of Hashimoto thyroiditis (HashT)
- Background evidence of previous HashT: Echogenic fibrous streaks in lobulated, hypoechoic gland
- Focal lymphomatous mass/nodule: "Pseudocystic" appearance with posterior enhancement
- Focal lymphomatous mass/nodule: Well-defined, solid, hypoechoic, heterogeneous, non-calcified
- Diffuse involvement: Hypoechoic, rounded gland with heterogeneous echo pattern
- Diffuse involvement: Simple thyroid enlargement, minimal change in echo pattern (often missed)
- Lymphadenopathy: "Reticulated" echo pattern or "pseudocystic" echo pattern

- Color Doppler: Thyroid nodules: Non-specific, nodules may be hypovascular or have chaotic intranodular vessels
- Color Doppler: Nodes: Hypervascular nodes, central & peripheral vascularity

Top Differential Diagnoses

- Anaplastic Thyroid Carcinoma (ATCa)
- Differentiated Thyroid Carcinoma (DTCa)
- Metastases to Thyroid

Diagnostic Checklist

- Rapidly enlarging thyroid mass in elderly patient is usually due to thyroid NHL or anaplastic carcinoma
- Absence of calcification, invasion & necrosis, while not specific, are suggestive of NHL

- o Presence of adjacent lymphomatous nodes & background HashT may be the only clue to diagnosis
- Lymphadenopathy: "Reticulated" echo pattern or "pseudocystic" echo pattern
  - o Usually multiple nodes, ± bilateral involvement
  - o Nodes are invariably solid, necrosis is not a feature
  - o Nodes cause mass effect on adjacent vessels but do not infiltrate carotid or jugular vein
- Color Doppler: Thyroid nodules: Non-specific, nodules may be hypovascular or have chaotic intranodular vessels
- Color Doppler: Nodes: Hypervascular nodes, central & peripheral vascularity

CT Findings

- CECT
  - o Primary tumor appearance
    - Homogeneous, solid, hypodense mass most common
    - Diffusely infiltrated gland results in hypodense thyromegaly which cannot reliably be differentiated from Hashimoto thyroiditis
    - Necrosis & calcification are uncommon
  - o Lymphadenopathy
    - Multiple, solid, nonenhancing, hypodense nodes typical

MR Findings

- T1WI: Isointense to normal surrounding thyroid gland
- T2WI: Hyperintense to normal surrounding thyroid gland
- T1 C+
  - o Primary tumor lower signal than surrounding residual thyroid gland
  - o Nodes do not significantly enhance

Nuclear Medicine Findings

- Gallium-67 scintigraphy
  - o Thyroid lymphoma is only thyroid malignancy in which intense uptake of gallium is reported

- o Useful for follow-up to differentiate whether any residual abnormality contains active lymphoma or scar tissue

Imaging Recommendations

- Best imaging tool
  - o Thyroid NHL is often picked up/suspected on routine serial follow up US of HashT
  - o Development of focal hypoechoic nodules or ill-defined hypoechoic areas in patients with HashT is suspicious for NHL
  - o Presence of lymphomatous nodes on US during examination of patient with HashT should raise suspicion of thyroid NHL
  - o US-guided biopsy of thyroid, ± neck nodes help to confirm diagnosis
  - o CECT of neck, chest, abdomen & pelvis required for staging when diagnosis is known
- Protocol advice
  - o Lymphomatous nodules & nodes were previously described to have "pseudosolid" appearance: Anechoic with posterior enhancement but solid on biopsy
  - o With modern transducers such appearance is rare in thyroid & nodes & internal solid nature is clearly identified
    - Lymphomatous nodes have a heterogeneous, reticulated appearance using modern high resolution transducers

DIFFERENTIAL DIAGNOSIS

Anaplastic Thyroid Carcinoma (ATCa)

- Rapidly enlarging, invasive thyroid mass in elderly patient against a background of multinodular goiter
- Calcification, necrosis, heterogeneous tumor with vascular & soft tissue extension & necrotic nodes common

THYROID NON-HODGKIN LYMPHOMA

Differentiated Thyroid Carcinoma (DTCa)
- Unilateral, ill-defined, solid, hypoechoic mass with abnormal vascularity, ± punctate calcification & adjacent characteristic adenopathy
- Large, invasive tumor may be indistinguishable from anaplastic carcinoma or lymphoma

Metastases to Thyroid
- May mimic thyroid lymphoma, but invariably there is evidence of disseminated disease and a known primary
- Focal, solid, solitary/multiple, well-defined nodules with hypervascularity or diffuse thyroid enlargement with adjacent characteristic adenopathy

Multinodular Goiter
- Multiple, hypoechoic, heterogeneous, cystic/septated nodules with perinodular vascularity, coarse calcification, ± comet tail artifact
- Rapid increase in size: Spontaneous hemorrhage

PATHOLOGY

General Features
- General path comments
  - Three forms of NHL in head and neck
    - Nodal NHL
    - Extranodal, lymphatic NHL (Waldeyer ring)
    - Extranodal, extralymphatic NHL (sinonasal, orbit, thyroid most common)
- Etiology: Primary hypothesis: Chronic stimulation from autoimmune lymphocytic thyroiditis leads to proliferation of lymphoid tissue, which undergoes mutation resulting in thyroid NHL
- Epidemiology
  - Chronic lymphocytic thyroiditis (Hashimoto thyroiditis) is associated in 40–80% of cases
    - Patients with chronic lymphocytic thyroiditis have a 70-fold increased risk of developing primary thyroid NHL
  - Primary thyroid NHL is 2-5% of all thyroid malignancies
    - Most are poorly differentiated non-Hodgkin B-cell tumors
    - Less common is low grade malignant lymphoma of mucosa-associated lymphoid tissue (MALT)
    - Rarely Hodgkin lymphoma, Burkitt cell lymphoma & T-cell lymphoma

CLINICAL ISSUES

Presentation
- Most common signs/symptoms
  - Rapidly enlarging thyroid mass, frequently with associated neck adenopathy in patient with HashT
    - Low grade NHL have a slower growth rate
  - Other signs/symptoms
    - Compression of, or local extension into surrounding tissues may cause dysphagia, dyspnea or pressure symptoms
    - Vocal cord paralysis & hoarseness suggest involvement of recurrent laryngeal nerve

- Regional & distant lymphadenopathy common
- Clinical Profile: Older female with rapidly growing lower, paramedian neck mass
- Approach to diagnosis
  - Fine needle biopsy usually performed first
    - Less reliable than for other thyroid malignancies
    - May be difficult to differentiate thyroid NHL from chronic lymphocytic thyroiditis
  - Surgical biopsy performed in patients when fine needle biopsy indeterminate
  - Most important distinction is between thyroid lymphoma & anaplastic carcinoma

Demographics
- Age: Peak incidence occurs in sixth decade
- Gender: M:F = 1:4

Natural History & Prognosis
- Thyroid NHL is highly curable
- Most thyroid lymphomas have an 85% 5 year survival rate
- Spread beyond thyroid gland reduces 5 year survival rate to about 35%

Treatment
- Diffuse large B-cell lymphoma
  - Combined-modality therapy with radiation & combined IV chemotherapy
- Low-grade malignant MALT lymphoma
  - Radiation therapy, oral chlorambucil or IV chemotherapy
- Surgery only when present with obstructive symptoms requiring acute palliative intervention

DIAGNOSTIC CHECKLIST

Image Interpretation Pearls
- Rapidly enlarging thyroid mass in elderly patient is usually due to thyroid NHL or anaplastic carcinoma
- Absence of calcification, invasion & necrosis, while not specific, are suggestive of NHL

SELECTED REFERENCES

1. Wong KT et al: Ultrasound of thyroid cancer. Cancer Imaging. 5:157-66, 2005
2. Harnsberger HR et al: Diagnostic Imaging: Head & Neck. 1st ed. Salt Lake City, Amirsys. III-11-40-43, 2004
3. Ahuja AT et al: Imaging in Head & Neck Cancer: A Practical Approach. 1st ed. London, Greenwich Medical Media. 143-66, 2003
4. Kim HC et al: Primary thyroid lymphoma: CT findings. Eur J Radiol. 46(3):233-9, 2003
5. Cha C et al: Primary thyroid lymphoma: can the diagnosis be made solely by fine-needle aspiration? Ann Surg Oncol. 9(3):298-302, 2002
6. Wirtzfeld DA et al: Clinical presentation and treatment of non-Hodgkin's lymphoma of the thyroid gland. Ann Surg Oncol. 8(4):338-41, 2001

IMAGE GALLERY

Typical

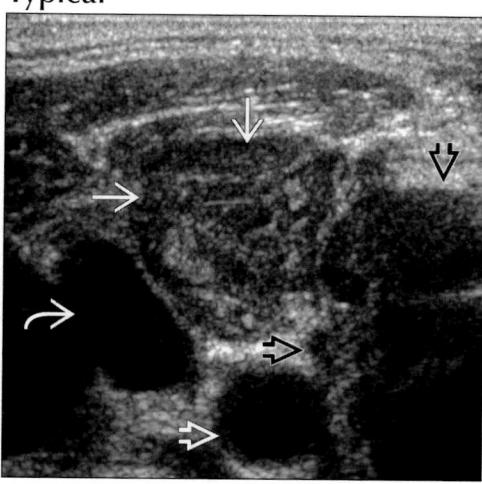
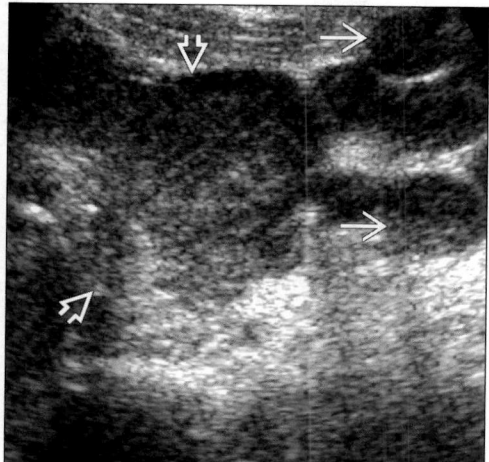

(Left) Transverse grayscale US shows a thyroid with sonographic evidence of HashT ➡ & an associated large, solid, hypoechoic mass ➡. Biopsy showed NHL. Note patent jugular vein ➡, carotid artery ➡. (Right) Transverse grayscale US shows a diffusely hypoechoic thyroid ➡ with lobulated contour & adjacent, round, solid hypoechoic nodes ➡. Biopsy thyroid & node: NHL. Nodes raised suspicion of NHL.

Typical

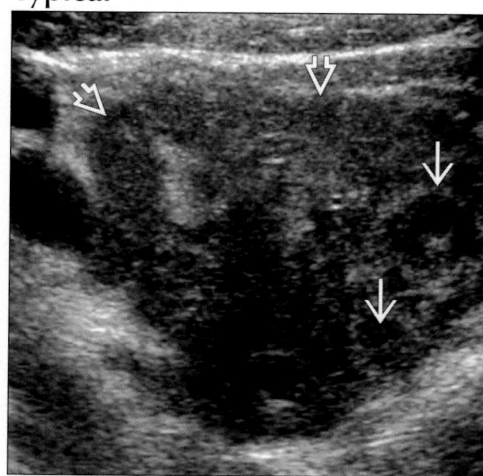
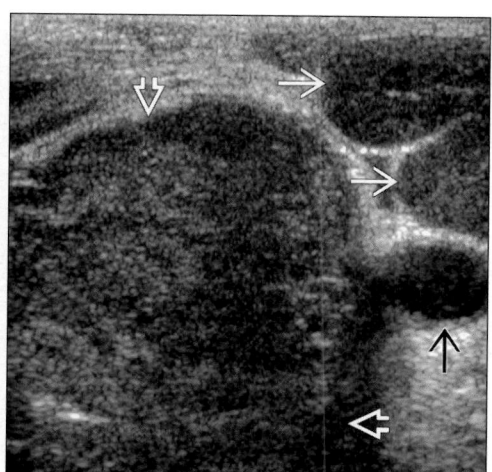

(Left) Transverse grayscale US of the thyroid ➡ shows sonographic evidence of HashT & focal, hypoechoic nodules ➡. Biopsy confirmed NHL. This was found on serial sonography in patient with HashT. (Right) Transverse grayscale US shows a diffusely enlarged, hypoechoic thyroid ➡ with a rounded contour & multiple associated hypoechoic nodes ➡. A biopsy confirmed NHL. Note patent carotid artery ➡.

Typical

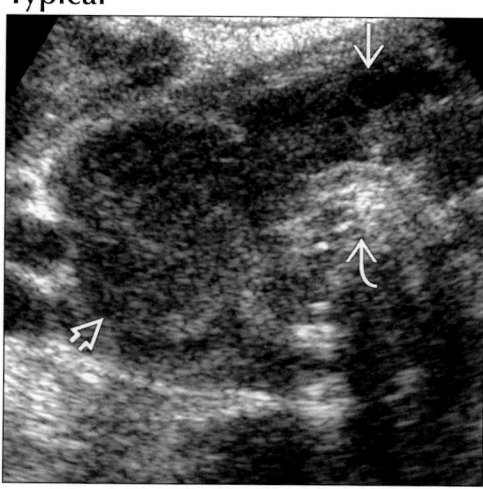
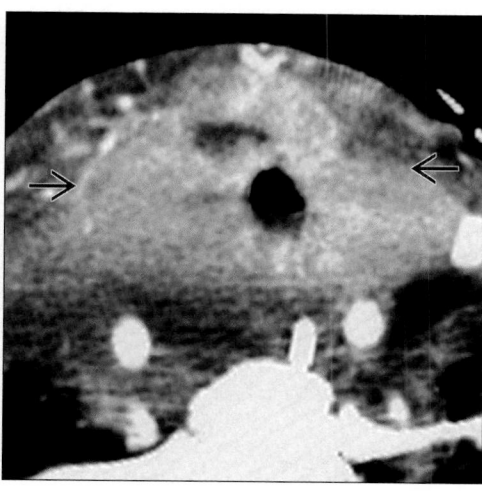

(Left) Transverse grayscale US shows a diffuse, hypoechoic, thyroid parenchymal echoes involving the right lobe ➡ & the isthmus ➡ with extension to left. Biopsy showed NHL. Trachea ➡. (Right) Corresponding axial CECT shows diffuse enlargement of the thyroid ➡ due to NHL involvement.

HASHIMOTO THYROIDITIS

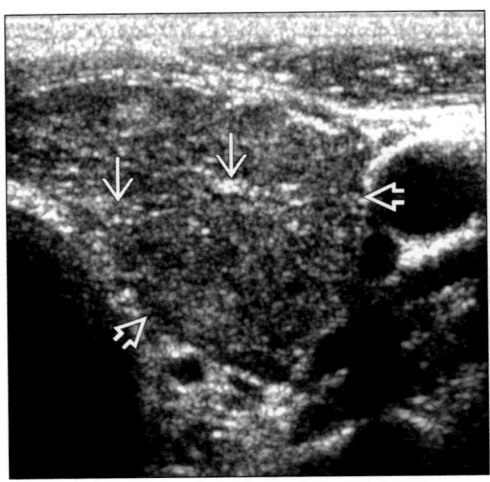

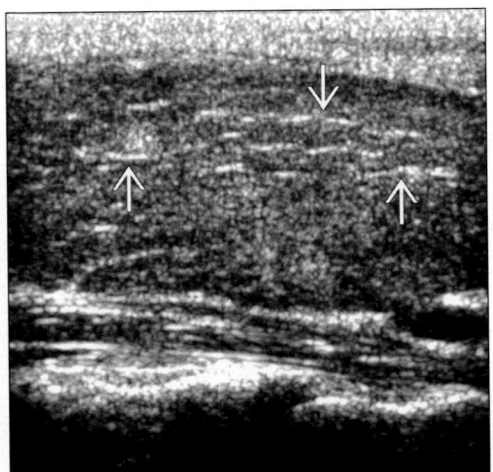

Transverse US an shows an enlarged thyroid ➡ with diffuse, hypoechoic, heterogeneous parenchyma & bright fibrotic streaks ➡. Note no focal bulge or hypoechoic nodules are seen to suggest NHL.

Corresponding longitudinal US shows the fibrotic streaks ➡ clearly. Note the clear visualization of thyroid parenchyma with high-resolution US, ideal for follow-up of HashT patients.

TERMINOLOGY

Abbreviations and Synonyms
- Hashimoto thyroiditis (HashT)
- Chronic lymphocytic thyroiditis, sclerosing lymphocytic thyroiditis

Definitions
- HashT: Chronic, autoimmune-mediated lymphocytic inflammation of thyroid gland

IMAGING FINDINGS

General Features
- Best diagnostic clue
  - Diffuse moderately enlarged, hypoechoic gland with lobulated outlines & heterogeneous echo pattern with fine bright fibrotic streaks within
    - Vascularity depends on stage & type of involvement
- Size: Moderate increase in thyroid gland size
- Morphology: Heterogeneous internal architecture with accentuation of lobular architecture by fibrosis

Ultrasonographic Findings
- Grayscale Ultrasound
  - Acute focal HashT: Ill-defined focal hypoechoic areas representing areas of lymphocytic infiltration
  - Acute diffuse HashT: Diffuse, hypoechoic, heterogeneous, micronodular echo pattern involving the whole gland
  - Chronic HashT: Enlarged, hypoechoic, heterogeneous gland with lobulated outlines
  - Chronic HashT: Hypoechoic areas separated by echogenic fibrous septa
  - Atrophic/end stage HashT: Small gland with heterogeneous echo pattern
- Color Doppler
  - **Color Doppler**: Acute focal/diffuse thyroiditis: Avascular gland
  - Chronic: Hypervascular when patient is hypothyroid reflecting hypertrophic action of TSH
  - Chronic: Following treatment when TSH returns to normal, hypervascularity decreases
  - Atrophic: Avascular/hypovascular gland
  - Hypervascularity is never as marked as Graves disease and flow velocities are within normal limits

---

DDx: Hashimoto Thyroiditis

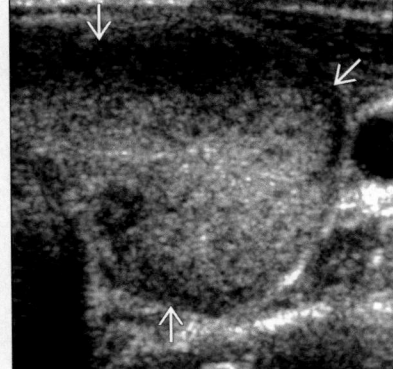

Thyroid NHL

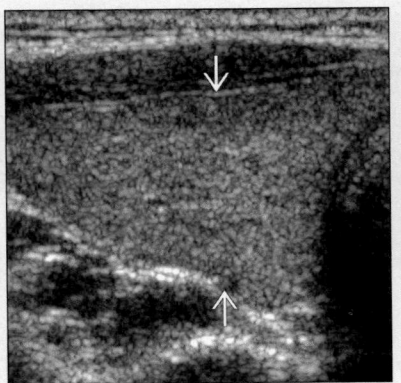

Graves Disease

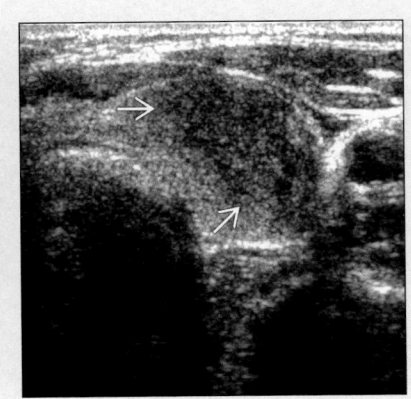

De Quervain Thyroiditis

HASHIMOTO THYROIDITIS

Key Facts

Imaging Findings
- Acute focal HashT: Ill-defined focal hypoechoic areas representing areas of lymphocytic infiltration
- Acute diffuse HashT: Diffuse, hypoechoic, heterogeneous, micronodular echo pattern involving the whole gland
- Chronic HashT: Enlarged, hypoechoic, heterogeneous gland with lobulated outlines
- Chronic HashT: Hypoechoic areas separated by echogenic fibrous septa
- Atrophic/end stage HashT: Small gland with heterogeneous echo pattern
- **Color Doppler**: Acute focal/diffuse thyroiditis: Avascular gland
- Chronic: Hypervascular when patient is hypothyroid reflecting hypertrophic action of TSH

- Chronic: Following treatment when TSH returns to normal, hypervascularity decreases
- Atrophic: Avascular/hypovascular gland
- There is an increased risk of non-Hodgkin lymphoma (NHL) in Hashimoto thyroiditis
- **When scanning patients with HashT always evaluate thyroid (± FNAC) for developing NHL, seen as**
- Focal bulge in the contour of the gland
- Developing areas of ill-defined hypoechogenicity, focal or diffuse, ± mass effect
- Lymphomatous adenopathy in adjacent neck

Top Differential Diagnoses
- Thyroid Non-Hodgkin Lymphoma (NHL)
- Graves Disease
- De Quervain Thyroiditis

CT Findings
- CECT
  - Nonspecific findings: Symmetric enlargement of thyroid, diffuse decreased density, typical
  - No necrosis or calcification evident

MR Findings
- Nonspecific findings with heterogeneous signal intensity
- On T2WI, parenchymal signal may be diffusely increased with lower intensity fibrotic bands

Nuclear Medicine Findings
- PET
  - Normal thyroid can have moderate diffuse FDG uptake
  - HashT may show thyroidal uptake
- Tc-99m pertechnetate and iodine 123 most commonly used agents
  - Early: Diffuse uniform increased activity mimicking Graves disease
  - Later: Coarse patchy activity mimicking multinodular goiter

Imaging Recommendations
- Best imaging tool
  - Diagnosis of HashT is made on clinical & biochemical tests of thyroid function & imaging is not necessary for diagnosis
  - There is an increased risk of non-Hodgkin lymphoma (NHL) in Hashimoto thyroiditis
    - US is ideal imaging modality to monitor the gland & for early detection of NHL
    - US evaluates thyroid gland and adjacent neck nodes & is readily combined with fine needle aspiration cytology (FNAC) for further evaluation
- Protocol advice
  - **When scanning patients with HashT always evaluate thyroid (± FNAC) for developing NHL, seen as**
    - Focal bulge in the contour of the gland

- Developing areas of ill-defined hypoechogenicity, focal or diffuse, ± mass effect
- Lymphomatous adenopathy in adjacent neck

DIFFERENTIAL DIAGNOSIS

Thyroid Non-Hodgkin Lymphoma (NHL)
- Focal/diffuse hypoechoic parenchymal echo pattern with extrathyroid spread & associated lymphomatous adenopathy
- Most patients with primary thyroid lymphoma have history of Hashimoto

Graves Disease
- Diffuse, hypoechoic, spotty, heterogeneous parenchymal echo pattern with increased vascularity

De Quervain Thyroiditis
- Focal, ill-defined hypoechoic area within thyroid, ± increased vascularity; progressive change on serial examination
- Patient has fever, raised white cell count & present with painful thyroid lump, ± thyrotoxicosis

Reidel Thyroiditis (Invasive Fibrosing Thyroiditis)
- Benign fibrosis of part or all of thyroid gland with diffuse enlargement & extension to surrounding soft tissues

Anaplastic Thyroid Carcinoma
- Heterogeneous, ill-defined, hypoechoic infiltrative mass against a background of multinodular goiter, with associated necrotic nodes

PATHOLOGY

General Features
- General path comments: Diffuse lymphocytic infiltration of thyroid

HASHIMOTO THYROIDITIS

- Genetics: Familial predisposition: ≤ 50% first-degree relatives have elevated thyroid autoantibodies
- Etiology
  - Anti-thyroid autoantibodies produce anti-thyroglobulin, anti-thyroperoxidase, anti-TSH-receptor ± anti-mitochondrial antibody
  - Functional organification defect
- Epidemiology
  - Most common cause goitrous hypothyroidism in USA
  - 10% population have detectable anti-thyroid autoantibodies
  - 3-4% have degree of autoimmune thyroiditis
- Associated abnormalities
  - Thyroid non-Hodgkin lymphoma
    - Patients with HashT have 70-80x risk of developing thyroid NHL
    - > 85% patients with primary thyroid lymphoma have coexistent Hashimoto
  - Hashimoto encephalopathy
    - Rare association, responds well to corticosteroids
    - Subacute encephalopathy with seizures or movement disorder in association with intrathecal antithyroid antibodies
  - Juvenile Hashimoto
    - Associated with type 1 diabetes; other autoimmune endocrine diseases
    - Down & Turner syndromes

Gross Pathologic & Surgical Features
- Firm, symmetrically enlarged gland
- Tan-yellow parenchyma; lymphocytic infiltration produces "fish-flesh" texture
- Fibrosis can accentuate thyroid lobular architecture

Microscopic Features
- Classic HashT diagnosis requires presence of 4 features
  - Diffuse infiltration of stroma between follicles with lymphocytes & plasma cells
  - Hürthle cell metaplasia; may form nodules
  - Atrophic, small thyroid follicles without colloid
  - Fibrosis
- Fibrosing variant of HashT seen in 10%; elderly patients typically, males > females
  - Atrophic thyroid with dense keloidal fibrosis
- Juvenile form of HashT
  - Prominent lymphocytic infiltrate without prominent Hürthle cells or glandular atrophy
  - Hyperplasia often present; may have hyperthyroidism

CLINICAL ISSUES

Presentation
- Most common signs/symptoms
  - Gradual painless enlargement of thyroid
    - Patients most often euthyroid with normal T3 and T4 hormones ("subclinical HashT")
  - Other signs/symptoms
    - 20% present with hypothyroidism
    - 5% have early stage "hashitoxicosis" = thyrotoxicosis with release of excess thyroid hormone

- Clinical Profile: Female over age of 40 with gradual moderate enlargement of thyroid

Demographics
- Age
  - Peak incidence: 4th-5th decades
  - Juvenile form predominantly in adolescents
- Gender
  - M:F = 1:9
  - Juvenile form
    - M:F = 1:2

Natural History & Prognosis
- Slow progression to hypothyroid state at rate of 5% per year
- Most important complication is increased incidence of thyroid malignancy
  - Non-Hodgkin lymphoma most frequent, especially MALT-type
  - Also papillary and Hürthle cell tumors, leukemia and plasmacytoma

Treatment
- Nonsurgical unless enlarged gland impedes airway
- Thyroid hormone replacement as necessary
- Corticosteroids if painful, tender gland or with encephalopathy
- Long term follow-up of any nodules & to detect development of NHL

DIAGNOSTIC CHECKLIST

Consider
- Rapid enlargement of thyroid in patient with history of Hashimoto = NHL until proven otherwise

Image Interpretation Pearls
- Important to follow-up ± aspirate under ultrasound any focal nodules because of increased risk of malignancy

SELECTED REFERENCES

1. Harnsberger HR et al: Diagnostic Imaging: Head & Neck. Salt Lake City, Amirsys. III-11-4 -7, 2004
2. Loy M et al: Correlation of computerized gray-scale sonographic findings with thyroid function and thyroid autoimmune activity in patients with Hashimoto's thyroiditis. J Clin Ultrasound. 32(3):136-40, 2004
3. Hegedus L: Thyroid ultrasound. Endocrinol Metab Clin North Am. 30(2):339-60, viii-ix, 2001
4. Langer JE et al: Sonographic appearance of focal thyroiditis. AJR Am J Roentgenol. 176(3):751-4, 2001
5. Solbiati L et al: Ultrasound of thyroid, parathyroid glands and neck lymph nodes. Eur Radiol. 11(12):2411-24, 2001
6. Ahuja AT et al: Practical Head & Neck Ultrasound. London, Greenwich Medical Media. 35-64, 2000
7. Weber AL et al: The thyroid and parathyroid glands. CT and MR imaging and correlation with pathology and clinical findings. Radiol Clin North Am. 38(5):1105-29, 2000

HASHIMOTO THYROIDITIS

IMAGE GALLERY

Typical

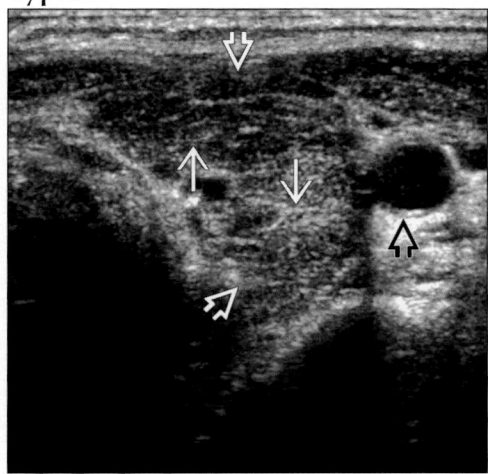

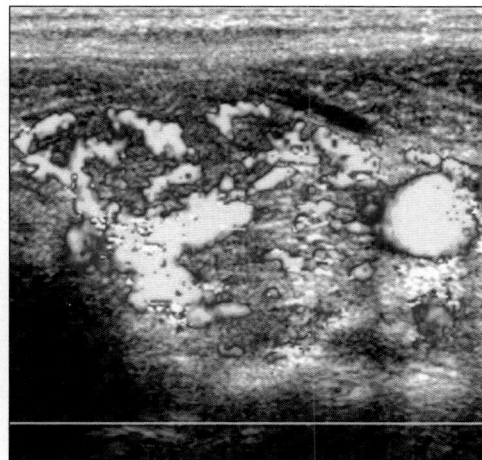

(Left) Transverse US shows a hypoechoic, heterogeneous, thyroid ➡ echo pattern with multiple fine fibrotic ➡ streaks. No focal contour bulge or mass to suggest NHL. Carotid artery ➡. *(Right)* Corresponding power Doppler US shows a marked increase in thyroid parenchymal vascularity, suggesting hypertrophic influence of TSH.

Typical

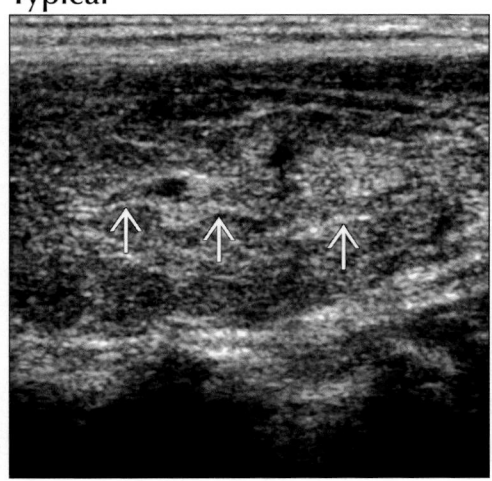

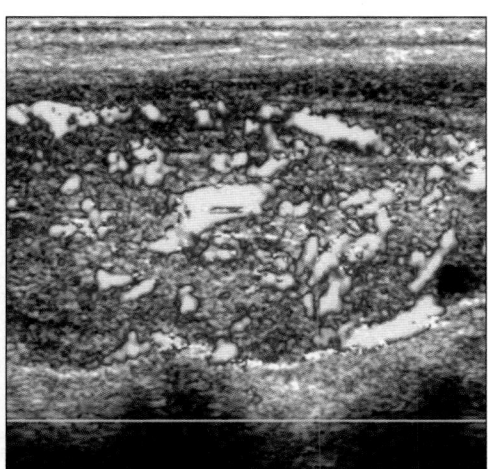

(Left) Longitudinal US shows a heterogeneous thyroid parenchymal echo pattern with multiple fine bright fibrotic streaks ➡. *(Right)* Corresponding power Doppler US shows a marked increase in parenchymal vascularity (hypertrophic action of TSH). This vascularity diminishes as TSH levels return to normal following treatment.

Typical

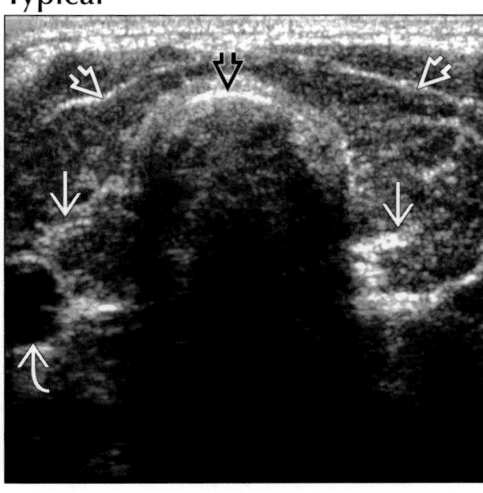

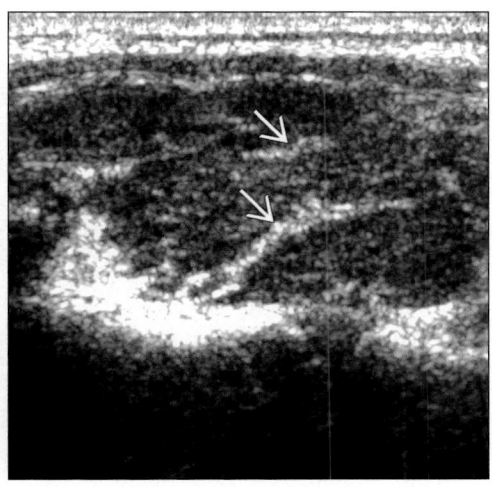

(Left) Transverse US shows a small, atrophic thyroid ➡ with hypoechoic echo pattern & fibrosis ➡ indicative of end stage HashT. Trachea ➡, right carotid artery ➡. *(Right)* Corresponding longitudinal US in end stage HashT shows hypoechoic, heterogeneous thyroid parenchymal echoes & fibrosis ➡. Note the absence of any focal hypoechoic nodules to suggest NHL.

MULTINODULAR GOITER

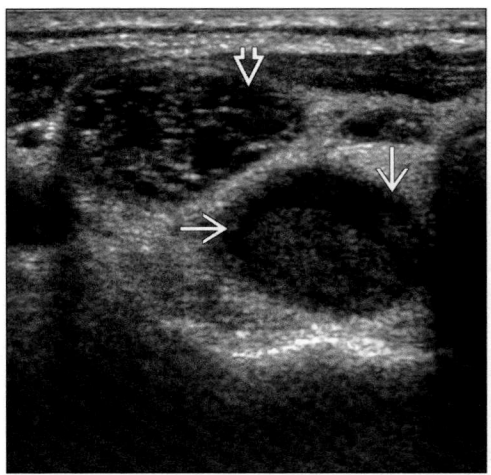

Longitudinal grayscale US shows multiple, well-defined, non-calcified, heterogeneous nodules ➡ with cystic change, against a coarse thyroid parenchymal echo pattern ➡; typical findings of MNG.

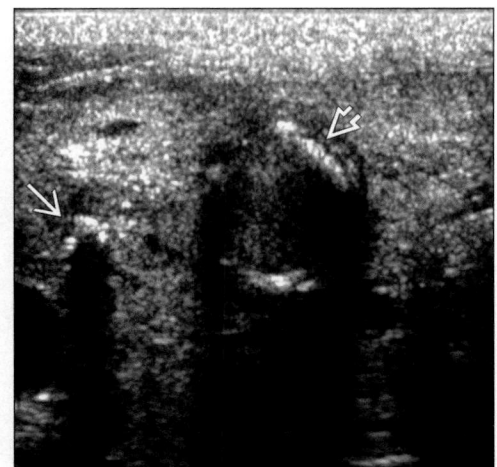

Grayscale US shows curvilinear ➡ & dysmorphic ➡ calcifications, with dense posterior shadowing, in a thyroid with coarse heterogeneous parenchymal echoes. These calcification are typical for MNG.

TERMINOLOGY

Abbreviations and Synonyms
- Multinodular goiter (MNG)
- Simple nodular goiter, nontoxic goiter

Definitions
- MNG: Diffuse, multi-nodular enlargement of thyroid gland in response to chronic TSH stimulation
- Plunging/substernal/retrosternal goiter: Inferior extension of MNG into mediastinum

IMAGING FINDINGS

General Features
- Best diagnostic clue
  - Well-margined, diffuse enlargement of thyroid gland, with a heterogeneous, nodular appearance
  - Calcifications, fibrosis, degenerative cysts & hemorrhage result in heterogeneous imaging appearance
- Location: Visceral space, thyroid bed; substernal extension occurs in 37% of patients

- Morphology
  - Well-margined, diffuse thyroid enlargement within visceral space of infrahyoid neck; may become very large (> 15 cm)
    - Carotid spaces displaced away from midline; trachea compressed between enlarged thyroid lobes

Ultrasonographic Findings
- Grayscale Ultrasound
  - Multiplicity of nodules, bilateral diffuse involvement
  - Solid nodules are often isoechoic with small proportion being hypoechoic (5%)
  - Despite being unencapsulated, nodules are sharply defined with halo
    - Halo composed of adjacent vessels & compressed thyroid
  - Heterogeneous internal echo pattern with internal debris, septa, solid/cystic portions
    - Solid portion within often represents blood clot
  - Dense shadowing calcification (curvilinear, dysmorphic, coarse)

DDx: Nodular Goiter

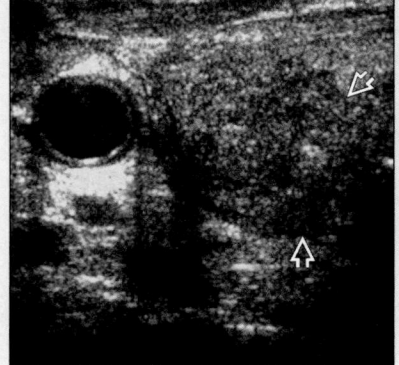

Papillary Carcinoma

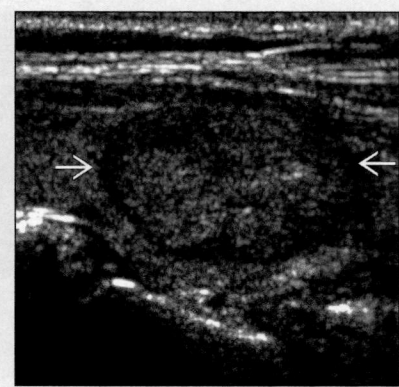

Follicular Carcinoma

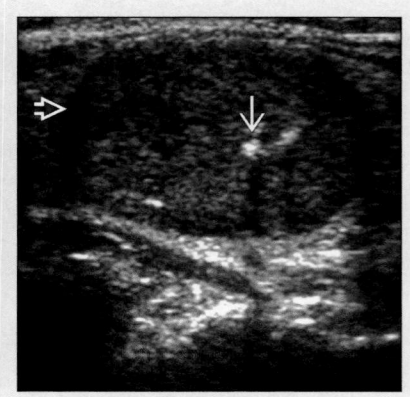

Medullary Carcinoma

MULTINODULAR GOITER

Key Facts

Imaging Findings

- Solid nodules are often isoechoic with small proportion being hypoechoic (5%)
- Despite being unencapsulated, nodules are sharply defined with halo
- Heterogeneous internal echo pattern with internal debris, septa, solid/cystic portions
- Dense shadowing calcification (curvilinear, dysmorphic, coarse)
- Nodules with comet tail artifact, highly suggestive of colloid nodule
- Cystic component due to hemorrhage or colloid within nodule
- Background thyroid parenchymal echoes are coarse & heterogeneous (fine bright echoes in normal gland)
- Color Doppler: Peripheral vascularity > intranodular vascularity
- Color Doppler: Septa, intranodular solid portions are avascular (organizing blood, clot)
- Look for papillary carcinoma in MNG: Search for solid, ill-defined, hypoechoic nodule, punctate microcalcification & chaotic intranodular vessels
- Main role of US in MNG is to identify presence of suspicious nodule & guide biopsy
- Evaluate neck for suspicious/metastatic nodes & for any retrosternal extension

Top Differential Diagnoses

- Papillary Carcinoma
- Follicular Carcinoma
- Medullary Carcinoma

- Nodules with comet tail artifact, highly suggestive of colloid nodule
- Cystic component due to hemorrhage or colloid within nodule
- Background thyroid parenchymal echoes are coarse & heterogeneous (fine bright echoes in normal gland)
- Color Doppler: Peripheral vascularity > intranodular vascularity
- Color Doppler: Septa, intranodular solid portions are avascular (organizing blood, clot)

Radiographic Findings

- Radiography
  - Chest X-ray findings
    - If suprasternal, may be normal or show mild tracheal deviation or narrowing
    - If substernal, superior mediastinal mass with tracheal deviation & narrowing

CT Findings

- NECT
  - Low attenuation areas of degenerative & colloidal cysts
  - Intermediate attenuation areas of solid adenomatous nodules & fibrosis
  - High attenuation areas from hemorrhage & calcification (90%, amorphous, focal ring-like)
- CECT
  - Thyroid parenchyma replaced with multiple, variably sized, heterogeneous, solid & cystic masses
  - Diffuse, inhomogeneous enhancement

MR Findings

- T1WI
  - Cystic degeneration, fibrosis & calcification contribute to hypointense foci
  - Hemorrhage within MNG may yield areas of high T1 signal
  - Coronal images show "cradling" of inferior margin of substernal MNG by brachiocephalic vessels
- T2WI
  - Fibrosis & calcification low signal on T2 sequences
  - Cystic degeneration, hemorrhage seen as high signal foci
- T1 C+: Diffuse markedly inhomogeneous enhancement

Nuclear Medicine Findings

- Radioiodine scintigraphy (Tc-99m pertechnetate or I-123)
  - No role in initial evaluation of nontoxic nodular goiter
  - Effective in recognizing a mediastinal mass as thyroid in nature
  - Heterogeneously iodine avid, with suppression of surrounding parenchyma

Imaging Recommendations

- Best imaging tool
  - US is ideal imaging modality of choice as it evaluates thyroid nodules, adjacent mass effect, helps to identify suspicious nodule
  - US is ideal to follow-up of patients who are otherwise asymptomatic but apprehensive about thyroid nodules
  - Risk of malignancy in MNG is 1-5%, most common cancer being papillary thyroid cancer
    - Anaplastic carcinoma is usually seen against a background of multinodularity, less common than papillary carcinoma
  - Look for papillary carcinoma in MNG: Search for solid, ill-defined, hypoechoic nodule, punctate microcalcification & chaotic intranodular vessels
    - Evaluate neck for metastatic nodes: Solid/cystic, hyperechoic, punctate microcalcification, abnormal vascularity, pre/paratracheal & deep cervical chain
  - US used to guide needle biopsy of suspicious nodules
  - US is unable to evaluate large goiters, particularly their mediastinal extent, CT/MR are better
  - CT/MR better evaluate extent, severity of airway compression & retrosternal extension
- Protocol advice

MULTINODULAR GOITER

- ○ Main role of US in MNG is to identify presence of suspicious nodule & guide biopsy
- ○ Evaluate neck for suspicious/metastatic nodes & for any retrosternal extension

DIFFERENTIAL DIAGNOSIS

Papillary Carcinoma
- Ill-defined, solid, hypoechoic nodule with punctate microcalcification & chaotic intranodular vessels
- Abnormal nodes: Solid/cystic, hyperechoic, punctate microcalcification, abnormal vessels, characteristic distribution

Follicular Carcinoma
- Ill-defined/well-defined, hypoechoic, solid nodule with abnormal vascularity & no calcification
- Unilateral with normal thyroid tissue seen; other small heterogeneous nodules to suggest MNG may be seen

Medullary Carcinoma
- Ill-defined/well-defined, hypoechoic, solid nodule with abnormal vascularity & coarse shadowing calcification
- Abnormal nodes: Solid, hypoechoic, coarse shadowing focus, abnormal vessels, characteristic distribution

Anaplastic Thyroid Carcinoma
- Rapidly enlarging, heterogeneous, ill-defined, coarse calcification, invasive tumor originating from thyroid gland
- Esophagus, trachea, carotid space may be invaded

PATHOLOGY

General Features
- General path comments
  - ○ MNG most common cause of asymmetric thyroid enlargement; 3-5% general population affected in developed countries
  - ○ MNG encompasses wide spectrum from incidental asymptomatic small solitary nodule to large intrathoracic goiter
  - ○ Substernal extension in 37%
    - Majority anterior mediastinum, rarely posterior mediastinum
    - Most common cause of anterior mediastinal mass
  - ○ 95% MNG benign; 5% malignant
    - Incidence of malignancy in MNG is same as a single nodule
- Etiology
  - ○ Environmental iodine deficiency leads to TSH elevation; thyroid hyperplasia results with gradual, diffuse glandular enlargement
  - ○ Areas of involution & fibrosis interspersed with areas of focal hyperplasia develop; results in development of multiple nodules
- Epidemiology
  - ○ Sporadic goiter
    - Generally adequate dietary iodine intake
    - Incidence of sporadic MNG estimated at approximately 5% in US
    - Prevalence of palpable nodules is approximately 5-6% in people aged 60 years
    - At ultrasound & autopsy incidence of small nonpalpable nodules approaches 50% in people aged 60 years
  - ○ Endemic goiter
    - Associated with iodine deficiency
    - More than 13% of world's population affected
    - Mild iodine deficiency associated with a goiter prevalence of 5-20%
    - Moderate iodine deficiency associated with a goiter prevalence of 20-30%
    - Severe iodine deficiency associated with a goiter prevalence of > 30%
- Associated abnormalities: Papillary carcinoma & anaplastic thyroid carcinoma may be seen with MNG

CLINICAL ISSUES

Presentation
- Most common signs/symptoms
  - ○ Large, multinodular lower neck mass
  - ○ Airway compression (55%); hoarseness (15%); dysphagia & superior vena cava syndrome (10%)
- Clinical Profile: Most euthyroid (normal TSH), but can become hyperthyroid or, rarely, hypothyroid

Demographics
- Age
  - ○ Sporadic goiter has no specific age incidence
  - ○ Endemic goiter from iodine deficiency occurs during childhood, continues to ↑ in size with age
- Gender: 2-4:1 female predominance

Natural History & Prognosis
- Growth & nodule production → functional autonomy; functional autonomy rarely results in thyrotoxicosis
- Spontaneous regression vs. gradually increasing size with development of multiple nodules, local compression symptoms ± cosmetic complaints
- Risk of cancer in MNG (5%)
  - ○ Risk factors for malignancy: Radiation exposure, family history of thyroid carcinoma, rapid growth

Treatment
- No treatment for asymptomatic, non-palpable MNG identified on neck imaging done for other reasons, ± US for FU
- Patients with prominent, growing, hard nodule may have US + FNA for cytology to exclude malignancy
- Large, non-toxic, compressive MNG: Surgical removal
  - ○ Post-operative thyroid hormone replacement
- Toxic MNG: Surgery or radioiodine therapy
- Substernal MNG: Suprasternal collar incision alone
  - ○ Median sternotomy rarely necessary (< 2%)

SELECTED REFERENCES

1. Harnsberger HR et al: Diagnostic Imaging: Head & Neck. 1st ed. Salt Lake City, Amirsys. III-11-8-11, 2004

IMAGE GALLERY

Typical

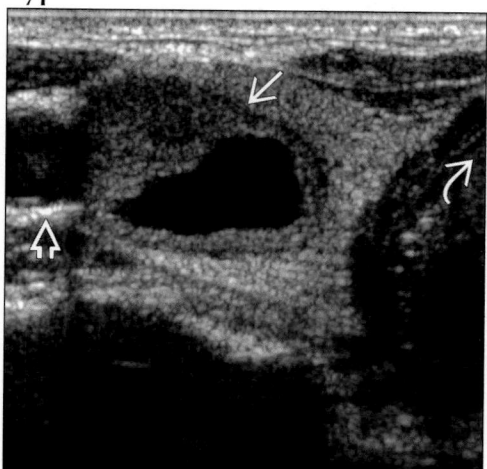
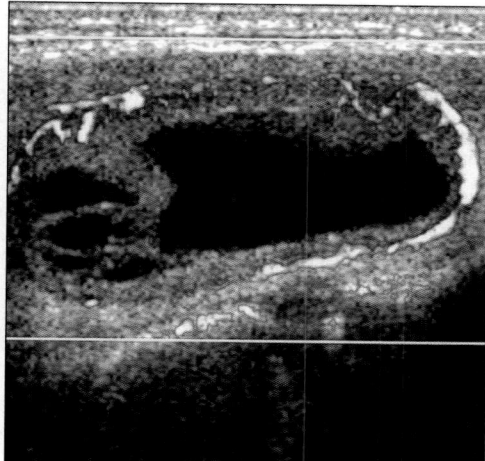

(Left) Transverse grayscale US shows a haloed, non-calcified nodule ➡, with cystic & solid components. Note the relationship to the carotid artery ➡ and trachea ➡. There is no extrathyroid spread. (Right) Corresponding longitudinal power Doppler shows perinodular vascularity with absence of vascularity in the septa & solid portions, suggesting it may be organizing blood clot in a MNG nodule.

Typical

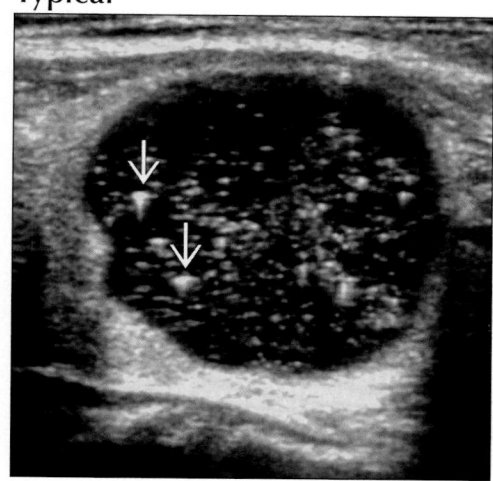
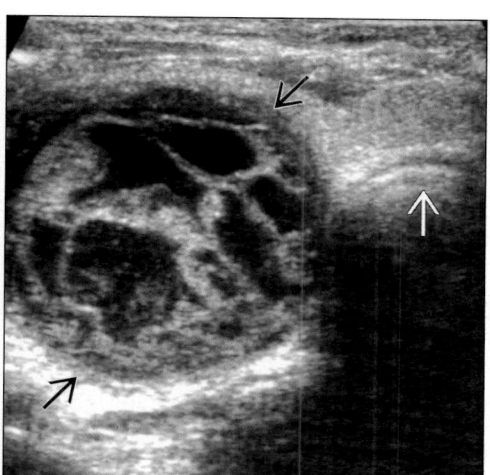

(Left) Grayscale US shows a well-defined, cystic thyroid nodule with echogenic debris & comet tail ➡ artifact in the cystic portion; features highly suggestive of colloid nodule. (Right) Transverse grayscale US shows septations in a well-defined, cystic thyroid nodule ➡, suggesting previous hemorrhage in a nodule in MNG. Such nodules are commonly seen in MNG. Trachea ➡.

Typical

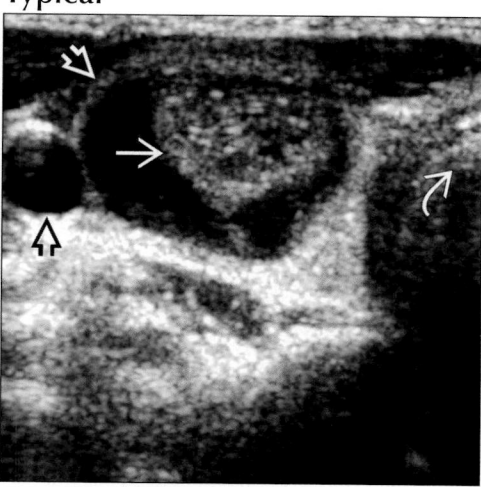
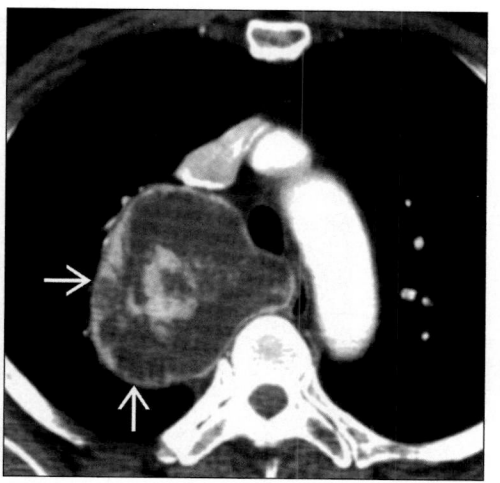

(Left) Transverse grayscale US of a MNG shows a cystic nodule ➡ with a solid portion ➡. It was avascular on Doppler, suggesting, a blood clot. Trachea ➡, carotid artery ➡. (Right) CECT shows a large nodule ➡ with a cystic & enhancing solid portion in the mediastinum. This was continuous with a large thyroid MNG in the neck. US is unable to evaluate such mediastinal extension.

GRAVES DISEASE

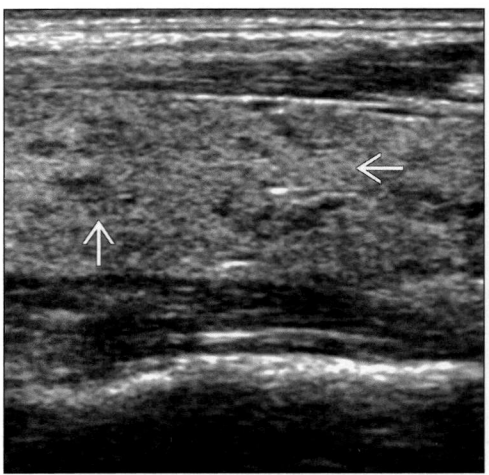

Longitudinal grayscale US shows a hypoechoic, heterogeneous spotty parenchymal echo pattern ➡ in a patient with Graves disease. Normal thyroid shows a fine bright, homogeneous echo pattern.

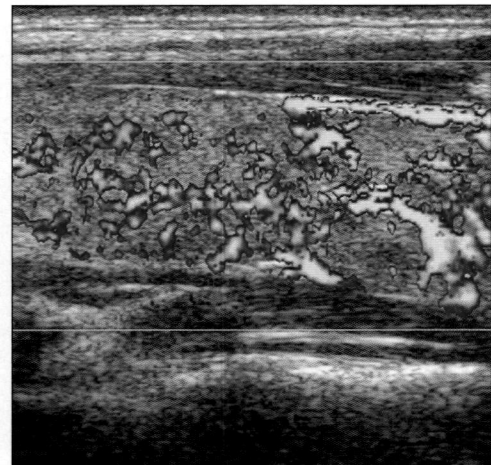

Corresponding power Doppler US shows a marked increase in thyroid vascularity ("thyroid inferno"). Spectral Doppler in such vessels will reveal increased flow velocities.

TERMINOLOGY

Abbreviations and Synonyms
- Graves disease (GD), diffuse toxic goiter

Definitions
- Autoimmune disorder with late acting thyroid stimulating antibodies (LATS) producing hyperplasia + hypertrophy of thyroid gland

IMAGING FINDINGS

General Features
- Best diagnostic clue: Moderately enlarged gland, hypoechoic with heterogeneous echo pattern and increase in parenchymal vascularity
- Size: Mild/moderate increase in thyroid gland size

Ultrasonographic Findings
- Grayscale Ultrasound
  - Mild/moderate diffuse, symmetric enlargement of thyroid gland, including isthmus
  - Increase in volume of thyroid up to 90 mL

- Normal volume: Neonate 0.4-1.4 mL, increasing by 1.0-1.3 mL for each 10 kg weight up to normal volume of 10-11 ± 3-4 mL in adults
  - Hypoechoic, heterogeneous, "spotty" parenchymal echo pattern
- Color Doppler
  - Marked increase in parenchymal vascularity (turbulent flow with A-V shunts), "thyroid inferno"
  - Increased vascularity does not correlate with thyroid function but is a reflection of inflammatory activity
  - Increased vascularity tends to decrease in response to treatment
  - Such increase in vascularity is also seen in patients with recurrence
  - Spectral Doppler: Increase in peak flow velocity (up to 120 cm/s) as measured in inferior thyroid artery

Imaging Recommendations
- Best imaging tool
  - Diagnosis of Graves disease is based on clinical signs & symptoms and laboratory findings
  - Imaging in Graves disease is usually not required for patient management

DDx: Graves Disease

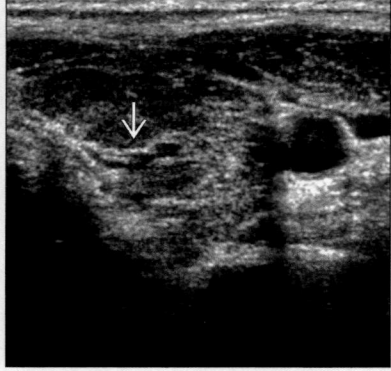

Hashimoto Thyroiditis

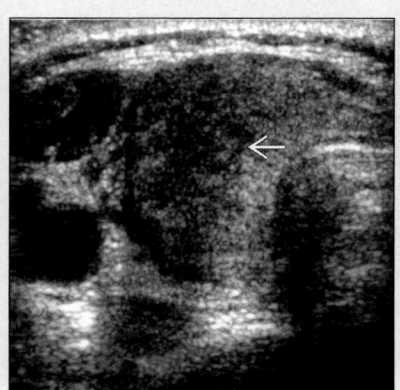

De Quervain Thyroiditis

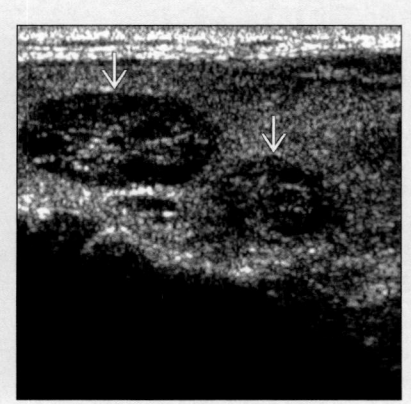

Nodular Goiter

GRAVES DISEASE

Key Facts

Imaging Findings
- Increase in volume of thyroid up to 90 mL
- Hypoechoic, heterogeneous, "spotty" parenchymal echo pattern
- Marked increase in parenchymal vascularity (turbulent flow with A-V shunts), "thyroid inferno"
- Such increase in vascularity is also seen in patients with recurrence
- Spectral Doppler: Increase in peak flow velocity (up to 120 cm/s) as measured in inferior thyroid artery
- Imaging in Graves disease is usually not required for patient management
- Imaging of thyroid may be necessary in patients who fail medical treatment and in whom other types of thyroiditis are considered

- Thyroid US may also be indicated in patients who undergo radioactive iodine treatment, to establish thyroid volume
- Patients with Graves disease may present with thyroid associated ophthalmopathy (TAO)
- Patients have exopthalmos with bilateral enlargement of external ocular muscles (EOM)

Top Differential Diagnoses
- Hashimoto Thyroiditis
- De Quervain Thyroiditis
- Nodular Goiter

Diagnostic Checklist
- In patients with TAO, CT or MR may be indicated to confirm diagnosis if it cannot be established clinically

---

- Imaging of thyroid may be necessary in patients who fail medical treatment and in whom other types of thyroiditis are considered
- In such instances, US of thyroid is the only imaging necessary
- Thyroid US may also be indicated in patients who undergo radioactive iodine treatment, to establish thyroid volume
- Some institutions may choose to do technetium thyroid scans; however, these involve use of radioactive pharmaceuticals and use ionizing radiation; US has no such disadvantages
  - Patients are advised to refrain from any iodine-containing food (seafood, fish, seaweed) cough syrup, iodine drug or antithyroid drugs for two weeks prior to procedure
  - Technetium thyroid scan: Marked uptake of radiopharmaceutical within hyperactive gland in Graves disease: "Superscan"
- Patients with Graves disease may present with thyroid associated ophthalmopathy (TAO)
  - Patients have exopthalmos with bilateral enlargement of external ocular muscles (EOM)
  - In patients with TAO, CT or preferably MR of orbit may be indicated to firmly establish diagnosis
  - Predilection for muscle bellies, sparing tendons (may be involved in acute phase)
  - Other features include: Enlarged lacrimal glands, increased orbital fat, enlarged superior opthalmic vein, stretched optic nerve
  - CT findings: NECT: Increased orbital fat, isodense enlargement of EOMs (inferior ≥ medial ≥ superior ≥ lateral ≥ oblique)
  - CECT: EOM enhancement greater than normal
  - MR findings: T1WI: Isointense enlargement of EOMs
  - T2WI: Acute: Increased EOM signal (edema), late stage: Decreased EOM signal (fibrosis)
  - T1 C+: EOM enhancement greater than normal

- Nuclear medicine finding: In-111 Octeotride: Retrobulbar uptake which indicates active inflammation, decreases with immunosuppressive therapy
- Protocol advice
  - Use of high resolution transducer is essential, scanning frequency ≥ 7.5 MHz
  - Scan in longitudinal and transverse planes including Doppler examination

DIFFERENTIAL DIAGNOSIS

Hashimoto Thyroiditis
- Rounded contours, hypoechoic, heterogeneous echo pattern with bright fibrotic streaks in parenchyma; atrophic gland in end stage disease
- High risk of developing NHL, which is seen as hypoechoic nodules in thyroid, ± associated lymphomatous nodes

De Quervain Thyroiditis
- Ill-defined, focal hypoechoic areas within thyroid, ± increased vascularity; raised white cell count (WCC), fever & tender thyroid
- Appearances evolve over time to subsequently involve the entire gland; thyroid may revert to normal echo pattern on successful treatment

Nodular Goiter
- Multiple, heterogeneous nodules, cystic change, septa, comet tail artifact, dense shadowing calcification
- Biochemical tests are usually normal & patients present with thyroid enlargement, ± palpable nodules

PATHOLOGY

General Features
- Genetics
  - Patients with GD show a genetic predisposition to the disease & increased association with certain HLA haplotypes

GRAVES DISEASE

- Unusually high incidence of other autoimmune diseases in their relatives
- Etiology: Autoimmune disorder; late acting thyroid stimulator (LATS) or thyroid stimulating autoantibodies (TSAb)
- Associated abnormalities: Concurrent development of Hashimoto disease & Graves disease is termed as Hashitoxicosis

Gross Pathologic & Surgical Features
- Diffuse & usually symmetrical enlargement of thyroid
- Weight; 50-150 g

Microscopic Features
- Focal collections of lymphocytes that occasionally show lymphoid germinal centers
  - Lymphoid cells in the interfollicular stroma & do not encroach upon follicles themselves
- Follicles show marked epithelial hyperplasia
- Increased vascularity & microvascularity with congestion

CLINICAL ISSUES

Presentation
- Most common signs/symptoms
  - Patients often present with palpitations, loss of weight despite increased appetite, sweating and wet palms
  - Cardiovascular: Hypermetabolic state → hyperdynamic circulatory state
    - Cardiomegaly, pulmonary edema, peripheral edema, tachycardia, mitral valve prolapse & increased cardiac output
  - Thyroid associated ophthalmopathy (TAO); periorbital edema, lid retraction, ophthalmoplegia, proptosis, malignant exophthalmos
    - Extraoccular muscle & orbital connective tissue inflammation, swelling due to autoimmune response
  - Muscular weakness & fatigue; common complaints, rarely muscle wasting
- Other signs/symptoms
  - Dermopathy; pretibial myxedema (5%), generalized inflammation of connective tissues & muscles
  - Temporary parathyroid suppression; increases both bone resorption & bone formation (resorption > formation)
- Lab data
  - Elevated T_3 + T_4 levels
  - Depressed TSH level
  - Antithyroperoxidase (circulating antithyroid) antibodies in 80% of GD
  - Organ nonspecific antibodies; antinuclear antibodies (ANA), smooth muscle & mitochondrial antibodies

Demographics
- Age: 3rd-4th decade
- Gender: M:F = 1:7

Natural History & Prognosis
- GD may undergo spontaneous remission

- Complication: 10-30% develop hypothyroidism within 1st year + 3% per year rate thereafter
  - Development of thyroid carcinoma in GD

Treatment
- Choice of treatment includes medical therapy as first line followed by radioactive iodine ablation or surgery in patients who do not respond to medical therapy
- Principles of treatment include: Immediate symptom control & eventual elimination of excessive glandular synthesis of thyroid hormone
- Beta blockers quickly control thyrotoxic symptoms of Graves disease
- Antithyroid drugs, radioactive ablation or thyroid surgery deal with eliminating excessive thyroid hormone production
- Childhood GD: Medical treatment (thionamides, iodine & beta-blockers) as first line of therapy
- Pregnancy & neonate: Medical treatment (thionamides) as first line of therapy
- Surgery: Thyroidectomy, reliable cure with small chance of recurrent hyperthyroidism
  - Reserved for patients with very large goiters, severe local symptoms, allergy to thionamides

DIAGNOSTIC CHECKLIST

Image Interpretation Pearls
- In patients with clinical & laboratory evidence of Graves disease imaging is usually not required
- US thyroid may be indicated if the goiter is nodular or if other thyroiditis is suspected
- Some institutions may choose technetium thyroid scans over US, depending on expertise available
- In patients with TAO, CT or MR may be indicated to confirm diagnosis if it cannot be established clinically

SELECTED REFERENCES

1. Abraham P et al: A systematic review of drug therapy for Graves' hyperthyroidism. Eur J Endocrinol. 153(4):489-98, 2005
2. Harnsberger HR et al: Diagnostic Imaging: Head & Neck. Salt Lake City, Amirsys. II-1-70-73, 2004
3. Felz MW et al: The many 'faces' of Graves' disease. Part 2. Practical diagnostic testing and management options. Postgrad Med. 106(5):45-52; quiz 158, 1999
4. LiVolsi VA: Thyroid Disease: Endocrinology, Surgery, Nuclear Medicine & Radiotherapy. USA, Lippincott-Raven. 65-104, 1997
5. Solbiati L et al: Ultrasound of Superficial Structures. UK, Churchill Livingstone. 49-86, 1995

GRAVES DISEASE

Typical

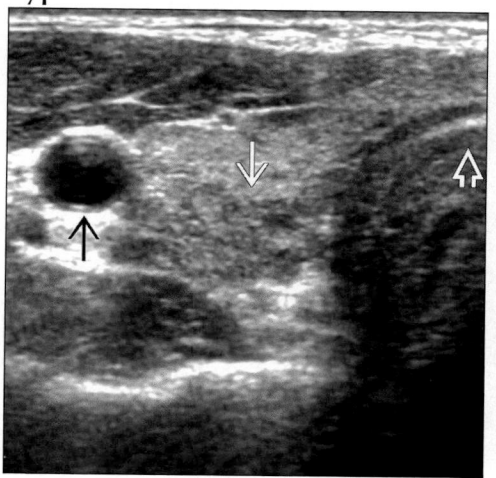

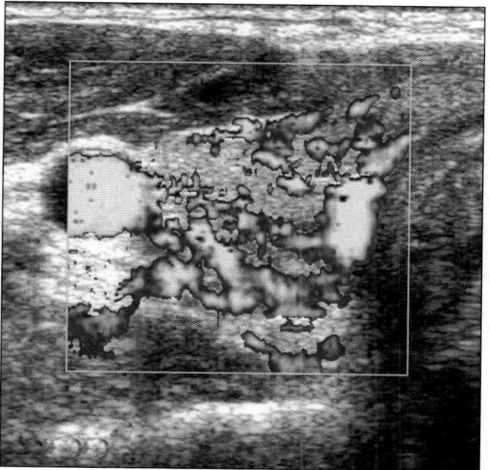

(Left) Transverse grayscale US of the thyroid in Graves disease shows a hypoechoic, heterogeneous spotty echo pattern ➡. In this patient the thyroid maintains its normal contour. Trachea ➡, carotid artery ➡. (Right) Corresponding power Doppler shows marked intrathyroid vascularity. Increase in vascularity does not correlate with thyroid function but is a reflection of inflammatory activity.

Typical

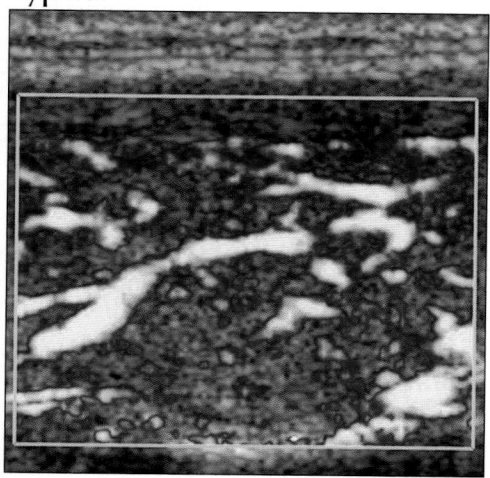

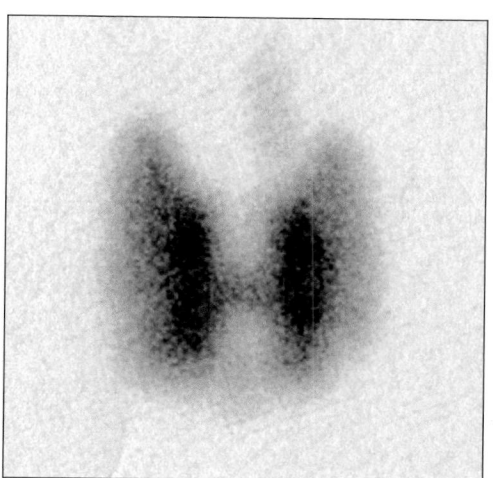

(Left) Power Doppler shows marked intrathyroid vascularity in Graves disease. In patients who respond to treatment such vascularity diminishes. It will increase again in recurrent disease. (Right) Technetium scintigraphy in Graves disease shows an increased, uniform uptake in the thyroid gland including isthmus ("superscan"). Some institutions may choose scintigraphy over US if imaging of thyroid is indicated.

Typical

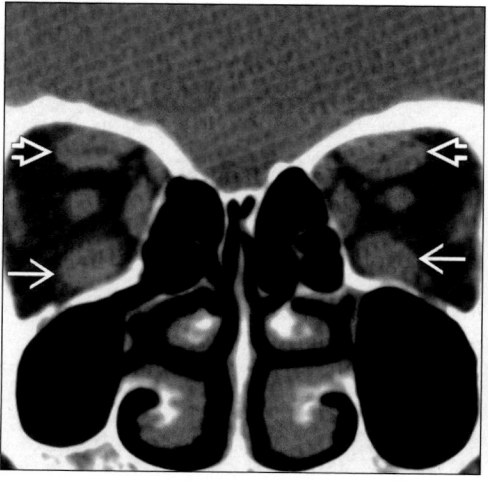

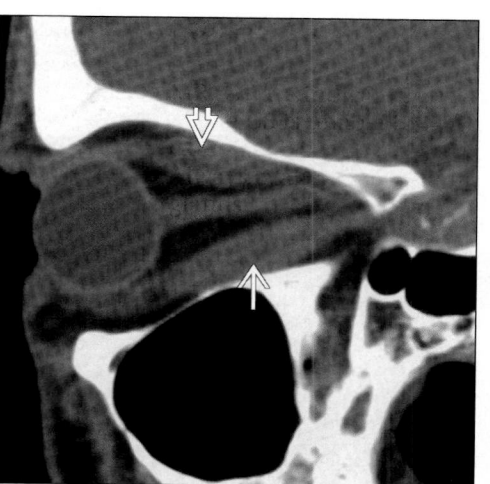

(Left) Coronal NECT in a patient with Graves disease with TAO. Note inferior ➡ & superior rectii ➡ are uniformly enlarged bilaterally. (Right) Sagittal NECT in a patient with Graves disease & TAO shows the enlarged muscle bellies of the superior ➡ & inferior ➡ recti. Note the tendoninous attachments are spared.

PARATHYROID ADENOMA, VISCERAL SPACE

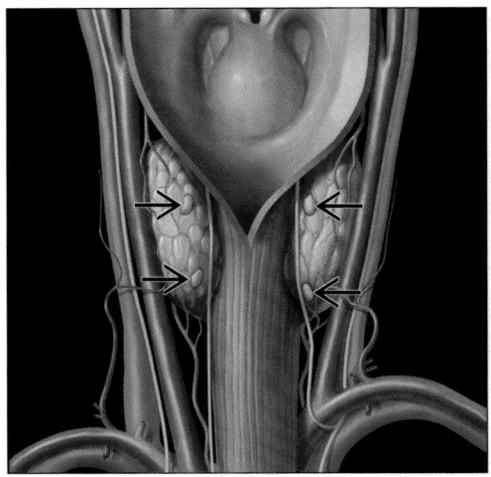

Graphic shows the normal location of the parathyroid glands ➡ and their relationship to the thyroid gland. PTAs in these locations are readily evaluated by grayscale and color Doppler US.

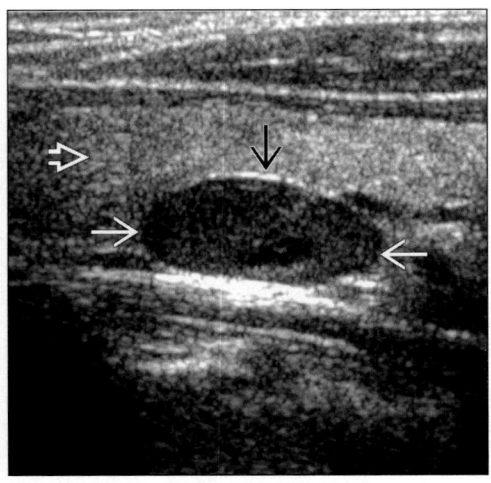

Longitudinal grayscale US shows a well-circumscribed, hypoechoic PTA ➡ behind the thyroid gland ➡. Note the sharp echogenic line ➡ separating it from thyroid.

TERMINOLOGY

Abbreviations and Synonyms
- Parathyroid adenoma (PTA)
- Hyperparathyroidism (HPT)
- Parathyroid hormone (PTH)

Definitions
- PTA: Benign neoplasm of parathyroid gland producing excess PTH

IMAGING FINDINGS

General Features
- Best diagnostic clue
  - Ultrasound (US) shows well-defined, hypoechoic extrathyroid nodule with bright capsule and parenchymal vascularity in vicinity of thyroid gland
  - Nuclear scintigraphy shows focal uptake of isotope (sestamibi or thallium) within PTA
- Location
  - Upper parathyroid glands
    - Posterior to upper-mid pole of thyroid
    - Rarely located posterior to pharynx or esophagus
  - Lower parathyroid glands
    - 65% inferior, lateral to lower pole of thyroid
    - 35% of lower parathyroid glands variably located along thymopharyngeal duct tract, extending from angle of mandible to lower anterior mediastinum
  - Intrathyroid location rare
- Size: Typically 1-3 cm in size
- Morphology
  - Round or oval, well-circumscribed, solid mass
  - Usually homogeneous, but cystic degeneration & hemorrhage may occur

Ultrasonographic Findings
- PTA: Well-circumscribed mass adjacent to thyroid gland, which are more common than ectopic PTAs
- Infrathyroid PTAs are usually round; retrothyroid PTAs may be oval or flat as parathyroid glands in this position develop within longitudinally aligned fascial planes; typically medial to common carotid artery
- Infrathyroid PTAs may demonstrate an arrowhead appearance pointing superiorly (seen on longitudinal scans)

DDx: Parathyroid Adenoma

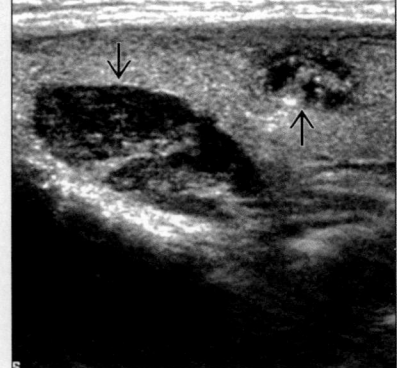

Thyroid Nodule

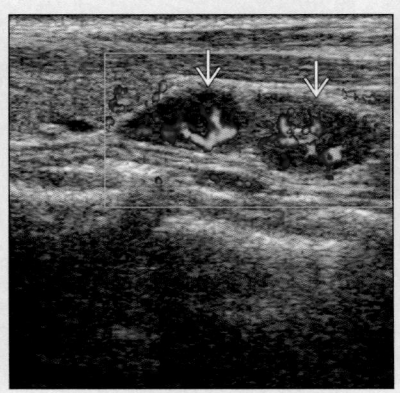

Paratracheal Lymph Node

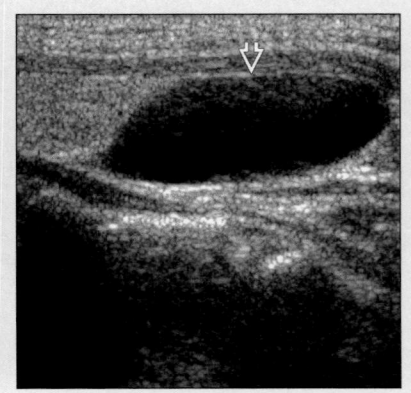

Thymic Cyst

REACTIVE ADENOPATHY

Key Facts

Imaging Findings

- Hypoechoic cortex compared to adjacent muscle, with normal echogenic hilus
- Oval in shape except for submandibular and parotid nodes which are usually round
- Color Doppler: Reactive nodes show hilar vascularity
- Spectral Doppler: Low vascular resistance (resistive index (RI) < 0.8, pulsatility index (PI) < 1.6)

- US is unable to evaluate retropharyngeal nodes and upper mediastinal nodes
- Nodes in the anterior compartment may be obscured by shadowing/artifact from tracheal rings & air in trachea

Top Differential Diagnoses

- Metastatic Node
- Tuberculous Node
- Metastatic Node from Papillary Thyroid Carcinoma

Imaging Recommendations

- Best imaging tool
  - US is unable to evaluate retropharyngeal nodes and upper mediastinal nodes
  - Nodes in the anterior compartment may be obscured by shadowing/artifact from tracheal rings & air in trachea
  - MR & CT overcome these limitations

DIFFERENTIAL DIAGNOSIS

Metastatic Node

- Hypoechoic, round, ± necrosis, absent hilus, peripheral vascularity and RI > 0.8, PI > 1.6

Tuberculous Node

- Round, hypoechoic, intranodal necrosis, nodal matting, soft tissue edema, displaced vascularity

Metastatic Node from Papillary Thyroid Carcinoma

- Hyperechoic, ± intranodal necrosis, punctate calcification, peripheral vascularity

PATHOLOGY

General Features

- General path comments

- Enlarged node may be due to nonspecific or specific histologic reaction to both non-infectious or infectious agents
- Most children 2-12 years have lymphadenopathy at some time

CLINICAL ISSUES

Presentation

- Clinical Profile: Most frequently, enlarged nodes in young patient with pharyngeal or systemic viral infection

Treatment

- Primary infectious source should be treated
- Monitor clinically for progression of symptoms

DIAGNOSTIC CHECKLIST

Consider

- Oval-shaped nodes likely to be benign & reactive
- Supraclavicular nodes are often neoplastic (60%) & the primary infraclavicular in location

SELECTED REFERENCES

1. Ahuja AT et al: Sonographic evaluation of cervical lymph nodes. AJR Am J Roentgenol. 184(5):1691-9, 2005
2. Ahuja A et al: Sonography of neck lymph nodes. Part II: abnormal lymph nodes. Clin Radiol. 58(5):359-66, 2003

IMAGE GALLERY

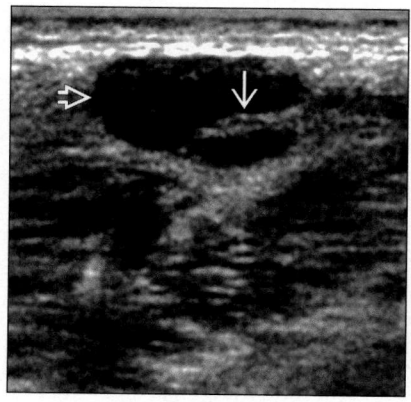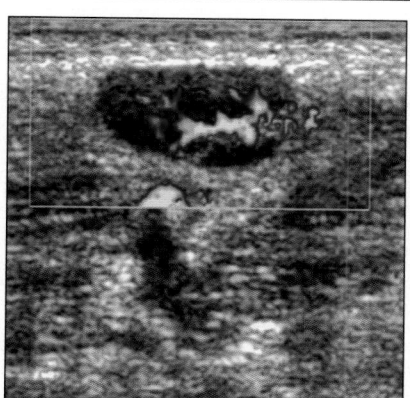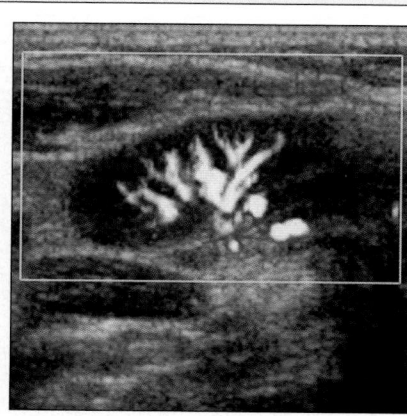

(Left) Grayscale US shows an oval, solid, hypoechoic node ⇨ with normal echogenic hilar ⇨ echo pattern. Note exquisite intranodal detail is obtained by using a high-resolution transducer. *(Center)* Corresponding power Doppler clearly shows hilar vascularity. Note the complete absence of vessels at the periphery of the node. Presence of peripheral vessels should raise suspicion of malignancy. *(Right)* Power Doppler US shows hilar vascularity in a reactive node. Spectral Doppler to measure RI & PI is not routinely indicated.

SQUAMOUS CELL CARCINOMA NODES

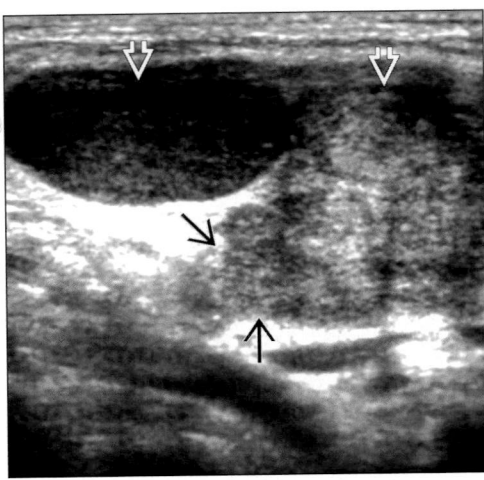

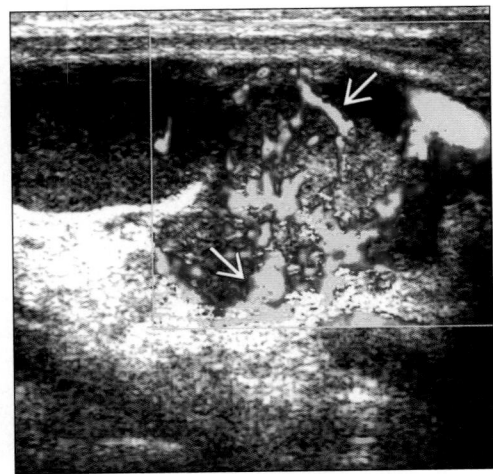

Grayscale US shows multiple metastatic nodes ⇨ in a patient with known HN SCCa. Note the absence of an echogenic hilum in both & ill-defined edges ⇨ in one, suggesting extracapsular spread.

Corresponding power Doppler US shows multiple prominent abnormal intranodal vessels. Note the large peripheral vessels ⇨, typical of metastatic nodes.

TERMINOLOGY

Abbreviations and Synonyms
- Squamous cell carcinoma (SCCa) nodes
- SCCa nodal metastases

Definitions
- Nodal metastasis from primary H&N SCCa

IMAGING FINDINGS

General Features
- Best diagnostic clue
  - Round, hypoechoic, heterogeneous node in expected nodal drainage level(s) of primary H&N SCCa
  - New neck mass in adult patient with H&N SCCa should raise suspicion of malignant node
- Location
  - Levels I-VI of neck, retropharyngeal space & parotid space
  - Level IIA (jugulodigastric group) is most frequently involved nodal group

- Size
  - Size alone cannot be used as absolute criteria as inflammatory nodes may be large and malignancy may be found in small nodes
    - In patients with known HN SCCa, an increase in nodal size on serial examination is highly suggestive of metastatic involvement
- Morphology
  - Rounded contour; loss of fatty hilum, eccentric cortical hypertrophy & large peripheral vessels suggest malignant node
  - Intranodal cystic/coagulation necrosis is often seen in metastases from HN SCCa
  - Extranodal spread suggested by indistinct nodal margins, infiltration of adjacent fat ± invasion of adjacent structures

Ultrasonographic Findings
- Metastatic nodes are commonly round
  - However, if there is focal intranodal tumor deposition, the node may show eccentric cortical hypertrophy
- Malignant nodes tend to have sharp borders

DDx: Squamous Cell Carcinoma Nodes

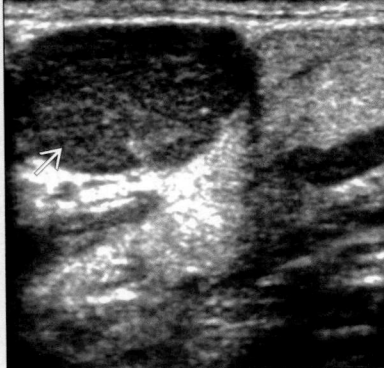

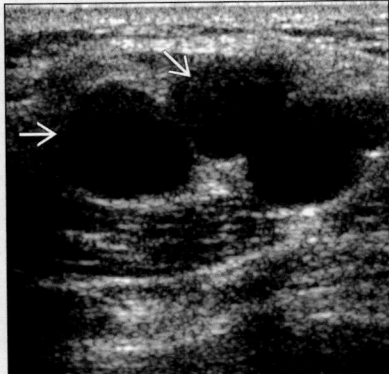

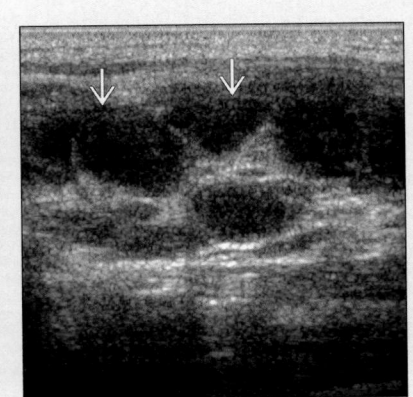

Non-Hodgkin Lymphoma Node

Papillary Carcinoma Thyroid Nodes

Tuberculous Lymph Nodes

SQUAMOUS CELL CARCINOMA NODES

Key Facts

Imaging Findings

- In patients with known HN SCCa, an increase in nodal size on serial examination is highly suggestive of metastatic involvement
- Metastatic nodes are commonly round
- Malignant nodes tend to have sharp borders
- In a proven metastatic node, presence of an unsharp nodal border suggests extracapsular spread
- Loss of normal echogenic hilar architecture (69-95%)
- Metastatic nodes from HN SCCa are hypoechoic, compared to adjacent muscle
- Calcification in metastatic HN SCCa nodes is rare
- Intranodal cystic necrosis is commonly found in metastatic nodes from HN SCCa
- Color Doppler: Metastatic nodes may have both peripheral or mixed (hilar & peripheral) vascularity

- US is unable to evaluate the primary tumor site

Top Differential Diagnoses

- Non-Hodgkin Lymphoma Nodes
- Neoplastic Nodes from Papillary Thyroid Cancer
- Tuberculous Nodes

Clinical Issues

- Nodal metastasis is single most important prognostic factor for H&N SCCa
- Single unilateral node reduces prognosis by 50%; bilateral nodes reduces prognosis by 75%
- Presence of extranodal spread reduces prognosis by further 50%; risk of recurrence ↑ 10 x
- Carotid artery encasement ~ 100% mortality

- Tumor deposition in nodes results in greater difference in acoustic impedance between node and surrounding soft tissues leading to sharp nodal border
- In a proven metastatic node, presence of an unsharp nodal border suggests extracapsular spread
- Loss of normal echogenic hilar architecture (69-95%)
- Metastatic nodes from HN SCCa are hypoechoic, compared to adjacent muscle
  - Metastatic nodes from thyroid papillary carcinoma tend to be hyperechoic to adjacent muscle
- Calcification in metastatic HN SCCa nodes is rare
  - Calcification is common in metastatic nodes from thyroid papillary & medullary carcinoma
- Intranodal cystic necrosis is commonly found in metastatic nodes from HN SCCa
  - Intranodal coagulation necrosis (seen as echogenic area) may be found in both malignant & inflammatory nodes
- Color Doppler: Metastatic nodes may have both peripheral or mixed (hilar & peripheral) vascularity
  - Presence of peripheral vascularity regardless of hilar vascularity is highly suggestive of metastases
- Spectral Doppler: High intranodal vascular resistance (resistive index [RI] > 0.8, pulsatility index [PI] > 1.6)
  - Evaluation of intranodal vascular resistance is time consuming & not routinely indicated in clinical practice

CT Findings

- CECT: Diffuse or rim-enhancement of node(s)

MR Findings

- T1WI: Isointense to muscle; necrosis seen as hypointense focus
- T2WI: Hyperintense; focal marked hyperintensity with necrosis or cystic change
- DWI: Early work suggests greater ADC values in metastatic SCCa nodes than benign adenopathy
- T1 C+
  - Inhomogeneous enhancement if there is necrosis
  - Dynamic T1 C+ MR may help to distinguish normal from neoplastic nodes

- Superparamagnetic iron oxide contrast agents
  - Accumulate in normal nodes making them markedly hypointense on T2* sequence

Nuclear Medicine Findings

- PET
  - FDG PET: Focal areas of metabolic activity are seen in larger nodal deposits
    - Accuracy ~ 75% for detection of positive nodes
    - Useful with positive nodal SCCa & unknown primary tumor site

Imaging Recommendations

- Best imaging tool
  - US is ideal imaging modality to screen neck nodes below angle of mandible & is readily combined with guided fine needle aspiration cytology (FNAC)
  - US is unable to evaluate the primary tumor site
    - Does not evaluate retropharyngeal & mediastinal nodes
  - Either CECT or MR stage primary tumor & nodes simultaneously
- Protocol advice
  - Always evaluate both sides of neck and be familiar with neck anatomy
  - Mandatory to use high resolution transducer, scanning frequency ≥ 7.5 MHz

---

DIFFERENTIAL DIAGNOSIS

Non-Hodgkin Lymphoma Nodes

- Multiple, round, hypoechoic, well-defined, pseudocystic or reticulated echo pattern with marked hilar and peripheral vascularity

Neoplastic Nodes from Papillary Thyroid Cancer

- Hyperechoic, solid/cystic, punctate calcification & peripheral vascularity

SQUAMOUS CELL CARCINOMA NODES

Tuberculous Nodes
- Multiple, hypoechoic, heterogeneous nodes with intranodal necrosis, nodal matting, soft tissue edema, avascular or displaced hilar vessels

2nd Branchial Cleft Cyst (2nd BCC)
- Anechoic, +/- pseudosolid pattern, thin/thick walls with faint internal debris, +/- septa & characteristic location in neck

PATHOLOGY

General Features
- General path comments
  - AJCC and AAO-HNS nodal level classification scheme
    - Level IA: Submental between anterior digastrics group; level IB: Submandibular, anterior to posterior margin submandibular gland (SMG)
    - Level II: High internal jugular group; IIA anterior, lateral or posterior and touching jugular; IIB posterior but not touching jugular
    - Level III: Mid internal jugular group; between inferior hyoid and cricoid cartilage
    - Level IV: Low internal jugular group; below inferior aspect of cricoid, anterior to oblique line (anterior scalene to sternocleidomastoid)
    - Level V: Spinal accessory group posterior to sternocleidomastoid; VA above cricoid, VB below inferior aspect cricoid
    - Level VI: Between internal carotids, below hyoid
  - Named nodal groups
    - Retropharyngeal: Between internal carotids from skull base to C3; medial & lateral groups
    - Supraclavicular: On same slice as clavicle; note these "merge" with levels IV and VB
    - Superior mediastinal: Below superior aspect of manubrium; sometimes called level VII
    - Parotid: Within parotid gland
    - Superficial groups: Occipital, pre- & post-auricular, facial
- Etiology: Lymphatic spread of primary SCCa to nodes
- Epidemiology
  - Presence of nodal metastasis at time of diagnosis varies by primary tumor site
    - Nasopharyngeal most with ~ 85%, laryngeal (glottic) primary least with < 10%

Gross Pathologic & Surgical Features
- Enlarged round pale nodes; frequently multiple
- Extracapsular spread seen as "naked tumor" in perinodal fat, adherent to vessels or invading muscles

Microscopic Features
- Metastases 1st lodge in subcapsular sinus then spread through whole node
- Squamous differentiation frequently with keratinizing morphology

Staging, Grading or Classification Criteria
- AJCC cervical node classification for all H&N SCCa (except nasopharyngeal carcinoma)
  - N1: Single ipsilateral node ≤ 3 cm
  - N2a: Single ipsilateral 3-6 cm; N2b: Multiple ipsilateral ≤ 6 cm; N2c: Bilateral or contralateral nodes ≤ 6 cm
  - N3: Any nodal mass > 6 cm
    - Note: N2 classifies tumor as stage IVa regardless of T stage
- Nasopharyngeal carcinoma nodal staging
  - N1: Unilateral nodes ≤ 6 cm; N2: Bilateral nodes ≤ 6 cm; N3: > 6 cm or supraclavicular node

CLINICAL ISSUES

Presentation
- Most common signs/symptoms
  - Painless firm neck mass, may be fixed to adjacent tissues especially if large
  - "Neck mass" (enlarged node) may be presenting feature of H&N SCCa
  - If no primary seen, imaging for "unknown primary"

Demographics
- Age: > 40 years
- Gender: M > F reflecting smoking propensity

Natural History & Prognosis
- Nodal metastasis is single most important prognostic factor for H&N SCCa
  - Single unilateral node reduces prognosis by 50%; bilateral nodes reduces prognosis by 75%
  - Presence of extranodal spread reduces prognosis by further 50%; risk of recurrence ↑ 10 x
- Carotid artery encasement ~ 100% mortality

Treatment
- Surgical resection at time of primary tumor resection ± XRT, primary XRT or chemotherapy plus XRT
- Classification of neck dissection
  - Radical neck dissection (RND): Resection of levels I-V plus sternocleidomastoid, IJV & CN11
  - Modified radical neck dissection: RND with preservation of SCM, IJV ± CN11
  - Selective neck dissection: One or more of nodal groups I-V preserved

SELECTED REFERENCES

1. Ahuja A et al: Sonographic evaluation of cervical lymph nodes. AJR. 184:1691-9, 2005
2. Harnsberger HR et al: Diagnostic Imaging Head & Neck. Salt Lake City, Amirsys. III-2-28-31, 2004
3. King AD et al: Necrosis in metastatic neck nodes: diagnostic accuracy of CT, MR imaging, and US. Radiology. 230(3):720-6, 2004
4. Ahuja A et al: Sonography of neck lymph nodes. Part II: abnormal lymph nodes. Clin Radiol. 58(5):359-66, 2003
5. Fischbein NJ et al: Assessment of metastatic cervical adenopathy using dynamic contrast-enhanced MR imaging. AJNR Am J Neuroradiol. 24(3):301-11, 2003
6. Som PM et al: Imaging-based nodal classification for evaluation of neck metastatic adenopathy. AJR Am J Roentgenol. 174(3):837-44, 2000

SQUAMOUS CELL CARCINOMA NODES

IMAGE GALLERY

Typical

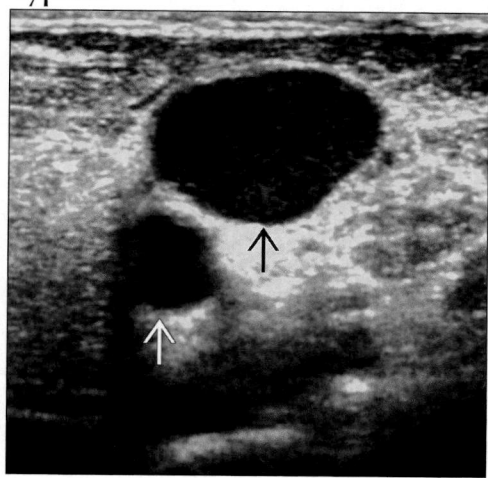

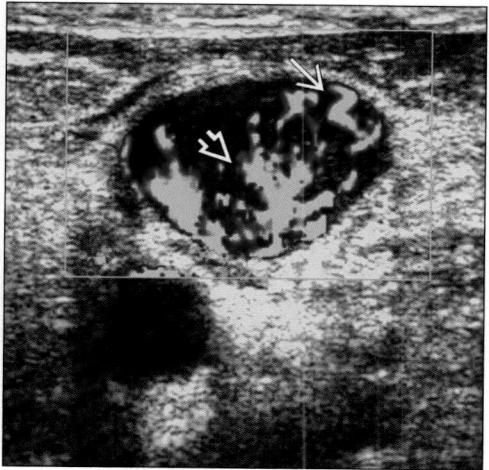

(Left) Transverse grayscale US shows a round, well-defined, hypoechoic node ➡ with loss of echogenic hilum in a patient with HN SCCa. Typical appearance of metastatic node. Carotid artery ➡. (Right) Corresponding power Doppler sonogram shows abnormal peripheral vessels ➡ consistent with a metastatic node. Note prominent hilar vessels ➡.

Typical

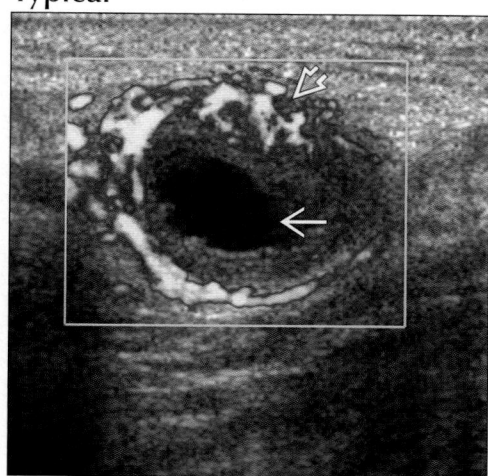

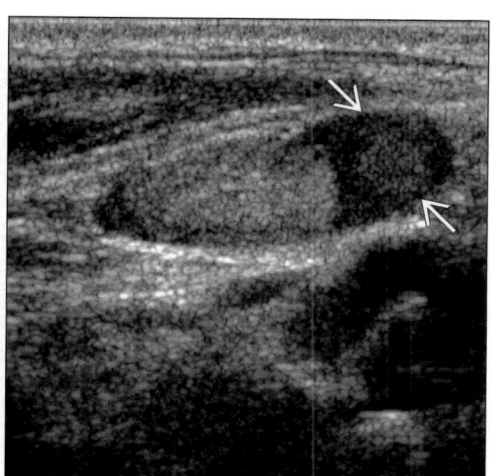

(Left) Power Doppler US shows abnormal peripheral ➡ vessels in a metastatic node from HN SCCa. Note intranodal cystic necrosis ➡, often seen in metastases from HN SCCa. (Right) Transverse grayscale US shows a focal area of hypertrophy ➡ (eccentric cortical hypertrophy) in a metastatic node from HN SCCa. US helps to guide needle into appropriate site for FNAC.

Typical

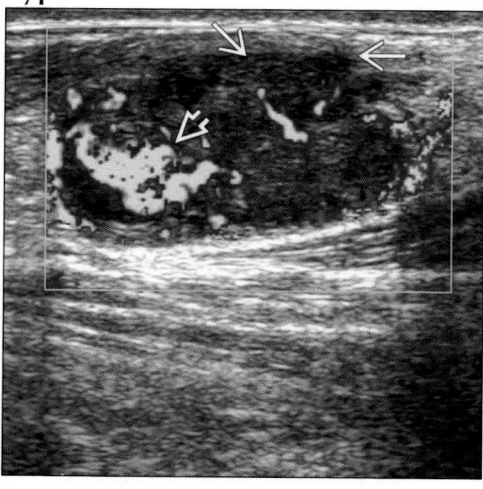

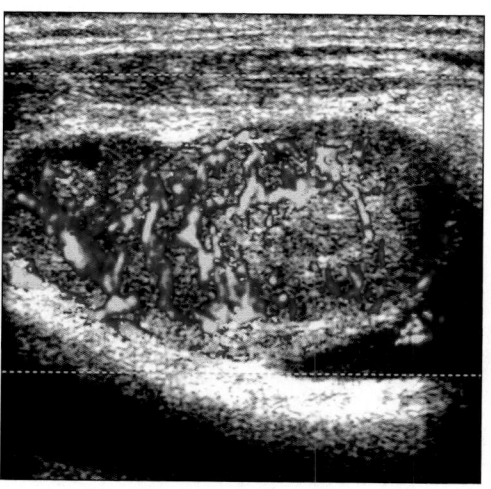

(Left) Power Doppler US shows abnormal peripheral vascularity ➡ in a metastatic node from HN SCCa. Note ill-defined edges ➡ anteriorly suggesting extracapsular involvement. (Right) Power Doppler US shows multiple abnormal vessels in a metastatic node from HN SCCa. Grayscale and vascular distribution suffice in predicting malignancy. Spectral Doppler is not used routinely.

TUBERCULOUS ADENOPATHY

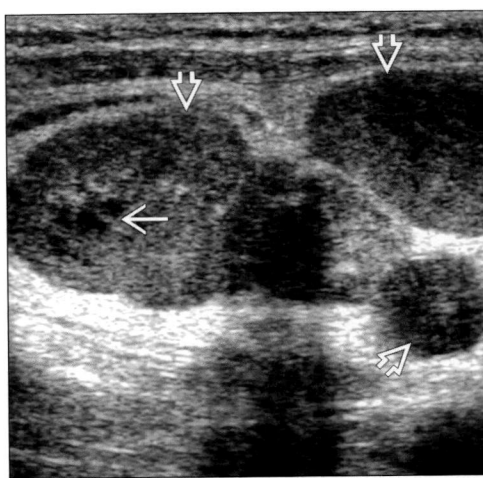

Longitudinal grayscale US shows multiple, matted nodes ⇥ in the posterior triangle. Note intranodal necrosis → & absence of normal soft tissues between some nodes. Features suggest TB.

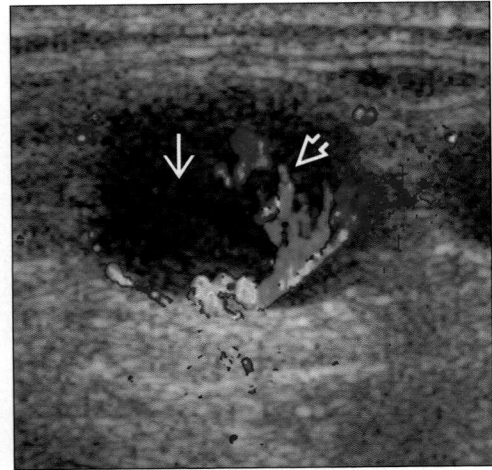

Power Doppler US shows displaced hilar vessels ⇥ due to a focal area of necrosis →. This is the most common intranodal distribution of vessels in TB infected nodes.

TERMINOLOGY

Abbreviations and Synonyms
- Tuberculous (TB) cervical lymphadenitis, scrofula

Definitions
- Enlargement of one or more cervical lymph nodes due to tuberculous infection

IMAGING FINDINGS

General Features
- Location: Usually unilateral, involving level V nodes

Ultrasonographic Findings
- Grayscale Ultrasound
  - Multiple, hypoechoic, round nodes in posterior triangle, supraclavicular fossa
  - Intranodal cystic/caseous necrosis, producing posterior enhancement
  - Multiple matted nodes with no normal intervening soft tissues between involved nodes
    - Tuberculous adenitis produces a periadenitis resulting in the affected nodes being clumped/matted together
  - Associated adjacent soft tissue edema, response to adjacent inflamed node
  - Nodal calcification is not seen in acute disease
    - Calcification may be seen in nodes following treatment or in recurrent disease in a previously affected/treated node
- Power Doppler
  - Hilar vascularity in 50%, but such vessels are displaced by focal areas of necrosis: "Displaced hilar vascularity"
  - No vascularity detected on power Doppler (19%)
    - Necrotizing granulomatous lesions may obliterate intranodal vessels
    - During healing phase, fibrosis & hyalinization obliterate intranodal vessels
  - Capsular (12%) vascularity due to supply from perinodal inflammatory tissues
- Spectral Doppler: Low intranodal vascular resistance
  - Intranodal vascular resistance: Malignant nodes > tuberculous nodes > reactive nodes

DDx: Tuberculous Adenopathy

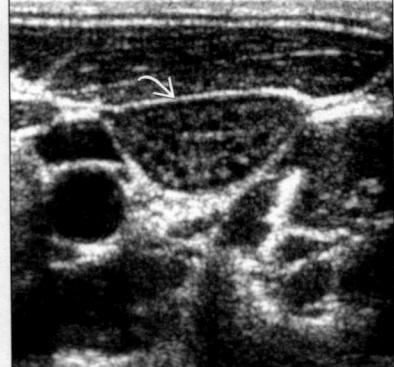

Non-Hodgkin Lymphoma Node

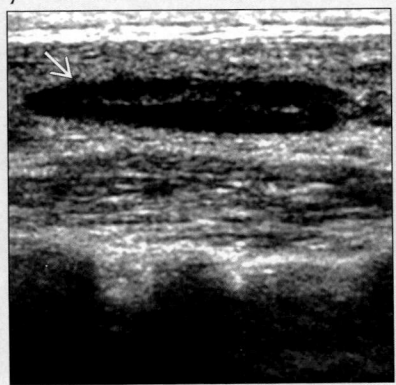

Reactive Adenopathy

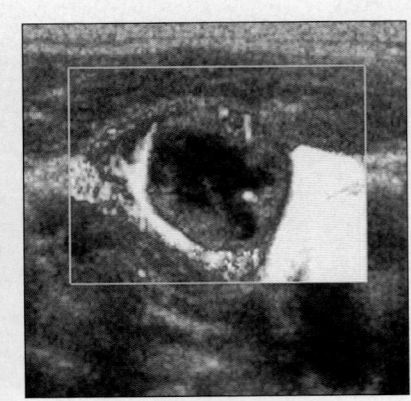

SCCa Nodal Metastasis

TUBERCULOUS ADENOPATHY

Key Facts

Imaging Findings

- Multiple, hypoechoic, round nodes in posterior triangle, supraclavicular fossa
- Intranodal cystic/caseous necrosis, producing posterior enhancement
- Multiple matted nodes with no normal intervening soft tissues between involved nodes
- Associated adjacent soft tissue edema, response to adjacent inflamed node

- Nodal calcification is not seen in acute disease
- Hilar vascularity in 50%, but such vessels are displaced by focal areas of necrosis: "Displaced hilar vascularity"
- No vascularity detected on power Doppler (19%)
- Capsular (12%) vascularity due to supply from perinodal inflammatory tissues
- Intranodal vascular resistance: Malignant nodes > tuberculous nodes > reactive nodes

Imaging Recommendations

- Best imaging tool: US is ideal imaging modality of choice as it identifies abnormal nodes, suggests diagnosis & guides cytology/biopsy for confirmation

DIFFERENTIAL DIAGNOSIS

NHL Nodes

- Hypoechoic, solid, non-necrotic, reticulated with posterior enhancement & abnormal vascularity

SCCa Nodal Metastases

- Round, hypoechoic nodes with intranodal necrosis, peripheral vascularity and known primary tumor

Reactive Nodes

- Multiple, solid, elliptical, hypoechoic with normal hilar echo pattern and vascularity

PATHOLOGY

General Features

- Etiology: Infection due to Mycobacterium tuberculosis & other members of M. tuberculosis complex: M. bovis, M. africanum and M. microti
- Epidemiology
  - More common in developing & south east Asian countries due to overcrowding, poverty, poor living conditions, malnutrition

- Now with increased incidence of HIV & AIDS; often encountered in developed countries

CLINICAL ISSUES

Presentation

- Most common signs/symptoms
  - Enlarged cervical solitary or multiple masses in posterior triangle & supraclavicular fossa, unilateral or bilateral
  - Constitutional symptoms & concomitant pulmonary tuberculosis; frequently absent

Demographics

- Age: Any age group, especially young children are more prone, M = F

Treatment

- Anti tuberculous therapy
- Surgery: LN excision by functional lymph node dissection
  - Nodes that do not respond despite adequate anti-tuberculous therapy, probably due to drug resistance

SELECTED REFERENCES

1. Ahuja A et al: Power Doppler sonography to differentiate tuberculous cervical lymphadenopathy from nasopharyngeal carcinoma. AJNR Am J Neuroradiol. 22(4):735-40, 2001

IMAGE GALLERY

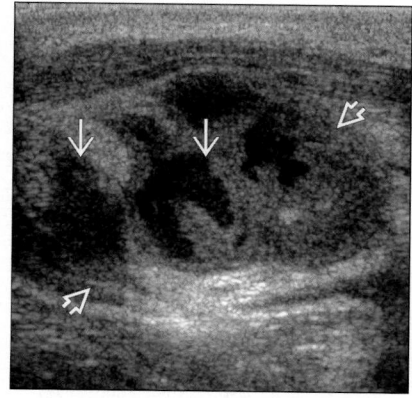 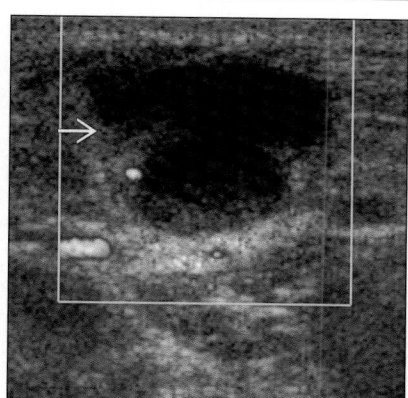 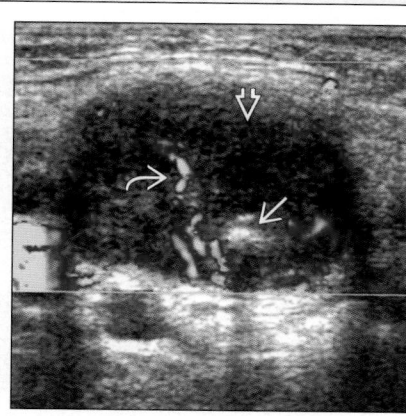

(Left) Longitudinal grayscale US shows a conglomerate of TB nodes ➡ clumped together in the posterior triangle with focal areas of cystic necrosis ➡. *(Center)* Power Doppler sonogram shows a necrotic node ➡ ("collar stud" appearance) with no internal vascularity, features typical of TB. *(Right)* Power Doppler sonogram of TB node shows displaced vascularity ➡ due to focal necrosis ➡. Note shadowing calcification ➡ suggesting recurrence in a previously treated node.

NON-HODGKIN LYMPHOMA NODES

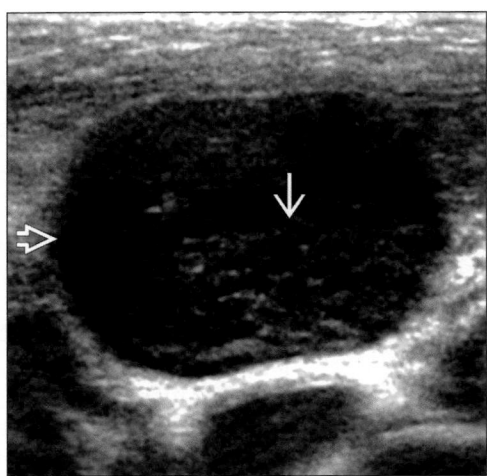

Grayscale US shows a solid, well-defined, hypoechoic NHL node ⇒ with a reticulated ➡ intranodal echo pattern. High-resolution US exquisitely shows the reticulated pattern helping in diagnosis.

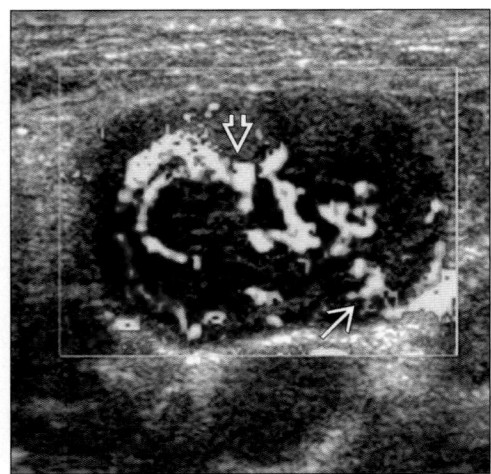

Corresponding power Doppler US shows markedly prominent hilar vessels ⇒ and peripheral vessels ➡ in a NHL node. Peripheral vessels alone are rare in NHL nodes.

TERMINOLOGY

Abbreviations and Synonyms
- Nodal non-Hodgkin lymphoma (NHL)

Definitions
- NHL: Cancer that develops in lymphoreticular system, thought to arise from lymphocytes & their derivatives

IMAGING FINDINGS

General Features
- Best diagnostic clue
  - Multiple, bilateral, non-necrotic enlarged nodes in usual & unusual (RPS, SMS, occipital) nodal chains
  - May also present as single dominant non-necrotic node with multiple smaller surrounding nodes
- Location
  - Nodal disease occurs in cervical chains
    - Levels II, III, & IV often involved
    - Superficial adenopathy or level V also common

- Non-nodal lymphatic disease occurs in palatine tonsil (most common), lingual tonsillar tissue & adenoids
  - Non-nodal extralymphatic disease occurs in paranasal sinuses, skull base & thyroid gland
- Morphology: Nodes round or oval, generally with no extracapsular extension
- If nodes show necrosis ± extranodal spread, aggressive NHL is implied
  - AIDS-associated lymphomas often aggressive

Ultrasonographic Findings
- NHL nodes are commonly round with sharp borders
- (blank)
  - Tumor deposition in nodes produces greater acoustic impedance between node & adjacent soft tissue leading to sharp nodal border
  - If unsharp border, it suggests extracapsular extension implying aggressive disease
- Loss of normal echogenic hilus (72-73%)
- Commonly hypoechoic compared to adjacent muscle
  - Previously described as "pseudocystic" nodes with posterior enhancement

DDx: Non-Hodgkin Lymphoma Nodes

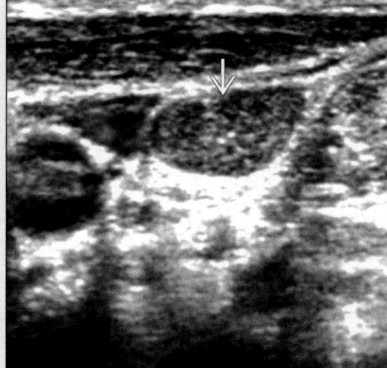

Systemic Metastatic Lymph Node

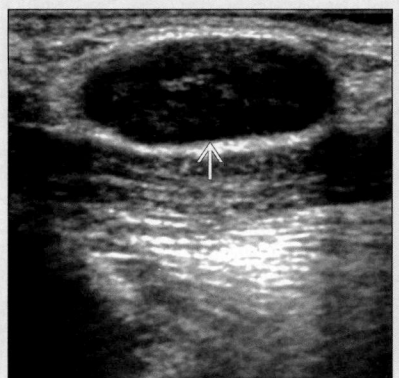

Reactive Lymph Nodes

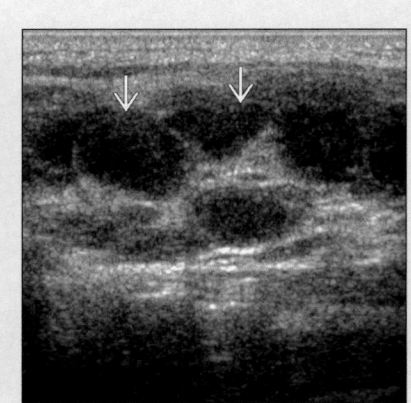

Tuberculous Lymph Nodes

SYSTEMIC METASTASES, NECK NODES

Key Facts

Imaging Findings
- Solid, hypoechoic, well-defined node with loss of normal echogenic hilus
- Intranodal coagulation/cystic necrosis, eccentric cortical hypertrophy may be seen
- Color Doppler: Peripheral or hilar & peripheral vascularity
- Spectral Doppler: High intranodal vascular resistance (resistive index [RI] > 0.8, pulsatility index [PI] > 1.6)
- If a node is confirmed as malignant on FNAC & has ill-defined borders, it suggests extracapsular spread
- Protocol advice: Do not mistake neck nodes for normal brachial plexus trunks/divisions

Top Differential Diagnoses
- Reactive Adenopathy
- Metastatic Adenopathy, Head & Neck Primary Squamous Cell Carcinoma (SCC)
- Non-Hodgkin Lymphoma, Nodal

Imaging Recommendations
- Best imaging tool
  - US is ideal imaging modality as it evaluates the most commonly involved part of neck & readily combines with guided fine needle aspiration cytology (FNAC)
  - If a node is confirmed as malignant on FNAC & has ill-defined borders, it suggests extracapsular spread
- Protocol advice: Do not mistake neck nodes for normal brachial plexus trunks/divisions

DIFFERENTIAL DIAGNOSIS

Reactive Adenopathy
- Elliptical, solid, hypoechoic nodes with normal echogenic hilus & low resistance hilar vascularity

Metastatic Adenopathy, Head & Neck Primary Squamous Cell Carcinoma (SCC)
- Round, hypoechoic, cystic necrosis, absent echogenic hilus & high resistance peripheral/mixed vascularity

Non-Hodgkin Lymphoma, Nodal
- Large, round, solid hypoechoic nodes, reticulated or pseudosolid pattern with abnormal vascularity

PATHOLOGY

General Features
- Etiology: Represents disseminated malignancy
- Epidemiology: Metastatic nodes from H&N primary more common than nodes from systemic malignancy

CLINICAL ISSUES

Presentation
- Most common signs/symptoms: Low cervical neck mass in patient with known systemic malignancy

Natural History & Prognosis
- Disseminated disease associated with poor prognosis

Treatment
- If cervical node is the only metastatic disease, selective neck dissection may be performed
- Otherwise chemotherapy ± XRT

DIAGNOSTIC CHECKLIST

Consider
- Cervical nodal metastases if patient with known primary presents with new infrahyoid neck mass
- Extend imaging through chest if no known primary, looking for esophageal or lung tumor

SELECTED REFERENCES
1. Ahuja AT et al: Sonographic evaluation of cervical lymph nodes. AJR Am J Roentgenol. 184(5):1691-9, 2005

IMAGE GALLERY

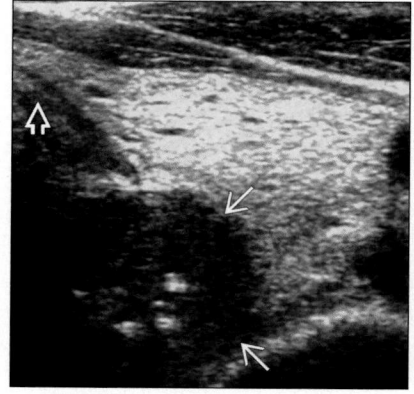 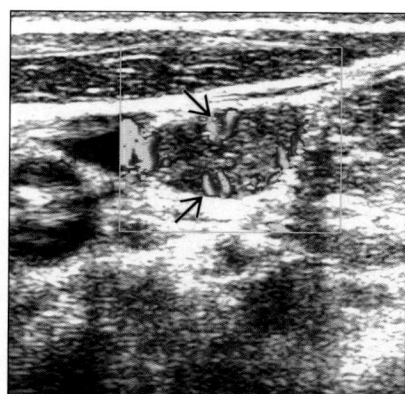 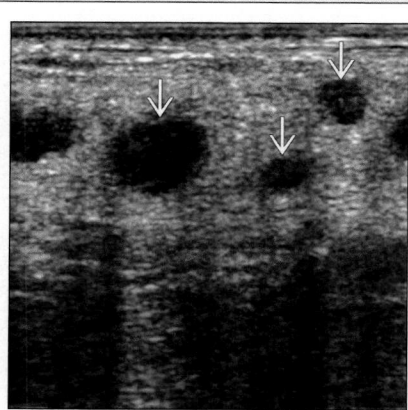

(Left) Transverse grayscale US shows a circumferential esophageal carcinoma ➡ with echogenic gas in lumen. Trachea ➡. *(Center)* Transverse power Doppler shows abnormal peripheral vascularity ➡ within a small node suggesting its malignant nature. FNAC confirmed metastatic esophageal carcinoma. *(Right)* Grayscale US shows multiple, small, round nodes ➡ in the supraclavicular fossa. Presence of such nodes in SCF in a patient with breast cancer suggests metastases, irrespective of nodal size. FNAC is indicated.

SIALADENITIS

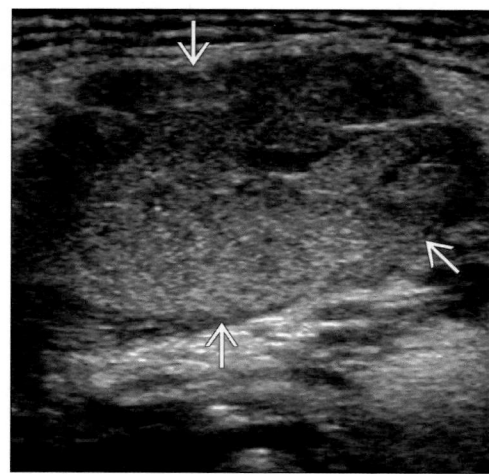

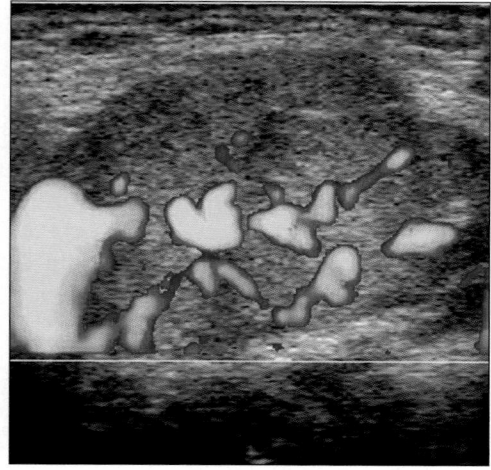

Transverse grayscale US of acute acalculous sialadenitis shows an enlarged SMG ➡ with rounded contours. It is diffusely hypoechoic with no duct dilatation. The gland was tender on transducer pressure.

Corresponding power Doppler US shows marked prominence of intraglandular vessels. Together with previous grayscale images, the appearance is typical of acute acalculous sialadenitis.

TERMINOLOGY

Abbreviations and Synonyms
- Submandibular gland (SMG) sialadenitis
- SMG sialadenosis

Definitions
- SMG sialadenitis: SMG inflammation ± submandibular duct calculus or stenosis
- Acute sialadenitis (AS): Acute SMG inflammation
  - Most common organism is Staphylococcus aureus
  - Others include Streptococcus viridans, Haemophilus influenzae & Escherichia coli
- Chronic sialadenitis(CS): Chronic SMG inflammation
  - Associated with conditions linked to ↓ salivary flow, including calculi & salivary stasis
- Chronic sclerosing sialadenitis (CSS), Kuttner tumor
  - Tumor-like condition of salivary glands, submandibular > parotid involvement
  - Periductal sclerosis, lymphocytic infiltration, reduction of secretory gland parenchyma, fibrosis, associated sialolithiasis (30-83%)

- Secondary SMG sialadenitis: SMG inflammation resulting from ductal obstruction from anterior floor of mouth (FOM) SCCa
  - Swollen SMG often mistaken for malignant node
- Sialolithiasis: Formation & deposition of concretions within SMG ductal system
  - Secondary to salivary stagnation, precipitation of calcium salts ± epithelial injury along duct leading to sialolith formation (nidus for stone formation)
- Autoimmune sialadenitis: Sialadenitis associated with autoimmune diseases
  - Autoimmune diseases (e.g., Sjögren syndrome) associated with salivary gland enlargement, keratoconjunctivitis sicca & xerostomia (dry mouth)
- Sialadenosis: Non-neoplastic noninflammatory swelling with acinar hypertrophy ± ductal atrophy
  - Can be inflammatory, autoimmune, drug induced, endocrine or metabolic

IMAGING FINDINGS

General Features
- Best diagnostic clue

DDx: Submandibular Sialadenitis

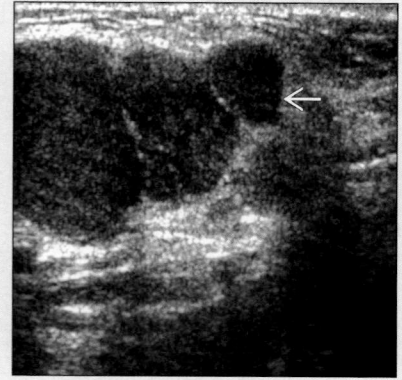

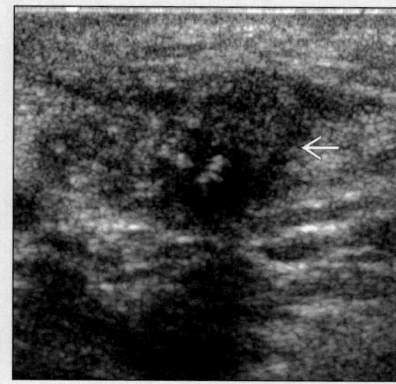

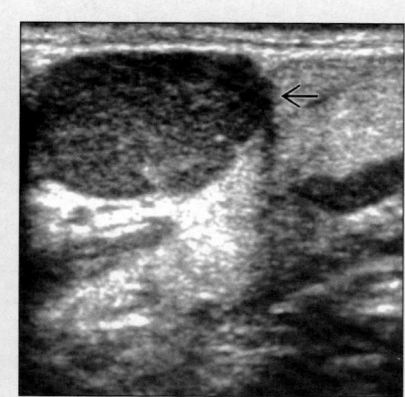

Benign Mixed Tumor SMG

SMG Carcinoma

Enlarged NHL Lymph Node

SIALADENITIS

Key Facts

Imaging Findings
- **Acute sialadenitis, acalculus**: Unilateral, enlarged hypoechoic gland with rounded contours
- No duct dilatation or calculi
- Tender on transducer pressure & increased intraglandular vascularity
- **Acute sialadenitis, calculus**: Unilateral enlarged, hypoechoic gland, normal contour
- Intra/extra glandular ductal dilatation and visualized calculus
- No obvious increase in vascularity
- **Chronic sclerosis sialadenitis**: Hypoechoic, heterogeneous "nodules"/"cirrhotic" appearance, bilateral, SMG > parotid
- Prominent intraglandular vessels running through "nodules" with no mass effect/displacement

- US is ideal imaging modality for SMG sialadenitis as it fully evaluates SMG, identifies calculus, duct dilatation & complications, such as abscess formation
- Use of high resolution transducer essential
- Always trace entire length of SM duct in multiple planes and compare with contralateral side
- Enlarged SM duct is often best clue to presence of calculus/stenosis
- Evaluate adjacent nodes as they may be enlarged during an acute episode

Top Differential Diagnoses
- Benign Mixed Tumor, Submandibular Gland
- Submandibular Gland Carcinoma
- Enlarged Submandibular Lymph Node

- Acute: Unilateral enlarged, hypoechoic SMG, increased vascularity, ± associated ductal dilatation ± calculus
- Chronic: Unilateral atrophic, hypoechoic, heterogeneous, hypovascular, ± associated ductal dilatation ± calculus
- Location
  - Submandibular space (SMS); SMG stones can be divided by location
    - Distal: Towards ductal opening in anterior sublingual space (SLS)
    - Proximal: Towards SMG hilum in SMS
  - SMG calculi are more likely to occur within duct than within SMG parenchyma

Ultrasonographic Findings
- **Acute sialadenitis, acalculus**: Unilateral, enlarged hypoechoic gland with rounded contours
  - No duct dilatation or calculi
  - Tender on transducer pressure & increased intraglandular vascularity
- **Acute sialadenitis, calculus**: Unilateral enlarged, hypoechoic gland, normal contour
  - Intra/extra glandular ductal dilatation and visualized calculus
  - No obvious increase in vascularity
- **Chronic sclerosis sialadenitis**: Hypoechoic, heterogeneous "nodules"/"cirrhotic" appearance, bilateral, SMG > parotid
  - Prominent intraglandular vessels running through "nodules" with no mass effect/displacement

Radiographic Findings
- Radiography: Stones are radio-opaque in 90% of plain film series (occlusal views)

CT Findings
- CECT
  - Acute sialadenitis secondary to calculus
    - Unilateral enhancing enlarged SMG with large duct behind intraductal calculus
    - Intraglandular ductal radicles & hilus also enlarged

- Chronic sialadenitis ± calculus
  - SMG small, fatty infiltrated ± intraductal calculus

MR Findings
- T2WI
  - Acute sialadenitis with calculus
    - Large, mixed high signal SMG with large duct ± stone
    - Stones may be missed
- T1 C+: Unilateral enhancing SMG with large duct

Other Modality Findings
- MR sialography possible but stone visualization is marginal
- Submandibular sialography no longer used
- CECT identifies calculus, soft tissue changes, complications, but involves use of contrast & ionizing radiation

Imaging Recommendations
- Best imaging tool
  - US is ideal imaging modality for SMG sialadenitis as it fully evaluates SMG, identifies calculus, duct dilatation & complications, such as abscess formation
    - For detection of salivary calculi, US has sensitivity of 94%, specificity 100%, accuracy 96%
- Protocol advice
  - Use of high resolution transducer essential
    - Scanning frequency ≥ 7.5 MHz
  - Always trace entire length of SM duct in multiple planes and compare with contralateral side
  - Enlarged SM duct is often best clue to presence of calculus/stenosis
  - Evaluate adjacent nodes as they may be enlarged during an acute episode

DIFFERENTIAL DIAGNOSIS

Benign Mixed Tumor, Submandibular Gland
- Well-defined, solid, hypoechoic, homogeneous mass with posterior enhancement, ± lobulated

SIALADENITIS

Submandibular Gland Carcinoma
- Ill-defined, solid, hypoechoic, heterogeneous mass in extraglandular infiltration, ± adjacent abnormal node

Enlarged Submandibular Lymph Node
- Reactive: Oval/round, hypoechoic with hilar architecture & vascularity
- Lymphoma: Round, solid, hypoechoic node with reticulated appearance & marked vascularity (hilar > peripheral)
- Metastatic SCCa: Round, hypoechoic, cystic necrosis, peripheral vascularity & absence of hilum

PATHOLOGY

General Features
- General path comments
  - SMG sialadenitis results from ductal obstruction from calculus, stenosis or anterior floor of mouth tumor
  - Calculi are more common in SMG duct than parotid gland duct
    - SMG saliva is thicker, more mucinous & more alkaline (calcium oxalate & phosphate are more likely to precipitate)
    - SMG duct courses superiorly, compared to inferior parotid duct; prone to stasis
    - SMG duct has larger diameter
- Etiology
  - Most common etiology: Calculus obstructs SMG duct with secondary sialadenitis that becomes suppurative sialadenitis
  - Less common etiology: Suppurative sialadenitis causes stenosis leading to chronic sialadenitis
  - Rare etiology: Primary glandular inflammation in Sjögren, AIDS or bacterial or viral infection
- Epidemiology
  - Major salivary ductal calculi
    - 85% in SMG duct; 15% in parotid ductal system
  - 90% of all SMG inflammatory disease is sialadenitis
  - SMG accounts for 10% of all cases of sialadenitis of major salivary glands

Gross Pathologic & Surgical Features
- Acutely inflamed gland is enlarged & annealed to surrounding soft tissue structures

Microscopic Features
- Acute sialadenitis: Parenchymal inflammation & lymphoid germinal centers
- Chronic sialadenitis: Mostly atrophy & fibrosis

CLINICAL ISSUES

Presentation
- Most common signs/symptoms
  - Unilateral, painful SMG swelling associated with eating or psychological gustatory stimulation = "salivary colic"
  - Other signs/symptoms
    - 30% SMG duct stones present with painless SMS mass
    - 80% present with painful SMG mass are secondary to calculus disease
    - Physical examination: If calculus in anterior duct, may be palpable to bimanual examination

Demographics
- Age: Older, debilitated, dehydrated patient

Natural History & Prognosis
- Protracted dilatation of duct may lead to SLS-SMS abscess

Treatment
- Treatment focused on eliminating sialadenitis causative factor
- Standard surgical technique in unrelenting obstructive SMG sialadenitis is extirpation of SMG
  - If calculus in anterior duct, may be removed by intraoral approach, without SMG removal
- When gland is inflamed without ductal dilatation, antibiotics may prevent surgery

DIAGNOSTIC CHECKLIST

Image Interpretation Pearls
- SMG sialadenitis imaging questions
  - If stone seen, is it in anterior or posterior SMG duct?
    - Anterior stones are removed per oral route
    - Posterior stones removed with SMG & duct
  - Is SMG affected without ductal pathology?
    - Consider Sjögren, AIDS or primary SMG infection

SELECTED REFERENCES

1. Harnsberger HR et al: Diagnostic Imaging: Head & Neck. 1st ed. Salt Lake City, Amirsys. III-4-22-25, 2004
2. Ahuja AT et al: Kuttner tumour (chronic sclerosing sialadenitis) of the submandibular gland: sonographic appearances. Ultrasound Med Biol. 29(7):913-9, 2003
3. Kalinowski M et al: Comparative study of MR sialography and digital subtraction sialography for benign salivary gland disorders. AJNR Am J Neuroradiol. 23(9):1485-92, 2002
4. Ching AS et al: Comparison of the sonographic features of acalculous and calculous submandibular sialadenitis. J Clin Ultrasound. 29(6):332-8, 2001
5. Williams HK et al: Chronic sclerosing sialadenitis of the submandibular and parotid glands: a report of a case and review of the literature. Oral Surg Oral Med Oral Pathol Oral Radiol Endod. 89(6):720-3, 2000
6. Ahuja AT: How I image the salivary glands. CME Journal Radiology. 1(2):76:81, 1999
7. Sekine S et al: Chronic sclerosing sialadenitis of the submandibular gland associated with idiopathic retroperitoneal fibrosis. Pathol Int. 49(7):663-7, 1999
8. Tighe JV et al: Relation of preoperative sialographic findings with histopathological diagnosis in cases of obstructive sialadenitis of the parotid and submandibular glands: retrospective study. Br J Oral Maxillofac Surg. 37(4):290-3, 1999

IMAGE GALLERY

Typical

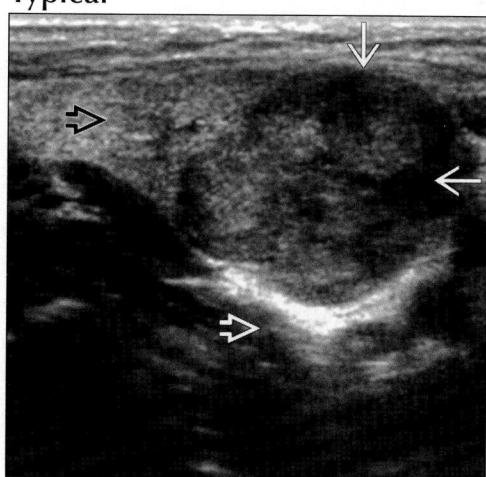

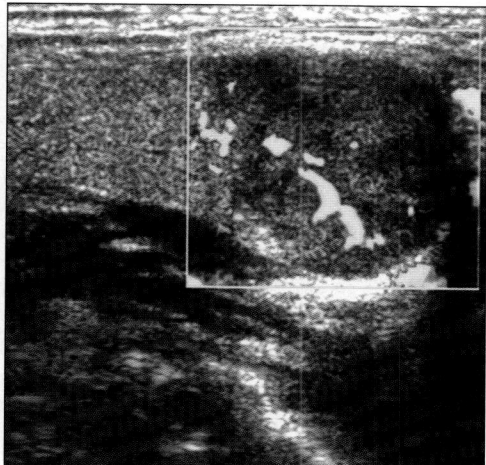

(Left) Transverse grayscale US shows a well-defined, lobulated submandibular BMT ➡ with homogeneous echoes & posterior enhancement ➡. Note its origin from the SMG ➡. US clearly evaluates mass. (Right) Corresponding power Doppler shows a large vessel within the BMT. Presence & distribution of vessels in benign salivary tumors is sparse. Benign lesions: RI < 0.8 & PI < 2.0 on spectral Doppler.

Typical

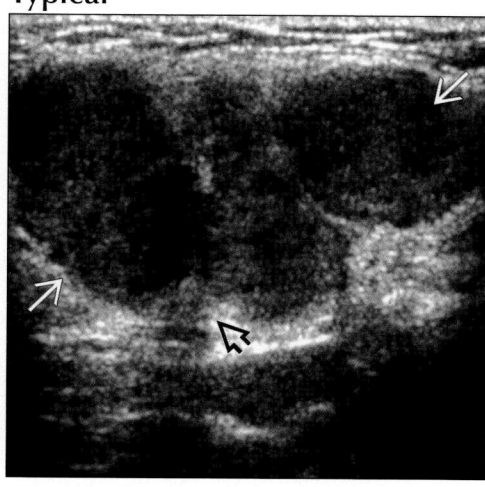

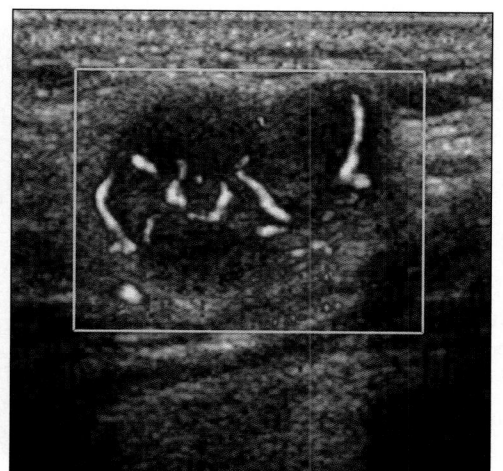

(Left) Transverse grayscale US shows a large, lobulated SMG BMT ➡. Some of its edges are ill-defined ➡ (due to hemorrhage) & appear suspicious. Note normal overlying subcutaneous tissue. (Right) Power Doppler US shows multiple vessels within a lobulated SMG BMT. Vascularity in benign lesions is sparse compared to malignant lesions which may have florid vascularity.

Typical

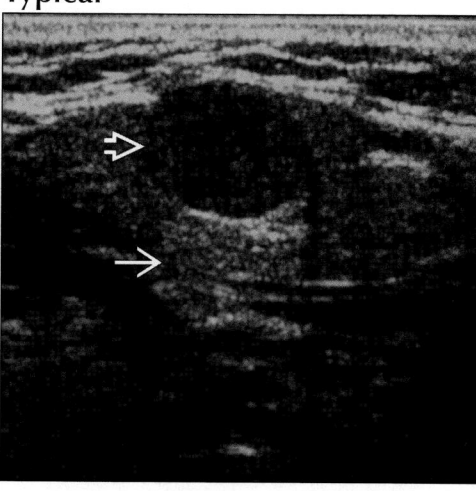

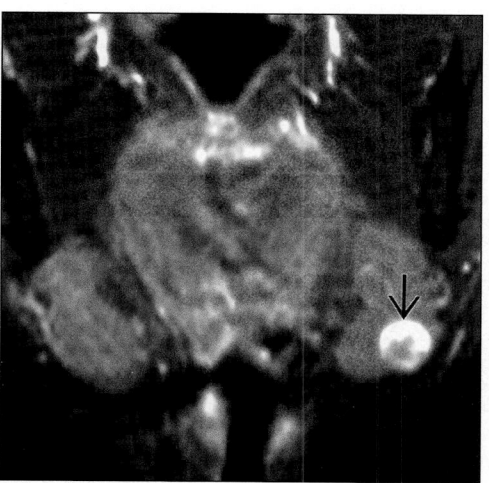

(Left) Transverse grayscale US shows a well-defined, homogeneous, solid, non-calcified SMG BMT ➡, with posterior enhancement ➡. US fully evaluates the tumor, associated nodes, & soft tissue. (Right) Corresponding coronal fat suppressed gadolinium enhanced T1WI MR shows intense enhancement in the SMG BMT ➡. No additional information is obtained on this MR compared to the previous US.

SUBMANDIBULAR GLAND CARCINOMA

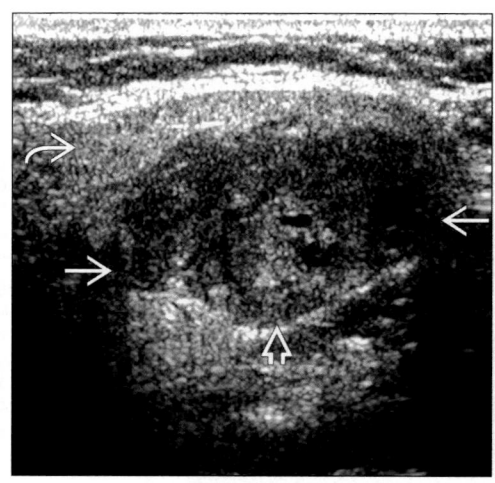

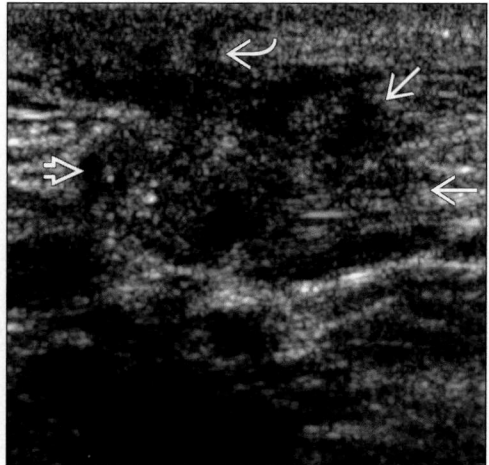

Transverse grayscale US shows a solid, hypoechoic, heterogeneous SMG mass ➡. Note its ill-defined edges ➡. US suggested its malignant nature; ACCa found at surgery. Normal SMG parenchyma ➡.

Transverse grayscale US of a SMG ACCa ➡ seen as an ill-defined, solid, hypoechoic heterogeneous mass. Note its ill-defined edges ➡ & extension to the subcutaneous tissue ➡.

TERMINOLOGY

Definitions
- Two major carcinomas of submandibular gland (SMG): Adenoid cystic carcinoma (ACCa) & mucoepidermoid Ca (MECa)

IMAGING FINDINGS

General Features
- Best diagnostic clue: Ill-defined, hypoechoic mass +/- invasion of extraglandular soft tissues/perineural, +/- nodal involvement

Ultrasonographic Findings
- Grayscale Ultrasound
  ○ Ultrasound is unable to differentiate between various malignant tumors
  ○ Small tumors may be well-defined & have homogeneous internal architecture
  ○ Large tumors are ill-defined with invasive edges & heterogeneous areas of necrosis/hemorrhage
  ○ +/- Extraglandular invasion of soft tissues

  ○ +/- Adjacent nodal, disseminated metastases
- Color Doppler
  ○ Pronounced intratumoral vascularity
  ○ Spectral Doppler: Increased intravascular resistance
    ■ Resistive index (RI) > 0.8, pulsatility index (PI) > 2.0

CT Findings
- NECT: Asymmetry of size & heterogeneous SMG
- CECT
  ○ Small tumor: Well-circumscribed, ovoid mass
  ○ Large tumor: Enhancing mass arising from SMG into SMS with invasive margins

MR Findings
- T1WI: Inhomogeneous signal intensity
- T2WI: Intermediate-high mixed signal intensity
- T1 C+
  ○ Small tumor: Ovoid intraglandular enhancing mass with sharp borders
  ○ Large tumor: Enhancing mass emerging from SMG into SMS with poorly defined margins

Imaging Recommendations
- Best imaging tool

DDx: Submandibular Carcinoma

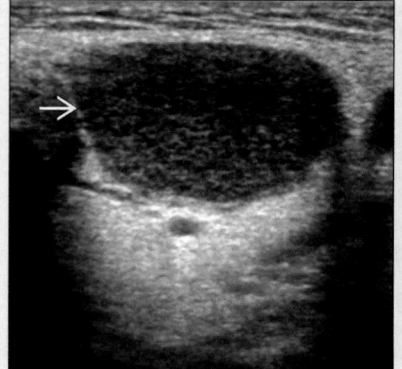

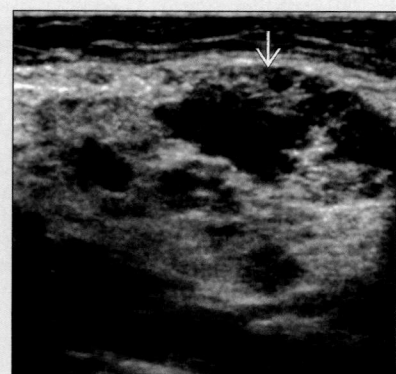

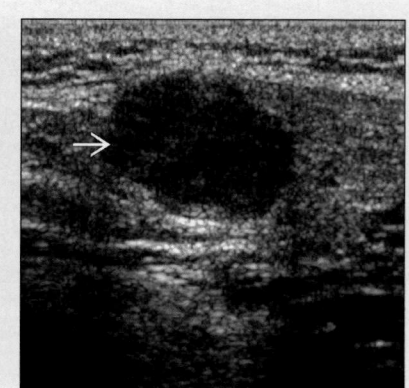

Submandibular Node, NHL

Kuttner Tumor

BMT, Submandibular Gland

SUBMANDIBULAR GLAND CARCINOMA

Key Facts

Terminology
- Two major carcinomas of submandibular gland (SMG): Adenoid cystic carcinoma (ACCa) & mucoepidermoid Ca (MECa)

Imaging Findings
- Small tumors may be well-defined & have homogeneous internal architecture
- Large tumors are ill-defined with invasive edges & heterogeneous areas of necrosis/hemorrhage

- +/- Extraglandular invasion of soft tissues
- +/- Adjacent nodal, disseminated metastases
- US is useful in identifying tumor, suggesting its malignant nature & guiding biopsy

Pathology
- 45% of SMG tumors are malignant; 55% benign
- Most common SMG carcinoma is ACCa (40%), MECa is 10% of all salivary gland malignancies

---

- ○ US is ideal imaging modality to evaluate SMG tumors due to their superficial location
- ○ US readily combines with fine needle aspiration cytology which has sensitivity of 83%, specificity 86% & accuracy of 85% for salivary gland tumors
- Protocol advice
  - ○ Evaluate tumor edge, extraglandular/nodal involvement, internal heterogeneity
  - ○ US cannot evaluate entire extent of large tumors & delineate perineural spread
    - ▪ US is useful in identifying tumor, suggesting its malignant nature & guiding biopsy
  - ○ MR ideally evaluates tumor, its local extent, perineural spread & nodal involvement if any

DIFFERENTIAL DIAGNOSIS

Malignant Node, Submandibular Space (SMS)
- Hypoechoic, well-defined, +/- multiple, abnormal vascularity, reticulated in NHL

Chronic Sclerosing Sialadenitis, Kuttner Tumor
- Bilateral involvement; multiple, hypoechoic areas in SMG with no mass effect or vascular displacement; end stage: Cirrhotic pattern

Benign Mixed Tumor (BMT) of SMG
- Well-defined, solid, hypoechoic, homogeneous with posterior enhancement

PATHOLOGY

General Features
- General path comments: Malignant tumors include ACCa, MECa & other rare lesions
- Epidemiology
  - ○ 45% of SMG tumors are malignant; 55% benign
  - ○ Most common SMG carcinoma is ACCa (40%), MECa is 10% of all salivary gland malignancies

CLINICAL ISSUES

Natural History & Prognosis
- 50% 5 year survival for all cancers
- Metastatic disease accounts for 30% of deaths

Treatment
- Surgical removal, node dissection, post-op XRT

SELECTED REFERENCES

1. Ahuja AT et al: Imaging in Head & Neck Cancer: A Practical Approach. 1st ed. London, Greenwich Medical Media. 115-41, 2003

IMAGE GALLERY

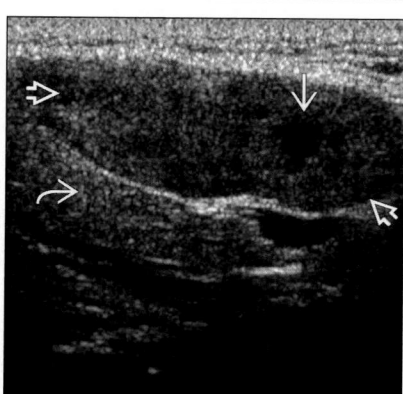 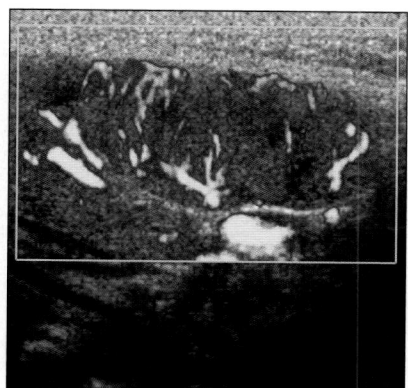 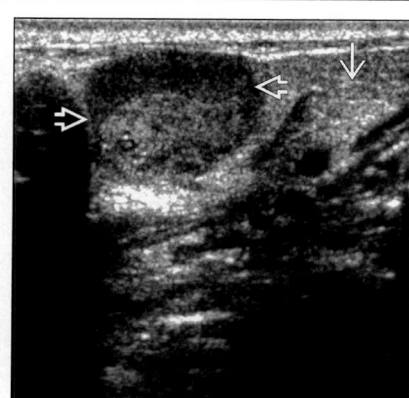

(Left) Transverse grayscale US shows intermediate grade MECa ➡. Note it is slightly hypoechoic to SMG parenchyma ➡ but fairly well-defined with focal internal heterogeneity/necrosis ➡. *(Center)* Corresponding power Doppler US showed marked tumor vascularity raising suspicion of malignancy. Intermediate MECa at surgery. *(Right)* Longitudinal grayscale US shows a well-defined, solid, hypoechoic, mass ➡ arising from the SMG ➡. Note it is fairly well-defined & simulates BMT. Confirmed low grade MECa at surgery.

KIMURA DISEASE

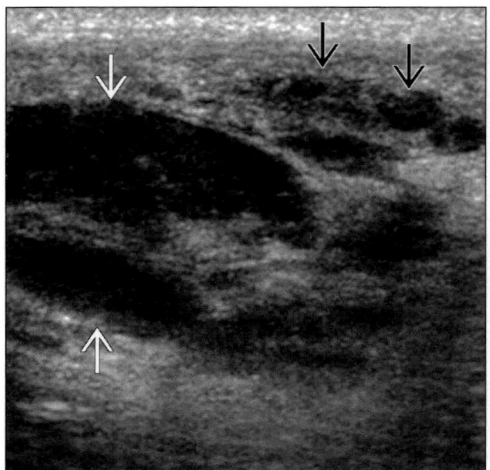

Transverse grayscale US shows a large, solid, hypoechoic node ➡ with hilar architecture in an Asian male. Note small, hypoechoic nodules ➡ in the adjacent parotid gland. Biopsy confirmed KimDs.

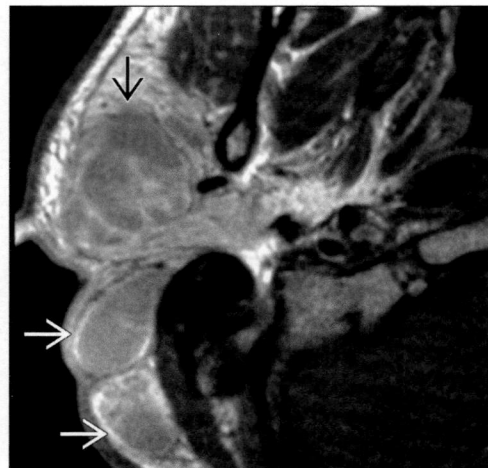

Corresponding, gadolinium enhanced, axial T1WI shows heterogeneous enhancement in the parotid mass ➡ & extraparotid nodes ➡ simulating malignancy. Biopsy confirmed KimDs.

TERMINOLOGY

Abbreviations and Synonyms
- Kimura disease (KimDs)
- Eosinophilic lymphogranuloma, eosinophilic hyperplastic lymphogranuloma

Definitions
- KimDs: Chronic inflammatory disorder of head & neck, primarily in young Asian males
  - Triad of painless unilateral cervical adenopathy or subcutaneous nodules, blood & tissue eosinophilia & markedly elevated serum IgE

IMAGING FINDINGS

General Features
- Best diagnostic clue: Lymphadenopathy & subcutaneous nodules ± salivary mass
- Location
  - Most commonly involves unilateral lymph nodes & subcutaneous tissues of head & neck

- Most have involvement of parotid gland or submandibular gland; rarely lacrimal gland
- Occasionally axillary or inguinal lymph nodes or subcutaneous forearm lesions
- Morphology
  - Enlarged lymph nodes & ipsilateral subcutaneous mass lesions
  - Salivary gland involvement may be diffuse infiltration, ill-defined mass or focal (intraparotid) nodes

Ultrasonographic Findings
- **Nodal**: Well-defined, enlarged, & hypoechoic
- Homogeneous internal architecture & preserved echogenic hilum
- No nodal matting or adjacent soft tissue edema
- Color Doppler: Hilar vascularity (87%), mixed hilar & peripheral (13%)
- Spectral Doppler: Low resistance vascularity, resistive index (RI) < 0.8, pulsatility index (PI) < 1.6
- **Extranodal**: Well/ill-defined hypoechoic masses, homogeneous or heterogeneous internal architecture
  - Hypoechoic areas interspersed with hyperechoic areas; "wooly" appearance

DDx: Kimura Disease

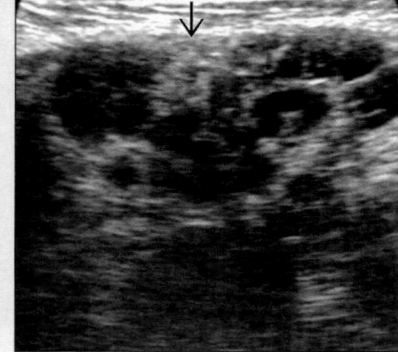

Sjögren Syndrome

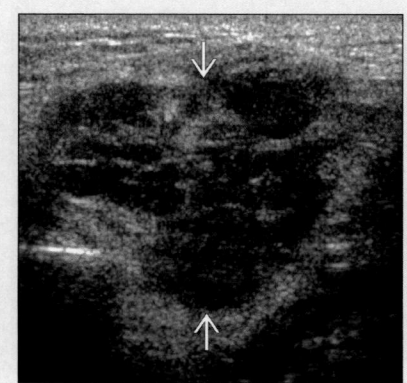

Parotid Carcinoma

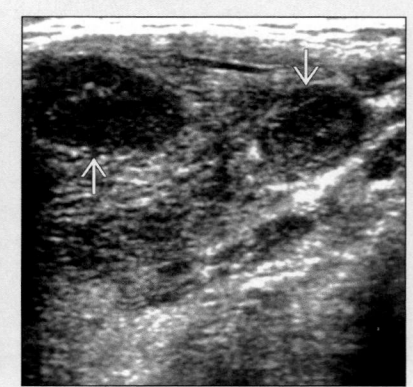

Parotid Metastases

KIMURA DISEASE

Key Facts

Terminology
- KimDs: Chronic inflammatory disorder of head & neck, primarily in young Asian males
- Triad of painless unilateral cervical adenopathy or subcutaneous nodules, blood & tissue eosinophilia & markedly elevated serum IgE

Imaging Findings
- Best diagnostic clue: Lymphadenopathy & subcutaneous nodules ± salivary mass
- **Nodal**: Well-defined, enlarged, & hypoechoic
- Homogeneous internal architecture & preserved echogenic hilum
- No nodal matting or adjacent soft tissue edema
- Color Doppler: Hilar vascularity (87%), mixed hilar & peripheral (13%)

- **Extranodal**: Well/ill-defined hypoechoic masses, homogeneous or heterogeneous internal architecture
- Hypoechoic areas interspersed with hyperechoic areas; "wooly" appearance
- Color Doppler: Arterial & venous flow throughout soft tissue masses
- US is unable to evaluate deep lobe parotid involvement and in such cases MR is modality of choice (preferred over CT)
- Always evaluate salivary & lacrimal glands and soft tissues of the neck

Top Differential Diagnoses
- Sjögren Syndrome
- Parotid Primary Malignancy
- Parotid Nodal Metastases

- ○ Color Doppler: Arterial & venous flow throughout soft tissue masses
- ○ Spectral Doppler: Low resistance vascularity, RI < 0.8, PI < 1.6

CT Findings
- CECT
  - ○ Multiple nodal masses
  - ○ Irregularly shaped subcutaneous masses ± salivary gland masses
  - ○ Moderate to intense nodal/lesional contrast-enhancement is characteristic, parotid lesion enhancement is heterogeneous
  - ○ Chronic cases may show less enhancement due to fibrosis

MR Findings
- T1WI: Isointense or hypointense nodal masses compared to parotid glands
- T2WI: Usually hyperintense; chronic fibrotic lesions may be hypointense
- T1 C+
  - ○ Enhancing nodes & masses characteristic
  - ○ Less enhancement expected with fibrotic lesions

Nuclear Medicine Findings
- Uptake of In-111pentetreotide, Tc-99m labeled autologous granulocytes
- Uptake of Tl-201 SPECT on early & delayed images

Imaging Recommendations
- Best imaging tool
  - ○ US is ideal initial modality of choice
    - ■ It evaluates nodal as well as extranodal manifestations of KimDs
  - ○ US is readily combined with guided biopsy and this helps to confirm diagnosis of KimDs
  - ○ US is unable to evaluate deep lobe parotid involvement and in such cases MR is modality of choice (preferred over CT)
- Protocol advice
  - ○ Always evaluate salivary & lacrimal glands and soft tissues of the neck

- ○ Use of high-resolution transducer is essential (≥ 7.5 MHz)

DIFFERENTIAL DIAGNOSIS

Sjögren Syndrome
- Hypoechoic, heterogeneous gland, reticulated pattern, microcysts/macrocysts, ± solid component, multiple glands involved

Parotid Primary Malignancy
- Ill-defined, solid, hypoechoic mass with intranodal vascularity, ± extraglandular extension, facial nerve involvement & associated malignant nodes

Parotid Nodal Metastases
- Solitary/multiple, ill-defined, hypoechoic masses with abnormal vascularity & known associated primary (SCCa, adjacent melanoma)

Sarcoidosis, Head & Neck
- Primary manifestation is multiple enlarged nodes
- Can involve entire parotid gland or intraparotid nodes, diffuse hypoechoic gland, submandibular involvement > parotid

Non-Hodgkin Lymphoma Nodes
- Multiple, solid, hypoechoic nodes with reticulated echo pattern, hilar > peripheral vascularity, ± posterior enhancement

PATHOLOGY

General Features
- General path comments: Abnormal proliferation of lymphoid follicles & vascular endothelium with dense eosinophilic infiltrate
- Etiology
  - ○ Unknown, though allergic and autoimmune theories favored because of elevated serum IgE
    - ■ Possibly post-infectious: Candida, parasite, virus
- Epidemiology: Rare disease, especially in non-Asians

KIMURA DISEASE

- Associated abnormalities
  - Renal dysfunction including nephrotic syndrome associated in 15-60%
    - Occasionally can precede development of subcutaneous lesions

Gross Pathologic & Surgical Features
- Tumorous masses of lymph nodes, subcutaneous tissues & salivary glands
  - Other unusual sites of involvement
    - Oral mucosa, auricle, scalp, lacrimal gland & orbit
- Vascular, rubbery, fibrotic masses
- Nodes may form confluent mass ± adherent to overlying dermis

Microscopic Features
- Lymphoid hyperplasia with germinal centers containing cellular, vascular & fibrous components
  - Dense eosinophilic infiltrates & eosinophilic microabscesses with central necrosis
  - Abundant plasma cells & lymphocytes (proliferation of HLA-DR CD4 cells)
  - Vascular proliferation and variable fibrosis around & within lesion
- Immunofluorescence studies
  - Germinal centers contain heavy IgE deposits
  - Variable IgG, IgM and fibrinogen

CLINICAL ISSUES

Presentation
- Most common signs/symptoms
  - Insidious onset of solitary or multiple painless swellings of head & neck, predominantly in preauricular and submandibular regions
  - Marked lymphadenopathy (periauricular, cervical, axillary, inguinal)
  - Other signs/symptoms
    - Occasional pruritus or pigmentation of skin overlying nodules
  - Facial nerve palsy not reported with parotid involvement
  - Laboratory
    - Peripheral eosinophilia & elevated serum IgE
    - Evaluate for renal dysfunction with creatinine, BUN & urinary protein
- Clinical Profile: 30 year old Asian male with painless nodal neck masses ± parotid mass

Demographics
- Age: Predominately 2nd & 3rd decades
- Gender: M:F = 3:1
- Ethnicity: Endemic in Asians, particularly Chinese and Japanese

Natural History & Prognosis
- Chronic benign course with nodules present for years
- Potentially disfiguring
  - Large (≥ 5 cm) subcutaneous lesions may ulcerate
- No malignant potential

Treatment
- Conservative surgical excision favored for initial diagnosis & treatment
  - Up to 25% recur
- Observation alone if not symptomatic or disfiguring
- Intralesional or oral steroids may temporize though not cure
  - Oral prednisolone for renal involvement
- Cyclosporine reported to induce remission
- Radiotherapy for persistent/recurrent problematic lesions

DIAGNOSTIC CHECKLIST

Image Interpretation Pearls
- Look for combination of imaging findings, particularly in Asian males
  - Unilateral cervical adenopathy
  - Subcutaneous well/ill-defined mass
  - Salivary gland abnormality: Intraparotid nodes or ill-defined or infiltrative mass

SELECTED REFERENCES

1. Harnsberger HR et al: Diagnostic Imaging: Head & Neck. 1st ed. Salt Lake City, Amirsys. III-2-32-35, 2004
2. Arshad AR: Kimura's disease of parotid gland presenting as solitary parotid swelling. Head Neck. 25(9):754-7, 2003
3. Chartapisak W et al: Steroid-resistant nephrotic syndrome associated with Kimura's disease. Am J Nephrol. 22(4):381-4, 2002
4. Ching AS et al: Extranodal manifestation of Kimura's disease: ultrasound features. Eur Radiol. 12(3):600-4, 2002
5. Shetty AK et al: Kimura's disease: a diagnostic challenge. Pediatrics. 110(3):e39, 2002
6. Ahuja A et al: Gray scale and power Doppler sonography in cases of Kimura disease. AJNR Am J Neuroradiol. 22(3):513-7, 2001
7. von Sivers K et al: Uptake of 111In-pentetreotide and 99mTc-labeled autologous granulocytes in Kimura's disease. Eur Radiol. 10(6):1026-8, 2000
8. Buggage RR et al: Kimura disease of the orbit and ocular adnexa. Surv Ophthalmol. 44(1):79-91, 1999
9. Hiwatashi A et al: Kimura's disease with bilateral auricular masses. AJNR Am J Neuroradiol. 20(10):1976-8, 1999
10. Armstrong WB et al: Kimura's disease: two case reports and a literature review. Ann Otol Rhinol Laryngol. 107(12):1066-71, 1998
11. Chusid MJ et al: Kimura's disease: an unusual cause of cervical tumour. Arch Dis Child. 77(2):153-4, 1997
12. Goldenberg D et al: Computerized tomographic and ultrasonographic features of Kimura's disease. J Laryngol Otol. 111(4):389-91, 1997
13. Nagamachi S et al: Tl-201 SPECT in Kimura's disease involving the parotid glands and cervical nodes. Clin Nucl Med. 21(2):125-8, 1996
14. Takahashi S et al: Kimura disease: CT and MR findings. AJNR Am J Neuroradiol. 17(2):382-5, 1996
15. Ahuja AT et al: Ultrasound of Kimura's disease. Clin Radiol. 50(3):170-3, 1995
16. Som PM et al: Kimura disease involving parotid gland and cervical nodes: CT and MR findings. J Comput Assist Tomogr. 16(2):320-2, 1992

KIMURA DISEASE

Typical

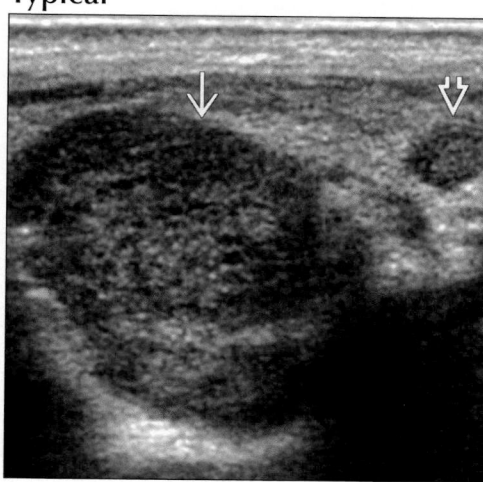 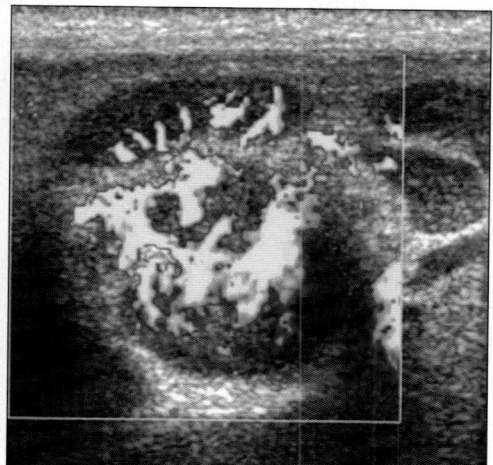

(Left) Transverse grayscale US shows a well-defined, solid, hypoechoic homogeneous mass in the superficial parotid ➡ in a patient with KimDs. There is no necrosis. Note another smaller adjacent nodule ➡. *(Right)* Corresponding power Doppler shows marked vascularity within the mass with a hilar distribution of vessels. In an Asian male consider nodal KimDs in a intraparotid node. Diagnosis confirmed at biopsy.

Typical

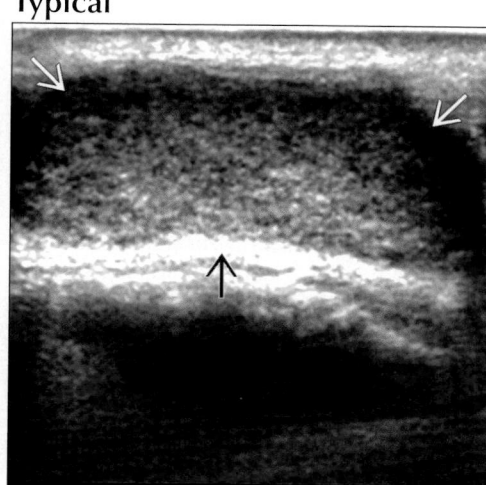 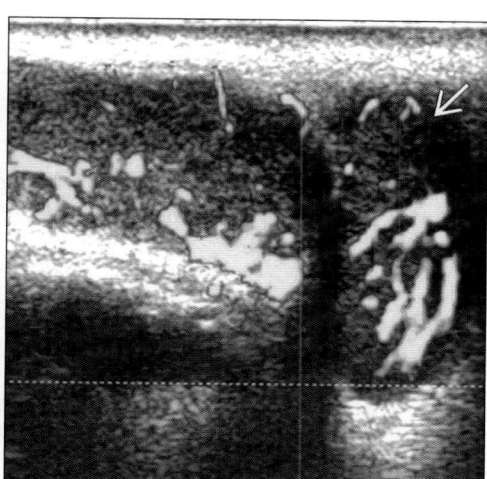

(Left) Longitudinal grayscale US shows an extrasalivary soft tissue mass ➡ in a patient with KimDs. It is well-defined, solid, hypoechoic with a homogeneous echo pattern & no necrosis. Mandible ➡. *(Right)* Corresponding power Doppler shows marked vascularity within the mass. Such vascularity is usually low resistance on spectral Doppler. Note another adjacent vascular nodule ➡. Biopsy confirmed KimDs.

Typical

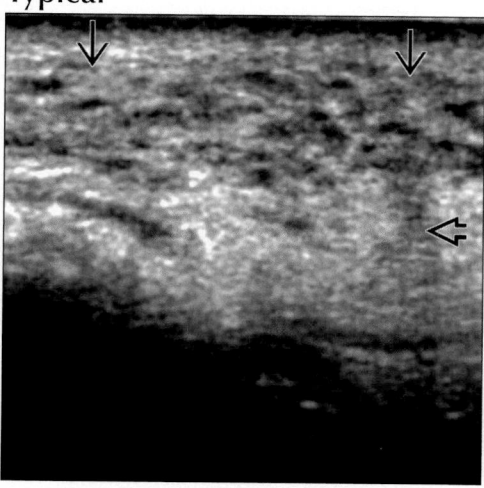 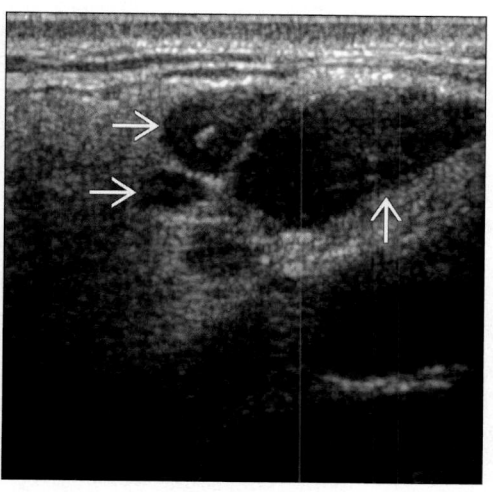

(Left) Longitudinal grayscale US shows ill-defined, solid, heterogeneous tissue ➡ overlying the parotid ➡ in an Asian male. Appearances raised suspicion of soft tissue KimDs. Biopsy confirmed. *(Right)* Longitudinal grayscale US shows multiple, well-defined nodules ➡ in the superficial lobe of the parotid gland in an Asian male. Differential diagnosis must include nodal KimDs. Biopsy confirmed the diagnosis.

SJOGREN SYNDROME, PAROTID

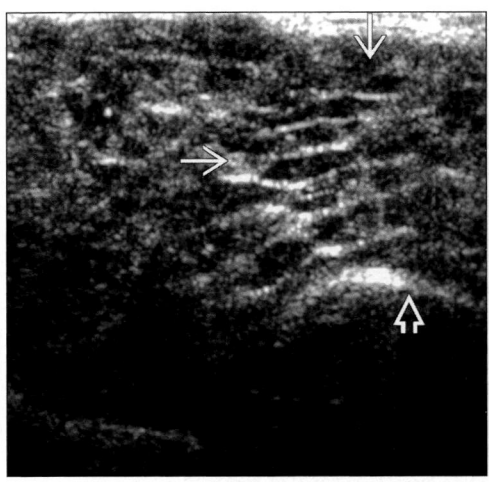

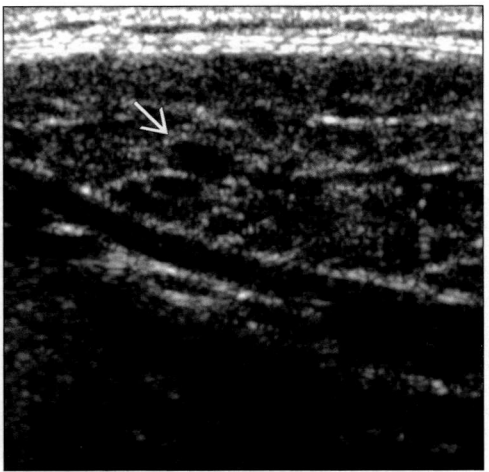

Transverse grayscale US shows the typical US appearance of the parotid gland in SjS. It is enlarged, with diffuse, heterogeneous, hypoechoic areas ➡ involving the superficial & deep lobes. Mandible ⬌.

Transverse grayscale US of the submandibular gland with diffuse hypoechoic areas ➡ within the enlarged gland. Same patient as in previous image. US of the lacrimal glands will often show similar changes.

TERMINOLOGY

Abbreviations and Synonyms
- Abbreviation: Sjögren syndrome (SjS)
- Synonym: Sicca syndrome

Definitions
- SjS: Chronic systemic autoimmune exocrinopathy that causes salivary & lacrimal gland tissue destruction
  - Primary SjS: Dry eyes & mouth; no collagen vascular disease (CVD)
  - Secondary SjS: Dry eyes & mouth with CVD, most commonly rheumatoid arthritis

IMAGING FINDINGS

General Features
- Best diagnostic clue: US shows bilateral enlarged parotids, +/- submandibular & lacrimal glands, multiple micro/macro cystic intraparotid solid lesions ± intraglandular calcifications
- Location: Bilateral salivary & lacrimal glands

- Size: Range from < 1 mm microcysts to macrocysts, +/- mixed solid-cystic masses > 2 cm
- Imaging appearance depends on stage of disease & presence or absence of lymphocyte aggregates within parotid
  - Earliest stage SjS: Parotids may appear normal
  - Intermediate stage SjS: "Miliary pattern" of small cysts diffusely throughout both parotids
  - Late stage SjS: Larger cystic (parenchymal destruction) & solid masses (lymphocyte aggregates) in both parotids
  - Any stage may have solid intraparotid masses secondary to lymphocytic accumulation that mimic tumor
  - Invasive parotid mass ± cervical adenopathy may signal malignant non-Hodgkin lymphoma (NHL) transformation

Ultrasonographic Findings
- Grayscale Ultrasound
  - Early stage "miliary" (≤ 1 mm punctate cystic changes) may be missed
  - Later stages of SjS are readily seen on US

DDx: Sjogren Syndrome, Parotid

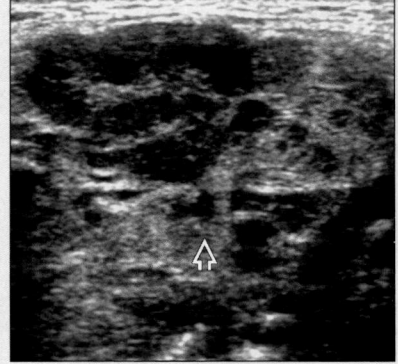

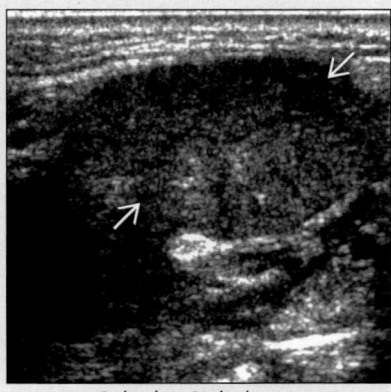

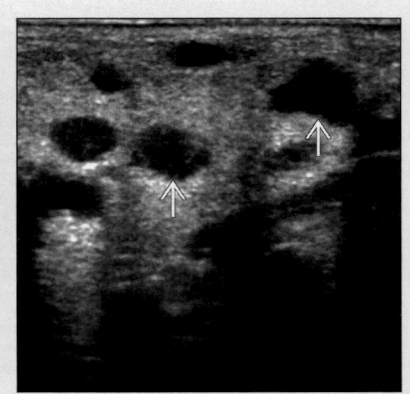

Kuttner Tumor　　　*Calculus Sialadenitis*　　　*Intra Parotid NHL Nodes*

SJOGREN SYNDROME, PAROTID

Key Facts

Terminology
- SjS: Chronic systemic autoimmune exocrinopathy that causes salivary & lacrimal gland tissue destruction

Imaging Findings
- Early stage "miliary" (≤ 1 mm punctate cystic changes) may be missed
- Later stages of SjS are readily seen on US
- Diffuse hypoechogenicity of salivary & lacrimal glands may be the only clue in early SjS
- Heterogeneous parenchymal echoes in salivary glands, +/- lacrimal glands
- Multiple discrete hypoechoic foci scattered throughout lacrimal & salivary glands
- Macrocysts in salivary & lacrimal glands

- Diffuse reticulated appearance of salivary & lacrimal glands with hypoechoic septa
- Lymphomatous change is seen as ill-defined, solid, hypoechoic areas within salivary glands +/- associated nodal disease
- Diagnosis of SjS is based on clinical, serologic & histologic evidence
- Primary role of imaging is to confirm or exclude salivary gland involvement & surveillance for lymphomatous change
- Sialography (conventional or MR) demonstrate earliest findings of SjS in peripheral ducts & acini

Top Differential Diagnoses
- Chronic Sclerosing Sialadenitis, Kuttner Tumor
- Calculus Sialadenitis
- NHL, Parotid Nodes

- Diffuse hypoechogenicity of salivary & lacrimal glands may be the only clue in early SjS
- Heterogeneous parenchymal echoes in salivary glands, +/- lacrimal glands
- Multiple discrete hypoechoic foci scattered throughout lacrimal & salivary glands
  - Correlates with lymphocytic aggregates
- Macrocysts in salivary & lacrimal glands
- Diffuse reticulated appearance of salivary & lacrimal glands with hypoechoic septa
- Lymphomatous change is seen as ill-defined, solid, hypoechoic areas within salivary glands +/- associated nodal disease
- Color Doppler
  - Increased parenchymal vascularity in SjS
    - Correlates with severity of disease

CT Findings
- NECT
  - Bilateral parotid enlargement, increased CT density & heterogeneity
  - Punctate calcification may be diffusely present in both parotids
- CECT
  - Wide range of appearances based on SjS stage
    - Early diffuse millimeter fluid density cystic lesions
    - Late macrocystic change ± solid nodules that may mimic BLL-HIV or tumor
  - Heterogeneous enhancement of solid & mixed cystic-solid lesions

MR Findings
- T1WI: Discrete collections of low signal intensity, reflecting watery saliva contained within them
- T2WI
  - Diffuse, bilateral high T2 1-2 mm foci (early stages, I & II)
  - Multiple high T2 signal > 2 mm foci (late stages, III & IV)
- STIR: Lesions more conspicuous
- T1 C+: Heterogeneous mild enhancement of nodular parenchyma & fibrosis with non-enhancing cystic changes

- MR sialography
  - Sensitive to diagnosis of SjS (approaching 95% sensitivity & specificity)
  - Stages severity of SjS & is replacing conventional sialography
  - Display punctate, globular, cavitary or destructive parotid distal ductal changes of SjS as focal high T2 signal

Imaging Recommendations
- Best imaging tool
  - Diagnosis of SjS is based on clinical, serologic & histologic evidence
    - Primary role of imaging is to confirm or exclude salivary gland involvement & surveillance for lymphomatous change
  - Sialography (conventional or MR) demonstrate earliest findings of SjS in peripheral ducts & acini
  - US is cost effective in surveillance of SjS patients
- Protocol advice
  - Use high frequency transducers (≥ 7.5 MHz)
  - Evaluate salivary & lacrimal glands at same time

DIFFERENTIAL DIAGNOSIS

Chronic Sclerosing Sialadenitis, Kuttner Tumor
- Submandibular > parotid, bilateral, hypoechoic heterogeneous nodules with no mass effect, cirrhotic looking gland

Calculus Sialadenitis
- Usually solitary gland involved, hypoechoic enlarged gland with increased vascularity, duct dilatation & calculus

NHL, Parotid Nodes
- Bilateral, solid, hypoechoic, round nodes with prominent vascularity, hilar > peripheral; other evidence of NHL seen

SJOGREN SYNDROME, PAROTID

Benign Lymphoepithelial Lesions-HIV (BLL-HIV)
- Mixed cystic & solid lesions enlarging both parotids may exactly mimic SjS
- Tonsillar hyperplasia & cervical reactive-appearing adenopathy

Sarcoidosis
- Rare manifestation of sarcoidosis; cervical & mediastinal lymph nodes
- Diffuse hypoechogenicity of salivary glands, submandibular > parotid

Warthin Tumors
- 20% multicentric; hypoechoic, solid/cystic elements with thick walls, septa in parotid apex
- Spares lacrimal & submandibular glands (SMG)

PATHOLOGY

General Features
- General path comments
  - Periductal lymphocyte aggregates extend into & destroy salivary acinar parenchyma
  - Autoimmune dysregulation leads to destruction of acinar cells & ductal epithelia of lacrimal & salivary glands
  - Activated lymphocytes selectively injure lacrimal & salivary glands leading to tissue damage
- Etiology
  - Poorly understood immune-mediated disease
  - Viral infection has been proposed as initiating event
- Epidemiology
  - Incidence of SjS is ~ 0.5%
  - 2nd most common autoimmune disorder after rheumatoid arthritis

Gross Pathologic & Surgical Features
- Enlarged parotid glands with multiple small to large cysts & lymphocyte aggregates

Microscopic Features
- Labial biopsy: CD4 positive T-cell lymphocytes
- Periductal lymphocyte & plasma cell infiltration & epimyoepithelial islands
  - Early stages: Lymphocyte-plasma cell infiltration obstructs intercalated ducts with enlarged distal ducts throughout parotids
  - Late stages: Activated lymphocytes destroy salivary tissue, leaving larger cysts & solid lymphocyte aggregates

Staging, Grading or Classification Criteria
- Based on conventional sialography or MR sialography
  - Stage I: Punctate contrast/high signal ≤ 1 mm
  - Stage II: Globular contrast/high signal 1-2 mm
  - Stage III: Cavitary contrast/high signal > 2 mm
  - Stage IV: Complete destruction of parotid gland parenchyma

CLINICAL ISSUES

Presentation
- Most common signs/symptoms: Tender bilateral parotid gland swelling
- Clinical Profile
  - Patient complains of recurrent acute episodes of tender glandular swelling
  - Less common chronic glandular enlargement with superimposed acute attacks, to non-tender, non-painful parotid enlargement
  - Other signs/symptoms
    - Dry eyes, dry mouth, dry skin
    - Rheumatoid arthritis > > systemic lupus erythematosus > progressive systemic sclerosis
- Laboratory
  - Requires positive labial/parotid biopsy or autoantibody against Sjögren-associated A or B antigen for diagnosis to be assigned
  - Rheumatoid factor positive in up to 95%
  - ANA positive in up to 80%
  - Schirmer test is positive (decreased tear production)

Demographics
- Age: 50-70 year old
- Gender
  - Striking female predominance (90-95%)
  - Most common in menopausal women
- Juvenile SjS
  - < 20 year old males
  - High rate of recurrent parotitis
  - Most resolve spontaneously at puberty

Natural History & Prognosis
- Slowly progressive syndrome that evolves over years
- NHL may complicate this otherwise chronic illness
- Parotid or GI locations most common NHL sites

Treatment
- Symptomatic moisture replacing therapy
- If systemic disease, immunotherapy may be used

DIAGNOSTIC CHECKLIST

Image Interpretation Pearls
- Large solid, hypoechoic lesions & cervical lymphadenopathy should raise concern for NHL or alternative diagnosis

SELECTED REFERENCES

1. Harnsberger HR et al: Diagnostic Imaging Head & Neck. 1st ed. Salt Lake City, Amirsys. III-7-12-15, 2004
2. Ohbayashi N et al: Sjogren syndrome: comparison of assessments with MR sialography and conventional sialography. Radiology. 209:683-8, 1998
3. Tonami H et al: MR sialography in patients with Sjogren syndrome. AJNR Am J Neuroradiol. 19(7): 1199-203, 1998
4. Ahuja et al: Ultrasound features of Sjogren syndrome. Australsian Radiology. 40:10-4, 1996
5. Takashima S et al: Sjogren syndrome: comparison of sialography and ultrasonography. J Clin Ultrasound. 20:99-109, 1992

IMAGE GALLERY

Typical

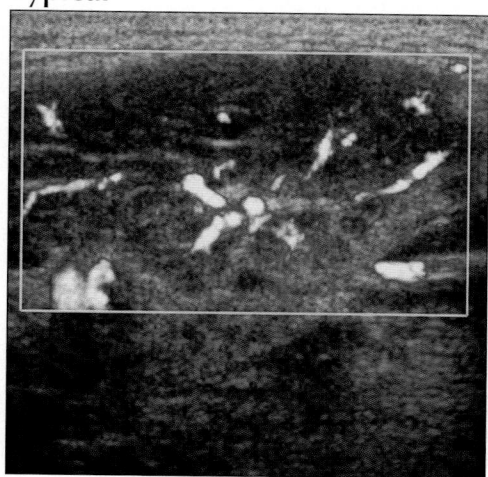

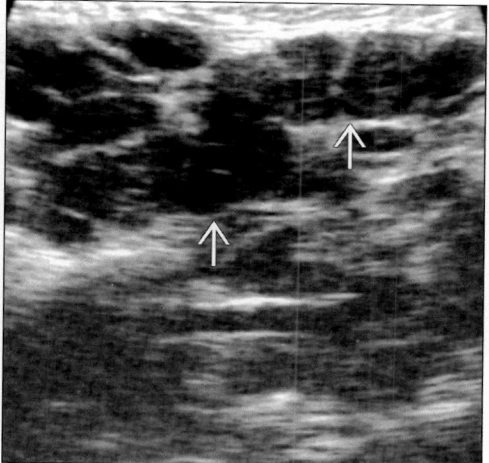

(Left) Power Doppler US shows prominent vascularity in the parotid gland in a patient with SjS. Presence & prominence of glandular vascularity correlates with severity of disease. (Right) Grayscale US shows multiple macrocysts ➡ diffusely involving the superficial & deep parotid lobes in SjS. US may miss changes in early disease but later stages are readily seen.

Typical

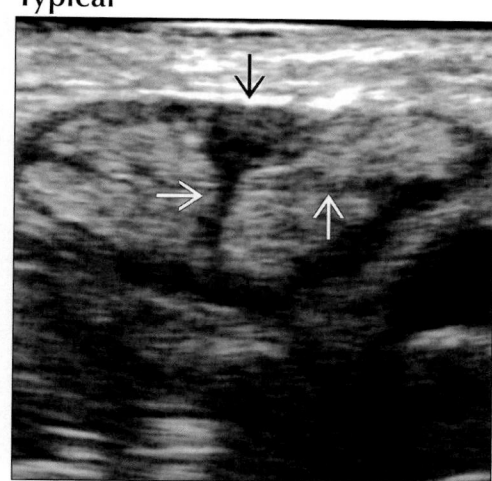

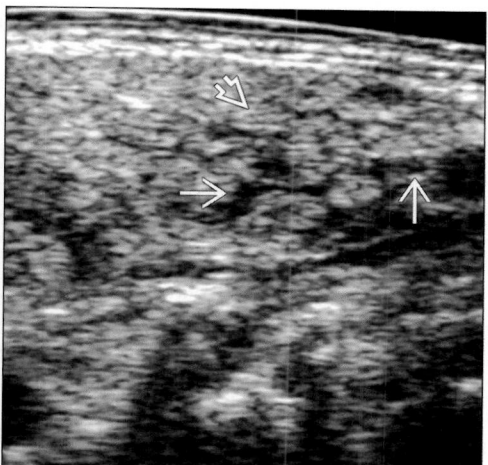

(Left) Grayscale US of the submandibular gland ➡ in a patient with SjS. Note reticulated appearance of the SMG with hypoechoic septa ➡. Similar changes were seen in the parotid & lacrimal glands. (Right) Grayscale US in patient with SjS showing typical reticulated ➡ change in the parotid gland with intervening hypoechoic septa ➡. Same patient as previous image.

Typical

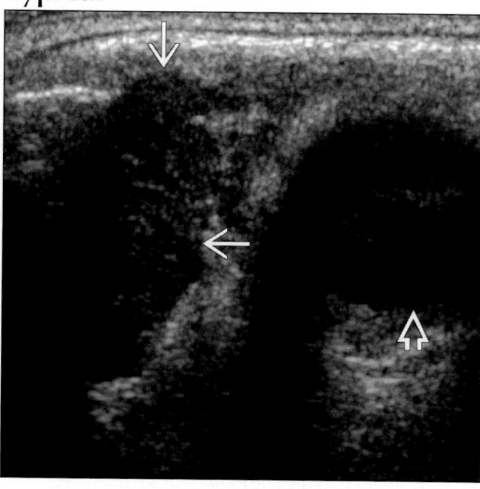

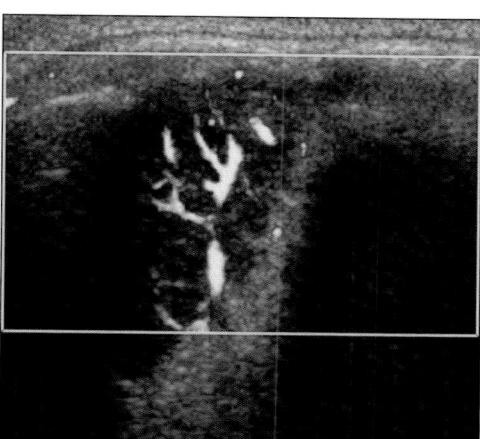

(Left) Transverse US of the orbit showing an enlarged, hypoechoic, heterogeneous lacrimal gland ➡ in a patient with SjS. Salivary glands showed similar change. Globe ➡. (Right) Corresponding power Doppler US of the lacrimal gland shows marked vascularity. High-resolution US readily evaluates the superficially located lacrimal gland.

BENIGN MIXED TUMOR, PAROTID

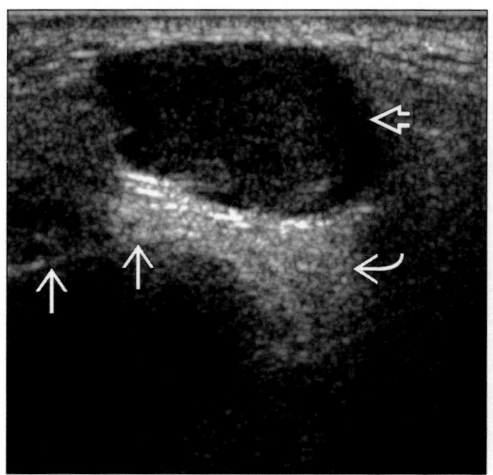

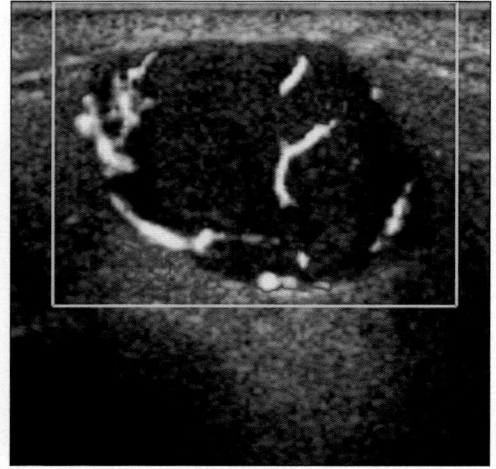

Transverse grayscale US shows a solid, well-defined, hypoechoic, homogeneous parotid BMT ➜ with posterior enhancement ➜ in the superficial lobe. US cannot evaluate the deep lobe. Mandible ➜.

Corresponding power Doppler US shows a few prominent vessels within the BMT. Malignant tumors often have profuse vascularity with high RI & PI. Benign tumors: RI < 0.8, PI < 2.0.

TERMINOLOGY

Abbreviations and Synonyms
- Abbreviation: Benign mixed tumor (BMT)
- Synonym: Pleomorphic adenoma

Definitions
- BMT: Benign heterogeneous tumor of parotid gland made up of an admixture of epithelial, myoepithelial & stromal components

IMAGING FINDINGS

General Features
- Best diagnostic clue
  - Small BMT: Sharply-marginated, intraparotid ovoid mass with homogeneous, hypoechoic echo pattern & posterior enhancement
  - Large BMT (> 2 cm): Lobulated mass with heterogeneous, hypoechoic echo pattern, +/- ill-defined edges
- Location: Parotid space

Ultrasonographic Findings
- Grayscale Ultrasound
  - Specificity 87%, accuracy 89%
  - Well-defined, solid, & hypoechoic compared to adjacent salivary tissue
  - Homogeneous internal echoes + posterior enhancement
    - Tumor offers few interfaces & allows sound to penetrate easily producing posterior enhancement
  - Large tumors may show heterogeneous internal echo pattern due to hemorrhage & necrosis
  - Heterogeneous BMT may have ill-defined edges mimicking malignant mass
  - Calcification is unusual, seen in long standing BMT
  - Calcification is dense, dysmorphic with posterior shadowing
  - No abnormal looking adjacent intra/peri parotid lymph node
  - No infiltration of overlying skin/subcutaneous tissue
- Color Doppler
  - Increase in peripheral vessels, mainly venous; often sparse

DDx: Benign Mixed Tumors, Parotid

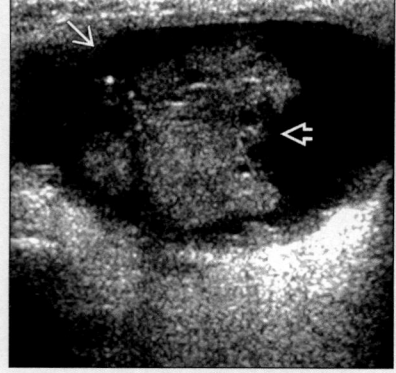

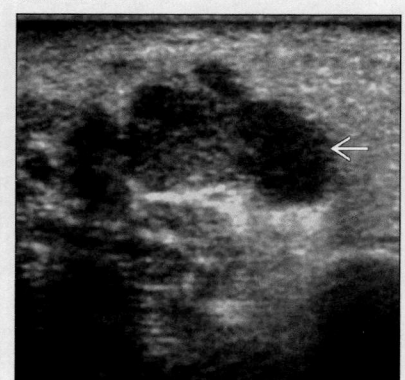

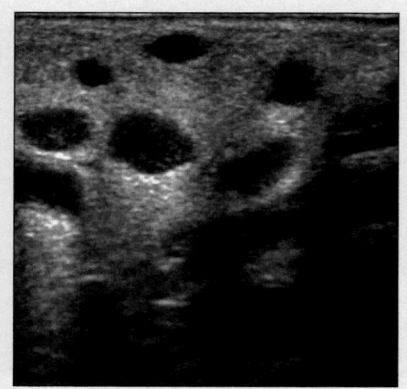

Warthin Tumor

Parotid Carcinoma

Intra Parotid NHL Nodes

BENIGN MIXED TUMOR, PAROTID

Key Facts

Imaging Findings

- Homogeneous internal echoes + posterior enhancement
- Large tumors may show heterogeneous internal echo pattern due to hemorrhage & necrosis
- Heterogeneous BMT may have ill-defined edges mimicking malignant mass
- Calcification is unusual, seen in long standing BMT
- No abnormal looking adjacent intra/peri parotid lymph node
- Increase in peripheral vessels, mainly venous; often sparse
- Spectral Doppler: Low intraBMT vascular resistance (resistive index [RI] < 0.8, pulsatility index [RI] < 2.0)
- US is unable to evaluate deep lobe masses or deep lobe extension of superficial lobe masses

- CECT, or preferably MR, indicated to fully evaluate parotid masses, their deep extension, and with high-resolution MR, their relationship to facial nerve
- If left untreated, 10-25% BMTs will undergo malignant transformation
- Intratumoral calcification implies long standing tumor & should raise suspicion
- BMT from apex of superficial lobe of parotid at angle of mandible is in close proximity to submandibular gland & should not be mistaken for SMG BMT

Top Differential Diagnoses

- Warthin Tumor
- Primary Parotid Carcinoma
- Non-Hodgkin Lymphoma, Parotid

- Spectral Doppler: Low intraBMT vascular resistance (resistive index [RI] < 0.8, pulsatility index [RI] < 2.0)

CT Findings

- CECT
  - Small BMT
    - Smoothly marginated, homogeneously enhancing, ovoid mass
  - Large BMT
    - Inhomogeneously enhancing, lobulated mass with areas of lower attenuation representing foci of degenerative necrosis & old hemorrhage
    - Dystrophic calcification may be present, distinguishing from Warthin tumor

MR Findings

- T1WI
  - Small BMT: Sharply marginated intraparotid mass with uniform hypointensity
  - Large BMT: Lobulated intraparotid mass with heterogeneous signal
  - Hyperintense signal can be seen in hemorrhagic lesions
- T2WI
  - Small BMT: Well-circumscribed intraparotid mass with uniform intermediate to high signal
  - Large BMT: Lobulated intraparotid mass with heterogeneous high signal
  - May demonstrate low signal intensity capsule
- STIR: Lesions more conspicuous
- T1 C+: Variable mild to moderate enhancement

Nuclear Medicine Findings

- Tc-99m Pertechnetate
  - Cold lesion; helps differentiate from Warthin tumor (hot)
    - All other lesions, including malignancy, present as cold defect

Imaging Recommendations

- Best imaging tool

- As majority of parotid BMTs are located in superficial parotid, US is ideal initial imaging modality for such lesions
- US is readily combined with guided fine needle aspiration cytology (FNAC) which has sensitivity of 83%, specificity 86% & accuracy of 85% for salivary gland tumors
- Although on ultrasound facial nerve cannot be seen, its location is inferred by identifying retromandibular vein (RMV) or external carotid artery (ECA) as they run together in parotid gland
- US is unable to evaluate deep lobe masses or deep lobe extension of superficial lobe masses
- CECT, or preferably MR, indicated to fully evaluate parotid masses, their deep extension, and with high-resolution MR, their relationship to facial nerve
- Protocol advice
  - In evaluating parotid masses, carefully assess
    - Edge: Benign lesions have well-defined edges & malignant tumors are ill-defined
    - Internal architecture: Benign tumors have homogeneous internal echo pattern, malignant tumors have heterogeneous architecture
    - Malignant tumors are more likely associated with skin, subcutaneous and nodal involvement
    - Malignant tumors show prominent vessels with high resistance, RI > 0.8, PI > 2.0
    - If left untreated, 10-25% BMTs will undergo malignant transformation
    - Intratumoral calcification implies long standing tumor & should raise suspicion
  - BMT from apex of superficial lobe of parotid at angle of mandible is in close proximity to submandibular gland & should not be mistaken for SMG BMT
    - Always identify origin of tumor as surgical incisions for parotid BMT & SMG BMT are different
    - Pattern of displacement of adjacent structures/vessels help in differentiating the two
  - Use of high resolution transducer is essential; scanning frequency ≥ 7.5 MHz

BENIGN MIXED TUMOR, PAROTID

- For large masses, one may have to use low resolution transducer (5 MHz) with standoff gel to evaluate its size and extent
  - Always evaluate both parotid and submandibular glands

DIFFERENTIAL DIAGNOSIS

Warthin Tumor
- Adult male smoker, 20% multicentric
- Hypoechoic, heterogeneous with solid & cystic component in superficial lobe of parotid gland

Primary Parotid Carcinoma
- Pain, facial nerve palsy & skin/subcutaneous induration.
- Ill-defined, heterogeneous internal echoes, +/- associated nodes, +/- extraglandular infiltration
- Low grade malignancy may be well defined, homogeneous & mimic BMT

Non-Hodgkin Lymphoma, Parotid
- Chronic systemic NHL may already be present
- Solitary, multiple or bilateral, round, solid, hypoechoic nodes with prominent hilar vascularity

Parotid Nodal Metastasis (Systemic or Skin SCCa or Melanoma)
- Clinical: Known primary or primary periauricular skin lesion
- Multiple, round, solid, +/- cystic nodes with abnormal peripheral vascularity

PATHOLOGY

General Features
- General path comments: Benign tumor arising from distal portions of parotid ductal system, including intercalated ducts & acini
- Etiology: Unknown; thought to arise from minor salivary gland rests
- Epidemiology
  - Most common parotid space tumor (80%)
  - 80% BMT arise in parotid glands
    - 8% in submandibular glands; 6.5% arise from minor salivary glands in nasopharyngeal mucosa
  - 80-90% of parotid BMTs involve superficial lobe
  - Multicentric BMT rare (< 1%)

Gross Pathologic & Surgical Features
- Lobulated heterogeneous mass with fibrous capsule
- Soft tan lobules representing epithelial component interspersed among lobulated firm, white, gritty chondromyxoid component

Microscopic Features
- Interspersed epithelial, myoepithelial & stromal cellular components must be identified to diagnose BMT
- BMT of major salivary glands is encased in fibrous capsule

- Sites of necrosis, hemorrhage, hyalinization & calcification may be present

CLINICAL ISSUES

Presentation
- Most common signs/symptoms
  - Painless cheek mass
  - Location dependent symptoms & signs
    - Superficial lobe or accessory parotid: "Cheek" mass
    - Parotid tail: Angle of mandible mass
    - Deep lobe: "Parapharyngeal space" mass pushing tonsil into pharyngeal airway
  - Facial nerve paralysis is rare

Demographics
- Age
  - Most common > 40 years
  - Age range is 30-60 years
- Gender: M:F = 1:2
- Ethnicity: Most common in Caucasians, rare in African-Americans

Natural History & Prognosis
- Slowly-growing, painless, benign tumor
- Recurrent tumor typically from incomplete resection or cellular "spillage" at surgery
- Recurrent BMT tends to be multifocal
- Malignant transformation reported up to 25% if left untreated
  - Degenerate to carcinoma, ex-pleomorphic adenoma (adenocarcinoma), malignant mixed tumor or metastasizing benign mixed tumor

Treatment
- Complete surgical resection of encapsulated mass within "adequate margin" of surrounding parotid gland tissue to avoid cellular spillage & "seeding"
- Radiation treatment of recurrent tumor, utility remains uncertain

SELECTED REFERENCES

1. Harnsberger HR et al: Diagnostic Imaging Head & Neck. 1st ed. Salt Lake City, Amirsys. III-7-16-19, 2004
2. Ahuja AT et al: Imaging in Head & Neck Cancer: A Practical Approach. London, Greenwich Medical Media. 115-41, 2003
3. Bialek EJ et al: Role of ultrasonography in diagnosis and differentiation of pleomorphic adenomas: work in progress. Arch Otolaryngol Head Neck Surg. 129(9):929-33, 2003
4. Evans RM: Salivary Glands. Bull. Br. Med. Ultrasound Soc. 9:20-5, 2001
5. Lamont JP et al: Prospective evaluation of office-based parotid ultrasound. Ann Surg Oncol. 8(9):720-2, 2001
6. Bradley MJ et al: Practical Head & Neck Ultrasound. London, Greenwich Medical Media. 17-33, 2000
7. Shimizu M et al: Statistical study for sonographic differential diagnosis of tumorous lesions in the parotid gland. Oral Surg Oral Med Oral Pathol Oral Radiol Endod. 88(2):226-33, 1999

BENIGN MIXED TUMOR, PAROTID

IMAGE GALLERY

Typical

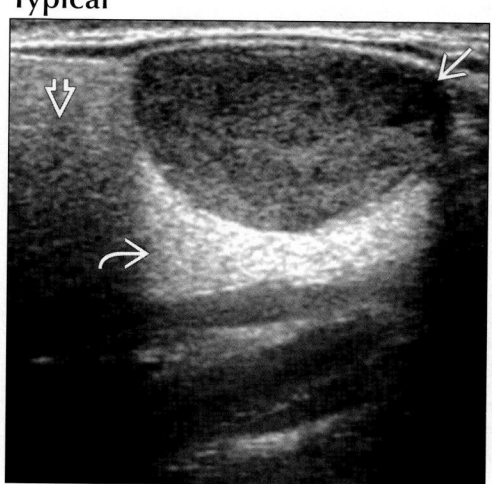
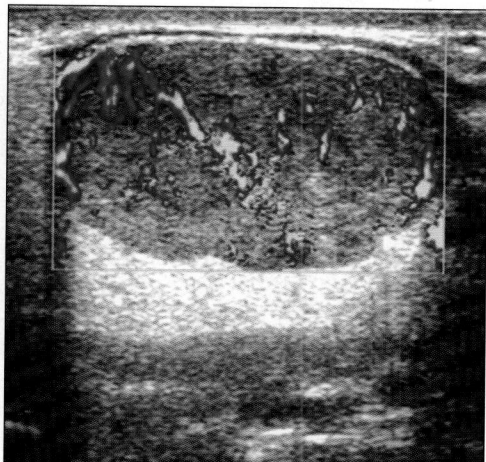

(Left) Longitudinal grayscale US shows a solid, hypoechoic, homogeneous, well-defined superficial lobe, parotid BMT ➡. Note intense posterior enhancement ➡, a feature of BMT. Normal parotid ➡. *(Right)* Corresponding power Doppler US shows intranodular vascularity. Vascularity is slightly prominent mimicking a malignant lesion. Malignant lesion: RI > 0.8, PI > 2.0.

Typical

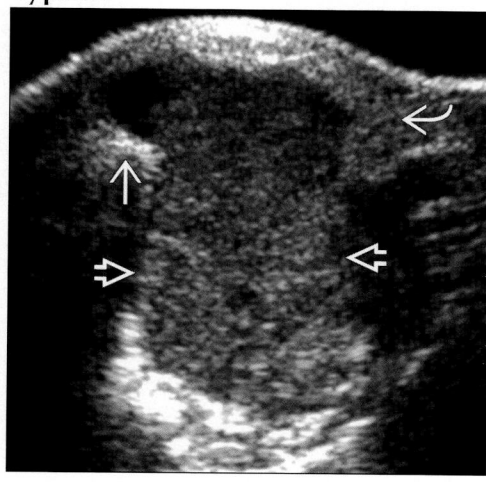
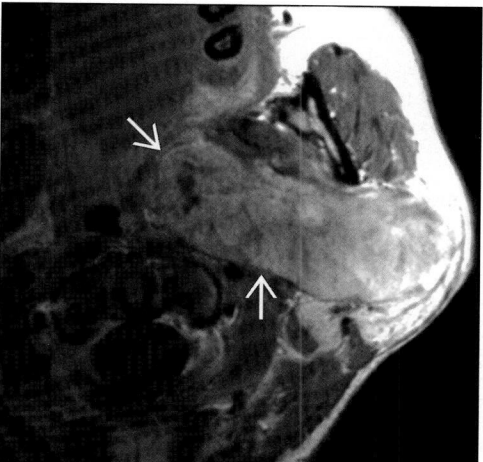

(Left) Transverse grayscale US with 5 MHz transducer & standoff gel shows a large, homogeneous parotid BMT ➡. Note US cannot define its deep anatomical relationships. Mandible ➡, parotid gland ➡. *(Right)* Corresponding, axial, gadolinium enhanced T1WI MR shows the full extent of a large parotid BMT ➡. In such a large tumor, the role of US is limited as it cannot see the deep lobe, but it helps to guide FNAC.

Typical

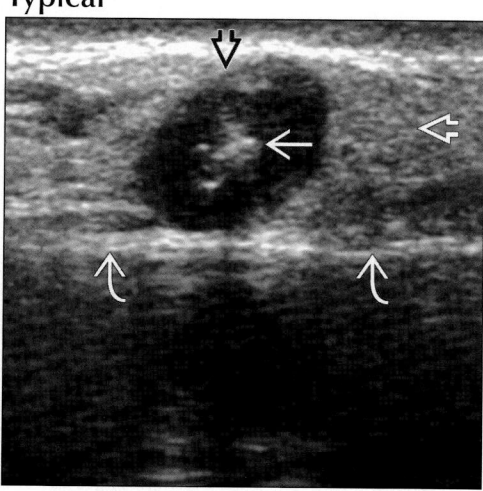
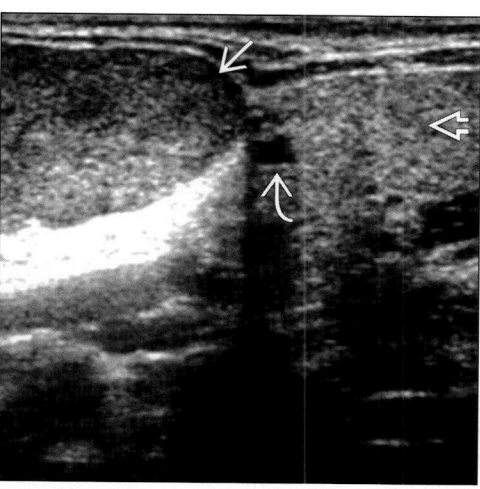

(Left) Longitudinal grayscale US shows a parotid BMT ➡ with dense calcification ➡. Presence of calcification suggests a long-standing lesion & is viewed with suspicion. Mandible ➡, normal parotid ➡. *(Right)* Transverse grayscale US shows a parotid BMT in the apex of the superficial lobe ➡. Note its close proximity to the submandibular gland ➡. Facial vessel ➡ helps to separate them.

WARTHIN TUMOR

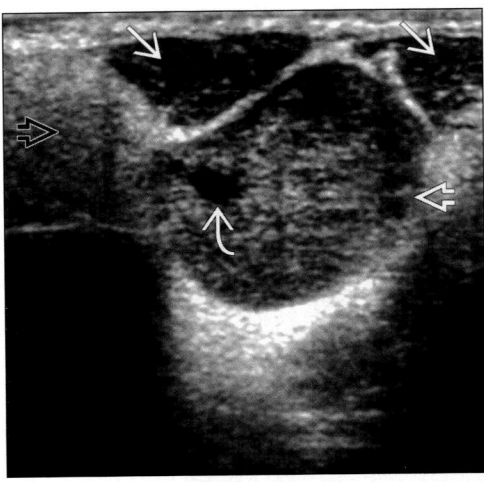

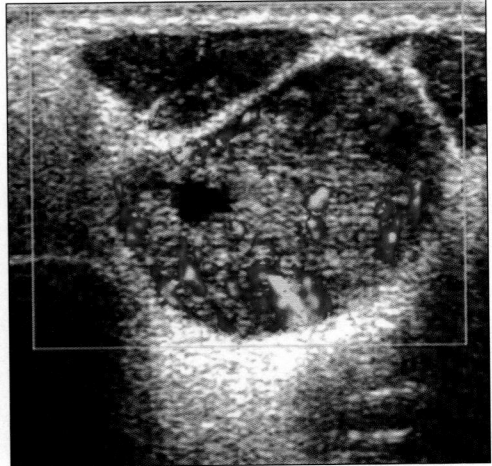

Transverse grayscale US shows a well-defined, hypoechoic Warthin tumor ➡ in the tail of the parotid gland with a focal intranodular cystic area ➡. Note adjacent smaller lesions ➡. Normal parotid ➡.

Corresponding power Doppler shows multiple prominent intranodular vessels. Vascularity may be striking, mimicking malignant tumors, but grayscale features help in diagnosis.

TERMINOLOGY

Abbreviations and Synonyms
- Papillary cystadenoma lymphomatosum; adenolymphoma; lymphomatous adenoma

Definitions
- Benign parotid tumor with characteristic histopathologic appearance composed of papillary structures, mature lymphocytic infiltrate & cystic changes

IMAGING FINDINGS

General Features
- Best diagnostic clue: Sharply-marginated parotid tail mass with heterogeneous echo pattern, solid & cystic components within
- Location
  - Intraparotid > > periparotid > upper cervical nodal location
  - When intraparotid, most commonly within parotid tail superficial to angle of mandible

Ultrasonographic Findings
- Grayscale ultrasound (specificity 91%, accuracy 89%)
  - Well-defined, hypoechoic, non-calcified mass in apex of superficial lobe of parotid
  - Heterogeneous internal architecture with cystic & solid components
  - May be multiseptated with thick walls, +/- posterior enhancement
  - Multiplicity of lesions, unilateral or bilateral (20%)
  - No abnormal associated intra/periparotid node
  - No skin & subcutaneous tissue infiltration
- Color Doppler: Prominent vessels, particularly "hilar" & septal (may be striking)
  - Spectral Doppler: Low resistance vessels (resistive index [RI] < 0.8, pulsatility index [PI] < 2.0)

CT Findings
- CECT
  - Solitary small, ovoid, non-calcified smoothly marginated masses in posterior aspect of superficial lobe of parotid
  - Cystic component in 30% with thin, uniform walls, & septae
  - Minimal enhancement of solid components

DDx: Warthin Tumor

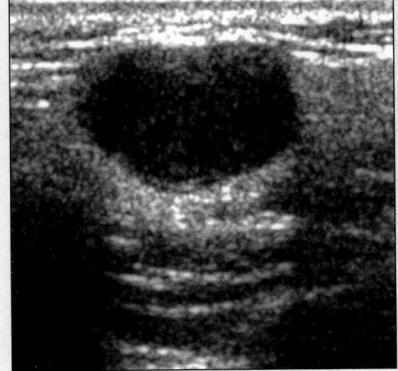

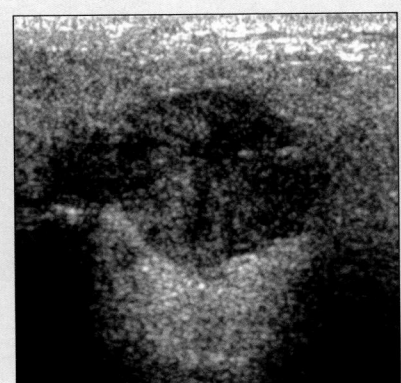

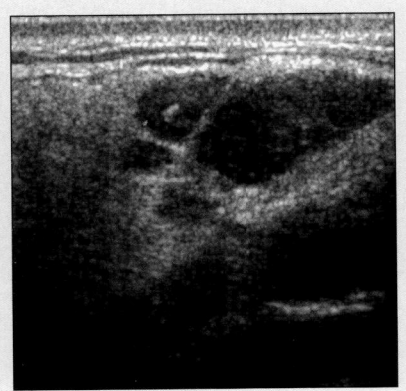

Benign Mixed Tumor, Parotid

Parotid Carcinoma

Lymph Node

WARTHIN TUMOR

Key Facts

Imaging Findings
- Well-defined, hypoechoic, non-calcified mass in apex of superficial lobe of parotid
- Heterogeneous internal architecture with cystic & solid components
- May be multiseptated with thick walls, +/- posterior enhancement
- Multiplicity of lesions, unilateral or bilateral (20%)
- No abnormal associated intra/periparotid node
- No skin & subcutaneous tissue infiltration
- Color Doppler: Prominent vessels, particularly "hilar" & septal (may be striking)
- Spectral Doppler: Low resistance vessels (resistive index [RI] < 0.8, pulsatility index [PI] < 2.0)
- As most of Warthin tumors are in superficial lobe, US is ideal initial imaging modality

- For large tumors, US may be unable to evaluate their entire extent, anatomical relationship
- As these lesions rarely turn malignant (< 1%), US is ideal for surveillance in patients who refuse surgery
- US is readily combined with fine needle aspiration cytology (FNAC) which has sensitivity of 83%, specificity 86% & accuracy of 85% for salivary gland tumors
- Use of high resolution transducer is essential; scanning frequency ≥ 7.5 MHz
- For large masses, use low resolution transducer (5 MHz) with standoff gel to evaluate its size & extent

Top Differential Diagnoses
- Benign Mixed Tumor, Parotid
- Malignant Tumor, Parotid
- Nodal Metastasis

- Multiple lesions, unilateral or bilateral, synchronous or metachronous in 20%

MR Findings
- T1WI
  - Low signal in both solid & cystic components
  - Cystic areas may show high signal secondary to proteinaceous debris ± hemorrhage
- T2WI
  - Intermediate to high T2 signal in solid component
  - High T2 signal in cystic foci
- STIR: Lesions more conspicuous, especially cystic component
- T1 C+: Minimal contrast-enhancement of solid components

Nuclear Medicine Findings
- PET: Increased uptake of FDG PET; may be incidentally diagnosed while looking for malignancy
- Tc-99m
  - Increased uptake within mitochondrial-rich oncocytes of Warthin tumors

Imaging Recommendations
- Best imaging tool
  - As most of Warthin tumors are in superficial lobe, US is ideal initial imaging modality
  - For large tumors, US may be unable to evaluate their entire extent, anatomical relationship
  - As these lesions rarely turn malignant (< 1%), US is ideal for surveillance in patients who refuse surgery
  - US is readily combined with fine needle aspiration cytology (FNAC) which has sensitivity of 83%, specificity 86% & accuracy of 85% for salivary gland tumors
  - Although on US, facial nerve cannot be seen, its location is inferred by identifying retromandibular vein (RMV) or external carotid artery (ECA) as they run together in parotid gland
- Protocol advice
  - Use of high resolution transducer is essential; scanning frequency ≥ 7.5 MHz

- For large masses, use low resolution transducer (5 MHz) with standoff gel to evaluate its size & extent
  - Always evaluate both parotid and submandibular glands
  - In evaluating salivary masses note
    - Edge: Benign lesions are well-defined & malignant lesions ill-defined
    - Malignant tumors are more likely associated with abnormal nodes, skin & subcutaneous infiltration
- MR best delineates intra- vs. extraparotid location, relationship to facial nerve plane, deep tissue extent for large tumors

DIFFERENTIAL DIAGNOSIS

Benign Mixed Tumor, Parotid
- Well-circumscribed, homogeneous, solid intraparotid mass with posterior enhancement
- Larger lesions may show cystic change (hemorrhage & necrosis) & mimic Warthin tumor

Malignant Tumor, Parotid
- Ill-defined, solid, hypoechoic, heterogeneous echo pattern, +/- nodes & extraglandular infiltration
- Low grade parotid malignancy may be well defined & homogeneous

Nodal Metastasis
- Primary malignancy on or around skin of ear
- Single or multiple hypoechoic, heterogeneous intraparotid nodes with abnormal vascularity

Benign Lymphoepithelial Lesions-HIV (BLL-HIV)
- When unilateral & singular, may strongly mimic Warthin tumor
- Tonsillar enlargement & cervical lymphadenopathy help differentiate

WARTHIN TUMOR

PATHOLOGY

General Features
- General path comments
  - Embryology
    - Parotid gland undergoes "late encapsulation", incorporating lymphoid tissue-nodes within superficial layer of deep cervical fascia
    - Warthin tumor arises within this lymphoid tissue
- Etiology
  - Smoking-induced, benign tumor arising from salivary-lymphoid tissue in intraparotid and periparotid lymph nodes
  - Theorized heterotopic salivary gland parenchyma present in pre-existing intra- or peri-parotid lymph nodes
  - Reported association with Epstein-Barr virus, most commonly in patients with multifocal or bilateral lesions
- Epidemiology
  - 2nd most common benign parotid tumor
  - 10% of all salivary gland epithelial tumors
  - 12% of benign parotid gland tumors
  - 20% multicentric, unilateral or bilateral, synchronous or metachronous
  - 5-10% may arise in extra-parotid locations (peri-parotid & upper neck lymph nodes)
- Associated abnormalities: Increased incidence in patients with autoimmune disorders

Gross Pathologic & Surgical Features
- Encapsulated, soft, ovoid mass with a smooth but lobulated surface
- Tan tissue with cystic spaces which contain a tenacious, mucoid, brown fluid or a thin, yellow fluid with cholesterol crystals
  - Papillary projections can also be seen within these cystic areas

Microscopic Features
- Papillary projections are lined with double epithelial layer
  - Inner-luminal layer: Tall columnar cells with their nuclei oriented toward lumen
  - Outer-basal layer: Cuboidal or polygonal cells with vesicular nuclei
- Inner lymphoid component of papillary projection is composed of mature lymphoid aggregates with germinal centers

CLINICAL ISSUES

Presentation
- Most common signs/symptoms
  - Angle of mandible (tail of parotid) mass
  - Mass is painless; multiple masses ~ 20%
- Clinical Profile
  - 90% of patients with this tumor smoke
  - Increased incidence associated with radiation exposure

Demographics
- Age: Mean age at presentation = 60 years
- Gender
  - M:F = 3:1
  - More recent reports show more equal gender incidence due to increasing number of women who smoke

Natural History & Prognosis
- Slowly-growing, benign tumor
- Malignant transformation (carcinoma or lymphoma) reported in < 1%
- "Recurrent" Warthin tumor may be from inadequate resection or from metachronous second lesion

Treatment
- Resection of mass within a collar of normal parotid tissue without injury to intraparotid facial nerve is treatment goal

DIAGNOSTIC CHECKLIST

Image Interpretation Pearls
- Always carefully examine for multiplicity & bilaterality
- Well-defined, hypoechoic, heterogeneous mass with cystic, solid component, septae and thick walls in tail of parotid in asymptomatic patient should be considered Warthin tumor

SELECTED REFERENCES

1. Harnsberger HR et al: Diagnostic Imaging Head & Neck. Salt Lake City, Amirsys. III-7-20-23, 2004
2. Ahuja AT et al: Imaging in Head & Neck Cancer: A Practical Approach. London, Greenwich Medical Media. 115-41, 2003
3. Hamilton BE et al: Earring lesions of the parotid tail. AJNR Am J Neuroradiol. 24(9):1757-64, 2003
4. Marioni G et al: Facial nerve paralysis secondary to Warthin's tumour of the parotid gland. J Laryngol Otol. 117(6):511-3, 2003
5. Parwani AV et al: Diagnostic accuracy and pitfalls in fine-needle aspiration interpretation of Warthin tumor. Cancer. 99(3):166-71, 2003
6. Steinhart H et al: Contrast-enhanced color Doppler sonography of parotid gland tumors. Eur Arch Otorhinolaryngol. 260(6):344-8, 2003
7. Raymond MR et al: Accuracy of fine-needle aspiration biopsy for Warthin's tumours. J Otolaryngol. 31(5):263-70, 2002
8. Shah GV: MR imaging of salivary glands. Magn Reson Imaging Clin N Am. 10(4):631-62, 2002
9. Webb AJ et al: Parotid Warthin's tumour Bristol Royal Infirmary (1985-1995): a study of histopathology in 33 cases. Oral Oncol. 38(2):163-71, 2002
10. Evans RM: Salivary Glands. Bull. Br. Med. Ultrasound Soc. 9:20-5, 2001
11. Bradley MJ et al: Practical Head & Neck Ultrasound. London, Greenwich Medical Media. 17-33, 2000
12. Joe VQ et al: Tumors of the parotid gland: MR imaging characteristics of various histologic types. AJR. 163:433-8, 1994
13. Minami M et al: Warthin tumor of the parotid gland: MR-pathologic correlation. AJNR. 14:209-14, 1993

WARTHIN TUMOR

IMAGE GALLERY

Typical

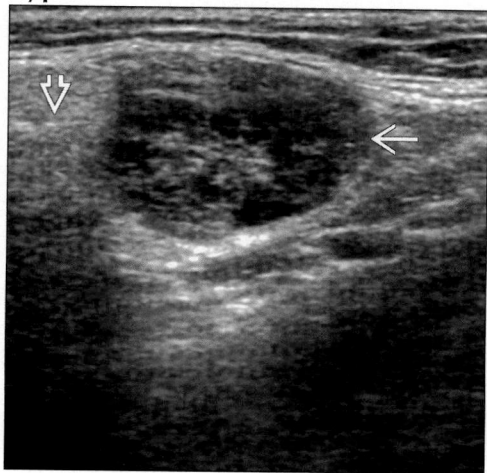 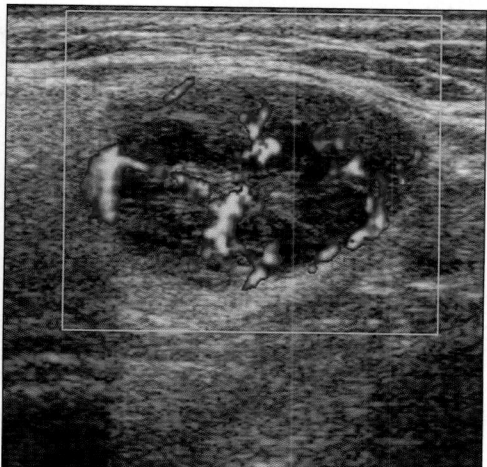

(Left) Longitudinal grayscale US shows a well-defined, hypoechoic, heterogeneous Warthin tumor ➡ in the superficial lobe parotid ➡. US fully examines such small tumors & aids in guided FNAC. *(Right)* Corresponding power Doppler US shows prominent intranodular vascularity. Note Warthin tumor has striking vascularity but RI < 0.8, PI < 2.0.

Typical

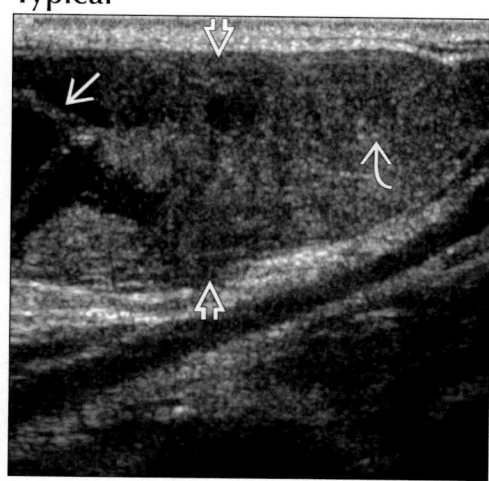 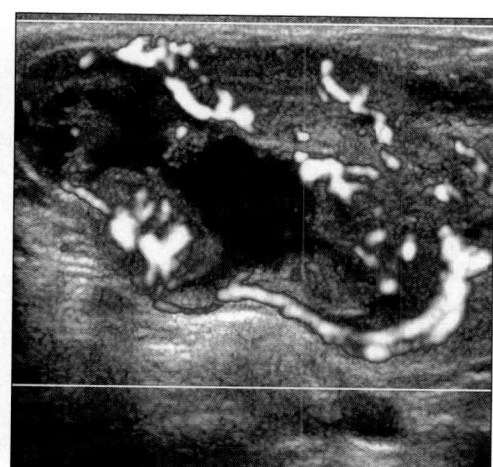

(Left) Longitudinal grayscale US shows a large Warthin tumor ➡ in the parotid tail. Note solid ➡, and cystic components, & septa ➡ within the tumor. No extraglandular extension seen. *(Right)* Power Doppler US of a Warthin tumor shows marked vascularity in the solid portion of the tumor. Presence of such vascularity may mimic malignancy but FNAC & grayscale features help in diagnosis.

Typical

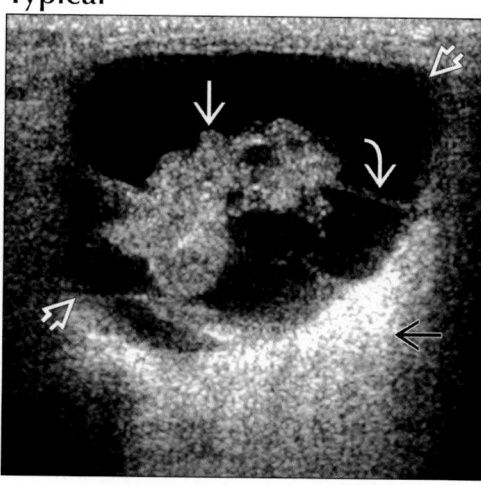 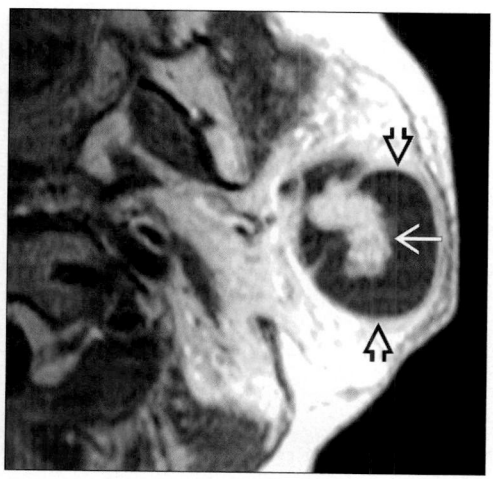

(Left) Transverse grayscale US shows a typical Warthin tumor ➡ with a cystic component, solid papillary portion ➡ & septa ➡. Presence of a cystic component produces posterior enhancement ➡. *(Right)* Corresponding gadolinium enhanced axial T1WI clearly shows cystic & enhancing solid ➡ elements of the Warthin tumor ➡. MR has the advantage of being able to evaluate deep lobe.

11

79

MUCOEPIDERMOID CARCINOMA, PAROTID

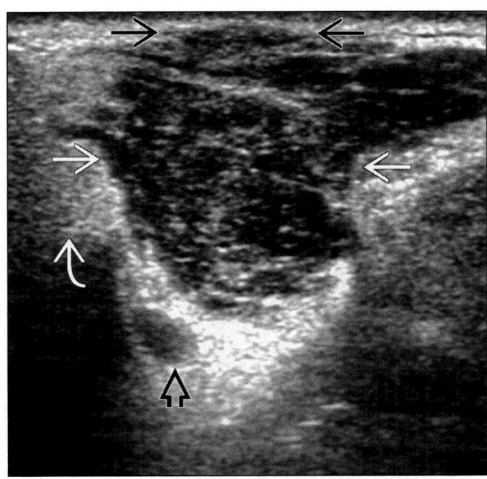

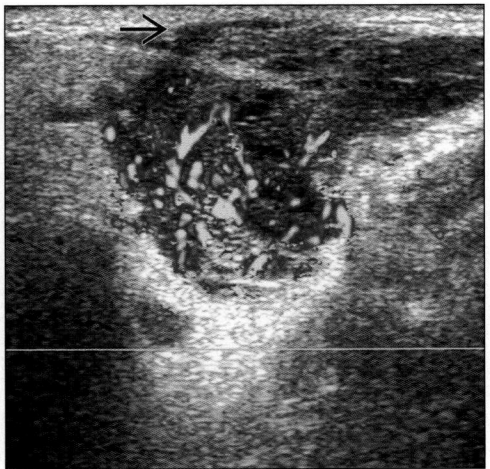

Transverse grayscale US shows an ill-defined, solid, hypoechoic MECa ➡ in the superficial parotid. Note the heterogeneous architecture & superficial extraglandular extension ➡. RMV ➡, mandible ➡.

Corresponding power Doppler shows a profuse vascularity within the MECa. Note extraglandular extension ➡ into overlying soft tissues. High grade MECa confirmed at histology.

TERMINOLOGY

Abbreviations and Synonyms
- Mucoepidermoid carcinoma (MECa)

Definitions
- MECa: Malignant epithelial salivary gland neoplasm composed of a variable admixture of both epidermoid & mucous-secreting cells arising from ductal epithelium

IMAGING FINDINGS

General Features
- Best diagnostic clue
  - Imaging appearance based on MECa histologic grade
  - Low grade MECa: Well-defined, solid, hypoechoic, homogeneous/heterogeneous parotid mass
  - High grade MECa: Ill defined, hypoechoic, heterogeneous mass, +/- infiltration into adjacent soft tissues & associated malignant nodes
  - Malignant adenopathy often present with high grade tumors
    - 1st order nodes = jugulodigastric nodes (level 2)
    - Intrinsic parotid nodes & parotid tail nodes also involved
- Location: Superficial lobe > > deep lobe parotid

Ultrasonographic Findings
- Grayscale Ultrasound
  - Low grade MECa may be well-defined, solid with predominantly homogeneous echo pattern
  - High grade MECa is ill-defined, hypoechoic with heterogeneous architecture due to necrosis & hemorrhage
  - Low grade MECa: No extraglandular invasion or lymphadenopathy
  - High grade MECa: Extraglandular invasion of adjacent soft tissue, skin
  - High grade MECa: +/- Associated intraparotid & jugulodigastric lymph node metastases
- Color Doppler
  - Color Doppler: Pronounced intratumoral vascularity
  - Spectral Doppler: Increased intravascular resistance
    - Resistive index RI > 0.8, pulsatility index PI > 2.0

CT Findings
- CECT

DDx: Mucoepidermoid Carcinoma, Parotid

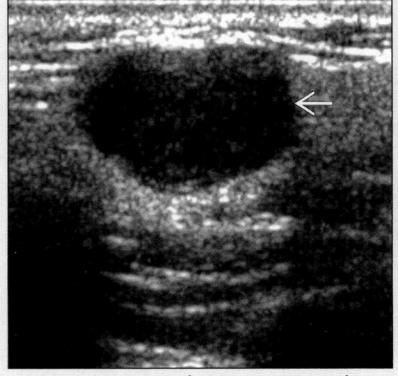

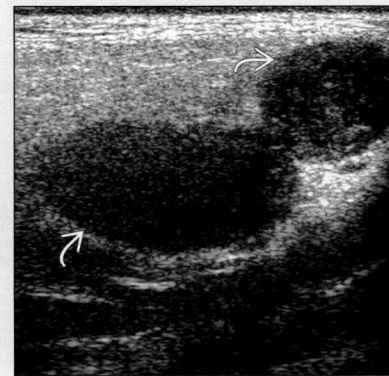

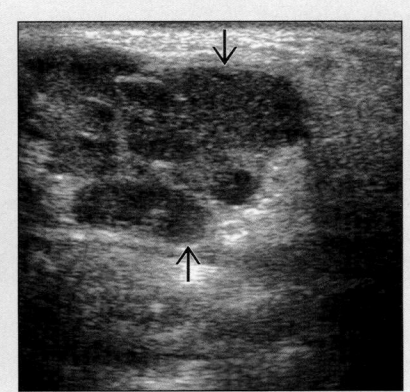

Benign Mixed Tumor, Parotid

Warthin Tumor

Parotid Metastases

11

80

MUCOEPIDERMOID CARCINOMA, PAROTID

Key Facts

Imaging Findings
- Imaging appearance based on MECa histologic grade
- Location: Superficial lobe > > deep lobe parotid
- Low grade MECa may be well-defined, solid with predominantly homogeneous echo pattern
- High grade MECa is ill-defined, hypoechoic with heterogeneous architecture due to necrosis & hemorrhage
- Low grade MECa: No extraglandular invasion or lymphadenopathy
- High grade MECa: Extraglandular invasion of adjacent soft tissue, skin
- High grade MECa: +/- Associated intraparotid & jugulodigastric lymph node metastases
- Color Doppler: Pronounced intratumoral vascularity
- Resistive index RI > 0.8, pulsatility index PI > 2.0

- As MECa commonly involves superficial lobe of parotid, US is ideal initial imaging modality
- US identifies malignancy, guides biopsy but cannot differentiate between various types of malignant parotid lesions
- US cannot evaluate deep extent of superficial lobe MECa and may miss a deep lobe tumor
- MR best delineates MECa local/regional extension & perineural spread
- Malignant tumors are more likely associated with adjacent soft tissue & nodal involvement

Top Differential Diagnoses
- Benign Mixed Tumor (BMT)
- Warthin Tumor
- Metastases to Parotid Nodes

- Low grade MECa
  - Enhancing inhomogeneous mass with sharp margins
  - Mucous cystic deposits create inhomogeneous enhancement
- High grade MECa
  - Enhancing invasive mass with shaggy margins
  - Intraparotid & cervical metastatic nodes

MR Findings
- T1WI
  - Low grade MECa: Heterogeneous well-defined mass with predominantly low signal
  - High grade MECa: Solid, infiltrative mass with tissue signal
- T2WI
  - Low grade MECa: Heterogeneous signal mass with predominantly low signal; cystic high signal foci commonly visible
  - High grade MECa: Intermediate signal infiltrating mass
- T1 C+
  - Heterogeneous enhancement
  - If lesion high grade, infiltrative or in high parotid near stylomastoid foramen, perineural spread on CN7 may occur

Nuclear Medicine Findings
- No pertechnetate uptake (unlike Warthin tumor)

Imaging Recommendations
- Best imaging tool
  - As MECa commonly involves superficial lobe of parotid, US is ideal initial imaging modality
  - US identifies malignancy, guides biopsy but cannot differentiate between various types of malignant parotid lesions
  - US is readily combined with guided fine needle aspiration cytology (FNAC)
    - FNAC has sensitivity of 83%, specificity 86% & accuracy of 85% for salivary gland tumors

  - US cannot visualize facial nerve: Position is inferred by identifying retromandibular vein (RMV) or external carotid artery as they run together in parotid gland
  - US cannot evaluate deep extent of superficial lobe MECa and may miss a deep lobe tumor
  - MR best delineates MECa local/regional extension & perineural spread
- Protocol advice
  - Use of high resolution transducer is essential
    - Scanning frequency > 7.5 MHz
  - In evaluating parotid masses, assess
    - Edge: Benign tumors have well-defined edges & malignant tumors have ill-defined edges; low grade MECa may have well-defined edges mimicking benign lesions
    - Internal architecture: Benign tumors have homogeneous internal echoes whereas malignant tumors have heterogeneous echo pattern due to necrosis & hemorrhage; but low grade MECa may have homogeneous echo pattern
    - Malignant tumors are more likely associated with adjacent soft tissue & nodal involvement
    - Malignant tumors have prominent vessels & high resistance (RI > 0.8, PI > 2.0)

DIFFERENTIAL DIAGNOSIS

Benign Mixed Tumor (BMT)
- Well-defined, lobulated, solid, hypoechoic mass with homogeneous echo pattern, posterior enhancement & sparse vascularity

Warthin Tumor
- Multicentric 20%, well-defined, hypoechoic with solid & cystic elements, thick wall septa, in parotid tail

Adenoid Cystic Carcinoma (ACCa)
- Well-defined/ill-defined, hypoechoic, homogeneous/heterogeneous echo pattern with prominent vascularity
- Prone to perineural spread

Non-Hodgkin Lymphoma (NHL)

- Primary parotid lymphoma: Invasive parenchymal tumor indistinguishable from high grade MECa or ACCa
- Primary nodal lymphoma: Multiple bilateral, solid hypoechoic nodes with prominent hilar vascularity

Metastases to Parotid Nodes

- Primary lesion usually on or around skin of ear (SCCa, melanoma)
- Solitary/multiple parotid masses, ill-defined, hypoechoic, heterogeneous architecture

PATHOLOGY

General Features

- Etiology: Exposure risk: Radiation, latency: 7-32 years
- Epidemiology
  - MECa represents 10% of all salivary gland tumors
  - MECa represents 30% of all salivary gland malignancies
  - Majority (60%) occur in parotid
  - Larger salivary gland → mass more likely benign
    - Parotid gland: 20% of masses malignant
    - Submandibular gland: 50% malignant
    - Sublingual gland: 80% malignant

Gross Pathologic & Surgical Features

- Gray, tan-yellow, or pink

Microscopic Features

- Mixture of epidermoid & mucous-secreting cells, with some cells intermediate between these
- Cellular atypia & pleomorphism
- Arises in glandular ductal epithelium

CLINICAL ISSUES

Presentation

- Most common signs/symptoms
  - Palpable parotid mass, usually rock-hard
  - Other signs/symptoms
    - Facial pain, otalgia, facial nerve paralysis, other cranial nerve involvement (V3)
  - Clinical presentation depends on tumor grade
    - Low grade: Painless, mobile, slowly-enlarging
    - High grade: Painful, non-mobile, rapidly-enlarging

Demographics

- Age: Usually 35-65 years old

Natural History & Prognosis

- Recurrence & survival rates depend on histologic grade
  - Low grade: 6% local recurrence; 90% 10 year survival rate
  - Intermediate grade: 20% local recurrence; 80% 10 year survival
  - High grade: 78% local recurrence; 27% 10 year survival rate
  - Distant metastases common in high grade; uncommon in low/intermediate

- 50% risk of occult cervical metastases in high grade MECa
- Poor prognostic signs
  - Male gender, age > 40
  - Fixed tumor, invasion of surrounding structures
  - Higher TNM stage or histologic grade

Treatment

- Low grade MECa
  - Wide local excision with preservation of facial nerve
  - Superficial parotidectomy if possible
  - Total parotidectomy may be necessary if tumor involves deep lobe
  - Post-operative radiotherapy
- High grade MECa
  - Wide local excision, usually requires extended total parotidectomy
  - Facial nerve sacrifice often necessary
  - Neck dissection routine
  - Post-operative radiotherapy with large port

DIAGNOSTIC CHECKLIST

Image Interpretation Pearls

- Low grade MECa may exactly mimic BMT
- High grade MECa has nonspecific invasive mass appearance
- General evaluation of parotid space masses
  - 1st decide whether lesion is intraparotid or extraparotid
  - If intraparotid, distinguish superficial vs. deep lobe
    - Divided by facial nerve plane, just lateral to retromandibular vein
  - Sharpness of margin, internal architecture, vascularity helps distinguish benign from malignant lesions
  - Remember to look for nodal metastases

SELECTED REFERENCES

1. Harnsberger HR et al: Diagnostic Imaging Head & Neck. 1st ed. Salt Lake City, Amirsys. III-7-24-27, 2004
2. Ahuja AT et al: Imaging in Head & Neck Cancer: A Practical Approach. 1st ed. London, Greenwich Medical Media. 115-41, 2003
3. Sakamoto M et al: Usefulness of heavily T(2) weighted magnetic resonance images for the differential diagnosis of parotid tumours. Dentomaxillofac Radiol. 32(5):295-9, 2003
4. Shah GV: MR imaging of salivary glands. Magn Reson Imaging Clin N Am. 10(4):631-62, 2002
5. Bradley MJ: Practical Head & Neck Ultrasound. London, Greenwich Medical Media. 17-33, 2000
6. Schlakman BN et al: MR of intraparotid masses. AJNR. 14:1173-80, 1993

IMAGE GALLERY

Typical

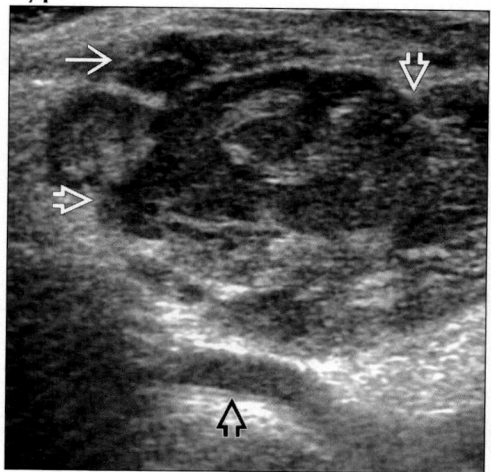
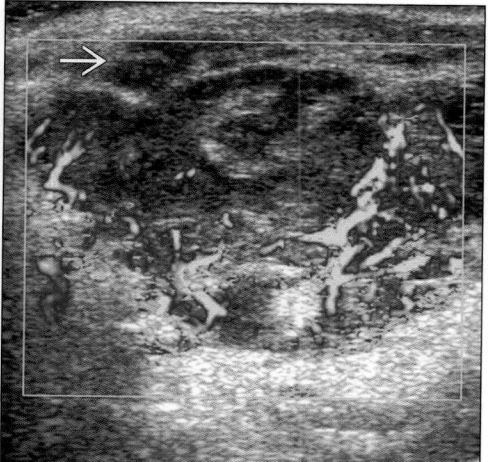

(Left) Longitudinal grayscale US shows a high grade MECa ➡ with heterogeneous internal architecture & extraglandular extension ➡. Note its relation to the RMV ➡, which is in close proximity to CN VII. (Right) Corresponding power Doppler US shows marked intra-tumoral vascularity often seen in malignant parotid tumors. Note extraglandular extension ➡.

Typical

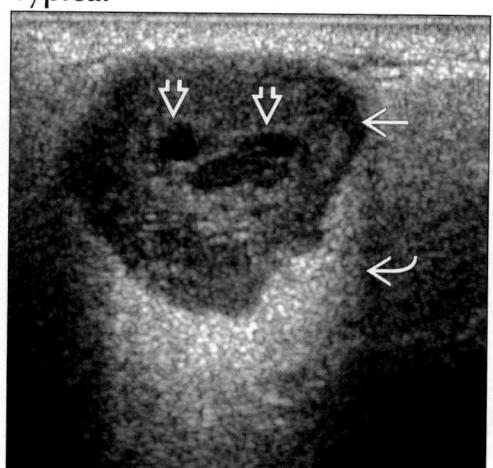
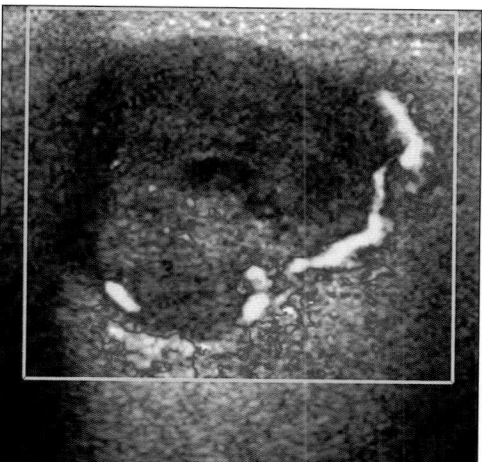

(Left) Transverse grayscale US shows a low grade MECa ➡ in the superficial parotid. Note it is fairly well-defined & has posterior enhancement ➡. The appearance mimics a BMT but cystic/necrotic areas ➡ raise suspicion of malignancy. (Right) Corresponding power Doppler US shows sparse vascularity within this low grade MECa mimicking BMT. Heterogeneous architecture and cystic necrosis should always raise suspicion of malignancy.

Typical

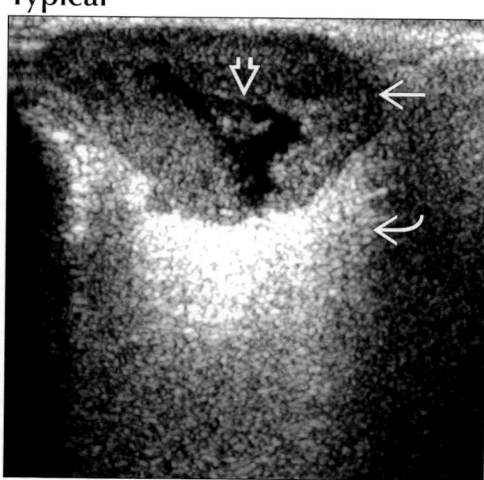
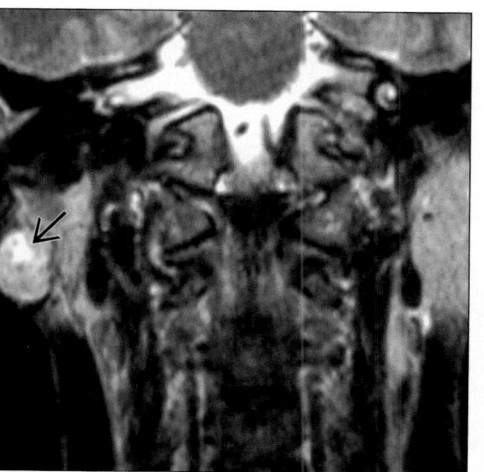

(Left) Transverse grayscale US shows a low grade MECa ➡, in the superficial parotid gland. The well-defined borders & posterior enhancement ➡ mimics a BMT, but intratumoral necrosis ➡ raised suspicion. (Right) Corresponding coronal T2WI MR shows a well-defined, high-signal MECa with cystic necrosis ➡. It could be easily mistaken for BMT.

ADENOID CYSTIC CARCINOMA, PAROTID

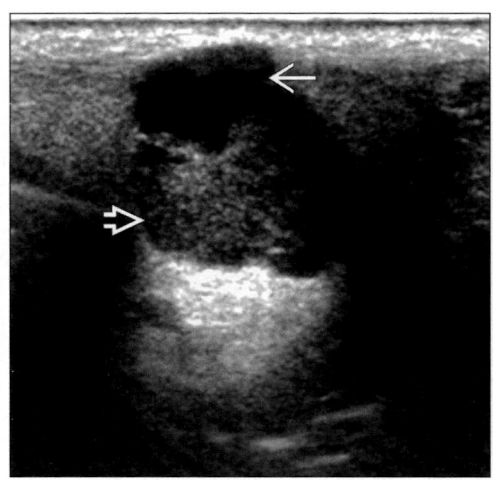

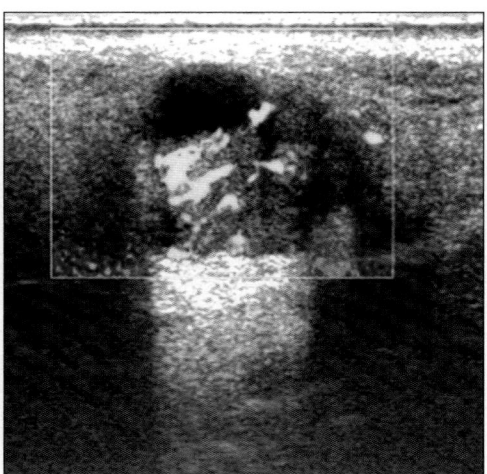

Longitudinal grayscale US shows low grade ACCa as a hypoechoic, heterogeneous tumor ⇨ with cystic necrosis ➡, which just bulges out of glandular contour. It is fairly well-defined & simulates a BMT.

Corresponding power Doppler US shows prominent vessels in the solid portion of the tumor raising suspicion of a malignancy. ACCa confirmed at surgery.

TERMINOLOGY

Abbreviations and Synonyms
- Adenoid cystic carcinoma (ACCa)

Definitions
- Malignant salivary gland neoplasm arising in peripheral parotid ducts

IMAGING FINDINGS

General Features
- Best diagnostic clue
  - Low grade ACCa: Well-defined, homogeneous, hypoechoic mass
  - Higher grade ACCa: Ill-defined, heterogeneous, hypoechoic mass with extraglandular invasion

Ultrasonographic Findings
- Grayscale Ultrasound
  - US is unable to differentiate ACCa from other salivary gland malignancies
  - Low grade tumors may be well-defined with homogeneous internal architecture
  - High grade tumors are ill-defined with invasive edges & heterogeneous areas of necrosis/hemorrhage
  - +/- Extraglandular invasion of soft tissues
  - +/- Adjacent nodal, disseminated metastases
- Color Doppler
  - Color Doppler: Pronounced intratumoral vascularity
  - Spectral Doppler: Increased intravascular resistance
    - Resistive index > 0.8, pulsatility index > 2.0

CT Findings
- CECT
  - Low grade: Enhancing homogeneous well-circumscribed mass
  - High grade: Enhancing mass with poorly-defined margins

MR Findings
- T1WI: Low to intermediate signal intensity
- T2WI: Moderate signal intensity; high grade tend to be lower in signal intensity
- T1 C+
  - Solid enhancement of mass
  - Perineural tumor on CN7 ± CN5

DDx: Adenocystic Carcinoma, Parotid

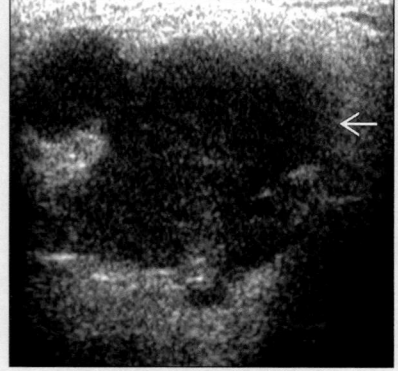

Benign Mixed Tumor, Parotid

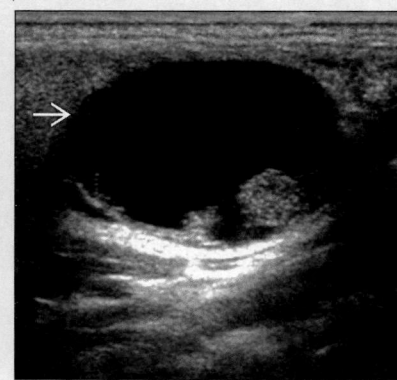

Warthin Tumor

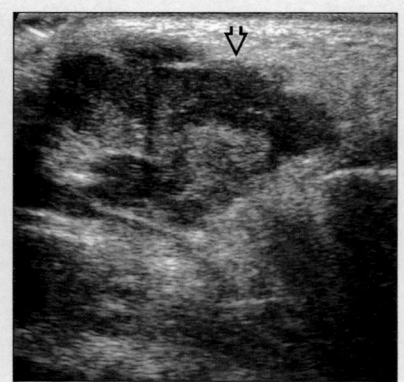

Parotid Metastases

ADENOID CYSTIC CARCINOMA, PAROTID

Key Facts

Imaging Findings
- Low grade tumors may be well-defined with homogeneous internal architecture
- High grade tumors are ill-defined with invasive edges & heterogeneous areas of necrosis/hemorrhage
- +/- Extraglandular invasion of soft tissues
- +/- Adjacent nodal, disseminated metastases
- Color Doppler: Pronounced intratumoral vascularity

- US cannot delineate extent of large tumors & detect perineural spread
- MR best delineates tumor extent & perineural extension

Clinical Issues
- Painful hard parotid mass; present months to years
- 33% present with pain & CN7 paralysis
- Favorable short term but poor long term prognosis

Imaging Recommendations
- Best imaging tool
  - US clearly evaluates superficial parotid but is unable to evaluate deep lobe masses or deep extension of superficial lobe lesions
  - US is readily combined with guided fine needle aspiration cytology (FNAC) with sensitivity of 83%, specificity 86% & accuracy of 85% for salivary gland masses
- Protocol advice
  - Carefully evaluate tumor edge, extraglandular/nodal involvement, internal heterogeneity
  - US cannot delineate extent of large tumors & detect perineural spread
    - US is useful in identifying tumor, predicting malignancy & guiding biopsy
- MR best delineates tumor extent & perineural extension

DIFFERENTIAL DIAGNOSIS

Benign Mixed Tumor (BMT)
- Well-defined, homogeneous, hypoechoic mass with posterior enhancement; lobulated when large

Warthin Tumor
- Well-defined, hypoechoic, solid + cystic component & septa in parotid tail; may be multicentric

Nodal Metastasis from Skin Neoplasm
- Ill-defined, solid, hypoechoic mass, +/- multiple nodes

PATHOLOGY

General Features
- General path comments: Superficially located, slow growing neoplasm with propensity for perineural extension & late recurrence

CLINICAL ISSUES

Presentation
- Most common signs/symptoms
  - Painful hard parotid mass; present months to years
  - 33% present with pain & CN7 paralysis

Natural History & Prognosis
- Favorable short term but poor long term prognosis

Treatment
- Surgical plan is wide resection with negative margins
- Post-operative radiotherapy for all but lowest grade

SELECTED REFERENCES
1. Ahuja AT et al: Imaging in Head & Neck Cancer: A Practical Approach. 1st ed. London, Greenwich Medical Media. 115-41, 2003

IMAGE GALLERY

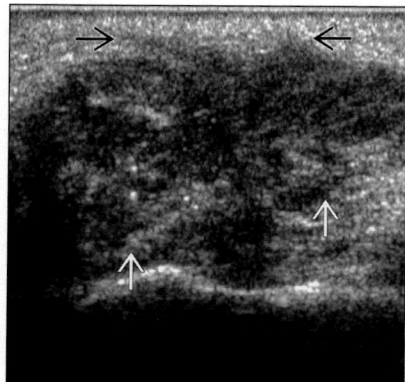 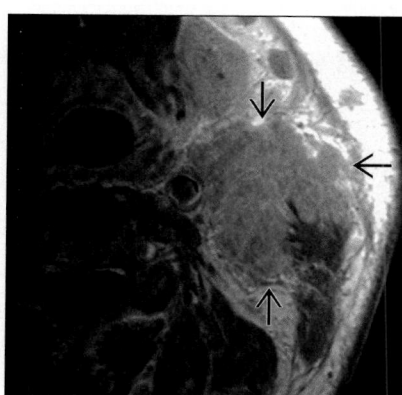 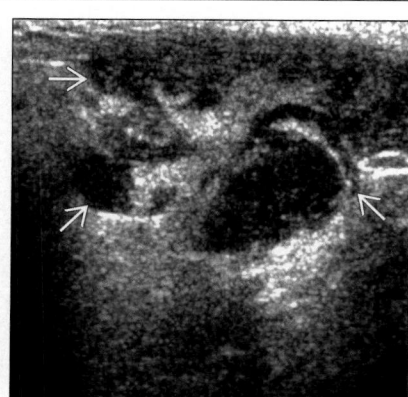

(Left) Transverse grayscale US shows a high grade ACCa ➡ seen as a solid, ill-defined, hypoechoic mass w/extraglandular extension ⇨. US predicts malignancy but can't differentiate between types. *(Center)* Corresponding, gadolinium enhanced axial T1WI MR shows an ill-defined parotid ACCa & its extent ⇨. MR best detects perineural spread & anatomical extent of tumor. *(Right)* Longitudinal grayscale US of a high grade ACCa ➡ shows an ill-defined, hypoechoic, heterogeneous mass. US predicts nature of lesion but can't delineate its extent & perineural spread.

BENIGN MASSETER MUSCLE HYPERTROPHY

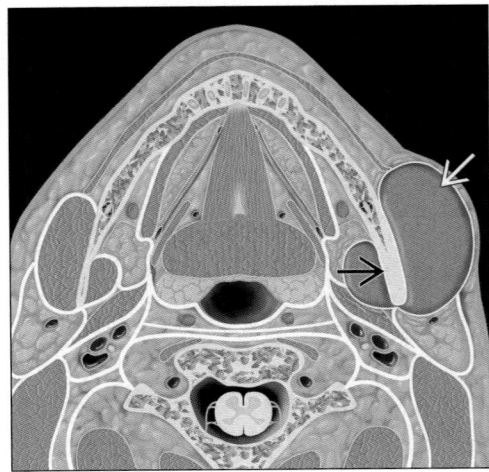

Transverse graphic shows unilateral masseter muscle hypertrophy →. Note underlying mandibular cortical thickening →. Compare with the contralateral normal masseter & mandible.

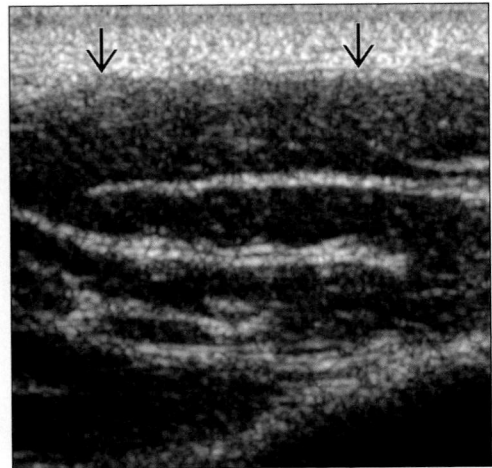

Transverse grayscale US shows an enlarged (> 13.5 mm) masseter muscle →. Always compare with the opposite side at similar landmarks. Note US clearly evaluates the muscle & rules out focal mass.

TERMINOLOGY

Abbreviations and Synonyms
- Benign masticator muscle hypertrophy (BMMH)
- Benign masseteric hypertrophy (BMH)

IMAGING FINDINGS

General Features
- Location
  - Masticator space; masseter most obviously affected
  - 50% bilateral, usually asymmetric
- Size
  - Muscles enlarge up to 3 times normal size
  - Normal transverse diameter of masseter muscle on ultrasound < 13.5 mm

Ultrasonographic Findings
- Enlarged masseter muscle with normal echogenicity
- No focal mass lesion, heterogeneity, calcification, cystic area within muscle
- Underlying mandibular cortex may be irregular suggesting bony hyperostosis

- Color Doppler: No abnormal vessels seen in muscle

CT Findings
- NECT: Enlarged masticator muscles with normal attenuation; cortical thickening affecting mandible & zygomatic arch
- CECT: Enlarged masticator muscles enhance normally

MR Findings
- T1WI: Enlarged masticator muscles isointense to normal muscle; decreased marrow signal in areas of cortical thickening (mandible, zygomatic arch)
- T2WI: Enlarged masticator muscles isointense to normal muscle
- T1 C+: Enlarged masticator muscles enhance normally

Imaging Recommendations
- Best imaging tool
  - As masseter is superficial in location, US is ideal imaging modality
  - Always compare at fixed landmarks: Angle of mandible, level of ear lobule, point between these two locations

DDx: Benign Masseter Muscle Hypertrophy

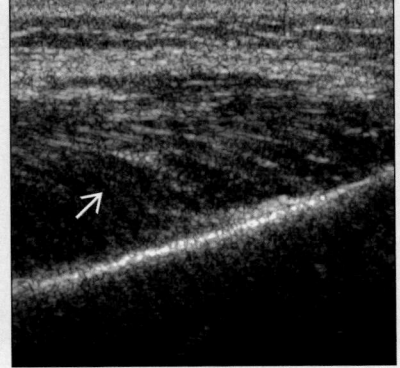

Masseter Muscle Inflammation

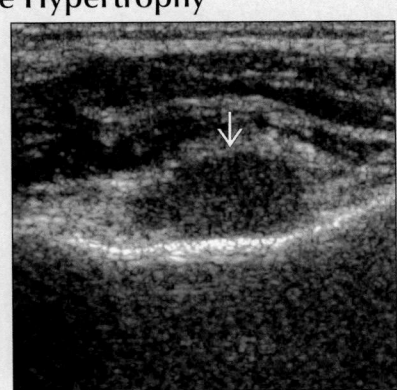

Masseter Muscle Metastases

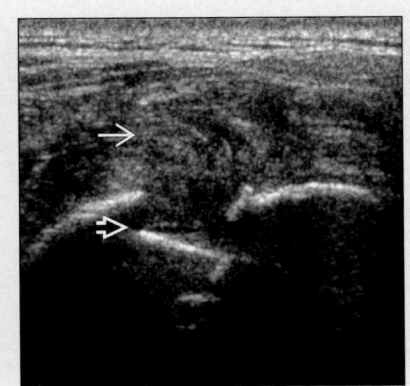

Mandibular Metastases

BENIGN MASSETER MUSCLE HYPERTROPHY

Key Facts

Imaging Findings
- Enlarged masseter muscle with normal echogenicity
- No focal mass lesion, heterogeneity, calcification, cystic area within muscle
- Color Doppler: No abnormal vessels seen in muscle
- US ideally guides position of needle for Botulinum toxin A injection used to treat BMH & for FU following treatment
- Always evaluate underlying salivary glands to rule out a salivary lesion simulating BMH

Clinical Issues
- Most common signs/symptoms: Nontender lateral facial mass that enlarges with jaw clenching
- Botulinum toxin A injection
- Surgery only for cosmetic reasons

- ○ US ideally guides position of needle for Botulinum toxin A injection used to treat BMH & for FU following treatment
- Protocol advice
  - ○ On US always compare both sides to evaluate masseter muscle
  - ○ If bilateral BMH it may be difficult to appreciate hypertrophy; evaluate with known US measurements (< 13.5 mm on transverse scans)
  - ○ Always evaluate underlying salivary glands to rule out a salivary lesion simulating BMH
  - ○ Other masticator muscles (medial & lateral pterygoids, temporalis) may also be involved; these are not evaluated by US due to their location

DIFFERENTIAL DIAGNOSIS

Masseter Muscle Inflammation
- Edematous, hypoechoic masseter +/- vascularity

Masseter Muscle Metastases
- Solitary/multiple hypoechoic mass along long axis of muscle & evidence of disseminated disease

Mandibular Metastases
- Focal bone destruction with mass infiltrating masseter

PATHOLOGY

General Features
- Etiology
  - ○ Bruxism (nocturnal teeth grinding), gum chewing, temporomandibular joint dysfunction
  - ○ Anabolic steroids ± unilateral chewing

CLINICAL ISSUES

Presentation
- Most common signs/symptoms: Nontender lateral facial mass that enlarges with jaw clenching

Treatment
- Botulinum toxin A injection
- Surgery only for cosmetic reasons

SELECTED REFERENCES

1. To EWH et al: A prospective study of effect of Botulinum toxin A on masseteric muscle hypertrophy with ultrasonographic & electromyographic measurement. Br J of Plastic Surgery. 54:197-200, 2001
2. Ahuja AT et al: Sonographic findings in masseter muscle metastases. JCU. 28(6):299-302, 2000

IMAGE GALLERY

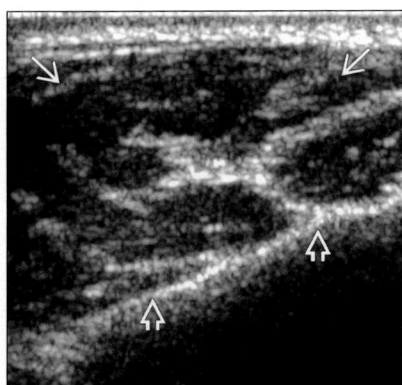 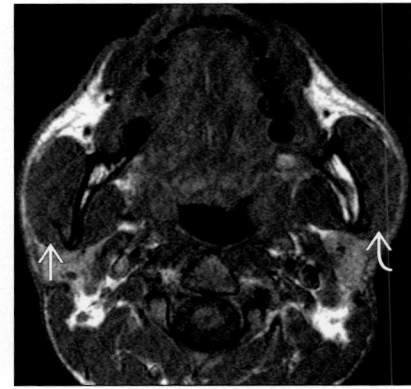 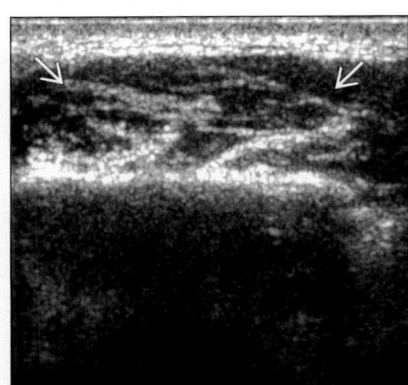

(Left) Transverse grayscale US shows enlarged (> 13.5 mm) masseter muscle ➡. US is ideal for guiding Botulinum toxin A injection & for follow-up for efficacy of treatment. Mandible ➡. *(Center)* Corresponding axial T1WI MR shows a hypertrophied right masseter muscle ➡ compared to the left ➡. MR better evaluates bone changes in the underlying mandible. *(Right)* Transverse US shows reduction in the size of the masseter muscle ➡ following Botulinum toxin A injection (same patient as in previous two images).

RANULA

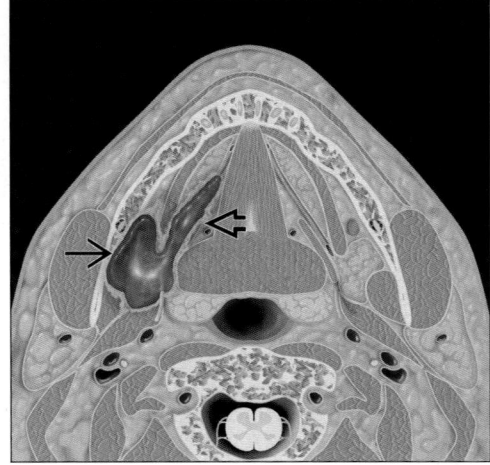

Axial graphic shows a diving ranula herniating from the sublingual to the submandibular space ⇨. The "tail sign" ⇨ is the collapsed cyst in the sublingual space.

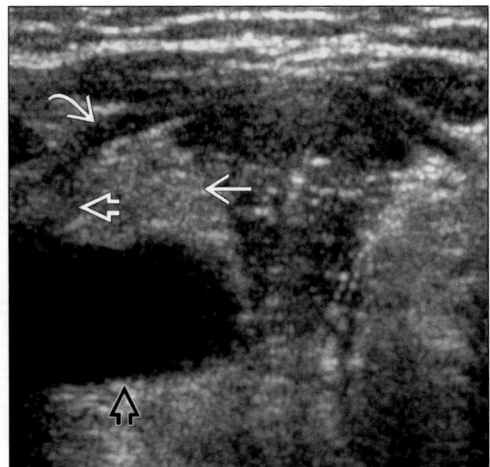

Transverse ultrasound shows an anechoic cystic lesion ⇨ in SLS. Identify its relation to sublingual gland ⇨ and mylohyoid muscle ⇨. Note it passes posterior ⇨ to the mylohyoid into the SMS, making it a diving ranula.

TERMINOLOGY

Abbreviations and Synonyms
- Abbreviations: Simple ranula (SR), diving ranula (DR)
- Term ranula derive from Latin "rana" = frog
  - Sublingual blebs in mouth of frog resemble simple ranula
- Synonyms: Sublingual gland mucocele, mucous retention cyst
  - DR also called plunging ranula

Definitions
- Ranula: Retention cyst resulting from trauma or inflammation of sublingual gland or minor salivary glands in sublingular space (SLS)
  - SR: Post-inflammatory retention cyst of sublingual or SLS minor salivary glands with epithelial lining
    - Located above mylohyoid muscle, near sublingual gland
  - DR: Extravasation pseudocyst; term used when SR becomes large, ruptures out posterior SLS into submandibular space (SMS) creating pseudocyst lacking epithelial lining

IMAGING FINDINGS

General Features
- Best diagnostic clue
  - Simple ranula: Well-defined, cystic, thin-walled SLS mass
  - Diving ranula: SLS + SMS cyst extension
- Location
  - SR: Sublingual space
  - DR: SLS + SMS
- Size
  - SR: < 3 cm
  - DR: < 6 cm; may be giant
- Morphology
  - SR: Oval-lenticular unilocular SLS mass
  - DR: Unilocular mass with one component in SLS with extension into SMS
    - When large will involve inferior parapharyngeal space (PPS)
    - If plunges through mylohyoid muscle vascular cleft, may end up anterior to submandibular gland (SMG)

DDx: Ranula

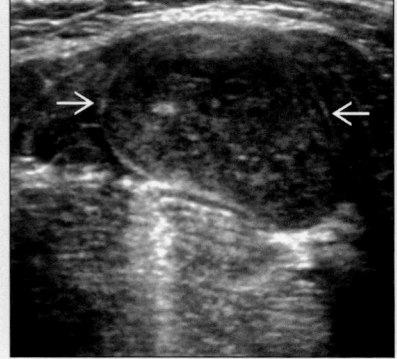

Dermoid

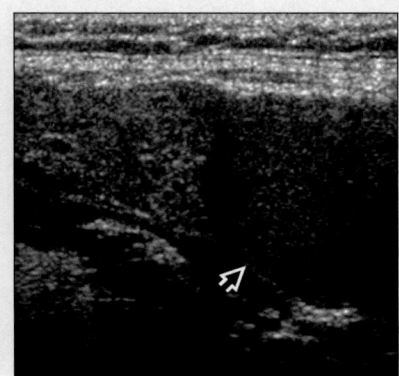

2nd Branchial Cleft Cyst

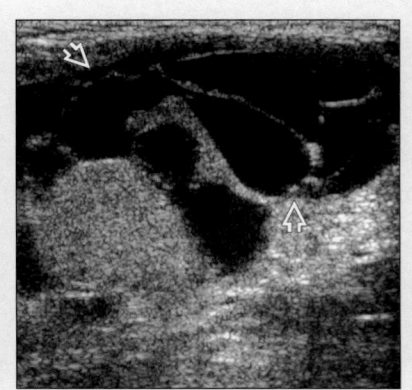

Lymphangioma

LYMPHANGIOMA

Key Facts

Imaging Findings
- May be detected on prenatal US or MR
- If no hemorrhage or infection: Unilocular/multilocular, anechoic compressible cysts with thin walls and intervening septa
- If no hemorrhage or infection: Despite large size they do not cause mass effect, in fact, adjacent muscles and vessels indent the lesion
- Color Doppler: No vascularity seen if uninfected
- If hemorrhage or infection: Unilocular or multilocular heterogeneous cysts with irregular walls, internal debris
- If hemorrhage or infection: Non-compressible hypoechoic, heterogeneous mass with thick walls, thick septa and mass effect

- Fluid-fluid levels due to separation of different fluids (suggests prior hemorrhage)
- Color Doppler: If infected, vascularity may be seen in the soft tissues around the lesion and within septa and walls
- Infiltrate between and around neurovascular structures
- While US can diagnose lymphangiomas, MR or CT are necessary to map their entire extent
- US is the ideal modality to guide injection of sclerosing agent and follow-up after treatment

Top Differential Diagnoses
- 2nd Branchial Cleft Cyst
- Thymic Cyst
- Neck Abscess

- o Color Doppler: No vascularity seen if uninfected
- Hemorrhagic/infected
  - o If hemorrhage or infection: Unilocular or multilocular heterogeneous cysts with irregular walls, internal debris
  - o If hemorrhage or infection: Non-compressible hypoechoic, heterogeneous mass with thick walls, thick septa and mass effect
  - o Fluid-fluid levels due to separation of different fluids (suggests prior hemorrhage)
  - o Color Doppler: If infected, vascularity may be seen in the soft tissues around the lesion and within septa and walls
- Infiltrate between and around neurovascular structures

Radiographic Findings
- Radiography: Retropharyngeal lymphangiomas may cause mass effect on pediatric airway, seen on AP or lateral neck film

CT Findings
- NECT
  - o Low density, often poorly-circumscribed cystic neck mass
  - o Fluid-fluid levels may be seen in multi-loculated lesions
- CECT
  - o No significant enhancement in cystic uni- or multilocular neck mass
  - o In absence of infection or complex lesion, wall imperceptible & does not enhance
  - o If complex lesion with venous vascular components, area of enhancing tissue or veins may be seen

MR Findings
- T1WI
  - o Primarily hypointense, but may be hyperintense if prior hemorrhage or high proteinaceous component
  - o Fluid-fluid level often seen within multiple compartments
- T2WI
  - o Best sequence to map lesion, as lymphangioma is hyperintense throughout

- o Trans-spatial, often poorly marginated
- T1 C+
  - o Most often, no significant enhancement or subtle rim-enhancement
  - o If areas of enhancement seen, most likely a mixed rest with venous vascular or hemangiomatous components

Imaging Recommendations
- Best imaging tool
  - o While US can diagnose lymphangiomas, MR or CT are necessary to map their entire extent
  - o Larger lesions best evaluated with MR
    - T2 high signal improves definition of local extension, proximity to normal structures, including vessels
- Protocol advice
  - o In large neck lesions, always evaluate axilla and mediastinum as they may be involved
  - o Lesions are superficial & compressible; try & avoid applying transducer pressure as this may compress the lesion
  - o Prior to treating with sclerosing agent always perform pre-procedure baseline imaging (US & MR)
  - o US is the ideal modality to guide injection of sclerosing agent and follow-up after treatment
  - o For small superficial lesions, sclerosant may be injected following sedation in children & under US guidance
    - This reduces procedure time and increases safety of procedure

DIFFERENTIAL DIAGNOSIS

2nd Branchial Cleft Cyst
- Ovoid unilocular mass at angle of mandible with characteristic displacement pattern
- Anechoic cyst or heterogeneous thick walled cyst or cyst with pseudosolid echo pattern

LYMPHANGIOMA

Thymic Cyst
- Unilocular, anechoic, well-defined infrahyoid lateral neck cyst with thin walls

Neck Abscess
- Thick, ill-defined, heterogeneous content with debris, +/- air within, and rim vascularity on Doppler
- Adjacent soft tissues have cellulitis, myositis fasciitis

Thyroglossal Duct Cyst
- Ovoid unilocular cystic mass in midline in vicinity of hyoid bone
- Embedded in infrahyoid strap muscles
- Anechoic cyst, or heterogeneous thick walled cyst or cyst with pseudosolid echo pattern

PATHOLOGY

General Features
- General path comments
  - Embryology: Multiple etiologic theories exist; best 2 below
    - Failure of embryologic fusion between primordial lymph sac & central venous system
    - May arise from sequestrations of embryonic lymph sacs
- Genetics
  - More common associated syndromes
    - Turner syndrome, Noonan syndrome, fetal alcohol syndrome

Microscopic Features
- Dilated endothelial lined lymphatic spaces
- Internal septations with varying thickness
- May have dilated, thin-walled vessels within mass
- 4 types of lymphangioma based on microscopic size of dilated lymphatic channels
  - Cystic hygroma, cavernous lymphangioma, capillary lymphangioma & vasculolymphatic malformation
  - Both lymphatic & venous vascular malformation may occur in same lesion (vasculolymphatic malformation)
  - Size of lymphatic spaces within lesion, at microscopy, differentiates one from another
- Imaging cannot differentiate subtypes of lymphangioma

Staging, Grading or Classification Criteria
- Lymphangioma grading based on microscopic, not radiologic, appearance
- Cystic hygroma is most common form
  - Consists of markedly dilated lymphatic spaces
  - Posterior cervical space & submandibular space are most common locations
- Cavernous lymphangioma composed of mildly dilated lymphatic spaces
- Capillary lymphangioma composed of smallest lymphatic spaces, least common form
- Vasculolymphatic malformation have venous component

CLINICAL ISSUES

Presentation
- Most common signs/symptoms
  - Soft, doughy neck mass detected within first 2 years of life
  - Other signs/symptoms
    - Large lymphangiomas can present with airway obstruction
- Clinical Profile
  - Usually incidental lesion in otherwise normal child
  - Turner most common syndromic association
- Physical exam: Soft, compressible, painless neck mass, usually in the posterior cervical or submandibular space

Demographics
- Age
  - Most commonly present at birth or within first 2 years of life (> 80%); small early adult group
  - Adult presentation unusual & suggests lymphangioma in adult may be acquired, probably post-traumatic

Natural History & Prognosis
- High local recurrence rate due to incomplete surgical resection
- No malignant potential

Treatment
- Surgical resection if lesion is isolated, unilocular & not associated with major vessels or nerves
- Percutaneous sclerosing agents may be used with extensive, trans-spatial lesions with significant vascular component

DIAGNOSTIC CHECKLIST

Consider
- T2 MR images are best to map extent of lymphangioma

Image Interpretation Pearls
- Trans-spatial multicystic neck mass with septation, debris, fluid level is most likely lymphangioma

SELECTED REFERENCES
1. Harnsberger HR et al: Diagnostic Imaging Head & Neck. 1st ed. Salt Lake City, Amirsys. IV-1-30-33, 2004
2. Ahuja AT et al: Practical Head & Neck Ultrasound. London, Greenwich Medical Media. 85-104, 2000

IMAGE GALLERY

Typical

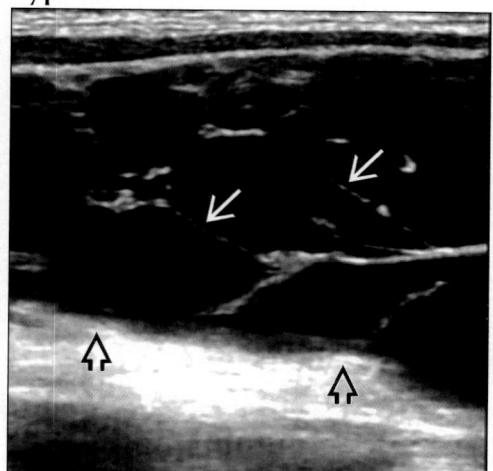
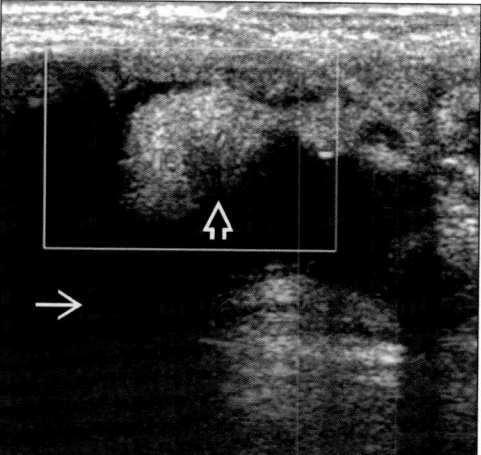

(Left) Ultrasound shows a large multiloculated lymphangioma ➢ with multiple thin septa ➡, the typical appearance of uninfected/nonhemorrhagic lesion. *(Right)* Color Doppler shows no significant vascularity in the solid "papilliferous" portion ➢ floating in the large cystic lesion ➡. The appearance suggests blood clot within a lymphangioma.

Typical

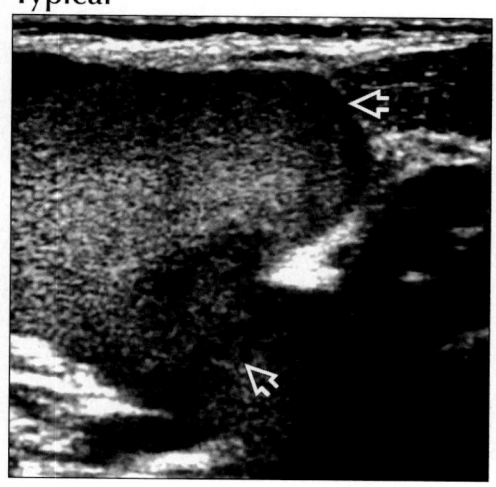
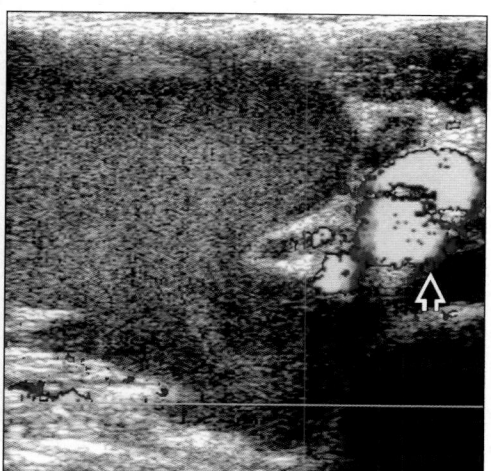

(Left) US shows a large lymphangioma ➢ with diffuse, homogeneous internal echoes, suggestive of previous hemorrhage or infection. *(Right)* Corresponding power Doppler shows relationship of the lymphangioma to adjacent major vessels ➢. Note the absence of vascularity within the lymphangioma. The deep extent of this lesion could not be evaluated by US.

Typical

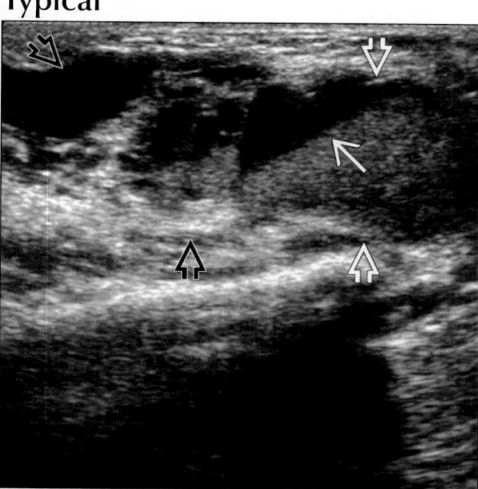
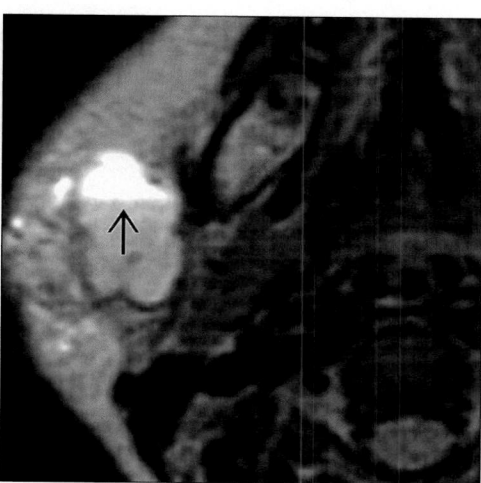

(Left) US shows a multiloculated parotid lymphangioma ➢ with a fluid level ➡ in the largest locule ➢. This appearance suggests a hemorrhage within and a separation of fluid based on specific gravity. *(Right)* Corresponding axial T2WI MR shows the fluid level ➡ within the parotid lymphangioma suggestive of a hemorrhage.

(Left) US shows a multiloculated lymphangioma with intervening septa ⮞ and internal debris ➡. Diffuse presence of debris and thick septa may suggest a previous infection. *(Right)* Corresponding power Doppler shows vascularity within the septa suggestive of an infective/inflammatory episode.

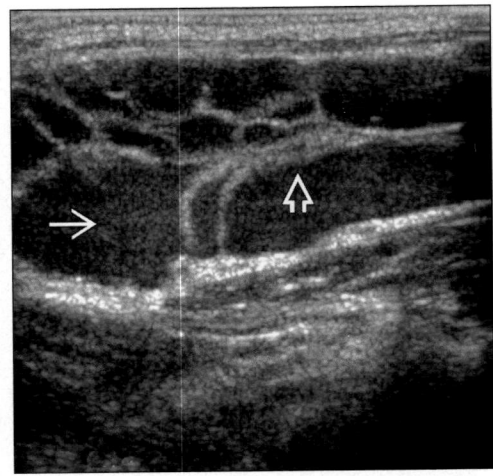
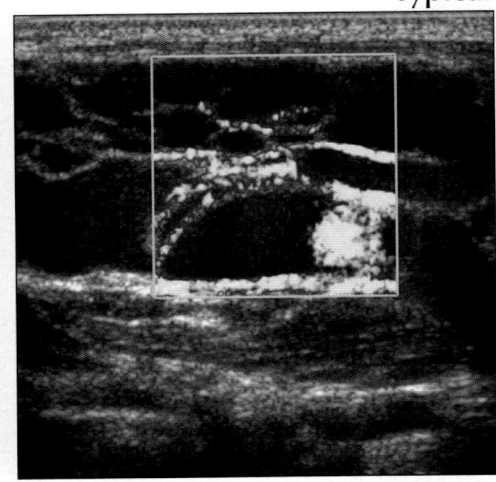

(Left) Transverse US shows an anechoic lymphangioma ⮞ with thin walls. Note its relation to the thyroid ⮞ and the CCA ➡. US clearly maps the anatomical extent of small lesions. *(Right)* Corresponding axial T2WI MR confirms the presence of a lymphangioma ⮞ and its anatomical extent. Note the similarity in appearance and extent of lesion between US and MR.

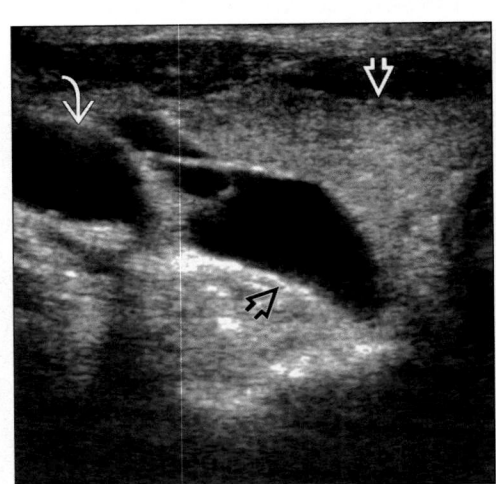
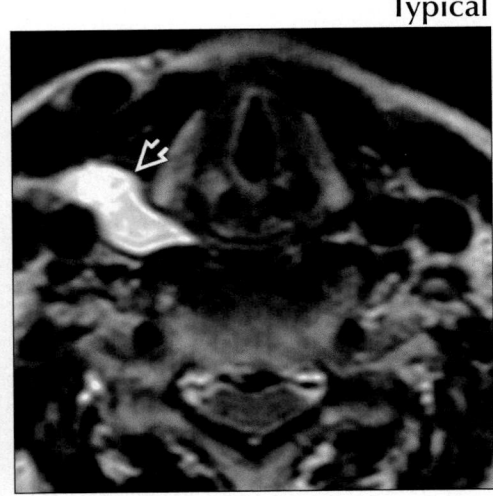

(Left) US shows a multiloculated lymphangioma ⮞ with thick septa ➡ and internal debris. Note US is unable to map its anatomical extent and relationship to the adjacent structures. *(Right)* Corresponding T2WI MR clearly defines extent of the lymphangioma ➡. Although US predicts the nature of a lesion it is necessary to do MR/CT to delineate extent, especially for large lesions.

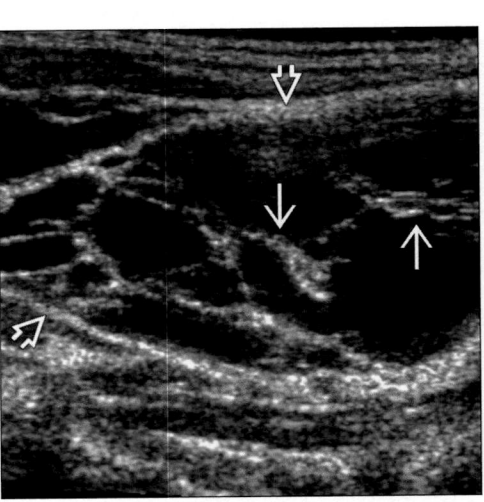
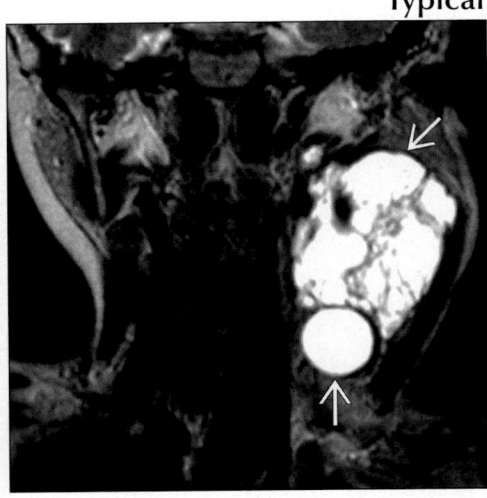

11

96

LYMPHANGIOMA

Typical

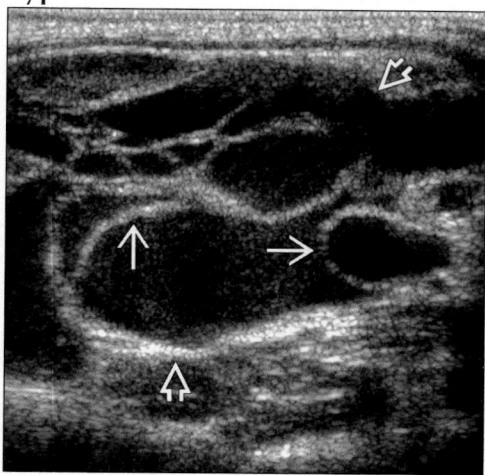

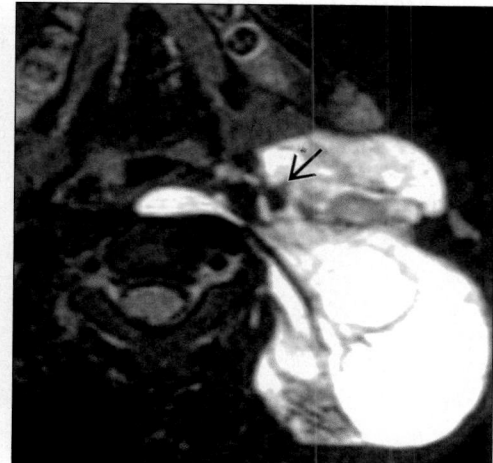

(Left) US shows a multiloculated lymphangioma ⊃ with multiple cystic spaces, thick intervening septa ➔, and fine internal echoes. Note the entire anatomical extent cannot be mapped by US. *(Right)* Corresponding axial T2WI MR, prior to OK-432 (sclerosing agent) injection, maps the extent of the lymphangioma and its proximity to the airway. The lesion invaginates around the normal structures ➔. T2 high signal helps delineate the lesion clearly.

Typical

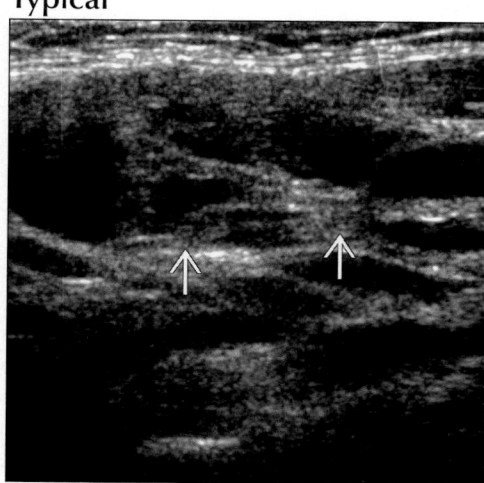

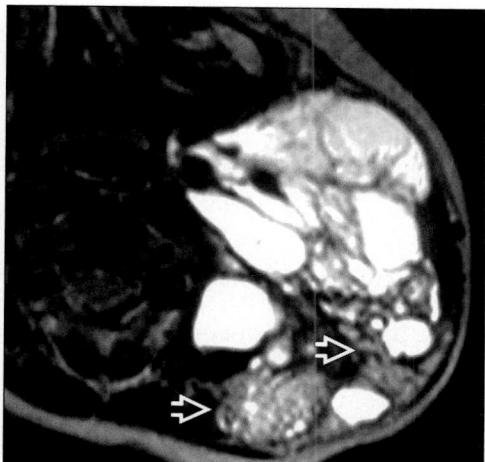

(Left) US (same patient as in previous 2 images) after first OK-432 injection shows a reduction in size and in number of cystic spaces in the lesion ➔. US is ideal to guide an interventional procedure and for a serial follow-up. *(Right)* Corresponding axial T2WI MR after first injection of OK-432 shows the obliteration of some loculi ⊃ within the lymphangioma. MR provides an objective assessment of the response to treatment.

Typical

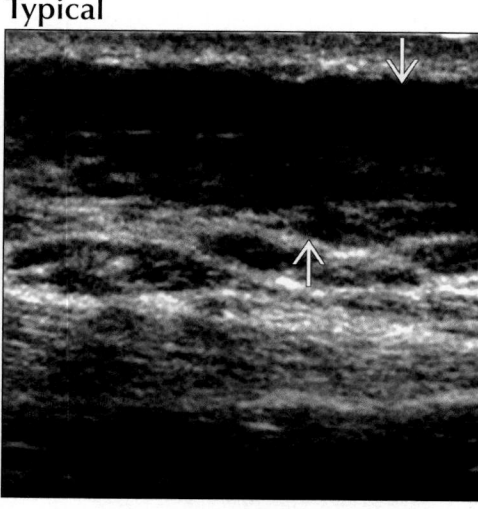

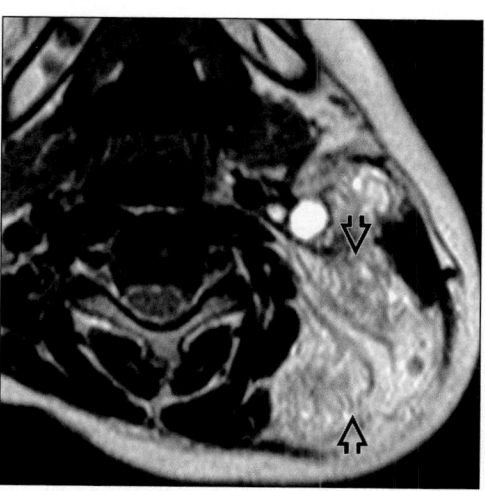

(Left) US (same patient as previous 4 images) after 2nd injection of OK-432 shows further reduction of the cystic spaces, with replacement by fatty tissue ➔. *(Right)* Corresponding axial T2WI MR after 2nd injection of OK-432 shows further reduction of cystic spaces and replacement by fatty tissue ⊃.

2ND BRANCHIAL CLEFT CYST

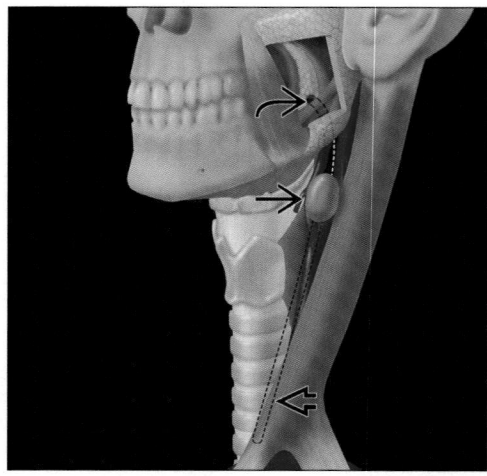

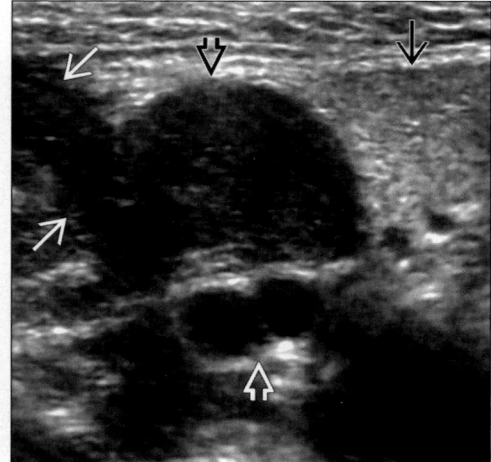

Graphic shows the 2nd BCC ➡ anterior to the sternomastoid muscle & lateral to the carotid space. The 2nd branchial cleft tract extends from the palatine tonsil ➡ to low neck ➡.

Grayscale US shows an infected 2nd BCC as a hypoechoic, cystic mass ➡ with internal debris. Note an infected tract in the soft tissue ➡. Carotid ➡, submandibular gland ➡.

TERMINOLOGY

Abbreviations and Synonyms
- Second branchial cleft cyst (2nd BCC)
- Second branchial cleft remnant or branchial cleft anomaly

Definitions
- Cystic remnant related to developmental alterations of 2nd branchial apparatus
  - 2nd branchial remnants may be fistula, sinus or cyst or any combination of these three

IMAGING FINDINGS

General Features
- Location
  - Characteristic location (most at or caudal to angle of mandible)
    - Posterolateral to submandibular gland
    - Lateral to carotid space
    - Anteromedial to sternocleidomastoid muscle (SCM)

  - Other unusual locations of 2nd BCC
    - Superiorly into parapharyngeal space or carotid space
    - Inferior along anterior surface of infrahyoid carotid space
    - Fistulous track may extend between external & internal carotid arteries to palatine tonsil
  - Can occur anywhere along line from tonsillar fossa to supraclavicular region
- Size: Variable, may range from several cm to > 5 cm
- Morphology
  - Ovoid or rounded well-circumscribed cyst
  - Focal rim of cyst extending to carotid bifurcation: "Notch sign" pathognomonic for 2nd BCC

Ultrasonographic Findings
- Typical location of cyst in relation to carotid sheath, submandibular gland and sternomastoid muscle is the first clue to its diagnosis
- Non-hemorrhagic/uninfected 2nd BCC
  - If no hemorrhage or infection: Unilocular, anechoic cyst with thin walls, posterior enhancement, faint internal debris

DDx: 2nd Branchial Cleft Cyst

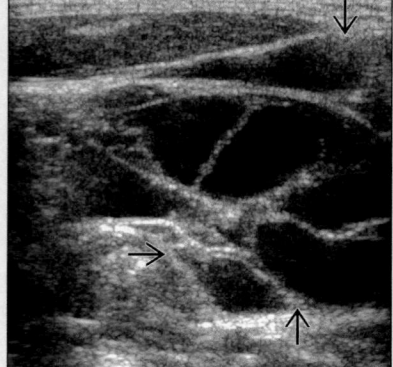

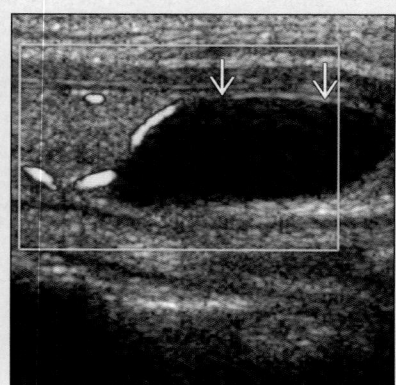

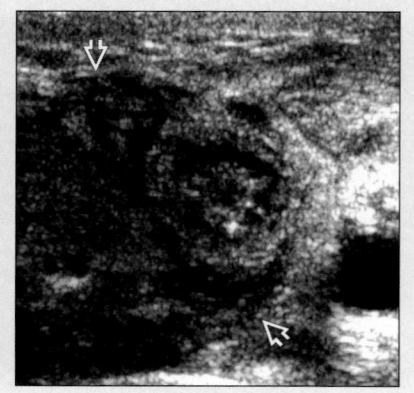

| Lymphangioma | Thymic Cyst | Neck Abscess |

2ND BRANCHIAL CLEFT CYST

Key Facts

Imaging Findings

- Typical location of cyst in relation to carotid sheath, submandibular gland and sternomastoid muscle is the first clue to its diagnosis
- If no hemorrhage or infection: Unilocular, anechoic cyst with thin walls, posterior enhancement, faint internal debris
- If no hemorrhage or infection: "Pseudosolid" appearance: Well-defined cyst with uniform, homogeneous internal echoes due to presence of mucus, debris, cholesterol crystals and epithelial cells within cyst
- Color Doppler: No vascularity seen within the cyst if uninfected; relationship with carotid artery clearly defined

- If hemorrhage/infection: Ill-defined, thick walls, septa, internal debris & inflammatory changes in adjacent soft tissue
- Color Doppler: If infected, vascularity may be seen within the thick walls, septa and adjacent soft tissues
- Hemorrhagic/infected 2nd BCC completely simulates a necrotic nodal metastases from SCC or papillary carcinoma of thyroid and in such cases fine needle aspiration cytology (FNAC) is essential for diagnosis
- US may show focal extension of cyst between ICA-ECA bifurcation; pathognomonic of 2nd BCC

Top Differential Diagnoses
- Lymphangioma
- Thymic Cyst
- Neck Abscess

- If no hemorrhage or infection: "Pseudosolid" appearance: Well-defined cyst with uniform, homogeneous internal echoes due to presence of mucus, debris, cholesterol crystals and epithelial cells within cyst
- Clue to cystic nature of a "pseudosolid" cyst is
  - Posterior acoustic enhancement, swirling motion of debris within cyst after applying intermittent transducer pressure or increasing power on Doppler; this swirling motion is evaluated only in real time and not on static images
  - Color Doppler: No vascularity seen within the cyst if uninfected; relationship with carotid artery clearly defined
- Hemorrhagic/infected 2nd BCC
  - If hemorrhage/infection: Ill-defined, thick walls, septa, internal debris & inflammatory changes in adjacent soft tissue
  - Color Doppler: If infected, vascularity may be seen within the thick walls, septa and adjacent soft tissues
  - Hemorrhagic/infected 2nd BCC completely simulates a necrotic nodal metastases from SCC or papillary carcinoma of thyroid and in such cases fine needle aspiration cytology (FNAC) is essential for diagnosis
- Cysts may have a cranial, parapharyngeal extension which may not be completely demonstrated by US and CT or MR is required
- US may show focal extension of cyst between ICA-ECA bifurcation; pathognomonic of 2nd BCC
- US may demonstrate the presence of a track or fistula associated with cyst

CT Findings
- NECT: Low density cyst with no discernible wall, unilocular, septated if infected
- CECT
  - Low density cyst with nonenhancing wall & surrounding soft tissues, unless infected
  - If infected, wall is thicker & enhances with surrounding soft tissues appearing "dirty" (cellulitis)

MR Findings
- T1WI
  - Cyst is usually isointense to CSF
  - Recurrently infected cysts may have hyperintense contents due to ↑ protein concentration
- T2WI: Hyperintense cyst, no discernible wall
- FLAIR: Cyst is iso- or slightly hyperintense to CSF
- T1 C+: Peripheral wall enhancement if cyst is infected, cyst contents generally do not enhance

Imaging Recommendations
- Best imaging tool
  - Ultrasound (combined with FNAC) is ideal for making the diagnosis and differentiating it from a metastatic lymph node
  - Pre-operative ultrasound adequately evaluates adjacent anatomical relations; for larger cysts CT or MR may be necessary
- Protocol advice: Bear in mind the "pseudosolid" nature of these cysts; intermittent application of transducer pressure and increasing power on Doppler will demonstrate swirling motion within cyst on real time examination

DIFFERENTIAL DIAGNOSIS

Lymphangioma
- Multilocular, trans-spatial, fills available spaces; may appear anechoic or "pseudosolid" on US with internal septation
- If unilocular, may be difficult to differentiate from 2nd BCC if it occurs in location typical for 2nd BCC

Thymic Cyst
- Cyst is inferior in cervical neck, centered in lateral visceral space and anechoic with thin walls

Neck Abscess
- Ill-defined, hypoechoic, heterogeneous echo pattern with debris, gas and vascularity in abscess wall

2ND BRANCHIAL CLEFT CYST

Cystic Malignant Adenopathy

- Necrotic mass with thick, ill-defined walls, hypoechoic, heterogeneous architecture and abnormal vascularity
- Metastases from SCC and papillary carcinoma of thyroid may have cystic appearance very similar to 2nd BCC

PATHOLOGY

General Features

- General path comments
  - Embryology
    - Branchial apparatus is precursor of many H&N structures
    - 2nd branchial arch overgrows 2nd, 3rd & 4th clefts and overgrowth forms a cavity called the "cervical sinus"
    - Failure of obliteration of cervical sinus results in 2nd branchial cleft remnants, either a cyst, sinus or fistula
    - Full 2nd branchial cleft fistula extends from SCM, through carotid artery bifurcation & terminates in tonsillar fossa
- Etiology: Failure of obliteration of cervical sinus, leading to a 2nd BCC, sinus or fistulae
- Epidemiology: 2nd BCC account for > 90% of all branchial cleft anomalies in teens and adults, 66-75% in children

Gross Pathologic & Surgical Features

- Well-defined cyst, lateral to carotid sheath
- Filled with cheesy material or serous, mucoid or purulent fluid
- If associated fistulous tract is present, cutaneous opening typically at anterior border of SCM near mid or lower portion

Microscopic Features

- Squamous epithelial-lined cyst
- Lymphoid infiltrate in wall, often in form of germinal centers
  - Lymphoid tissue suggests epithelial rests may be entrapped within cervical lymph nodes during embryogenesis

Staging, Grading or Classification Criteria

- Four subtypes have been described by Bailey
  - Type I is anterior to SCM, beneath platysma muscle
  - Type II is adjacent to ICA & often adherent to IJV; most common
  - Type III extends between ICA & ECA to lateral pharyngeal wall
  - Type IV lies against lateral pharyngeal wall & may extend to skull base

CLINICAL ISSUES

Presentation

- Most common signs/symptoms: Painless, recurrent, compressible lateral neck mass in child or young adult increasing in size following upper respiratory tract infection
- Clinical Profile: 2nd BCC often enlarge during upper respiratory infection, probably due to response of lymphoid tissue
- Other symptoms
  - Intermittent, soft, painless, compressible lateral neck mass; painful if infected

Demographics

- Age: Two peak ages of presentation, under 5 years old child or in 2nd or 3rd decade (less common)

Natural History & Prognosis

- If untreated, may become repeatedly infected & inflamed
- Recurrent inflammation makes surgical resection more difficult
- Excellent prognosis if lesion is completely resected

Treatment

- Complete surgical resection is treatment of choice
- Surgeon must dissect around cyst bed to exclude the possibility of an associated fistula or tract
  - If a tract goes superomedially, it passes through carotid bifurcation into crypts of palatine (faucial) tonsil
  - If a tract goes inferiorly, it passes along anterior carotid space, reaching skin in supraclavicular area
    - If fistula present, it is seen at birth; mucoid secretion emitted from skin opening

DIAGNOSTIC CHECKLIST

Consider

- Is the cyst thick walled, ill-defined, with septa, vascularity & heterogeneous echo pattern to suggest infection
- Could "cyst" be cystic papillary carcinoma nodal met?

Image Interpretation Pearls

- Beware an adult with first presentation of "2nd BCC"
  - Mass may be metastatic node from head & neck SCCa primary tumor
  - US guided FNAC necessary to confirm diagnosis

SELECTED REFERENCES

1. Ahuja AT et al: Second branchial cleft cysts: variability of sonographic appearances in adult cases. AJNR Am J Neuroradiol. 21(2):315-9, 2000
2. Ahuja A et al: Solitary cystic nodal metastasis from occult papillary carcinoma of the thyroid mimicking a branchial cyst: a potential pitfall. Clin Radiol. 53(1):61-3, 1998
3. Harnsberger HR et al: Branchial cleft anomalies and their mimics: computed tomographic evaluation. Radiology. 152(3):739-48, 1984

2ND BRANCHIAL CLEFT CYST

IMAGE GALLERY

Typical

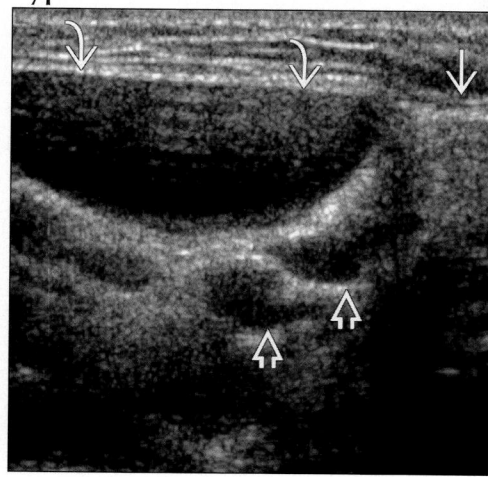
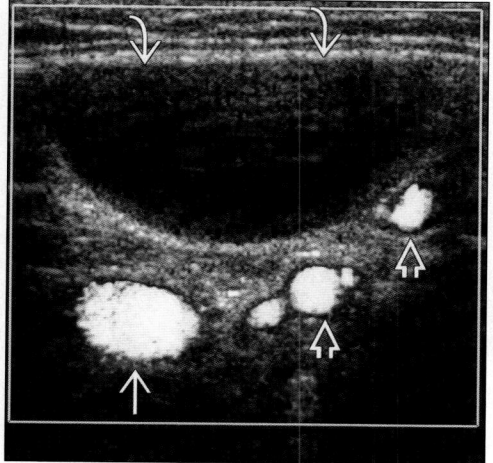

(Left) Transverse grayscale US shows a cystic, anechoic mass ➡ with thin walls related to the carotid artery ➡ and the submandibular gland ➡. Appearances and location typical for 2nd BCC. *(Right)* Corresponding power Doppler shows the avascular nature of the mass ➡ and confirms its relationship to the carotid artery ➡ and the internal jugular vein ➡.

Typical

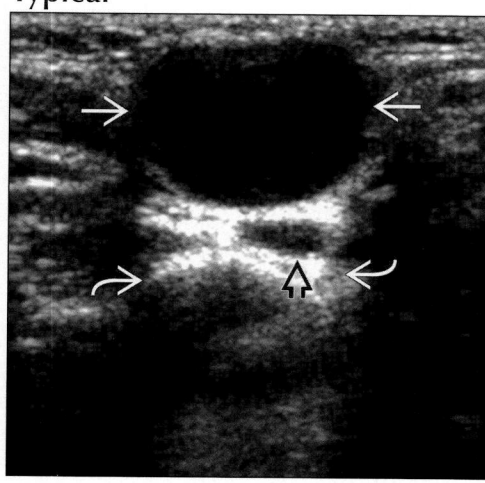
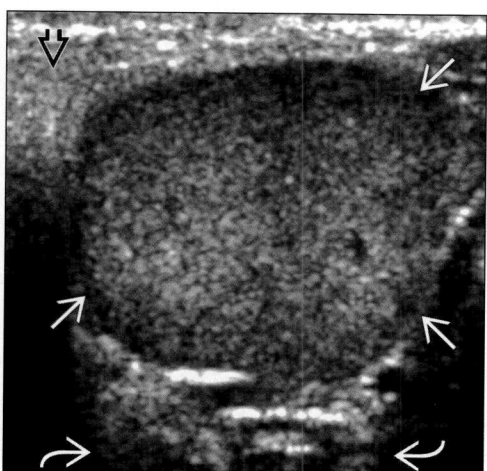

(Left) Transverse grayscale US shows a well-defined, anechoic cystic mass ➡ with thin walls & posterior enhancement ➡. Note its relationship to the carotid artery ➡. This appearance is typical of 2nd BCC at this location. *(Right)* Grayscale US shows a well-defined 2nd BCC ➡ with uniform, homogeneous internal echoes and posterior enhancement ➡. Typical "pseudosolid" appearance of a 2nd BCC. ➡ Submandibular gland.

Typical

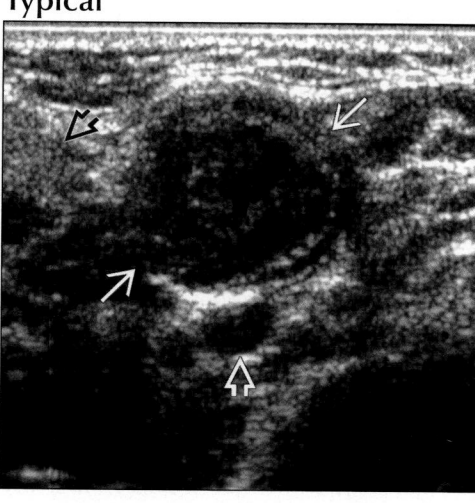
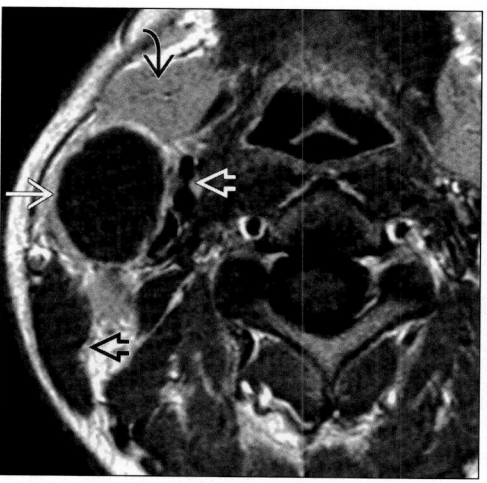

(Left) Grayscale US shows an ill-defined, thick-walled 2nd BCC ➡ with internal debris, simulating a metastatic node from SCC or papillary thyroid carcinoma. FNAC confirms diagnosis. Submandibular gland ➡, carotid artery ➡. *(Right)* Axial T1 C+ MR shows a typical 2nd BCC ➡ with no central enhancement & a thin cyst wall. Note its relationship to the submandibular gland ➡, carotid ➡ and sternomastoid muscle ➡.

CAROTID BODY PARAGANGLIOMA

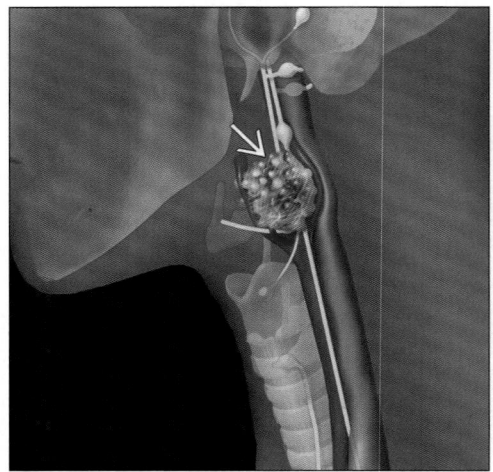

Graphic shows the characteristic location of a CBP ➡ in the crotch of ECA & ICA at the carotid bifurcation.

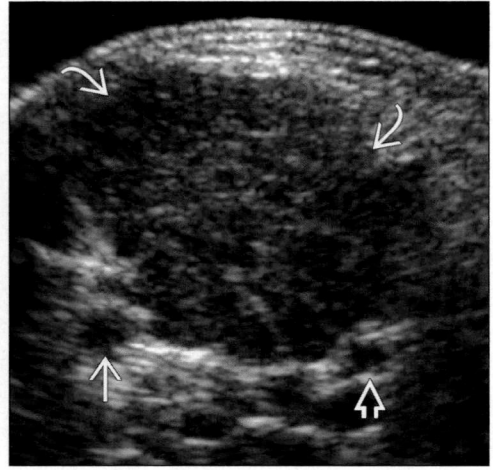

Transverse grayscale US shows a solid, hypoechoic, well-defined mass ➡ splaying the carotid bifurcation. Note its typical location in the crotch of the ICA ➡ & ECA ➡. Typical location & features of a CBP.

TERMINOLOGY

Abbreviations and Synonyms
- Carotid body paraganglioma (CBP)
- Carotid body tumor; chemodectoma; non-chromaffin paraganglioma

Definitions
- CBP: Benign vascular tumor arising in glomus bodies in carotid body found in crotch of ECA & ICA at carotid bifurcation

IMAGING FINDINGS

General Features
- Best diagnostic clue: Vascular mass splaying ECA and ICA
- Location
  ○ Carotid space just above hyoid bone
  ○ Mass centered in crotch of carotid bifurcation
- Size
  ○ Variable
  ○ 1-6 cm typical

- Morphology: Ovoid, mass with broad lobular surface contour

Ultrasonographic Findings
- Location of tumor at carotid bifurcation is the first clue to its diagnosis
- CBP is usually solid, well-defined & hypoechoic with splaying of ICA, ECA
- Parenchymal echo pattern is homogenous, +/- serpigeneous vessels within
- Large tumors may show heterogeneous architecture due to necrosis or hemorrhage within
- No evidence of calcification or internal necrosis
- Large tumors may completely encase the bifurcation
- Color Doppler: Confirms the relationship of the tumor to carotid bifurcation & splaying of ICA, ECA
  ○ CBPs commonly are hypervascular with prominent tortuous vessels within
  ○ CBPs may appear to be avascular, particularly the deeper components which are not well interrogated by Doppler
  ○ Color power angiogram demonstrates vascular tumor in "Y" of carotid bifurcation

DDx: Carotid Body Paraganglioma

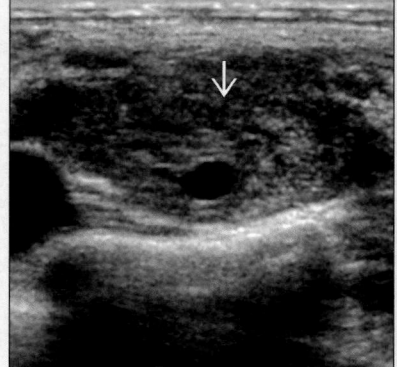

Vagal Nerve Schwannoma

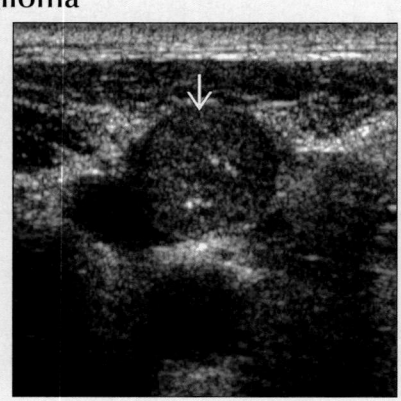

Metastatic Lymph Node

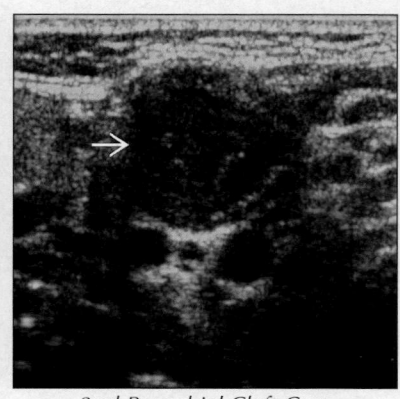

2nd Branchial Cleft Cyst

CAROTID BODY PARAGANGLIOMA

Key Facts

Imaging Findings

- Location of tumor at carotid bifurcation is the first clue to its diagnosis
- CBP is usually solid, well-defined & hypoechoic with splaying of ICA, ECA
- Parenchymal echo pattern is homogenous, +/- serpigeneous vessels within
- Large tumors may show heterogeneous architecture due to necrosis or hemorrhage within
- No evidence of calcification or internal necrosis
- Large tumors may completely encase the bifurcation
- Color Doppler: Confirms the relationship of the tumor to carotid bifurcation & splaying of ICA, ECA
- CBPs commonly are hypervascular with prominent tortuous vessels within
- CBPs may appear to be avascular, particularly the deeper components which are not well interrogated by Doppler
- Color power angiogram demonstrates vascular tumor in "Y" of carotid bifurcation
- Always evaluate/compare with opposite side as the tumors may be bilateral
- US is unable to evaluate other paragangliomas such as glomus vagale, glomus jugulare
- During real time scanning use gentle transducer pressure to prevent compression of vessels within tumor

Top Differential Diagnoses

- Vagal Schwannoma/Neurofibroma
- Metastatic Node
- 2nd Brachial Cleft Cyst (BCC)

CT Findings

- CTA: Oblique sagittal reconstruction shows enhancing tumor in "Y" of carotid bifurcation
- NECT
  - Lobular mass splaying ICA & ECA
  - Density similar to neck muscles
- CECT
  - Avidly-enhancing mass in crotch between ECA and ICA at carotid bifurcation
  - Enhancement is usually rapid compared to carotid space schwannoma
    - Dynamic CECT can distinguish CBP & schwannoma
  - CBP extends from carotid artery bifurcation cephalad

MR Findings

- T1WI
  - Mass signal similar to muscle
  - "Salt & pepper" appearance if bigger than 1.5 cm
  - "Salt": Rare finding in CBP; secondary to subacute hemorrhage
    - High signal areas within tumor parenchyma
    - Seen only in larger tumors
  - "Pepper": Expected MR finding in CBP > 2 cm
    - Hypointense serpentine or punctate flow channels due to high vascularity in fibrous matrix of CBP
    - May be seen on tumor margin or within parenchyma
- T2WI: Mass signal slightly above that of muscle
- T1 C+
  - Intense enhancement
  - Larger high velocity flow voids still seen
- MRA
  - MRA without contrast: Splayed ECA-ICA; tumor not seen
  - MRA with contrast: Splaying plus enhancing CBP

Angiographic Findings

- Prolonged, intense tumor blush between ICA & ECA
- Arteriovenous shunting creates "early vein" phenomenon
- Main feeding branch is ascending pharyngeal artery

Imaging Recommendations

- Best imaging tool
  - US is the ideal initial modality to identify and diagnose a CBP
  - US readily evaluates the opposite side for CBP but is unable to adequately evaluate other paragangliomas in the neck
  - CECT or MR plus angiography done before surgery, coverage should extend from temporal bones to lower neck
- Always evaluate/compare with opposite side as the tumors may be bilateral
- US is unable to evaluate other paragangliomas such as glomus vagale, glomus jugulare
- During real time scanning use gentle transducer pressure to prevent compression of vessels within tumor
- Angiography goals
  - Provide vascular road map for surgeon
  - Searches for multicentric tumors
  - Pre-operative embolization for prophylactic hemostasis
  - Evaluate collateral arterial & venous circulation of brain
    - Important knowledge if sacrifice of major vessel become necessary
- In familial patient group, screening CECT or MR beginning at 20 years old

DIFFERENTIAL DIAGNOSIS

Vagal Schwannoma/Neurofibroma

- Clinical: Sporadic or NF2 or NF1 associated
- Fusiform, hypoechoic mass in carotid space (+/- displacement of carotid bifurcation) in continuity with vagus nerve, +/- thickened vagus nerve
- May demonstrate well-defined cystic areas within tumor & posterior enhancement
- Prominent vascularity within mass, may disappear with transducer pressure

CAROTID BODY PARAGANGLIOMA

Metastatic Node
- Clinical: Asymptomatic "pulsatile mass", +/- known head & neck primary tumor
- On US: Hypoechoic/hyperechoic mass, +/- cystic necrosis, +/- punctate calcification, abnormal vascularity, pulsates against carotid bulb

2nd Brachial Cleft Cyst (BCC)
- Cystic mass closely related to carotid artery, submandibular gland, sternomastoid muscle
- Non infected/infected/hemorrhagic: Anechoic/"pseudosolid" pattern, thin/thick walls, internal debris, posterior enhancement, avascular/vascularity in wall

Carotid Bulb Ectasia
- Clinical: Older patient with atherosclerosis
- US shows an ectatic, thick walled, calcified carotid bulb; often bilateral involvement

PATHOLOGY

General Features
- Genetics
  - All paraganglioma occur in sporadic & familial form
    - Familial paraganglioma is autosomal dominant
- Etiology
  - Arise from Glomus bodies (paraganglia) in carotid body
    - Composed of chemoreceptor cells derived from primitive neural crest
    - Found in temporal bone, jugular foramen, upper carotid space & carotid bifurcation
- Epidemiology
  - CBP is most common location for head & neck paragangliomas (60-67% of total)
  - 2-10% of paragangliomas are multicentric in non-familial group
  - Familial incidence of multicentricity may reach 50-90%
  - Considerable more frequent in high altitudes (Peru, Mexico, Colorado)
- Associated abnormalities
  - Paragangliomas have tendency to occur multifocally
    - CBP may occur with jugulare or vagale paragangliomas
  - Thyroid carcinoma
  - Other visceral neoplasms
  - Familial MEN syndromes

Gross Pathologic & Surgical Features
- Lobulated, reddish-purple mass with fibrous pseudocapsule

Microscopic Features
- Chief cells & sustentacular cells are surrounded by a fibromuscular stroma
- Nests of chief cells are characteristic (zellballen)
- Electromicroscopy shows neurosecretory granules

CLINICAL ISSUES

Presentation
- Most common signs/symptoms
  - Pulsatile, painless angle of mandible mass
  - 20% have vagal ± hypoglossal neuropathy
  - Catecholamine-secreting CBP is rare
  - Other signs/symptoms
    - If tumor is functional, clinical picture may include paroxysmal hypertension, palpitations, flushing & irritability
- Clinical Profile: Slow growing painless angle of mandible mass

Demographics
- Age
  - Occur at all ages
  - Most common in 4th and 5th decade with a mean age 50 years

Natural History & Prognosis
- Surgical cure without lasting post-operative cranial neuropathy is expected in CBP < 5 cm
- Larger CBP (> 5 cm) may have surgical complications
  - Permanent vagal ± hypoglossal neuropathy

Treatment
- Surgical excision is treatment of choice
- Radiotherapy is used for lesion control in poor surgical candidates
- Malignant transformation is extremely rare

DIAGNOSTIC CHECKLIST

Consider
- US/CT/MR appearances are diagnostic

Image Interpretation Pearls
- When imaging diagnosis of CBP made, radiologist must look for 2nd lesion
  - Check jugular foramen (Glomus jugulare) & nasopharyngeal carotid space (glomus vagale): these are best evaluated by CT/MR

SELECTED REFERENCES

1. Alkadhi H et al: Evaluation of topography and vascularization of cervical paragangliomas by magnetic resonance imaging and color duplex sonography. Neuroradiology. 44(1):83-90, 2002
2. Persky MS et al: Combined endovascular and surgical treatment of head and neck paragangliomas--a team approach. Head Neck. 24(5):423-31, 2002
3. Stoeckli SJ et al: Evaluation of paragangliomas presenting as a cervical mass on color-coded Doppler sonography. Laryngoscope. 112(1):143-6, 2002
4. Mafee MF et al: Glomus faciale, glomus jugulare, glomus tympanicum, glomus vagale, carotid body tumors, and simulating lesions. Role of MR imaging. Radiol Clin North Am. 38(5):1059-76, 2000
5. Dobson MJ et al: MR angiography and MR imaging of symptomatic vascular malformations. Clin Radiol. 52(8):595-602, 1997
6. Jansen JC et al: Color Doppler imaging of paragangliomas in the neck. J Clin Ultrasound. 25(9):481-5, 1997

CAROTID BODY PARAGANGLIOMA

IMAGE GALLERY

Typical

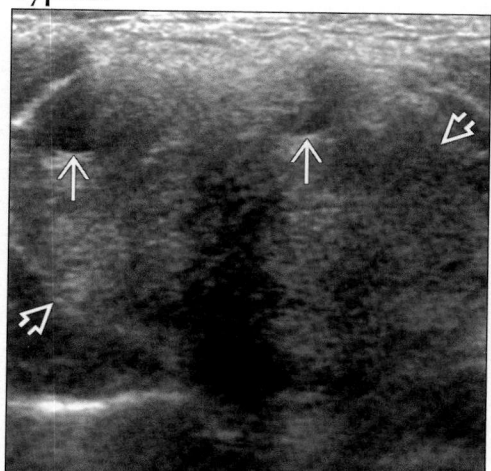
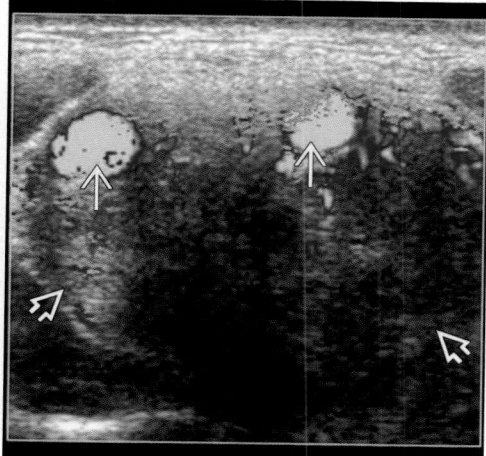

(Left) Transverse grayscale US shows a solid, well-defined, hypoechoic mass ⮞ insinuating between the carotid bifurcation ➡. This is the typical location of a CBP. *(Right)* Corresponding power Doppler clearly identifies the carotid bifurcation ➡ & its relationship to the CBP ⮞.

Typical

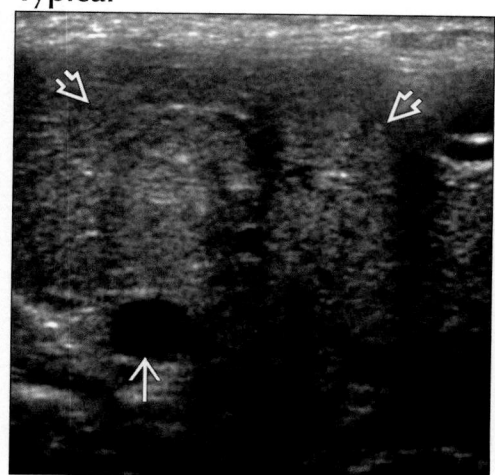
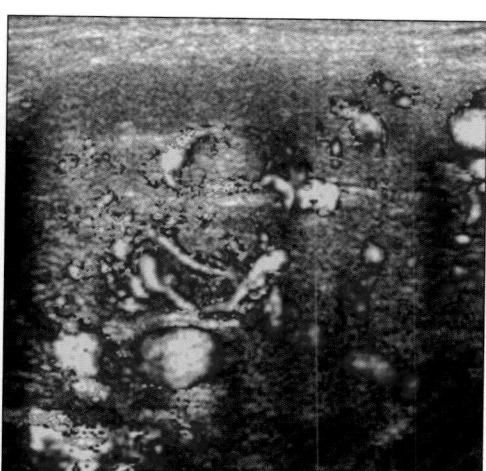

(Left) Grayscale US shows a large, hypoechoic, well-defined, non-calcified, homogeneous CBP ⮞ in close relation to the carotid artery ➡. *(Right)* Corresponding power Doppler US shows prominent vascularity in the tumor parenchyma & its relationship to the carotid vessels.

Typical

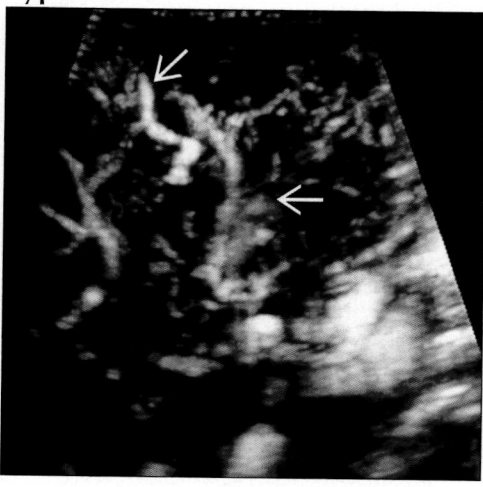
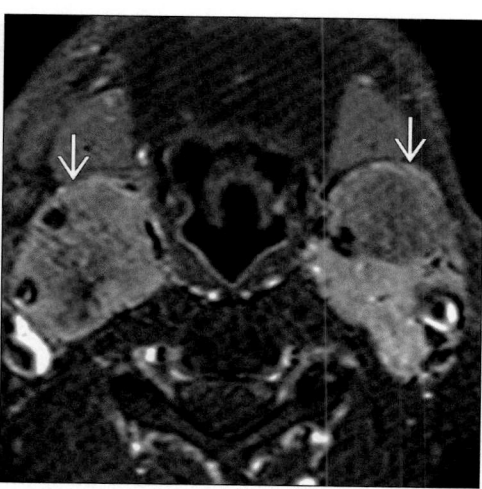

(Left) Color power angiogram shows multiple, large, tortuous tumor vessels ➡ in a mass at the carotid bifurcation. A similar mass was seen on the opposite side. *(Right)* Corresponding fat suppressed, contrast enhanced T1WI MR shows bilateral CBP ⮞ & their relationship to the carotid bifurcation (same patient as previous image).

THYROGLOSSAL DUCT CYST

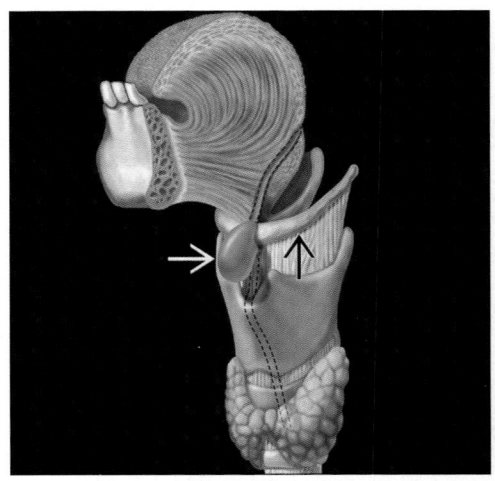

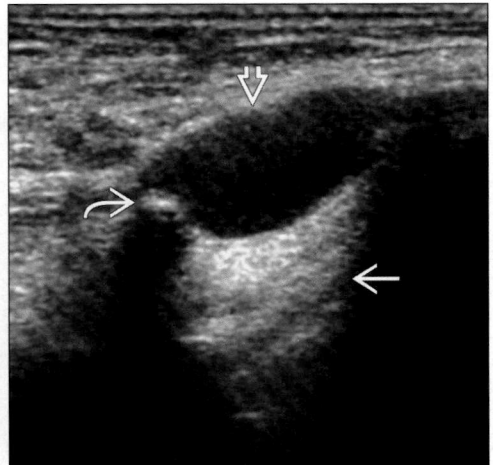

Graphic shows the course of the TGDC from the foramen cecum to the thyroid bed. Note the close relationship of the cyst ➡ to the hyoid bone ➡. A cyst may occur anywhere along the tract.

Longitudinal grayscale US shows a well-defined, anechoic, infrahyoid, TGDC ➡ with thin walls & posterior enhancement ➡. Note close relationship to the hyoid bone seen as echogenic shadowing focus ➡.

TERMINOLOGY

Abbreviations and Synonyms
- Thyroglossal duct cyst (TGDC)
- Thyroglossal duct remnant

Definitions
- TGDC: Remnant of thyroglossal duct found between foramen cecum of tongue base & thyroid bed in infrahyoid neck

IMAGING FINDINGS

General Features
- Best diagnostic clue: Midline cystic neck mass embedded in infrahyoid strap muscles ("claw sign")
- Location
  - 20-25% in suprahyoid neck
  - Almost 50% at hyoid bone
  - About 25% in infrahyoid neck
  - Most in suprahyoid neck are midline
  - May be paramedian in infrahyoid neck
- Size: Usually between 2-4 cm, but may be smaller

- Morphology: Round or ovoid cyst

Ultrasonographic Findings
- Relationship of cyst to hyoid bone and its location along the expected course from foramen cecum to thyroid bed is first clue to its diagnosis
- Non-hemorrhagic/uninfected TGDC
  - If no hemorrhage/infection: Unilocular, well-defined, anechoic cyst with posterior enhancement, faint internal debris
  - No evidence of mural nodule/mass or calcification
  - If no hemorrhage/infection: "Pseudosolid" appearance: Well-defined cyst with uniform, homogeneous internal echoes due to proteinaceous content secreted by lining
  - Clue to cystic nature of a "pseudosolid" TGDC is
    - Posterior acoustic enhancement, swirling motion of debris within cyst after applying intermittent transducer pressure or increasing power on Doppler; this swirling motion is evaluated only in real time and not on static images
  - Color Doppler: No vascularity seen within cyst if uninfected
- Hemorrhagic/infected TGDC

DDx: Thyroglossal Duct Cyst

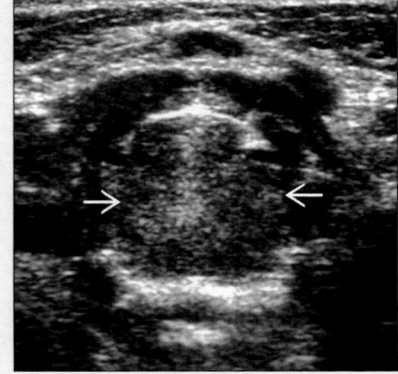

Sublingual Thyroid

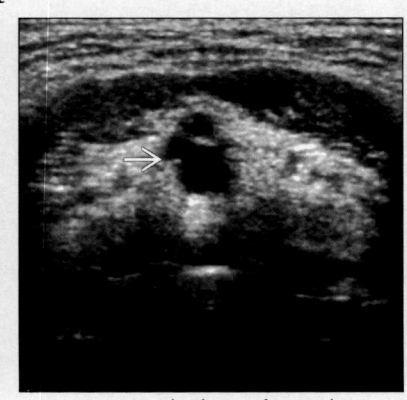

Dermoid, Floor of Mouth

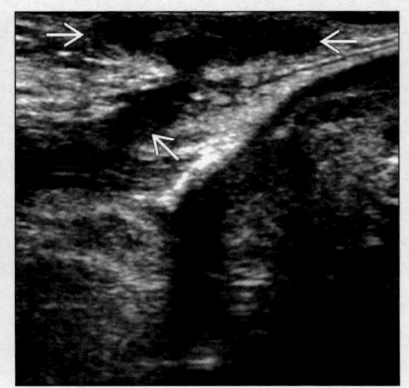

Subcutaneous Abscess

THYROGLOSSAL DUCT CYST

Key Facts

Imaging Findings

- If no hemorrhage/infection: Unilocular, well-defined, anechoic cyst with posterior enhancement, faint internal debris
- No evidence of mural nodule/mass or calcification
- If no hemorrhage/infection: "Pseudosolid" appearance: Well-defined cyst with uniform, homogeneous internal echoes due to proteinaceous content secreted by lining
- Color Doppler: No vascularity seen within cyst if uninfected
- If hemorrhage/infection: Ill-defined, thick walls, internal debris, septa & inflammatory changes in soft tissues
- Color Doppler shows no vascularity within intracystic blood clots; infected walls and septa may show vascularity
- Thyroid carcinoma can develop in a TGDC (1% in adults) and these appear as vascular solid nodules within cyst, +/- calcification
- Ultrasound-guided fine needle aspiration cytology (FNAC) is recommended in presence of solid nodule within TGDC
- Nuclear scintigraphy only if unable to identify normal thyroid gland

Top Differential Diagnoses

- Lingual or Sublingual Thyroid
- Dermoid or Epidermoid at Floor of Mouth
- Submandibular or Sublingual Space or Subcutaneous Abscess

- If hemorrhage/infection: Ill-defined, thick walls, internal debris, septa & inflammatory changes in soft tissues
- Color Doppler shows no vascularity within intracystic blood clots; infected walls and septa may show vascularity
- Thyroid carcinoma can develop in a TGDC (1% in adults) and these appear as vascular solid nodules within cyst, +/- calcification
- Ultrasound-guided fine needle aspiration cytology (FNAC) is recommended in presence of solid nodule within TGDC

CT Findings

- NECT: Low density (cystic) midline neck mass
- CECT
  - Benign-appearing, cystic neck mass
  - Low density mass, occasionally septated
  - Cystic midline neck mass with thin rim of peripheral enhancement
    - Wall may enhance if infected
  - Suprahyoid TGDC: Occurs at base of tongue or within posterior floor of mouth
  - At level of hyoid bone, found in midline abutting hyoid
    - May project into pre-epiglottic space
    - Usually anterior or ventral to hyoid bone
  - Infrahyoid TGDC: Embedded in strap muscles
    - The more inferior the TGDC, the more paramedian
  - If associated thyroid carcinoma, solid eccentric mass, often with calcification within cyst

MR Findings

- T1WI
  - Cyst usually with decreased signal intensity
  - May be hyperintense if filled with proteinaceous secretions
- T2WI: Homogeneously hyperintense
- T1 C+
  - Nonenhancing cyst is norm
  - Rim-enhancement if infected

Imaging Recommendations

- Best imaging tool
  - TGDCs are diagnosed clinically and role of imaging is to
    - Confirm diagnosis
    - Assess its relation to hyoid bone
    - Identify presence/absence of suspicious thyroid carcinoma
    - Evaluate presence of normal thyroid tissue in thyroid bed
  - US is the ideal imaging modality as it readily provides appropriate preoperative information
- Protocol advice
  - Scans in longitudinal plane clearly evaluate the relation of TGDC to hyoid bone
  - Scans in transverse plane identify cyst embedded within strap muscles, any pre-epiglottic component and presence of normal thyroid tissue in thyroid bed
- Nuclear scintigraphy only if unable to identify normal thyroid gland

DIFFERENTIAL DIAGNOSIS

Lingual or Sublingual Thyroid

- Identify normal thyroid tissue in ectopic location; empty thyroid bed
- Well-defined nodule with fine bright parenchymal echo pattern with vascularity within, +/- changes of nodular hyperplasia

Dermoid or Epidermoid at Floor of Mouth

- Neither directly involves hyoid bone; well-defined cystic mass, anechoic, +/- pseudosolid pattern, moves independently of the tongue

Submandibular or Sublingual Space or Subcutaneous Abscess

- Not embedded in strap muscles; ill-defined, thick walls with septa, internal debris, vascularity in inflamed walls and adjacent soft tissues

THYROGLOSSAL DUCT CYST

Malignant Delphian Chain Necrotic Node

- May be difficult to differentiate necrotic node from infected TGDC, not embedded in strap muscle

PATHOLOGY

General Features

- General path comments
  - Embryology-anatomy
    - Thyroglossal duct (TGD) originates near foramen cecum, at posterior third of tongue
    - Thyroid anlage arises at base of tongue, then descends to final location (thyroid bed) along TGD
    - Descends through base of tongue, floor of mouth, around or through hyoid bone, anterior to strap muscles, to final position in thyroid bed anterior to thyroid or cricoid cartilage
    - At 5-6 gestational weeks, TGD involutes, with foramen cecum & pyramidal thyroid lobe normal remnants
    - Failure of involution, with persistent secretory activity, results in TGDC
- Genetics
  - Familial cases occur (rare); usually autosomal dominant
  - Thyroid developmental anomalies often occur in same family
- Etiology
  - Failure of involution of TGD & persistent secretion of epithelial cells lining duct result in TGDC
  - TGDC can occur anywhere along route of descent of TGD
  - Ectopic thyroid tissue can also occur anywhere along this course
- Epidemiology
  - Most common congenital neck lesion
    - 90% of non-odontogenic congenital cysts
    - 3 times as common as branchial cleft cysts
  - At autopsy, > 7% of population will have TGD remnant somewhere along course of tract
  - < 1% TGDC have associated thyroid carcinoma
- Associated abnormalities
  - Thyroid agenesis, ectopia, pyramidal lobe
  - Occasionally associated with carcinoma
    - Most commonly papillary carcinoma of the TGD

Gross Pathologic & Surgical Features

- Smooth, benign-appearing cyst, with tract to hyoid bone ± foramen cecum

Microscopic Features

- Cyst lined by respiratory or squamous epithelium
- Small deposits of thyroid tissue with colloid commonly associated

CLINICAL ISSUES

Presentation

- Most common signs/symptoms
  - Midline or paramedian doughy, compressible painless neck mass in child or young adult
  - Other signs/symptoms
    - Recurrent appearance of midline neck mass with upper respiratory tract infections or trauma
  - Physical examination
    - If TGDC around hyoid bone, cyst elevates when tongue is protruded

Demographics

- Age
  - Age of presentation
    - < 10 years (90%), 10% are 20-35 years
- Gender: M < F if hereditary form

Natural History & Prognosis

- Recurrent, intermittent swelling of mass, usually following a minor upper respiratory infection
- Rapid enlarging mass suggests either infection or associated differentiated thyroid carcinoma
  - Carcinoma is associated with TGDC (< 1%)
  - Differentiated thyroid Ca (85% papillary carcinoma)

Treatment

- Complete surgical resection, termed a "Sistrunk procedure"
  - Entire cyst & midline portion of hyoid bone is resected
  - Tract to foramen cecum dissected free, to prevent recurrence
  - Sistrunk procedure is treatment of choice
    - Even if imaging shows no obvious connection to hyoid bone
    - Exception is low infrahyoid neck TGDC
- Sistrunk procedure decreases recurrence rate from 50% to < 4%
- Prognosis is excellent with complete surgical resection

DIAGNOSTIC CHECKLIST

Consider

- Relationship to hyoid bone important to note: Suprahyoid, hyoid or infrahyoid in location
- Any associated nodularity or chunky calcification suggests associated thyroid carcinoma
- Thyroid bed should be imaged, to be sure there is a thyroid gland present

SELECTED REFERENCES

1. Harnsberger HR et al: Diagnostic Imaging Head & Neck. 1st ed. Salt Lake City, Amirsys. IV-1-22-25, 2004
2. Ahuja et al: Sonographic evaluation of thyroglossal duct cysts in children. Clin Radiol. 55;770-4, 2000
3. Glastonbury CM et al: The CT and MR imaging features of carcinoma arising in thyroglossal duct remnants. AJNR Am J Neuroradiol. 21(4):770-4, 2000
4. Ahuja AT et al: Thyroglossal duct cysts: sonographic appearances in adults. AJNR Am J Neuroradiol. 20:579-82, 1999
5. Reede DL et al: CT of thyroglossal duct cysts. Radiology. 157:121-5, 1985

LIPOMA

Typical

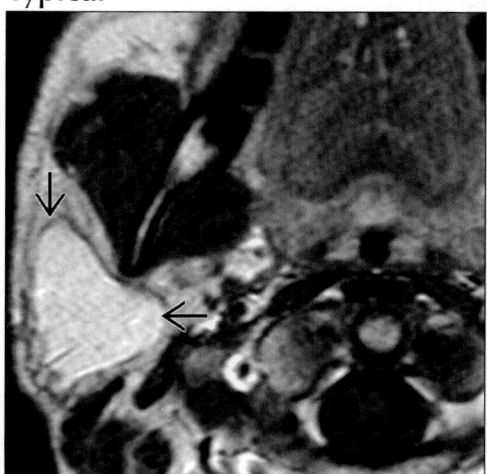 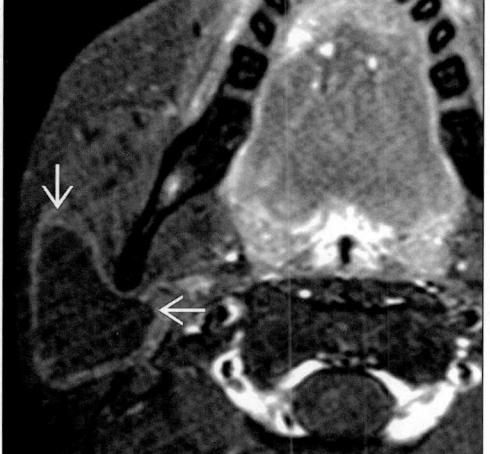

(Left) Axial T1WI MR shows a well-circumscribed, hyperintense mass ⟹ in the right parotid. Note the absence of soft tissue stranding & nodularity; typical appearance of a benign lipoma. (Right) Corresponding axial T1WI MR with fat saturation shows complete signal suppression in the lipoma ⟹, similar to subcutaneous fat. MR is better than US in showing entire extent of large lipomas.

Typical

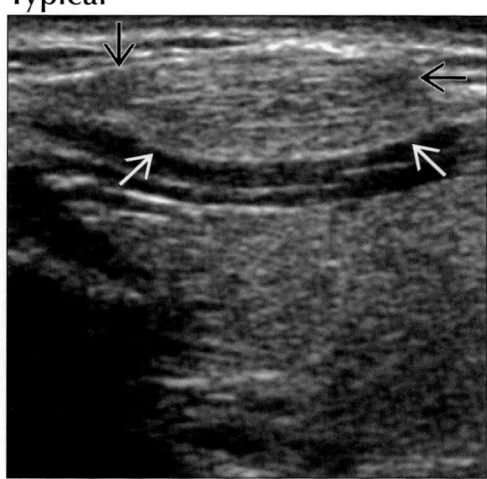 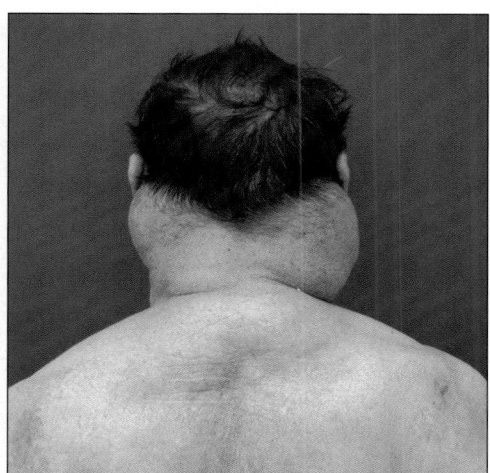

(Left) Grayscale US shows a well-defined, hyperechoic benign lipoma ⟹ with bright echogenic lines within it. Note its mass effect on the strap muscles ⟹ but no infiltration, nodularity or stranding. (Right) Clinical photograph of a patient with Madelung disease (BSL). Note diffuse fatty accumulation involving the cervical & dorsal regions. US identifies unencapsulated fat but cannot delineate extent.

Typical

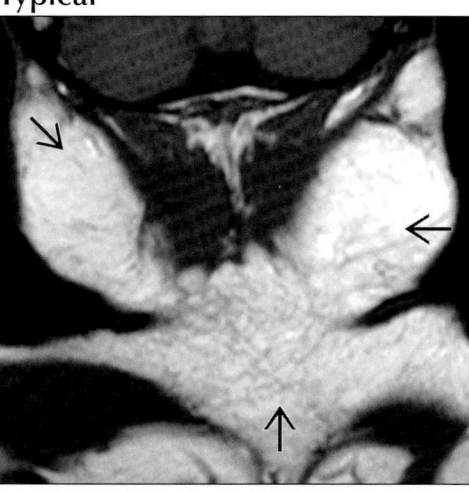 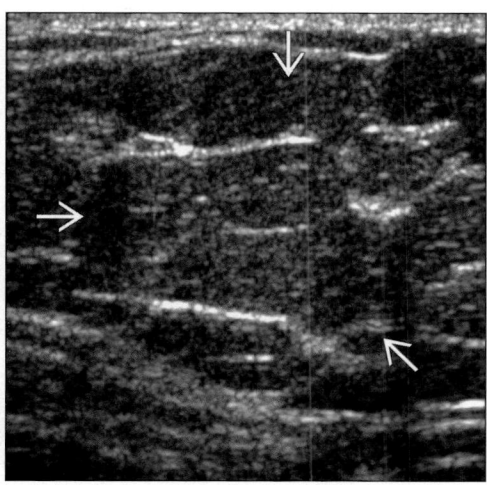

(Left) Coronal T1WI MR shows a diffuse, symmetric, unencapsulated fatty accumulation ⟹ in the cervical & upper dorsal regions in BSL. US is unable to define extent of fat deposition & underlying neck lesion if any. (Right) Corresponding grayscale US shows a lobular, diffuse infiltration of fat ⟹ in the soft tissues of neck. As fat deposition in BSL is diffuse and unencapsulated, US is unable to define exact extent.

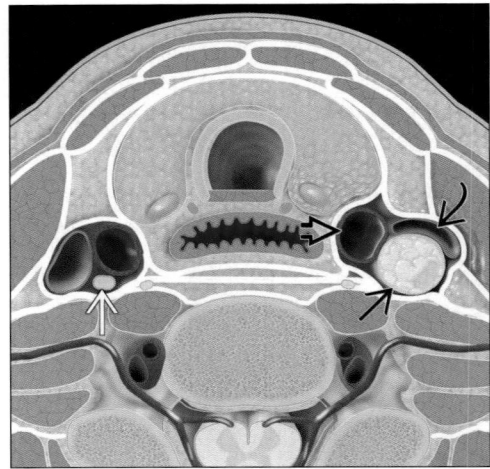

Transverse graphic shows the relationship of a vagal schwannoma ⇒ to the CCA ⊳ & IJV ⇒. Compare with the normal vagus nerve ➡ on contralateral side. US can clearly delineate these structures.

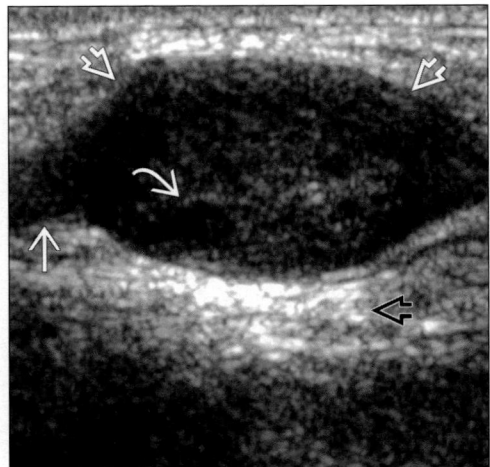

Longitudinal grayscale US shows a well-defined, solid mass ➡ with focal cystic area ➡ & posterior enhancement ⊳. Note its continuity with the adjacent nerve ➡. Findings typical of a nerve sheath tumor.

TERMINOLOGY

Abbreviations and Synonyms
- Neuroma; neurilemmoma

Definitions
- Benign tumor of Schwann cells that wrap around vagus nerve in carotid space (CS)

IMAGING FINDINGS

General Features
- Size
  - Lesions are usually large when clinically detected
  - 2-8 cm range
- Morphology
  - Ovoid to fusiform
  - Tumor margins are smooth, sharply-circumscribed
- In infrahyoid neck, mass displaces thyroid & trachea to contralateral side, common carotid artery (CCA) anteromedially

Ultrasonographic Findings
- Ultrasound is able to evaluate/visualize nerve sheath tumors only in infrahyoid neck, vagal nerve schwannoma being most common
- Vagal nerve schwannomas are often fusiform in shape/oval with tapering ends
- Schwannomas are hypoechoic with heterogeneous echo pattern & often show posterior enhancement (despite being solid)
- Sharply defined focal cystic areas may be seen within schwannomas
- Continuity with nerve/thickening of adjacent nerve - diagnostic
- Color Doppler shows increased vascularity within tumor, prominent tortuous vessels
- Vascularity is sensitive to pressure & may "disappear" with increasing transducer pressure
- Mass effect with flattening/occlusion of jugular vein

CT Findings
- NECT
  - Well-circumscribed CS soft tissue density mass
  - Mass density similar to adjacent neck muscles
- CECT

DDx: Vagus Schwannoma, Infrahyoid Carotid Space

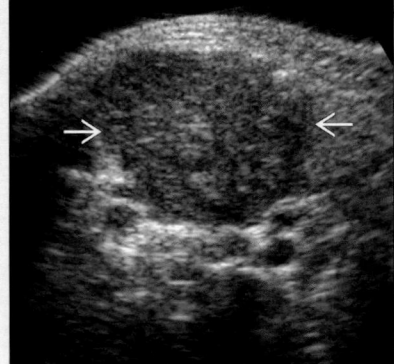

Carotid Body Paraganglioma

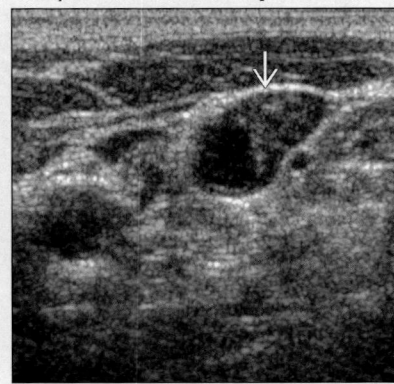

Malignant Lymph Node

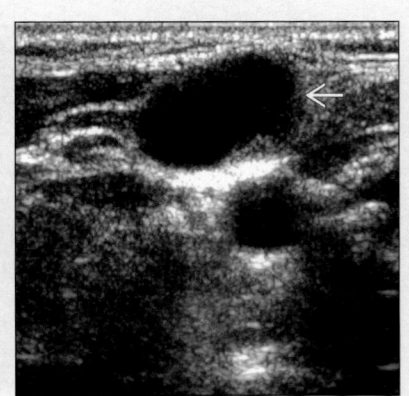

2nd Branchial Cleft Cyst

VAGUS SCHWANNOMA, INFRAHYOID CAROTID SPACE

Key Facts

Imaging Findings
- Ultrasound is able to evaluate/visualize nerve sheath tumors only in infrahyoid neck, vagal nerve schwannoma being most common
- Vagal nerve schwannomas are often fusiform in shape/oval with tapering ends
- Schwannomas are hypoechoic with heterogeneous echo pattern & often show posterior enhancement (despite being solid)
- Sharply defined focal cystic areas may be seen within schwannomas
- Continuity with nerve/thickening of adjacent nerve - diagnostic
- Color Doppler shows increased vascularity within tumor, prominent tortuous vessels

- Vascularity is sensitive to pressure & may "disappear" with increasing transducer pressure
- Mass effect with flattening/occlusion of jugular vein
- Neurofibromas may be lobulated, do not show posterior enhancement & show less vascularity compared to schwannomas
- Aspiration cytology/biopsy triggers excruciating pain (considered diagnostic by some); important to recognize nature of these lesions to prevent biopsy
- Transverse scans identify tumor & longitudinal scans evaluate continuity/nerve thickening

Top Differential Diagnoses
- Carotid Body Paraganglioma
- Malignant Lymph Node
- 2nd Branchial Cleft Cyst

- Uniform enhancement is rule on CECT
  - Minority are low density even with enhancement
- Focal areas of absent enhancement seen on CECT if intramural cystic change present

MR Findings
- T1WI
  - Variable T1 signal ranging from low to high
  - No high velocity flow voids even when large
- T2WI
  - Tumor signal higher than muscle
  - Intramural cysts, if present, are high signal foci within tumor
- T1 C+
  - Dense uniform enhancement is typical
  - Intratumoral cysts/nonenhancing cysts often present in larger lesions

Angiographic Findings
- Angiography is usually unnecessary unless tumor histopathology in doubt
- Scattered contrast "puddles" typical of schwannoma
- No dominant feeding arteries seen; no arteriovenous shunting or vascular encasement is seen

Imaging Recommendations
- Best imaging tool
  - Ultrasound is ideal imaging modality for infrahyoid schwannomas as it adequately demonstrates tumor & adjacent relations
  - Ultrasound is unable to distinguish schwannomas from neurofibromas
    - Neurofibromas may be lobulated, do not show posterior enhancement & show less vascularity compared to schwannomas
  - Aspiration cytology/biopsy triggers excruciating pain (considered diagnostic by some); important to recognize nature of these lesions to prevent biopsy
- Protocol advice
  - Location of tumor in close proximity of carotid & internal jugular vein (IJV) is a clue to its diagnosis

- Normal vagus nerve is always seen with high-resolution transducers, therefore compare with contralateral side
- Transverse scans along carotid artery/internal jugular vein readily identify vagus nerve
- Vagus nerve typically shows a "fibrillar" pattern on high-resolution US with bright streaks within
- Transverse scans identify tumor & longitudinal scans evaluate continuity/nerve thickening
- Apply gentle transducer pressure as intra-tumoral vessels are very sensitive to pressure
- FNAC/biopsy is painful, therefore recognize nature of lesion to prevent biopsy
- CECT or MR can be used to confirm this diagnosis & evaluate anatomical extent of large tumors

DIFFERENTIAL DIAGNOSIS

Carotid Body Paraganglioma
- Mass center: Nestled in common carotid artery bifurcation with splaying of ICA, ECA
- Bilateral with prominent intratumoral vessels; solid, hypoechoic, well defined with no posterior enhancement

Malignant Lymph Node
- History of known head & neck primary tumor
- Hypoechoic, heterogeneous, well-defined mass with peripheral vascularity, +/- intranodal necrosis, +/- multiple

2nd Branchial Cleft Cyst
- Location in relation to carotid, submandibular gland & sternomastoid is key
- Anechoic, thin walled with posterior enhancement/pseudosolid/heterogeneous mass; avascular +/- vessels in wall if infected

Internal Jugular Vein Thrombosis
- History of IJV instrumentation usually present
- Non-compressible IJV with heterogeneous echoes within; vascularity in thrombus if tumor thrombus

VAGUS SCHWANNOMA, INFRAHYOID CAROTID SPACE

Carotid Artery Pseudoaneurysm, Neck
- Ovoid outpouching of carotid artery; Doppler identifies the connection with carotid artery & demonstrates abnormal flow
- Well-defined, thin walled anechoic structure +/- flow within

PATHOLOGY

General Features
- Etiology
  - Arises from Schwann cells wrapping around cranial nerve in carotid space of extracranial H&N
  - Nerve of origin
    - Infrahyoid carotid space to aortic arch: Vagus nerve
- Epidemiology
  - Rare tumor of extracranial H&N
  - Suprahyoid CS schwannoma > > infrahyoid CS schwannoma
- Associated abnormalities: Neurofibromatosis type 2

Gross Pathologic & Surgical Features
- White-tan, smooth, encapsulated, sausage-shaped mass

Microscopic Features
- Differentiated neoplastic Schwann cells
  - Malignant transformation is exceedingly rare
  - Melanotic malignant schwannomas have been described as distinct entity
- Spindle cells with elongated nuclei
  - Alternating areas of organized, compact cells (Antoni A) & loosely arranged, relatively acellular tissue (Antoni B)
  - Both cell types present in all tumors
- Immunochemistry
  - Strong, diffuse, immuno-staining for S-100 protein
    - S-100 protein = neural-crest marker antigen present in supporting cell of nervous system

CLINICAL ISSUES

Presentation
- Most common signs/symptoms
  - Asymptomatic palpable mass
    - Vagus nerve schwannoma: Anterolateral neck mass
  - Vagus nerve schwannomas may present with
    - Dysphagia, dysphonia
    - Hoarseness, arrhythmia
    - Pain occurs with large tumors
- Clinical Profile: Healthy 45 year old male with asymptomatic infrahyoid lateral neck mass

Demographics
- Age
  - Age range: 18-63 years
  - Average age at presentation = 45 years
- Gender: Male predominance

Natural History & Prognosis
- Delay in diagnosis is frequent, due to nonspecific symptoms
- Slow but persistent tumor growth until airway compromise or cosmetic issues supervene
- Vagus nerve preservation is not always possible at surgery
  - If vagus nerve resection required, partial vagal neuropathy present even if successful reconnection completed

Treatment
- Gross total resection without sacrifice of vagus nerve is treatment of choice
  - Enucleation of tumor with CN10 preservation possible in most cases
  - Infrequently nerve resection occurs at time of tumor removal
    - End-to-end anastomosis of vagus nerve used if short segment removed
    - Nerve graft interposition used if long segment vagus nerve is removed
  - Severe transient bradycardia may occur during removal

DIAGNOSTIC CHECKLIST

Image Interpretation Pearls
- Fusiform, sharply circumscribed, solid CS mass with posterior enhancement, sharp cystic spaces & vascularity within, in continuity with thickened vagus nerve suggests vagus nerve schwannoma

SELECTED REFERENCES
1. Harnsberger HR et al: Diagnostic Imaging Head & Neck. 1st ed. Salt Lake City, Amirsys. III-8-24-27, 2004
2. Evans RM et al: Imaging in Head and Neck Cancer: A Practical Approach. London, Greenwich Medical Media. 199-214, 2003
3. Leu YS et al: Extracranial head and neck schwannomas: a review of 8 years experience. Acta Otolaryngol. 122(4):435-7, 2002
4. Colreavy MP et al: Head and neck schwannomas--a 10 year review. J Laryngol Otol. 114(2):119-24, 2000
5. Gilmer-Hill HS et al: Neurogenic tumors of the cervical vagus nerve: report of four cases and review of the literature. Neurosurgery. 46(6):1498-503, 2000
6. King AD et al: Sonography of peripheral nerve tumours of the neck. AJR. 169:1695-8, 1997
7. Yumoto E et al: Parapharyngeal vagal neurilemmoma extending to the jugular foramen. J Laryngol Otol. 110(5):485-9, 1996
8. Park CS et al: Neurilemmomas of the cervical vagus nerve. Head Neck. 13(5):439-41, 1991
9. Heitmiller RF et al: Vagal schwannoma. Ann Thorac Surg. 50(5):811-3, 1990
10. Silver AJ et al: Computed tomography of the carotid space and related cervical spaces. Part II: Neurogenic tumors. Radiology. 150(3):729-35, 1984

VAGUS SCHWANNOMA, INFRAHYOID CAROTID SPACE

Typical

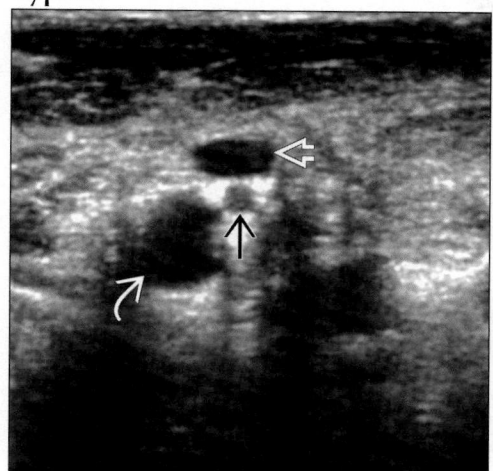
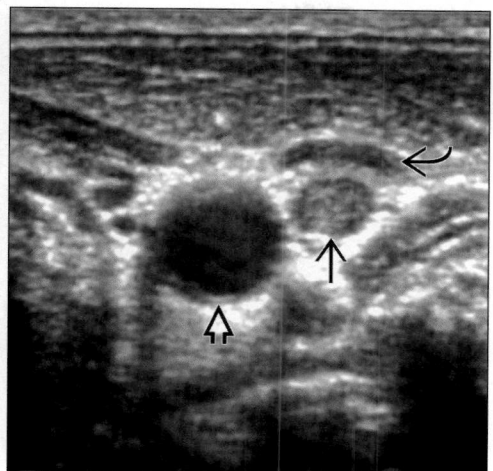

(Left) Transverse grayscale US shows a normal vagus nerve ➡ & its relationship to the CCA ➡ and IJV ➡. A normal vagus nerve is always seen on high-resolution US. *(Right)* Transverse grayscale US shows a vagal schwannoma ➡ & its relationship to the CCA ➡ & IJV ➡. Note the mass effect on the IJV. High-resolution US is ideal for demonstrating such nerve sheath tumors.

Typical

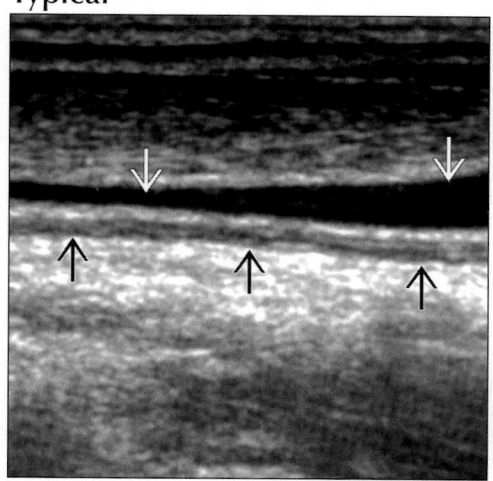
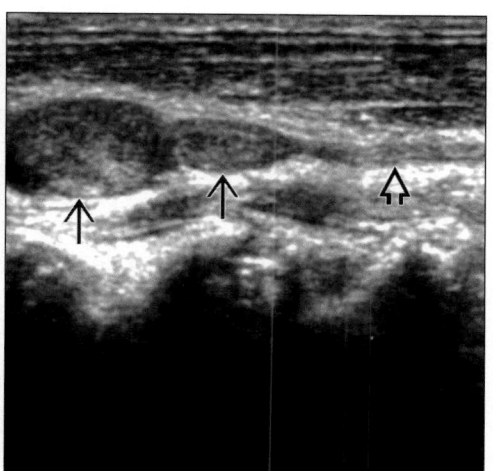

(Left) Longitudinal grayscale US shows a normal vagus nerve ➡ with its fibrillary pattern. Note its relationship to IJV the ➡. Longitudinal US allows the visualization of the length of the nerve & its internal pattern. *(Right)* Longitudinal grayscale US shows multiple small nerve sheath tumors ➡ in continuity with the vagus nerve ➡. Note US clearly demonstrates the nature of the mass and prevents a painful biopsy.

Typical

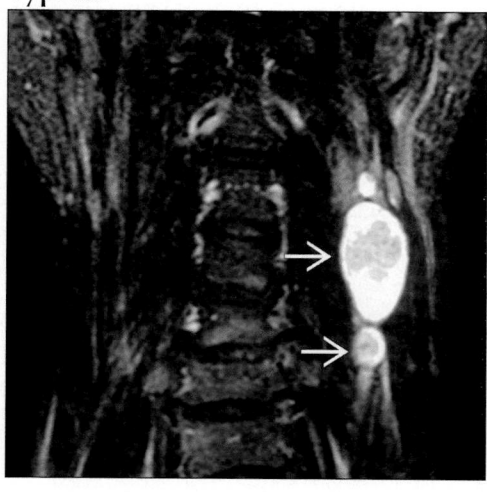
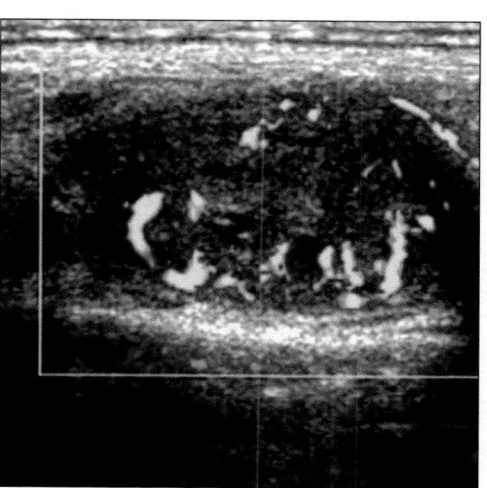

(Left) Coronal fat-suppressed T2WI MR shows multiple, fusiform vagal schwannomas ➡. Same patient as previous image. *(Right)* Power Doppler shows prominent vessels within a vagal schwannoma. Note, the vessels are sensitive to pressure & may disappear with increasing transducer pressure.

BRACHIAL PLEXUS SCHWANNOMA

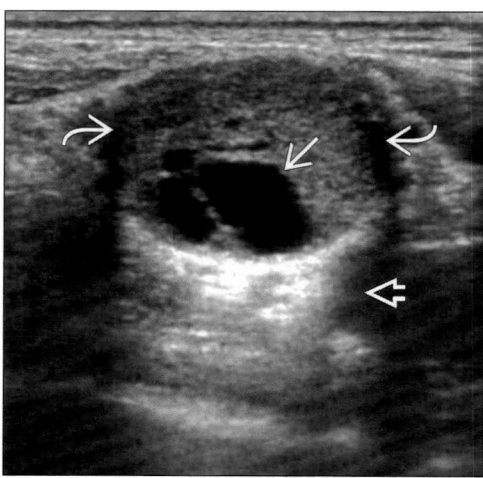

Grayscale US demonstrates a well-defined, hypoechoic mass ➡ with sharp cystic areas ➡ & posterior enhancement ⏩. Typical findings of nerve sheath tumor; location suggested BP schwannoma.

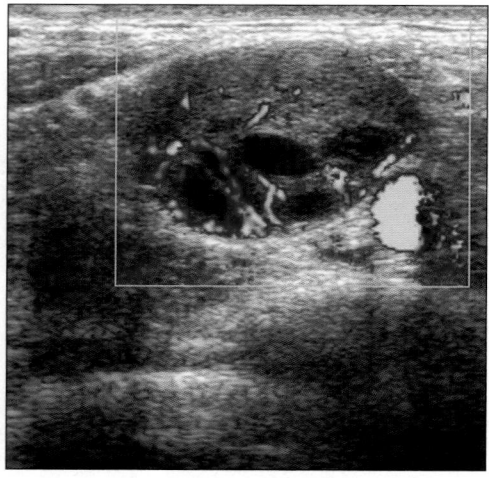

Corresponding color Doppler (CD) shows prominent vascularity within the tumor. Grayscale/CD appearance & location between the anterior & middle scalene muscles is typical of a BP schwannoma.

TERMINOLOGY

Definitions
- Benign neoplasm of Schwann cells that wrap brachial plexus (BP) nerves in perivertebral space (PVS)

IMAGING FINDINGS

General Features
- Best diagnostic clue: Well-circumscribed, fusiform, hypoechoic mass, +/- intratumoral cystic spaces, vascularity & in continuity with brachial plexus between anterior & middle scalene muscles in posterior cervical space
- Location
  ○ May arise anywhere along course of BP including intra- & extradural spaces, neural foramen, PVS, posterior cervical space to axillary apex
  ○ Lesions within PVS are situated between anterior & middle scalene muscles
  ○ Ultrasound is only able to fully evaluate lesions in posterior cervical space/lateral neck

Ultrasonographic Findings
- Fusiform/oval shape +/- tapering ends, +/- sharply defined cystic/hemorrhagic areas within
- Hypoechoic, well-defined with heterogeneous echo pattern & posterior enhancement (despite being solid)
- In continuity with brachial plexus trunks, divisions
- Color Doppler shows prominent vascularity within, +/- mass effect on adjacent vessels

CT Findings
- NECT
  ○ Typically isodense to muscle
  ○ Calcification is uncommon
- CECT: Moderate to strong enhancement

MR Findings
- T1WI: Isointense to muscle
- T2WI
  ○ Hyperintense, approaching signal of regional vessels
  ○ "Target" sign: Central hypo-, peripheral hyperintense signal commonly seen in benign peripheral nerve sheath tumor (PNST)
  ○ "Fascicular" sign: Multiple, irregular, central hypointense foci typical of benign PNST

DDx: Brachial Plexus Schwannoma

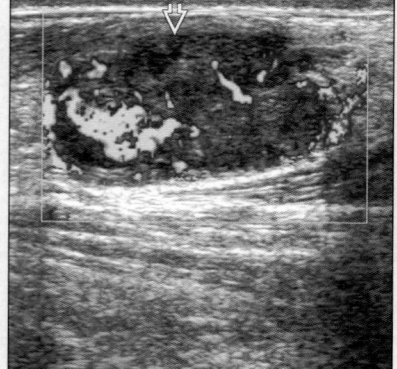

Metastatic Node

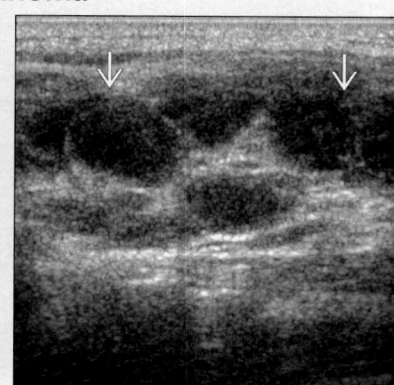

Tuberculous Lymph Node

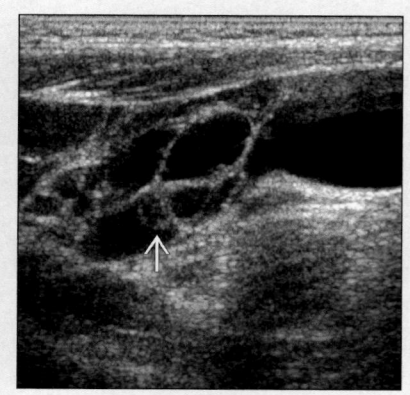

Lymphangioma

BRACHIAL PLEXUS SCHWANNOMA

Key Facts

Imaging Findings

- Best diagnostic clue: Well-circumscribed, fusiform, hypoechoic mass, +/- intratumoral cystic spaces, vascularity & in continuity with brachial plexus between anterior & middle scalene muscles in posterior cervical space
- Ultrasound is only able to fully evaluate lesions in posterior cervical space/lateral neck

- Fusiform/oval shape +/- tapering ends, +/- sharply defined cystic/hemorrhagic areas within
- Hypoechoic, well-defined with heterogeneous echo pattern & posterior enhancement (despite being solid)
- In continuity with brachial plexus trunks, divisions
- Color Doppler shows prominent vascularity within, +/- mass effect on adjacent vessels

---

- T1 C+: "Reverse target" sign: Central enhancement > peripheral enhancement

Imaging Recommendations

- Best imaging tool
  - High-resolution US clearly identifies nature of lesion in lateral neck but is unable to delineate proximal & distal extent of large lesions
  - MR confirms extent of large PNST after US has made the diagnosis
- Protocol advice
  - Transverse scans clearly identify normal brachial plexus trunks as three round, hypoechoic structures between anterior and middle scalene
  - Longitudinal scans identify trunks & divisions along their course
  - Transverse scans help to quickly identify the tumor & longitudinal scans, their continuity with trunks, divisions
  - Intratumoral vascularity is sensitive to pressure, so hold transducer gently
  - Pressure/manipulating the mass with transducer may cause symptoms of radiculopathy

DIFFERENTIAL DIAGNOSIS

Neurofibroma

- May be indistinguishable from schwannoma; cystic degeneration, hemorrhage uncommon; less vascular & show no posterior enhancement

Metastatic Nodes

- Multiple, heterogeneous, hypoechoic, round nodes with necrosis, peripheral vascularity, known primary

Tuberculous Nodes

- Multiple, matted, necrotic nodes with adjacent soft tissue edema; avascular/displaced vascularity within

Lymphangioma

- Transpatial, cystic, septated, avascular mass with negligible mass effect

CLINICAL ISSUES

Presentation

- Most common signs/symptoms: Painless, slow growing mass in lateral neck ± radiculopathy; malignant degeneration rare

Treatment

- Surgical excision

SELECTED REFERENCES

1. Harnsberger HR et al: Diagnostic Imaging Head & Neck. 1st ed. Salt Lake City, Amirsys. III-10-14-15, 2004
2. King AD et al: Sonography of peripheral nerve tumors of the neck. AJR. 169:1695-8, 1997

IMAGE GALLERY

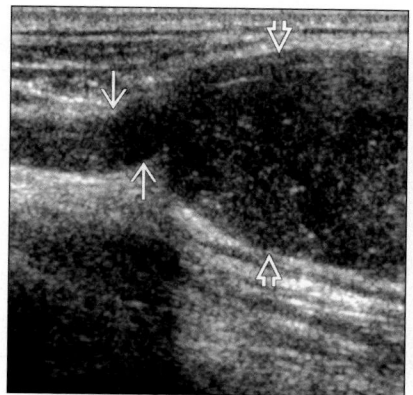
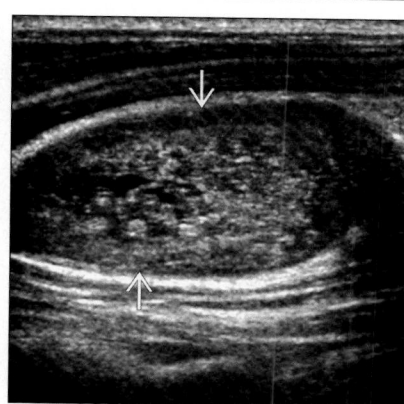
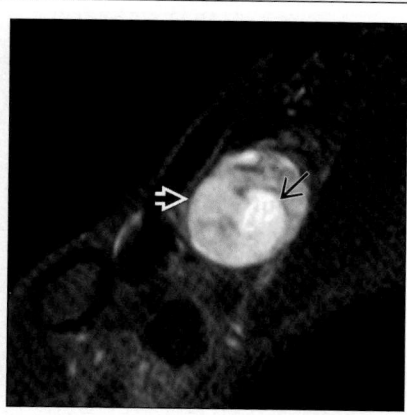

(Left) Longitudinal grayscale US of a BP schwannoma ➡. Note its continuity with the BP trunk ➡. High-resolution US consistently demonstrates such continuity & internal echo pattern. *(Center)* US shows a well-defined, oval, hypoechoic BP schwannoma ➡, with focal areas of cystic/hemorrhagic change. *(Right)* Sagittal T2WI FS MR shows a hyperintense BP schwannoma ➡ with an area of cystic necrosis ➡. MR is useful in evaluating full extent of large lesions, which are not amenable to US.

VENOUS VASCULAR MALFORMATION

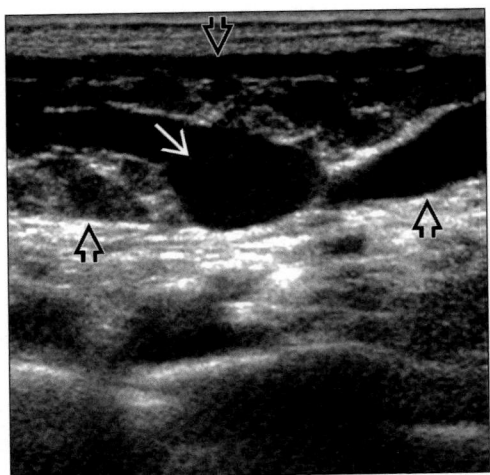

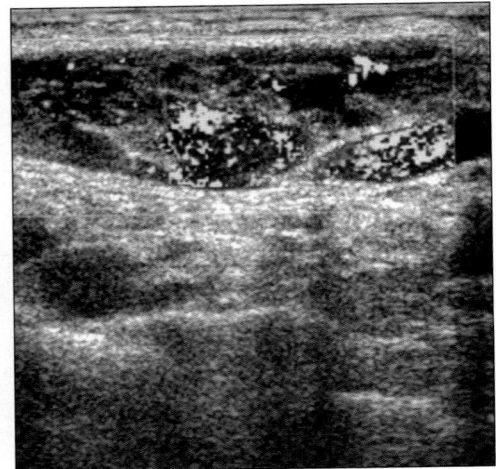

Grayscale US shows multiple, hypoechoic, serpigeneous sinusoidal spaces in a superficial mass ⊳. Note the faint internal echoes ➡. These often show slow "to & fro" movement on real time US.

Corresponding power Doppler shows flow within the sinusoidal/vascular spaces. Flow is usually slow, so use a low wall filter & PRF to increase sensitivity. Hold the transducer gently over the lesion.

TERMINOLOGY

Abbreviations and Synonyms
- Venous vascular malformation (VVM)
- Cavernous malformation, cavernous hemangioma (this latter term should be avoided)

Definitions
- Slow-flow post-capillary lesion composed of endothelial-lined vascular sinusoids

IMAGING FINDINGS

General Features
- Best diagnostic clue: Lobulated soft tissue "mass" with phleboliths
- Location
  - Most commonly in buccal region
  - Masticator space, sublingual space, tongue, orbit & dorsal neck are other common locations
  - May be superficial or deep, diffuse or localized
- Size: Variable, may be very large
- Morphology
  - Multilobulated; solitary or multiple
  - May be circumscribed or trans-spatial, infiltrating adjacent soft tissue compartments

Ultrasonographic Findings
- Soft compressible mass with multiple serpigeneous sinusoidal spaces within
- Mass and sinusoidal spaces increase in size on Valsalva, crying & in dependent position
- Slow moving debris ("to & fro") on real time US within dilated channels suggestive of vascular flow
- Hypoechoic with heterogeneous echo pattern
  - Lesions with small vascular channels are more echogenic & less compressible than lesions with large vascular lumens
- Phleboliths are seen as focal echogenic focus/foci with dense posterior shadowing
  - Using high resolution transducers, phleboliths can be seen in almost 60% of cases
- Spectral Doppler: No arterial flow on Doppler, but venous flow may be observed & augmented by compression with transducer
- Color Doppler: Slow flow within venous, sinusoidal spaces

DDx: Venous Vascular Malformation

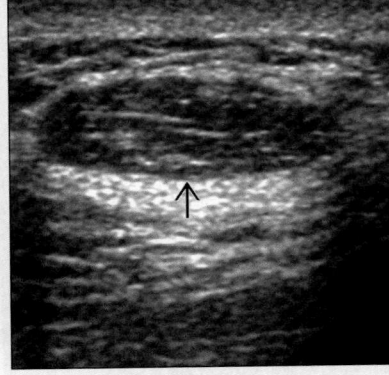

Lipoma

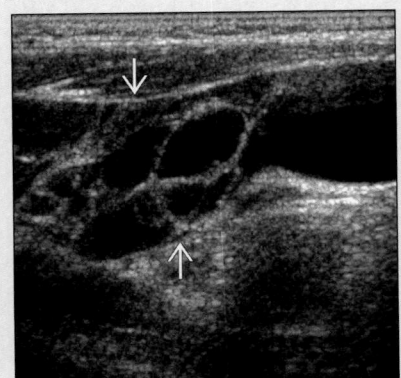

Lymphangioma

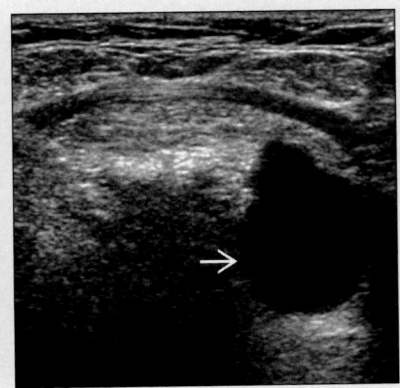

Ranula

DERMOID AND EPIDERMOID

IMAGE GALLERY

Typical

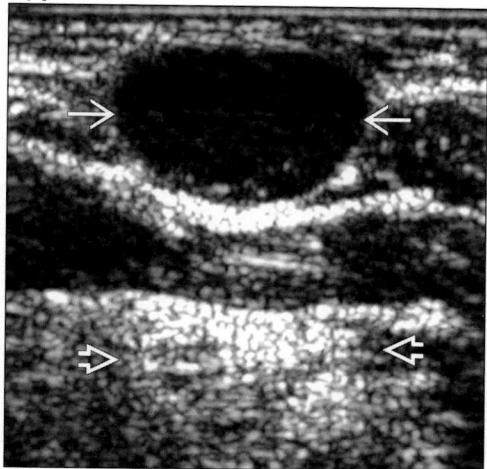 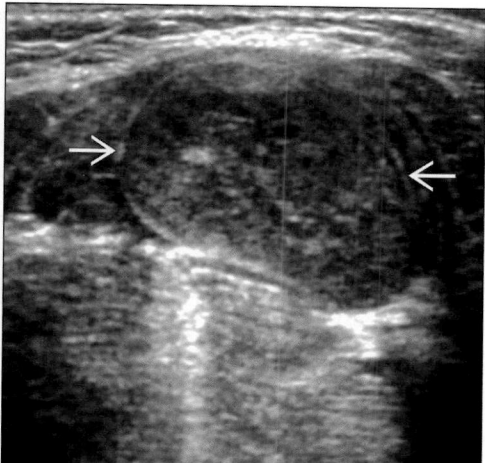

(Left) Transverse grayscale US shows a submental epidermoid ➡. It is anechoic with posterior enhancement ⇨, faint internal debris & thin walls. US adequately evaluates such small superficial lesions. *(Right)* Transverse grayscale US shows a well-defined, hypoechoic mass in the SLS with a heterogeneous internal echo pattern suggesting a dermoid ➡. Diagnosis confirmed at surgery. No additional imaging was necessary.

Typical

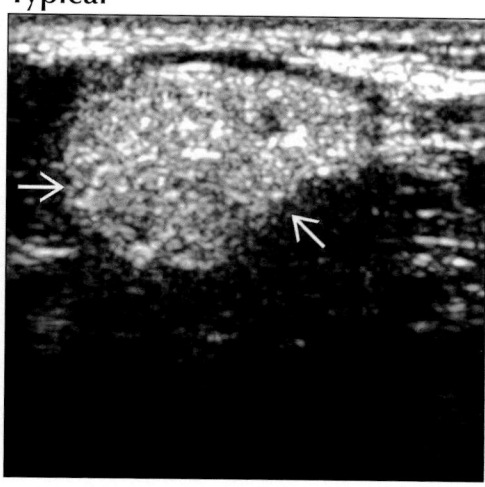 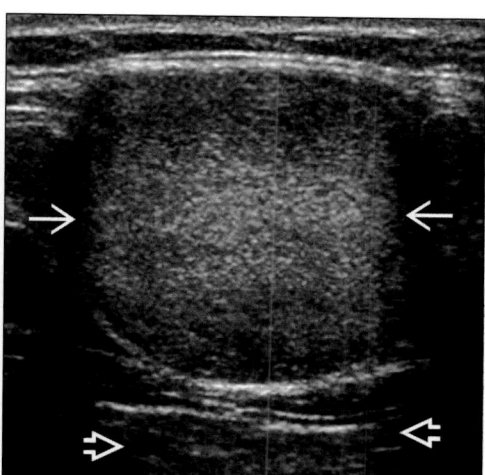

(Left) Grayscale US shows a well-defined mass with uniform bright internal echoes ➡. Transducer pressure elicited a swirling motion of contents suggesting its cystic nature. Histology confirmed epidermoid. *(Right)* Grayscale US shows the typical pseudosolid pattern of an epidermoid ➡, i.e., homogeneous internal echoes. Note the faint posterior enhancement ⇨. Swirling contents were noted with transducer pressure.

Typical

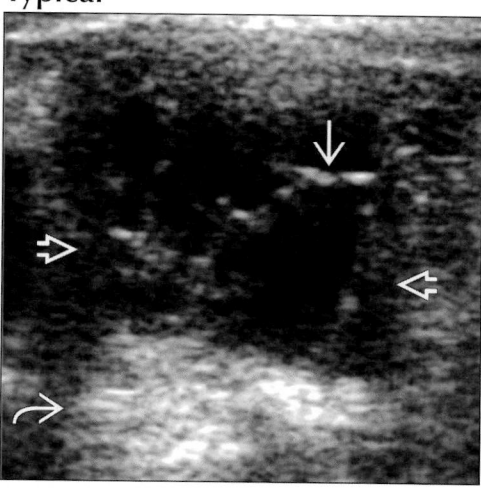 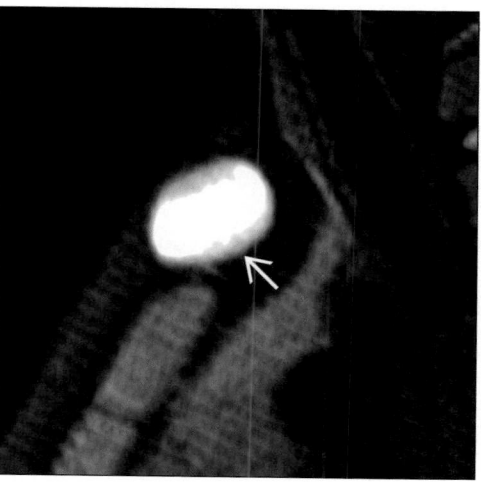

(Left) Grayscale US shows a heterogeneous cystic mass ⇨ with internal septa ➡, debris & posterior enhancement ⇨ located superficially in the submental region. A dermoid was found at surgery. *(Right)* Sagittal fat suppressed T2WI MR shows a well-defined, cystic mass ➡ in the sternal notch. Note no suppression of signal within the mass suggests it is fluid rather than fat. Sugery showed a sternal notch epidermoid.

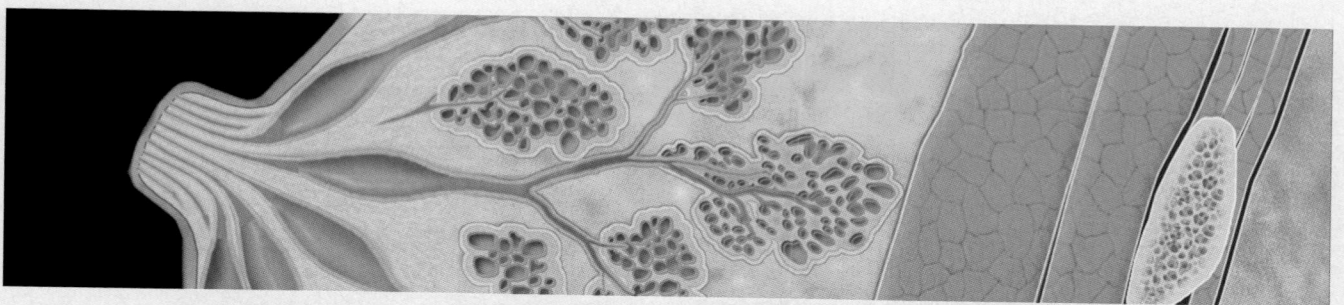

SECTION 12: Breast

Introduction and Overview

BREAST SONOGRAPHY

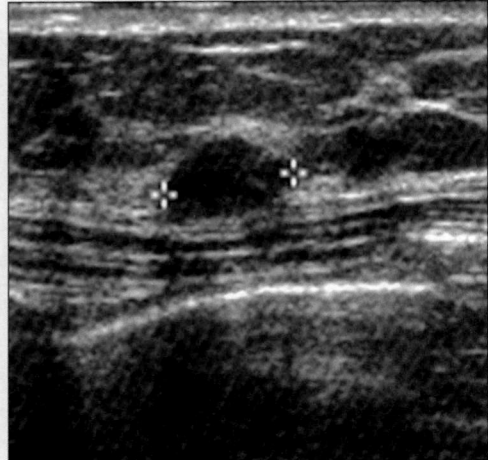

Transverse ultrasound in a patient with a palpable mass. The field of view is too big ➡, the focal zone ➤ is set too low & the overall gain is too high. The study was read as negative.

Transverse ultrasound in the same patient with the same transducer and correct settings shows a solid mass (calipers), biopsy proven fibroadenoma. Incorrect technique will lead to missed diagnosis of cancer.

TERMINOLOGY

Abbreviations
- Ultrasound (US)
- Time gain compensation curve (TGC)
- Terminal duct lobular unit; anatomic subunit of breast tissue (TDLU)

IMAGING ANATOMY

Anatomic Relationships
- Breast fat appears hypoechoic, glandular tissue echogenicity > fat

ANATOMY-BASED IMAGING ISSUES

Imaging Protocols
- Indications for breast ultrasound
  - Primary evaluation of palpable mass in young patient (< 30 y)
  - Evaluation of mammographic mass
    - Cystic vs. solid vs. asymmetric breast tissue
    - Determine extent of breast cancer: Useful for multicentric/multifocal tumor especially in dense breast tissue
  - Evaluation of mammographic density
    - Asymmetric breast tissue without focal mass vs. dominant lesion lesion requiring intervention
  - Evaluation of lesion seen on one view
    - Mammogram will show medial/lateral or superior/inferior
    - Look for sonographic correlate, if seen place BB on skin
    - Repeat mammogram → confirm sonographic finding is mammographic finding
    - Cyst aspiration/core biopsy/marker deployment as indicated
  - Evaluation of axilla
    - Palpable lymph nodes can be assessed ± biopsied with US guidance
    - Examination of axilla in patients with cancer → FNA suspicious nodes → if positive, full axillary node dissection rather than sentinel node biopsy
  - Evaluation of palpable mass
    - Specific benign diagnosis is possible e.g., simple cyst
    - Negative ultrasound is reassuring
  - Implant evaluation
    - "Snowstorm" appearance highly specific for extracapsular silicone
  - "Second look" scan for MR findings not seen mammographically
    - Focussed US in area of MR abnormality
    - Reports indicate 2nd look scan may be positive even if negative "screening" US
  - Evaluation of nipple discharge
    - Particularly helpful if galactography fails: If intraductal mass seen use US to localize for excision
  - Diagnosis and treatment of breast abscess
    - US identifies fluid collection, provides guidance for aspiration → symptomatic relief, culture
    - Serial aspirations and catheter drainage less invasive than surgery
  - "Screening" ultrasound
    - Particularly useful for patients with dense breast tissue
    - ACRIN 6666 study in progress to evaluate screening breast US
  - Guidance for intervention
    - Cyst aspiration
    - Core biopsy: Standard core needle or vacuum assisted
    - Pre-operative wire localization for excisional biopsy/lumpectomy
  - Intraoperative
    - May be helpful to surgeon in multifocal tumors to ensure complete excision/margin clearance
- Technique
  - High frequency linear array transducer with center of frequency 10 MHz preferred

BREAST SONOGRAPHY

Breast Ultrasound

Key Concepts and Questions
- Is a mass cystic or solid?
- Does a solid mass have malignant features?
- Is there a correlate to a palpable mass in a patient with negative mammogram?
- Is there a correlate to mammographically occult abnormality detected on breast MR?
  - "Second look" ultrasound may show lesions identified by MR
  - Allows US guide biopsy/localization for excision
- Is there an occult cancer in a high-risk patient with dense breast tissue?
  - High-risk women 2-3x more likely to have cancer seen only sonographically
  - In one series detection rate of cancer in 50 y/o with dense tissue = 50% for mammography, 79% for US

Breast Ultrasound is Highly Operator Dependent
- Poor technique → misinterpretation of findings → incorrect management decisions
- Poor technique will result in missed/delayed cancer diagnosis

Images Should be Saved Even if Study is Negative
- Screening: Radial images at 12, 3, 6, and 9 clockface + subareolar view
- Palpable/mammographic finding: Annotated radial and antiradial at site of finding

---

- Position patient so that area of interest is as thin as possible
  - Supine for medial breast
  - Oblique with arm above head for lateral breast
  - Patient can elevate breast for inferior lesions
- Field of view to reach chest wall but not beyond
- Overall gain set so that fat is grey
  - Too much gain creates artifactual echoes → cysts look complex or solid
  - Too little gain → masses look cystic, hypoechoic masses may "disappear"
- Gradually increase TGC with increasing field of view
  - Compensates for absorption of sound by tissues
  - Aim for equivalent shades of gray throughout image
- Set focal zone at lesion
  - Most current transducers allow realtime scanning with multiple focal zones
  - Once lesion identified set single focal zone at that depth for maximum resolution
- Vary transducer pressure while scanning
  - Some shadowing is artifactual: Will ↓ or resolve with ↑ transducer pressure
  - Pressure → ↓ tissue thickness → ↑ increased resolution
  - Light pressure better when evaluating flow
- Change angle of insonation
  - Important to see borders of masses, evaluate subareolar area
- "Rolled nipple" technique important in evaluation of nipple discharge
  - Roll nipple over examiner's finger
  - Scan long axis of superficial aspect of nipple-areola complex to look for distal intraductal mass
- Use standoff pad/large amount of gel for superficial lesions
  - Superficial lesion may be obscured by near field artifact
- Mark palpable lesions: "Paperclip trick"
  - Trap palpable mass between limbs of an unfolded paperclip

- Ring-down artifact from limbs of clip marks mass margins on images
- Confirms that sonographic finding is the palpable finding
- Documents absence of sonographic mass if scan negative
- Color Doppler
  - Vocal fremitus: Tissues vibrate when patient hums; movement → "color"
    - Mass vibrates < normal tissue → defect in color-filled background
  - Internal vascularity: Proves mass is solid, not complex cyst
    - May help with identification of papilloma in distended duct
- Scan planes
  - Breast ducts are arranged radially from the nipple
  - Scan in radial and antiradial (orthogonal to radial) planes
  - Images labeled with scan plane, clock face, distance from nipple
  - Distance can be annotated as
    - Anterior, middle, posterior depth dividing breast into thirds from nipple to chest wall or distance from nipple in cms

Imaging Pitfalls
- Wrong depth
  - Too much depth → loss of resolution in breast tissue → potential to miss small masses
  - Insufficient depth → deep lesions will be missed
- Incorrect contrast (overall gain)
  - May miss hypoechoic masses
  - May mask true nature of lesion
- Incorrect assumption that ↑ through transmission ⇒ cyst
  - Means that lesion reflects less ultrasound than surrounding tissues
  - Cellular carcinoma/fibroadenoma often have ↑ through transmission
- Incorrect assumption that distal acoustic shadowing ⇒ carcinoma

BREAST SONOGRAPHY

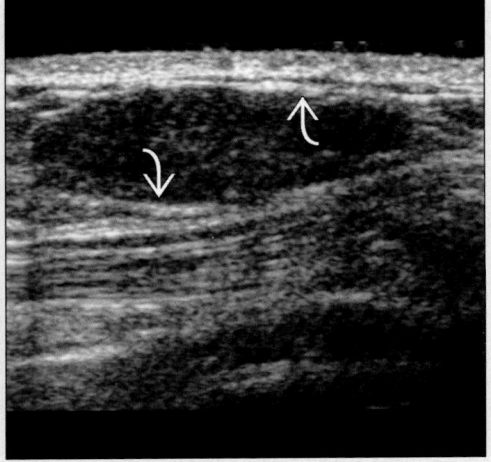

Transverse ultrasound shows typical sonographic features of cancer. There are spiculated margins ➡, microcalcifications ➡ and distal acoustic shadowing ➡. Also note the irregular shape and echogenic rim.

Transverse ultrasound in contrast to the previous case shows a well-circumscribed oval mass with thin echogenic margin ➡ orientated parallel to the skin i.e. wider than tall. Biopsy: Benign fibroadenoma.

- ○ Means that lesion reflects more ultrasound than surrounding tissues
- ○ Fibrosis/calcification are reflective
  - Desmoplastic reaction in cancer
  - Scar tissue post lumpectomy/radiation therapy/trauma/implant complication
  - Calcified mass or high calcium content fluid e.g., galactocele
- • Mistaking cross section of rib for solid mass
  - ○ Any lesion must be scanned in two planes → ribs elongate as transducer is rotated
  - ○ Ribs are deep to pectoral muscle therefore not in breast tissue
- • Failure to appreciate diffuse changes in echogenicity
  - ○ Use split screen/extended field of view and comparison side to side
  - ○ Invasive lobular carcinoma in particular may cause subtle diffuse alterations in echotexture

PATHOLOGY-BASED IMAGING ISSUES

Key Concepts or Questions
- • Breast cyst
  - ○ Well defined margin, sharp posterior wall echo, increased through transmission
  - ○ Proteinaceous debris → low level internal echoes
  - ○ Thin avascular septations
  - ○ Clustered microcysts reflect breast TDLU anatomy and are benign
- • Ultrasound not used instead of pathologic diagnosis, rather allows triage of patient, avoidance of low yield biopsy
  - ○ Solid mass malignant features
    - Irregular shape
    - Angular margins, duct extension
    - Taller than wide
    - Distal acoustic shadowing
  - ○ Solid mass benign features
    - Oval shape
    - Well circumscribed margins
    - Uniformly echogenic
    - Wider than tall
- • Lymph node evaluation
  - ○ Reactive: May be seen with infection including HIV
    - Large nodes with symmetrically thickened cortex
  - ○ Neoplastic: Metastatic breast cancer, lymphoma commonest
    - Indistinct margin
    - Diffuse or nodular cortical thickening
    - Diminutive echogenic hilum

CLINICAL IMPLICATIONS

Clinical Importance
- • US essential in evaluation of mammographic mass or density
- • US may reveal a mass in association with mammographic calcifications
  - ○ Allow US-guided biopsy: Quicker and simpler than stereotactic
  - ○ Sampling solid component ↑ likelihood of accurate diagnosis
- • Negative mammogram + negative ultrasound of palpable mass → 98% negative predictive value
  - ○ Clinical findings dictate need for biopsy

RELATED REFERENCES

1. Berg WA: Sonographically depicted breast clustered microcysts: is follow-up appropriate? AJR Am J Roentgenol. 185(4):952-9, 2005
2. Berg WA: Supplemental screening sonography in dense breasts. Radiol Clin North Am. 42(5):845-51, vi, 2004
3. Berg WA: Rationale for a trial of screening breast ultrasound: American College of Radiology Imaging Network (ACRIN) 6666. AJR Am J Roentgenol. 180(5):1225-8, 2003
4. Dennis MA et al: Breast biopsy avoidance: the value of normal mammograms and normal sonograms in the setting of a palpable lump. Radiology. 219(1):186-91, 2001
5. Stavros AT et al: Solid breast nodules: use of sonography to distinguish between benign and malignant lesions. Radiology. 196(1):123-34, 1995

CYSTS & CYST-LIKE LESIONS

Typical

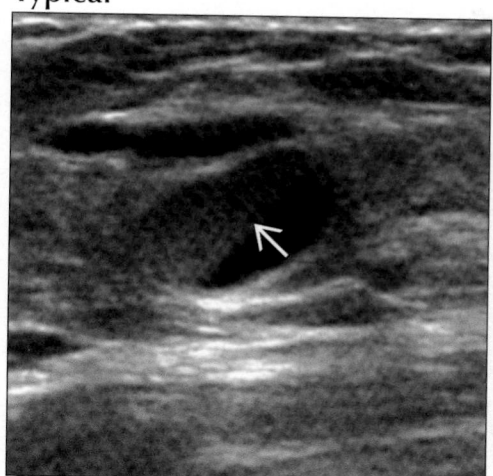
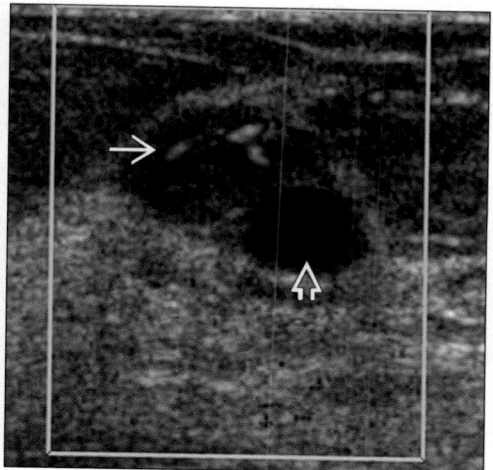

(Left) Radial ultrasound shows a circumscribed oval mass with fluid-debris level ➡ consistent with a complicated cyst. On anti-radial imaging homogeneous low level echoes were seen mimicking a solid mass. *(Right)* Ultrasound shows a complex cystic circumscribed, oval mass with solid vascular components ➡ and eccentric cystic areas ➡. US-guided core biopsy showed benign complex fibroadenoma.

Typical

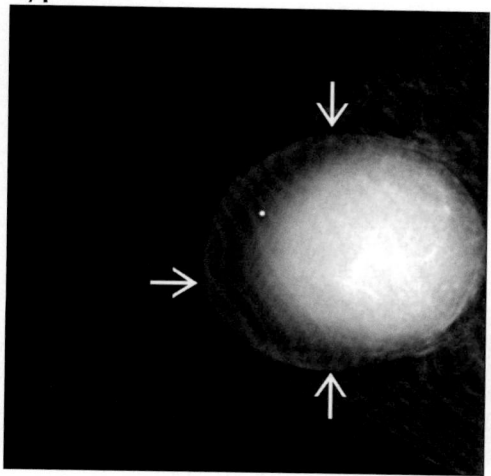
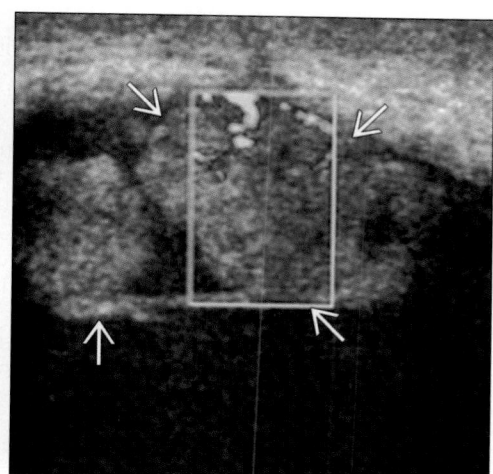

(Left) CC mammogram in a 52 year old patient shows a large well-circumscribed mass ➡ encompassing the entire central aspect of the breast. The patient stated that the mass had recently increased in size. *(Right)* Ultrasound evaluation in the same patient shows the lesion to be predominantly cystic, but with a solid vascular intraluminal mass ➡ along part of the cyst wall. Biopsy revealed papillary DCIS.

Variant

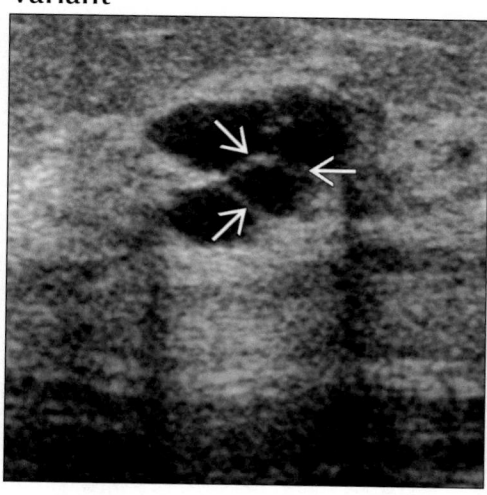
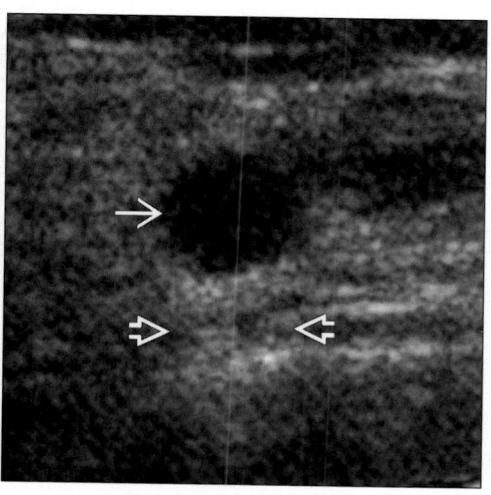

(Left) Ultrasound shows a simple anechoic cyst with multiple thin internal septae ➡ consistent with multiple small adjacent simple cysts. No Doppler flow was noted within septations confirming benignity. *(Right)* Ultrasound shows a round, hypoechoic mass ➡ with indistinct margins & minimal posterior enhancement ➡. The lesion was difficult to distinguish from a solid mass. US-guided biopsy showed cyst wall & proteinaceous cyst contents, compatible with complicated cyst.

BREAST CANCER, DCIS

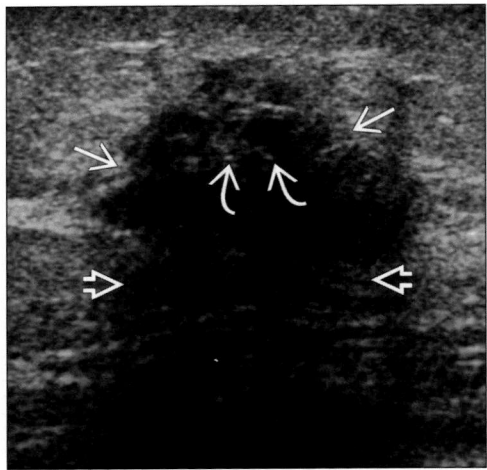 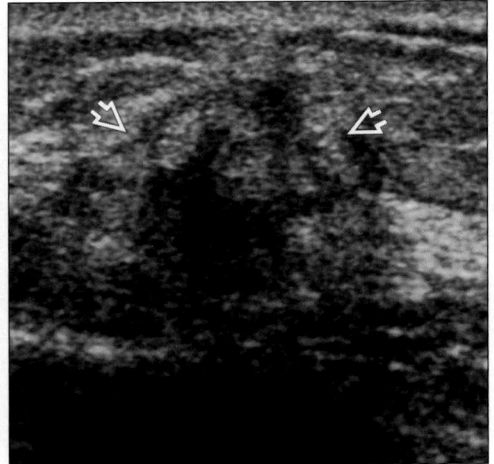

Transverse ultrasound of palpable tumor shows typical irregular hypoechoic mass ➜ with posterior shadowing ⇥ and microcalcifications ⇗.

Transverse ultrasound of (same patient as previous image) the axilla shows markedly abnormal lymph node ⇥, which has lost its architecture due to metastatic tumor. US biopsy prior to surgery aids in staging.

TERMINOLOGY

Definitions
- Neoplastic growth in the breast

IMAGING FINDINGS

General Features
- Location
  - 50% occur in upper outer quadrant
    - Due to tendency for greatest volume of glandular tissue in the upper outer breast
  - 20% subareolar/central region
  - Remainder in other quadrants of breast
- Morphology: Ranges widely from spiculated mass to circumscribed nodule to pleomorphic calcifications

Ultrasonographic Findings
- Grayscale Ultrasound
  - Most often hypoechoic irregular mass
    - With some degree of posterior acoustic shadowing
  - Margins
    - Angular
    - Microlobulated
    - Spiculated
  - Thick echogenic halo
  - Growth perpendicular to plane of breast tissue (taller than wide)
  - Associated findings
    - Foci of calcification
    - Satellite solid tumors adjacent to primary
    - Surrounding tissue edema
    - Duct extension
  - Can be isoechoic, circumscribed and/or lobulated
    - DCIS
    - Medullary
  - Uniformly hyperechoic lesions most often benign
    - However beware of isoechoic or hypoechoic areas within the main mass, especially if palpable
- Power Doppler: Variable internal blood flow

Imaging Recommendations
- Best imaging tool
  - Mammography combined with sonography
    - Identify multifocal and multicentric tumors
    - Ultrasound can localize solid component in area of mammographic calcifications

DDx: Suspicious-Appearing Benign Masses

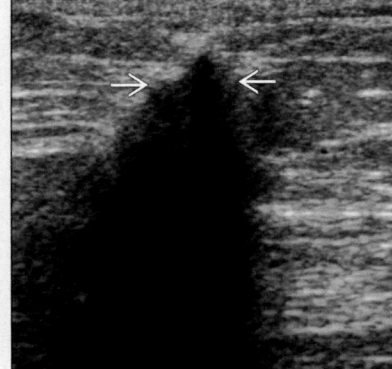 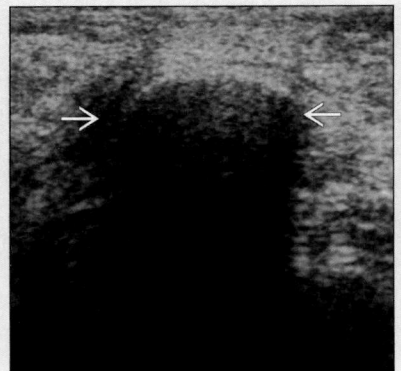 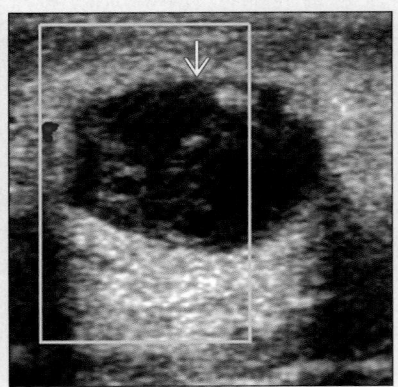

Postlumpectomy Scar *Fat Necrosis* *Hematoma*

BREAST CANCER, DCIS

Key Facts

Imaging Findings
- 50% occur in upper outer quadrant
- Most often hypoechoic irregular mass
- Can be isoechoic, circumscribed and/or lobulated
- Uniformly hyperechoic lesions most often benign
- Ultrasound can localize solid component in area of mammographic calcifications
- Breast MR becoming more widely used to increase sensitivity of detection
- Ultrasound can be used to assess for pathologic lymph nodes in axilla

Top Differential Diagnoses
- Post-Operative Scar
- Fat Necrosis
- Hematoma

Pathology
- Invasive ductal: 65-80% of all breast cancers
- Mucinous, medullary and tubular generally have better prognosis

Clinical Issues
- Prevalence of ~ 2.3 million women in the USA
- Survival distinctly related to stage at diagnosis
- Pre-op percutaneous core biopsy preferred to confirm diagnosis
- Treatment regimen depends on the type and stage of tumor as well as patient factors

Diagnostic Checklist
- Breast MR in high-risk patients or those with dense tissue to assess for multicentric or multifocal disease
- Circumscribed masses can be malignant

- Use ultrasound-guided biopsy to pre-operatively diagnose invasive cancer vs DCIS
  - Breast MR becoming more widely used to increase sensitivity of detection
    - Dense tissue can obscure details on mammogram and ultrasound
    - Check for other tumors in same breast
    - Screen contralateral breast
    - Follow tumor size in neoadjuvant chemotherapy
    - Consider in a high-risk patient
- Check axillary regions on mammogram
  - Ultrasound can be used to assess for pathologic lymph nodes in axilla
  - Biopsy of suspicious lymph nodes aids in clinical staging

DIFFERENTIAL DIAGNOSIS

Post-Operative Scar
- Can be difficult to distinguish from recurrence if at lumpectomy site
  - Appears suspicious by ultrasound
    - Central apparent "mass"
    - Posterior acoustic shadowing
    - Dystrophic calcifications
- May require biopsy to be certain
- Scars should ↓ over time
  - Most scars remodel over the first 2 years post lumpectomy
  - Most recurrences 2-5 years post lumpectomy
- Look for evidence of underlying growth to prove recurrence
  - Convex margins
  - Internal Doppler flow
  - Increasing size over short interval follow-up

Fat Necrosis
- Can be difficult to distinguish from recurrence if at lumpectomy site
  - Dystrophic calcifications can appear initially heterogeneous
  - Can be a solid-appearing mass on ultrasound

- Oil cysts can appear solid on ultrasound but are clearly fat containing on mammography
- If not associated with lumpectomy, correlate with clinical history
  - Should have history of trauma

Hematoma
- Correlate with history of acute trauma
  - Should resolve over short interval follow-up
- Can be homogeneously hypoechoic or heterogeneous
- May have surrounding echogenic halo of edema
- Look for fluid-debris level
  - No soft tissue component
- No internal vascularity

Breast Abscess
- Clinical exam should show erythema and tenderness
- May have a history of prior breast intervention
  - Cyst aspiration
  - Percutaneous biopsy
  - Surgical excision
- Often with homogeneous internal echoes
- Surrounding echogenic halo of edema may be present

PATHOLOGY

General Features
- Genetics
  - Breast cancer related genes may account for up to 5-10% of all breast cancers
  - Hereditary breast cancer syndromes
    - BRCA-1
    - BRCA-2
    - Li-Fraumeni syndrome - p53 tumor-suppressor mutations
    - Cowden disease
    - Peutz-Jeghers syndrome
- Etiology
  - Multifactorial
    - Nongenetic associations range from dietary factors to weight to levels of physical activity

- Common theme of prolonged or increased estrogen exposure
- Epidemiology: 1:8 lifetime risk of developing breast cancer for women today
- Risk factors
  - Early menarche
  - Late menopause
  - Nulliparous women
  - Older age at time of first pregnancy
  - Radiation to the breast at a young age
    - Hodgkin disease treatment
    - Atomic bomb survivors

Gross Pathologic & Surgical Features
- Invasive ductal usually palpable firm mass
- Invasive lobular often difficult to palpate at surgery and in gross specimen

Microscopic Features
- Invasive ductal: 65-80% of all breast cancers
  - Malignant duct cells invading connective tissue stroma
  - Graded according to nuclear atypia, histologic differentiation, mitotic activity
- Invasive lobular
  - Typical single-file appearance of monoclonal cells
  - May be missed on FNA if few cells sampled
- DCIS
  - Low, intermediate, high nuclear grade
- Multiple other cell types exist
  - Mucinous, medullary and tubular generally have better prognosis
    - Tubular usually < 2 cm
    - Medullary presents as circumscribed mass with lymphocytic infiltrate
  - Invasive papillary rare

CLINICAL ISSUES

Presentation
- Most common signs/symptoms
  - Suspicious finding on screening mammogram
  - Palpable lump
- Other signs/symptoms
  - Bloody nipple discharge
  - Rarely pain

Demographics
- Age
  - Median age at diagnosis: 61 years old
  - Median age at death: 69 years old
- Gender: Much more common in women than men
- Ethnicity
  - 134:100,000 in Caucasian women
  - 118:100,000 in African-American women
- Prevalence of ~ 2.3 million women in the USA
  - Includes breast cancer survivors and those currently being treated

Natural History & Prognosis
- Overall 5 year survival rate 88.5%
  - 89.7% for Caucasian women
  - 77.3% for African-American women

- Survival distinctly related to stage at diagnosis
  - 61% diagnosed when cancer is localized
    - Survival at 5 years: 98.1%
  - 31% diagnosed after spread to regional lymph nodes or beyond primary site
    - Survival at 5 years: 83.1%
  - 6% diagnosed after metastasized
    - Survival at 5 years: 26%

Treatment
- Pre-op percutaneous core biopsy preferred to confirm diagnosis
  - Often able to perform with ultrasound guidance
- Treatment regimen depends on the type and stage of tumor as well as patient factors
- Surgical
  - Lumpectomy with sentinel node/axillary dissection
  - Mastectomy with sentinel node/axillary dissection
- Medical
  - Chemotherapy
    - Usually following surgical resection
    - Can consider neoadjuvant chemotherapy; shrink tumor prior to surgical intervention
  - Hormonal therapy
    - Tamoxifen: Blocks estrogen receptors
    - Arimidex: Blocks estrogen production in peripheral tissue
    - Herceptin: Blocks Her2/neu protein
- Radiation
  - External beam
  - Interstitial
    - Multiple catheters with radioactive seeds placed into breast around lumpectomy site
  - Localized
    - Balloon and catheter inserted into lumpectomy cavity with outpatient delivery of radioactive seeds

DIAGNOSTIC CHECKLIST

Consider
- Breast MR in high-risk patients or those with dense tissue to assess for multicentric or multifocal disease

Image Interpretation Pearls
- Circumscribed masses can be malignant

SELECTED REFERENCES

1. Ries LAG wt al: SEER Cancer Statistics Review, National Cancer Institute, 1975-2003. Bethesda, MD, posted to the SEER web site, 2006
2. Shoma A et al: Ultrasound for accurate measurement of invasive breast cancer tumor size. Breast J. 12(3):252-6, 2006
3. van Rijk MC et al: Ultrasonography and fine-needle aspiration cytology can spare breast cancer patients unnecessary sentinel lymph node biopsy. Ann Surg Oncol. 13(1):31-5, 2006
4. Ohta T et al: Ultrasonographic findings of invasive lobular carcinoma differentiation of invasive lobular carcinoma from invasive ductal carcinoma by ultrasonography. Breast Cancer. 12(4):304-11, 2005

IMAGE GALLERY

Typical

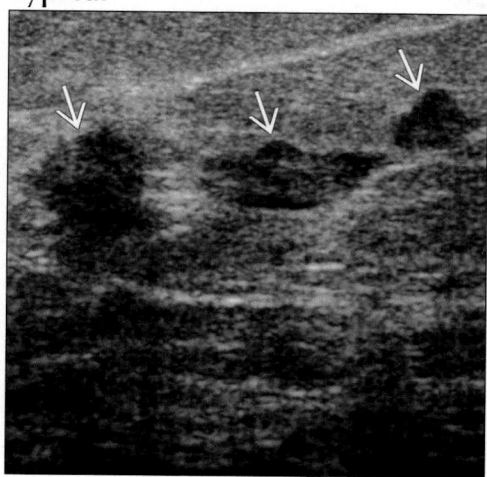 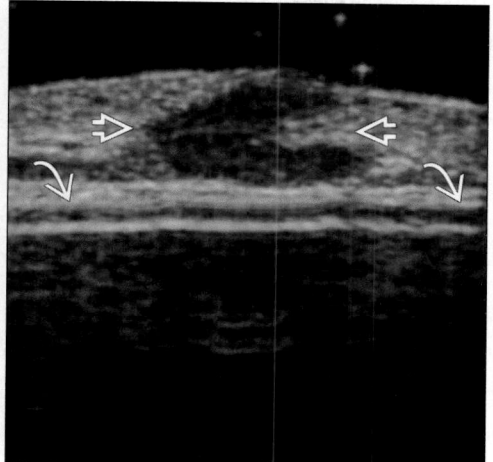

(Left) Longitudinal ultrasound shows multifocal tumors growing along ductal system ➡. Largest mass was subareolar, with these masses extending radially from nipple at 9 o'clock. Given extent and location, mastectomy was performed. *(Right)* Longitudinal ultrasound shows solid palpable mass ➡ at site of red skin bump in patient with prior mastectomy and reconstruction (implants) ➡ for high grade DCIS. This was an invasive tumor.

Typical

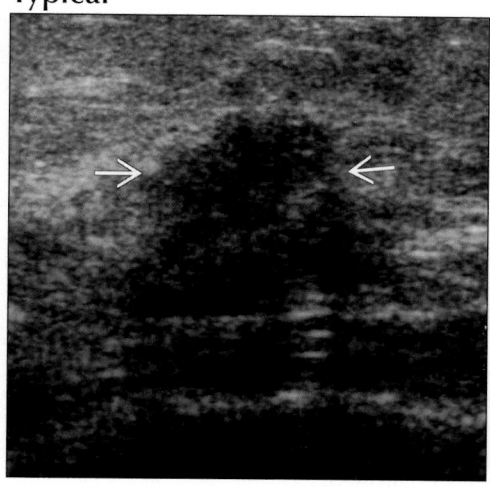 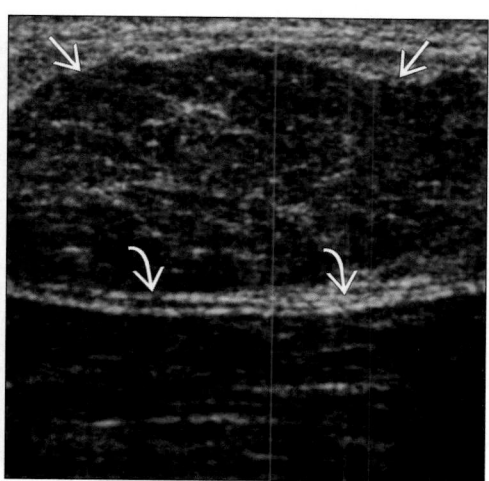

(Left) Transverse ultrasound shows typical hypoechoic mass with indistinct margins ➡, consistent with breast cancer in a male patient presenting with a palpable mass. The appearance of breast cancer in men is not significantly different from that in women. *(Right)* Transverse ultrasound of a palpable lump in a woman with implants ➡ shows solid circumscribed mass ➡. Core biopsy showed DCIS.

Variant

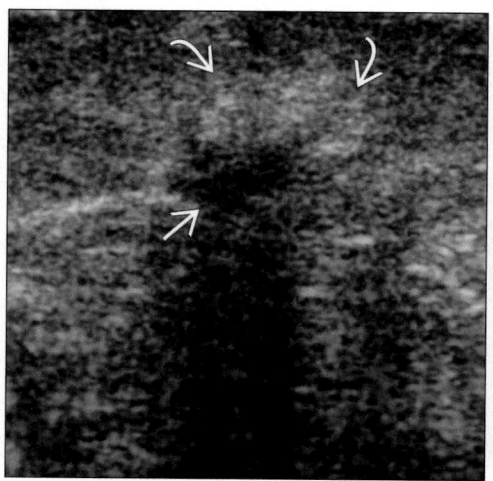 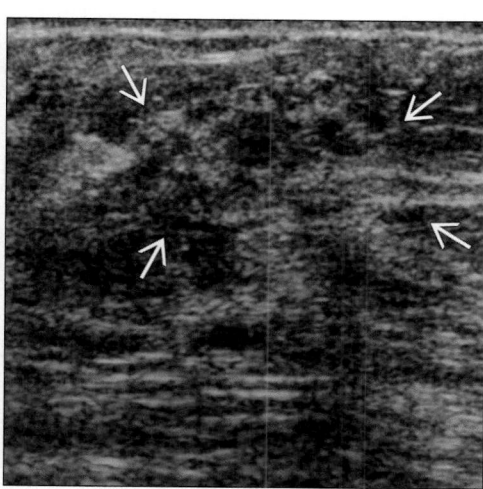

(Left) Transverse ultrasound shows a 4 mm invasive cancer ➡, with an echogenic halo ➡. At lumpectomy this was only a small part of a 7 cm invasive lobular cancer. Sonographic size estimates can be deceiving. *(Right)* Transverse ultrasound shows architectural distortion and heterogeneity ➡, within a mostly echogenic palpable area. Core biopsy revealed invasive ductal carcinoma with lobular features.

SOLID NON-MALIGNANT BREAST MASSES

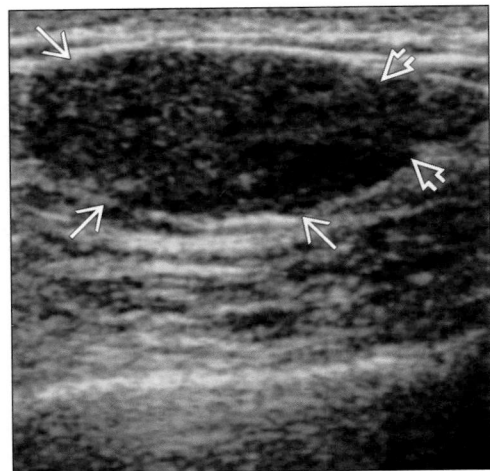

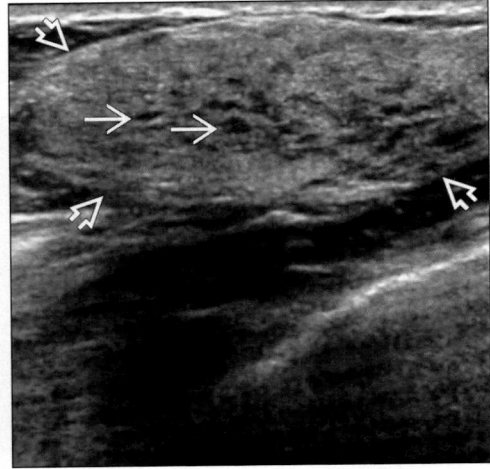

Ultrasound shows a uniformly hypoechoic solid mass ➡ with smooth margins, two smooth, gentle lobulations ➡, and a thin echogenic capsule. Biopsy proved benign fibroadenoma.

Ultrasound of a palpable abnormality shows a hyperechoic mass ➡ with small areas of interspersed decreased echogenicity ➡. Biopsy showed dense stromal fibrosis.

TERMINOLOGY

Definitions
- Benign solid breast lesion

IMAGING FINDINGS

General Features
- Degree of suspicion based on mammographic and sonographic appearance
- Biopsy often necessary to prove benignity
- BI-RADS classification of sonographic appearance depends on suspicious vs benign findings
  - If any suspicious findings → biopsy
  - Biopsy if findings indeterminate

Ultrasonographic Findings
- **Sonographic features highly predictive of benignity**
  - Diffusely/markedly hyperechoic
  - Shape
    - Elliptical/oval
    - Lesion wider than it is tall, orientation parallel to skin
  - Margins
    - Smooth, circumscribed
    - Gently lobulated (fewer than four lobulations)
  - Capsule
    - Thin, echogenic capsule
    - Capsule completely encompasses margin
- **Features concerning for malignancy**
  - Markedly hypoechoic
  - Shape
    - Irregular
    - Architectural distortion
    - Lesion taller than wide
  - Margins
    - Microlobulated
    - Spiculated
    - Angular
  - Thick echogenic halo
  - Distal acoustic shadowing
  - Microcalcifications
  - Duct extension
- **Indeterminate sonographic features**
  - Isoechoic or mildly hypoechoic
  - Increased through transmission
  - Heterogeneous or homogeneous texture

DDx: Circumscribed Malignant Breast Lesions

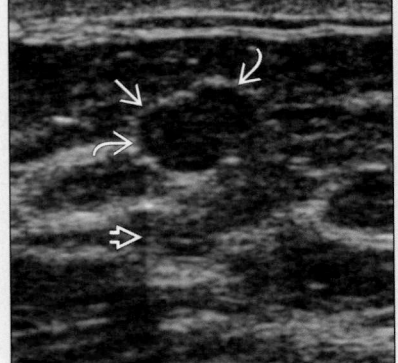

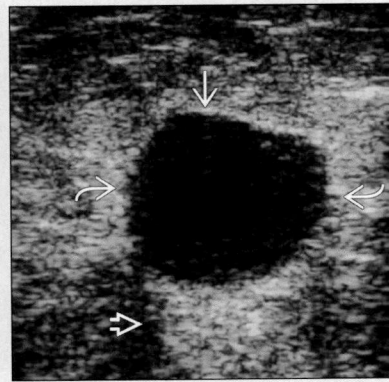

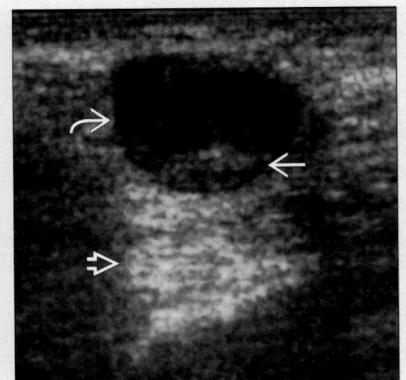

Low Grade DCIS

Medullary Carcinoma

Lymph Node Metastasis

SOLID NON-MALIGNANT BREAST MASSES

Top Differential Diagnoses
- Fibroadenoma
- Lymph Node
- Lipoma
- Fat Necrosis
- Sclerosing Adenosis - Nodular
- Stromal Fibrosis
- Fibroadenolipoma
- Lactating Adenoma
- Tubular Adenoma
- Diabetic Mastopathy
- Granular Cell Tumor
- Pseudoangiomatous Stromal Hyperplasia (PASH)
- Malignant Breast Mass

Clinical Issues
- Palpable breast mass

Key Facts
- Mass/asymmetry on mammogram
- Like mammography, the risk of malignancy for a sonographically benign appearing mass should be less than 2% (BI-RADS 3)

Diagnostic Checklist
- Excisional biopsy is mandatory if core biopsy pathology benign yet imaging characteristics suspicious
- Biopsy is often necessary to distinguish benign from malignant masses
- Goal of sonography is to identify those lesions where suspicion of malignancy is so low that biopsy can be avoided
- Negative predictive value of classification of a lesion as sonographically benign reported as high as 99.5%

Mammographic Findings
- Mammographic features highly predictive of benignity
  - Circumscribed margins
  - Equal or low density
  - Stability over time

Imaging Recommendations
- Best imaging tool
  - Ultrasound
    - Initial evaluation of palpable lesions for those under 35 years old
    - Sonographic characterization of lesions is superior to mammographic in premenopausal breast tissue
    - Further evaluation of mammographic masses
  - For patients over 35 years with palpable breast mass start with mammography
    - Problem solving/lesion characterization with ultrasound
- Protocol advice
  - If even one suspicious sonographic feature present → biopsy
  - If sonographic features are indeterminate → biopsy
  - If mammographic features are suspicious, biopsy even if sonographic features benign
  - If interval mammographic or sonographic enlargement → biopsy
  - Consider MR for further evaluation if
    - Mammographically dense breast tissue
    - Multiple indeterminate lesions
    - Strong family history of breast cancer
  - MR findings should not negate biopsy if mammographic or sonographic features suspicious

DIFFERENTIAL DIAGNOSIS

Fibroadenoma
- Circumscribed or gently lobulated margins
- Hypo- to isoechoic
- Homogeneous low-level internal echogenicity
  - May contain echogenic internal septations
- Long axis parallel to skin surface
- May contain large coarse shadowing calcifications

Lymph Node
- Hypoechoic circumscribed mass with hyperechoic hilum
  - Hilum may be vascular
- Oval or reniform shape
- Increasing size with loss of hilum is suspicious → biopsy

Lipoma
- Ovoid or round circumscribed mass
- Iso- or slightly hyperechoic to subcutaneous fat
- Circumscribed radiolucent mass on mammogram

Fat Necrosis
- Ill-defined irregular complex sonographic mass - may have cystic areas
- Anechoic to mixed hyper and hypoechoic
- Round, oval, or lobulated lucent mammographic mass
- Develop peripheral rim calcifications

Sclerosing Adenosis - Nodular
- Oval, circumscribed, hypoechoic solid mass
- May contain calcifications
- Appearance may mimic cancer
- Circumscribed, indistinct, or partially obscured mass on mammogram

Stromal Fibrosis
- Hypoechoic, heterogeneous, or isoechoic mass with variable margins
- May have dense posterior shadowing - biopsy to verify diagnosis
- Variable sonographic and mammographic appearance

Fibroadenolipoma
- Mix of echogenic fat and sonolucent glandular elements
- Oval shape and usually circumscribed
- Compressible
- "Breast-within-a-breast" appearance on mammogram

SOLID NON-MALIGNANT BREAST MASSES

Lactating Adenoma
- Occurs in pregnant, lactating, or post-partum women
- Oval or gently lobulated well-circumscribed mass
- Homogeneously hypo- or isoechoic with posterior acoustic enhancement
- May contain echogenic septations

Tubular Adenoma
- Similar mammographic and sonographic appearance to fibroadenoma
- Circumscribed oval or lobulated mass
- Homogeneously hypoechoic
- May contain microcalcifications

Diabetic Mastopathy
- Hypoechoic region or mass with indistinct margins
- May have marked posterior acoustic shadowing
- Suspect in long-standing diabetics with palpable fixed, hard breast mass
- Symmetric areas of homogeneous dense parenchyma on mammogram

Granular Cell Tumor
- Irregular, hypoechoic shadowing sonographic mass
- Spiculated, lobulated, or circumscribed high density mammographic mass
- Can occur anywhere in the body, most frequently in the head and neck

Pseudoangiomatous Stromal Hyperplasia (PASH)
- Round or oval solid mass with variable margins
  - Usually circumscribed or macrolobulated
- Mixed internal echogenicity

Malignant Breast Mass
- Most often hypoechoic, irregular mass with posterior acoustic shadowing
  - Margins usually angular, microlobulated, or spiculated but can be circumscribed or lobulated
  - Growth perpendicular to plane of breast tissue (taller than wide)
  - Thick echogenic halo
- Most common pathology invasive ductal carcinoma, invasive lobular carcinoma or DCIS

CLINICAL ISSUES

Presentation
- Most common signs/symptoms
  - Palpable breast mass
  - Mass/asymmetry on mammogram

Natural History & Prognosis
- Like mammography, the risk of malignancy for a sonographically benign appearing mass should be less than 2% (BI-RADS 3)
- Excellent prognosis for lesions characterized as sonographically benign

Treatment
- No treatment is usually necessary for benign lesions
  - Patient may request excision for reassurance

- Excision occasionally required for "benign" lesions
  - Granular cell tumor
  - Large PASH lesion
  - Enlarging biopsy proven fibroadenoma (risk of phyllodes)

DIAGNOSTIC CHECKLIST

Consider
- Excisional biopsy is mandatory if core biopsy pathology benign yet imaging characteristics suspicious
- Biopsy is often necessary to distinguish benign from malignant masses
  - Substantial overlap in sonographic characteristics
  - Pathology is gold standard for benign diagnosis
  - Goal of sonography is to identify those lesions where suspicion of malignancy is so low that biopsy can be avoided

Image Interpretation Pearls
- Negative predictive value of classification of a lesion as sonographically benign reported as high as 99.5%

SELECTED REFERENCES

1. Cho N et al: Differentiating benign from malignant solid breast masses: comparison of two-dimensional and three-dimensional US. Radiology. 240(1):26-32, 2006
2. Costantini M et al: Characterization of solid breast masses: use of the sonographic breast imaging reporting and data system lexicon. J Ultrasound Med. 25(5):649-59; quiz 661, 2006
3. Hong AS et al: BI-RADS for sonography: positive and negative predictive values of sonographic features. AJR Am J Roentgenol. 184(4):1260-5, 2005
4. Mainiero MB et al: Characterization of breast masses with sonography: can biopsy of some solid masses be deferred? J Ultrasound Med. 24(2):161-7, 2005
5. Graf O et al: Follow-up of palpable circumscribed noncalcified solid breast masses at mammography and US: can biopsy be averted? Radiology. 233(3):850-6, 2004
6. Tardivon AA et al: Imaging and management of nonpalpable lesions of the breast. Eur J Radiol. 42(1):2-9, 2002
7. Stavros AT et al: Solid breast nodules: use of sonography to distinguish between benign and malignant lesions. Radiology. 196(1):123-34, 1995

SOLID NON-MALIGNANT BREAST MASSES

IMAGE GALLERY

Typical

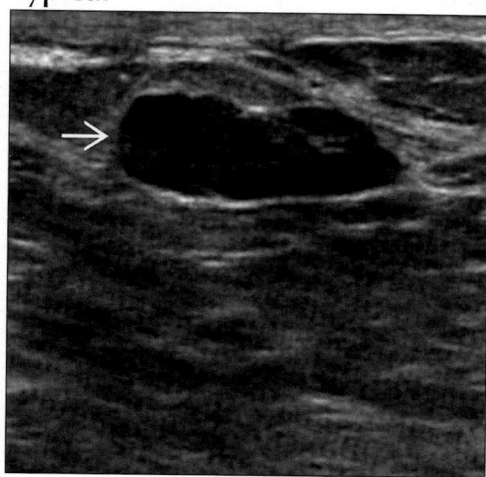 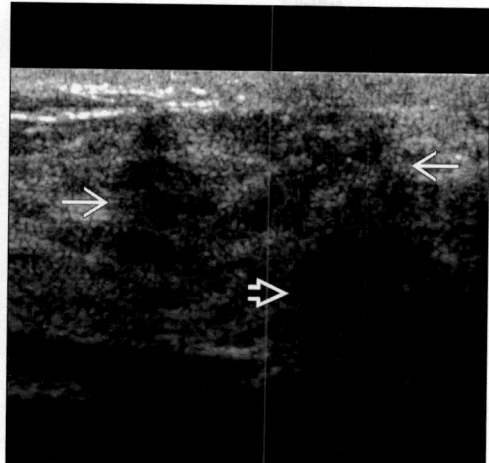

(Left) Longitudinal ultrasound shows a circumscribed hypoechoic mass ➡ with gently lobulated margins and neither posterior enhancement nor shadowing. US-guided biopsy showed nodular adenosis. *(Right)* Transverse ultrasound of a new palpable mass shows an irregular ill-defined hypoechoic mass ➡ with posterior shadowing ➡. US-guided core biopsy revealed diabetic mastopathy.

Typical

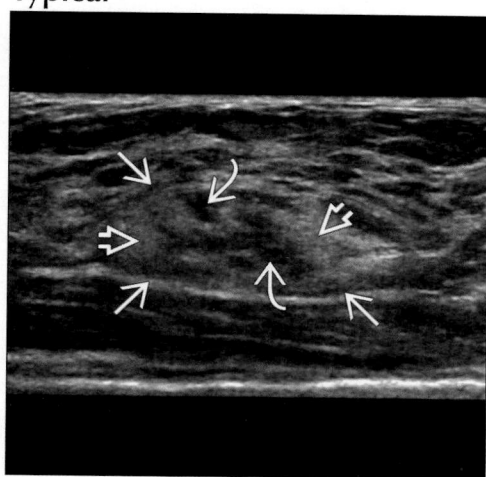 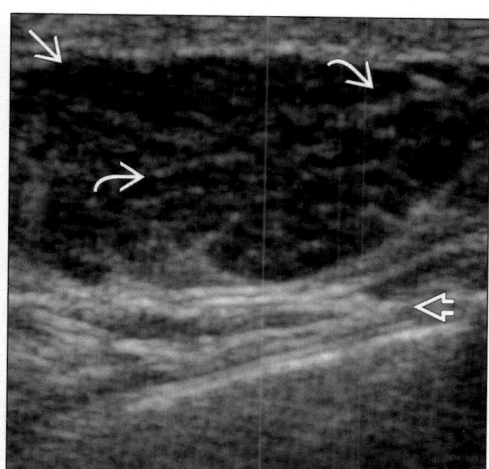

(Left) Longitudinal ultrasound shows a circumscribed lesion ➡ with mixed areas of echogenic fat ➡ & sonolucent glandular elements ➡. Mammography showed a stable, encapsulated fat-containing lesion diagnostic for fibroadenolipoma. *(Right)* Longitudinal ultrasound of a palpable mass shows a circumscribed slightly hypoechoic mass ➡ with echogenic internal septations ➡ & posterior enhancement ➡. Biopsy showed a lactating adenoma.

Typical

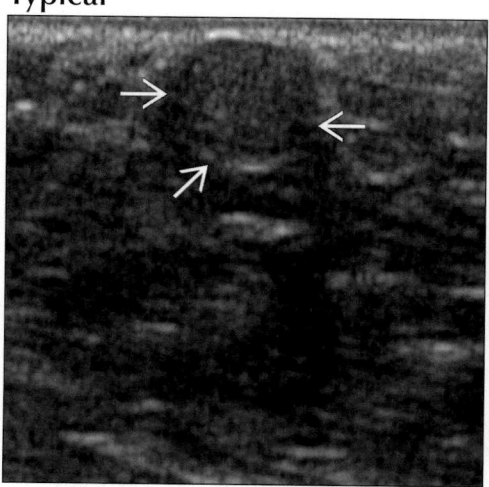 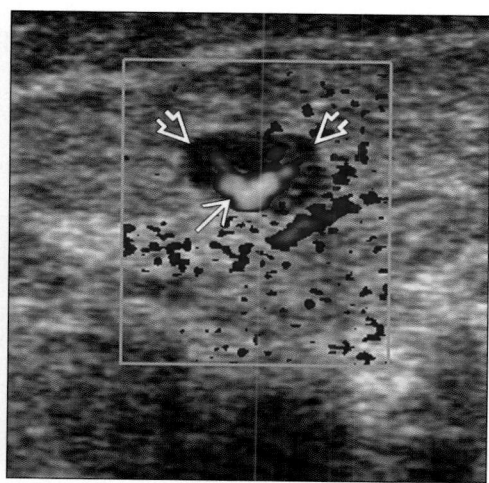

(Left) Transverse ultrasound of a palpable mass shows a superficial, circumscribed mass ➡ slightly hypoechoic to surrounding fat. She had multiple prior lipomas resected from this area. This is compatible with benign lipoma. *(Right)* Longitudinal power Doppler ultrasound shows a well-circumscribed hypoechoic mass ➡ with central vascular hilum ➡ characteristic of benign lymph node.

FAT NECROSIS

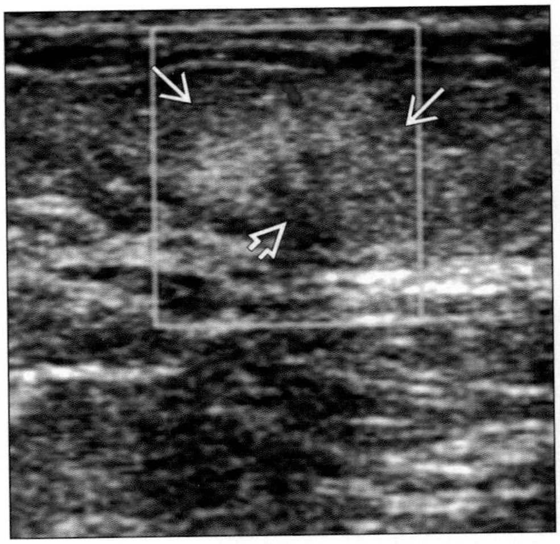

Ultrasound shows a hyperechoic mass ➔ with central hypoechoic focus ➲, typical of fat necrosis. The patient had history of trauma to this region 1 month prior. Biopsy, requested by patient, showed fat necrosis.

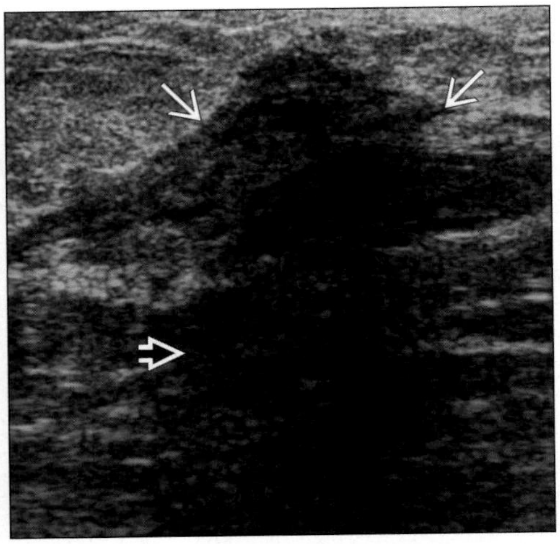

Ultrasound shows a hypoechoic mass-like lesion ➔ with irregular margins and shadowing ➲. The patient had car a accident 1 year prior with extensive airbag injury in this region. Biopsy showed fat necrosis.

TERMINOLOGY

Definitions

- Result of injury to breast fat
- Benign nonsuppurative process related to breast trauma/surgery
- May have other etiologies such as ischemia
  - Post-radiation vasculitis
  - Extensive surgery: Quadrantectomy, multiple re-excisions for margins
  - After autologous reconstruction, e.g., transverse rectus abdominis musculocutaneous (TRAM) flap
    - Entire blood supply to flap dependent on microvascular anastomosis
    - Fat necrosis most common in upper outer portion of flap where blood supply is most tenuous
- Chemical irritation
  - Ruptured cyst or ectatic ducts: Cholesterol crystals
  - Plasma cell mastitis

IMAGING FINDINGS

General Features

- Best diagnostic clue: Oil cyst(s) ± rim calcification on mammography
- Location
  - Most common in subareolar & superficial areas near skin
    - More vulnerable to trauma
- Size: Ranges from a few mm to several cm

Ultrasonographic Findings

- Sonographic appearances evolve over time
  - Acute phase: Within days of event
    - Edema of breast fat → increased echogenicity
    - Use split screen to compare with unaffected side if large area is involved
  - Subacute: Complex cystic phase
    - Ill-defined complex cystic areas within edematous fat: Mixed hypo/hyper to anechoic mass
    - Thin echogenic cyst wall develops: May be multi-loculated
    - Diffuse low level internal echoes
    - Posterior enhancement

DDx: Fat-Containing Masses

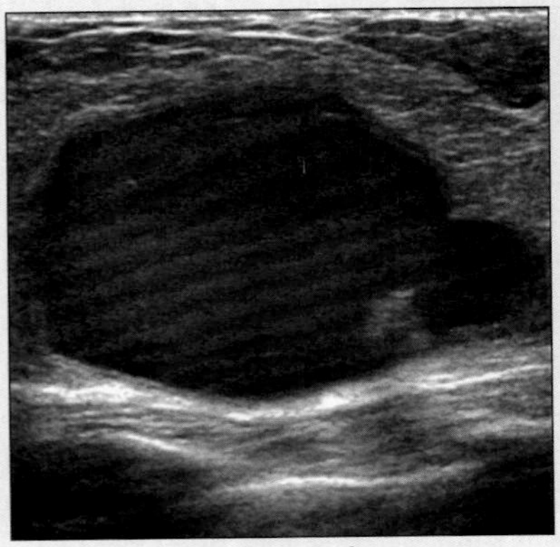

Galactocele

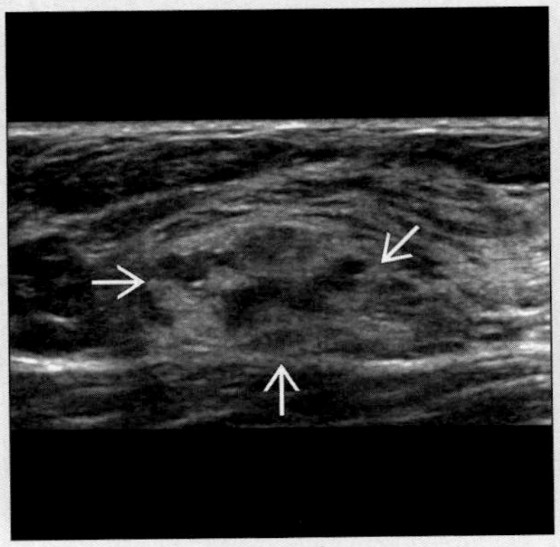

Fibroadenolipoma

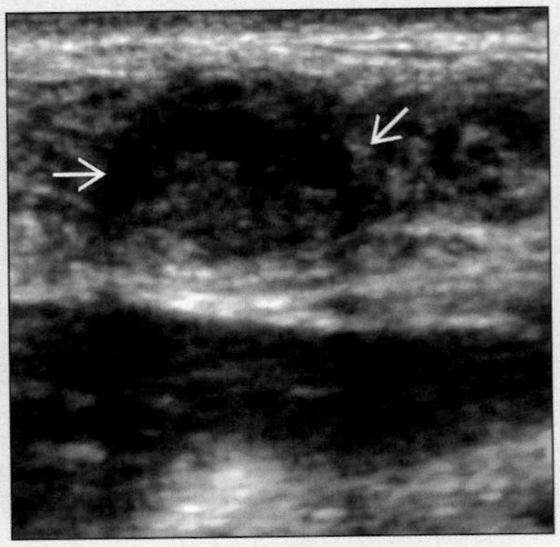

Lipoma

FAT NECROSIS

Key Facts

Terminology
- Benign nonsuppurative process related to breast trauma/surgery

Imaging Findings
- Round, oval, or lobulated lucent mass
- Isolated calcifications
- Spiculated or irregular mass/asymmetry
- Band-like density
- Sonographic appearances evolve over time
- Protocol advice: Perform ultrasound if mammogram negative, inconclusive, or shows asymmetry or ill-defined mass

Top Differential Diagnoses
- Encapsulated Fat-Containing Lesions
- Infiltrating Ductal or Lobular Carcinoma

- DCIS

Pathology
- No history of prior trauma or surgery in 35-50%

Clinical Issues
- No treatment usually necessary

Diagnostic Checklist
- Imaging findings overlap with malignancy
- Proper clinical history helpful: Trauma, surgery
- Fat necrosis mass should decrease over time
- Calcifications develop 1.5-5 yrs (or later) post-trauma, coarsen over time
- Calcification at lumpectomy site within first 1.5 yrs more likely residual carcinoma

---

- Late phase: 18 months or more after event
  - Wall calcifies: Posterior enhancement changes to intense acoustic shadowing
  - May look thick walled or even solid
  - If secondary to surgical cavity more likely to have angular margins
- Sonographic spectrum therefore includes
  - Anechoic mass
  - Irregular hypoechoic mass
  - Complex mass
  - Architectural distortion
- Posterior features change with time: Enhancement to shadowing once fibrosis & calcifications develop
- Color Doppler
  - Internal flow increases concern for recurrent tumor in lumpectomy patient
    - May see flow in granulation tissue within 6 months of surgery
    - Hyperemia post-radiation therapy persists longer; generally settles within a year

Mammographic Findings
- Round, oval, or lobulated lucent mass
  - Oil cyst(s) when round, oval
  - Develop peripheral rim of calcifications
  - Inner aspect of mass appears circumscribed
  - Indistinct interface with breast tissue may be due to surrounding edema, fibrosis, inflammation
- Isolated calcifications
  - Fine linear or pleomorphic
    - Early manifestation
    - May be confused with ductal carcinoma in situ (DCIS)
  - Fat necrosis calcifications become dystrophic over time
  - Lucent-centered, eggshell at edge of oil cysts
  - Calcifications unusual before at least 18 months post-trauma
- Spiculated or irregular mass/asymmetry
  - Due to fibrosis/desmoplastic reaction
  - Should decrease over time
- Band-like density
  - Ask patient about prior seatbelt injury

MR Findings
- T1WI: High signal central fat
- T2WI
  - Low signal with fat-suppression
  - May see surrounding increased signal due to edema
- T1 C+
  - Thin rim of peripheral enhancement may persist up to 18 months post-trauma
    - Rarely fat necrosis will enhance years later

Imaging Recommendations
- Best imaging tool
  - Mammography
    - Magnification views for subtle calcifications
- Protocol advice: Perform ultrasound if mammogram negative, inconclusive, or shows asymmetry or ill-defined mass

DIFFERENTIAL DIAGNOSIS

Encapsulated Fat-Containing Lesions
- Lipoma
  - No history of trauma: No calcifications
- Fibroadenolipoma
  - Encapsulated fat & glandular elements
  - "Breast-within-a-breast" mammographic appearance
- Galactocele
  - Associated with lactation
  - Echogenic, usually with fluid-debris layer (nondependent debris due to fat content)
  - Aspiration yields milky fluid or creamy inspissated secretions

Infiltrating Ductal or Lobular Carcinoma
- Some fat necrosis may mimic carcinoma particularly if it is densely fibrotic or inflamed
- Review old films for evolution of fat necrosis changes
- No history of trauma
- If in doubt → biopsy

FAT NECROSIS

DCIS
- Fine linear or pleomorphic calcifications may appear similar to fat necrosis
- Only associated with a mass in about 10% of cases

PATHOLOGY

General Features
- General path comments
  - Inflammation/hemorrhage into fat → damage to adipocytes
  - Damaged cells leak fat → breakdown to fatty acids (FA) → more inflammation
  - Fibrous capsule forms to encapsulate process
  - Saponification of fatty acids in capsule → calcium deposition
  - Non-encapsulated fatty acids incite granulomatous foreign body-like reaction
  - Chronic foreign body-like reaction → fibrosis, skin retraction
    - Can be hard to differentiate from desmoplastic reaction in cancer
- Etiology
  - Accidental injury
    - Blunt or penetrating trauma: Direct blow to the thorax, seatbelt injury, stab or gunshot wound
  - Iatrogenic injury
    - Surgery: Biopsy, lumpectomy, flap reconstruction, reduction, augmentation, explantation
    - Post-lumpectomy adjuvant radiation therapy
    - Direct silicone injection
  - Spontaneous development reported in patients with diabetes or collagen vascular disease
  - No history of prior trauma or surgery in 35-50%

Gross Pathologic & Surgical Features
- Firm or hard nodular yellowish-white mass
- May be associated with recent or old hemorrhage

Microscopic Features
- Loss of nuclei, fusion of adipocytes
  - Damaged cells coalesce
  - Creation of expanded fatty spaces
- Accumulation of foamy histiocytes
  - Fuse into multinucleated giant cells
- Inflammatory reaction
  - Accumulation of lymphocytes, polymorphonucleocytes, plasma cells
- Peripheral fibrosis with central necrosis

CLINICAL ISSUES

Presentation
- Can occur at any age
- Highly variable clinical presentation
  - May be asymptomatic on screening
  - Tender or non-tender, palpable mass or masses
  - Occasional skin thickening, retraction
- Imaging findings may be preceded by ecchymosis ± erythema

Natural History & Prognosis
- Excellent - no malignant potential

Treatment
- No treatment usually necessary
- Rarely requires excision for painful mass

DIAGNOSTIC CHECKLIST

Consider
- Differentiation of fat necrosis from tumor recurrence in cancer patients treated with breast conservation may be difficult
- Fat necrosis findings are complicated by those of the underlying process e.g., post-op seroma/hematoma, ischemia
- Imaging findings overlap with malignancy
  - Biopsy required if diagnosis unclear

Image Interpretation Pearls
- Proper clinical history helpful: Trauma, surgery
- Ultrasound technique
  - Use compression
    - Fat necrosis not tense therefore compressible
    - Invasive cancer is not compressible
  - Scan plane parallel to scar
    - Mass like appearance due to orientation along surgical dissection planes
  - Scan plane perpendicular to scar
    - Linear appearance, less mass-like
    - Track to skin scar usually evident
- Spot compression mammography may be very helpful
  - Demonstration of oil cysts within a spiculated mass reassuring for diagnosis of fat necrosis
  - Invasive tumor invades fat, does not engulf it
- Fat necrosis mass should decrease over time
  - Rarely inflammatory fat necrosis mass will increase → biopsy
- Calcifications develop 1.5-5 yrs (or later) post-trauma, coarsen over time
- Calcification at lumpectomy site within first 1.5 yrs more likely residual carcinoma

SELECTED REFERENCES

1. Gatta G et al: Clinical, mammographic and ultrasonographic features of blunt breast trauma. Eur J Radiol. 2006
2. Crystal P et al: Sonographic findings of palpable isoechoic breast fat necrosis: look for skin integrity. J Ultrasound Med. 24(1):105-7, 2005
3. Cawson JN et al: False-positive breast screening due to fat necrosis following mammography. Australas Radiol. 48(2):217-9, 2004
4. Chala LF et al: Fat necrosis of the breast: mammographic, sonographic, computed tomography, and magnetic resonance imaging findings. Curr Probl Diagn Radiol. 33(3):106-26, 2004
5. Kinoshita T et al: Fat necrosis of breast: a potential pitfall in breast MRI. Clin Imaging. 26(4):250-3, 2002
6. Williams HJ et al: Imaging features of breast trauma: a pictorial review. Breast. 11(2):107-15, 2002

FAT NECROSIS

Typical

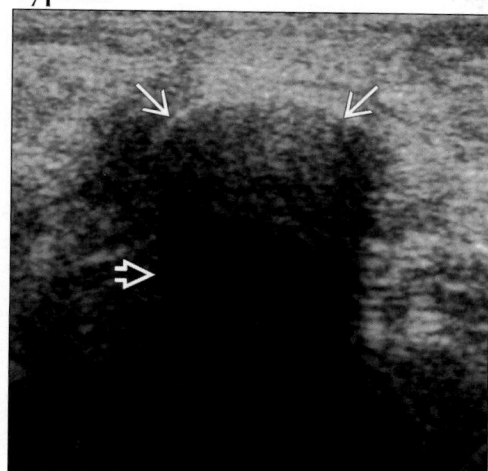

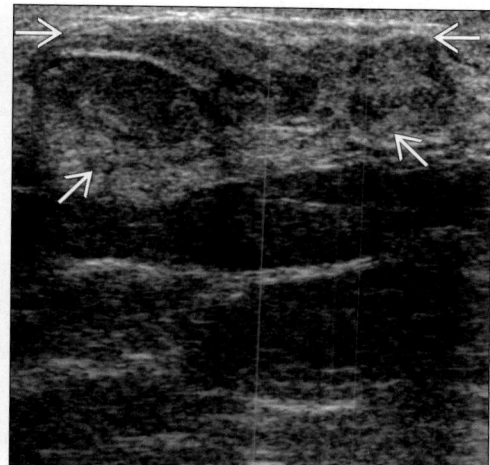

(Left) Ultrasound shows a palpable, intensely shadowing ➡ mass with anterior echogenic rim ➡ at the lumpectomy site in a 38 y/o. The patient requested excision which showed fat necrosis. *(Right)* Ultrasound shows a mixed echogenicity mass ➡ at the site of a mammographically suspicious asymmetry. This 69 y/o sustained breast injury one year earlier. Biopsy showed fat necrosis.

Typical

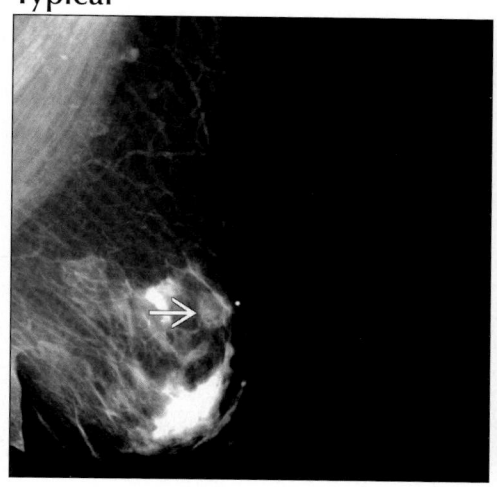

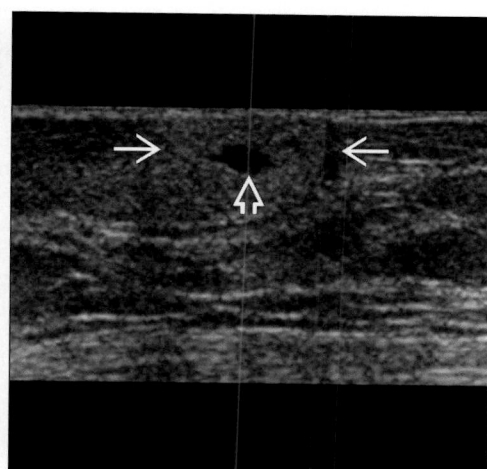

(Left) MLO mammographic view shows a round, well-circumscribed and fat-containing mass ➡. This palpable mass is consistent with fat necrosis by mammographic characteristics alone. *(Right)* Ultrasound in the same patient as previous image shows oval, well circumscribed primarily hyperechoic mass ➡ with areas of internal hypo- to anechogenicity ➡. US findings are also consistent with fat necrosis, which was confirmed by biopsy.

Typical

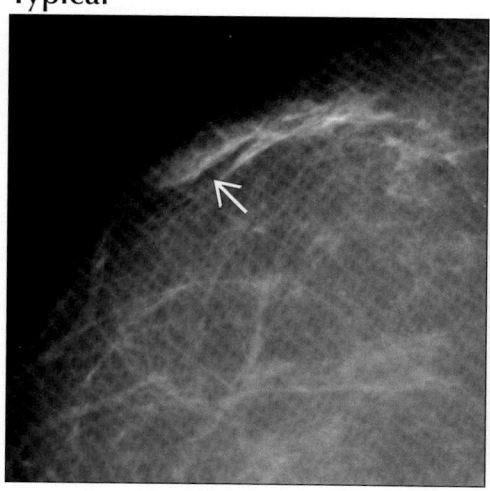

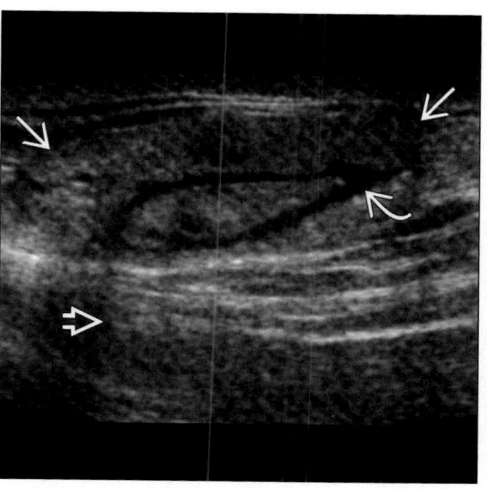

(Left) CC mammogram shows band-like asymmetry ➡ in an area of palpable abnormality which appeared after a fall several weeks earlier. *(Right)* Ultrasound in the same patient as left shows an ovoid area of increased echogenicity ➡ with some anechoic fluid component ➡ & minimal posterior enhancement ➡. The sonographic findings, together with the history, are typical of fat necrosis. In this case, findings resolved on follow-up.

BREAST ABSCESS

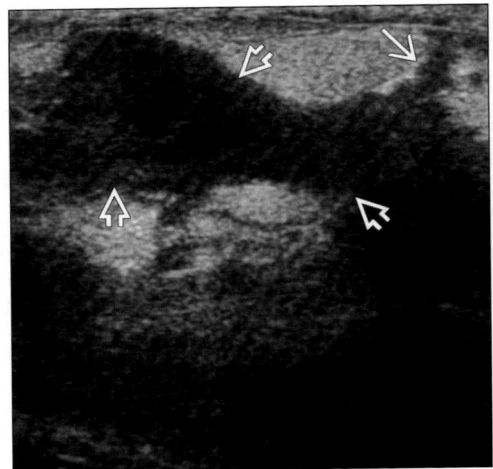

Longitudinal ultrasound shows an irregular hypoechoic abscess with both circumscribed and irregular margins ➡ and a tract extending towards the skin surface ➡.

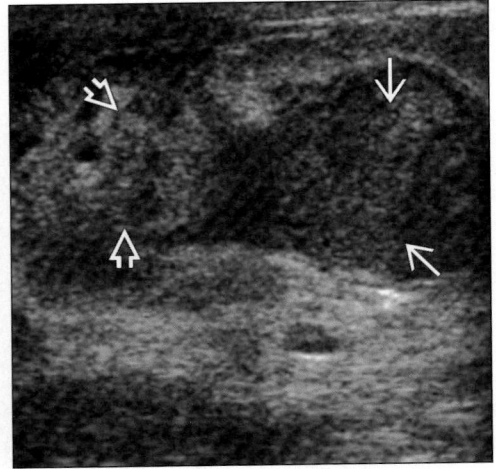

Transverse ultrasound shows an abscess with heterogeneous, hypo- ➡ and hyperechoic ➡ mass-like appearance. Clinical history helps differentiate between solid mass and abscess.

TERMINOLOGY

Abbreviations and Synonyms
- Focal breast infection

Definitions
- Localized pus collection within breast tissue
- Puerperal or lactational breast abscess

IMAGING FINDINGS

General Features
- Best diagnostic clue
  - Hypoechoic, irregular, complex sonographic mass with surrounding increased echogenicity (edema)
  - Clinical history and physical exam suggests infection
- Location: Subareolar most common but may be peripheral
- Size: Variable: Often 2-4 cm but may be up to 10 cm
- Morphology
  - Sonographic ill-defined mass with irregular margins
    - Usually hypoechoic and heterogeneous
  - Focal density on mammogram

Ultrasonographic Findings
- Grayscale Ultrasound
  - Hypoechoic, irregular, complex sonographic mass
  - Heterogeneous texture, may have solid components
  - Surrounding increased echogenicity (edema)
  - Variable margins: Irregular, thick-walled, circumscribed
  - May have fluid/debris level or septation
  - Gentle probe pressure may show movement of thick, purulent fluid within the cavity
  - Air may be present within the abscess cavity
    - Bright specular reflectors
  - May see tract extending from the abscess cavity toward skin surface or into deeper tissues
- Power Doppler
  - Hyperemia in surrounding tissue common
  - Inspissated fluid may be isoechoic
    - Ballottement to show color from sloshing of contents
- Ultrasound: Modality of choice for diagnosis and treatment

DDx: Complex Fluid Collections

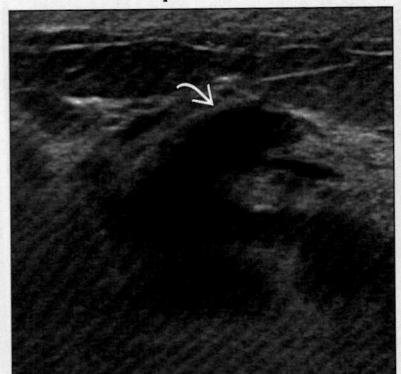

Inflammatory Carcinoma

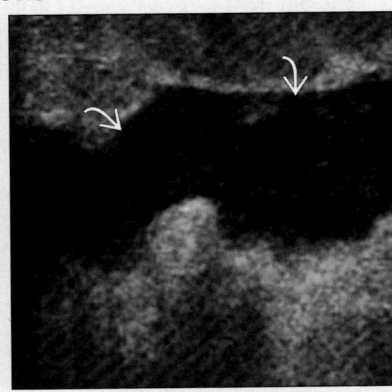

Post-Operative Seroma

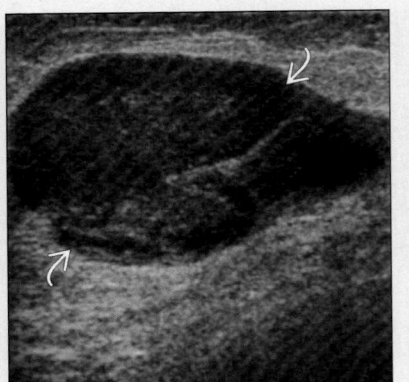

Hematoma

BREAST ABSCESS

Key Facts

Terminology
- Localized pus collection within breast tissue
- Puerperal or lactational breast abscess

Imaging Findings
- Hypoechoic, irregular, complex sonographic mass with surrounding increased echogenicity (edema)
- May have fluid/debris level or septation
- Gentle probe pressure may show movement of thick, purulent fluid within the cavity
- May see tract extending from the abscess cavity toward skin surface or into deeper tissues
- Hyperemia in surrounding tissue common
- Ultrasound: Modality of choice for diagnosis and treatment

Top Differential Diagnoses
- Inflammatory Carcinoma
- Seroma
- Hematoma

Pathology
- Duct ectasia → stasis → obstruction → inflammation
- Puerperal abscess: Nipple fissure causes sub-areolar inflammation, duct obstruction, milk stasis, infection

Clinical Issues
- Inflamed, erythematous, indurated, painful area on breast

Diagnostic Checklist
- Clinical presentation key to selecting appropriate imaging

Mammographic Findings
- Ill-defined, noncalcified mass or focal asymmetry
  - Variable margins (ill-defined, irregular, spiculated)
- Pain may limit use of mammography
- Mammography often not performed in younger women when history and physical exam suggests infection

MR Findings
- Usually not required for diagnosis
- Abscess cavity may show intense rim enhancement due to hyperemia
- May show adjacent edema (high signal on T2WI) and skin thickening

Imaging Recommendations
- Best imaging tool: Ultrasound is most beneficial
- Protocol advice
  - Start with ultrasound in young patients
  - Use lower frequency transducer for larger abscess
  - Use color Doppler to show surrounding hyperemia

DIFFERENTIAL DIAGNOSIS

Inflammatory Carcinoma
- Simulates infectious process
  - May appear to respond to antibiotics
  - May lead to delay in diagnosis
- Skin biopsy is diagnostic, but may have false negative results

Seroma
- No signs/symptoms of infection

Hematoma
- May be echogenic if acute
- Subacute may show fluid-fluid level

Invasive Ductal or Lobular Carcinoma
- Hypoechoic, irregular sonographic mass
- Clinical presentation and history helps differentiate

Mastitis
- Diffuse infection may harbor a focal abscess
- Infectious agent enters through nipple during lactation

Necrotic Tumor
- Squamous cell metastases may manifest as a largely necrotic mass

Epidermal Inclusion or Sebaceous Cyst
- Can be distinguished clinically

PATHOLOGY

General Features
- Etiology
  - Duct ectasia → stasis → obstruction → inflammation
  - Skin/nipple abrasion with breastfeeding
  - Squamous metaplasia of lactiferous ducts (SMOLD)
    - Recurrent mastitis which can result in abscess
    - High association with smoking
  - Infective organisms
    - Staphylococcus aureus and epidermidis most common
    - Streptococcus: More diffuse inflammation ± cellulitis, if abscess forms may become chronic
    - Anaerobic or microaerophilic organisms
    - Less common agents: Fungal, viral, parasitic, mycobacterium, cat scratch disease
  - Non-puerperal abscess
    - Peri-menopausal: Etiology less clear, multifactorial, possibly related to hormonal changes
    - Late teens/early twenties: Associated with underlying congenital nipple inversion and squamous metaplasia
    - 90% of women with non-puerperal peri-ductal mastitis are smokers
  - Infection in post-lumpectomy seroma cavity
- Puerperal abscess: Nipple fissure causes sub-areolar inflammation, duct obstruction, milk stasis, infection

BREAST ABSCESS

- o Peripheral, central, or non-specific pattern of involvement
- o Peripheral
  - ▪ Infection in sub-lobar ducts or pre-existing galactocele
  - ▪ Abscess forms early
  - ▪ Often multiloculated
- o Central
  - ▪ Rapid lobar spread with hyperemia
  - ▪ Infection in dilated central ducts
  - ▪ Usually unilocular, parallel to ducts
- o Non-specific pattern
  - ▪ Ill-defined hyperemia and edema
  - ▪ Poorly distinguished ducts
  - ▪ Diagnosis difficult until abscess forms
- Non-puerperal or peri-areolar abscess
  - o Underlying duct ectasia, less often cysts
  - o Nipple inversion may precede or be caused by periductal inflammation, fibrosis
  - o Pathogenesis
    - ▪ Stasis → inflammation → infection
  - o Weakened, inflamed duct wall ruptures releasing fatty secretions → inflammation
  - o Migratory focal abscesses
    - ▪ Different lobar ducts affected
  - o Prone to fistula formation
- Epidemiology: Puerperal abscess: 4.8-11% incidence in lactating women

Gross Pathologic & Surgical Features
- Focal mass
- Inflammation

Microscopic Features
- Mixed acute and chronic inflammation
- May have fat necrosis

CLINICAL ISSUES

Presentation
- Most common signs/symptoms
  - o Painful focal or diffuse skin thickening and edema
  - o Inflamed, erythematous, indurated, painful area on breast
  - o Focal abscess
    - ▪ May present as painful palpable mass ("red, hot, tender lump")
- Other signs/symptoms
  - o Mastitis
  - o Nipple inversion: May be intermittent
  - o Nipple discharge
  - o Mammary fistula (also known as milk fistula)
- Most common during reproductive years
- Peripheral location more common in groups at increased risk: Diabetic, HIV, steroid use, recent surgery

Natural History & Prognosis
- May resolve spontaneously
- Non-puerperal sub-areolar abscesses often indolent, chronic, and recurrent
  - o Recurrence rate: 10-38%
- Nipple retraction or inversion may become permanent

- If untreated
  - o "Pointing" of abscess with subsequent drainage through skin
  - o Mammary/milk fistula formation
  - o May lead to rupture of multiple ducts

Treatment
- Local and systemic treatment necessary
  - o Systemic antibiotics directed to skin organisms
    - ▪ Cephalexin 250-500 mg qid x 10 d or Zithromycin (Z-pak)
  - o Percutaneous US guided drainage of cavity
    - ▪ Thick pus may require 18 gauge needle or larger
    - ▪ Culture not usually necessary unless refractory to treatment
  - o Cavities < 3 cm may be completely evacuated with aspiration
    - ▪ 50-60% require repeat aspiration
  - o May require indwelling catheter drainage
    - ▪ Cavities > 3-4 cm or complex
  - o Surgical incision and drainage may be required
  - o Surgical excision rarely required for refractory cases
- Exclude malignancy
  - o Especially in older women
  - o May need short interval follow-up exam if clinical picture is not typical
- Puerperal abscess
  - o Encourage continued breast emptying by breast feeding or pumping
- Non-puerperal abscess
  - o Recurrent subareolar abscess may require surgical excision of plugged lactiferous ducts
  - o Wedge excision of affected area of nipple in chronic cases

DIAGNOSTIC CHECKLIST

Consider
- Clinical presentation key to selecting appropriate imaging

Image Interpretation Pearls
- Complex fluid in an abscess may mimic a solid mass
  - o Ballottement useful to distinguish fluid from solid mass

SELECTED REFERENCES
1. Christensen AF et al: Ultrasound-guided drainage of breast abscesses: results in 151 patients. Br J Radiol. 78(927):186-8, 2005
2. Eryilmaz R et al: Management of lactational breast abscesses. Breast. 14(5):375-9, 2005
3. Varey AH et al: Treatment of loculated lactational breast abscess with a vacuum biopsy system. Br J Surg. 92(10):1225-6, 2005
4. Versluijs-Ossewaarde FN et al: Subareolar breast abscesses: characteristics and results of surgical treatment. Breast J. 11(3):179-82, 2005
5. Ulitzsch D et al: Breast abscess in lactating women: US-guided treatment. Radiology. 232(3):904-9, 2004

BREAST ABSCESS

IMAGE GALLERY

Typical

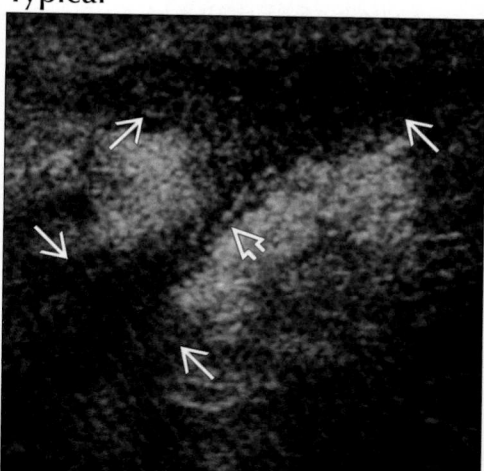
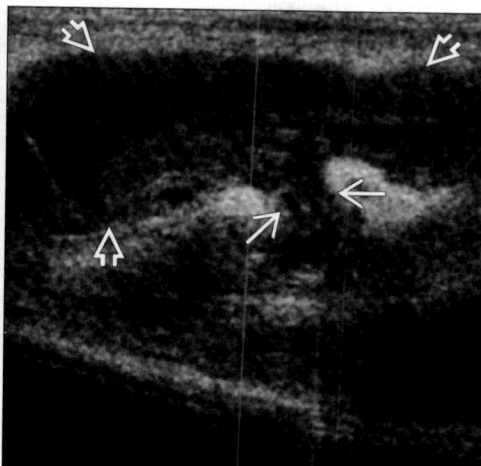

(Left) Transverse ultrasound shows two irregular hypoechoic cavities ➡ connected by a sinus tract ⇒. *(Right)* Transverse ultrasound shows circumscribed hypoechoic abscess ⇒ with a sinus tract ➡ extending towards the deeper tissues.

Typical

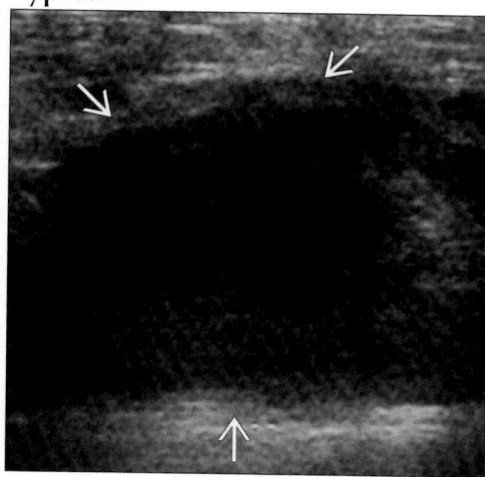
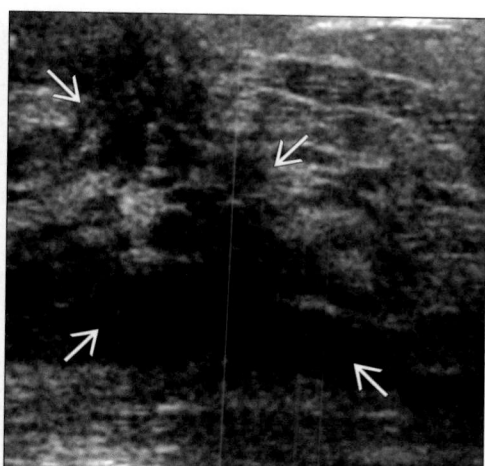

(Left) Longitudinal ultrasound shows a hypoechoic abscess with subtle internal echoes and slightly irregular margins. The borders are somewhat thickened ➡. *(Right)* Transverse ultrasound shows a subtle heterogeneous abscess with ill-defined margins ➡. Aspiration yielded frank pus.

Typical

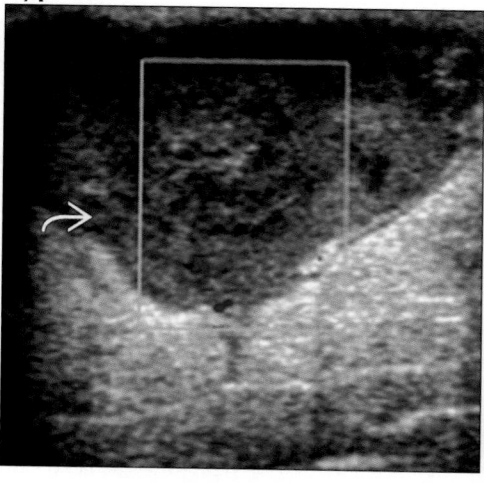
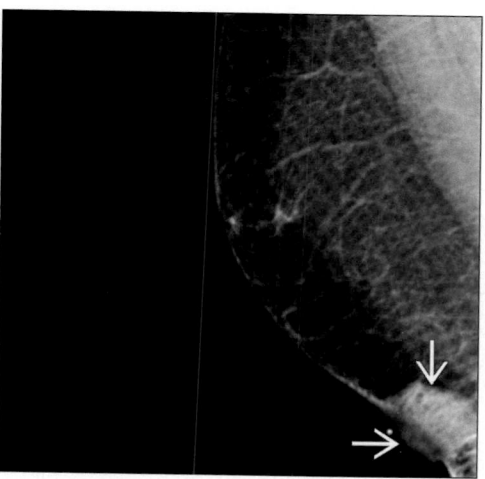

(Left) Longitudinal color Doppler ultrasound shows a circumscribed hypoechoic abscess ➡ with heterogeneous internal echoes and little peripheral flow, mimicking a solid mass. Peripheral hyperemia is more typical. *(Right)* Oblique (MLO) mammogram shows a mass in the inferior breast ➡. This appears to extend beyond the skin surface. Pus was expressed from the lesion during mammographic compression.

INTRACTAL PAPILLOMA

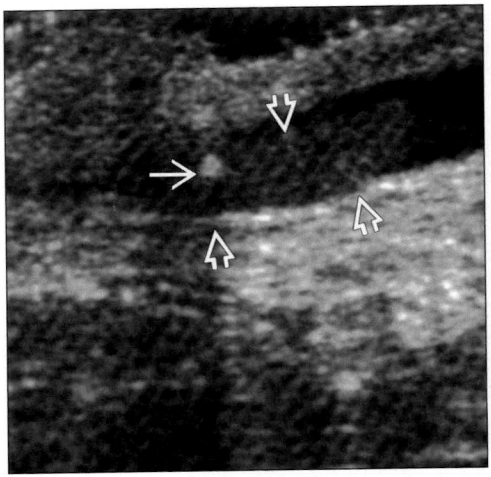

Longitudinal ultrasound shows a mass within a dilated subareolar duct, seen in a patient with exuberant serous nipple discharge ➤. A single calcification is present ➡.

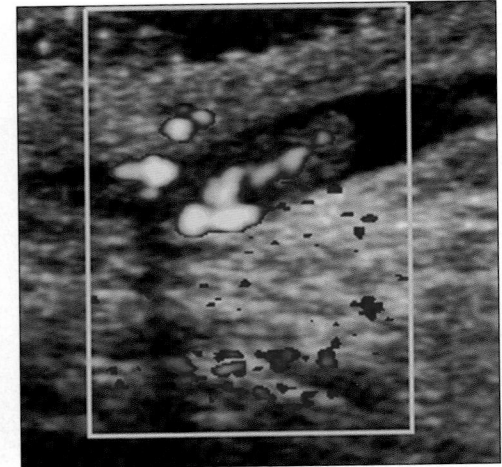

Longitudinal power Doppler ultrasound shows marked vascularity in the intraductal mass. Surgical excision yielded benign papilloma.

TERMINOLOGY

Definitions
- Papillary growth within a duct

IMAGING FINDINGS

General Features
- Best diagnostic clue: Solid mass within a dilated duct or cyst
- Location
  - Usually large ducts
  - Subareolar

Ultrasonographic Findings
- Grayscale Ultrasound
  - Lobulated solid mass
    - Within dilated duct
    - May also be seen in a cystic lesion
    - If associated with hemorrhage then increased concern for papillary carcinoma
  - Most often homogeneously hypoechoic
  - If peripheral may have ill-defined margins
  - Associated coarse calcifications may be seen
  - Difficult to identify the lesion if involved duct is not dilated
    - Especially true of peripheral papillomas
- Power Doppler: Often has visible internal vascularity

Mammographic Findings
- Mammography frequently shows no abnormality
- Galactography may also be useful to assess for intraductal lesion
  - Intraluminal filling defect
  - Expansion of duct around lesion
  - Ductal dilation up to the lesion

Imaging Recommendations
- Use ultrasound to evaluate for intraductal mass in subareolar region
  - Attempt to localize discharging duct orifice
    - Focused scan in that quadrant helps increase sensitivity
  - Scan radially around nipple
  - Use generous gel to provide a relative standoff pad for imaging superficially
  - Attempt to visualize subareolar ducts by angling transducer along long axis of duct

DDx: Intraductal Lesions

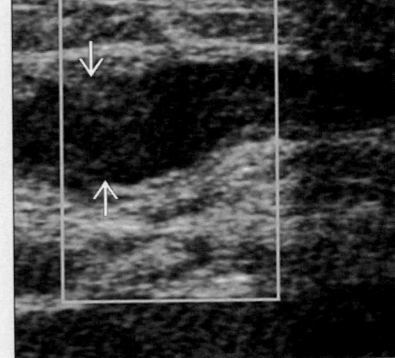

Debris

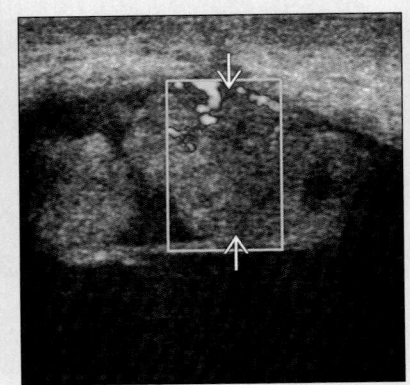

Papillary Carcinoma

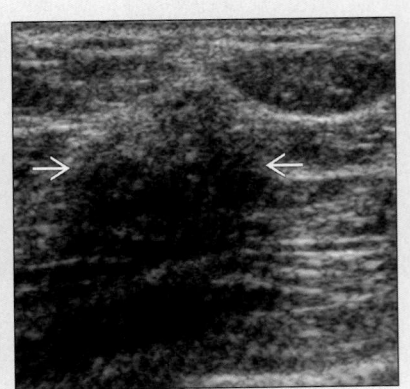

Ductal Carcinoma in Situ (DCIS)

INTRADUCTAL PAPILLOMA

Key Facts

Terminology
- Papillary growth within a duct

Imaging Findings
- Best diagnostic clue: Solid mass within a dilated duct or cyst
- Difficult to identify the lesion if involved duct is not dilated
- Power Doppler: Often has visible internal vascularity
- Attempt to localize discharging duct orifice
- Scan radially around nipple
- Use "rolled nipple" imaging technique
- Confirm intraductal lesion in radial and antiradial views

Top Differential Diagnoses
- Duct Ectasia/Ductal Debris

- Invasive Papillary Carcinoma
- Breast Cancer/DCIS
- Nipple Adenoma

Clinical Issues
- Any atypia on core biopsy requires surgical excision
- Many now recommend surgical excision of all papillary intraductal lesions

Diagnostic Checklist
- Negative ultrasound in a patient with nipple discharge does not exclude papilloma as mass may not be seen if duct not distended with fluid at time of scan
- Attempt to straighten duct to avoid false positives
- Image along long axis of duct for best resolution

- ○ Use "rolled nipple" imaging technique
  - ▪ Nipple "rolled" over examiner's finger
  - ▪ Transducer applied to elongated superficial surface
  - ▪ Allows visualization of distal intraductal/intra nipple lesions
- ○ Confirm intraductal lesion in radial and antiradial views
  - ▪ Ducts are tortuous; periductal tissue or branch points may simulate intraductal lesion on 1 view

DIFFERENTIAL DIAGNOSIS

Duct Ectasia/Ductal Debris
- No internal Doppler flow
- Up to 25% of patients have nipple discharge
- Usually yellow-greenish or milky
  - ○ May be bloody
- May see floating debris or fluid-debris level
  - ○ Attempt to induce positional changes, similar to evaluation of complicated cysts
- If acutely inflamed may rupture and cause abscess

Invasive Papillary Carcinoma
- Uncommon
  - ○ 1-2% of all breast cancers
- Older patients than solitary benign papillomas
- Palpable, often large subareolar mass
  - ○ Many have associated nipple discharge
- Complex partly cystic mass on ultrasound
  - ○ Variable solid component
  - ○ Fluid may be hemorrhagic

Breast Cancer/DCIS
- Solid hypoechoic mass
- Posterior acoustic shadowing
- DCIS may present as a solid, relatively circumscribed mass

Nipple Adenoma
- Primary tumor of the nipple
- Papillary hyperplasia of duct epithelium with fibrosis

PATHOLOGY

General Features
- Papillary growth within ductal system
- Most are solitary and in large subareolar duct
- Need to differentiate intraductal papilloma from multiple peripheral papillomas and papillomatosis
  - ○ Multiple peripheral papillomas
    - ▪ Tend to occur in younger patients
    - ▪ Less likely to present with nipple discharge
    - ▪ Peripherally located intraductal lesions originate in terminal duct lobular unit
    - ▪ More likely to recur
    - ▪ More often bilateral
    - ▪ Multiple peripheral nodules on mammography/ultrasound
    - ▪ Increased risk of developing carcinoma; more likely to undergo malignant transformation
  - ○ Papillomatosis refers to a type of epithelial hyperplasia
    - ▪ Papillary epithelial projections into ductal lumen
    - ▪ In the spectrum of fibrocystic changes/parenchymal hyperplasia (florid duct hyperplasia of usual type)
    - ▪ No discrete radiologic correlate

Gross Pathologic & Surgical Features
- Rarely > 1 cm
  - ○ Usually under 5 mm
- Most often in a dilated major duct close to nipple
  - ○ May also be within a cyst
- Soft, friable tumors

Microscopic Features
- Composed of multiple branching papillae
  - ○ Central core of connective tissue
  - ○ Covered by cuboidal or columnar epithelial cells
  - ○ Intervening myoepithelial layer
- Only epithelial and myoepithelial cells present
- No atypical cells when benign
  - ○ Epithelial hyperplasia or fibrosis may make differentiation from papillary carcinoma difficult

INTRADUCTAL PAPILLOMA

- o Papilloma infarction may simulate invasive carcinoma

CLINICAL ISSUES

Presentation
- Most common signs/symptoms
  - o Spontaneous nipple discharge
    - Clear, bloody, or serous
- Other signs/symptoms
  - o Palpable subareolar mass
  - o May be incidental finding during sonogram of adjacent area

Demographics
- Age: Most frequent in women 30-50 years old

Natural History & Prognosis
- Subsequent risk of breast cancer may be increased
  - o If atypical ductal hyperplasia (ADH) or limited DCIS seen within papilloma
  - o Similar to risk with parenchymal atypical ductal hyperplasia
  - o Risk mostly to the same breast in the area of the papilloma
- Some data suggest even solitary papillomas without atypia are associated with increased risk of breast cancer
  - o If true would warrant surgical excision of all papillary lesions
    - Up to 26% of lesions upgraded to ADH or DCIS when excised
  - o Consider short interval follow-up if excision not performed
    - Use BI-RADS category 3: Follow-up at 6 month intervals for two years to ensure stability
    - Only if imaging findings are concordant with benign pathologic diagnosis
    - Caveat is that imaging alone cannot reliably predict malignancy

Treatment
- Biopsy
  - o Fine needle aspiration (FNA)
    - Sensitivity as low as 44%
  - o Core biopsy
    - Sensitivity 82%
    - Much higher specificity than FNA
    - Negative predictive value up to 94%
    - Any atypia on core biopsy requires surgical excision
    - Need to exclude higher grade lesion if atypia present
    - Sensitivity improves with larger needle size, number of samples, and use of vacuum-assisted biopsy devices
- Surgical excision
  - o Removal of the duct has been the most reliable method of obtaining a diagnosis
    - Vacuum-assisted core biopsy techniques have improved percutaneous diagnosis

- Not conclusive if "excision" by coring until all visible mass removed truly equal to surgical excision of intact mass
- o Many now recommend surgical excision of all papillary intraductal lesions
  - More accurate histologic evaluation possible as mass is not fragmented
  - Will catch smaller foci of carcinoma in situ or atypia
  - Can include wider margin in case of solitary papilloma associated with carcinoma
- Breast endoscopy
  - o Can visualize intraluminal defect
  - o Aid for guiding surgical resection
  - o May be beneficial as blind resection can miss multiple or more peripheral lesions
    - Typical blind resection extends for first 2-3 cm of retroareolar duct
    - Will miss lesions beyond that margin

DIAGNOSTIC CHECKLIST

Consider
- Surgical excision of all papillary lesions to avoid histologic underestimation
- Negative ultrasound in a patient with nipple discharge does not exclude papilloma as mass may not be seen if duct not distended with fluid at time of scan

Image Interpretation Pearls
- Attempt to straighten duct to avoid false positives
- Image along long axis of duct for best resolution

SELECTED REFERENCES

1. Al Sarakbi W et al: Breast papillomas: current management with a focus on a new diagnostic and therapeutic modality. Int Semin Surg Oncol. 3:1, 2006
2. Ganesan S et al: Ultrasound spectrum in intraductal papillary neoplasms of breast. Br J Radiol. 2006
3. Lam WW et al: Role of radiologic features in the management of papillary lesions of the breast. AJR Am J Roentgenol. 186(5):1322-7, 2006
4. Mercado CL et al: Papillary lesions of the breast at percutaneous core-needle biopsy. Radiology. 238(3):801-8, 2006
5. Georgountzos V et al: Benign intracystic papilloma in the male breast. Breast J. 11(5):361-2, 2005
6. Gutman H et al: Are solitary breast papillomas entirely benign? Arch Surg. 138(12):1330-3, 2003
7. Dooley WC: Routine operative breast endoscopy for bloody nipple discharge. Ann Surg Oncol. 9(9):920-3, 2002
8. Francis A et al: Breast papilloma: mammogram, ultrasound and MRI appearances. Breast. 11(5):394-7, 2002
9. Rosen EL et al: Imaging-guided core needle biopsy of papillary lesions of the breast. AJR Am J Roentgenol. 179(5):1185-92, 2002
10. Vargas HI et al: Management of bloody nipple discharge. Curr Treat Options Oncol. 3(2):157-61, 2002
11. Mercado CL et al: Papillary lesions of the breast: evaluation with stereotactic directional vacuum-assisted biopsy. Radiology. 221(3):650-5, 2001

INTRADUCTAL PAPILLOMA

Typical

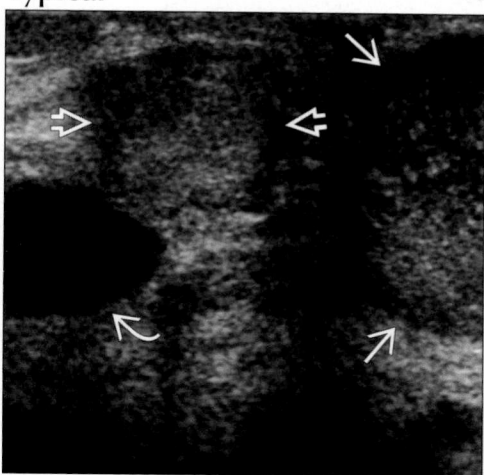
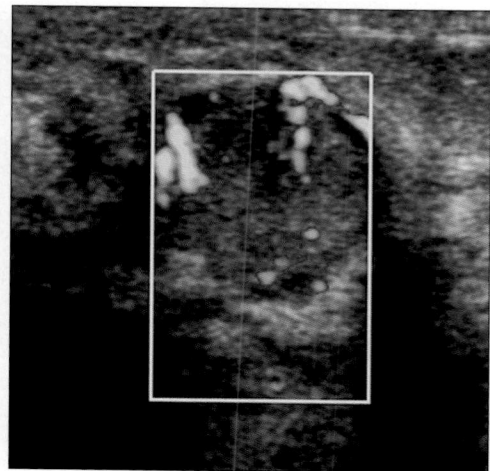

(Left) Transverse ultrasound of the subareolar region shows a symptomatic complicated cyst ➡, a simple cyst ➡ and an incidental 1.5 cm lobulated subareolar mass ➡. *(Right)* Transverse power Doppler ultrasound in the same case as previous image shows significant vascularity within the subareolar mass, shown to be a benign papilloma on core biopsy and surgical excision.

Typical

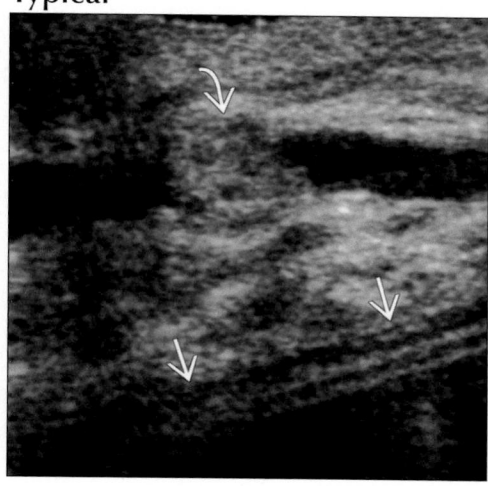
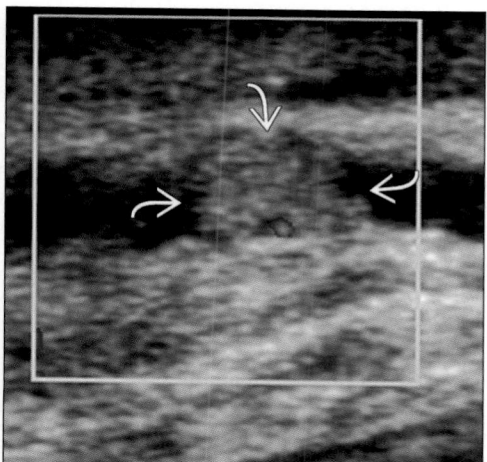

(Left) Longitudinal ultrasound shows a 4 mm intraductal mass ➡ in a patient with bloody nipple discharge. Implants are partially seen ➡. *(Right)* Longitudinal power Doppler ultrasound shows that the lesion had only minimal visible internal vascularity. However the lobulated margins and convex contours ➡ aid in distinguishing this from debris. This was an intraductal papilloma on surgical excision.

Variant

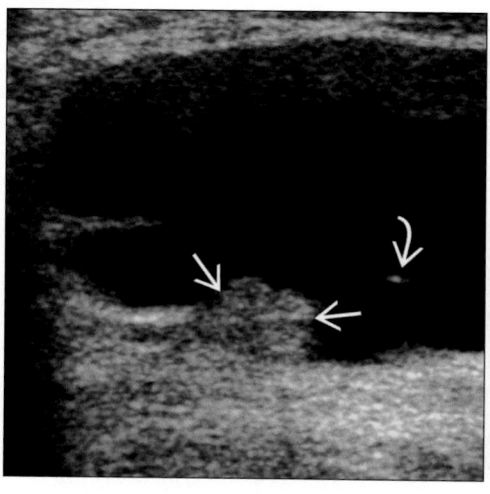
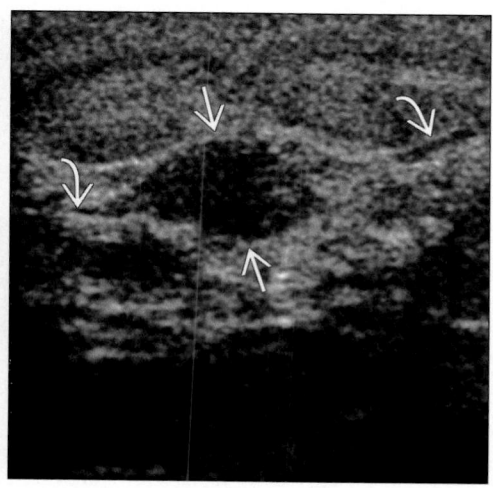

(Left) Transverse ultrasound shows a lobulated intracystic papilloma ➡ in a patient with a palpable lump. Minimal floating debris is present ➡. *(Right)* Longitudinal ultrasound shows a solid subareolar intraductal mass ➡, correlating with a mammographic density (not shown). Note minimal ductal dilation ➡. This was a papilloma at biopsy.

DUCTAL ECTASIA

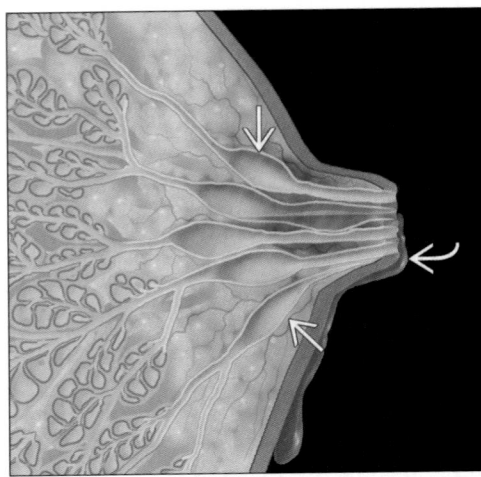

Graphic shows dilated major subareolar ducts ➡ and nipple discharge ➡. Duct ectasia may be secondary to inflammation, obstruction, or glandular atrophy and stasis.

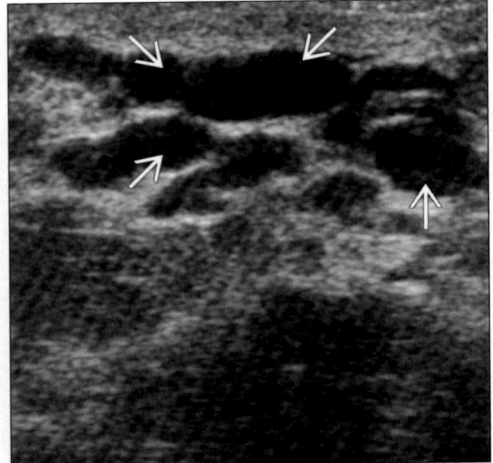

Ultrasound in the subareolar region of a woman with bloody nipple discharge shows duct ectasia ➡ without intraluminal mass. Further evaluation may include galactography or surgery.

TERMINOLOGY

Abbreviations and Synonyms
- Mammary duct ectasia, mastitis obliterans

IMAGING FINDINGS

General Features
- Best diagnostic clue
  - Tubular or branching structure(s) most commonly in the subareolar regions of both breasts on mammography
  - One or more tubular structures may be seen away from the nipple
- Location
  - Subareolar
    - Of no clinical concern when bilateral, symmetric and asymptomatic

Ultrasonographic Findings
- Grayscale Ultrasound
  - US: Anechoic fluid, or hypoechoic debris in dilated subareolar ducts
    - Debris may be mobile
    - Repositioning the patient and waiting 2-5 minutes may be beneficial in demonstrating mobility
  - Intraluminal masses may be demonstrated
    - Debris may be difficult to differentiate from masses
  - Color or power Doppler may be beneficial, debris is non-vascular
  - Compression
    - Inspissated secretions or intraluminal blood collapse with transducer pressure
    - Intraluminal mass will not compress with pressure
    - Mass may be obscured by surrounding secretions
- Color Doppler
  - Vascular stalk may be seen with papillomas, papillary lesions
    - Internal flow distinguishes mass from inspissated secretions
    - Flow is within fibrovascular stalk supplying lesion

Mammographic Findings
- Tubular radiopaque retroareolar structures
- Bilateral tubular/branching retroareolar ducts benign unless symptomatic e.g., spontaneous nipple discharge

DDx: Tubular Structures

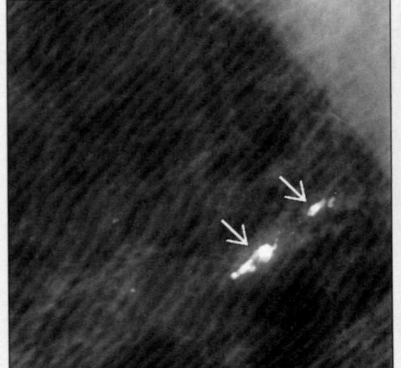

Solitary Dilated Duct, DCIS

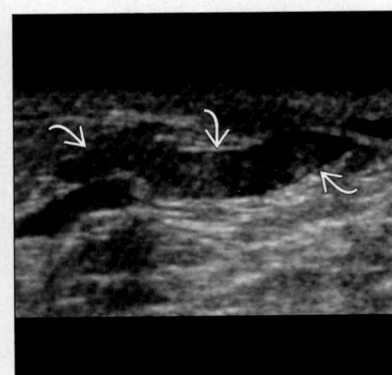

Multiple Papillomas

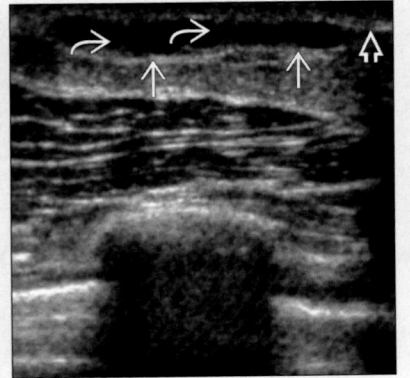

Mondor Disease

DUCTAL ECTASIA

Key Facts

Imaging Findings

- Tubular or branching structure(s) most commonly in the subareolar regions of both breasts on mammography
- Calcifications may be present within or around ducts
- US: Anechoic fluid, or hypoechoic debris in dilated subareolar ducts
- Debris may be mobile
- Intraluminal masses may be demonstrated
- Debris may be difficult to differentiate from masses
- Inspissated secretions or intraluminal blood collapse with transducer pressure
- Intraluminal mass will not compress with pressure
- Internal flow distinguishes mass from inspissated secretions

Top Differential Diagnoses

- Normal Variant
- Ductal Carcinoma in Situ (DCIS)
- Papilloma
- Secretory Calcifications

Clinical Issues

- Most common signs/symptoms: Asymptomatic screening mammogram finding
- Palpable retroareolar tubular structures
- Nipple discharge, spontaneous or with manipulation
- No known increased risk for breast cancer
- No further imaging when asymptomatic, multiple and without suspicious calcifications, masses or distortion
- Biopsy may be recommended if suspicious clinical or imaging characteristics

---

○ Further work-up may include magnification views; US, ductography, MR
  - Orthogonal magnification mammography to look for microcalcifications
○ US: Fluid-filled ducts without evidence of intraluminal mass
  - If mass present most likely papilloma
- Unilateral or single dilated duct may require further assessment
  ○ Comparison with old films to determine if it is a new finding
  ○ Orthogonal magnification mammography
  ○ US: Assess for intraluminal mass(es)
- Calcifications may be present within or around ducts
  ○ Benign secretory rod-like calcifications, some with lucent centers within or around ducts are benign
  ○ Suspicious forms (fine linear, pleomorphic, amorphous, punctate) suggesting a ductal distribution must be further evaluated
  ○ Possibly suspicious microcalcifications should be evaluated with orthogonal magnification mammography
- Tubular radiopaque structure away from the retroareolar region
  ○ May require magnification mammography, US
  ○ May be the presenting feature of papilloma, ductal carcinoma in situ (DCIS)

MR Findings

- T1WI: Retroareolar tubular structures may be bright when filled with proteinaceous or bloody fluid
- T2WI: Intraductal fluid may be bright
- T1 C+
  ○ May enhance
  ○ Intensity less than the normal nipple
  ○ Intraductal masses may enhance, some intensely
    - Papilloma
    - DCIS

DIFFERENTIAL DIAGNOSIS

Normal Variant

- Asymptomatic
- Symmetric bilateral dilatation typically of no clinical significance in postmenopausal women
- Dilatation may be somewhat asymmetric

Ductal Carcinoma in Situ (DCIS)

- Isolated single or multiple dilated duct(s) an uncommon presentation of DCIS
  ○ 4 of 300 nonpalpable breast cancers detected as single dilated duct in one series
- Usually has associated calcifications (fine linear, pleomorphic, amorphous, punctate) in a linear distribution

Papilloma

- May be central or peripheral
- Central lesions often present with spontaneous bloody nipple discharge
- Often multiple
- May appear as a mammographic mass with or without calcifications
  ○ Calcifications usually punctate or amorphous
- US: Intraluminal mass(es) within ectatic duct
  ○ Doppler may demonstrate vascular stalk
- MR patterns of enhancing papillomas variable
  ○ Small, smooth enhancing masses at ends of ectatic ducts
  ○ Irregular enhancing masses, some reported with rim-enhancement or spiculations
  ○ Occult on MR; not seen either with fat-suppressed T2 or following contrast injection
- May degenerate into atypical or malignant papillary lesions

Mondor Disease

- Thrombophlebitis of the superficial veins
- Self limiting process
- Typically associated with pain and a palpable cord

DUCTAL ECTASIA

Secretory Calcifications
- Benign, rod-like, coarse, linear mammographic calcifications
- Form either within ducts (may have lucent centers) or around ducts
- Unusual under the age of 60 years
- Typically bilateral
- Plasmacytic reaction to ductal retained secretion
- May present with a palpable mass

Abscess
- Clinical constellation includes tenderness and palpable mass near the nipple
- Often begins in the subareolar ducts
- More common in pregnant and nursing women
- US demonstrates thick indistinct wall surrounding echogenic debris
- Clinical setting and aspiration usually diagnostic

Granulomatous Lobular Mastitis
- No specific pathogenic organism
- Ducts filled with debris
- Associated irregular mass(es)

PATHOLOGY

General Features
- General path comments
  - Dilated major subareolar ducts
    - Occasional involvement of smaller ducts
  - Thick or granular secretions
- Etiology
  - May be secondary to inflammation, obstruction, glandular atrophy and stasis
  - Not related to parity or breast-feeding
- Epidemiology
  - Tissue atrophy
  - Cigarette smoking
  - Hyperprolactinemia
  - Prolonged phenothiazine exposure

Gross Pathologic & Surgical Features
- Grossly dilated, thick-walled ducts; thick or granular secretions

Microscopic Features
- Eosinophilic proteinaceous material, foam cells
- Inflammatory changes in ducts and surrounding tissue
- Epithelium may be thin; may be replaced by scar

CLINICAL ISSUES

Presentation
- Most common signs/symptoms: Asymptomatic screening mammogram finding
- Other signs/symptoms
  - Palpable retroareolar tubular structures
  - Pain
  - Nipple discharge, spontaneous or with manipulation
    - Yellow, green, brown, greenish-black → likely benign

- Bloody → 10-13% association malignancy, with most cases caused by benign papillomas
- Clear → < 1% association with DCIS when uniductal and spontaneous

Natural History & Prognosis
- No known increased risk for breast cancer

Treatment
- No further imaging when asymptomatic, multiple and without suspicious calcifications, masses or distortion
- Spontaneous bloody or clear nipple discharge requires further assessment in the evaluation for potential malignancy
  - Clinical assessment
  - Spot and/or magnification mammographic views
  - US, grayscale and color Doppler
  - Ductography: Requires visibility of discharging duct on the day of the procedure to allow cannulation
  - MR
- Biopsy may be recommended if suspicious clinical or imaging characteristics

DIAGNOSTIC CHECKLIST

Consider
- Duct ectasia is common and almost always benign

Image Interpretation Pearls
- Presence of a peripheral tubular mammographic structure should lead to further investigation
  - Finding may require biopsy
  - Papilloma, DCIS may manifest with this appearance

SELECTED REFERENCES
1. Daniel BL et al: Magnetic resonance imaging of intraductal papilloma of the breast. Magn Reson Imaging. 21(8):887-92, 2003
2. Ammari FF et al: Periductal mastitis. Clinical characteristics and outcome. Saudi Med J. 23(7):819-22, 2002
3. Rosen PP et al: Rosen breast pathology. Philadelphia, Lippincott Williams & Wilkins. Chapter 3, 33-9, 2001
4. Bassett LW et al: Diagnosis of diseases of the breast. Philadelphia, WB Saunders Co. Chapter 25, 413-4, 1997
5. Cardenosa G: Breast imaging companion. Philadelphia, Lippincott-Raven. 184-7, 1997
6. Huynh PT et al: Dilated duct pattern at mammography. Radiology. 204(1):137-41, 1997
7. Sickles EA: Mammographic features of "early" breast cancer. AJR Am J Roentgenol. 143(3):461-4, 1984

DUCTAL ECTASIA

IMAGE GALLERY

Typical

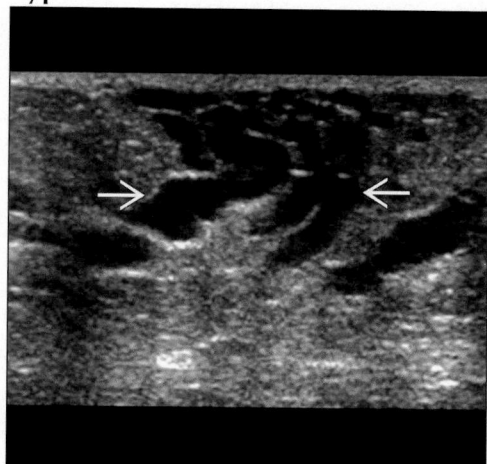
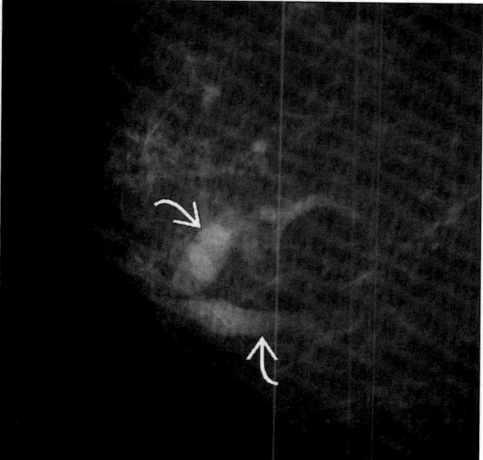

(Left) Ultrasound in a young nursing mother shows anechoic tubular structures ➡ representing dilated milk filled ducts extending close to the skin surface. (Right) MLO mammogram shows the typical mammographic appearance of duct ectasia. Two dilated tubular structures ➡ are noted in the subareolar region in an asymptomatic woman. US showed fluid-filled ducts consistent with ectasia.

Typical

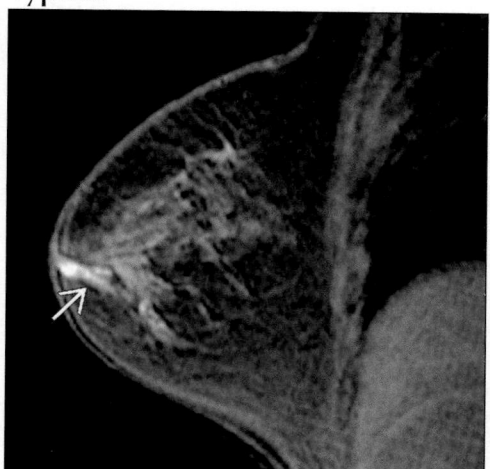
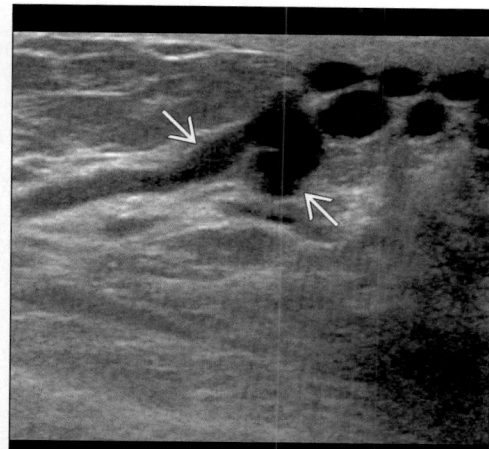

(Left) Sagittal pre-contrast T1WI FS MR shows a hyperintense retroareolar duct ➡ in a 56 year old with ipsilateral invasive lobular cancer. No enhancement was evident on subtraction images. US is shown in the next image. (Right) Ultrasound shows no intraluminal filling defects in these mildly ectatic ducts ➡ in the retroareolar area. No further evaluation was performed.

Typical

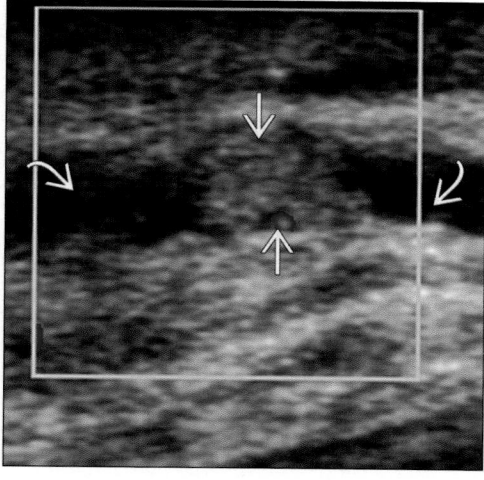
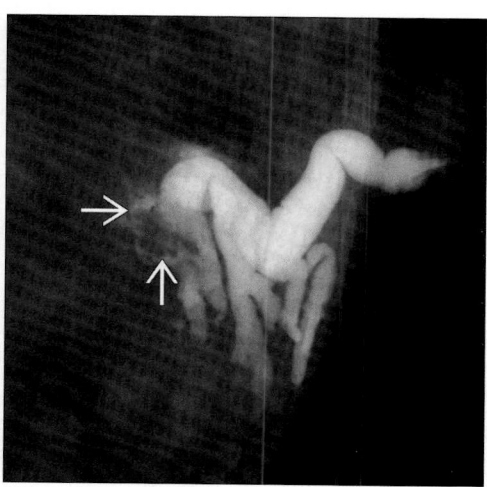

(Left) Ultrasound shows an intraductal papilloma ➡ with a vascular stalk within a dilated duct ➡. US is useful to evaluate for intraductal mass in patients with bloody or clear nipple discharge, (Right) Galactography in a patient with bloody nipple discharge shows a benign papilloma ➡ in a dilated duct 2 cm from the nipple. Galactography helps to evaluate suspicious nipple discharge if US fails to show an intraductal mass.

GYNECOMASTIA

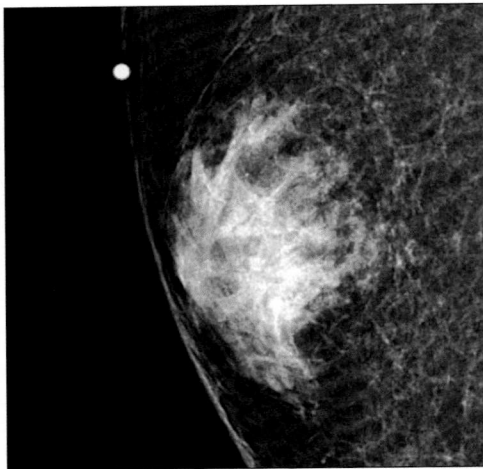

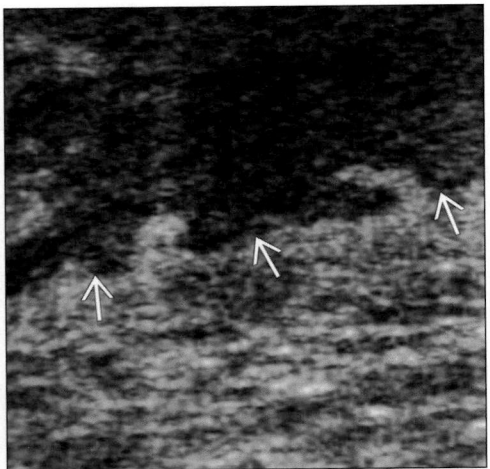

Mediolateral oblique mammogram shows typical case of palpable (note skin marker) asymmetric gynecomastia.

Longitudinal ultrasound shows typical hypoechoic appearance of subareolar gynecomastia. Margins are undulating but not spiculated ➡, and there is no posterior shadowing.

TERMINOLOGY

Definitions
- Male breast enlargement
  - Secondary to ductal and stromal proliferation
  - Result from imbalance of androgens and estrogens
    - Relative increase in estrogen levels causes stimulation of breast tissue
    - Overcomes inhibitory effects of androgens

IMAGING FINDINGS

General Features
- Best diagnostic clue
  - Glandular tissue in the subareolar region(s) on mammogram
  - Subareolar hypoechogenicity on ultrasound
- Location
  - Subareolar
  - Asymmetric in ~ 70%
- Morphology
  - Nodular
  - Dendritic
  - Diffuse glandular

Ultrasonographic Findings
- Grayscale Ultrasound
  - Hypoechoic area at the site of the palpable lump
    - Early nodular phase: Circumscribed subareolar mass, usually with a lobulated border
    - Late fibrous dendritic phase: Stellate margin, "finger-like" projections
  - Hyperechoic tissue in diffuse glandular pattern
    - Similar appearance to normal female glandular tissue
    - Most often associated with exogenous hormone use for sex reassignment
    - Can also be seen with hormone therapy used to treat prostate cancer
- Power Doppler: May have vascularity within the area

Imaging Recommendations
- Best imaging tool
  - Mammography may be only exam required
  - Ultrasound used as adjunct
    - Use to exclude underlying mass
    - Can appear malignant due to shadowing
    - Difficult to image subareolar tissues

DDx: Palpable Male Breast Lumps

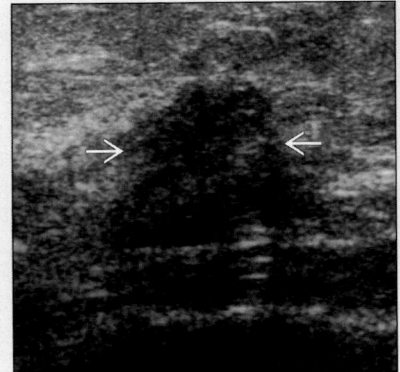

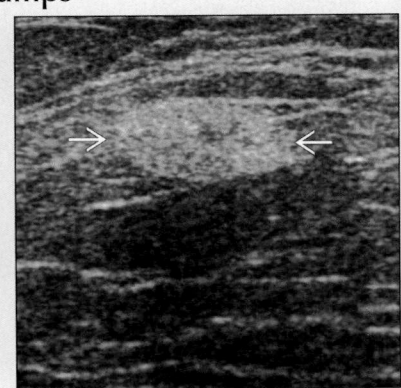

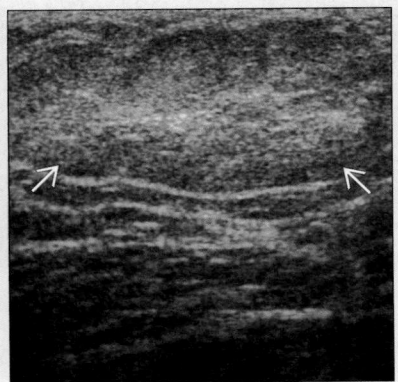

Male Breast Cancer

Myoepithelioma

Lipoma

GYNECOMASTIA

Key Facts

Terminology
- Male breast enlargement

Imaging Findings
- Asymmetric in ~ 70%
- Early nodular phase: Circumscribed subareolar mass, usually with a lobulated border
- Late fibrous dendritic phase: Stellate margin, "finger-like" projections
- Hyperechoic tissue in diffuse glandular pattern
- Power Doppler: May have vascularity within the area
- Mammography may be only exam required
- Ultrasound used as adjunct

Top Differential Diagnoses
- Breast Cancer
- Other Neoplasm, Non-Breast Origin
- Lipoma

Pathology
- Epidemiology: Most common etiology of male breast mass

Clinical Issues
- Pain or tenderness
- Palpable lump
- May be unilateral or bilateral

Diagnostic Checklist
- Testicular or other neoplasm causing secondary gynecomastia
- Mammography often is the only study required in evaluating suspected gynecomastia

---

- Protocol advice
  - Bilateral mammogram
    - Compare left and right sides
    - Can often see gynecomastia on the asymptomatic side as well
  - Ultrasound useful if questionable mammographic findings
    - Density is not subareolar
    - Palpable area appears mass-like

DIFFERENTIAL DIAGNOSIS

Breast Cancer
- Usually painless eccentric palpable lump
  - Associated skin and nipple changes common
    - Likely due to relatively late presentation
- Sonography similar to female breast cancer

Other Neoplasm, Non-Breast Origin
- Metastatic disease to the breast
- Chest wall tumors

Lipoma
- Mammographic findings should be diagnostic
  - Fat-containing encapsulated mass at palpable lump
- Ultrasound shows a benign lesion
  - May be difficult to distinguish from adjacent fatty tissue
    - Circumscribed nodule
    - Isoechoic to adjacent fat

Pseudogynecomastia
- May be seen with obesity and/or rapid weight gain
- Usually can be distinguished with clinical exam

Hematoma
- Rapid clinical onset following trauma
- Ultrasound shows a complicated cystic collection or solid lesion
  - Should resolve over time
- No internal blood flow

Fat Necrosis
- Palpable nontender lump
- Correlate with history of trauma
- Usually fat containing on mammogram
  - Unless associated with fibrosis in chronic setting
- Can be cystic or solid in appearance on ultrasound

Abscess
- Complicated cyst with internal debris on ultrasound
  - May contain air
  - Can be seen on ultrasound and mammogram
- Should have associated clinical findings
  - Fever
  - Skin erythema
- Drainage yields pus

Lipomastia
- Seen in HIV patients on antiretroviral therapy
  - Enlargement of the male breasts occur
- Sonography shows hypoechoic subareolar areas
  - Both for gynecomastia and lipomastia
- MR may be useful to distinguish

PATHOLOGY

General Features
- Genetics
  - Most cases not related to genetic transmission
  - Associated with Klinefelter syndrome (47 XXY)
    - Due to hypogonadism with androgen deficiency
- Etiology
  - Idiopathic
    - ~ 25% have no underlying abnormality found
    - Inherent sensitivity to estrogen/androgen activity may predispose despite normal hormone levels
  - Physiologic
    - Neonatal: Transplacental estrogen
    - Pubertal: Up to 60% of adolescent males due to hormone surge
    - Elderly: Decreased testosterone levels
  - Relative estrogen excess

GYNECOMASTIA

- Cirrhosis: Inhibited metabolism of estrogen
- Obesity: Peripheral estrogen conversion
  - Relative androgen deficiency
    - Aging
    - Hypogonadism (Klinefelter syndrome)
  - Drugs with estrogenic activity
    - Alcohol
    - Cimetidine
    - Spironolactone
    - Thiazide diuretics
    - Verapamil
    - Amiodarone
    - Captopril
    - Marijuana
    - Heroin
    - Anabolic steroids
  - Testicular carcinoma
    - Gynecomastia occurs in up to 10% of patients with malignant testicular tumors
    - Functioning tumors only: Increase serum estrogens
    - Leydig cell or germ cell most commonly
  - Other nontesticular hormone-producing neoplasms
    - Adrenal, liver, lung, renal
- Epidemiology: Most common etiology of male breast mass

Microscopic Features
- Male breast tissue
  - Major ducts only
    - Minimal secondary branching
  - No lobular units
- Gynecomastia
  - Nodular pattern
    - Early pattern of duct and stromal proliferation
    - Marked hyperplasia of ductal epithelium
    - Reversible
  - Dendritic pattern
    - Late pattern of fibrosis and hyalinization replacing duct
    - Irreversible with evolution of fibrosis

CLINICAL ISSUES

Presentation
- Most common signs/symptoms
  - Pain or tenderness
  - Palpable lump
    - Breast exam can distinguish from pseudogynecomastia
    - Usually a firm lump; differentiate from hard, fixed neoplastic process
  - Generalized swelling without discrete lump
  - May be unilateral or bilateral

Demographics
- Age
  - Trimodal age distribution
    - Neonatal
    - Pubertal
    - Elderly
- Gender: Male

Natural History & Prognosis
- Increasing prevalence with age
  - Highest between age 50-80 years
  - Ranges from 24-65%
- Biopsy can be performed if clinical diagnosis in question
  - Fine needle aspiration (FNA)
  - Core biopsy can be used for diagnosis if necessary
  - More often surgical excision if desire removal anyway

Treatment
- Reassurance
  - Obtain thorough clinical history to assess for exogenous causes
  - Exclude possibility of cirrhosis
  - Examine for signs of hypogonadism
    - Consider hormone-producing tumors
- Revise medication list
  - Replace or switch medication
- Surgical excision
  - If not reversible and symptomatic
    - Can be used to treat persistent pubertal gynecomastia as well
  - Subcutaneous mastectomy
- Medication
  - Tamoxifen
  - Danozal

DIAGNOSTIC CHECKLIST

Consider
- Testicular or other neoplasm causing secondary gynecomastia

Image Interpretation Pearls
- Mammography often is the only study required in evaluating suspected gynecomastia

SELECTED REFERENCES
1. Hanavadi S et al: The role of tamoxifen in the management of gynaecomastia. Breast. 15(2):276-80, 2006
2. Caruso G et al: High-frequency ultrasound in the study of male breast palpable masses. Radiol Med (Torino). 108(3):185-93, 2004
3. Welch ST et al: Sonography of pediatric male breast masses: gynecomastia and beyond. Pediatr Radiol. 34(12):952-7, 2004
4. Busch JM et al: Cancer mimicked on sonography: lipomastia in an HIV-positive man undergoing antiretroviral therapy. AJR Am J Roentgenol. 181(1):187-9, 2003
5. Daniels IR et al: How should gynaecomastia be managed? ANZ J Surg. 73(4):213-6, 2003
6. Fruhstorfer BH et al: A systematic approach to the surgical treatment of gynaecomastia. Br J Plast Surg. 56(3):237-46, 2003
7. Gunhan-Bilgen I et al: Male breast disease: clinical, mammographic, and ultrasonographic features. Eur J Radiol. 43(3):246-55, 2002
8. Weinstein SP et al: Spectrum of US findings in pediatric and adolescent patients with palpable breast masses. Radiographics. 20(6):1613-21, 2000

GYNECOMASTIA

Typical

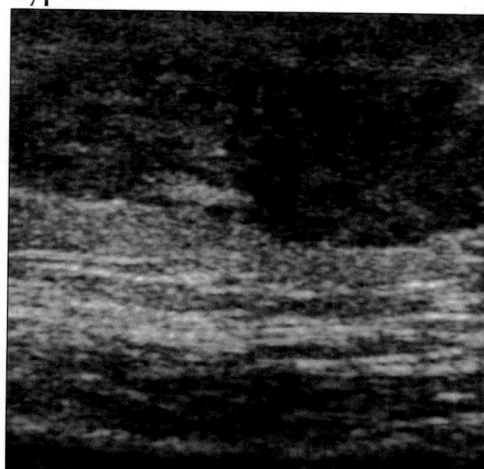
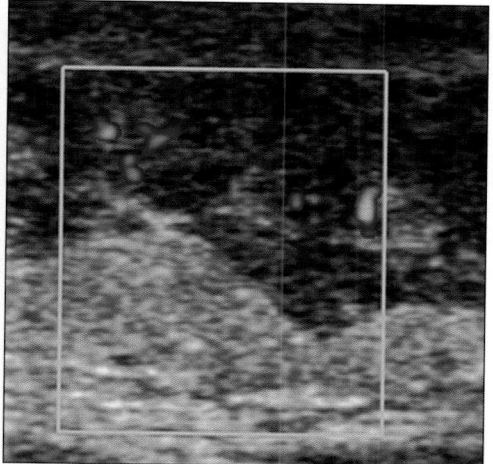

(Left) Transverse ultrasound shows more nodular appearing area of gynecomastia, which can be confused with focal mass. *(Right)* Transverse power Doppler ultrasound of same patient as previous image, shows remainder of the gynecomastia has typical appearance, with regional vascularity demonstrated.

Typical

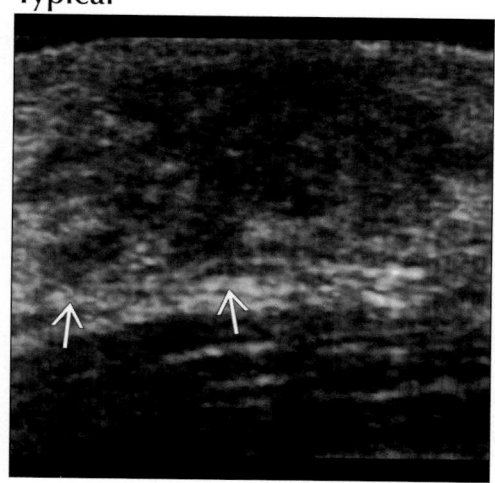
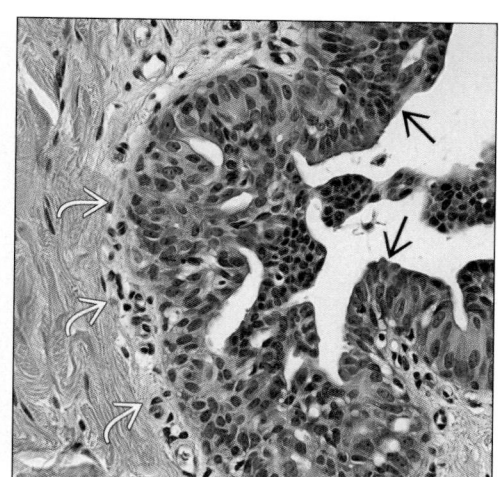

(Left) Longitudinal ultrasound shows typical appearance of gynecomastia in an adolescent male with breast bud development. Some margins are spiculated ➡, but without discrete mass. In females this should not be removed or breast tissue will not develop. *(Right)* Histology of 17 year old male with gynecomastia shows florid hyperplasia ➡ in transition to inactive stage, with early periductal fibrosis ➡.

Variant

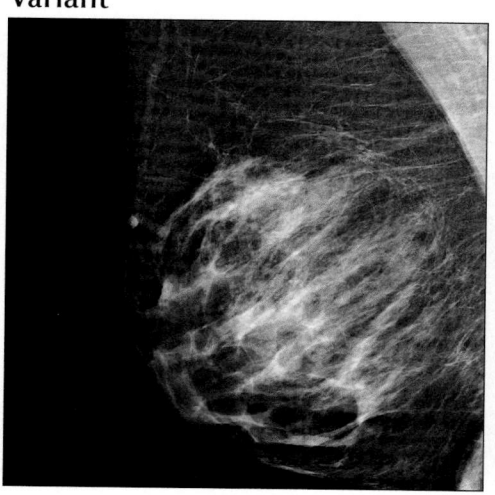
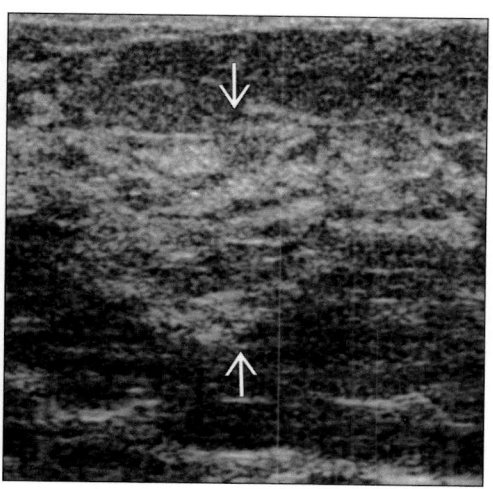

(Left) Mediolateral oblique mammogram of the right breast shows overall appearance of breast tissue in a male on exogenous hormonal stimulation for gender reassignment. *(Right)* Transverse ultrasound of the same patient as the previous image shows an island of glandular breast tissue ➡ in right breast. Note glandular tissue is indistinguishable from female parenchyma.

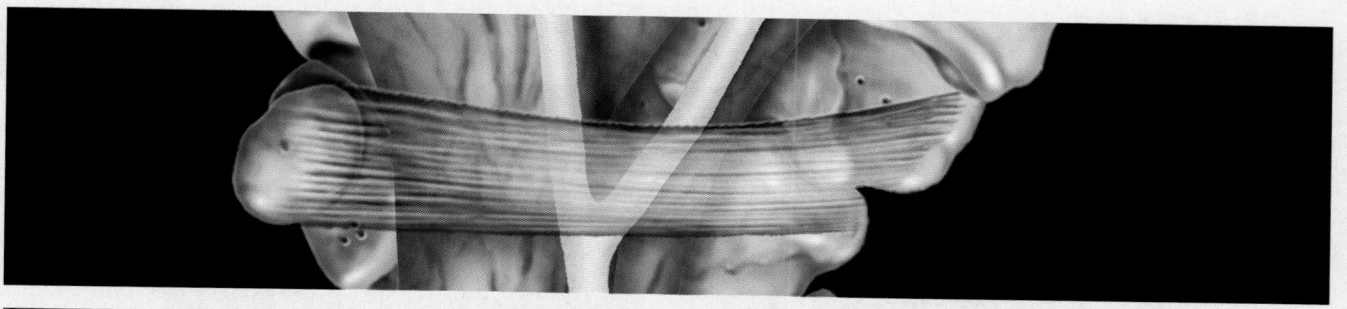

SECTION 13: Musculoskeletal

MUSCULOSKELETAL SONOGRAPHY

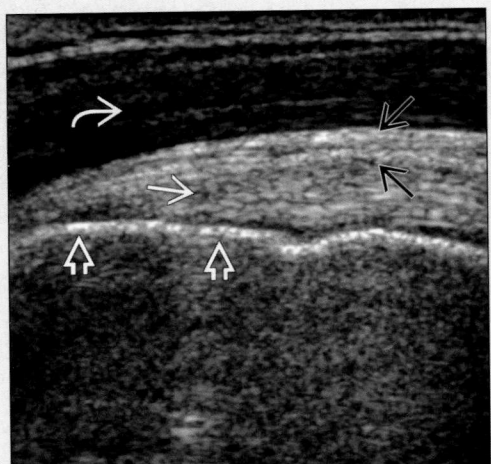

Longitudinal ultrasound shows normal supraspinatus tendon ➡ & insertional area ⇒ onto the greater tuberosity of the humerus. (Deltoid muscle ⟱). The bursa lies between two layers ⇨ of peribursal fat.

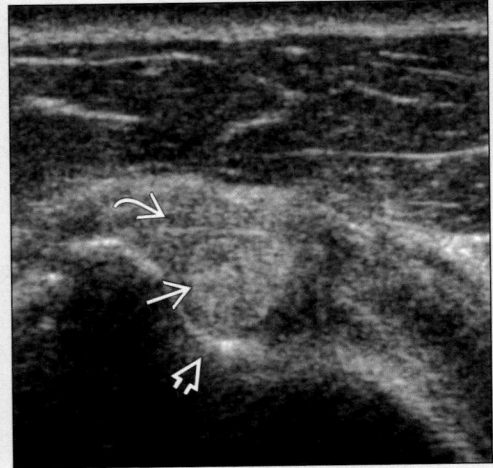

Transverse ultrasound shows moderate biceps tendinosis ➡ within the proximal bicipital groove ⇒. Normal biceps tendon is ovoid rather than round. Note thickening of surrounding synovial sheath ➡.

IMAGING ANATOMY

Critical Anatomic Structures

- **Shoulder region:** Supraspinatus, infraspinatus, subscapularis tendons & insertional areas; long head of biceps & bicipital groove; rotator cuff interval; subacromial-subdeltoid bursal area; acromioclavicular joint; coracoacromial ligament; glenohumeral joint
  - Insertional areas of supraspinatus, infraspinatus, teres minor tendons cannot be separated
  - Origin & proximal intracapsular portion long head of biceps not visible
  - Small amount of fluid in biceps tendon sheath is normal
  - Rotator cuff interval = between supraspinatus & subscapularis tendons (contains biceps tendon, coracohumeral & superior glenohumeral ligaments)
  - Normal subacromial-subdeltoid bursa not visible; peribursal fat inseparable from thin bursal wall
  - Posterior aspect of glenohumeral joint better depicted than anterior aspect
- **Elbow joint:** Radiohumeral & ulnohumeral articulations; joint capsule; triceps tendon; ulnar nerve; common extensor tendon origin, antecubital fossa contents including biceps insertion; common flexor tendon origin
  - Ulnar nerve caliber normally slightly ↑ in cubital tunnel
  - Individual tendons cannot be separated at common flexor & extensor tendon origins
- **Wrist joint:** Distal radioulnar joint, radiocarpal & ulnocarpal articulations; Lister tubercle & six extensor compartments dorsum of wrist; flexor tendons; median nerve; flexor retinaculum; carpal tunnel; ulnar nerve & Guyon canal
  - Extensor pollicis longus tendon crosses over extensor carpi radialis longus & brevis tendons → thumb
  - Abductor pollicis longus larger than extensor pollicis brevis tendon in first compartment
  - Extensor carpi radialis brevis tendon ulnar to extensor carpi longus tendon

- Carpal tunnel defined by proximal & distal boundaries of flexor retinaculum
- Median nerve lies between flexor digitorum superficialis & profundus distal forearm
  - Becomes more superficial just proximal to carpal tunnel
  - Lies just beneath retinaculum in line with ring finger
  - Usually divides → digital branches just beyond tunnel
- **Hip joint:** Proximal femur, hip capsule, iliopsoas tendon, sartorius & rectus femoris muscles, anterosuperior labrum, greater trochanter, tensor fascia lata, insertional area of gluteus minimus & medius tendons; gluteus maximus muscle
  - Hip capsule attached to acetabular rim & intertrochanteric line
    - Iliopsoas bursa communicates with hip joint in 15% normal subjects
  - Gluteus minimus is inserted more anteriorly on greater trochanter than gluteus medius
    - Trochanteric bursa lies between gluteus maximus muscle & greater trochanter
- **Knee joint:** Patella; patellar tendon; medial & lateral retinacula & recesses; suprapatellar pouch; quadriceps tendon; medial femorotibial articulation; medial collateral ligament; body medial meniscus; lateral femorotibial articulation; lateral collateral ligament, popliteal fossa; semimembranosus, semitendinosus & pes anserinus tendons
  - Normally, a small amount of fluid is apparent in medial or lateral recesses
    - Medial or lateral recesses distend with ↑ fluid before suprapatellar recess
  - Gastrocnemius-semimembranosus bursa lies between medial belly gastrocnemius & semimembranosus tendon (distended → Baker cyst)

MUSCULOSKELETAL SONOGRAPHY

Musculoskeletal Sonography

Key Concepts

- Good quality musculoskeletal ultrasound is dependent on a good understanding of musculoskeletal anatomy
- Most tissues (tendons, nerves etc.) have same appearance irrespective of location
- Another pre-requisite is knowledge of pathologies which occur at specific sites
  - Most musculoskeletal pathology is site-specific
  - "You only find what you look for; you only look for what you know"
  - Tissue-specific pathology (e.g., tendinosis, tendon tears, tenosynovitis) has similar appearance irrespective of location
- Musculoskeletal ultrasound is most useful when symptoms are focal e.g. point tenderness

Technique

- Develop systematic examination & checklist for each joint or region which at least includes all critical anatomical structures
- Contralateral side available for comparison
- For soft tissue masses, evaluate location, extent, internal structure, consistency, vascularity, relationship to adjacent structures, surrounding tissues ± regional nodes
- Ultrasound & MR are very complimentary examinations
- MR examination, if necessary, can be tailored to yield specific answers not provided by ultrasound
- Ultrasound is the best first-line investigation for most soft tissue pathology

---

- **Ankle joint:** Tibia-talar articulation; anterior recess ankle joint; structures posterior to medial malleolus (**T**om, **D**ick and **H**arry - **t**ibialis posterior tendon, flexor **d**igitorum tendon, posterior tibialis **a**rtery, vein & tibial **n**erve, flexor **h**allucis longus tendon); structures posterior to lateral malleolus (peroneus brevis & longus tendons) anterior talofibular ligament; calcaneofibular ligament; anterior tibiofibular ligament; Achilles tendon
  - Peroneus brevis musculotendinous junction is more distal & tendon → base of fifth metatarsal
  - Peroneus longus tendon passes obliquely across sole of foot → base first metatarsal & medial cuneiform
    - Tendons separated by peroneal tubercle lateral aspect calcaneus
  - Small amount of fluid in retrocalcaneal bursa normal

ANATOMY-BASED IMAGING ISSUES

Imaging Approaches

- High resolution transducer (≥ 7.5 MHz) essential for most musculoskeletal ultrasound
  - For deeper areas (gluteal region, proximal thigh) & large masses, a 5 Mhz transducer is necessary
- Ensure both you & patient are in comfortable position to examine part under investigation
  - Use plenty of coupling gel for superficial lesions
- Tendons, nerves & ligaments are prone to anisotropy; frequent transducer angulation necessary to view all portions
  - For example, anterior, mid- & posterior fibers supraspinatus, medial & lateral aspects may need to be assessed separately
- Develop systematic examination & checklist for each joint or region which at least includes all critical anatomical structures
  - Start with area of suspected primary pathology & then evaluate rest of joint or region
  - ± Dynamic examination

- For soft tissue masses, evaluate location, extent, internal structure, consistency, vascularity, relationship to adjacent critical structures, surrounding tissues ± regional nodes
- In children, full examination may not be possible before child becomes restless
  - Concentrate on most critical area prior to examining rest of joint or region
    - Sedation not usually necessary or beneficial for children
- Good quality musculoskeletal ultrasound is dependent on a good understanding of musculoskeletal anatomy
- Another pre-requisite is knowledge of likely pathologies which occur in specific areas
  - Most musculoskeletal pathology is site-specific
    - "You only find what you look for; you only look for what you know"
- Most tissues (tendons, nerves, ligaments) have same appearance irrespective of location
  - Also, tissue-specific pathology has similar appearance irrespective of location
    - For example, ultrasound appearances of tendinosis, tendon tears, or tenosynovitis similar irrespective of location

CLINICAL IMPLICATIONS

Clinical Importance

- Ultrasound is the best first-line investigation for most soft tissue pathology
  - Explanation for patient symptoms can usually be obtained with ultrasound examination
    - Good way of planning subsequent investigations, if necessary
  - Most soft tissue masses can be accurately diagnosed with ultrasound
    - Many common soft tissue masses (e.g., lipoma, nerve sheath tumor) are optimally imaged by ultrasound

MUSCULOSKELETAL SONOGRAPHY

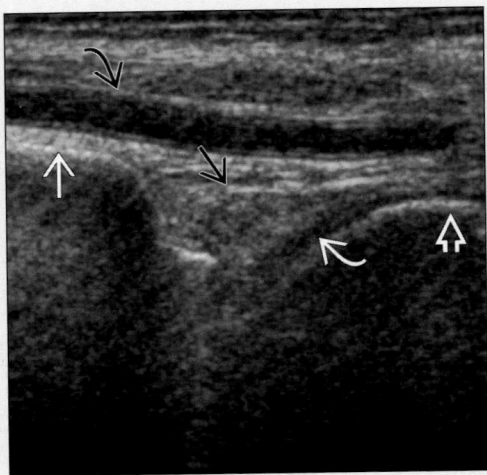

Longitudinal ultrasound shows normal ankle joint with distal tibia ➡, talus ➡, articular cartilage on talar dome ➡, thin anterior capsule ➡ & anterior tibial artery ➡.

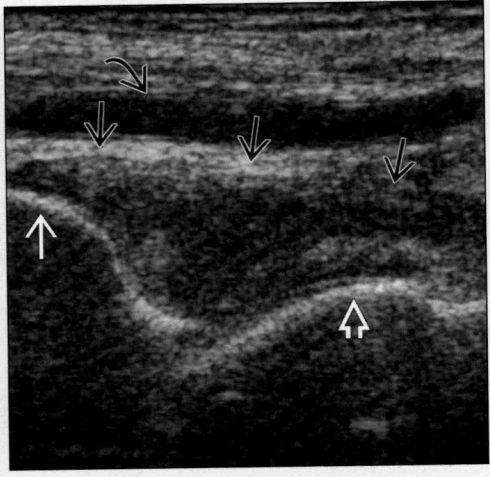

Longitudinal ultrasound shows ankle joint distended ➡ with echogenic fluid due to acute inflammatory arthropathy. Tibia ➡, talus ➡, anterior tibial artery ➡.

- ■ If findings non-specific → ± ultrasound-guided biopsy (or fine needle aspiration for cytology, FNAC)
- If satisfactory explanations for symptoms not found on ultrasound examination → ± proceed to further investigation, usually MR
  - ○ Little benefit to repeating ultrasound generally except to follow longitudinal progress of disease
- Musculoskeletal ultrasound most useful when symptoms localized to specific area e.g. point tenderness
  - ○ Less useful when symptoms not well-localized e.g., related to whole knee or whole ankle joint
- Contralateral side available for comparison, if necessary
  - ○ However, subclinical disease commonly occurs on contralateral side in some disease entities (e.g., tendinosis, entrapment neuropathy, fasciitis, synovitis)
  - ○ Be wary of indiscriminately using contralateral side as normal standard, especially for comparative measurements
- Ultrasound & MR are very complimentary investigations
  - ○ In addition to the general benefits of ultrasound (quicker, less expensive, more readily available etc.), it also
    - ■ Provides very high resolution of near-field structures
    - ■ Enables assessment of several anatomical regions during same examination (e.g., both shoulders; groin nodes & calf tumor)
    - ■ Allows dynamic assessment of tissues during movement (e.g., tendon, nerve subluxation)
    - ■ Not prone to metallic artifact (soft tissue infection, tumor recurrence alongside metallic fixation devices)
    - ■ Provides ready assessment of vascularity
    - ■ Facilitates image-guided diagnostic (biopsy, FNAC, aspiration for culture) or therapeutic (injection, drainage) intervention

- MR also has advantages over ultrasound & in these situations either proceed directly to MR (or perform MR after ultrasound assessment)
  - ○ Visualization of areas not accessible to ultrasound
    - ■ Intraarticular pathology (e.g., superior labral tears)
    - ■ Intraosseous abnormality (reactive bone change or bone involvement)
  - ○ Improved perception of large objects (particularly deep margins & ill-defined lesions)
    - ■ Including anatomical relationships (surgical roadmap)
  - ○ Better characterization of tissue type & also internal structure of large masses
  - ○ More reliable volume assessment of ill-defined structures (e.g., synovial volume)
  - ○ More sensitive at depicting soft tissue edema (particularly muscle)
- Ultrasound should ideally precede MR for most soft tissue problems
  - ○ MR examination, if necessary, can be tailored to yield specific answers not provided by ultrasound
  - ○ MR examination time can be shortened
    - ■ For example, no need to examine regional lymph nodes if ultrasound assessment already performed
    - ■ May not need intravenous contrast if tumor vascularity has been assessed on ultrasound

RELATED REFERENCES

1. Bianchi S et al: Ultrasound appearance of tendon tears. Part 2: lower extremity and myotendinous tears. Skeletal Radiol. 35(2):63-77, 2006
2. Bianchi S et al: Ultrasound of tendon tears. Part 1: general considerations and upper extremity. Skeletal Radiol. 34(9):500-12, 2005
3. McNally EG: Lower limb: anatomy and techniques. In: Practical Musculoskeletal Ultrasound. Philadelphia, Elsevier, 23-42, 2005
4. McNally EG: Upper limb: anatomy and techniques. In: Practical Musculoskeletal Ultrasound. Philadelphia, Elsevier, 1-21, 2005
5. Martinoli C et al: US of the shoulder: non-rotator cuff disorders. Radiographics. 23(2):381-401; quiz 534, 2003

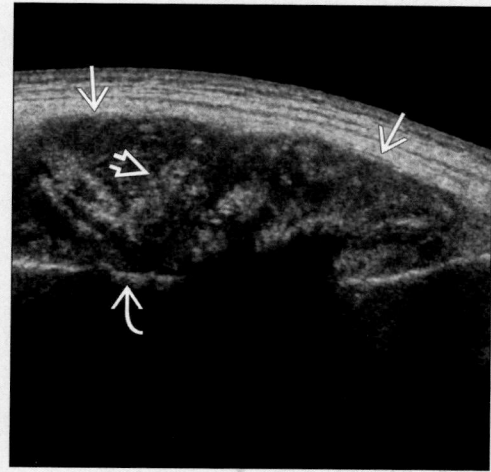
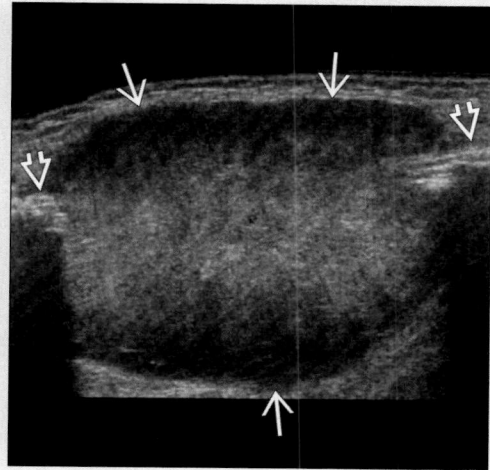

(Left) Longitudinal ultrasound shows a large extraosseous osteosarcoma ➡ arising from the distal femur ➡. Note spicules of osteoid ➡ within the hypoechoic tumor matrix. *(Right)* Longitudinal ultrasound shows an osseous metastatic deposit ➡ breaching the cortex of the tibia ➡. Cortical disruption allows intramedullary extent & size of the metastatic deposit to be appreciated.

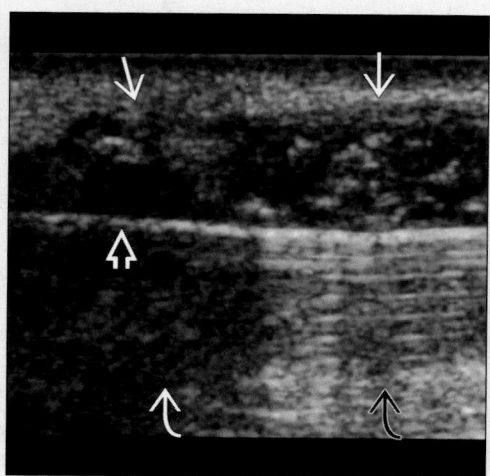
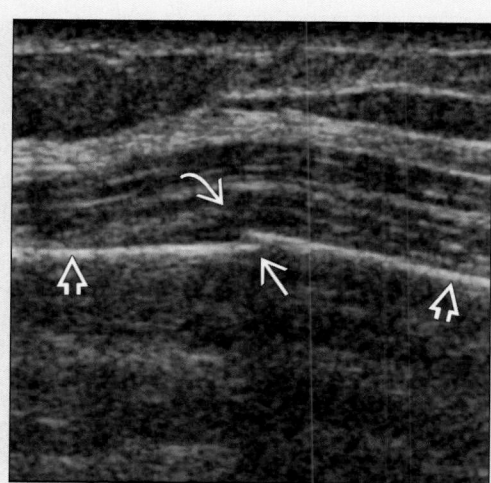

(Left) Longitudinal ultrasound shows a giant cell tumor recurrence ➡ next to a fixation plate ➡ of the radius, not appreciated on MR (metallic artifact). Artifact changes from shadowing ➡ to reverberation ➡ with ↑ plate angulation. *(Right)* Transverse ultrasound shows a mildly displaced rib fracture ➡ with a break in the anterior cortex ➡ of the rib & slight angulation. Mild soft tissue swelling is seen ➡ alongside the fracture site.

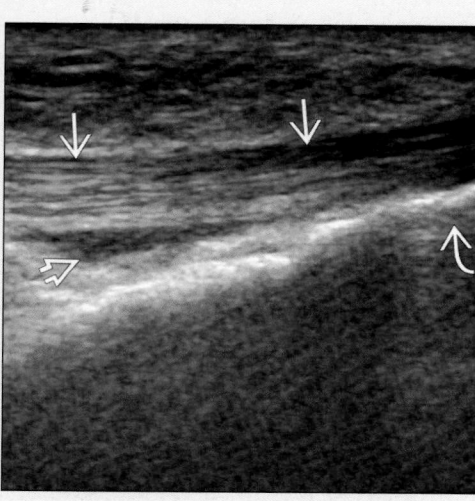
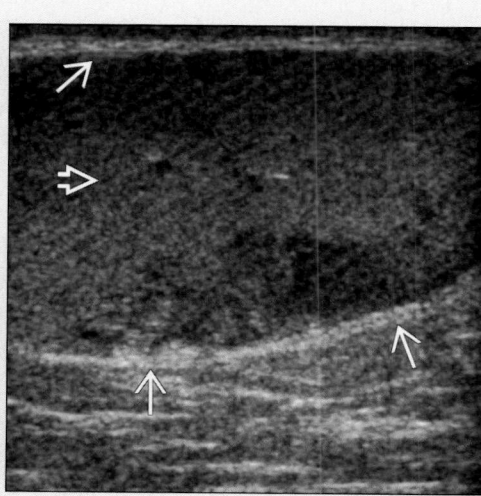

(Left) Longitudinal ultrasound shows the normal fibrillar pattern of the patellar tendon ➡ at its insertion onto the proximal tibia ➡. A small amount of fluid in deep infrapatellar bursa ➡ is normal. *(Right)* Transverse ultrasound shows a subcutaneous sebaceous cyst of the thigh. The thin capsule ➡, echogenic internal contents ➡ & consistency of the cyst can be appreciated.

ROTATOR CUFF TENDINOSIS

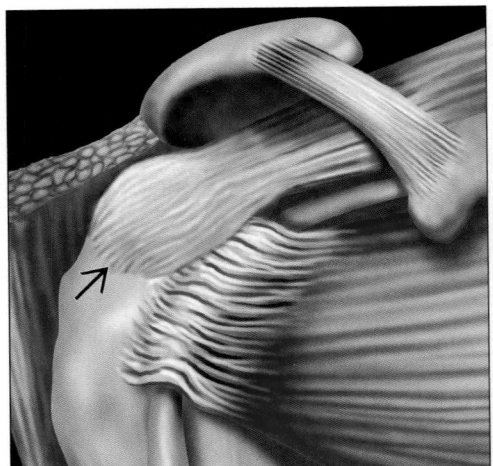

Oblique graphic shows a diffusely thickened supraspinatus tendon ➡ indicative of tendinosis.

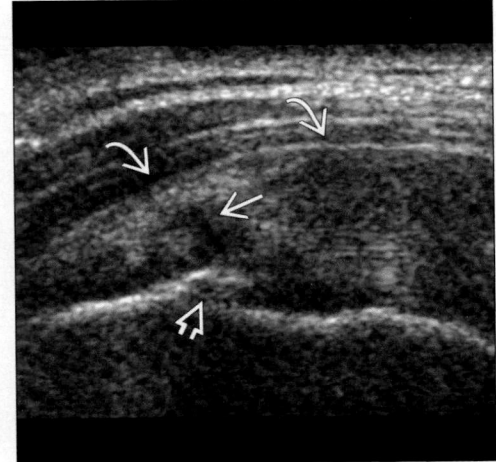

Longitudinal ultrasound shows a diffusely thickened, hypoechoic supraspinatus tendon ➡ with a linear tear ➡ extending inferiorly to the insertional area. The insertional area cortex is irregular ➡.

TERMINOLOGY

Abbreviations and Synonyms
- Rotator cuff tendinosis, rotator cuff tendinopathy, supraspinatus tendinosis
- Rotator cuff impingement, subacromial impingement, supraspinatus impingement

Definitions
- Collagenous degeneration of the rotator cuff tendons with proteoglycan deposition, most commonly of supraspinatus tendon

IMAGING FINDINGS

General Features
- Best diagnostic clue: Diffusely thickened tendon with variable hypoechogenicity and loss of normal fibrillar pattern
- Location: Supraspinatus tendon most commonly affected
- Size: Diffusely thickened tendon
- Morphology

- ○ Thickened, inhomogeneous tendon +/- surface fraying
- ○ Tendon torn or partially torn in advanced cases with fluid entering defect

Ultrasonographic Findings
- Thickened inhomogeneous rotator cuff tendon with areas of hypoechogenicity
  - ○ Graded as mild, moderate or severe based on degree of thickening and hypoechogenicity
  - ○ Focal hypoechoic areas can be difficult to distinguish from intrasubstance tears; tears tend to be more linear
  - ○ Non-intrasubstance tears are discernible through changes in tendon contour (contour flattening, retraction, fluid gap)
- In severe cases, tendon is severely thickened and diffusely hypoechoic
- Tendinosis generally affects all rotator cuff tendons to some degree with supraspinatus most affected
  - ○ Biceps tendinosis usually accompanies rotator cuff tendinosis
- Tendon hyperemia is not a feature of rotator cuff tendinosis

DDx: Rotator Cuff Tendinosis

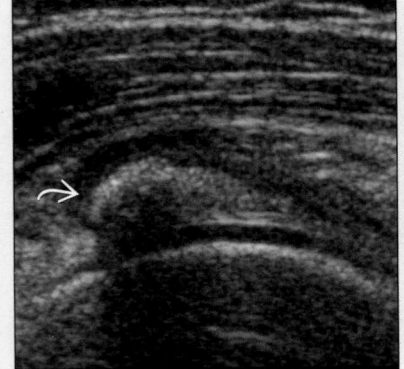

Calcific Tendinitis

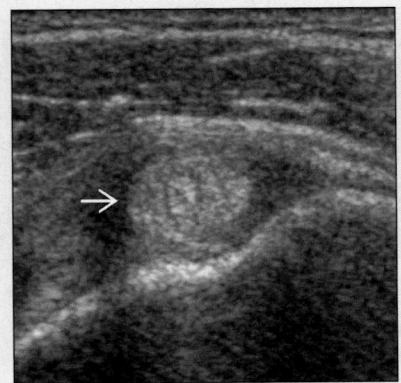

Biceps Tendinosis

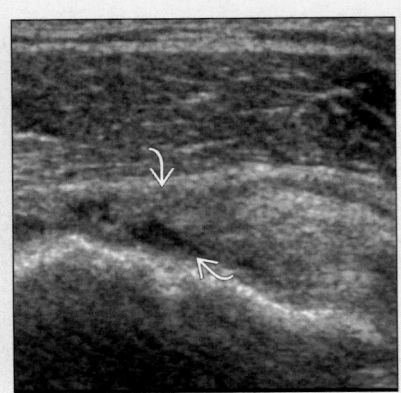

Supraspinatus Tear

ROTATOR CUFF TENDINOSIS

Key Facts

Terminology
- Collagenous degeneration of the rotator cuff tendons with proteoglycan deposition, most commonly of supraspinatus tendon

Imaging Findings
- Best diagnostic clue: Diffusely thickened tendon with variable hypoechogenicity and loss of normal fibrillar pattern
- Focal hypoechoic areas can be difficult to distinguish from intrasubstance tears; tears tend to be more linear
- Non-intrasubstance tears are discernible through changes in tendon contour (contour flattening, retraction, fluid gap)
- In severe cases, tendon is severely thickened and diffusely hypoechoic

- Tendinosis generally affects all rotator cuff tendons to some degree with supraspinatus most affected
- Biceps tendinosis usually accompanies rotator cuff tendinosis
- Tendon hyperemia is not a feature of rotator cuff tendinosis
- Cortical defects and irregularity in and around tendon insertional area commonly associated

Top Differential Diagnoses
- Calcific Tendinitis
- Tendon Tears

Diagnostic Checklist
- Systematic examination; look especially at edges for contour deformity; confirm suspected abnormalities in orthogonal plane

---

- Cortical defects and irregularity in and around tendon insertional area commonly associated
  - + Subacromial-subdeltoid bursitis
- MR better than ultrasound at showing structural abnormality that may precipitate impingement
  - MR better at depicting tendon delamination and subacromial-subdeltoid bursitis
- Ultrasound better than MR at showing milder degrees of tendinosis and biceps tendinosis
  - Ultrasound allows ready comparison with opposite side; subclinical disease of similar severity often present on opposite side

Radiographic Findings
- Radiography
  - Flat-undersurface acromion; anteriorly-hooked acromion; anterior or lateral downsloping acromion; os acromiale
  - Hypertrophic osteoarthropathy acromio-clavicular joint; acromial spurs
  - Sclerosis or subcortical cysts around greater tuberosity

MR Findings
- T1WI
  - Thickened tendon with intermediate signal intensity
    - Heterogeneous tendon(s) signal
  - Hypointense to intermediate signal intensity in thickened or fluid containing subacromial-subdeltoid bursa
- T2WI
  - Increased signal intensity of tendon on PD FSE, FS PD FSE, STIR & T2* GRE
    - Heterogeneous tendon(s) signal
  - +/- Hyperintense bursitis or glenohumeral joint effusion
  - +/- Anterolateral osteophytic acromial spurs or acromioclavicular osteoarthropathy
    - +/- Type II (curved undersurface) or type III (anterior hook) acromion shape
    - +/- Thickening of coracoacromial ligament insertional area

- Irregularity and hypointensity of greater tuberosity insertional area
- Subcortical cyst formation around insertional area
- MR arthrography
  - More sensitive for small articular surface tears

Imaging Recommendations
- Best imaging tool: Ultrasound
- Protocol advice
  - Patient sitting; systematic examination; tendons examined taut and non-taut
    - Extension and internal rotation for supraspinatus
    - Abduction and internal rotation for infraspinatus and teres minor
    - External rotation for subscapularis

DIFFERENTIAL DIAGNOSIS

Calcific Tendinitis
- Occurs in association with tendinopathy
- Tendon thickened with intrasubstance echogenicity (small deposits) or acoustic shadowing (large deposits)
  - Calcium hydroxyapatite deposition within tendon
- Hypointense calcium deposit on all pulse sequences
  - +/- Hyperintense surrounding edema on T2WI

Tendon Tears
- Partial or full-thickness depending on whether all (complete) or part of (partial) tendon affected
  - Most commonly affect supraspinatus tendon
  - Less common in normal tendons; usually occur with background tendinosis
  - Hypoechoic sharply demarcated defect
    - +/- Retraction or blunting of tendon edge
    - +/- Flattening of tendon
    - +/- Non-visualization of tendon if complete and retracted
  - Intrasubstance tears difficult to detect in presence of tendinosis
    - Articular or bursal surface tears seen though contour deformity

ROTATOR CUFF TENDINOSIS

Posterosuperior Glenoid Impingement
- Internal impingement
- Posterosuperior cuff, labrum, humeral head

Magic Angle Artifact
- Leads to artifactual increased signal at curved portion of supraspinatus and biceps tendon without thickening on short TE sequences
- Ultrasound not susceptible to magic angle affect

PATHOLOGY

General Features
- General path comments
  - Common degenerative, pain producing disorder
    - Relationship between pain and severity of tendinosis is variable
- Genetics: Familial predisposition
- Etiology
  - Intrinsic theory: Overuse, degeneration and tearing of the rotator cuff
  - Extrinsic theory: Secondary to impingement syndrome
    - Spurs, acromial shape, os acromiale, anterior, lateral downsloping acromion, thickened coracoacromial ligament
  - Eccentric tensile overload of the rotator cuff tendons
  - Combination of extrinsic, intrinsic, and biomechanical factors
  - Collagen vascular diseases along with tendinosis of other tendons
- Epidemiology
  - Tendinosis extremely common especially with advancing age
  - Shoulder pain is third most common cause of chronic musculoskeletal pain
    - After low back and cervical pain

Gross Pathologic & Surgical Features
- Thickened, indurated tendon
- Loss of integrity of tendon in partial or full-thickness tears
- Partial tear may be on the bursal surface, articular surface or interstitial

Microscopic Features
- Collagen degeneration without influx of inflammatory cells: "Tendinosis" is preferred term over tendinitis
- Increase in glycosaminoglycan and proteoglycan
- Tendon cell apoptosis (cell death) within supraspinatus
- Mucoid/eosinophilic/fibrillary degeneration and scarring
- Angiofibroblastic hyperplasia

Staging, Grading or Classification Criteria
- Impingement
  - Stage I: Reversible edema & hemorrhage typically in active patient ≤ 25 years
  - Stage II: Fibrosis and tendinitis
  - Stage III: Degeneration & rupture often associated with osseous changes in patients > 40 years

CLINICAL ISSUES

Presentation
- Most common signs/symptoms
  - Often subclinical; usually bilateral in older patients
  - Slowly progressive, poorly localized shoulder pain
    - Pain, weakness, and loss of shoulder motion
    - Pain anterolateral aspect of shoulder aggravated by overhead activity
    - Night pain
    - Majority have no single precipitating event
- Clinical Profile
  - Young athletes (precipitating event, os acromiale)
  - Older athletes or older non-athletic population (insidious onset, degenerative-type structural abnormality)
- Pain even without tendon tear
- Most common referral indication for shoulder ultrasound or MR

Demographics
- Age: Peak: > 40 years for impingement, most common 55 years
- Gender: M:F = 1:1 or slight female predominance

Natural History & Prognosis
- Insidious onset of pain in adult patient with impingement syndrome
- +/- Progression to tear

Treatment
- Physical therapy
- Corticosteroids via injection to treat associated bursitis
- Subacromial decompression for impingement

DIAGNOSTIC CHECKLIST

Consider
- Small tear if no abnormality on first inspection with ultrasound in patient with tendinosis and sudden deterioration in symptoms; check again

Image Interpretation Pearls
- Systematic examination; look especially at edges for contour deformity; confirm suspected abnormalities in orthogonal plane
- FS PD FSE may overestimate cuff pathology (tendinosis mistaken for cuff tear)

SELECTED REFERENCES

1. Bianchi S et al: Ultrasound of tendon tears. Part 1: general considerations and upper extremity. Skeletal Radiol. 34(9):500-12, 2005
2. Sanders TG et al : A systematic approach to magnetic resonance imaging interpretation of sports medicine injuries of the shoulder. Am J Sports Med. 33(7): 1088-105, 2005
3. Teefey SA et al: Ultrasonography of the rotator cuff. A comparison of ultrasonographic and arthroscopic findings in one hundred consecutive cases. J Bone Joint Surg Am. 82(4):498-504, 2000
4. Seibold CJ et al: Rotator cuff: evaluation with US and MR imaging. Radiographics. 19(3):685-705, 1999

ROTATOR CUFF TENDINOSIS

IMAGE GALLERY

Typical

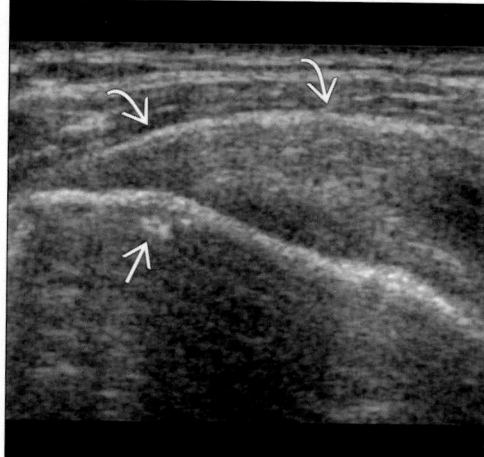
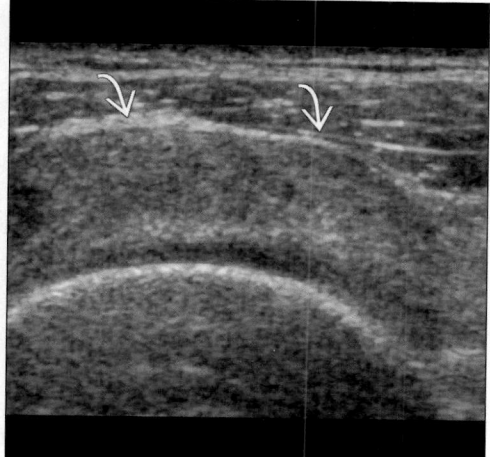

(Left) Longitudinal ultrasound shows a hypoechoic, supraspinatus tendon ➔ with loss of the normal fibrillar pattern indicative of tendinosis. There are minimal bony changes at the insertional area ➔. *(Right)* Transverse ultrasound in the same patient as previous image shows a diffusely thickened, hypoechoic supraspinatus tendon indicative of tendinosis ➔.

Typical

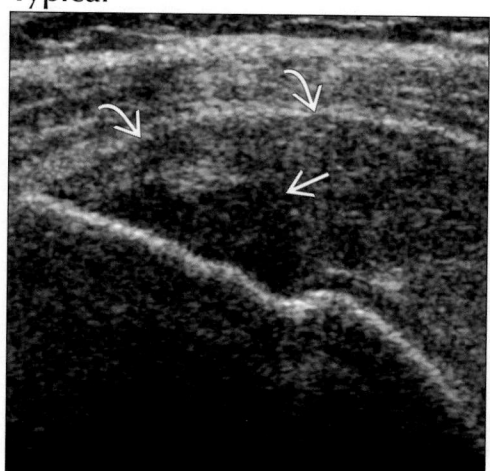
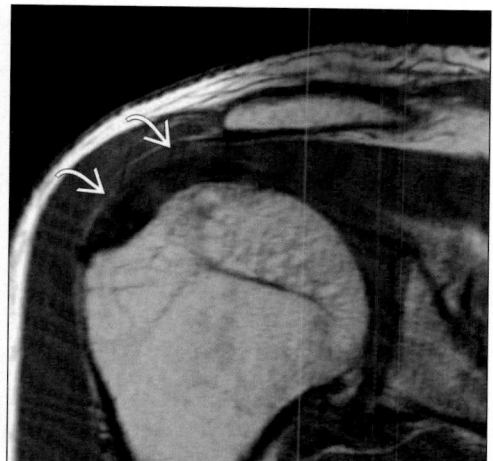

(Left) Longitudinal ultrasound shows a very thickened, hypoechoic supraspinatus tendon ➔. There is a focal, more hypoechoic area ➔ at the insertional area. This was due to proteoglycan deposition and not a tear. *(Right)* Coronal T1WI MR shows a diffusely thickened supraspinatus tendon ➔ with variable intermediate signal intensity indicative of supraspinatus tendinosis.

Typical

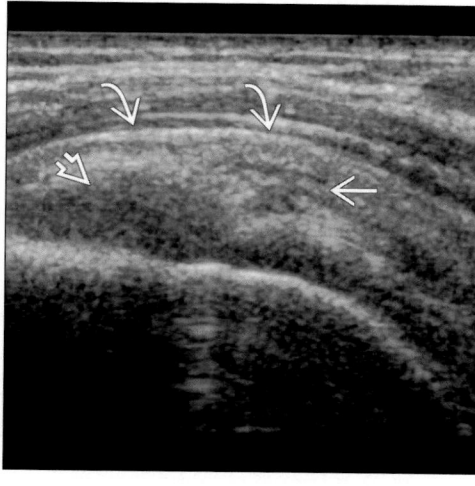
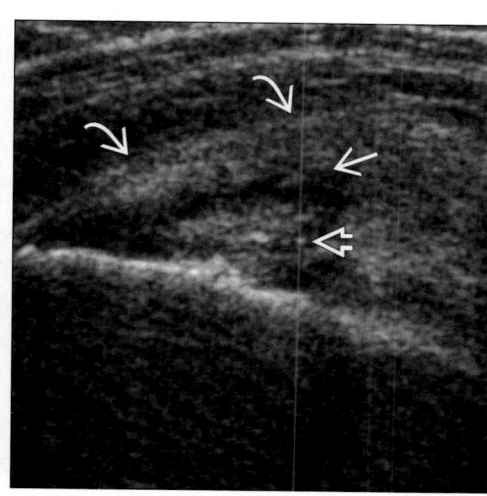

(Left) Longitudinal ultrasound shows a thickened supraspinatus tendon ➔ with a linear longitudinally orientated intrasubstance tear ➔. The focal hypoechoic area ➔ adjacent to the tendon insertion is a feature of tendinosis & does not represent a tear. *(Right)* Longitudinal US shows a thickened supraspinatus tendon ➔ with an avulsive-type tear ➔ from the insertional area. Small echogenic foci ➔ within the tear are due to gas loculi.

ROTATOR CUFF TEAR

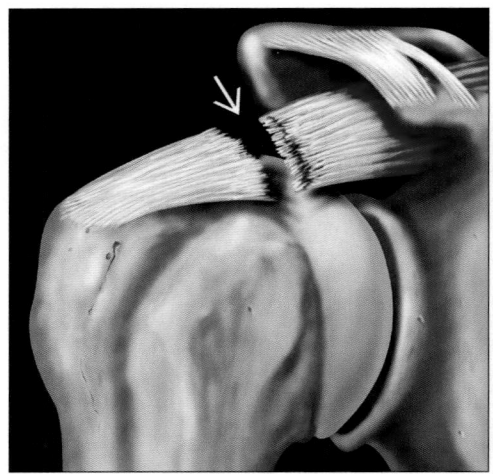

Longitudinal graphic shows a complete tear ➡️ of the supraspinatus tendon just proximal to the insertion ("critical area").

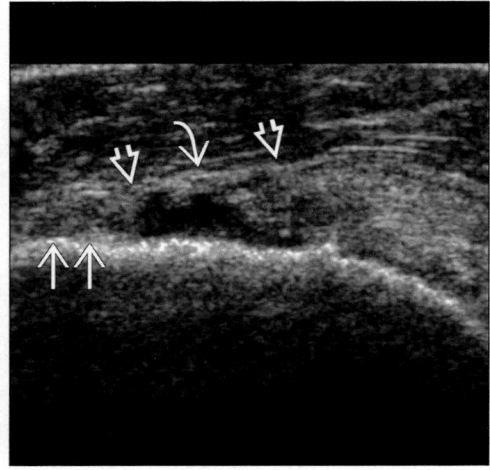

Transverse ultrasound shows a full-thickness tear ➡️ of the supraspinatus tendon just proximal to the insertional area ➡️. The gap is filled with fluid. Note flattening of the bursal convexity of the tendon ➡️.

TERMINOLOGY

Abbreviations and Synonyms
- Partial-thickness, full-thickness or complete rotator cuff tendon tear
- "Massive" rotator cuff tear

Definitions
- "Massive" tear: Complete tear of supraspinatus and infraspinatus tendons
- Complete or incomplete (partial) tear of rotator cuff tendon
  - Supraspinatus tendon most common, followed by infraspinatus tendon
    - Complete tear: All fibers of tendon torn
    - Incomplete (partial) tear: Some fibers of tendon torn
  - Two types of partial tear
    - Full-thickness tear: Only part of the tendon is torn (e.g., anterior fibers, mid- or posterior fibers of supraspinatus)
    - Partial-thickness: Only part of the depth of the tendon is torn (bursal surface, mid-substance, articular surface)

IMAGING FINDINGS

General Features
- Best diagnostic clue: Discontinuity of tendon filled with fluid
- Location
  - Supraspinatus tendon tears close to or at insertional area
  - Anterior fibers most commonly torn
  - Many tears are avulsive in type at junction of tendon to Sharpey fibers
  - Isolated tear of infraspinatus tendon uncommon
    - Since the supraspinatus insertion is 15 mm wide, tears extending posteriorly of length > 15 mm must involve infraspinatus tendon
- Size: Varies from fraying to complete tear
- Morphology: Irregularity (fraying) to complete absence of tendon

Ultrasonographic Findings
- Discontinuity or gap within tendon filled with clear fluid (primary sign)
  - Gap filled with echogenic fluid or blood +/- gas locules (comet tail artifacts)

DDx: Rotator Cuff Tear

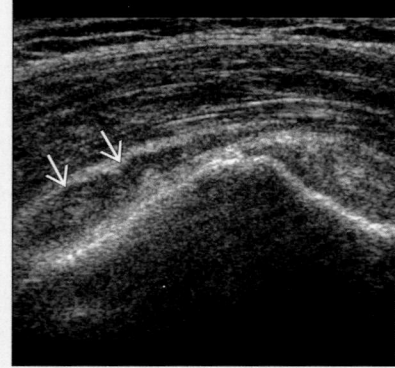

Bursitis

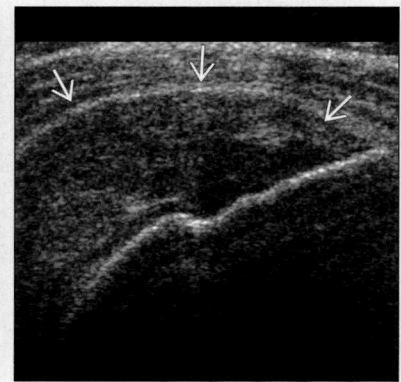

Tendinosis

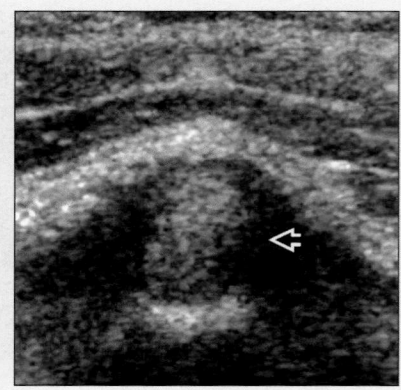

Biceps Tendinosis

ROTATOR CUFF TEAR

Key Facts

Terminology
- Partial-thickness, full-thickness or complete rotator cuff tendon tear

Imaging Findings
- Best diagnostic clue: Discontinuity of tendon filled with fluid
- Supraspinatus tendon tears close to or at insertional area
- Anterior fibers most commonly torn
- Gap filled with echogenic fluid or blood +/- gas locules (comet tail artifacts)
- Focal flattening of convex bursal surface
- Retraction of tendon from insertional area or blunting of edge of tendon insertion
- Intrasubstance tear: Linear irregular sharp hypoechoic area within tendon substance

- Recognition of intrasubstance tears difficult in moderate to severe tendinosis
- Complete tear with retraction: Non-visualization of tendon
- Fluid within subacromial-subdeltoid bursa
- Muscle atrophy assessed at level of scapular spine (better by MR)

Top Differential Diagnoses
- Bursitis
- Rotator Cuff Tendinopathy
- Bicipital Tendinosis

Diagnostic Checklist
- Systematic examination for secondary signs as well as primary sign of tear

---

- ○ Focal flattening of convex bursal surface
- ○ Retraction of tendon from insertional area or blunting of edge of tendon insertion
- ○ Undulation of smooth tendon contour
- Intrasubstance tear: Linear irregular sharp hypoechoic area within tendon substance
- Recognition of intrasubstance tears difficult in moderate to severe tendinosis
  - ○ Look especially for contour deformity or marginal retraction of tendon
  - ○ Pay particular attention to anterolateral aspect of supraspinatus tendon
- Complete tear with retraction: Non-visualization of tendon
  - ○ Approximation of humeral head to acromion
- Fluid within subacromial-subdeltoid bursa
- Muscle atrophy assessed at level of scapular spine (better by MR)

Radiographic Findings
- Radiography
  - ○ Findings associated with impingement
    - Acromial spurs; type III (hooked) acromion; acromioclavicular (AC) degenerative change
    - Cortical irregularity and sclerosis of greater tuberosity
    - Approximation of humerus to acromion with complete tears

MR Findings
- T1WI: Thickening of rotator cuff tendons, of intermediate signal intensity
- T2WI
  - ○ Fluid signal intensity filling an incomplete gap in the tendon
    - Gap: Articular surface or bursal surface
    - Intrasubstance, gap not-communicating with surface
    - Intrasubstance tears not seen at arthroscopy
  - ○ +/- Fluid within subacromial bursa (more consistently seen with MR than ultrasound)
  - ○ +/- Associated bicipital tendinosis (intermediate high signal within biceps tendon)

- ○ FS PD FSE
  - Sensitive for evaluating partial tears
- ○ +/- Retraction of the tendon edge
- ○ T1 sagittal +/- muscle atrophy of at level of scapular spine
  - MR proton spectroscopy more sensitive than MR or ultrasound to mild degrees of atrophy
  - Muscle atrophy is predictor of negative outcome after surgery
- ○ Predisposing structural abnormality better shown by MR than ultrasound
- MR arthrography
  - ○ Possibly more sensitive for articular surface tears

Imaging Recommendations
- Best imaging tool
  - ○ Ultrasound
    - As a first line investigation
- Protocol advice: High frequency transducer; patient sitting; systematic examination.

DIFFERENTIAL DIAGNOSIS

Bursitis
- Very similar symptomatology
- Fluid distension of subacromial-subdeltoid bursa
- Fluid distension is a common feature of tendon tears
  - ○ Fluid accumulates preferentially adjacent to acromion, lateral aspect of upper arm, medial to coracoid
    - Examine with arm in different positions

Rotator Cuff Tendinopathy
- Thickened tendon with loss of fibrillar pattern and increasing hypogenicity
- Can be difficult to distinguish from partial thickness tears
- Prevalence increases with age

Bicipital Tendinosis
- Commonly accompanies rotator cuff tendinosis

ROTATOR CUFF TEAR

Calcific Tendinitis
- Calcium hydroxyapatite
  - Echogenic foci within tendon substance +/- acoustic enhancement

PATHOLOGY

General Features
- General path comments
  - Three types partial tears of rotator cuff tear
    - Articular surface
    - Interstitial: Not seen at arthroscopy
    - Bursal surface
  - Partial thickness tears cause muscle contraction pain similar to other partial tendon injuries (Achilles tendon, extensor carpi radialis brevis)
  - Pain with reflex inhibition of muscle action and loss of strength
  - Altered cuff function: Humeral head ascends under deltoid contraction
  - Impinging cuff between humeral head & coracoacromial arch
  - Abrasion of cuff occurs with altered humeroscapular motion = cuff degeneration
- Etiology
  - Acute strain
  - Chronic microtrauma/persistent strain
  - Impingement syndromes
  - Collagen vascular diseases along with tears of other tendons
- Epidemiology: Incidence of partial thickness tears 32-37% after 40 years
- Associated abnormalities
  - Posterosuperior labral tears or fraying with internal impingement
  - Posterosuperior humeral head chronic impaction internal impingement
  - Superior labrum anterior to posterior (SLAP) tears associated with articular surface partial tears

Gross Pathologic & Surgical Features
- Thickened, indurated tendon edges
- Loss of integrity of tendon collagen fibers
- Hemorrhage in interstitial tears
- Associated subacromial-subdeltoid bursitis

Microscopic Features
- Collagen degeneration without influx of inflammatory cells
- Inflammatory cells in adjacent bursa = bursitis
- Increased levels of smooth muscle actin (SMA)
  - SMA-positive cells + glycosaminoglycan and proteoglycan promote retraction of torn fibers

Staging, Grading or Classification Criteria
- Type I: Superficial capsular fraying, small local area, < 1 cm
- Type II: Mild fraying, some failure of tendon fibers, < 2 cm
- Type III: Moderate fragmentation and fraying, often involves entire supraspinatus surface, usually < 3 cm
- Type IV: Severe tear with fraying, fragmentation and flap
  - Often involves more than one tendon

CLINICAL ISSUES

Presentation
- Most common signs/symptoms
  - Pain with abduction flexion maneuvers/impingement tests
  - Shoulder pain with use of rotator cuff
  - Partial tears are more painful than full thickness tears
- Clinical Profile: Athlete, patient after 40 years of age with impingement

Demographics
- Age
  - Younger athlete in case of internal impingement
  - Older than 40 years in subacromial impingement
- Gender: M = F, M > F in throwing athletes and heavy laborers

Natural History & Prognosis
- Insidious onset of pain in adult patient with impingement syndrome
- Sudden onset of pain in acute traumatic event
- Many partial-thickness tears progress to full thickness tears within 2 years
- May heal with cessation of impingement activities/physical therapy (P/T)

Treatment
- Autologous blood injection under ultrasound guidance for partial tears
  - Physiotherapy for minor partial tears
- Arthroscopic debridement and subacromial decompression for larger tears

DIAGNOSTIC CHECKLIST

Consider
- A small surface tear if you see unexplained bursal fluid
  - Pay particular attention to tendon contour and margins of insertional area

Image Interpretation Pearls
- Systematic examination for secondary signs as well as primary sign of tear

SELECTED REFERENCES

1. Bianchi S et al: Ultrasound of tendon tears. Part 1: general considerations and upper extremity. Skeletal Radiol. 2005
2. Prasad N et al: Outcome of open rotator cuff repair. An analysis of risk factors. Acta Orthop Belg. 71(6):662-6, 2005
3. Schulz CU et al: Coracoid tip position on frontal radiographs of the shoulder: a predictor of common shoulder pathologies? Br J Radiol. 78(935):1005-8, 2005
4. Read JW et al: Shoulder ultrasound: Diagnostic accuracy for impingement syndrome, rotator cuff tear, and biceps tendon pathology. J Shoulder Elbow Surg 7(3):264-71, 1998

ROTATOR CUFF TEAR

IMAGE GALLERY

Typical

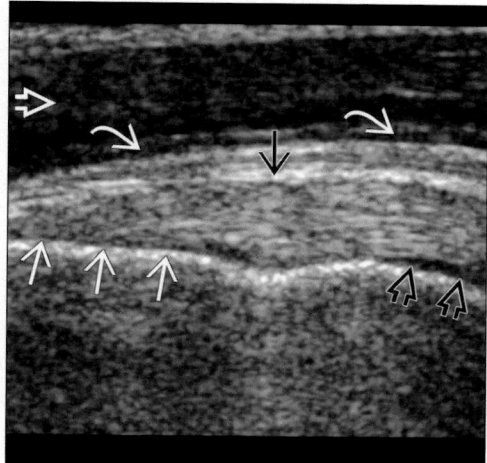

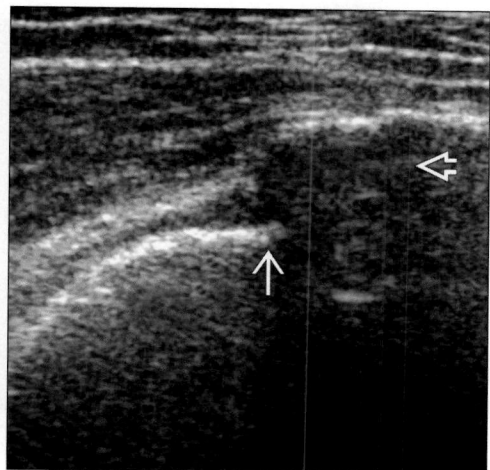

(Left) Transverse ultrasound shows a normal supraspinatus tendon ➡. Note the intrinsic fibrillar pattern, insertional area ➡, articular cartilage ➡, echogenic bursa ➡ and deltoid muscle ➡. *(Right)* Transverse ultrasound shows a chronic complete supraspinatus (and infraspinatus) tendon tear. Both are torn and retracted medially (i.e., no tendon visible). The humeral head ➡ is subluxed superiorly, and located just beneath the acromion ➡.

Variant

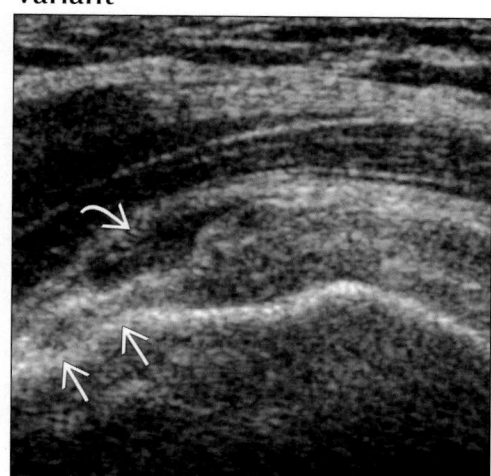

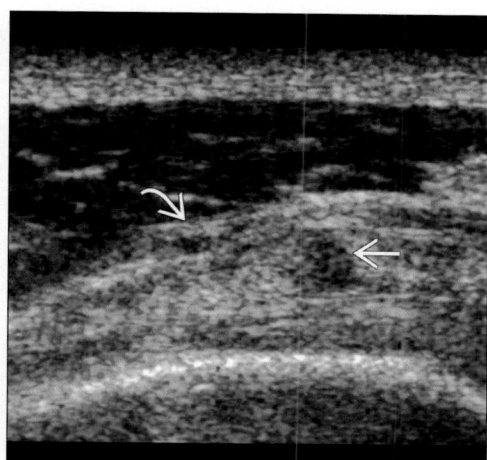

(Left) Longitudinal ultrasound shows a large, bursal surface, partial-thickness tear ➡ of the supraspinatus tendon just above the insertional area ➡. *(Right)* Longitudinal ultrasound shows mild tendinosis with a sharp, focal hypoechoic area within the supraspinatus tendon ➡ compatible with the bursal surface partial tear. There is mild flattening of the bursal convexity and a small amount of fluid in the subacromial-subdeltoid bursa ➡.

Typical

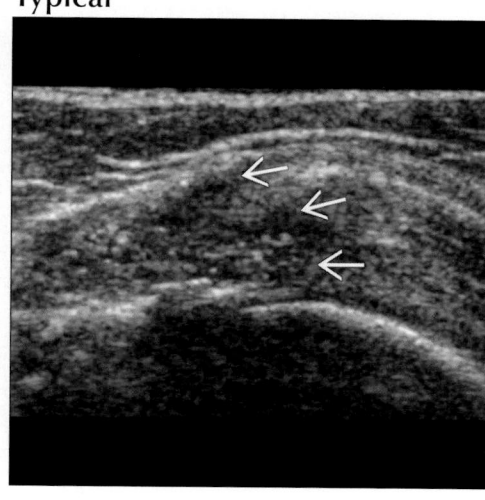

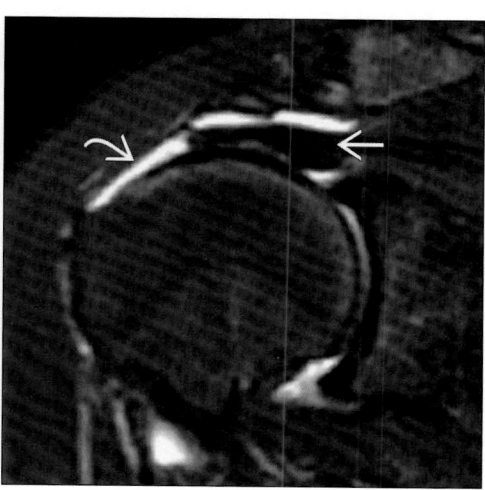

(Left) Longitudinal ultrasound shows a large, acute, full-thickness supraspinatus tendon tear just proximal to insertion. As the gap is filled with echogenic blood, the tendon edge ➡ is difficult to delineate and there is no bursal convexity depression. *(Right)* Coronal T2WI FS MR shows a large, full-thickness, avulsive-type tear ➡ of the supraspinatus tendon ➡ with retraction.

(Left) Longitudinal ultrasound shows a complete acute tear of the supraspinatus tendon. There is no tendon visible with fluid filling the space between the acromion ➡, bursa ⇢ and humeral head ⮞. *(Right)* Coronal T2WI FS MR shows an acute complete tear of the supraspinatus (and infraspinatus) tendons. The supraspinatus tendon ➡ is retracted deep to the acromioclavicular joint.

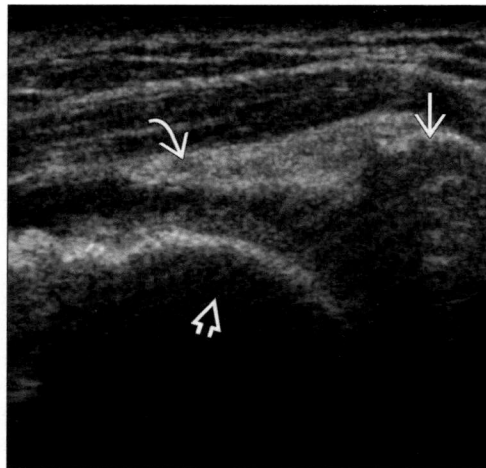

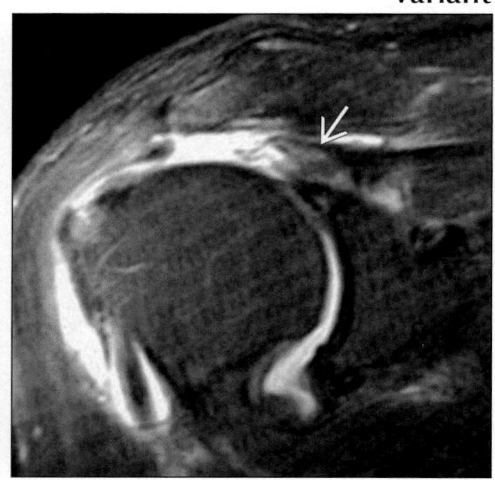

(Left) Longitudinal ultrasound shows a shallow, bursal surface tear (fraying) ⇢ of the supraspinatus tendon ➡. Note the finely serrated bursal contour ⇢ with mild bursal distension. There is cortical irregularity of the supraspinatus insertional area ⮞. *(Right)* Longitudinal ultrasound shows a flap-like, linear, bursal surface, and supraspinatus tear ➡. There is blood and clot in the moderately distended bursa ➡.

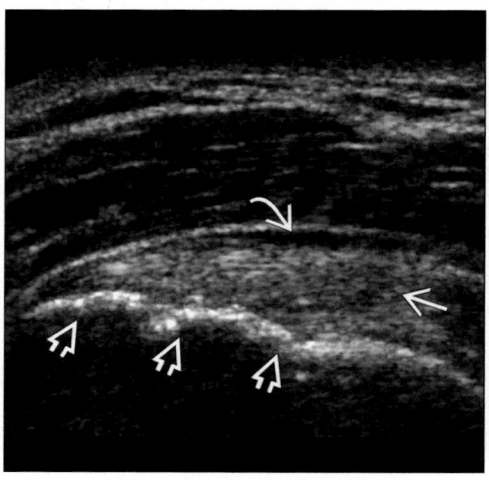

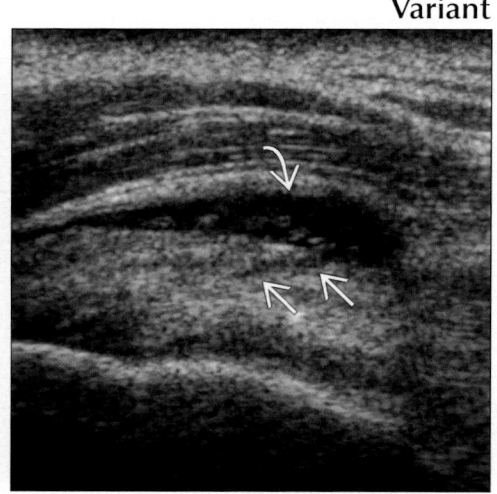

(Left) Oblique ultrasound shows moderate severity tendinosis with a partial-thickness, bursal surface tear ➡. Mild distension of the subacromial-subdeltoid bursa is present ⇢. *(Right)* Transverse ultrasound shows a large, avulsive-type tear of the supraspinatus tendon from its insertional area ➡ with retraction. Only a few Sharpey fibers ⮞ remain attached at the insertion. The bursal convexity of the tendon is mildly flattened ➡.

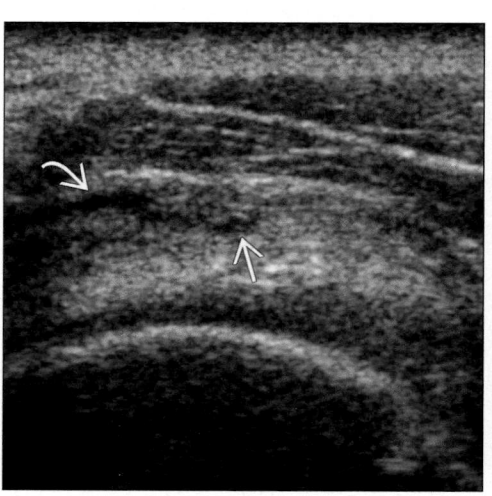

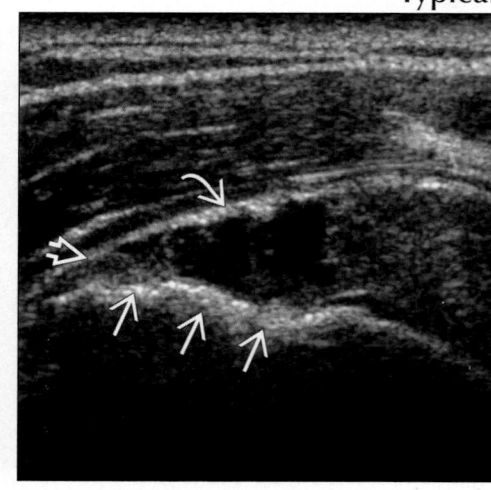

ROTATOR CUFF TEAR

Typical

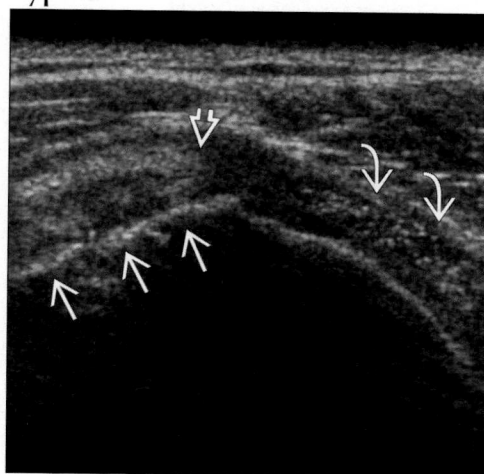

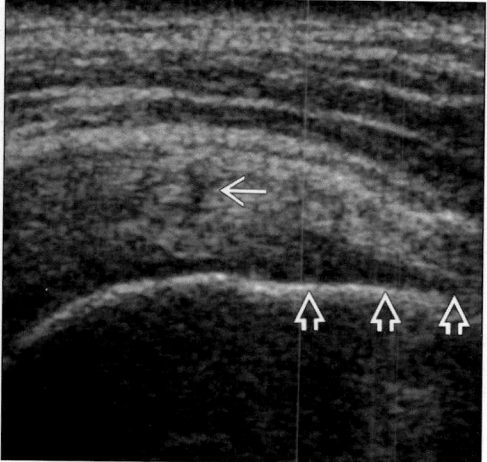

(Left) Longitudinal ultrasound shows a complete tear of the supraspinatus tendon just proximal to the insertion ➡. Only the lateral end of the torn tendon is visible ➡. The medial end has retracted, with the gap filled with echogenic blood (comet-tail artifacts) ➡. *(Right)* Longitudinal ultrasound shows a sharp, branching, vertical, intrasubstance, supraspinatus tendon tear ➡ just proximal to the insertion ➡.

Typical

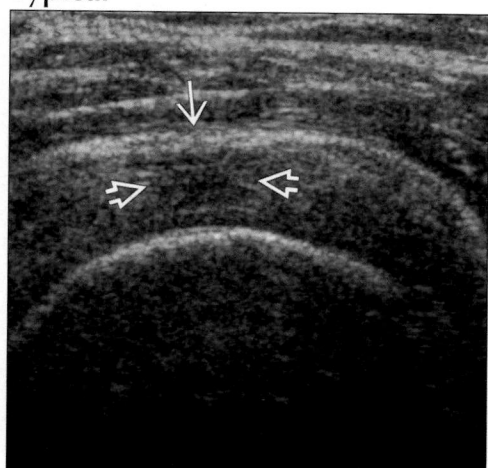

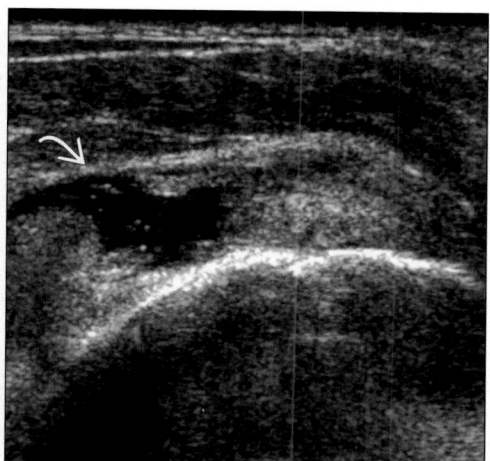

(Left) Transverse ultrasound shows moderate severity tendinosis with a full-thickness tear of the anterior fibers of the infraspinatus tendon. The gap is filled with echogenic fluid, making tendon ends ➡ difficult to see clearly. Note mild flattening of the bursal convexity ➡. *(Right)* Transverse ultrasound shows a large, acute, full-thickness tear of the supraspinatus tendon ➡. The gap is filled with fluid with a few comet-tail artifacts, probably due to blood.

Typical

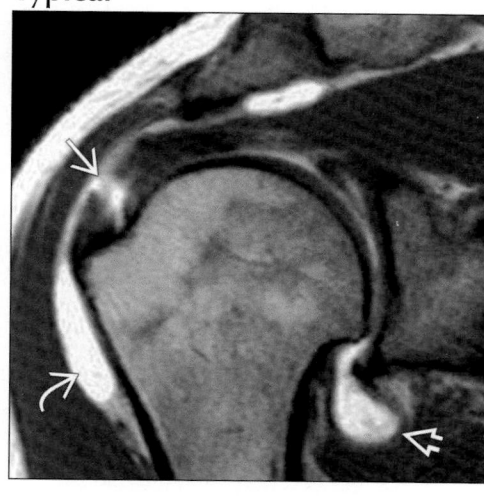

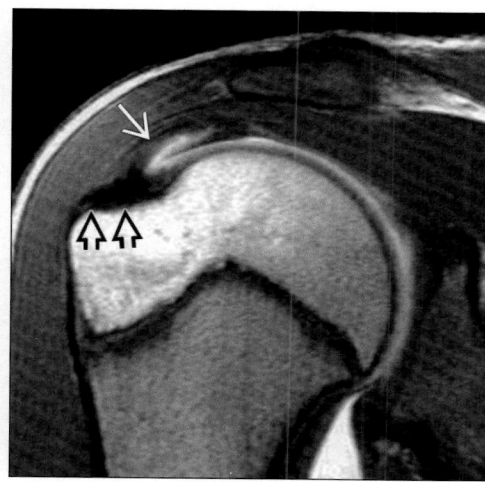

(Left) Coronal T2WI shows a full-thickness acute tear of the supraspinatus tendon at its insertion ➡. There is fluid distension of both the subacromial-subdeltoid bursa ➡ and the glenohumeral joint ➡. *(Right)* Coronal T2WI MR of a young patient shows a large, bursal surface, partial tear ➡ of the supraspinatus tendon just proximal to the insertion ➡.

NON-ROTATOR CUFF TENDINOSIS

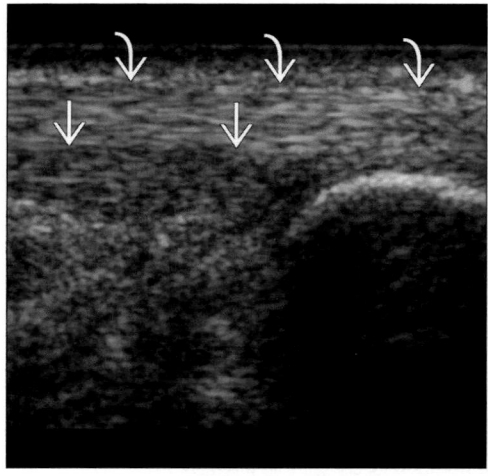

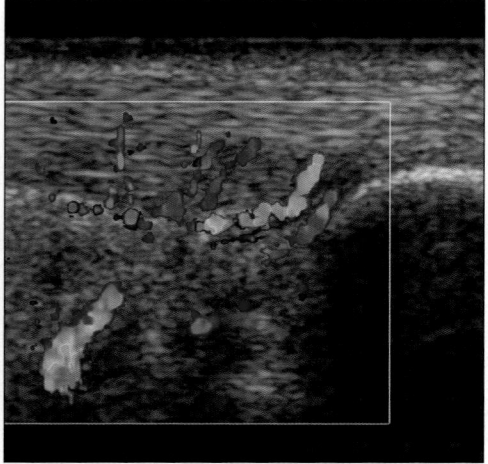

Longitudinal ultrasound shows a thickened Achilles tendon ➔ with a hypoechoic area ➔ on the deeper aspect associated with loss of the normal fibrillar pattern indicative of tendinosis.

Longitudinal color Doppler ultrasound (same patient as previous image) shows marked hyperemia of the hypoechoic area. The vessels are regularly distributed.

TERMINOLOGY

Abbreviations and Synonyms
- Tendinosis or tendinopathy, Achilles tendinosis, patellar tendinosis, posterior tibialis tendinosis etc.

Definitions
- Tendinosis or tendinopathy represents collagenous tendon degeneration with proteoglycan deposition
- Paratenon-connective tissue envelope incompletely surrounds Achilles and patellar tendon (also referred to as peritenon)
- Paratenonitis is inflammation of connective tissue envelope (paratenon)
- Paratendinitis is generalized inflammation of tissues surrounding the tendon

IMAGING FINDINGS

General Features
- Best diagnostic clue: Focal, nodular or diffuse tendon enlargement with loss of normal fibrillar echotexture
- Location

- ○ Achilles tendon
  - ■ Calcaneal insertional area more frequently than mid-portion of tendon
- ○ Patellar tendon
  - ■ Inferior pole of patella more frequently than tibial insertion
- ○ Posterior tibialis tendon
  - ■ Navicular insertion more frequently than remainder of tendon
- Size: Variable in longitudinal extent: Tends to affect areas of decreased perfusion
- Morphology
  - ○ Focal or nodular or diffuse tendon thickening
  - ○ Anterior convexity of mid-third Achilles tendon

Ultrasonographic Findings
- Increased tendon thickening with hypoechogenicity and progressive loss of normal fibrillar pattern
  - ○ Some tendons (Achilles, patellar, posterior tibialis, rotator cuff tendon, common extensor tendons of forearm) are more susceptible to tendinosis
- Cross-sectional area of tendon routinely measured at specific locations

DDx: Non-Rotator Cuff Tendinosis

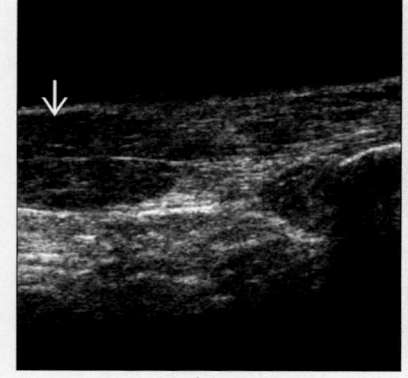

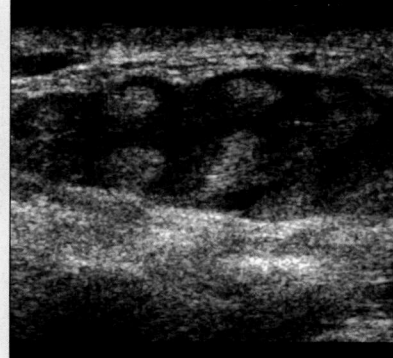

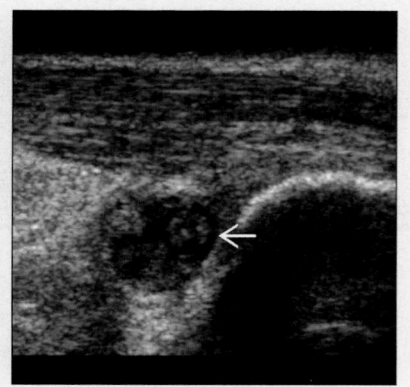

Xanthomata

Tenosynovitis

Retrocalcaneal Bursitis

NON-ROTATOR CUFF TENDINOSIS

Key Facts

Imaging Findings
- Best diagnostic clue: Focal, nodular or diffuse tendon enlargement with loss of normal fibrillar echotexture
- Increased tendon thickening with hypoechogenicity and progressive loss of normal fibrillar pattern
- Some tendons (Achilles, patellar, posterior tibialis, rotator cuff tendon, common extensor tendons of forearm) are more susceptible to tendinosis
- Cross-sectional area measurements useful for follow-up rather than diagnosis
- Level of hyperemia correlates with disease activity
- **Partial tears** seen as sharp linear hypoechoic defect within area of tendinosis
- May be difficult to detect in severe tendinosis
- Should not be confused with vascular channels within tendon

- Secondary signs include adjacent bursitis (Achilles, common extensor), reactive bone changes, paratenon (Achilles, patella) and synovial inflammation

Top Differential Diagnoses
- Xanthoma
- Tenosynovitis
- Retrocalcaneal Bursitis

Clinical Issues
- Most common signs/symptoms: Pain with stretching of tendon

Diagnostic Checklist
- Examine paratenon or synovial sheath and paratendinous tissues for inflammatory change separate from tendinosis
- Routinely examine with color Doppler

- ○ Cross-sectional area measurements useful for follow-up rather than diagnosis
  - ▪ Area measurements take a long time to change
- Intra- or paratendinous hyperemia is a common feature
  - ○ Level of hyperemia correlates with disease activity
- **Partial tears** seen as sharp linear hypoechoic defect within area of tendinosis
  - ○ Occur with moderate to severe tendinosis
  - ○ Partial tears tend to run longitudinally in tendon
  - ○ May be difficult to detect in severe tendinosis
  - ○ Should not be confused with vascular channels within tendon
    - ▪ Examine with color Doppler ultrasound
- Proteoglycan accumulation seen as focal hypoechoic area which may bulge beyond margins of tendon
- Dystrophic calcification within area of tendinosis (particularly in Achilles and patellar tendons)
- Secondary signs include adjacent bursitis (Achilles, common extensor), reactive bone changes, paratenon (Achilles, patella) and synovial inflammation
  - ○ More common with more severe degrees of tendinosis
  - ○ Marrow bone change not seen on ultrasound (seen with MR)
  - ○ Effusions may occur in tendons with complete synovial sheaths (e.g., posterior tibialis)

Radiographic Findings
- Radiography
  - ○ Sclerosis, cortical irregularity, hyperostosis for insertional tendinosis
  - ○ Accessory navicular bone
  - ○ Intrasubstance dystropic calcification
  - ○ Enlarged Achilles tendon

MR Findings
- T1WI
  - ○ Increased cross sectional area on axial images
  - ○ Increased signal intensity
  - ○ Thickening + intermediate signal of peritendinous tissue dorsal, medial, & lateral to Achilles tendon
- T2WI

- ○ Intermediate signal within enlarged tendon
- ○ Hyperintense inflammatory fluid around tendon
- ○ Partial tears hyperintense on FS PD FSE or STIR images
- ○ Haglund deformity: Insertional tendinosis with reactive calcaneal marrow edema and hyperostosis + retrocalcaneal bursitis
- T1 C+: Enhancement of hyperemic area of tendinosis, peritendinous tissues and marrow at bony insertional site

Imaging Recommendations
- Best imaging tool: Ultrasound as all tendons are readily accessible and is of higher resolution than MR
- Protocol advice
  - ○ Examine both symptomatic and contralateral side
    - ▪ As contralateral subclinical disease is common, do not use asymptomatic contralateral side as a normal standard

---

DIFFERENTIAL DIAGNOSIS

Xanthoma
- Nodular or diffuse involvement of tendon
- Primarily affects Achilles tendon and, to a lesser extent, the patellar tendon
- Affected areas tend to to be more nodular and less hyperemic than tendinosis
- Differentiation can be difficult on imaging (xanthomata are feature of severe hypercholesterolemia)

Tenosynovitis
- Affects tendon with complete synovial sheath
- Synovial rather than tendon thickening predominates

Retrocalcaneal Bursitis
- Isolated bursitis is uncommon: Usually occurs in conjunction with Achilles tendinosis

NON-ROTATOR CUFF TENDINOSIS

PATHOLOGY

General Features
- General path comments
  - Relevant anatomy
    - Achilles or patellar tendon have no synovial sheath
    - Retrocalcaneal bursae between Achilles insertion and Kager fad pad
  - Posterior tibialis inserts into accessory navicular (when present), medial pole of navicular and cuneiform bones
    - Cornuate navicular is elongated medial pole of navicular
- Etiology
  - Achilles: Hypovascular watershed zone 2-6 cm proximal to calcaneal insertion
    - Eccentric loading of fatigued muscle-tendon unit
    - Overtraining
    - Runners susceptible in both acceleration (sprinting) and deceleration (eccentric contraction)
  - Posterior tibialis: Pes planus and accessory navicular (posterior tibialis)
  - Patellar tendon: Running and jumping
  - Systemic arthropathy
    - Enthesopathies
    - Rheumatoid arthritis
- Epidemiology
  - Achilles and patellar tendinosis commonly though not always associated with overuse
  - Posterior tibialis tendinosis usually associated with pes planus

Gross Pathologic & Surgical Features
- Inadequate healing
- Loss of normal tendon luster
- Nodular thickening
- Calcification
- Inflamed peritenon

Microscopic Features
- Chronic paratendinitis
  - Hypertrophic connective tissue
  - Increased capillary infiltration
  - Fibrinogen deposition and fibrinoid necrosis
  - Round cell infiltrate
  - Increase in glycosaminoglycans (chondroitin sulfate) and mucoid degeneration
  - Leakage of plasma proteins secondary to disruption of local blood flow
  - Absence of tendon inflammatory response (separate from inflammatory disease of peritendinous tissues and peritenon)

CLINICAL ISSUES

Presentation
- Most common signs/symptoms: Pain with stretching of tendon
- Other signs/symptoms
  - Achilles: Morning heel stiffness

- Tendinosis is often visible on ultrasound with minimal or no symptoms (subclinical)
  - Subclinical disease common on contralateral side in patients with unilateral symptoms
- Clinical Profile
  - Chronic dull to sharp pain, aggravated by onset of exercise
    - Gradually subsides in hours to days after exercise
    - Improvement with prolonged rest
    - Tenderness to deep palpation
    - Posterior tibialis pain aggravated by prolonged standing or walking

Demographics
- Age
  - Adult ages 25-40 most at risk
  - Also young athletes, sedentary individuals and older population
- Gender: More common in males

Natural History & Prognosis
- Established ultrasound features bodes for chronic relapsing remitting symptomatology
- Minimal to mild ultrasound features bodes for a favorable outcome if managed correctly

Treatment
- Conservative
  - Therapeutic rest
  - Controlled slow stretching exercise
  - Cross training or alternative exercise
  - Antiinflammatory medication
  - Immobilization
  - Shoe supports for posterior tibialis tendinosis
- Non-conservative
  - Focal proteoglycan accumulation treated with debridement
  - Suturing of large partial tears
  - Autologous blood injection for partial tears
  - Release ± excision paratenon in paratenonitis
  - Excision of calcaneal prominence or accessory navicular bone in insertional tendinopathy

DIAGNOSTIC CHECKLIST

Consider
- Examine paratenon or synovial sheath and paratendinous tissues for inflammatory change separate from tendinosis
- Routinely examine with color Doppler
- Look for secondary features
- Measurement useful for follow-up

SELECTED REFERENCES
1. Bianchi S et al: Ultrasound appearance of tendon tears. Part 2: lower extremity and myotendinous tears. Skeletal Radiol. 35(2):63-77, 2006
2. Paavola M et al: Achilles tendinopathy. J Bone Joint Surg Am 84-A(11):2062-76, 2002
3. Myerson M: Foot and ankle disorders. vol 2. Philadelphia PA, Lippincott Raven, (55):1367-98, 2000

IMAGE GALLERY

Typical

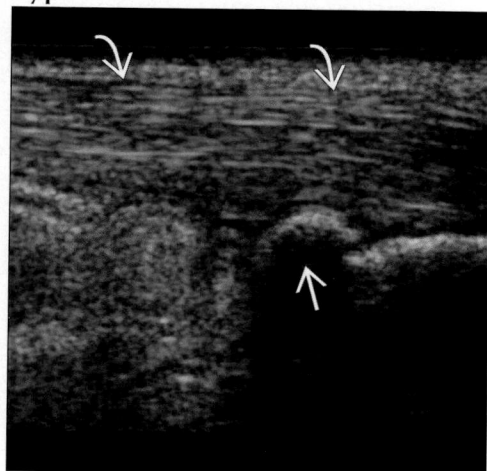 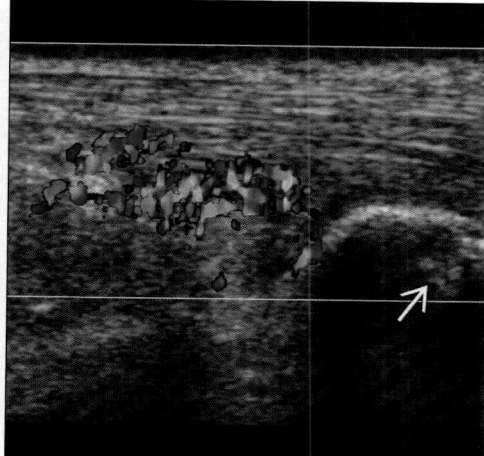

(Left) Longitudinal ultrasound shows a thickened Achilles tendon ➔. The fibrillar pattern is poorly defined, but there is no discrete abnormal area. Mild calcaneal hyperostosis is present ➔. *(Right)* Longitudinal color Doppler ultrasound (same patient as previous image) clearly shows an abnormal hyperemic area on the inferior surface of the Achilles tendon. Mild calcaneal irregularity ➔ is again seen.

Typical

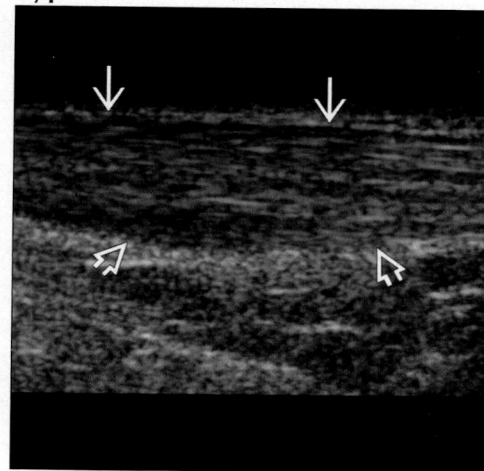 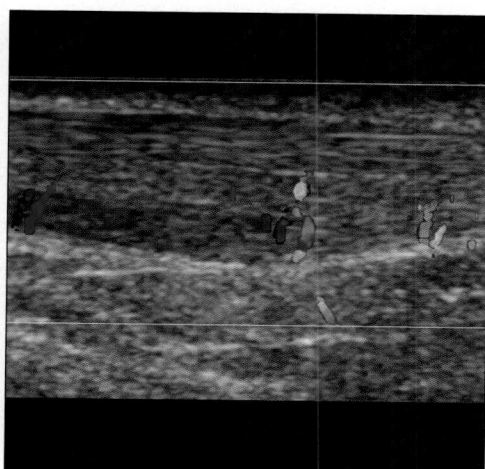

(Left) Longitudinal ultrasound shows a thickened mid-segment of the Achilles tendon ➔ with a convex anterior border ➔ indicative of mid-segment tendinosis. *(Right)* Longitudinal color Doppler ultrasound (same patient as previous image) shows moderate hyperemia extending into the deeper half of the mid-segment of the Achilles tendon.

Variant

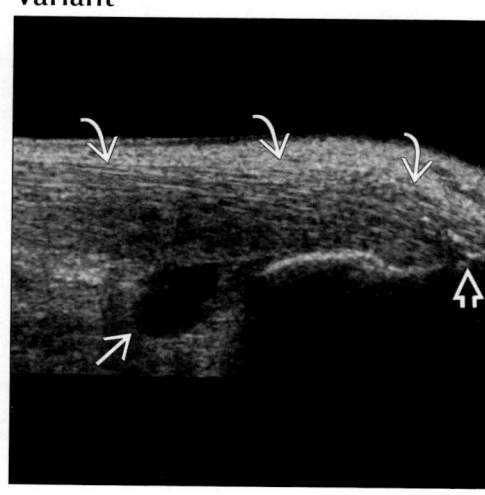 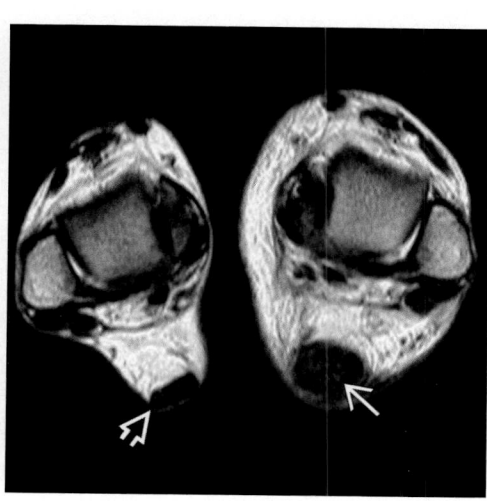

(Left) Longitudinal ultrasound shows a thickened Achilles tendon ➔ indicative of tendinosis with retrocalcaneal bursal distension ➔ and early insertional calcification ➔. *(Right)* Transverse T2WI MR shows a thickened, left Achilles tendon with increased signal intensity ➔ indicative of Achilles tendinosis compared to the normal right side ➔.

Variant

(Left) Transverse ultrasound shows a thickened, hypoechoic Achilles tendon ➡ indicative of tendinosis. There are large foci of dystrophic calcification ➡ with acoustic shadowing within the tendon substance. *(Right)* Transverse ultrasound shows a thickened, heterogeneous Achilles tendon ➡ with a thickened paratenon ➡ overlying the superficial aspect of the tendon.

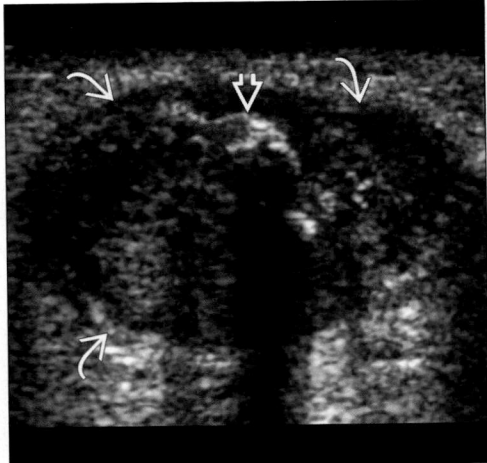
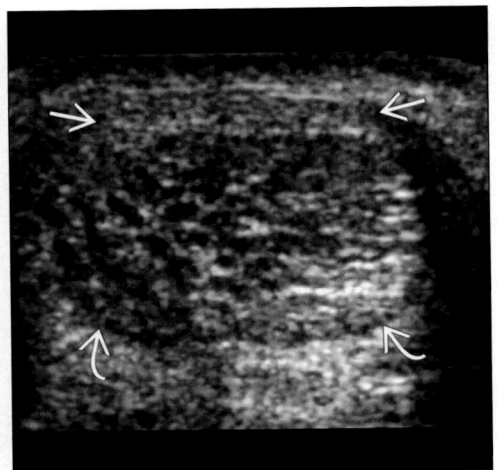

Typical

(Left) Longitudinal ultrasound shows a thickened patellar tendon ➡ just distal to the inferior pole of the patella, indicative of tendinosis. There is some intratendinous dystropic calcification ➡. *(Right)* Longitudinal color Doppler ultrasound (same patient as previous image) shows marked hyperemia of the tendinosis affected area.

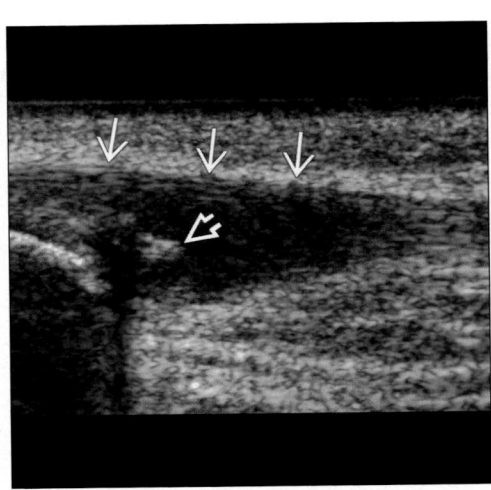
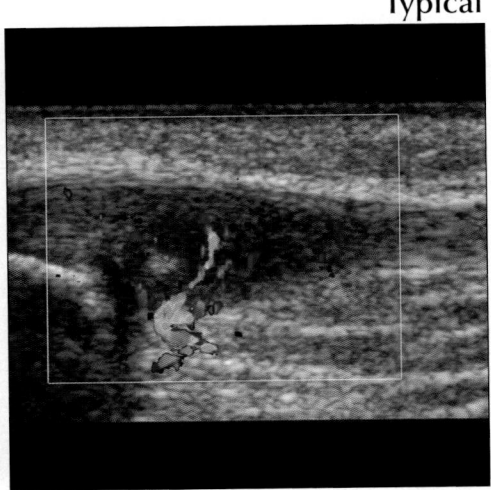

Typical

(Left) Transverse ultrasound (same patient as previous image) shows measurement of the cross-sectional area of the patellar tendon. The central portion of the patella tendon is particularly thickened and hypoechoic ➡. *(Right)* Sagittal T2WI MR shows a thickened patellar tendon with some central intermediate signal intensity ➡, just distal to the inferior pole of the patella compatible with tendinosis.

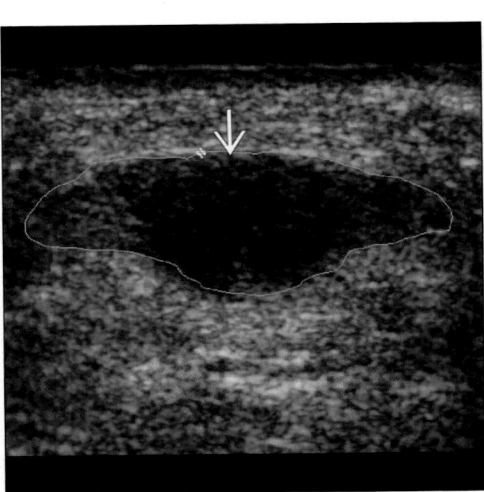
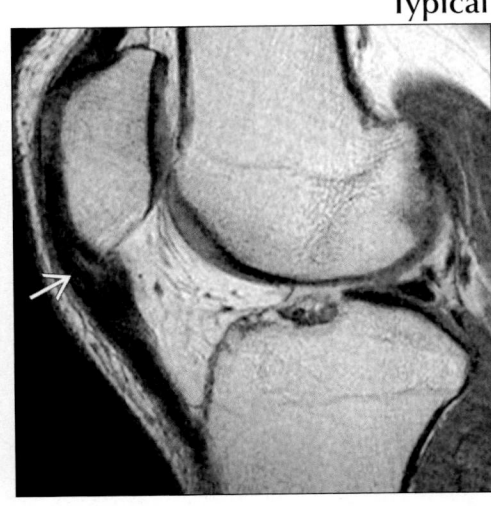

Typical

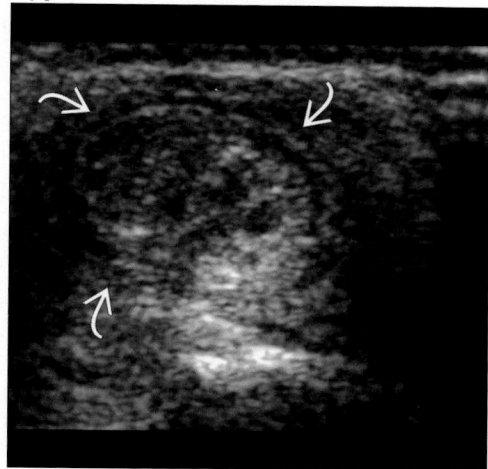

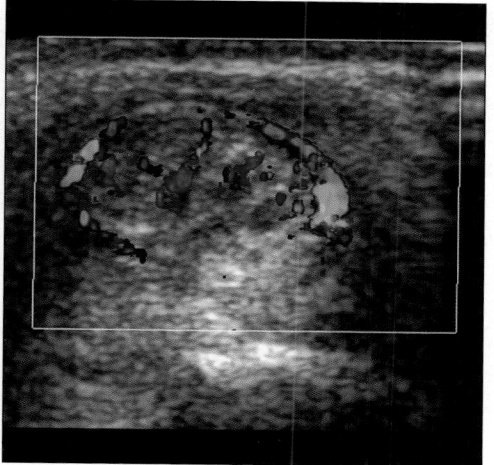

(Left) Transverse ultrasound at the hindfoot level shows a thickened, hypoechoic, heterogeneous, posterior tibialis tendon ➡ indicative of tendinosis. (Right) Transverse color Doppler ultrasound (same location as previous image) shows intratendinous and peritendinous hyperemia. These intratendinous vascular channels can, on grayscale, be misinterpreted as tears.

Typical

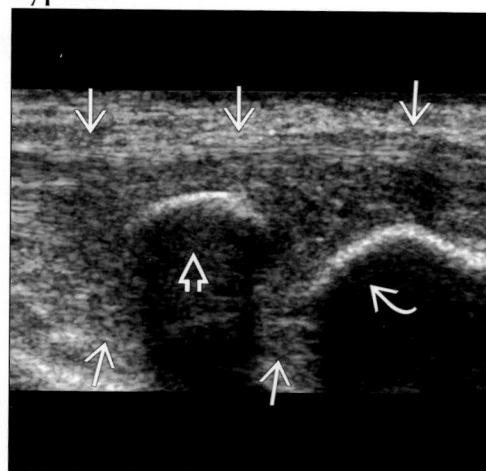

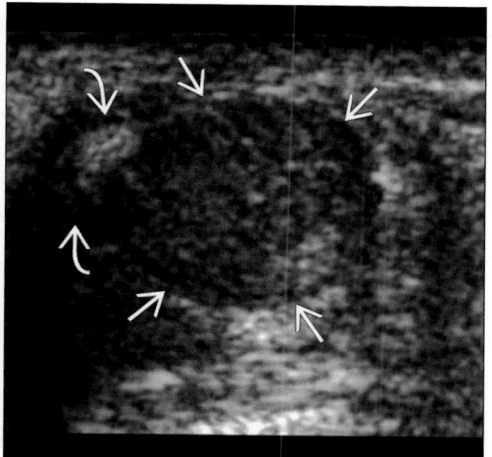

(Left) Longitudinal ultrasound shows a thickened, hypoechoic, posterior tibialis tendon ➡ indicative of insertional tendinosis near the insertion into the accessory navicular ➡ & the medial pole of the navicular bone ➡. (Right) Transverse ultrasound of the hindfoot shows a thickened, hypoechoic peroneus longus tendon ➡ overlying a normal peroneus brevis ➡ tendon. Normally, the peroneus longus & brevis tendons are the same caliber.

Typical

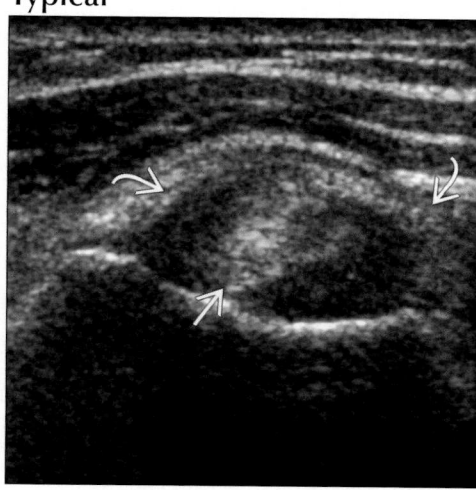

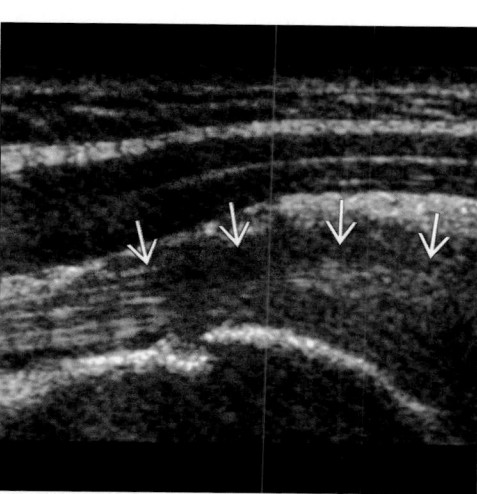

(Left) Transverse ultrasound shows a thickened, poorly marginated, biceps tendon ➡ at the uppermost aspect of the bicipital groove, indicative of tendinosis. There is swelling and hypoechogenicity of the surrounding tendon sheath ➡. (Right) Longitudinal ultrasound (same patient as previous image) shows how tendinosis affects the biceps tendon ➡ principally as it leaves the bicipital groove and turns to a horizontal course. The surrounding synovial sheath is swollen.

NON-ROTATOR CUFF TENDON TEARS

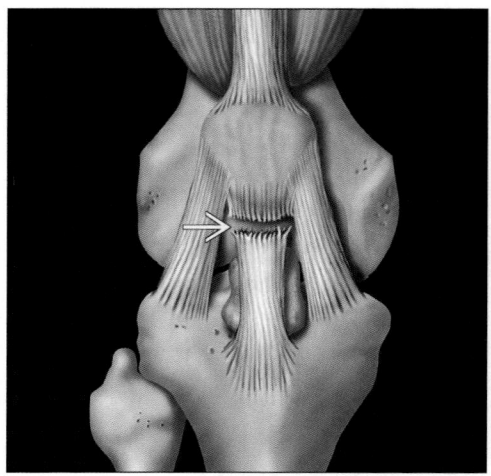

Longitudinal graphic shows a tear of the patellar tendon ➡ just distal to the inferior pole of the patella.

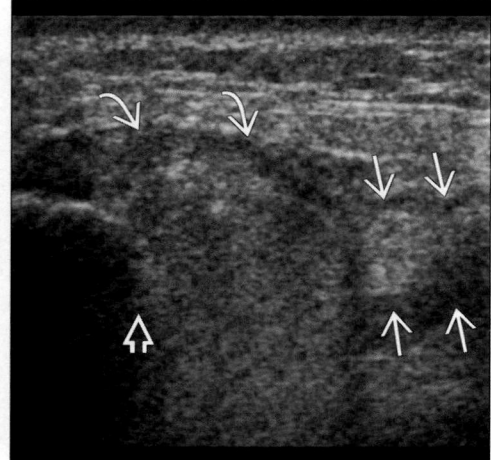

Longitudinal ultrasound of the knee shows a complete tear (avulsion) of the patellar tendon ➡ from the inferior pole of the patella ➡. The gap is filled with blood ➡.

TERMINOLOGY

Abbreviations and Synonyms
- Tendon rupture, tendon tear, tendon sprain, tendon strain

Definitions
- Tendon tear is a partial or complete discontinuity in tendon
- Tendon sprain or strain both refer to microscopic tendon tear (i.e., tendon distraction injury in the absence of identifiable macroscopic tear)

IMAGING FINDINGS

General Features
- Best diagnostic clue: Fluid-filled gap in tendon
- Location
  - Achilles tendon mid-way between calcaneum and musculotendinous junction
  - Patellar tendon just distal to patella
  - Quadriceps tendon just proximal to patella
  - Finger tendons at carpometacarpal level
  - Biceps tendon at upper end of bicipital groove
- Size: Variable based on tendon retraction
- Morphology: Enlarged retracted tendon ends in complete tear

Ultrasonographic Findings
- Fluid-filled gap within tendon, either partial thickness, full-thickness/complete
  - Gap usually filled with anechoic or hypoechoic fluid
  - In acute phase, gap may be filled with blood +/- gas locules making tendon ends difficult to see
    - Especially true for tears of large tendons
    - Look for depressed tendon edges at site of tear
    - Passively contracting and relaxing tendon during ultrasound examination may aid identification of tendon gap
  - Larger tendons tend to tear transversely while smaller tendons tend to tear either longitudinally or transversely
  - Tendon ends often swollen, especially finger tendons, improving visibility on ultrasound examination

DDx: Non-Rotator Cuff Tendon Tears

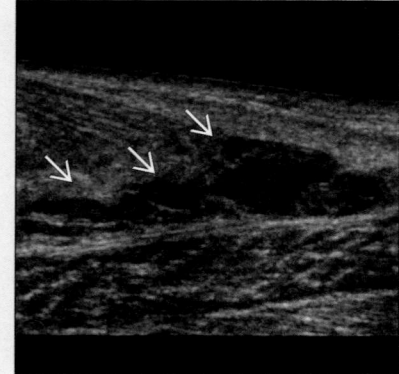

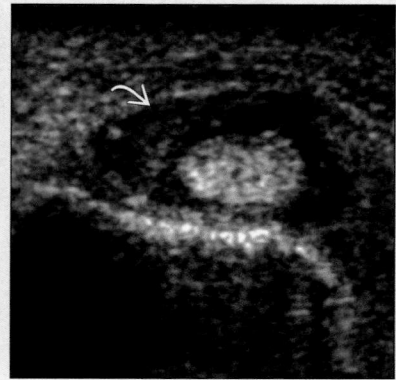

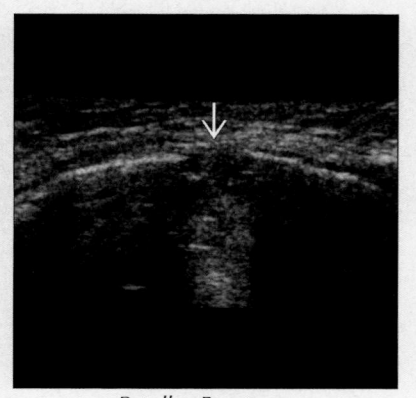

Myofascial Tear   Tenosynovitis   Patellar Fracture

NON-ROTATOR CUFF TENDON TEARS

Key Facts

Imaging Findings

- Fluid-filled gap within tendon, either partial thickness, full-thickness/complete
- In acute phase, gap may be filled with blood +/- gas locules making tendon ends difficult to see
- Look for depressed tendon edges at site of tear
- Larger tendons tend to tear transversely while smaller tendons tend to tear either longitudinally or transversely
- Tendon ends often swollen, especially finger tendons, improving visibility on ultrasound examination
- Swelling of tendon ends can impede ultrasound assessment regarding presence and severity of pre-existing tendinosis
- Collapsed synovial sheath may be mistaken for attenuated tendon

- Reparative hypoechoic granulation tissue and fibrosis may bridge gap in chronic complete tendon tears
- Incomplete tendon tears also heal by hypoechoic reparative granulation tissue
- Ultrasound accurate at detecting re-tear or defining cause of limitation of movement following repair
- Tendon remains swollen and hyperemic long after tendon integrity and strength has returned
- Best imaging tool: Ultrasound confirms tendon tears with high accuracy and precision
- For small tendons, examine first in transverse plane along length of tendon

Top Differential Diagnoses

- Myofascial Tear
- Tenosynovitis
- Patellar Fracture

- Examine along course of tendon (in transverse plane) from distal to proximal until both ends identified
- Swollen finger tendon ends may give rise to ovoid-shaped mass in mid-palm mimicking tumour
- Swelling of tendon ends can impede ultrasound assessment regarding presence and severity of pre-existing tendinosis
  - Intratendinous calcification and hyperemia are good clues to pre-existing tendinosis
  - Ultrasound depiction of contralateral tendinosis may also help
- Collapsed synovial sheath may be mistaken for attenuated tendon
  - Applies to smaller tendons (i.e., finger flexors and biceps tendons)
  - Many tendons (e.g., Achilles, patella, quadriceps, triceps) do not have complete synovial sheath)
- If bicipital or extensor carpi ulnaris grooves empty, check that the tendons have not subluxed
- Reparative hypoechoic granulation tissue and fibrosis may bridge gap in chronic complete tendon tears
  - Especially true for Achilles tendon
- Incomplete tendon tears also heal by hypoechoic reparative granulation tissue
  - Granulation tissue vascularity appreciated on color Doppler imaging
- Ultrasound accurate at detecting re-tear or defining cause of limitation of movement following repair
  - Suture material often seen traversing gap
  - Limitation in movement of small tendons (finger tendons) may be due to tendon adhesions and not re-tear
- Tendon remains swollen and hyperemic long after tendon integrity and strength has returned
  - Especially true for larger tendons
  - Speed of rehabilitation should be gauged clinically and not by serial ultrasound examination

MR Findings

- T1WI

- Assess morphology of tendon edges
- Assess tendon enlargement + retraction
- T2WI
  - Disruption with discontinuity ± wavy retracted tendon
  - Hemorrhage or edema in and around tendon gap: Hyperintense (FS PD FSE)
  - Enlarged tendon with intratendinous fluid or scar tendon may be seen for up to 12 months post-surgery treatment
- T1 C+: FS T1 C+ to enhance granulation tissue at tear site and define margins

Imaging Recommendations

- Best imaging tool: Ultrasound confirms tendon tears with high accuracy and precision
- Protocol advice
  - For small tendons, examine first in transverse plane along length of tendon
  - For quadriceps and patella, examine with knee flexed to 45°
  - For Achilles, examine prone with foot over end of bed
  - For finger tendons, mark retracted ends of tendons on skin to aid surgical exploration

DIFFERENTIAL DIAGNOSIS

Myofascial Tear

- No tendon gap
- Junction of medial gastrocnemius with Achilles tendon is the most common site of myofascial tear

Tenosynovitis

- Many also lead to pain, swelling and limitation of movement
- No tendon gap

Patellar Fracture

- Patella may fracture due to direct trauma in young patients or indirect trauma in elderly osteoporotic patients

NON-ROTATOR CUFF TENDON TEARS

- May clinically mimic quadriceps or patellar tendon fracture

PATHOLOGY

General Features
- General path comments
  - Relevant anatomy
  - Tendons tear at quite distinctive locations
    - Close to bony attachment (patellar, quadriceps, gluteus medius)
    - Changing direction (biceps, posterior tibialis)
    - Crossing joints (extensor carpi ulnaris, tibialis anterior)
    - Areas of relative hypovascularity (Achilles)
  - Quadriceps tendon made up of three laminae
    - Superficial lamina (from rectus femoris), intermediate lamina (vastus lateralis and medialis) and deep lamina (vastus intermedialis)
- Etiology
  - Repetitive microtrauma and indirect trauma common
    - Direct trauma uncommon
  - Younger patients tear large tendons during severe exertion
    - Typically, affected tendon normal or has a mild tendinosis
  - Older patients tear large or medium-sized tendons during modest exertion
    - Typically, affected tendon has moderate or severe tendinosis
  - Elderly patients tear medium-sized or small tendons spontaneously or with minimal exertion
    - Typically, affected tendon has severe tendinosis
- Epidemiology
  - Gluteus medius, quadriceps, patella, Achilles, posterior tibialis and tibialis anterior are lower limb tendons prone to tear
  - Biceps, triceps, extensor carpi ulnaris and long finger flexor and extensor tendons are upper limb non-rotator cuff tendons prone to tear
- Associated abnormalities: Underlying tendinosis is a usual accompaniment especially in older patients

Gross Pathologic & Surgical Features
- Achilles tendon
  - Achilles tears 3-4 cm proximal to calcaneal insertion
  - Posterior fibers of Achilles tear first as anterior fibers are under less tension during dorsiflexion
  - Plantaris tendon usually remains intact as it has a more anterior calcaneal insertion
- Quadriceps tendon
  - Partial tears usually involve superficial or superficial and intermediate laminae

Microscopic Features
- Degeneration with decreased collagen cross-linking
  - Loss of viscoelasticity and increased stiffness

Staging, Grading or Classification Criteria
- Achilles type 1: Tear involving less than 50% of tendon cross-sectional area
- Achilles type 2: Complete tear with gap 3 cm or less

- Achilles type 3: Complete tear with gap 3-6 cm
- Achilles type 4: Complete tear with gap greater than 6 cm

CLINICAL ISSUES

Presentation
- Most common signs/symptoms
  - Acute onset of pain +/- swelling during exertion
  - Clinical assessment can be incorrect up to 25%
  - Up to 40% of quadriceps tears are undiagnosed initially as weak knee extension is preserved by the patellar retinacular expansions
    - Usually occurs during slip or fall
- Clinical Profile
  - Exertional activity in young/middle-aged subjects
  - Non-exertional activity in elderly subjects
  - Palpable tendon defect
  - For Achilles tendon, squeezing calf muscles normally causes plantar flexion (Thompson test)

Demographics
- Age: After age 30 (30 to 50 years most common)
- Gender: M:F = 5:1

Natural History & Prognosis
- Achilles tendon
  - Non-surgical rate of re-rupture 21%
  - Surgical rate of re-rupture 2%

Treatment
- Achilles tendon tear:
  - Cast immobilization
    - Above knee cast with plantar flexion for 4 weeks followed by below knee cast with decreased plantar flexion
    - Indicated for acute tears and when ultrasound shows good approximation of tendon ends with plantar flexion
- Surgical repair usually required
  - Type 1 and 2 tears; end-to-end anastomosis
  - Type 3 tear; autogenous tendon graft flap
  - Type 4 tear; free tendon graft or synthetic graft
- Other tendons tears: Surgical repair or no specific treatment

DIAGNOSTIC CHECKLIST

Image Interpretation Pearls
- Examine entire of length of tendon looking for fluid-filled gap, empty tendon sheath (small tendons) or focal depression of tendon surface

SELECTED REFERENCES

1. Bianchi S et al: Ultrasound appearance of tendon tears. Part 2: lower extremity and myotendinous tears. Skeletal Radiol. 35(2):63-77, 2006
2. Bianchi S et al: Ultrasound of tendon tears. Part 1: general considerations and upper extremity. Skeletal Radiol. 34(9):500-12, 2005

IMAGE GALLERY

Typical

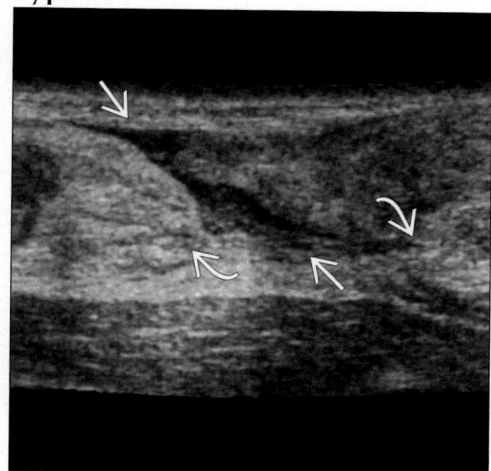 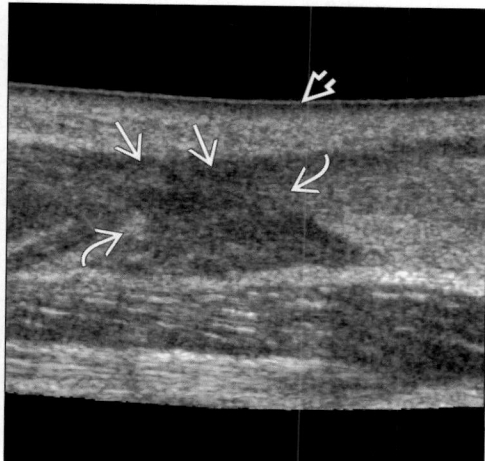

(Left) Longitudinal ultrasound shows an acute, mid-segment, complete tear ➡ of the Achilles tendon. The tendon gap and retracted tendon ends ➡ are clearly demarcated. *(Right)* Longitudinal ultrasound shows an acute tear ➡ of the mid-segment Achilles tendon. The tear is filled with blood. The ends of the tendon ➡ are less distinct than in the previous image. Note the subcutaneous tissue swelling ➡.

Variant

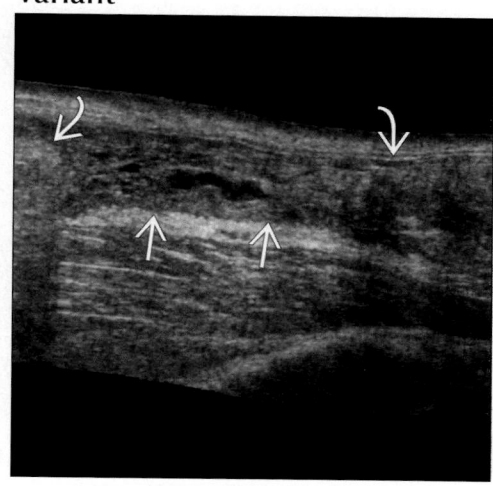 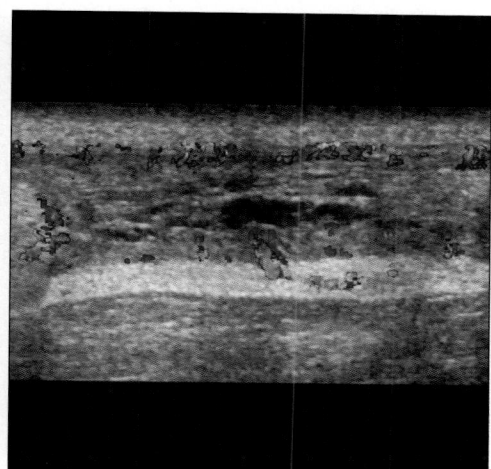

(Left) Longitudinal ultrasound shows a chronic, non-treated, complete tear of the Achilles tendon with retraced tendon ends ➡. The tendon gap ➡ is bridged by reparative granulation tissue. *(Right)* Longitudinal color Doppler ultrasound (at same location as previous image) shows characteristic peripheral hyperemia of granulation tissue bridging the tendon gap. This is an indication of lesion chronicity.

Typical

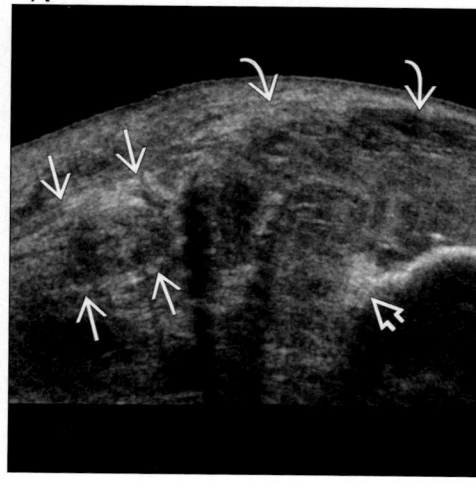 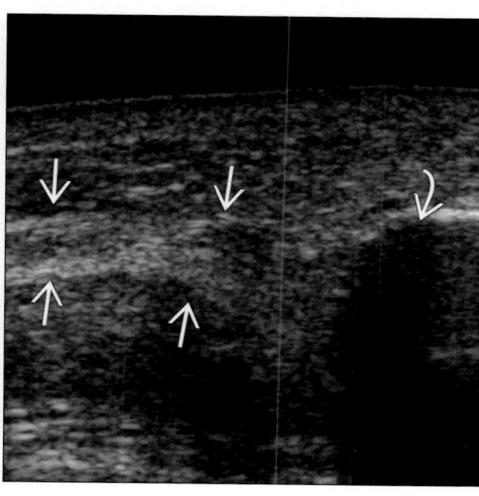

(Left) Longitudinal ultrasound of acute, complete, quadriceps rupture shows large hematoma ➡ between the retracted swollen quadriceps tendon ➡ and the superior pole of the patella where some short fibers remain attached ➡. *(Right)* Longitudinal ultrasound of chronic, complete, quadriceps tendon tear shows non-swollen quadriceps tendon ➡ retracted proximally from the superior pole of the patella ➡.

13

25

Variant

(Left) Longitudinal ultrasound of the hindfoot shows an attenuated posterior tibialis tendon segment ➡ with a central linear hypoechoic area ➡. The latter may represent an intrasubstance tear or linear proteoglycan accumulation. *(Right)* Longitudinal ultrasound of the foot shows an acute, complete, tear of the posterior tibialis tendon ➡ just proximal to the navicular insertion ➡. There is insertional tendinosis ➡.

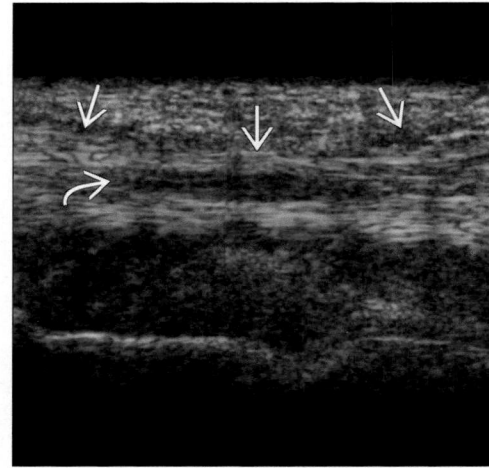
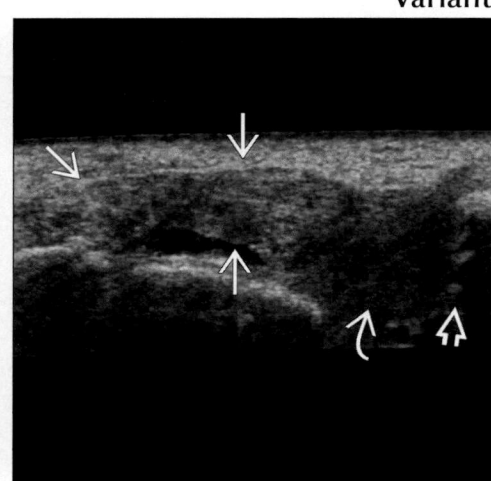

Variant

(Left) Transverse ultrasound of posterior tibialis tendon shows linear hypoechoic areas ➡ within the tendon suggestive of partial-thickness tears. *(Right)* Transverse color Doppler ultrasound (at same level as previous image) shows linear hypoechoic areas that represent either hypertrophied vascular channels or healed tears containing hyperemic granulation tissue.

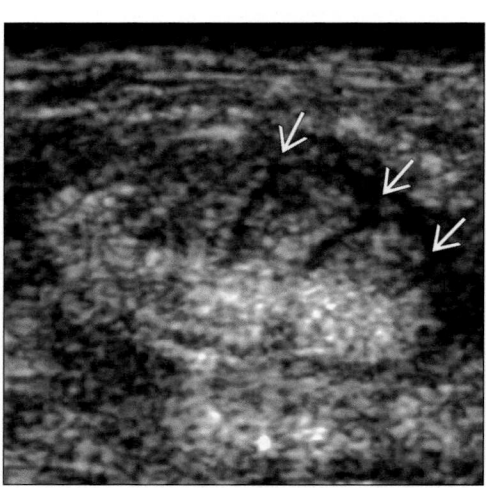
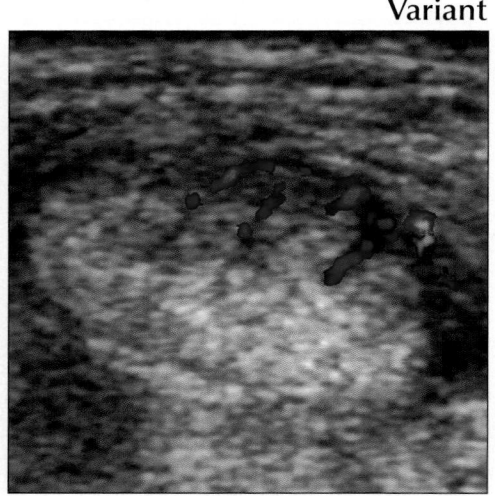

Typical

(Left) Transverse ultrasound just proximal to ankle shows a longitudinal full-thickness tear ➡ of the tibialis tendon ➡. The tibia ➡ lies deep to tendon. *(Right)* Transverse ultrasound of the hindfoot shows a full-thickness longitudinal tear ➡ of the swollen peroneus brevis tendon. The peroneus longus tendon ➡ is normal. The calcaneofibular ligament lies deep to tendons ➡.

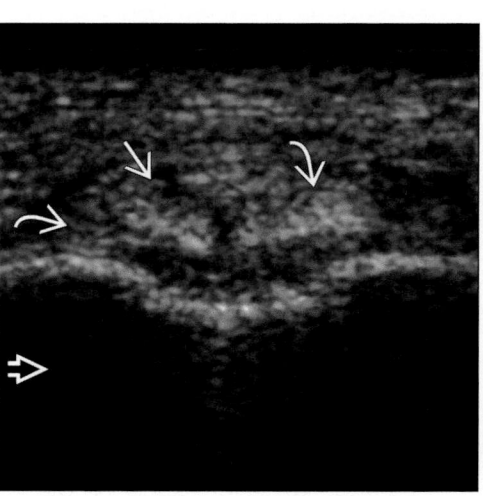
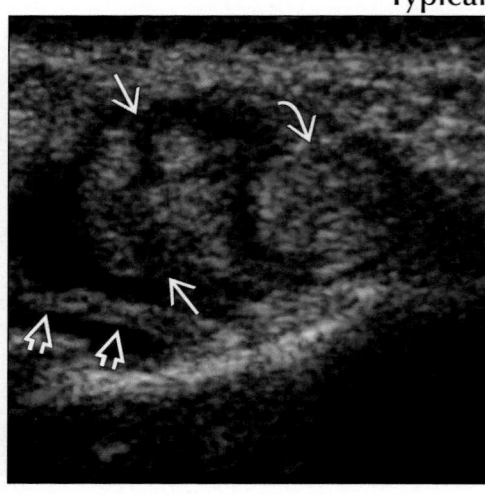

NON-ROTATOR CUFF TENDON TEARS

Typical

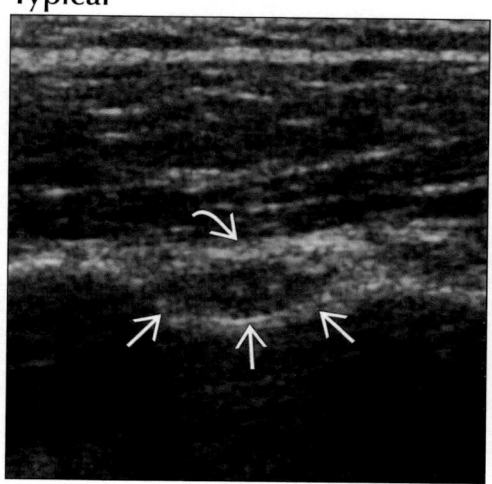

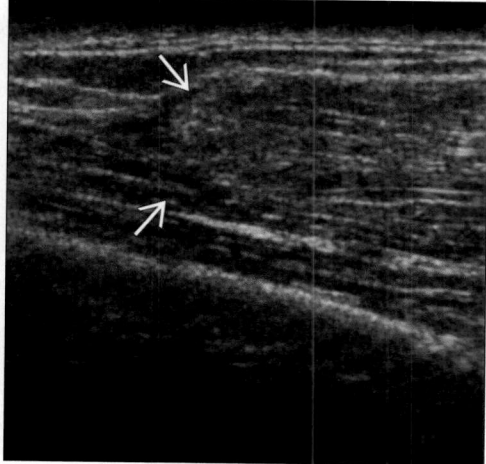

(Left) Transverse ultrasound of the upper arm shows a largely empty bicipital groove ⮕ indicative of a complete tear of the long head of the biceps tendon. Note overlying intact transverse ligament ⮕. *(Right)* Longitudinal ultrasound of the mid-arm shows the retracted belly of the biceps muscle ⮕.

Typical

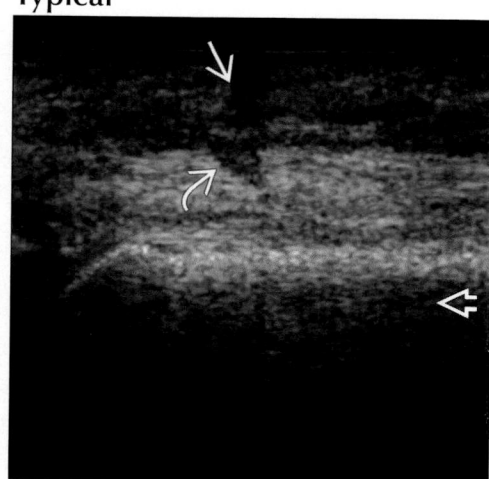

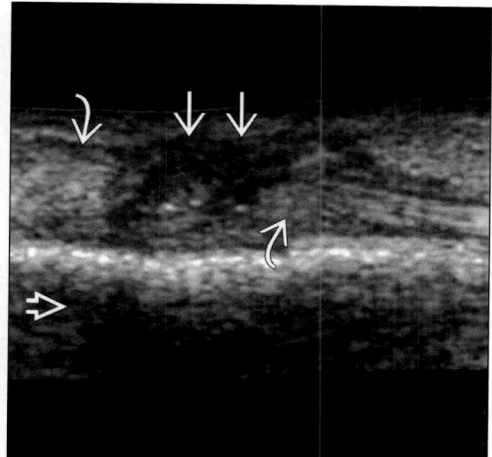

(Left) Longitudinal ultrasound of the hand one week following a penetrating injury shows a partial-thickness tear ⮕ on dorsal surface of the swollen middle finger extensor tendon. Note skin wound ⮕ and metacarpal bone ⮕. *(Right)* Longitudinal ultrasound of a hand one month following blunt trauma shows a complete tear ⮕ of the middle finger extensor tendon overlying the metacarpal bone ⮕. Retracted tendon ends ⮕ are swollen.

Variant

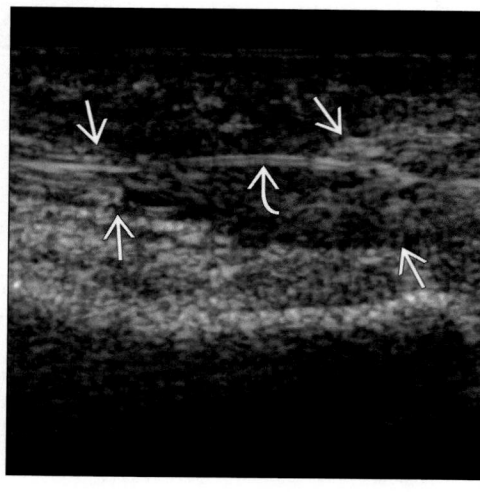

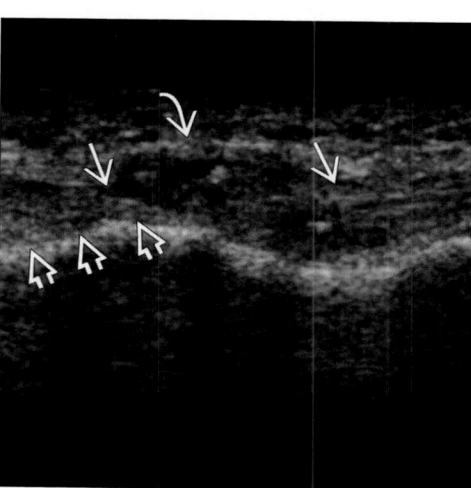

(Left) Longitudinal ultrasound of the thumb two months following surgical repair shows a complete re-tear of the flexor pollicis longus tendon. Suture material ⮕ transverses the gap between retracted tendon ends ⮕. *(Right)* Longitudinal ultrasound of the middle finger six months following a penetrating trauma shows a fibrotic-type mass ⮕ between the flexor tendon ends ⮕. The distal tendon is adherent to the irregular, previously injured, proximal phalanx ⮕.

TENOSYNOVITIS

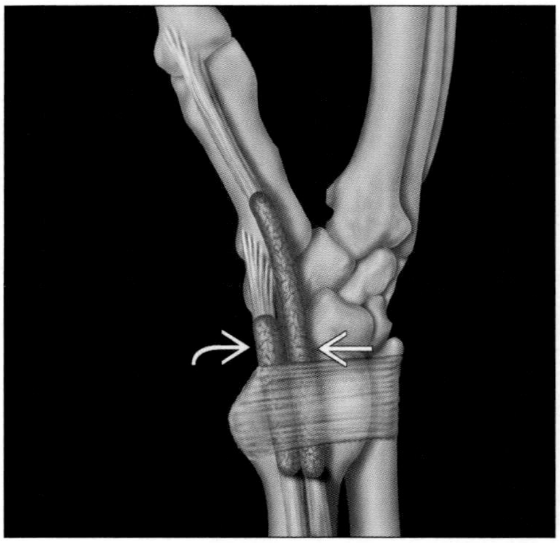

Longitudinal graphic shows tenosynovitis of abductor pollicis longus (APL) ➡ and extensor pollicis brevis (EPB) ➡ tendons indicative of de Quervain tenosynovitis.

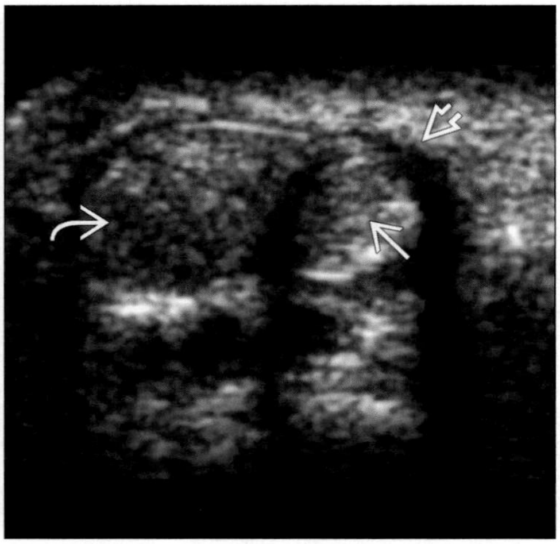

Transverse ultrasound of the wrist shows diffuse swelling of larger APL ➡ and smaller EPB ➡ tendons indicative of de Quervain tenosynovitis. Note mild synovial thickening of EPB ➡.

TERMINOLOGY

Abbreviations and Synonyms

- Acute exudative tenosynovitis, acute tenosynovitis, chronic tenosynovitis, de Quervain disease, tendinitis, tendonitis, stenosing tenosynovitis, intersection syndrome, repetitive strain injury, infective tenosynovitis, inflammatory tenosynovitis

Definitions

- Acute exudative tenosynovitis refers to purulent distension of synovial sheath, usually synonymous with infection
- De Quervain disease refers to tenosynovitis of first extensor compartment (abductor pollicis longus (APL) and extensor pollicis brevis (EPB))
- Tendinitis or tendonitis are arbitrary terms
  - Tendon inflammation (tendinitis or tendonitis) does not occur without synovial inflammation
  - Inflammation is not a recognized feature of tendon degeneration (i.e. tendinosis)
- Stenosing tenosynovitis is chronic tenosynovitis associated with tendon sheath adhesions or stenosis entrapping synovial fluid
- Intersection syndrome is distal forearm pain, about 5 cm proximal to Lister tubercle, where first and second dorsal extensor compartment tendons cross
- Repetitive strain injury is considered to be due to low grade tenosynovitis of wrist tendons
  - Imaging usually normal in repetitive strain injury

IMAGING FINDINGS

General Features

- Best diagnostic clue: Distension of tenosynovium (tendon sheath) due to fluid or synovitis with variable tendon swelling
- Location
  - Only occurs in tendons encased by synovium
    - Wrist tendons more common than ankle tendons
- Size: Variable, depending on cause, severity, duration
- Morphology: Distension of tendon sheath and tendon

Ultrasonographic Findings

- Can vary depending on capacity of tendon sheath to distend
- **Acute exudative tenosynovitis**
  - Usually due to acute infection

DDx: Tenosynovitis

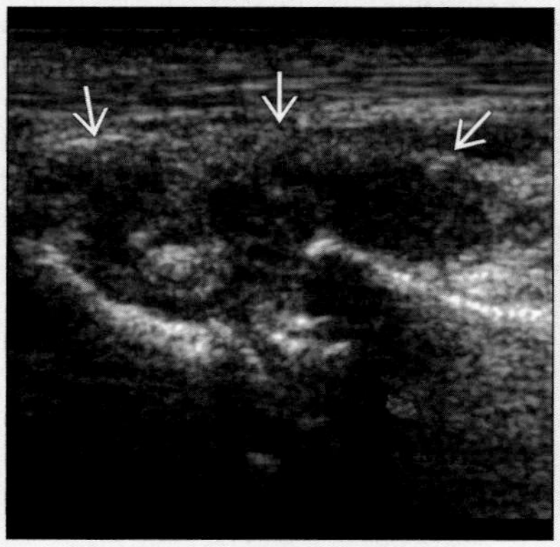

Joint Synovitis

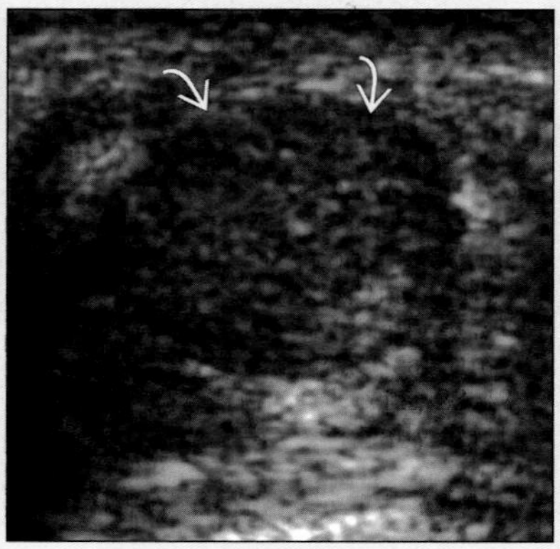

Tendinosis

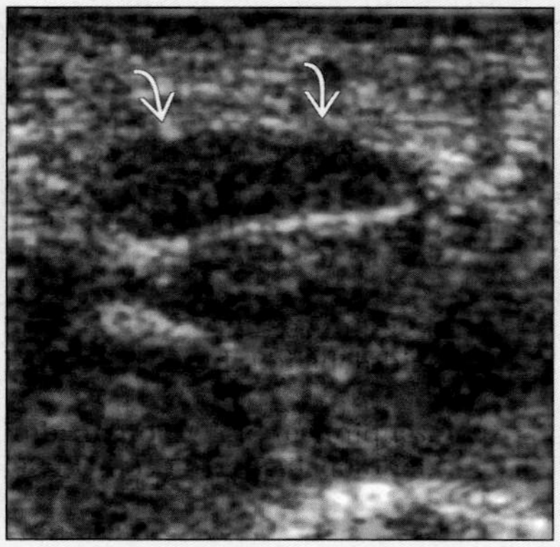

Carpal Tunnel Syndrome

TENOSYNOVITIS

Key Facts

Imaging Findings

- Best diagnostic clue: Distension of tenosynovium (tendon sheath) due to fluid or synovitis with variable tendon swelling
- Only occurs in tendons encased by synovium
- **Acute exudative tenosynovitis**
- Usually due to acute infection
- Fluid accumulation within sheath with little or no synovial proliferation
- Fluid usually has speckled appearance due to aggregation of purulent debris
- **Acute non-exudative tenosynovitis**
- Synovial proliferation within sheath predominates over fluid accumulation
- **Chronic tenosynovitis (active)**
- Similar to acute non-exudative tendon synovitis expect that hyperemia is predominantly within sheath
- **Chronic tenosynovitis (inactive)**
- Clear fluid accumulation within mildly thickened sheath

Top Differential Diagnoses

- Synovitis
- Tendinosis

Diagnostic Checklist

- Tendinosis rather than tenosynovitis, if tendon predominantly swollen with intratendinous hyperemia
- Use color Doppler to distinguish synovial inflammation from synovial effusion

---

- Fluid accumulation within sheath with little or no synovial proliferation
- Fluid usually has speckled appearance due to aggregation of purulent debris
- Tendon usually mild or moderately thickened, +/- indistinct margins on transverse imaging (if severe infection)
- Hyperemia around, rather than within, tendon sheath
- Infection may spread from tendon sheath into peritendinous tissues
- May detect foreign body following penetrating trauma
- Ultrasound-guided fluid aspiration helpful to isolate organism
- Acute non-exudative tenosynovitis
  - May be due to inflammation or infection
    - Synovial proliferation within sheath predominates over fluid accumulation
    - Hyperemia predominantly around rather than within tendon sheath
  - Chronic tenosynovitis (active)
    - May be due to inflammation or infection
    - Similar to acute non-exudative tendon synovitis expect that hyperemia is predominantly within sheath
    - Rice bodies may develop in radial and ulnar volar bursa in chronic infection or inflammation; MR better at detecting than ultrasound
  - Chronic tenosynovitis (inactive)
    - Clear fluid accumulation within mildly thickened sheath
    - In stenosing tenosynovitis, fluid not readily compressible, if entrapped
  - Mild secondary tenosynovial swelling can occur in presence of severe cellulitis or edema

Radiographic Findings

- Radiography
  - Soft tissue swelling
  - Radio-opaque foreign body following penetrating injury
  - Signs of erosive or septic arthropathy

MR Findings

- T1WI
  - Hypo to intermediate signal intensity of fluid in distended sheath
  - Debris within sheath = intermediate signal
  - Intermediate signal within swollen tendon indicates tendinosis
- T2WI
  - Intermediate to hyperintense fluid within distended synovial sheath
  - Intermediate signal within swollen tendon indicates tendinosis
- T1 C+ FS: Differentiates fluid from synovitis of tendon sheath

Imaging Recommendations

- Best imaging tool
  - Ultrasound is accurate at revealing presence and extent of tenosynovitis
    - Facilitates fine needle aspiration (for culture, crystals) or biopsy to determine cause
- Protocol advice
  - Examine length of tendon or group of tendons in axial plane
  - Minimal transducer pressure will avoid effacing tendon sheath effusion
  - Always include evaluation with color Doppler
  - Examine nearby joints for synovitis or effusion

DIFFERENTIAL DIAGNOSIS

Synovitis

- Synovial swelling and hyperemia

Tendinosis

- Inflammation is not a recognized feature of tendinosis
- Tendon swelling, disruption of fibrillar echotexture and intratendinous hyperemia predominate in tendinosis
- Intratendinous neovascularization is not a usual feature of tenosynovitis

TENOSYNOVITIS

- Distinction between tenosynovitis and tendinosis not always clear-cut as mixed patterns may exist
  - Particularly with de Quervain disease which often has element of tendinosis

Carpal Tunnel Syndrome
- Compression of median nerve in carpal tunnel
- Swelling of median nerve

Gouty Tophi
- Mixed echogenic nodules alongside tendon sheath
- Gout may also precipitate tenosynovitis

PATHOLOGY

General Features
- General path comments
  - Relevant anatomy: Wrist flexor tendons
    - Flexor tendon sheaths of thumb and little finger communicate with radial and ulnar bursa respectively on volar aspect of wrist and carpus
    - In 50% cases, radial and ulnar bursae communicate via intermediate bursa
  - Relevant anatomy: Wrist extensor tendons
    - Six discrete extensor tendon sheath which do not communicate with each other or with flexor tendon sheaths
    - Finger extensor tendon expansions do not have tendon sheath
  - Relevant anatomy: De Quervain disease
    - First compartment, radial side of anatomical snuff box
    - Larger abductor pollicis longus and smaller extensor pollicis brevis
    - Longitudinal septum separates both tendons in 25% patients
    - Superficial branch radial nerve branch overlies first extensor compartment
  - Relevant anatomy: Extensor carpi ulnaris
    - Sixth compartment - near ulnar styloid process
- Etiology
  - Overuse injury
  - Infection, acute or chronic
  - Systemic arthropathies, e.g. rheumatoid arthritis or psoriasis
  - Crystal deposition disease e.g. uric acid, calcium pyrophosphate
  - Often, no specific cause found
- Epidemiology
  - Extensor carpi ulnaris and de Quervain tenosynovitis common in athletes
  - Infective tenosynovitis more common in immunosuppressed patients, or in persons with occupations prone to penetrating injury

Gross Pathologic & Surgical Features
- Tenosynovium and tendon inflammation

Microscopic Features
- Inflammatory cells infiltrate tenosynovium
- Tenosynovitis predominantly affects tenosynovium

CLINICAL ISSUES

Presentation
- Most common signs/symptoms
  - Pain, swelling and tenderness of affected tendons
  - Limitation of movement
- Other signs/symptoms
  - Crepitus (subjective, palpable or audible)
  - Tendon triggering

Demographics
- Age: Most common in middle-aged to elderly
- Gender
  - Inflammatory tenosynovitis, de Quervain disease, and repetitive strain injury have female predominance
  - Infective tenosynovitis has no sex predominance

Natural History & Prognosis
- Majority (80%) improve with conservative treatment
- Fibrosis and adhesions may occur within tendon sheath

Treatment
- Acute exudative tenosynovitis
  - Surgical drainage
  - Elevation, appropriate antibiotics
- Non-infective tenosynovitis and chronic infective tenosynovitis
  - Rest, splinting, physiotherapy
    - Anti-inflammatory medication +/- steroid injection (ultrasound guidance)
    - Appropriate antibiotics
    - Synovectomy, if failed conservative treatment

DIAGNOSTIC CHECKLIST

Consider
- Tendinosis rather than tenosynovitis, if tendon predominantly swollen with intratendinous hyperemia
- Secondary tenosynovial swelling if there is severe surrounding cellulitis or edema

Image Interpretation Pearls
- Use color Doppler to distinguish synovial inflammation from synovial effusion

SELECTED REFERENCES

1. Chau CL et al: Musculoskeletal infections: ultrasound appearances. Clin Radiol. 60(2):149-59, 2005
2. Daenen B et al: Sonography in wrist tendon pathology. J Clin Ultrasound. 32(9):462-9, 2004
3. Chau CL et al: Rice-body formation in atypical mycobacterial tenosynovitis and bursitis: findings on sonography and MR imaging. AJR Am J Roentgenol. 180(5):1455-9, 2003
4. Silvestri E et al: Power Doppler analysis of tendon vascularization. Int J Tissue React. 25(4):149-58, 2003
5. Clarke MT et al: The histopathology of de Quervain's disease. J Hand Surg [Br]. 23(6):732-4, 1998

TENOSYNOVITIS

IMAGE GALLERY

Typical

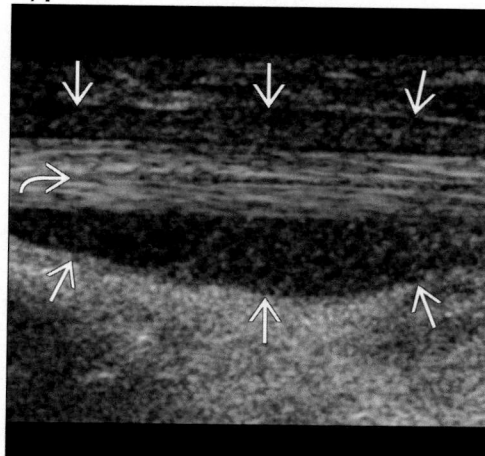
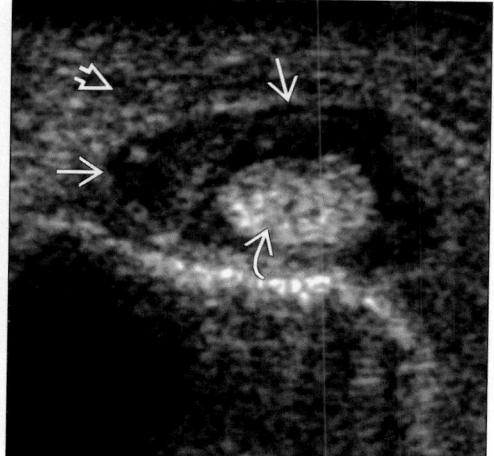

(Left) Longitudinal ultrasound shows acute exudative tenosynovitis with distension ➡ of the extensor digitorum tendon sheath by echogenic fluid. The middle finger tendons ➡ are moderately swollen. (Right) Transverse ultrasound shows acute tenosynovitis of the extensor carpi ulnaris tendon with moderate tendon thickening ➡, severe tendon sheath thickening ➡ and moderate peritendinous edema ➡.

Typical

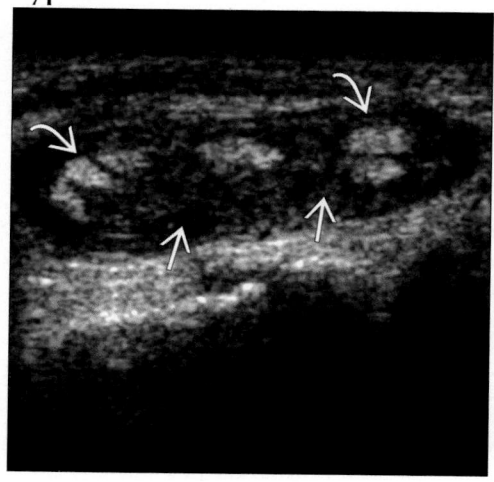
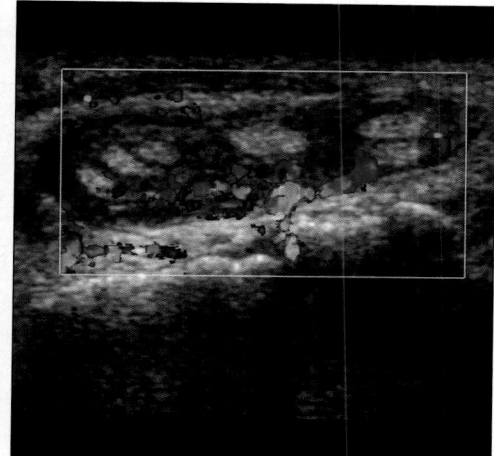

(Left) Transverse ultrasound shows active chronic tenosynovitis of extensor digitorum tendons with mild tendon thickening ➡ and moderate synovial proliferation ➡. (Right) Transverse color Doppler ultrasound (at same location as previous image) shows moderate hyperemia, predominantly located within the tendon sheath, indicative of active chronic tenosynovitis.

Typical

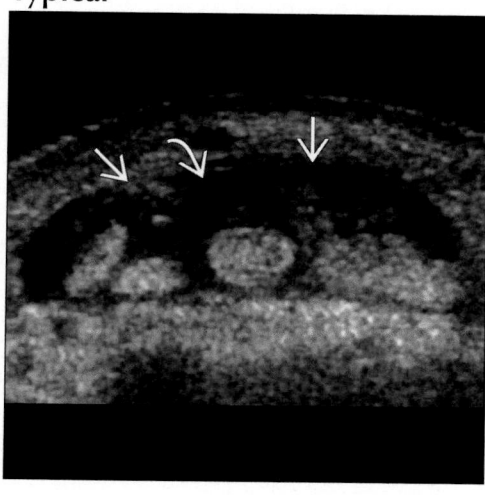
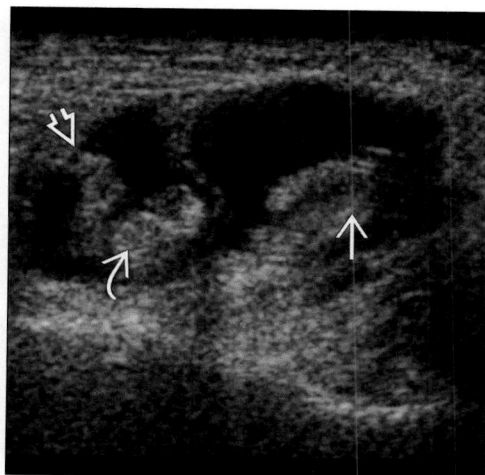

(Left) Transverse ultrasound shows chronic tenosynovitis of the extensor digitorum tendons with combination of tendon sheath effusion ➡ and synovial proliferation ➡ leading to distension of the tendon sheath. (Right) Transverse ultrasound shows inactive chronic tenosynovitis of the posterior tibialis ➡ and flexor digitorum ➡ tendons. Note fluid distension of tendon sheaths with aggregations of synovial proliferation ➡.

ELBOW EPICONDYLITIS

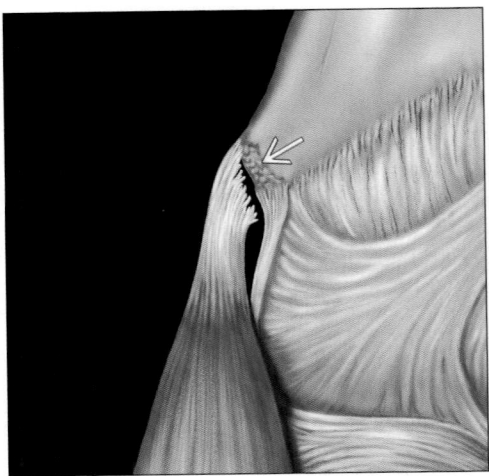

Longitudinal graphic shows an almost complete tear (avulsion) ➡ of the common extensor tendon origin from the lateral epicondyle (lateral epicondylitis or tennis elbow).

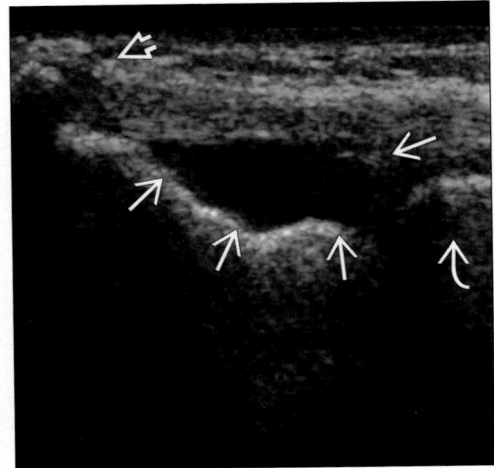

Longitudinal ultrasound shows an almost complete tear (avulsion) ➡ of the common extensor origin from the lateral epicondyle. Note insertional cortical hyperostosis ➡. (Radial head ➡).

TERMINOLOGY

Abbreviations and Synonyms
- Tennis elbow, lateral epicondylitis, golfer's elbow, medial epicondylitis

Definitions
- Chronic microtrauma of extensor tendons originating from the lateral epicondyle (tennis elbow)
- Chronic microtrauma of flexor tendons originating from the medial epicondyle (golfer's elbow)

IMAGING FINDINGS

General Features
- Best diagnostic clue: Thickening and fibrillar disruption of common extensor tendon (lateral epicondylitis) or common flexor tendon (medial epicondylitis) origin
- Location
  - Common extensor tendon origin from lateral epicondyle
    - Usually first affects extensor carpi radialis brevis followed by anterior fibers of extensor digitorum
    - +/- Tear of underlying radial collateral ligament
  - Common flexor tendon origin from medial epicondyle
    - Usually first affects flexor carpi radialis, pronator teres, and palmaris longus
- Size: Varies from fibrillar disruption to tendon thickening to intrasubstance tear to complete avulsion
- Morphology
  - Diffuse tendon thickening to tear or avulsion
    - Smaller tears tend to be linear and intrasubstance in type while larger tears tend to be avulsive in type

Ultrasonographic Findings
- Thickened, hypoechogenic tendon with surface bowing and disruption of normal fibrillar pattern
  - Tendon hypoechogenicity usually affects deeper aspects of tendon initially spreading to more superficial aspects as disease progresses
  - Sharp, linear hypoechoic areas within tendon indicative of intrasubstance tendon tears

DDx: Elbow Epicondylitis

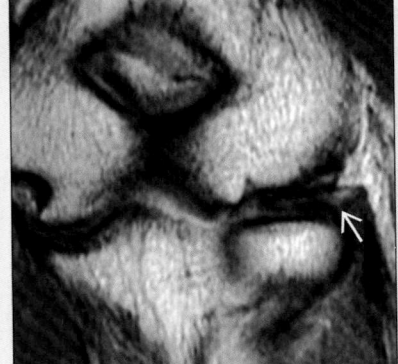

Synovial Flange

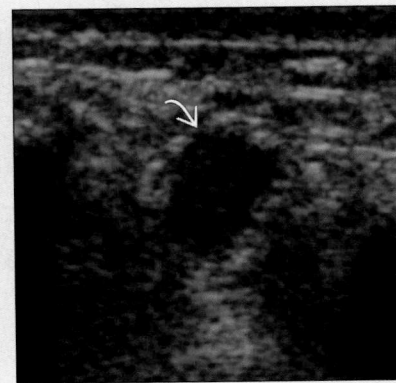

Cubital Tunnel Syndrome

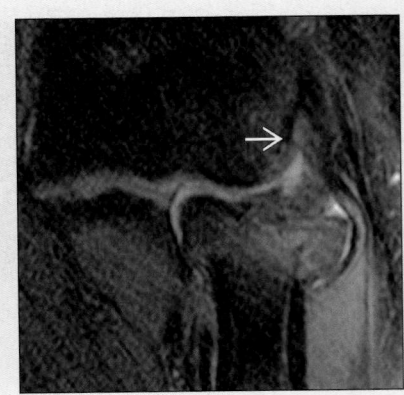

Lateral Collateral Ligament Tear

ELBOW EPICONDYLITIS

Key Facts

Terminology
- Tennis elbow, lateral epicondylitis, golfer's elbow, medial epicondylitis

Imaging Findings
- Best diagnostic clue: Thickening and fibrillar disruption of common extensor tendon (lateral epicondylitis) or common flexor tendon (medial epicondylitis) origin
- Usually first affects extensor carpi radialis brevis followed by anterior fibers of extensor digitorum
- Sharp, linear hypoechoic areas within tendon indicative of intrasubstance tendon tears
- Deeper, anechoic areas indicative of avulsive-type tear
- Hypoechoic areas with internal echoes indicative of focal proteoglycan deposition

Top Differential Diagnoses
- Hypertrophy of Radiohumeral Synovial Flange
- Cubital Tunnel Syndrome
- Radial Collateral Ligament Injury

Pathology
- Lateral epicondylitis is the most common cause of elbow pain
- Lateral epicondylitis is about twenty times more common than medial epicondylitis

Diagnostic Checklist
- Ligament injury if post-traumatic onset
- Look to deep margin of tendon for small tendon tears
- Severe pain or acute exacerbation is usually due to tendon tear

---

- ○ Deeper, anechoic areas indicative of avulsive-type tear
- ○ Hypoechoic areas with internal echoes indicative of focal proteoglycan deposition
- Compare with contralateral side
  - ○ Contralateral subclinical or clinical disease can often occur
- Measure either cross-sectional area of tendon or maximum depth of mid-portion of tendon origin
- Fluid around tendon is not commonly seen in intrasubstance or avulsive tears
- Routinely assess tendon vascularity with color Doppler imaging and grade subjectively i.e. absent, minimal, mild, moderate or severe
  - ○ Normal tendons do not display intrinsic vascularity
  - ○ Cross-sectional area, degree of hypoechogenicity and vascularity are useful measures for follow-up ultrasound study
- Radial collateral ligament can be injured with more advanced lateral epicondylitis
- Dystrophic intrasubstance calcification occurs commonly though is usually mild in degree
- Patients may have characteristic symptoms of epicondylitis but no abnormality on ultrasound
  - ○ Conversely, patients may have no symptoms of epicondylitis and mild to moderate disease on ultrasound

Radiographic Findings
- Radiography
  - ○ Cortical irregularity and hyperostosis of common tendon origin area
  - ○ Dystrophic calcification within common tendon origin
  - ○ Soft tissue swelling at common tendon origin

MR Findings
- T1WI
  - ○ Thickening and increased signal intensity within the common extensor (or flexor) tendon origin at the lateral (and medial) epicondyle respectively

- ○ For tennis elbow, swelling and intermediate signal intensity of lateral collateral ligament indicates sprain or tear
- T2WI FS
  - ○ Thickening and increased signal intensity of common extensor (of flexor) tendon origin
    - Hyperintensity usually seen in deeper aspect of tendon
    - Peritendinitis is feature of severe cases
    - Insertional subcortical marrow changes are not usually seen
  - ○ In advanced tennis elbow, increased signal +/- discontinuity of radial collateral ligament may be seen

Imaging Recommendations
- Best imaging tool: Ultrasound
- Protocol advice
  - ○ Examination with shoulder and elbow flexed; elbow internally rotated for lateral epicondylitis and externally rotated for medial epicondylitis
  - ○ Examine with transducer aligned both at right angles to and parallel to long axis of tendons
  - ○ Always include evaluation with color Doppler and compare with contralateral side

DIFFERENTIAL DIAGNOSIS

Hypertrophy of Radiohumeral Synovial Flange
- Synovial fold projecting into posterolateral aspect of the joint
- Fold can hypertrophy with repetitive pronation and supination
  - ○ Symptomatic folds show hypertrophy and increased innervation

Cubital Tunnel Syndrome
- Compression of ulnar nerve in cubital tunnel
- Inflammation of ulnar nerve may occur with lateral epicondylitis

ELBOW EPICONDYLITIS

Radial Collateral Ligament Injury
- Usually history of moderate to severe trauma

Elbow Synovitis
- Thickened inflamed synovium with effusion

PATHOLOGY

General Features
- General path comments
  - Relevant anatomy
  - Extensor carpi radialis brevis, extensor digitorum, extensor carpi ulnaris arise from lateral epicondyle
    - Extensor carpi radialis brevis lies deep to extensor digitorum and extensor carpi ulnaris tendons
    - Lateral collateral ligament lies immediately deep to common extensor tendon and runs in a slightly different direction
  - Bursa may exist between common extensor tendons and radial collateral ligament at level of elbow joint line
  - Pronator teres, flexor carpi radialis, flexor digitorum superficialis, palmaris longus and flexor carpi ulnaris arise from medial epicondyle
    - Flexor digitorum superficialis lies deep to flexor carpi radialis, palmaris longus and flexor carpi ulnaris
- Etiology: Repetitive microtrauma with repeated varus stress (tennis elbow) or valgus stress (golfer's elbow)
- Epidemiology
  - Lateral epicondylitis is the most common cause of elbow pain
  - Lateral epicondylitis is about twenty times more common than medial epicondylitis
  - Most patients with tennis elbow do not play tennis
  - Tennis elbow is more common in golfers than golfer's elbow

Gross Pathologic & Surgical Features
- Tendinosis with tendon thickening +/- macroscopic partial tear or full-thickness tears
  - Cortical hyperostosis can occur as feature of reactive change in underlying periosteum

Microscopic Features
- Angiofibroblastic degeneration with disrupted collagen fibers, neovascularization and tenocyte proliferation
  - Tendon tears with reparative granulation tissue
  - Maturation of fibrous tissue to scar-like tendon tissue
- Epicondylitis is not an inflammatory condition
- Pathology is similar for both medial and lateral epicondylitis

Staging, Grading or Classification Criteria
- Tennis elbow stage 1. Reversible inflammatory change
- Tennis elbow stage 2. Non-reversible pathologic change to origin of extensor carpi radialis brevis (ECRB) muscle
- Tennis elbow stage 3. Tear of ECRB tendon
- Tennis elbow stage 4. Secondary changes such as fibrosis

CLINICAL ISSUES

Presentation
- Most common signs/symptoms
  - Adult patients present with lateral or medial elbow pain
    - Pain aggravated by vigorous exercise and gradually lessens with rest over several days
    - Lateral epicondylitis aggravated by forced wrist extension; medial epicondylitis aggravated by forced wrist flexion
    - Tenderness of tendon origin
- Clinical profile
  - Tennis player or other activity resulting in chronic, repeated varus stress
  - Pain on chair test or resisted long finger extension for lateral epicondylitis

Demographics
- Age: Adults
- Gender: M = F depending on level of physical activity

Natural History & Prognosis
- Will usually improve with rest or change in type of physical activity
  - Chronic symptoms or relapse more likely if established tendinosis on ultrasound
  - For subacute or chronic disease, level of tendon vascularity on ultrasound corresponds to level of disease activity

Treatment
- Conservative
  - Rest affected tendons
    - Most patients respond to conservative treatment
    - Combination of dry needling and autologous blood injection under ultrasound guidance is effective for refractory cases
- Surgical
  - Unhealthy amorphous tissue excised
  - Tendon tear repair or tendon release

DIAGNOSTIC CHECKLIST

Consider
- Ligament injury if post-traumatic onset

Image Interpretation Pearls
- Look to deep margin of tendon for small tendon tears
- Severe pain or acute exacerbation is usually due to tendon tear

SELECTED REFERENCES

1. Connell DA et al: Ultrasound-guided autologous blood injection for tennis elbow. Skeletal Radiol. 35(6):371-7, 2006
2. Levin D et al: Lateral epicondylitis of the elbow: US findings. Radiology. 237(1):230-4, 2005
3. Miller TT et al: Comparison of sonography and MRI for diagnosing epicondylitis. J Clin Ultrasound. 30(4):193-202, 2002
4. Connell D et al: Sonographic examination of lateral epicondylitis. AJR Am J Roentgenol. 176(3):777-82, 2001

ELBOW EPICONDYLITIS

Typical

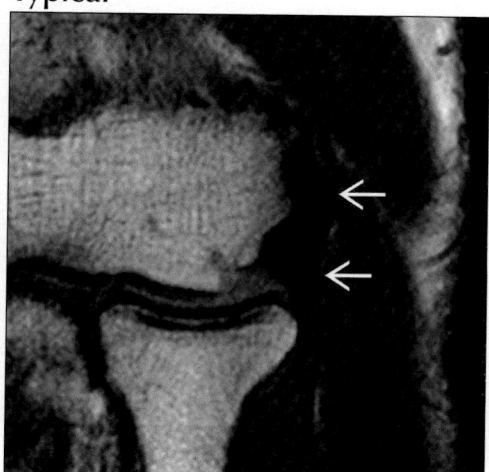
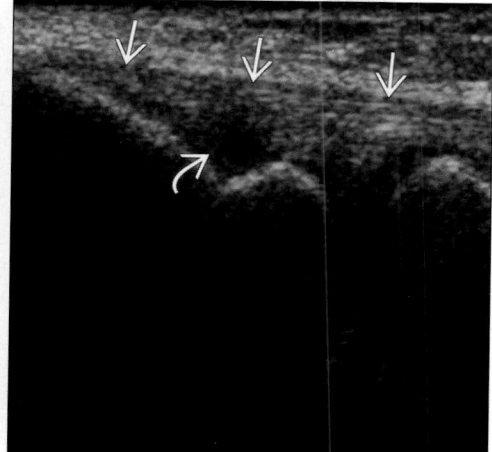

(Left) Coronal T1WI MR shows a thickened common extensor tendon origin ➡ at the lateral epicondyle indicative of lateral epicondylitis (tennis elbow). (Right) Longitudinal ultrasound shows disruption of the fibrillar pattern of the common extensor insertion ➡ indicative of moderate tendinosis ➡. There is a focal area of proteoglycan deposition on the deeper aspect of the tendon.

Typical

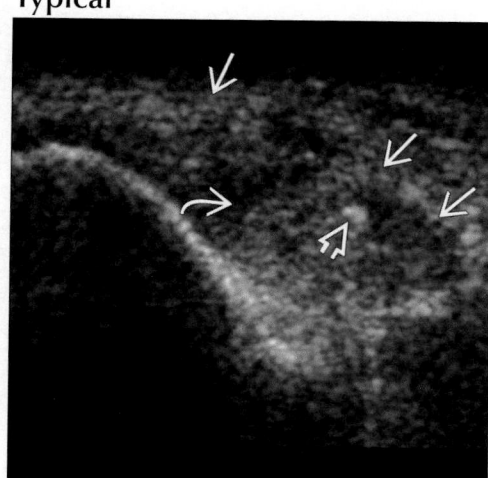
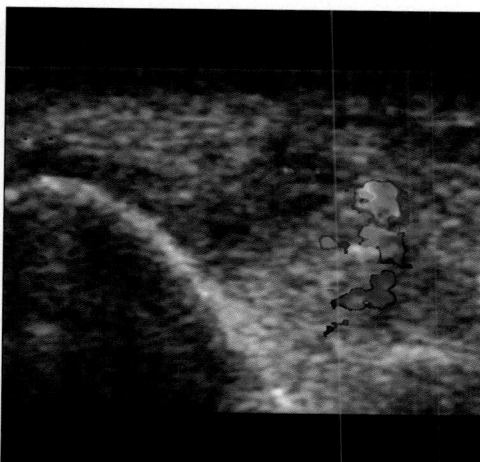

(Left) Transverse ultrasound shows mild tendinosis of the common extensor tendon insertion ➡. There is a thin tear extending through the substance of the tendon ➡. Note early intratendinous calcification ➡. (Right) Transverse color Doppler ultrasound (at same location as previous image) shows mild intratendinous hyperemia.

Typical

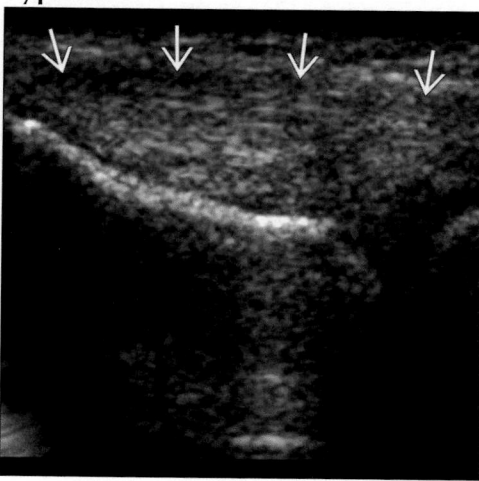
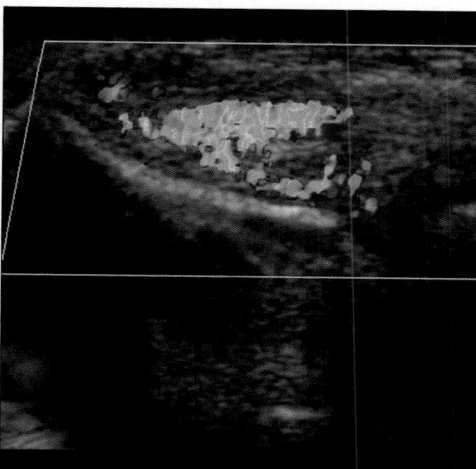

(Left) Longitudinal ultrasound shows moderate thickening and fibrillar disruption of the common extensor tendon insertion ➡, indicative of moderate tendinosis. No tear is visible. Note slight surface convexity. (Right) Longitudinal color Doppler ultrasound (at same location as previous image) shows marked hyperemia of the common extensor tendon insertion, indicative of active disease.

ELBOW EPICONDYLITIS

Typical

(Left) Transverse ultrasound in same patient as previous image, shows thickening of the common extensor tendon ➡ origin at the lateral epicondyle, indicative of moderate tendinosis.
(Right) Transverse color Doppler ultrasound at same location as previous image, shows marked hyperemia indicative of active disease.

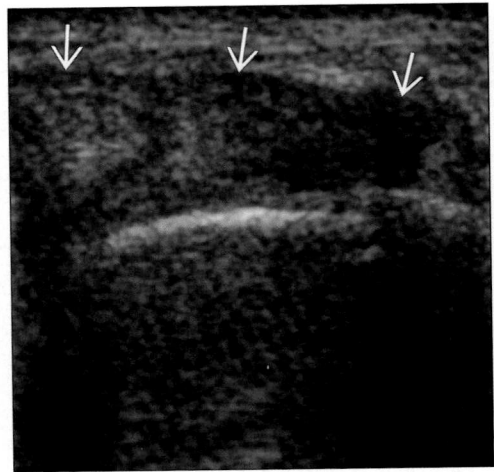
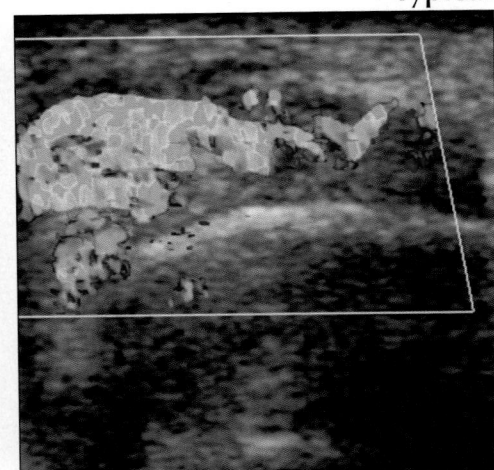

Variant

(Left) Longitudinal ultrasound shows small tear (localized avulsion) ➡ at the common extensor tendon origin from the lateral epicondyle. *(Right)* Longitudinal ultrasound shows focal proteoglycan deposition with "comet-tail" artifacts ➡ deep in the common extensor tendon origin with small intrasubstance tear ➡. "Comet-tail" artifacts are due to gas or calcific foci.

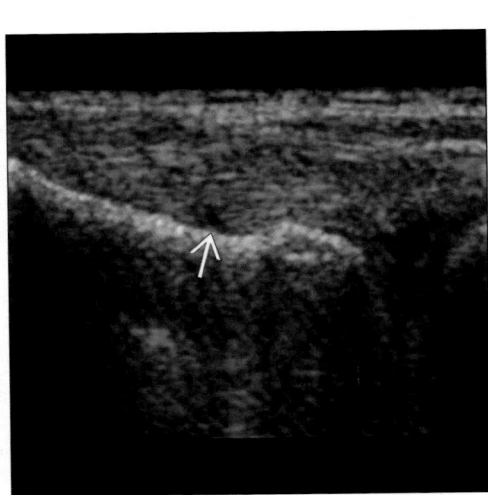
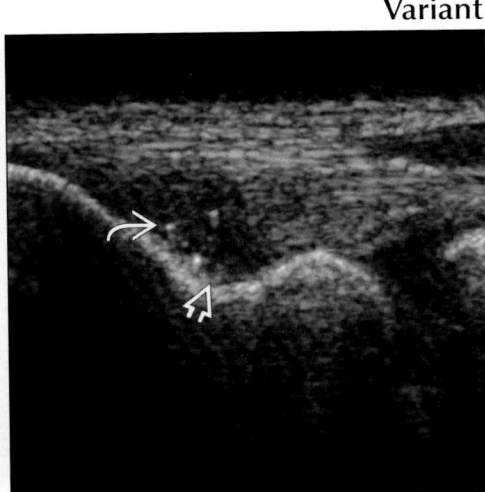

Typical

(Left) Longitudinal ultrasound shows thickening of the common extensor tendon ➡ near the insertion, with a large tear of the deeper aspect of the tendon ➡. *(Right)* Transverse ultrasound of the same patient as previous image, shows a tear ➡ involving mid-fibers of the thickened common extensor tendon origin ➡.

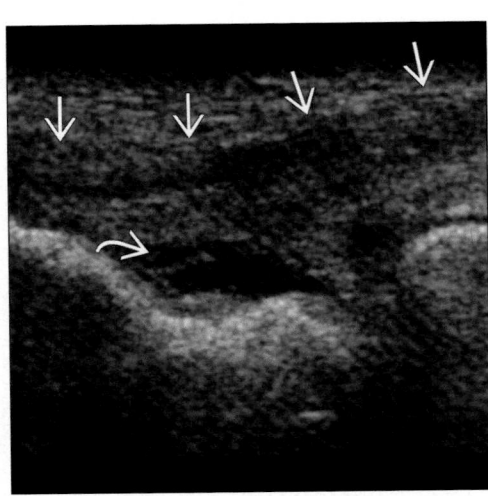
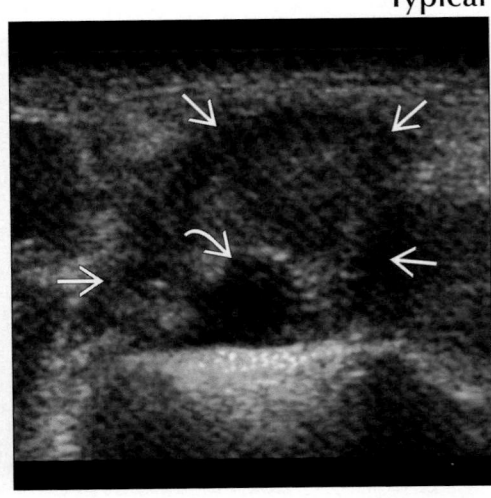

Typical

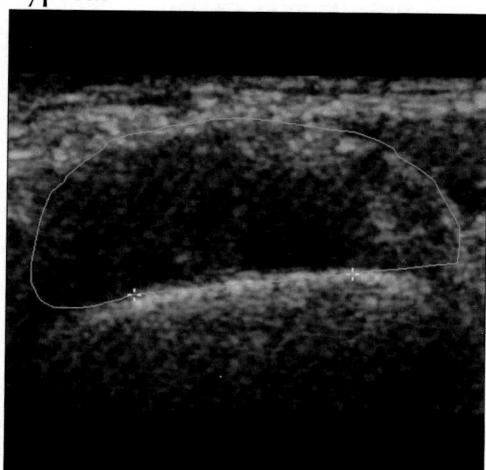
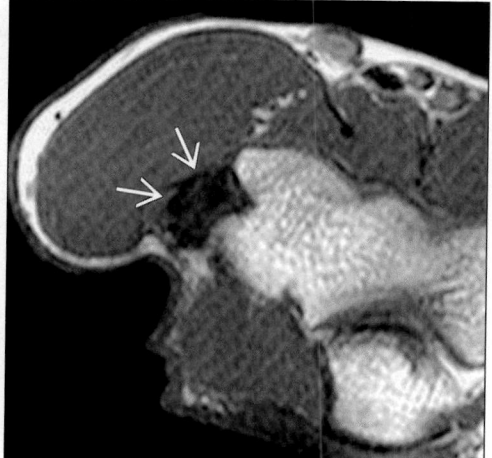

(Left) Transverse ultrasound shows measurement of the cross-sectional area of the common extensor tendon at the bony attachment. *(Right)* Axial T1WI MR in the same patient as the previous image, shows a thickened common extensor tendon origin ➡. Variable signal intensities (hypo and isointense to muscle) indicate tendinosis.

Typical

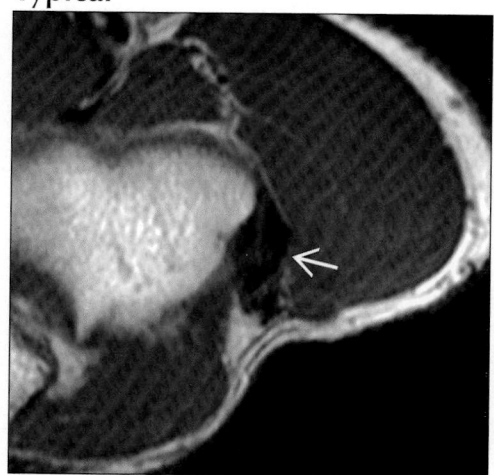
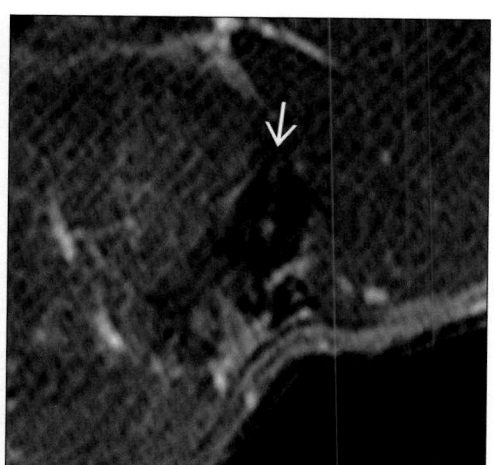

(Left) Axial T1WI MR shows thickening and signal heterogenicity of the common extensor tendon origin ➡ from the lateral epicondyle, indicative of lateral epicondylitis. *(Right)* Axial T1WI MR with fat-suppression shows a small linear hyperintensity ➡ extending through the mid-portion of the common extensor tendon origin, indicative of a small intrasubstance tear.

Typical

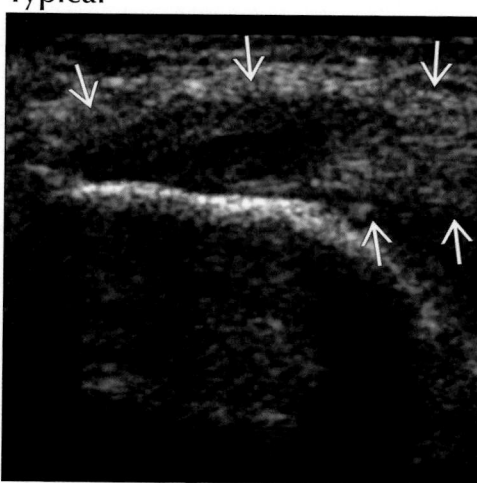
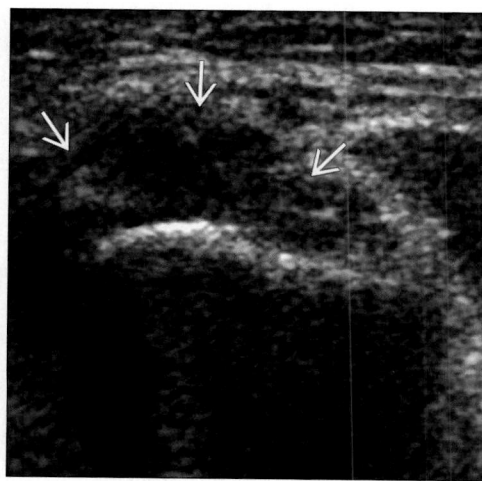

(Left) Longitudinal ultrasound shows a thickened common flexor tendon ➡ with fibrillar disruption at the origin from the medial epicondyle, indicative of moderate-severity medial epicondylitis (golfer's elbow). *(Right)* Transverse ultrasound in the same patient as the previous image, shows moderate thickening and hypoechogenicity of the common flexor tendon origin ➡ from the medial epicondyle (golfer's elbow).

13

37

FAT INJURY

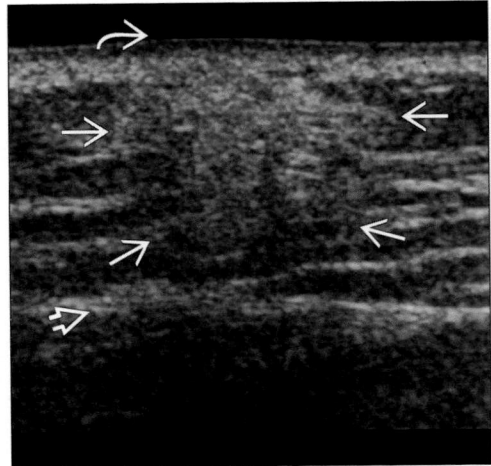

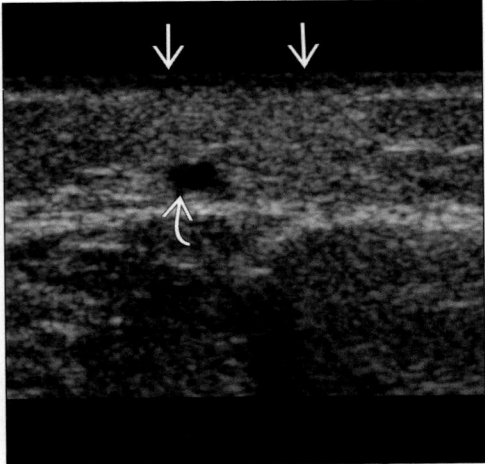

Transverse ultrasound shows a localized area of subcutaneous fat echogenicity with loss of striation ➡ following recent trauma. There is mild swelling ➡. The investing fascia ➡ is normal.

Longitudinal ultrasound shows discrete echogenic area with loss of striation ➡ indicative of subcutaneous fat necrosis. There is mild reduction in subcutaneous fat depth. No prior trauma. Note subcutaneous vein ➡.

TERMINOLOGY

Abbreviations and Synonyms
- Post-traumatic fat necrosis, post-traumatic lipoatrophy, panniculitis, lipoatrophic panniculitis, Weber-Christian disease

Definitions
- Focal inflammation +/- necrosis of subcutaneous fat
- Fat necrosis may occur secondary to either direct trauma or inflammation (panniculitis)
- Weber-Christian disease is a non-specific disease that embraces several specific types of panniculitis

IMAGING FINDINGS

General Features
- Best diagnostic clue: Localized increased echogenicity of subcutaneous fat with loss of normal fat striation
- Location
  - Subcutaneous fat often over bony protuberances
    - Majority involve lower limbs or gluteal region
- Size
  - From 3-7 cm
  - Usually full depth of subcutaneous tissue is affected
- Morphology: Focal swelling of subcutaneous tissues progressing to induration and atrophy

Ultrasonographic Findings
- Grayscale Ultrasound
  - Localized increased echogenicity of subcutaneous fat
    - Loss of normal subcutaneous fat striation
    - Irregular poorly defined margins without discrete mass
    - +/- Localized swelling +/- lobulation of subcutaneous fat due to edema
  - Swelling of subcutaneous fat in early disease
    - Subcutaneous fat in affected area becomes better defined and more hypoechoic with increasing chronicity
  - +/- Fluid accumulation within affected fat
    - Linear fluid collections located superficial to investing fascia
    - Larger, more rounded fluid collections in areas with more abundant subcutaneous fat e.g., buttock
  - +/- Calcification of affected subcutaneous fat

DDx: Fat Injury and Inflammation

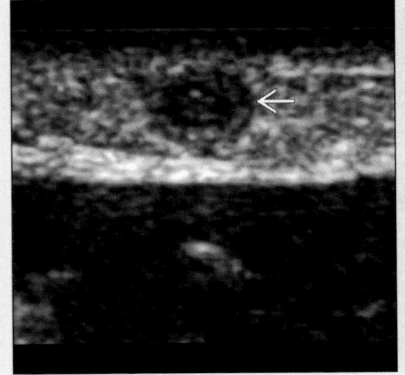

Superficial Thrombophlebitis

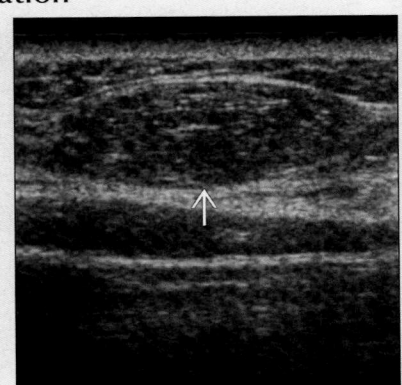

Subcutaneous Lipoma

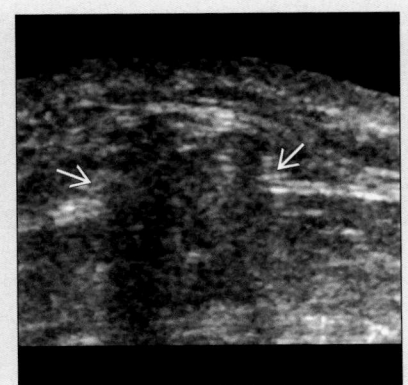

Muscle Hernia

FAT INJURY

Key Facts

Terminology
- Focal inflammation +/- necrosis of subcutaneous fat
- Fat necrosis may occur secondary to either direct trauma or inflammation (panniculitis)

Imaging Findings
- Best diagnostic clue: Localized increased echogenicity of subcutaneous fat with loss of normal fat striation
- Irregular poorly defined margins without discrete mass
- +/- Localized swelling +/- lobulation of subcutaneous fat due to edema
- Subcutaneous fat in affected area becomes better defined and more hypoechoic with increasing chronicity
- +/- Fluid accumulation within affected fat
- +/- Calcification of affected subcutaneous fat

- Minimal to mild hyperemia seen with active panniculitis

Top Differential Diagnoses
- Superficial Thrombophlebitis
- Subcutaneous Lipoma
- Muscle Hernia

Clinical Issues
- Evolving lesion over weeks or months
- May have relapsing/remitting course

Diagnostic Checklist
- Look for pancreatic disease in patient presenting with unexplained panniculitis or fat necrosis

---

- May vary from mild speckled calcification to dense calcification
- Calcification more frequent and more dense with increasing duration of disease
- Shadowing artifact may impede lesion depiction
- Less severe shadowing artifact can result from aggregations of fibrosis without calcification
- Area of subcutaneous fat necrosis become better defined and more hypoechoic with increasing chronicity
  - Subcutaneous fat atrophy may develop at later stage of disease
  - Compare with adjacent normal subcutaneous fat and comparable area on contralateral side
- Usually fascia and muscle deep to affected area are normal
  - May rarely show disruption if prior trauma
- Color Doppler
  - Usually no hyperemia
  - Minimal to mild hyperemia seen with active panniculitis

Radiographic Findings
- Focal swelling or atrophy of subcutaneous soft tissues
- Subcutaneous calcification
- Gas locules within subcutaneous tissues following high pressure trauma

MR Findings
- T1WI
  - Focal hyperintense subcutaneous fat swelling
  - Spiculated areas of linear hypointensity within subcutaneous fat due to reactive fibrosis
    - +/- Nodular areas of subcutaneous hypointensity due to calcification
    - +/- Larger hypointense areas within subcutaneous fat due to fluid
  - Investing fascia, muscle and bone normal
- T2WI FS
  - Focal hyperintense subcutaneous fat swelling with edema
    - +/- Nodular areas of subcutaneous hypointensity due to calcification

- +/- Larger hyperintense areas within subcutaneous fat due to fluid
- +/- Focal lipoatrophy of subcutaneous fat
  - Investing fascia, muscle and bone normal
- T1 C+ FS: None or minimal contrast-enhancement

Imaging Recommendations
- Best imaging tool
  - Ultrasound allows a definitive diagnosis in majority of cases
    - Better at depicting associated calcification than MR
- Protocol advice
  - Minimal transducer pressure to avoid effacement of adjacent fat
  - Ample acoustic gel to fill any skin depression
  - Use color Doppler to access vascularity

DIFFERENTIAL DIAGNOSIS

Superficial Thrombophlebitis
- Localized swelling wall of subcutaneous vein
- +/- Perivenous edema
- +/- Intraluminal thrombosis

Subcutaneous Lipoma
- Discrete non-tender lipomatous mass within subcutaneous tissues
- Fine linear striations parallel to long axis of mass
- Minimal or no internal vascularity on color Doppler imaging

Muscle Hernia
- Localized disruption of investing fascia
- Protrusion of muscle into subcutaneous tissues, especially during muscle exertion

Subcutaneous Vascular Anomaly
- Visible vascular channels or lakes
- Mild to moderate hyperemia
- +/- Calcified phleboliths
- Very slow evolution and non-tender

FAT INJURY

PATHOLOGY

General Features
- Etiology
  - Following trauma
    - About 50% patients report prior trauma
  - Following panniculitis (inflammation) of subcutaneous fat
    - Panniculitis may be idiopathic or secondary to infection, systemic inflammatory disorders, myeloproliferative disorders, pancreatic disease or drugs
    - Panniculitis may present de novo or as erythema nodosum or Weber-Christian disease
    - Weber-Christian disease: Systemic manifestations (fever, arthralgia, anemia, leucopenia, deranged liver function) and subcutaneous panniculitis
  - Erythema nodosum
    - Streptococcal infection
    - Pulmonary tuberculosis
    - Rheumatic fever
  - Systemic inflammatory disorders
    - Polyarteritis nodosa
    - Systemic lupus erythematosus
    - Dermatomyositis
    - Morphea
    - Takayasu arteritis
    - Necrotizing vasculitis
  - Myeloproliferative disorders
    - Lymphoma
  - Pancreatic disease
    - Either pancreatitis (50%) or pancreatic carcinoma (50%)
    - May precede recognition of pancreatitis disease in 50%
    - Thought to be due to hematogenous-borne pancreatic enzymes trypsin and lipase
    - Arthritis, (especially ankle) may be associated as pancreatitis, panniculitis, polyarthralgia (PPP) syndrome
    - Multiple sites of fat necrosis ("metastatic fat necrosis") including intraosseous involvement may occur
    - Intraosseous fat necrosis not visible on ultrasound, best seen on MR
  - Drug hypersensitivity

Gross Pathologic & Surgical Features
- Vary according to changing evolutionary nature of the lesion
- Lobular thickening of subcutaneous fat surrounded by fibrous septa
- Later stages may show more dense fibrosis and atrophy of subcutaneous fat

Microscopic Features
- Large scalpel incisional biopsy rather than needle biopsy required
- Inflammatory infiltrate predominantly involving subcutaneous septa or lobules
  - Septal panniculitis +/- vasculitis
  - Lobular panniculitis +/- vasculitis
- Aggregates of foamy phagocytic macrophages
- Reactive fibrous tissue enveloping and separating areas of fat necrosis
  - May give rise to "bunch of grapes" appearance
- Cytology of cystic aspirate may reveal anuclear fat cells (vacuolated fat cells or "ghost cells")

CLINICAL ISSUES

Presentation
- Most common signs/symptoms
  - Evolving lesion over weeks or months
  - Tender subcutaneous swelling
    - Progressing to induration and later atrophy
- Other signs/symptoms
  - Pain and tenderness in about 50%
  - May be asymptomatic
  - May present de novo as focal depression in subcutaneous tissues

Demographics
- Age: Young to middle-aged
- Gender: No sex predilection

Natural History & Prognosis
- Resolves over weeks or months with induration +/- atrophy
- Indurated subcutaneous tissue either returns to normal, remains slightly indurated or undergoes progressive fat atrophy leading to a focal depression in the skin surface
- May have relapsing/remitting course

Treatment
- Often no specific treatment
- +/- Antiinflammatory medication, if lesions painful and tender
- +/- Corticosteroids +/- immunosuppressants, if Weber-Christian disease

DIAGNOSTIC CHECKLIST

Consider
- Look for pancreatic disease in patient presenting with unexplained panniculitis or fat necrosis

Image Interpretation Pearls
- Ill-defined localized echogenicity of subcutaneous fat, clinically evolving over weeks or months is usually due to either panniculitis, subcutaneous fat injury or necrosis

SELECTED REFERENCES

1. Diaz Cascajo C et al: Panniculitis: definition of terms and diagnostic strategy. Am J Dermatopathol. 22(6):530-49, 2000
2. Lopez JA et al: MRI diagnosis and follow-up of subcutaneous fat necrosis. J Magn Reson Imaging. 7(5):929-32, 1997
3. Canteli B et al: Fat necrosis. Skeletal Radiol. 25(3):305-7, 1996

FAT INJURY

IMAGE GALLERY

Typical

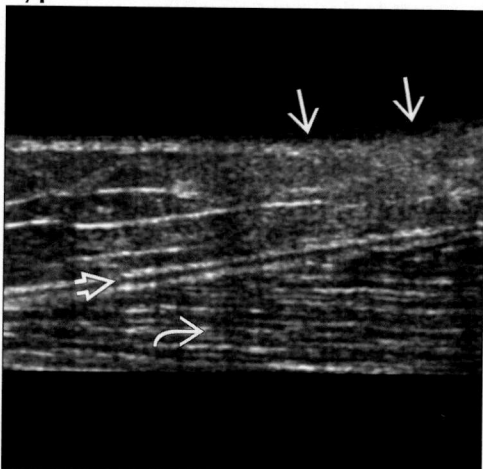 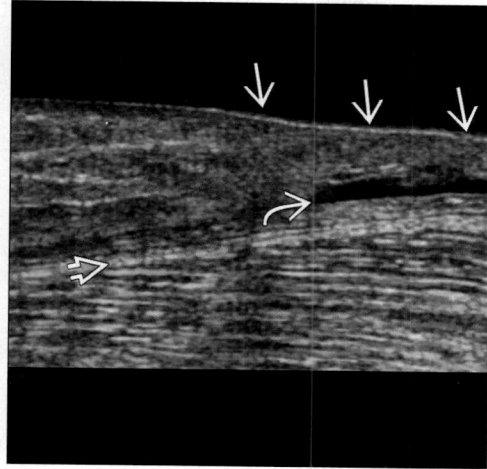

(Left) Longitudinal ultrasound of the calf shows focal echogenicity with loss of striation of subcutaneous fat ⇨ indicative of fat necrosis. Note normal investing fascia ⇨ and calf muscle ➡. *(Right)* Longitudinal ultrasound of the calf shows subcutaneous fat necrosis of the calf region with reduced bulk of subcutaneous fat ➡ and fluid accumulation ➡ superficial to investing fascia ⇨.

Variant

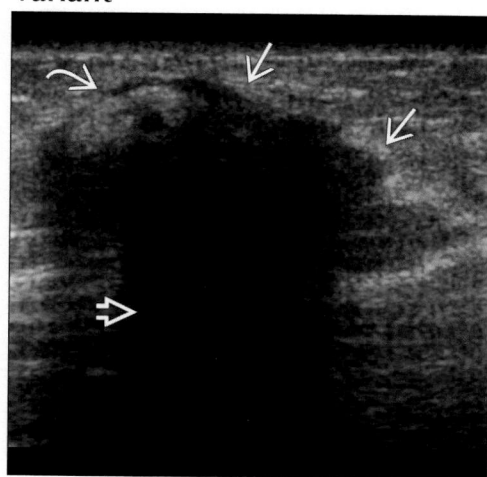 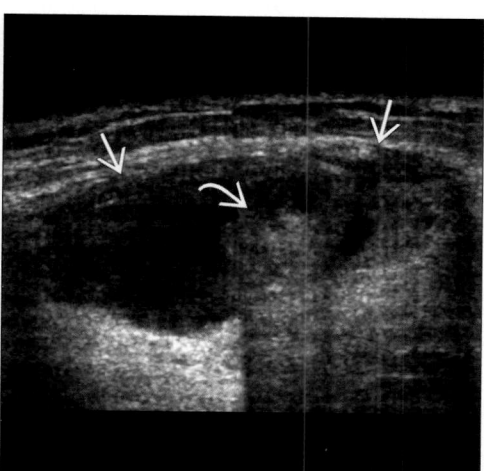

(Left) Transverse ultrasound of the buttock region shows a well-defined hypoechoic mass ➡ due to fat necrosis within the subcutaneous tissues. There is prominent calcification ➡ with acoustic shadowing ⇨. *(Right)* Longitudinal ultrasound of buttock region shows a well-defined, largely cystic mass ➡ with early calcification ➡. This is in an area of blunt trauma.

Typical

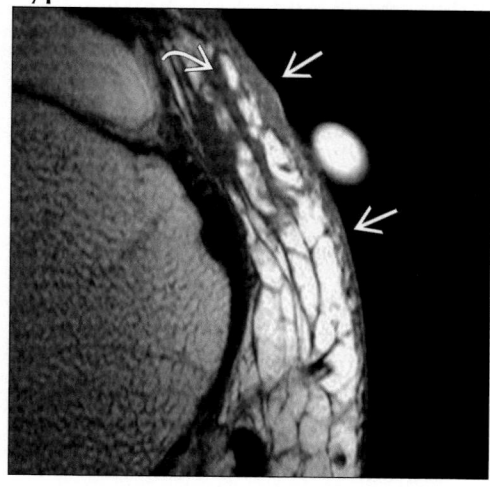 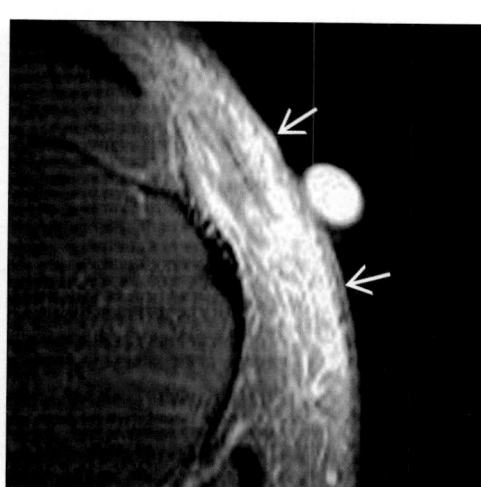

(Left) Axial T1WI MR of the knee region shows swelling of subcutaneous tissues ➡, with hypointense thickening of subcutaneous striations ⇨ due to fat necrosis. *(Right)* Axial fat-suppressed T2WI in the same patient shows moderate focal edema of the subcutaneous tissues ➡ due to fat necrosis. Note how edema is better shown on this sequence than T1WI.

MUSCLE INFARCTION

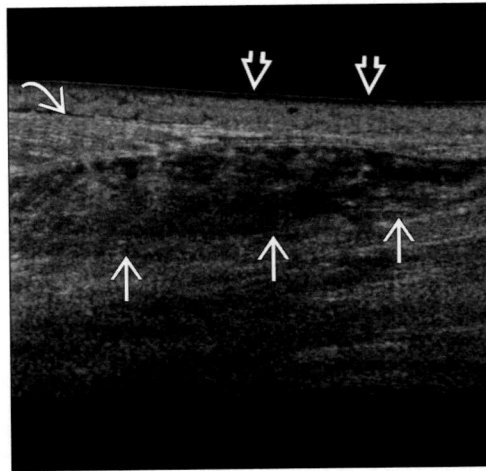

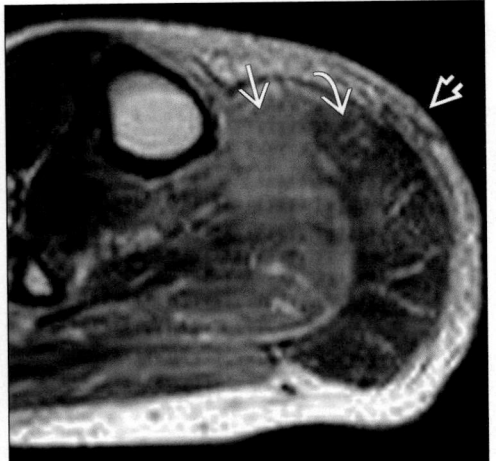

Longitudinal ultrasound shows an ill-defined, hypoechoic area ➡ within the soleus muscle, indicative of diabetic muscle infarction. Note normal overlying gastrocnemius muscle ➡ and subcutaneous edema ➡.

Axial T2WI MR at the same location as the previous image, shows edema and swelling of the soleus muscle ➡, normal gastrocnemius muscle ➡ and overlying subcutaneous edema ➡.

TERMINOLOGY

Abbreviations and Synonyms
- Diabetic muscle infarction, aseptic myonecrosis, ischemic myonecrosis, tumoriform focal muscular degeneration

Definitions
- Muscle infarction leading to muscle cell death

IMAGING FINDINGS

General Features
- Best diagnostic clue: Focal muscle edema in susceptible diabetic patient
- Location
  - Most commonly affects thigh (80%), especially vastus lateralis (24%) and vastus medialis (22%)
  - Calf muscle infarction less common (20%)
  - Upper limb muscle infarction rare (1%)
  - Located deep within affected muscle
  - Usually involves single muscle though occasionally more than one muscle within same area may be affected
  - Bilateral muscle involvement uncommon (8%)
- Size: Variable, though typically 3-5 cm
- Morphology
  - Initially affected muscle is swollen
  - Later firm muscle mass may develop at affected site

Ultrasonographic Findings
- Grayscale Ultrasound
  - Focal ill-defined swelling and hypoechogenicity of affected muscle
  - Effacement and disruption of normal muscular architecture
  - Acoustic enhancement posterior to the area of infarction is often present
  - +/- Fluid superficial to infarcted area (subfascial fluid)
    - No internal motion of fluid on transducer ballotment
  - +/- Gas within infarcted area, echogenic foci with reverberation artifact

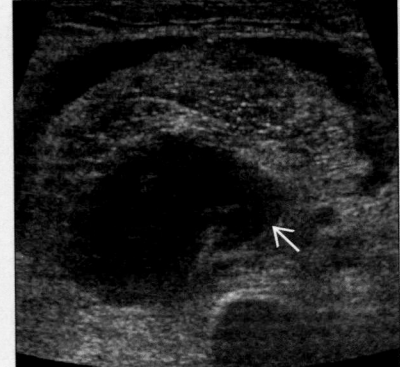

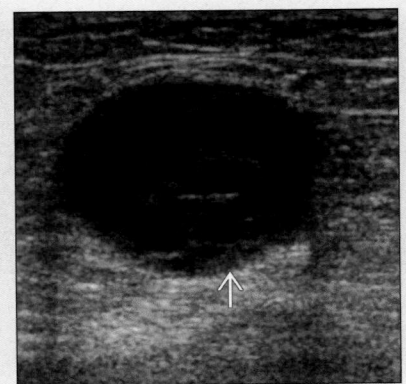

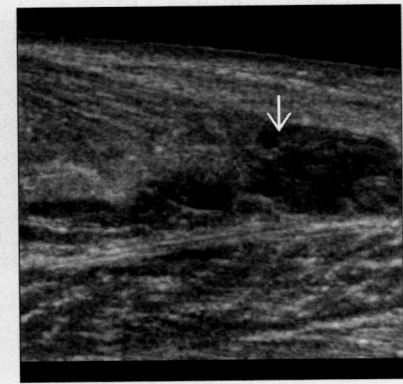

DDx: Muscle Infarction

Muscle Abscess

Muscle Tumor

Muscle Tear

MUSCLE INFARCTION

Key Facts

Imaging Findings

- Best diagnostic clue: Focal muscle edema in susceptible diabetic patient
- Most commonly affects thigh (80%), especially vastus lateralis (24%) and vastus medialis (22%)
- Located deep within affected muscle
- Focal ill-defined swelling and hypoechogenicity of affected muscle
- Effacement and disruption of normal muscular architecture
- Acoustic enhancement posterior to the area of infarction is often present
- +/- Fluid superficial to infarcted area (subfascial fluid)
- +/- Gas within infarcted area, echogenic foci with reverberation artifact
- Subcutaneous tissue edema overlying infarcted area
- Infarcted area may resolve or evolve into medium-sized discrete hypoechoic mass
- Affected area is iso- or hypovascular initially relative to surrounding non-affected muscle
- Later becomes mildly hypervascular compared to surrounding unaffected muscle
- Perform early examination followed by serial examinations at 3-4 weekly intervals for 9-12 weeks to observe changing nature of lesion
- Routinely compare vascularity of affected muscle with contralateral non-affected muscle

Top Differential Diagnoses

- Muscle Abscess
- Muscle Tumor
- Deep Venous Thrombosis

- ○ Hemorrhage within affected area cannot be identified on ultrasound: Best seen by MR
- ○ Subcutaneous tissue edema overlying infarcted area
  - ■ Varies proportional to extent, severity and duration of infarction
  - ■ Degree of subcutaneous edema may provide clue to duration of infarction
- ○ Infarcted area may resolve or evolve into medium-sized discrete hypoechoic mass
  - ■ Mass appears during reparative phase and is not a feature of acute phase
  - ■ Mass may have linear internal echoes due to muscle fibers
  - ■ Mass slowly resolves
  - ■ Mass tends to become more well-defined and firmer with time
- ○ Calcification not a feature
- ○ Ultrasound can exclude deep venous thrombosis more readily than MR or CT
- Color Doppler
  - ○ Affected area is iso- or hypovascular initially relative to surrounding non-affected muscle
    - ■ Later becomes mildly hypervascular compared to surrounding unaffected muscle

Radiographic Findings

- Radiography: Arterial calcification indicative of diabetic vasculopathy

CT Findings

- Contrast-enhanced CT shows swollen affected muscle +/- hypodense ring-enhancing lesion

MR Findings

- T1WI
  - ○ Swollen isointense affected muscle
  - ○ +/- Focal hyperintensity within affected muscle due to hemorrhage
- T2WI FS
  - ○ Focally edematous muscle
    - ■ Degree of muscle edema more pronounced on MR than ultrasound
  - ○ +/- Subfascial fluid collection

- ○ Edema of overlying subcutaneous fat
- ○ +/- Discrete mass at site of infarction
- T1 C+
  - ○ No muscle enhancement in early infarction
  - ○ Mild to moderate muscle enhancement in later stages of infarction

Imaging Recommendations

- Best imaging tool: Ultrasound to help confirm diagnosis of diabetic muscle infarction and exclude likely differential diagnoses
- Protocol advice
  - ○ Perform early examination followed by serial examinations at 3-4 weekly intervals for 9-12 weeks to observe changing nature of lesion
  - ○ Routinely compare vascularity of affected muscle with contralateral non-affected muscle

DIFFERENTIAL DIAGNOSIS

Muscle Abscess

- Very painful and tender +/- fever
- Predominant fluid component
- Deteriorates and becomes more liquefied with time
- Purulent fluid on aspiration

Muscle Tumor

- Discrete mass usually
- Mass effect usually appreciable with displacement of adjacent musculature
- Mass usually has intrinsic vascularity
- Muscle edema not a strong feature
- Does not resolve with time

Muscle Tear

- Focal muscle fibre retraction or discontinuity
- Initial onset of pain during exercise

Deep Venous Thrombosis

- Non-compressibility of affected vein
- Visible thrombus within veins
- Lack of distal augmentation

MUSCLE INFARCTION

PATHOLOGY

General Features
- General path comments: Evolving lesion with infarction followed by repair
- Etiology
  - Probably caused by vascular occlusion from
    - Arteriosclerosis obliterans
    - Embolization of arteriosclerotic plaque
    - Thrombosis related to altered coagulation-fibrinolysis system
    - Anti-phospholipid antibodies may be contributory
- Epidemiology
  - Diabetes mellitus = 5.9% population
  - Muscle infarction is an uncommon complication of diabetes

Gross Pathologic & Surgical Features
- Gross pathology and surgical exploration usually avoided
  - Biopsy often not necessary
  - Biopsy should be undertaken when presentation and/or clinical course is atypical
    - Percutaneous biopsy preferable over open biopsy
- Swollen, non-hemophagic, pale, whitish muscle

Microscopic Features
- Large areas of muscle necrosis (myonecrosis) and edema
  - Phagocytosis of necrotic muscle fibers
  - Granulation tissue repair with fibrosis
  - Muscle fibre replacement by fibrous tissue
    - +/- Myofiber replacement of infarcted muscle
- Small arteries of infarcted area may have thickened hyalinized walls and be occluded with fibrin or calcium fragments
- Inflammatory infiltrate not a notable feature

CLINICAL ISSUES

Presentation
- Most common signs/symptoms
  - Acute onset of painful swelling of affected muscle
  - Pre-existing diabetes
- Other signs/symptoms
  - Resolution of swelling with appearance of painful palpable mass (33%) over three weeks
  - Fever (10%)
  - Often delay between onset of symptoms and presentation (average 4 weeks)
- Clinical Profile
  - Mean duration of diabetes prior to diabetic muscle infarction is 15 years
  - 2/3 have type 1 diabetes, 1/3 have type 2 diabetes
  - Accompanying diabetic complications common
    - Nephropathy (72%)
    - Retinopathy (57%)
    - Neuropathy (55%)
    - Peripheral vascular disease (6%)
    - Hypertension (6%)
  - Laboratory tests inconclusive
    - Elevated creatine kinase (52%)
    - Elevated white cell count (8%)
    - Elevated erythrocyte sedimentation rate (53%)
  - Muscle infarction may also occur in patients with chronic renal failure or angiopathy and no diabetes

Demographics
- Age: Average 42 years (range 19-81 years)
- Gender: More frequent in diabetic women (62%)

Natural History & Prognosis
- Settles in about 5-8 weeks with conservative treatment
- About 1/3 of patients experience second episode of muscle infarction
  - Most commonly involves different muscle (85%) rather than the same muscle (15%)
- Overall, diabetic muscle infarction is a poor prognostic sign
  - About 20% patients die within two years due to other accompanying diabetic complications

Treatment
- Conservative
  - Bedrest initially
  - Analgesia and symptomatic treatment
  - Leg elevation
  - Gradual resumption of activity as pain resolves
  - Careful metabolic control of diabetes (may reduce likelihood of recurrence)
  - Usually resolves spontaneously
    - Antiplatelet therapy, if hypercoagulable state
    - Steroids, if antiphospholipid antibodies present
- Complications
  - Bleeding into the infarcted area may be induced by biopsy
  - No other reported complications

DIAGNOSTIC CHECKLIST

Consider
- Diabetic muscle infarction in any patient with known diabetic complication presenting with muscle pain

Image Interpretation Pearls
- Diagnosis based on occurrence of typical ultrasonographic findings in at-risk patient
- Serial examination showing evolving changes will allow definitive diagnosis without need for biopsy

SELECTED REFERENCES

1. Chow KM et al: Muscle infarction in peritoneal dialysis patients. Am J Kidney Dis. 42(5):1102-3, 2003
2. Trujillo-Santos AJ: Diabetic muscle infarction: an underdiagnosed complication of long-standing diabetes. Diabetes Care. 26(1):211-5, 2003
3. Delaney-Sathy LO et al: Sonography of diabetic muscle infarction with MR imaging, CT, and pathologic correlation. AJR Am J Roentgenol. 174(1):165-9, 2000
4. Sharma P et al: Diabetic muscle infarction: atypical MR appearance. Skeletal Radiol. 29(8):477-80, 2000

MUSCLE INFARCTION

IMAGE GALLERY

Typical

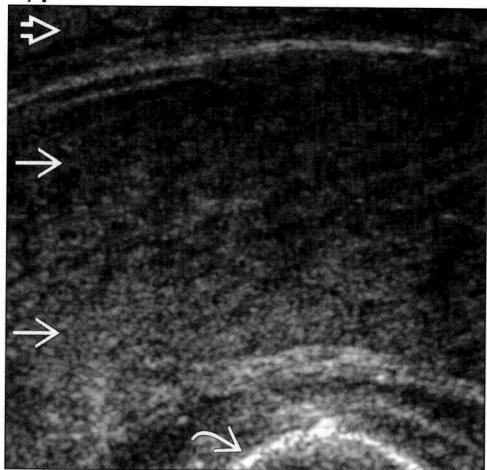

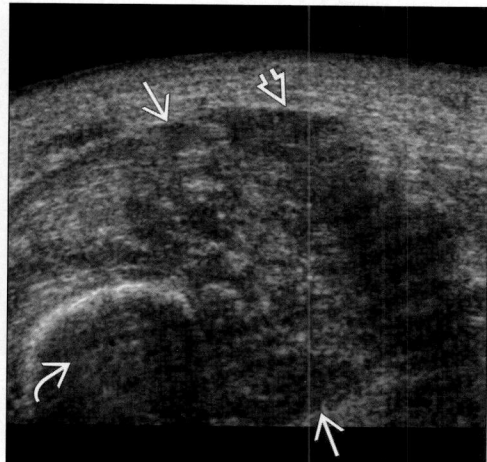

(Left) Transverse ultrasound shows a severely swollen and hypoechoic vastus intermedius muscle ➡ in a diabetic patient, indicative of muscle infarction. Note femoral shaft ➡ and edematous subcutaneous fat ➡. (Right) Transverse ultrasound shows edema, hypoechogenicity, and swelling of the vastus lateralis ➡, indicative of diabetic muscle infarction. Note area of edematous tissue laterally ➡. Femoral shaft ➡.

Typical

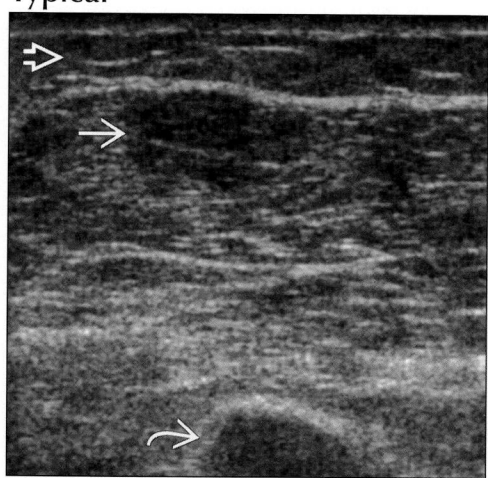

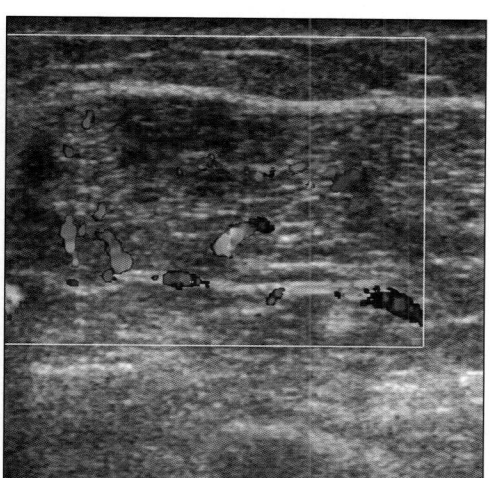

(Left) Transverse ultrasound shows a focal, well-defined hypoechoic area ➡ within the biceps brachii, indicative of a resolving diabetic muscle infarction. Note lack of overlying subcutaneous edema ➡. Humeral shaft is also visible ➡. (Right) Transverse color Doppler ultrasound at the same location, shows moderate hyperemia surrounding the hypoechoic muscle mass.

Variant

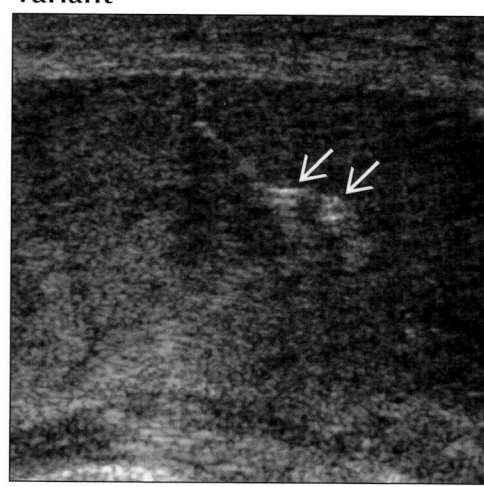

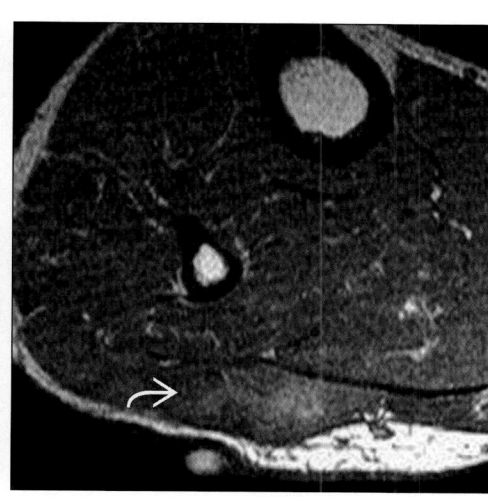

(Left) Transverse ultrasound in a case of diabetic muscle infarction shows small echogenic reverberation artifacts ➡ suggestive of gas formation within the vastus intermedius muscle. (Right) Axial T1WI MR shows a swollen lateral belly of the gastrocnemius muscle with ill-defined hyperintensity centrally ➡, indicative of hemorrhage within an area of diabetic muscle infarction.

MUSCLE INJURY

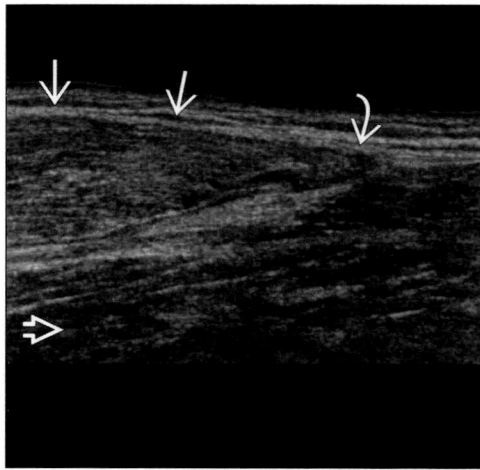
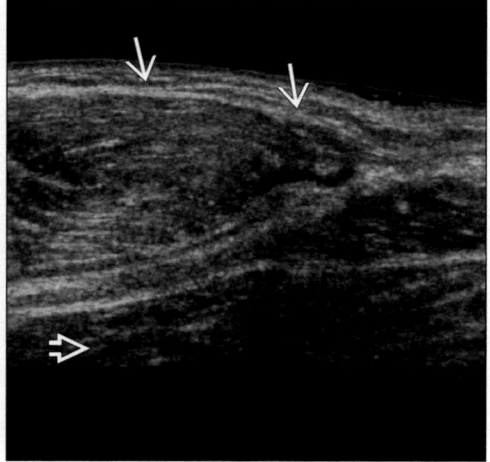

Longitudinal ultrasound at rest shows a relaxed, retracted, rectus femoris muscle ➡ due to a complete tear at the myofascial junction distally ➡. Normal vastus intermedius muscle ➡.

Transverse ultrasound during contraction (at same location) shows a contracted, completely torn rectus femoris muscle ➡. Note normal vastus intermedius muscle ➡.

TERMINOLOGY

Abbreviations and Synonyms
- Muscle pull, muscle strain, tennis leg, plantaris tear, muscle contusion, muscle hematoma, delayed onset muscle soreness, muscle hernia

Definitions
- Tear, pull, strain: Stretch injury of muscle with tear of muscle or myofascial fibers
- Contusion: Direct blunt compressive trauma to muscle without definable tear
- Hernia: Abnormal protrusion of muscle or part of muscle out of investing fascia in which it is normally contained

IMAGING FINDINGS

General Features
- Best diagnostic clue: Muscle tear; hypoechoic area within muscle or at myofascial junction
- Location

- o Usually affects lower limb muscles (quadriceps, gastrocnemius, soleus)
  - ▪ Myofascial junction (most common), intramuscular
- Morphology: Muscle fiber discontinuity with local hemorrhage and edema

Ultrasonographic Findings
- **Muscle tear (MT)**
  - o Discontinuity +/- retraction of muscle fibers either within muscle or at myofascial junction
  - o Tear filled with hematoma or fluid
  - o +/- Mild muscle and subcutaneous edema
- **Muscle hematoma (MH)**
  - o Typically associated with grade II tears
  - o Appearance varies with duration of hematoma, severity and location
  - o Hypoechoic, usually well-defined mass +/- hyperechoic hematoma
  - o +/- Acoustic enhancement
  - o Liquefaction seen as anechoic areas, initially either at rim of hematoma or centrally
  - o +/- Peripheral hyperemia during reparative phase (reparative fibrovascular granulation tissue)

DDx: Muscle Injury

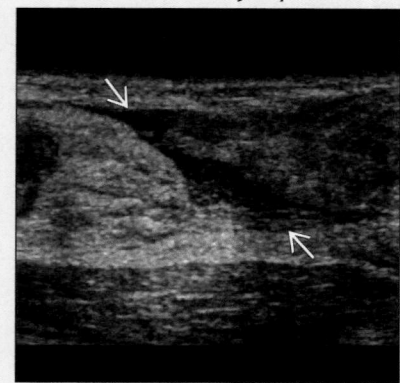
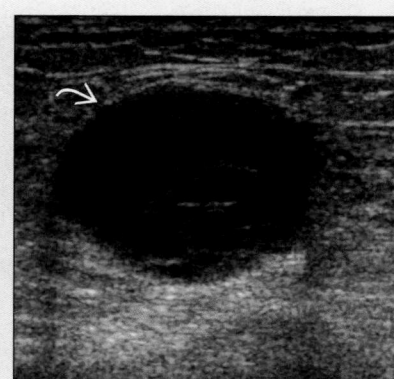
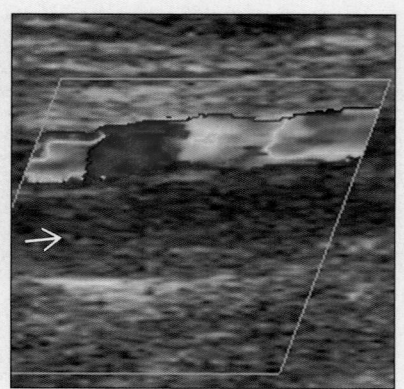

Tendon Tear

Muscle Tumor

Deep Venous Thrombosis

MUSCLE INJURY

Key Facts

Imaging Findings
- Morphology: Muscle fiber discontinuity with local hemorrhage and edema
- **Muscle tear (MT)**
- Discontinuity +/- retraction of muscle fibers either within muscle or at myofascial junction
- Tear filled with hematoma or fluid
- **Muscle hematoma (MH)**
- Typically associated with grade II tears
- Appearance varies with duration of hematoma, severity and location
- Hypoechoic, usually well-defined mass +/- hyperechoic hematoma
- +/- Acoustic enhancement
- Liquefaction seen as anechoic areas, initially either at rim of hematoma or centrally

- +/- Peripheral hyperemia during reparative phase (reparative fibrovascular granulation tissue)
- Peripheral granulation tissue usually hyperechoic and hyperemic
- **Muscle contusion (MC)**
- Ill-defined hyperechogenicity of muscle which may cross fascial boundary
- No fiber discontinuity
- **Muscle hernia**
- Focal protrusion of muscle or part of muscle through investing fascia
- Accentuated by muscle contraction or standing

Top Differential Diagnoses
- Tendon Tear
- Soft Tissue Tumor
- Deep Venous Thrombosis

- Peripheral granulation tissue usually hyperechoic and hyperemic
- No central vascularity
- **Delayed onset muscle soreness (DOMS)**
  - DOMS: Affected muscle may be normal or, if severe, diffusely hyperechoic
- **Muscle contusion (MC)**
  - Ill-defined hyperechogenicity of muscle which may cross fascial boundary
  - No fiber discontinuity
  - Hyperemia during reparative phase
- **Muscle hernia**
  - Focal protrusion of muscle or part of muscle through investing fascia
  - Accentuated by muscle contraction or standing

Radiographic Findings
- Radiography
  - Usually normal
  - Soft tissue mass in tears associated with large amount of hemorrhage and deranged architecture

CT Findings
- NECT
  - Normal in small tears
  - Low attenuation area due to edema
  - High attenuation area due to hemorrhage
  - Affected muscle enlarged compared to contralateral side
  - Soft tissue mass in intra-substance or retracted tears
- CECT: +/- Enhancement during reparative phase

MR Findings
- T1WI
  - Muscle tears
    - Low to intermediate signal intensity hemorrhage
    - +/- Hyperintense subacute hemorrhage
    - Peripheral hypointense hemosiderin
    - Loss of normal muscle striations +/- retracted muscle belly
  - DOMS
    - Muscle swelling of intermediate signal intensity
  - Muscle hernia

- Focal defect in investing fascia +/- muscle protrusion
- Often accompanying vessel
- T2WI
  - Muscle tear
    - Hyperintense edema in affected muscle
    - Inhomogeneous signal intensity mass in mid-substance tears due to hemorrhage and edema
    - Perimuscular hyperintense fluid
  - DOMS
    - Diffuse homogeneous hyperintensity
- T2* GRE: Susceptibility artifact due to hemorrhage
- T1 C+
  - Variable peripheral enhancement of intramuscular hematoma
  - "Bulls-eye lesion": Peripheral enhancement around intramuscular tear

Imaging Recommendations
- Best imaging tool: Ultrasound since most muscle tears are accessible
- Protocol advice
  - Examine mainly with muscle at rest & compare with contralateral side
  - Look closely at myofascial junction

DIFFERENTIAL DIAGNOSIS

Tendon Tear
- Quadriceps, patella or Achilles

Soft Tissue Tumor
- May mimic mid-substance tear with palpable mass
- Tumor usually has central enhancement as opposed to peripheral enhancement of hematoma
- Hemosiderin less pronounced with tumor

Deep Venous Thrombosis
- Non-compressibility of affected vein, lack of distal augmentation
- Thrombus visible within vein

MUSCLE INJURY

PATHOLOGY

General Features
- General path comments
  - Relevant anatomy
    - Plantaris muscle and tendon originates medial to lateral belly gastrocnemius and inserts anteromedial to Achilles tendon
    - In mid-calf, plantaris tendon is located deep to medial belly of gastrocnemius muscle
    - Seen as small ovoid structure within myofascia deep to medial belly gastrocnemius
    - Near insertion is barely distinguishable from Achilles tendon
    - Plantaris is absent in 10% legs (two-thirds absent bilaterally)
- Etiology
  - Muscle tear and hematoma
    - Strenuous athletic activity
    - Inadequate stretching & warm-up exercises (possibly)
    - Violent eccentric contraction
  - DOMS
    - Reversible structural damage at cellular level with temporary reduced muscle strength following unaccustomed exertion
- Epidemiology
  - Muscle injury: 30% of sports-related injuries
  - Rectus femoris: Most frequently injured quadriceps muscle
  - Medial belly gastrocnemius myofascial tear much more common than plantaris tendon tear

Gross Pathologic & Surgical Features
- Musculotendinous junction tear
- Intrasubstance tear
- Tear at deep intramuscular tendon

Microscopic Features
- Muscle edema, hemorrhage and phagocytosis
- Muscle fiber necrosis, edema with macrophagic infiltrate
- Fibroblastic response

Staging, Grading or Classification Criteria
- Grade 1: Small tear involving a few (< 5%) of muscle or myofascial unit
- Grade 2: Partial (5% - < 100%) tear of muscle or myofascial unit
- Grade 3: Complete (100%) tear of muscle or myofascial unit & retraction

CLINICAL ISSUES

Presentation
- Most common signs/symptoms
  - Tear and hematoma: Sudden onset of limb pain at time of exertion; "pop" sensation
    - Localized swelling and tenderness ± later, a discrete mass
    - Complete rupture: Palpable defect with retracted mass

  - DOMS: Swelling and pain beginning 1-2 days after exercise, peaking at 3 days and resolving by day 7
  - Muscle hernia: Chronic pin-point pain and tenderness
    - Usually has well-developed musculature

Demographics
- Age
  - Young athlete
    - In children, apophyseal avulsion fractures tend to predominate
    - In older patients, tendon tears predominate

Natural History & Prognosis
- Majority of muscle injuries improve with conservative treatment
  - Serial ultrasound examination not useful for guiding speed of rehabilitation
  - Speed of rehabilitation should be gauged clinically
- Surgery indicated for compartment syndrome, complete tear, hernia and troublesome reparative fibrosis
  - Compartment syndrome occurs with severe tears

Treatment
- Conservative
  - RICE (rest, ice, compression, elevation)
  - Physical therapy: Stretching & exercises
  - Non-steroidal anti-inflammatory drugs (NSAIDs)
  - Gradual increase in activity
- Surgery
  - Decompression for compartment syndrome
  - Hematoma evacuation
  - Suturing of complete muscle rupture
  - Repair of investing fascia defect (if muscle hernia)
  - Resection of fibrotic mass

DIAGNOSTIC CHECKLIST

Consider
- Muscle hernia in any muscular patient with pinpoint muscle pain and tenderness

Image Interpretation Pearls
- Pay particular attention to distal myofascial junction of medial belly gastrocnemius for small tears

SELECTED REFERENCES
1. Connell DA et al: Longitudinal study comparing sonographic and MRI assessments of acute and healing hamstring injuries. AJR Am J Roentgenol. 183(4):975-84, 2004
2. Bianchi S et al: Central aponeurosis tears of the rectus femoris: sonographic findings. Skeletal Radiol. 31(10):581-6, 2002
3. Delgado GJ et al: Tennis leg: clinical US study of 141 patients and anatomic investigation of four cadavers with MR imaging and US. Radiology. 224(1):112-9, 2002

13

48

MUSCLE INJURY

IMAGE GALLERY

Typical

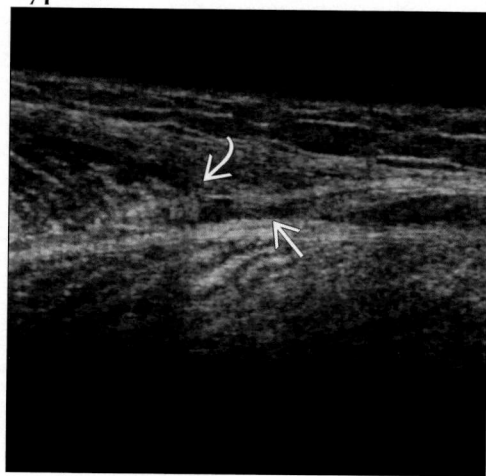
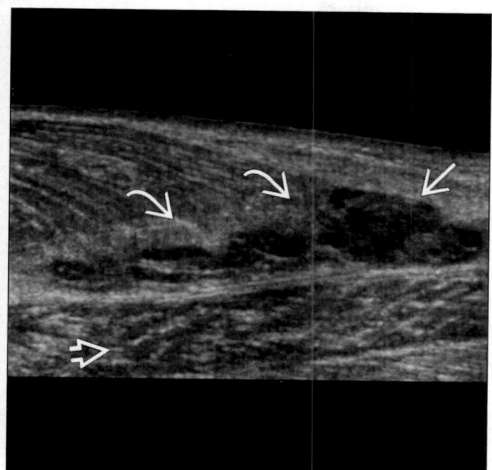

(Left) Longitudinal ultrasound shows a small myofascial tear ➥ of the medial belly of the distal gastrocnemius. Note the retracted muscle belly with a blunted edge ➥. *(Right)* Longitudinal ultrasound shows a more extensive tear ➥ of the medial belly of the gastrocnemius at the myofascial function. A hematoma is filling the gap ➥. Soleus muscle ➥.

Typical

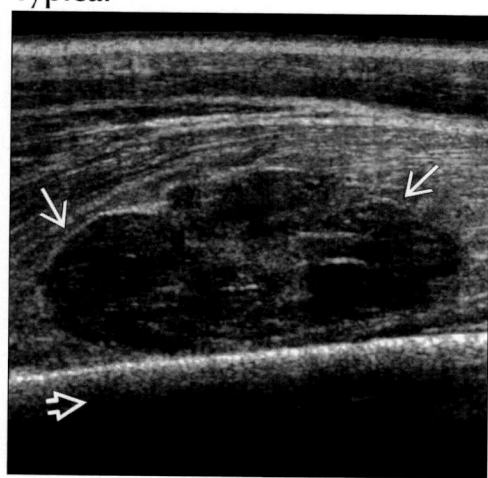
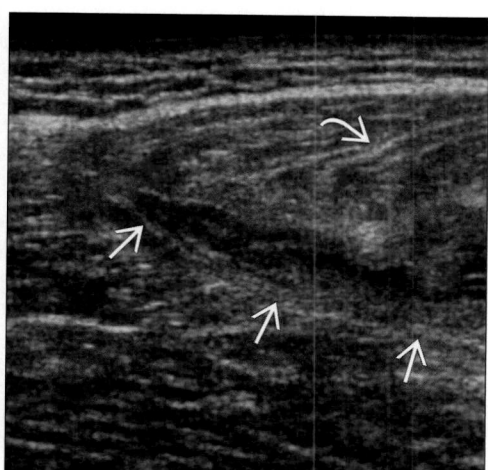

(Left) Oblique ultrasound shows a well-defined hematoma ➥ deep in the thigh musculature, just superficial to the femur ➥. No color flow was present on Doppler. *(Right)* Transverse ultrasound shows a large tear ➥ in the hamstring muscles, with localized retraction of muscle fibers ➥.

Variant

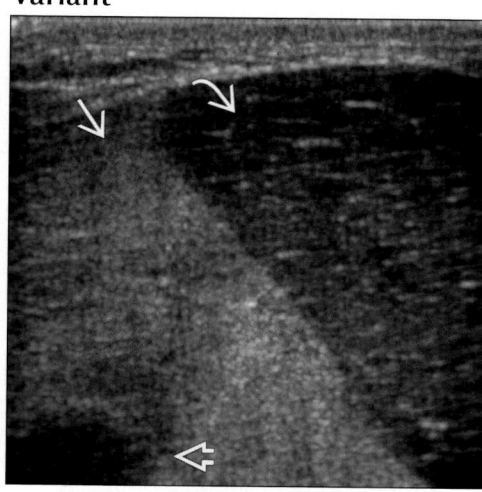
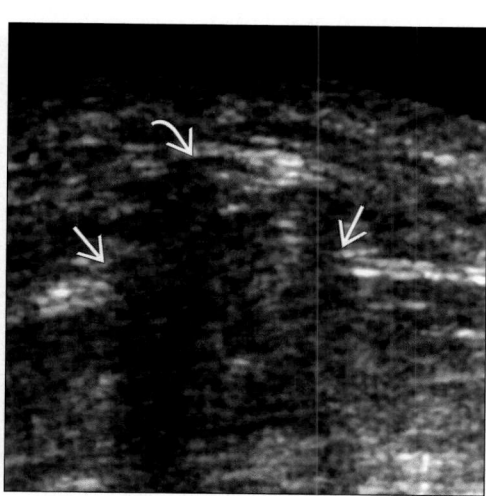

(Left) Transverse ultrasound shows diffuse echogenicity of the brachialis muscle ➥, one day following excessive exertion on a rowing machine, indicative of delayed onset muscle soreness. Normal biceps brachii ➥. Humeral shaft ➥. *(Right)* Transverse ultrasound shows herniation ➥ of the peroneal muscle into the subcutaneous tissues through a defect ➥ in the investing fascia.

OSTEOARTHROSIS

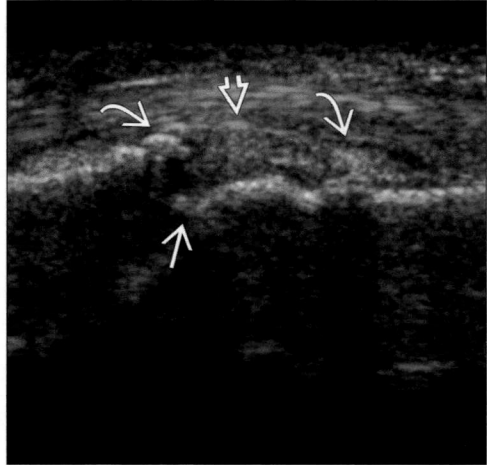

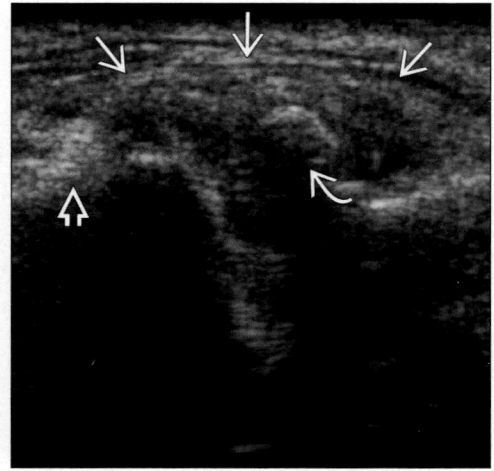

Longitudinal ultrasound shows joint space narrowing ➡, *marginal osteophytosis* ➡ *& capsular swelling* ➡ *on the volar aspect of the proximal interphalangeal joint, middle finger, indicative of osteoarthrosis.*

Longitudinal ultrasound shows marginal osteophytosis of the trapezium ➡ *and first metacarpal* ➡ *with capsular swelling* ➡ *of the first carpometacarpal joint, indicative of osteoarthrosis.*

TERMINOLOGY

Abbreviations and Synonyms
- Osteoarthritis, degenerative joint disease, osteoarthropathy, primary or secondary osteoarthrosis

Definitions
- Primary: Progressive loss of articular cartilage with associated bone & soft tissue abnormalities
- Secondary: Accelerated degenerative joint disease due to joint deformity resulting from congenital, traumatic, infective, inflammatory or metabolic disorder

IMAGING FINDINGS

General Features
- Best diagnostic clue: Articular cartilage thinning accompanied by osteophytosis, subchondral sclerosis, subchondral cyst formation ± synovial hypertrophy, capsular swelling & periarticular edema

- Location: Knee (particularly medial femorotibial & patellofemoral), hip, fingers, first carpometacarpal joint
- Size: May affect localized area, compartment, or whole of joint
- Morphology: Progressive loss of articular cartilage with marginal new bone formation & capsular swelling

Ultrasonographic Findings
- Usually used to exclude infective, inflammatory or crystal deposition disease rather than diagnose osteoarthrosis
- Joint space narrowing, marginal osteophytosis ± capsular swelling & effusion are the ultrasound signs of osteoarthrosis
  - Joint space narrowing for some joints (e.g., patellofemoral joint) may not be readily appreciable on US
  - Cartilage thinning or defects cannot be fully evaluated with ultrasound
- Medial meniscal extrusion common feature of moderate to severe medial femorotibial osteoarthrosis
- Joint effusion (may be anechoic or slightly echogenic)

DDx: Osteoarthrosis

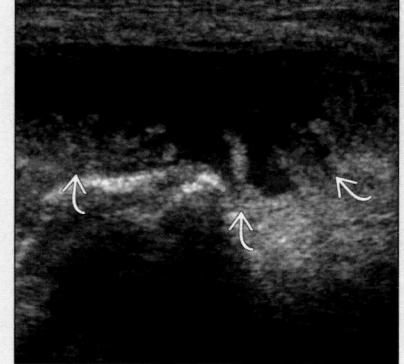

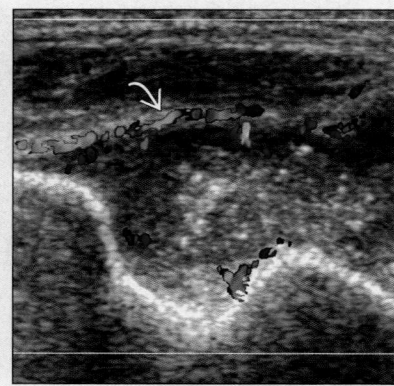

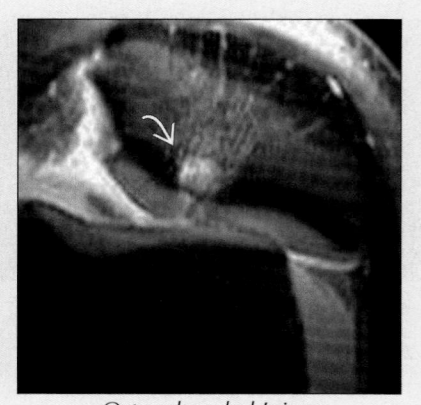

| *Inflammatory Synovitis* | *Crystal Deposition* | *Osteochondral Injury* |

OSTEOARTHROSIS

Key Facts

Imaging Findings
- Best diagnostic clue: Articular cartilage thinning accompanied by osteophytosis, subchondral sclerosis, subchondral cyst formation ± synovial hypertrophy, capsular swelling & periarticular edema
- High-field strength MR imaging has high sensitivity & specificity for cartilage thinning & defects
- Joint space narrowing, marginal osteophytosis ± capsular swelling & effusion are the ultrasound signs of osteoarthrosis
- Cartilage thinning or defects cannot be fully evaluated with ultrasound
- Medial meniscal extrusion common feature of moderate to severe medial femorotibial osteoarthrosis
- Joint effusion (may be anechoic or slightly echogenic)
- Medial & lateral parapatellar recess (retinacular recesses) often distend prior to suprapatellar recess
- Mild synovial proliferation is a common finding
- Particulate debris may be visible within joint fluid
- Associated Baker cysts identified by ultrasound with high level of accuracy
- Ultrasound-guided joint aspiration helpful to exclude infective, inflammatory or crystal deposition disease

Top Differential Diagnoses
- Inflammatory Arthritis
- Crystal Deposition Synovitis
- Chondral Injury

Pathology
- Primary & secondary osteoarthrosis may be different diseases with a common final pathway

---

- ○ Medial & lateral parapatellar recess (retinacular recesses) often distend prior to suprapatellar recess
- Mild synovial proliferation is a common finding
- Acute exacerbation characterized by
  - ○ Capsular swelling
  - ○ Mild to moderate synovial capsular hyperemia
    - Low resistance (resistive index < 8.0) flow
    - Capsular-synovial hyperemia difficult to depict at hip joint
  - ○ Joint effusion
  - ○ Synovial hypertrophy
  - ○ Edema of periarticular tissues (better seen with MR)
- Particulate debris may be visible within joint fluid
  - ○ Ultrasound can detect radiographically occult intra-articular debris
  - ○ Ultrasound cannot usually determine whether particular debris is free or attached
  - ○ Central aspects of joint cannot be visualized with ultrasound (better seen with MR)
- Joint subluxation can be exaggerated on ultrasound as dependent on transducer angulation & alignment
- Associated Baker cysts identified by ultrasound with high level of accuracy
- Ultrasound-guided joint aspiration helpful to exclude infective, inflammatory or crystal deposition disease
  - ○ Specimen for crystal should be sent fresh as alcohol will dissolve crystals

Radiographic Findings
- Radiography
  - ○ Primary screening modality for osteoarthrosis
  - ○ Joint space narrowing, subchondral sclerosis, subchondral cysts, & osteophyte formation
    - Mild subluxation, especially in small joints
  - ○ Significant cartilage loss may be present with normal radiographic appearances

CT Findings
- Plain CT not useful for evaluating cartilage
- CT-arthrography has high sensitivity, specificity for cartilage thinning & focal defects (comparable or better than MR imaging)

MR Findings
- T1WI
  - ○ Joint space narrowing, subchondral cysts, marrow fat signal extending into osteophytes
    - Subchondral decreased signal indicating sclerosis or edema
- T2WI
  - ○ Subchondral edema demonstrated with fat saturation
    - Joint effusion ± intra-articular particulate debris
    - Reactive-type synovitis
  - ○ ± Baker cyst
  - ○ Diffuse periarticular edema with acute exacerbation
- PD/Intermediate
  - ○ PD variable thinning of articular cartilage
    - Capsular & synovial thickening
    - Associated abnormalities such as meniscal degeneration (flattening), meniscal extrusion & tears
    - Subchondral sclerosis difficult to appreciate without T1 contrast
    - Edema difficult to appreciate without fat suppression
  - ○ High-field strength MR imaging has high sensitivity & specificity for cartilage thinning & defects

Imaging Recommendations
- Best imaging tool: MR for cartilage visualization
- Protocol advice: FSE PD FS

DIFFERENTIAL DIAGNOSIS

Inflammatory Arthritis
- Systemic, other symmetrical disease
- Serological markers
- Synovitis ± erosions

Crystal Deposition Synovitis
- Can appear similar to acute exacerbation of osteoarthrosis
  - ○ Effusion predominates ± para-articular tophi

OSTEOARTHROSIS

- ○ Joint space narrowing & osteophytosis will be present if there is pre-existing primary or secondary osteoarthrosis
- ○ Ultrasound-guided aspiration for crystals, cytology, & culture

Chondral Injury
- Ultrasound assessment limited
  - ○ Best seen by MR imaging
  - ○ Chondral or osteochondral injury on PD FS imaging as chondral swelling/defect ± subchondral marrow edema
- Prior trauma history common

PATHOLOGY

General Features
- General path comments
  - ○ Progressive destruction of articular cartilage
  - ○ Primary & secondary osteoarthrosis may be different diseases with a common final pathway
  - ○ Secondary osteoarthrosis can be explained by overload paradigm ("wear and tear")
  - ○ Primary osteoarthrosis profile does not reconcile in many respects with overload paradigm e.g., it occurs commonly in chair sitting Caucasians & osteophytosis can occur without cartilage loss
    - Primary osteoarthrosis may be purely catabolic with destruction of articular cartilage due to overload or enzymatic action
    - Primary osteoarthrosis more likely to be bimodal with anabolic phase following by catabolic phase
    - Anabolic phase characterized by hypertrophy of bone (osteophytosis), cartilage (reduplicated tidemark) & synovium
    - Catabolic phase characterized by articular cartilage loss
    - Diminished synovial clearance of normal joint enzymes may be contributory
    - Closed, positive feedback loop may modulate joint enzymatic level & activity
- Epidemiology: Affects 90% of patients older than 40 years
- Associated abnormalities: Deformity, subluxation, loose bodies with catching & locking, ankylosis

Gross Pathologic & Surgical Features
- Degraded cartilage with fissured and/or ulcerated cartilage surface, loss of surface sheen

Microscopic Features
- Diminution of chondrocytes in superficial zones with chondrocyte swelling
- Cartilage matrix loses its ability to stain for proteoglycans with Alcian blue or safranin-O
- Matrix chondrocytes demonstrate proliferation in clusters (brood capsules)
- Neovascularity penetrates layer of calcified cartilage & new chondrocytes extend up from deeper layers
- Hypertrophied synovium becomes folded into villous folds with variable infiltration of plasma cells & lymphocytes

Staging, Grading or Classification Criteria
- Primary osteoarthrosis
  - ○ Knee, hip, first metacarpophalangeal & interphalangeal articulations
- Secondary osteoarthrosis (due to underlying joint deformity)
- Articular cartilage damage (stages)
  - ○ I: Edema (chondromalacia)
  - ○ II: Surface fibrillation with superficial defects
  - ○ III: Deep fibrillation with large deep defects
  - ○ IV: Full thickness defect & subchondral sclerosis, cyst formation ± bony attenuation

CLINICAL ISSUES

Presentation
- Most common signs/symptoms: Pain on movement (or at rest) with joint swelling (due to effusion, capsular-synovial thickening, periarticular edema)
- Clinical Profile: Catching, locking or grinding in older patient

Demographics
- Age: Typically older patients (> 50 years)
- Gender: Female predominance

Natural History & Prognosis
- Progressively debilitating disease without medical intervention

Treatment
- Conservative
  - ○ Minimize overloading e.g., weight loss
  - ○ Muscle strengthening
  - ○ Pain management by analgesics or NSAIDs
  - ○ Hyaluronic acid injections, glucosamine & chondroitin supplements
- Surgical
  - ○ For patients with persistent symptoms & pain
  - ○ Arthroscopy (debridement)
  - ○ Resurfacing procedure (for hip osteoarthrosis)
  - ○ Arthroplasty
  - ○ Realignment osteotomies for younger patients to redistribute weight bearing load

DIAGNOSTIC CHECKLIST

Consider
- Secondary osteoarthrosis if osteoarthrosis of shoulder, elbow, wrist, ankle or foot in young (< 50 yrs) patient
- Joint aspiration to help exclude infective or crystal deposition disease

Image Interpretation Pearls
- On MR utilize FS PD FSE to visualize chondral erosions & subchondral edema

SELECTED REFERENCES

1. Alexander CJ: Idiopathic osteoarthritis: time to change paradigms? Skeletal Radiol. 33(6):321-4, 2004

OSTEOARTHROSIS

IMAGE GALLERY

Typical

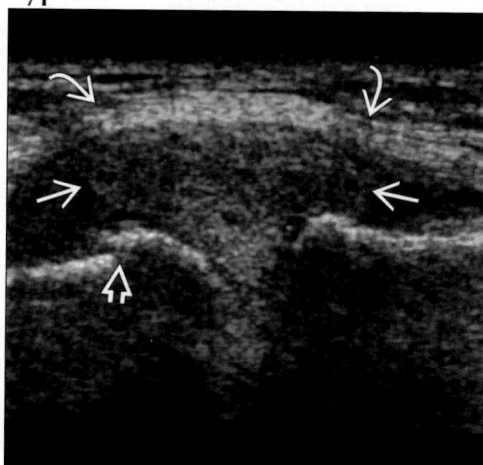
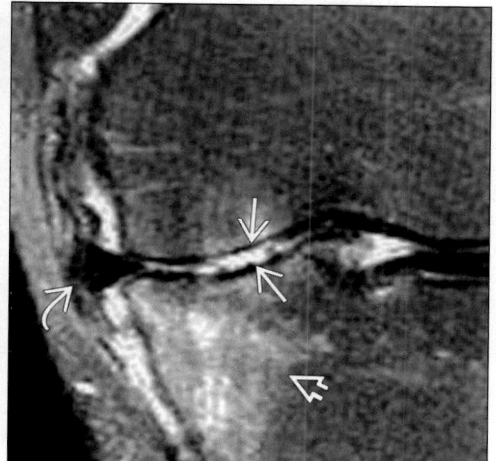

(Left) Longitudinal ultrasound shows an extruded medial meniscus ➡, displacing the medial collateral ligament ➡. Note medial femorotibial joint space narrowing and marginal osteophytosis ➡. *(Right)* Coronal T2WI with fat-suppression shows complete loss of articular cartilage ➡, extrusion of the medial meniscus ➡, subchondral intramedullary edema ➡, and pericapsular edema with increase in joint fluid.

Variant

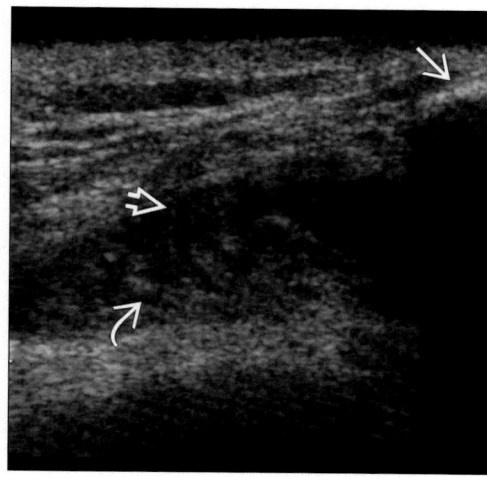
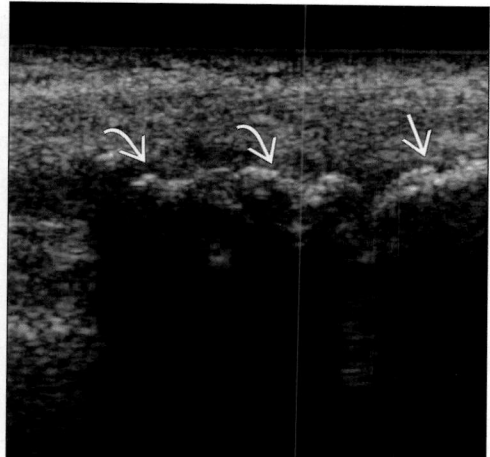

(Left) Transverse ultrasound shows prominent synovial hypertrophy ➡ in the medial patellar recess, with a small increase in joint fluid ➡. These findings are due to acute exacerbation of osteoarthrosis. Patella ➡. *(Right)* Longitudinal ultrasound shows a large, calcified mass ➡ within the suprapatellar pouch just proximal to the patella ➡. The deep component of this calcified mass is not visible.

Typical

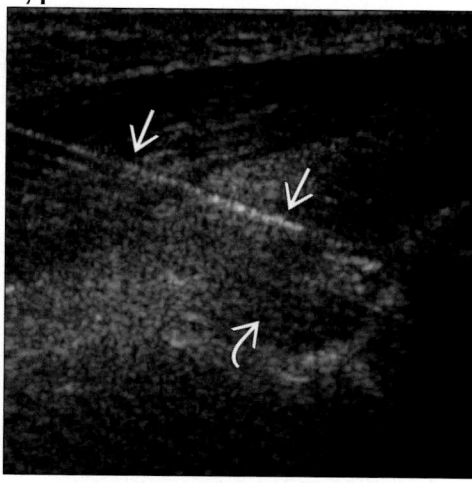
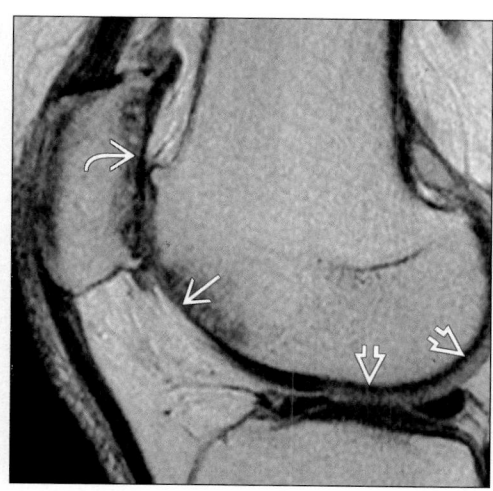

(Left) Grayscale ultrasound shows fine-needle ➡ aspiration of an echogenic elbow joint effusion ➡ due to acute exacerbation of osteoarthrosis. *(Right)* Sagittal T1WI MR shows severe patellofemoral osteoarthrosis, with full-thickness cartilage loss of the patella ➡ and femoral trochlea ➡. Note normal cartilage on the mid- and posterior aspects of the medial femoral condyle ➡.

INFLAMMATORY ARTHRITIS

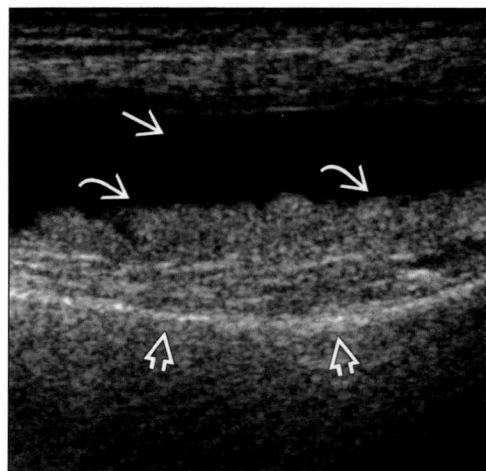

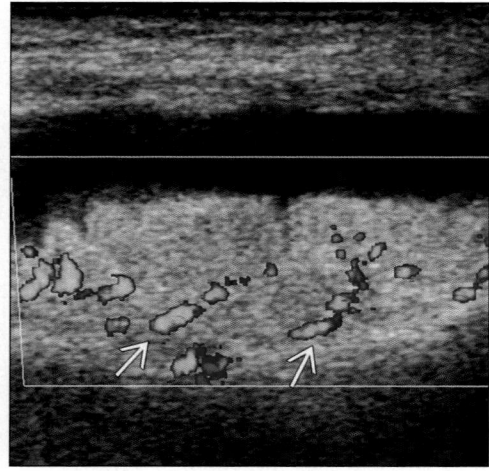

Longitudinal ultrasound of the suprapatellar region shows an anechoic joint effusion ➡, with thickened synovium ➡, just superficial to the distal femur ➡.

Power Doppler ultrasound of the thickened synovium, in the same region as the previous image, shows moderate hyperemia ➡ indicative of moderate inflammatory activity.

TERMINOLOGY

Abbreviations and Synonyms
- Rheumatoid arthritis, inflammatory arthritides, polyarthritis or polyarthropathy, connective tissue disease, juvenile inflammatory arthropathy

Definitions
- Systemic autoimmune inflammatory disorders, primarily affecting synovial membrane with secondary involvement of articular surface & bone

IMAGING FINDINGS

General Features
- Best diagnostic clue: Thickened hyperemic synovium
- Location
  - Wrist joint
  - Intercarpal joints, carpometacarpal, metacarpophalangeal (MCP), metatarsophalangeal (MTP) & interphalangeal joints
  - Elbow, shoulder, hip, knee, ankle, intertarsal joints
  - Any synovial-lined joint

- Size: From single (monoarthopathy), to few (oligoarthropathy), to many (polyarthropathy) joint involvement
- Morphology: Synovial thickening, effusion, erosions, joint space narrowing, deformity, subluxation, bony attrition, ankylosis

Ultrasonographic Findings
- Grayscale Ultrasound
  - **Effusion**
    - Sensitive, nonspecific indicator of synovitis
  - **Thickened hypoechoic synovium (pannus) commonest finding**
    - May be hyperechoic or hypoechoic depending on fluid content
    - Synovial thickening → diffuse, frond-like, or nodular
    - May resemble echogenic or hypoechoic synovial fluid
    - Joint fluid is normally anechoic
    - Precipitated fibrin seen as very small floating hyperechoic foci/debris

DDx: Inflammatory Arthritis

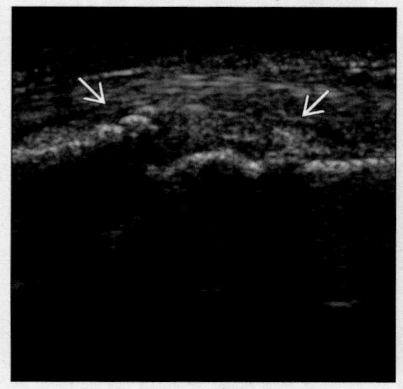

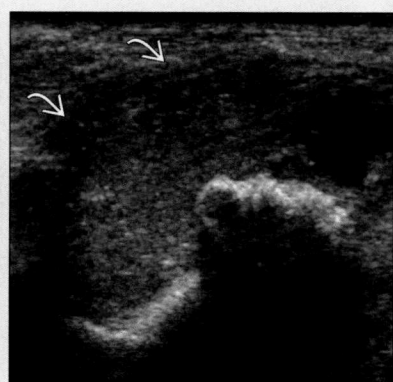

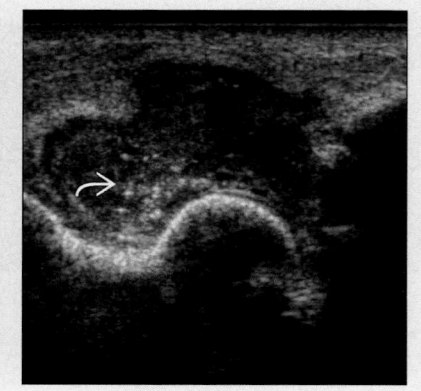

Osteoarthrosis

Septic Arthritis

Crystal Deposition

INFLAMMATORY ARTHRITIS

Key Facts

Imaging Findings
- Best diagnostic clue: Thickened hyperemic synovium
- Any synovial-lined joint
- Size: From single (monoarthopathy), to few (oligoarthropathy), to many (polyarthropathy) joint involvement
- Pattern of disease more important than individual radiographic signs
- **Thickened hypoechoic synovium (pannus) commonest finding**
- Synovial thickening → diffuse, frond-like, or nodular
- May resemble echogenic or hypoechoic synovial fluid
- Precipitated fibrin seen as very small floating hyperechoic foci/debris
- **Marginal bony erosions**

- 6.5 times more MCP erosions detected with ultrasound than radiography
- US-guided joint aspiration or injection very useful
- US accurate at detecting associated tenosynovitis, bursal distension, entrapment neuropathy
- **Color Doppler (CD) helpful in distinguishing synovial proliferation from joint fluid**
- Allows level of disease activity to be assessed
- Active pannus shows high flow on CD
- Inactive synovial proliferation → low/absent flow
- Spectral analysis: Active disease associated with decreased resistive index (RI)

Top Differential Diagnoses
- Osteoarthrosis
- Septic Arthritis
- Crystal Deposition Disease

- Ultrasound 10 times more sensitive than clinical examination at detecting early MTP joint synovitis
  - **Marginal bony erosions**
    - Ultrasound much more sensitive than radiography
    - 6.5 times more MCP erosions detected with ultrasound than radiography
    - Reproducibility of ultrasound in erosion detection is high
  - US-guided joint aspiration or injection very useful
  - US accurate at detecting associated tenosynovitis, bursal distension, entrapment neuropathy
- Color Doppler
  - **Color Doppler (CD) helpful in distinguishing synovial proliferation from joint fluid**
  - Allows level of disease activity to be assessed
    - Active pannus shows high flow on CD
    - Inactive synovial proliferation → low/absent flow
    - Grade level of synovial vascularity semiquantitatively (as absent, mild, moderate or severe) or quantitatively with computer-assisted measurement
    - Quantitative or semiquantitative assessment of synovial vascularity with micro-bubble contrast-enhanced Doppler ultrasound
    - Spectral analysis: Active disease associated with decreased resistive index (RI)

Radiographic Findings
- Radiography
  - Often negative in early stages of disease
  - Soft tissue swelling, juxta-articular osteopenia (demineralization), joint space narrowing (erosion of cartilage), marginal bony erosions, & focal bone outgrowths (protuberances)
    - Pattern of disease more important than individual radiographic signs
  - Joint subluxation (particularly small joints of fingers & toes) & distal ulna (dorsal subluxation)
  - Joint obliteration & ankylosis - particularly of carpus
  - Arthritis mutilans & joint deformity (swan-neck, buttoniere) less commonly seen nowadays with disease-modifying therapy

MR Findings
- T1WI
  - More sensitive at depicting early erosions against background of hyperintense marrow fat
  - Hypertrophied hypointense synovium
- T2WI FS
  - Shows fluid & edematous tissue (synovium, erosions, subchondral marrow, para-articular soft tissues)
  - Effusions & pannus both hyperintense & may not be readily distinguishable
  - T1-weighted & T2-fat suppressed sequences provide most information on bone erosions & edema
    - Joint space narrowing, erosions, edema graded semi-quantitatively (Outcome Measures in Rheumatology Clinical Trials, OMERACT score)
- T1 C+
  - Effusions or fluid will not enhance while pannus & acute or subacute erosions will enhance vigorously
  - Contrast-enhancement necessary to appreciate degree of synovitis
    - Segmentation subtraction of pre- & post-contrast examinations allows volume of enhancing synovium to be quantified
    - Dynamic perfusion imaging allows perfusion indices to be quantified

Imaging Recommendations
- Best imaging tool
  - Ultrasound
    - As most joints accessible & multiple joints can be examined at the same examination
- Protocol advice
  - High-resolution (≥ 10 MHz) transducer, schematic examination of each joint
    - Passive movement of joint may displace fluid not previously demonstrable
    - As well as color Doppler, probe compression can help differentiate fluid from synovium
    - Fluid displaces rather than compresses by probe compression

INFLAMMATORY ARTHRITIS

DIFFERENTIAL DIAGNOSIS

Osteoarthrosis
- Joint space narrowing with marginal osteophytosis & absence of erosions
  - Synovial proliferation & hyperemia not as pronounced in osteoarthrosis as in inflammatory arthritis
- Inflammatory osteoarthropathy characterized by small joint involvement, erosions & synovial proliferation similar to other inflammatory arthritides
  - Clinical course, radiography & laboratory tests helpful to distinguish

Septic Arthritis
- Very similar to acute inflammatory monoarthropathy
- Joint aspiration helpful

Crystal Deposition Disease
- Very similar to acute inflammatory monoarthropathy
- ± Rounded or linear echogenic foci within joint fluid, synovium or articular cartilage due to crystal deposition
- Joint aspiration helpful
  - Aspirate should be fresh & unmixed as alcohol or water will dissolve crystals

PATHOLOGY

General Features
- Epidemiology: RA incidence = 1% of population

Gross Pathologic & Surgical Features
- Bilateral, symmetrical joint involvement
- Rheumatoid arthritis primarily a disease of synovial inflammation
- Synovial inflammatory mass (pannus) leads to marginal erosions at junction of articular cartilage & bare area of bone
- Chronic synovitis/inflammation: → Capsular, ligamentous laxity & tendon attrition/rupture
- Caput ulnar syndrome
  - Laxity of ulnar carpal ligaments
  - → Dorsal subluxation of ulna → tendon attrition & tearing

Microscopic Features
- Synovial inflammation
  - Hyperplasia of synovial cells with lymphocytic & plasma cells infiltrate
  - Synovial membrane exudes fibrinous exudate
- Rheumatoid factor
  - Serum IgM antibody 70% of RA patients
  - Directed against Fc fragment of IgG
  - High titers associated with severe disease

CLINICAL ISSUES

Presentation
- Most common signs/symptoms
  - Rheumatoid arthritis: 4 of 7 criteria must be met for diagnosis

- Morning stiffness lasting > one hour
- Arthritis of three or more joints
- Arthritis of hand joints
- Symmetric arthritis
- Positive serum rheumatoid factor
- Rheumatoid nodules
- Radiographic changes
- Other signs/symptoms: Malaise, weakness, weight loss, myalgia, fever, anemia, leukopenia, thrombocytosis

Demographics
- Age
  - 25-60 years most common
  - 40-60 years - peak incidence
- Gender: M:F = 1:3

Natural History & Prognosis
- Progressive disease with exacerbations
- Progressive joint destruction
- Complications
  - Progressive joint malalignment with secondary osteoarthropathy
  - Tendon attrition & rupture
  - Median & ulnar nerve neuropathy
  - Rheumatoid nodules at pressure sites
  - Avascular necrosis
  - Pulmonary (granulomas, fibrosis, pleuritis), ocular, (episcleritis), stromal (Sjögren syndrome) & renal complications
  - Lymphadenopathy, splenomegaly (Felty syndrome)

Treatment
- Conservative
  - Non-steroidal anti-inflammatory agents
    - Inhibit prostaglandin synthesis by blocking cyclooxygenase enzymes, COX-1 & COX-2
  - Corticosteroids
    - Systemic or intra-articular
  - Disease-modifying agents
    - Methotrexate, leflunomide, etanercept, infliximab, antimalarials, gold salts, sulfasalazine, d-penicillamine, cyclosporin-A, cyclophosphamide, azathioprine
- Surgical
  - Synovectomy & tenosynovectomy
  - Tendon rupture & repair
  - Arthroplasty or arthrodesis

DIAGNOSTIC CHECKLIST

Image Interpretation Pearls
- Use Color Doppler, movement and compression to distinguish hypoechoic proliferative synovium from fluid
- Aspirate any joint fluid if septic arthritis or crystal deposition disease suspected

SELECTED REFERENCES
1. Wang SC et al: Joint sonography. Radiol Clin North Am. 37(4):653-68, 1999

INFLAMMATORY ARTHRITIS

IMAGE GALLERY

Typical

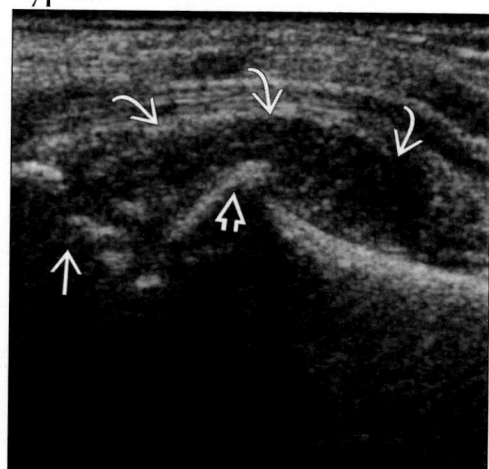
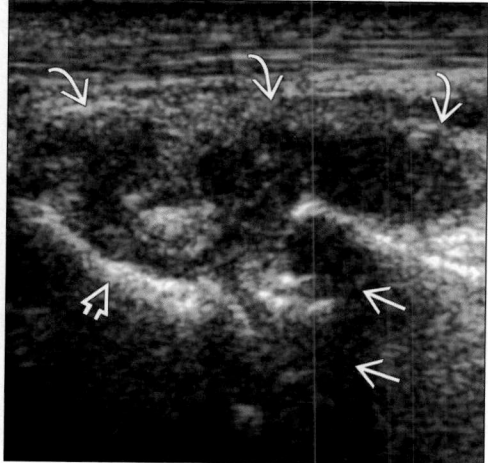

(Left) Longitudinal ultrasound shows distended capsule ⇨ on the ulnocarpal aspect of the wrist. The capsule is filled with echogenic synovium (confirmed by color Doppler imaging). Note triquetral erosion ➡ (ulnar head ➡). *(Right)* Longitudinal ultrasound shows distension of the radioscaphoid aspect of the wrist capsule ⇨ by echogenic synovium. Note erosion ➡ of the distal radial articular surface and joint space narrowing (scaphoid ➡).

Typical

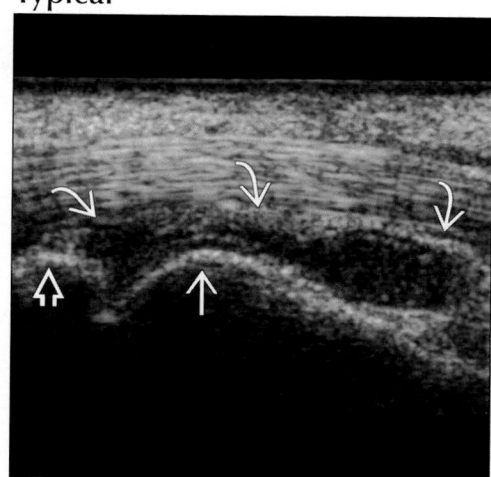
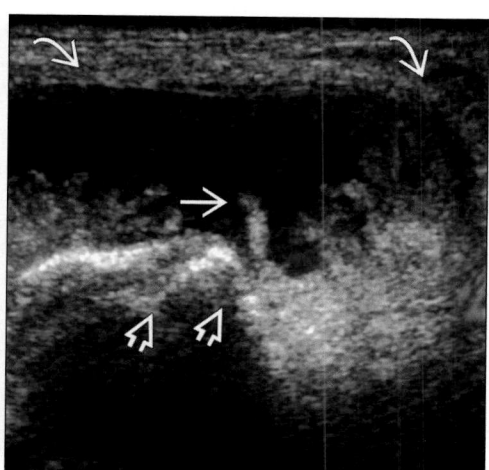

(Left) Longitudinal ultrasound shows distension of the index finger MCP joint capsule ⇨ deep to the flexor tendons. Note the metacarpal head ➡ and proximal phalanx ➡. No erosions are present. *(Right)* Oblique ultrasound shows markedly distended elbow capsule ⇨ with effusion and frond-like synovial proliferation ➡ (lateral humeral condyle ➡).

Typical

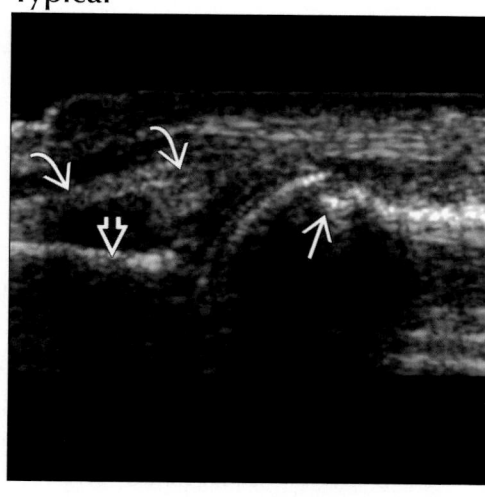
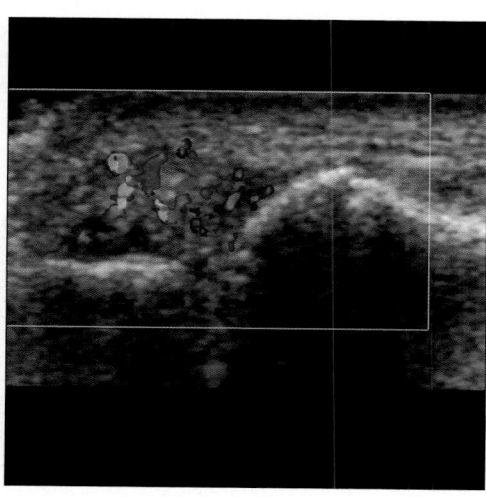

(Left) Longitudinal ultrasound of the index finger MCP joint shows erosion of the metacarpal head ➡ (not visible on radiography), mild capsular distension ⇨ and volar subluxation of the proximal phalanx ➡. *(Right)* Longitudinal color Doppler ultrasound at almost the same level as the previous image, confirms distended capsule is filled with hyperemic synovium indicating disease activity.

DEVELOPMENTAL HIP DYSPLASIA

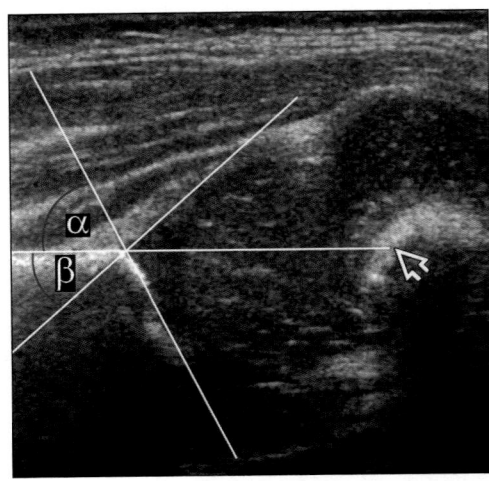

Longitudinal ultrasound shows the standard coronal view of a non-dysplastic hip, with iliac line ➡, and alpha (α) and beta (β) angles.

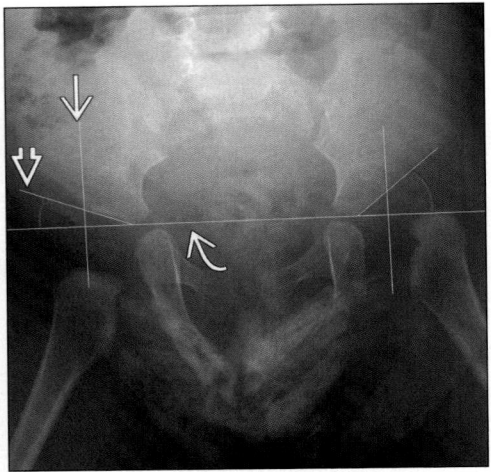

Frontal radiograph shows Hilgenreiner ➡, Perkins ➡, acetabular roof ➡ lines and acetabular index angles. There is a left acetabular dysplasia with dislocation of the femoral head.

TERMINOLOGY

Abbreviations and Synonyms
- Developmental dysplasia of hip (DDH), congenital dysplasia of hip (CDH)

Definitions
- Dysplasia of hip: Abnormal development of acetabular and femoral components of hip joint

IMAGING FINDINGS

General Features
- Best diagnostic clue: Shallow acetabulum ± malposition of femoral head
- Location
  - Left hip involvement: 60%
  - Bilateral involvement: 20%
- Size: Mild subluxation to complete dislocation
- Morphology: Ranges from shallow acetabulum to complete dislocation and false acetabulum

Ultrasonographic Findings
- Ultrasound most useful between birth & six months
  - Both static and dynamic evaluation
  - Three lines drawn to assess acetabular morphology
    - Line along straight contour of ilium
    - Line from promontory along acetabular roof for α angle
    - Line from promontory to tip of labrum for β angle
- Normal hip
  - Sharp edge to ossified acetabular roof (promontory)
  - > 50% of femoral head covered by bony acetabulum (bony coverage)
  - α angle > 60°, β angle < 55°
    - α angle more critical than β angle
- Capsular laxity: > 50% bony coverage femoral head at rest, with < 50% bone coverage on stress examination or normal movement
- Subluxation: < 50% bony coverage at rest
  - Some centres define subluxation as < 33% bony coverage and 33% → 50% as indeterminate
- Dislocation: Femoral head lies completely outside of bony acetabulum at rest

DDx: Developmental Hip Dysplasia

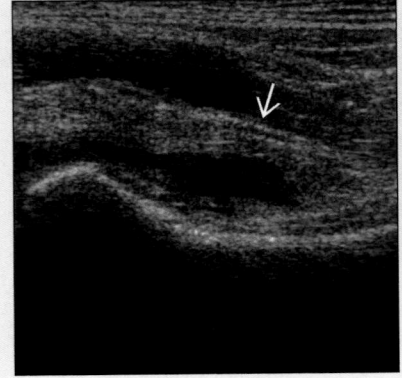

Septic Arthritis

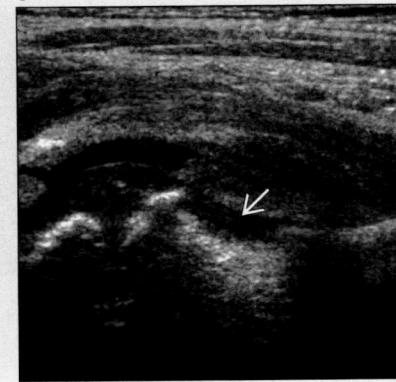

Osteomyelitis

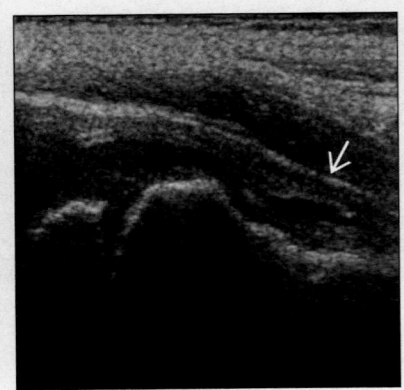

Transient Synovitis

DEVELOPMENTAL HIP DYSPLASIA

Key Facts

Imaging Findings
- Best diagnostic clue: Shallow acetabulum ± malposition of femoral head
- Several lines and angles help determine correct position of femoral head and shape of acetabulum
- Ultrasound most useful between birth & six months
- Sharp edge to ossified acetabular roof (promontory)
- α angle > 60°, β angle < 55°
- Capsular laxity: > 50% bony coverage femoral head at rest, with < 50% bone coverage on stress examination or normal movement
- Subluxation: < 50% bony coverage at rest
- Dislocation: Femoral head lies completely outside of bony acetabulum at rest

Top Differential Diagnoses
- Septic Arthritis
- Osteomyelitis
- Transient Synovitis

Pathology
- Hourglass joint capsule
- Femoral head flattened medially

Clinical Issues
- Most common signs/symptoms: Palpable clunk using Ortolani & Barlow maneuvers
- Age: Newborns
- M:F = 1:4
- Positive family history, breech presentation, oligohydramnios, torticollis, foot deformity
- Early treatment = good result with harness or splint
- Delayed treatment = irreversible dysplasia
- Decreased range of motion, adductor spasm

Radiographic Findings
- Radiography
  - Supine frontal projection with hips in neutral position
    - Only reliable after femoral capital epiphysis begins to ossify at 3-5 months
  - Hip dysplasia associated with relatively shallow acetabulum with slanting roof and relatively small superolaterally placed femoral head
    - Several lines and angles help determine correct position of femoral head and shape of acetabulum
  - Hilgenreiner line links tops of both triradiate cartilages
    - Femoral metaphysis should lie below Hilgenreiner line
  - Perkin line is perpendicular to Hilgenreiner through lateral margin of the bony acetabulum
    - Femoral capital epiphysis should lie within inner lower quadrant of intersection between Perkin and Hilgenreiner line
  - Acetabular index is angle between acetabular roof and Hilgenreiner line
    - In newborn is 30-32°, becoming smaller in older in children
  - Van Rosen line bisects axis of femoral shafts
    - Should pass though acetabula
  - Center-edge angle of Wiberg: Used for older children

MR Findings
- T2WI
  - Inverted limbus of acetabular roof seen on coronal images
    - Hypertrophy of hypointense ligamentum teres and fibrofatty pulvinar
    - Hypointense interposed iliopsoas tendon
  - Acetabular index calculation from coronal MR

Imaging Recommendations
- Best imaging tool: Ultrasound up to 6 months of age
- Protocol advice
  - Linear transducer ≥ 10 Mhz (0-2 months) and 7.5 MHz (2-6 months plus)
  - Lateral decubitus (or supine) position with standard orthogonal views
  - Coronal view: Most important view
    - Align transducer 10-15° obliquely (usually posteriorly) from coronal plane to obtain straight iliac line
    - Image showing deepest part of acetabulum, triradiate cartilage, center of femoral head and straight iliac contour: "egg in spoon" view
  - Transverse view:
    - Image showing femoral head over triradiate cartilage: "ice cream cone" view
  - Dynamic-testing (optional): Apply Barlow maneuver in attempt to displace femoral head from acetabulum during real-time imaging
    - ⇒ ± Reduced coverage of femoral head
  - Ensure that definitions of capsular laxity, subluxation and dislocation are clear to all interpreting results
  - If in doubt ⇒ repeat ultrasound in 2-4 weeks
  - ± MR helpful in situations where dislocated femoral head fails to reduce

DIFFERENTIAL DIAGNOSIS

Septic Arthritis
- Clinical signs of infection
- Hip effusion + variable capsular-synovial thickening
- Ultrasound-guided hip joint aspiration to confirm

Osteomyelitis
- Clinical signs of infection
- Effusion, if proximal femur involved
- Medullary canal edema and hyperemia on MR imaging

Transient Synovitis
- Older age group
- Capsular-synovial thickening + variable effusion

DEVELOPMENTAL HIP DYSPLASIA

PATHOLOGY

General Features
- General path comments
  - Relevant anatomy
    - Acetabulum and femoral head develop from same block of primitive mesenchymal cells
    - Cleft separates both components at 7-8 weeks
    - Hip joint separation is complete by 11 weeks
    - Acetabular and hip joint development continues after birth
    - Acetabulum particularly susceptible to remodeling first ten weeks post-natally
    - Contact between the femoral head and acetabulum necessary for acetabular development
- Genetics
  - Familial predisposition
    - 6% risk with affected sibling
    - 12% risk with affected parent
    - 26% risk with affected parent + affected sibling
- Etiology
  - Laxity of joint capsule
  - Inadequate contact between acetabulum and femoral head
- Epidemiology: Dysplasia: 0.8% newborn (0.3% boys; 1.4% girls)

Gross Pathologic & Surgical Features
- Hourglass joint capsule
- Femoral head flattened medially
- Thick + tight transverse ligament
- Deficient superior + posterior acetabular rim

Microscopic Features
- Hyperplastic ligamentum teres
- Hypertrophic pulvinar

Staging, Grading or Classification Criteria
- Modified Graf staging
  - Type Ia = mature hip, angular bony promontory, $\alpha > 60°$; $\beta < 55°$
  - Type Ib = mature hip, roundish bony promontory, $\alpha > 60°$; $\beta < 55°$
  - Type IIa = physiologic immaturity < 3 months with $\alpha = 50\text{-}60°$; $\beta = 55\text{-}77°$
  - Type IIb = immaturity > 3 months with alpha $\alpha = 50\text{-}60°$; $\beta = 55\text{-}77°$
  - Type IIc = critical hip, subluxation with $\alpha = 43\text{-}49°$; $\beta > 77°$
  - Type III = dislocated hip, $\alpha < 43°$
  - Type IV = dislocated hip, inverted labrum, $\alpha < 43°$

CLINICAL ISSUES

Presentation
- Most common signs/symptoms: Palpable clunk using Ortolani & Barlow maneuvers
- Clinical Profile
  - Ortolani maneuver
    - Hip is flexed to 90° and gently abducted while lifting thigh anteriorly
    - "Clunk" felt as dislocated femoral head reduces
  - Barlow maneuver
    - Hip is flexed to 90° and gently adducted while pushing thigh posteriorly
    - "Clunk" felt as femoral head dislocates

Demographics
- Age: Newborns
- Gender
  - M:F = 1:4
    - Females particularly susceptible to female hormone, relaxin, which may contribute to ligamentous laxity
  - Left hip 3 times as commonly affected as right hip
    - Possibly related to left occiput anterior position of most non-breech babies in utero
    - In this position, left hip lies against maternal spine which may limit abduction
- Risk factors
  - Positive family history, breech presentation, oligohydramnios, torticollis, foot deformity
    - 3% of births are breech; 8% of girls with breech birth have developmental hip dysplasia
    - Due of hip flexed, knee extended position of breech babies in utero

Natural History & Prognosis
- Prognosis
  - Early treatment = good result with harness or splint
  - Delayed treatment = irreversible dysplasia
- Decreased range of motion, adductor spasm
- Limb shortening, osteoarthrosis, avascular necrosis

Treatment
- Conservative
  - Pavlik harness +/- closed reduction (if dislocated)
- Surgical for dislocation or subluxation failing to respond to conservative treatment
  - Open reduction + spica cast
  - Adductor tenotomy + release of iliopsoas
  - Varus (derotational) vs. reconstructive osteotomy

DIAGNOSTIC CHECKLIST

Consider
- On ultrasound examination, incorrect orientation can make a deep hip appear shallow
  - Though not possible to make shallow hip appear deep
- Prognosis excellent if diagnosed & treated early, even for severe degrees of DDH

Image Interpretation Pearls
- Key to diagnosis rests on obtaining correct coronal (longitudinal) view
- Be clear with respect to your definitions of capsular laxity, subluxation and dislocation
- If in doubt, repeat ultrasound in 2-4 weeks

SELECTED REFERENCES

1. American Institute of Ultrasound in Medicine: AIUM Practice Guideline for the performance of the ultrasound examination for detection of developmental dysplasia of the hip. J Ultrasound Med. 22(10):1131-6, 2003

DEVELOPMENTAL HIP DYSPLASIA

IMAGE GALLERY

Typical

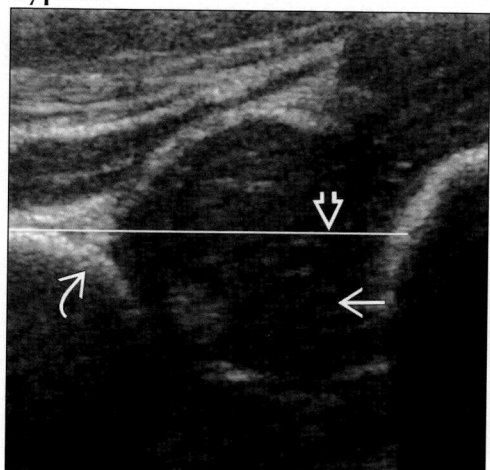

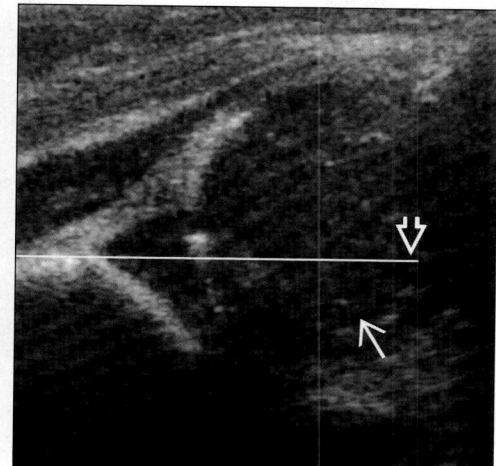

(Left) Longitudinal ultrasound shows an immature acetabulum with roundish acetabular promontory ➔. The majority of the unossified femoral head ➔ lies below the iliac line ➔. *(Right)* Longitudinal ultrasound on same patient as previous image with active hip motion, shows the majority of the femoral head ➔ lying above the iliac line ➔. This indicates capsular laxity and is common in newborns.

Typical

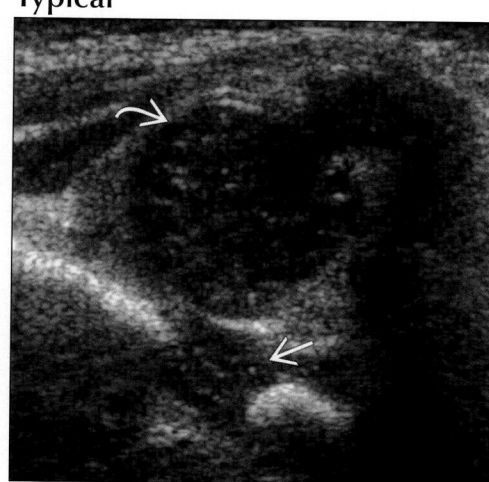

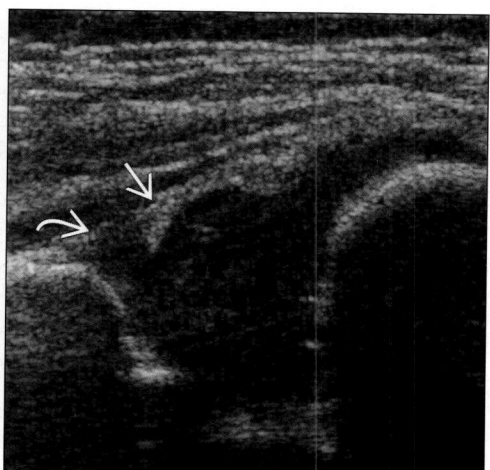

(Left) Longitudinal ultrasound of neonate shows completely dislocated femoral head ➔ lying superior to the acetabulum. The acetabulum as depicted by the triradiate cartilage ➔ is flat and has not developed. *(Right)* Longitudinal ultrasound in same patient as previous image, shows normally developed acetabulum after two months treatment in Pavlik harness. Note unossified component of the acetabulum ➔ and labrum ➔.

Typical

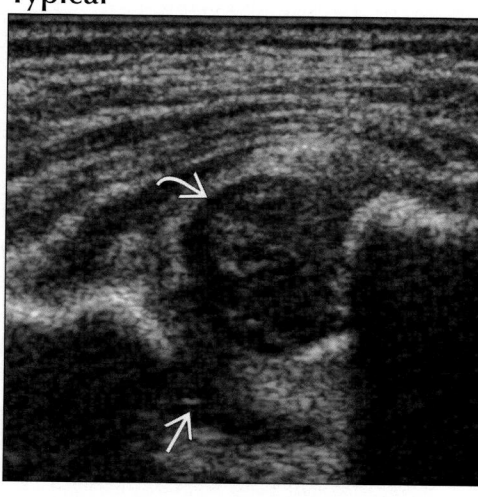

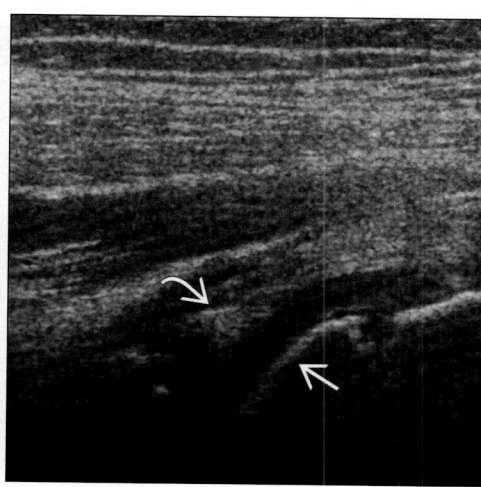

(Left) Longitudinal ultrasound shows subluxed small femoral head ➔ located primarily outside of the acetabulum. The unossified bony component of the acetabulum can be seen ➔. *(Right)* Longitudinal ultrasound of 7 month old child shows almost fully ossified femoral capital epiphysis ➔. Ultrasound does not confer much advantage over radiography at this stage. Note labrum ➔.

NERVE INJURY

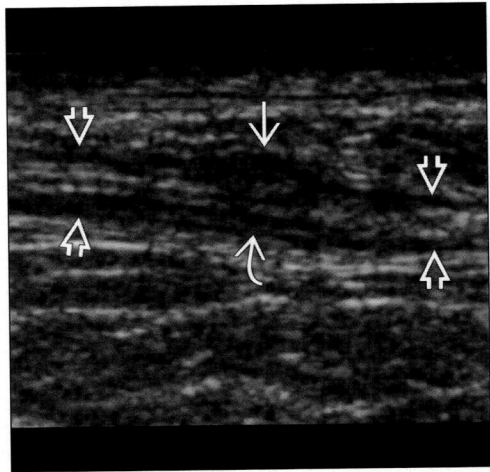

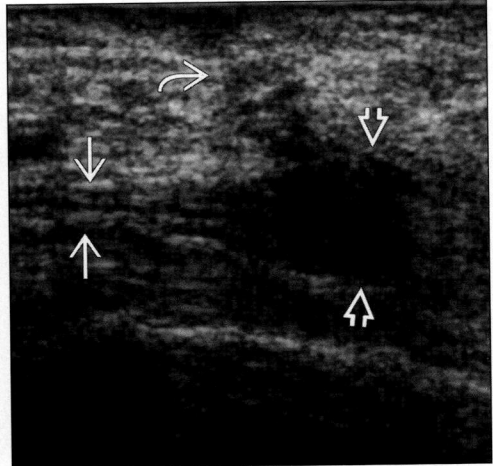

Longitudinal ultrasound shows disruption & swelling of the superficial epineurium ⇨ of the median nerve ⇨ indicating axonotmesis (~ 30% of nerve caliber affected). Deep epineurium ⇨ is intact.

Longitudinal ultrasound shows transection of the tibial nerve ⇨ following a laceration ⇨ near the ankle with a medium-sized neuroma ⇨ of the nerve stump.

TERMINOLOGY

Abbreviations and Synonyms
- Saturday night palsy, honeymooner syndrome, crutch syndrome, wheelchair syndrome = neurapraxia

Definitions
- Neurapraxia ⇒ ↓ nerve function ⇔ ion conduction block
  - Praxis = function (Greek)
- Axonotmesis = "axon-cutting" ⇒ ↓ nerve function due to disruption of axon ± sheath
  - Variable according to whether endo-, peri- or epineurium affected
- Neurotmesis = "nerve-cutting" ⇒ loss of nerve function due to disruption of entire nerve

IMAGING FINDINGS

General Features
- Best diagnostic clue: Disruption of normal fibrillar pattern of nerve + focal nerve swelling
- Location: Digital > median > ulnar > sciatic > radial

- Size
  - Ranging from marginally swollen nerve → up to about four times normal size
    - Chronic denervation → muscle atrophy
- Morphology
  - Ranges from focal nerve swelling to complete discontinuity with retraction ± neuroma
    - Slightly enlarged muscle in acute denervation → fatty atrophy with chronic denervation

Ultrasonographic Findings
- Detection of injury
  - Neurapraxia
    - Appearance of nerve & surrounding tissues usually normal
    - ± Focal swelling of nerve
  - Axonotmesis or neurotmesis
    - Disruption of continuity of nerve
    - Disruption of fibrillar pattern
    - ± Surrounding hemorrhage or edema
    - Detection in acute stage may be limited due to artifact caused by overlying wound
- Localization of injury
  - Nerves divide at inconstant levels

DDx: Nerve Injury

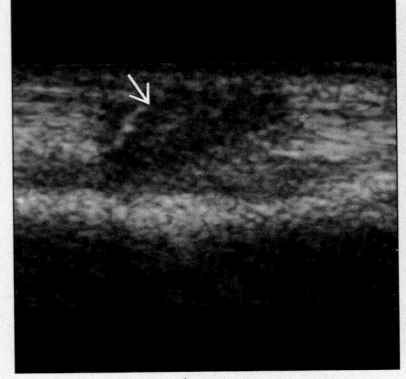

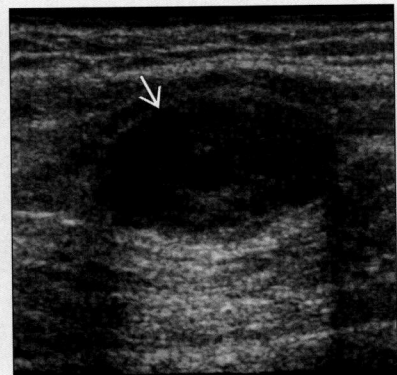

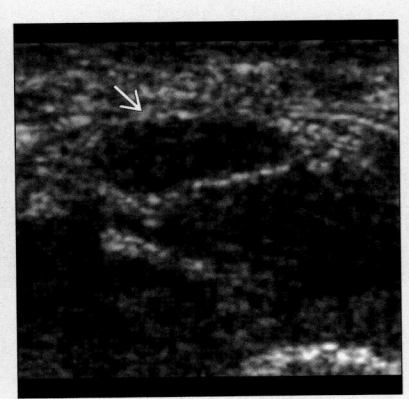

Tendon Injury   *Nerve Sheath Tumor*   *Nerve Entrapment*

NERVE INJURY

Key Facts

Terminology
- Neurapraxia ⇒ ↓ nerve function ⇔ ion conduction block
- Axonotmesis = "axon-cutting" ⇒ ↓ nerve function due to disruption of axon ± sheath
- Neurotmesis = "nerve-cutting" ⇒ loss of nerve function due to disruption of entire nerve

Imaging Findings
- Best diagnostic clue: Disruption of normal fibrillar pattern of nerve + focal nerve swelling
- Location: Digital > median > ulnar > sciatic > radial
- Acute/subacute denervation → ± mild muscle swelling
- Chronic denervation → muscle atrophy
- Ultrasound best to show nerve injury
- MR best to show effect of denervation on muscle

- Observe caliber, integrity of nerve, echogenicity & stiffness of perineural fat
- If nerve abnormality evident → align transducer along long axis of nerve
- Observe nerve movement when passively moving adjacent joints

Top Differential Diagnoses
- Tendon Injury
- Nerve Sheath Tumor
- Nerve Entrapment

Diagnostic Checklist
- In general, ultrasound probably slightly overestimates rather than underestimates nerve injury
- Check for integrity of epineurium followed by integrity of individual fascicles, if visible

---

- ○ Ultrasound can depict bifurcation level & confirm if main or distal branch affected
- Type of injury
  - ○ Axonotmesis = incomplete discontinuity of nerve
  - ○ Neurotmesis = complete discontinuity of nerve ± retraction
    - Retraction of nerves < tendon retraction
    - Up to few cm
    - Nerve injury overlying mobile joint → > retraction
- Presence of perineural fibrosis
  - ○ Irregular hypoechoic tissue replacing echogenic perineural fat
  - ○ Focal swelling of nerve
  - ○ ± Tethering of nerve
  - ○ ± Reduced motility of nerve on moving part
- Continuity of nerve post-operatively
  - ○ Continuity of epineurial sheath
    - ± Continuity of nerve fascicles
- Presence of neuroma
  - ○ Quite common finding
  - ○ Hypoechoic rounded or ovoid mass at site of disrupted nerve
  - ○ Connected to proximal end of severed nerve
  - ○ Largely avascular
  - ○ May be small & intraneural
    - Small neuromas may be difficult to distinguish from nodular fibrosis
- Muscle denervation
  - ○ Mild swelling & increased echogenicity of affected muscle seen after two weeks
    - Due to capillary dilatation & muscle edema
  - ○ Later → decreased muscle bulk & increased echogenic fat within & between muscle bundles
    - Due to muscle atrophy & fatty replacement

MR Findings
- T1WI
  - ○ Acute/subacute denervation → ± mild muscle swelling
  - ○ Chronic denervation → muscle atrophy
- T2WI FS
  - ○ Acute/subacute denervation → hyperintense muscle
    - ± Mild increase in muscle size

- T1 C+: Acute/subacute denervation → enhancement of denervated muscle
- Muscle edema & enhancement may be seen 24 hours after denervation
  - ○ Increasing muscle edema parallels increase in muscle enhancement
    - Both probably reflect ↑ capillary engorgement & ↑ blood volume within affected muscle
  - ○ Pattern of muscle involvement can predict likely nerve injury
- Muscle edema & enhancement reverse with reinnervation of muscle

Imaging Recommendations
- Best imaging tool
  - ○ Ultrasound best to show nerve injury
    - High resolution
    - Easy orientation along long & short axes of nerve
  - ○ MR best to show effect of denervation on muscle
- Protocol advice
  - ○ Scan transversely along course of nerve
    - Easiest plane to trace course of nerve
  - ○ Observe caliber, integrity of nerve, echogenicity & stiffness of perineural fat
  - ○ If nerve abnormality evident → align transducer along long axis of nerve
    - Best plane to appreciate continuity & discontinuity of epineurium & fascicles
    - If incomplete discontinuity → estimate degree of transection (e.g., 10%, 40%, 90%)
    - Measure gap, if present
  - ○ Observe nerve movement when passively moving adjacent joints

---

DIFFERENTIAL DIAGNOSIS

Tendon Injury
- Sometimes torn in conjunction with nerve
- Discontinuity of tendon fibers

Nerve Sheath Tumor
- May mimic traumatic neuroma

NERVE INJURY

- Entering & exiting nerve
- Traumatic neuromas less vascular

Nerve Entrapment
- Typical locations
- Nerve swelling proximal to level of entrapment
- Leads to demyelination (neurapraxia) & secondary changes in affected muscle

PATHOLOGY

General Features
- General path comments
  - Relevant anatomy
    - Axon ± covered by myelin (nerve fiber)
    - Endoneurium = loose connective tissue between fibers
    - Perineurial sheath groups fibers into fascicles
    - Epineurium encircles & runs between fascicles; outer layers of epineurium condensed into sheath
  - Fascicles within large peripheral nerve continually divide & reunite (fascicular plexus)
    - Particularly in lumbar & brachial plexuses
- Etiology
  - Blunt or penetrating trauma
    - ± Iatrogenic; fracture repair & fixation, arthroscopy, carpal tunnel release, surgical exploration
- Epidemiology
  - 2-3% patients admitted to level I trauma center
  - > Dominant limb

Gross Pathologic & Surgical Features
- Axonal injury → Wallerian degeneration → regeneration

Microscopic Features
- Axonal apoptosis followed by phagocytosis
- Schwann cell proliferation (bands of Bunger)
- Sprouting axonal filopodia → growth cone, regulated by neurotrophic & neurotopic mediators

Staging, Grading or Classification Criteria
- Sunderland grading system
- Grade 1: Neurapraxia
  - Neural tubes intact
    - No axonal regeneration required
- Grade 2-4: Axonotmesis
  - Grade 2: Axon disrupted but endo-, peri- & epineurium intact
    - Regenerating axons always reach original motor & sensory targets
  - Grade 3: Axons & endoneurium disrupted but peri- & epineurium intact
    - Regenerating axons may not reach original motor & sensory targets
  - Grade 4: Axons, endo- & perineurium disrupted but epineurium intact
    - Regenerating axons usually do not reach original motor & sensory targets
- Grade 5: Neurotmesis
  - Complete transection of all neural tubes

- Regenerating axons invariably do not reach original motor & sensory targets
  - Classification system difficult to apply clinically as mixed injury common

CLINICAL ISSUES

Presentation
- Most common signs/symptoms: Weakness ± numbness ± pain
- Other signs/symptoms
  - Type of transection, nerve function fails sequentially
  - Motor → proprioception → touch → temperature → pain → autonomic
    - Recovery in reverse order

Demographics
- Age: > Young adults
- Gender: M:F = 2.2:1

Natural History & Prognosis
- Neurapraxia ⇒ excellent prognosis
- Axonotmesis & neurotmesis ⇒ variable prognosis depending on extent of injury
- Axons regenerate at ~ 1 mm/day (slower in older patients)

Treatment
- Neurapraxia: Supportive treatment
- Axonotmesis or neurotmesis
  - Immediate or delayed repair
    - Immediate requires clean wound, no crush injury, good vascular supply & soft tissue coverage
  - End-to-end closure
  - Nerve graft ± vascularization
  - Nerve transfer

DIAGNOSTIC CHECKLIST

Consider
- Ultrasound is very good at localizing site of injury in axonotmesis/neurotmesis & detecting perineural fibrosis/neuroma
  - In general, ultrasound probably slightly overestimates rather than underestimates nerve injury

Image Interpretation Pearls
- Check for integrity of epineurium followed by integrity of individual fascicles, if visible

SELECTED REFERENCES

1. Peer S et al: Sonographic evaluation of primary peripheral nerve repair. J Ultrasound Med. 22(12):1317-22, 2003
2. Lee SK et al: Peripheral nerve injury and repair. J Am Acad Orthop Surg. 8(4):243-52, 2000
3. Martinoli C et al: Ultrasonography of peripheral nerves. Semin Ultrasound CT MR. 21(3):205-13, 2000

IMAGE GALLERY

Typical

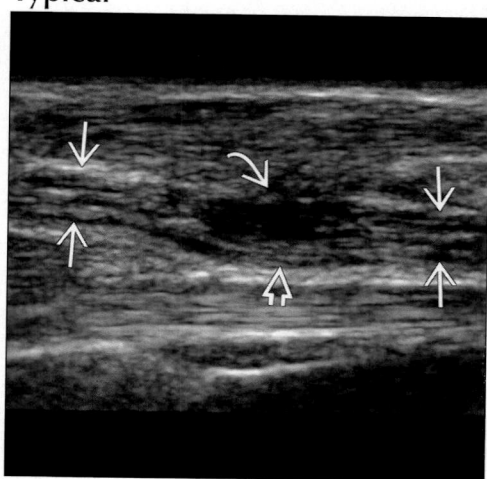
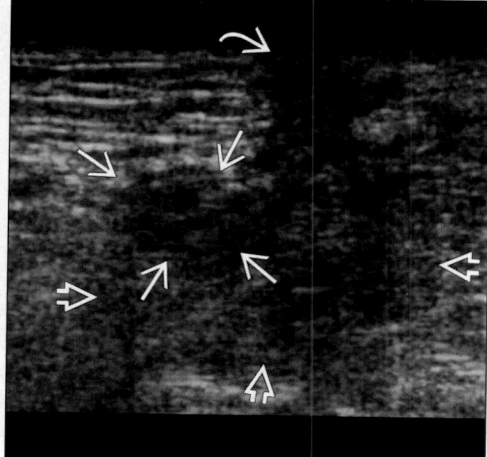

(Left) Longitudinal ultrasound shows axonotmesis of the median nerve ➡ with disruption of the superficial aspect of the nerve ➡. About 50% of the nerve caliber is affected. The deep epineurium ➡ is intact. *(Right)* Transverse ultrasound shows a large amount of fibrosis ➡ partially encasing the swollen ulnar nerve ➡ in mid-arm region. Path of the laceration ➡.

Typical

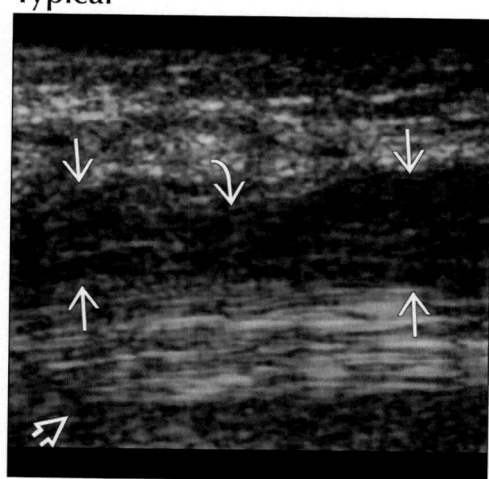
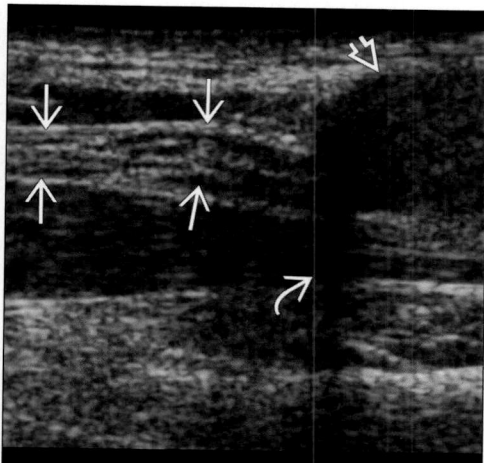

(Left) Longitudinal ultrasound shows swollen median nerve with indistinct fascicles ➡ and focal disruption ➡. Oblique incomplete laceration involved 70% of the nerve fascicles at surgery (flexor tendon ➡). *(Right)* Longitudinal ultrasound shows a neuroma ➡ at the distal end of the transected median nerve ➡. Note edge shadowing ➡ at the proximal end of the neuroma.

Typical

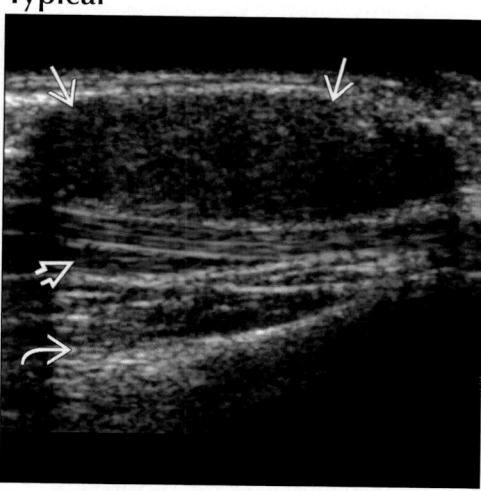
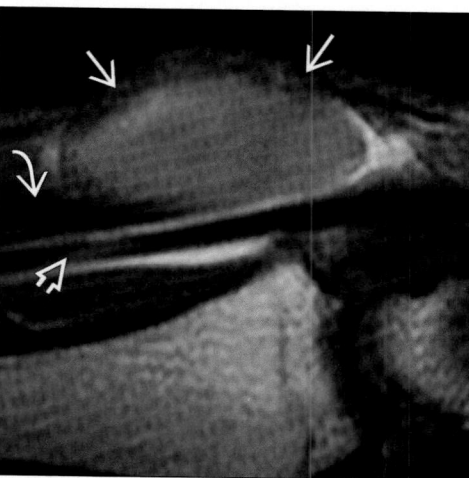

(Left) Longitudinal ultrasound immediately distal to the previous image shows an ovoid neuroma ➡ of the proximal transected median nerve. Note mild posterior enhancement ➡ (underlying flexor tendon ➡). *(Right)* Longitudinal T2WI MR at the same location shows the stump neuroma ➡ of the median nerve ➡. A normal underlying flexor tendon ➡ is seen.

13

65

PERIPHERAL NERVE SHEATH TUMOR

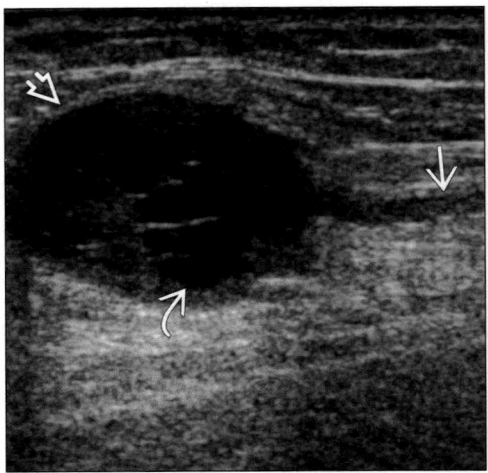

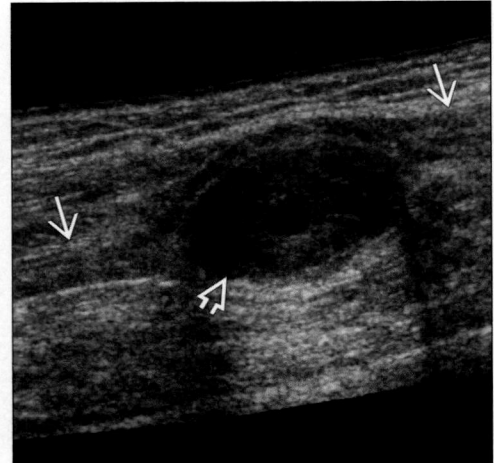

Longitudinal ultrasound shows a tumor ➡ of the medial sural cutaneous nerve with several cystic areas ➡. The nerve ➡ courses distally from tumor.

Longitudinal ultrasound of the posterior tibial nerve ➡ shows a tumor ➡ with central cystic areas. The tumor lies eccentric to the main bulk of the nerve. Histology: Schwannoma.

TERMINOLOGY

Abbreviations and Synonyms
- Peripheral nerve sheath tumors divided into
  - Schwannoma (i.e., neurilemmoma)
  - Neurofibroma

Definitions
- Benign tumors arising from peripheral nerves

IMAGING FINDINGS

General Features
- Best diagnostic clue: Well-defined hypoechoic mass arising from nerve, occasionally heterogeneous
- Location: Along any peripheral nerve, intermuscular > subcutaneous > intramuscular
- Size
  - Usually < 5 cm
    - Larger tumors from large nerves (up to 20 cm)
  - Nerve tumors usually grow slowly until critical mass reached and then largely stop growing

- Morphology: Soft tissue mass located alongside vascular bundle

Ultrasonographic Findings
- Well-defined, largely homogeneous, hypoechoic mass
  - Occasionally heterogeneous
    - Heterogenicity related to myxoid stroma, hemorrhage, fibrosis or calcification
    - Hemorrhage may lead to sudden increase in tumor size clinically
- Arise from nerve
  - Typically fusiform, oblong or lobulated shape and orientated along long axis of nerve
    - Nerve sheath tumors may appear to align centrally or eccentrically along course of nerve
  - Nerve entering or exiting from tumor seen in majority (90%) using high resolution transducers
    - Nerve often shows slight enlargement just proximal and distal to tumor
    - When nerve sheath tumor arises from small peripheral nerves, entering/exiting nerve may not be seen

DDx: Nerve Tumors

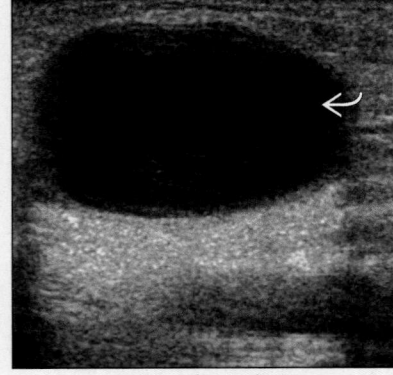

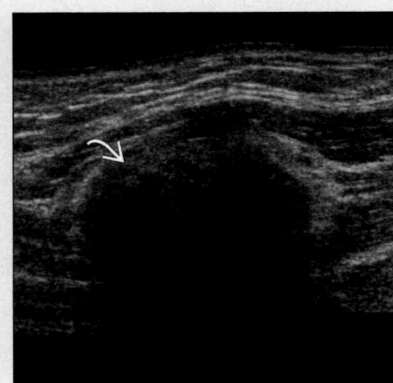

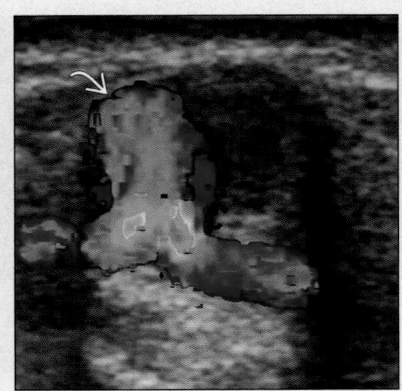

Lymph Node

Soft Tissue Tumor

Pseudoaneurysm

PERIPHERAL NERVE SHEATH TUMOR

Key Facts

Imaging Findings

- Best diagnostic clue: Well-defined hypoechoic mass arising from nerve, occasionally heterogeneous
- Heterogenicity related to myxoid stroma, hemorrhage, fibrosis or calcification
- Typically fusiform, oblong or lobulated shape and orientated along long axis of nerve
- Nerve sheath tumors may appear to align centrally or eccentrically along course of nerve
- Nerve entering or exiting from tumor seen in majority (90%) using high resolution transducers
- Nerve often shows slight enlargement just proximal and distal to tumor
- Tumors often contain "cystic" areas
- Posterior enhancement very common (70%)

- Occasionally tumor has echogenic rim due to fibrous capsule, fibrous pseudocapsule or compression of surrounding fat
- Usually are moderately vascular with central irregular vascular pattern
- Ultrasound diagnosis of nerve sheath tumor is based on consortium of features rather than single feature
- Ultrasound appearances of schwannoma and neurofibroma overlap considerably
- Best imaging tool: Ultrasound since diagnosis is generally feasible based on ultrasound findings alone

Top Differential Diagnoses

- Lymph Node
- Soft Tissue Tumor (Non-Neurogenic)
- Pseudoaneurysm

- Compressed fascial planes may simulate a nerve on longitudinal imaging; always confirm on transverse plane
- Arises within neurovascular bundle
  - Some small nerves do not have readily identifiable accompanying vascular bundle
- Tumors often contain "cystic" areas
  - Degenerative "ancient" schwannomas are predominantly "cystic"
  - "Cystic" areas can be due to myxoid accumulation, previous hemorrhage or necrosis
    - Hemorrhage into "cystic" or solid part of tumor may lead to sudden increase in tumor size
- Posterior enhancement very common (70%)
  - ± "Edge-shadowing" at edge of tumor
    - Pseudo "edge-shadowing" results from posterior enhancement through main part of tumor
- Occasionally tumor has echogenic rim due to fibrous capsule, fibrous pseudocapsule or compression of surrounding fat
- Vascular pattern varied
  - Usually are moderately vascular with central irregular vascular pattern
    - Some display predominantly peripheral vascularity
    - Some do not have any demonstrable vascularity on color Doppler imaging
  - Vascularity may blanch with transducer pressure
- Ultrasound diagnosis of nerve sheath tumor is based on consortium of features rather than single feature
  - Ultrasound features are nearly always typical enough to make diagnosis without need for biopsy
    - Biopsy may be very painful
- Ultrasound appearances of schwannoma and neurofibroma overlap considerably
  - Do not focus on making this histological distinction on imaging
  - Report on centric/eccentric location of tumor to parent nerve, if visible, rather than likely cell type

MR Findings

- T1WI: Soft tissue mass isointense to muscle
- T2WI

- Well-defined fusiform mass hyperintense to muscle and fat
- "Target sign": Center of low signal (due to collagen and condensed Schwann cells)
- Neural tail
- T1 C+
  - Variable enhancement
  - Often peripheral enhancement
- Nerve root involvement
  - Intradural extramedullary mass
  - Well-defined dumbbell shaped mass (extradural component extends through neural foramen)
    - Only extradural component seen on ultrasound
  - Widening of neural foramen
- Peripheral nerve involvement
  - Related to neurovascular bundle, nerve entering and exiting mass
  - Peripheral rim of fat ("split-fat" sign)
  - May cause displacement of associated neurovascular bundle
  - Large masses may cause venous obstruction and hypertrophy of feeding vessels
- MR appearances of schwannoma and neurofibroma overlap considerably

Imaging Recommendations

- Best imaging tool: Ultrasound since diagnosis is generally feasible based on ultrasound findings alone
- Protocol advice
  - High frequency (10 MHz) transducer
    - Use copious gel and stand-off transducer technique when assessing vascularity of more superficial tumors

DIFFERENTIAL DIAGNOSIS

Lymph Node

- Reactive node usually has distinguishing features
- Malignant or lymphomatous node may simulate nerve sheath tumor
  - Nodes do not have entering or exiting nerve

PERIPHERAL NERVE SHEATH TUMOR

○ Nerve sheath tumors arising from small nerves do not occur at sites of adenopathy

Soft Tissue Tumor (Non-Neurogenic)
• Does not have entering or exiting nerve
• Does not have consortium of features typical of neural tumor

Pseudoaneurysm
• Color Doppler features distinguish with certainty

PATHOLOGY

General Features
• General path comments
  ○ Schwannoma thought to arise from Schwann cells; myelin-producing neuroglial cells present along peripheral axons
  ○ Neurofibroma thought to arise from loose connective tissue between nerve fibers, especially endoneurium
• Genetics
  ○ Neurofibromatosis type 1 (NF-1), Von Recklinghausen disease
    ▪ Autosomal dominant, common genetic disorder
    ▪ High rate of penetrance
    ▪ 50% cases arise from new mutation
    ▪ Genetic mutation on Nf1 gene chromosome 17
    ▪ Nf1 gene encodes for neurofibromin, which suppresses growth stimulator Ras
• Epidemiology
  ○ Schwannoma: 5% of all benign soft tissue tumors
  ○ Neurofibroma: Slightly more than 5% of all benign soft tissue tumors
• Associated abnormalities
  ○ NF-1: Neurofibromatosis
    ▪ Skeletal abnormalities, kyphoscoliosis, tibial pseudoarthrosis, rib deformity, meningocele, optic nerve glioma, astrocytoma

Gross Pathologic & Surgical Features
• Schwannoma
  ○ True capsule composed of epineurium
  ○ For large nerves, tumor tends to lie eccentric to parent nerve with nerve displaced to periphery of mass
    ▪ For small nerves, tumor may visually obliterate parent nerve
  ○ Tend to be more prone to myxoid degeneration, hemorrhage and calcification
• Neurofibroma
  ○ Firm, gray-white shiny mass often without capsule
  ○ Lesion often cannot be separated from parent nerve
  ○ Extension of tumor outside epineurium of small nerves
  ○ Plexiform neurofibroma: Multifocal myxoid lesions, "bag of worms", diagnostic of NF-1

Microscopic Features
• Schwannoma
  ○ Intermixed Antoni A cells: Cellular, arranged in short bundles or interlacing fascicles

○ Antoni B cells: Less cellular and organized, more myxoid component
• Neurofibroma
  ○ Does not contain Antoni A or B cells
  ○ Composed of interlacing bundles of spindle cells, fibroblasts, with involvement of nerve fibers
  ○ Immunohistochemistry: S-100 expression typically positive

CLINICAL ISSUES

Presentation
• Most common signs/symptoms: Slowly growing painless mass with positive Tinel sign
• Clinical Profile
  ○ Neurofibroma associated with NF-1: Neurofibromatosis, Lisch nodules, café-au-lait spots
    ▪ Only 10% of patients with neurofibroma have NF-1

Demographics
• Age: 20-30 years
• Gender: M:F = 1:1

Natural History & Prognosis
• Schwannoma: Recurrence unusual
  ○ Malignant change extremely rare
• Neurofibroma
  ○ Malignant change occurs in 4% of NF-1 patients
    ▪ Occurs in plexiform neurofibromas, rare in solitary tumors
  ○ Increase in size, pain, neurological deficit clinically and heterogenicity on ultrasound or MR imaging used as predictors of malignancy
    ▪ Not accurate predictors since may result from active growth or bleeding into benign tumor
  ○ PET imaging more accurate in predicting malignancy in plexiform neurofibromas

Treatment
• Surgical excision of symptomatic lesions
• Schwannoma
  ○ Resection with sparing of associated nerve
• Neurofibroma
  ○ Resection with excision of parent nerve
    ▪ Excision of parent nerve necessary as inseparable from tumor
  ○ Incomplete excision of neurologically important nerves to minimize neurological impairment

DIAGNOSTIC CHECKLIST

Consider
• Nerve sheath tumor, even if parent nerve not seen, provided other ultrasound features are compatible

SELECTED REFERENCES
1. Beggs I: Pictorial review: imaging of peripheral nerve tumours. Clin Radiol. 52(1):8-17, 1997

PERIPHERAL NERVE SHEATH TUMOR

IMAGE GALLERY

Typical

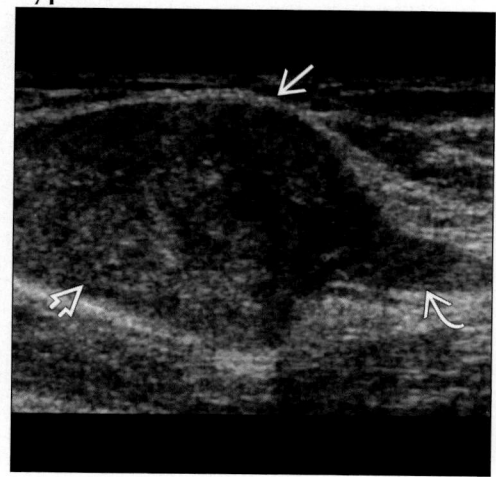
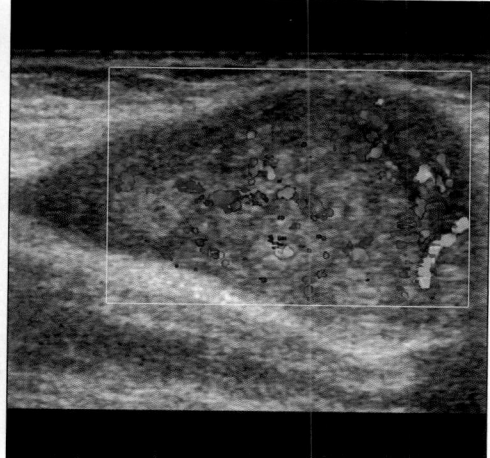

(Left) Longitudinal ultrasound shows a large tumor of the ulnar nerve ⮞ in the forearm. The tumor seems to lie eccentric to the nerve ⮞. Surrounding compressed tissues ⮞ are echogenic. *(Right)* Longitudinal color Doppler ultrasound of the same ulnar nerve tumor, shows typical prominent chaotic vascularity of a nerve sheath tumor.

Typical

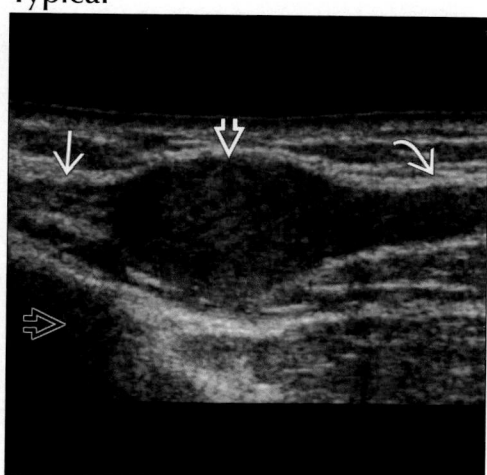
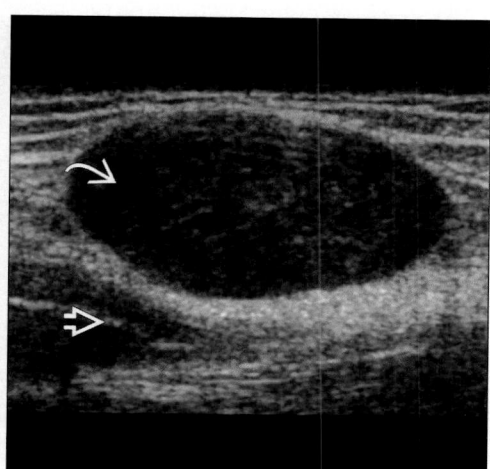

(Left) Longitudinal ultrasound shows an ulnar nerve schwannoma posterior to the medial epicondyle ⮞. Note the normal caliber fibrillar nerve proximal ⮞, and thickened hypoechoic nerve ⮞ distal to the tumor ⮞. *(Right)* Oblique ultrasound shows a schwannoma of subcutaneous nerve of the thigh. No nerve is visible proximally or distally. Shape, hypoechogenicity, cystic areas ⮞ and posterior enhancement ⮞ are nevertheless typical.

Typical

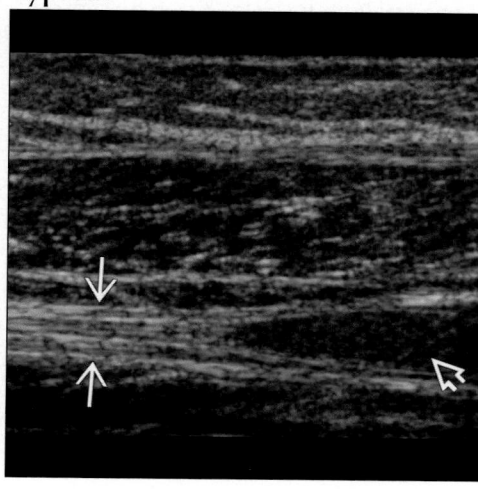
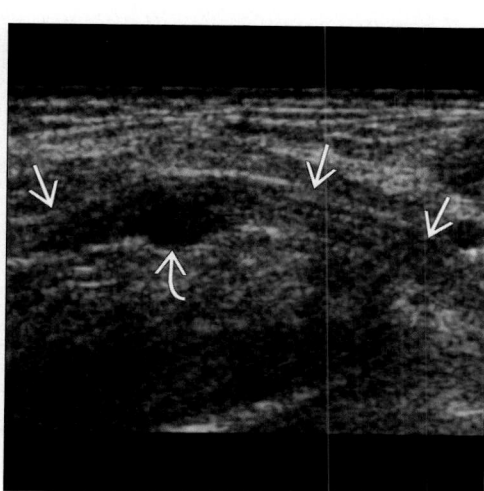

(Left) Longitudinal ultrasound in a young patient with neurofibromatosis shows a tumor ⮞ extending centrally within the tibial nerve ⮞ in the calf. *(Right)* Oblique ultrasound in a patient with tarsal tunnel syndrome shows a small nerve sheath tumor ⮞, arising eccentrically from the tibial nerve ⮞ at the ankle.

Typical

(Left) Transverse ultrasound shows a large extraforaminal schwannoma ➡ of the C7 nerve with a neural tail ➡ extending into C6/7 neural foramen. *(Right)* Longitudinal ultrasound with extended scan plane shows a lobulated schwannoma ➡ extending along and expanding the tibial nerve ⇶ in the calf.

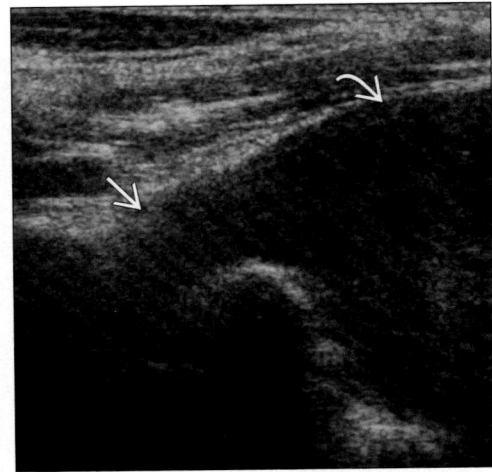
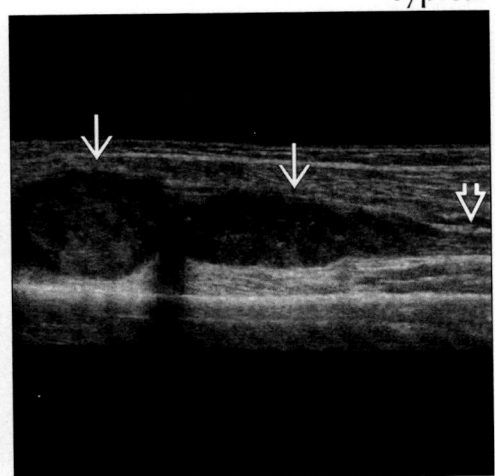

Typical

(Left) Longitudinal ultrasound shows several small to medium-sized cystic areas ➡ within the matrix of a sciatic nerve sheath tumor. These areas of myxoid accumulation are typical of nerve sheath tumors. *(Right)* Transverse color Doppler ultrasound of the axilla shows a schwannoma of the median nerve with minimal demonstrable vascularity ➡. Adjacent vascular bundle ➡.

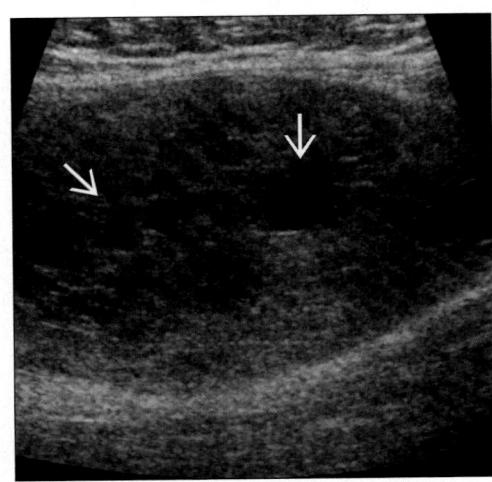
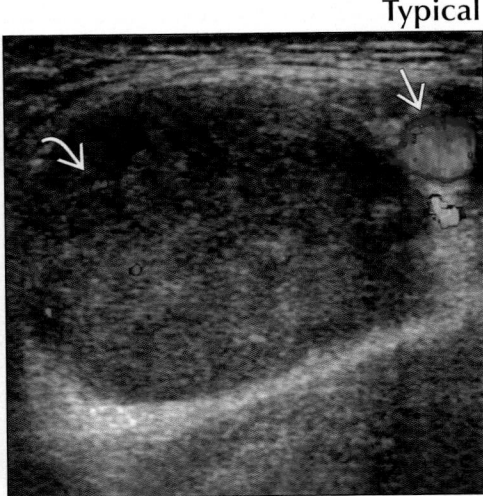

Variant

(Left) Longitudinal ultrasound shows speckled ➡ echotexture within an ulnar neurofibroma. Shape, location, hypoechogenicity, cystic areas ➡ and posterior enhancement ⇶ are typical. *(Right)* Longitudinal ultrasound in a patient with neurofibromatosis shows a tumor of the posterior interosseous nerve, with featureless echotexture and a distinct echogenic rim ➡.

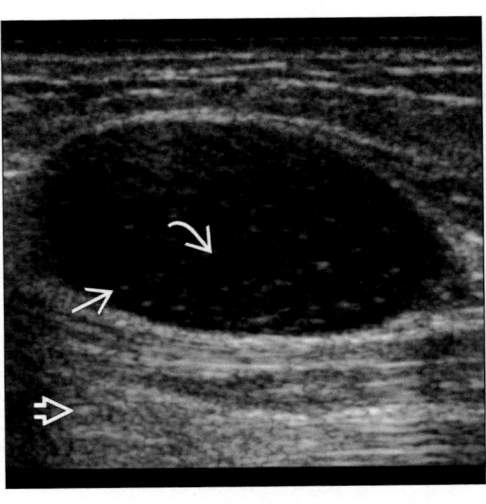
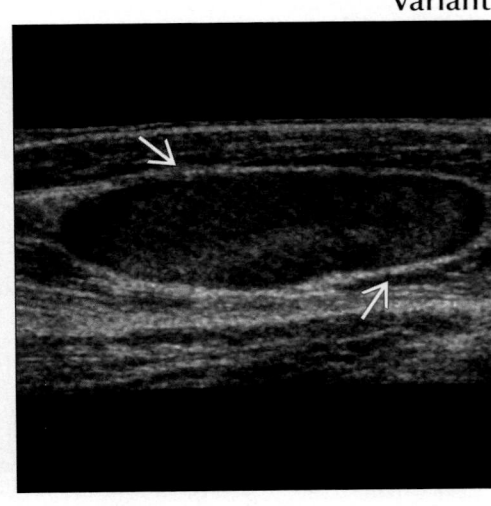

PERIPHERAL NERVE SHEATH TUMOR

Typical

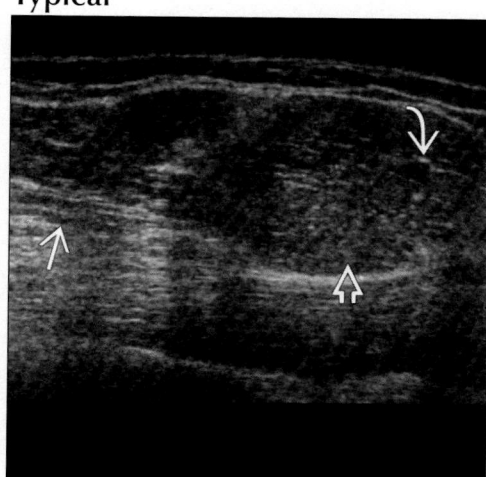
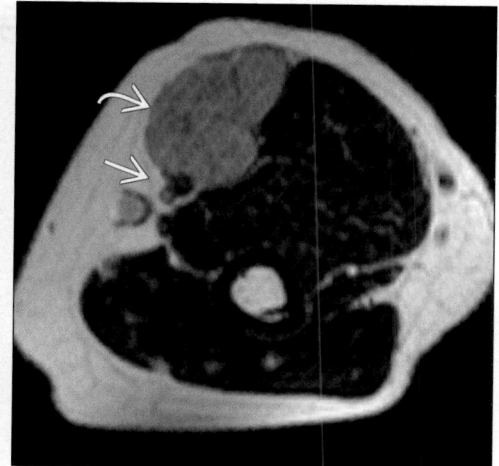

(Left) Longitudinal ultrasound shows an isoechoic, slightly lobulated tumor ➡ of the median nerve in the arm. The nerve ➡ enters the deep aspect of the tumor. Note cystic area ➡ and minimal posterior enhancement. *(Right)* Axial T2WI MR shows a large lobulated median nerve tumor ➡ located alongside the vascular bundle ➡ in the mid-arm.

Variant

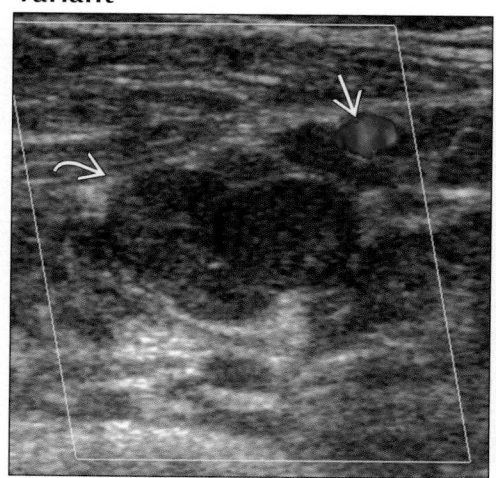
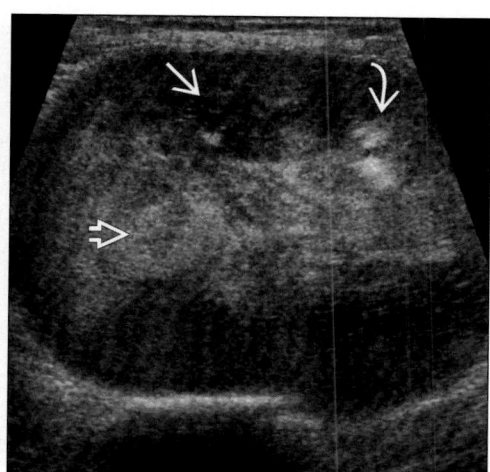

(Left) Transverse ultrasound shows a lobulated schwannoma of the tibial nerve ➡ at the distal calf. No tumor vascularity demonstrable. *(Vascular bundle ➡). (Right)* Longitudinal ultrasound shows a large heterogeneous peroneal nerve schwannoma with hypoechoic cystic areas ➡. Hyperechoic areas represent calcification ➡ and hemorrhage ➡.

Variant

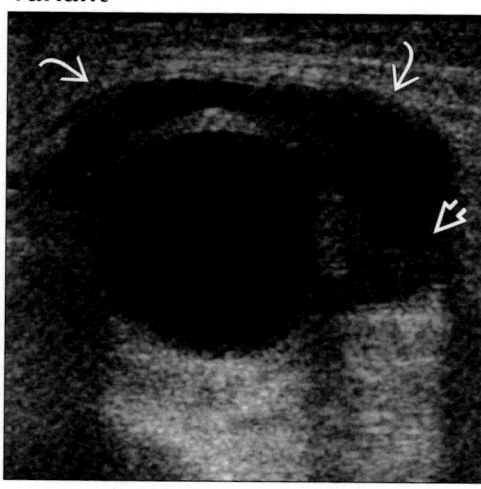
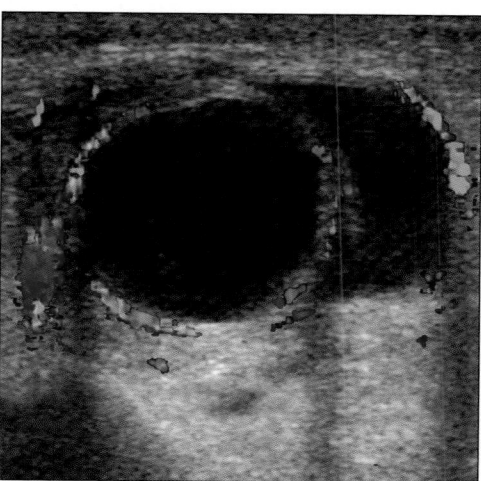

(Left) Transverse ultrasound shows a largely degenerated, cystic nerve sheath tumor ➡ of the peroneal nerve, with recent increase in size due to hemorrhage. Note hemorrhagic debris at the base of the cyst ➡. *(Right)* Transverse ultrasound at the same location as the previous image, shows moderate peripheral vascularity of the tumor.

CARPAL TUNNEL SYNDROME

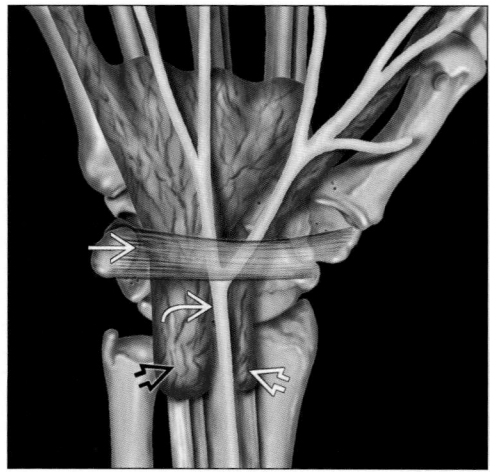

Longitudinal graphic shows the median nerve ⇒ deep to the flexor retinaculum ⇒ and superficial to tendons contained within the ulnar ⇒ and radial ⇒ bursae. The nerve usually divides just beyond the tunnel outlet.

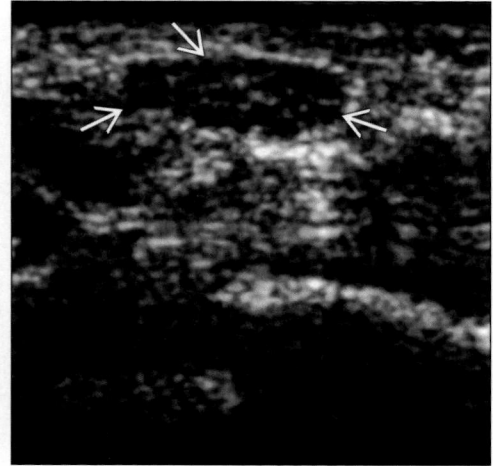

Transverse ultrasound shows an enlarged (14 mm²) median nerve ⇒, located just proximal to the carpal tunnel. Nerve area ≥ 12 mm² is a positive predictor for CTS.

TERMINOLOGY

Abbreviations and Synonyms
- Carpal tunnel syndrome (CTS)

Definitions
- Symptoms secondary to compression of median nerve at carpal tunnel
  - Most common entrapment neuropathy

IMAGING FINDINGS

General Features
- Best diagnostic clue: Swollen median nerve proximal to and within carpal tunnel
- Location: Immediately adjacent to, and deep to flexor retinaculum
- Size: Nerve cross-sectional area varies from 5 mm² to 25 mm² or greater
- Morphology: Hourglass-type appearance of median nerve due to alternating swelling and compression

Ultrasonographic Findings
- Swelling of median nerve just proximal to, within and just beyond carpal tunnel
- Measurements obtained at three points; proximal to tunnel, at tunnel inlet, and outlet
  - More swollen median nerve, more likely possibility of carpal tunnel syndrome
- No agreed cutoff point to define enlarged cross-sectional area of median nerve
  - Rigid criteria not likely to be useful in clinical practice
    - Especially when subject to known inter- and intra-observer measurement error ± inter-population variation
  - Most reliable measures yet to be established
    - Combination of several criteria may prove most useful
- If median nerve cross-sectional area ≥ 12 mm², at any measurement point, strong positive predictor of CTS
- If median nerve cross-sectional area ≤ 9 mm², at all measurement points, strong negative predictor of CTS

DDx: Carpal Tunnel Syndrome

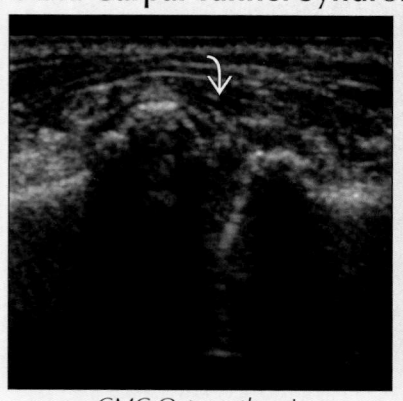

CMC Osteoarthrosis

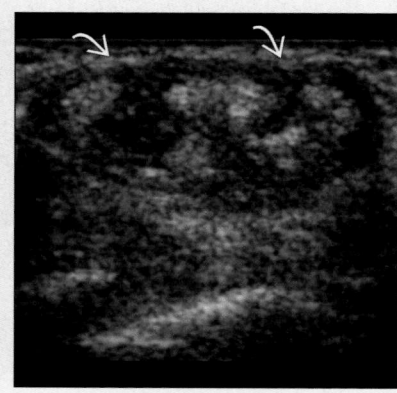

Tenosynovitis

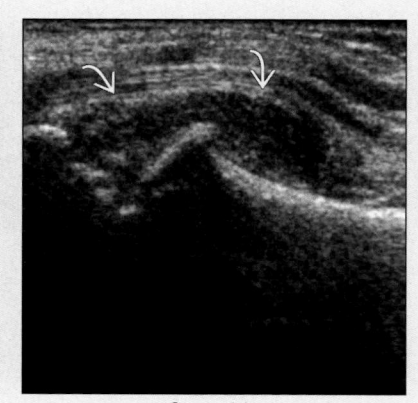

Synovitis

CARPAL TUNNEL SYNDROME

Key Facts

Terminology
- Symptoms secondary to compression of median nerve at carpal tunnel
- Most common entrapment neuropathy

Imaging Findings
- Best diagnostic clue: Swollen median nerve proximal to and within carpal tunnel
- Measurements obtained at three points; proximal to tunnel, at tunnel inlet, and outlet
- If median nerve cross-sectional area ≥ 12 mm², at any measurement point, strong positive predictor of CTS
- If median nerve cross-sectional area ≤ 9 mm², at all measurement points, strong negative predictor of CTS
- If median nerve cross-sectional area between 9 mm² and 12 mm² at all measurement points, predictive value less

- ± Retinacular bowing > 2.5 mm
- Best imaging tool: Ultrasound as accurate, quick, comfortable and relatively inexpensive
- Wrist supported on flat surface with fingers relaxed
- High resolution (≥ 10 MHz) linear transducer

Pathology
- Nerve compression or ischemia leads to fluid leakage and increase in endoneural pressure
- Leads to fibrosis deep to perineurium between nerve fibers, followed by demyelination and finally Wallerian degeneration

Diagnostic Checklist
- More swollen median nerve, more likely possibility of carpal tunnel syndrome

---

- If median nerve cross-sectional area between 9 mm² and 12 mm² at all measurement points, predictive value less
  - For cutoff 9 mm² proximal to tunnel and 12 mm² at outlet, sensitivity 94%, specificity 65%, false positive rate 12%, false negative rate 19%
  - For cut-off 10 mm² proximal to tunnel, sensitivity 83%, specificity 73%, false positive rate 15%, false negative rate 31%
- ± Retinacular bowing > 2.5 mm

MR Findings
- T1WI
  - Swelling of median nerve
    - Palmar bowing of flexor retinaculum
- T2WI
  - Swollen median nerve
  - Hyperintensity of enlarged median nerve
    - Median nerve may normally be hyperintense on T2WI FS
    - May be more hyperintense than usual in carpal tunnel syndrome
- T1 C+: Useful for depicting tenosynovitis, especially if fat-suppression used

Imaging Recommendations
- Best imaging tool: Ultrasound as accurate, quick, comfortable and relatively inexpensive
- Protocol advice
  - Wrist supported on flat surface with fingers relaxed
    - Hand-wrist exercises should not precede examination as they may increase nerve caliber
  - High resolution (≥ 10 MHz) linear transducer
  - Identify nerve in distal forearm in transverse plane
    - In transverse plane, trace course of nerve distally to wrist
  - Measure nerve caliber just proximal to carpal tunnel, at tunnel inlet and tunnel outlet
    - Proximal defined as just proximal to flexor retinaculum
    - Inlet defined as deep to proximal border of flexor retinaculum

- Outlet defined as deep to distal border of flexor retinaculum
- Nerve may be difficult to see at outlet in persons with thick palmar skin
  - ± Measure nerve immediately beyond tunnel outlet
    - Defined as just distal to distal border retinaculum
    - This measurement has wide variation as nerve usually splits into digital branches here
  - ± Measure retinacular bowing from line joining medial and lateral attachments of retinaculum
    - No agreement on location (inlet, mid-portion, outlet) to measure retinacular bowing though outlet probably most discriminatory
    - Degree of retinacular bowing is of questionable discriminatory value
  - General tips
    - Try to keep transducer aligned at right angles and not oblique to nerve
    - Still, slight angulation of transducer can utilize anisotropy to improve nerve delineation
    - Best to make measurements immediately after freezing image
    - Measure cross-sectional area of nerve by trace rather than ellipsoid calipers
  - Non-discriminatory measures
    - Flattening ratio of nerve, retinacular thickness
    - Carpal tunnel depth or volume

DIFFERENTIAL DIAGNOSIS

First Carpometacarpal Osteoarthrosis
- Osteoarthrosis of joint between trapezium and first metacarpal bone
- Pain from this joint often poorly localized

Tenosynovitis
- Tendon sheath effusion and hyperemia predominates
  - May induce secondary CTS

Synovitis
- Synovial swelling and hyperemia predominates
  - Many induce secondary CTS

CARPAL TUNNEL SYNDROME

PATHOLOGY

General Features
- General path comments
  - Most likely results from ischemia or compression of median nerve within carpal tunnel
  - Anatomy of flexor retinaculum
    - Attached on radial side to scaphoid, trapezium & fascia overlying thenar muscles
    - Attached on ulnar side to pisiform, hook of hamate & fascia overlying hypothenar muscles
  - Ten structures pass through carpal tunnel
    - Median nerve
    - Eight tendons of flexor digitorum superficialis and profundus muscles (within ulnar bursa)
    - Flexor pollicis longus tendon (within radial bursa)
  - Narrowest level of carpal tunnel is tunnel outlet
    - Normal carpal tunnel pressure is about 2.5 mmHg
    - Cross-sectional area of carpal tunnel diminishes and tunnel pressure increases with wrist flexion/extension, and finger flexion
    - Lumbrical muscles, which originate from flexor tendons distal to carpal tunnel, can move into distal tunnel during finger flexion
- Etiology
  - Majority primary with no specific structural cause found
  - Increased risk in
    - Females, increasing age, increasing body mass index
    - Repetitive physical work
    - Pregnancy, estrogen replacement, diabetes, myxoedema
    - Inflammatory or degenerative wrist arthropathy
  - Also may occur with
    - Previous Colles fracture or carpal bone dislocation
    - Tenosynovitis, median nerve tumors, ganglia or accessory muscles decreasing functional volume of carpal tunnel
- Epidemiology
  - Cumulative lifetime incidence rate of 8%
    - 0.5 million carpal tunnel decompressions performed yearly in USA

Gross Pathologic & Surgical Features
- Swollen nerve compressed deep to retinaculum

Microscopic Features
- Nerve compression or ischemia leads to fluid leakage and increase in endoneural pressure
  - Leads to fibrosis deep to perineurium between nerve fibers, followed by demyelination and finally Wallerian degeneration

Staging, Grading or Classification Criteria
- No widely used grading scheme

CLINICAL ISSUES

Presentation
- Most common signs/symptoms: Paresthesia ± pain in one or more radial three and a half digits
- Other signs/symptoms

- Paresthesia ± pain in palm, wrist or proximal to wrist
- Occasionally may affect ulnar two digits
- ± Abductor pollicis brevis and opponens pollicis weakness (early finding) followed by atrophy (late finding)
- Clinical Profile
  - Nocturnal exacerbation
    - Attributed to physiological increase in carpal tunnel pressure at nighttime and tendency of wrists to flex during sleep
  - Positive Tinel and Phalen signs
  - Electrodiagnostic studies (EDS) test functional integrity of nerve
    - Median nerve sensory conduction over 8 cm is compared to ipsilateral ulnar nerve sensory conduction over 8 cm
    - Main diagnostic parameter is median-ulnar sensory latency delay of > 0.5 msec
    - Natural tendency for nerve conduction to decrease with age
    - In population with high prevalence of CTS, specificity of EDS is over 90%
    - In population with low prevalence of CTS, positive predictive value of EDS is only 33% with 20% false positive rate

Demographics
- Age: Peak: 50 years ± 15 years
- Gender: M:F = 1:6

Natural History & Prognosis
- Symptoms usually remain over months or years
  - Tendency to improve clinically and electrophysiologically over time even without specific treatment
    - Minority of patients will progress

Treatment
- Conservative
  - Neutral position wrist splint
  - Steroid injections into carpal canal, oral steroids, ultrasound therapy
- Surgical
  - Flexor retinaculum release; open vs. endoscopic ± ultrasound-guided

DIAGNOSTIC CHECKLIST

Consider
- CTS in all patients with unexplained hand, wrist or distal forearm paresthesia ± pain even though symptoms not typical of CTS

Image Interpretation Pearls
- More swollen median nerve, more likely possibility of carpal tunnel syndrome

SELECTED REFERENCES
1. Wong SM et al: Carpal tunnel syndrome: diagnostic usefulness of sonography. Radiology. 232(1):93-9, 2004

IMAGE GALLERY

Typical

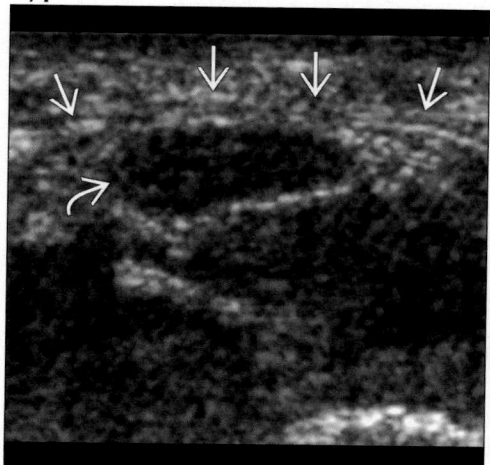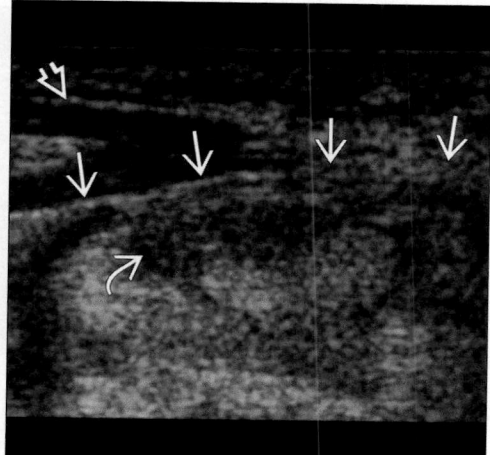

(Left) Transverse ultrasound shows an enlarged (15 mm²) median nerve ➡ at the tunnel inlet. Note proximal border of the flexor retinaculum ➡ overlying the nerve at the tunnel inlet. *(Right)* Transverse ultrasound shows an enlarged (13 mm²) median nerve ➡ at the tunnel outlet. Note distal border of the flexor retinaculum ➡ and the thenar muscles ➡.

Typical

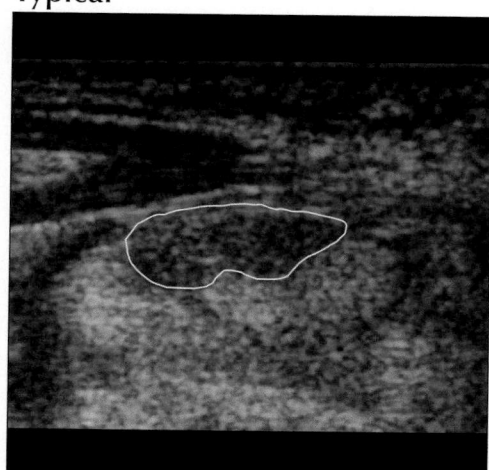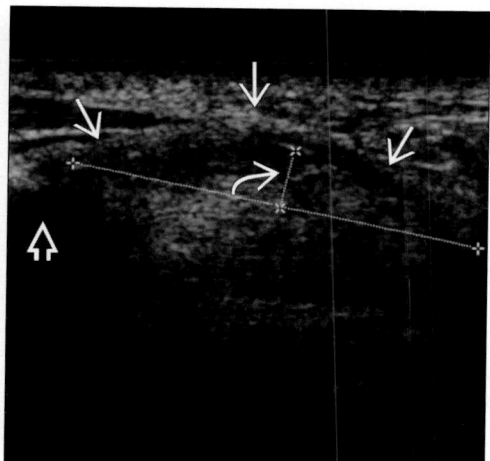

(Left) Transverse ultrasound at the same location as the previous image, shows the median nerve outline at the tunnel outlet (cross-sectional area - 13 mm²). *(Right)* Transverse ultrasound shows the degree of retinacular bowing ➡ being measured at the tunnel outlet. The distance ➡ between the line joining the retinacular attachments and the highest point of the palmar bowing is measured. Trapezium ➡.

Typical

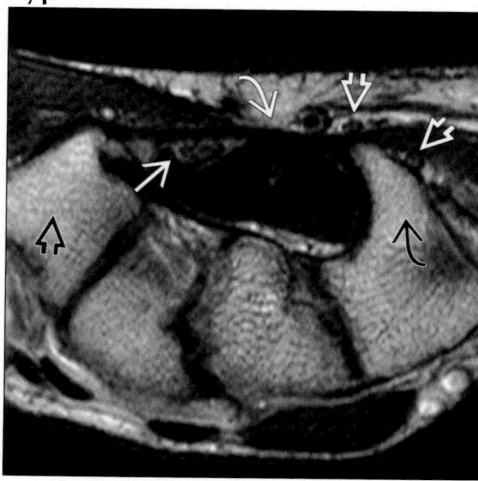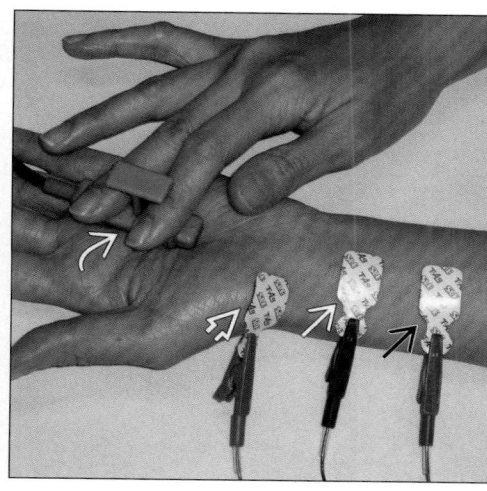

(Left) Axial T2WI MR shows a normal caliber median nerve ➡ deep to the flexor retinaculum ➡ at the tunnel outlet. Note the trapezium ➡, hook of hamate ➡ and superficial/deep ulnar nerve branches ➡. *(Right)* Clinical photograph shows electrodiagnostic studies testing median nerve sensory conduction over 8 cm, with stimulating ➡, ground ➡, active recording ➡ and reference ➡ electrodes.

SOFT TISSUE INFECTION

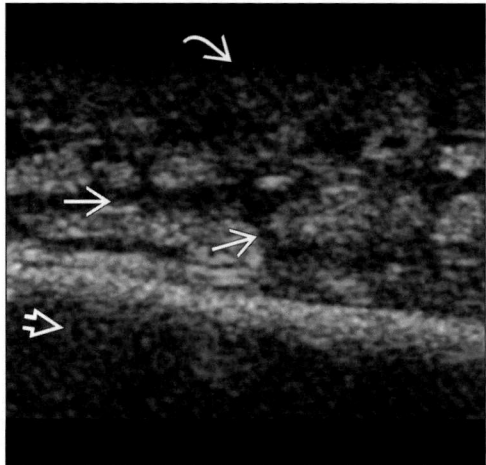

Longitudinal ultrasound shows swollen echogenic subcutaneous fat ➡ and thickening of the interlobular septa ➡, indicative of subcutaneous edema. Tibia ➡.

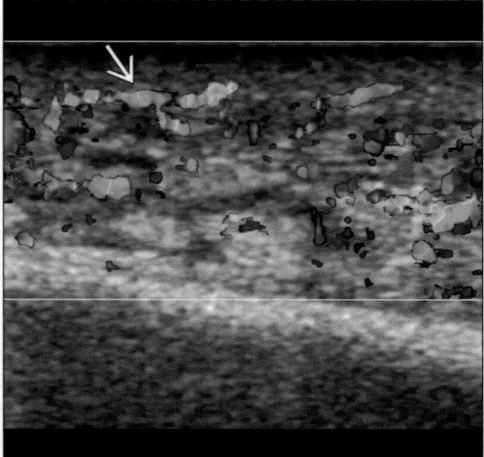

Longitudinal color Doppler ultrasound at the same location, shows diffuse hyperemia ➡ of the edematous subcutaneous tissue and absence of discrete mass. Findings are indicative of cellulitis.

TERMINOLOGY

Abbreviations and Synonyms
- Cellulitis, necrotizing fasciitis, pyomyositis, infectious myositis, phlegmon, abscess

Definitions
- Cellulitis = inflammation of cells = spreading inflammation of subcutaneous and deeper tissues
- Necrotizing fasciitis: Severe spreading cellulitis of investing and deep fascia with vascular occlusion and necrosis
- Pyomyositis = infective myositis = suppurative bacterial infection of muscle
- Phlegmon: Localized intense inflammation prior to development of abscess or ulceration
- Abscess: Localized collection of pus

IMAGING FINDINGS

General Features
- Best diagnostic clue: Edema and hyperemia of affected tissues ± fluid accumulation

- Location
  - Any soft tissue tissue can become infected
  - Most common sites
    - Cellulitis: Dorsum hand and feet
    - Necrotizing fasciitis: Thigh and leg
    - Pyomyositis: Large muscles of pelvis and lower limb; frequently multifocal
- Size: Varies from small localized abscess to multi-compartmental disseminated infection
- Morphology: Inflammation ± fluid ± abscess

Ultrasonographic Findings
- **Cellulitis**
  - Edema and hyperemia of subcutaneous fat
    - Edematous fat is echogenic on ultrasound
    - Thickened interlobular septa
    - ± Periseptal fluid & fluid above investing fascia
    - Need combination of edema & hyperemia to diagnose cellulitis
  - Edema alone = non-specific feature of many non-infectious conditions (venous insufficiency, heart failure, lymphoedema)
    - Hyperemia not feature of non-infectious edema

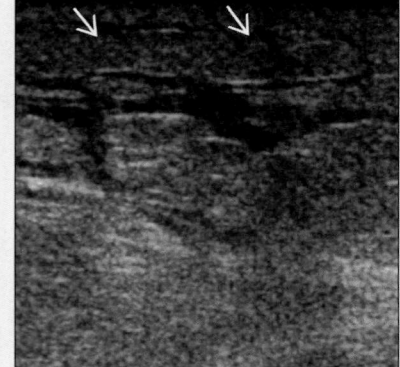 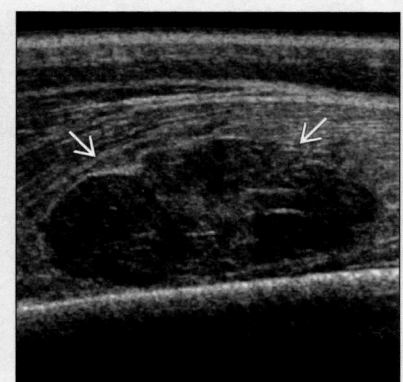 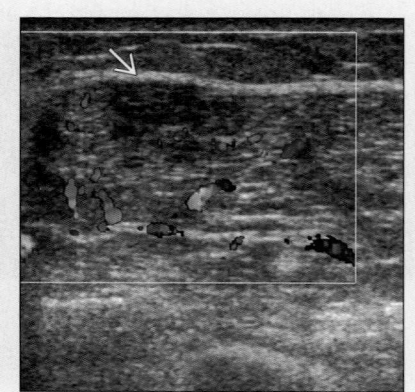

DDx: Soft Tissue Infection

| Subcutaneous Edema | Muscle Hematoma | Diabetic Muscle Infarction |

SOFT TISSUE INFECTION

Key Facts

Terminology
- Cellulitis = inflammation of cells = spreading inflammation of subcutaneous and deeper tissues
- Necrotizing fasciitis: Severe spreading cellulitis of investing and deep fascia with vascular occlusion and necrosis
- Pyomyositis = infective myositis = suppurative bacterial infection of muscle

Imaging Findings
- **Cellulitis**
- Edema and hyperemia of subcutaneous fat
- Edematous fat is echogenic on ultrasound
- Thickened interlobular septa
- ± Periseptal fluid & fluid above investing fascia
- **Necrotizing fasciitis**
- Affects subcutaneous fat, fascia and muscle

- Thickened disrupted fascia with perifascial fluid (fluid above and below investing fascia)
- Severe associated subcutaneous and muscle edema
- ± Muscle necrosis (difficult to detect)
- **Pyomyositis**
- Diffuse muscle swelling with edema ± hyperemia
- Edematous muscle is echogenic on ultrasound
- ± Focal hypoechoic areas due to abscess, necrosis or serous exudate
- Best imaging tool: Ultrasound ± ultrasound-guided aspiration gives sufficient information to make prompt diagnosis and guide treatment

Top Differential Diagnoses
- Subcutaneous Edema
- Muscle Hematoma
- Muscle Infarction

- Appearance of subcutaneous edema varies according to severity and architecture of subcutaneous fat
  - Amorphous swelling with indistinct lobules/cobblestone with accentuated lobules/windswept appearance
  - ± Aspiration of fluid for culture
- **Necrotizing fasciitis**
  - Affects subcutaneous fat, fascia and muscle
  - Thickened disrupted fascia with perifascial fluid (fluid above and below investing fascia)
  - Severe associated subcutaneous and muscle edema
  - ± Muscle necrosis (difficult to detect)
  - ± Aspiration of fluid for culture
- **Pyomyositis**
  - Diffuse muscle swelling with edema ± hyperemia
  - Edematous muscle is echogenic on ultrasound
    - ± Focal hypoechoic areas due to abscess, necrosis or serous exudate
- **Abscess**
  - Posterior enhancement characteristic
  - Depending on maturity and content, echogenicity of fluid may vary from hypoechoic → isoechoic → hyperechoic
    - If thick fluid/debris present; may mimic solid mass ⇒ low threshold for aspiration as fluid not readily discernible
  - Echo movement on real-time imaging
  - ± Gas locules
    - → Comet-tail artifacts or larger shadowing artifact
  - ± Septations
  - Wall thickness proportional to chronicity of abscess
  - ± Peripheral hyperemia

Radiographic Findings
- Often non-contributory
- Soft tissue swelling with obliteration of fascial planes
  - ± Gas locules within soft tissues
  - ± Radio-opaque foreign body
  - ± Concomitant osteitis or osteomyelitis

CT Findings
- Especially for iliopsoas abscesses, other pelvic abscesses and large complex abscesses of limbs

- Contrast-enhancement useful at differentiating cellulitis/myositis, serous exudate or abscess
  - Rough guide
  - No fluid collection = cellulitis/myositis
    - Fluid collection without rim-enhancement = serous exudate
    - Fluid collection with rim-enhancement = abscess

MR Findings
- T1WI
  - Cellulitis: Swelling, hypointensity & increased reticulation of subcutaneous fat
    - No discrete mass
  - Necrotizing fasciitis: Thickening of investing and deep fascial planes
    - ± Hypointense gas locules
  - Pyomyositis: Hyperintensity with loss of muscle definition compared to unaffected muscle
    - ± Hyperintense rim around fluid collections
  - Abscess: Well-defined intermediate to low signal intensity area
- T2WI FS
  - Cellulitis: Diffuse hyperintensity of subcutaneous tissues
    - ± Feathery edema of adjacent tissues
  - Necrotizing fasciitis: Swelling of fascia with perifascial fluid
    - Edema of adjacent musculature
    - ± Fluid areas indicative of necrosis, exudate or abscess
  - Pyomyositis: Diffuse hyperintensity of muscle ± overlying subcutaneous tissues
    - Highly hyperintense area ⇒ fluid collection
    - ± Edematous changes in adjacent structures: Subcutaneous tissues > fascial planes > bone & joints
  - Abscess: High signal intensity area with surrounding edema ± hyperemia
- T1 C+
  - Useful at delineating fluid collection/abscess/necrosis
  - Cannot differentiate septic from aseptic fluid on imaging

SOFT TISSUE INFECTION

Imaging Recommendations
- Best imaging tool: Ultrasound ± ultrasound-guided aspiration gives sufficient information to make prompt diagnosis and guide treatment
- Protocol advice
  - Routinely assess with color Doppler imaging
  - Observe possible fluid collections at rest ± after compression to detect moving echoes indicative of fluid
    - If fluid present, consider aspiration for culture
  - Occasionally, little or no fluid can be aspirated despite visibly moving echoes

DIFFERENTIAL DIAGNOSIS

Subcutaneous Edema
- Similar to cellulitis
- Hyperechoic fat and thickened interlobular septa
  - Hyperemia present with cellulitis
- Usually readily distinguished clinically

Muscle Hematoma
- Similar to muscle abscess
- Hypoechoic mass with posterior enhancement, variable liquefaction & surrounding edema
- Usually readily distinguished clinically

Muscle Infarction
- Similar to focal pyomyositis
- Hypoechoic mass with surrounding edema and hyperemia
- Usually readily distinguished clinically

PATHOLOGY

General Features
- Etiology
  - Predisposing factors
  - General: Poor health, venous/lymphatic stasis, skin laceration/ulceration or exfoliation, obesity, immunosuppression (including diabetes), infection elsewhere
    - Cellulitis: ± Penetrating trauma
    - Pyomyositis: ± Blunt muscle trauma
  - Causative organisms
    - Cellulitis = Streptococcus pyogenes, Staphylococcus aureus
    - Necrotizing fasciitis = Group A β-hemolytic Streptococci
    - Pyomyositis = Staphylococcus aureus, Mycobacterium tuberculosis, Nocardia asteroides, Streptococcus pyogenes, Streptococcus viridans, Cryptococcus neoformans
- Epidemiology
  - Frequency of occurrence
    - Cellulitis (common) > > pyomyositis > necrotizing fasciitis (uncommon)

Gross Pathologic & Surgical Features
- Cellulitis
  - Acute inflammatory reaction

- Necrotizing fasciitis
  - Facilitated by enzymes, bacteria spread from subcutaneous tissues → investing & deep fascia → muscle
    - Induces vascular thrombosis → tissue necrosis
    - Superficial nerve ischaemia → characteristic local anesthesia
- Pyomyositis
  - Bacterial infection of skeletal muscle ± necrosis or abscess

Microscopic Features
- Cellulitis: Acute inflammatory infiltrate, capillary dilatation ± abscess formation
- Necrotizing fasciitis: Fascial inflammation and necrosis, subcutaneous fat necrosis, arterial thrombi, vasculitis and myonecrosis
- Pyomyositis: Acute inflammatory infiltrate, capillary dilatation ± abscess formation

CLINICAL ISSUES

Presentation
- Most common signs/symptoms
  - Cellulitis
    - Inflammation: Redness (rubor), heat (calor), swelling (tumor), pain (dolor) and dysfunction (functio laesa) ± lymphangitis, blistering necrosis ± lymphadenopathy
  - Necrotizing fasciitis
    - Rapidly progressive condition with severe inflammation of tissues
    - ± Blistering necrosis, cyanosis, severe tenderness, high fever, tachycardia, hypotension and impaired consciousness
  - Pyomyositis
    - Deep pain, tenderness ± mass

Demographics
- Age: More common in older patients
- Gender: M:F = 1:1

Natural History & Prognosis
- Cellulitis: Responds well to treatment
- Necrotizing fasciitis: Mortality up to 25%
- Pyomyositis: Less favorable response in immunocompromised patient

Treatment
- Cellulitis: Elevation, splinting + antibiotic therapy
- Necrotizing fasciitis: Early radical surgical debridement + irrigation + antibiotic therapy
- Pyomyositis: Antibiotic therapy
  - Abscess: Ultrasound-guided percutaneous aspiration or catheter drainage; surgical incision & drainage

SELECTED REFERENCES
1. Chau CL et al: Musculoskeletal infections: ultrasound appearances. Clin Radiol. 60(2):149-59, 2005
2. Struk DW et al: Imaging of soft tissue infections. Radiol Clin North Am. 39(2):277-303, 2001

SOFT TISSUE INFECTION

IMAGE GALLERY

Typical

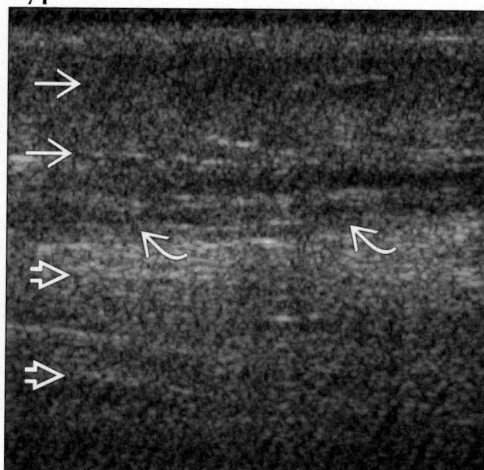

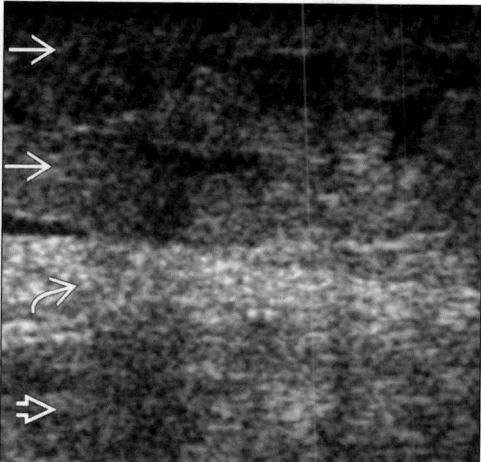

(Left) Longitudinal ultrasound shows amorphous pattern of echogenic, edematous, subcutaneous tissues ➡ without discrete mass. The muscle ➡ and investing fascia ➡ are also edematous. *(Right)* Longitudinal ultrasound shows cobblestone pattern of edematous subcutaneous tissues ➡. Investing fascia ➡ and muscle ➡ are also edematous.

Typical

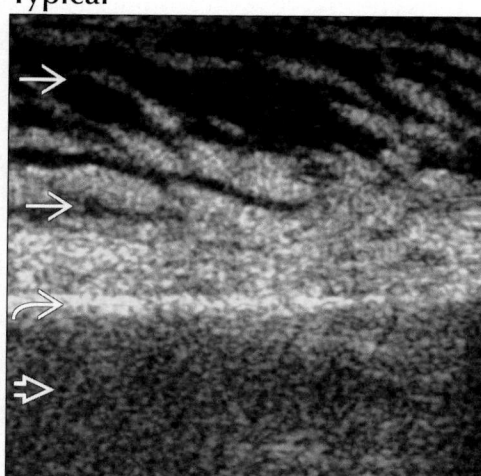

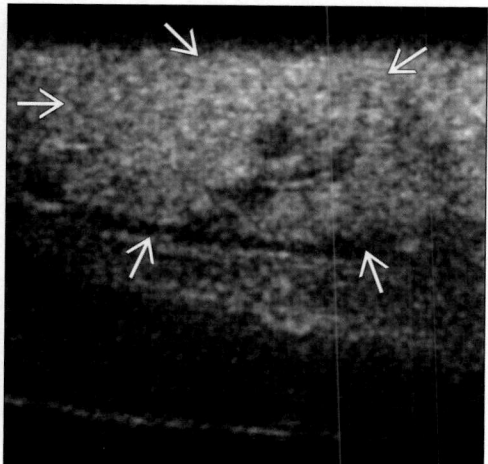

(Left) Longitudinal ultrasound shows windswept pattern ➡ of edematous pre-tibial subcutaneous fat (tibia ➡ with echogenic anterior cortex ➡). *(Right)* Longitudinal ultrasound in a child with thigh swelling, erythema and central punctum for three days shows thickening and increased echogenicity of the subcutaneous fat ➡. Peripheral hyperemia was present consistent with phlegmon.

Typical

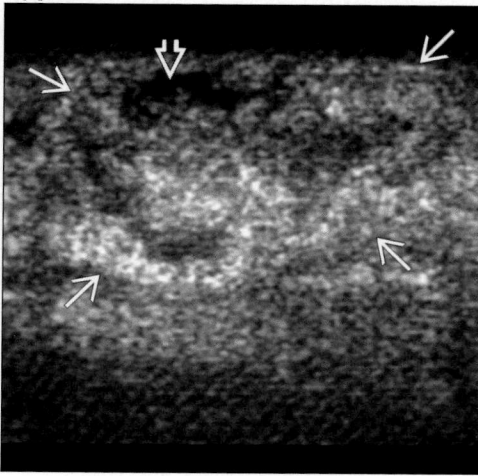

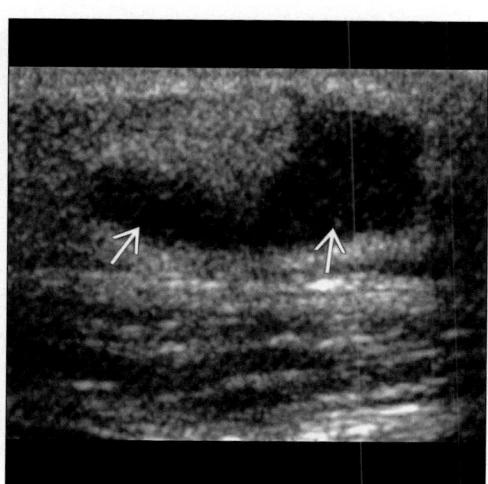

(Left) Longitudinal ultrasound (same region as previous image) three days later, shows coalescence of inflammation ➡ and early liquefaction ➡. *(Right)* Longitudinal ultrasound (same region as previous image) two days later, shows increased liquefaction ➡ with reduced swelling of subcutaneous tissues. 1 mL purulent blood-stained fluid was aspirated.

(Left) Longitudinal ultrasound of thigh shows a lobulated ischemic subcutaneous abscess ➡ extending through the investing fascia ⮞ into the vastus lateralis muscle ➡. Surgical exploration revealed necrotizing fasciitis. *(Right)* Transverse ultrasound of an adult with systemic lupus erythematosus, shows a large abscess ➡ within the brachialis muscle with perimuscular fluid exudate ⮞. Humeral shaft ➡.

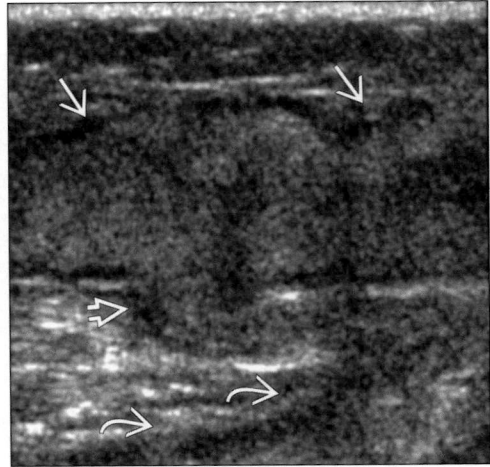
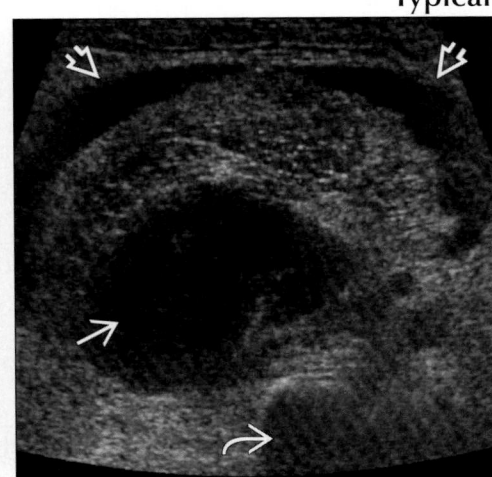

(Left) Longitudinal ultrasound shows hypoechoic area ➡ within the soleus muscle consistent with pyomyositis and small abscess ⮞. Gastrocnemius muscle ➡. *(Right)* Longitudinal ultrasound of the same patient as previous image, shows a larger abscess cavity ➡ with surrounding hypoechoic edema ➡ within the contralateral gastrocnemius muscle. Purulent fluid was aspirated.

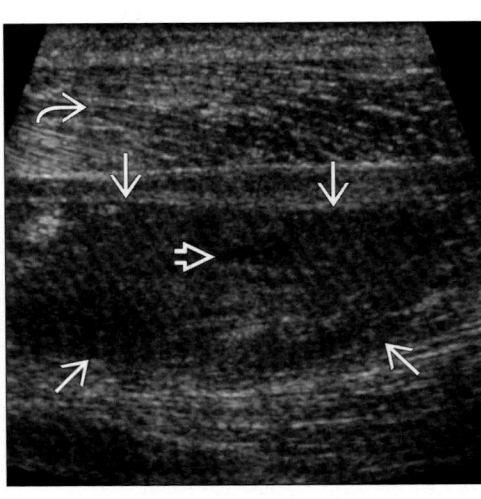
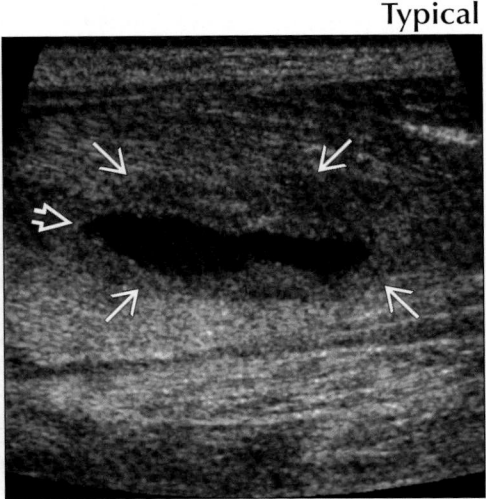

(Left) Longitudinal ultrasound in an intravenous drug addict shows a large isoechoic abscess ➡ within the subcutaneous fat of the proximal thigh. Note small area of more distinct liquefaction ⮞. Purulent fluid was aspirated. *(Right)* Transverse ultrasound of the thigh in an intravenous drug addict shows a large, hypoechoic, intramuscular abscess ➡ with a gas locule ⮞. Purulent fluid was drained surgically.

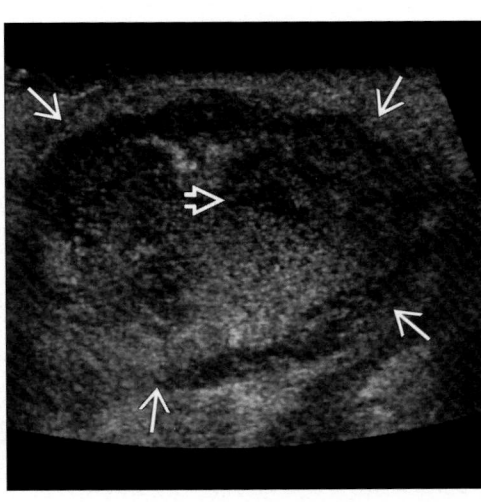
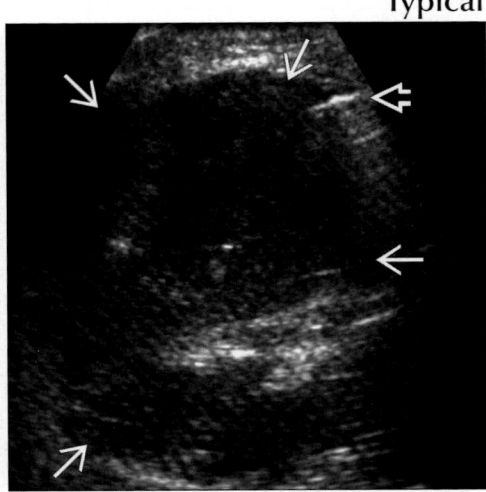

Typical

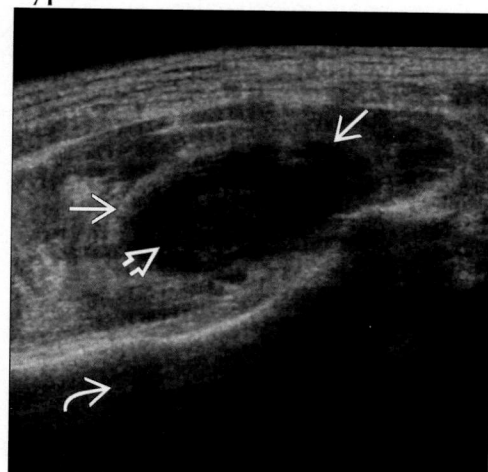
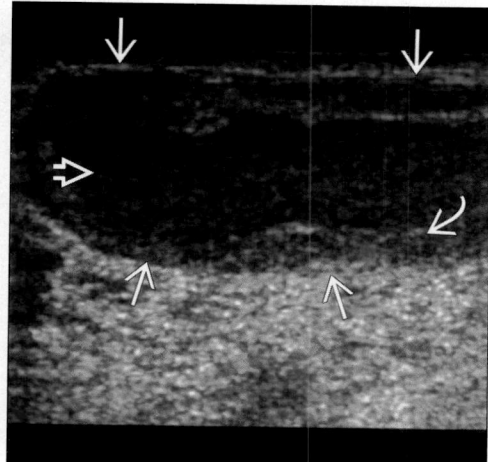

(Left) Transverse ultrasound shows a large abscess cavity ➡ containing echogenic debris ⇨ within swollen infraspinatus muscle. Scapula ➡. *(Right)* Longitudinal ultrasound of an adult patient with renal tuberculosis shows a well-defined ➡, thick-walled ⇨, subcutaneous thigh abscess with finely echogenic fluid ⇨ due to tuberculosis.

Typical

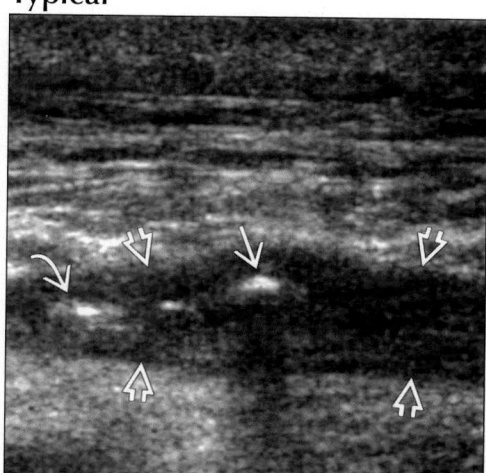
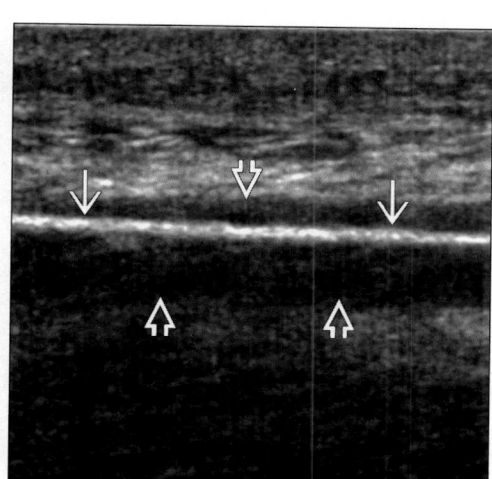

(Left) Transverse ultrasound of an adult patient with tuberculous empyema, fistula to skin and retained wooden probe. Echogenic wooden probe ➡ with surrounding fistula ⇨ and gas loculi ➡. *(Right)* Longitudinal ultrasound of chest wall in same patient as previous image, shows echogenic wooden probe ➡ within hypoechoic fistula ⇨.

Typical

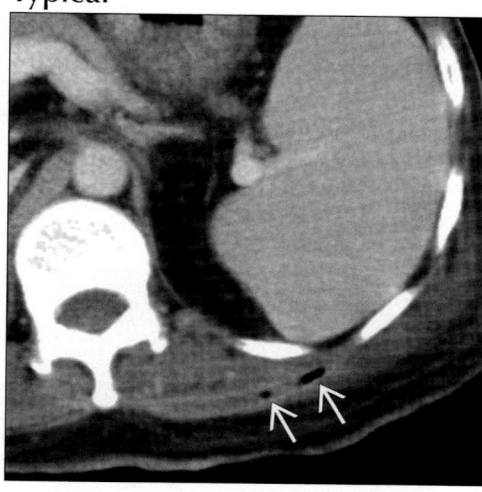
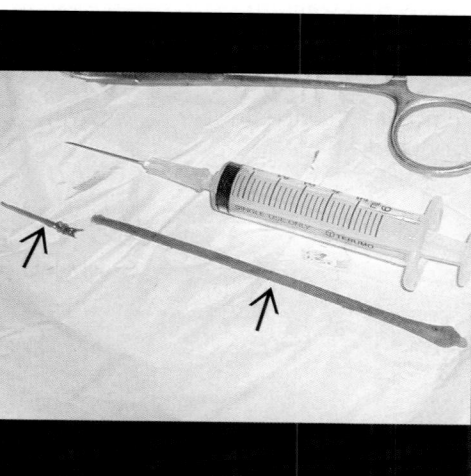

(Left) Transverse CECT in same patient as previous image, shows hypodense wooden probe ➡ within the chest wall. Wood can simulate air on both CT and ultrasound. *(Right)* Clinical photograph in same patient as previous image, shows a wooden probe (broken) ➡ following removal under ultrasound guidance.

13

BONE INFECTION

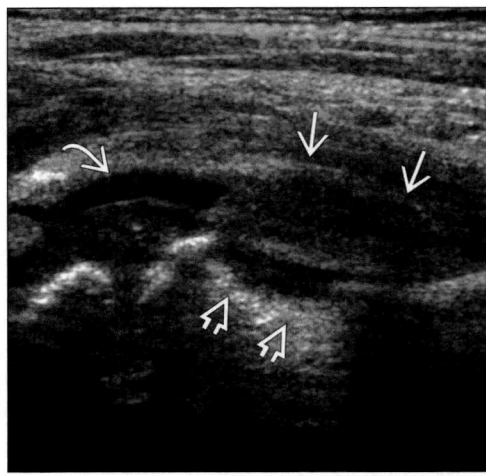

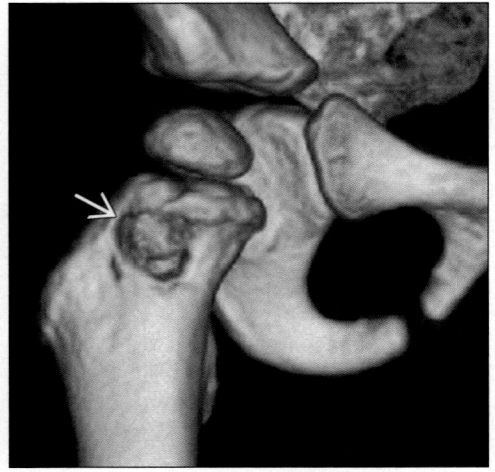

Longitudinal ultrasound shows marked synovial thickening of the hip joint ➡, small effusion ➡ and large cortical defect ➡ in the anterolateral aspect of femoral metaphysis. Percutaneous biopsy revealed TB.

NECT with 3-dimensional reconstruction of the same patient as the previous image, confirms the cortical defect ➡ in the anterolateral aspect of femoral metaphysis.

TERMINOLOGY

Abbreviations and Synonyms
- Acute osteomyelitis, chronic osteomyelitis, osteitis, Brodie abscess

Definitions
- Osteomyelitis = infection of bone marrow
- Acute osteomyelitis = symptomatic osteomyelitis < six weeks duration
- Chronic osteomyelitis = symptomatic osteomyelitis > six weeks duration
- Infective osteitis = infection of bone cortex (usually contiguous with juxtacortical infection)
- Sequestrum = fragment of dead bone surrounded by granulation tissue (literally = separated)
- Involucrum = layer of living periosteal new bone formed around dead bone (literally = to wrap in)
- Cloaca = opening in cortex or involucrum through which sequestra, fluid or granulation tissue is discharged (literally = drain)
- Brodie abscess = focal area of chronic osteomyelitis with abscess and surrounding sclerosis

IMAGING FINDINGS

General Features
- Best diagnostic clue
  - Periosteal thickening and hyperemia with juxta-cortical edema
    - Ultrasound can suggest diagnosis of osteomyelitis but sensitivity/specificity limited compared to MR
  - If clinical suspicion of osteomyelitis, MR should be performed following radiography
    - Prominent bone marrow hyperintensity on T2WI FS without discrete mass
- Location
  - Acute osteomyelitis ⇒ metaphyses of long tubular bones
  - Chronic osteomyelitis ⇒ diaphyses of long tubular bones
  - Osteitis ⇒ alongside area of chronic soft tissue infection or ulceration
- Size: Acute osteomyelitis usually less extensive than chronic osteomyelitis
- Morphology
  - Acute osteomyelitis ⇒ bony resorption

DDx: Bone Infection

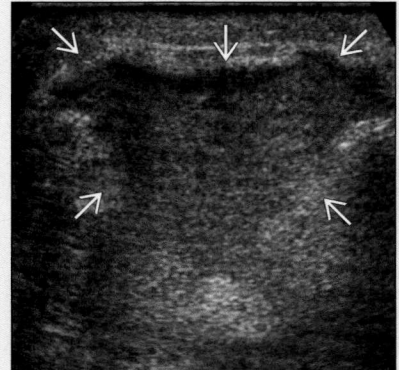

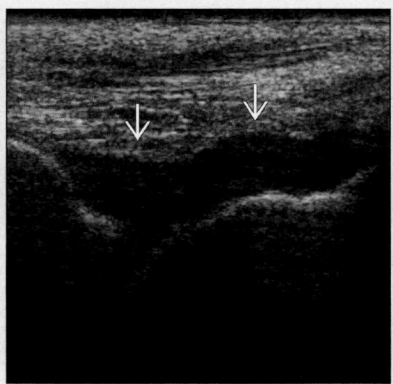

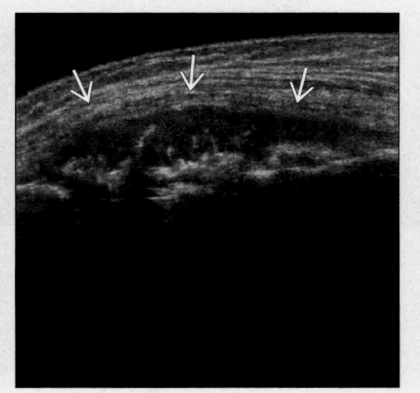

Soft Tissue Infection

Septic Arthritis

Bone Sarcoma

BONE INFECTION

Key Facts

Imaging Findings
- Periosteal thickening and hyperemia with juxta-cortical edema
- Ultrasound can suggest diagnosis of osteomyelitis but sensitivity/specificity limited compared to MR
- Acute osteomyelitis ⇒ bony resorption
- Chronic osteomyelitis ⇒ simultaneous bony resorption, draining infection (sequestra, cloaca, sinus tract) and bony repair (bone deposition, expansion)
- Ultrasound useful in neonates & young infants, when clinical signs are often non-specific and absent
- US shows features of acute osteomyelitis several days earlier than radiography
- Ultrasound less sensitive than MR or scintigraphy

- Ultrasound sensitivity highest in suspected osteomyelitis of tubular bones in children where propensity to develop periosteal reaction is highest
- Ultrasound also useful in post-operative patients when metallic implants limit MR assessment
- **Ultrasound only depicts outer cortical, periosteal and extraosseous changes**
- Periosteal thickening
- ± Juxtacortical soft tissue edema and hyperemia
- ± Cortical irregularity
- ± Sympathetic joint effusion

Top Differential Diagnoses
- Soft Tissue Infection
- Septic Arthritis
- Bone Sarcoma

- o Chronic osteomyelitis ⇒ simultaneous bony resorption, draining infection (sequestra, cloaca, sinus tract) and bony repair (bone deposition, expansion)

Ultrasonographic Findings
- Ultrasound useful in neonates & young infants, when clinical signs are often non-specific and absent
  - o US shows features of acute osteomyelitis several days earlier than radiography
    - Ultrasound less sensitive than MR or scintigraphy
- Ultrasound sensitivity highest in suspected osteomyelitis of tubular bones in children where propensity to develop periosteal reaction is highest
  - o Check bone detail if performing ultrasound for suspected soft tissue or joint infection
- Ultrasound also useful in post-operative patients when metallic implants limit MR assessment
- **Ultrasound only depicts outer cortical, periosteal and extraosseous changes**
  - o Periosteal thickening
  - o ± Juxtacortical soft tissue edema and hyperemia
  - o ± Cortical irregularity
  - o ± Sympathetic joint effusion
- Severe infection may show
  - o Subperiosteal exudate, or less commonly, abscess
  - o Soft tissue abscess
    - Amiable to ultrasound-guided aspiration
  - o Cortical disruption ± extra-osseous inflammatory mass
    - Amiable to ultrasound-guided biopsy
- Chronic osteomyelitis may show
  - o Sinus tracts
  - o Cloaca
  - o Sequestra
- Ultrasound appearances of acute bone infection are non-specific
  - o Periosteal thickening ± subperiosteal fluid ± soft tissue edema also seen in
    - Stress reaction of bone
    - Sickle cell disease with medullary infarction
    - Bone sarcoma

- In neonates and young children, pure chondral infection may occur
  - o ± Difficult to detect on ultrasound as hypoechoic fluid is of similar echogenicity to hypoechoic cartilage

Radiographic Findings
- Radiography
  - o Insensitive for early acute osteomyelitis
  - o Radiographic bony changes occur 10-14 days after symptom-onset depending on severity of infection
    - Soft tissue edema, periosteal elevation, focal osteolysis
  - o Sensitive for chronic osteomyelitis
    - Sclerosis, periosteal thickening, sequestra, cloaca, expansion ± bowing
    - Involucrum rarely seen nowadays

CT Findings
- NECT
  - o Useful when MR not available
    - More sensitive than radiography
    - Good bone detail, periosteal thickening
  - o Useful in chronic osteomyelitis at depicting cloaca, sequestra and sinus tracts
    - Sequestra may be difficult to see on MR (hypointense) or radiography (if marked sclerosis and cortical thickening)
- CECT: Abscesses and sinus tracts enhance peripherally

MR Findings
- T1WI: Hypointense marrow edema ± cortical destruction
- T2WI FS
  - o Acute osteomyelitis: Hypointense marrow edema without discrete mass
    - ± Focal cortical destruction
    - ± Periosteal thickening (lamellar, Codman triangle)
    - ± Juxtacortical edema, inflammation or inflammatory mass
    - MR = most sensitive and specific imaging investigation for acute osteomyelitis

BONE INFECTION

o Chronic osteomyelitis; additional findings include
  - ± Cortical thickening
  - ± Intra-osseous, transcortical, or extra-osseous sinus tracts
  - ± Hypointense sequestra
  - ± Periosteal thickening (lamellar immature ⇔ thick mature)
  - Appearances vary with level of inflammatory activity
o Brodie abscess (intramedullary abscess cavity): Hyperintense + hypointense sclerotic rim
  - Abscess surrounded by reactive sclerotic bone and inflammation
- T1 C+
  o Differentiates abscess (rim-enhancement) from inflammatory tissue (diffuse enhancement)
    - Sequestra, in chronic osteomyelitis, may also enhance peripherally and simulate abscess
    - Enhancing tissue, in chronic osteomyelitis, may represent reparative or inflammatory tissue

Nuclear Medicine Findings
- Bone Scan: Increased activity on all three phases

Imaging Recommendations
- Best imaging tool
  o MR: High sensitivity & specificity for both acute and chronic osteomyelitis
    - Very high negative predictive value i.e., a normal MR excludes osteomyelitis
- Protocol advice: T1 + FS PD FSE or STIR axial, coronal & sagittal, pre- and post-contrast

DIFFERENTIAL DIAGNOSIS

Soft Tissue Infection
- Soft tissue edema and inflammation ± inflammatory mass ± abscess
- Check bone surface for signs of osteomyelitis

Septic Arthritis
- Similar clinical picture to acute osteomyelitis
- Medium to large joint effusion ± hyperemia ± positive joint aspiration

Bone Sarcoma
- No clinical signs of infection
- Cortical destruction ± extraosseous soft tissue mass ± spiculated new bone formation

PATHOLOGY

General Features
- General path comments
  o For acute osteomyelitis
    - Metaphysis/epiphysis: Infants
    - Metaphysis: > 1 year to skeletal maturity
- Etiology
  o Staphylococcus aureus = most common infecting organism in all age groups
  o Common organisms = Streptococcus, Pseudomonas, Haemophilus, Enterobacter, Tuberculosis

o ± No organism isolated or mixed organisms
  - Especially chronic osteomyelitis
- Epidemiology: Chronic osteomyelitis in adults usually 2° to trauma

Gross Pathologic & Surgical Features
- Hematogenous seeding
- Direct contamination
- Contiguous spread

Microscopic Features
- Inflammation of marrow
- Vascular compromise
- Necrosis, abscesses, sequestra

CLINICAL ISSUES

Presentation
- Most common signs/symptoms: Pain, tenderness, fever with signs of inflammation
- Other signs/symptoms: Restricted motion, constitutional symptoms
- Clinical Profile
  o Acute osteomyelitis progresses over days to weeks
    - ± Positive blood cultures
  o Chronic osteomyelitis usually presents de-novo without pre-existing acute osteomyelitis
    - Typically established at time of presentation
    - Early disease is subclinical

Demographics
- Age
  o Acute osteomyelitis ⇔ young children
  o Chronic osteomyelitis ⇔ older age group
- Gender: M = F

Natural History & Prognosis
- Good prognosis for acute osteomyelitis if treated early
- Chronic osteomyelitis difficult to fully eradicate
  o ∴ Relapsing-remitting course

Treatment
- Conservative
  o Rest, elevation, intravenous antibiotics
- Surgical
  o Debridement ± antibiotic-impregnated beads

DIAGNOSTIC CHECKLIST

Consider
- Bone infection if you detect unexplained periosteal thickening or juxtacortical inflammatory mass even though cortex seems intact

SELECTED REFERENCES
1. Van Holsbeeck MT et al: Musculoskeletal Ultrasound. 2nd ed. Philadelphia PA, Mosby. 265-8, 2001

BONE INFECTION

Typical

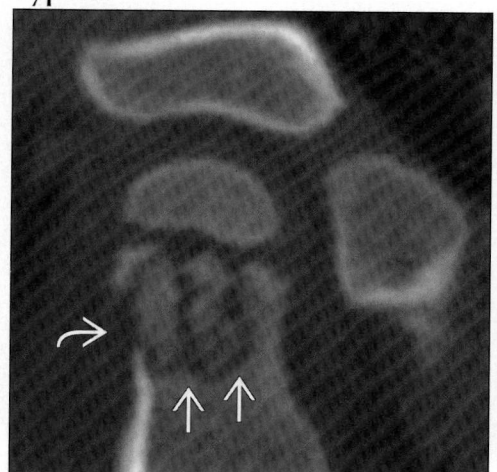

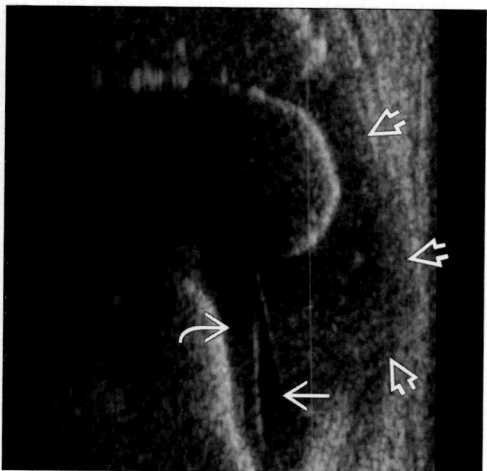

(Left) CECT of the proximal femur shows an anterior cortical defect ➡ and intramedullary, channel-like defects ➡ indicative of infection (tuberculous osteomyelitis). *(Right)* Longitudinal ultrasound in a child with suspected septic arthritis shows a small ankle joint effusion ➡. Note the unossified medial malleolus ➡ and incompletely ossified talus ➡.

Typical

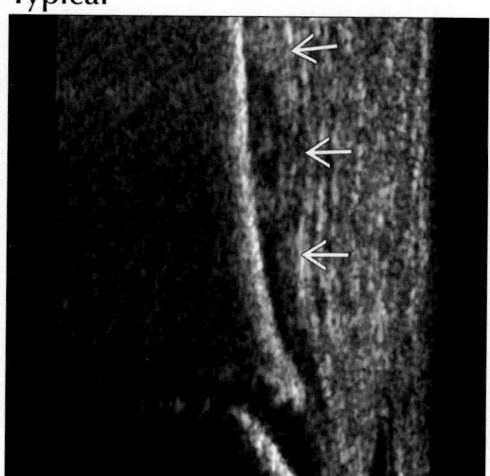

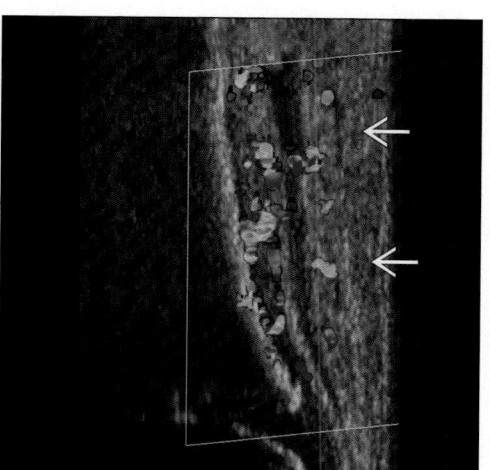

(Left) Longitudinal ultrasound just proximal to the previous image shows periosteal thickening ➡ along the medial aspect of the distal tibial metaphysis, suggestive of osteomyelitis. *(Right)* Longitudinal color Doppler ultrasound at same location as the previous image shows marked hyperemia of the periosteum and juxtacortical tissue ➡. MR examination revealed osteomyelitis of the distal tibia.

Typical

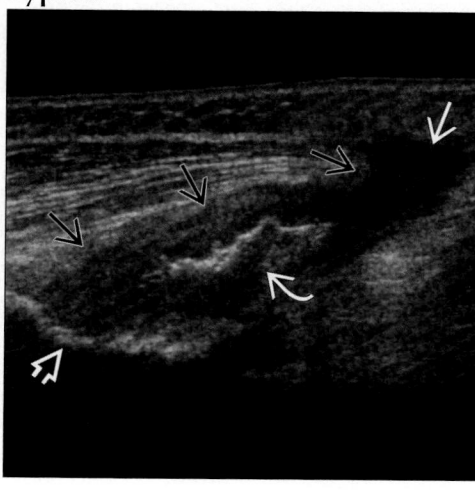

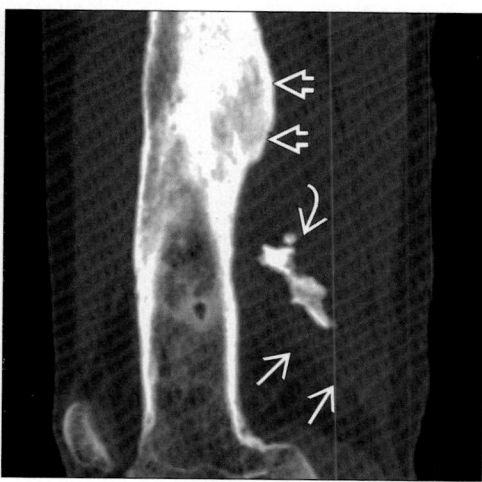

(Left) Longitudinal ultrasound with extended field-of view shows a large sequestrum ➡ within the sinus tract ➡, which extends from the femoral cortex ➡ to the investing fascia ➡ of the thigh. *(Right)* NECT with sagittal reconstruction at the same location as the previous image shows the sequestrum ➡, sinus tract ➡ and thickened sclerotic femoral diaphysis ➡ indicative of chronic osteomyelitis.

(Left) Longitudinal ultrasound of immature sinus tract ➡ from bone shows disruption of investing fascia ➡ and permeations ➡ along the fascia and into the subcutaneous fat. Such permeations are indicative of infection. *(Right)* Longitudinal ultrasound shows a mature sinus tract ➡ extending from the cortex ➡ to the skin in chronic osteomyelitis. Cortex at the point of contact often appears intact on ultrasound.

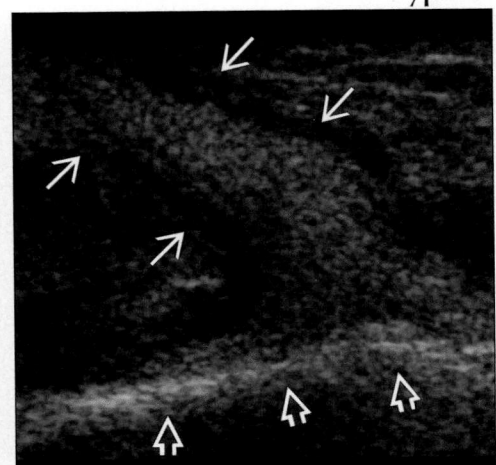

(Left) AP radiograph shows mild expansion, mixed sclerosis/lysis of mid-humeral shaft ➡ with soft tissue mass distally ➡, suggestive of chondrosarcoma or chronic osteomyelitis. *(Right)* Longitudinal ultrasound at same location as previous image, shows focal cortical disruption ➡, and a large extramedullary inflammatory-type mass ➡ with small cystic area ➡, indicating osteomyelitis.

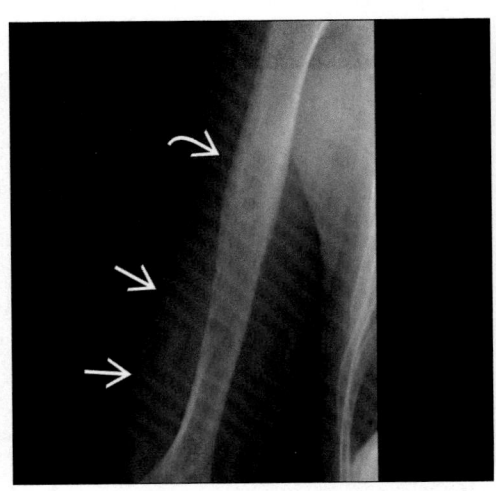

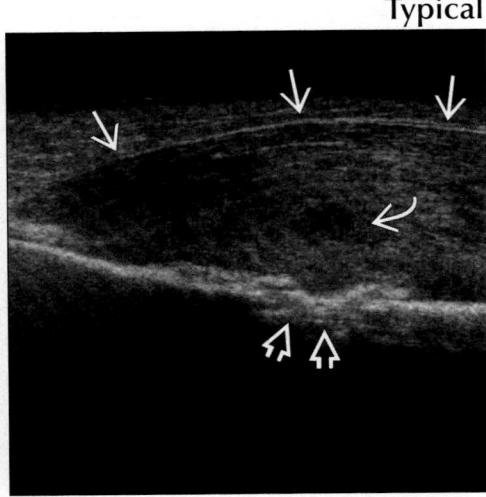

(Left) Transverse ultrasound at same location as previous image, shows cystic area ➡ within the inflammatory mass. Ultrasound-guided aspiration of the cyst yielded purulent fluid which grew Staphylococcus aureus. *(Right)* Coronal T1 C+ MR in same patient as previous image, shows several small intramedullary abscesses ➡ with large juxtacortical inflammatory mass ➡, compatible with chronic osteomyelitis.

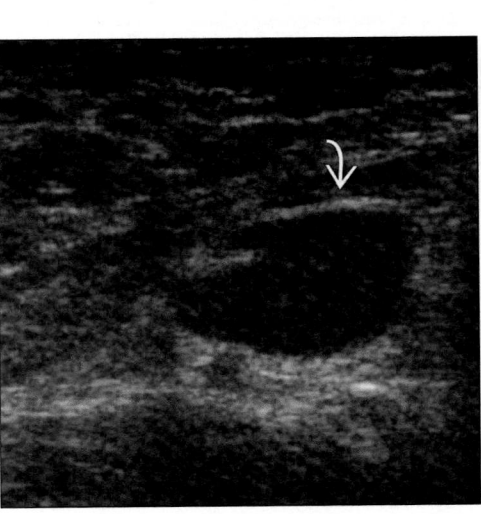

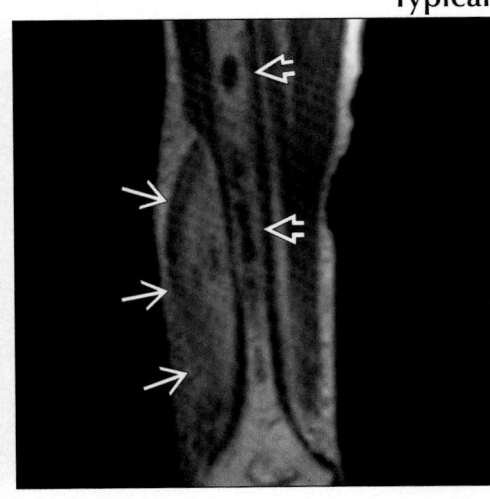

BONE INFECTION

Typical

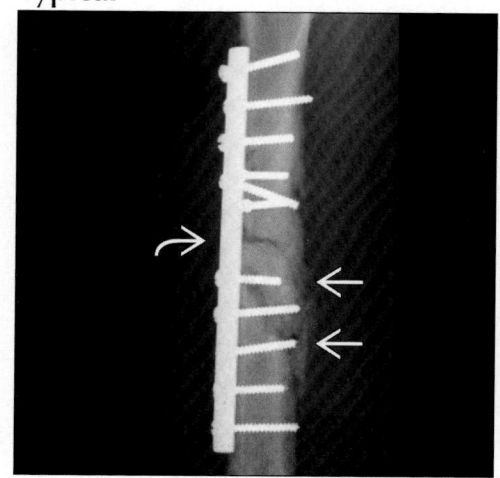

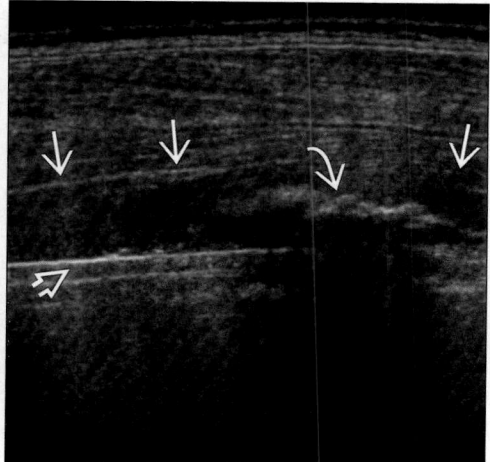

(Left) Radiograph shows a non-united fracture ➡ of the femoral shaft, with interrupted lamellar periosteal new bone ➡ indicative of osteomyelitis. Plate and screw fixation seen. *(Right)* Longitudinal ultrasound at the same location, with extended field-of-view, shows inflammatory tissue ➡ alongside the fixation plate ➡ and periosteal new bone formation ➡.

Typical

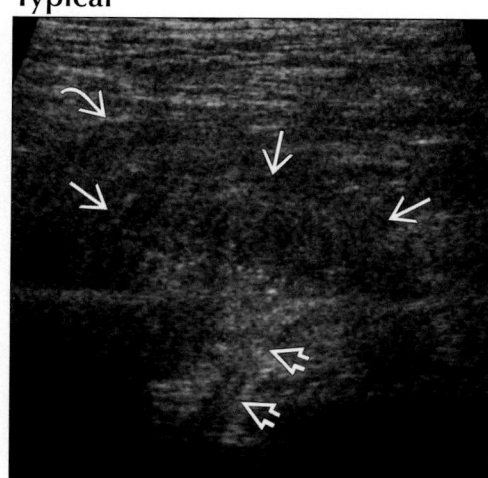

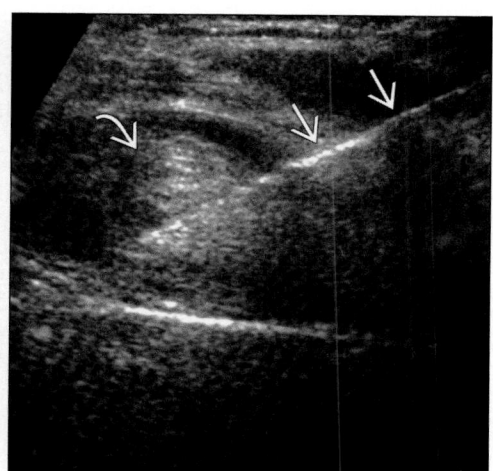

(Left) Longitudinal ultrasound of the same patient as the previous image, shows inflammatory exudate ➡ exuding from the fracture site ➡. Note generalized edema of juxtacortical tissues ➡. *(Right)* Longitudinal ultrasound in the same patient, shows percutaneous biopsy ➡ of the inflammatory tissue ➡. Culture yielded Staphylococcus aureus. Histology revealed acute on chronic inflammation.

Typical

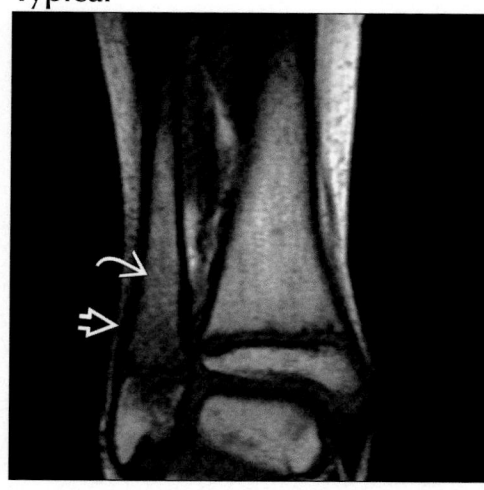

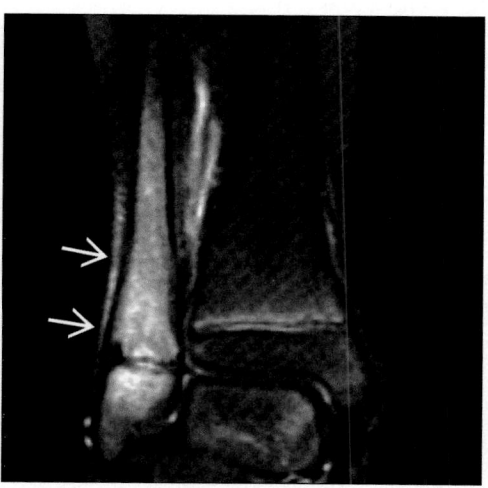

(Left) Coronal T1WI MR shows mild periosteal thickening ➡ and hypointensity of the medullary canal of the distal fibular metaphysis ➡. Note absence of discrete mass. *(Right)* Coronal T2WI MR with fat-suppression at the same location shows marked medullary canal and juxtacortical edema ➡. The appearances are compatible with early acute osteomyelitis.

JOINT INFECTION

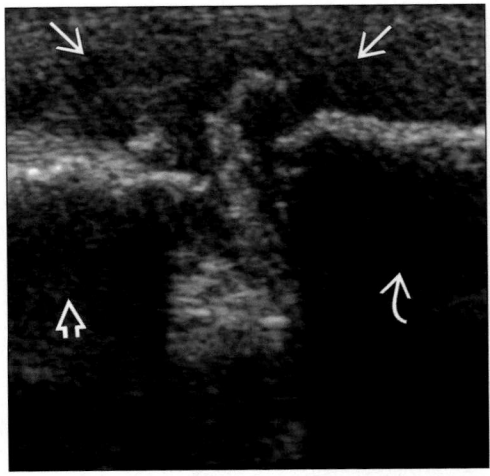 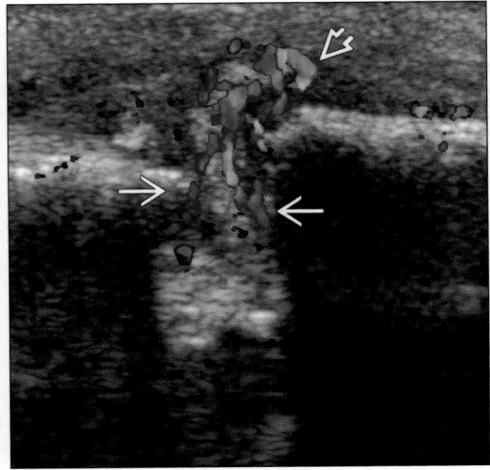

Longitudinal ultrasound in a diabetic patient, shows chronic septic arthritis with widening and irregularity of medial cuneiform ➡, first metatarsal ➡ joint. The capsule is distended ➡ with echogenic contents.

Longitudinal color Doppler ultrasound at same location as previous image, shows marked hyperemia ➡ within and alongside the joint ➡ indicating that the joint is filled with hyperemic granulation tissue.

TERMINOLOGY

Abbreviations and Synonyms
- Joint infection, infective arthritis

Definitions
- Bacterial infection of joint fluid

IMAGING FINDINGS

General Features
- Best diagnostic clue: Echogenic joint effusion with positive aspirate ± synovial/capsular thickening and hyperemia
- Location
  - Hip = knee > shoulder, ankle, wrist, elbow, small joints of hands and feet, sternoclavicular joint, acromioclavicular joint
    - May be multifocal; especially in at-risk patient
    - Gonococcal arthritis ⇒ predilection for small joints of hand and feet (disseminated gonococcal infection)

Ultrasonographic Findings
- Normal ultrasound examination excludes septic arthritis
- **Joint effusion**
  - Cardinal sign of septic arthritis
  - ± Clumps of echoes or multiple fine echoes within joint fluid
    - Swirling or moving echoes on real-time imaging
  - Anechoic joint fluid does not exclude septic arthritis
    - Joint aspiration & analysis of joint fluid only way to truly exclude joint infection
  - In some non-distensible joints (e.g., acromioclavicular, sternoclavicular, sacroiliac joints) effusion is minimal
  - **Findings in more chronic infections**
    - Synovial proliferation
    - ± Central hyperemia of joint
    - Capsular thickening
    - Viscosity of joint fluid increases
    - Amount of joint fluid decreases
    - ± Residual small pockets of fluid
    - Progressive joint space narrowing (chondrolysis)
    - Marginal erosions (osteolysis)

DDx: Joint Infection

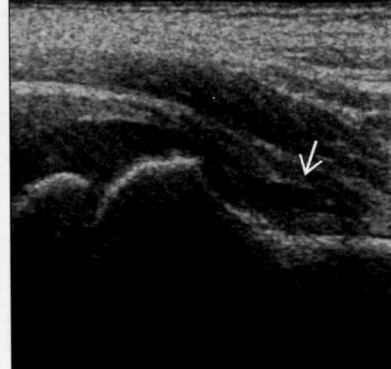 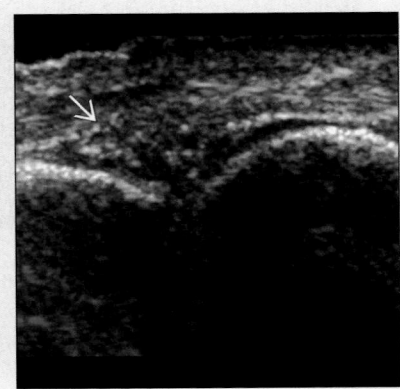 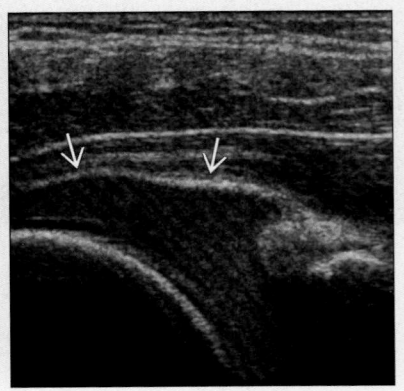

| *Transient Synovitis* | *Crystal Arthropathy* | *Hemarthrosis* |

JOINT INFECTION

Key Facts

Terminology
- Bacterial infection of joint fluid

Imaging Findings
- **Joint effusion**
- Cardinal sign of septic arthritis
- ± Clumps of echoes or multiple fine echoes within joint fluid
- Swirling or moving echoes on real-time imaging
- Anechoic joint fluid does not exclude septic arthritis
- **Findings in more chronic infections**
- Synovial proliferation
- Viscosity of joint fluid increases
- Amount of joint fluid decreases
- Progressive joint space narrowing (chondrolysis)
- Marginal erosions (osteolysis)
- Peri-articular soft tissue extension

Top Differential Diagnoses
- Transient Synovitis Hip
- Crystal Arthropathy
- Hemarthrosis

Clinical Issues
- Non-gonococcal septic arthritis: Prognosis good if detected and treated early
- Gonococcal septic arthritis: Good prognosis

Diagnostic Checklist
- Ultimate diagnosis rests on isolating pathogens from aspirated joint fluid
- Early diagnosis and treatment = key to success
- Normal ultrasound excludes septic arthritis

- Secondary degenerative change
  - Peri-articular soft tissue extension
  - ± Visible capsular rupture
    - Infective tenosynovitis
    - Abscess
    - Inflammatory mass

Radiographic Findings
- Radiography
  - Early stages
    - Usually normal
    - ± Joint effusion, widening of affected joint
    - ± Periarticular swelling & obliteration of fat planes
    - ± Periarticular osteopenia
  - Late stages
    - ± Narrowing of joint space (chondrolysis), marginal erosions (osteolysis), secondary osteoarthrosis, ankylosis

MR Findings
- T1WI
  - Hypointense or isointense joint effusion
  - ± Hypointense periarticular marrow edema
  - ± Hypointense para-articular soft tissue extension
- T2WI
  - Hyperintense joint effusion with capsular distension
    - ± Synovial proliferation
    - ± Periarticular edema, inflammation or abscess
- T1 C+: Enhancement of synovium, capsule, pericapsular tissues

Imaging Recommendations
- Best imaging tool: Ultrasound
- Protocol advice
  - Aspirate → cytology, culture & crystals (adults)
    - Prior to initiation of antibiotic therapy
  - Cytology: Turbid, low viscosity fluid with leucocyte count > 50,000 mm³
    - ~ 90% polymorphs
  - Compensated polarized light microscopy sample should be fresh (i.e., not mixed with water or alcohol, as these will dissolve crystals)
    - Uric acid crystals (negatively birefringent)

- Calcium pyrophosphate dihydrate crystals (positively birefringent)
    - Simultaneous crystalline and bacterial arthritis may occur
  - Gram stain and culture
    - Send sample for culture stat
    - Higher yield than if sample left standing or kept in fridge overnight
    - Aerobic, anaerobic, mycobacterial & fungal culture
    - Aspirate culture positive in 90%
    - Aspirate gram stain positive in 50%
  - Percutaneous synovial biopsy
    - Tru-cut core biopsy
    - Forceps biopsy via though dilated entry portal

DIFFERENTIAL DIAGNOSIS

Transient Synovitis Hip
- Children
- Self-limiting
- Anechoic or mildly echogenic fluid ± synovial/capsular thickening
  - Tendency for subclinical disease of contralateral hip
- If doubt → aspirate

Crystal Arthropathy
- Synovitis ± effusion ± crystalline particles (seen as comet-tail artifacts)
  - ± Periarticular tophi
  - ± Serum uric acid
- If doubt → aspirate

Hemarthrosis
- Traumatic or spontaneous onset ± underlying coagulopathy
- Finely echogenic fluid similar to acute septic arthritis
  - Synovial/capsular thickening not a feature
- If doubt → aspirate

JOINT INFECTION

PATHOLOGY

General Features
- Etiology
  - Most commonly due to hematogenous seeding of synovium from bacteremia
  - Less common causes
    - Complication of surgery (hip or knee arthroplasty)
    - Spread from adjacent osteomyelitis focus
    - Inoculation during joint injection or aspiration
    - Penetrating trauma (bite or knife puncture)
- Epidemiology
  - 2-10 per 100,000/year incidence
  - > Patients over 60 years age
    - > Degenerative joint disease and reduced immunity
    - ↓ Thymic & T-lymphocytic function and ↓ B-cell antibody production
  - > Rheumatoid arthritis (x 10 general incidence)
  - > Diabetics, poor general health, corticosteroids
- Associated abnormalities: Tenosynovitis, osteomyelitis, pyomyositis, endocarditis
- Organisms
  - Staphylococcus aureus
    - Most common organism especially in diabetics and rheumatoid arthritis patients
    - Late (> 3 months) infection of prosthesis
    - Early infection of prosthesis ⇔ surgical contamination ⇔ Staphylococcus epidermidis
  - Streptococcus pyogenes
  - Gram-negative organisms (Pseudomonas aeruginosa, Escherichia coli, Neisseria gonorrhoeae)
    - Especially intravenous drug users, extremes of age and immunosuppressed
    - Neisseria gonorrhoeae ⇔ disseminated gonococcal infection (> USA)
    - Gonococcal infection also ⇒ reactive arthritis

Gross Pathologic & Surgical Features
- Hyperemic synovium
- Bacterial seeding of synovium
- Synovium membrane ⇒ no limiting basement plate under well-vascularized synovium
  - Facilitates bacterial entry to joint
- ⇒ Bacterial adherence & colonization
- ⇒ Bacterial proliferation → acute inflammatory response
- ⇒ Cytokine & acute phase protein release → tissue damage

Microscopic Features
- Acute inflammatory response
- Synovitis
- Tissue damage

CLINICAL ISSUES

Presentation
- Most common signs/symptoms: Mono-articular pain, swelling and limitation of movement
- Other signs/symptoms: Fever, malaise

- Clinical Profile: At-risk patient with recent onset of joint inflammation

Demographics
- Age: Extremes of age, especially elderly
- Gender
  - Non-gonococcal arthritis; M:F = 1:1
  - Gonococcal arthritis; M:F= 1:10

Natural History & Prognosis
- Depends on immunocompetency of host, virulence of organism, rapidity of detection, treatment response
  - Non-gonococcal septic arthritis: Prognosis good if detected and treated early
    - Early = < 7 days after onset of symptoms
  - Poor prognostic indicators
    - > 6 days to make joint (clinically) sterile after onset of treatment
    - Virulent organism
    - Elderly
    - Immunosuppressed
    - Osteoarthrosis & rheumatoid arthritis; prone to delayed diagnosis with symptoms of infection wrongly attributed to underlying disease
- Impairment of joint function results in 50%
- Morbidity 5-20% due to bacteremia
  - Septic oligoarthritis (30% mortality)
  - Septic oligoarthritis + rheumatoid arthritis or Staphylococcus aureus infection = 50% mortality
- Gonococcal septic arthritis: Good prognosis
  - Symptoms ↓ rapidly without sequelae

Treatment
- Conservative
  - IV antibiotics
  - Splinting to prevent contractures
  - ± Repeated ultrasound-guided percutaneous aspiration
  - ± Percutaneous ultrasound-guided tidal irrigation
    - Irrigation of joint through closed system
  - Physiotherapy once ↓ symptoms
- Arthroscopic debridement
- Arthrotomy and wound irrigation/debridement
- Infected prosthesis usually requires replacement
  - Removal & debridement (stage 1)
  - Reimplantation (stage 2)

DIAGNOSTIC CHECKLIST

Consider
- Ultimate diagnosis rests on isolating pathogens from aspirated joint fluid
  - Early diagnosis and treatment = key to success
- Normal ultrasound excludes septic arthritis
- Ultrasound & aspiration ⇒ diagnosis
  - MR ⇒ damage assessment

SELECTED REFERENCES
1. Chau CL et al: Musculoskeletal infections: ultrasound appearances. Clin Radiol. 60(2):149-59, 2005
2. Shirtliff ME et al: Acute septic arthritis. Clin Microbiol Rev. 15(4):527-44, 2002

JOINT INFECTION

IMAGE GALLERY

Typical

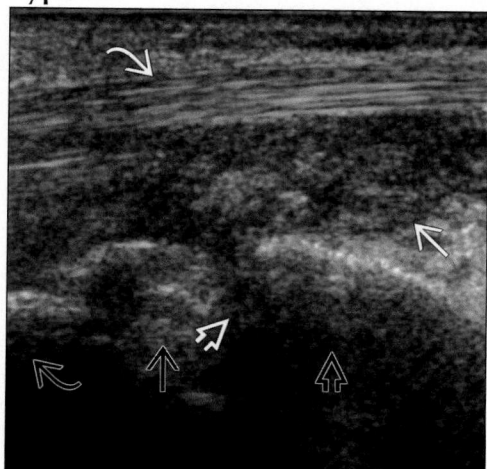 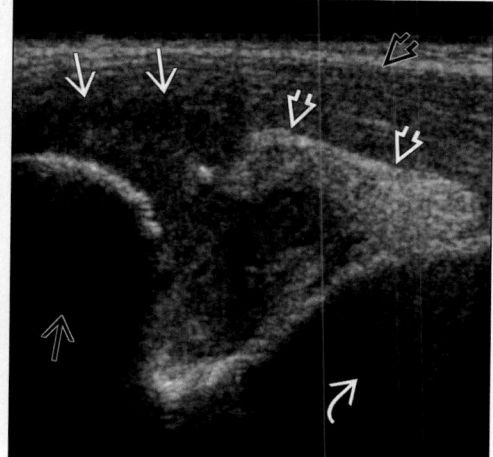

(Left) Longitudinal ultrasound shows chronic septic arthritis with an inflammatory infiltrate ➡ extending from the wrist joint ⊳, deep to the extensor tendons ➡. Radius ⊳, lunate ➡ and capitate ➡. *(Right)* Longitudinal ultrasound of septic arthritis of the elbow shows an echogenic effusion ➡ and rupture of the posterior aspect of the elbow capsule ➡. Triceps muscle-tendon ➡, olecranon ➡ and distal humerus ➡.

Typical

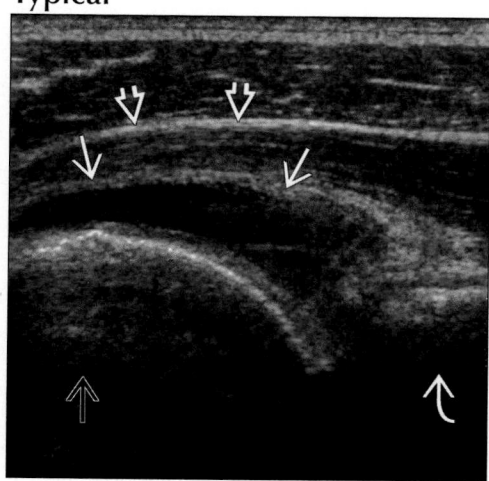 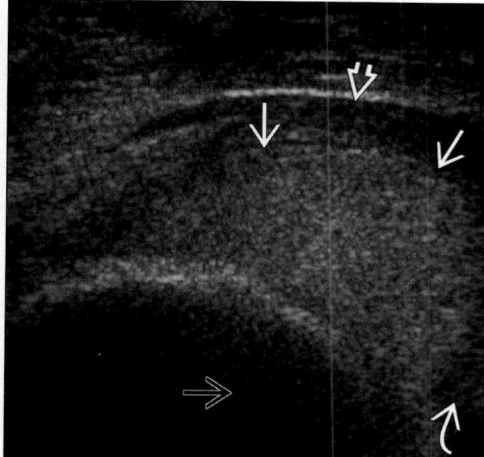

(Left) Transverse ultrasound of acute septic arthritis of the shoulder shows distention of the posterior aspect of the glenohumeral joint by hypoechoic fluid ➡. Infraspinatus muscle-tendon ➡, humeral head ➡ and glenoid ➡. *(Right)* Transverse ultrasound of acute septic arthritis of the shoulder with the posterior aspect of the glenohumeral joint distended by echogenic fluid ➡. Infraspinatus muscle-tendon ➡, humeral head ➡ and glenoid ➡.

Typical

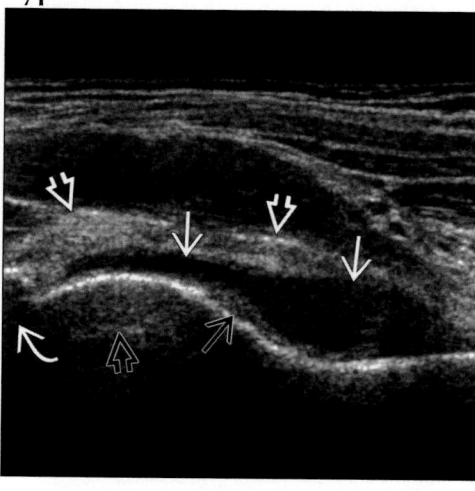 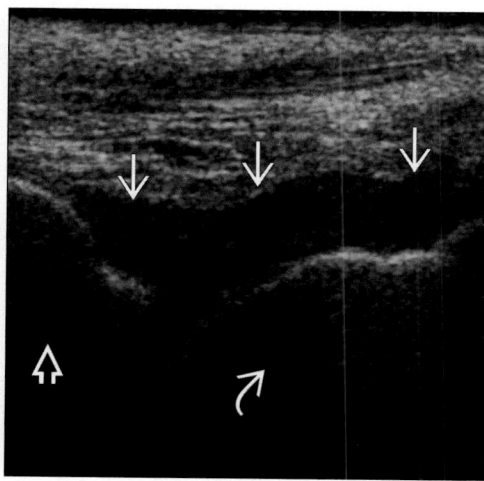

(Left) Longitudinal ultrasound of the hip shows a large joint effusion ➡ due to acute septic arthritis. The capsule is thickened and distended ➡ with little synovial thickening ➡. Acetabulum ➡, femoral head ➡. *(Right)* Longitudinal ultrasound shows acute septic arthritis of the ankle with distension of the ankle capsule by hypoechoic fluid ➡. Purulent fluid was aspirated. Distal tibia ➡ and talus ➡.

POST-OPERATIVE INFECTION

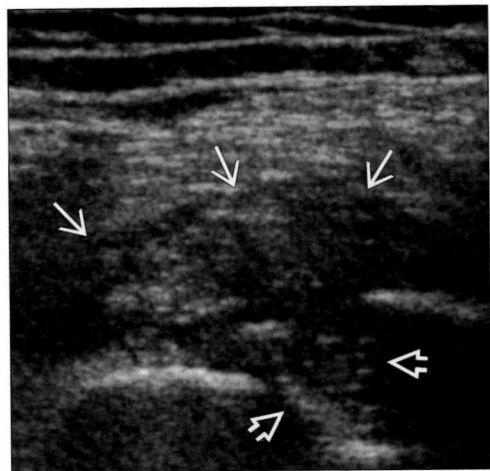
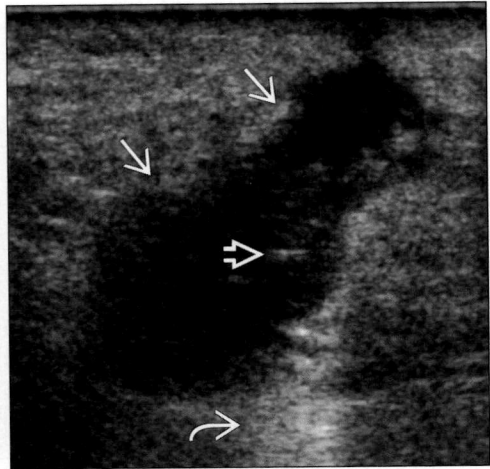

Longitudinal ultrasound following removal of an infected hip prosthesis shows intense inflammatory edema ➡, with small echogenic foci alongside the cortical defect in the proximal femur ⧑.

Longitudinal ultrasound of same patient as previous image, shows a thick channel of edematous tissue ➡ extending from deeper tissues to the skin surface. Note small gas locules ⧑ and acoustic enhancement ➡.

TERMINOLOGY

Abbreviations and Synonyms
- Post-surgical infection, wound infection

Definitions
- Infection at surgical site within one month of surgery
  - Or within one year if implant performed

IMAGING FINDINGS

General Features
- Best diagnostic clue: Inflammation ± collection persisting one week after surgery
- Location
  - Soft tissue, bone or joint
  - Hip, knee, spine or any operative site
  - Superficial infection = infection superficial to investing fascia
  - Deep infection = infection deep to investing fascia
- Size: Localized around surgical site
- Morphology: From localized wound infection to acute osteomyelitis

Ultrasonographic Findings
- Mild soft tissue edema, fluid and hyperemia = very common signs in early post-operative period
- Intensity and pattern of edema, fluid and hyperemia helps differentiate infectious from non-infectious inflammation
  - Inflammation from surgical disruption of tissues & subsequent repair follows expected pattern & is usually mild in degree
  - Inflammation from post-operative infection is more severe & does not follow expected pattern
- Degree of soft tissue edema, > amount of fluid, > degree of hyperemia ⇒ greater likelihood of post-operative infection
- Edematous tissue = hyperechoic if mildly edematous & hypoechoic if more intensely edematous
- Fluid may collect as discrete collection or as accumulation at fascial or tissue interface
  - Anechoic or hypoechoic
  - ± Echogenic fluid (often blood)
  - ± Debris
- ± Gas

DDx: Post-Operative Infection

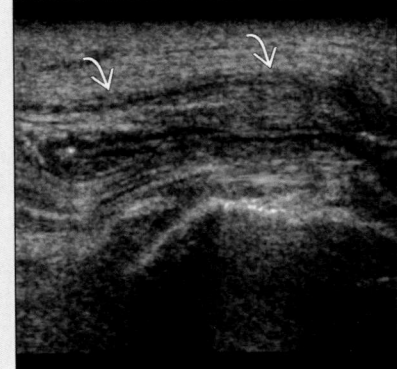
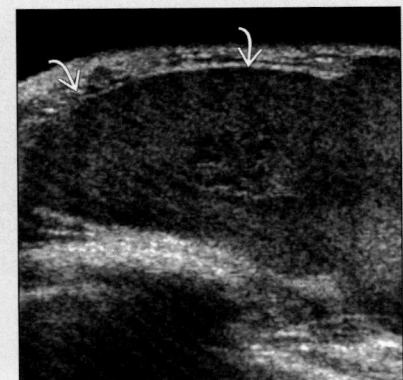
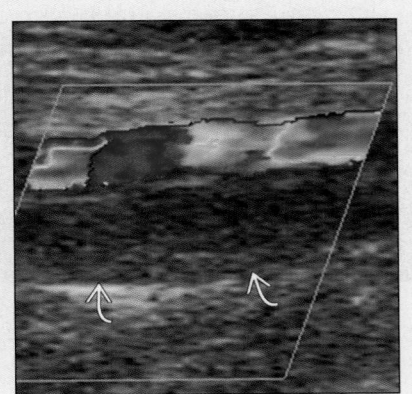

Non-Infective Inflammation

Hematoma

Deep Venous Thrombosis

POST-OPERATIVE INFECTION

Key Facts

Terminology
- Infection at surgical site within one month of surgery
- Or within one year if implant performed

Imaging Findings
- Mild soft tissue edema, fluid and hyperemia = very common signs in early post-operative period
- Fluid may collect as discrete collection or as accumulation at fascial or tissue interface
- Usually not possible to distinguish infected fluid, non-infected seroma or liquefied hematoma
- Ultrasound not prone to metallic artifact
- Ultrasound accessible to post-operative patient
- Examine dependent areas carefully since collections will develop/accumulate here preferentially

Top Differential Diagnoses
- Post-Operative Inflammation
- Hematoma
- Deep Venous Thrombosis

Diagnostic Checklist
- Accurate & timely recognition is key to successful eradication of post-operative infection
- Most post-operative infections evident clinically
- Ultrasound helps to define site of soft tissue infection, isolate fluid & provide aspirate for culture
- Integrity of recently operated bone is impaired
- If juxtacortical infection present, high probability bone is also affected
- Intensity and pattern of edema, fluid and hyperemia helps differentiate infectious from non-infectious inflammation

---

- ○ May be present normally in first few days after surgery
- ○ Longer if open wound or drain present
- Usually not possible to distinguish infected fluid, non-infected seroma or liquefied hematoma
  - ○ ⇒ Need to aspirate
- Synovial-capsular thickening common after surgery
  - ○ Joint capsule disruption during arthroplasty
    - ▪ Limits development of post-operative effusion
    - ▪ Allows drainage of fluid into periarticular tissues
- Ultrasound not prone to metallic artifact
  - ○ Good visualization of juxtacortical tissues
- Ultrasound accessible to post-operative patient
- Helps localize site of infection (superficial/deep), isolate fluid and provide aspirate to identify organism
- Limitations of ultrasound
  - ○ Cannot differentiate mild post-operative infection from non-infective post-operative inflammation
  - ○ Transducer access occasionally limited by external fixators, bandaging or cutaneous wound
  - ○ Not sensitive at detecting osteomyelitis

Radiographic Findings
- Best initial investigation
  - ○ Aids interpretation of subsequent ultrasound & other investigations

CT Findings
- CECT
  - ○ Multidetector CT less prone to metallic artifact
    - ▪ CT (or MR) → most useful in re-assessment of infection after implant has been removed
  - ○ Delineates bony abnormality and soft tissue infection
    - ▪ ± CT-guided aspiration or drainage
  - ○ Information from plain CT limited, especially with respect to abscess formation

MR Findings
- T1WI: Hypointense soft tissue swelling
- T2WI FS: Hyperintense soft tissue swelling ± hyperintense fluid or fluid collection
- T1 C+

- ○ Infective, non-infective inflammatory and reparative tissue all enhance
  - ▪ Pattern and intensity of enhancement allows discrimination
  - ▪ Generally > enhancement ⇒ greater likelihood of infection
- ○ Useful at delineating fluid collections
  - ▪ Wall enhancement > with abscesses than with sterile collections
- ○ MR imaging severely limited by metallic susceptibility artifact

Nuclear Medicine Findings
- Bone Scan
  - ○ Diagnosis of periprosthetic infection ± combined with labeled leukocyte scintigraphy
  - ○ No periprosthetic uptake = no infection
  - ○ Periprosthetic uptake = loosening or infection
    - ▪ + Uptake at same site on labeled leukocyte scintigraphy ⇒ infection most likely
    - ▪ + No uptake at same site in labeled leukocyte scintigraphy ⇒ loosening most likely
  - ○ High sensitivity with moderate specificity
    - ▪ Repair can simulate infection
  - ○ Low sensitivity for spinal infection (poor uptake)
- PET CT
  - ○ Combines high sensitivity of PET imaging with high-resolution of CT imaging
    - ▪ ↓ Specificity, particularly in post-operative cases
    - ▪ Glucolysis also feature of non-infectious inflammation & repair
  - ○ Activity around shaft & tip of hip prosthesis → > likelihood of infection compared to activity around head & neck of prosthesis

Imaging Recommendations
- Best imaging tool: Ultrasound
- Protocol advice
  - ○ Remove bandaging; cover suture line with thin polyurethane adhesive dressing
  - ○ Copious gel to maximize contact at surgical incision
  - ○ Examine dependent areas carefully since collections will develop/accumulate here preferentially

POST-OPERATIVE INFECTION

- For example, following hip arthroplasty, roll patient to lateral decubitus position to examine gluteal and posterior thigh regions
  - If performing aspiration, ensure aseptic technique, as damaged tissues susceptible to inoculation

DIFFERENTIAL DIAGNOSIS

Post-Operative Inflammation
- Difficult to distinguish from post-operative infection
- Pattern & intensity of edema, fluid accumulation, hyperemia important

Hematoma
- Discrete hematoma uncommon
  - Hypoechoic mass with fixed fine internal echoes
- Partially liquefied hematoma with blood clot more common

Deep Venous Thrombosis
- Limb swelling & fever
- May co-exist with post-operative infection
- Non-compressible vein

PATHOLOGY

General Features
- Etiology
  - Incidence of infection following knee or hip arthroplasty = 0.5-2%
    - Early infection (< 3 months after surgery) = mostly due to surgical contamination
    - Late infection (within one year of surgery) = mostly due to hematogenous seeding of operative site
    - Prostheses; disrupt integrity of tissues, affect blood supply & provide surface for bacterial adherence
  - Staphylococcus aureus
    - Responsible organism in half of cases
  - Gram-negative bacilli (Bactcrioides, Escherichia coli, Pseudomonas, Proteus, Klebsiella, Enterococcus)
- Epidemiology
  - Risks related to procedure
    - Long operation time (> 3 hours)
    - High blood loss (> 1,000 mL)
    - Instrumentation
    - Multiple surgical sites (e.g., fixation + bone grafting)
    - Staged operation or repeat operation
  - Risks related to patient
    - Frailty
    - Co-existent morbidity
    - Co-existent remote site infection
    - Obesity
    - Smoking

Gross Pathologic & Surgical Features
- Cellulitis
- Pyomyositis
- Abscess

Microscopic Features
- Acute or acute-on-chronic inflammatory infiltrate, capillary dilatation ± abscess formation

CLINICAL ISSUES

Presentation
- Most common signs/symptoms: Pain & swelling
- Other signs/symptoms: Wound oozing, inflammation, fever
- Clinical Profile: Leukocytosis, raised inflammatory markers

Demographics
- Age: Less common in young patients
- Gender: M:F = 1:1

Natural History & Prognosis
- Superficial infection can usually be treated successfully with antibiotic therapy
- Established deep infection often difficult to eradicate without removing implant

Treatment
- Antibiotic therapy
- Aspiration or drainage (image-guided) of collections
- ± Debridement
- ± Implant removal

DIAGNOSTIC CHECKLIST

Consider
- Accurate & timely recognition is key to successful eradication of post-operative infection
  - Ultrasound very helpful in this respect
- Most post-operative infections evident clinically
  - Ultrasound helps to define site of soft tissue infection, isolate fluid & provide aspirate for culture
  - Nuclear medicine studies help identify bone infection around prostheses
- Integrity of recently operated bone is impaired
  - If juxtacortical infection present, high probability bone is also affected
- Polymerase chain reaction (PCR) techniques may play increasing role in organism identification
  - Isolate organism by identification of specific genetic sequences rather than culture

Image Interpretation Pearls
- Intensity and pattern of edema, fluid and hyperemia helps differentiate infectious from non-infectious inflammation
- Search dependent areas for collections in post-operative patients
- Imaging appearances & nuclear medicine study results are influenced by concurrent antibiotic therapy

SELECTED REFERENCES

1. Peterson JJ: Postoperative infection. Radiol Clin North Am. 44(3):439-50, 2006

POST-OPERATIVE INFECTION

Typical

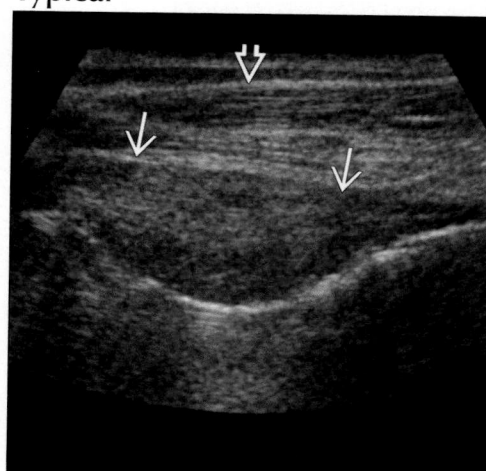
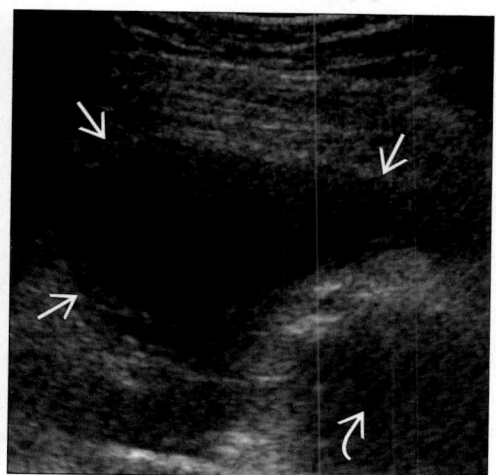

(Left) Longitudinal ultrasound shows marked synovial/capsular thickening ➡ of the hip joint five days post-arthroplasty. Such distension (12 mm) is not uncommon & does not imply infection. Note clean peri-articular soft tissues ➡.
(Right) Transverse ultrasound of the thigh following hip arthroplasty shows hypoechoic fluid collection ➡ posterior to proximal femur ➡. Aspiration yielded mildly blood-stained fluid. No growth.

Typical

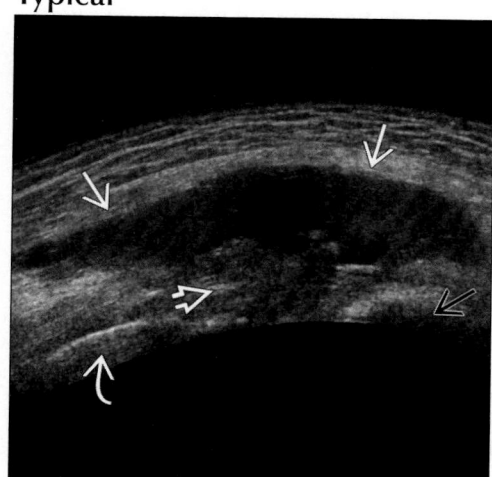
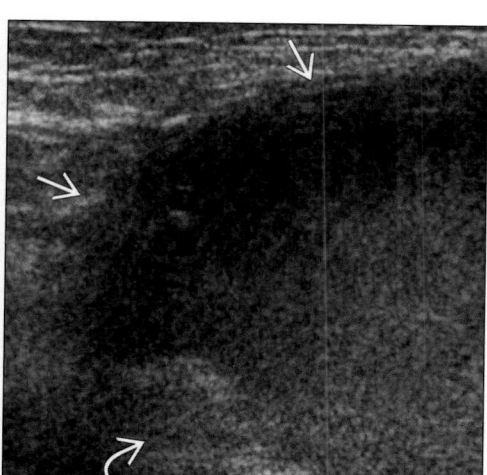

(Left) Longitudinal ultrasound following hip arthroplasty shows edematous tissue ➡ and hypoechoic fluid collection ➡ posterior to proximal femur ➡ and ischium ➡. Aspirate grew Staphylococcus aureus.
(Right) Longitudinal ultrasound of thigh following excision of soft tissue tumor shows a large echogenic collection ➡ postero-medial to femur ➡. Aspirate yielded blood-stained fluid (no growth) though wound swab grew Pseudomonas.

Typical

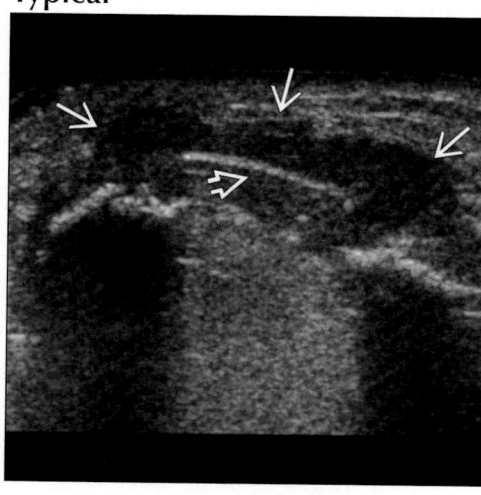
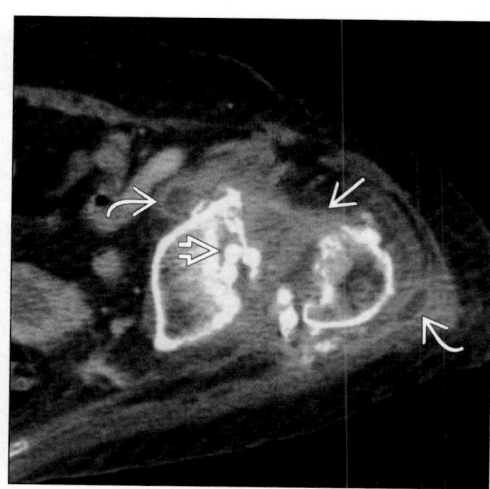

(Left) Transverse ultrasound of tibial fracture shows thick-rim of viscous-type fluid ➡ around the fixation plate ➡. Aspirate yielded only small amount (needle-hub) of material which grew Staphylococcus aureus. *(Right)* Transverse CECT of the left hip region following removal of hip prosthesis shows enhancing inflammatory tissue ➡ of hip region with small rim-enhancing abscesses ➡ and gentamicin beads ➡.

HEMARTHROSIS & LIPOHEMARTHROSIS

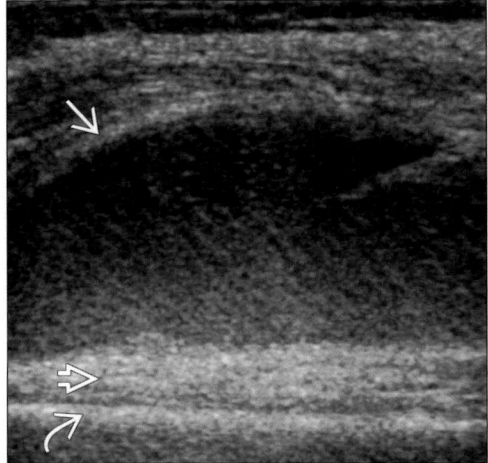

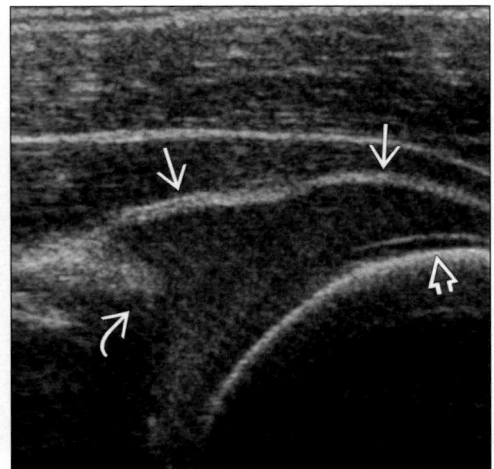

Longitudinal ultrasound of the suprapatellar pouch shows an acute hemarthrosis ➡, with sedimentation evidenced by graded ↑ echogenicity from superficial to deep. Juxtacortical fat ⬎. Femoral cortex ⬎.

Transverse ultrasound along the posterior aspect of the shoulder shows an acute hemarthrosis with a distended joint capsule ➡. No layering is present. Glenoid labrum ⬎. Articular cartilage of humeral head ⬎.

TERMINOLOGY

Abbreviations and Synonyms
- Post-traumatic hemarthrosis or lipohemarthrosis, spontaneous hemarthrosis, hemophilic arthropathy

Definitions
- Hemarthrosis = blood in joint cavity
- Lipohemarthrosis = blood & fat in joint cavity
  - Very specific for intra-articular fracture
- Spontaneous hemarthrosis = hemarthrosis developing in absence of predisposing trauma, synovial tumor or hemophilia
- Hemophilic arthropathy = arthropathy secondary to repeated hemarthrosis due to inherited clotting disorder

IMAGING FINDINGS

General Features
- Best diagnostic clue: Layered joint effusion
- Location: Knee > ankle > elbow > shoulder > hip
- Size: Large effusion

- Morphology: Joint cavity distended with blood ± fat

Ultrasonographic Findings
- Acute stage
  - Large effusion
    - Finely speckled echogenic joint fluid
    - Minimal or no synovial thickening or hyperemia
  - ± Graded ↑ echogenicity from more hypoechoic (superficial) → more hyperechoic (deep)
    - Due to early sedimentation of cellular elements
  - ± Layering of different fluid components
    - Specific for hemarthrosis or lipohemarthrosis
    - Seen after part under examination is static for few minutes
  - **Hemarthrosis initially ⇒ finely speckled echogenic joint fluid**
  - After ~ 5 minutes ⇒ ± two-layered appearance of joint effusion
    - Superficial hypoechoic layer representing supernatant serum
    - Inferior hyperechoic layer representing dependent RBCs
  - **Lipohemarthrosis initially ⇒ finely speckled echogenic joint fluid**

DDx: Hemarthrosis & Lipohemarthrosis

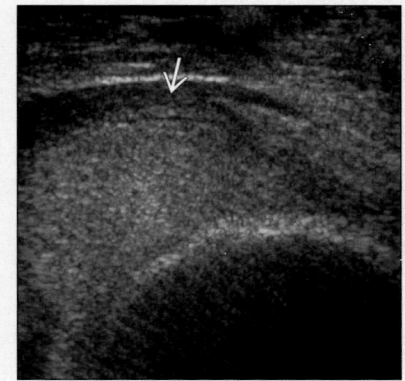

Septic Arthritis

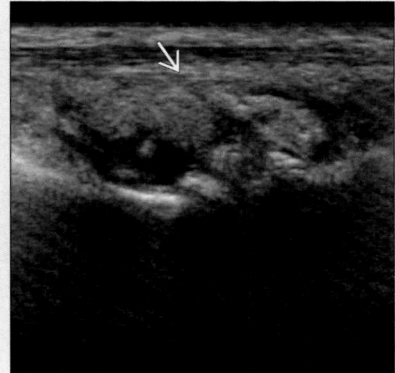

Gout

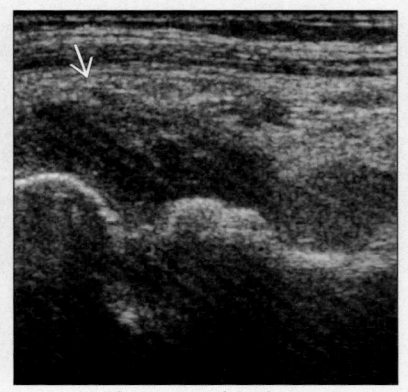

Rheumatoid Arthritis

HEMARTHROSIS & LIPOHEMARTHROSIS

Key Facts

Terminology
- Hemarthrosis = blood in joint cavity
- Lipohemarthrosis = blood & fat in joint cavity

Imaging Findings
- Best diagnostic clue: Layered joint effusion
- **Hemarthrosis initially ⇒ finely speckled echogenic joint fluid**
- After ~ 5 minutes ⇒ ± two-layered appearance of joint effusion
- Superficial hypoechoic layer representing supernatant serum
- **Lipohemarthrosis initially ⇒ finely speckled echogenic joint fluid**
- After ~ 10 minutes ⇒ three-layered appearance of joint effusion
- Superior hyperechoic layer representing floating fat

- Central hypoechoic layer representing supernatant serum
- Inferior hyperechoic layer representing dependent RBCs
- ± Hypoechoic areas within floating fat due to trapped blood

Top Differential Diagnoses
- Septic Arthritis
- Gout
- Inflammatory Synovitis

Diagnostic Checklist
- Fine specked echogenic effusion → two-layer appearance (hemarthrosis) or three-layer appearance (lipohemarthrosis)

- ○ After ~ 10 minutes ⇒ three-layered appearance of joint effusion
  - ▪ Superior hyperechoic layer representing floating fat
  - ▪ Central hypoechoic layer representing supernatant serum
  - ▪ Inferior hyperechoic layer representing dependent RBCs
- ○ ± Hypoechoic areas within floating fat due to trapped blood
- ○ Demonstration of layers probably dependent on three factors
  - ▪ Amount of blood or fat in joint
  - ▪ Time part under examination is static prior to imaging
  - ▪ Time after fracture
- Subacute stage
  - ○ Blood clots → discrete echogenic foci within joint
  - ○ Joint fluid → more anechoic
  - ○ ± Fibrinous adhesions
- Repeated hemarthrosis
  - ○ Early hemophiliac arthropathy ⇒ ↑ joint fluid, mild to moderate synovial proliferation with synovial hyperemia
  - ○ Late hemophiliac arthropathy ⇒ less joint fluid, severe synovial thickening with ↓ intensity of synovial hyperemia
    - ▪ Hemosiderin deposition not apparent on ultrasound
  - ○ Secondary osteoarthrosis
    - ▪ Joint space narrowing
    - ▪ Marginal osteophytosis
    - ▪ ± Meniscal extrusion
    - ▪ Chondral, subchondral bony erosions & subchondral cysts not usually visible on ultrasound
  - ○ ± Baker cyst
  - ○ ± Pseudotumor (expanding hematoma)
    - ▪ Hypoechoic ± hyperechoic areas (recent bleeding) ± anechoic areas (liquefaction)

Radiographic Findings
- Hyperdense joint effusion

- ○ Density of hemorrhage > synovial fluid
- Horizontal beam radiography → fat-fluid level due to differences in attenuation fat; blood components
  - ○ Fat less dense & floats on surface of blood
  - ○ Lipohemarthrosis present in 35% of intra-articular fractures about knee
    - ▪ High specificity but low sensitivity for intra-articular fractures

CT Findings
- NECT
  - ○ Hemarthrosis: Two distinct layers
    - ▪ Superior isodense layer (~ 30 HU) = serum
    - ▪ Inferior hyperdense layer (~ 70 HU) = RBCs
  - ○ Lipohemarthrosis: Three distinct layers
    - ▪ Superior hypodense (~ -70 HU) layer = fat
    - ▪ Central intermediate (~ 20 HU) = serum
    - ▪ Inferior hyperdense (~ 90 HU) = RBCs

MR Findings
- T2WI
  - ○ Hemarthrosis: Two distinct signal bands
    - ▪ Superior hypointense band (serum)
    - ▪ Inferior isodense band (dependent RBCs)
  - ○ Lipohemarthrosis: Three distinct signal bands
    - ▪ Superior hyperintense band (floating fat)
    - ▪ Central hyperintense band (serum)
    - ▪ Inferior isointense band (dependent RBCs)
  - ○ ± Thin hypointense band due to chemical shift artifact at serum-fat interface

Imaging Recommendations
- Best imaging tool: Ultrasound
- Protocol advice
  - ○ Minimize movement of part under examination
  - ○ Repeat examination at 5-20 minutes (layering)

DIFFERENTIAL DIAGNOSIS

Septic Arthritis
- Gradual onset joint swelling over 1-2 days
  - ○ More insidious onset if non-pyogenic infection

HEMARTHROSIS & LIPOHEMARTHROSIS

- Very tender with marked limitation of movement
  - ± Larger aggregates than hemarthrosis/lipohemarthrosis
  - ± Aspiration (if doubt)

Gout
- Severe inflammation
- Echogenic crystal aggregates ± tophi
- ± Aspiration (if doubt)

Inflammatory Synovitis
- Marked synovial proliferation & hyperemia
- ± Polyarticular ± marginal erosions
- ± Joint space narrowing
- ± Aspiration (if doubt)

PATHOLOGY

General Features
- Genetics: Hemophilia A or B: X-linked recessive
- Etiology
  - Post-traumatic hemarthrosis/lipohemarthrosis
    - Bleeding from laceration of synovial vessels or leakage from marrow cavity
    - Lipohemarthrosis always signifies intra-articular fracture
    - Only way marrow fat can enter joint
  - Spontaneous hemarthrosis
    - Due to spontaneous bleeding from synovium
- Epidemiology
  - Relative frequency; hemophilia A (85%), hemophilia B (14%), other clotting disorders (1%)
    - 1 in 5,000 males; 60% cases severe

Gross Pathologic & Surgical Features
- Synovial proliferation & inflammation

Microscopic Features
- Acute on chronic inflammation
- Hemosiderin-laden macrophages; fibrosis

Staging, Grading or Classification Criteria
- Arnold-Hilgartner scale (for hemophiliac arthropathy of knee)
  - Stage 0: Normal joint
  - Stage I: Soft-tissue swelling present
  - Stage II: Osteoporosis & overgrowth of epiphysis
  - Stage III: Early subchondral bone cysts, squaring of patella, intercondylar notch widened
  - Stage IV: As per stage III but joint space narrowed
  - Stage V: Fibrous joint contracture, loss of joint space, severe enlargement of epiphysis & substantial joint disorganization of joint

CLINICAL ISSUES

Presentation
- Most common signs/symptoms: Rapid onset joint effusion
- Other signs/symptoms
  - Tense, warm joint
    - Arterial or venous bleeding

Demographics
- Age
  - Post-traumatic hemarthrosis/lipohemarthrosis: ↑ 20-30 years
  - Spontaneous hemarthrosis: ↑ Middle-aged or elderly
  - Hemophilic arthropathy: Neonate → throughout life
- Gender
  - Hemarthrosis & lipohemarthrosis > males
    - Related to increased trauma prevalence in males
  - Hemophilia almost exclusively in males

Natural History & Prognosis
- Acute hemorrhage resolves over 1-2 weeks
- Hemophiliac arthropathy
  - Repeated hemarthrosis → progressive arthropathy

Treatment
- Rest & analgesia
  - ± Aspiration if very painful (distension)
- Immobilization of associated fracture
- Hemophilic arthropathy
  - Acute hemorrhage: Rest & ice
  - Correct coagulation factor deficiency
    - Infusion of factor VIII (hemophilia A) or factor IX (hemophilia B)
  - Repeated hemarthroses
  - Chemical synovectomy with intra-articular administration of rifampicin or osmic acid (± ultrasound-guided)
  - Radiosynovectomy with intra-articular administration of yttrium, gold or phosphorus (± ultrasound-guided)
    - Induces synovial fibrosis → reduced bleeding
    - Extra-articular injection or leakage → radiation burn ± inflammatory reaction
    - Contraindicated if leaking Baker cyst
  - Intra-articular administration of hyaluronic acid (± ultrasound-guided)
  - Surgery: Joint replacement (severe arthropathy)

DIAGNOSTIC CHECKLIST

Consider
- Lipohemarthrosis ⇒ single fluid level (fat-fluid) on radiography though ⇒ double fluid level (fat-serum-RBCs) on ultrasound, CT & MR
  - Because cross-sectional imaging can also separate serous & cellular components of blood

Image Interpretation Pearls
- Fine specked echogenic effusion → two-layer appearance (hemarthrosis) or three-layer appearance (lipohemarthrosis)

SELECTED REFERENCES

1. Lugo-Olivieri CH et al: Fluid-fluid levels in injured knees: do they always represent lipohemarthrosis? Radiology. 198(2):499-502, 1996
2. Bianchi S et al: Sonographic evaluation of lipohemarthrosis: clinical and in vitro study. J Ultrasound Med. 14(4):279-82, 1995

HEMARTHROSIS & LIPOHEMARTHROSIS

IMAGE GALLERY

Typical

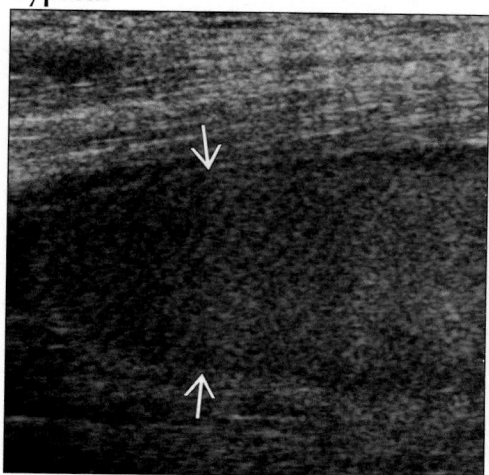 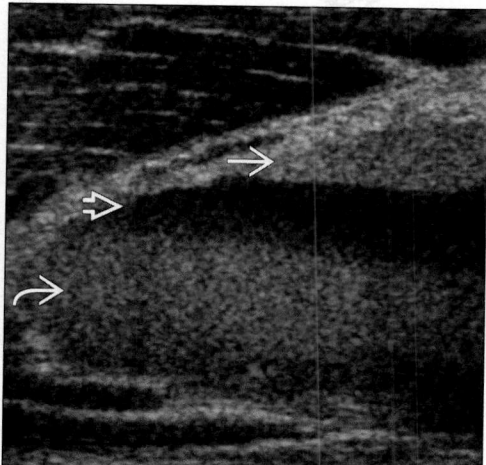

(Left) Longitudinal ultrasound of the suprapatellar pouch shows an acute lipohemarthrosis. The joint capsule is distended ➡ with echogenic fluid. No layering or sedimentation is present. *(Right)* Longitudinal ultrasound (same location as previous image) repeated 15 minutes later, shows a three layer appearance of a lipohemarthrosis. Fat layer ➡, serum layer ⇒ and cellular (RBC) layer ➡.

Typical

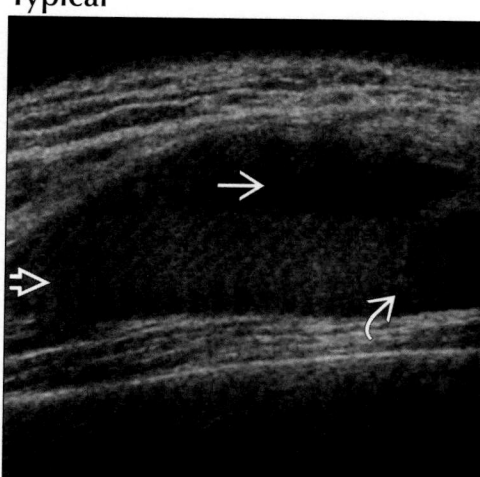 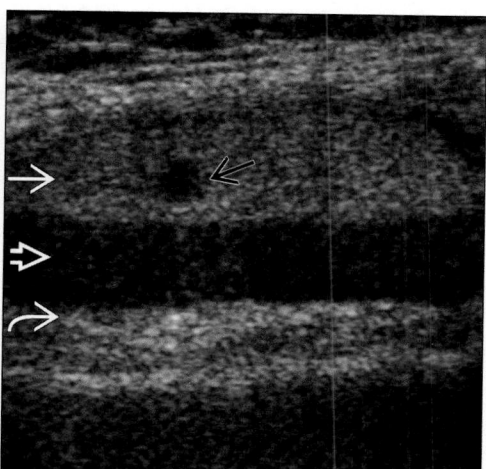

(Left) Longitudinal ultrasound of the suprapatellar pouch shows an acute hemarthrosis with a two layer appearance. Serum layer ➡ and cellular (RBC) layer ⇒. Note synovial plica (fold) ➡ traversing the suprapatellar pouch. *(Right)* Transverse ultrasound of the suprapatellar pouch shows a lipohemarthrosis with fat ➡, serum ⇒ and cellular ➡ layers. The hypoechoic area ⇒ in the fat layer is due to the entrapped blood.

Typical

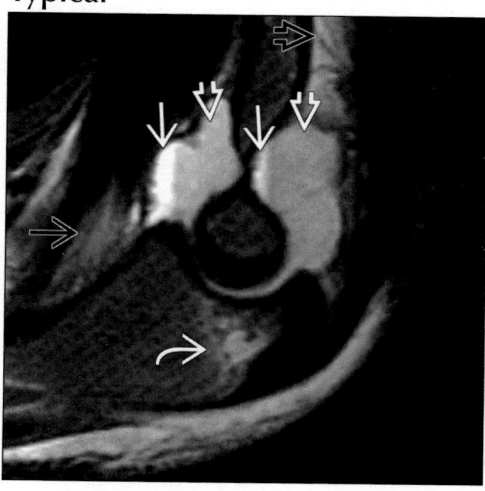 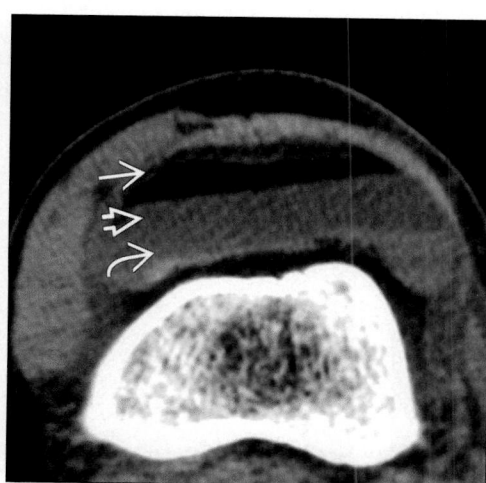

(Left) Sagittal T2WI MR with fat-suppression shows a hemarthrosis of the elbow. Two-layers, with serum ➡ and cellular ⇒ components, are seen in both the anterior and posterior recesses. Note edema in the olecranon ➡. (Triceps ⇒, brachialis ➡). *(Right)* Axial NECT shows a lipohemarthrosis in the suprapatellar pouch of the knee. The three-layered appearance is composed of fat ➡, serum ⇒, and cellular (RBC) ➡ components.

GOUT AND PSEUDOGOUT

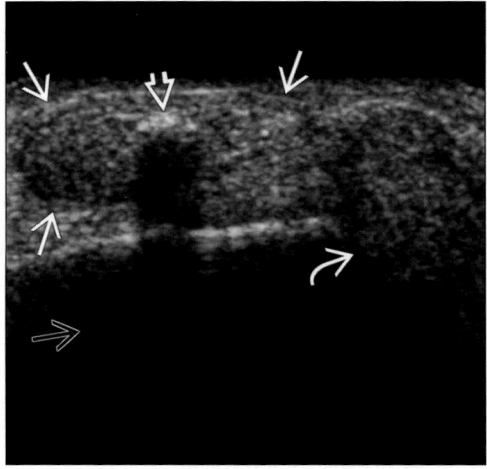

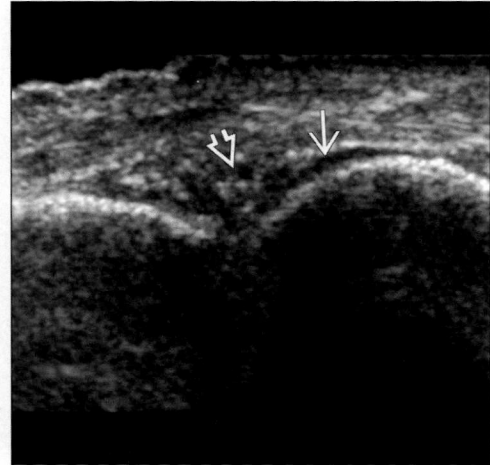

Longitudinal ultrasound of gouty arthropathy shows the elbow joint capsule distended with finely echogenic fluid "urate sand" ➡ and larger echogenic crystal aggregate ⇨. Ulna ⇨. Elbow joint ⇨.

Longitudinal ultrasound shows thin echogenic band ➡ on the surface of the metacarpal head articular cartilage with small echogenic foci ⇨ in joint ("snowstorm appearance") indicative of gouty arthropathy.

TERMINOLOGY

Abbreviations and Synonyms
- Gout, gouty arthropathy, crystalline arthropathy, metabolic arthritis, tophaceous gout, podagra, gouty tophi, pseudogout

Definitions
- Inflammatory arthropathy due to urate crystal deposition (gout) or calcium pyrophosphate dihydrate (CPPD) crystal deposition (pseudogout)

IMAGING FINDINGS

General Features
- Best diagnostic clue: Identification of echogenic foci (crystals) in joint or soft tissues
- Location
  - Gout most commonly affects first metatarsophalangeal joint (podagra) (50%) → later becomes polyarticular
    - Gouty tophi → adjacent to metatarsophalangeal joint of hallux, other toes, fingers, helix of ear, olecranon bursae
  - Pseudogout → any joint especially knee, wrist, scapho-trapezium-triquetral joints
    - Extra-chondral involvement (synovium, tendons, ligaments, soft tissues) less common in pseudogout than gout
- Size: Gouty tophi range from few mm → 5 cm
- Morphology
  - Monoarticular swelling → deforming polyarthropathy
    - Tophi → hard discrete nodules in subcutaneous, para-articular, & other tissues

Ultrasonographic Findings
- More accurate than clinical examination or radiography at detecting gouty tophi
- Soft tissue
  - Soft tophi (no acoustic shadowing) → hard tophi (intense acoustic shadowing)
    - Depends on compactness of crystals within tophaceous deposits

DDx: Gout & Pseudogout

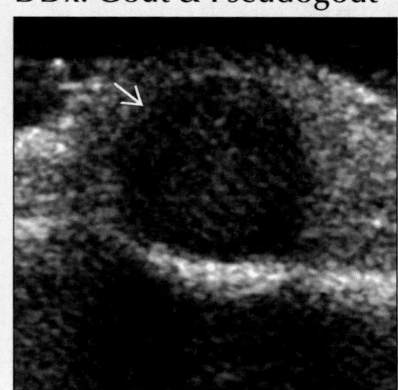

Rheumatoid Nodule

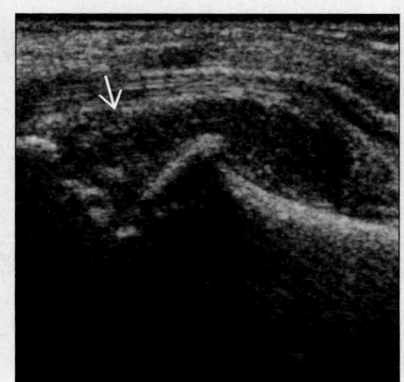

Rheumatoid Arthritis

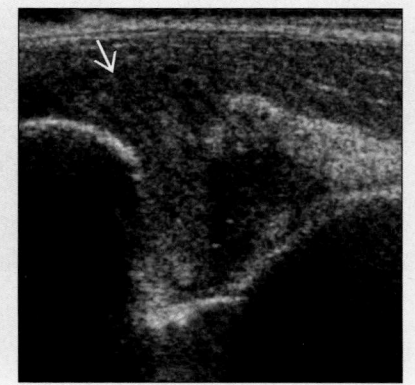

Septic Arthritis

GOUT AND PSEUDOGOUT

Key Facts

Terminology
- Inflammatory arthropathy due to urate crystal deposition (gout) or calcium pyrophosphate dihydrate (CPPD) crystal deposition (pseudogout)

Imaging Findings
- **Soft tissue**
- Soft tophi (no acoustic shadowing) → hard tophi (intense acoustic shadowing)
- Ranges from microdeposits with small hyperechoic foci within tendon → large hyperechoic foci with intense acoustic shadowing
- Fibrillar pattern disrupted, tendon stretched & displaced
- **Synovial fluid**
- ↑ Anechoic fluid ± few echogenic foci
- Fine punctuate echogenicity ("urate sand")

- Large echogenic aggregates ("snowstorm appearance")
- **Articular (hyaline) cartilage**
- Gout → thin echogenic band on surface of cartilage (urate deposition)
- Pseudogout → thin echogenic band mid-zone of cartilage (CPPD deposition)
- **Fibrocartilage**
- Pseudogout ⇒ punctuate echogenic foci within hypoechoic fibrocartilaginous disc (wrist) or menisci (knee) due to CPPD deposition
- ± Synovial fluid aspiration for analysis by polarizing light microscopy (sensitivity 84%, specificity 100%)

Top Differential Diagnoses
- Rheumatoid Nodule
- Rheumatoid Arthritis
- Septic Arthritis

- ○ Acoustic shadowing limits measurement of tophus volume
- ○ Even with dense shadowing, echogenic foci (from crystal aggregation) evident at periphery
- **Tendons (& ligaments)**
  - ○ Ranges from microdeposits with small hyperechoic foci within tendon → large hyperechoic foci with intense acoustic shadowing
    - Fibrillar pattern disrupted, tendon stretched & displaced
    - ± Tendon rupture (uncommon)
    - Acoustic shadowing with larger (> 5 mm) masses
- **Synovial fluid**
  - ○ Gout → variable appearance of joint fluid
    - ↑ Anechoic fluid ± few echogenic foci
    - Fine punctuate echogenicity ("urate sand")
    - Large echogenic aggregates ("snowstorm appearance")
  - ○ Pseudogout → ± echogenic aggregates in joint fluid
- **Articular (hyaline) cartilage**
  - ○ Gout → thin echogenic band on surface of cartilage (urate deposition)
    - No acoustic shadowing
  - ○ Pseudogout → thin echogenic band mid-zone of cartilage (CPPD deposition)
    - No acoustic shadowing
- **Fibrocartilage**
  - ○ Pseudogout ⇒ punctuate echogenic foci within hypoechoic fibrocartilaginous disc (wrist) or menisci (knee) due to CPPD deposition
- **Bone**
  - ○ Marginal erosions
    - May be obscured by acoustic shadowing of overlying tophus

Radiographic Findings
- Eccentric soft tissue hyperdense swelling ± calcification ⇒ tophi
- Asymmetrical arthropathy
  - ○ Absence of osteopenia
  - ○ Joint space preserved until late
  - ○ Marginal erosions with overhanging edges & thin sclerotic edge

- Larger than erosions of rheumatoid arthritis

MR Findings
- T1WI: Tophi: Well-defined masses, iso-intense (to muscle)
- T2WI
  - ○ Tophi: Low to high signal intensity
    - Variable intensity reflects amount of urate deposition, edema & maturity of granulation tissue
  - ○ Useful to quantify volume of tophi
    - Average percentage difference for tophus volume measurement = 14% (inter-reader), 17% (intra-reader)
- T1 C+
  - ○ Tophi: Honeycomb-like heterogeneous to near-homogeneous enhancement
    - Honeycomb appearance due to avascular urate surrounded by vascularized granulation tissue
    - Variable enhancement reflects varying amount of vascularized granulation tissue
  - ○ Contrast-enhancement not necessary to demonstrate tophi

Imaging Recommendations
- Best imaging tool: Ultrasound to inspect joint & adjacent tissues & aid joint aspiration
- Protocol advice
  - ○ Assess all aspects of joint (cartilage, fluid, synovium) & periarticular structures (ligaments, tendons, bone)
  - ○ ± Synovial fluid aspiration for analysis by polarizing light microscopy (sensitivity 84%, specificity 100%)
    - Only small amount of fluid required for analysis
    - Send fresh specimen (crystals dissolved by water, alcohol, formalin)
    - Urate crystals ⇒ needle-like, negatively birefringent
    - CPPD crystals ⇒ rod-like, positively birefringent
  - ○ Urate & CPPD crystals may co-exist
  - ○ Also send fluid for Gram-stain, culture & cell count

GOUT AND PSEUDOGOUT

DIFFERENTIAL DIAGNOSIS

Rheumatoid Nodule
- Hypoechoic, well-defined ± hyperemia
  - No echogenic foci
  - Typical locations (over bony prominences)

Rheumatoid Arthritis
- Symmetrical polyarthropathy
- Proteinaceous aggregates of inflammatory arthropathy less echogenic than crystal aggregates
- Absence of crystals on synovial fluid analysis

Septic Arthritis
- Distinction from acute gout can be difficult
  - Septic arthritis & crystal arthropathy may co-exist
  - Synovial fluid analysis helpful

PATHOLOGY

General Features
- General path comments
  - Uric acid = end product of purine catabolism
    - ↓ Excretion uric acid in urine (90% cases)
    - ↑ Production uric acid (10% cases)
  - Only fraction of patients with hyperuricemia develop clinical gout
  - Urate solubility affected by other factors other than concentration
    - Cold, pH, tissue composition & turnover
    - Uric acid preferentially deposits in synovium, around joints, tendons, ligaments
  - Urate crystals coated with apolipoprotein E or B
    - Protein coating may stop crystals from triggering inflammation
    - Immunoglobulins bind to bare areas on crystals & initiate phagocytosis by neutrophils
    - ∴ Exposure of bare areas on crystals (flux in uric acid level or trauma) may trigger acute inflammation
- Etiology
  - Genetic
  - Diet ("disease of kings")
  - Diabetes, thiazide diuretics, renal impairment
- Epidemiology: 1% general population
- Associated abnormalities
  - Hypertension, diabetes mellitus, metabolic syndrome, abdominal obesity, hyperlipidemia
  - Renal stones (x 1,000 increased incidence)
    - Pure uric acid stones (80%); mixed stones i.e., calcium oxalate or calcium phosphate deposition on uric acid core (20%)

Gross Pathologic & Surgical Features
- Tophi; multilobulated locules containing white, chalky material

Microscopic Features
- Multicentric urate crystals surrounded by vascularized granulation tissue & inflammatory infiltrate

CLINICAL ISSUES

Presentation
- Most common signs/symptoms
  - Acute monarticular arthritis (90%)
    - Severe inflammation reaching maximum intensity in 8-12 hours
- Other signs/symptoms
  - Gouty tophi
    - Arthritis usually precedes development of tophi
    - Tophi slowly enlarge over years

Demographics
- Age
  - Peak onset = 30-50 years (males) & 50-70 years (females)
    - Earlier with renal insufficiency or genetic predisposition
- Gender
  - Gout; male:female = 9:1
    - Estrogen ⇒ mildly uricosuric
    - ∴ Gout unusual in premenopausal women
  - Pseudogout; male:female = 1.5:1

Natural History & Prognosis
- Acute attack resolves spontaneously in < 2 weeks, if untreated
  - Joint normal between attacks (early disease)
  - ⇒ Polyarticular involvement with attacks become less intense, more frequent & lasting longer
  - ⇒ More proximal & upper limb joint involvement
  - ⇒ Chronic polyarthropathy (± almost symmetrical)
- Gouty nephropathy

Treatment
- Limiting acute attack
  - Rest
  - Non-steroidal anti-inflammatory agents
- Prevention or reversal of crystal deposition
  - Diet modification
  - Weight reduction
  - Drug therapy: Allopurinol, probenecid or colchicine
- Surgery
  - Excision of tophi (cosmetic, chronically discharging)

DIAGNOSTIC CHECKLIST

Consider
- Ultrasound evaluation should include assessment of synovial fluid, articular cartilage, tendons, ligaments as well as soft tissue tophi
  - Distinction between gout & pseudogout rests on site of crystal deposition & synovial fluid analysis

Image Interpretation Pearls
- Demonstration of echogenic crystals in typical sites

SELECTED REFERENCES

1. Grassi W et al: "Crystal clear"-sonographic assessment of gout and calcium pyrophosphate deposition disease. Semin Arthritis Rheum. 36(3):197-202, 2006

GOUT AND PSEUDOGOUT

IMAGE GALLERY

Typical

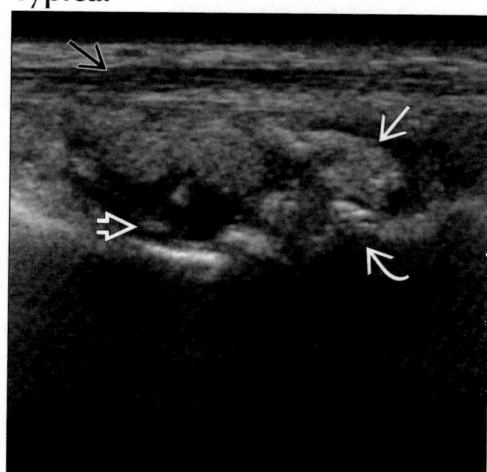

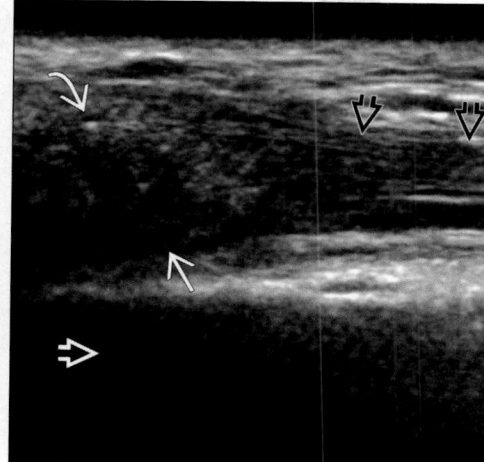

(Left) Longitudinal ultrasound shows soft tophus ➡ and smaller crystal aggregates ➡ within the distended interphalangeal joint of the hallux. Marginal osteophytosis ➡. Extensor hallucis longus tendon ➡. *(Right)* Longitudinal ultrasound of the distal forearm shows soft tophaceous deposit ➡ in the substance of the flexor digitorum profundus tendon ➡. Note small echogenic foci ➡ within the tophus. Radius ➡.

Typical

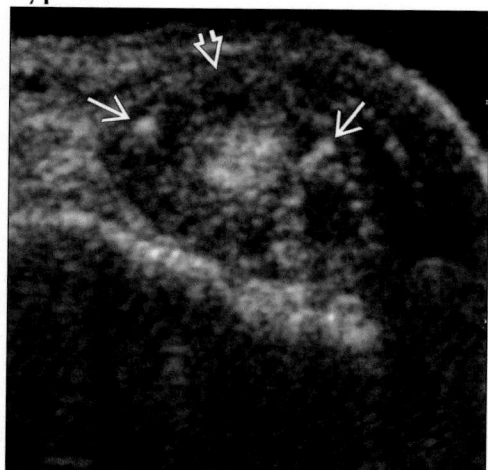

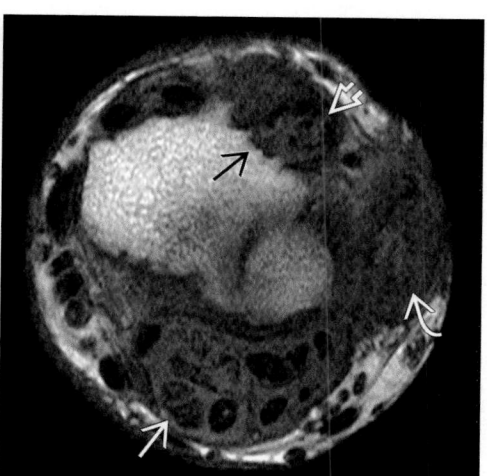

(Left) Transverse ultrasound shows thickened extensor carpi ulnaris tendon ➡ containing small ➡, and some larger, echogenic foci (crystals) indicative of gouty tendinopathy. *(Right)* Transverse T2WI MR of the wrist shows tophaceous gout affecting several flexor ➡ and extensor ➡ tendons, including the extensor carpi ulnaris ➡. Surface bone erosions are present ➡.

Typical

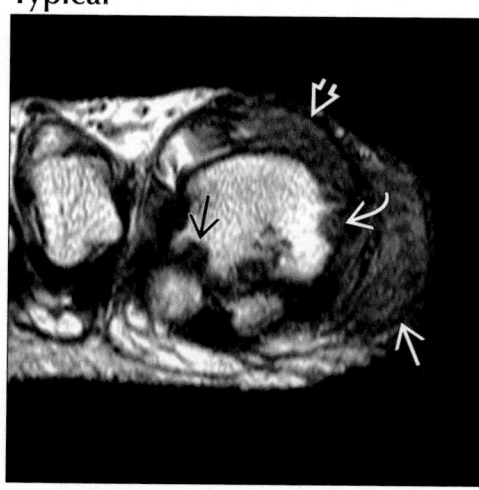

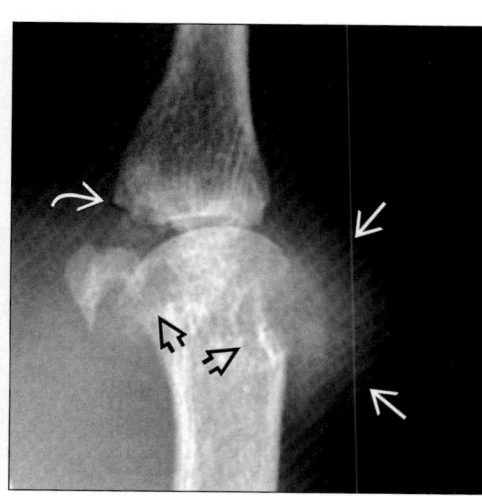

(Left) Transverse T2WI MR of 1st metatarsophalangeal joint shows gouty tophi on medial ➡ and extensor aspects ➡ of the metatarsal head with intraosseous extension ➡. Note erosions ➡ deep to sesamoid bones. *(Right)* Radiograph of the thumb shows gouty arthropathy of the 1st metacarpophalangeal joint with joint space narrowing, articular ➡ and marginal erosions ➡, and hyperdense soft tissue tophus ➡.

BAKER CYST

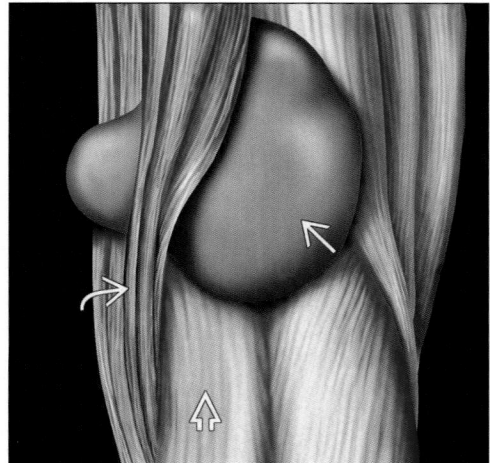

Longitudinal graphic shows a Baker cyst ➡ located between the semimembranosus tendon ➡ and the medial belly of the gastrocnemius ⇨.

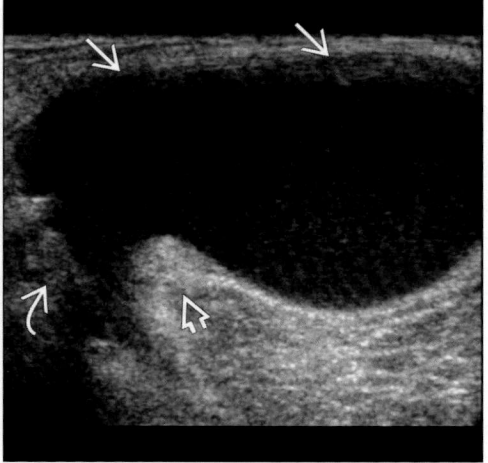

Transverse ultrasound shows a typical Baker cyst ➡ with a "talk-bubble" configuration. The neck extends between the semimembranosus tendon ➡ and the medial belly of the gastrocnemius ⇨.

TERMINOLOGY

Abbreviations and Synonyms
- Baker cyst, popliteal cyst, gastrocnemius-semimembranosus bursa
  - Baker cyst preferred term since popliteal cyst can also refer to para-articular ganglion cysts, para-meniscal cysts etc.

Definitions
- Fluid distension of gastrocnemius-semimembranosus bursa

IMAGING FINDINGS

General Features
- Best diagnostic clue: Fluid-filled sac with neck arising from interspace between gastrocnemius muscle and semimembranosus tendon
- Location: Posterior to medial femoral condyle
- Size: Range from 1-30 cm long axis or greater
- Morphology: Small non-distended sac to large multiloculated sac extending to mid-third of calf

Ultrasonographic Findings
- Fluid-filled popliteal fossa mass
  - Anechoic with posterior enhancement
  - Must see neck arising from medial gastrocnemius-semimembranosus tendon interspace to make diagnosis of Baker cyst
    - Characteristic "talk-bubble" configuration on transverse scans
  - Extension through knee capsule not seen
- Cysts typically well-defined and thin-walled
  - No wall hyperemia
- Thick-walled cysts suggest inflammatory knee arthropathy or intra-cystic hemorrhage
  - Thick-walled cysts often have hyperemic walls
- Cyst may be septated
  - Usually bi-locular or tri-locular
- Contain anechoic synovial fluid, typically gelatinous in consistency
  - Swirling fluid artifact not a feature
  - ± Fine echogenic speckles
  - ± Comet-tail artifacts
  - ± Fibrinous-type exudate (particularly with inflammatory arthropathy)

DDx: Baker Cyst

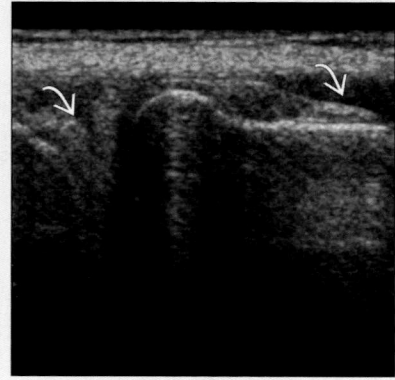

Parameniscal Cyst

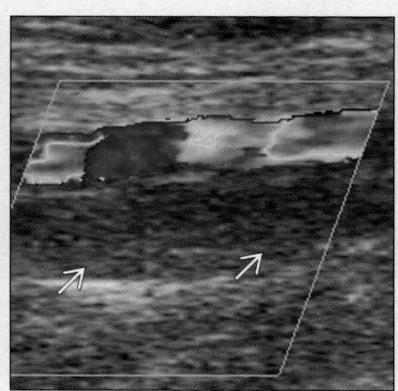

Deep Venous Thrombosis

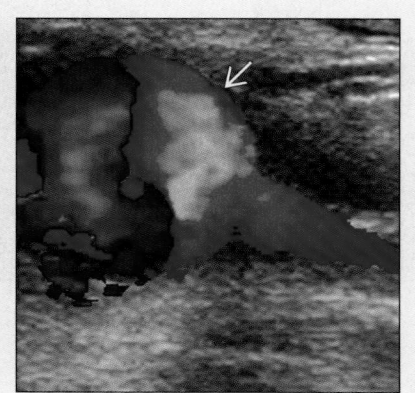

Popliteal Artery Aneurysm

BAKER CYST

Key Facts

Imaging Findings

- Best diagnostic clue: Fluid-filled sac with neck arising from interspace between gastrocnemius muscle and semimembranosus tendon
- Characteristic "talk-bubble" configuration on transverse scans
- Cysts typically well-defined and thin-walled
- Thick-walled cysts suggest inflammatory knee arthropathy or intra-cystic hemorrhage
- Thick-walled cysts often have hyperemic walls
- Cyst may be septated
- Contain anechoic synovial fluid, typically gelatinous in consistency
- Free fluid tracking adjacent to cyst indicates recent leakage

- Irregular and multiloculated cysts may result from repeated cyst leakage and re-collection
- Cysts usually extend distally superficial to medial belly gastrocnemius muscle
- Contralateral subclinical Baker cysts common
- US accurately confirms presence, location and extent
- Examine with patient prone, knees extended
- Follow medial belly of gastrocnemius proximally and locate interspace between medial gastrocnemius head and semimembranosus tendon
- Routinely examine contralateral side

Top Differential Diagnoses

- Parameniscal Cyst
- Deep Venous Thrombosis
- Popliteal Artery Aneurysm

- ○ ± Calcific particulate matter
- ○ ± Blood clots
- Free fluid tracking adjacent to cyst indicates recent leakage
  - ○ Irregular and multiloculated cysts may result from repeated cyst leakage and re-collection
- Cysts usually extend distally superficial to medial belly gastrocnemius muscle
  - ○ ± Extension deep to medial belly gastrocnemius
  - ○ ± Extension to distal thigh
  - ○ ± Intramuscular extension
    - Medial belly gastrocnemius, vastus medialis
    - Through muscular fascia weakened by trauma, perforating vessels or distension
- Contralateral subclinical Baker cysts common
  - ○ Routinely examine both popliteal fossae

Radiographic Findings

- Radiography
  - ○ Soft tissue swelling posteromedial knee
    - +/- Calcified debris
    - +/- Displacement of calcified popliteal artery

MR Findings

- T1WI
  - ○ Decreased signal intensity well-defined mass in expected location
  - ○ Subacute hemorrhage in cyst seen as areas of hyperintensity
- T2WI
  - ○ Increased signal intensity mass: Gastrocnemius-semimembranosus bursa
    - ± Debris
    - ± Hemorrhage (fluid level/hypointensity foci-hemosiderin)
    - ± Calcified bodies (hypointense)
    - ± Thick synovial wall
  - ○ ± Hyperintense surrounding fluid
    - = Leakage/rupture
- T2* GRE: Sensitive to hypointense foci of hemosiderin
- T1 C+
  - ○ ± Rim-enhancement
    - Hyperemic synovial lining

- Recommended when evaluating atypical cyst contents

Imaging Recommendations

- Best imaging tool
  - ○ Ultrasound
    - US accurately confirms presence, location and extent
- Protocol advice
  - ○ Examine with patient prone, knees extended
  - ○ Follow medial belly of gastrocnemius proximally and locate interspace between medial gastrocnemius head and semimembranosus tendon
    - Baker cyst arises from interspace between these two structures
  - ○ Routinely examine contralateral side

DIFFERENTIAL DIAGNOSIS

Parameniscal Cyst

- Associated meniscal tear, typically horizontal tear
- Cyst extends proximally to meniscus
- Not in typical location for Baker cyst

Deep Venous Thrombosis

- Similar clinical picture to cyst extension, rupture or hemorrhage
- Both conditions common and may coexist-exist
- Non-compressible venous thrombosis

Popliteal Artery Aneurysm

- Saccular or fusiform dilation of popliteal artery
- Color Doppler imaging confirms vascular flow in aneurysm

PATHOLOGY

General Features

- General path comments

BAKER CYST

o Slit-like capsular opening into gastrocnemius-semimembranosus bursa (Baker cyst) behind posterior horn medial meniscus
  ▪ Slit = 15-20 mm vertically-orientated opening
o Capsule unsupported at this location
  ▪ Between expansions of semimembranosus tendon medially and posterior cruciate ligament laterally
o Slit present on cadaveric study in 50% subjects over 50 years age
  ▪ Prevalence increases with age
  ▪ Probably due to degenerative thinning of joint capsule
o Synovial fluid extruded through slit into bursa (cyst)
o Wall of bursa composed of fibrous tissue lined by synovium
  ▪ Synovium of bursa in continuity with synovium of knee joint
o Synovial disorders of knee also affect Baker cyst
  ▪ Synovitis, synovial osteochondromatosis, pigmented villonodular synovitis (PVNS)
  ▪ Infected cysts (uncommon)
  ▪ Synovial sarcoma (rare)
o Other mechanisms whereby Baker cysts may potentially develop are
  ▪ Accumulation of fluid within non-communicating gastrocnemius-semimembranosus bursa
  ▪ Herniation of posterior joint capsule due to increased intra-articular pressure
• Etiology
o Fluid from joint effusion extending into cyst
o Fluid may communicate freely or be restricted with ball valve-like mechanism
• Epidemiology
o Most commonly encountered cyst around knee
  ▪ ~ 15% general population
  ▪ ~ 5% pediatric MR knee studies → ~ 15% asymptomatic middle-aged knees → ~ 50% elderly MR knee studies
• Associated abnormalities
o Associated with intra-articular pathology in ~ 85-98% cases
  ▪ Meniscal tears, arthritis (degenerative, inflammatory), chondral defects, cruciate ligament tears
o In children, usually not associated with intra-articular pathology or joint effusion
  ▪ Possibly related to unrecognized trauma or congenital predisposition
  ▪ Frequently bilateral

Gross Pathologic & Surgical Features
• Fluid-filled bursal sac in popliteal space

Microscopic Features
• Lined by synovium, similar to knee joint
• Four histopathologic types of Baker cyst
  o Fibrous
  o Synovial
  o Inflammatory
  o Transitional

CLINICAL ISSUES

Presentation
• Most common signs/symptoms
  o Painless mass medial side of popliteal fossa
  o Symptoms from underlying internal derangement (meniscal tear, osteoarthrosis, chondral defect etc.)
• Other signs/symptoms
  o Sudden onset of calf pain due to
    ▪ Extension of cyst
    ▪ Leakage/rupture of cyst
    ▪ Bleeding into cyst
  o Anticoagulation for clinically suspected deep venous thrombosis may aggravate bleeding or induce calf hematoma in cyst rupture
  o Symptoms from pressure on popliteal artery, vein or tibial nerve are uncommon

Demographics
• Age: Prevalence increases with age
• Gender: More common in males

Natural History & Prognosis
• Cyst may regress or enlarge
  o Overall, good prognosis, especially children
• In children, if cysts treated conservatively, ~ ½ disappear and ~ ½ regress

Treatment
• Conservative
  o Treatment of associated internal derangement
  o Nonsteroidal anti-inflammatory agents, ice, assisted weight-bearing
  o Cyst aspiration with intracystic steroid injection
    ▪ High rate of recurrence
  o Trial of conservative treatment optimal in children
• Surgical
  o Excision ± closure of joint-bursal communication
    ▪ Recurrence common

DIAGNOSTIC CHECKLIST

Consider
• Intra-articular pathology as this is very frequently associated with Baker cysts in adults

Image Interpretation Pearls
• Look for characteristic "talk-bubble" configuration of cyst on transverse imaging

SELECTED REFERENCES
1. Labropoulos N et al: New insights into the development of popliteal cysts. Br J Surg. 91(10):1313-8, 2004
2. McCarthy CL et al: The MRI appearance of cystic lesions around the knee. Skeletal Radiol. 33(4):187-209, 2004
3. Torreggiani WC et al: The imaging spectrum of Baker's (popliteal) cysts. Clin Radiol. 57(8):681-91, 2002

IMAGE GALLERY

Typical

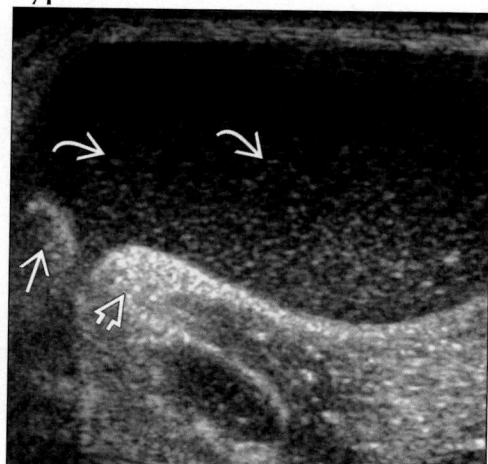
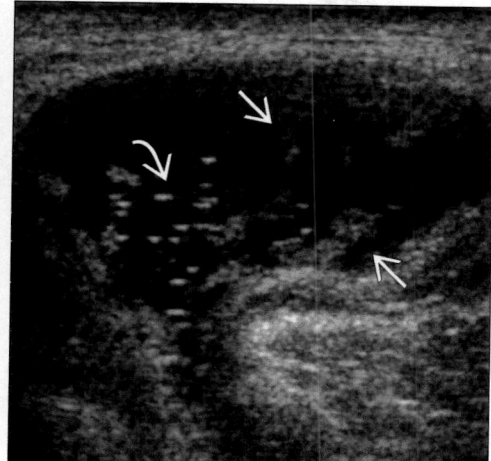

(Left) Transverse ultrasound shows Baker cyst with neck arising between semimembranosus tendon ➡ and medial belly gastrocnemius muscle ➡. Note finely speckled fluid within the cyst ➡. *(Right)* Transverse ultrasound shows Baker cyst with thick synovial fronds ➡ and comet-tail artifacts ➡.

Variant

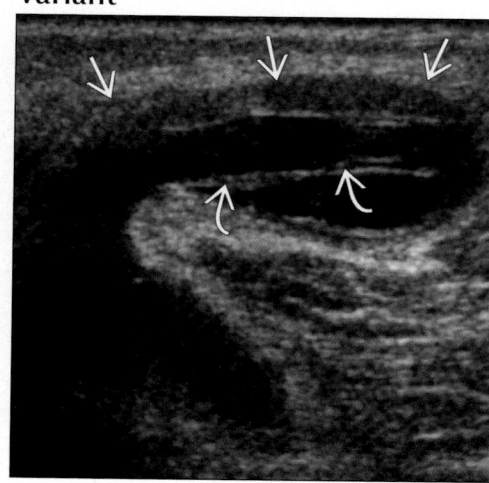
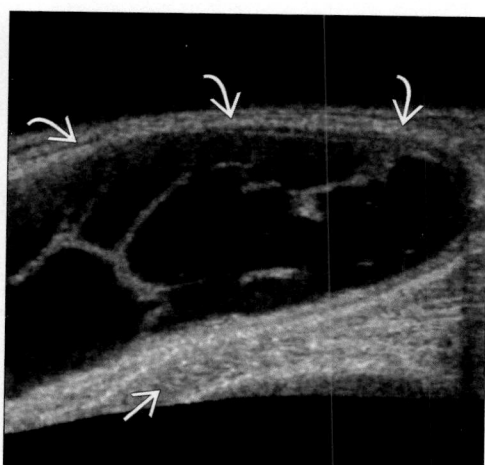

(Left) Transverse ultrasound shows thick-walled Baker cyst ➡ with fibrinous stranding ➡. *(Right)* Longitudinal ultrasound with extended field-of-view, shows multiloculated Baker cyst ➡ extending distally in typical location superficial to medial belly of gastrocnemius muscle ➡.

Variant

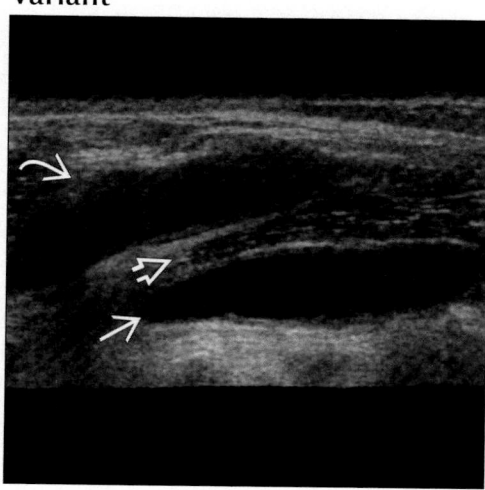
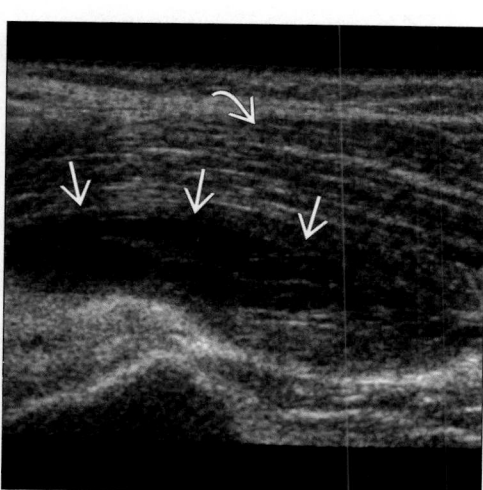

(Left) Longitudinal ultrasound shows mainly anechoic Baker cyst extending distally both superficial to ➡, and deep to ➡, medial belly gastrocnemius muscle ➡. *(Right)* Longitudinal ultrasound shows thick-walled Baker cyst ➡ extending distally deep to medial belly gastrocnemius muscle ➡.

Variant

(Left) Longitudinal ultrasound shows a largely anechoic Baker cyst ➥, which has ruptured into the medial belly of the gastrocnemius muscle ➡. *(Right)* Transverse ultrasound at same location, shows a well-defined Baker cyst ➥ located within the medial belly of the gastrocnemius muscle ➡.

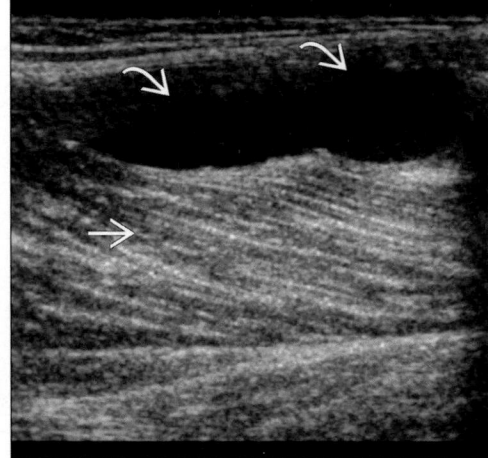
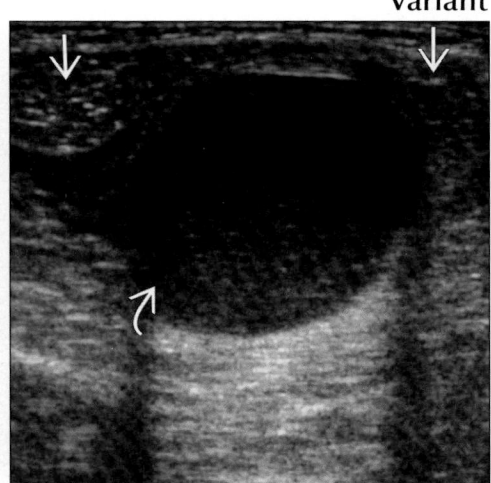

Variant

(Left) Longitudinal ultrasound with extended field-of view, shows recent hemorrhage into a Baker cyst ➡ with finely echogenic fluid ➥ and thrombus ➡ within the cyst. *(Right)* Transverse ultrasound shows a Baker cyst distended with a more organized echogenic hemorrhage ➥, containing hypoechoic areas ➡ and a gas loculus ➡. A fibrinous exudate may have a similar appearance.

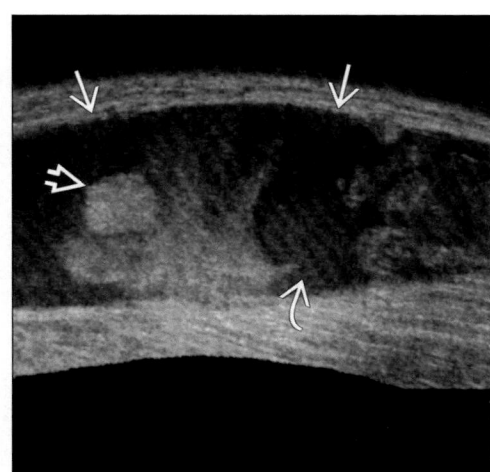
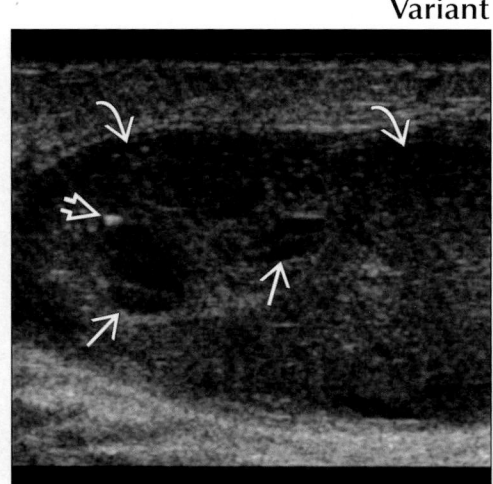

Variant

(Left) Longitudinal ultrasound with extended field-of-view, shows cyst leakage, with fluid ➡ tracking over the gastrocnemius muscle distal to the contained Baker cyst ➥. Note the lack of a wall around the free fluid. *(Right)* Transverse ultrasound shows leakage, from Baker cyst ➥. Echogenic fluid is tracking laterally ➡ over the gastrocnemius muscle. Note the cyst fluid is composed of echogenic fibrinous-type exudate.

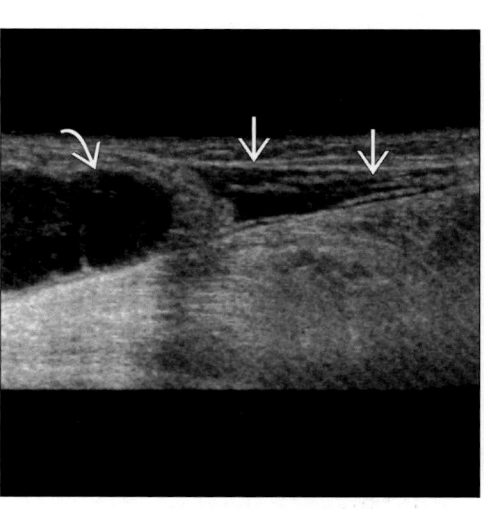
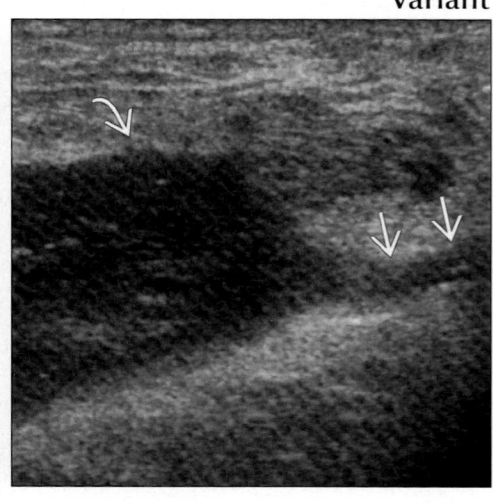

13

BAKER CYST

Typical

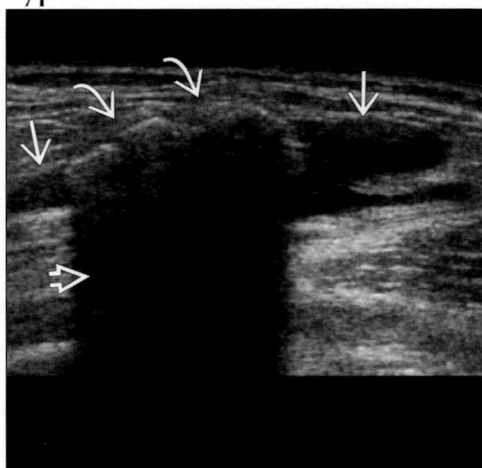

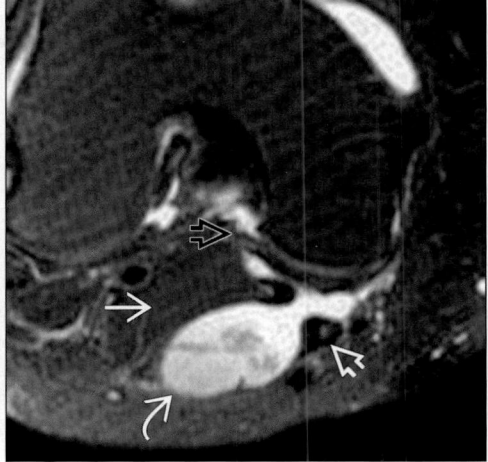

(Left) Longitudinal ultrasound shows calcific debris ➡, with acoustic shadowing ➡, contained within a Baker cyst ➡. There was also calcified particulate debris within the knee joint and popliteal fossa on radiography (not shown). *(Right)* Axial T2WI MR with fat-suppression shows a distended Baker cyst ➡ containing a fibrinous-type exudate. Note medial belly gastrocnemius ➡, semimembranosus tendon ➡ and posterior knee capsule ➡.

Variant

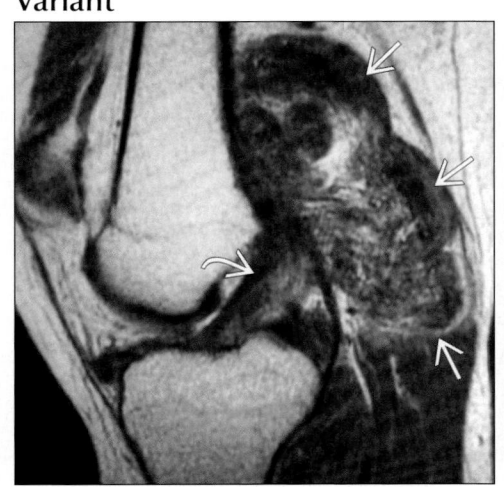

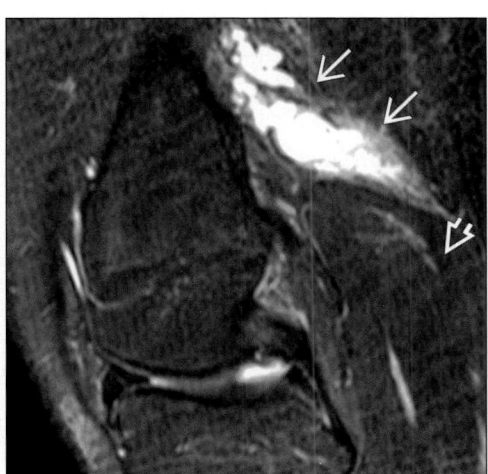

(Left) Sagittal T1WI MR shows synovial proliferation due to PVNS, affecting the posterior aspect of the knee joint ➡ and the distended Baker cyst ➡. *(Right)* Sagittal T2WI MR with fat-suppression shows irregular proximal extension ➡ of a Baker cyst to the distal thigh. Medial belly gastrocnemius muscle ➡.

Variant

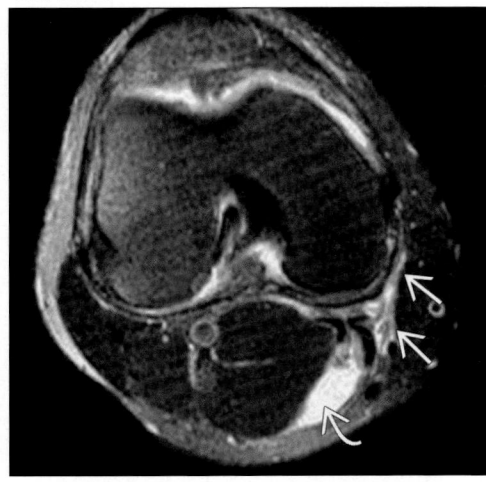

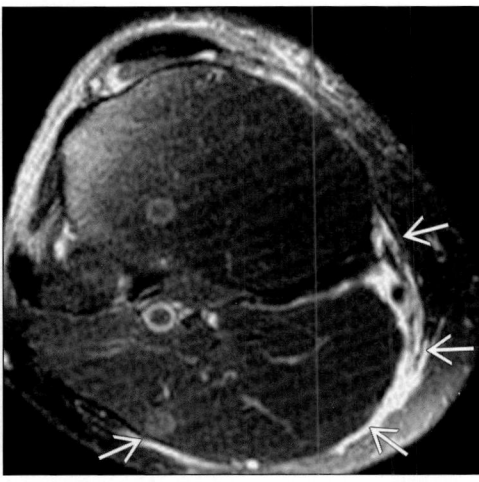

(Left) Axial T2WI MR with fat-suppression shows recent rupture of a Baker cyst ➡, with free fluid tracking away from the cyst along the posteromedial aspect of the knee ➡. *(Right)* Transverse T2WI MR with fat-suppression slightly more distal to previous image, shows fluid ➡ from the ruptured Baker cyst tracking over the calf muscle posteromedially and posteriorly.

BURSITIS

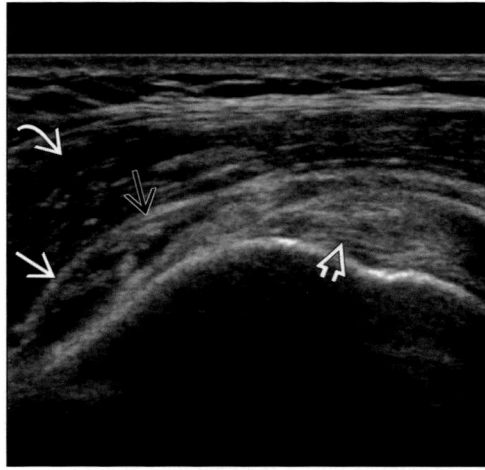
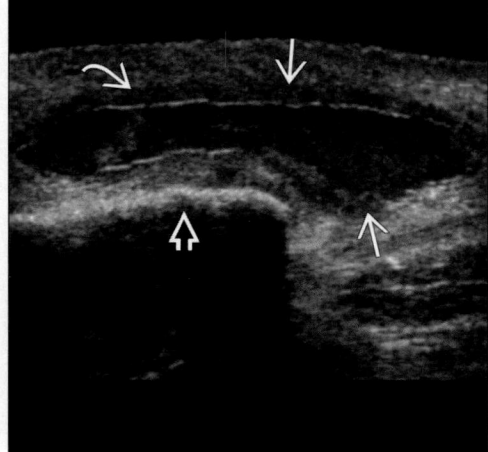

Transverse ultrasound of the shoulder shows distended subacromial-subdeltoid bursa ➡ with intrabursal debris. Normal supraspinatus tendon ➡, deltoid muscle ➡ and peribursal fat ➡.

Longitudinal ultrasound of the elbow shows olecranon bursa ➡ distended with echogenic fluid and some debris and mild bursal wall thickening ➡. Olecranon ➡.

TERMINOLOGY

Abbreviations and Synonyms
- Subacromial-subdeltoid bursitis, olecranon bursitis, ischial tuberosity (ischiogluteal) bursitis, trochanteric bursitis (hip bursitis), iliopsoas bursitis, semimembranous bursitis, pes anserinus bursitis, prepatellar bursitis (housemaid's knee), infrapatellar bursitis (preacher's knee), retrocalcaneal bursitis

Definitions
- Inflammation of lining of bursae
- Two types of bursae
  - Synovial bursae: Constant synovial-lined bursae which occur in defined anatomical locations
  - Adventitial bursae: Non-synovial-lined bursae which are acquired due to friction between opposing parts

IMAGING FINDINGS

General Features
- Best diagnostic clue: Fluid distended sac in typical location

- Location
  - Commonly inflamed synovial bursae
  - Subacromial-subdeltoid bursa: Large bursa overlying rotator cuff tendons
    - Communicates with glenohumeral joint if supraspinatus/infraspinatus tendons torn
  - Olecranon bursa: Superficially located between olecranon & overlying skin
  - Ischial tuberosity bursa: Between ischial tuberosity (hamstring tendon attachment) & gluteus maximus muscle
  - Iliopsoas bursa: Large bursa between iliopsoas tendon & anterior part of hip joint
    - Communicates with hip joint in 15% subjects
    - > 20 bursae described around hip joint
  - Trochanteric bursa: Overlies insertion of gluteus medius & minimus tendons into greater trochanter femur
  - Semimembranous bursa: Posteromedial to semimembranous musculotendinous junction & tendon distal thigh
  - Pes anserine bursa: Between sartorius, gracilis, & semitendinosus tendons & proximal tibia

DDx: Bursitis

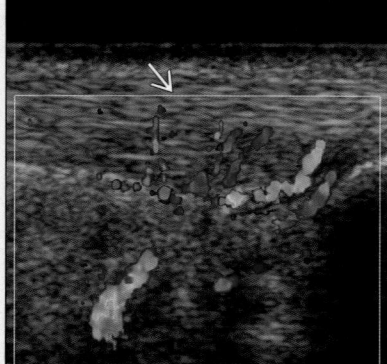
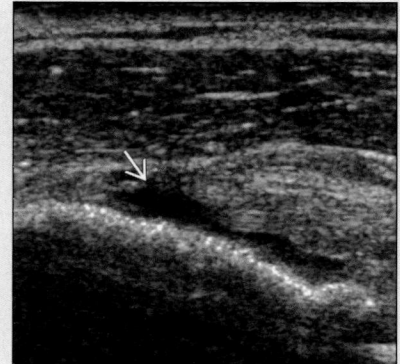
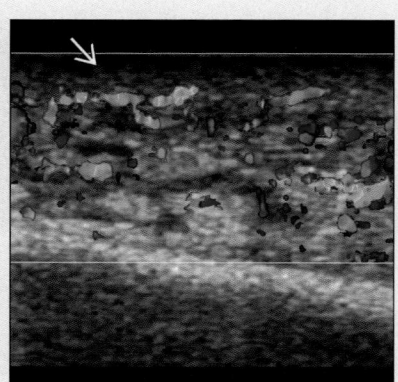

Tendinosis

Tendon Tear

Soft Tissue Infection

BURSITIS

Key Facts

Terminology
- Inflammation of lining of bursae
- Synovial bursae: Constant synovial-lined bursae which occur in defined anatomical locations
- Adventitial bursae: Non-synovial-lined bursae which are acquired due to friction between opposing parts

Imaging Findings
- Bursae: Synovial-lined sacs not visualized on ultrasound unless distended with fluid
- Most bursae accessible to ultrasound
- US facilitates image-guided aspiration or injection
- High resolution (~ 10 MHz) linear transducer for superficial bursae
- Lower resolution (~ 7 MHz) for deeper bursae
- ↓ Transducer pressure to avoid bursal effacement
- ± Comparison with opposite side

- ± Aspiration (cytology, crystals, Gram stain & culture including fungal, TB culture)

Top Differential Diagnoses
- Tendinosis
- Tendon Tear
- Subcutaneous Cellulitis

Diagnostic Checklist
- Small amount of fluid may be normal in subacromial-subdeltoid bursa, deep infrapatellar bursa, retrocalcaneal bursa
- Bursitis is common; infective bursitis is uncommon
- Chronic bursitis often associated with wall-thickening & internal debris

---

- Prepatellar bursa: Overlies inferior pole patella & proximal patellar tendon
- Infrapatellar bursa: Overlies distal aspect patellar tendon
- Retrocalcaneal bursa: Between calcaneus, Achilles tendon & Kager fat
- Size: Few mms to several cms depending on distension of involved bursae
- Morphology
  - Bursae: Synovial-lined sacs not visualized on ultrasound unless distended with fluid
    - Small amount of fluid → flattened
    - Moderate amount of fluid → oval-shaped
    - Large amount of fluid → rounded

Ultrasonographic Findings
- Subacromial-subdeltoid (SASD) bursa
  - Fluid collects in dependent positions
    - Lateral aspect greater tuberosity (teardrop configuration) over biceps, near coracoid & also deep to acromion
    - Fluid in bursa over biceps groove is separate from intra-articular fluid in long head biceps tendon sheath
    - MR marginally more sensitive than ultrasound at detecting SASD fluid (transducer effacement, subacromial location)
  - Bursal fluid strongly associated with supraspinatus tendon tears
  - Bursal wall thickening & hyperemia generally not a feature
    - If present, consider inflammatory arthropathy (e.g., SLE)
    - Bursa most commonly affected by inflammatory arthropathy
    - ± Rice bodies
    - Small rice bodies better seen by MR
- Olecranon bursitis: Thick-walled + hyperemic ± peribursal edema
  - ± Hemorrhage
  - Consider gout/pseudogout, inflammatory arthropathy, infection

- Ischial tuberosity bursitis: Large irregular bursa with moderate wall thickening ± fronding ± debris
  - ± Hemorrhage
  - ± Hyperemia (uncommon) or calcification (uncommon)
- Greater trochanteric bursitis: Uncommon
  - Most cases of trochanteric bursitis due to gluteus medius, minimus insertional tendinosis
- Semimembranous bursitis: Thin-walled, mild to moderate distension
  - No hyperemia or debris
    - Very small degrees of bursal distension better seen with MR
  - Infection very uncommon
- Pes anserinus bursitis: Large bursa
  - Distended bursa indented by three tendons looks like goose's foot (hence "anserine")
  - Prone to synovial proliferation
- Prepatellar bursitis: Mild wall thickening
  - ± Hyperemia or debris
  - Occasionally infected
- Infrapatellar bursitis: Mild wall thickening
  - ± Hyperemia or debris
- Retrocalcaneal bursitis: Varies from marked synovial proliferation with hyperemia (common) to fluid distension without synovial proliferation (uncommon)
  - Nearly always associated with Achilles tendinosis

Radiographic Findings
- Radiography: Soft tissue swelling

MR Findings
- T1WI: Homogeneous decreased signal intensity mass at typical location
- T2WI
  - Fluid signal intensity
  - ± Inflammatory debris (isointense) or calcification (hypointense)
  - ± Associated tendinosis (thickening with variable increased signal intensity)
  - ± Rice bodies (intense)
    - Rice-shaped fibrin aggregates (multiple)

BURSITIS

- Associated with inflammatory arthropathy, mycobacterium infection
- MR more sensitive than ultrasound at detecting small rice bodies
- T1 C+: ± Wall enhancement: ↑ Enhancement with synovial thickening greater

Imaging Recommendations
- Best imaging tool
  - Ultrasound
  - Most bursae accessible to ultrasound
    - US facilitates image-guided aspiration or injection
- Protocol advice
  - High resolution (~ 10 MHz) linear transducer for superficial bursae
    - Lower resolution (~ 7 MHz) for deeper bursae
  - ↓ Transducer pressure to avoid bursal effacement
    - Use sufficient acoustic gel
  - Transducer palpation or movement of part may allow fluid to be appreciated
    - Transducer angulation (anisotropy, tendon visualization)
  - ± Comparison with opposite side
  - ± Aspiration (cytology, crystals, Gram stain & culture including fungal, TB culture)
  - Small amount of fluid in some bursae (deep infrapatellar, retrocalcaneal, subacromial-subdeltoid) may be normal
  - Check hip & iliopsoas muscle for tuberculous infection when iliopsoas bursa distended
  - Subacromial-subdeltoid bursal fluid & no obvious tear
    - ⇒ Pay particular attention to anterior leading edge supraspinatus tendon for small avulsive-type tear

DIFFERENTIAL DIAGNOSIS

Tendinosis
- Insertional tendinosis common accompaniment of bursitis
  - Tendon thickening, ± avulsive-type tears
  - ± Hyperemia & bony proliferation or resorption

Tendon Tear
- Tendon discontinuity
  - May precipitate bursal distension
  - Especially rotator cuff tear

Subcutaneous Cellulitis
- Soft tissue edema & hyperemia
- No discrete collection

PATHOLOGY

General Features
- Etiology
  - Chronic frictional trauma or overuse
  - Acute trauma
  - Crystalline deposit (gout/pseudogout) uncommon
  - Infection (± penetrating trauma) uncommon
- Epidemiology: Common disorder, especially subacromial-subdeltoid bursitis

Gross Pathologic & Surgical Features
- Bursal sac inflammation with variable thickening of synovial-like lining
  - Variable amount of fluid

Microscopic Features
- Thickened synovial lining with inflammatory reaction
  - Exudate ± hemorrhagic by-products ± rice bodies

CLINICAL ISSUES

Presentation
- Most common signs/symptoms: Pain ± mass
- Clinical Profile
  - Overuse phenomenon
  - ± Index traumatic event

Demographics
- Age: Typically middle-aged
- Gender: Overall M = F

Natural History & Prognosis
- Insidious onset
  - ± Resolution with cessation of aggravating activity

Treatment
- Conservative
  - Rest
  - Anti-inflammatory agents
  - Local corticosteroids ± long-acting local anesthetic injection (± ultrasound-guided)
  - Antibiotics if infectious
- Surgical
  - Excision for resistant cases

DIAGNOSTIC CHECKLIST

Consider
- Small amount of fluid may be normal in subacromial-subdeltoid bursa, deep infrapatellar bursa, retrocalcaneal bursa
  - MR more sensitive to very small amounts of fluid than ultrasound
- Bursitis is common; infective bursitis is uncommon
- Chronic bursitis often associated with wall-thickening & internal debris
- Inflammatory arthropathy if SASD bursa thick-walled ± hyperemic

Image Interpretation Pearls
- Fluid distended sac in typical location

SELECTED REFERENCES

1. Connell DA et al: Sonographic evaluation of gluteus medius and minimus tendinopathy. Eur Radiol. 13(6):1339-47, 2003

BURSITIS

IMAGE GALLERY

Typical

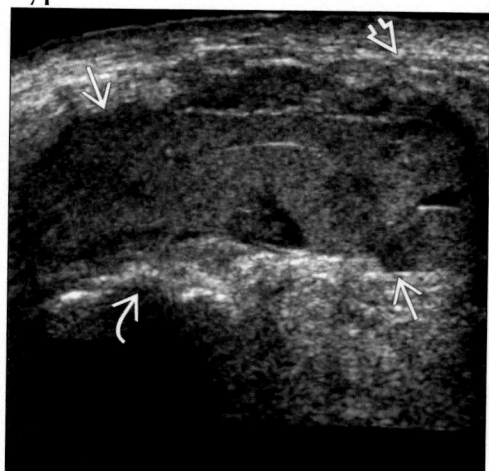
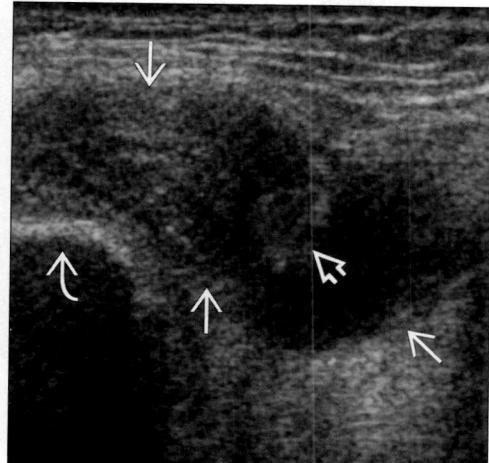

(Left) Longitudinal ultrasound shows ischial tuberosity bursa ➡ distended with hemorrhage. The gluteal muscle ➡ is atrophic. Ischial tuberosity ➡. *(Right)* Transverse ultrasound shows distended pes anserinus bursa ➡ and semitendinous tendon ➡. The gracilis and sartorius tendons are not shown. Synovial proliferation gives bursitis a solid appearance. Medial tibial condyle ➡.

Typical

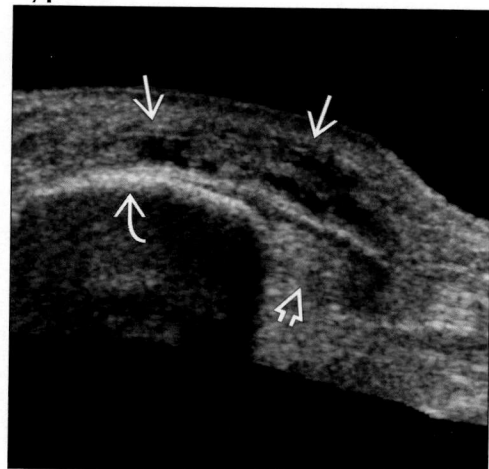
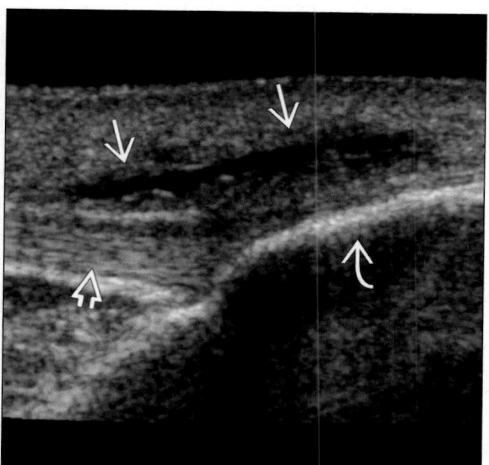

(Left) Longitudinal ultrasound shows distended pre-patellar bursa ➡ with thickened irregular walls and some internal debris. Note normal patella ➡ and patellar tendon ➡. *(Right)* Longitudinal ultrasound shows distended infra-patellar bursa ➡ with thickened irregular walls and some internal debris. Normal patellar tendon ➡ and tibial tuberosity ➡.

Typical

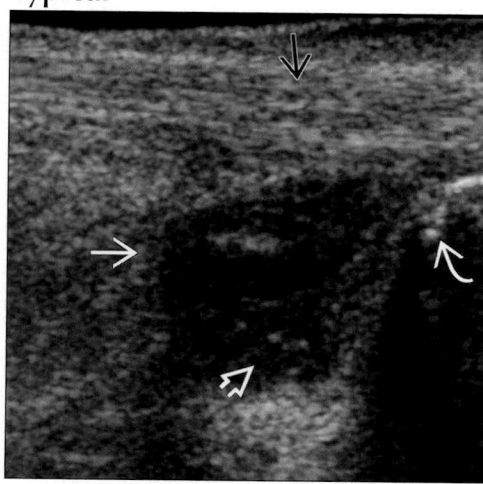
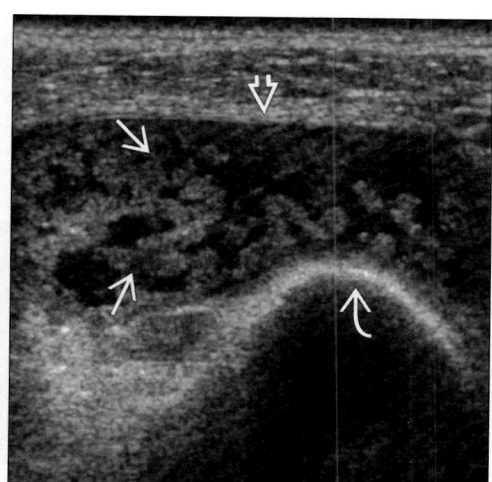

(Left) Longitudinal ultrasound shows distended retrocalcaneal bursa ➡ with synovial proliferation of the bursal wall ➡. There is minimal surface irregularity of the calcaneus ➡ (normal Achilles tendon ➡). *(Right)* Transverse ultrasound of the proximal arm in a patient with rheumatoid arthritis shows the subacromial-subdeltoid bursa distended with multiple rice bodies ➡. Minimal bursal wall thickening ➡. Humeral shaft ➡.

GANGLION CYST

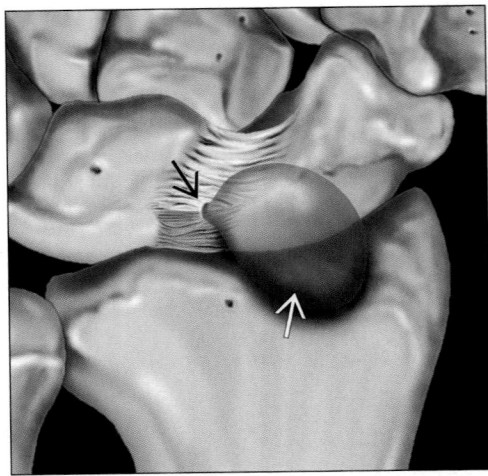

Graphic shows the typical location of a dorsal wrist ganglion cyst ➡ arising from a defect in the dorsal capsule of the scapholunate ligament ➡.

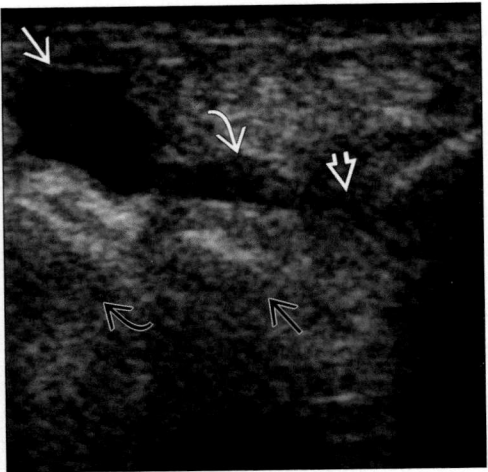

Longitudinal ultrasound shows a typical dorsal ganglion cyst ➡ with a stalk ➡ extending towards the radiolunate articulation ➡. Lunate ➡ and capitate ➡.

TERMINOLOGY

Abbreviations and Synonyms
- Ganglion, ganglia, carpal ganglion, dorsal wrist ganglion, palmar wrist ganglion, occult ganglia, bible bump, Gideon disease

Definitions
- Mucinous soft tissue mass occurring in predictable location
- Occult ganglion: Ganglion not clinically apparent

IMAGING FINDINGS

General Features
- Best diagnostic clue: Fluid-filled mass with stalk extending towards joint
- Location
  - Dorsal wrist ganglia are more common clinically
    - Palmar wrist ganglia are more common overall (i.e., most palmar ganglia are asymptomatic)
  - Dorsal wrist ganglia
    - Scapholunate joint
    - Radioscaphoid joint
    - Scapho-trapezio-trapezoid joint (triscaphe joint)
    - Ulnocarpal joint
  - Volar wrist ganglia
    - Arising between radioscaphocapitate and long radiolunate ligament
    - Radioscaphoid joint
    - Scapho-trapezio-trapezoid joint (triscaphe joint)
    - Ulnocarpal joint
    - Pisiform-triquetral joint
  - Finger
    - Flexor tendon sheaths near A1 pulley (focal anchoring of tendon sheath at level of metacarpophalangeal joint)
    - Between dorsal aspect distal interphalangeal joint and nail bed (digital mucous cysts)
  - Foot & ankle
    - Navicular-cuneiform joint
    - Inter-cuneiform joint
    - Subtalar joint
    - Talo-navicular joint
  - Proximal tibiofibular syndesmosis
  - Facet joint (spine) (not usually demonstrable by ultrasound)

DDx: Ganglion Cyst

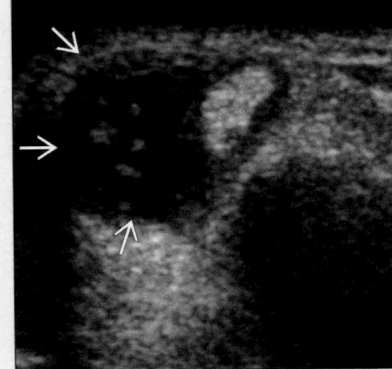

Tenosynovitis

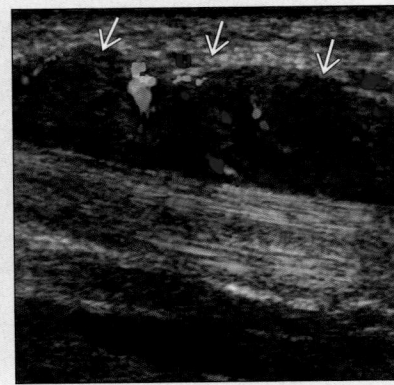

Tenosynovial Giant Cell Tumor

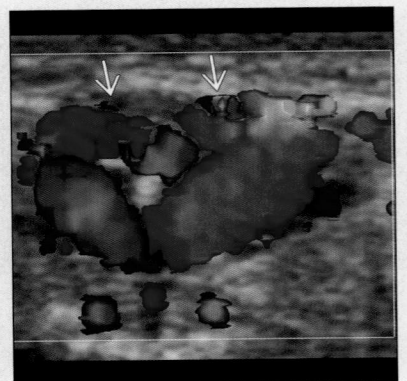

Vascular Anomaly

GANGLION CYST

Key Facts

Imaging Findings
- Best diagnostic clue: Fluid-filled mass with stalk extending towards joint
- Morphology: Ovoid or irregular configuration with stalk connecting to joint of origin
- Elongated neck allows cyst to surface at distance from joint of origin
- Hypoechoic with clear fluid
- ± Septations
- ± Comet-tail artifacts
- Not compressible
- No hyperemia except with recent leakage when surrounding tissues may be mildly hyperemic and edematous
- Ultrasound will allow diagnosis of most ganglion cysts
- Multidirectional capability allows stalk to be traced towards joint
- Locate tell-tale stalk of cyst and tract it back towards joint of origin
- Evaluate with color Doppler to exclude vascular anomaly, nerve sheath tumor

Top Differential Diagnoses
- Tenosynovitis
- Giant Cell Tumor (GCT) of Tendon Sheath
- Vascular Anomaly

Clinical Issues
- In adults, up to 50% of wrist ganglia will resolve without treatment within six years
- In children, > 90% ganglion cysts will resolve without treatment within one year

---

- Hip
  - Anterosuperior
  - Associated with labral tear
- Shoulder
  - Posterosuperior
  - Associated with labral tear
- Acromioclavicular joint
- Knee
  - Anterior and posterior cruciate ligaments
  - Para-articular
- Proximal tibiofibular joint
- Size
  - Average 5 mm; ganglia from large joint may reach > 50 mm maximum dimension
  - Size may increase with activity
- Morphology: Ovoid or irregular configuration with stalk connecting to joint of origin

Ultrasonographic Findings
- Hypoechoic fluid-filled mass with stalk extending towards joint
  - Typical location
  - Elongated neck allows cyst to surface at distance from joint of origin
  - Hypoechoic with clear fluid
  - ± Septations
  - ± Comet-tail artifacts
  - Not compressible
  - No hyperemia except with recent leakage when surrounding tissues may be mildly hyperemic and edematous
- Stalk may be thin and serpiginous
  - Location of entry site of stalk into joint will help surgical planning
- Ganglia close to A1 pulley have no visible communication with tendon sheath

Radiographic Findings
- Radiography
  - Usually normal
  - ± Soft tissue density
  - ± Intraosseous carpal ganglion

MR Findings
- T1WI: Hypointense to intermediate signal intensity mass
- T2WI
  - Uniformly hyperintense soft tissue cystic mass
  - Narrow stalk connecting cyst to joint
  - Intraosseous carpal ganglions, hyperintense
  - MR very sensitive at detecting occult ganglia
  - Distension of capsular recesses may simulate cysts
    - Capsular recesses occur in expected locations
    - Wide communication with joint cavity
    - If capsular "recess" is unusually distended for given amount of joint effusion, consider ganglion
    - Cysts persist with change in joint position

Imaging Recommendations
- Best imaging tool
  - Ultrasound will allow diagnosis of most ganglion cysts
    - Multidirectional capability allows stalk to be traced towards joint
- Protocol advice
  - Locate tell-tale stalk of cyst and tract it back towards joint of origin
  - Extension through joint capsule often not seen
    - Examination of wrist in flexion ± extension may occasionally help
  - Note important relationships of cyst (i.e., relationship to adjacent tendons and neurovascular bundle)
  - Evaluate with color Doppler to exclude vascular anomaly, nerve sheath tumor

DIFFERENTIAL DIAGNOSIS

Tenosynovitis
- Common wrist swelling
- Less well-defined
- Distension of tendon sheath

GANGLION CYST

Giant Cell Tumor (GCT) of Tendon Sheath
- Soft tissue mass, usually hyperemic
- Eccentrically located to tendon sheath

Vascular Anomaly
- Compressible ± phleboliths ± flow on color Doppler imaging
- Lymphangiomas may appear similar to ganglion cysts
  - Tend to occur in areas where ganglion cysts do not occur
  - Do not have stalk communicating with joint

PATHOLOGY

General Features
- Etiology
  - Typical locations presumably due to weakness in capsule
    - Possibly due to degenerative or traumatic tear in capsule
    - History of trauma usually not present
    - Joint fluid pumped (one way valve) between collagen bundles
  - Post-traumatic ganglia may occasionally develop acutely over a few hours to days
- Epidemiology
  - 80% of all soft tissue masses of wrist & hand
    - Most (80%) wrist ganglia presenting clinically are on dorsal surface
    - Yet, MR of asymptomatic subjects → most (80%) ganglia occur on volar surface
    - Most volar ganglia are asymptomatic
- Associated abnormalities
  - Intraosseous ganglia more common in subject with soft tissue ganglia
  - Possibly reflection of underlying joint pathology
  - Single ganglion may simultaneously have both intraosseous and extracapsular components

Gross Pathologic & Surgical Features
- Cystic mucinous fluid contained in pseudocapsule
- Dorsal ganglia close to where dorsal interosseous nerve approaches joint capsule

Microscopic Features
- Capsular lining = compressed loose areolar tissue = pseudocapsule
- No inner cell lining
  - Not lined by synovial tissue

CLINICAL ISSUES

Presentation
- Most common signs/symptoms: Slowly growing soft tissue mass
- Clinical Profile
  - Localized pain ± firm mass ± weakness
    - Typically pain on attempted full dorsiflexion of wrist e.g., getting out of chair
    - Cyst transilluminates
  - Neurologic findings with extension into carpal tunnel or Guyon canal and nerve compression (uncommon)

Demographics
- Age: 20-50 years
- Gender: M < F

Natural History & Prognosis
- In adults, up to 50% of wrist ganglia will resolve without treatment within six years
  - In children, > 90% ganglion cysts will resolve without treatment within one year

Treatment
- Observe
  - High rates of spontaneous resolution both in adults & children
- Active treatment
  - Indicated if cyst painful, if cosmetic disfiguration or if fails to resolve after one year
- Manual rupture by hitting with large book
  - Not recommended (soft tissue injury)
- Aspiration (ultrasound-guided)
  - Useful for cysts alongside flexor tendon sheath: > 70% complete resolution
  - < 50% complete resolution less for other cysts though they may become smaller and less symptomatic (incomplete resolution)
  - Aspiration ± steroid injection
    - Offers no advantage over aspiration alone
- Surgical
- Open resection
- Excision of stalk + small portion joint capsule
  - ~ 5-15% recurrence rate
  - Similar for dorsal or volar wrist ganglia
  - Up to 30% may have persistent pain or limitation of movement ± recurrence
- Arthroscopic resection: Less scarring
  - Capsular defect, stalk and cyst débrided from intra-articular approach
  - Similar recurrence rate to open resection

DIAGNOSTIC CHECKLIST

Consider
- Clinically ⇒ most common on dorsal aspect wrist
- MRI ⇒ more common volar aspect of wrist
- Contain gelatinous material of variable consistency

Image Interpretation Pearls
- Locate stalk of ganglion & trace to joint of origin
- Always examine with color Doppler
  - Occasionally nerve sheath tumor, giant cell tumor and vascular anomalies may simulate cysts

SELECTED REFERENCES
1. Lowden CM et al: The prevalence of wrist ganglia in an asymptomatic population: magnetic resonance evaluation. J Hand Surg [Br]. 30(3):302-6, 2005
2. Bianchi S et al: Ultrasonographic evaluation of wrist ganglia. Skeletal Radiol. 23(3):201-3, 1994

GANGLION CYST

IMAGE GALLERY

Typical

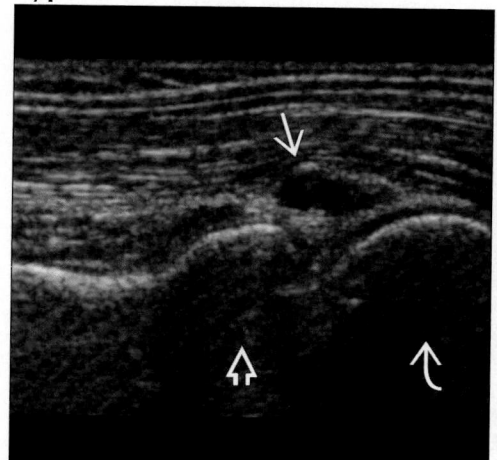
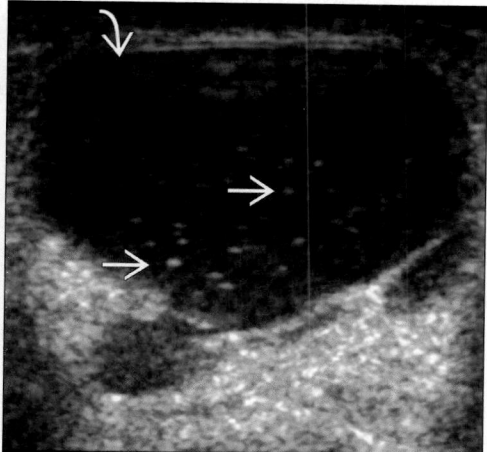

(Left) Longitudinal ultrasound of the elbow joint shows a small ganglion cyst ➡ bulging out from the anterior capsule between the capitellum ➡ and the radial head ➡. *(Right)* Transverse ultrasound shows a large ganglion cyst ➡ on the volar aspect of the wrist containing small comet-tail artifacts ➡.

Typical

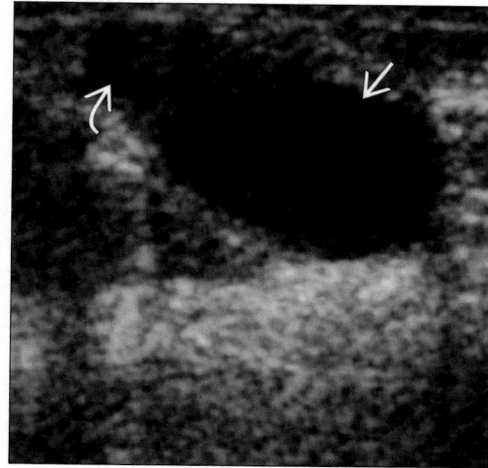
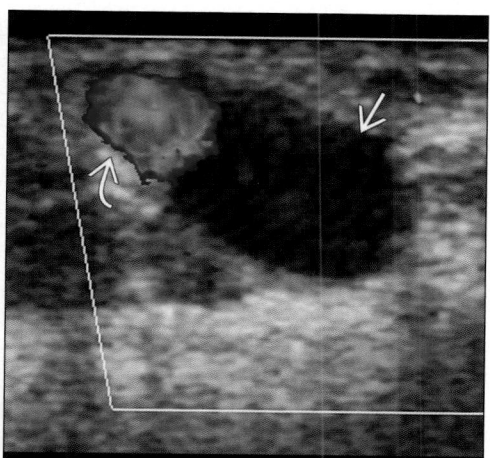

(Left) Transverse ultrasound shows a volar wrist ganglion cyst ➡ located just proximal to the wrist crease. The radial artery ➡ is inseparable from the ganglion cyst. *(Right)* Transverse color Doppler ultrasound at the same location as previous image clearly shows the radial artery ➡ located at the edge of the ganglion cyst ➡.

Typical

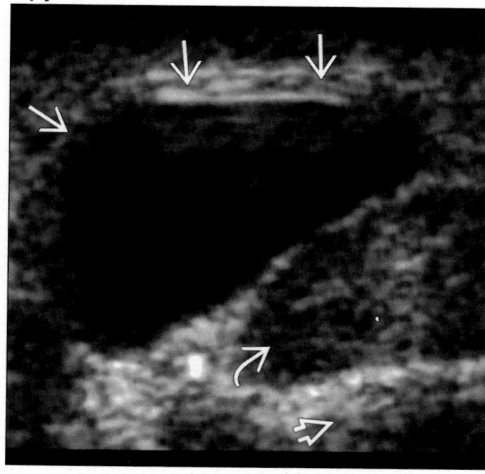
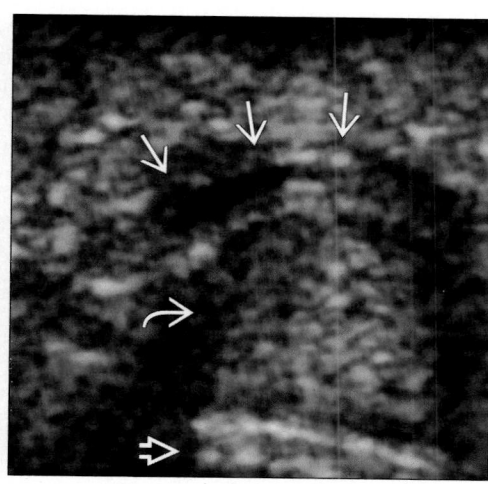

(Left) Transverse ultrasound shows a hypoechoic ganglion cyst ➡ located alongside the flexor tendon ➡ just distal to the metacarpophalangeal joint and A1 pulley. Metacarpal bone ➡. *(Right)* Transverse ultrasound at the same location as previous image, shows a collapsed ganglion cyst ➡ following needle aspiration. Flexor tendon ➡. Metacarpal bone ➡.

PARAMENISCAL CYST

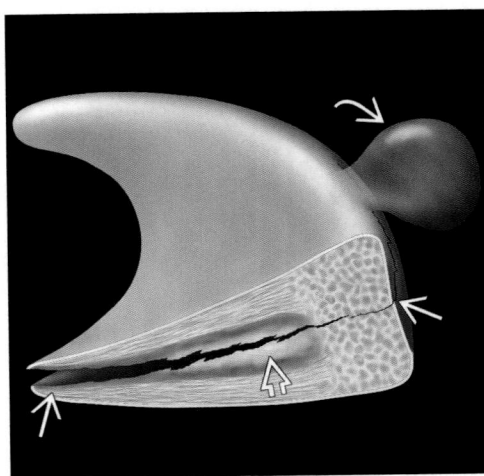

Graphic shows a horizontal meniscal tear ("fish-mouth" tear) →, with some mucoid degeneration → and small parameniscal cyst → arising from the peripheral aspect of the tear.

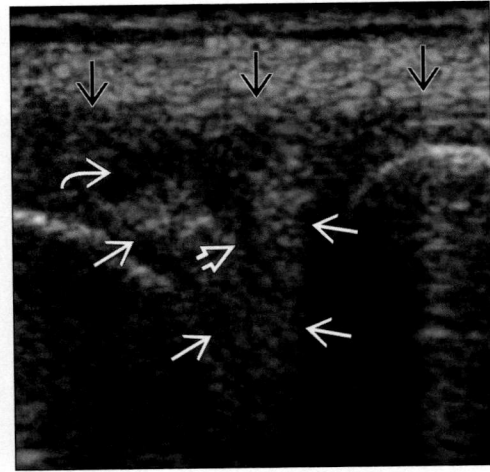

Longitudinal ultrasound shows a triangular-shaped medial meniscus → with a mid-substance, peripheral, horizontal tear → and small parameniscal cyst → lying deep to the medial collateral ligament →.

TERMINOLOGY

Abbreviations and Synonyms
- Parameniscal cyst, meniscal cyst

Definitions
- Cyst extending from meniscal tear
  - Horizontal tear most common

IMAGING FINDINGS

General Features
- Best diagnostic clue: Cystic mass in continuity with horizontal meniscal tear
- Location
  - Can arise from any part of meniscus
  - Most common locations
    - Posterior horn medial meniscus
    - Anterior horn lateral meniscus
  - Medial meniscus = lateral meniscus tears
- Size: Few mm → large extra-articular cyst (> 10 cm)
- Morphology

- Direction of extension from parameniscal area subject to capsuloligamentous anatomy on medial and lateral aspects of knee
- Cysts from posterior horn medial meniscus penetrate capsule and often extend either
  - Inferiorly deep to semimembranous and pes anserinus tendons
  - Anteriorly superficial to medial collateral ligament
- Cysts from anterior horn lateral meniscus penetrate capsule and extend
  - Deep to iliotibial tract or lateral collateral ligament
- Lateral cysts tend to remain closer to knee capsule
  - More likely to be clinically apparent and clinically palpable

Ultrasonographic Findings
- Horizontal meniscal tear + parameniscal cyst ± extra-articular component with communicating stalk
- Menisci seen as diffusely echogenic, sharply-defined structures within medial and lateral femora-tibial compartments of knee
  - Medial meniscus easier to see on ultrasound
    - Only peripheral ¾ → ¼ of menisci seen on ultrasound

DDx: Parameniscal Cyst

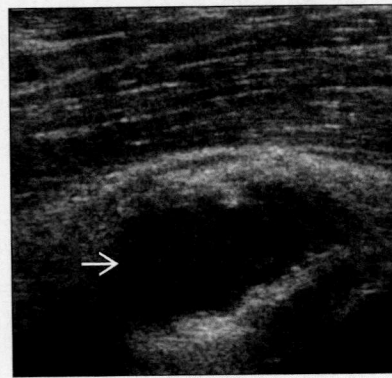

Ganglion

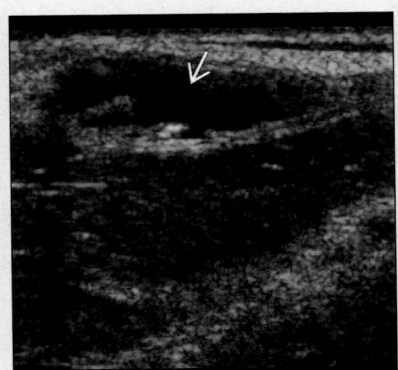

Bursitis

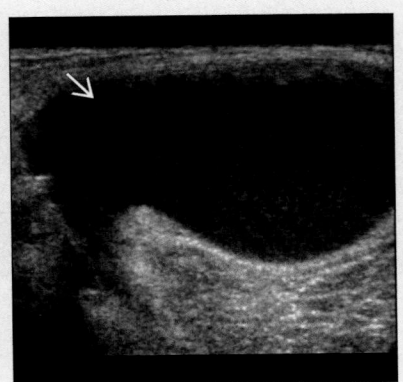

Baker Cyst

PARAMENISCAL CYST

Key Facts

Imaging Findings

- Best diagnostic clue: Cystic mass in continuity with horizontal meniscal tear
- Horizontal meniscal tear + parameniscal cyst ± extra-articular component with communicating stalk
- Menisci seen as diffusely echogenic, sharply-defined structures within medial and lateral femora-tibial compartments of knee
- Meniscal tear = linear or wedge-shaped hypoechogenicity within meniscus extending to meniscal periphery or articular surface
- Cyst may lie in direct continuity with meniscus or connect via connecting stalk
- Stalk of parameniscal cyst, if present, must be seen to connect with meniscal tear

- Cyst and contents of parameniscal cyst similar to para-articular ganglia and Baker cyst: All three contain synovial fluid
- If meniscal communication not seen, then parameniscal cyst can only be suggested as diagnosis

Top Differential Diagnoses

- Ganglion Cyst
- Bursitis
- Baker Cyst

Diagnostic Checklist

- Not every para-articular cyst with stalk extending to knee joint is a parameniscal cyst
- Demonstration of meniscal tear extending to articular surface is relevant as this will effect operative approach

---

- Meniscal tear = linear or wedge-shaped hypoechogenicity within meniscus extending to meniscal periphery or articular surface
- Para-meniscal cyst
  - Usually well-defined and filled with hypoechoic gelatinous-type fluid
  - ± Multiloculated
  - ± Septated
  - ± Comet-tail artifacts
    - Similar to those seen in Baker cyst or ganglion cysts
  - ± Echogenic debris (proteinaceous content or previous hemorrhage)
- Cyst usually thin-walled
  - Wall usually not hyperemic
- Cyst may lie in direct continuity with meniscus or connect via connecting stalk
- Stalk of parameniscal cyst, if present, must be seen to connect with meniscal tear
  - Stalk usually serpiginous and narrow
    - → Cyst may be located some length from meniscal tear
  - Stalk contents may be echogenic and thus difficult to see
  - In order to diagnose parameniscal cyst, need to see cyst connecting with meniscal tear
- Cyst and contents of parameniscal cyst similar to para-articular ganglia and Baker cyst: All three contain synovial fluid
  - Main difference is
    - Stalk in parameniscal cyst → meniscal tear
    - Stalk in para-articular ganglion → joint
    - Stalk in Baker cyst → between semimembranous tendon - medial gastrocnemius muscle → joint
- If meniscal communication not seen, then parameniscal cyst can only be suggested as diagnosis
  - Not sufficient to detect intra-articular origin as intra-articular ganglia with extra-articular extension will also have this characteristic
  - In these situations, consider MR to assess intra-articular origin and meniscal integrity

MR Findings

- T1WI
  - Intermediate to low signal intensity mass = cyst
  - If proteinaceous, cyst may be of higher signal intensity
- T2WI
  - Rounded, hyperintense mass
    - Lobulation and septation
  - Linear hyperintense meniscal signal extending to articular surface = tear
    - Occasionally associated peripheral meniscal tear does not visibly connect with meniscal surface (non-communicating tear)

Imaging Recommendations

- Best imaging tool
  - Ultrasound first line of investigation
    - Very accurate at detecting cystic nature of para-articular mass
    - In about one-half of cases will be able to depict meniscal origin of cyst
    - In remaining cases, → MR to confirm meniscal origin
- Examine with knee extended
- Determine whether cyst in continuity with meniscus
  - Determine whether meniscal tear present in meniscus at contact point with cyst
- If extra-articular cyst, locate stalk of cyst
  - Track stalk of cyst to knee joint
  - Determine if stalk originates from meniscal tear
- Note relationship of cyst to adjacent structures
  - Medially
    - Medial collateral ligament
    - Pes anserinus (sartorius, gracilis, semitendinous) tendons
  - Laterally
    - Ileo-tibial band
    - Lateral collateral ligament
- ± Examine with varying degrees of flexion to accentuate visualization of meniscal tear ± stalk

PARAMENISCAL CYST

DIFFERENTIAL DIAGNOSIS

Ganglion Cyst
- Can extend from intra-articular to extra-articular compartment
- Does not originate from meniscal tear
- ± Osteoarthrosis

Bursitis
- Medial parameniscal cyst mimicked by
  - Semimembranosus bursitis
  - Pes anserinus bursitis
- Lateral parameniscal cyst mimicked by
  - Deep infrapatellar bursa (anteriorly located lateral parameniscal cyst)

Baker Cyst
- Distension of semimembranous-gastrocnemius bursa
  - Cyst with "talk-bubble" configuration in popliteal fossa
  - Stalk arises from interspace between semimembranous tendon and medial belly gastrocnemius
  - No connection with meniscus

PATHOLOGY

General Features
- General path comments
  - Results from extrusion of synovial fluid from tear into cyst
    - "Ball valve" mechanism
  - Most commonly associated with horizontal peripheral tears
    - Or radial split tear with horizontal component
- Etiology
  - Forcing of joint fluid through horizontal meniscal tear into cyst
    - Compression/decompression of horizontal tear with knee flexion/extension may explain association with this type of tear
    - Cyst may enlarge after period of exercise
    - Hemorrhage into cyst may also result in enlargement
  - Occasionally peripheral horizontal tear associated with parameniscal cyst may not visibly communicate with articular surface
  - Possible explanations include
    - Articular extension minute and too small to see
    - Articular extension may have healed
    - Articular extension not present; cyst arising from mucopolysaccharide produced within meniscus
- Epidemiology
  - Relatively common
    - 7% in surgically removed menisci

Gross Pathologic & Surgical Features
- Cyst filled with mucinous-type fluid
  - In continuity with horizontal cleavage meniscal tear or flap (oblique) tear with predominately horizontal component
  - Associated with discoid menisci

Microscopic Features
- Cyst wall within meniscus formed by
  - Compressed meniscal collagen with areas of mucinous degeneration in adjacent meniscus
- Cyst wall outside meniscus (parameniscal) formed by
  - Compressed, loose areolar tissue

CLINICAL ISSUES

Presentation
- Most common signs/symptoms
  - Palpable mass ± pain near joint line
  - Size varies with knee position
    - Palpable cyst at 15-30° of flexion, disappearing at full extension and flexion (Pisani sign)
  - Lateral parameniscal cyst more readily palpable
    - Lateral cysts tend to present earlier and more frequently than medial cysts

Demographics
- Age: Seen in age groups in which meniscal tears occur
- Gender: M:F = 1:1

Natural History & Prognosis
- Mass enlarges with time

Treatment
- Arthroscopic resection of cyst and repair of tear
  - Tear must be closed to prevent growth or re-emergence of cyst
- Open resection of cyst if meniscal tear not communicating with articular surface

DIAGNOSTIC CHECKLIST

Consider
- Not every para-articular cyst with stalk extending to knee joint is a parameniscal cyst
  - Intra-articular ganglion cyst with para-articular extension can look very similar
- Demonstration of meniscal tear extending to articular surface is relevant as this will effect operative approach
  - Arthroscopic if communicating meniscal tear present
  - Open if non-communicating meniscal tear present

Image Interpretation Pearls
- Cyst alongside meniscus in continuity with meniscal tear = parameniscal cyst
  - Meniscal tear usually has horizontal component
  - Anywhere along meniscus but anterior horn lateral meniscus and posterior horn medial meniscus most common

SELECTED REFERENCES
1. McCarthy CL et al: The MRI appearance of cystic lesions around the knee. Skeletal Radiol. 33(4):187-209, 2004

PARAMENISCAL CYST

IMAGE GALLERY

Typical

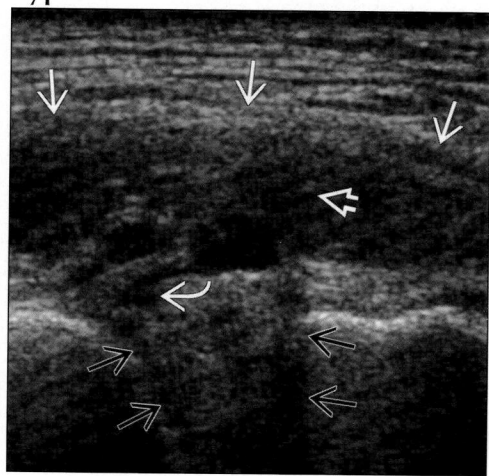 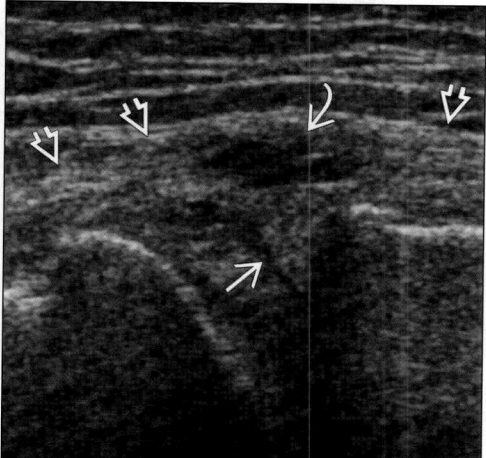

(Left) Longitudinal ultrasound shows a parameniscal cyst ➡, with mixed echogenicity content, displacing the medial collateral ligament ➡. The cyst is continuous with the tear ➡ in the peripheral aspect medial meniscus ➡. *(Right)* Longitudinal ultrasound shows a tear ➡ in the peripheral aspect medial meniscus with a parameniscal cyst ➡ extending into the medial collateral ligament ➡.

Typical

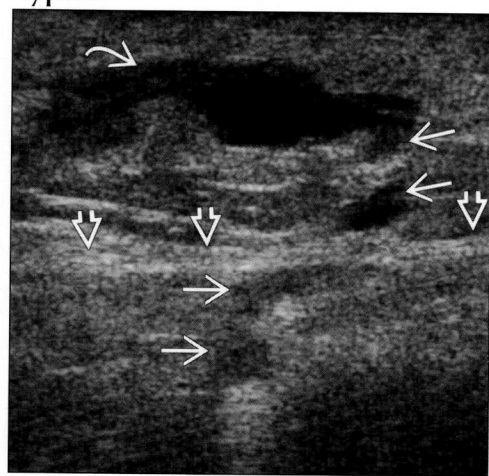 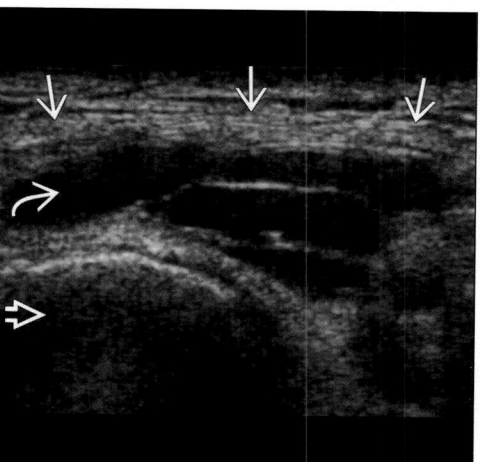

(Left) Transverse ultrasound shows a mixed echogenicity parameniscal cyst ➡ on the lateral side of the knee. The stalk ➡ extends through the lateral collateral ligament ➡ towards the lateral meniscus. *(Right)* Longitudinal ultrasound shows a multiseptated parameniscal cyst ➡, deep to the lateral collateral ligament ➡. Femoral condyle ➡.

Typical

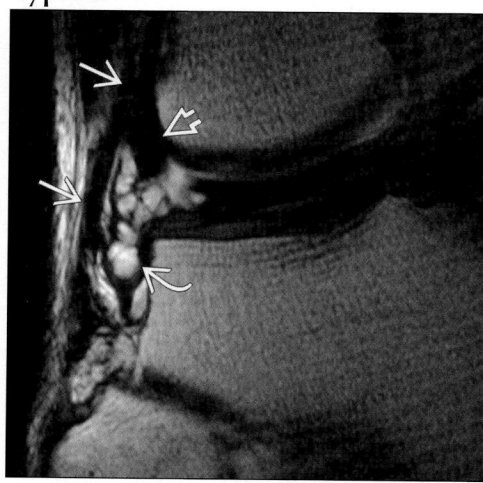 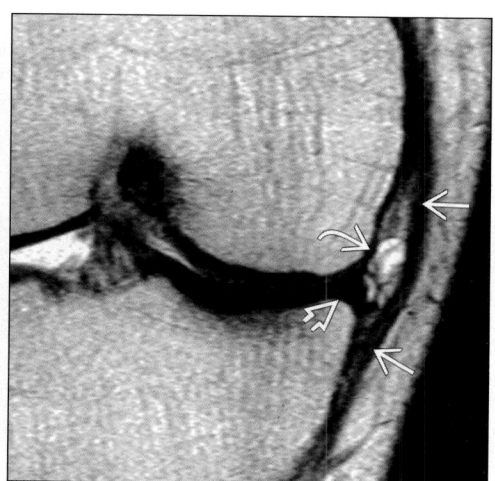

(Left) Coronal T2WI MR shows a multiseptated parameniscal cyst ➡, deep to the lateral collateral ligament ➡. Note heterogenicity of the cyst contents are indicative of proteinaceous fluid or hemorrhage. Popliteus tendon ➡. *(Right)* Coronal T2WI MR shows extension of a multiseptated parameniscal cyst ➡ deep to the medial collateral ligament ➡. The cyst arose from a horizontal meniscal tear (not shown). Body medial meniscus ➡.

SYNOVIAL TUMOR

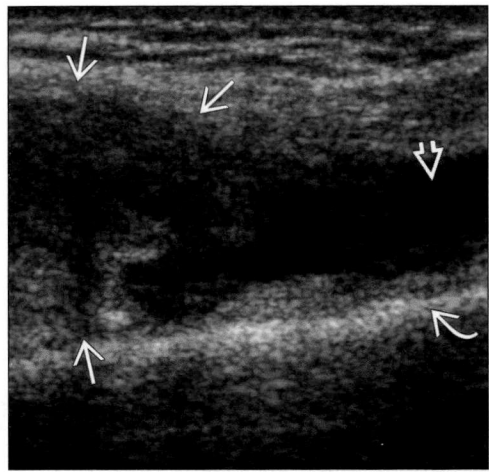

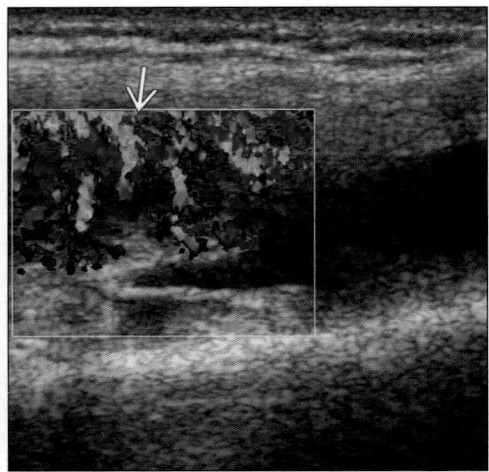

Longitudinal ultrasound shows focally thickened synovium ➡ at the upper end of the suprapatellar pouch, indicative of PVNS. Note joint effusion ➡. No calcified nodules present. Femoral cortex ➡.

Corresponding longitudinal color Doppler ultrasound shows marked hyperemia ➡ of focally thickened synovium, indicative of PVNS.

TERMINOLOGY

Abbreviations and Synonyms
- Pigmented villonodular synovitis (PVNS), giant cell tumor of tendon sheath (GCTTS), tenosynovial giant cell tumor, focal nodular synovitis, synovial osteochondromatosis
- Synovial sarcoma, misnomer since not derived from true synovial cells; re-categorized as "malignant tumor of uncertain differentiation"

Definitions
- Pigmented villonodular synovitis (PVNS) (diffuse/focal) & giant cell tumor of tendon sheath (GCTTS) recently re-categorized as fibrohistiocytic tumors
  - GCTTS & focal PVNS also known as focal nodular synovitis
- Synovial osteochondromatosis = synovial metaplasia characterized by cartilaginous loose bodies which later ossify

IMAGING FINDINGS

General Features
- Best diagnostic clue
  - PVNS: Tumor-like hypoechoic hypervascular synovium
  - GCTTS: Eccentric nodular mass along tendon sheath ± hyperemia
  - Synovial osteochondromatosis: Thickened synovium with discrete echogenic foci ± hyperemia
- Location
  - Occurs in synovial-lined joints, tendon sheaths & bursae
    - PVNS: Knee (80%) followed by hip, ankle, shoulder & elbow; polyarticular rare
    - GCTTS: Most common in tendons of hand
    - Synovial osteochondromatosis: Knee followed by elbow, hip & shoulder; polyarticular (5%)
- Size
  - PVNS & GCTTS: Thickened synovium masses ranging from few cm to 20 cm
  - Synovial osteochondromatosis: Nodules from few mm to about 20 mm
- Morphology

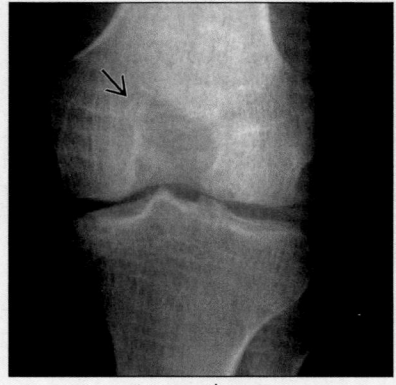

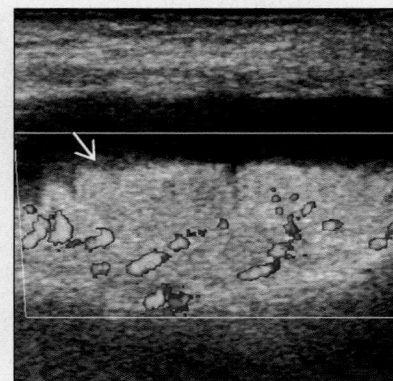

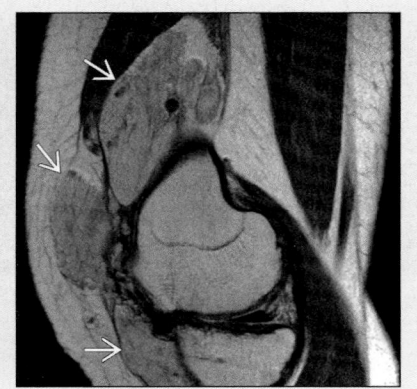

DDx: Synovial Tumor

Hemarthrosis

Synovitis

Synovial Hemangioma

SYNOVIAL TUMOR

Key Facts

Terminology
- Pigmented villonodular synovitis (PVNS) (diffuse/focal) & giant cell tumor of tendon sheath (GCTTS) recently re-categorized as fibrohistiocytic tumors
- GCTTS & focal PVNS also known as focal nodular synovitis
- Synovial osteochondromatosis = synovial metaplasia characterized by cartilaginous loose bodies which later ossify

Imaging Findings
- PVNS: Tumor-like hypoechoic hypervascular synovium
- GCTTS: Eccentric nodular mass along tendon sheath ± hyperemia

- Synovial osteochondromatosis: Thickened synovium with discrete echogenic foci ± hyperemia
- Occurs in synovial-lined joints, tendon sheaths & bursae
- PVNS: Knee (80%) followed by hip, ankle, shoulder & elbow; polyarticular rare
- GCTTS: Most common in tendons of hand
- Synovial osteochondromatosis: Knee followed by elbow, hip & shoulder; polyarticular (5%)
- PVNS & GCTTS: Thickened synovium masses ranging from few cm to 20 cm
- Synovial osteochondromatosis: Nodules from few mm to about 20 mm

Top Differential Diagnoses
- Hemophilic Arthropathy
- Synovitis

- PVNS & GCTTS: Thickened synovium, diffuse or focal
- Synovial osteochondromatosis: Synovial thickening & intra-articular nodules

Ultrasonographic Findings
- PVNS (diffuse)
  - Effusion
  - Thickened synovium with mass-like areas
  - Severe synovial hyperemia
  - Hemosiderin not visible on ultrasound
  - ± Intra-articular bony erosion
- PVNS (focal)
  - Well-defined hypoechoic intra-articular nodule
  - Infrapatellar > suprapatellar location
  - ± Mild hyperemia
  - ± Effusion
- GCTTS
  - Eccentric hypoechoic tendon sheath mass
  - ± Mild hyperemia
  - Otherwise normal tendon & tendon sheath
- Synovial osteochondromatosis
  - Mild to moderate synovial thickening
  - Joint effusion
  - Multiple echogenic nodules, typically small (up to 20 mm) in size
  - Non-ossified cartilaginous nodules may be difficult to see on ultrasound
    - Hypoechoic; similar to joint fluid
  - ± Mild hyperemia
- All synovial tumors
  - → Ultrasound guided core biopsy for confirmation
  - Especially PVNS and GCTTS

Radiographic Findings
- Radiography
  - PVNS
    - Dense soft tissue swelling
    - ± Erosions with sclerotic margins, especially hip
    - Preservation of joint space till late
    - No juxta-articular osteopenia
  - Synovial osteochondromatosis
    - Multiple small ossified bodies within joint

- Cartilage nodules not ossified in 20%
- ± Intra-articular erosions, especially hip
- Preservation of joint space till late
- No juxta-articular osteopenia

MR Findings
- T1WI
  - PVNS
    - Intermediate to decreased signal intensity masses
- T2WI
  - PVNS
    - Hypointense to intermediate signal secondary to paramagnetic effect of iron
    - ± Intermediate signal erosions with hypointense margin
    - ± Surrounding hyperintense edema
    - Hyperintense effusion
- T2* GRE
  - PVNS
    - Foci of hypointensity due to hemosiderin deposits
    - Hemosiderin present in only about 85% of PVNS cases i.e., absence of hemosiderin does not exclude diagnosis
- T1 C+
  - PVNS
    - Inflamed synovium enhances

Imaging Recommendations
- Best imaging tool
  - Ultrasound for nodular PVNS & GCTTS
  - MR for diffuse PVNS
    - Ultrasound can suggest diagnosis of diffuse PVNS though MR more specific & better defines extent
  - Radiography followed by MR for synovial osteochondromatosis
- Protocol advice: GRE sequences for hemosiderin

DIFFERENTIAL DIAGNOSIS

Hemophilic Arthropathy
- Clinical history
- Familial (X-linked)

SYNOVIAL TUMOR

- ± Polyarticular
- ± Hemarthrosis (& hemosiderin)

Synovitis
- Systemic inflammatory disorder
- ± Polyarticular
- + RA factor usually

Synovial Hemangioma
- Vascular anomaly involving synovium
- Phleboliths, venous lakes
- ± Hemarthrosis (& hemosiderin)

PATHOLOGY

General Features
- General path comments
  - PVNS
    - Synovial proliferative disorder
    - Diffuse or nodular (focal) forms
    - Nodular PVNS (which also includes GCTTS) known as focal nodular synovitis
    - Although histologically almost identical, focal nodular synovitis may be separate entity from diffuse PVNS
  - Focal nodular synovitis
    - Is localized to one area of synovium
    - Does not have frond-like projections
    - Has less hemosiderin deposition
    - Tends to become more pedunculated with growth
  - Synovial osteochondromatosis
    - Synovial metaplasia
- Etiology: Idiopathic disorders
- Epidemiology: Approximately two/million

Gross Pathologic & Surgical Features
- PVNS
  - Diffuse or focal (nodular) form
  - ± Joint filled with non-clotted blood
  - Yellow-brown cut-surface (fat and hemosiderin)
- GCTTS
  - Rubbery, encapsulated, multinodular mass
  - Yellow-brown cut-surface
- Synovial osteochondromatosis
  - Synovial thickening
  - Multiple bodies, both free and attached to synovium

Microscopic Features
- PVNS & GCTTS
  - Synovial mass
  - Fibrohistiocytic cells, foamy histiocytes, giant cells with hemosiderin
  - ± Sclerotic rimmed bone erosions
- Synovial osteochondromatosis
  - Initial active phase of synovial proliferation without loose bodies
    - → Late inactive phase with inactive synovial disease and loose bodies
  - Multiple nodules of hyaline cartilage formed within subsynovial connective tissue
  - Nodules hypercellular with varying cellular atypia
  - Later ossify (endochondral ossification)

- Nodules may contain cartilage, cartilage and bone, or mature bone with fatty marrow

CLINICAL ISSUES

Presentation
- Most common signs/symptoms: Joint swelling
- Other signs/symptoms
  - Pain
  - Limitation of movement

Demographics
- Age: 30-50 years typically
- Gender
  - PVNS: M:F = 2: 1
  - GCTTS: M:F = 1:1
  - Synovial osteochondromatosis: M:F = 2:1

Natural History & Prognosis
- PVNS (diffuse): → Progressive arthropathy
- PVNS (focal) & GCTTS: Good response to excision
- Synovial osteochondromatosis: Active → inactive phase

Treatment
- PVNS (diffuse)
  - Synovectomy
  - Recurrence
    - 20% after complete (open) synovectomy
    - 50% after incomplete (arthroscopic) synovectomy
  - Intra-articular yttrium-90 radiation synovectomy
- GCTTS & focal PVNS
  - Limited synovectomy
- Synovial osteochondromatosis
  - Synovectomy
  - Recurrence 15%

DIAGNOSTIC CHECKLIST

Consider
- Diffuse PVNS and focal PVNS (focal nodular synovitis) may represent separate entities

Image Interpretation Pearls
- PVNS ⇒ hyperemic, hypoechoic synovial mass
  - T2* GRE identifies hemosiderin (hypointense)
    - Not imperative to see hemosiderin on gradient echo MR imaging to make diagnosis of PVNS
- GCTTS presents as eccentric, rather than concentric, tendon sheath mass
- Calcified bodies not invariably present in synovial osteochondromatosis
- Ultrasound-guided biopsy will confirm diagnosis of most synovial tumors

SELECTED REFERENCES

1. Sheldon PJ et al: Imaging of intraarticular masses. Radiographics. 25(1):105-19, 2005
2. Huang GS et al: Localized nodular synovitis of the knee: MR imaging appearance and clinical correlates in 21 patients. AJR Am J Roentgenol. 181(2):539-43, 2003

SYNOVIAL TUMOR

IMAGE GALLERY

Typical

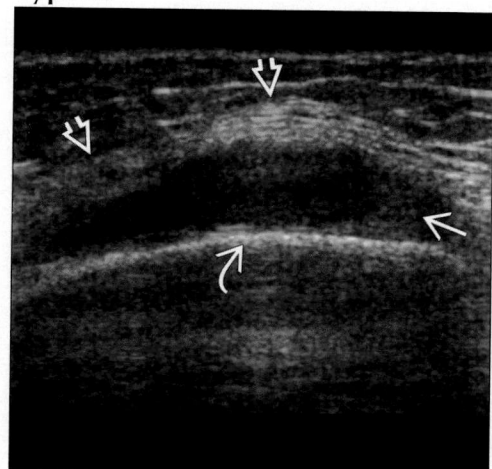
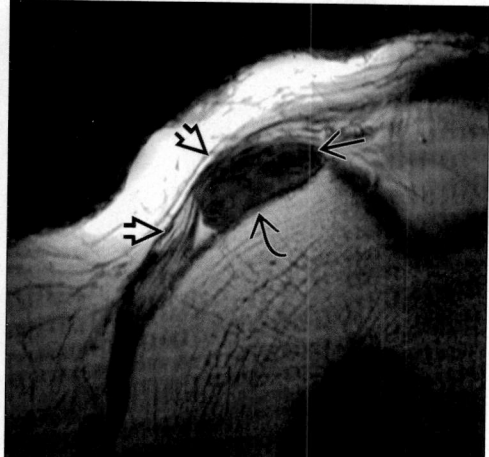

(Left) Transverse ultrasound shows a focal hypoechoic mass ➡ located between the retinaculum ⮞ and the femoral cortex ➡. The mass was mildly hyperemic. Appearances are suggestive of focal PVNS (focal nodular synovitis). *(Right)* Corresponding transverse T2WI MR shows a focal heterogeneous hypointense mass ➡ located between the retinaculum ⮞ and the femoral cortex ➡, due to focal PVNS (focal nodular synovitis).

Typical

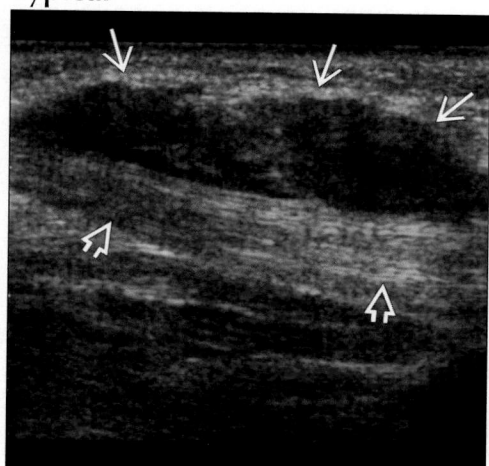
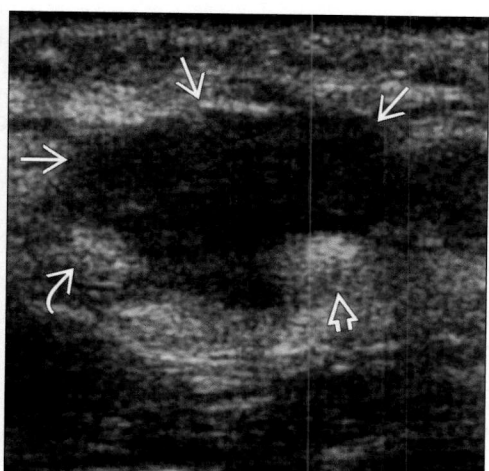

(Left) Longitudinal ultrasound shows a hypoechoic mass ➡ alongside the flexor pollicis longus tendon ⮞, indicative of GCTTS. No tendon sheath effusion is present. Tendon is normal. *(Right)* Corresponding transverse ultrasound shows eccentric location of hypoechoic GCTTS ➡ contacting the flexor pollicis longus tendon ⮞ and the flexor tendon to the index finger ➡.

Typical

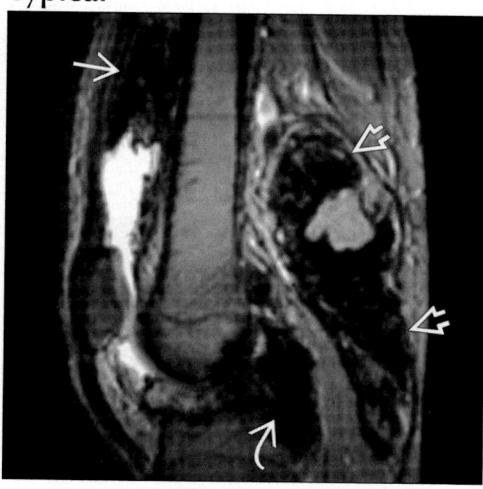
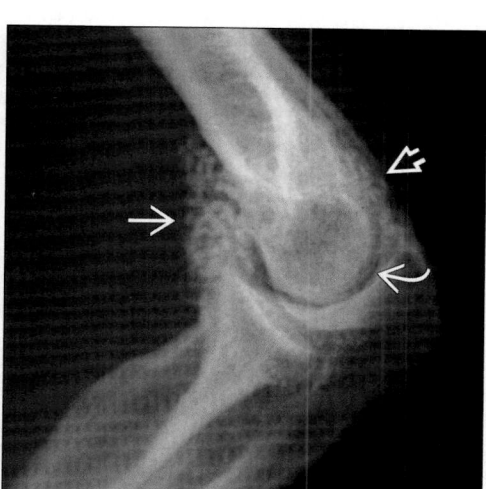

(Left) Longitudinal gradient-echo T2 WI MR of the knee shows hypointense masses of the suprapatellar pouch ➡, posterior aspect the knee ➡ and popliteal fossa ⮞, due to PVNS. Note hypointensity due to hemosiderin deposition. *(Right)* Lateral radiograph of the elbow shows many small calcified nodules in the anterior ➡ and posterior ⮞ joint recesses due to synovial osteochondromatosis. Moderate joint space narrowing ➡ is present.

PLANTAR FASCIITIS & FIBROMATOSIS

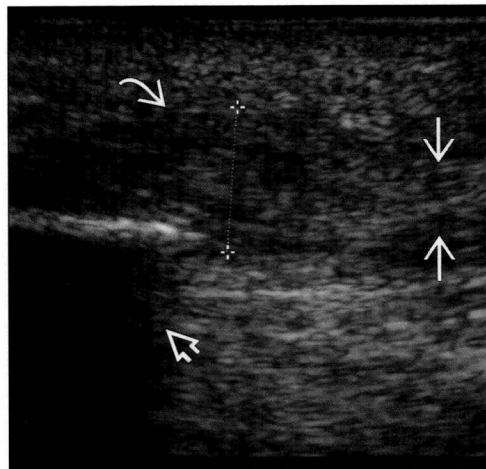

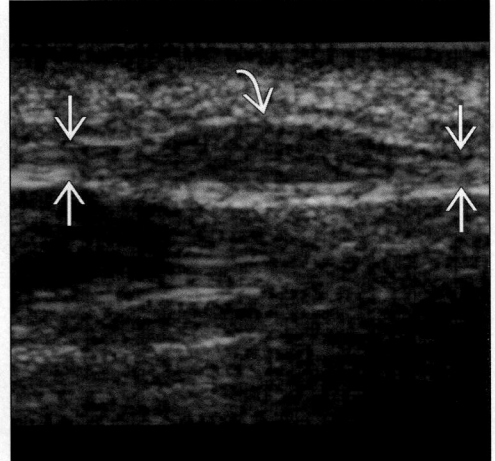

Longitudinal ultrasound shows thickened (8.6 mm, calipers) plantar fascia ➡ at calcaneal insertion. This merges with normal caliber fascia ➡. Calcaneus ▷.

Longitudinal ultrasound shows a fusiform-shaped, hypoechoic nodule ➡ arising within the plantar fascia ➡ consistent with plantar fibromatosis. Note well-defined, superficial and deep margin of nodule.

TERMINOLOGY

Abbreviations and Synonyms
- Plantar fasciitis: Jogger's heel, tennis heel, policeman's heel, heel spur syndrome, calcaneal spur syndrome
- Plantar fibromatosis: Ledderhose disease

Definitions
- Plantar fasciitis: Degeneration ± chronic inflammation ± fibroblastic proliferation of plantar fascia insertion to medial tuberosity calcaneus
- Plantar fibromatosis: Nodular fibroblastic proliferation of plantar fascia separate from calcaneus

IMAGING FINDINGS

General Features
- Best diagnostic clue
  - **Plantar fasciitis**: Thickened plantar fascial insertion
  - Plantar fibromatosis: Nodular thickening of plantar fascia
- Location
  - Plantar fasciitis: Medial tuberosity calcaneus

- Bilateral in one-third
  - ○ Plantar fibromatosis: Affects medial (60%) or mid-portion (40%) of fascia
    - Bilateral in one-third
    - Several nodules may co-exist in same fascia
- Size
  - ○ Plantar fasciitis: Fascial thickness varies from 2-12 mm
  - ○ Plantar fibromatosis
    - Average length 13 mm (range 4-17 mm)
    - Average width 10 mm (range 4-22 mm)
    - Average depth 4 mm (range 2-10 mm)
- Morphology
  - ○ Plantar fasciitis: Fascial thickening at insertion, merges with plantar fascia
  - ○ Plantar fibromatosis: Discrete well-defined nodule

Ultrasonographic Findings
- **Plantar fasciitis**
  - ○ Plantar fascia thickness > 4.5 mm (most useful sign)
  - ○ ± Hypoechogenicity of plantar fascia
  - ○ ± Lack of fascial definition
  - ○ ± Peri-fascial edema
  - ○ Calcaneal spur

DDx: Plantar Fasciitis & Fibromatosis

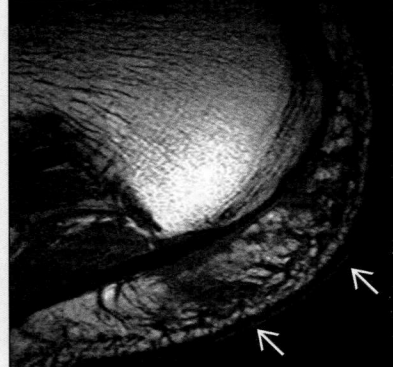

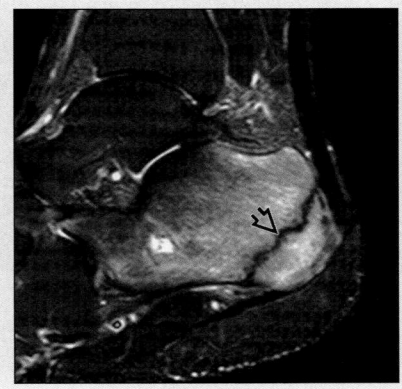

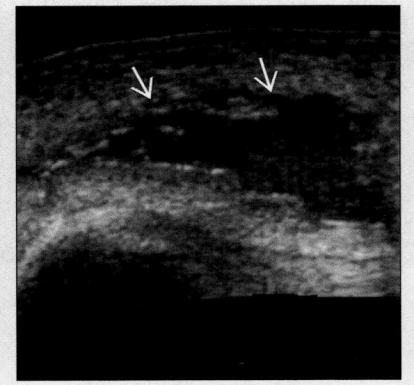

Subcutaneous Fat Necrosis

Calcaneal Fracture

Plantar Bursitis

PLANTAR FASCIITIS & FIBROMATOSIS

Key Facts

Imaging Findings
- **Plantar fasciitis**: Thickened plantar fascial insertion
- Plantar fascia thickness > 4.5 mm (most useful sign)
- ± Hypoechogenicity of plantar fascia
- ± Lack of fascial definition
- ± Peri-fascial edema
- Spur is located deep to (& not within) fascia
- May simulate anterior edge of calcaneus
- **Plantar fibromatosis**
- Discrete fusiform-shaped nodule of plantar fascia separated from calcaneal insertion
- Hypoechoic to plantar fascia (75%)
- Posterior acoustic enhancement (20%)
- Intrinsic vascularity (10%)
- Majority located within mid-substance or plantar aspect of plantar fascia

Top Differential Diagnoses
- Subcutaneous Fat Necrosis
- Calcaneal Stress or Insufficiency Fracture
- Plantar Bursitis

Diagnostic Checklist
- MR if ultrasound negative for plantar fasciitis
- Aggressive plantar fibromatosis likely if plantar fascia nodule has indistinct/infiltrative superficial or deep margins
- Likliness of fasciitis increases with thickness of calcaneal insertion
- Plantar fibromatosis = distinct plantar fascial nodule separate from calcaneal insertion

---

- ■ Spur is located deep to (& not within) fascia
- ■ May simulate anterior edge of calcaneus
- ○ Calcification not a feature
- **Plantar fibromatosis**
  - ○ Discrete fusiform-shaped nodule of plantar fascia separated from calcaneal insertion
  - ○ Hypoechoic to plantar fascia (75%)
    - ■ Isoechoic to plantar fascia (25%)
  - ○ Posterior acoustic enhancement (20%)
  - ○ Intrinsic vascularity (10%)
  - ○ Majority located within mid-substance or plantar aspect of plantar fascia
    - ■ If nodule has indistinct ± infiltrative superficial or deep margin, consider aggressive plantar fibromatosis
  - ○ Co-existent thickening of ipsilateral calcaneal insertion present in one-third of patients without related symptoms

Radiographic Findings
- Radiography
  - ○ Plantar fasciitis: Plantar calcaneal spur present in about 50% of patients with plantar fasciitis
    - ■ Also found in asymptomatic subjects
    - ■ Fluffy periostitis, erosion, sclerosis → ± enthesopathy
  - ○ Useful in atypical cases to exclude other causes of heel pain

MR Findings
- T1WI
  - ○ Plantar fasciitis: Thickening of plantar fascia at calcaneal insertion
  - ○ Plantar fibromatosis: Low intensity nodule along plantar fascia
- T2WI: Plantar fibromatosis: Low to intermediate signal intensity nodule along plantar fascia
- STIR
  - ○ Plantar fasciitis
    - ■ Thickness > 4.5 mm (almost 100%)
    - ■ Subcutaneous or perifascial edema (90%)
    - ■ Insertional marrow edema (40%)

- ■ Markedly increased insertional marrow edema, erosions and sclerosis suggestive of inflammatory enthesopathy (associated with spondyloarthropathy)

Nuclear Medicine Findings
- Bone Scan
  - ○ Plantar fasciitis: Positive in 60-98% cases
    - ■ Increased blood flow ± blood pooling ± increased activity on delayed images

Imaging Recommendations
- Best imaging tool: Plantar fasciitis & fibromatosis; ultrasound is accurate, quick and accessible
- Protocol advice
  - ○ Examine fascia in transverse and longitudinal planes
    - ■ Routinely examine both sides as subclinical contralateral disease is common in both diseases

DIFFERENTIAL DIAGNOSIS

Subcutaneous Fat Necrosis
- Focal subcutaneous edema ± swelling ± perifascial fluid
- Trauma history
- MR probably more sensitive than ultrasound

Calcaneal Stress or Insufficiency Fracture
- Stress Fx: Normal bone ↔ abnormal stress
- Insufficiency Fx: Abnormal bone ↔ normal stress
- Not apparent on ultrasound; best assessed by MR

Plantar Bursitis
- Fluid-filled bursa or flat hypoechoic area superficial to plantar fascia
- Typically forefoot region

PATHOLOGY

General Features
- General path comments
  - ○ Plantar fascia = multilayered fibrous aponeurosis, 1-2 mm thick, with medial, central and lateral bands

PLANTAR FASCIITIS & FIBROMATOSIS

- Central cord largest; originates from medial calcaneal tuberosity
- Divides in forefoot into five bands which insert onto plantar plates of metatarsophalangeal joints and bases of proximal phalanges
- Etiology
  - Plantar fasciitis: Possibly caused by repetitive microtrauma or microvascular injury
  - Plantar fibromatosis: Unknown etiology; not knowingly related to trauma
    - Possibly genetic
    - Possibly related to collagen profile
- Epidemiology
  - Plantar fasciitis: Most common cause of heel pain
    - 10% of running injuries (excessive running, faulty shoes, running on uneven surfaces, high arched foot or short Achilles tendon)
    - Additional risk factors: Obesity, prolonged weightbearing, pes planus, reduced ankle dorsiflexion)
  - Plantar fibromatosis: Less common than plantar fasciitis
    - No specific risk factors identified
- Associated abnormalities
  - May be related to other fibroproliferative diseases (Dupuytren contracture, Peyronie disease etc.)
    - Onset of other fibromatoses may be delayed for 5-10 years after onset of plantar fibromatosis

Gross Pathologic & Surgical Features
- Plantar fasciitis: Firm thickening of plantar fascia at calcaneal insertion
- Plantar fibromatosis: Firm whitish nodule
  - No capsule or pseudocapsule
  - Although macroscopically circumscribed, microscopically has ill-defined borders

Microscopic Features
- Plantar fasciitis: Degeneration of plantar fascia ± fibroblastic proliferation ± chronic inflammatory change
- Plantar fibromatosis: Three phases of fibroblastic proliferation within plantar fascia
  - Proliferative phase: Nodular fibroblastic proliferation
  - Active phase: Collagen synthesis and deposition
  - Mature phase: Reduced fibroblastic proliferation, collagen maturation

CLINICAL ISSUES

Presentation
- Most common signs/symptoms
  - Plantar fasciitis: Heel pain ↑ by weightbearing
    - Pain worse on first few steps in morning
  - Plantar fibromatosis: Sole pain ± palpable firm lump
    - Pain ↑ by prolonged weightbearing
- Clinical Profile
  - Plantar fasciitis: Tenderness on deep palpation medial calcaneal tuberosity
  - Plantar fibromatosis: Sole lump usually non-tender or mildly tender

Demographics
- Age
  - Plantar fasciitis: 40-60 years
    - Younger in predisposed individuals (runners, military personnel)
  - Plantar fibromatosis: 50 years (30-80 years)
- Gender: Plantar fasciitis & fibromatosis: M:F = 1:1

Natural History & Prognosis
- Plantar fasciitis
  - Symptoms resolve in 80% within 12 months with conservative treatment
- Palmar fibromatosis
  - Similar tendency to improve with time
    - Nodules become smaller and lesser painful

Treatment
- Plantar fasciitis
  - Conservative: Start treatment soon after onset
    - Anti-inflammatory agents
    - ± Padding and strapping, shoe inserts
    - ± Stretching of plantar fascia
    - ± Night splints to keep ankle in neutral position
  - Steroid ± long-acting local anesthetic injection (± ultrasound guidance)
    - Usually not possible to inject directly into plantar fascia → inject to perifascial tissues
    - ± Only provides temporary relief for about 4 weeks
  - Extracorporal shock wave therapy
    - No substantive evidence of benefit
  - Surgery (for patients with persistent symptoms)
    - Open or endoscopic partial or complete release of plantar fascia
    - Persistent pain in ¼
- Plantar fibromatosis
  - Conservative
    - Shoe inserts
    - ± Steroid ± long-acting local anesthetic injection (± ultrasound guidance) to nodule
  - Surgery (for very painful nodules)
    - Recurrence common after surgery

DIAGNOSTIC CHECKLIST

Consider
- MR if ultrasound negative for plantar fasciitis
- Aggressive plantar fibromatosis likely if plantar fascia nodule has indistinct/infiltrative superficial or deep margins

Image Interpretation Pearls
- Likeliness of fascitis increases with thickness of calcaneal insertion
- Plantar fibromatosis = distinct plantar fascial nodule separate from calcaneal insertion

SELECTED REFERENCES

1. Buchbinder R: Clinical practice. Plantar fasciitis. N Engl J Med. 350(21):2159-66, 2004
2. Griffith JF et al: Sonography of plantar fibromatosis. AJR Am J Roentgenol. 179(5):1167-72, 2002

PLANTAR FASCIITIS & FIBROMATOSIS

IMAGE GALLERY

Typical

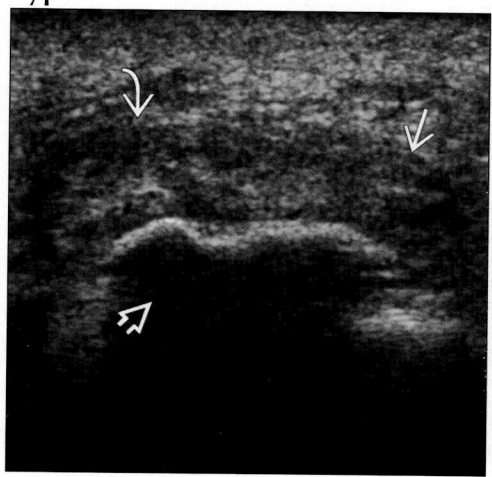
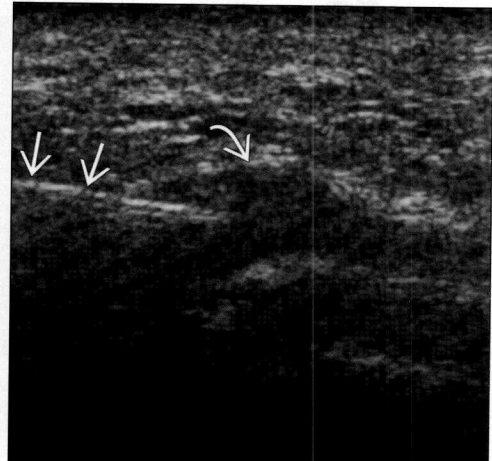

(Left) Transverse ultrasound shows a thickened plantar fascia insertion onto the calcaneus. The plantar fascia is more thickened medially ➡ than laterally ➡. Note the ill-defined fascial margin and calcaneal spur ➡. *(Right)* Transverse ultrasound shows needle insertion ➡ into the medial aspect of the plantar fascia ➡ at the calcaneus for the therapeutic injection. Usually a perifascial rather than intrafascial injection is performed.

Typical

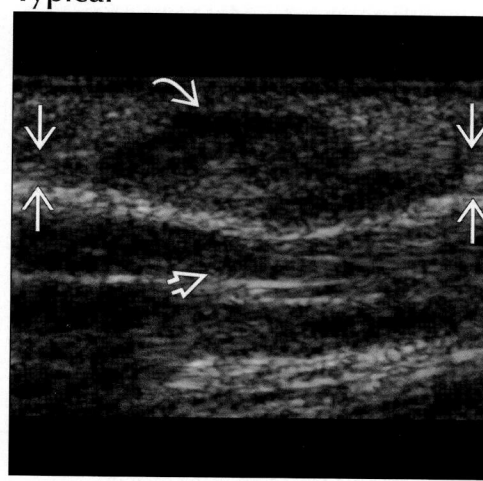
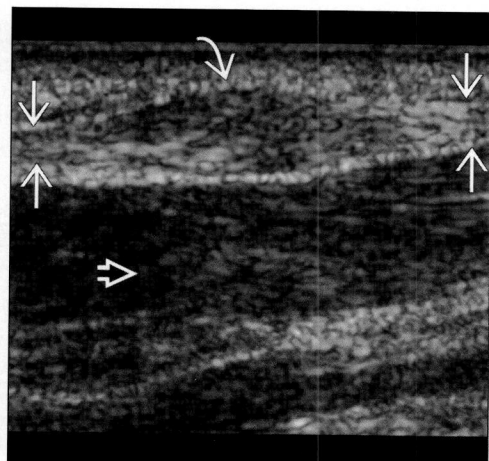

(Left) Longitudinal ultrasound shows an irregular hypoechoic nodule ➡ arising from the plantar fascia ➡, consistent with plantar fibromatosis. Note indentation of underlying muscle ➡. *(Right)* Longitudinal ultrasound shows a fusiform shaped plantar fascia nodule ➡, almost isoechoic to the plantar fascia ➡, consistent with plantar fibromatosis. Note mild posterior acoustic enhancement ➡.

Typical

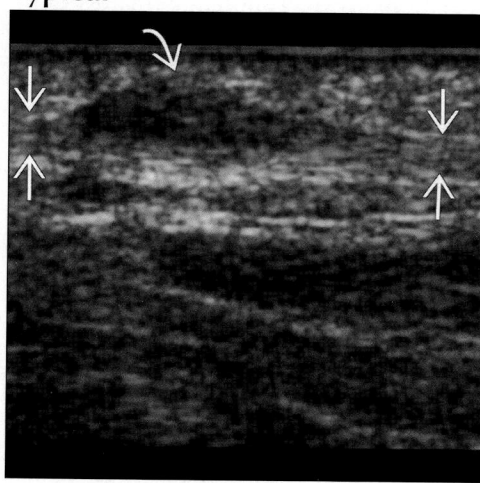
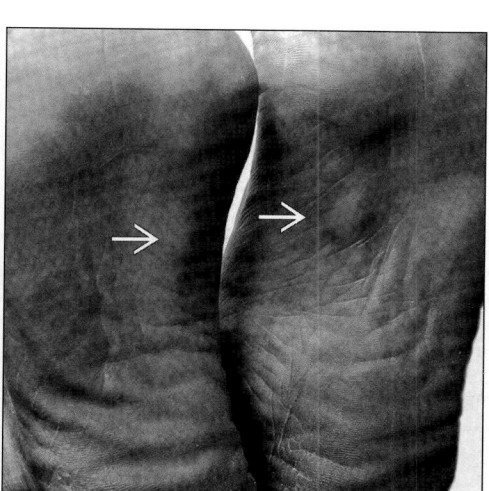

(Left) Longitudinal ultrasound shows a hypoechoic nodule ➡ arising from the superficial aspect of the plantar fascia ➡, consistent with plantar fibromatosis. *(Right)* Clinical photograph shows small nodules ➡ of plantar fibromatosis on the medial aspect of both soles.

PERIPHERAL LIPOMA

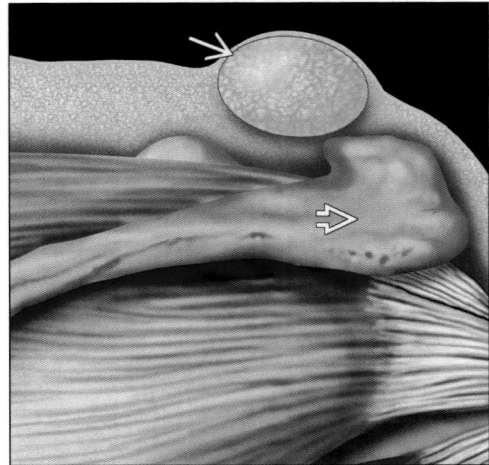

Graphic shows a well-defined lipoma ➡ located in the subcutaneous tissues overlying the acromion ➡.

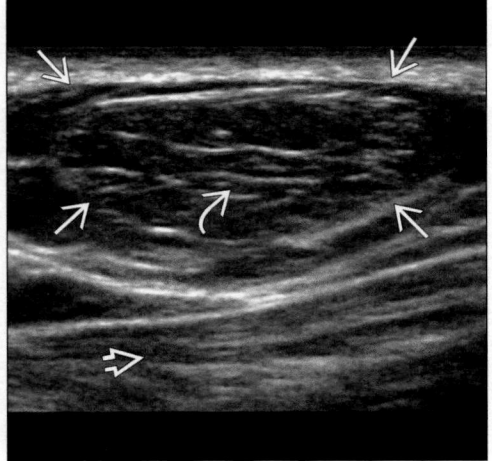

Transverse ultrasound shows a well-defined slightly echogenic lipoma ➡ within the subcutaneous fat of the scapular region. Note the fine internal striations parallel to the skin ➡. Muscle layer ➡.

TERMINOLOGY

Abbreviations and Synonyms
- Fatty tumor
  - Nine distinct types of benign fatty tumor
    - Lipoma
    - Lipomatosis
    - Lipomatosis of nerve
    - Lipoblastoma/lipoblastomatosis
    - Angiolipoma
    - Myolipoma of soft tissue (rare)
    - Chondroid lipoma (rare)
    - Spindle-cell lipoma/pleomorphic lipoma
    - Hibernoma

Definitions
- Lipoma: Benign soft tissue tumor composed of mature adipose tissue
- Lipomatosis: Diffuse overgrowth of mature adipose tissue that infiltrates soft tissues of affected part; > children
- Angiolipoma: Lipoma variant containing thin-walled blood-vessels; > subcutaneous

- Lipoblastoma/lipoblastomatosis: Admixture of mature and immature adipocytes; > children
- Spindle-cell lipoma/pleomorphic lipoma: Mixture of fat & spindle cells; > subcutaneous, > adult males
- Hibernoma: Brown fat similar to that found in hibernating animals; > subcutaneous, > adults, > trunk

IMAGING FINDINGS

General Features
- Best diagnostic clue: Echogenic mass with fine internal echoes aligned parallel to long axis of tumor
- Location
  - Superficial i.e., subcutaneous; most common
    - Posterior trunk, extremities, neck
    - Multifocal: 10%
  - Deep i.e., subfascial (deep to investing fascia)
    - Intermuscular
    - Intramuscular; inclusive of supramuscular & submuscular (i.e., juxtacortical) locations
  - Lipomas do not transverse investing fascia
    - Subcutaneous lipomas remain confined to subcutaneous layer

DDx: Lipoma

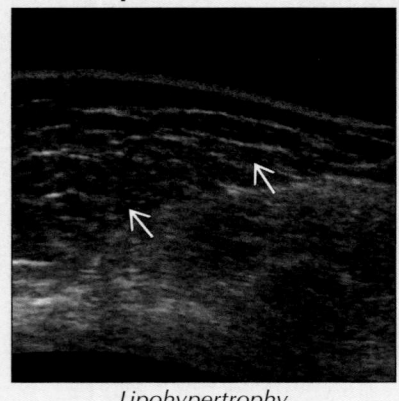

Lipohypertrophy

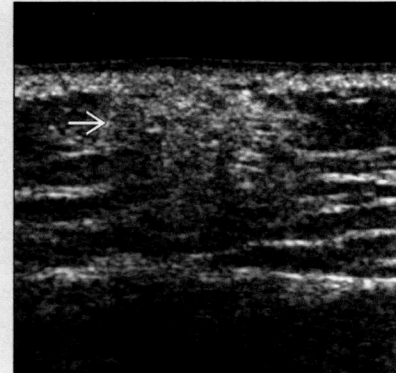

Fat Injury

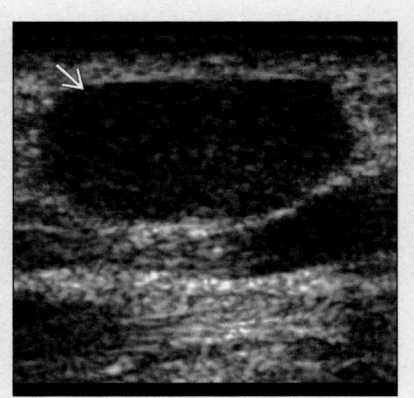

Nerve Sheath Tumor

SOFT TISSUE SARCOMA

Key Facts

Imaging Findings
- Large heterogeneous hypoechoic mass
- Usually located in deep (subfascial) tissues
- Well-encapsulated
- ± Myxoid tissue: Well-defined, intra-tumoral anechoic or hypoechoic areas
- ± Necrosis: Poorly-defined hypoechoic areas
- ± Calcification: Discrete intra-tumoral echogenic foci with acoustic shadowing
- ± Hemorrhage: Ill-defined intra-tumoral echogenic areas without acoustic shadowing
- Usually hypervascular with disorganized vascular pattern on color Doppler imaging
- 16-gauge or 14-gauge Tru-cut core biopsy with co-axial system necessary for tissue typing & histological staging

- Fine-needle aspiration for cytology (FNAC) is not sufficient for initial diagnosis
- FNAC useful for detecting residual disease, recurrence or deep-seated retroperitoneal lesions
- Concentrate on defining tumor extent
- Assess relation to neurovascular bundle & bone
- Evaluate involvement of regional nodes

Top Differential Diagnoses
- Benign Soft Tissue Tumor
- Muscle Metastasis
- Muscle Hematoma

Diagnostic Checklist
- Nearly all STS are well-defined (i.e. sharp definition does not equate to benign tumor)

- ± Hemorrhage: Ill-defined intra-tumoral echogenic areas without acoustic shadowing
- Usually hypervascular with disorganized vascular pattern on color Doppler imaging
  - Vacular pattern may be orderly
  - May be hypovascular or avascular
- Ultrasound-guided biopsy
  - Consult orthopedic surgeon regarding biopsy site
  - 16-gauge or 14-gauge Tru-cut core biopsy with co-axial system necessary for tissue typing & histological staging
    - Several cores from non-cystic areas of tumor
    - Fine-needle aspiration for cytology (FNAC) is not sufficient for initial diagnosis
    - FNAC useful for detecting residual disease, recurrence or deep-seated retroperitoneal lesions

Radiographic Findings
- Radiography
  - Deep soft tissue mass
  - ± Calcification
    - Synovial sarcoma (30%)
    - Malignant fibrous histiocytoma (10%)
    - Liposarcoma (5%)
  - ± Ossification (liposarcoma)
  - ± Cortical erosion of adjacent bone

MR Findings
- Large, well-defined soft tissue mass
- Malignant fibrous histiocytoma
  - Heterogeneous pattern variably isointense on T1-weighted & hyperintense on T2-weighted images
    - Cystic areas & hemorrhage common
    - ± Fat (T1, T2 hyperintense)
    - ± Calcification (T1, T2 hypointense)
- Liposarcoma
  - Variable amount of fat
    - ± Thick (> 2 mm) hypointense septations
    - ± Cystic (myxoid) component (T2 hyperintense)
    - ± Nodular or globular non-fatty (hypointense) component
- Synovial sarcoma
  - Para-articular mass

- Largely T1-isointense; T2 hyperintense
  - ± Hemorrhage (T1 hyperintense)
  - ± Cystic areas (T2 hyperintense)
  - ± Calcification (T1, T2 hypointense) (30%)
  - ± Bone invasion (20%)

Imaging Recommendations
- Best imaging tool: Ultrasound followed by MR
- Protocol advice
  - Concentrate on defining tumor extent
    - Identify muscle compartment involved
    - Confirm that tumor is well-marginated
  - Assess relation to neurovascular bundle & bone
    - Neurovascular bundle may be either separate from, in contact with or encased (partial or complete) by tumor
  - Evaluate involvement of regional nodes
  - Final diagnosis depends on histological assessment following biopsy

DIFFERENTIAL DIAGNOSIS

Benign Soft Tissue Tumor
- Lipoma, ganglion, nerve sheath tumor & vascular anomalies all have characteristic ultrasound appearances

Muscle Metastasis
- Smaller & less well-defined than STS
- ± More peritumoral edema
- ± Known primary tumor (majority), disseminated disease

Muscle Hematoma
- ± Trauma history
- No intrinsic vascularity
  - Peripheral vascularity (healing stage)
- Acoustic enhancement

SOFT TISSUE SARCOMA

PATHOLOGY

General Features
- General path comments
  - Classified according to tissue type rather than anatomical origin
    - For example; fibrosarcoma may not arise from fibrous tissue but histologically most resembles fibrous tissue
  - Most STS are of high grade histologically
  - Grow centrifugally from single focus
    - Pseudocapsule formed by host reaction & compression of adjacent connective tissues
    - Reactive zone peripheral to pseudocapsule contains tiny extensions (pseudopods) of tumor
    - Pseudopods may detach to give satellite nodules
  - STS respects fascial and anatomical boundaries
    - Usually grow within compartment of origin
    - Do not become extrafascial or invade bone/neurovascular bundle unless very aggressive
- Etiology
  - Idiopathic
  - ± Radiation-induced
- Epidemiology
  - < 1% of adult cancer
  - 6% of childhood cancer
  - Benign: Malignant soft tissue tumor > 100:1

Gross Pathologic & Surgical Features
- Multilobulated, mass ± attached to adjacent structures
- Focal cyst formation, hemorrhage, necrosis
- Pseudocapsule

Microscopic Features
- Malignant fibrous histiocytoma
  - Pleomorphic variety: 60%
    - Fibroblast-like spindle cells & giant cells resembling histiocytes, arranged in pleomorphic-storiform pattern
  - Myxoid variety (30%): Abundant cyst-like gelatinous areas (now termed myxofibrosarcoma)
  - Giant cell variety (5%): Osteoclast-like giant cells ± osteoid (50%)
  - Inflammatory variety (5%): Inflammatory cells, foam cells
- Liposarcoma
  - Well-differentiated variety: 40%
    - Mainly fat with pathognomic lipoblasts that confer malignancy
    - Thick (> 2 mm) septations
    - Nodular areas of non-lipomatous tissue
  - Myxoid variety (40%): Myxoid component > round cell component
  - Round cell variety (10%): Round cell component > myxoid component
  - Pleomorphic variety (5%): Little fat
  - De-differentiated variety (5%): Little fat

Staging, Grading or Classification Criteria
- Histological grading (as high, intermediate or low grade) depends on
  - Degree of cellularity
  - Cellular pleomorphism anaplasia
  - Mitotic activity
  - Degree of necrosis
  - Infiltrative growth
- Surgical staging system
  - Stage Ia: Low grade, intracompartmental
  - Stage Ib: Low grade, extracompartmental
  - Stage IIa: High grade, intracompartmental
  - Stage IIb: High grade, extracompartmental
  - Stage IIIa: Low/high grade, intracompartmental, metastases
  - Stage IIIb: Low/high grade, extracompartmental, metastases

CLINICAL ISSUES

Presentation
- Most common signs/symptoms: Painless soft tissue mass enlarging over several months
- Clinical Profile: Often indistinguishable from benign tumor

Demographics
- Age: 10-90 years, peak: 50 years
- Gender: M:F = 1.1:1
- Ethnicity: More common in Caucasians

Natural History & Prognosis
- Depends of histological grade & surgical resectability
  - 50% of high grade tumor develop metastases despite adequate treatment
    - < 10% of those with metastases survive > 2 years

Treatment
- Most adult STS are chemoresistant (overall < 25% response rate)
- Surgical resection with wide margins
  - Resection margins should ↑ with high grade tumor
  - Aim to excise all peritumoral satellite nodules
  - Satellite nodules present in about 20% STS
  - Microscopic satellite nodules not apparent on pre-operative imaging
- ± Adjuvant radiotherapy to tumor bed
- Local recurrence rate ~ 10% for limb or limb-girdle STS
  - 80% of recurrences occur within two years of surgery

DIAGNOSTIC CHECKLIST

Consider
- Biopsies should be planned with tumor excision in mind

Image Interpretation Pearls
- Any large deep-seated mass without features characteristic of benign tumor
- Nearly all STS are well-defined (i.e. sharp definition does not equate to benign tumor)

SELECTED REFERENCES

1. Moskovic E: Soft tissue sarcomas In: Imaging in Oncology (2nd ed.) London, Taylor and Francis. 537-57, 2004

SOFT TISSUE SARCOMA

IMAGE GALLERY

Typical

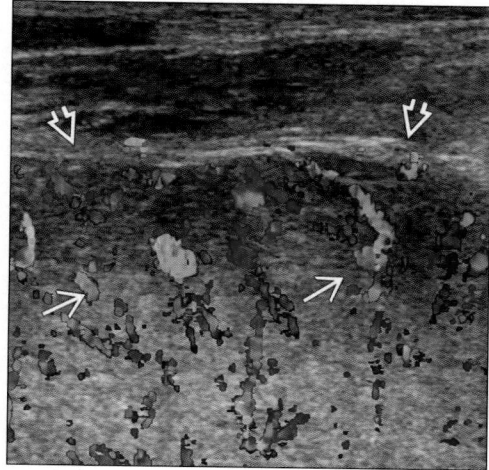
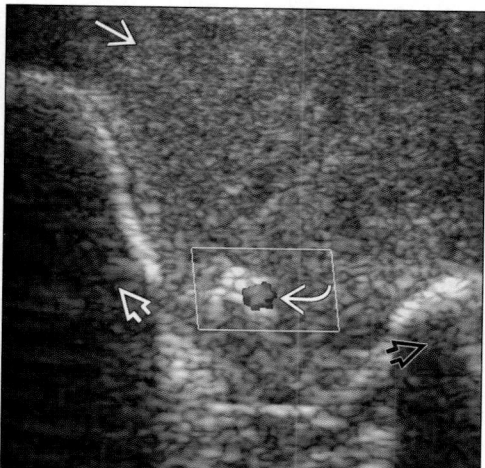

(Left) Transverse color Doppler ultrasound of the forearm shows the hypervascular nature ➡ of STS (myxoid MFH) ➡. The pattern of vascularity is not discriminatory for benign versus malignant soft tissue tumor. *(Right)* Transverse ultrasound shows a soft tissue sarcoma (alveolar rhabdomyosarcoma) ➡ encasing the anterior tibial artery ➡ and bulging between the tibia ➡ and fibula ➡.

Typical

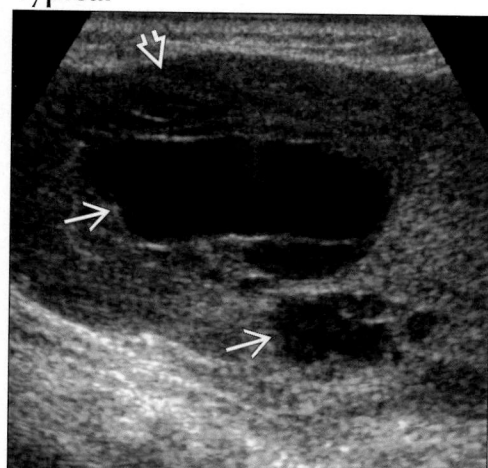
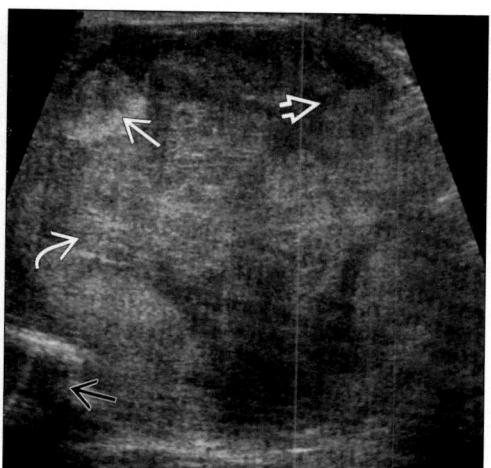

(Left) Longitudinal ultrasound of the arm shows well-defined, anechoic areas representing intratumoral myxoid tissue ➡ within a soft tissue sarcoma (pleomorphic MFH) ➡. *(Right)* Transverse ultrasound of the forearm shows a large heterogeneous STS (pleomorphic MFH) ➡. Fluid-fluid areas ➡ and echogenic areas ➡ are indicative of intratumoral hemorrhage. Radius ➡.

Typical

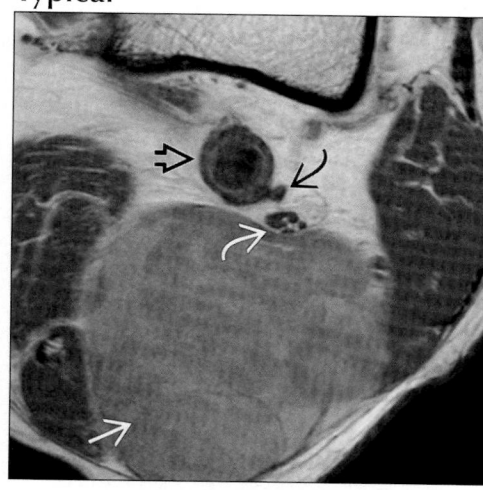
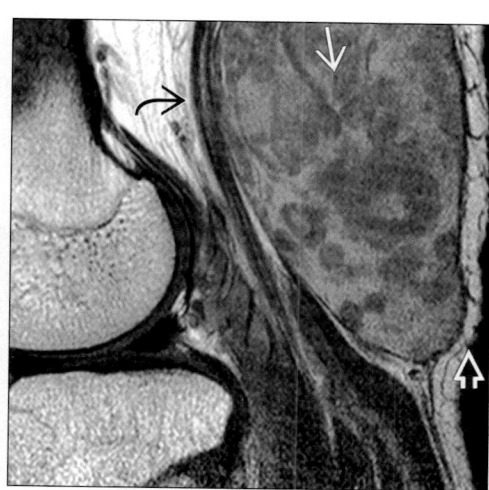

(Left) Axial intermediate-weighted MR image of popliteal fossa shows a well-defined STS (myxoid/round cell liposarcoma) ➡ contacting the tibial nerve ➡ but separate from the popliteal vein ➡ and artery ➡. *(Right)* Corresponding sagittal intermediate-weighted MR image shows a well-defined, oblong-shaped tumor ➡, located between the subcutaneous fat ➡ and the neurovascular bundle ➡.

PERIPHERAL VASCULAR ANOMALY

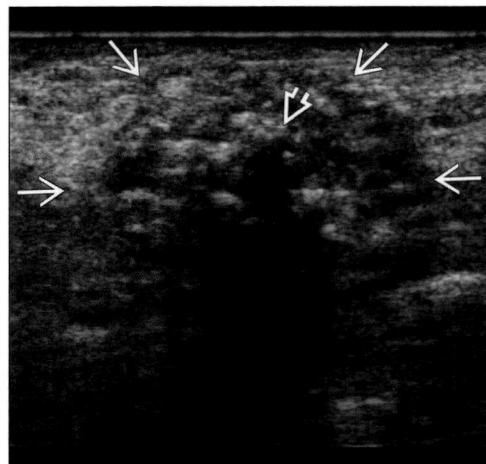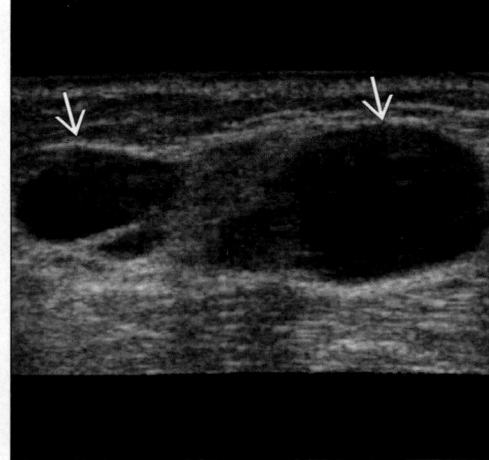

Transverse ultrasound shows a vascular malformation ➡ containing phleboliths ⇨ within the abductor hallucis muscle. Doppler analysis showed predominant venous flow compatible with venous malformation.

Longitudinal ultrasound of the shoulder region shows a well-defined multicystic subcutaneous mass ➡, indicative of lymphatic vascular malformation. Doppler showed minimal peripheral blood flow.

TERMINOLOGY

Abbreviations and Synonyms
- Hemangioma
- Kaposiform hemangioendothelioma
- Vascular malformation comprising venous, capillary, lymphatic, arteriovenous & mixed malformations
- Many other synonyms: Port-wine stain, strawberry angioma, cavernous hemangioma, cystic hygroma

Definitions
- Vascular anomaly: Inclusive term comprising hemangioma, Kaposiform hemangioendothelioma & vascular malformation
- Hemangioma: Childhood
  - Characterized by proliferation → involution
    - "Hemangioma" not applicable to adult vascular lesion
- Kaposiform hemangioendothelioma; early infancy
  - Vascular tumor histologically different from hemangioma (rare)
- Vascular malformation: Childhood & adulthood
  - Neither proliferation nor involution are features
  - Venous malformation: Mainly venous
  - Capillary malformation: Mainly capillary
  - Lymphatic malformation: Mainly lymphatic
  - Arteriovenous malformation or arteriovenous fistula: Mainly arterial (high-flow)
  - Mixed malformation = mixed components = capillary-venous, lymphatic-venous etc.

IMAGING FINDINGS

General Features
- Best diagnostic clue: ↑ Vascular channels ± discrete mass ± phleboliths
- Location
  - Head, including intracranial, & neck (40%)
  - Trunk (20%) & extremities (40%)
  - ± Multifocal, uni- or multi-compartmental
- Size: < 1 cm → > 100 cm
- Morphology: From single vessel ectasia ⇒ discrete well-defined mass ⇒ large ill-defined advancing collection of anomalous vessels

Ultrasonographic Findings
- Hemangiomas
  - Solid intensely hypervascular mass ± lobulated

DDx: Peripheral Vascular Anomaly

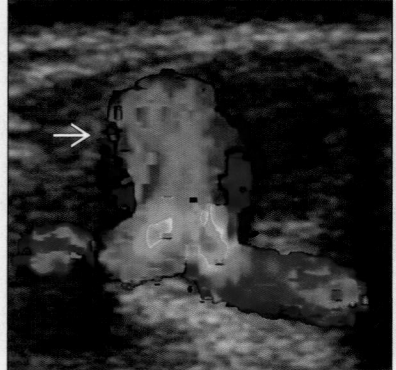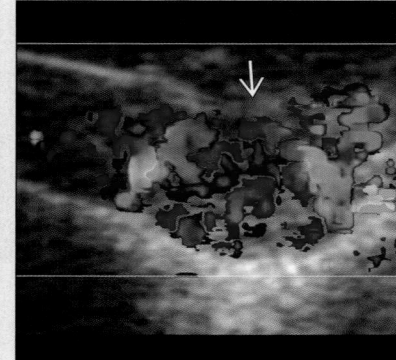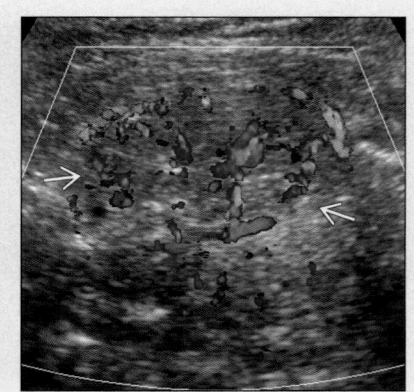

Pseudoaneurysm   *Glomus Tumor*   *Alveolar Soft Part Sarcoma*

PERIPHERAL VASCULAR ANOMALY

Key Facts

Terminology

- Vascular anomaly: Inclusive term comprising hemangioma, Kaposiform hemangioendothelioma & vascular malformation
- Hemangioma: Childhood
- Kaposiform hemangioendothelioma; early infancy
- Vascular malformation: Childhood & adulthood
- Venous malformation: Mainly venous
- Capillary malformation: Mainly capillary
- Lymphatic malformation: Mainly lymphatic
- Arteriovenous malformation or arteriovenous fistula: Mainly arterial (high-flow)
- Mixed malformation = mixed components = capillary-venous, lymphatic-venous etc.

Imaging Findings

- Best diagnostic clue: ↑ Vascular channels ± discrete mass ± phleboliths
- Use ultrasound to make diagnosis & assess flow
- Use MR to define extent

Top Differential Diagnoses

- Pseudoaneurysm
- Glomus Tumor
- Alveolar Soft Part Sarcoma (ASPS)

Diagnostic Checklist

- Classification not always clear-cut despite imaging, clinical & even histological evaluation
- Age of onset, behavior, site, size, margination, vascular vs. stroma component, & high- vs. low-flow = important parameters to note

---

- ○ ± Peripheral draining veins ± feeding arteries
- Venous malformation
  - ○ Slow-flow channels ± venous lakes ± cavernous veins
    - Slow or no flow on color Doppler examination
    - Moving echoes on real time imaging
    - ± Thrombosed vessels
    - ± Venous lakes = large, irregular spaces not conforming to vascular channel
    - ± Cavernous veins = more tubular
  - ○ ± Phleboliths (very common); acoustic shadowing
  - ○ Supporting stroma
- Capillary malformation
  - ○ Thickening and increased echogenicity of dermis
    - Ultrasound excludes underlying vascular anomaly
- Lymphatic malformation
  - ○ Microcystic: Multiple tiny cysts within matrix
    - Cysts may be too small to resolve with ultrasound ⇒ appears as solid lesion
    - Largely avascular
  - ○ Macrocystic; i.e., cystic hygroma: Thin-walled, septated, fluid-filled cystic spaces
    - ± Internal echoes (hemorrhage or infection)
    - Largely avascular
- Arteriovenous malformation
  - ○ High velocity flow and pulsatile ± mass
  - ○ Phleboliths uncommon

Radiographic Findings

- Radiography
  - ○ Nonspecific soft tissue mass ± phleboliths
  - ○ ± Mature periosteal new bone formation

MR Findings

- T2WI FS
  - ○ Extent of involvement well demonstrated
    - Skin, subcutaneous fat, muscle, neurovascular bundle, bone, synovium
    - Focal, multifocal or diffuse
    - Extent may be underestimated as vascular channels not distended or thrombosed
  - ○ Low-flow: No signal voids nor large feeding arteries
  - ○ High-flow: Signal voids ± large feeding arteries
  - ○ Connection with normal vasculature

- ± Dominant feeding artery or draining vein
- MRA
  - ○ Better at revealing nidus than ultrasound or MR
    - Nidus = feature of arteriovenous malformation = point or points of arteriovenous communication
    - Not a feature of other vascular anomalies

Angiographic Findings

- Prelude to sclerotherapy or embolization
  - ○ Best investigation at demonstrating nidus

Imaging Recommendations

- Best imaging tool
  - ○ Use ultrasound to make diagnosis & assess flow
  - ○ Use MR to define extent
- Protocol advice
  - ○ ↓ Transducer pressure to avoid compression
  - ○ Note following features
  - ○ Location, size, extent and margin
    - Size: ± Panoramic imaging
    - Extent: ± Skin ± subcutaneous fat ± muscle
  - ○ Vascular channel type
    - Small, medium or large channels ± venous lakes ± cavernous veins
  - ○ Flow: Spectral analysis
    - Categorized as slow- or high-flow depending on predominant flow pattern
    - High-flow = arterial; low-flow or no flow = venous
    - One artery does not imply high-flow lesion
    - Moving grayscale echoes in very slow-flowing lesion
  - ○ Amount of stroma vs. vascular component
    - Example: 10% stroma: 90% vascular component or 40% stroma: 60% vascular
    - More difficult when lesion ill-defined
  - ○ Phleboliths

DIFFERENTIAL DIAGNOSIS

Pseudoaneurysm

- Arterial "to and fro" pattern
- Surrounding hematoma

PERIPHERAL VASCULAR ANOMALY

Glomus Tumor
- Usually subungual
- Other location in hand and wrist

Alveolar Soft Part Sarcoma (ASPS)
- 2nd or 3rd decade, lower limbs
- ± Intramuscular mass with intra- ± extra-tumoral hypervascularity
- Metastases (nodal, lung) in 20% at presentation

PATHOLOGY

General Features
- General path comments
  - Hemangioma: Derangement in angiogenesis
    - Endothelial proliferation followed by involution
  - Vascular malformation: Error of vascular morphogenesis
    - No endothelial proliferation nor involution
- Epidemiology
  - Prevalence: 1.5% general population
  - Hemangioma: Most common tumor of childhood
  - Vascular malformation: Venous (40%), capillary (5%), lymphatic (35%), arteriovenous (10%) and mixed (10%)
- Associated abnormalities
  - Maffucci syndrome
    - Enchondromas + soft tissue venous malformations
  - Osler-Weber-Rendu syndrome
    - Arteriovenous malformations in skin, mucosa, lung and brain
  - Klippel-Trenaunay-Weber syndrome
    - Low-flow vascular malformations ± large aberrant lateral vein ± limb hypertrophy
  - Gorham-Scott syndrome
    - Intraosseous venous and lymphatic malformations

Gross Pathologic & Surgical Features
- Hemangioma: More lobulated, mass-like
- Vascular malformation: More ill-defined

Microscopic Features
- Hemangioma: Plump endothelial cells, especially during proliferative phase
  - Extracellular matrix contains growth promoting proteins
- Vascular malformation: Flat endothelial cells
  - Patchy deficiency of smooth muscle in wall → dilatation
  - Extracellular matrix does not contain growth promoting proteins
  - Arteries and arterioles (with elastic lamina in walls) integral part of arteriovenous malformations
- Even histologically, distinction between vascular anomalies can be difficult

CLINICAL ISSUES

Presentation
- Most common signs/symptoms: Pain, swelling
- Other signs/symptoms

- Bluish discoloration, mass ± engorges with gravity
- Pain after exercise, edema, hemorrhage, local hypertrophy, ulceration, contractures

Demographics
- Age
  - Vascular anomalies are present at birth ⇒ become clinically apparent at varying times
    - Hemangioma: First month of life
    - Capillary, lymphatic malformation: First two years of life
    - Venous malformation: Birth ⇒ early adulthood
    - Arteriovenous malformation: Early teens

Natural History & Prognosis
- Hemangioma
  - Proliferation (months) → stabilization (years) → spontaneous involution
  - ± Biphasic proliferative phase
    - Involute at rate of 10% per year
  - Residual cometic deformity in ~ 50%
    - Comprising atrophied or excessive fibrofatty tissue
    - Later involution has greater cosmetic deformity
- Vascular malformation
  - Grow slowly proportional to patient growth
    - ± More rapid growth precipitated by puberty, pregnancy, infection, trauma or unknown factor
    - Arteriovenous malformation very unpredictable
    - Limb and life-threatening
  - Lymphatic malformation may spontaneously regress

Treatment
- Hemangioma: Wait & see, steroids, laser or surgery
- Vascular malformation
  - Sclerotherapy
    - Angiography → fluoroscopic guidance → percutaneous sclerosing agent (alcohol) → nidus
    - Contraindicated if high flow (risk of shunting to systemic circulation)
  - Coil embolotherapy
- Wide surgical excision
  - ± Pre-operative or post-operative emblo/sclerotherapy
  - High morbidity & recurrence rates

DIAGNOSTIC CHECKLIST

Consider
- Treatment based on clinical & imaging features
  - Classification not always clear-cut despite imaging, clinical & even histological evaluation
    - Still try to make best-guess prediction

Image Interpretation Pearls
- Age of onset, behavior, site, size, margination, vascular vs. stroma component, & high- vs. low-flow = important parameters to note

SELECTED REFERENCES
1. Fayad L et al: Vascular malformations in the extremities: emphasis on MR imaging features that guide treatment options. Skeletal Radiol. 35(3):127-37, 2006

IMAGE GALLERY

Typical

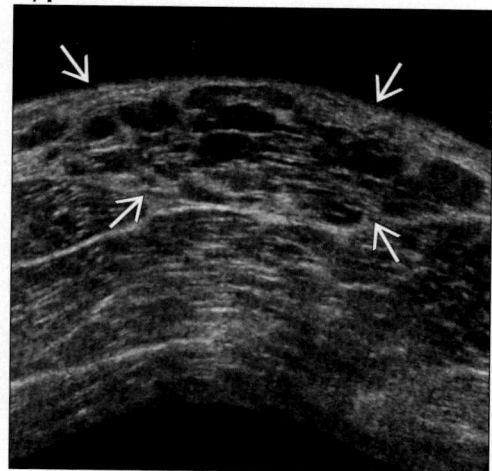 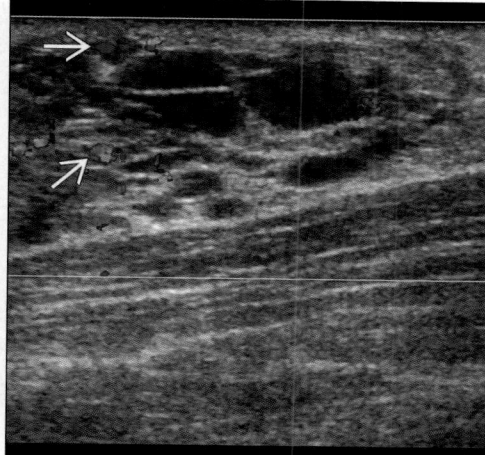

(Left) Transverse ultrasound of the thigh with extended field-of-view shows a well-defined subcutaneous mass ➡ with cystic spaces and no phleboliths. *(Right)* Corresponding transverse color Doppler ultrasound shows small vessels ➡ between cystic spaces. Spectral analysis showed predominantly venous flow. Overall appearance indicative of mixed lympho-venous malformation.

Typical

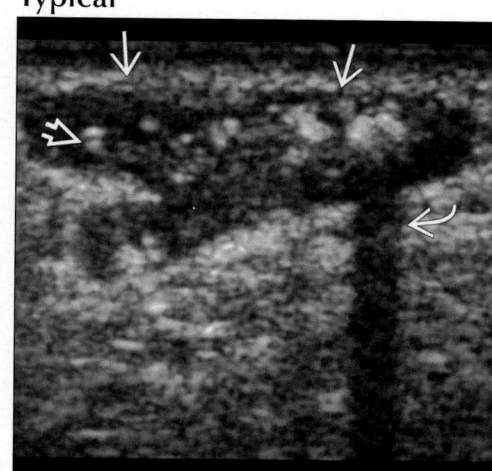 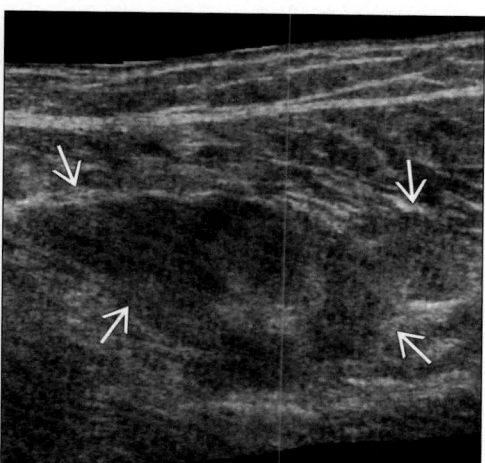

(Left) Transverse ultrasound shows a well-defined, subcutaneous, venous malformation ➡ of the heel, with phleboliths as indicated by echogenic foci with acoustic shadowing ➡ and comet-tail artifacts ➡ respectively. *(Right)* Longitudinal ultrasound with extended field-of-view shows a large venous lake ➡ as part of a venous malformation within the gastrocnemius muscle. Echogenic contents represent slow-flowing blood.

Typical

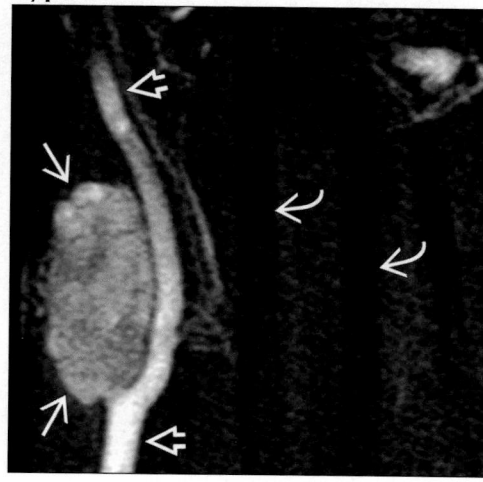 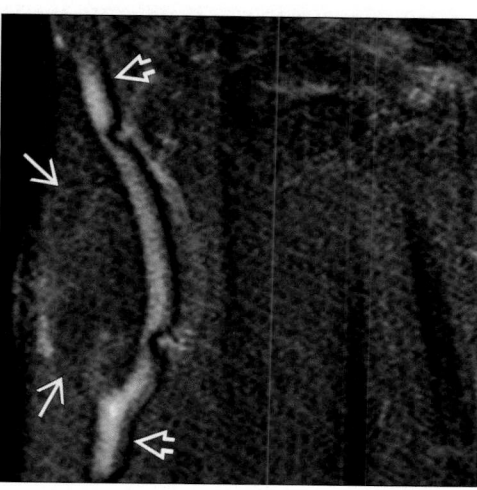

(Left) Coronal T2WI MR with fat-suppression shows a well-defined venous malformation ➡ by the radial artery ➡. Note lack of flow voids. Flexor tendons ➡. *(Right)* Coronal T1 post-gadolinium MR with fat-suppression shows nonenhancement of the venous malformation ➡ indicating very slow-flow. Radial artery ➡.

(Left) Axial T2WI MR with fat-suppression shows a large intramuscular and subcutaneous venous malformation ➡ of the proximal arm extending through the quadrigeminal space ➡. Signal voids = phleboliths ➡. Humerus ➡. *(Right)* Axial T1 post-gadolinium MR with fat-suppression shows that only the central aspects of the malformation enhance ➡, indicative of brisk blood flow centrally.

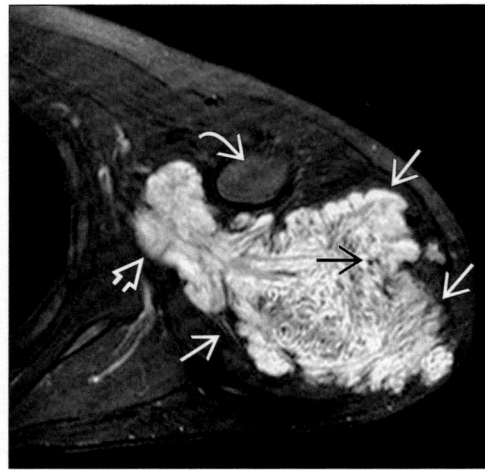

(Left) Axial T2WI MR with fat-suppression shows a deep, irregular, venous malformation of the hand with some venous lakes ➡ and fluid-fluid levels ➡ due to stagnant blood. Signal voids ➡ = extensor tendons. *(Right)* Transverse ultrasound in a six year old, shows a well-defined, subcutaneous, solid mass ➡ of the shoulder. The mass was present from birth and static for several years, suggestive of hemangioma. No phleboliths. Muscle ➡.

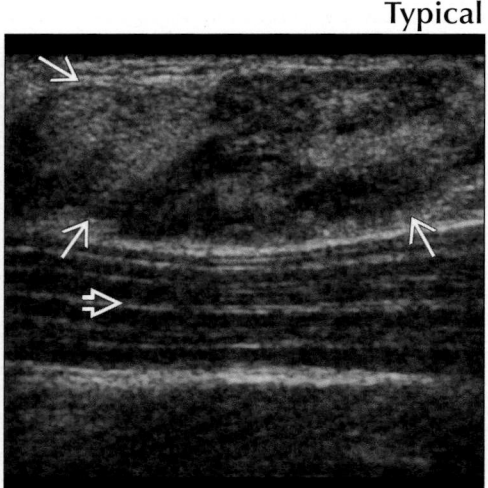

(Left) Transverse ultrasound of the same lesion as previous image, shows many vascular channels ➡ within the mass. *(Right)* Corresponding transverse pulsed Doppler ultrasound of a vascular channel shows high velocity arterial flow indicative of a high-flow hemangioma.

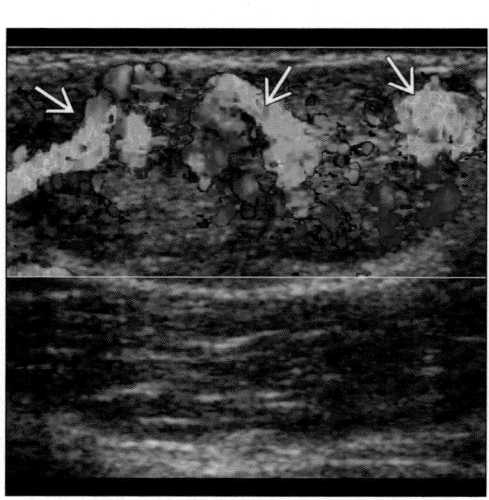
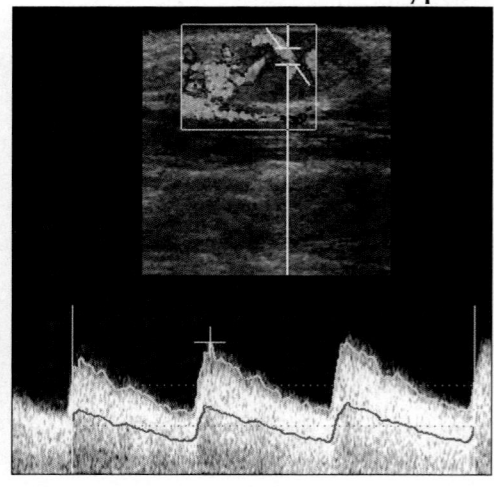

PERIPHERAL VASCULAR ANOMALY

Typical

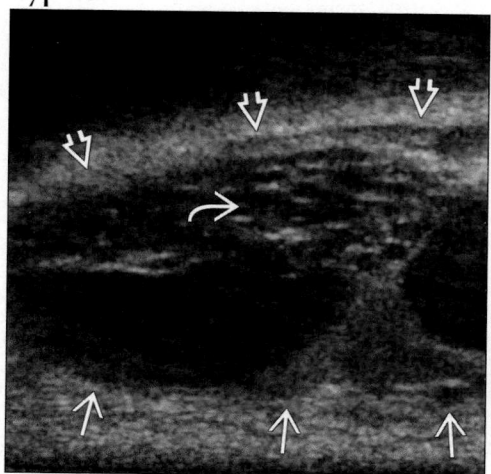
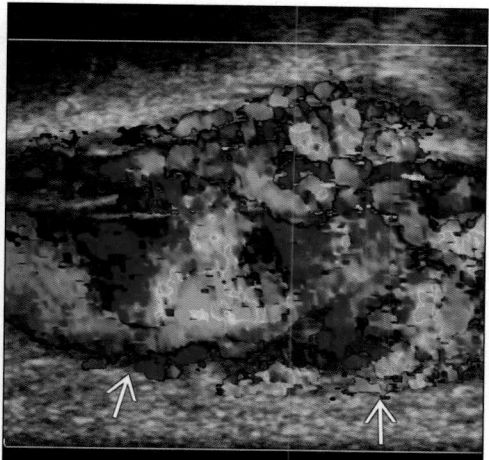

(Left) Longitudinal ultrasound of forefoot shows a vascular malformation with large ➡ and small ➡ vascular spaces adjacent to the metatarsal shaft ➡. *(Right)* Corresponding longitudinal color Doppler ultrasound shows color Doppler signal throughout the mass ➡. Spectral analysis showed predominant arterial flow indicative of a high-flow arteriovenous malformation.

Typical

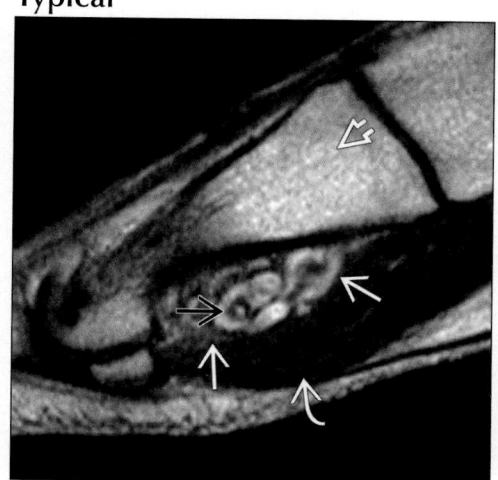
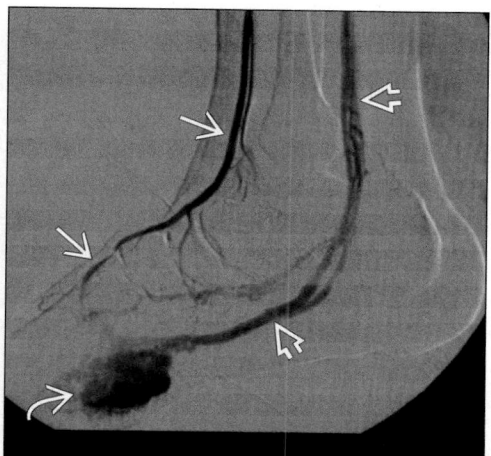

(Left) Sagittal T2WI MR of same lesion as previous image, shows the arteriovenous malformation ➡ adjacent to the metatarsal shaft ➡. Note flow-voids ➡ within the lesion. Flexor hallucis brevis muscle ➡. *(Right)* Corresponding angiogram shows feeding dorsalis pedis artery ➡, arteriovenous malformation ➡ and draining posterior tibialis vein ➡.

Variant

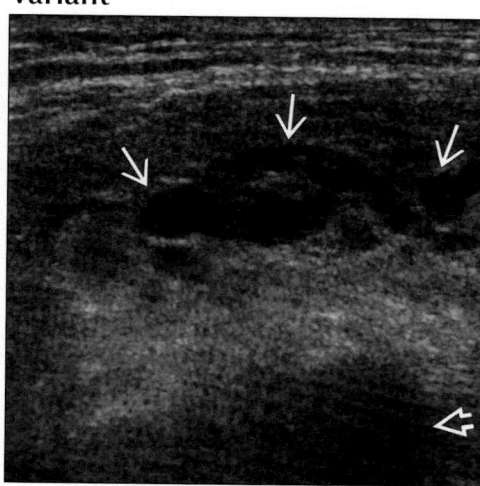
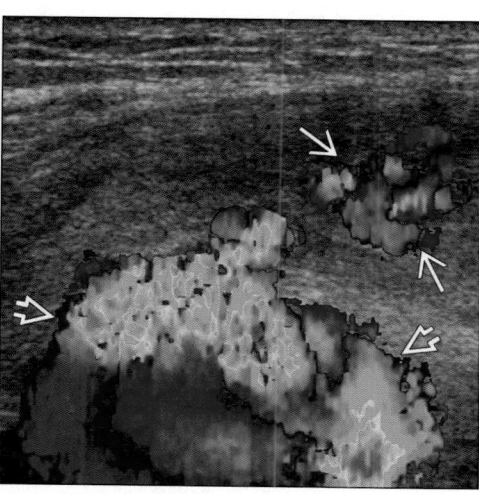

(Left) Transverse ultrasound of an adult with spontaneous thigh swelling shows an irregular intramuscular collection of vessels ➡ superficial to the hypoechoic mass ➡. *(Right)* Corresponding transverse color Doppler ultrasound shows both an arteriovenous malformation ➡ and a large pseudoaneurysm ➡. Surgery revealed arteriovenous malformation complicated by spontaneous bleeding and pseudoaneurysm.

FOREIGN BODY AND INJECTION GRANULOMAS

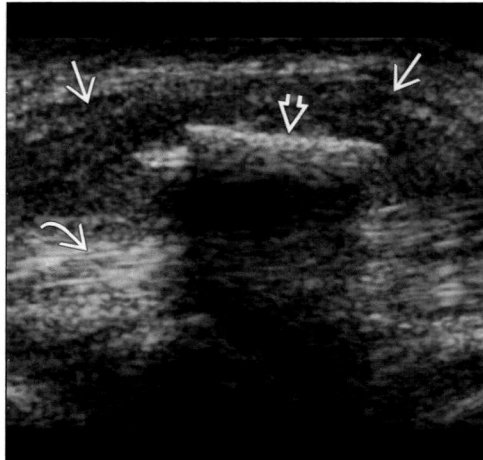

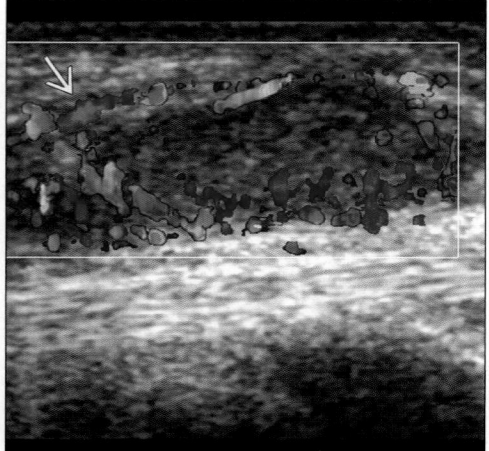

Longitudinal ultrasound of the palm shows a wood fragment ➡ in subcutaneous tissue, superficial to the flexor tendons ➡. Note the thick rim of the granulation tissue ➡. Entry site was proximal to the wrist crease.

Longitudinal color Doppler ultrasound just medial to the previous image, shows typical peripheral hyperemia ➡ of the granulation tissue surrounding the wood fragment.

TERMINOLOGY

Abbreviations and Synonyms
- Foreign body granuloma (FBG), injection granuloma (IG), pseudotumor

Definitions
- Foreign body granuloma = localized tissue reaction to foreign body within tissues
- Injection granuloma = localized tissue reaction to material injected into tissues

IMAGING FINDINGS

General Features
- Best diagnostic clue
  - Foreign body granuloma: Echogenic material with posterior artifact ± hyperemic hypoechoic rim
  - Injection granuloma: Localized swelling subcutaneous tissues → ill-defined mass with peripheral hyperemia → well-defined mass ± calcification
- Location
  - Foreign body granuloma: Subcutaneous tissue hand, wrists, feet
  - Injection granulomas: Subcutaneous tissue gluteal region, proximal arm
- Size
  - Foreign body granuloma: Usually small (1-3 cm) though can be large (10 cm plus)
    - Dependent on size of foreign body
  - Injection granuloma: Usually small (2-5 cm)
    - Dependent on amount & dispersion of injection
- Morphology
  - Foreign body granuloma: Depends on size & shape of foreign body & inflammatory response
  - Injection granuloma: Firm → hard subcutaneous nodule

Ultrasonographic Findings
- **Foreign body granuloma (FBG)**
  - Echogenic object with posterior artifact (reverberation/comet-tail artifact or posterior shadowing)
  - Echogenicity dependent on acoustic impedance between retained foreign body & surrounding tissue

DDx: Foreign Body & Injection Granulomas

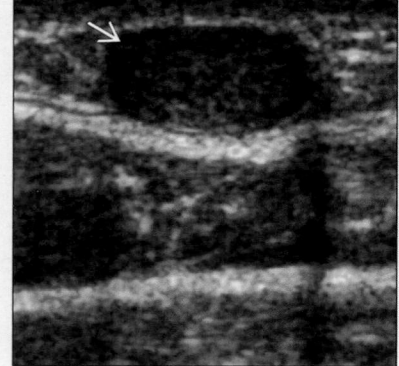

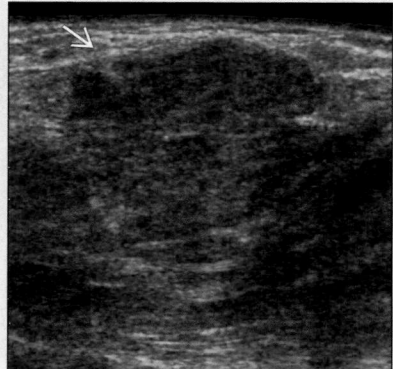

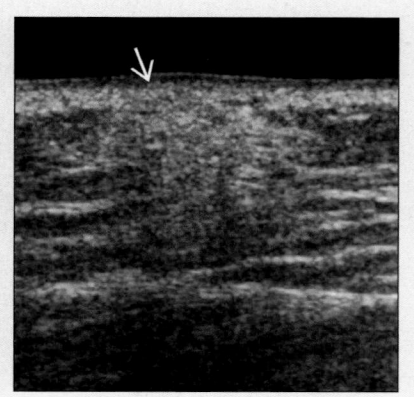

Subcutaneous Fibroma

Subcutaneous Metastasis

Subcutaneous Fat Necrosis

FOREIGN BODY AND INJECTION GRANULOMAS

Key Facts

Terminology
- Foreign body granuloma = localized tissue reaction to foreign body within tissues
- Injection granuloma = localized tissue reaction to material injected into tissues

Imaging Findings
- **Foreign body granuloma (FBG)**
- Reflectivity for some objects (wood, metal, glass, plastic) > others (bamboo)
- ± Hypoechoic rim of inflammatory tissue, granulation tissue or fibrosis
- False positive ultrasound with gas in soft tissues or fresh hematoma, calcification
- ± Sinus tract to foreign body
- **Injection granuloma (IG)**
- Focal swelling, disruption of subcutaneous fat

- Swelling may progress to ill-defined/well-defined hypoechoic mass
- Deep margin of mass often cannot be seen
- Ultrasound: Modality of choice to detect radiolucent foreign bodies & diagnose injection granulomas
- Foreign body may be located some distance from entry wound
- Assess presence, thickness (& vascularity) of hypoechoic rim (influences retrieval method)
- Look for associated complications (soft tissue infection, neurovascular or tendon injury)

Diagnostic Checklist
- In the right clinical context, ultrasound appearances of injection granulomas are specific enough not to warrant further investigation

---

- ■ Reflectivity for some objects (wood, metal, glass, plastic) > others (bamboo)
- ■ Posterior artifact dependent on smooth versus rough surface of foreign body & alignment to ultrasound beam
- ○ ± Hypoechoic rim of inflammatory tissue, granulation tissue or fibrosis
  - ■ Dependent on intensity of inflammatory response & duration of retention
  - ■ May be apparent within 24 hours of retention (inflammatory response)
  - ■ Improves sensitivity & specificity of ultrasound detection
  - ■ Variable hyperemia of hypoechoic rim
- ○ False positive ultrasound with gas in soft tissues or fresh hematoma, calcification
  - ■ Calcification is radiopaque
- ○ ± Sinus tract to foreign body
  - ■ Along tract of penetrating wound
  - ■ Developing de novo from retained foreign body
- Injection granuloma (IG)
  - ○ Focal swelling, disruption of subcutaneous fat
    - ■ Similar to early stages of fat necrosis
    - ■ ± Small areas of liquefaction
    - ■ ± Mild peripheral hyperemia
  - ○ Swelling may progress to ill-defined/well-defined hypoechoic mass
    - ■ ± Mild peripheral hyperemia
    - ■ ± Dense calcification
    - ■ Deep margin of mass often cannot be seen

Radiographic Findings
- Foreign body granuloma: Detects radiopaque foreign bodies
  - ○ ≤ 15% wood foreign bodies radiopaque
  - ○ Limited information on exact location of foreign body & associated soft tissue response or injury
- Injection granuloma: ± Calcified subcutaneous mass

CT Findings
- NECT
  - ○ Foreign body granuloma

- ■ Typically seen as hyperdense object within subcutaneous mass with variable surrounding inflammation or fibrosis
- ■ Wood may appear hypoechoic & simulate air
- ○ Injection granuloma: Well-defined subcutaneous mass
  - ■ ± Calcification (often dense), lobulated or rim

MR Findings
- Less accurate than US at detecting foreign body
  - ○ Good visualization of inflammatory reaction

Nuclear Medicine Findings
- Injection granuloma may accumulate tracer on FDG PET imaging
  - ○ False positive for subcutaneous metastases

Imaging Recommendations
- Best imaging tool
  - ○ Ultrasound: Modality of choice to detect radiolucent foreign bodies & diagnose injection granulomas
    - ■ Sensitivity, specificity > 90% for foreign body detection
- Protocol advice
  - ○ Foreign body
    - ■ Examine beyond entry wound
    - ■ Foreign body may be located some distance from entry wound
    - ■ For example, hand entry wound may give rise to foreign body distal forearm
    - ■ Note size, shape, location & orientation of foreign body
    - ■ Relate size, shape to likely foreign body
    - ■ Assess presence, thickness (& vascularity) of hypoechoic rim (influences retrieval method)
    - ■ Look for associated complications (soft tissue infection, neurovascular or tendon injury)
    - ■ ± Ultrasound-guided retrieval or localization
    - ■ Repeat ultrasound in 2-10 days if clinical history suspicious & ultrasound findings negative or equivocal
  - ○ Injection granuloma
    - ■ Assess location, size & margination of granuloma

FOREIGN BODY AND INJECTION GRANULOMAS

- Assess vascularity
- Determine presence of calcification
- Fine needle aspiration for cytology, biopsy or additional imaging not necessary

DIFFERENTIAL DIAGNOSIS

Subcutaneous Fibroma
- Hypoechoic well-defined subcutaneous nodule
  - No linear echogenic material within mass
- No history of penetrating trauma or injection

Subcutaneous Metastasis
- Hypoechoic well-defined vascular nodule
  - No linear echogenic material within mass
- No history of penetrating trauma or injection
- Usually known disseminated malignancy

Subcutaneous Fat Necrosis
- Localized swelling, ↑ echogenicity & disruption of subcutaneous fat
  - No linear echogenic material within mass
- ± Recollection of prior blunt trauma

PATHOLOGY

General Features
- Etiology
  - Foreign body granuloma
    - Penetrating foreign body (wood, glass, metal sliver, bamboo etc.)
    - Retained foreign body (gauze, cotton swab etc.)
  - Injection granuloma
    - Injection of drug into subcutaneous fat
    - Many "intramuscular" injections → subcutaneous tissue
    - Granulomas much less frequent with intramuscular injection
    - Tissue reaction dependent on site, composition & amount of injected drug

Gross Pathologic & Surgical Features
- Foreign body granuloma: Foreign body with variable rim of inflammatory or fibrous tissue
- Injection granuloma: Tissue necrosis with mass comprised of inflammatory or fibrous tissue

Microscopic Features
- Injection granuloma
  - Necrosis of fat cells
  - Dense fibrous tissue reaction with inflammation
  - ± Foreign-body giant cells
    - Inflammation may persist > one year after injection

CLINICAL ISSUES

Presentation
- Most common signs/symptoms
  - Foreign body granuloma
    - History of penetrating injury

  - Palpable mass, initially tender becoming less tender over ensuring weeks
  - Injection granuloma
    - History of injection
    - Tender area → palpable mass
- Other signs/symptoms
  - Original trauma or injection may be forgotten
    - May present as unexplained mass

Demographics
- Age
  - Foreign body granuloma > young or middle-aged
  - Injection granuloma > elderly
- Gender: M = F

Natural History & Prognosis
- Foreign body granuloma
  - Inert tissue → persists as non-tender mass
  - Reactive tissue → persistent tender mass
    - Continuing inflammation → ± sinus tract develops to skin
  - Injection granuloma
    - Mass becomes less tender, smaller & harder
    - Usually persists as small hard nodule

Treatment
- Foreign body granuloma
  - Percutaneous removal with forceps through puncture wound or small incision
  - Cutaneous or needle location → surgical excision
- Injection granuloma
  - Treatment rarely necessary

DIAGNOSTIC CHECKLIST

Consider
- Routine use of ultrasound has dramatically ↑ detection rate of soft tissue foreign bodies & ↓ number of unnecessary operations
- In the right clinical context, ultrasound appearances of injection granulomas are specific enough not to warrant further investigation

Image Interpretation Pearls
- Foreign body granuloma: Echogenic material with posterior artifact ± rim of hyperemic hypoechoic tissue near site of penetrating trauma
- Injection granuloma = localized fat necrosis or fibrotic-type mass ± calcification at infection site.

SELECTED REFERENCES

1. Prosch H et al: Case report: Gluteal injection site granulomas: false positive finding on FDG-PET in patients with non-small cell lung cancer. Br J Radiol. 78(932):758-61, 2005
2. Boyse TD et al: US of soft-tissue foreign bodies and associated complications with surgical correlation. Radiographics. 21(5):1251-6, 2001

FOREIGN BODY AND INJECTION GRANULOMAS

IMAGE GALLERY

Typical

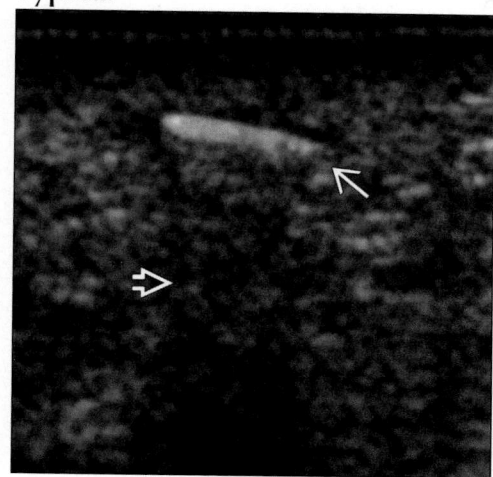 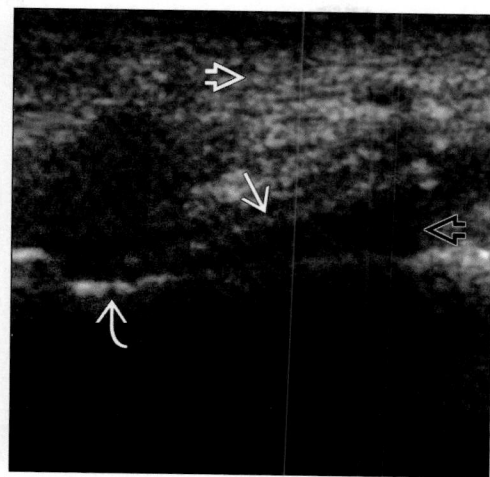

(Left) Longitudinal ultrasound shows a small glass fragment ➡ in the subcutaneous tissue. Note minimal surrounding hypoechogenicity and mild posterior shadowing ➡.
(Right) Longitudinal ultrasound shows a bamboo splinter ➡, volar aspect metacarpal bone ➡. Note how the fragment is isoechoic to the subcutaneous fat ➡ but is accentuated by a thin hypoechoic rim and posterior shadowing ➡.

Typical

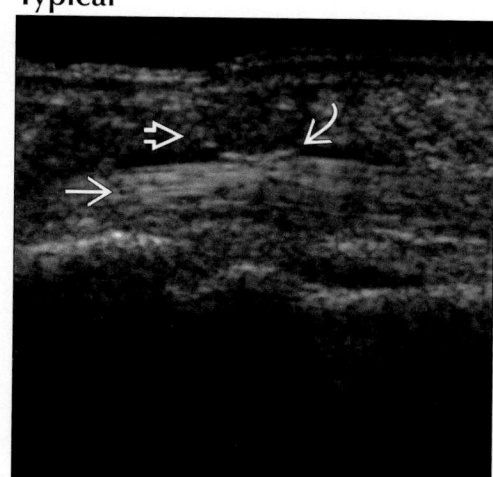 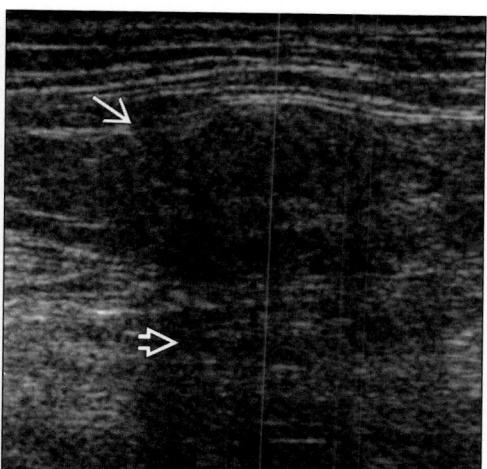

(Left) Longitudinal ultrasound in a patient with a glass bulb laceration, shows curved echogenic foci ➡ due to gas alongside tendon ➡ and in puncture wound ➡. A repeat ultrasound the next day confirmed no foreign body. *(Right)* Transverse ultrasound of the gluteal region shows an ill-defined hypoechoic area ➡ representing fat necrosis and inflammation at the site of a previous injection. Mild posterior shadowing ➡ is present.

Typical

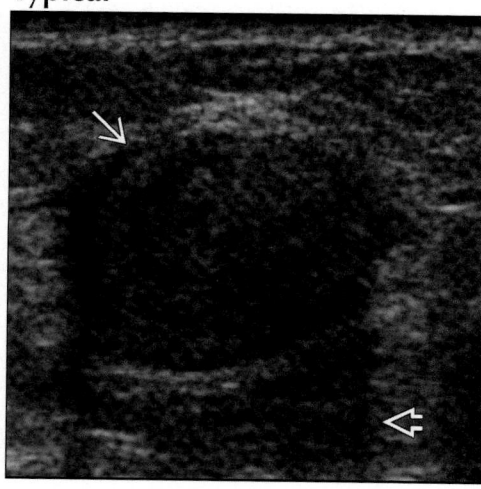 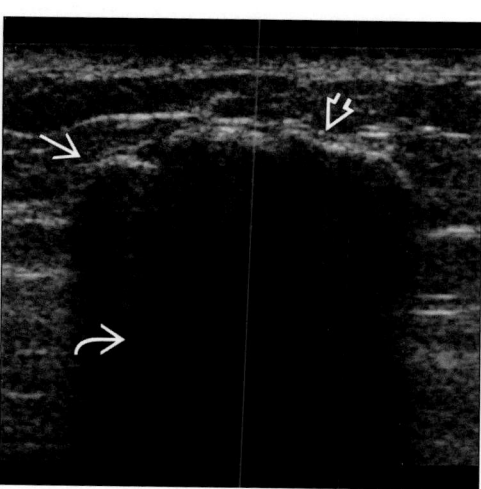

(Left) Longitudinal ultrasound of a gluteal injection granuloma shows a well-defined hypoechoic mass ➡ in the subcutaneous tissue. No calcification is visible although there is moderate posterior shadowing ➡. *(Right)* Transverse ultrasound of a gluteal injection granuloma shows a well-defined, hypoechoic, subcutaneous mass ➡. Calcification is present ➡ with intense posterior shadowing ➡, obscuring the posterior margin of the mass.

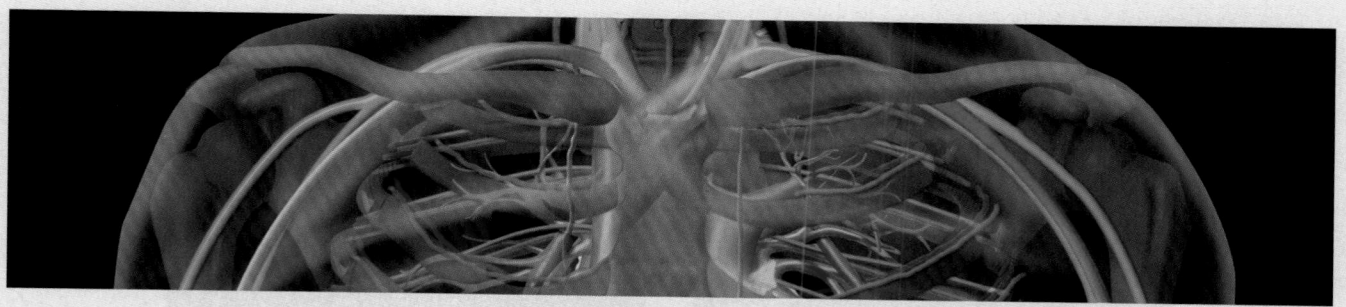

SECTION 14: Vascular

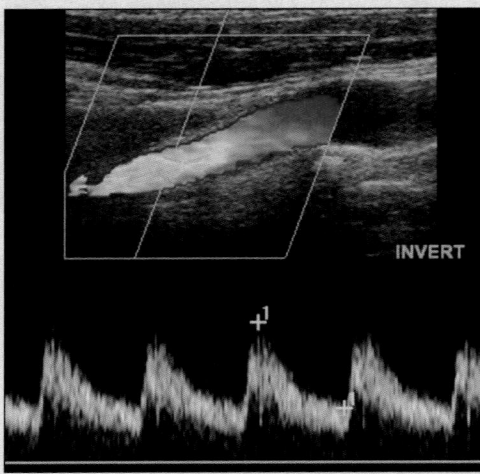

Longitudinal color Doppler ultrasound of an internal carotid artery (ICA) shows a low pulsatility Doppler arterial waveform.

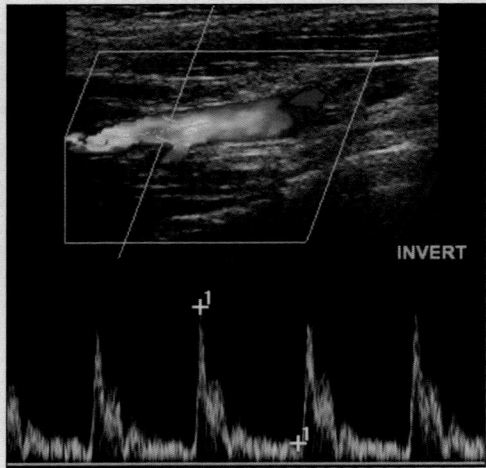

Longitudinal color Doppler ultrasound of an external carotid artery (ECA) shows a moderate pulsatility arterial waveform.

IMAGING ANATOMY

General Anatomic Considerations

- "Proximal" and "distal" in arterial and venous systems apply to position of arterial or venous segment in relation to heart (rather than direction of flow)

Critical Anatomic Structures

- Main arteries of the neck
  - Aortic arch → brachiocephalic trunk then right common carotid artery or left common carotid artery → internal carotid artery and external carotid artery
  - Aortic arch → brachiocephalic trunk right subclavian artery or left subclavian artery → vertebral artery
- Main arteries of the upper limbs
  - Aortic arch → brachiocephalic trunk then right subclavian artery or left subclavian artery → axillary artery → brachial artery → radial artery and ulnar artery → common interosseous artery (continuation of ulnar artery) → anterior and posterior interosseous arteries
- Main arteries of the lower limbs
  - Abdominal aorta → common iliac artery → internal and external iliac arteries → common femoral artery (continuation of EIA) → superficial femoral artery (SFA) and profunda femoris artery → popliteal artery (continuation of SFA) → anterior tibial artery (ATA) and tibioperoneal (TP) trunk → posterior tibial artery and peroneal artery (continuation of TP trunk) and dorsalis pedis artery (continuation of ATA)
- Main visceral arteries of the abdominal aorta
  - Celiac artery, superior mesenteric artery, inferior mesenteric artery, renal arteries
- Main veins of the neck
  - Internal jugular vein → brachiocephalic vein → superior vena cava (SVC)
  - External jugular vein → subclavian vein → brachiocephalic vein → SVC
  - Anterior jugular vein → external jugular vein → subclavian vein → brachiocephalic vein → SVC

- Vertebral vein → brachiocephalic vein → SVC
- Main superficial veins of the upper limbs
  - Cephalic vein (radial side) → gives median cubital vein to join basilic vein while continuing to ascend up lateral aspect of arm → axillary vein (usually paired)
  - Basilic vein → brachial vein → axillary vein
- Main deep veins of upper limbs
  - Brachial vein → axillary vein → subclavian vein → brachiocephalic vein → SVC
- Main superficial veins of lower limbs
  - Long saphenous vein (LSV) (ascends medially starting on dorsum of foot passing anterior to medial malleolus) → common femoral vein
  - Short saphenous vein (SSV) (ascends laterally starting on dorsum of foot passing posterior to lateral malleolus) → popliteal vein
- Main deep veins of lower limbs
  - Below knee calf veins: Anterior tibial veins, posterior tibial veins, peroneal veins (often paired), gastrocnemius vein, soleal vein → popliteal vein
  - Above knee veins: Popliteal vein (Pop V) → superficial femoral vein (continuation of Pop V and deep femoral vein → common femoral vein (CFV) → external iliac vein (continuation of CFV) and internal iliac vein → common iliac vein → inferior vena cava (IVC)
- Main perforator veins of lower limbs
  - Perforator veins connect superficial veins to deep veins of lower limbs
  - Thigh perforators connecting to LSV: Hunterian perforators (proximal thigh); Dodd perforator(s) (distal thigh)
  - Calf perforators connecting to the LSV: Typically located at 6, 12, 18, 24, 28 and 32 cm from heel
  - Cockett perforators (distal medial calf); Boyd perforators (proximal medial calf)
  - Calf perforators connecting SSV to gastrocnemius vein: 2 proximal lateral calf perforators

VASCULAR IMAGING & DOPPLER

Key Facts

General Anatomic Considerations
- "Proximal" and "distal" in the arterial and venous systems apply to the position of the arterial or vein segment in relation to the heart

Doppler Spectral Analysis
- Low pulsatility Doppler arterial waveforms
  - Have broad systolic peaks and forward flow throughout diastole
  - This waveform is seen in low resistance circulatory systems such as carotid, vertebral, renal and celiac axis
- Moderate pulsatility Doppler arterial waveforms
  - Systolic peak is tall and sharp but forward flow is present throughout diastole (may be interrupted by early diastole flow reversal)

- This waveform is seen in moderate resistance circulatory systems such as external carotid artery and superior mesenteric artery (during fasting)
- High pulsatility Doppler waveforms arterial waveforms
  - Systolic peak is tall, arrow and sharp with reversed or absent diastolic flow
  - This waveform is seen in high resistance circulatory systems such as extremity arteries in a resting individual
- Normal venous waveforms
  - Spontaneous and phasic with respiration
  - More proximal IVC and hepatic veins show pulsatile flow pattern due to right atrial pressure changes during cardiac cycle

ANATOMY-BASED IMAGING ISSUES

Key Concepts or Questions
- Doppler effect
  - Change in observed frequency of wave because of motion of source or observer
- Doppler shift
  - Doppler shift frequency fD is defined as difference between received and transmitted frequencies
    - $fD = fr - f_0 = 2f_0 v \cos\theta / c$ where
    - fr: Received frequency
    - F_0: Frequency of the transmitted beam
    - v: Flow velocity
    - Θ: Doppler angle which is angle between direction of flow and axis of ultrasound beam
    - c: Seed of ultrasound
  - Thus when $\theta = 90°$, $\cos\theta = 0$ giving no Doppler shift
  - Transducer beam should therefore be oriented to make an angle of 30-60° with the arterial lumen to receive a reliable Doppler signal
- Continuous wave Doppler (CW) units and pulsed wave (PW) Doppler units can be used for detection of Doppler shift
  - PW Doppler is subject to aliasing artifacts in measurement of high velocities, CW Doppler is not
  - Final result in many cases should be a distinct display of a "sonogram" with clearly defined maximum-velocity trace
  - Real time imager and a Doppler instrument can be combined to give duplex ultrasound instrument
- Pulse repetition frequency (PRF)
  - Transducer repeated emits brief pulses of sound at a fixed rate which is called the PRF
  - **Maximum PRF possible is $1/Td = c/2d$**
    - Td is minimum time needed for ultrasound pulses to propagate to range of interest and return
    - d is depth at which sample volume is set or distance to tissue of interest
    - c is speed of ultrasound
    - Note that $d = cTd/2$ (distance equation)
- Aliasing

- With a pulsed wave Doppler instrument, a limitation referred to as "aliasing" exists on the maximum Doppler frequency that can be detected for a given depth and on the set of operating conditions
- If present may lead to anomalies in the detected spectral waveform
- Maximum velocity detectable with pulsed Doppler (Vmax)
  - **$Vmax = c^2/8f_0 d$**
    - c: Speed of ultrasound
    - F_0: Frequency of the transmitted beam
    - d: Depth at which the sample volume is set or distance to tissue of interest
- **Doppler spectral analysis**
  - This is a way to separate a complicated signal (composed of many single frequency signals) into its individual frequency components so that the relative contribution of each frequency to the original signal can be determined
  - Relative contribution is denoted by signal power in a given frequency interval and spectrum is referred to as power spectrum
  - Information of a spectral Doppler display includes
    - Doppler frequency (or reflector velocity) is plotted on the vertical y axis
    - Doppler frequency shift can be converted to velocity once the Doppler angle is known using the Doppler formula
    - Time is plotted on the horizontal x axis
    - For each time segment, the amount of signal within specific frequency bins is indicated by a shade of gray
    - Amount of signal corresponds to amount of blood flowing at the corresponding velocity
  - **Waveforms and pulsatility**
    - Distinct wave on the Doppler frequency spectrum can be seen with each cardiac cycle beginning with systole and ending with diastole; waveform refers to the shape of this wave
    - Pulsatility is an important flow property which is defined by the waveform

VASCULAR IMAGING & DOPPLER

Longitudinal pulsed Doppler ultrasound of a CCA shows a low pulsatility arterial waveform.

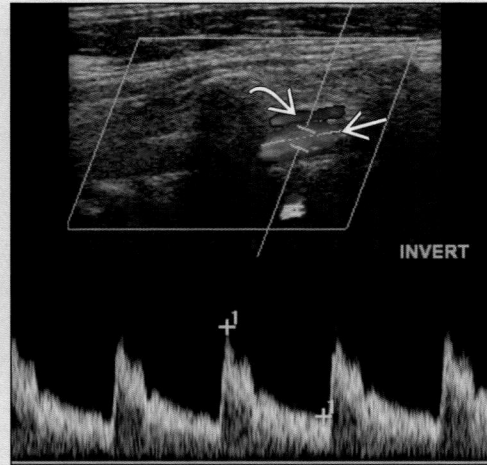

Longitudinal color Doppler ultrasound of normal VA ➡ with VV ⇒ running parallel to it. Note low pulsatility arterial waveform from the vertebral artery.

- ○ **Low pulsatility Doppler arterial waveforms**
  - ■ Have broad systolic peaks and forward flow throughout diastole
  - ■ Low pulsatility waveforms are also monophasic meaning that flow is always forwards
  - ■ Low resistance circulatory systems such as carotid, vertebral, renal and celiac axis
- ○ **Moderate pulsatility Doppler arterial waveforms**
  - ■ Appearance somewhere between low and high resistance pattern
  - ■ Systolic peak is tall and sharp but forward flow is present throughout diastole (may be interrupted by early diastole flow reversal)
  - ■ Moderate resistance circulatory systems such as external carotid artery and superior mesenteric artery (during fasting)
- ○ **High pulsatility Doppler waveforms arterial waveforms**
  - ■ Systolic peak is tall, narrow and sharp with reversed or absent diastolic flow
  - ■ Classical triphasic waveform, sharp systolic peak (1st phase); brief flow reversal (2nd phase); brief forward flow (3rd phase)
  - ■ High resistance circulatory systems such as extremity arteries in a resting individual
- ○ **Normal venous waveforms**
  - ■ Spontaneous and phasic with respiration
  - ■ More proximal IVC and hepatic veins show pulsatile flow pattern due to right atrial pressure changes during cardiac cycle
- • Color Doppler (CD) imaging (or color-velocity imaging)
  - ○ Done by estimating and displaying the mean velocity relative to the ultrasound beam direction of scatterers and reflectors in a scanned region
  - ○ Echo signals from moving reflectors are generally displayed so that the color hue, saturation or brightness indicates the relative velocity
  - ○ Color flow image data are superimposed on B-mode data from stationary structures to obtain a composite image

- ○ Aliasing can occur in color Doppler imaging commonly seen as a wraparound artifact on the display resulting in apparent flow reversal
- • Power Doppler (PD) imaging (or energy mode imaging)
  - ○ Alternative processing method ignores the velocity and simply estimates the strength (or power or energy) of the Doppler signal detected from each location
  - ○ Main advantages when compared with CD imaging
    - ■ PD is more sensitive to low and weak flow states than CD
    - ■ Angle effects on the Doppler frequency are ignored unless the angle becomes so close to perpendicular that the Doppler signals are below the flow detectability thresholds of the color processor
    - ■ Aliasing does not affect PD imaging, thus a more continuous display of flow in tortuous vessels can be provided
  - ○ Main disadvantages when compared with CD imaging
    - ■ Flow direction is not displayed which may be a useful diagnostic feature
    - ■ Image build up tends to be slower and frame rates lower because of the use of more signal averaging in PD imaging when compared with CD imaging

RELATED REFERENCES

1. Zwiebel WJ et al: Introduction to Vascular Ultrasonography. 5th edition. Philadelphia, Elsevier Saunders,, 1-89, 2005

IMAGE GALLERY

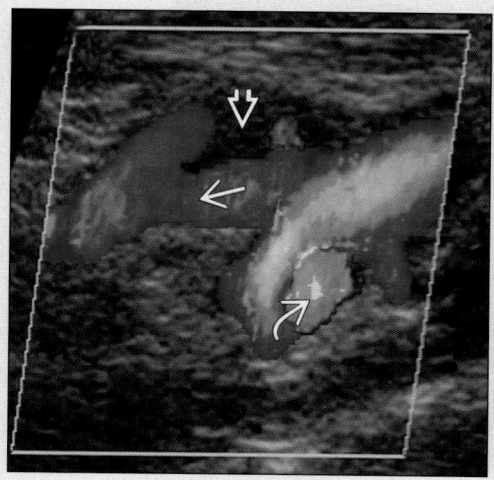
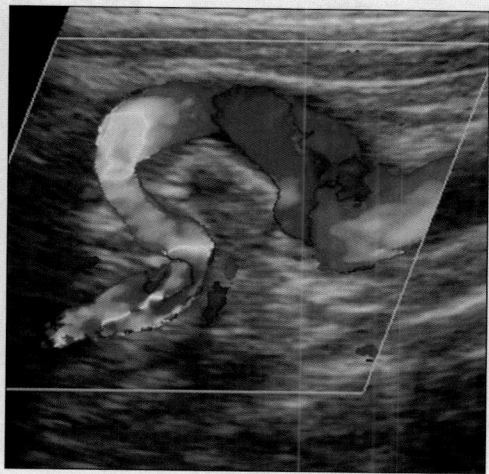

(Left) Oblique color Doppler ultrasound of normal carotid bulb shows "bizarre" color pattern: Antegrade ➡, retrograde ➡ & stagnant ➡ flow may be seen simultaneously during a cardiac cycle. (Right) Oblique color Doppler ultrasound shows a normal tortuous ICA, which is a common finding in the elderly. Note the complex color flow pattern created due to vessel tortuosity.

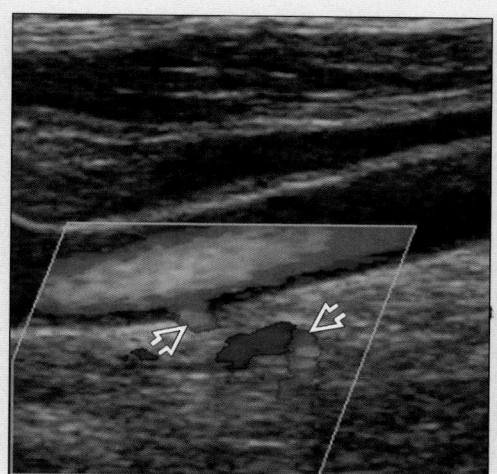
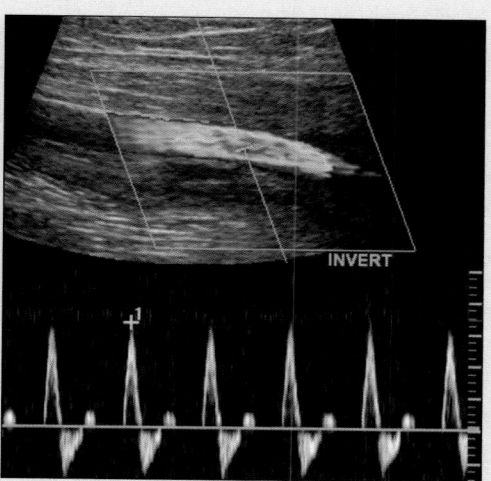

(Left) Longitudinal color Doppler ultrasound shows a small aberrant branch ➡ arising from distal CCA. (Right) Longitudinal color Doppler ultrasound of normal superficial femoral artery shows typical triphasic waveform (high pulsatility arterial waveform).

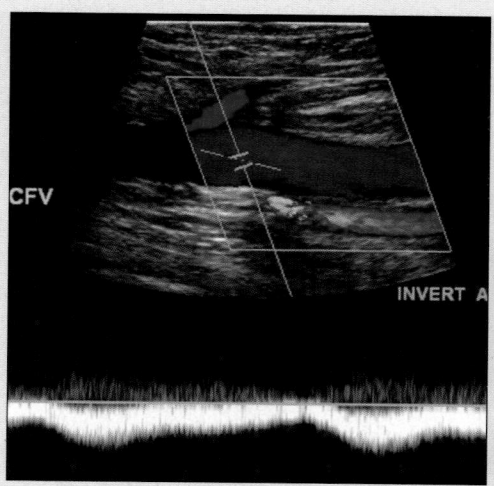
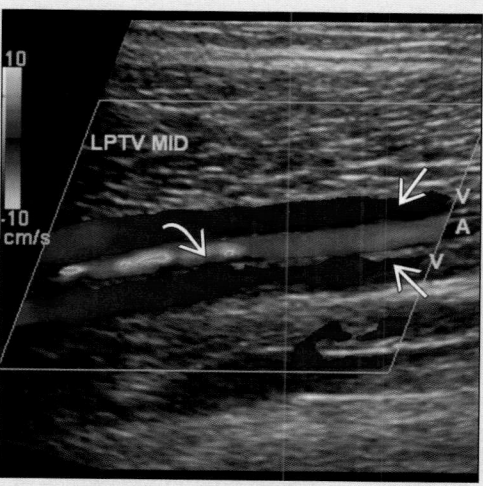

(Left) Longitudinal color Doppler ultrasound of a normal common femoral vein shows normal spontaneous and phasic flow varying with respiration. (Right) Longitudinal color Doppler ultrasound shows normal anatomy of calf vessels. Paired posterior tibial veins ➡ normally run parallel to posterior tibial artery ➡. This configuration helps to locate calf veins.

14

CAROTID STENOSIS/OCCLUSION

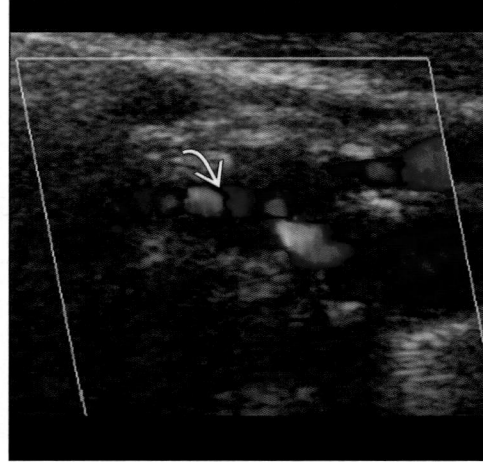

Longitudinal color Doppler ultrasound shows high grade ICA stenosis. Arterial lumen is significantly narrowed with "aliasing" flow artifact seen ➔ due to increased flow velocity.

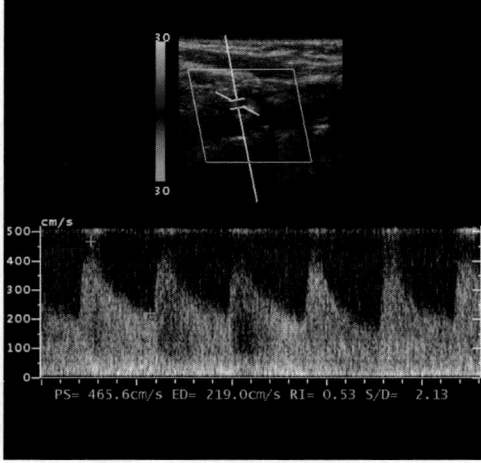

PS= 465.6cm/s ED= 219.0cm/s RI= 0.53 S/D= 2.13

Corresponding spectral Doppler analysis shows findings of stenosis. Both PSV and EDV are markedly increased, suggesting degree of stenosis ≥ 70%.

TERMINOLOGY

Definitions
- Stenosis = narrowing; occlusion = complete blockage

IMAGING FINDINGS

General Features
- Best diagnostic clue
  - Stenosis: Elevated blood flow velocity on spectral Doppler ultrasonography (US)
  - Occlusion: Absence of blood flow on color or spectral Doppler US
- Location
  - Predominantly internal carotid artery (ICA) origin
  - Less frequent: Common carotid artery (CCA); except as complication following radiotherapy for neck cancer
- Size: Stratification of obstruction: < 50%; ≥ 50-69%; ≥ 70% stenosis; near occlusion; occlusion
- Morphology
  - Residual lumen varies: Concentric, eccentric, irregular

  - Possible plaque ulceration

Ultrasonographic Findings
- Grayscale Ultrasound
  - Atherosclerotic plaque
    - Fatty or "soft": Hypoechoic or slightly echogenic; ↑ risk of embolization
    - Fibrous: Mildly echogenic; stable; ↓ risk of embolization
    - Calcified: Highly echogenic with distal shadowing; focal/diffuse; dystrophic; ↓ risk of embolization
    - Ulcerated: Focal crypt in plaque with sharp or overhanging edges; ↑ risk of embolization
    - Homogeneous: Uniform medium level echotexture; ↓ risk of embolization
    - Heterogeneous: Focal or scattered areas of hypoechogenicity; ↑ risk of embolization
  - Stenosis: Plaque formation + luminal narrowing
  - Occlusion: Echogenic material filling lumen
- Color Doppler: Useful for guiding angle correction during velocity measurement
  - May depict blood flow in crypt of ulcerated plaque

DDx: Carotid Stenosis/Occlusion

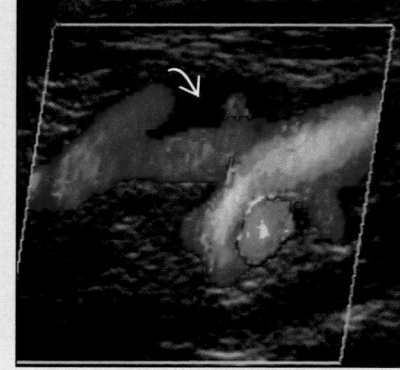

Bulb Flow Artifact

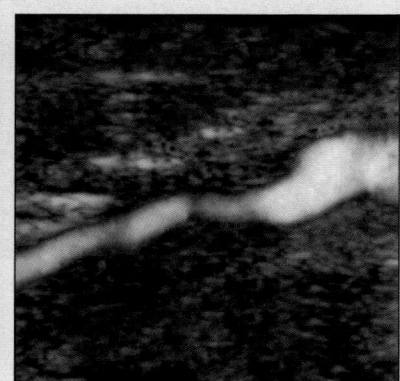

ICA Dissection

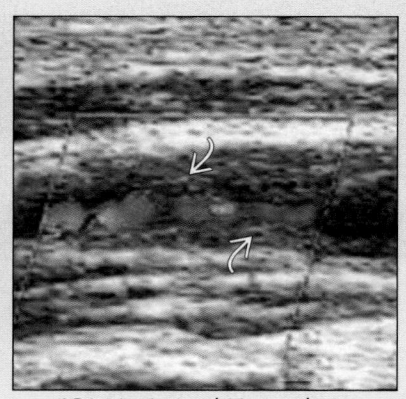

ICA Neointimal Hyperplasia

CAROTID STENOSIS/OCCLUSION

Key Facts

Imaging Findings
- Predominantly internal carotid artery (ICA) origin
- Size: Stratification of obstruction: < 50%; ≥ 50-69%; ≥ 70% stenosis; near occlusion; occlusion
- Color Doppler: Useful for guiding angle correction during velocity measurement
- Power Doppler: Useful for detecting low velocity flow at and distal to pre-occlusive stenoses
- Spectral Doppler: Useful for estimating degree of stenosis with velocity parameters
- < 50% ICA stenosis: PSV < 125 cm/s (EDV < 40 cm/s; SVR < 2.0)
- 50-69% ICA stenosis: PSV 125-229 cm/s (EDV 40-99 cm/s; SVR 2-3.9)
- ≥ 70% diameter ICA stenosis: PSV ≥ 230 cm/s (EDV ≥ 100 cm/s; SVR ≥ 4.0)

- Near-occlusion: Variable velocity
- Occlusion: Absent flow on color/spectral Doppler
- CCA stenosis: No defined Doppler criteria but ICA criteria seem to work
- DSA: Gold standard for documentation of carotid stenosis/occlusion
- DSA may undercall degree of stenosis due to underestimation of outer luminal diameter at stenosis with post-bulbar diameter

Diagnostic Checklist
- Always correlate grayscale, color Doppler, and spectral Doppler findings when evaluating carotid stenosis

---

- ○ Stenosis < 50%: Relatively uniform intraluminal color hues at and distal to stenosis
- ○ Stenosis ≥ 50%: Mildly disturbed intraluminal color hues at and distal to stenosis
- ○ Stenosis ≥ 70%: Color scale shift or aliasing due to elevated velocity at stenosis with significant poststenotic turbulence
- ○ Occlusion: Absent color flow
- Power Doppler: Useful for detecting low velocity flow at and distal to pre-occlusive stenoses
  - ○ Differentiates between patent, pre-occlusive stenoses and occlusion
- Spectral Doppler: Useful for estimating degree of stenosis with velocity parameters
  - ○ Peak systolic velocity (PSV) most popular and recommended
  - ○ Systolic velocity ratio (SVR) = (ICA stenosis/normal CCA)
  - ○ End diastolic velocity (EDV)
  - ○ < 50% ICA stenosis: PSV < 125 cm/s (EDV < 40 cm/s; SVR < 2.0)
  - ○ 50-69% ICA stenosis: PSV 125-229 cm/s (EDV 40-99 cm/s; SVR 2-3.9)
  - ○ ≥ 70% diameter ICA stenosis: PSV ≥ 230 cm/s (EDV ≥ 100 cm/s; SVR ≥ 4.0)
  - ○ Near-occlusion: Variable velocity
    - ▪ May be much lower than expected due to high flow resistance
    - ▪ Diagnosis based on color Doppler appearance and damped Doppler waveforms distal to stenosis
  - ○ Occlusion: Absent flow on color/spectral Doppler
    - ▪ Carotid artery lumen filled with echogenic material on grayscale US
  - ○ Ancillary Doppler waveform findings secondary to ICA occlusion/high grade stenosis
    - ▪ Ipsilateral CCA: High resistance waveforms
    - ▪ Ipsilateral CCA: Low resistance waveforms if ECA is a collateral
    - ▪ Ipsilateral ECA: Low resistance waveforms if it is a collateral
    - ▪ Contralateral CCA: High velocity low resistance waveforms if crossover collateralization present

- ▪ Ipsilateral ICA: Damped/irregular waveforms distal to high grade stenosis
- CCA stenosis: No defined Doppler criteria but ICA criteria seem to work
  - ○ Often can measure stenosis directly from cross sectional US images
  - ○ Ancillary Doppler waveform findings secondary to CCA occlusion/high grade stenosis
    - ▪ Ipsilateral ICA: Low resistance low velocity waveforms; antegrade flow
    - ▪ Ipsilateral ECA: Low resistance low velocity waveforms; retrograde flow

MR Findings
- MRA
  - ○ Combination of MRA and US may replace DSA
  - ○ MRA may over or under estimate degree of carotid stenosis due to flow turbulence

Angiographic Findings
- DSA
  - ○ DSA: Gold standard for documentation of carotid stenosis/occlusion
  - ○ Accepted ICA stenosis measurement protocol
    - ▪ (1-least stenosis diameter on any imaging plane/diameter of post-bulbar ICA) x 100%
  - ○ DSA may undercall degree of stenosis due to underestimation of outer luminal diameter at stenosis with post-bulbar diameter
  - ○ Angiographic ≥ 70% diameter stenosis warrants carotid endarterectomy (CEA)

Imaging Recommendations
- Best imaging tool: Color Doppler US ± MRA
- Protocol advice
  - ○ Always correlate grayscale, color and power Doppler, and spectral Doppler findings
  - ○ Possible misdiagnoses using spectral Doppler alone
    - ▪ Pre-occlusive lesions with low flow velocity
    - ▪ Low stenosis velocity due to poor cardiac function or tandem stenoses
    - ▪ High stenosis velocity due to collateralization

CAROTID STENOSIS/OCCLUSION

DIFFERENTIAL DIAGNOSIS

Bulb Flow Artifacts
- May give rise to areas of static flow mimicking plaque formation
- Complex flow pattern in carotid bulb - normal finding
- Undisturbed flow in carotid bulb, sign of plaque filling

Carotid Dissection
- CCA: Extends from arch and ends at bifurcation
  - Two CCA lumens with blood flow in one or both
  - Possible oscillating membrane
- ICA: Begins near skull base and extends inferiorly; may not reach bifurcation
  - Long stenosis or occlusion on color/power Doppler
  - High resistance Doppler waveforms proximal to dissection

Neointimal Hyperplasia Post-CEA or Stenting
- Smooth, tapered narrowing in treated area
- Uniform medium echogenicity wall thickening

PATHOLOGY

General Features
- Genetics: Probably multi-genetic
- Etiology
  - Complex, multifactorial
    - Genetic: Lipid metabolism dyscrasia
    - Underlying disease; especially diabetes and hypertension
    - Lifestyle: Smoking, diet
    - Anatomic/mechanical factors: Most severe at ICA origin
    - Inflammation: ↑ Recognized pathogenic factors
    - Infection: Possible chlamydia/helicobacter association
- Epidemiology
  - Carotid atherosclerosis = major cause of morbidity/mortality
    - Up to 40% of deaths in elderly
    - 90% of large cerebral infarcts caused by embolization (not all carotid)
    - High grade carotid stenosis in 30% of carotid territory strokes

Gross Pathologic & Surgical Features
- Fatty/inflammatory material narrowing lumen

Microscopic Features
- Subendothelial deposition of lipid ("fatty streak")
- Lipid deposits incite inflammatory response
- Macrophages ingest lipid ⇒ foam cells
- Inflammation ⇒ migration/transformation of smooth muscle cells
  - Subendothelial "fibrous cap" is formed
- Continued plaque growth and inflammation damage fibrous plaque
  - Inflammation/damage to cap ⇒ platelet/thrombus aggregation ⇒ embolization

CLINICAL ISSUES

Presentation
- Most common signs/symptoms
  - Transient cerebral ischemia (TIA)
  - Stroke
  - Amaurosis fugax

Demographics
- Age
  - Elderly > age 60
    - Clinically significant stenosis uncommon < age 50
- Gender: Male predominance (possibly lifestyle and/or genetics)

Natural History & Prognosis
- TIA, by definition, has no permanent sequelae
- Stroke: Silent, permanent neurological defect, or with recovery

Treatment
- Current clinical practice (based on major carotid endarterectomy trials)
  - ≥ 70% or pre-occlusive ICA stenosis: CEA/carotid stenting, symptomatic or asymptomatic
  - ≥ 50% but < 70 % ICA stenosis: Intervention if symptomatic
  - < 50% stenosis: Medical treatment
  - Occlusion: No ipsilateral therapy; possible intervention for contralateral disease
- Supportive for stroke

DIAGNOSTIC CHECKLIST

Consider
- Stenosis ≥ 70% when abnormally high/low carotid flow velocity detected in presence of plaque
- Occlusion when carotid flow is absent

Image Interpretation Pearls
- Always correlate grayscale, color Doppler, and spectral Doppler findings when evaluating carotid stenosis

SELECTED REFERENCES

1. Wardlaw JM et al: Accurate, practical and cost-effective assessment of carotid stenosis in the UK. Health Technol Assess. 10(30):1-200, 2006
2. Zwiebel WJ et al: Ultrasound assessment of carotid plaque. In: Introduction to vascular ultrasonography. 5th ed. Philadelphia, Saunders/Elsevier. 155-69, 2005
3. Grant EG et al: Carotid artery stenosis: gray-scale and Doppler US diagnosis--Society of Radiologists in Ultrasound Consensus Conference. Radiology. 229(2):340-6, 2003
4. Gorelick PB: Carotid endarterectomy : where do we draw the line? Stroke. 30(9):1745-50, 1999
5. Lee DH et al: Duplex and color Doppler flow sonography of occlusion and near occlusion of the carotid artery. AJNR Am J Neuroradiol. 17(7):1267-74, 1996

IMAGE GALLERY

Typical

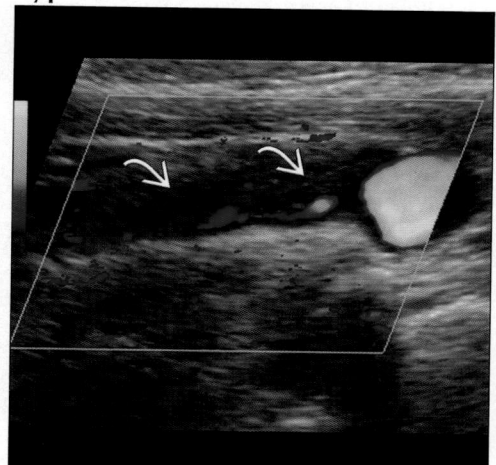
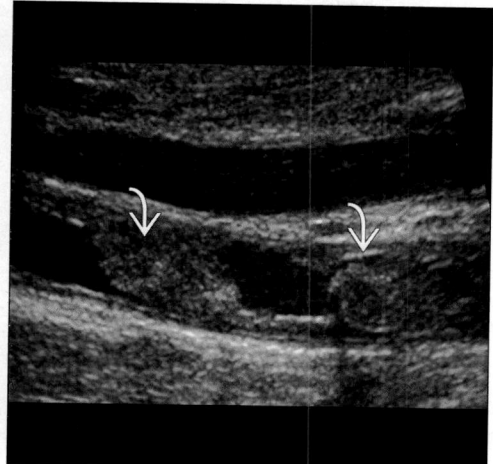

(Left) Longitudinal color Doppler ultrasound shows soft plaque ➶, which is typically hypoechoic. With grayscale imaging alone, it is easily missed. Such plaque has a high risk of embolization. (Right) Longitudinal ultrasound shows an irregular fibrous plaque ➶ in the CCA causing tight stenosis. Such plaque is relatively stable and carries a low risk of cerebral embolism.

Typical

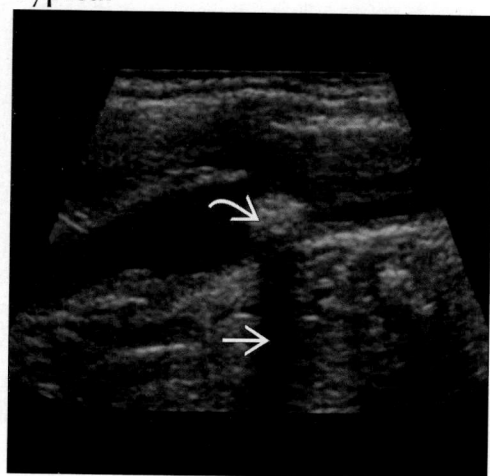
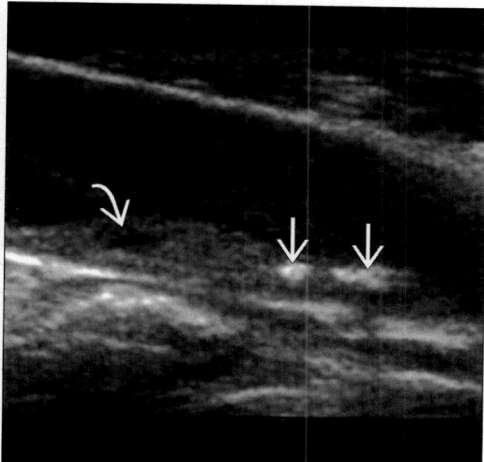

(Left) Longitudinal ultrasound shows calcified plaque ➶ characterized by its distal acoustic shadowing ➶. Such plaque has minimal risk of a cerebral embolic event. (Right) Longitudinal ultrasound shows heterogeneous plaque with areas of calcifications ➶ and hypoechogenicity ➶. Such plaque has increasing risk of a cerebral embolism.

Typical

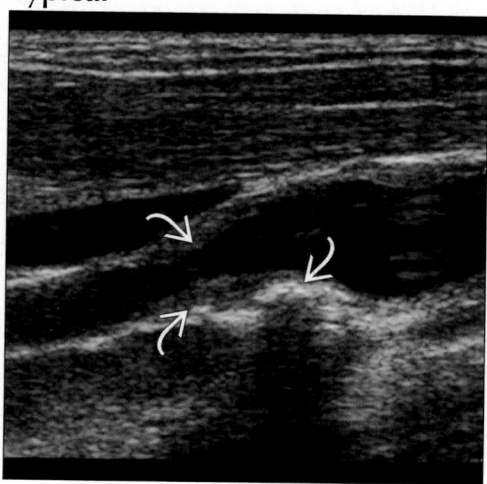
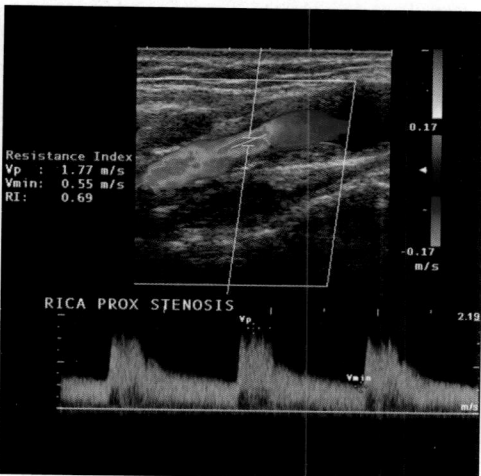

(Left) Longitudinal ultrasound shows ICA partially occluded by fibrous plaque with foci of calcifications ➶. With eye-balling technique, vessel diameter reduction is more than 50%. (Right) Corresponding spectral Doppler ultrasound shows ICA stenosis. At stenosis, PSV measures 177 cm/s, which is indicative of moderate stenosis of 50-69%.

(Left) Longitudinal power Doppler ultrasound shows echogenic plaque in the ICA causing near occlusion. Color signals are demonstrated in the small residual lumen ⇒ consistent with subtotal stenosis. *(Right)* Corresponding spectral Doppler ultrasound shows flow velocity findings. Note PSV is inconsistent with ≥ 70% stenosis which may be due to high flow resistance within narrowed lumen.

Typical

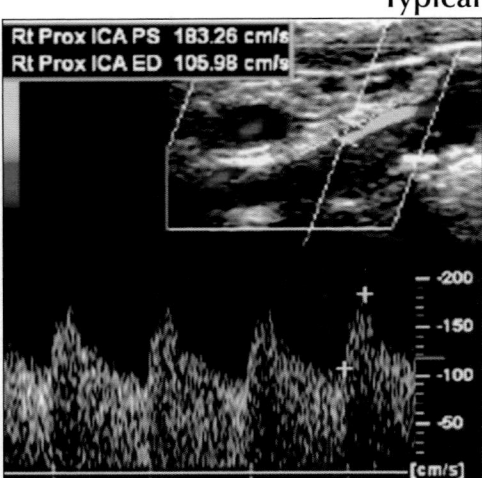

(Left) Longitudinal color Doppler ultrasound shows near ICA occlusion with slender residual lumen ➡ surrounded by echogenic plaque. Note color Doppler US is useful to assess patency of stenosis. *(Right)* Corresponding spectral Doppler ultrasound shows significantly damped flow in the residual lumen of near ICA occlusion. Note velocity is variable in near arterial occlusion.

Typical

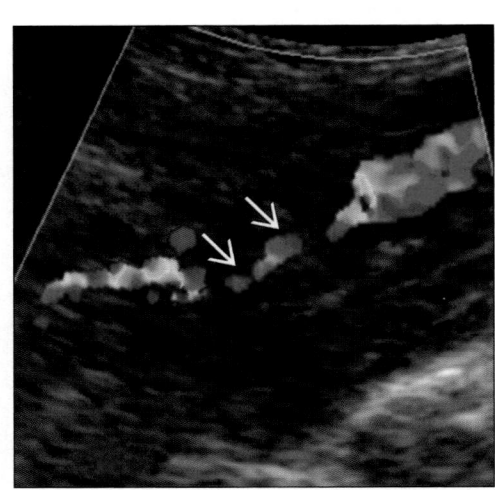
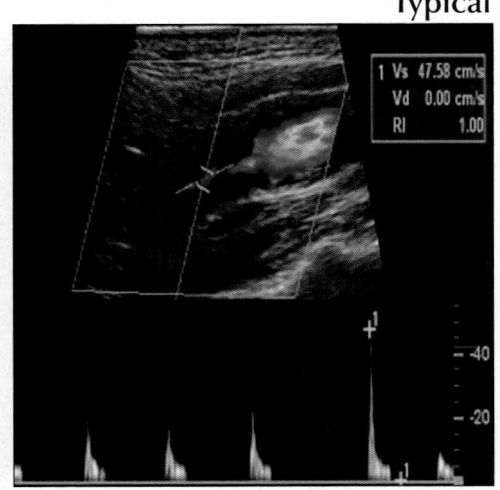

(Left) Spectral Doppler ultrasound shows high grade CCA stenosis. Although there is no defined Doppler criteria for grading CCA stenosis, ICA criteria work well in grading CCA stenosis. *(Right)* Corresponding spectral Doppler ultrasound shows flow velocity change in the post-stenotic segment. Note post-stenotic flow turbulence is seen as irregularities ➡ in the spectral display.

Typical

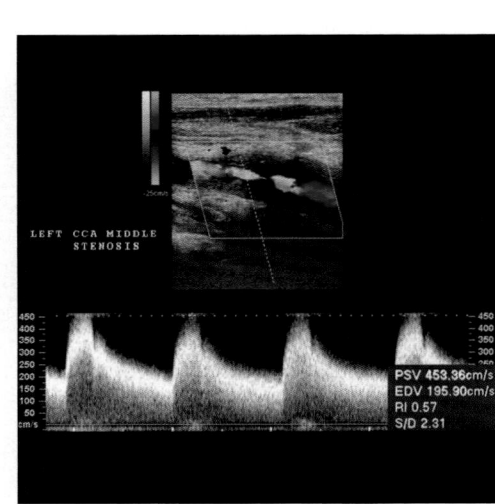
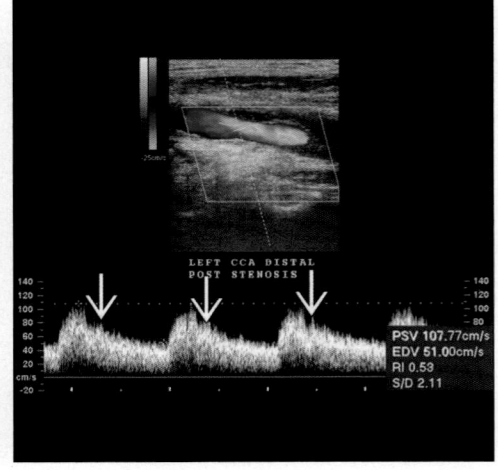

14

CAROTID STENOSIS/OCCLUSION

Typical

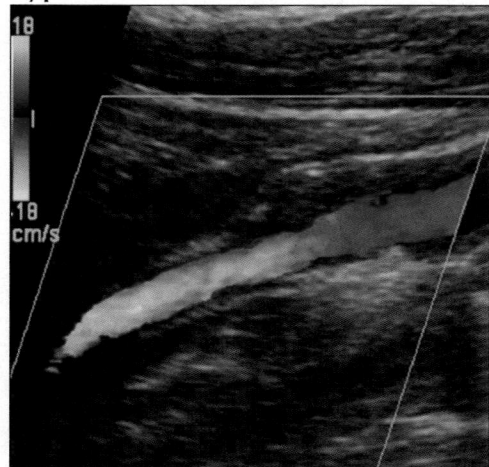
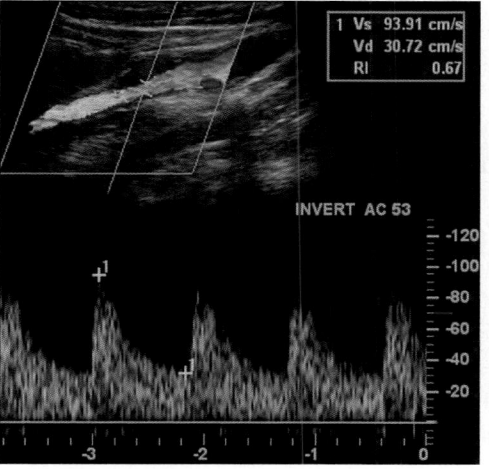

(Left) Longitudinal color Doppler ultrasound shows a bulb stenosis between 50-69% with normalization of color flow signal within the bulb. Note complex flow pattern is a normal finding in the carotid bulb. *(Right)* Corresponding spectral Doppler ultrasound shows bulb stenosis with normalization of flow velocity to below suggested cutoff (> 125 cm/s) for > 50% stenosis.

Typical

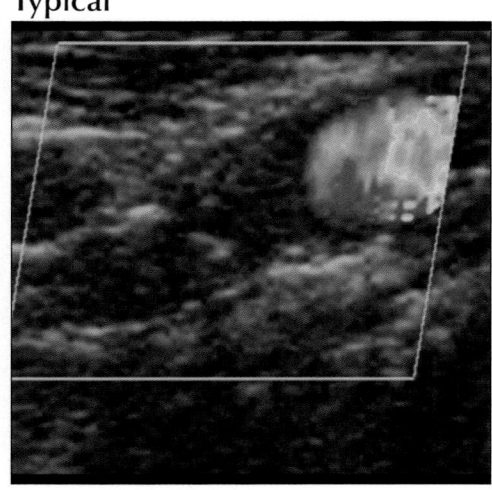
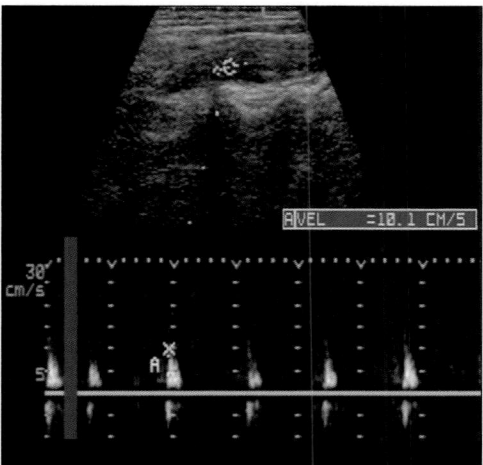

(Left) Longitudinal color Doppler ultrasound shows total ICA occlusion. The artery is occluded with echogenic plaque with absent color signal. *(Right)* Corresponding spectral Doppler ultrasound shows a low-velocity "to-and-fro" waveform just proximal to respective ICA occlusion. This waveform is typically seen in pre-occlusive arterial segment.

Typical

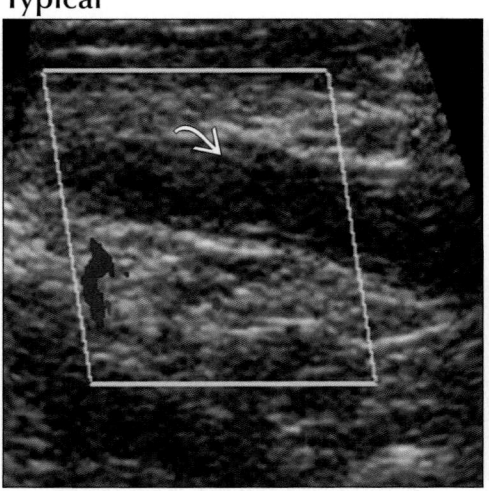
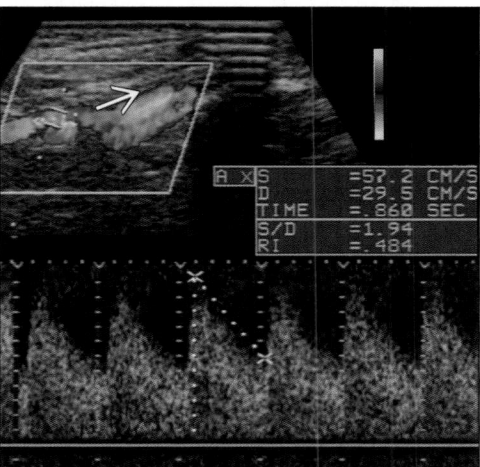

(Left) Longitudinal color Doppler ultrasound shows total CCA occlusion with absent intraluminal color flow ➢. Occlusive CCA disease is a well-known complication following radiotherapy for neck cancer. *(Right)* Corresponding spectral Doppler ultrasound shows retrograde ECA flow ➡ secondary to CCA occlusion. ECA Doppler waveform is of low resistance suggestive of collateral flow.

VERTEBRAL STENOSIS/OCCLUSION

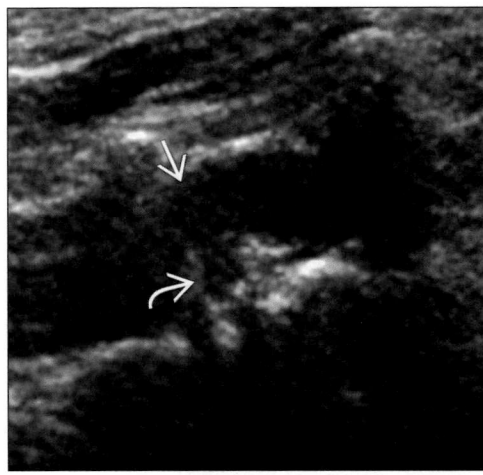
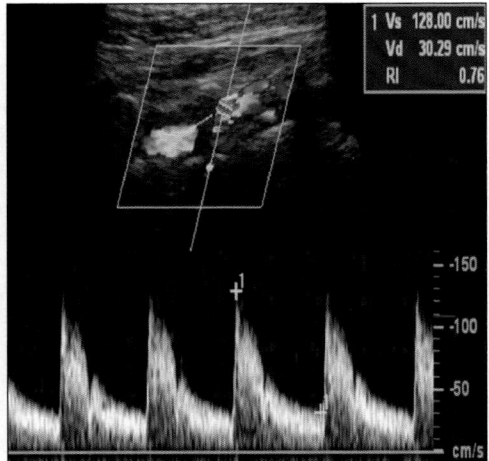

Longitudinal ultrasound shows a heterogeneous plaque ➘, in the VA, narrowing the vessel lumen ➡. Atherosclerosis is the primary cause for VA occlusive disease.

Corresponding longitudinal color Doppler ultrasound shows PSV at stenotic site is markedly elevated, suggestive of high grade stenosis.

TERMINOLOGY

Abbreviations and Synonyms
- Vertebral artery (VA) is divided into four segments
  - V1: Origin ↔ point before entering transverse foramen of sixth cervical vertebrae (C6)
  - V2: Interforaminal segment between C6 and C2
  - V3: Atlas loop
  - V4: Intracranial segment ↔ point before converging to basilar artery (BA)

Definitions
- Luminal narrowing or blockage due to plaque formation, thrombosis or dissection

IMAGING FINDINGS

General Features
- Best diagnostic clue
  - Stenosis: Focal ↑ in peak systolic velocity (PSV) at stenosis with poststenotic turbulent/dampened flow
  - Occlusion: Absence of Doppler flow signals
- Location
  - Plaque formation: Proximal VA > distal VA
    - Origin (commonest)
    - High grade stenosis in V2 and V3 is uncommon
  - Dissection: Distal V1 (commonest)
  - Thrombosis: Variable
- Size
  - Normal VA diameter: 2-4 mm
  - Hypoplasia: < 2 mm or side-side difference ≥ 1.2 mm

Ultrasonographic Findings
- Grayscale Ultrasound
  - Limited in depiction and characterization of plaque and detection of ostial stenosis
  - Stenosis: Intraluminal hypoechoic/heterogeneous material
  - Occlusion: Hypoechoic material filling arterial lumen
  - Long-standing occlusion: Contracted vessel caliber, extremely difficult to depict
- Pulsed Doppler: Indirect signs for stenosis/occlusion: Altered spectral Doppler waveform or flow resistance
- Color Doppler

DDx: VA Stenosis/Occlusion

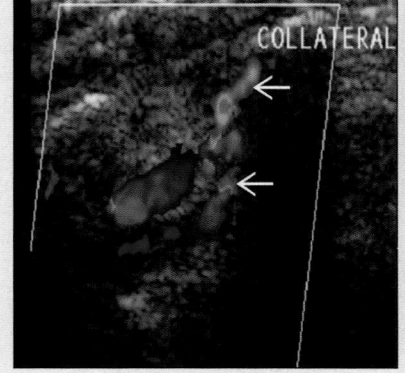

Collateral Artery

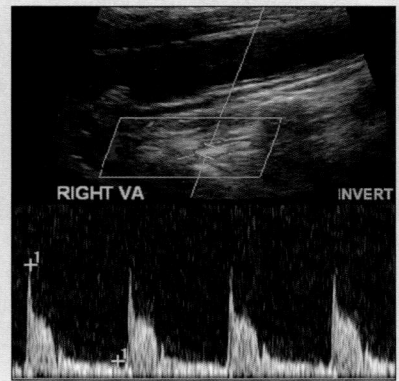

VA Hypoplasia

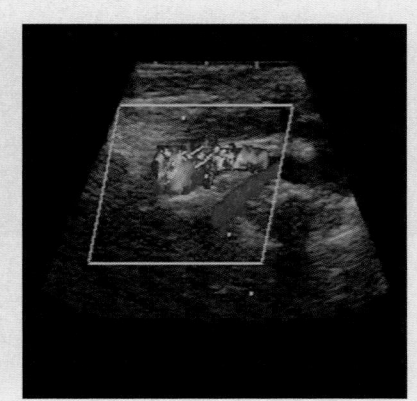

Arteriovenous Fistula

VERTEBRAL STENOSIS/OCCLUSION

Key Facts

Imaging Findings

- Stenosis: Focal ↑ in peak systolic velocity (PSV) at stenosis with poststenotic turbulent/dampened flow
- Occlusion: Absence of Doppler flow signals
- Stenosis: Intraluminal hypoechoic/heterogeneous material
- Occlusion: Hypoechoic material filling arterial lumen
- Long-standing occlusion: Contracted vessel caliber, extremely difficult to depict
- Pulsed Doppler: Indirect signs for stenosis/occlusion: Altered spectral Doppler waveform or flow resistance
- Color Doppler: Stenosis: Doppler signal resembles that of internal carotid artery
- No standardized flow velocity criteria available to document degree of stenosis
- Mild: US is insensitive for detection of mild stenosis

- Moderate: Focal flow velocity ↑ ± poststenotic disturbance
- High grade: Focal flow velocity markedly ↑ + aliasing + poststenotic disturbance/dampened flow ± prestenotic high-resistance flow
- Subtotal occlusion: Overall ↓ in flow velocity + prestenotic high-resistance flow
- Occlusion: Absent Doppler signals ± collaterals
- Color Doppler imaging is ideal for screening VA occlusive disease and evaluation of subclavian steal
- DSA is best to evaluate VA stenosis/occlusion

Diagnostic Checklist

- Presence of intraluminal plaque with abnormal ↑ or ↓ of PSV or flow resistance

---

- Valuable for evaluation of VA stenosis/occlusion and secondary collateralization
- Color Doppler: Stenosis: Doppler signal resembles that of internal carotid artery
  - No standardized flow velocity criteria available to document degree of stenosis
  - Mild: US is insensitive for detection of mild stenosis
  - Moderate: Focal flow velocity ↑ ± poststenotic disturbance
  - High grade: Focal flow velocity markedly ↑ + aliasing + poststenotic disturbance/dampened flow ± prestenotic high-resistance flow
- Subtotal occlusion: Overall ↓ in flow velocity + prestenotic high-resistance flow
- Occlusion: Absent Doppler signals ± collaterals
- Elevated VA flow velocity may indicate collateral pathway or compensatory increased flow due to contralateral VA hypoplasia or stenosis/occlusion
- Asymmetrical VA flow velocities may be due to difference in vessel caliber or unilateral occlusive disease
- Subclavian steal due to ipsilateral proximal subclavian artery stenosis/occlusion is best demonstrated by abnormal VA flow direction
  - Mild steal: Systolic deceleration
  - Moderate steal: Alternating flow
  - Complete steal: Flow reversal
- Dynamic tests with arm exercise or artificial arm hyperemia after cuff compression are recommended for investigating subclavian steal
- Transcranial color Doppler (TCCD)
  - Useful in assessing patency of V4 segment and BA
  - Acoustic window: Transoccipital approach through foramen magnum
  - Severe subclavian steal: Reversed flow in BA + VA

MR Findings

- MRA
  - Similar to ultrasound, both are limited in demonstrating ostial stenosis
  - Tends to overestimate ostial stenosis at VA

Angiographic Findings

- DSA
  - Selective angiography remains the gold standard
  - More sensitive than MRA & ultrasound for VA ostial stenosis
  - Delayed imaging performed to demonstrate reconstitution of VA through cervical collaterals

Imaging Recommendations

- Best imaging tool
  - Color Doppler imaging is ideal for screening VA occlusive disease and evaluation of subclavian steal
  - DSA is best to evaluate VA stenosis/occlusion
- Protocol advice
  - Ultrasound is always performed as initial test
  - Selective vertebral angiography as pre-operative investigation

DIFFERENTIAL DIAGNOSIS

Collateral Artery

- Occluded VA is usually reconstituted via cervical collaterals
- Flow in patent post-occlusive segment is variable and may be dampened, high-resistance or alternating

VA Hypoplasia

- ↑ Risk of ischemic posterior circulation stroke
- Flow resistance is higher than normal because
  - Flow friction ↑ in small vessel
  - Hypoplastic VA often supplies only ipsilateral posterior inferior cerebellar artery

Subclavian Steal

- Moderate steal with alternating flow may mimic "to-and-fro" flow in preocclusive segment

Arteriovenous Fistula (AVF)

- Abnormal communication between VA and Vertebral Vein (Vert V)

VERTEBRAL STENOSIS/OCCLUSION

- High velocity turbulent flow detected on color Doppler at the communication may be confused with high grade stenosis

Extrinsic Bony Compression
- Caused by osteophytes, edge of the transverse foramina, or the intervertebral joints

PATHOLOGY

General Features
- General path comments
  - VA stenosis accounts for 20% of posterior circulation ischemic stroke, mostly due to microembolization
  - VA stenosis rarely causes hemodynamic stroke
  - V4 stenosis is strongly associated with brainstem infarction
- Etiology
  - Atherosclerosis (primary)
  - Fibrous banding in the neck
  - Fibromuscular dysplasia
  - VA dissection
  - Vasculitis, giant-cell arteritis (most common)
  - Extrinsic compression by osteophytes, edge of the transverse foramina, or the intervertebral joints
    - V2 segment most commonly affected during rotation and extension of neck
- Epidemiology
  - No population-based prevalence data for extracranial VA stenosis
  - Japanese, Chinese and African Americans > Caucasians

Gross Pathologic & Surgical Features
- Very few pathological in-vivo specimens available, as endarterectomy for vertebral stenosis is rare

CLINICAL ISSUES

Presentation
- Most common signs/symptoms
  - Vertebrobasilar insufficiency (VBI)
    - Dizziness, vertigo, drop attack
    - Diplopia, perioral numbness
    - Alternating paresthesias, dysarthria, imbalance
    - Tinnitus, dysphasia
  - Stroke (cerebellar, brain stem, posterior hemispheric)

Demographics
- Age: Mean: 62.5 years
- Gender: M > F

Natural History & Prognosis
- Atherosclerosis
  - Atheroma formation with small lipid deposition in intima
  - Atheroma progression with ↑ lipid pool → narrowing of arterial lumen
  - Rupture of plaque → thrombus formation
    - Healing and fibrosis of rupture plaque → further luminal narrowing
    - Total arterial occlusion

- Thromboembolic stroke
- Prognosis is good after VA reconstruction, combined stroke and death rate < 4%
- Fair prognosis for acute vertebrobasilar occlusion; mortality rate ↓ from 90% to 60%

Treatment
- Symptomatic VBI but not fit for surgery: Long-term anticoagulation
- Acute VB occlusion
  - Atherothrombotic: Combined therapy of intravenous Abciximab and intra-arterial fibrinolysis + percutaneous transluminal angioplasty/stenting
  - Embolic occlusions: Mechanical catheter devices, such as basket or snare devices or rheolytic systems
- Chronic VB occlusion
  - Surgical intervention only considered in symptomatic patients
  - V1: Reconstruction with transposition of proximal VA onto common carotid artery (most common)
  - V1: Endarterectomy and bypass (less common)
  - V2: Elective surgical reconstruction rarely undertaken
  - V3 & V4: Surgical reconstruction, bypass or transposition

DIAGNOSTIC CHECKLIST

Consider
- Alteration of VA flow velocity, flow asymmetry and flow resistance as causes for stenosis/occlusion

Image Interpretation Pearls
- Presence of intraluminal plaque with abnormal ↑ or ↓ of PSV or flow resistance

SELECTED REFERENCES

1. Park JH et al: Hypoplastic vertebral artery; Frequency and associations with ischemic Stroke territory. J Neurol Neurosurg Psychiatry. 2006
2. Tian JW et al: Transcranial color Doppler flow imaging in detecting severe stenosis of the intracranial vertebral artery: a prospective study. Clin Imaging. 30(1):1-5, 2006
3. Eckert B: Acute vertebrobasilar occlusion: current treatment strategies. Neurol Res. 27 Suppl 1:S36-41, 2005
4. Jeng JS et al: Evaluation of vertebral artery hypoplasia and asymmetry by color-coded duplex ultrasonography. Ultrasound Med Biol. 30(5):605-9, 2004
5. Saito K et al: Vertebral artery occlusion in duplex color-coded ultrasonography. Stroke. 35(5):1068-72, 2004
6. Cloud GC et al: Diagnosis and management of vertebral artery stenosis. QJM. 96(1):27-54, 2003
7. Randoux B et al: Proximal great vessels of aortic arch: comparison of three-dimensional gadolinium-enhanced MR angiography and digital subtraction angiography. Radiology. 229(3):697-702, 2003
8. Berguer R et al: A review of 100 consecutive reconstructions of the distal vertebral artery for embolic and hemodynamic disease. J Vasc Surg. 27(5):852-9, 1998

IMAGE GALLERY

Typical

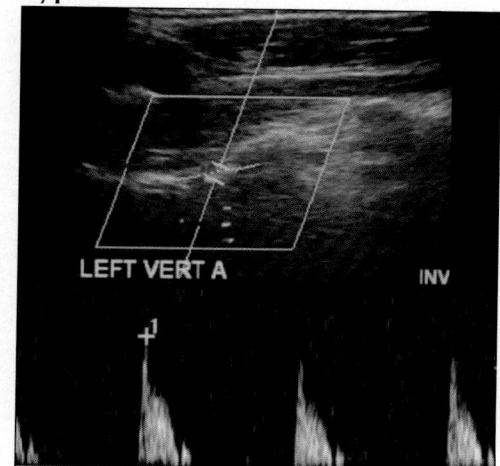

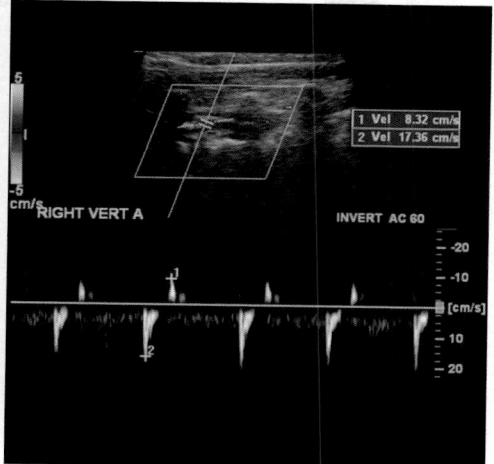

(Left) Longitudinal color Doppler ultrasound shows abnormal VA flow with monophasic waveforms. This finding is an indirect sign to suggest arterial occlusion distal to the site of interrogation. *(Right)* Longitudinal color Doppler ultrasound shows abnormal "to and fro" VA flow. Although oscillating flow is indicative of distal occlusion, it may mimic subclavian steal with alternating flow.

Typical

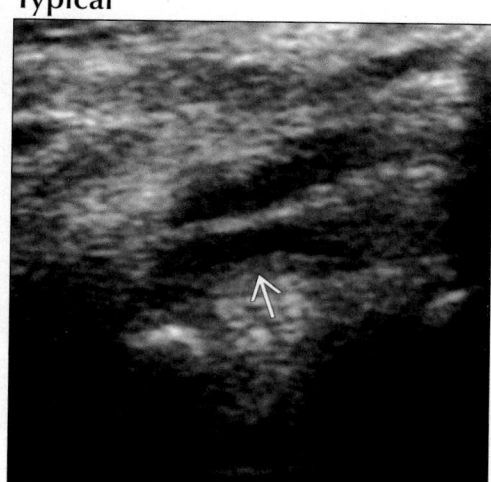

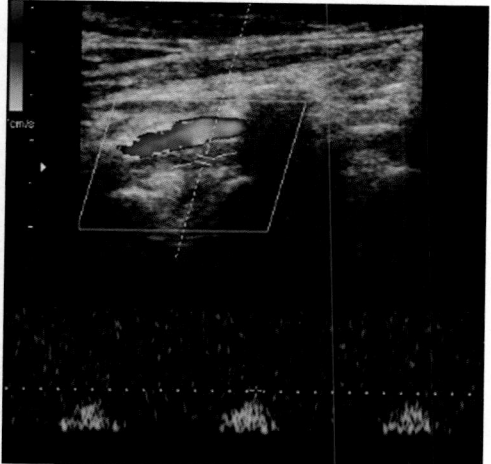

(Left) Longitudinal ultrasound shows plaque ➡ in the VA causing over 50% diameter reduction. *(Right)* Corresponding longitudinal color Doppler ultrasound shows spectral analysis. Note Doppler waveform is dampened with ↓ flow velocity, highly suggestive of tandem proximal tight stenosis.

Typical

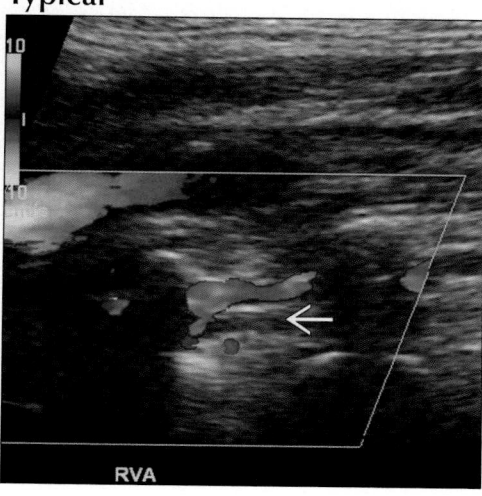

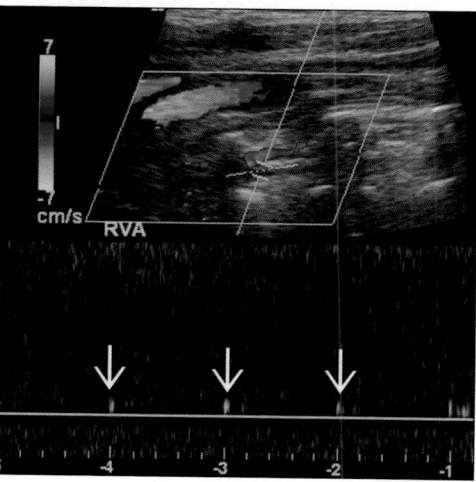

(Left) Longitudinal color Doppler ultrasound shows a small VA with absent color signal ➡. Findings are suggestive of total occlusion of a hypoplastic VA or a contracted VA due to chronic occlusion. *(Right)* Corresponding longitudinal color Doppler ultrasound shows spectral analysis of VA occlusion with artifactual signals ➡ detected due to adjacent arterial pulsations.

VERTEBRAL STENOSIS/OCCLUSION

(Left) Longitudinal ultrasound shows a patent VA segment distal to an occlusion, supplied by a collateral ➡. Collateralization is readily identified with color Doppler imaging. *(Right)* Corresponding longitudinal color Doppler ultrasound shows spectral analysis in a post-occlusive segment with a dampened monophasic pattern mimicking flow in subtotal stenosis.

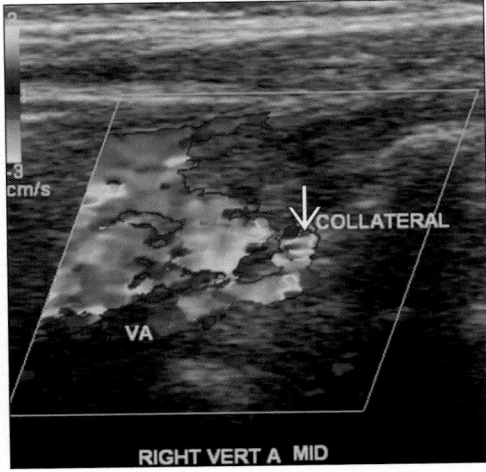

Typical

(Left) Longitudinal ultrasound shows a VA segment occluded by echogenic thrombus ➡. Color Doppler imaging should be used to assess patency of the distal segment maintained via collaterals. *(Right)* Longitudinal color Doppler ultrasound shows an alternating flow in the patent distal segment of the previous occlusion, probably maintained by cervical collateralization.

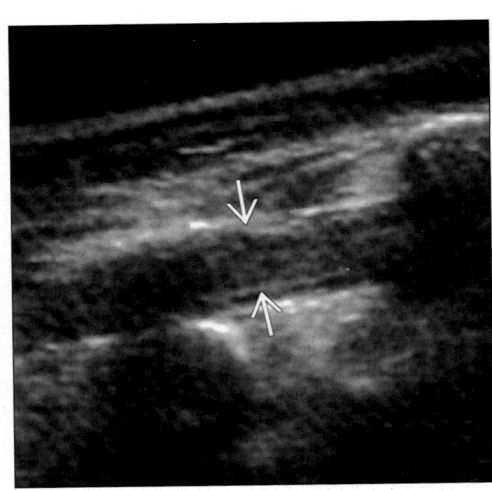
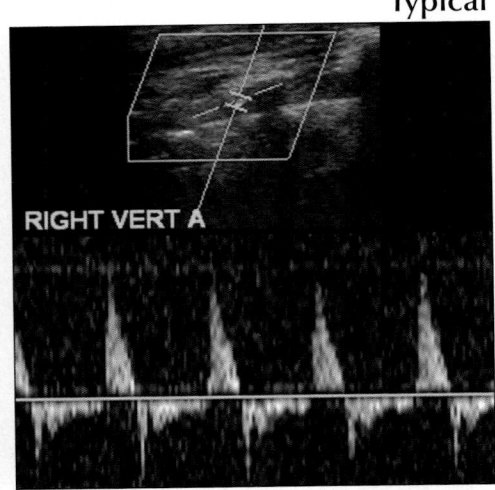

Typical

(Left) Longitudinal color Doppler ultrasound shows moderate subclavian steal with minimal antegrade flow ➡ evident only during end diastole of the cardiac cycle. *(Right)* Longitudinal color Doppler ultrasound shows abundant retrograde flow ➡ in the corresponding VA during systole. Note flow direction in VA is same as Vert V ➡, typical of subclavian steal.

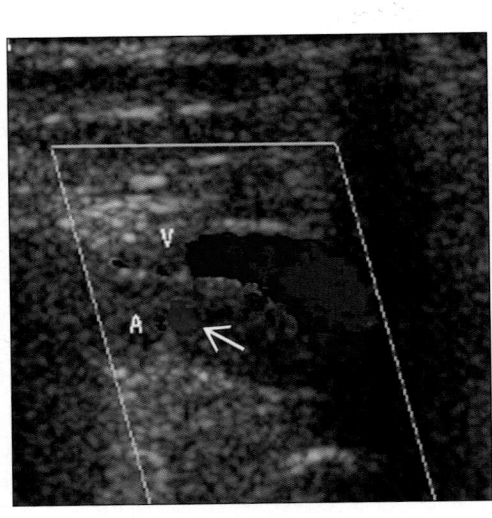
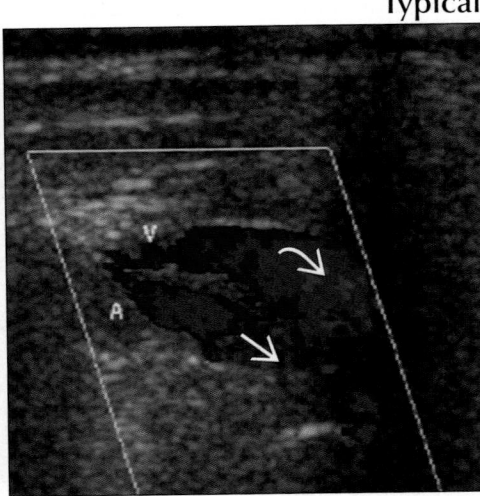

VERTEBRAL STENOSIS/OCCLUSION

Typical

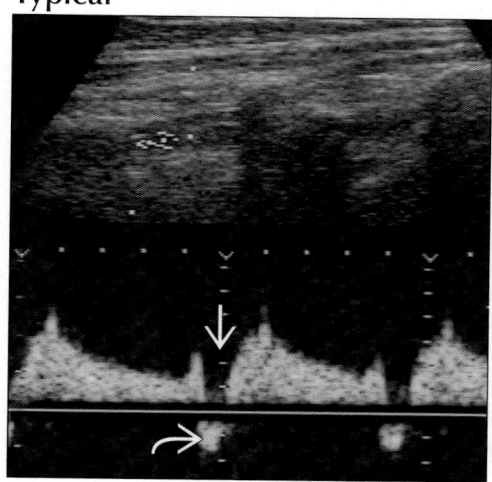
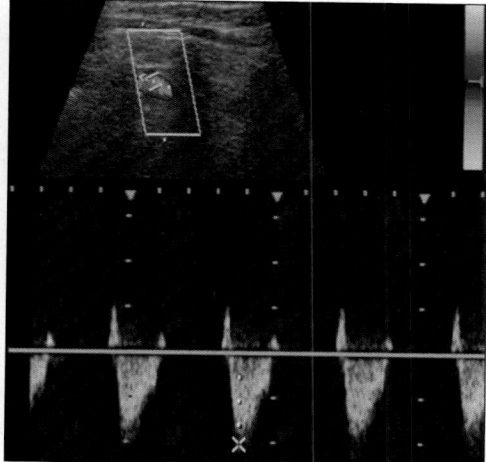

(Left) Longitudinal color Doppler ultrasound shows systolic deceleration in mild subclavian steal. A notch ➡ is seen in the Doppler waveform during systole with minimal flow reversal ➡. (Right) Longitudinal color Doppler ultrasound shows complete steal with VA flow reversal. This is due to presence of severe stenosis/occlusion at the origin of the ipsilateral subclavian artery.

Typical

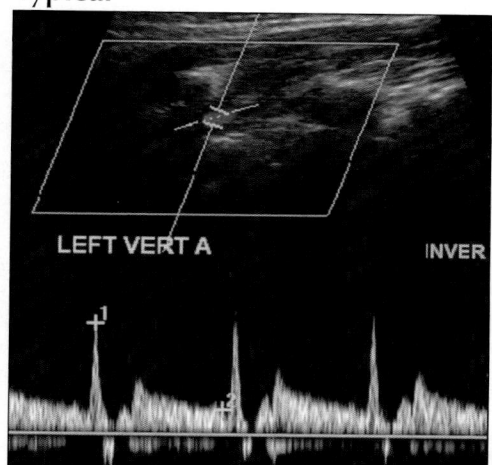
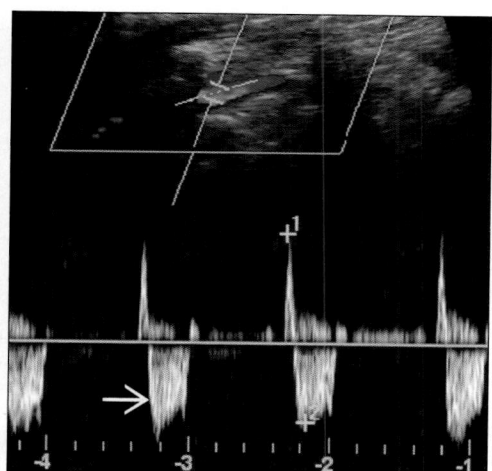

(Left) Longitudinal color Doppler ultrasound shows mild subclavian steal with arm resting. Note stealing of blood may be aggravated after arm exercise or artificial arm hyperemia. (Right) Longitudinal color Doppler ultrasound shows aggravation of steal in the corresponding VA after arm exercise. Note resulting Doppler waveform alternates with increasing retrograde flow ➡.

Typical

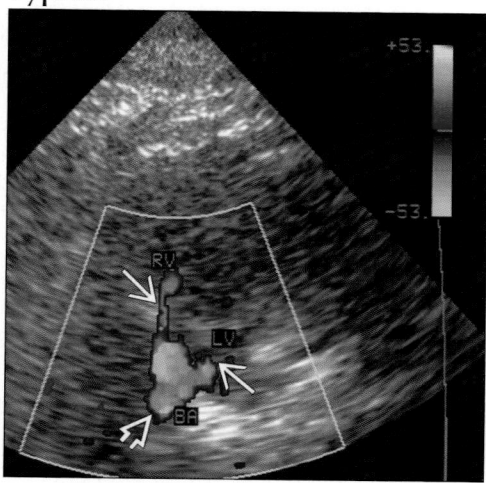
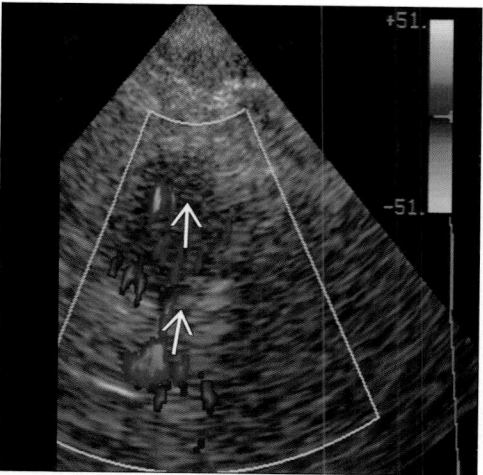

(Left) Transoccipital TCCD shows two VA ➡ terminate to form basilar artery (BA) ➡. Note flow direction of these arteries is away from the transducer, indicating normal antegrade flow. (Right) Transoccipital TCCD shows severe subclavian steal resulting in retrograde flow ➡ in both the VA and BA. Patients with intracranial steal are likely to be symptomatic.

AORTIC/ILIAC ANEURYSM

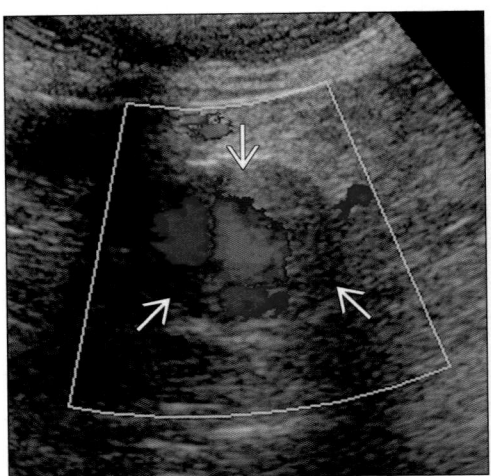 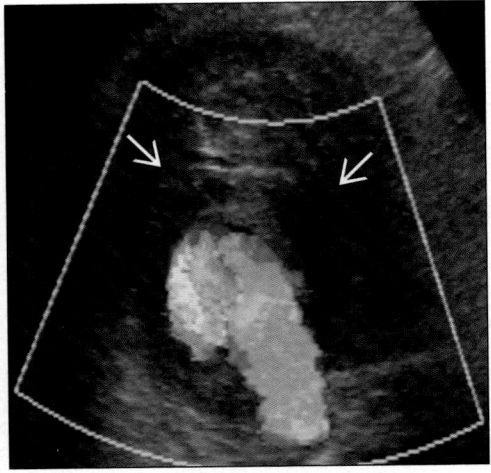

Transverse color Doppler ultrasound shows an AAA with circumferential mural thrombus in its lumen ➡.

Transverse color Doppler ultrasound shows an AAA with mural thrombus in the anterior wall ➡.

TERMINOLOGY

Definitions

- Aneurysm
  - An artery is considered aneurysmal when its diameter equals or exceeds 1.5 times the normal diameter (outer wall to outer wall)
- True aneurysm
  - Composite layers of the vessel wall are intact but stretched
  - Majority of aortic and iliac aneurysms are true aneurysms
- False aneurysm
  - Occurs when a hole in the arterial wall permits escape of blood which is subsequently confined by surrounding tissue
- Mycotic aneurysm
  - Refers to infection related aneurysms
- Arterial dissection
  - Occurs when blood enters the media through a defect (entry site) in the intima and dissects along the length of the artery
  - Intima may be stripped away in some parts and a new lumen (false lumen) may be formed

- Blood may flow freely through both the true and false lumens
- False lumen may compress the true lumen
- False lumen may end up supplying branch vessels and the branch vessels may occlude when the false lumen occludes
- Most aortic dissections originate from the thoracic aorta although localized abdominal dissection has been reported
- Aneurysm neck
  - When applied to infrarenal aortic aneurysm refers to the distance between the more inferior of the renal arteries and the origin of the aneurysm

IMAGING FINDINGS

General Features

- Best diagnostic clue: When the diameter of the aorta or an artery equals or exceeds 1.5 times the diameter of the normal portion of the artery
- Location
  - Aneurysm can occur anywhere in the aorta

DDx: Abdominal Aortic Aneurysm

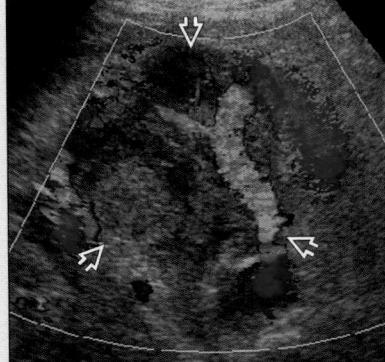 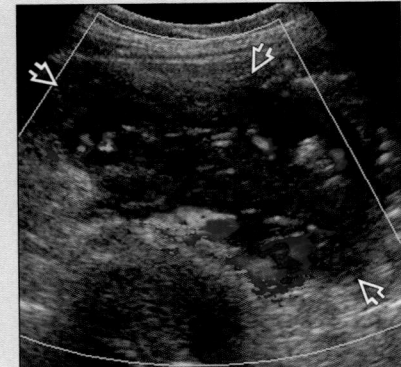 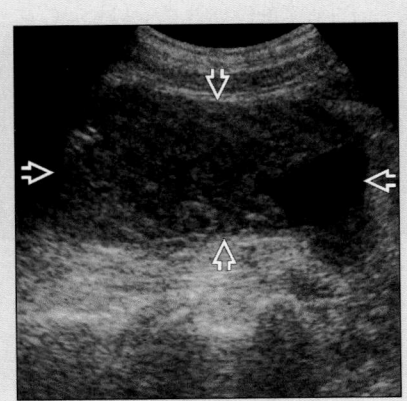

Paraaortic Lymphadenopathy *Paraaortic Sarcoma* *Paraaortic Hematoma*

AORTIC/ILIAC ANEURYSM

Key Facts

Terminology
- An artery is considered aneurysmal when its diameter equals or exceeds 1.5 times the normal diameter (outer wall to outer wall)

Imaging Findings
- **Grayscale ultrasound:** Bulbous or fusiform dilatation of the aorta/artery
- Concentric layers of thrombus may line the interior of large aneurysms which may act as a source for distal emboli
- Membrane or intimal flap may be present in dissection
- Retroperitoneal hematoma is highly suggestive of aortic rupture
- Hematoma is hypoechoic and asymmetrical and typically displaces ipsilateral kidney

- **Color Doppler:** Should be incorporated in all studies of abdominal aorta
- Confirm patency of celiac axis, superior mesenteric artery, renal arteries
- Look for flow disturbances associated with stenosis
- Measure distance between SMA and neck of aneurysm; renal arteries should be unaffected if the aneurysm begins > 2 cm inferior to the SMA
- Ultrasound is an excellent non invasive tool for aneurysm screening, follow-up and useful for assessment of endoleak post endovascular repair
- CT remains the gold standard and preferred imaging modality
- Examine aorta from diaphragm to bifurcation
- Interrogate iliac arteries

- o Most common site for aortic aneurysm is in the infrarenal aorta
- o Iliac artery aneurysm typically occurs in the common iliac artery
- o Extension into the internal iliac artery is not uncommon
- o Extension into the external iliac artery is almost never seen (except in mycotic aneurysm), reason unknown
- Size
  - o Abdominal aorta is considered aneurysmal when its outer wall to outer wall diameter reaches 3 cm
  - o Surgical or endovascular repair is usually recommended for abdominal aortic aneurysm (AAA) > 5.5 cm in diameter
  - o Common iliac artery is considered aneurysmal when its outer wall to outer wall diameter reaches 2 cm
  - o Surgical or endovascular repair is usually recommended for iliac aneurysm > 3 cm in diameter
- Morphology
  - o Saccular or fusiform
  - o Frequently tortuous and aorta may elongate and dilate
  - o Aorta may deviate to the left or anteriorly creating a significant kink at the aneurysm neck

Ultrasonographic Findings
- Grayscale Ultrasound
  - o **Grayscale ultrasound:** Bulbous or fusiform dilatation of the aorta/artery
  - o Concentric layers of thrombus may line the interior of large aneurysms which may act as a source for distal emboli
  - o Membrane or intimal flap may be present in dissection
  - o Retroperitoneal hematoma is highly suggestive of aortic rupture
  - o Hematoma is hypoechoic and asymmetrical and typically displaces ipsilateral kidney
  - o Intraperitoneal fluid may be present if there is leakage into the peritoneal space
- Color Doppler

- o **Color Doppler:** Should be incorporated in all studies of abdominal aorta
- o Particularly useful for demonstration of aortic dissection
- o Confirm patency of celiac axis, superior mesenteric artery, renal arteries
- o Look for flow disturbances associated with stenosis
- o Measure distance between SMA and neck of aneurysm; renal arteries should be unaffected if the aneurysm begins > 2 cm inferior to the SMA

Imaging Recommendations
- Best imaging tool
  - o Ultrasound is an excellent non invasive tool for aneurysm screening, follow-up and useful for assessment of endoleak post endovascular repair
  - o CT remains the gold standard and preferred imaging modality
    - For assessment of possible aortic rupture
    - For assessment of suitability for endovascular or surgical repair of the aortic aneurysm
    - For post endovascular repair follow-up, particularly for assessment of endoleak
- Protocol advice
  - o Low frequency 2-5 MHz probe should be used
  - o Examine in longitudinal, transverse and coronal planes
  - o Examine aorta from diaphragm to bifurcation
  - o Document anteroposterior (AP) and transverse diameter of the aortic aneurysm, outer wall to outer wall
  - o Note that interobserver variability for aortic diameter measurement ~ 5 mm, thus significant increase in size should be reported only when increase > 5 mm
  - o Interrogate iliac arteries
  - o Measure iliac artery aneurysms if present
  - o Document stenoses in iliac arteries if present (may affect suitability for endovascular repair)
  - o Measure the length of the neck of the aneurysm
  - o Document kidney length and hydronephrosis if present

AORTIC/ILIAC ANEURYSM

○ 6 month follow-up should be performed once an aneurysm is discovered
○ Follow-up may be yearly for small and stable aneurysms

DIFFERENTIAL DIAGNOSIS

Paraaortic Lymphadenopathy
• When extensive may mimic AAA, though contour usually more lobulated on GS

Paraaortic Tumor
• CD useful for differentiation and may demonstrate vasculature within tumour (not a feature of AAA)

Paraaortic Fluid Collection
• CD useful for differentiation as no flow should be present within the collection

Aortic Dissection
• May be present as an extension of a thoracic dissection or less commonly as a localized dissection within an AAA
• Intimal flap on GS is diagnostic of dissection

PATHOLOGY

General Features
• Etiology: Atherosclerosis
• Epidemiology
  ○ 4.5% at age 65 in Western nations
  ○ 10.8% at age 80

CLINICAL ISSUES

Presentation
• Most common signs/symptoms
  ○ Abdominal, back or leg pain
  ○ Sudden onset of severe abdominal or back pain may suggest leakage of aneurysm
  ○ Prostration, shock or death may be associated with frank rupture

Demographics
• Age: Most aortic aneurysms evolve between ages 60-70
• Gender: Male predominance; 76% aortoiliac aneurysms occur in men

Natural History & Prognosis
• Up to 60% asymptomatic, discovered incidentally on physical examination or imaging
• Leaking aortic aneurysm associated with a 50% mortality
• Risk of aneurysm rupture
  ○ For aneurysms < 5 cm, 3-5% over 10 yrs; for aneurysms > 5 cm, 5%/yr
• Risk of aneurysm development is very low if aorta < 2.5 cm at age 70
• Single screening ultrasound showing abdominal aorta < 2.5 cm virtually excludes aortic aneurysm for life
• Iliac aneurysms usually co-exist with distal aortic aneurysms

• Isolated iliac aneurysms are uncommon but can be deadly
  ○ Cannot be palpated until a large size is reached
  ○ May present non-specifically with abdominal or pelvic pain and delay diagnosis

Treatment
• Complications of aortic aneurysm
  ○ Renal artery obstruction
  ○ Hydronephrosis
  ○ Retroperitoneal fibrosis
  ○ Rupture
• Endovascular or surgical repair generally recommended
  ○ Aortic aneurysms > 5.5 cm; Iliac aneurysms > 3.0 cm
• Comparison of endovascular and open surgical aortic aneurysm repair
  ○ Endovascular repair
    ▪ 1.6% 30 day operative mortality
    ▪ 4% aneurysm related deaths at 4 years
    ▪ ~ 28% deaths from all causes at 4 years
    ▪ 41% post-operative complications within 4 years, endoleak being the main problem
    ▪ Higher cost when compared with open surgery
  ○ Open surgical repair
    ▪ 4.5% 30 day operative mortality
    ▪ 7% aneurysm related deaths at 4 years
    ▪ ~ 28% deaths from all causes at 4 years
    ▪ 9% post-operative complications within 4 years
  ○ Endovascular repair associated with lower 30 day operative mortality and aneurysm related deaths
  ○ No difference between endovascular repair and surgery in deaths from all causes
  ○ Endovascular repair is more expensive and has more post-operative complications requiring intervention

DIAGNOSTIC CHECKLIST

Image Interpretation Pearls
• Measure aortic/iliac aneurysm diameter from outer wall to outer wall
• Interobserver variability for aortic diameter measurement on ultrasound ~ 5 mm and thus significant increase in aortic diameter should only be reported when increase > 5 mm
• Renal arteries should be unaffected if the aneurysm begins > 2 cm inferior to the SMA

SELECTED REFERENCES

1. EVAR trial participants. Related Articles et al: Endovascular aneurysm repair versus open repair in patients with abdominal aortic aneurysm (EVAR trial 1): randomised controlled trial. Lancet. 365(9478):2179-86, 2005
2. Zwiebel WJ et al: Introduction to Vascular Sonography, 5th ed. Philadelphia, Elsevier Saunders. 529-69, 2005
3. Greenhalgh RM et al: Comparison of endovascular aneurysm repair with open repair in patients with abdominal aortic aneurysm (EVAR trial 1), 30-day operative mortality results: randomised controlled trial. Lancet. 364(9437):843-8, 2004

IMAGE GALLERY

Typical

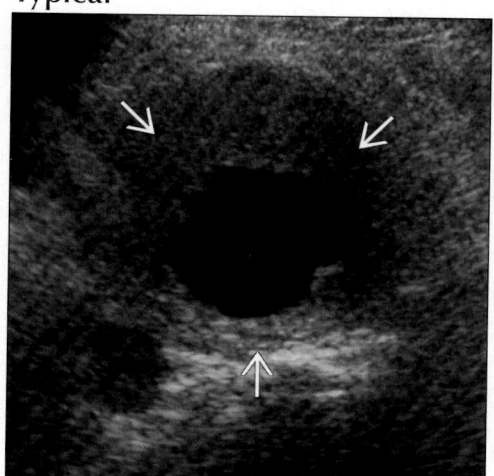 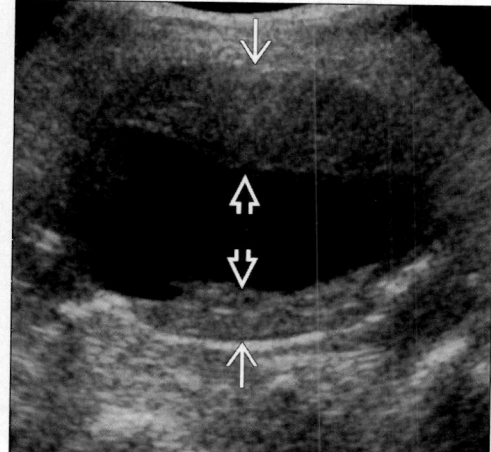

(Left) Transverse transabdominal ultrasound shows an AAA with a moderate amount of circumferential mural thrombus ➡. *(Right)* Corresponding longitudinal transabdominal ultrasound shows that the outer wall ➡ is substantially larger in diameter when compared with the lumen ➡.

Typical

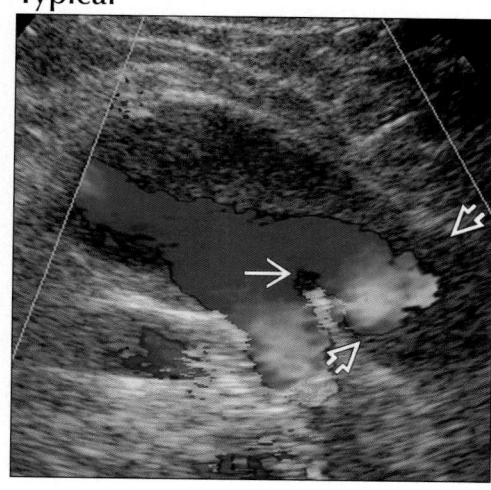 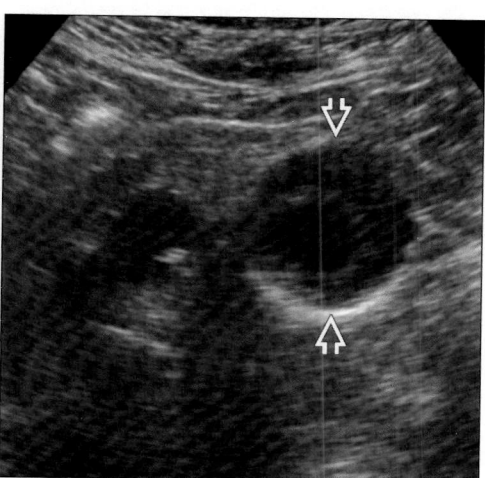

(Left) Longitudinal color Doppler ultrasound shows an AAA involving the bifurcation of the aorta ➡. Note the left common iliac artery also appears aneurysmal ➡. *(Right)* Corresponding transverse transabdominal ultrasound shows the left common iliac artery is dilated with intramural thrombus ➡.

Typical

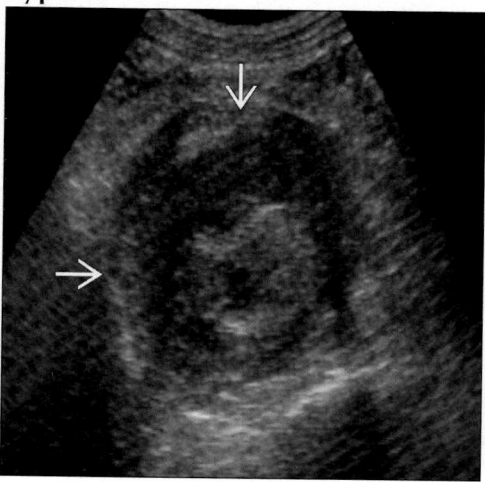 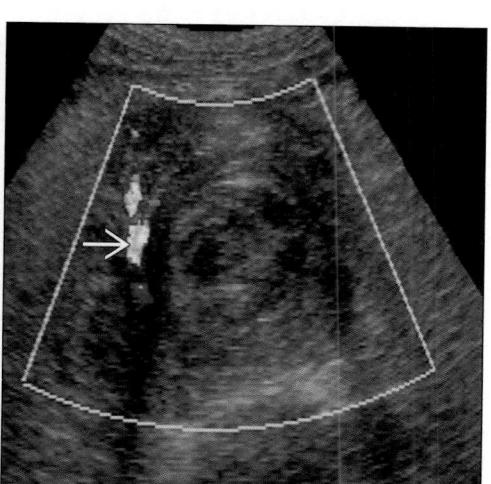

(Left) Transverse transabdominal ultrasound shows an AAA ➡ with intramural thrombus occluding the lumen. *(Right)* Corresponding transverse color Doppler ultrasound shows color signal detected in periaortic region likely representing flow in collaterals around the occluded aorta ➡.

AORTIC/ILIAC ANEURYSM

Typical

(Left) Longitudinal transabdominal ultrasound shows an AAA ➜ with mixed color turbulent flow within the aneurysm sac. *(Right)* Transverse transabdominal ultrasound shows a large AAA ➜ with no significant intramural thrombus.

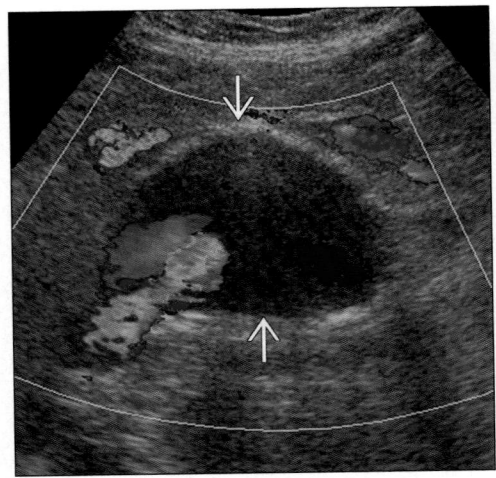
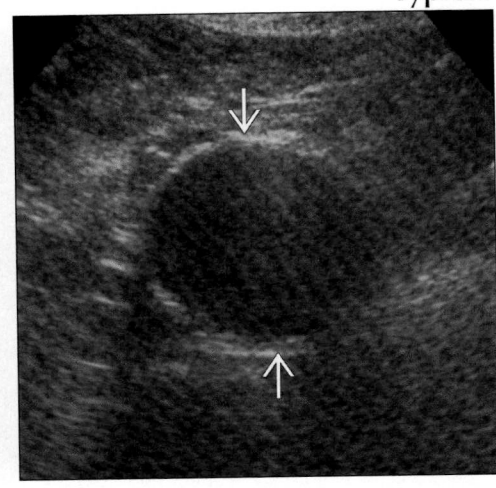

Typical

(Left) Oblique transabdominal ultrasound shows a suprarenal AAA ➜ starting close to the SMA ➜. As a general rule, if the distance between the SMA and AAA is < 2.0 cm it is suggestive of a suprarenal origin. *(Right)* Oblique transabdominal ultrasound shows a distal AAA ➜ with no involvement of the bifurcation.

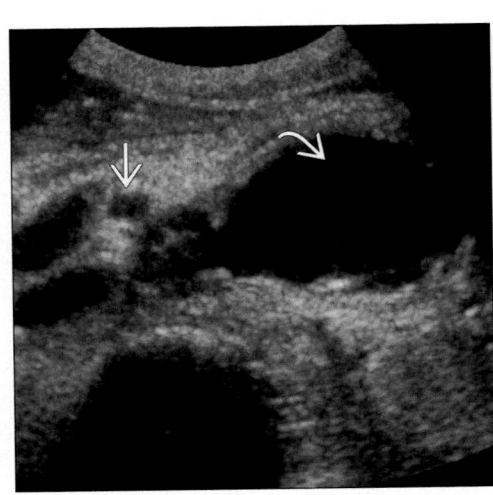
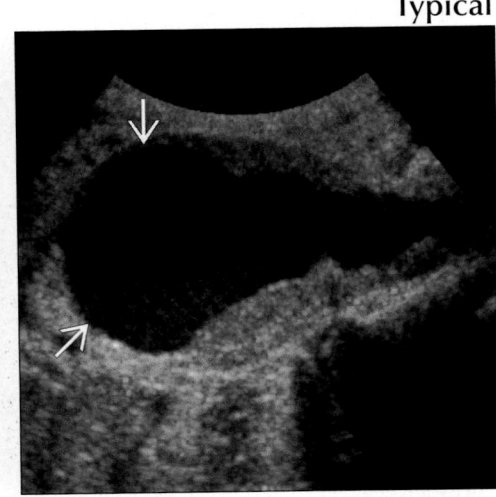

Typical

(Left) Transverse transabdominal ultrasound shows mural thrombus ➜ in a suprarenal AAA. *(Right)* Transverse transabdominal ultrasound shows renal arteries ➜ clearly identified from the corresponding suprarenal AAA.

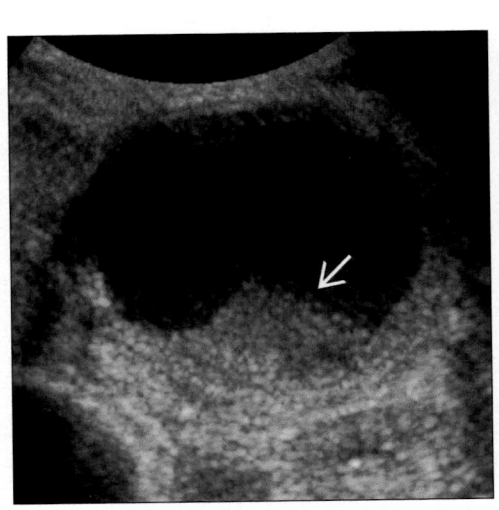
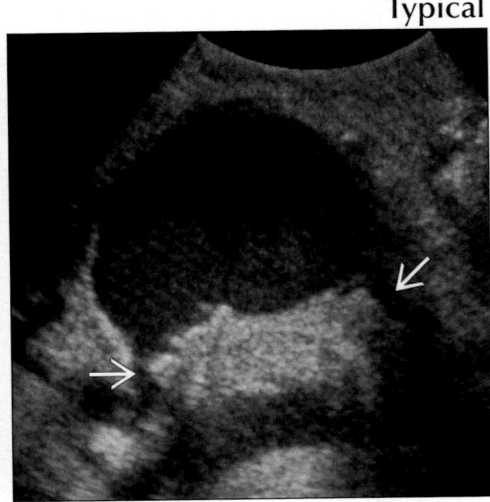

AORTIC/ILIAC ANEURYSM

Typical

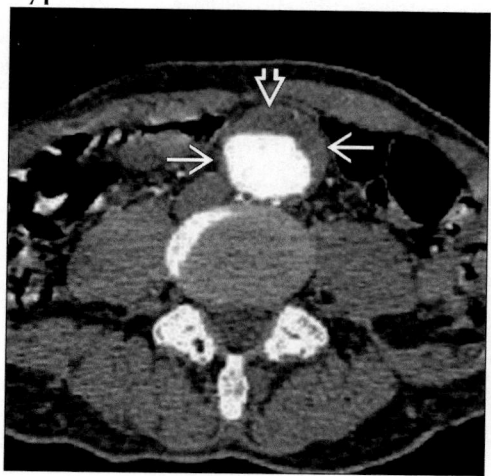

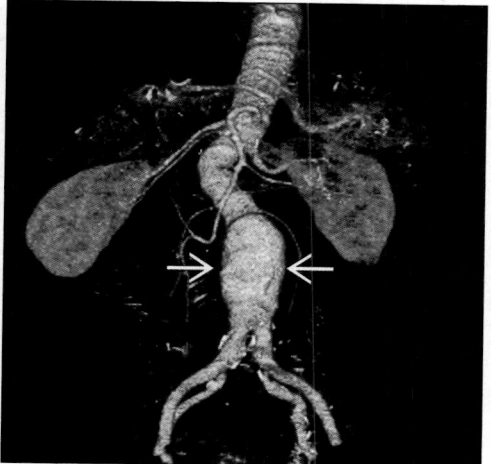

(Left) Transverse CECT shows a 5.5 cm infrarenal abdominal aortic aneurysm ➡ with low attenuation mural thrombus ➡. Note the outer diameter of the aneurysm is significantly larger than contrast-enhanced lumen. (Right) CT Angiogram (CTA) shows a volume rendered image of a infrarenal abdominal aortic aneurysm ➡ with an angulated neck.

Typical

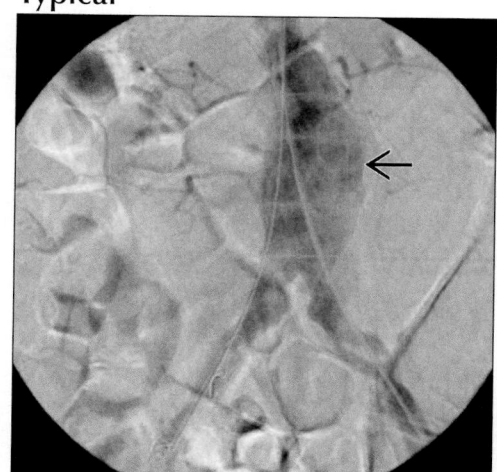

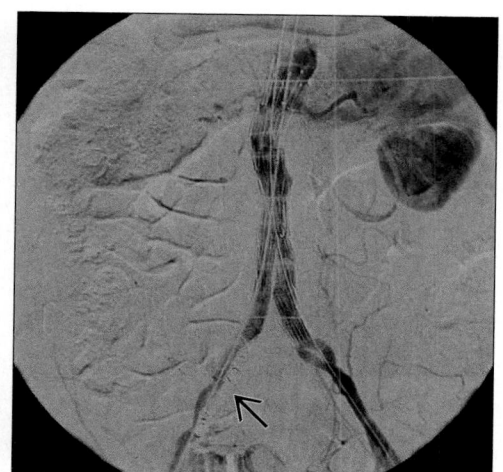

(Left) Digital substraction angiogram (DSA) shows the same infrarenal abdominal aortic aneurysm ➡ as above, pre-stenting. (Right) DSA shows exclusion of abdominal aortic aneurysm post-stenting. Note coils have been deliberately used to embolize the right internal iliac artery ➡ to prevent endoleak into the right limb extension (deployed to the external iliac artery).

Typical

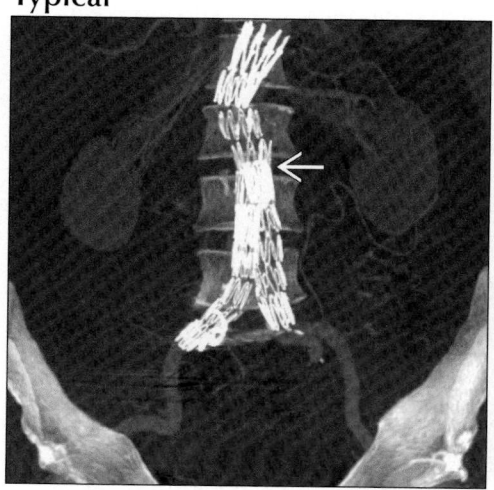

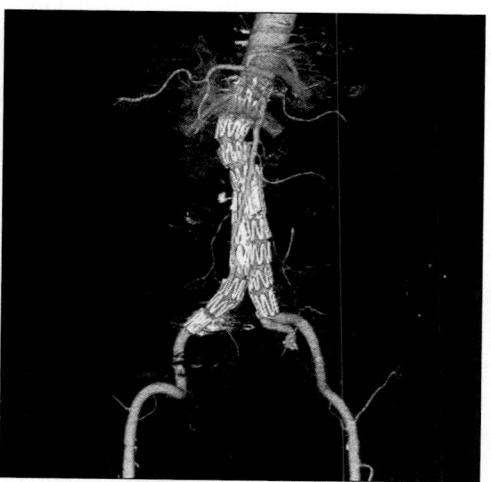

(Left) CTA shows a maximal intensity projection image of the endovascular stent ➡ in situ. (Right) CTA shows a volume rendered image of the endovascular stent in situ. Note that bones and soft tissue structures have been removed from the reconstructed model.

AORTO-ILIAC OCCLUSIVE DISEASE

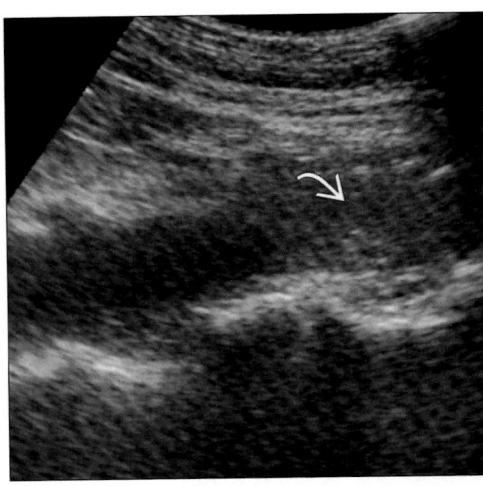 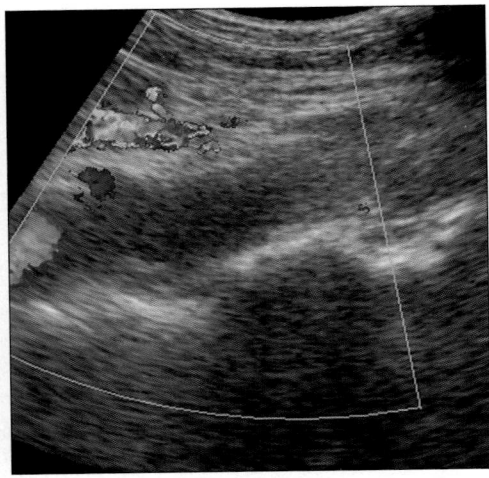

Longitudinal transabdominal ultrasound shows aortic occlusion with the aortic lumen filled with echogenic thrombus ➡.

Corresponding longitudinal CD ultrasound shows aortic occlusion, which is confirmed by absence of color Doppler signal within the aortic segment.

TERMINOLOGY

Definitions
- Stenosis
  - Area with diameter narrowing of arterial lumen; increasing peak systolic velocity is seen with increasingly narrowed lumen due to turbulent flow
- Occlusion
  - Area where lumen is completely blocked with absent flow

IMAGING FINDINGS

Ultrasonographic Findings
- Grayscale Ultrasound
  - **Grayscale (GS):** Useful for identifying plaques and calcification
  - Not possible to determine the degree of arterial narrowing on GS alone
  - Occlusive thrombus may be present in the lumen of the occluded aorta or iliac arteries
- Pulsed Doppler

- **Pulsed Doppler (PuD):** Useful for evaluating waveform & measuring peak systolic velocity (PSV)
- Normal waveform: Triphasic with no spectral broadening
- 1-19% diameter reduction
  - Triphasic waveform with minimal spectral broadening
  - PSV increase < 30% relative to adjacent proximal segment
  - Proximal and distal waveforms remain normal
- 20-49% diameter reduction
  - Triphasic waveform usually maintained, but reverse flow diminished
  - Spectral broadening prominent
  - Filling in of clear area under the systolic peak
  - PSV increase 30-100% relative to adjacent proximal segment
  - Proximal and distal waveforms remain normal
- 50-99% diameter reduction
  - Monophasic waveform, loss of reverse flow and forward flow throughout cardiac cycle
  - Extensive spectral broadening
  - PSV > 100% relative to adjacent proximal segment

14

24

DDx: Aorto-Iliac Occlusive Disease

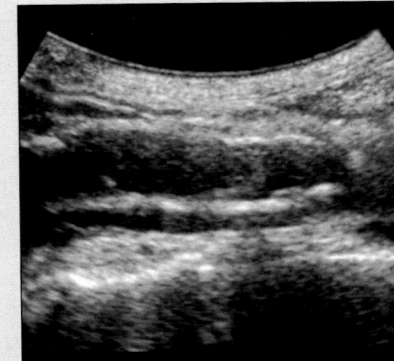 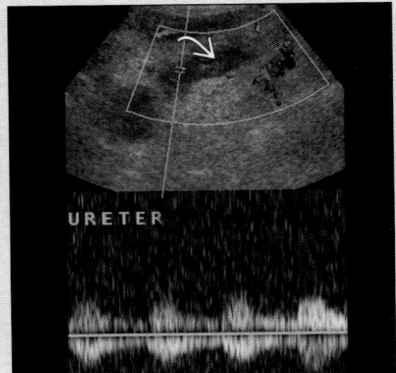 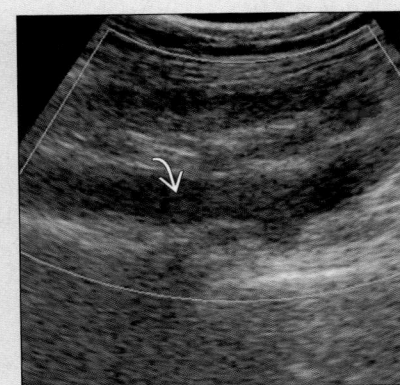

Dissecting AAA *Ureteric TCC* *Pelvic DVT*

AORTO-ILIAC OCCLUSIVE DISEASE

Key Facts

Imaging Findings

- **Grayscale (GS):** Useful for identifying plaques and calcification
- Not possible to determine the degree of arterial narrowing on GS alone
- Occlusive thrombus may be present in the lumen of the occluded aorta or iliac arteries
- **Pulsed Doppler (PuD):** Useful for evaluating waveform & measuring peak systolic velocity (PSV)
- Normal waveform: Triphasic with no spectral broadening
- **Color Doppler (CD):** Allows distinction of artery from vein (based on flow direction)
- Disturbance in flow usually apparent with ready demonstration of turbulent flow
- Helps in accurate PuD sampling

- **Power Doppler (PD):** More sensitive to low flow rates than CD
- Good for picking up slow flow distal to occlusions and collaterals
- Less dependent on flow rate and angle of ultrasound beam; does not depict flow direction
- Use 3.5-5 MHz transducer for the aorto-iliac segment
- Graded compression is useful when excessive bowel gas obscures aorta and iliac arteries
- Angle correction is crucial in spectral Doppler assessment

Diagnostic Checklist

- Use graded compression when excessive bowel gas obscures aorta and iliac arteries
- Arterial stenosis assessment should be based on the combined findings on GS, PuD, PD and CD

- Distal waveform monophasic with reduced systolic velocity
  - Occlusion
    - No flow
    - Preocclusive thump may be present just proximal to occlusion
    - Distal waveform is monophasic with reduced systolic velocity
- Color Doppler
  - **Color Doppler (CD):** Allows distinction of artery from vein (based on flow direction)
  - Disturbance in flow usually apparent with ready demonstration of turbulent flow
  - Helps in accurate PuD sampling
- Power Doppler
  - **Power Doppler (PD):** More sensitive to low flow rates than CD
  - Good for picking up slow flow distal to occlusions and collaterals
  - Less dependent on flow rate and angle of ultrasound beam; does not depict flow direction

Imaging Recommendations

- Best imaging tool
  - Magnetic resonance angiography is the preferred imaging modality in the author's institution because
    - Does not involve use of ionizing radiation
    - Provides good overall assessment of arterial tree with good correlation with conventional angiography
    - Excellent images for the lower limb run-off vessels
  - CT angiogram (CTA) also gives excellent depiction of aorto-iliac occlusive disease
- Protocol advice
  - Ultrasound
    - Use 3.5-5 MHz transducer for the aorto-iliac segment
    - Graded compression is useful when excessive bowel gas obscures aorta and iliac arteries
    - Assessment of the degree of aorta or arterial stenosis should be made by a combination of GS, PuD, CD and PD assessment

- Angle correction is crucial in spectral Doppler assessment
  - Multidetector CT (MDCT)
    - 100 mL of 350 mg iodine/mL contrast injected at 2.5-3 mL/s
    - Region of interest can be placed at the common femoral artery for smart preparation to guide start of acquisition
  - Magnetic resonance angiography (MRA)
    - Gadolinium contrast-enhanced 3D MRA superior to conventional time of flight or phase contrast technique; better signal to noise ratio and shorter scanning time
    - Moving table and appropriate software required
  - Digital subtraction angiography (DSA)
    - Usually reserved for patients undergoing endovascular intervention or have contraindications for the other non-invasive imaging modalities; e.g., cardiac pacemaker, metallic implants which may cause artifacts
    - Brachial or axillary artery puncture may be necessary in cases of bilateral iliac arteries or aortic occlusion; non invasive imaging with MRA or CTA usually preferred in such cases prior to intervention

DIFFERENTIAL DIAGNOSIS

Pelvic DVT
- May be mistaken for occluded iliac arteries unless CD or PuD assessment is made

Ureteric TCC
- May be mistaken for occluded aorta or iliac arteries unless CD or PuD assessment is made

Intraabdominal Lymphadenopathy
- May mimic occluded aorta or iliac arteries on GS
- Use of CD and PuD should allow correct identification of the aorta and iliac arteries

AORTO-ILIAC OCCLUSIVE DISEASE

PATHOLOGY

General Features
- Etiology
  - **Atherosclerotic occlusive disease**
    - Smoking, diabetes mellitus, hypertension, obesity, hypercoagulable states
  - **Non atherosclerotic occlusive disease**
    - Inflammatory: Takayasu arteritis, systemic giant cell arteritis, radiation induced arteritis, Behçet disease
    - Non-inflammatory: Adventitial cystic disease
    - Embolic: Acute onset usually in the presence of underlying stenosis, consider cardiac source (atrial fibrillation, endocarditis or atrial myxoma) and aortic source (thrombus in aneurysm)
    - Trauma: Acute onset, obstruction or obliteration of flow may be caused by dissection, tear or avulsion of vessel
    - Aneurysm: Accumulation of mural thrombus may cause narrowing of the lumen of aorta and iliac arteries

CLINICAL ISSUES

Presentation
- Most common signs/symptoms
  - Buttock claudication most common
  - Calf claudication, rest pain, arterial ulceration and gangrene may also be present if there is arterial occlusive disease distal to the iliac arteries

Treatment
- Multidisciplinary management approach advised
- **Medical**
  - Management of associated medical problems and treatment of modifiable risk factors
  - Antiplatelet therapy and anticoagulation may be considered
- Exercise therapy
  - Supervised graded exercise therapy has been shown to be useful in patients with intermittent claudication
- Choice of interventional radiological or surgical treatment in the iliac segment may be guided by the Transatlantic Inter-Society Consensus (TASC) groups A-D or Society of Interventional Radiology (SIR) categories 1-4 classification
  - TASC A/SIR Cat 1
  - Percutaneous endovascular treatment is the treatment of choice
  - Stenoses less than 3 cm in length that are concentric and non-calcified
  - TASC B/SIR Cat 2
  - Lesions well suited for percutaneous endovascular treatment
  - Stenoses 3-5 cm in length or calcified or eccentric stenosis less than 3 cm in length
  - TASC C/SIR Cat 3
  - Lesions amenable to percutaneous endovascular treatment but has a moderate chance of success compared with surgery

- Stenoses 5-10 cm in length or chronic occlusion less than 5 cm in length after thrombolytic therapy
- TASC D/SIR Cat 4
- Extensive vascular disease where percutaneous endovascular treatment has a limited role compared with surgical bypass
- Lesions are (a) stenoses greater than 10 cm in length, (b) chronic occlusions greater than 5 cm in length after thrombolytic therapy, (c) extensive bilateral aorto-iliac atherosclerotic disease, or (d) iliac stenoses in patients with abdominal aortic aneurysm or other lesions requiring aortic or iliac surgery
- **Interventional radiological**
- Infrarenal aorta
  - Bare metal stent (usually balloon mounted e.g., Palmaz stent) may be used for treatment of focal aortic stenosis
  - Surgery usually the treatment of choice when there is occlusion in the infrarenal aorta
- Iliac segment
  - Angioplasty or stenting (transluminal)
  - Technical success 95-99% for stenoses; 70-80% for occlusions
  - Stenting shown to have better long term patency with less requirement for long term intervention
- **Surgical**
- Endarterectomy may be required if there is occlusion in the infrarenal aorta
- Bypass options aorto-iliac occlusive disease
  - Aortobifemoral bypass
  - Iliofemoral bypass (ipsilateral or contralateral)
  - Axillofemoral bypass
  - Femorofemoral cross over graft

DIAGNOSTIC CHECKLIST

Consider
- Use graded compression when excessive bowel gas obscures aorta and iliac arteries

Image Interpretation Pearls
- Arterial stenosis assessment should be based on the combined findings on GS, PuD, PD and CD

SELECTED REFERENCES

1. Zwiebel WJ et al: Introduction to Vascular Ultrasonography. 5th ed. Philadelphia, Elsevier Saunders. 254-569, 2005
2. Dormandy JA et al: Management of peripheral arterial disease (PAD). TASC Working Group. TransAtlantic Inter-Society Consensus (TASC). J Vasc Surg. 31(1 Pt 2):S1-S296, 2000

IMAGE GALLERY

Typical

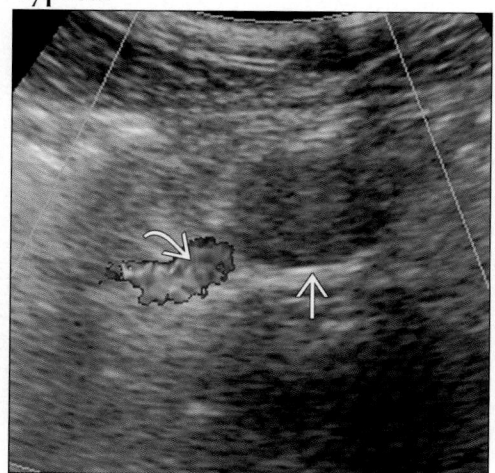
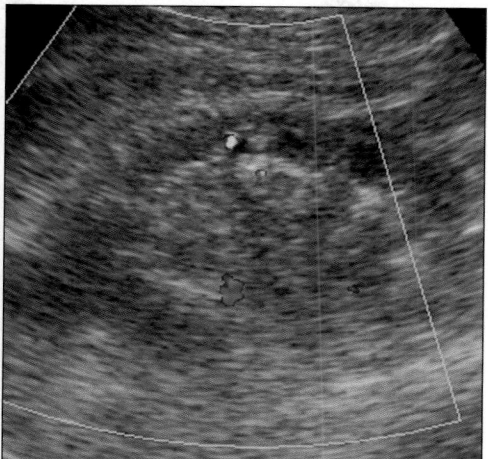

(Left) Transverse color Doppler ultrasound shows an aortic ➜ occlusion devoid of intraluminal color Doppler signal. However, color signal is clearly depicted in the IVC ➜ adjacent to it. *(Right)* Longitudinal color Doppler ultrasound of the left kidney shows scarce color flow detected intrarenally, concerning for left renal artery involvement. Same patient as previous image.

Typical

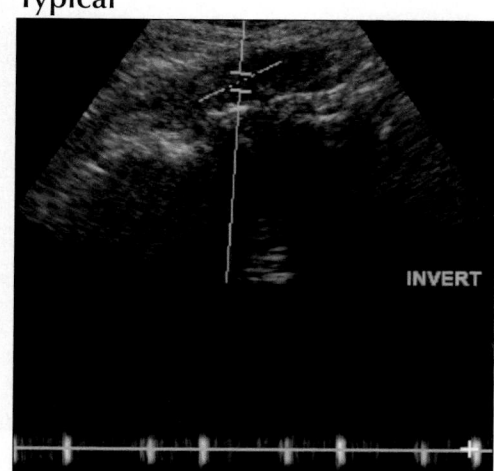
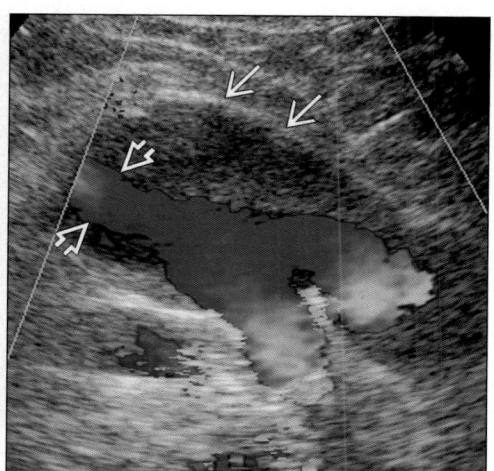

(Left) Longitudinal transabdominal ultrasound shows previous aortic total occlusion. Note there is no spectral Doppler signal detected. *(Right)* Longitudinal color Doppler ultrasound shows a moderate amount of mural thrombus ➜ in the infrarenal aorta just above the bifurcation, causing narrowing of the aortic lumen ➜.

Typical

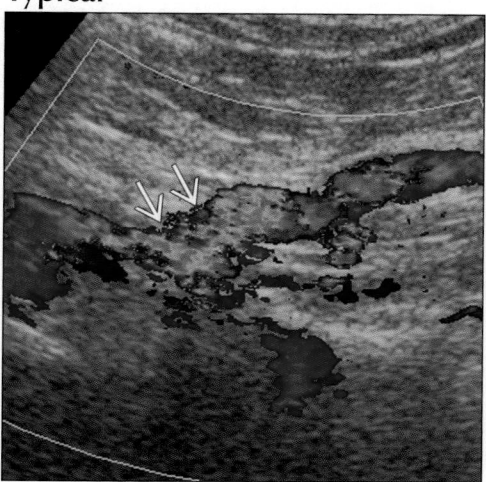
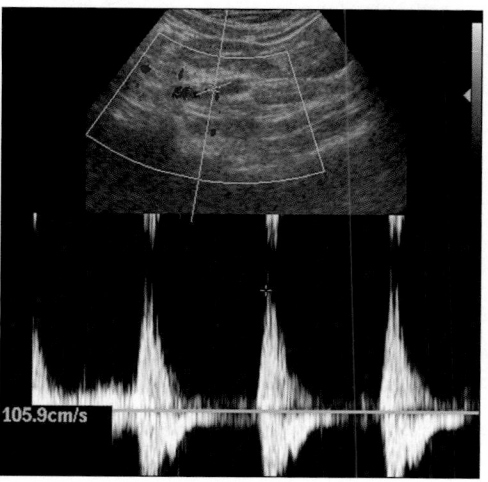

(Left) Oblique color Doppler ultrasound shows the common iliac artery (CIA) with > 50% diameter reduction. High-velocity turbulent flow ➜ is seen as "aliasing" artifact on color Doppler imaging at the stenotic segment. *(Right)* Corresponding oblique pulsed color Doppler ultrasound shows spectral Doppler trace at the CIA stenosis, with characteristic high-velocity bidirectional waveform.

Typical

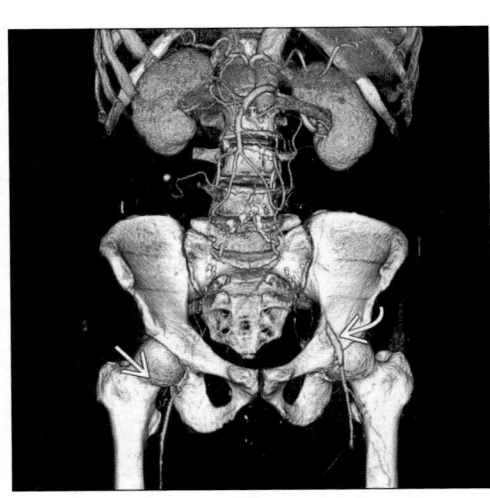
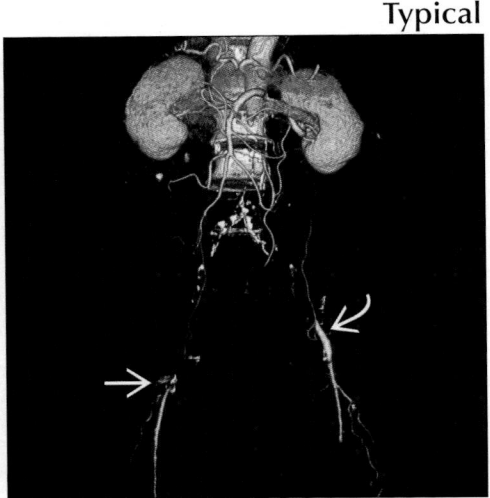

(Left) CTA shows a volume rendered image demonstrating complete occlusion of the left external iliac artery ➡. There is also an IVC filter in this image ➡. (Right) CTA shows maximal intensity projection (MIP) image of same patient as previous image, with demonstration of the left external iliac artery (EIA) occlusion ➡ and IVC filter ➡. A right nephrostomy catheter ➡ is also seen on this image.

Typical

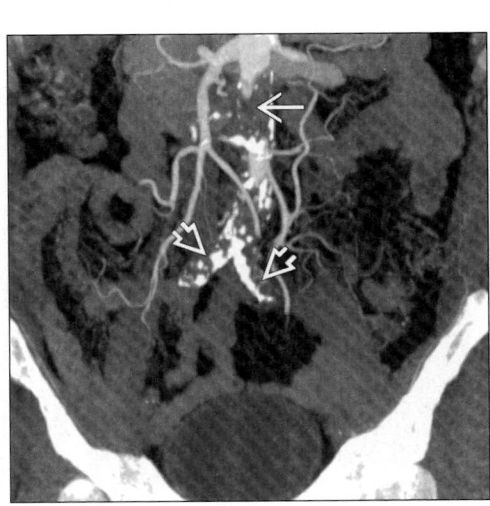
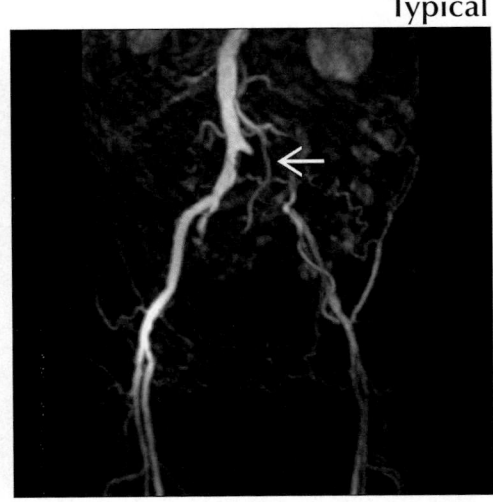

(Left) CTA shows a volume rendered image of a patient with complete occlusion of the infrarenal aorta and common iliac arteries. Note reconstitution of the profunda femoris artery (PFA) on the right ➡ and common femoral artery (CFA) on the left ➡. (Right) CTA shows a volume rendered image with bone removal. The reconstituted right PFA ➡ and left CFA ➡ are better seen.

Typical

(Left) CTA shows coronal reformatted image of the same patient as the previous image, with complete occlusion of the infrarenal aorta and common iliac arteries. Note hypodense thrombus within the infrarenal aorta ➡ and common iliac arteries ➡. (Right) MRA shows occlusion of the left common iliac artery ➡ in a different patient.

AORTO-ILIAC OCCLUSIVE DISEASE

Typical

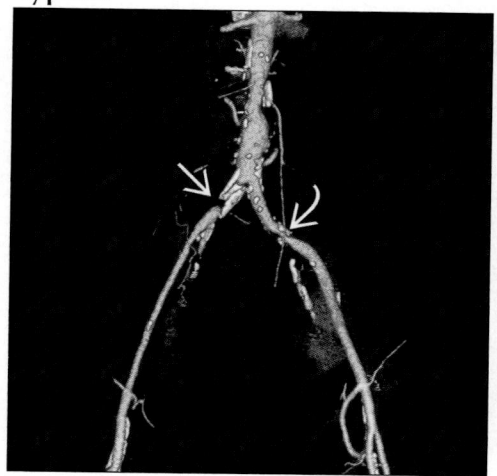
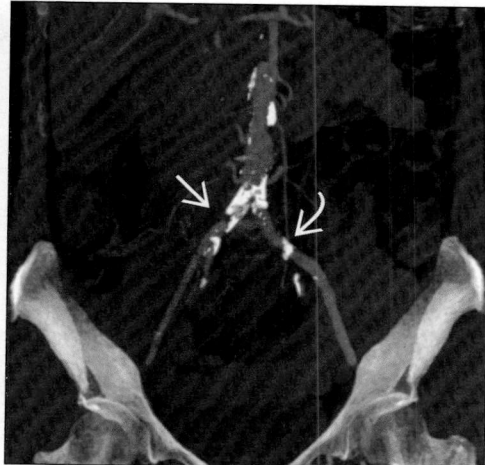

(Left) CTA shows a volume rendered image demonstrating occlusion of right CIA by calcified plaque ➔ and focal stenosis of the distal left CIA ➔. *(Right)* CTA shows a maximal intensity projection image of same patient as previous image, demonstrating occlusion of the right CIA by calcified plaque ➔ and focal stenosis of the distal left CIA ➔.

Typical

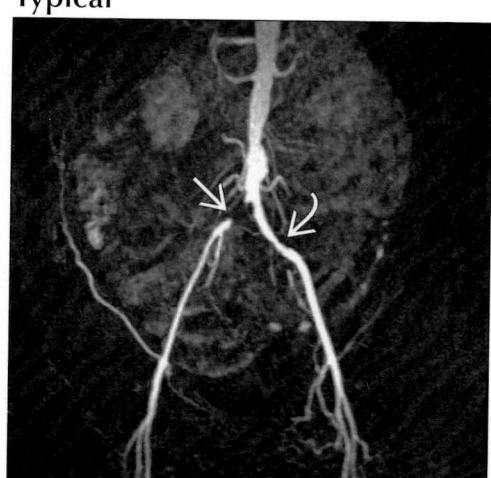
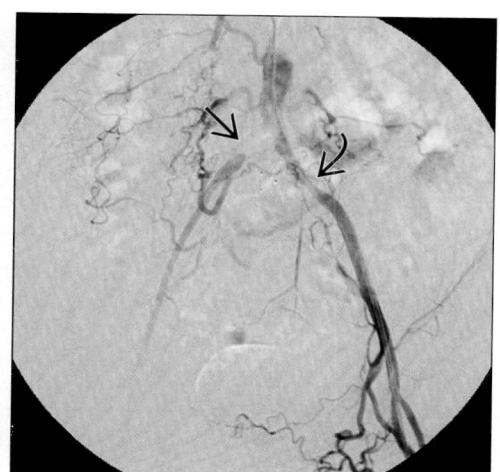

(Left) MRA shows occlusion of the right CIA ➔ and focal stenosis of the distal left CIA ➔ in the same patient as the previous image. *(Right)* DSA shows occlusion of the right CIA ➔ and focal stenosis of the distal left CIA ➔ in the same patient as previous image.

Typical

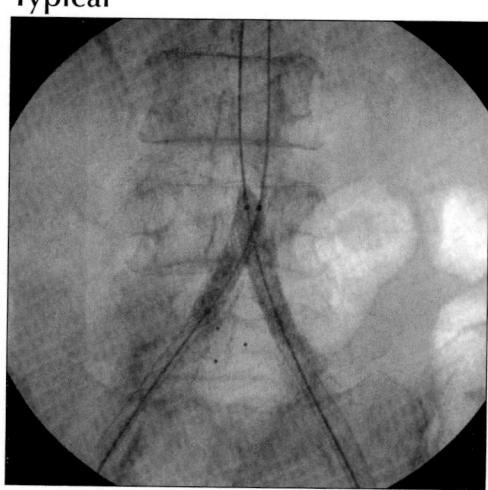
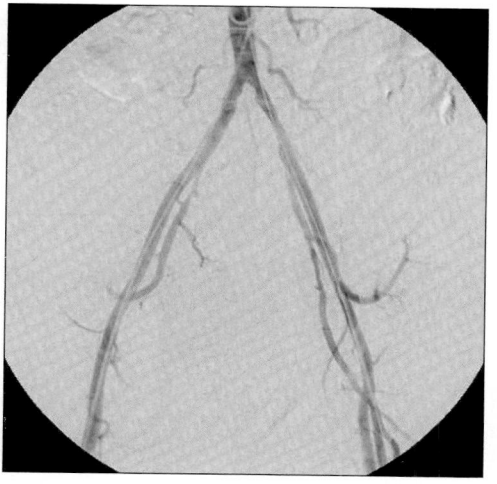

(Left) DSA shows an unsubtracted image demonstrating use of kissing balloon and kissing stent technique in treatment of right CIA occlusion and distal left CIA stenosis in the same patient as previous image. Note the simultaneous inflation of both angioplasty balloons within the deployed stents. *(Right)* DSA post bilateral CIA stenting shows restoration of flow through both CIAs.

IVC OBSTRUCTION

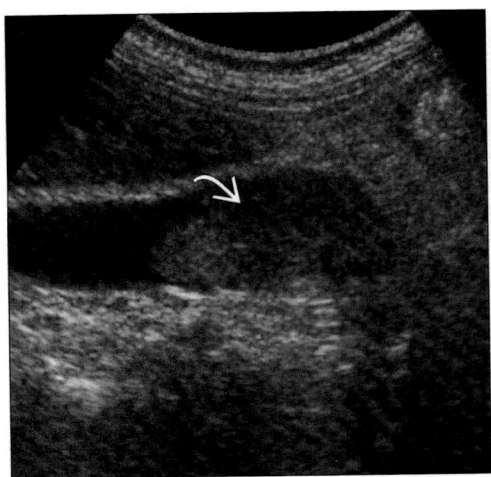 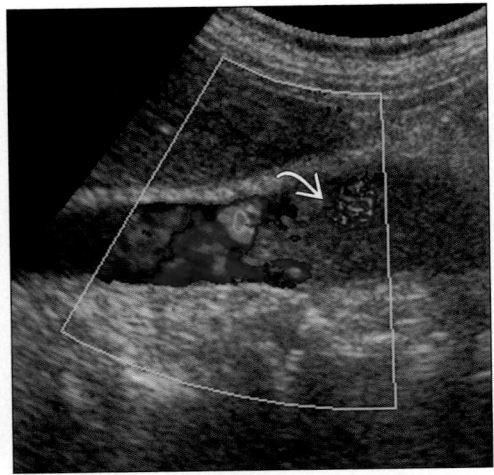

Longitudinal transabdominal ultrasound shows IVC thrombus ➡ in a patient with known sigmoid carcinoma.

Corresponding longitudinal color Doppler ultrasound shows IVC thrombosis ➡.

TERMINOLOGY

Abbreviations and Synonyms
- Inferior vena cava (IVC), obstruction, occlusion
- IVC thrombus

Definitions
- "Proximal" and "distal" in the venous system applies to the position of a vein segment in relation to the heart (rather than the flow direction of blood)

IMAGING FINDINGS

General Features
- Location
  - Thrombus usually propagates into the IVC from a tributary vessel
    - Common iliac veins (CIV), renal veins (RV), hepatic veins (HV)
  - Thrombus may also develop in the IVC secondary to obstructive processes that reduce flow
- Size

- Mean diameter of normal IVC is 17.2 mm (range 5-29 mm) just below renal veins during quiet respiration
- Diameter increases about 10% during deep inspiration
- Diameter of > 3 cm is a contraindication to IVC filter placement

Ultrasonographic Findings
- Grayscale Ultrasound
  - Acute IVC thrombosis
    - Presence of thrombus within the IVC
    - Echogenicity of thrombus varies with age: Fresh thrombus may be virtually anechoic while chronic thrombus tends to be more echogenic
    - Free-floating thrombus: Recently formed clot (is closer to the heart) may not adhere to the vein wall giving a tongue-like appearance
    - Distension of IVC
- Pulsed Doppler
  - Pulsed Doppler: Proximal portion has a pulsatile flow pattern due to right atrial pressure changes during cardiac cycle

DDx: IVC Obstruction

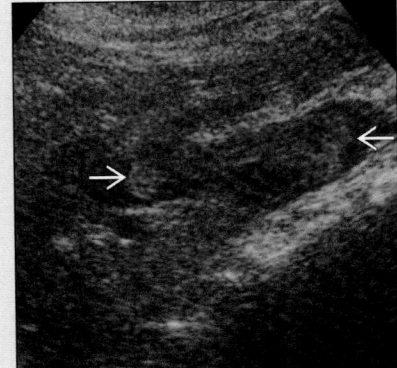 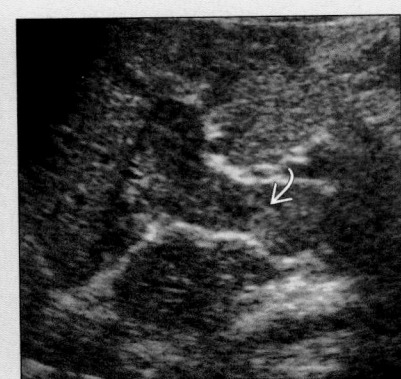 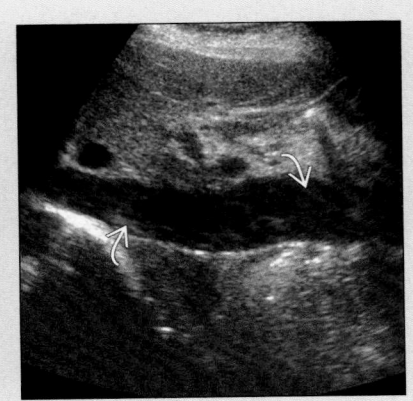

Renal Vein Thrombosis *Portal Vein Thrombosis* *Flow Artifact*

IVC OBSTRUCTION

Key Facts

Imaging Findings
- Presence of thrombus within the IVC
- Echogenicity of thrombus varies with age: Fresh thrombus may be virtually anechoic while chronic thrombus tends to be more echogenic
- Free-floating thrombus: Recently formed clot (is closer to the heart) may not adhere to the vein wall giving a tongue-like appearance
- Distension of IVC
- Pulsed Doppler: Proximal portion has a pulsatile flow pattern due to right atrial pressure changes during cardiac cycle
- In the more distal IVC above the CIV confluence, only respiratory variations may be seen

- Continuous flow (uniform flow without respiratory or cardiac variation) is a significant finding and should prompt investigation of more proximal obstruction in the IVC
- Color Doppler: Useful to detect low echo or anechoic thrombus, which may be missed on grayscale
- Useful for demonstration of recanalized lumen in the thrombus and collateralization
- May show flow within partially obstructed lumen and around free floating thrombus
- Power Doppler: Particularly useful to demonstrate slow flow in IVC

Diagnostic Checklist
- Acute IVC thrombosis may be hypoechoic and can be overlooked if color flow examination is not performed

---

- In the more distal IVC above the CIV confluence, only respiratory variations may be seen
- Partial obstruction may eliminate normal flow variation
- Continuous flow (uniform flow without respiratory or cardiac variation) is a significant finding and should prompt investigation of more proximal obstruction in the IVC
- Color Doppler
  - Color Doppler: Useful to detect low echo or anechoic thrombus, which may be missed on grayscale
  - Useful for demonstration of recanalized lumen in the thrombus and collateralization
  - May show absence of flow
  - May show flow within partially obstructed lumen and around free floating thrombus
- Power Doppler: Particularly useful to demonstrate slow flow in IVC

Imaging Recommendations
- Best imaging tool
  - Ultrasound
    - Good initial test to screen for IVC thrombus in cases of lower limb deep vein thrombosis
    - Look for causes of IVC obstruction
    - Useful for measurement of diameter of IVC and assessment of proximal extent of thrombus prior to intervention (e.g., IVC filter)
    - Visualization of infrahepatic portion of IVC and iliac veins, however, may be obscured by bowel gas
  - Multidetector CT (MDCT)
    - Probably best and most readily available imaging tool for IVC obstruction
    - Can demonstrate extent of IVC involvement
    - Provides excellent anatomical detail of abdomen and pelvis and delineates the cause of IVC obstruction
  - MR
    - MR venogram (MRV) useful for demonstrating patency of IVC

- Coupled with appropriate conventional sequences (e.g., T1 and T2 fat-saturation sequences) may also demonstrate cause of IVC obstruction
  - Digital subtraction venogram (DSV)
    - Usually performed as part of an interventional procedure, e.g., IVC filter or IVC stent placement
    - Useful for confirmation and exclusion of thrombus within the IVC
- Protocol advice
  - Ultrasound
    - Both longitudinal and transverse examination of the entire IVC (infrahepatic, intrahepatic and suprahepatic portions) should be carried out
    - Longitudinal scanning often more informative
    - Use 3.5-5 MHz transducer for the IVC
    - Graded compression may be useful when excessive bowel gas obscures the IVC and iliac veins
    - Angle correction is crucial for spectral Doppler assessment
    - Color flow Doppler examination mandatory to exclude hypoechoic acute thrombosis
    - Power Doppler may be useful in the detection of extremely low flow states
    - If IVC is thrombosed, involvement of tributaries and cause of obstruction (e.g., hepatic or tumors, extrinsic compression) should be ascertained

DIFFERENTIAL DIAGNOSIS

Renal Vein Thrombosis
- Renal vein thrombus may extend into the IVC

Portal Vein Thrombosis
- Careful tracing of the thrombosed vein to the pancreatic head should help to distinguish portal vein thrombosis from IVC thrombosis

Flow Artifact
- Due to sluggish flow in IVC

IVC OBSTRUCTION

IVC Anomalies
- Knowledge of congenital IVC variants such as duplication, interrupted IVC with azygous/hemiazygous continuation, transposition of the IVC (solitary left sided IVC) are important for correct diagnosis of IVC obstruction

PATHOLOGY

General Features
- **Intrinsic obstruction: Neoplastic**
  - Renal cell carcinoma (in 10%), Wilm tumor, hepatocellular carcinoma, hepatic adenocarcinoma, adrenal carcinoma, pheochromocytoma
  - Metastatic retroperitoneal lymph nodes (e.g., carcinoma of the ovaries, cervix and prostate)
- **Intrinsic obstruction: Non-neoplastic**
  - Proximally extending thrombus from iliofemoral deep vein thrombosis
  - Systemic disorders: Coagulopathy, Budd-Chiari syndrome, dehydration, nephrotic syndrome, infection (pelvic inflammatory disease), sepsis, congestive heart failure, nephrotic syndrome
  - Iatrogenic: IVC filter, IVC ligation or plication, surgical clip
  - Traumatic phlebitis
  - Severe exertion
- **Intrinsic caval disease: Neoplastic**
  - Leiomyoma, leiomyosarcoma, endothelioma
- **Intrinsic caval disease: Non-neoplastic**
  - Congental membrane
  - Interrupted IVC with azygous continuation
    - Incidence (0.6%), congenital failure to form subcardinohepatic anastomosis
    - Enlarged azygous and hemiazygous veins, paravertebral and retrocrural veins
    - No definable intrahepatic IVC
    - Iliac veins and renal veins drain via the azygous/hemiazygous system
    - Drainage of hepatic veins directly into the left atrium via the suprahepatic portion of the IVC
- **Extrinsic compression: Neoplastic**
  - Retroperitoneal lymphadenopathy due to metastatic disease or lymphoma
  - Renal or adrenal tumors (particularly in children, hepatic masses, pancreatic tumor)
  - Desmoplastic reaction to tumor (e.g., metastatic carcinoid)
- **Extrinsic compression: Non-neoplastic**
  - Hepatomegaly, massive ascites
  - Tortuous aorta/aortic aneurysm
  - Retroperitoneal hematoma, retroperitoneal lymphadenopathy (e.g., from granulomatous diseases such as TB), retroperitoneal fibrosis
- **Functional obstruction**
  - Pregnant uterus, Valsalva maneuver, straining/crying (in children), supine position with large abdominal mass
- Associated abnormalities
  - Interrupted IVC with azygous continuation
  - May be associated with congential heart disease, congenital pulmonary venolobar syndrome, indeterminate situs, polysplenia or asplenia (rare)

CLINICAL ISSUES

Presentation
- Most common signs/symptoms
  - Majority of cases (60-70%) in chronic obstruction may be asymptomatic as venous return is directed to the azygous/hemiazygous system and collaterals
  - In 20-30% of cases in chronic obstruction and in acute obstruction, patient may develop bilateral lower limb swelling and edema

Treatment
- Anticoagulation therapy with unfractioned and low molecular weight regimes followed by oral warfarinization as per treatment of deep vein thrombosis
- IVC filter insertion
  - Infrarenal placement of IVC filter preferred
  - Suprarenal placement shown to be reasonably safe, but theoretical risk of inducing renal vein thrombosis secondary to IVC thrombosis
  - IVC thrombosis/occlusion may occur secondary to IVC filter insertion
- Thrombolysis ± IVC filter placement to prevent pulmonary embolism has been advocated by some, though use limited by risk of major bleeding (11%) and stroke (3%)
- Surgery
  - IVC ligation used to be a surgical treatment option for recurrent pulmonary embolism from deep vein thrombosis
  - Surgical removal of the obstructing cause for the IVC obstruction
  - Venous bypasses may be considered in symptomatic chronic venous IVC obstruction

DIAGNOSTIC CHECKLIST

Image Interpretation Pearls
- Acute IVC thrombosis may be hypoechoic and can be overlooked if color flow examination is not performed

SELECTED REFERENCES

1. Zwiebel WJ et al: Introduction to Vascular Sonography. 5th edition. Philadelphia, Elsevier Saunders. 545-9, 2005
2. Ridwelski K et al: Primary sarcoma of the inferior vena cava: review of diagnosis, treatment, and outcomes in a case series. Int Surg. 86(3):184-90, 2001
3. Singh-Panghaal S et al: Inferior vena caval leiomyosarcoma: diagnosis and biopsy with color Doppler sonography. J Clin Ultrasound. 25(5):275-8, 1997

IMAGE GALLERY

Typical

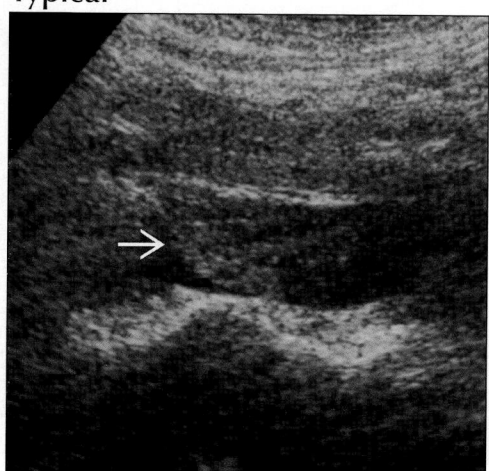
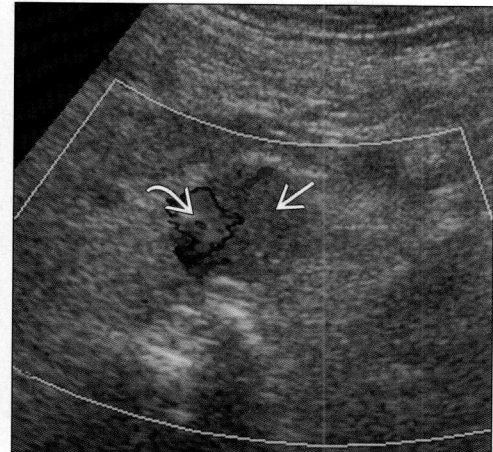

(Left) Longitudinal transabdominal ultrasound shows IVC tumor thrombus ➡ in a patient with known renal cell carcinoma (RCC). *(Right)* Transverse color Doppler ultrasound shows corresponding RCC tumor thrombus ➡ causing partial obstruction of IVC with incomplete color filling ➔ of lumen.

Typical

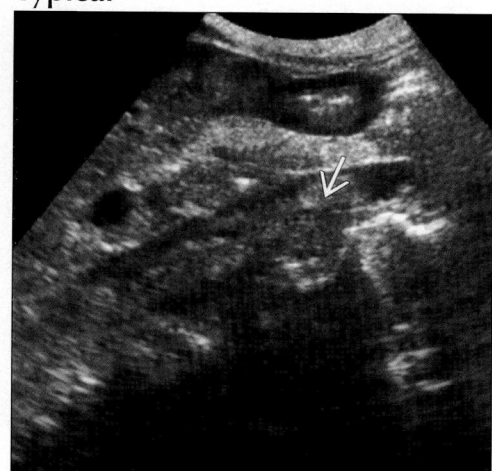
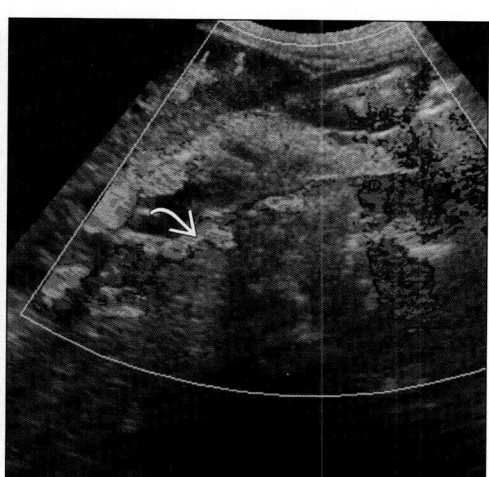

(Left) Longitudinal transabdominal ultrasound shows IVC partially filled with tumor thrombus ➡ in a patient with a history of colon cancer. *(Right)* Longitudinal color Doppler ultrasound shows color signals ➔ in the residual lumen of the IVC.

Typical

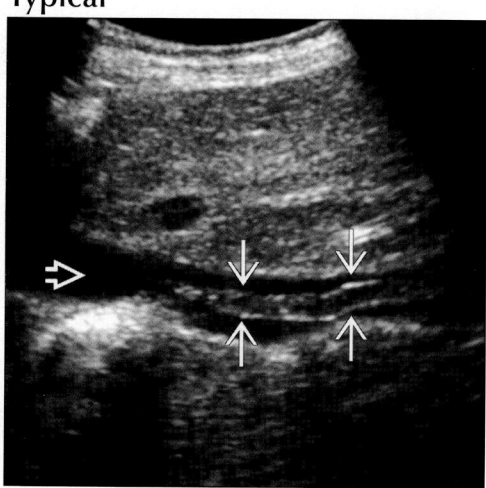
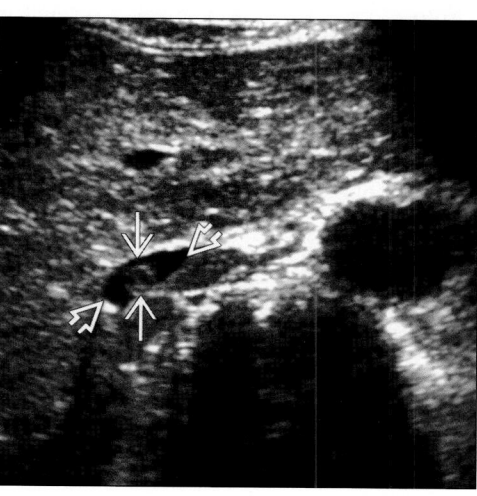

(Left) Longitudinal transabdominal ultrasound shows an echogenic "tongue" of thrombus ➔, extending from the iliac veins into the partially patent IVC ➔. *(Right)* Transverse transabdominal ultrasound shows corresponding thrombus ➡ within the partially patent IVC ➔.

(Left) Transverse transabdominal ultrasound shows a large complex cystic tumor ➡ compressing the IVC ➪. (Right) Transverse transabdominal ultrasound of the same patient as previous image demonstrates compressibility of the compressed IVC ➪ suggesting luminal patency.

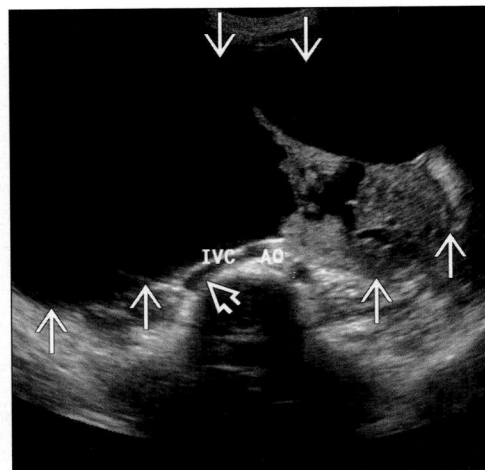
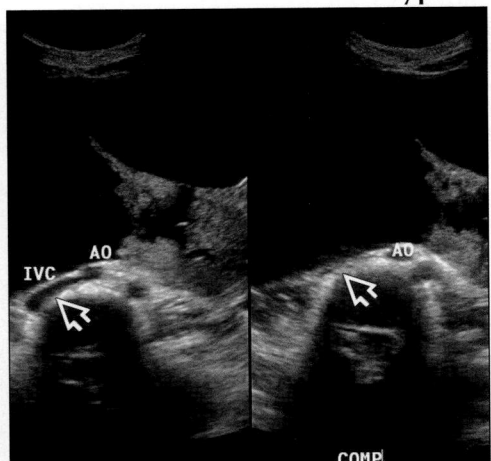

(Left) Longitudinal transabdominal ultrasound shows an echogenic IVC ➡ filter within the infrarenal IVC. Note echogenic material within the IVC filter, suggestive of thrombus. (Right) Corresponding longitudinal color Doppler ultrasound shows residual color flow through the partially thrombosed IVC (likely related to the in situ IVC filter).

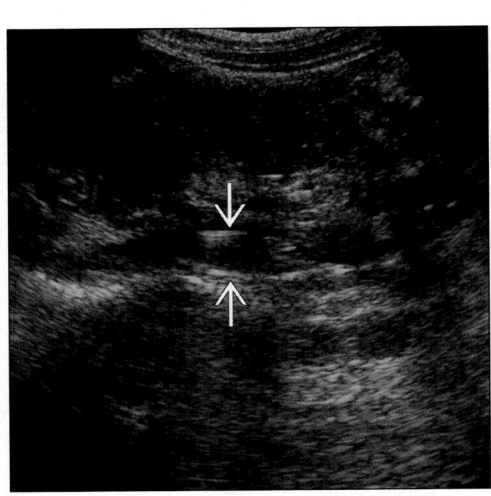
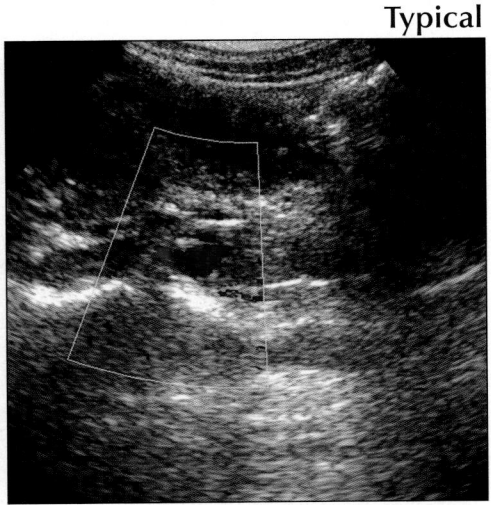

(Left) Nonsubtracted IVC cavogram in the same patient as above shows a filling defect within the IVC filter ➡. (Right) Corresponding subtracted IVC cavogram again demonstrates a filling defect (thrombus) within the IVC filter ➡.

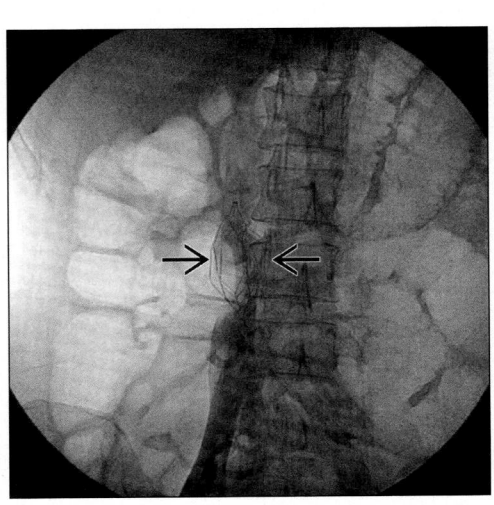
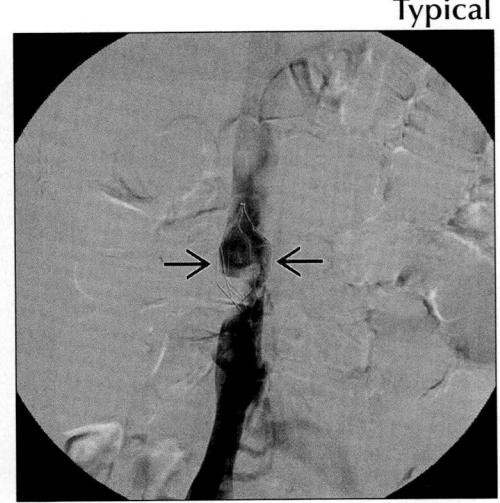

IVC OBSTRUCTION

Typical

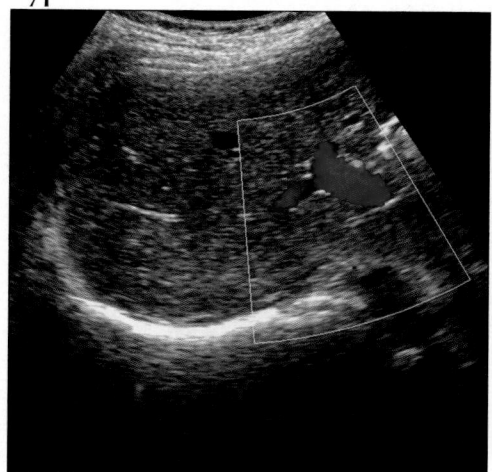
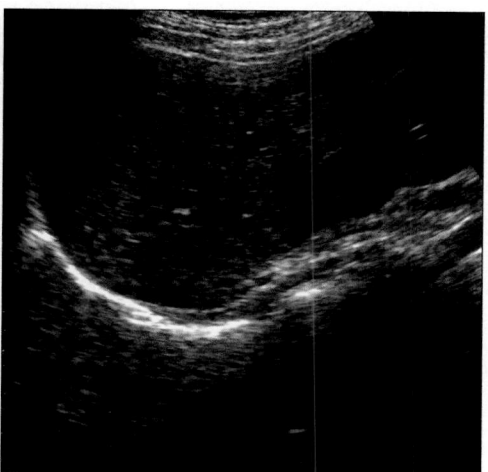

(Left) Transverse color Doppler ultrasound shows an absent intrahepatic IVC. This finding is suggestive of interrupted IVC with azygous/hemiazygous continuation. *(Right)* Longitudinal transabdominal ultrasound confirms absence of intrahepatic IVC.

Typical

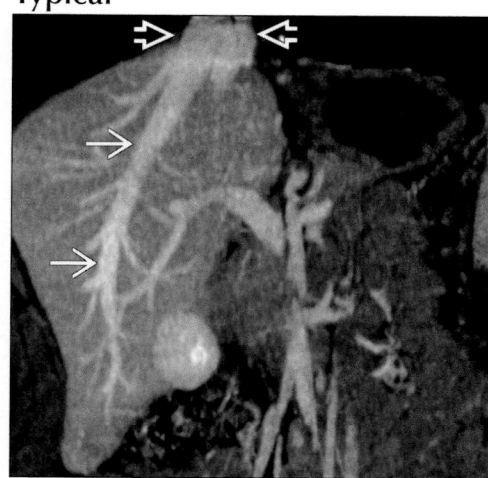
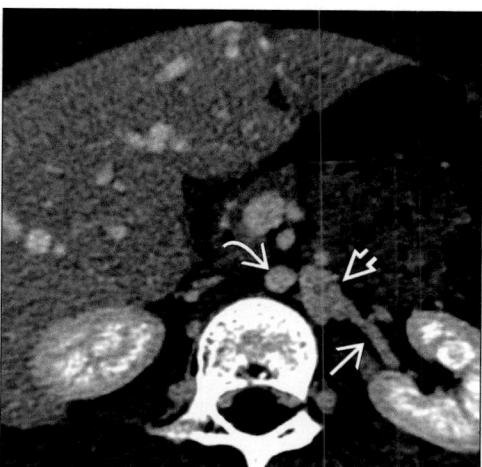

(Left) Coronal reformat multidetector contrast-enhanced CT image of the same patient as previous image, demonstrating absence of the intrahepatic and infrahepatic IVC. The right hepatic vein ➡ is seen to drain into the suprahepatic IVC ➡. *(Right)* Axial CECT of the same patient as the previous image at level of left renal vein ➡. Note absence of the IVC to the right of the aorta ➡ with the left renal vein drains into the dilated azygous vein ➡.

Typical

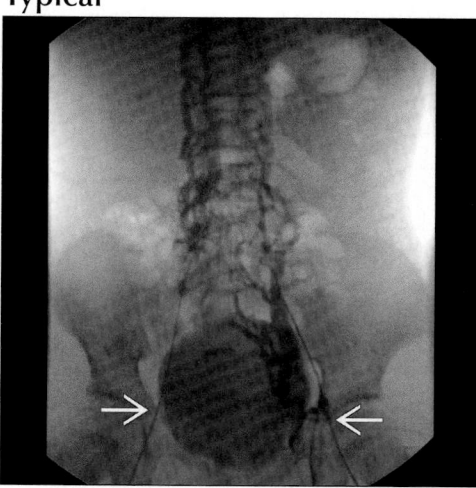
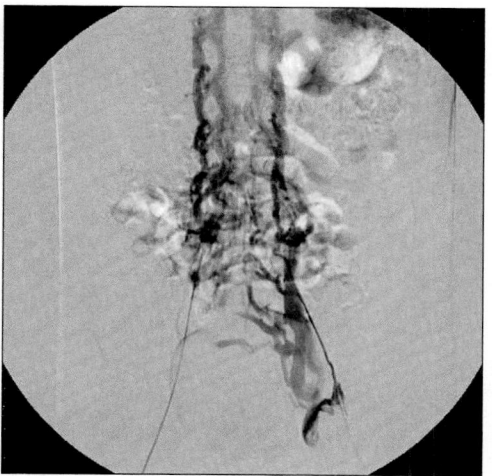

(Left) Unsubtracted venogram of the same patient as previous image with contrast injected via catheters ➡ inserted into both common femoral veins. Note absence of IVC and filling of the azygous/hemiazygous system and the paravertebral veins. *(Right)* Corresponding subtracted venogram again demonstrates contrast filling of the azygous/hemiazygous system and the paravertebral veins.

14

DEEP VEIN THROMBOSIS

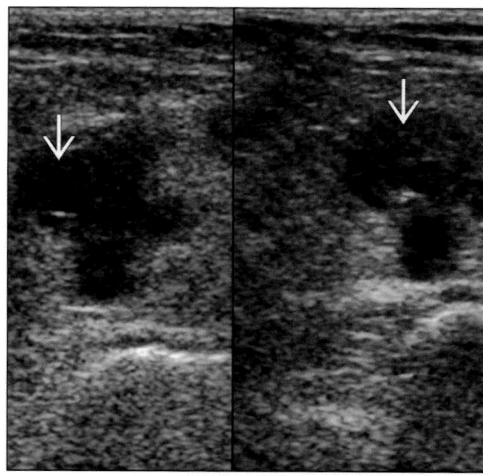

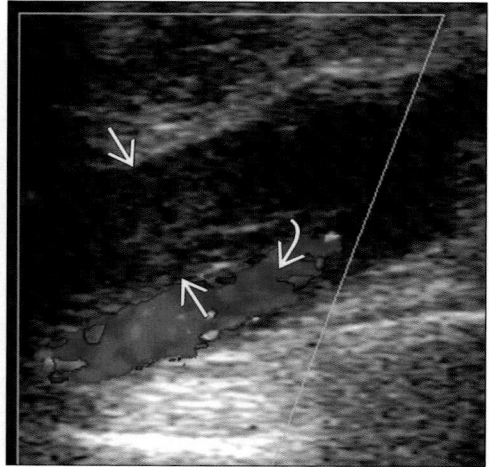

Transverse ultrasound shows acute DVT of the popliteal vein, filled with hypoechoic thrombus ➡️ (right) and incompressible with transducer pressure (left).

Corresponding longitudinal color Doppler ultrasound shows vein with absent intraluminal color signal ➡️, while the artery ➡️ posterior to it demonstrates complete color filling.

TERMINOLOGY

Abbreviations and Synonyms
- Deep vein thrombosis (DVT), pulmonary embolism (PE), venous thromboembolic disease (VTE)

Definitions
- Deep vein thrombosis is a condition by which blood changes from liquid to solid state and produces a blood clot (thrombus) within the deep venous system typically in the lower limbs
- It can also be seen in the upper limbs (especially related to central venous catheters)
- Pulmonary embolism is defined as obstruction of the pulmonary artery or one of its branches by an embolus, usually a blood clot derived from thrombosis of the leg veins
- Venous thromboembolic disease refers to deep vein thrombosis and pulmonary embolism, related aspects of the same disease process

IMAGING FINDINGS

Ultrasonographic Findings
- Grayscale Ultrasound
  - Acute thrombosis (~ 14 days)
    - Low echogenicity thrombus: May be virtually anechoic, flow may be seen within recanalized thrombus
    - Venous distension: Recently thrombosed veins are distended and substantially larger than accompanying artery
    - Loss of compressibility: Thrombus is excluded if vein can be completely compressed
    - Free floating thrombus: Most recently formed clot (usually on the end closer to the heart) may not adhere to the vein wall
    - Collateralization: Tortuous and braided collateral veins, usually smaller than the normal vein
  - Subacute thrombosis (~ 2 weeks to 6 months)
    - Thrombus becomes more echogenic, variable
    - Decrease thrombus and vein size: Retraction and lysis may reduce size of vein which may even be normal

DDx: Deep Vein Thrombosis

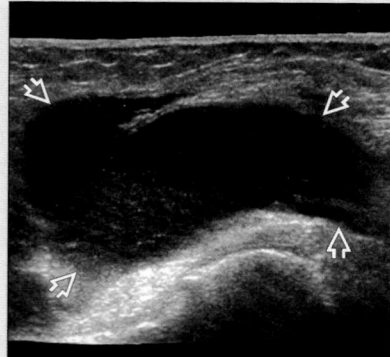

Baker Cyst

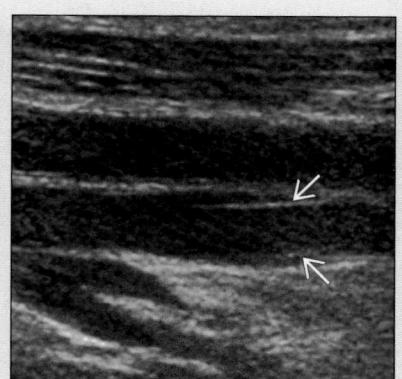

Thicken Valves

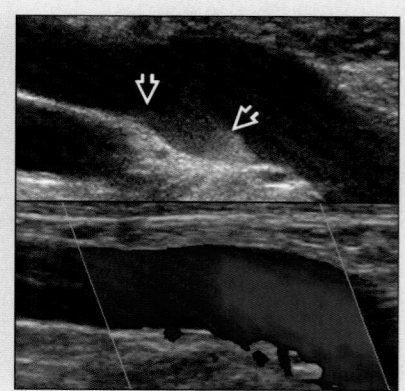

Artifactual "Echocontrast"

DEEP VEIN THROMBOSIS

Key Facts

Imaging Findings
- Acute thrombosis (~ 14 days)
- Low echogenicity thrombus: May be virtually anechoic, flow may be seen within recanalized thrombus
- Venous distension: Recently thrombosed veins are distended and substantially larger than accompanying artery
- Loss of compressibility: Thrombus is excluded if vein can be completely compressed
- Free floating thrombus: Most recently formed clot (usually on the end closer to the heart) may not adhere to the vein wall
- Collateralization: Tortuous and braided collateral veins, usually smaller than the normal vein

- Color Doppler: Useful to detect low echo or anechoic thrombus which may be missed on grayscale US
- Duplex Doppler ultrasound is first line imaging investigation with sensitivity and specificity for acute symptomatic DVT between 90-100%
- CECT and MR/MR venography are good non-invasive imaging tools for assessment of pelvic veins and IVC and for exclusion of pelvic and abdominal causes of DVT

Clinical Issues
- Acute DVT: Swollen and tender lower limb (extent of swelling depends on site of DVT), increased temperature
- Chronic leg swelling, ankle pigmentation, and ulceration in the lower calf and ankle (gaiter zone)

- Adherence of thrombus: Free floating thrombus becomes attached to vein wall
- Resumption of flow: Luminal flow may be restored; but vein may remain occluded
- Collateralization: Collateral venous channel continues to develop
  - Chronic phase (≥ 6 months)
    - Post-thrombotic scarring: Thrombus that has not lysed will be invaded by fibroblasts in process of becoming organized as fibrous tissue
    - Wall thickening: Scarred veins are thick-walled with reduced luminal diameter
    - Echogenic intraluminal material: Post thrombotic fibrous scars which appear as plaque-like areas along the vein and may occasionally calcify
    - Synechiae: Formed from unlysed thrombus that is attached to one side of the vein wall and gradually transformed into a fibrous band
    - Fibrous cord: In veins which fail to recanalize, vein may be reduced to an echogenic cord which is much smaller than normal vein
    - Valve abnormalities: Valve damage is frequently associated with venous thrombosis, and thickening of valve cusps and restricted cusp motion may result leading to reflux and venous stasis
- Pulsed Doppler
  - Spontaneous flow (any waveform present)
    - Expected in medium to large veins, but flow is often not spontaneous in smaller calf veins
  - Phasic flow (variation in flow velocity with respiration)
    - When phasic pattern is absent, flow is described as continuous, indicating the presence of obstruction closer to the heart
  - Valsalva maneuver
    - Causes abrupt cessation of blood flow in large and medium size veins documenting patency of venous system from point of examination to thorax
  - Augmentation (↑ in flow velocity with distal compression)

- Absence of this response indicates presence of obstruction further away from the heart to the site of examination
- Color Doppler
  - Color Doppler: Useful to detect low echo or anechoic thrombus which may be missed on grayscale US
  - Demonstration of recanalized lumen in the thrombus and collateralization
  - Demonstration of reflux in valvular incompetence
- Power Doppler: Particularly useful in the demonstration of slow flow through recanalized lumen and collaterals

Imaging Recommendations
- Best imaging tool
  - Duplex Doppler ultrasound is first line imaging investigation with sensitivity and specificity for acute symptomatic DVT between 90-100%
  - CECT and MR/MR venography are good non-invasive imaging tools for assessment of pelvic veins and IVC and for exclusion of pelvic and abdominal causes of DVT
  - Conventional venography has a false negative rate of 11% and should be reserved for use as problem solving aid

DIFFERENTIAL DIAGNOSIS

Interpretation Errors
- Baker cyst, artifactual "echocontrast" from slow flow, thickened valve mistaken for thrombus in chronic venous obstruction, failure to identify duplicated vein

Technical Errors
- Inadequate compression, improper use of color flow image, poor venous distension, misidentification of deep vs. superficial veins

DEEP VEIN THROMBOSIS

PATHOLOGY

General Features
- Genetics
  - A number of inherited prothrombotic disease states have been described
  - Antithrombin III deficiency, protein C and protein S deficiency, factor V Leiden, factor II G20210A, primary hyperhomocysteinemia, Dysfibrinogenemias and Hypofibrinolysis
- Etiology
  - Acquired prothrombotic states associated with DVT
  - Immobilization, surgery within 3 months (especially on legs/pelvis), stroke, paralysis of extremities, history of DVT (risk factor 2.5)
  - Obesity (risk factor 1.5), malignancy (risk factor 2.5; either as part of a paraneoplastic syndrome or by obstruction to the deep venous system), cigarette smoking, hypertension
  - Oral contraception and hormone replacement therapy (risk factor 3.2), pregnancy and puerperium, secondary homocystinemia
  - Antiphospholipid syndrome, congestive heart failure, myeloproliferative disorders, nephrotic syndrome, inflammatory bowel disease, sickle cell anemia, polycythemia, age > 40 (risk factor 2.2)
- Epidemiology
  - VTE: 70-113 cases/100,000/year; DVT: 48/100,000; PE: 23/100,000 in clinical studies in Caucasians with no post mortem data
  - Race/ethnicity: 2.5-4x lower risk of development of VTE amongst Hispanics and Asian-Pacific islanders compared with Caucasians and African-Americans
  - Seasonal variation: More common in winter than summer
  - About 25-50% idiopathic

CLINICAL ISSUES

Presentation
- Most common signs/symptoms
  - Acute DVT: Swollen and tender lower limb (extent of swelling depends on site of DVT), increased temperature
  - Post thrombotic syndrome: Sequelae of DVT resulting from chronic venous obstruction and/or acquired incompetence of valves
  - Chronic leg swelling, ankle pigmentation, and ulceration in the lower calf and ankle (gaiter zone)
- Other signs/symptoms: Signs and symptoms from pulmonary embolism: Shortness of breath, pleuritic chest pain, tachycardia, hypoxia, hypotension

Demographics
- Age: Exponential increase in VTE with age particularly over 40 yrs; 25-30 yr old ~ 30 cases/100,000; 70-79 yr old ~ 300-500 cases/100,000
- Gender: M = F

Natural History & Prognosis
- Tibial/peroneal thrombi resolve spontaneously in 40%, stabilize in 40%, propagate to popliteal vein in 20%
- Likelihood for pulmonary embolism: Iliac veins (77%), femoropopliteal veins (35-67%), calf veins (0-46%)
- Post thrombotic syndrome in 20% of DVT
- Death after treated VTE: 30 day incidence ~ 6% after incident DVT; 30 day incidence ~ 12% after PE; death associated with cancer, age and cardiovascular disease

Treatment
- Anticoagulation therapy indicated for above knee DVT and PE; treatment for calf vein DVT controversial
- Heparin anticoagulation, both unfractionated or low molecular weight regimes, are effective initial treatment for acute DVT
- Oral warfarin may be started once therapeutic levels of heparinization have been achieved; guided by International normalized ratio (INR)
- Warfarinization for DVT usually 3 months; generally longer for PE; maybe life long for recurrent DVT/PE or prothrombotic tendencies
- IVC filter considered for patients with high risk of PE (e.g., patients with fresh iliac vein or IVC thrombus) or patients who are not suitable for anticoagulation (e.g., recent surgery, bleeding peptic ulcer, bleeding diatheses)
- Thrombolysis reduces the prevalence and severity of post thrombotic syndrome and is considered in extensive ilio-femoral venous thrombosis and venous gangrene; but its use is limited by the contraindications, increased risk of major bleeding (11%) and stroke (3%)
- Surgery still has an important role in management of chronic venous obstruction: Valve repair or transplantation, perforator interruption or stripping of superficial venous system if deep venous system is patent, venous bypasses

DIAGNOSTIC CHECKLIST

Image Interpretation Pearls
- Thrombus is excluded if the vein is completely compressed

SELECTED REFERENCES

1. Zwiebel WJ et al: Introduction to Vascular Sonography. 5th edition. Philadelphia, Elsevier Saunders. 403-78, 2005
2. White RH. Related Articles et al: The epidemiology of venous thromboembolism. Circulation. 107(23 Suppl 1):I4-8, 2003
3. Dähnert W: Deep vein thrombosis. In: Radiology Review Manual. 3rd edition. Baltimore, William & Wilkins. 462-3, 1996

IMAGE GALLERY

Typical

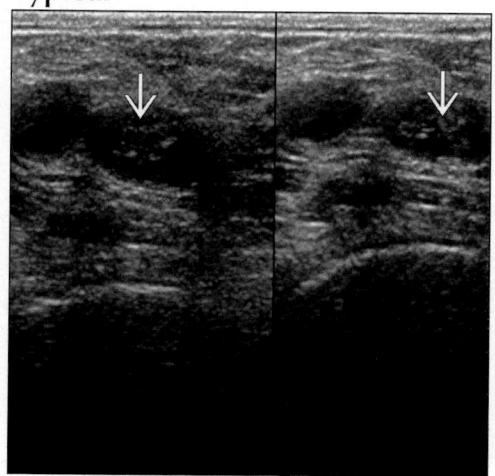 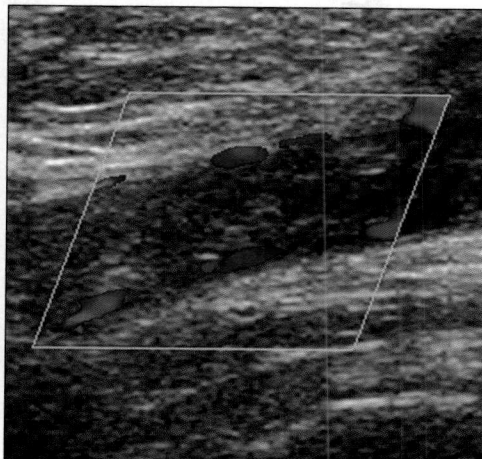

(Left) Transverse ultrasound shows thrombosis of the common femoral vein (CFV) ➡. The vessel is non-compressible (right side of image). *(Right)* Corresponding longitudinal color Doppler ultrasound shows DVT of CFV with partial color filling.

Typical

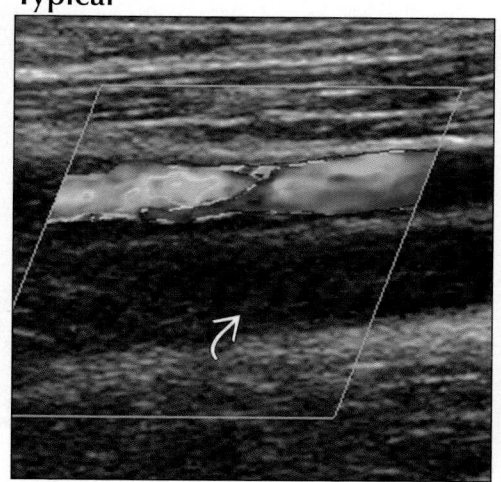 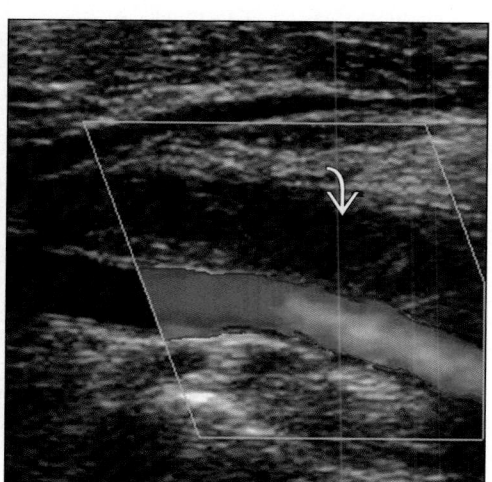

(Left) Longitudinal color Doppler ultrasound shows acute thrombosis of the superficial femoral vein (SFV) ➡. *(Right)* Longitudinal color Doppler ultrasound shows acute thrombosis of the popliteal vein ➡.

Typical

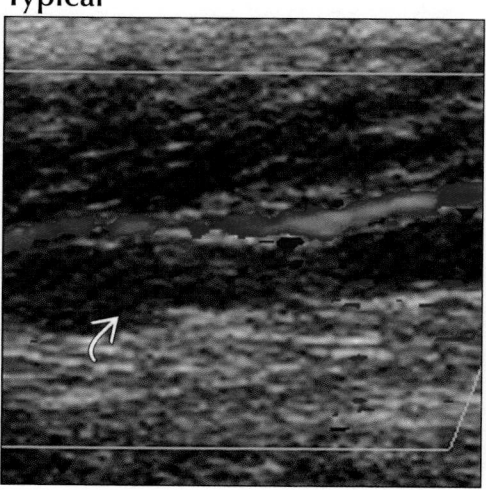 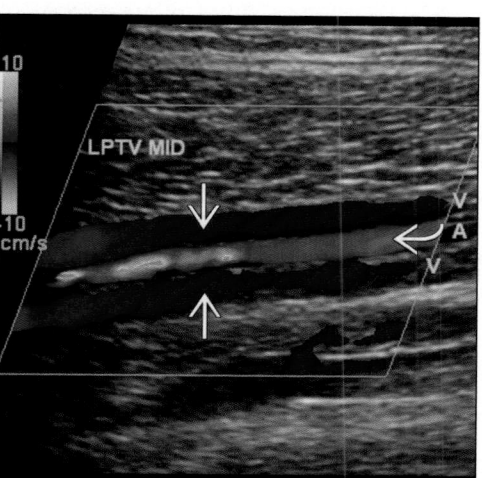

(Left) Longitudinal color Doppler ultrasound shows thrombosis of one of the posterior tibial veins (PTV) ➡. *(Right)* Longitudinal color Doppler ultrasound shows a normal posterior tibial artery ➡ accompanied by a pair of normal, patent, posterior tibial veins ➡. Note that calf veins are usually paired.

14

DEEP VEIN THROMBOSIS

(**Left**) Longitudinal color Doppler ultrasound shows acute thrombosis of the peroneal veins ➡. Note paired thrombosed peroneal veins ➡ are accompanied by small peroneal artery ➡. (**Right**) Transverse ultrasound shows chronic DVT of the SFV. The thrombosed vein ➡ is contracted and filled with echogenic thrombus.

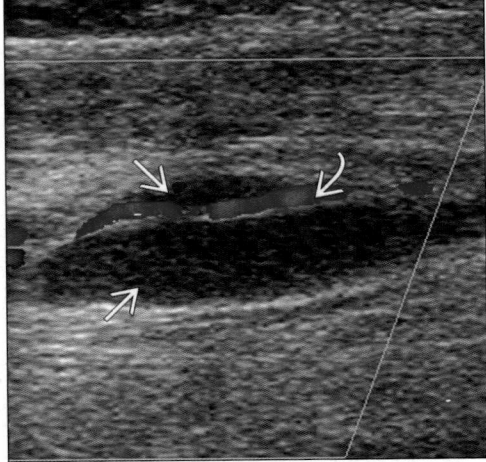
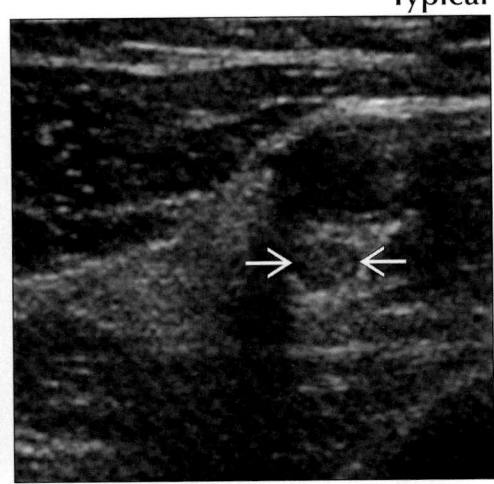

(**Left**) Longitudinal ultrasound shows a soleal vein thrombosis with intraluminal incompressible, hypoechoic thrombus ➡. Note sluggish flow in the soleal vein may mimic venous thrombosis. (**Right**) Longitudinal color Doppler ultrasound shows chronic DVT with partial recanalization of thrombus ➡.

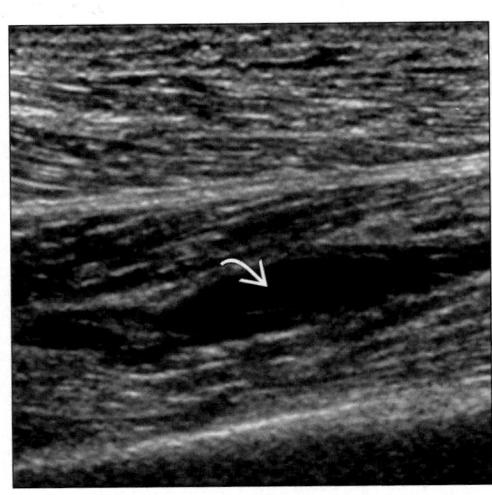
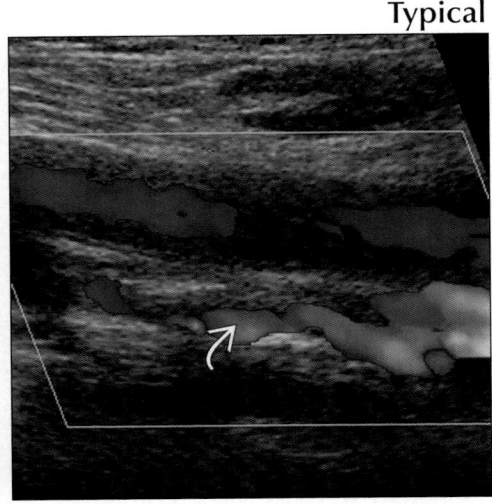

(**Left**) Transverse ultrasound shows chronic DVT with a contracted thrombus ➡. (**Right**) Longitudinal ultrasound shows chronic DVT within the CFV. Note the thrombosed vein ➡ contains multiple calcifications ➡ with acoustic shadowing.

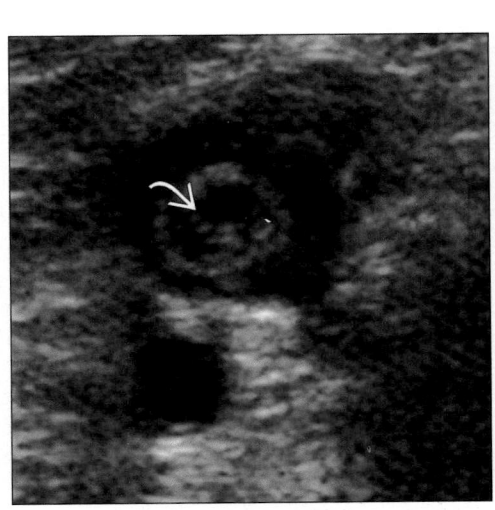
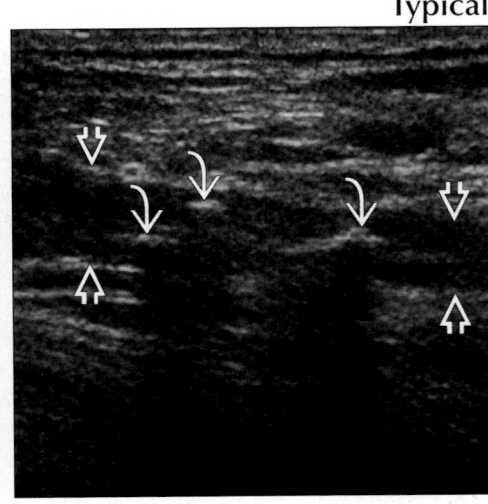

Typical

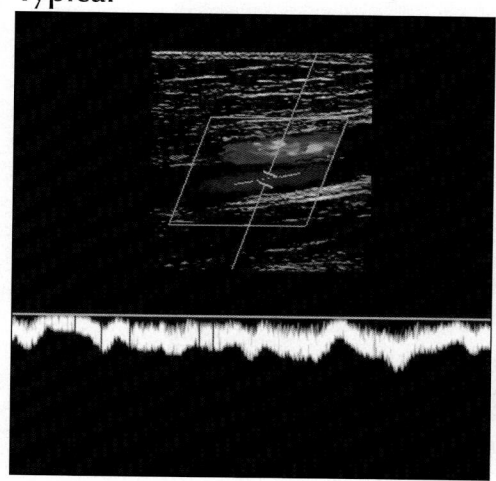
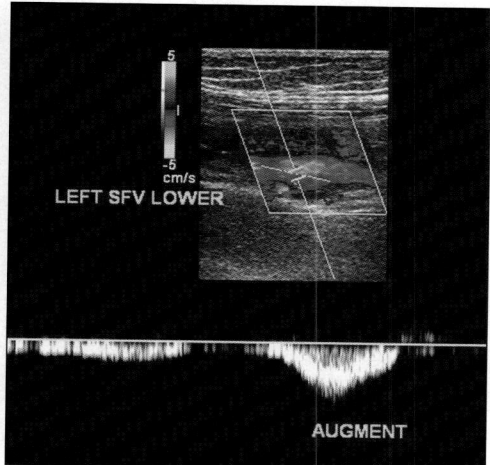

(Left) Longitudinal pulsed Doppler ultrasound shows the normal variation in phasic flow in the SFV. Note phasic variation is absent and becomes continuous if an obstructing lesion is present between the site of examination and heart. *(Right)* Longitudinal pulsed Doppler ultrasound shows normal augmentation in the SFV when the calf is compressed. This indicates there are no obstructing lesions between the site of examination and calf.

Typical

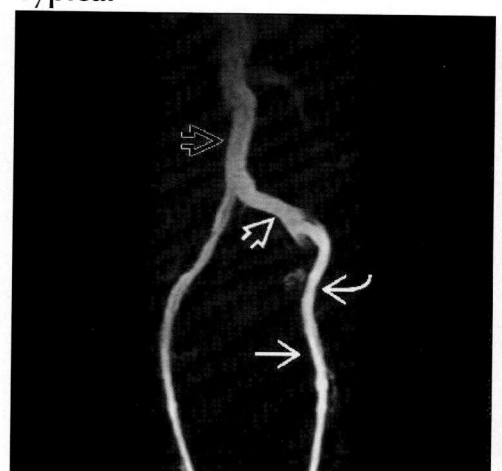
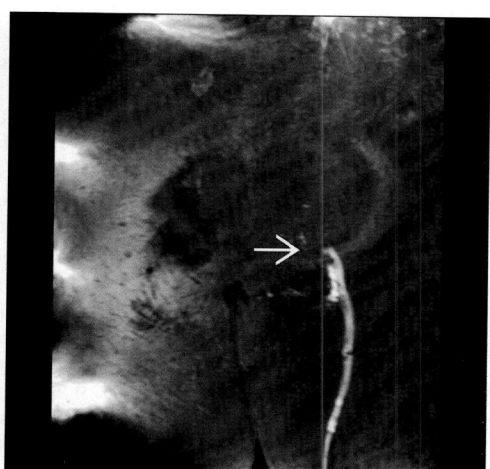

(Left) MR venogram of the common femoral veins ➡, external iliac veins ➡, common iliac veins ➡ and inferior vena cava ➡. Contrast was injected simultaneously via pedal veins in both feet. *(Right)* MRV shows obstruction to flow of contrast at the origin of the left external iliac vein (EIV) ➡ indicating thrombosis of the left EIV.

Other

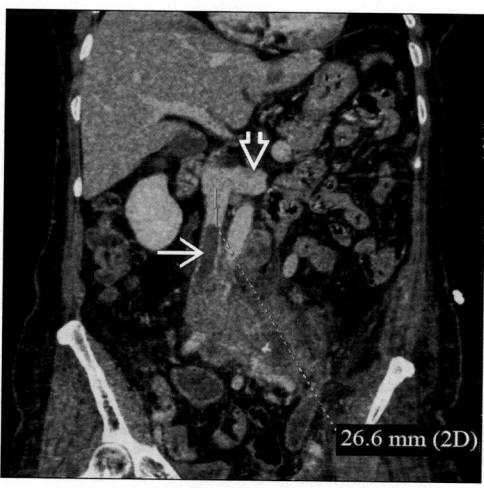
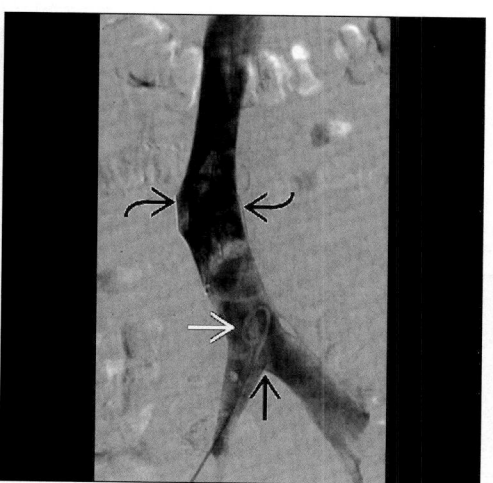

(Left) Oblique CECT shows nonenhancing thrombus within the infrarenal IVC ➡. Distance between the left renal vein ➡ and the top of the IVC thrombus was measured (26.3 mm) for assessment of suitability for IVC filter deployment. *(Right)* IVC cavogram with pigtail catheter ➡ positioned above the common iliac vein confluence ➡. An IVC filter ➡ is seen within the infrarenal IVC with thrombus (filling defects) trapped within it.

EXTREMITY ARTERIAL OCCLUSIVE DISEASE

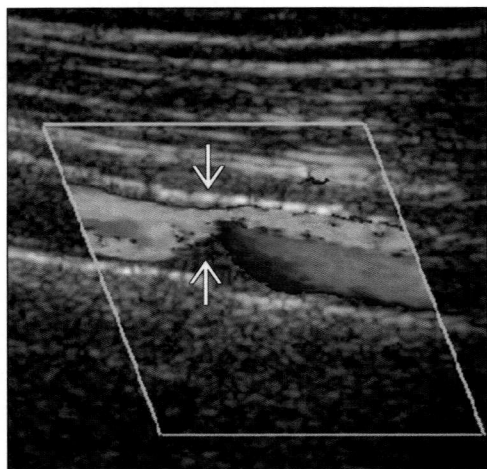

Longitudinal color Doppler ultrasound shows a turbulent flow at stenotic site in a superficial femoral artery ➡.

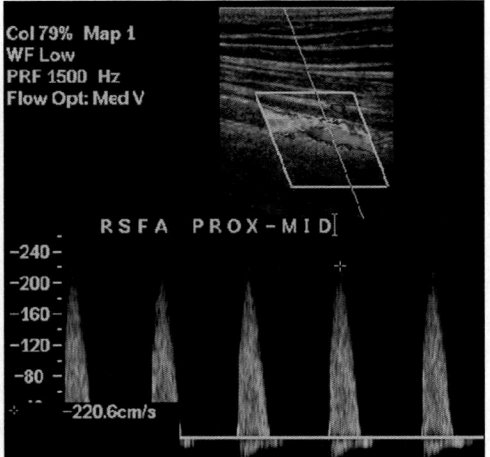

Longitudinal pulsed Doppler ultrasound shows markedly increased peak systolic velocity (220 cm/s), monophasic waveform, spectral broadening with loss of reverse phase flow suggestive of 50-99% stenosis.

TERMINOLOGY

Definitions
- Stenosis: Area with diameter narrowing of arterial lumen; increasing peak systolic velocity is seen with increasingly narrowed lumen due to turbulent flow
- Occlusion: Area where the lumen is completely blocked with no flow present

IMAGING FINDINGS

Ultrasonographic Findings
- Grayscale Ultrasound
  - **Grayscale (GS):** Useful for identifying plaques, calcification and anatomical variations
  - Not possible to determine the degree of arterial narrowing on grayscale alone
- Pulsed Doppler
  - **Pulsed Doppler (PuD):** Useful for evaluating waveform
  - Measures peak systolic velocity
  - Normal
    - Triphasic waveform
      - No spectral broadening
  - 1-19% diameter reduction
    - Triphasic waveform with minimal spectral broadening
    - Peak systolic velocity increase < 30% relative to adjacent proximal segment
    - Proximal and distal waveforms remain normal
  - 20-49% diameter reduction
    - Triphasic waveform usually maintained, but reverse flow diminished
    - Spectral broadening prominent
    - Filling in of clear area under the systolic peak
    - Peak systolic velocity increase 30-100% relative to adjacent proximal segment
    - Proximal and distal waveforms remain normal
  - 50-99% diameter reduction
    - Monophasic waveform, loss of reverse flow and forward flow throughout cardiac cycle
    - Extensive spectral broadening
    - Peak systolic velocity > 100% relative to adjacent proximal segment
    - Distal waveform monophasic with reduced systolic velocity
  - Occlusion

DDx: Extremity Arterial Occlusive Disease

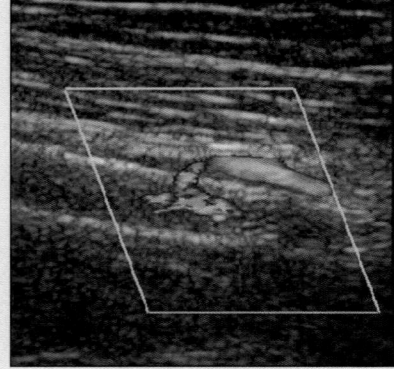

Arterial Collateral

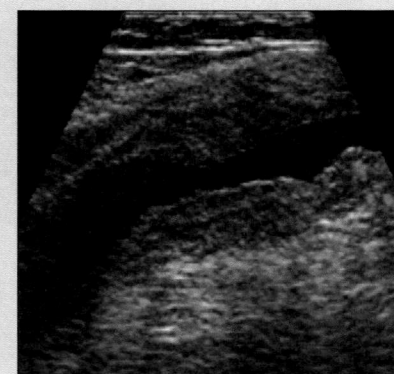

Popliteal Artery Aneurysm

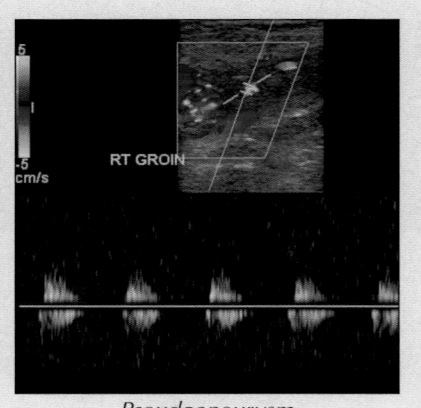

Pseudoaneurysm

EXTREMITY ARTERIAL OCCLUSIVE DISEASE

Key Facts

Imaging Findings
- **Grayscale (GS)**: Useful for identifying plaques, calcification and anatomical variations
- Not possible to determine the degree of arterial narrowing on grayscale alone
- **Pulsed Doppler (PuD)**: Useful for evaluating waveform
- Measures peak systolic velocity
- **Color Doppler**: Allows distinction of artery from veins (based on flow direction)
- Disturbance in flow usually apparent with ready demonstration of turbulent flow
- Allows pulsed Doppler flow samples to be accurately taken
- **Power Doppler**: More sensitive to low flow rates than CD

- Good for picking up slow flow distal to occlusions and collaterals
- Less dependent on flow rate and angle of ultrasound beam; does not depict flow direction
- Iliac segment: Use 3.5-5 MHz transducer
- Femoropopliteal and infrapopliteal segments: Use 5-10 MHz transducer
- Assessment of degree of arterial stenosis or occlusion should be made by a combination of grayscale, spectral Doppler, color and PD assessment
- Angle correction crucial in spectral Doppler assessment

Top Differential Diagnoses
- Collaterals
- Popliteal Aneurysm
- Pseudoaneurysm

- No flow
- Preocclusive thump may be present just proximal to occlusion
- Distal waveform is monophasic with reduced systolic velocity
- Color Doppler
  - **Color Doppler**: Allows distinction of artery from veins (based on flow direction)
  - Disturbance in flow usually apparent with ready demonstration of turbulent flow
  - Allows pulsed Doppler flow samples to be accurately taken
- Power Doppler
  - **Power Doppler**: More sensitive to low flow rates than CD
  - Good for picking up slow flow distal to occlusions and collaterals
  - Less dependent on flow rate and angle of ultrasound beam; does not depict flow direction

Imaging Recommendations
- Best imaging tool
  - Magnetic resonance angiography is the preferred imaging modality in the author's institution because
    - Does not involve the use of ionizing radiation
    - Gives good overall assessment of the arterial tree with good correlation with conventional angiography
    - Excellent images for the lower limb run-off vessels
- Protocol advice
  - Ultrasound
    - Iliac segment: Use 3.5-5 MHz transducer
    - Femoropopliteal and infrapopliteal segments: Use 5-10 MHz transducer
    - Assessment of degree of arterial stenosis or occlusion should be made by a combination of grayscale, spectral Doppler, color and PD assessment
    - Angle correction crucial in spectral Doppler assessment
  - Multidetector CT (MDCT)
    - 100 mL of 350 mg iodine/mL contrast injected at 2.5-3 mL

- For lower limb CT angiography (CTA), region of interest can be placed at common femoral artery for smart preparation to guide start of acquisition, second acquisition may be necessary from knee down for distal run-off
- For upper limb CTA, region of interest can be placed at aortic arch for smart preparation to guide start of acquisition, arm of interest should be raised above shoulder while contralateral arm can be kept by patient's side
  - Magnetic resonance angiography (MRA)
    - Gadolinium contrast-enhanced 3D MRA superior to conventional time of flight or phase contrast technique; better signal to noise ratio and shorter scanning time
    - Moving table and appropriate software required
    - If distal run-off is not well shown, repeat dedicated examination of the foot using head coil may be useful
  - Digital subtractive angiography (DSA)
    - Usually reserved for patient undergoing endovascular intervention or having contraindications for the other non-invasive imaging modalities; e.g., cardiac pacemaker, metallic implants which may cause artifacts

DIFFERENTIAL DIAGNOSIS

Collaterals
- Erroneous identification as narrowed artery with reduced flow

Popliteal Aneurysm
- Mimics atheromatous occlusion

Pseudoaneurysm
- Turbulent flow mistaken for stenosed artery

EXTREMITY ARTERIAL OCCLUSIVE DISEASE

PATHOLOGY

General Features
- Etiology
  - Atherosclerotic occlusive disease
    - Smoking, diabetes mellitus, hypertension, obesity, hypercoagulable states
  - Non atherosclerotic occlusive diseases
  - Large vessels
  - Inflammatory: Takayasu arteritis, systemic giant cell arteritis, radiation induced arteritis
  - Non-inflammatory: Popliteal entrapment, adventitial cystic disease
  - Small vessels
  - Inflammatory: Vasculitis of connective tissue disease; scleroderma, rheumatoid arthritis, SLE; Buerger disease
  - Vasospastic: Raynaud syndrome
  - Embolism: Acute onset, consider cardiac source (atrial fibrillation or endocarditis) and aortic source (thrombus in aneurysm)
  - Trauma: Acute onset, obstruction or obliteration of flow may be caused by dissection, tear or avulsion of vessel
  - Aneurysms: Popliteal artery aneurysms are often associated with occlusion of the popliteal artery

CLINICAL ISSUES

Presentation
- Most common signs/symptoms
  - Lower limb symptoms
    - Calf claudication, buttock claudication, rest pain, arterial ulceration, gangrene
  - Upper limb symptoms
    - Cold, painful hand worse on exercise, finger tip ulceration, gangrene
- Other signs/symptoms
  - Other signs of arterial occlusive disease
    - Subclavian steal

Treatment
- Medical
  - Management of associated medical problems and treatment of modifiable risk factors
- Choice of interventional radiological or surgical treatment in the lower limb may be guided by the TransAtlantic Inter-Society Consensus (TASC) groups A-D or Society of Interventional Radiology (SIR) categories 1-4 classification
  - TASC A/SIR Cat 1: Percutaneous endovascular treatment is the treatment of choice
  - TASC B/SIR Cat 2: Lesions well suited for percutaneous endovascular treatment
  - TASC C/SIR Cat 3: Lesions amenable to percutaneous endovascular treatment but has a moderate chance of success compared with surgery
  - TASC D/SIR Cat 4: Extensive vascular disease where percutaneous endovascular treatment has a limited role compared with surgical bypass
- Interventional radiological
- Iliac segment

- Angioplasty or stenting (transluminal)
- Technical success 95-99% for stenoses; 70-80% for occlusions
- Stenting shown to have better long term patency with less requirement for long term intervention
- Femoropopliteal segment
  - Angioplasty is mainstay; stenting may produce better longer patency with nitinol stents
  - Technical success ~ 90% for stenoses; 70-80% for occlusions (subintimal approach may be required)
  - Cryoplasty, drug-eluting stent may have lower restenosis rate due to reduction in elastic recoil and neointimal hyperplasia
- Infrapopliteal segment
  - Angioplasty is mainstay; stenting only suitable for focal lesions but disease often multilevel and diffuse
  - Technical success ~ 90% for focal stenoses
  - Clinical result better than radiological patency
  - Shown to be useful in treatment of diabetic foot and limb salvage
- Surgical
- Iliac segment
  - Aortobifemoral bypass
  - Iliofemoral bypass (ipsilateral or contralateral)
  - Axillobifemoral bypass
  - Femorofemoral cross over graft
- Femoropopliteal segment
  - Above knee femoropopliteal bypass graft (artificial graft material such as Poly Tetra Fluoro Ethylene (PTFE) can be used)
  - Below knee femoropopliteal bypass graft (only vein graft can be used because of poor long term patency of below knee PTFE graft)
- Infrapopliteal segment
  - Femorodistal bypass graft (only vein graft can be used)
  - Popliteodistal bypass graft (only vein graft can be used)
  - In situ long saphenous vein graft
- Choice between interventional radiological and surgical treatment in the upper limb not as clear cut
- Multidisciplinary management approach advised
- Interventional radiological
  - Angioplasty and stenting possible in the brachiocephalic and subclavian arteries
  - Covered stent may be useful in dissection or trauma
- Surgical
  - Appropriate bypass surgery
  - Repair of damaged artery: e.g., endarterectomy, vein patch

DIAGNOSTIC CHECKLIST

Image Interpretation Pearls
- Arterial stenosis assessment should be made on the combined findings on GS, PuD, PD and CD

SELECTED REFERENCES

1. Zwiebel WJ et al: Introduction to Vascular Ultrasonography, 5th ed. Philadelphia, Elsevier Saunders, 2005

IMAGE GALLERY

Typical

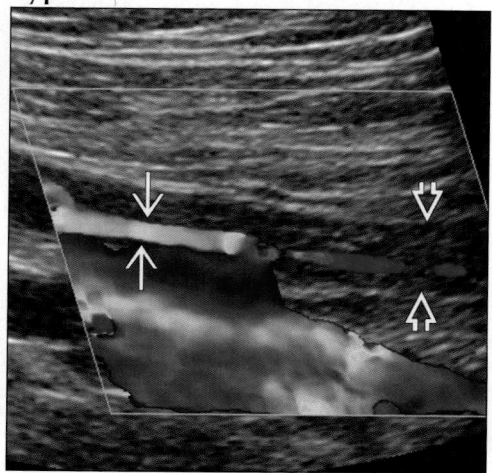

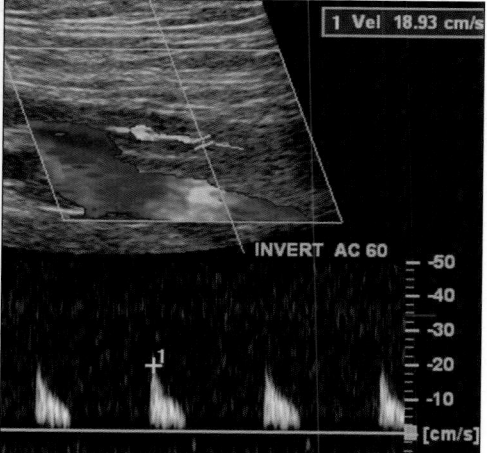

(Left) Longitudinal color Doppler ultrasound shows long stenotic superficial femoral artery (SFA) segment with trickle flow. Note that the patent lumen outlined by the red color ➔ is considerably narrower than the diameter of the artery ➔. *(Right)* Longitudinal pulsed Doppler ultrasound shows monophasic low velocity flow.

Typical

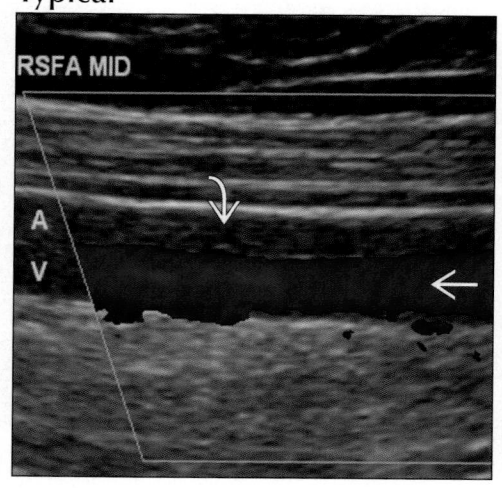

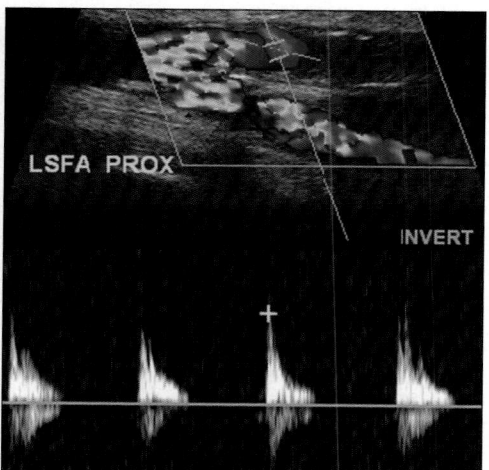

(Left) Longitudinal color Doppler ultrasound shows complete SFA occlusion ➔. The arterial segment is filled with hypoechoic material and there is absent of color flow signal. The SFV ➔ running parallel to it is normal. *(Right)* Longitudinal color Doppler ultrasound shows abnormal "to and fro" Doppler waveform in the segment just proximal to the previous arterial occlusion. Findings are typical of preocclusive segment.

Typical

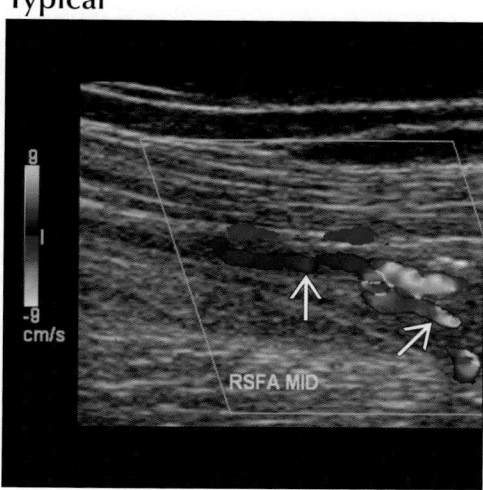

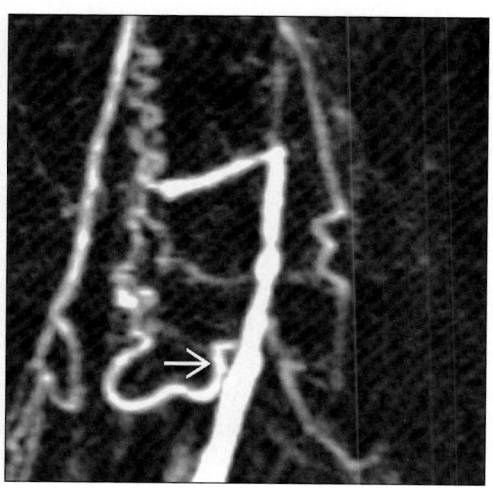

(Left) Longitudinal color Doppler ultrasound shows a collateral with retrograde flow ➔ reconstituting the segment distal to previous arterial occlusion. Note collaterals are common in arterial occlusion. *(Right)* Corresponding MRA of total SFA occlusion with distal segment reconstituted by a collateral ➔.

Typical

(Left) Longitudinal color Doppler ultrasound shows turbulent flow within a previously placed popliteal artery stent indicative of restenosis likely from neointimal hyperplasia.
(Right) Longitudinal pulsed Doppler ultrasound shows increased peak systolic velocity with "wrap around" artifact suggestive of turbulent flow and significant stenosis.

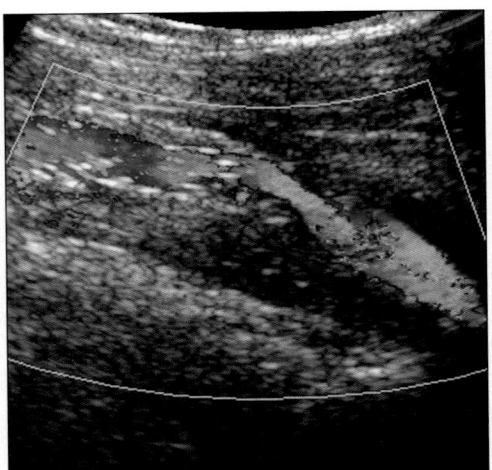

Typical

(Left) DSA shows balloon angioplasty of a new stent placed coaxially through a previously placed, stenosed stent (on two preceding ultrasound images). *(Right)* DSA performed after stenting and angioplasty shows no significant residual stenosis demonstrated.

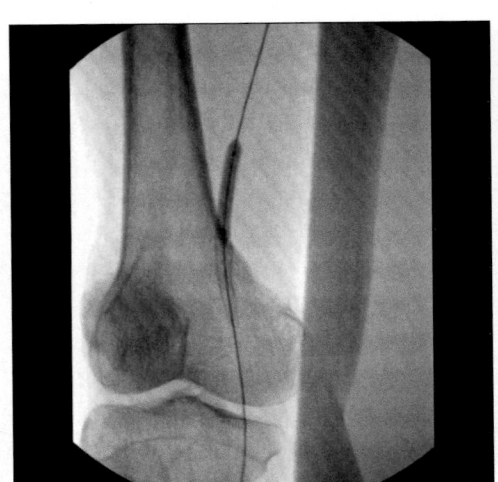
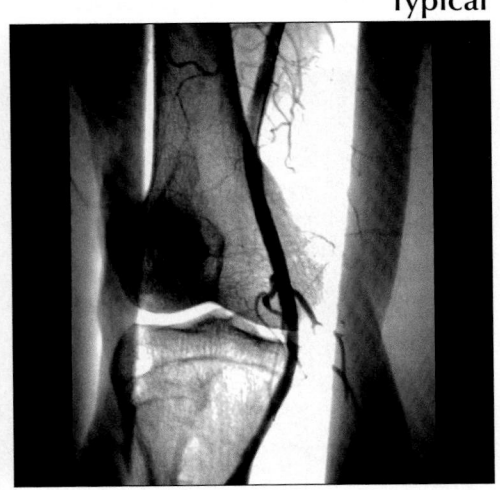

Typical

(Left) MRA shows long right SFA occlusion ➡ and multiple left SFA stenoses ➡. *(Right)* MRA shows good depiction of distal run-off vessels in the same patient as previous image. Note posterior patent tibial arteries ➡ can be seen to the feet. A few stenoses are seen in anterior tibial arteries ➡.

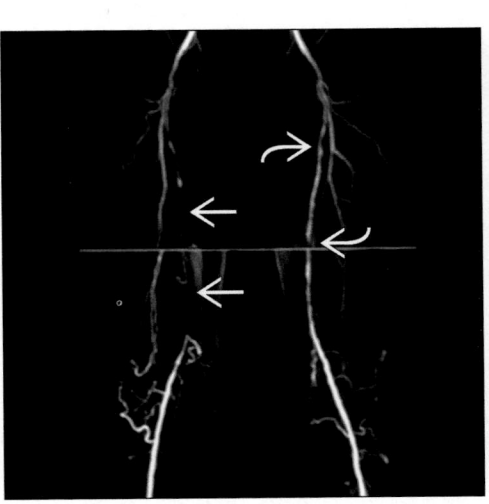
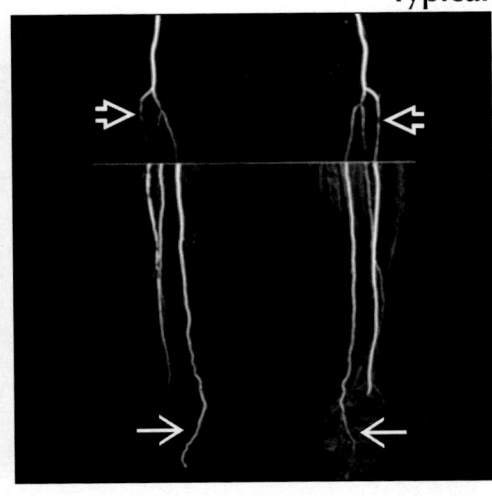

EXTREMITY ARTERIAL OCCLUSIVE DISEASE

Typical

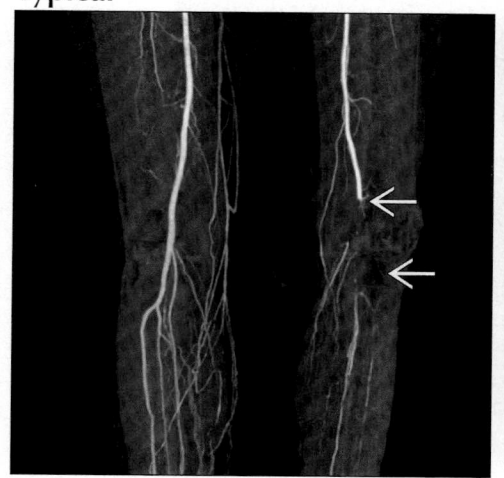
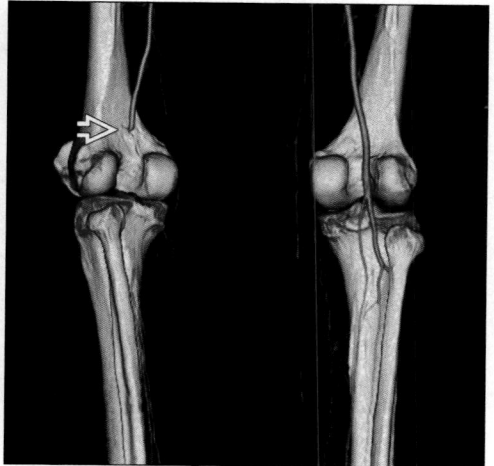

(Left) CTA shows frontal maximal intensity projection image demonstrating occlusion in the left popliteal artery ➡ just above the femoral condyles. *(Right)* CTA shows posterior volume rendered view from the same patient as previous image, again demonstrating occlusion of the left popliteal artery above the femoral condyles ➡.

Typical

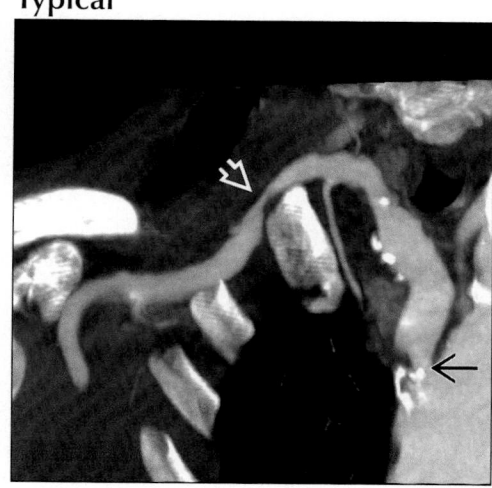
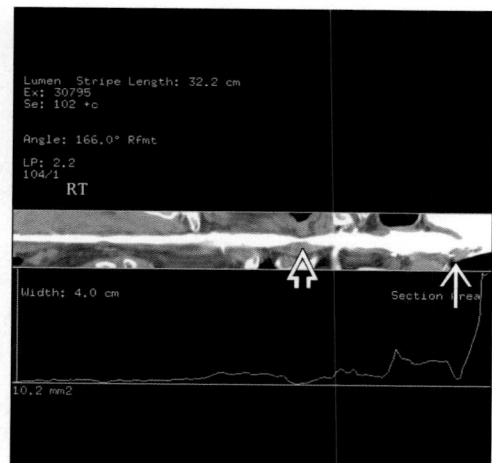

(Left) Oblique CTA shows an oblique view of the right brachiocephalic artery, subclavian artery and axillary artery. Note > 75% right subclavian/axillary artery junction stenosis ➡ and 50-75% right brachiocephalic artery origin stenosis ➡. *(Right)* CTA shows vessel analysis view in the same patient again showing a right brachiocephalic artery stenosis ➡ and right subclavian/axillary artery stenosis ➡.

Typical

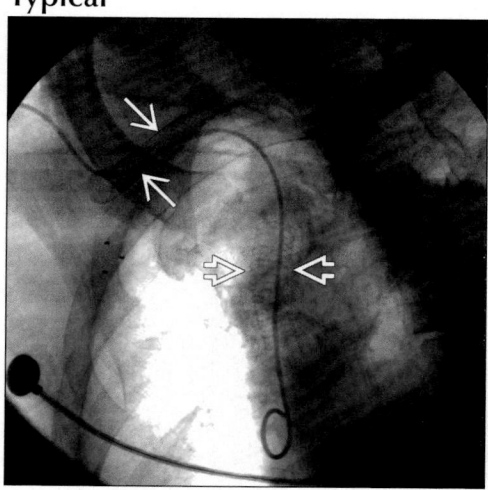
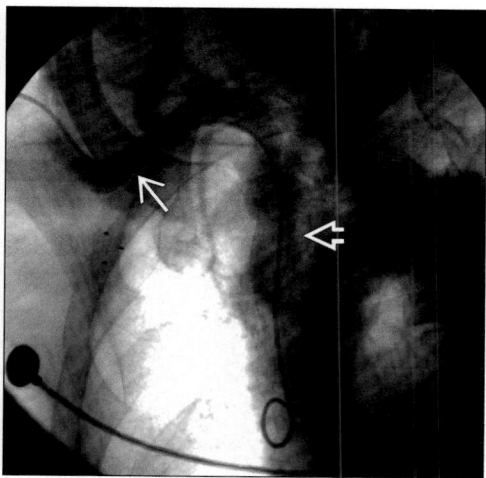

(Left) DSA shows stents placed across the right subclavian/axillary artery stenosis ➡ and right brachiocephalic artery stenosis ➡ of the same patient in previous image. *(Right)* DSA shows satisfactory post stenting angiogram of the right subclavian/axillary artery ➡ and right brachiocephalic artery ➡.

PERIPHERAL ARTERIAL PSEUDOANEURYSM

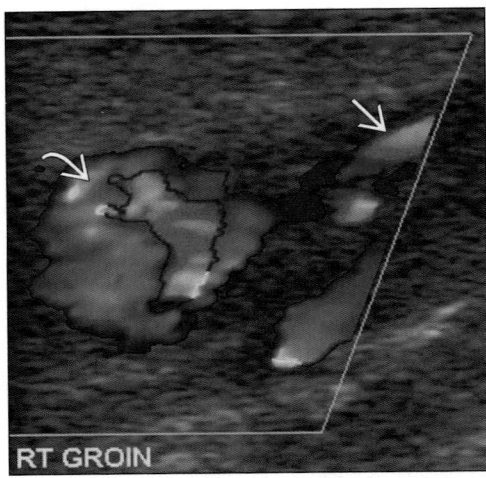

Longitudinal color Doppler ultrasound shows a vascular groin lesion ➔ arising from the CFA ➔ with internal swirling flow in a patient after an arterial puncture; classic features of pseudoaneurysm.

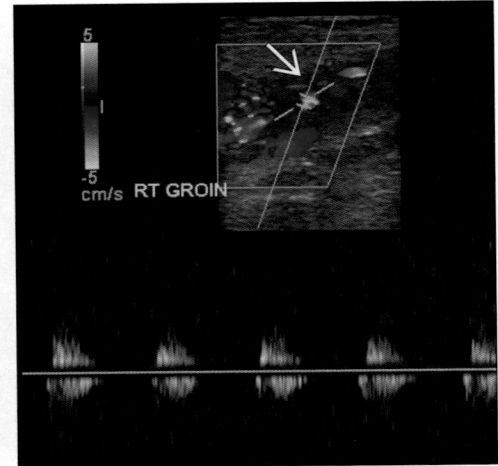

Corresponding longitudinal color Doppler ultrasound shows bidirectional flow demonstrated at the neck ➔ of the lesion, which is pathognomonic for a pseudoaneurysm.

TERMINOLOGY

Abbreviations and Synonyms
- Pseudoaneurysm; false aneurysm

Definitions
- Pseudoaneurysm defined as
  - Outpouching of a blood vessel, involving a defect in the 2 innermost layers (tunica intima and media) with continuity of the outermost layer (adventitia)
  - Alternatively, all three layers are damaged and bleeding is contained by blood clot or surrounding structures

IMAGING FINDINGS

General Features
- Best diagnostic clue: Characteristic "yin-yang" sign on color Doppler
- Location
  - Most commonly found involving the common femoral artery (CFA) where needle puncture is performed for angiographic examination
  - Usually arises from the superficial side of the artery that is punctured
- Size
  - Often 1-3 cm in diameter
  - Large pseudoaneurysms can exceed 5 cm
- Morphology
  - May have a narrow or wide neck
  - Presence of a string of aneurysms with multiple lumens is common

Ultrasonographic Findings
- Grayscale ultrasound
  - **Grayscale Ultrasound**: Usually hypoechoic or anechoic structure
  - Slow flow may occasionally be seen
  - Neck connects pseudoaneurysm to artery
  - String of aneurysms with multiple lumens is common
  - Thrombus may be seen in the lumen
- Pulsed Doppler
  - **Pulsed Doppler**: Characteristic "to and fro" flow is typically present in the neck of the aneurysm
  - Turbulent high velocity flow may be present if the neck is narrowed

DDx: Pseudoaneurysm

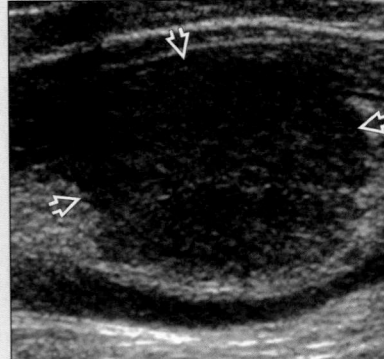

Muscle Tumor

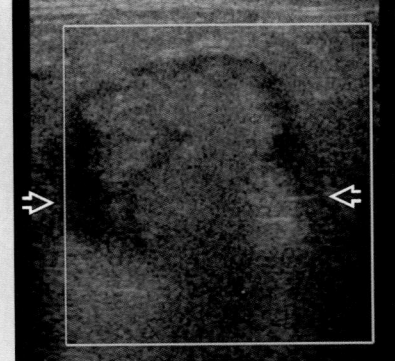

Inguinal Hernia

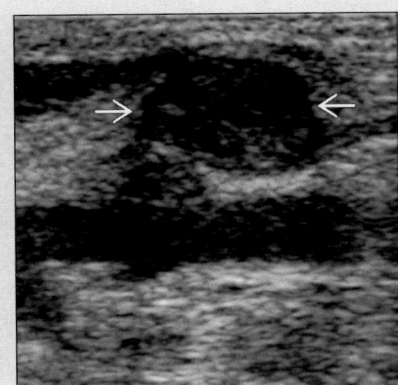

Groin Hematoma

PERIPHERAL ARTERIAL PSEUDOANEURYSM

Key Facts

Imaging Findings
- **Grayscale Ultrasound**: Usually hypoechoic or anechoic structure
- Slow flow may occasionally be seen
- Neck connects pseudoaneurysm to artery
- String of aneurysms with multiple lumens is common
- Thrombus may be seen in the lumen
- **Pulsed Doppler**: Characteristic "to and fro" flow is typically present in the neck of the aneurysm
- Turbulent high velocity flow may be present if the neck is narrowed
- **Power Doppler**: Demonstrates slow flow outside an artery
- May demonstrate slow flow into the pseudoaneurysm better than CD
- **Color Doppler**: Characteristic "yin-yang" sign

- Swirling flow seen as different color signals within lesion
- Lumen may not be fully filled with color due to partial thrombosis
- Flow can sometimes be detected in needle tract without an associated lumen

Top Differential Diagnoses
- Inguinal Hernia
- Groin Hematoma
- Muscle Tumor
- Distended Iliopsoas Bursa

Diagnostic Checklist
- "Yin-yang" sign on color Doppler and "to and fro" flow on pulsed Doppler

---

- ○ "To and fro" flow may be lost with only forward flow that increases towards end-diastole when an arteriovenous fistula is present
- Power Doppler
  - ○ **Power Doppler**: Demonstrates slow flow outside an artery
  - ○ May demonstrate slow flow into the pseudoaneurysm better than CD
- Color Doppler
  - ○ **Color Doppler**: Characteristic "yin-yang" sign
    - ■ Swirling flow seen as different color signals within lesion
  - ○ Lumen may not be fully filled with color due to partial thrombosis
  - ○ Flow can sometimes be detected in needle tract without an associated lumen
  - ○ Rarely an arteriovenous fistula may be demonstrated

CT Findings
- CTA
  - ○ Arterial enhancement of lumen of pseudoaneurysm
  - ○ Contrast extravasation may be present if there is rupture of the pseudoaneurysm
  - ○ Fresh hematoma around pseudoaneurysm may be slightly hyperdense
  - ○ Volume rendered and maximal intensity projections useful for delineation of anatomy and assessment for suitability for intervention

MR Findings
- T1WI
  - ○ Flow void may be seen within lumen of the pseudoaneurysm
  - ○ High signal may be seen in methemoglobin containing portions of hematoma surrounding pseudoaneurysm
- T1 C+: Lumen of pseudoaneurysm may enhance
- MRA
  - ○ Contrast-enhanced MRA preferred over conventional "time of flight" or phase contrast techniques because of superior signal to noise ratio
  - ○ Double to triple dose gadolinium typically used
  - ○ Pseudoaneurysm & supplying artery identified

- ○ Early venous filling may be seen if arteriovenous fistula is present

Imaging Recommendations
- Best imaging tool
  - ○ Duplex Doppler ultrasound
    - ■ Should be considered first line investigation
    - ■ Readily demonstrates pseudoaneurysm
    - ■ No ionizing radiation
- Protocol advice
  - ○ 5 MHz linear transducer or a 2-5 MHz curved array transducer
  - ○ 2-5 MHz curved array transducer may be required for the iliac arteries or in case of extensive hematoma
  - ○ MRA useful for delineating anatomy in complex cases and guiding intervention
  - ○ CT/MR useful for post treatment follow-up and exclusion of unsuspecting causes

DIFFERENTIAL DIAGNOSIS

Inguinal Hernia
- Peristalsis may be present
- CD and PD useful for differentiation

Groin Hematoma
- CD and PD useful for differentiation

Muscle Tumor
- May have increased vascularity on CD and PD
- Rarely associated with pseudoaneurysm

Distended Iliopsoas Bursa
- CD and PD useful for differentiation

PATHOLOGY

General Features
- Etiology
  - ○ Iatrogenic
    - ■ Needle puncture from angiography (typically CFA)

- Incidence increases with the use of: Large-bore sheaths, post-procedural anticoagulation therapy, antiplatelet therapy used during the intervention, post-surgery (inadvertent arterial injury)
  o Traumatic
    - Stab injuries
    - Direct blow
    - Fractures
  o Infection/inflammation
    - Infection or inflammation adjacent to the artery
  o Septic embolism
    - Endocarditis
    - Infective aortitis
  o Intravenous drug abuse
    - Inadvertent needle puncture of artery
    - Septic emboli from endocarditis
  o Idiopathic

CLINICAL ISSUES

Presentation
- Most common signs/symptoms: Increased swelling which may be pulsatile over site of previous needle puncture, surgery or trauma
- Other signs/symptoms
  o Pain at site of pseudoaneurysm
  o Anemia in cases of significant blood loss

Demographics
- Gender: No gender difference in incidence

Treatment
- Conservative
  o Small pseudoaneurysms < 1 cm may spontaneously thrombose
- US-guided compression
  o Can be time consuming (up to an hour may be required)
  o Success rate ~ 90%, but drops to 60-70% if anticoagulation is used
  o Less likely to succeed when
    - Aneurysm more than 7-10 days old
    - Associated infection
    - Severe pain/discomfort
    - Large hematoma
    - Aneurysm above the inguinal ligament
- US-guided thrombin injection
  o Human thrombin
    - Failure and complications are rare
    - 1st injection pseudoaneurysm thrombosis rate ~ 90%; overall success rate ~ 95%
    - Increments of 100 IU, typically up to 1,000 IU can be injected into the pseudoaneurysm sac
    - Injection at the neck controversial: Advocated by some authors for more complete thrombosis, but argued by some to cause arterial embolization; should only be done if the needle tip can be well visualized
    - Pseudoaneurysm geometry is the key determining factor for success; long and narrow neck more favorable
    - Not suitable for wide neck aneurysms

- Potential complications include distal ischemia (e.g., blue toes which tend to spontaneously resolve) < 1%, wound infection, and allergic reactions
  o Bovine thrombin
    - Typically 500-1,000 U
    - Replaced by human thrombin because of risk of allergy and prion infection
- Interventional radiology
  o Embolization
    - For pseudoaneurysms of an artery where flow can be sacrificed, metal coil embolization proximally and distally to "trap" the pseudoaneurysm may be performed
    - If access to artery distal to pseudoaneurysm is not possible despite use of microcatheter, particulate matter or glue can be considered for distal portion of artery
  o Covered stenting
    - For pseudoaneurysms of an artery where flow has to be preserved, covered stent may be used to seal off the pseudoaneurysm
    - Target artery needs to be of reasonable size (> 6 mm)
    - Contraindicated if there is infection
- Surgery
  o Surgical repair of the damaged artery
  o Bypass surgery with ligation proximal and distal to the pseudoaneurysm may occasionally be required
  o Surgery usually reserved as a last resort
  o Complications include
    - Wound-healing disorders
    - Permanent femoral neuralgias
    - Lymphatic leaks (up to 40%)

DIAGNOSTIC CHECKLIST

Image Interpretation Pearls
- "Yin-yang" sign on color Doppler and "to and fro" flow on pulsed Doppler

SELECTED REFERENCES

1. Krueger K et al: Postcatheterization pseudoaneurysm: results of US-guided percutaneous thrombin injection in 240 patients. Radiology. 236(3):1104-10, 2005
2. Zwiebel WJ et al: Introduction to Vascular Ultrasonography. 5th ed. Philadelphia, Elsevier Saunders. 391-9, 2005
3. Albrecht RJ et al: Traumatic peroneal artery pseudoaneurysm: use of preoperative coil embolization. J Vasc Surg. 39(4):912, 2004
4. Kruger K et al: Femoral pseudoaneurysms: management with percutaneous thrombin injections--success rates and effects on systemic coagulation. Radiology. 226(2):452-8, 2003
5. Allan PL et al: Clinical Doppler Ultrasound. London, Churchill Livingstone. 82-4, 2000
6. Vasseur MA et al: Coil embolization of a gluteal false aneurysm in a patient with Marfan syndrome. J Vasc Surg. 27(1):177-9, 1998

PERIPHERAL ARTERIAL PSEUDOANEURYSM

IMAGE GALLERY

Typical

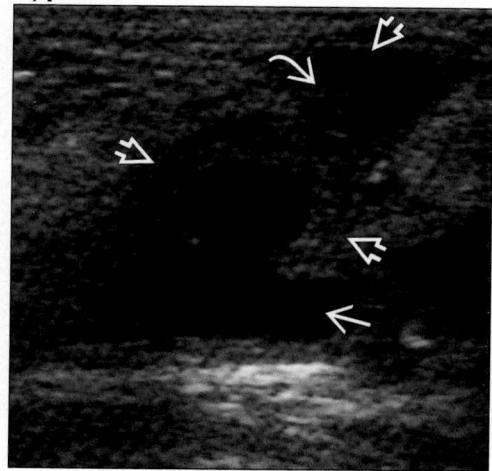 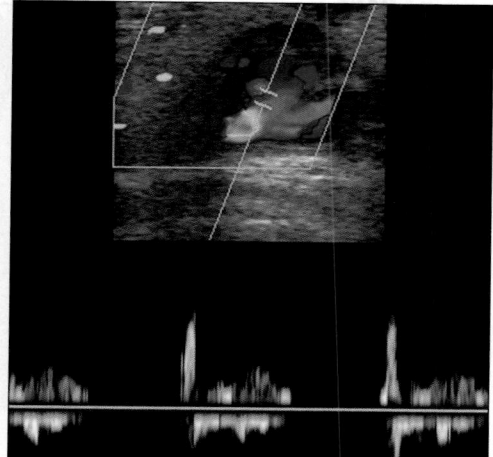

(Left) Longitudinal ultrasound shows wide based pseudoaneurysm ➡ arising from the CFA ➡. Note extravasated blood ➡ is enclosed by adjacent soft tissue indicative of contained arterial rupture. (Right) Corresponding longitudinal color Doppler ultrasound shows swirling flow within the wide neck pseudoaneurysm.

Typical

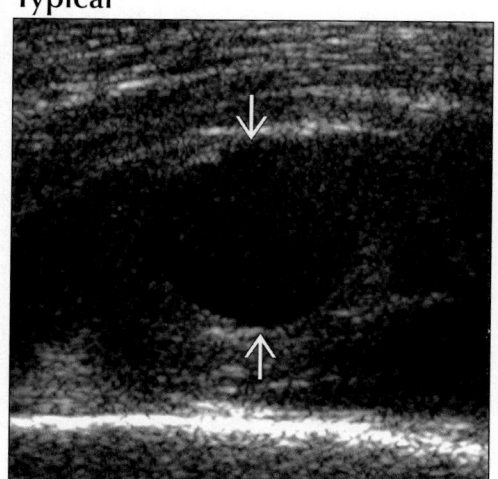 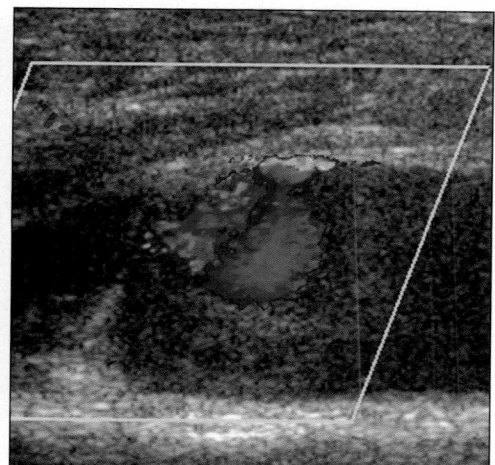

(Left) Transverse ultrasound shows a pseudoaneurysm ➡ in the lateral aspect of the left knee of a patient after knee replacement. (Right) Corresponding transverse color Doppler ultrasound shows the characteristic "yin-yang" sign within the same pseudoaneurysm.

Typical

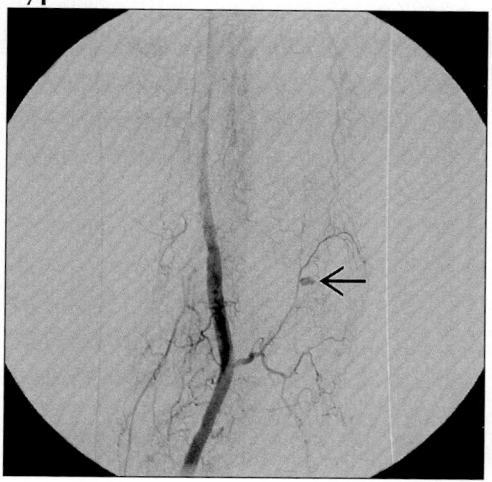 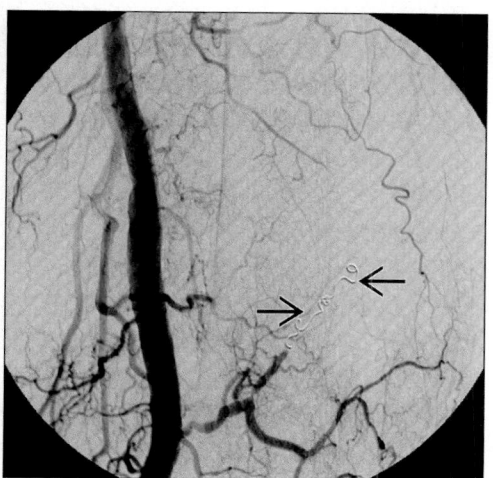

(Left) DSA shows a pseudoaneurysm ➡ arising from a branch of the left lateral geniculate artery (same image as previous two images). (Right) Corresponding post-embolization DSA shows successful embolization with coils ➡ within an arterial branch leading to the pseudoaneurysm.

Typical

(Left) Axial T1WI MR shows a flow void ➡ within a large heterogeneous mass in the posterior aspect of the left upper thigh, suspicious of pseudoaneurysm with a large surrounding hematoma. Note T1 high signal components ⇨ are likely to represent methemoglobin in the hematoma. *(Right)* Axial T1 C+ MR shows enhancement within the lumen of the pseudoaneurysm ➡ and along periphery of the hematoma ⇨.

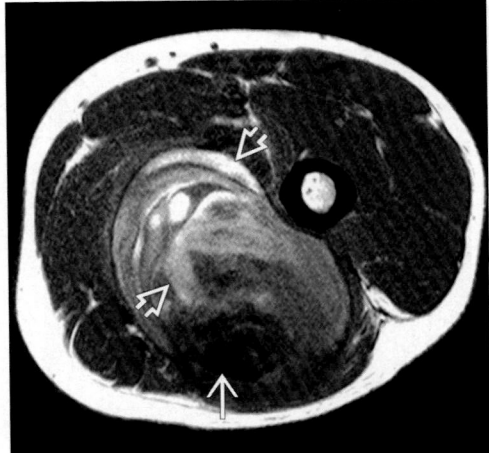
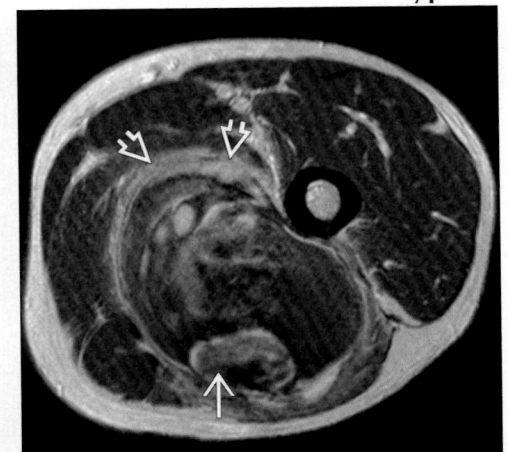

Typical

(Left) Axial FFE MR image, at the same level as the previous image, with "blooming" artifact ➡ from hemosiderin in the hematoma surrounding the pseudoaneurysm lumen ⇨. *(Right)* Oblique MRA shows the pseudoaneurysm ➡ arising from a branch of the left profunda femoris artery.

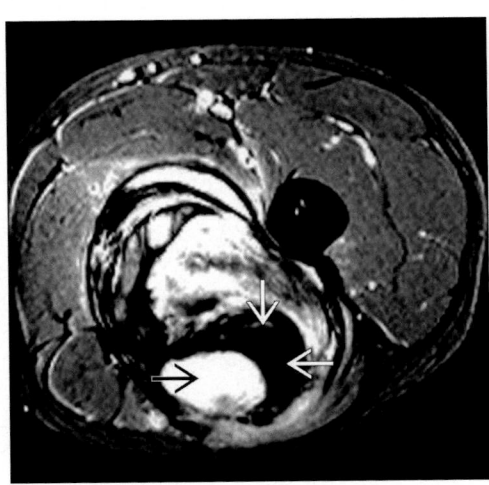
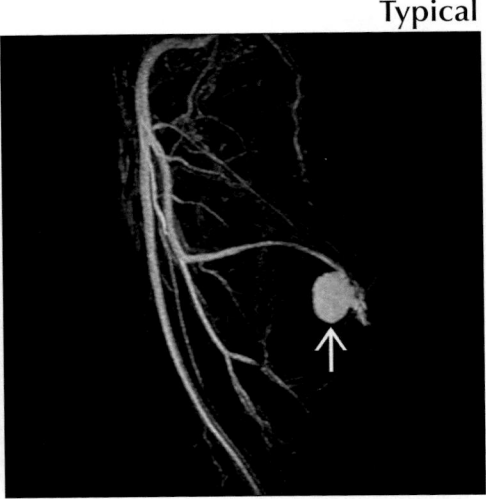

Typical

(Left) Transverse color Doppler ultrasound shows the characteristic "yin-yang" sign in a pseudoaneurysm (3 cm lumen). *(Right)* Corresponding transverse pulsed Doppler ultrasound shows characteristic "to and fro" flow in the neck of the same pseudoaneurysm.

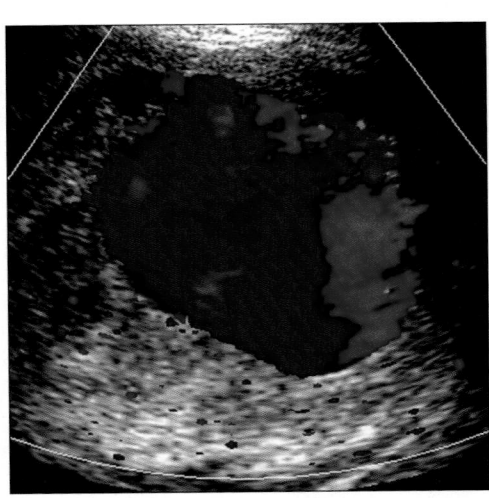
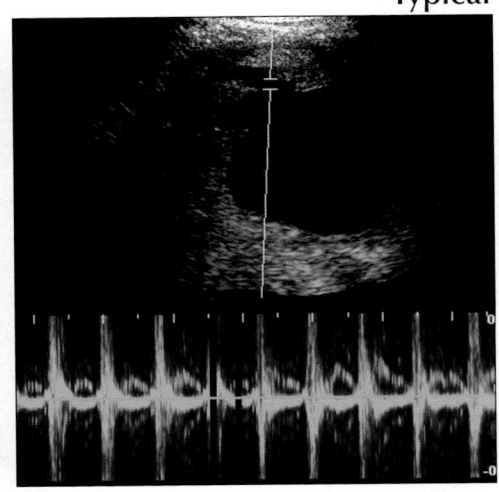

PERIPHERAL ARTERIAL PSEUDOANEURYSM

Typical

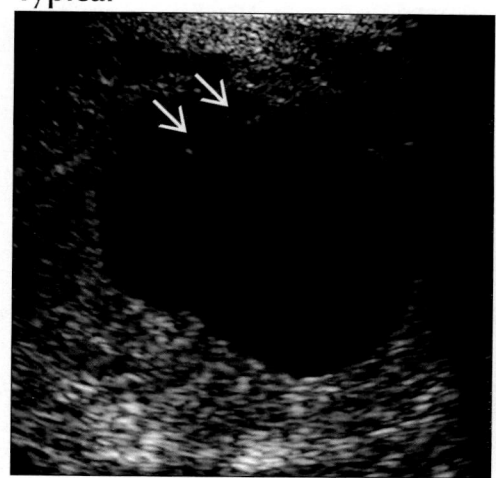 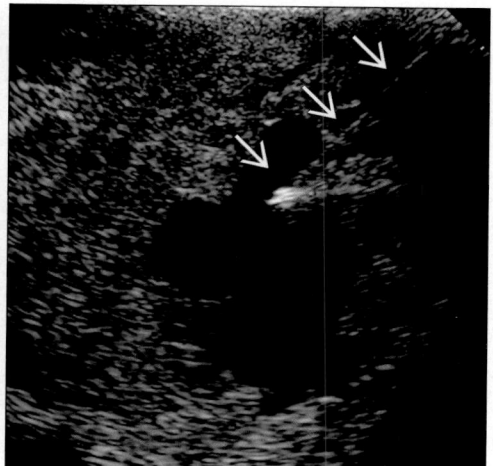

(Left) Transverse ultrasound shows a needle ➡ inserted into the pseudoaneurysm for thrombin injection. *(Right)* Transverse ultrasound shows partial thrombosis of same pseudoaneurysm with the needle ➡ in situ.

Typical

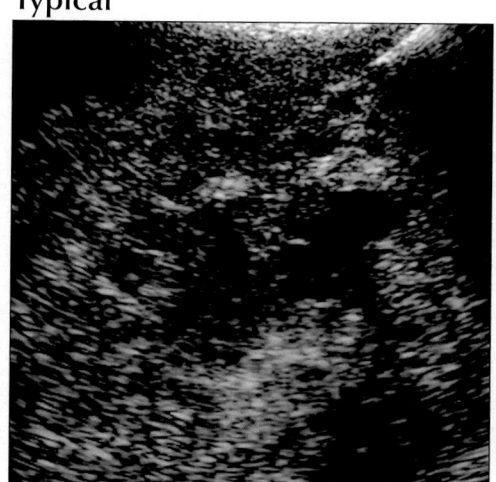 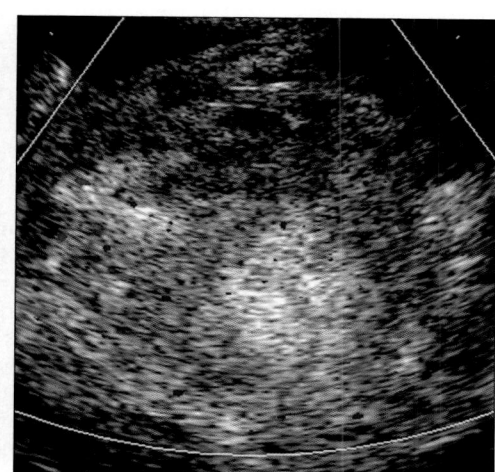

(Left) Transverse ultrasound shows near complete thrombosis of the same pseudoaneurysm. *(Right)* Transverse ultrasound shows complete thrombosis.

Typical

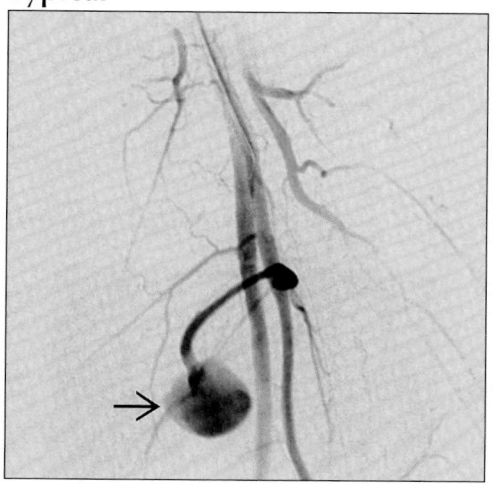 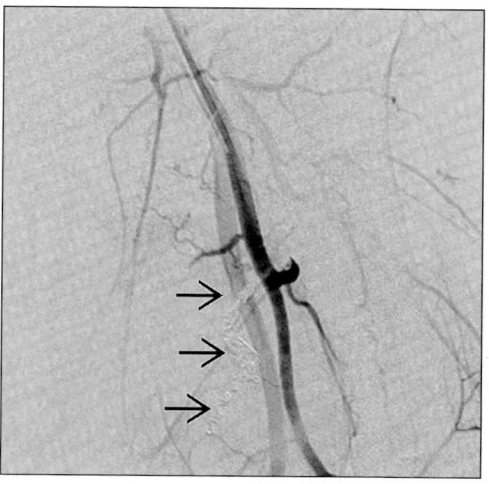

(Left) Oblique DSA shows reperfusion in the pseudoaneurysm ➡ despite thrombin injection (same as previous four US images). *(Right)* Oblique DSA shows successful embolization with coils ➡ of arterial branch of the left profunda femoris artery leading to pseudoaneurysm.

PERIPHERAL ARTERIOVENOUS FISTULA

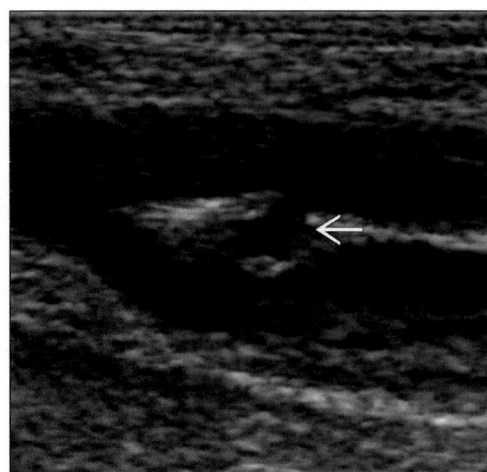

Longitudinal ultrasound shows a femoral AVF. Note the communicating channel between SFA and SFV ➔.

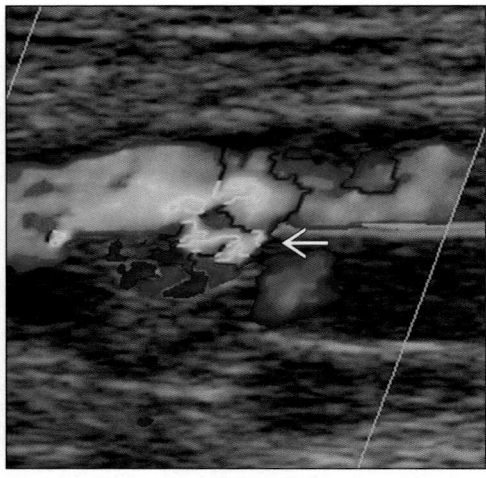

Corresponding longitudinal color Doppler ultrasound shows color Doppler flow through the communicating channel between the SFA and SFV ➔.

TERMINOLOGY

Definitions
- Arteriovenous fistula is usually defined as an abnormal direct communication between an artery and a vein

IMAGING FINDINGS

General Features
- Location
  - Congenital AV fistula
    - Any site
  - Acquired AV fistula
    - In post-traumatic cases, AV fistula usually found around site of injury
  - Surgically created AV fistula
  - Main types of AV fistula
    - Forearm: Radial artery to cephalic vein
    - Forearm vein transposition: Radial artery to ulnar, dorsal or volar vein transposition
    - Upper arm: Brachial artery to cephalic vein
    - Basilic vein transposition: Brachial artery to basilic vein

- Main graft types
  - Forearm loop: Brachial artery - antecubital vein
  - Upper arm straight: Brachial artery - basilic vein
  - Upper arm loop: Axillary artery - axillary vein
  - Thigh graft: Common femoral/superficial femoral artery - greater saphenous/common femoral vein
- Morphology
  - Congenital
    - Multiple arteriovenous connections are typically present
    - Single or multiple draining veins may be present
  - Acquired
    - Usually single arteriovenous connection seen
  - Surgically created
    - Perianastomotic stenosis may be seen in surgical fistulas

Ultrasonographic Findings
- Grayscale Ultrasound
  - **Grayscale ultrasound**: Arterial strictures may be seen proximal to site of fistula
  - Venous strictures may be seen in draining vein from fistula

---

DDx: Arteriovenous Fistula

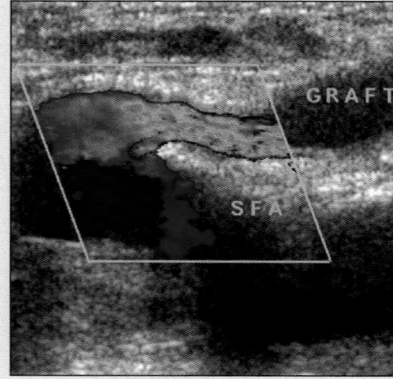

In-Situ Vein Graft

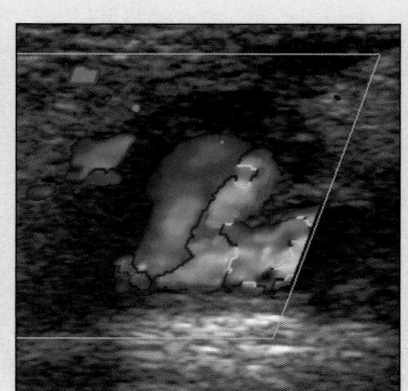

Pseudoaneurysm

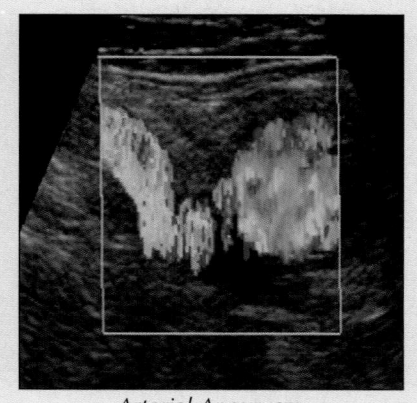

Arterial Aneurysm

PERIPHERAL ARTERIOVENOUS FISTULA

Key Facts

Imaging Findings
- **Grayscale ultrasound**: Arterial strictures may be seen proximal to site of fistula
- Venous strictures may be seen in draining vein from fistula
- Aneurysmal dilatation around puncture sites for dialysis is common
- Mural thrombus may be present
- Venous stenoses in central veins (e.g., subclavian vein, brachiocephalic vein) are common
- **Pulsed Doppler**: Peak systolic velocity (PSV) can be calculated at AVF and sites of visible stenosis
- PSV ≥ 2.0 m/s equals > 50% diameter reduction
- PSV ≥ 3.0 m/s equals ≥ 75% diameter reduction
- Wrap around artifact may be present in areas of high velocity flow

- **Color Doppler**: Useful for identification of flow direction for distinction of arteries and veins
- Useful for distinction of the arterial limb from the venous limb in loop grafts
- Turbulent flow seen in areas of significant stenoses
- Aliasing may be present at areas of turbulent flow
- Duplex Doppler allows quantification and assessment of flow through the AV fistula
- ≥ 7 MHz high-resolution transducer should be used to evaluate feeding artery and draining vein

Diagnostic Checklist
- **Ultrasound**: Transverse plane is useful to identify and evaluate vessel diameter, wall thickness and compressibility
- Longitudinal plane is useful for evaluation of flow direction

---

- ○ Aneurysmal dilatation around puncture sites for dialysis is common
- ○ Mural thrombus may be present
- ○ Venous stenoses in central veins (e.g., subclavian vein, brachiocephalic vein) are common
- Pulsed Doppler
  - ○ **Pulsed Doppler**: Peak systolic velocity (PSV) can be calculated at AVF and sites of visible stenosis
    - ■ PSV ≥ 2.0 m/s equals > 50% diameter reduction
    - ■ PSV ≥ 3.0 m/s equals ≥ 75% diameter reduction
  - ○ Wrap around artifact may be present in areas of high velocity flow
- Color Doppler
  - ○ **Color Doppler**: Useful for identification of flow direction for distinction of arteries and veins
  - ○ Useful for distinction of the arterial limb from the venous limb in loop grafts
  - ○ Turbulent flow seen in areas of significant stenoses
  - ○ Aliasing may be present at areas of turbulent flow

Imaging Recommendations
- Best imaging tool
  - ○ Duplex Doppler ultrasound
    - ■ May demonstrate the site of AV communication
    - ■ Duplex Doppler allows quantification and assessment of flow through the AV fistula
  - ○ MR
    - ■ Best tool for demonstrating full extent of involvement (demonstrates involvement in subcutaneous tissue, muscles and bones), particularly in congenital vascular AV fistula/AV malformations
  - ○ MRA
    - ■ May be used as a non invasive tool to demonstrate site of AV communication
  - ○ DSA
    - ■ Remains the gold standard for demonstrating precise site of AV communication
    - ■ Allows dynamic assessment of flow through AV fistula
    - ■ Usually performed as part of endovascular intervention
    - ■ Sometimes necessary for pre-operative assessment

- Protocol advice
  - ○ US
  - ○ ≥ 7 MHz high-resolution transducer should be used to evaluate feeding artery and draining vein
  - ○ For surgically created AV fistula for hemodialysis
    - ■ **Peak systolic velocities should be assessed at**
    - ■ 2 cm cranial to arterial anastomosis within feeding artery
    - ■ 2 cm caudal to venous anastomosis within graft
    - ■ At arterial and venous anastomoses
    - ■ At mid graft
  - ○ Transverse plane is useful to identify and evaluate vessel diameter, wall thickness and compressibility
  - ○ Longitudinal plane is useful for evaluation of flow direction
  - ○ **MR**
    - ■ T1 sequence should be included to demonstrate anatomy around AV fistula
    - ■ T2 fat-suppression sequence should be included and is usually the best sequence for demonstrating full involvement of AV fistula/vascular malformation
    - ■ T1 post-contrast sequence with fat-saturation also useful for demonstrating full extent of involvement and may help with distinction of vascular tumor from vascular malformations
  - ○ **MRA**
  - ○ Gadolinium contrast-enhanced sequences are preferred to conventional time of flight or phase contrast sequences
    - ■ Better signal to noise ratio and shorter imaging time
  - ○ Arterial and venous phase acquisition should be included
  - ○ **DSA**
  - ○ Conventional common femoral access may be used
  - ○ Direct puncture of the venous site of AV fistula may also be performed, especially for upper limb AV fistula
  - ○ Orthopaedic tourniquet or blood pressure cuff is a useful tool

PERIPHERAL ARTERIOVENOUS FISTULA

- Allows temporary occlusion of arterial flow such that arterial limb of AV fistula can be demonstrated by contrast reflux from venous limb
- Allows temporary occlusion of arterial flow such that liquid sclerosants can be used for embolization of AV fistula

DIFFERENTIAL DIAGNOSIS

In-Situ Vein Graft
- Proximal LSV anastomosed in situ to common femoral artery as the proximal end of a femoro-distal arterial bypass graft

Pseudoaneurysm
- In contrast to an AVF, a draining vein will not be seen

Arterial Aneurysm
- A draining vein should not be present in arterial aneurysm

PATHOLOGY

General Features
- Etiology
  - Congenital: Usually present with many small communications within a soft tissue mass
    - AV-fistula may be present as part of vascular malformation
    - AV vascular malformation is less common than venous vascular malformations
  - Acquired: Most commonly have a single connection
    - Traumatic: Stab or penetrating injury, gun shot wounds
    - Iatrogenic: Needle puncture from angiography, inadvertent damage to vessels during surgery
  - Surgically created
    - AV fistulae for hemodialysis
    - AV fistula for protection of flow through distal in situ bypasses, e.g., in situ long saphenous femoro-distal bypass graft

CLINICAL ISSUES

Presentation
- Most common signs/symptoms
  - Triad of birthmark, abnormal varicosities and limb enlargement are associated with congenital AV fistula/vascular malformation
  - Pain
  - Abnormal pigmented lesion and swelling
  - Abnormal throbbing sensation or pulsatile mass over site of AV fistula
  - Ischemic symptoms in tissue distal to the AV fistula
    - "Steal" effect causing reduction of arterial flow to distal soft tissues
    - Venous hypertension from AV fistula causing increase venous pressure and therefore, impairment in venous return from distal tissue
    - Ulcers and gangrene in severe cases

- Other signs/symptoms: Signs/symptoms of cardiac failure if high output cardiac failure develops

Demographics
- Age: At birth if congenital; any age for acquired causes
- Gender: No difference in incidence between male and female

Natural History & Prognosis
- Congenital AV fistulae or communications
  - Tend to grow proportionate to size of patient
  - May progress or increase in size with trauma, hormonal changes (e.g., puberty and pregnancy)
- Acquired AV fistulae
  - High output cardiac failure may result in severe cases
  - Ischemic symptoms of distal tissues may result in amputation in severe cases

Treatment
- Interventional radiology
  - Embolization of abnormal communication or nidus of AV fistula
    - Sclerosant (e.g., sodium tetradecyl sulphate 3% or alcohol can be used)
    - Glue (e.g., histoacryl butyrate)
  - Covered stent
    - Usually placed on arterial side to cover and occlude AV fistula
  - Coil embolization
    - Usually placed in venous side to completely occlude draining vein
    - Embolization of arterial supply not generally performed (unless artery can be sacrificed) because of risk of ischemia to distal tissue
  - Angioplasty or stenting
    - Useful for treatment of anastomotic stenosis and stenoses in venous or arterial limb of surgically created fistulae for use in hemodialysis until definitive surgery can be performed
    - Cutting balloon is particularly useful for angioplasty of venous limb stenoses
- Surgical
  - Surgical ligation of AV fistula
  - Complete surgical resection of AV communication and affected tissue

DIAGNOSTIC CHECKLIST

Image Interpretation Pearls
- **Ultrasound**: Transverse plane is useful to identify and evaluate vessel diameter, wall thickness and compressibility
- Longitudinal plane is useful for evaluation of flow direction

SELECTED REFERENCES
1. Zwiebel WJ et al: Introduction to Vascular Ultrasonography, 5th ed. Philadelphia, Elsevier Saunders. pp256; 325-340, 2005

14

56

IMAGE GALLERY

Typical

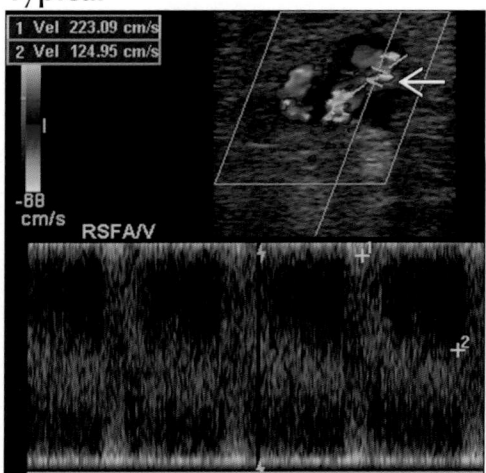
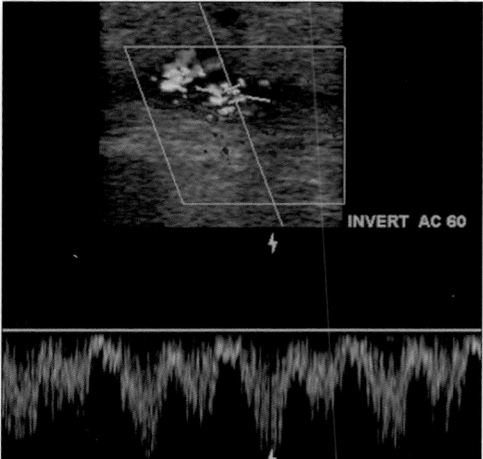

(Left) Longitudinal color Doppler ultrasound shows a femoral AVF ➔ with turbulent flow. *(Right)* Longitudinal color Doppler ultrasound shows arterialization of the venous signal of AVF. Same patient as previous image.

Typical

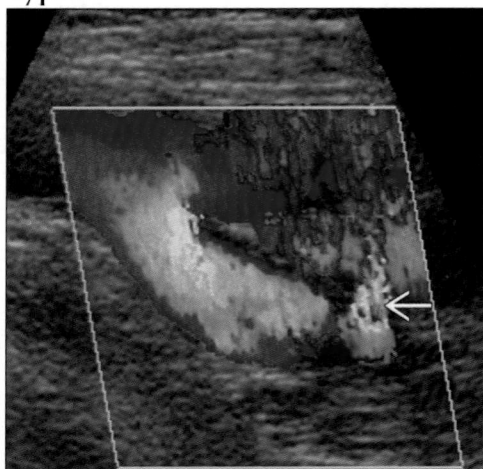
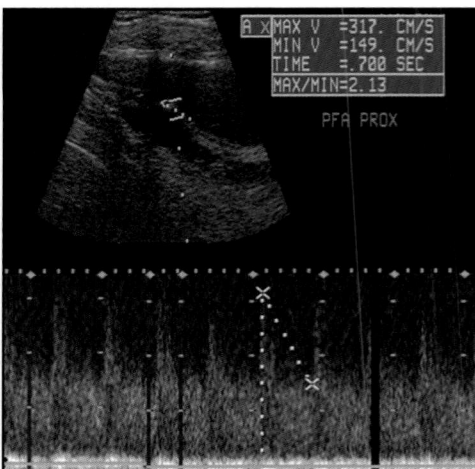

(Left) Longitudinal color Doppler ultrasound shows an AVF ➔ between the profunda femoris artery (PFA) and the superficial femoral vein (SFA). Turbulent flow with "aliasing" is demonstrated. *(Right)* Longitudinal pulsed Doppler ultrasound shows high velocity turbulent flow through the same AV fistula arising from the PFA.

Typical

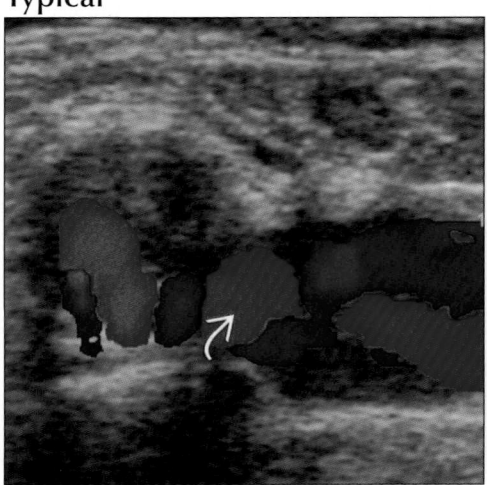
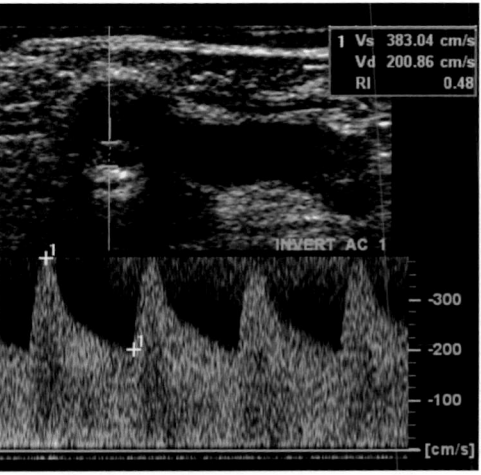

(Left) Transverse color Doppler ultrasound shows a large AVF ➔ between the common femoral artery (CFA) and common femoral vein (CFV). *(Right)* Transverse pulsed Doppler ultrasound shows high velocity flow through the same AV fistula as in previous image.

VARICOSE VEINS/INCOMPETENT PERFORATOR

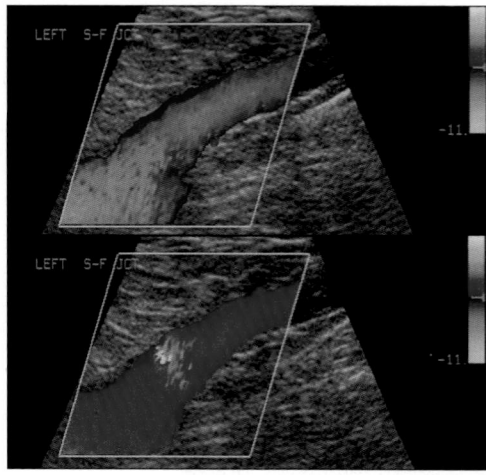

Longitudinal color Doppler ultrasound shows reflux at the saphenofemoral junction. Note change in color code from blue to red demonstrating reversal of flow at the saphenofemoral junction during Valsalva maneuver.

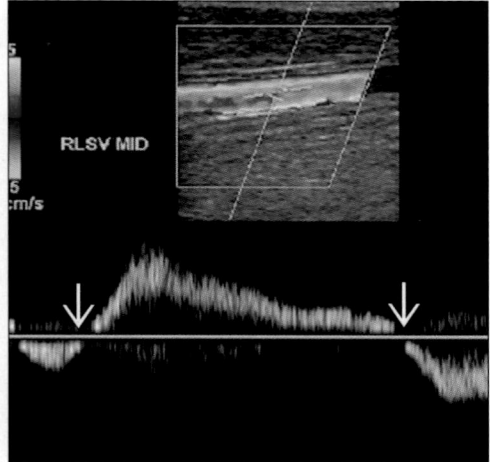

Longitudinal color Doppler ultrasound shows incompetent LSV with significant flow reflux > 2.0 s during Valsalva maneuver ➡. Findings are consistent with valvular incompetence.

TERMINOLOGY

Abbreviations and Synonyms
- Varicose veins (VV)

Definitions
- Chronic venous insufficiency refers to venous valvular incompetence in the superficial, deep, and/or perforating veins
- Venous reflux that persists for longer than 0.5 s at any level is considered clinically significant
- "Proximal" and "distal" in the venous system applies to the position of a vein segment in relation to the position of the heart (rather than the flow direction of blood)

IMAGING FINDINGS

Ultrasonographic Findings
- Grayscale Ultrasound
  - **Grayscale ultrasound**: Allows definition of vein lumen, vein valve leaflets and vein wall morphology
  - Assesses compressibility of the vein and acoustic properties of thrombus for evaluation of age of thrombus
- Pulsed Doppler
  - **Pulsed Doppler**: Differentiates venous from arterial flow
  - Documents venous flow pattern and flow direction
  - Allows timing of duration of venous reflux through incompetent valves
  - Normal venous flow signal should be
    - Spontaneous and phasic with respiration
  - In presence of obstruction by thrombus or extrinsic compression
    - Doppler spectral waveforms become continuous and nonphasic
    - Augmentation with distal limb compression is diminished (the contralateral limb can be used as a reference)
- Color Doppler
  - **Color Doppler**: Differentiates partial thrombosis from venous occlusion
  - Distinguishes reflux in the deep veins from reflux in the superficial system at the saphenofemoral junction and saphenopopliteal junction

DDx: Varicose Vein

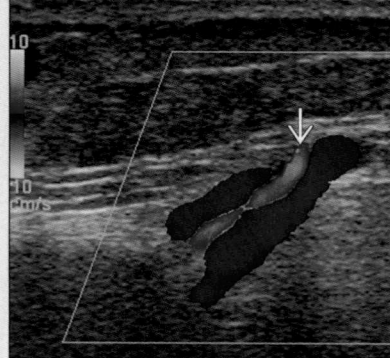

Arterial Perforator

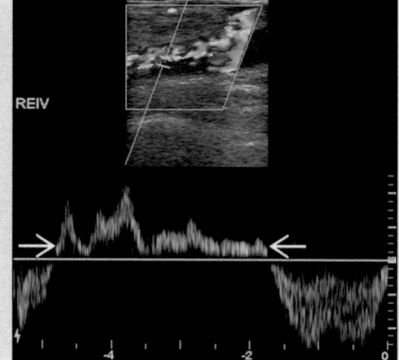

LSV Steal

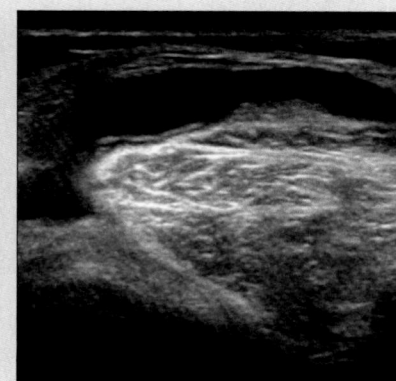

Baker Cyst

VARICOSE VEINS/INCOMPETENT PERFORATOR

Key Facts

Imaging Findings
- **Grayscale ultrasound**: Allows definition of vein lumen, vein valve leaflets and vein wall morphology
- Assesses compressibility of the vein and acoustic properties of thrombus for evaluation of age of thrombus
- **Pulsed Doppler**: Differentiates venous from arterial flow
- Documents venous flow pattern and flow direction
- Allows timing of duration of venous reflux through incompetent valves
- **Color Doppler**: Differentiates partial thrombosis from venous occlusion
- Distinguishes reflux in the deep veins from reflux in the superficial system at the saphenofemoral junction and saphenopopliteal junction

- Identifies incompetent perforating veins
- Demonstrates recanalization of chronically thrombosed venous segment and collateralization around thrombosed veins
- Best imaging tool: Combination of grayscale, pulsed Doppler and color Doppler ultrasound

Top Differential Diagnoses
- Calf Arterial Perforator
- LSV Steal
- Baker Cyst

Diagnostic Checklist
- When venous insufficiency is suggested during recumbent ultrasound examination, confirm findings by moving patient to standing position

---

- ○ Identifies incompetent perforating veins
- ○ Demonstrates recanalization of chronically thrombosed venous segment and collateralization around thrombosed veins

Imaging Recommendations
- Best imaging tool: Combination of grayscale, pulsed Doppler and color Doppler ultrasound
- Equipment
  - ○ High-resolution ultrasound system with 3-10 MHz pulsed Doppler and color Doppler transducers
  - ○ Tilting examination table (optional; useful for lowering feet below the heart)
  - ○ Platform 45-60 cm in height with support railing (optional for patient to stand during examination)
  - ○ Rapid cuff inflator and air source with selection of cuff (optional)
- Patient postioning
  - ○ Supine position
    - ■ Head slightly elevated, feet below level of heart (if tilting table available) to maximize venous pooling in the lower limbs
    - ■ Hips are externally rotated, with knees slightly flexed
    - ■ Permits easy access to the common femoral vein (CFV), superficial femoral vein (SFV), deep femoral vein (DFV), posterior tibial vein (PTV) and long saphenous vein (LSV)
  - ○ Lateral decubitus position
    - ■ Permits easy access to the common iliac vein (CIV), external iliac vein (EIV), popliteal vein (Pop V) and short saphenous vein (SSV)
  - ○ Prone position with feet slightly elevated with a pillow or a roll of towel
    - ■ Prevents hyperextension of knee which may cause compression of the popliteal vein and saphenopopliteal junction
    - ■ Useful for examination of the Pop V and SSV
- Technique
  - ○ Examination of the venous system includes the deep venous system, superficial venous system and perforator veins

- ○ Longitudinal imaging useful for assessment of flow direction and reflux
- ○ Transverse imaging useful for assessment of compressibility
- ○ Deep venous system examination starts with CFV, and includes DFV, SFV, Pop V and tibial veins to the level of the ankle
- ○ When grayscale imaging of the SFV is compromised in the distal thigh, transducer is moved to longitudinal imaging in the popliteal fossa for the distal SFV
- ○ Important to note tibial veins are often paired
- ○ Superficial venous system examination starts with the saphenofemoral junction and includes the LSV, saphenopopliteal junction and SSV
- ○ Perforator veins examination includes the mid thigh perforators, medial calf perforators and lateral thigh perforators
- ○ In thigh, identification of medially located perforators best accomplished beginning at the CFV level
- ○ Perforators connect the LSV to the deep veins
- ○ Hunterian perforator(s) (proximal thigh); Dodd perforator(s) (distal thigh)
- ○ Incompetent perforator veins are larger than competent perforator veins
- ○ Perforator veins > 4 mm are usually incompetent
- ○ Perforator veins < 3 mm are usually competent
- ○ In the calf, medially located perforators are typically located at 6, 12, 18, 24, 28 and 32 cm from heel
- ○ Cockett perforators (distal medial calf); Boyd perforators (proximal medial calf)
- ○ In calf, laterally located perforators vary in location
- ○ In proximal lateral calf, 2 perforators connect SSV to gastrocnemius vein (GV)
- ○ In distal calf, 2 perforators approximately 5 and 12 cm above the ankle
- ○ **Examination at each level should include**
- ○ Confirmation of flow by placing spectral Doppler sample volume over the vein lumen
- ○ Flow occurs in a forward cephalad direction when limb is compressed distal to the probe

VARICOSE VEINS/INCOMPETENT PERFORATOR

o There should be no evidence of retrograde flow with release of distal compression, with Valsalva maneuver or with limb compression proximal to the probe
o Recognition of flow direction with color Doppler
o Identification of anatomic landmarks and flow patterns
o Detection of morphologic and hemodynamic abnormalities
o Color flow imaging parameters should be optimized for detection of low velocity flow
o Decrease velocity scale and wall filters
o Use appropriately angled, narrow color box
o When venous insufficiency is suggested during recumbent ultrasound examination, confirm findings by moving patient to standing position

DIFFERENTIAL DIAGNOSIS

Calf Arterial Perforator
• Flow direction opposite to perforator vein and may mimic reflux in the calf perforators
• Important therefore to assess flow with spectral Doppler

LSV Steal
• Flow regurgitation in EIV/CFV due to blood stealing as a result of significant flow reflux in LSV
• Common association with LSV incompetence

Baker Cyst
• May mimic large varicose veins

PATHOLOGY

General Features
• Etiology
  o Primary valvular incompetence
  o Secondary valvular incompetence
    ▪ Extrinsic compression of vein
    ▪ Venous hypertension resulting from arteriovenous communications
  o Vascular malformations

CLINICAL ISSUES

Presentation
• Most common signs/symptoms
  o Edema, dilated veins, leg pain
  o Changes in skin around ankle region
    ▪ Pigmentation
    ▪ Skin-thickening
    ▪ Ulceration
  o Patients with incompetence involving the superficial, perforating and deep venous systems may get full spectrum of symptoms
  o Patients with segmental incompetence will have less symptoms

Demographics
• Age

o Visible tortuous varicose veins
  ▪ 10-15% of males > 15 yr old
  ▪ 20-25% of females > 15 yr old
o Moderate or chronic venous insufficiency
  ▪ 2-5% of adult males
  ▪ 3-7% of adult females

Treatment
• For venous insufficiency attributable to LSV incompetence
• Minimally invasive procedure performed as outpatient or day case procedure
  o Foam sclerosant ablation of the LSV
    ▪ Sodium tetradecyl sulphate 3% can be used
    ▪ Ultrasound used to guide treatment and compression of saphenofemoral junction
  o Radiofrequency ablation (RFA) or laser ablation of the LSV
    ▪ Conscious sedation and IV analgesia may be given
    ▪ Ultrasound used to guide catheter placement and injection of tumescent local anesthesia in the perivenous fascia around LSV
    ▪ RF or laser energy heats and contracts vein wall
    ▪ Catheter is withdrawn from 1.5 cm below the saphenofemoral junction to LSV around the knee region
    ▪ Denuded vein contracts and narrows
  o Conventional surgery
    ▪ Usually performed under general anesthesia
    ▪ LSV stripping and stab avulsion of varicosities

DIAGNOSTIC CHECKLIST

Image Interpretation Pearls
• When venous insufficiency is suggested during recumbent ultrasound examination, confirm findings by moving patient to standing position

SELECTED REFERENCES

1. Merchant RF et al: Long-term outcomes of endovenous radiofrequency obliteration of saphenous reflux as a treatment for superficial venous insufficiency. J Vasc Surg. 42(3):502-9; discussion 509, 2005
2. Neumyer MM: Ultrasound diagnosis of venous insufficiency. In: Zwiebel et al: Introduction to Vascular Sonography, 5th ed. Philadelphia, Elsevier Saunders. 479-510, 2005
3. Perala J et al: Radiofrequency endovenous obliteration versus stripping of the long saphenous vein in the management of primary varicose veins: 3-year outcome of a randomized study. Ann Vasc Surg. 2005
4. Min RJ et al: Endovenous laser treatment of saphenous vein reflux: long-term results. J Vasc Interv Radiol. 14(8):991-6, 2003

IMAGE GALLERY

Typical

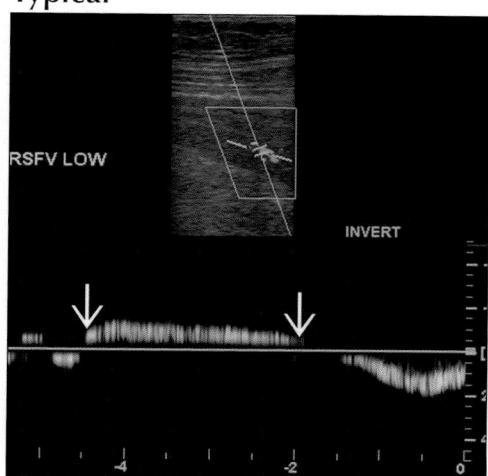 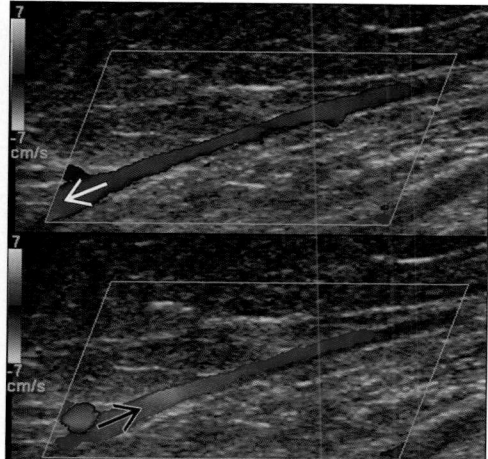

(Left) Longitudinal color Doppler ultrasound shows incompetent SFV with significant flow reflux ➡. Note abnormal reflux time is respectively taken as > 0.5 s and > 2.0 s with patient standing and supine. *(Right)* Longitudinal color Doppler ultrasound shows incompetent SSV with antegrade flow ➡ demonstrated during normal respiration (top), whereas flow reflux ➡ is noted during Valsalva maneuver (bottom).

Typical

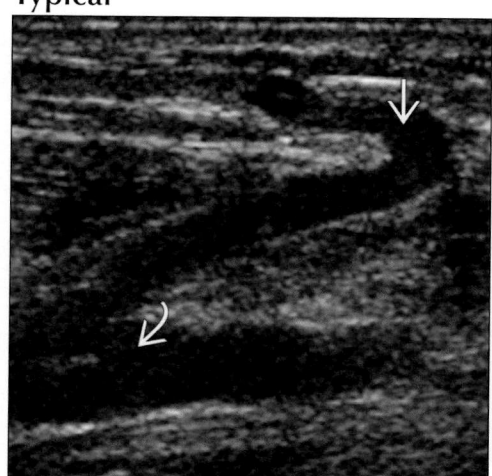 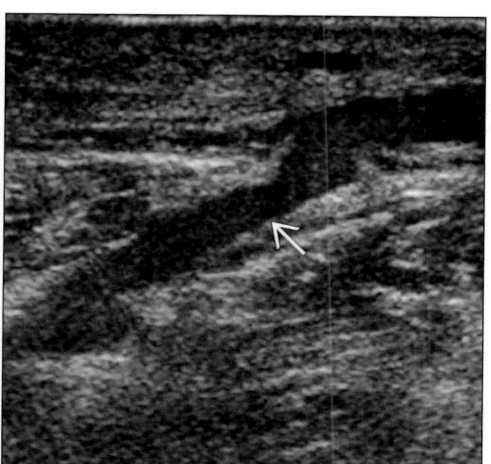

(Left) Longitudinal grayscale ultrasound shows a calf perforator ➡ penetrating the deep fascia and connecting to a deep vein ➡. *(Right)* Longitudinal grayscale ultrasound shows a large calf perforator ➡. Note incompetent perforators are usually larger than competent perforators.

Typical

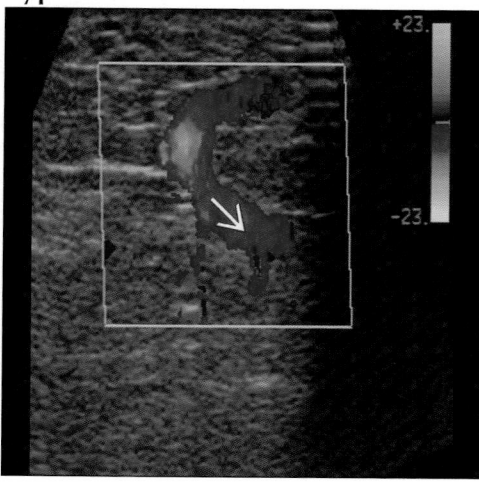 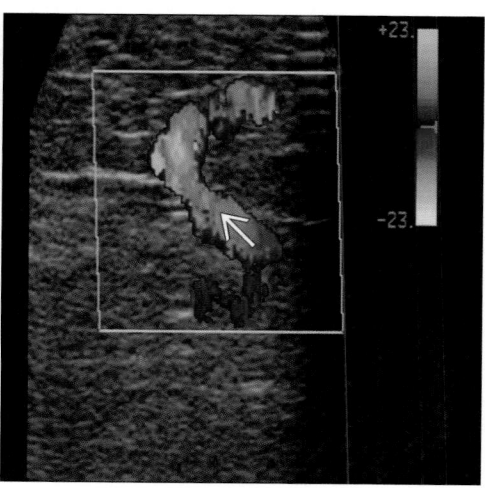

(Left) Longitudinal ultrasound shows a large calf perforator with antegrade flow ➡ to the deep venous system. *(Right)* Longitudinal color Doppler ultrasound shows the respective large calf perforator with retrograde flow ➡ after sudden cuff deflation.

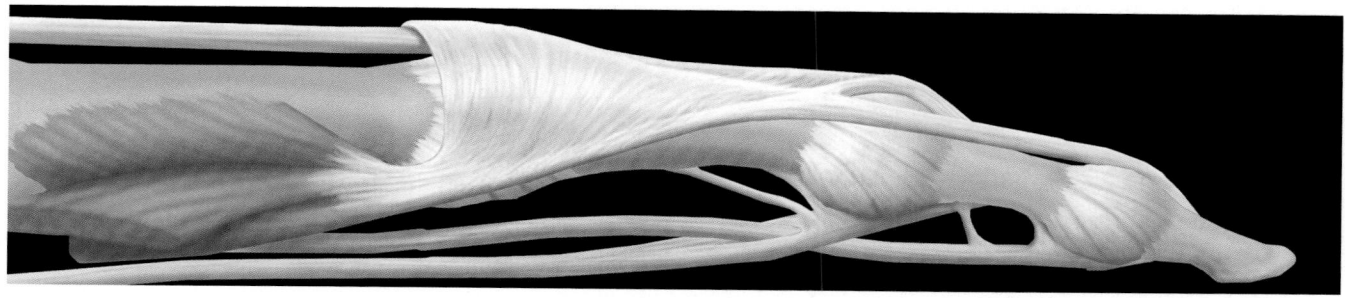

INDEX

INDEX

INDEX

i

iii

INDEX

i

iv

INDEX

INDEX

INDEX

INDEX

INDEX

i

x

INDEX

INDEX

INDEX

INDEX

INDEX

Myoepithelioma, **12:34i**, 12:35
Myofascial tear, **13:22i**, 13:23
Myometrial contraction, focal, **9:18i**, 9:20
Myometrial/endometrial calcification, 9:42–43
    differential diagnosis, **9:42i**, 9:43
    endometritis vs., 9:39
Myositis, infectious. *See* Soft tissue infection

N

Nabothian cyst, 9:6–8, **9:9i**
    differential diagnosis, **9:6i**, 9:7–8
    Gartner duct cyst vs., **9:108i**, 9:109
Neck abscess
    lymphangioma vs., **11:92i**, 11:94
    second brachial cleft cyst vs., **11:98i**, 11:99
Necrotic tumors, 12:23
Necrotizing fasciitis. *See* Soft tissue infection
Nephritis, focal bacterial, 5:72–73
    differential diagnosis, **5:72i**, 5:73
    renal lymphoma vs., 5:105
    renal metastasis vs., 5:93
    renal trauma vs., **5:62i**, 5:64
Nephrocalcinosis, 5:36–38, **5:39i**
    allograft rejection vs., **6:14i**, 6:15
    differential diagnosis, **5:36i**, 5:37
    emphysematous pyelonephritis vs., **5:74i**, 5:75
    urolithiasis vs., **5:30i**, 5:32
Nephrolithiasis. *See* Urolithiasis
Nerve entrapment. *See also* Carpal tunnel syndrome
    nerve injury vs., **13:62i**, 13:64
Nerve injury, 13:62–64, **13:65i**
    differential diagnosis, **13:62i**, 13:63–64
Nerve sheath tumor. *See* Peripheral nerve sheath tumor
Neurofibroma
    brachial plexus schwannoma vs., 11:119
    vagal nerve, vs. carotid body paraganglioma, **11:102i**, 11:103
Nodular goiter. *See* Multinodular goiter
Non-germ cell tumor, 10:22–23, **10:22i**
Non-Hodgkin lymphoma nodes, 11:48–50, **11:51i**
    differential diagnosis, **11:48i**, 11:49–50
    Kimura disease vs., 11:65
    mucoepidermoid carcinoma vs., 11:82
    parotid
        benign mixed tumor vs., **11:72i**, 11:74
        Sjogren syndrome vs., **11:68i**, 11:69
    squamous cell carcinoma node vs., **11:42i**, 11:43
    submandibular
        sialadenitis vs., **11:54i**, 11:55–56
        submandibular gland carcinoma vs., **11:62i**, 11:63
    systemic metastases vs., **11:52i**, 11:53
    thyroid. *See* Thyroid non-Hodgkin lymphoma
    tuberculous adenopathy vs., **11:46i**, 11:47

O

Oncocytoma, renal
    angiomyolipoma vs., 5:95
    renal cell carcinoma vs., 5:88
Oral cavity abscess, 11:90
Orchitis. *See* Epididymitis/orchitis
Osteitis. *See* Bone infection
Osteoarthrosis, 13:50–52, **13:53i**
    carpal tunnel syndrome vs., **13:72i**, 13:73
    differential diagnosis, **13:50i**, 13:51–52
    inflammatory arthritis vs., **13:54i**, 13:56
Osteochondral injury, **13:50i**, 13:52
Osteomyelitis. *See* Bone infection
Osteosarcoma, **13:82i**, 13:84
Ovarian cyst, functional, 9:66–68, **9:69i**
    differential diagnosis, **9:66i**, 9:67
    hemorrhagic cyst vs., **9:70i**
    parovarian cyst vs., **9:104i**, 9:105
    perigraft fluid collections vs., 6:11
Ovarian cystadenoma/carcinoma
    endometrioma vs., **9:124i**, 9:126
    fibrothecoma vs., **9:116i**, 9:117
    mucinous, 9:84–86, **9:87i**
        differential diagnosis, **9:84i**, 9:85
        functional ovarian cyst vs., 9:67
        ovarian hyperstimulation vs., 9:77
        serous cystadenoma/carcinoma vs., **9:80i**, 9:81
    perigraft fluid collections vs., **6:10i**, 6:11
    peritoneal inclusion cyst vs., **9:120i**, 9:121
    serous, 9:80–82, **9:83i**
        differential diagnosis, **9:80i**, 9:81
        functional ovarian cyst vs., 9:67
        mucinous cystadenoma/carcinoma vs., 9:85
    sex cord-stromal tumor vs., **9:112i**, 9:113
Ovarian teratoma, 9:88–90, **9:91i–93i**
    differential diagnosis, **9:88i**, 9:89
    ectopic pregnancy vs., **9:48i**, 9:49
    endometrioma vs., **9:124i**, 9:125
    fibrothecoma vs., **9:116i**, 9:117
    hemorrhagic cyst vs., **9:70i**, 9:71
    mucinous ovarian cystadenoma/carcinoma vs., **9:84i**, 9:85
    sex cord-stromal tumor vs., **9:112i**, 9:113
Ovarian torsion
    hemorrhagic cyst vs., 9:71
    ovarian teratoma vs., 9:89
    sex cord-stromal tumor vs., **9:112i**, 9:113
Ovarian vein thrombosis, 9:39
Ovary
    hyperstimulation, 9:76–78, **9:79i**
        differential diagnosis, **9:76i**, 9:77
    imaging issues, 9:3
    metastases vs. serous cystadenoma/carcinoma, **9:80i**, 9:81

xv

INDEX

INDEX

INDEX

xx

INDEX